Compliments,

Cardis Cardiology.

TEXTBOOK OF INTERVENTIONAL CARDIOLOGY

TEXTBOOK OF INTERVENTIONAL CARDIOLOGY

5TH EDITION

Eric J. Topol, MD

Director, Scripps Translational Science Institute
Chief Academic Officer, Scripps Health
Professor of Translational Genomics, The Scripps Research Institute
Senior Consultant, Division of Cardiovascular Diseases
Scripps Clinic
La Jolla, California

SAUNDERS

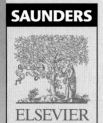

ELSEVIER

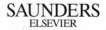

SAUNDERS
ELSEVIER

1600 John F. Kennedy Blvd.
Ste 1800
Philadelphia, PA 19103-2899

TEXTBOOK OF INTERVENTIONAL CARDIOLOGY   ISBN: 978-1-4160-4835-0

Notice

Knowledge and best practice in this field are constantly changing. As new research and
experience broaden our knowledge, changes in practice, treatment, and drug therapy may
become necessary or appropriate. Readers are advised to check the most current
information provided (i) on procedures featured or (ii) by the manufacturer of each
product to be administered, to verify the recommended dose or formula, the method and
duration of administration, and contraindications. It is the responsibility of the
practitioner, relying on his or her experience and knowledge of the patient, to make
diagnoses, to determine dosages and the best treatment for each individual patient, and to
take all appropriate safety precautions. To the fullest extent of the law, neither the
Publisher nor the Editor assumes any liability for any injury and/or damage to persons or
property arising out of or related to any use of the material contained in this book.

The Publisher

Library of Congress Cataloging-in-Publication Data

Textbook of interventional cardiology / [edited by] Eric J. Topol.—5th ed.
   p. ; cm
  Includes bibliographical references and index.
  ISBN 978-1-4160-4835-0
  1. Heart—Interventional radiology. 2. Angioplasty. 3. Cardiovascular system—Diseases—
Treatment. I. Topol, Eric J., 1954-
    [DNLM: 1. Cardiovascular Diseases—surgery. 2. Cardiovascular Diseases—drug
therapy. 3. Cardiovascular Surgical Procedures—methods. WG 168 T355 2008]
  RD598.35.I55T49 2008
  617.4'12059—dc22   2007018033

Executive Publisher: Natasha Andjelkovic
Developmental Editor: Agnes Hunt Byrne
Publishing Services Manager: Frank Polizzano
Project Manager: Michael H. Goldberg
Design Direction: Steven Stave

Printed in China

Last digit is the print number: 9 8 7 6 5 4 3 2 1

This book is dedicated to my family—my wife, Susan, and our kids, Sarah and Evan, who have been with me every step along the way.

Contributors

Jorge R. Alegria, MD
Fellow, Interventional Cardiology, Mayo Clinic College
of Medicine, Rochester, Minnesota
Balloon Angioplasty: Is It Still a Viable Intervention?

Alexandra Almonacid, MD
Research Associate, Harvard Medical School; Assistant
Director, Angiographic Core Laboratory, Brigham and
Women's Hospital, Boston, Massachusetts
Qualitative and Quantitative Coronary Angiography

R. David Anderson, MD, MS
Associate Professor of Medicine and Director of
Interventional Cardiology, Division of Cardiovascular
Medicine, University of Florida College of Medicine,
Gainesville, Florida
Elective Intervention for Chronic Coronary Syndromes

Paolo Angelini, MD
Clinical Professor of Medicine, Baylor College of
Medicine; Interventional Cardiologist, Texas Heart
Institute, St. Luke's Episcopal Hospital, Houston, Texas
Surgical Standby: State of the Art

Gary M. Ansel, MD
Assistant Clinical Professor of Medicine, Medical
University of Ohio, Toledo; Director, Peripheral
Vascular Intervention, Riverside Methodist Hospital;
Investigator, MidWest Cardiology Research Foundation,
Columbus, Ohio
Venous Interventions

Saif Anwaruddin, MD
Fellow, Cardiology, Cleveland Clinic, Cleveland,
Ohio
Inflammation Status

Christopher Bajzer, MD
Associate Director, Peripheral Intervention, Heart and
Vascular Institute, Cleveland Clinic, Cleveland, Ohio
Renal Artery Stenosis

Anthony A. Bavry, MD, MPH
Fellow, Interventional Cardiology, Cleveland Clinic,
Cleveland, Ohio
Late Stent Thrombosis

Matthew C. Becker, MD
Fellow, Cardiovascular Disease, Cleveland Clinic,
Cleveland, Ohio
Hypertrophic Cardiomyopathy

Robert H. Beekman III, MD
Professor of Pediatric Cardiology, University of
Cincinnati College of Medicine; Professor, Cincinnati
Children's Hospital Medical Center, Cincinnati, Ohio
Transcatheter Therapies for Congenital Heart Disease

Peter B. Berger, MD
Associate Chief Research Officer and Director of the
Center for Clinical Studies, Geisinger Health Systems,
Danville, Pennsylvania
Intervention in Complex Lesions and Multivessel Disease

Farzin Beygui, MD, PhD
Permanent University Hospital Staff, Faculté de
Médicine Pitié-Salpêtrière, Université Paris VI; Senior
Consultant, Pitié-Salpêtrière University Hospital, Paris,
France
*Transradial Percutaneous Coronary Intervention for a Major
Reduction of Bleeding Complications*

John A. Bittl, MD
Interventional Cardiologist, Munroe Regional Medical
Center, Ocala Heart Institute, Ocala, Florida
*Role of Adjunct Devices: Cutting Balloon, Thrombectomy,
Laser, Ultrasound, and Atherectomy*

Ashley B. Boam, MS
Chief, Interventional Cardiology Devices Branch,
Center for Devices and Radiological Health, U.S. Food
and Drug Administration, Rockville, Maryland
Regulatory Issues

Philipp Bonhoeffer, MD
Professor of Cardiology, Institute of Child Health; Chief
of Cardiology and Director of the Cardiac
Catheterisation Laboratory, Great Ormond Street
Hospital, London, United Kingdom
Pulmonary and Tricuspid Valve Interventions

Michael Brandle, MD, MS
Associate Professor of Endocrinology, Zurich School of Medicine, Zurich; Division Chief, Division of Endocrinology and Diabetes, Department of Internal Medicine, Kantonsspital St. Gallen, St. Gallen, Switzerland
Diabetes

Ralph G. Brindis, MD, MPH
Clinical Professor of Medicine, University of California, San Francisco, School of Medicine, San Francisco; Senior Advisor for Cardiovascular Diseases, Northern California Kaiser Permanente; Physician, Department of Cardiology, Kaiser Permanente Oakland Medical Center, Oakland, California
Quality of Care in Interventional Cardiology

David Buckles, PhD
Chief, Peripheral Vascular Devices Branch, Center for Devices and Radiological Health, U.S. Food and Drug Administration, Rockville, Maryland
Regulatory Issues

Heinz Joachim Büttner, MD
Director, Interventional Cardiology, Herz-Zentrum Bad Krozingen, Bad Krozingen, Germany
Evidence-Based Interventional Practice

Christopher P. Cannon, MD
Associate Professor of Medicine, Harvard Medical School; Associate Physician, Cardiovascular Division, Brigham and Women's Hospital, Boston, Massachusetts
Lipid Lowering in Coronary Artery Disease

Ivan P. Casserly, BSc, MB BCh
Assistant Professor of Medicine, University of Colorado School of Medicine and University of Colorado Hospital; Director of Interventional Cardiology, Denver Veterans Affairs Medical Center, Denver, Colorado
Carotid and Cerebrovascular Interventions

Matthews Chacko, MD
Assistant Professor of Medicine, Johns Hopkins University School of Medicine; Director of Peripheral Interventions, and Faculty, Interventional Cardiology, Coronary Care Unit, and the Thayer Firm, Division of Cardiology, Johns Hopkins Hospital, Baltimore, Maryland
Thrombolytic Intervention

Derek P. Chew, MBBS, MPH
Associate Professor of Medicine, Flinders University School of Medicine; Director of Cardiology, Flinders Medical Centre, Adelaide, South Australia, Australia
Anticoagulation in Percutaneous Coronary Intervention

Leslie Cho, MD
Director, Women's Cardiovascular Center; Medical Director, Preventive Cardiology and Rehabilitation, Cleveland Clinic, Cleveland, Ohio
Gender and Ethnicity Issues in Percutaneous Coronary Intervention

Ryan D. Christofferson, MD
Fellow, Interventional Cardiology, Cleveland Clinic, Cleveland, Ohio
Percutaneous Mitral Valve Repair

Louise Coats, MBBS, MRCP
Clinical Research Fellow, Institute of Child Health and Great Ormond Street Hospital, London, United Kingdom
Pulmonary and Tricuspid Valve Interventions

Antonio Colombo, MD
Faculty of Medicine and Surgery, Vita-Salute San Raffaele University; Director of Invasive Cardiology, San Raffaele Scientific Institute and Columbus Hospital, Milan, Italy
Ostial and Bifurcation Lesions

Bertrand Cormier, MD
Hospital Doctor, Service Médecine-Cardiologie, Institut Hospitalier Jacques Cartier, Massy, France
Mitral Valvuloplasty

Marco A. Costa, MD, PhD
Associate Professor of Medicine and Director of Research, Division of Cardiology, University of Florida College of Medicine Jacksonville, Jacksonville, Florida
Restenosis

Alain Cribier, MD
Professor of Medicine, University of Rouen; Chief, Department of Cardiology, Hôpital Charles Nicolle, Rouen, France
Percutaneous Aortic Valvular Approaches: Balloon Aortic Valvuloplasty and Percutaneous Valve Replacement with the Cribier-Edwards Bioprosthesis

Fernando Cura, MD, PhD
Vice Director, Interventional Cardiology and Endovascular Therapies, Instituto Cardiovascular de Buenos Aires, Buenos Aires, Argentina
Access Management and Closure Devices

Pranab Das, MD
Fellow, Interventional Cardiology, Loyola University Chicago Stritch School of Medicine, Maywood, Illinois
Bioabsorbable Stents

P. J. de Feyter, MD, PhD
Erasmus Medical Center, Rotterdam, The Netherlands
Percutaneous Intervention for Non-ST Segment Elevation Acute Coronary Syndromes

Robert S. Dieter, MD, RVT
Assistant Professor of Medicine, Loyola University Chicago Stritch School of Medicine, Maywood, Illinois
Upper Extremities and Aortic Arch

John S. Douglas, Jr., MD
Professor of Medicine, Emory University School of Medicine; Director of Interventional Cardiology and Cardiac Catheterization Laboratories, Emory University Hospital, Atlanta, Georgia
Percutaneous Intervention in Patients with Prior Coronary Bypass Surgery

Stephen G. Ellis, MD
Director, F. Mason Sones Cardiac Catheterization
Laboratory, Cleveland Clinic, Cleveland, Ohio
Drug-Eluting and Bare Metal Stents

Helene Eltchaninoff, MD
Professor of Medicine, University of Rouen; Chief,
Cardiac Catheterization Laboratory, Department of
Cardiology, Hôpital Charles Nicolle, Rouen, France
*Percutaneous Aortic Valvular Approaches: Balloon Aortic
Valvuloplasty and Percutaneous Valve Replacement with the
Cribier-Edwards Bioprosthesis*

Nezar Falluji, MD
Assistant Professor, Division of Cardiology,
Linda and Jack Gill Heart Institute,
University of Kentucky, Lexington,
Kentucky
Lower Extremity Interventions

Andrew Farb, MD
Medical Officer, Center for Devices and Radiological
Health, U.S. Food and Drug Administration, Rockville,
Maryland
Regulatory Issues

Peter J. Fitzgerald, MD, PhD
Professor of Medicine (Cardiology) and Engineering,
Stanford University School of Medicine; Director,
Center for Cardiovascular Technology, Stanford
University, Stanford, California
Intravascular Ultrasound

Shmuel Fuchs, MD
Associate Professor of Cardiology, Sackler School of
Medicine, Tel Aviv University, Tel Aviv; Director,
Catheterization Laboratory Service, Golda-Hasharon
Hospital, Rabin Medical Center, Petah Tikva, Israel
*Percutaneous Myocardial Revascularization: Lasers and
Biologic Compounds*

Valentin Fuster, MD, PhD
Professor of Medicine, Mount Sinai School of Medicine;
Director, Cardiovascular Institute, Mount Sinai Hospital,
New York, New York
Atherothrombosis and the High-Risk Plaque

Mario J. Garcia, MD
Professor of Medicine and Radiology, Mount Sinai
School of Medicine; Director of Cardiac Imaging,
Mount Sinai Hospital, New York, New York
*Functional Testing and Multidetector Computed
Tomography*

Lowell Gerber, MD
Chief of Cardiovascular Services, Florida Hospital
Heartland, Sebring, Florida
*Percutaneous Aortic Valvular Approaches: Balloon Aortic
Valvuloplasty and Percutaneous Valve Replacement with the
Cribier-Edwards Bioprosthesis*

Hussam Hamdalla, MD
Assistant Professor and Associate Program Director,
Interventional Cardiology Fellowship, University of
Kentucky College of Medicine, Lexington, Kentucky
*Role of Platelet Inhibitor Agents in Percutaneous Coronary
Intervention*

Hidehiko Hara, MD
Fellow, Preclinical Research, Minneapolis Heart Institute
and Foundation, Minneapolis, Minnesota
The Left Atrial Appendage

Motoya Hayase, MD
Associate Director, Interventional Cardiovascular
Therapy, The Skirball Center for Cardiovascular
Research, Cardiovascular Research Foundation,
Orangeburg, New York
Percutaneous Revascularization Procedures

Howard C. Herrmann, MD
Professor of Medicine, University of Pennsylvania
School of Medicine; Director, Interventional Cardiology
and Cardiac Catheterization Laboratories, Hospital of
the University of Pennsylvania, Philadelphia,
Pennsylvania
*Support Devices for High Risk Percutaneous Coronary
Intervention*

Russel Hirsch, MBChB
Associate Professor of Pediatric Cardiology, University
of Cincinnati College of Medicine; Director, Cardiac
Catheterization Laboratory, Cincinnati Children's
Hospital Medical Center, Cincinnati, Ohio
Transcatheter Therapies for Congenital Heart Disease

David R. Holmes, Jr., MD
Professor of Medicine, Mayo Clinic College of Medicine;
Consultant, Mayo Clinic, Rochester, Minnesota
*Balloon Angioplasty: Is It Still a Viable Intervention?; The
Left Atrial Appendage*

Yasuhiro Honda, MD
Co-Director, Cardiovascular Core Analysis Laboratory,
Center for Cardiovascular Technology, Stanford
University, Stanford, California
Intravascular Ultrasound

Hüseyin Ince, MD
Lecturer in Cardiology, University of Rostock School of
Medicine; Deputy Head, Division of Cardiology and
Angiology, University Hospital Rostock, Rostock,
Germany
Aortic Vascular Interventions (Thoracic and Abdominal)

Eduardo Infante de Oliveira, MD
Staff Cardiologist, Hospital de Santa Maria, Faculdade
de Medicina de Lisboa, Lisbon, Portugal
Renal Artery Stenosis

Bernard Iung, MD
Professor of Cardiology, University of Paris VII; Hospital
Doctor, Service de Cardiologie, Hôpital Bichat, Paris,
France
Mitral Valvuloplasty

Alice K. Jacobs, MD
Professor of Medicine, Boston University School of
Medicine; Director, Cardiac Catheterization Laboratories
and Interventional Cardiology, Boston Medical Center,
Boston, Massachusetts
*Regional Centers of Excellence for the Care of Patients with
Acute Ischemic Heart Disease*

Hani Jneid, MD
Division of Cardiology, University of Louisville, Louisville, Kentucky
Percutaneous Balloon Pericardiotomy for Patients with Pericardial Effusion and Tamponade

Samuel L. Johnston, MD
Fellow, Cardiology, Loyola University Chicago Stritch School of Medicine, Maywood, Illinois
Upper Extremities and Aortic Arch

Samir R. Kapadia, MD
Associate Professor of Medicine, Cleveland Clinic Lerner College of Medicine of Case Western Reserve University; Staff, Cleveland Clinic, Cleveland, Ohio
Imaging for Intracardiac Interventions; Mitral Valve Repair; Hypertrophic Cardiomyopathy

Adnan Kastrati, MD
Professor of Cardiology, Technische Universität; Director, Catheterization Laboratory, Department of Cardiology, Deutsches Herzzentrum, Munich, Germany
Percutaneous Coronary Interventions in Acute ST-Segment Elevation Myocardial Infarction

Dean J. Kereiakes, MD
Professor of Clinical Medicine, The Ohio State University College of Medicine, Columbus; Medical Director, Christ Cincinnati Heart and Vascular Center; Medical Director, Lindner Center for Research and Education, Cincinnati, Ohio
Regional Centers of Excellence for the Care of Patients with Acute Ischemic Heart Disease

Morton J. Kern, MD
Professor of Medicine, University of California, Irvine, School of Medicine, Irvine; Associate Chief of Cardiology and Director of the Cardiac Care Unit, UC Irvine Medical Center, Orange, California
Intracoronary Pressure and Flow Measurements

Matheen A. Khuddus, MD
Fellow, Cardiology, Division of Cardiology, University of Florida College of Medicine, Gainesville, Florida
Elective Intervention for Chronic Coronary Syndromes

Young-Hak Kim, MD
Assistant Professor of Medicine, Ulsan University; Attending Physician, Asan Medical Center, Seoul, South Korea
Percutaneous Intervention for Left Main Coronary Artery Stenosis

Ran Kornowski, MD
Associate Professor of Cardiovascular Medicine, Sackler School of Medicine, Tel Aviv University, Tel Aviv; Director, Interventional Cardiology and Cardiac Catheterization Laboratories, Beilinson and Golda-Hasharon Hospitals, Rabin Medical Center, Petah Tikva, Israel
Percutaneous Myocardial Revascularization: Lasers and Biologic Compounds

Alexandra J. Lansky, MD
Associate Professor of Clinical Medicine, Columbia University College of Physicians and Surgeons; Director of Clinical Services, Center for Interventional Vascular Therapy, New York–Presbyterian Hospital/Columbia University Medical Center, New York, New York
Qualitative and Quantitative Coronary Angiography

John M. Lasala, MD, PhD
Professor of Medicine, Washington University School of Medicine; Director, Interventional Cardiology, and Medical Director, Cardiac Catheterization Laboratory, Barnes-Jewish Hospital, St. Louis, Missouri
Percutaneous Closure of Patent Foramen Ovale and Atrial Septal Defect

Robert J. Lederman, MD
Investigator, Cardiovascular Branch, Division of Intramural Research, National Heart, Lung, and Blood Institute, National Institutes of Health, Bethesda, Maryland
Cardiovascular Interventional Magnetic Resonance Imaging

Michael J. Lim, MD
Assistant Professor of Medicine and Director, Interventional Cardiology Fellowship Training Program, Saint Louis University School of Medicine; Director, Cardiac Catheterization Laboratory, Saint Louis University Hospital, St. Louis, Missouri
Intracoronary Pressure and Flow Measurements

A. Michael Lincoff, MD
Professor of Medicine, Cleveland Clinic Lerner College of Medicine of Case Western Reserve University; Vice Chairman for Research, Department of Cardiovascular Medicine, and Director, Cleveland Clinic Cardiovascular Coordinating Center, Cleveland Clinic, Cleveland, Ohio
Abrupt Vessel Closure

Thomas R. Lloyd, MD
Professor of Pediatrics, University of Michigan Medical School; Director, Cardiac Catheterization Laboratory, C. S. Mott Children's Hospital, Ann Arbor, Michigan
Transcatheter Therapies for Congenital Heart Disease

Daniel B. Mark, MD, MPH
Professor of Medicine, Duke University School of Medicine; Co-Director, Coronary Care Unit, and Attending Physician, Duke University Medical Center, Durham, North Carolina
Medical Economics in Interventional Cardiology

Bernhard Meier, MD
Professor of Cardiology, Faculty of Medicine, University of Bern; Director of Cardiology, University Hospital, Bern, Switzerland
Chronic Total Occlusion

Victor M. Mejia, MD
Hospital of the University of Pennsylvania, Philadelphia, Pennsylvania
Support Devices for High Risk Percutaneous Coronary Intervention

Gilles Montalescot, MD, PhD
Professor of Cardiology, Institut de Cardiologie, Pitié-Salpétrière Hospital, Paris, France
Transradial Percutaneous Coronary Intervention for a Major Reduction of Bleeding Complications

Pedro R. Moreno, MD
Associate Professor of Medicine, Mount Sinai School of Medicine; Director, Interventional Cardiology Research, Mount Sinai Hospital, New York, New York
Atherothrombosis and the High-Risk Plaque

Douglass A. Morrison, MD, PhD
Interventional Cardiologist, Yakima Heart Center, Yakima, Washington
Extent of Atherosclerotic Disease and Left Ventricular Function

Debabrata Mukherjee, MD, MS
Gill Foundation Professor of Interventional Cardiology, University of Kentucky College of Medicine; Director, Cardiac Catheterization Laboratories, University of Kentucky Medical Center, Lexington, Kentucky
Periprocedural Myocardial Infarction and Embolism-Protection Devices; Bioabsorbable Stents; Lower Extremity Interventions

Srihari S. Naidu, MD
Director, Cardiac Catheterization Laboratory, Winthrop-University Hospital, Mineola, New York
Support Devices for High Risk Percutaneous Coronary Intervention

Brahmajee K. Nallamothu, MD, MPH
Assistant Professor of Internal Medicine, Division of Cardiology, University of Michigan Medical School, Ann Arbor, Michigan
Renal Dysfunction

Craig R. Narins, MD
Assistant Professor of Medicine and Cardiology and Assistant Professor of Vascular Surgery, University of Rochester School of Medicine and Dentistry, Rochester, New York
Preoperative Coronary Intervention

Gjin Ndrepepa, MD
Associate Professor of Cardiology, Technische Universität and Deutsches Herzzentrum, Munich, Germany
Percutaneous Coronary Interventions in Acute ST-Segment Elevation Myocardial Infarction

Franz-Josef Neumann, MD
Honorary Professor of Cardiology, Albert-Ludwgs-Universität, Frieburg; Medical Director and Chairman, Herz-Zentrum Bad Krozingen, Bad Krozingen, Germany
Evidence-Based Interventional Practice

Christoph A. Nienaber, MD, PhD
Professor of Internal Medicine and Cardiology, University of Rostock School of Medicine; Head, Division of Cardiology and Angiology, University Hospital Rostock, Rostock, Germany
Aortic Vascular Interventions (Thoracic and Abdominal)

Masakiyo Nobuyoshi, MD, PhD
Clinical Professor, Kyoto University Faculty of Medicine, Kyoto; Chairperson, Kokura Memorial Hospital, Kitakyushu, Fukuoka Prefecture, Japan
Small-Vessel and Diffuse Disease

Igor F. Palacios, MD
Associate Professor of Medicine, Harvard Medical School; Director, Knight Catheterization Laboratory, Massachusetts General Hospital, Boston, Massachusetts
Percutaneous Balloon Pericardiotomy for Patients with Pericardial Effusion and Tamponade

Seung-Jung Park, MD, PhD
Professor of Medicine, Ulsan University; Director, Asan Medical Center, Seoul, South Korea
Percutaneous Intervention for Left Main Coronary Artery Stenosis

Uptal D. Patel, MD
Assistant Professor of Medicine and Pediatrics, Divisions of Nephrology and Pediatric Nephrology, Duke University School of Medicine, Durham, North Carolina
Renal Dysfunction

Marc S. Penn, MD, PhD
Director, Bakken Heart-Brain Institute, Cleveland Clinic, Cleveland, Ohio
Stem Cell Therapy for Ischemic Heart Disease

Carl J. Pepine, MD
Eminent Scholar, American Heart Association–Suncoast Chapter Chair, Professor of Medicine, and Chief, Division of Cardiovascular Medicine, University of Florida College of Medicine, Gainesville, Florida
Elective Intervention for Chronic Coronary Syndromes

Marc A. Pfeffer, MD, PhD
Dzau Professor of Medicine, Harvard Medical School; Senior Physician, Cardiovascular Division, Brigham and Women's Hospital, Boston, Massachusetts
Angiotensin-Axis Inhibition

Jeffrey J. Popma, MD
Research Associate, Harvard Medical School; Director, Invasive Cardiovascular Services, St. Elizabeth's Medical Center; Director, Angiographic Core Laboratory, Brigham and Women's Hospital, Boston, Massachusetts
Qualitative and Quantitative Coronary Angiography

Mark J. Post, MD, PhD
Professor of Vascular Physiology and Chair of the Department of Physiology, University of Maastricht, Maastricht, The Netherlands
Angiogenesis and Arteriogenesis

Vivek Rajagopal, MD
Staff Cardiologist, Cardiac Disease Specialists, Piedmont Hospital, Atlanta, Georgia
Other Adjunctive Drugs for Coronary Intervention: β-Blockers and Calcium Channel Blockers

Stephen R. Ramee, MD
Section Head, Invasive/Interventional Cardiology, Ochsner Clinic Foundation, New Orleans, Louisiana
Chronic Mesenteric Ischemia: Diagnosis and Intervention; Acute Stroke Intervention

Kausik K. Ray, MD, MRCP
Senior Clinical Research Associate, University of
Cambridge; Honorary Consultant Cardiologist,
Addenbrookes Hospital, Cambridge, United Kingdom
Lipid Lowering in Coronary Artery Disease

Marco Roffi, MD
Associate Professor of Medicine, University of Geneva;
Director, Interventional Cardiology Unit, University
Hospital, Geneva, Switzerland
Diabetes

Javier Sanz, MD
Assistant Professor of Medicine, Mount Sinai School of
Medicine; Staff Cardiologist and Associate Director of
CT and MRI in Cardiology, Mount Sinai Hospital, New
York, New York
Atherothrombosis and the High-Risk Plaque

Wolf Sapirstein, MD
Medical Officer, Center for Devices and Radiological
Health, U.S. Food and Drug Administration, Rockville,
Maryland
Regulatory Issues

Albert Schömig, MD
Professor of Medicine, Technische Universität; Chief,
Department of Cardiology, Deutsches Herzzentrum,
Munich, Germany
*Percutaneous Coronary Interventions in Acute ST-Segment
Elevation Myocardial Infarction*

Daniel G. Schultz, MD
Director, Center for Devices and Radiological Health,
U.S. Food and Drug Administration, Rockville,
Maryland
Regulatory Issues

Robert S. Schwartz, MD
Medical Director of Pre-Clinical Research, Minneapolis
Heart Institute and Foundation, Minneapolis,
Minnesota
The Left Atrial Appendage

Mehdi H. Shishehbor, DO, MPH
Interventional Fellow, Department of Cardiovascular
Medicine, and National Institutes of Health K12
Scholar, Cleveland Clinic, Cleveland, Ohio
Imaging for Intracardiac Interventions

Mitchell J. Silver, DO
Associate Professor of Cardiology, Ohio University
College of Medicine, Athens; Staff Cardiologist/Vascular
Medicine, Riverside Methodist Hospital, Columbus,
Ohio
Venous Interventions

Daniel I. Simon, MD
Herman K. Hellerstein Professor of Cardiovascular
Research, and Director, Case Cardiovascular Center,
Case Western Reserve University School of Medicine;
Chief, Cardiovascular Medicine, and Director, Heart and
Vascular Institute, University Hospitals Case Medical
Center, Cleveland, Ohio
Restenosis

Michael Simons, MD
A.G. Huber Professor of Medicine and Director,
Angiogenesis Research Center, Dartmouth Medical
School, Hanover; Chief of Cardiology, Dartmouth-
Hitchcock Medical Center, Lebanon, New Hampshire
Angiogenesis and Arteriogenesis

B. Clay Sizemore, MD
Cardiology Fellow, Division of Cardiovascular Medicine,
University of Florida College of Medicine, Gainesville,
Florida
Elective Intervention for Chronic Coronary Syndromes

Goran Stankovic, MD
Assistant Professor of Medicine, University of Belgrade
School of Medicine; Interventional Cardiologist,
University Institute for Cardiovascular Diseases, Clinical
Center of Serbia, Belgrade, Serbia
Ostial and Bifurcation Lesions

Steven R. Steinhubl, MD
Associate Professor, University of Kentucky College of
Medicine, Lexington, Kentucky
*Role of Platelet Inhibitor Agents in Percutaneous Coronary
Intervention*

Srihari Thanigaraj, MD
Associate Professor of Medicine, Cardiology Division,
Washington University School of Medicine and Barnes-
Jewish Hospital, St. Louis, Missouri
*Percutaneous Closure of Patent Foramen Ovale and Atrial
Septal Defect*

Eric J. Topol, MD
Director, Scripps Translational Science Institute; Chief
Academic Officer, Scripps Health; Professor of
Translational Genomics, The Scripps Research Institute;
Senior Consultant, Division of Cardiovascular Diseases,
Scripps Clinic, La Jolla, California
Inflammation Status; Thrombolytic Intervention

Christophe Tron, MD
Chief, Intensive Care Unit, Department of Cardiology,
Hôpital Charles Nicolle, Rouen, France
*Percutaneous Aortic Valvular Approaches: Balloon Aortic
Valvuloplasty and Percutaneous Valve Replacement with the
Cribier-Edwards Bioprosthesis*

Alec Vahanian, MD
Professor of Cardiology, University of Paris VII; Head of
Cardiology Department, Hôpital Bichat, Paris, France
Mitral Valvuloplasty

Robert A. Van Tassel, MD
Senior Consultant, Cardiology, Minneapolis Heart
Institute and Foundation, Minneapolis, Minnesota
The Left Atrial Appendage

Ron Waksman, MD
Professor of Medicine, Georgetown University School of
Medicine; Associate Chief of Cardiology and Director of
Experimental Angioplasty and New Technologies,
Washington Hospital Center, Washington, DC
Vascular Brachytherapy for Restenosis

Christopher J. White, MD
Chair, Department of Cardiology, Ochsner Clinic
Foundation, New Orleans, Louisiana
*Chronic Mesenteric Ischemia: Diagnosis and Intervention;
Acute Stroke Intervention*

Paul G. Yock, MD
Martha Meier Weiland Professor of Medicine and
Bioengineering, Stanford University School of Medicine;
Director, Program in Biodesign, Stanford University,
Stanford, California
Intravascular Ultrasound

Hiroyoshi Yokoi, MD
Director of Clinical Section, Department of Cardiology,
Kokura Memorial Hospital, Kitakyusu, Fukuoka
Prefecture, Japan
Small-Vessel and Diffuse Disease

Alan Zajarias, MD
Assistant Professor of Medicine, Cardiology Division,
Washington University School of Medicine;
Interventional Cardiologist, Barnes-Jewish Hospital, St.
Louis, Missouri
*Percutaneous Closure of Patent Foramen Ovale and Atrial
Septal Defect*

Khaled M. Ziada, MD
Assistant Professor of Medicine, Division of
Cardiovascular Medicine, and Associate Director,
Interventional Cardiology Fellowship Program,
University of Kentucky College of Medicine, Lexington,
Kentucky
*Periprocedural Myocardial Infarction and Embolism-
Protection Devices*

Andrew A. Ziskind, MD, MBA
Professor of Medicine, Washington University School of
Medicine; President, Barnes-Jewish Hospital, St. Louis,
Missouri
*Percutaneous Balloon Pericardiotomy for Patients with
Pericardial Effusion and Tamponade*

Preface

Radical, maximally invasive surgery was performed for the preparation of this fifth edition of *Textbook of Interventional Cardiology*. There are over 30 new chapters and 70 new authors, for a complete revamping of the coverage of the ever-burgeoning field of interventional cardiology.

Section 1, Patient Selection, which is now considered highly important, is new to this edition. As percutaneous interventions have supplanted surgical ap-proaches for many types of patients and anatomical subsets, the risk and benefit assessment is critical. New chapters dedicated to arterial inflammation at baseline, which may be quite pivotal for long-term prognosis; functional testing, especially with multidetector CT angiography; and demographics, such as gender, ancestry, diabetes, and renal disease, have been added to help guide cardiologists in patient selection. An overview of evidence-based practice in interventional cardiology helps pull much of this together.

The complexity of coronary interventions has drastically changed, with approaches to left mainstem lesions that are unprotected, complex bifurcations, and diffuse disease now more common. Chapters on these topics, as is the case throughout the book, are written by international authorities. New chapters on transradial intervention and peri-access site management, which may be an important segue to facilitate outpatient intervention, are especially pragmatic.

The past year has been checkered in the field, with marked public attention given to late thrombosis of drug-coated stents and the results of the COURAGE trial. Late stent thrombosis, to which a new chapter is dedicated, is certainly a lingering concern that has led to more prolonged dual antiplatelet therapy and a shift in practice in the United States toward more bare metal stents. While the incidence of late stent thrombosis is quite low, we clearly need more information in order to prevent this dreaded complication. The COURAGE trial sparked debate as to whether percutaneous coronary intervention procedures were even warranted as compared with a pharmacologic-only strategy. The trial had major shortcomings, but the most important was the selection of the endpoint of death or myocardial infarction. No prior trial had shown benefit for this endpoint in the history of interventional cardiology, so to anticipate that this could be possible defies any Bayesian or *a priori* knowledge of the field. While interventional cardiology has been under

fire for these two issues, the hope is that this will settle with the realization that there has been truly remarkable and relentless progress in the field.

One of the most exciting frontiers is the transformation of select hospitals into interventional centers of excellence. Two new chapters address this opportunity. One tackles acute myocardial infarction and acute coronary syndromes. The other chapter deals with the concept of stroke centers, performing acute intervention on patients with evolving stroke.

What are the other new frontiers for this field? The book delves much more deeply into each type of "big artery," noncoronary intervention with the lower and upper extremities, mesenteric, renal, carotid, and cerebrovascular arterial beds, along with venous interventions. This is a major difference from the last edition—the practice of interventional cardiology now extends to virtually all of the major artery beds. Certainly intracardiac intervention is a promising new dimension, with intracardiac echo, left atrial appendage closure, and percutaneous repair of the mitral valve or aortic valve. Using catheter-based intervention for stem cell therapy, regeneration therapy, or angiogenesis are particularly topical and important research paths. And the same applies for detection of vulnerable plaque and the controversy of whether nonobstructive inflamed segments of arteries should undergo intervention to preempt plaque fissure, erosion, or rupture. All of these topics are covered in newly added chapters.

The chapters on quality of care and regulatory issues also are new and present salient perspectives on the practice and regulatory aspects of the field.

Cumulatively, this book not only has hopefully tracked the progress in the field but also has provided a futuristic perspective. Compared with the field when the first edition of this textbook was published in the 1980s, when all there was to work with were relatively primitive balloon angioplasty catheters and a bit of roulette as to whether a major coronary dissection would be induced, the practice of interventional cardiology today is unrecognizable. Rarely is just a balloon used, the procedure is almost invariably calm and predicable, and now the real interventional cardiologist is "pan-vascular" and evolving to practice an "intracardiac" genre, facile in all of the noncoronary vasculature procedures including the ability to close a patent foarmen ovale or left atrial appendage, or perform transcatheter valve repair.

Of the five editions of this book, I believe this one has captured and anticipated the field better than any other. I am especially grateful to the 125 authors from all over the world who shared their expertise and have put together an unprecedented reference source for our field. Michael Goldberg and his book production team at Elsevier have been formidable supporters, providing an exceptional layout; Natasha Andjelkovic, executive publisher, and Agnes Byrne, developmental editor, also at Elsevier, were most helpful in getting this project off the ground, along with my prior editorial assistant, Donna Wasiewicz-Bressan. I also want to express my deepest thanks to my friend and colleague Dr. Paul Teirstein, who has shown me a whole new level of interventional cardiology since my arrival in La Jolla. We all hope that the interventional cardiologist will find this a particularly useful reference source for what still remains the most remarkable discipline in medicine—one in which immediate gratification for patients can be achieved, and long-term imaginative solutions to complex challenges just keep accruing at a breakneck pace.

Eric J. Topol

Contents

DVD Contents

Patient Selection

CHAPTER

1 Inflammation Status

Saif Anwaruddin and Eric J. Topol

KEY POINTS

- Inflammation should be considered a risk factor for coronary atherosclerosis and acute coronary syndromes (ACS).
- Molecular biomarkers may help to define the inflammatory state and to describe characteristics such as plaque morphology and acute thrombosis.
- Within interventional cardiology, despite technologic advances, inflammation still remains a limiting factor in terms of restenosis, stent thrombosis, microembolization, and so on.
- Adjuvant medical therapy has improved outcomes in interventional cardiology, and this may, in part, be due to potent anti-inflammatory properties of these drugs.
- The optimal timing of pretreatment with adjuvant medical therapy in both elective and emergent percutaneous coronary intervention (PCI) has been shown to be of significance and may be related to controlling the inflammatory response to injury from PCI.
- Future directions in interventional cardiology will focus on device-based therapies, but there will also be a need to discover newer drug therapies that allow for more effective and efficient methods of modulating inflammation.

Although atherosclerosis and acute coronary syndromes (ACS) are related, they remain distinct entities from both a pathophysiologic and a clinical standpoint. Many patients develop severe atherosclerotic disease of coronary vessels but never experience an ACS, whereas others die of an ACS without symptomatic evidence of significant antecedent coronary atherosclerosis. This heterogeneity probably reflects differences in genetic heritability and environmental factors that, in turn, contribute to differences in both the predisposition and the response to injury.[1] As our understanding of these entities improves, evidence supporting the role of inflammation as a central component of both of these processes continues to accumulate.

Inflammation appears to be integral in the induction and propagation of atherogenesis and atherothrombosis. The perpetuation of atherosclerosis by inflammation is also a concept that has important implications, both for the identification of patients at risk and in the treatment of clinically apparent disease. The presence of clinically detectable levels of inflammation in otherwise asymptomatic patients should be considered a harbinger of potentially adverse outcomes.

Current emphasis on risk factor modification focuses primarily on the traditional coronary artery disease risk factors, including smoking, dyslipidemia, hypertension, and the presence of diabetes. Despite affecting the response of patients with atherosclerosis and ACS to various therapies and ultimately dictating their clinical course, inflammation has emerged as a risk factor that needs to be addressed and modi-

fied. How to accomplish this task is a question is of tremendous value, not only in terms of preventive strategies, but also for currently available percutaneous coronary interventions (PCI).

Controversy exists regarding the best way to define inflammation as a risk factor in otherwise healthy patients and in those with preexisting coronary artery disease. Although C-reactive protein (CRP) has been extensively studied, both as an independent marker of risk and as an active participant in the process, some researchers have questioned the clinical value of this marker.

The focus on a single vulnerable plaque is only the tip of the proverbial iceberg. The ACSs seem to be driven by inflammation, a process that more globally affects the entire coronary tree. Although treating individual "unstable" plaques remains enticing, a more complete approach to interventional therapy must be employed, with an emphasis on treating the vulnerable lesion in the context of the broader inflammatory component. As details of the underlying molecular and genetic mechanisms become more apparent, treatment of atherosclerosis and ACS may ultimately become more individually tailored.

Understanding the connection between inflammation and thrombosis is vital to achieving an appreciation of the pathophysiology behind ACS and coronary artery disease. To better serve our patients with this information, viable methods of quantifying arterial inflammation as a modifiable risk factor need to be developed and utilized. Ultimately, this information can help rationalize treatment strategies in order to overcome current obstacles within interventional

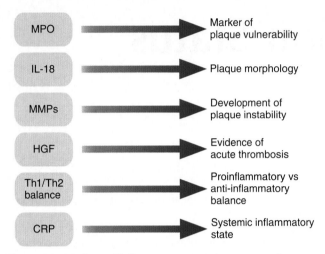

Figure 1-1. Markers of inflammatory status in coronary disease. CRP, C-reactive protein; HGF, hepatocyte growth factor; IL-18, interleukin-18; MMPs, matrix metalloproteinases; MPO, myeloperoxidase; Th, helper T cells.

cardiology. With the use of drug-eluting stents (DES) and adjuvant medical therapy, this process is already underway, but it continues to evolve. The challenge is to overcome the limitations, including restenosis and thrombosis, that have important inflammatory underpinnings. This chapter provides an overview of the complex inflammatory components that contribute to atherothrombosis and how percutaneous strategies induce or are influenced by arterial inflammation.

INFLAMMATION, ATHEROSCLEROSIS, AND ATHEROTHROMBOSIS

Quantifying Inflammatory Status

The evaluation and modification of clinical predictors in patients with known coronary atherosclerosis, or in those at risk for developing atherosclerosis or atherothrombosis, is well established. The limitation of these traditional clinical predictors lies in their inability to adequately incorporate other elements, such as inflammation. Attempts to quantify the degree of inflammation and its significance require understanding of the underlying molecular factors involved in the inflammatory and thrombotic processes (Fig. 1-1).

Molecular biomarkers of inflammation can be used to predict the future risk of clinical events or to evaluate an appropriate response to therapy. Their use may facilitate targeted therapeutic strategies based on a comprehensive molecular risk profile rather than simply on clinical characteristics. The challenge remains in being able to accurately define and measure the inflammatory state. Although many candidates have been considered, only a select number are supported by the available clinical data. Even fewer have been rigorously evaluated in large-

scale clinical studies to ensure their utility and to confirm their value. Candidate markers need to undergo a meticulous process of evaluation to examine their worth in the clinical context, including an assessment of their practicality, their cost-effectiveness, and whether they add information beyond that which is already known. Furthermore, whether specifically targeting these markers with medical therapy affects clinical outcomes remains to be seen.

C-reactive Protein

Traditionally defined as an acute phase reactant, CRP has achieved recognition as a marker of inflammation. The value of high-sensitivity CRP (hsCRP) as a marker of systemic inflammation is in its ability to predict cardiovascular risk. Extensive large-scale epidemiologic data exist that support the ability of CRP to predict the risk of future cardiovascular events in otherwise healthy individuals,[2,3] in those with unstable angina, and in patients who have undergone PCI procedures. The association between CRP and cardiovascular events only strengthens the importance of inflammation in ACS and atherosclerotic disease.

Although CRP is produced in the liver, there is ample evidence to suggest that it is actively involved in atherosclerotic disease. Its role in upregulation of adhesion molecule expression in endothelial cells and in controlling macrophage recruitment lend support to its involvement in atherosclerosis and ACS. In addition, autopsy studies have demonstrated CRP immunoreactivity in plaques with vulnerable morphology.[4] Therefore, CRP represents an attractive target for medical therapy, in both primary and secondary prevention strategies. However, studies have not addressed CRP as a treatable risk factor per se, but have focused instead on the secondary effects of treatment on CRP levels. An ongoing study, the Justification for the Use of Statins in Primary Prevention: an Intervention Trial Evaluating Rosuvastatin (JUPITER), is attempting to address this question.[5]

Platelets: Mediators Of Inflammation and Thrombosis

Platelets are central to the processes of atherosclerosis and ACS, because they provide a link between inflammation and thrombosis. In the context of ACS and PCI, the effect of platelet inhibition probably extends beyond the ability to inhibit thrombosis, involving regulation of platelet-mediated inflammation (Fig. 1-2). The interactions among platelets, endothelium, and leukocytes facilitate the process of platelet-mediated inflammation and thrombosis. Antiplatelet therapy continues to be an effective method of preventing thrombosis; however, a significant benefit may occur through modulation of the inflammatory properties inherent to platelet function.

Considerable interest has been generated for the platelet-derived CD40 ligand (CD40L) and soluble CD40 ligand (sCD40L) in the context of atherosclerosis and ACS. Although it was originally thought to

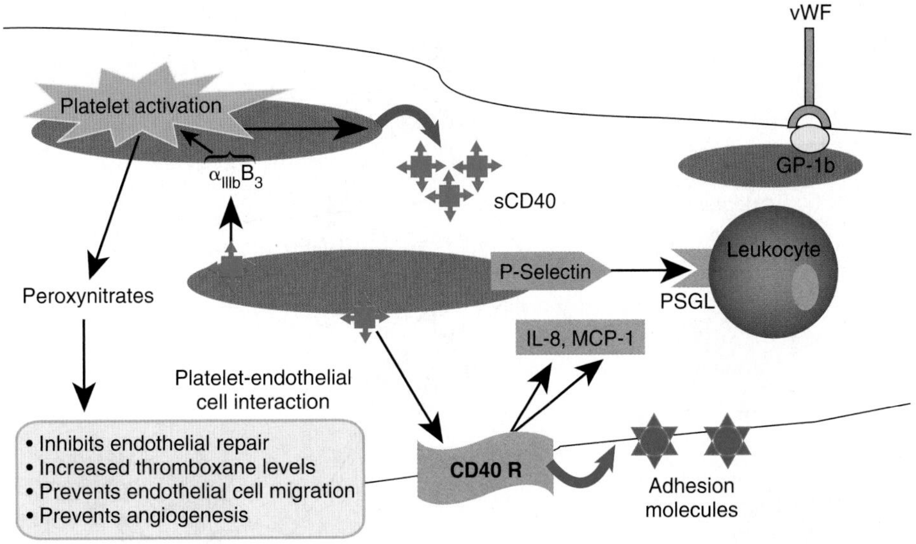

Figure 1-2. Platelets as mediators of inflammation. $\alpha_{IIb}\beta_3$, a glycoprotein receptor; CD40 R, CD40 receptor; GP-1b, glycoprotein-Ib; IL-8, interleukin-8; MCP-1, monocyte chemoattractant protein-1; PSGL, P-selectin glycoprotein ligand; sCD40, soluble CD40; vWF, von Willebrand factor. (From Anwaruddin S, Askari A, Topol EJ: Redefining risk in acute coronary syndromes using molecular medicine. J Am Coll Cardiol 2007;49:279-289.)

be involved in cellular development within the context of humoral immunity, CD40L has been found on other cell types, including eosinophils, T cells, basophils, and monocytes, in both bound and soluble forms. Commensurate with its widespread distribution is the myriad of functions CD40L participates in related to atherogenesis and ACS.

By facilitating direct interaction with endothelial cells, platelet-bound CD40L is pro-inflammatory and has been shown to upregulate cellular adhesion molecules, increase secretion of chemokines,[6] and increase tissue factor production. Facilitating the activation of monocytes,[7] in combination with its other roles, places CD40L in the center of the atherosclerotic process. In addition to potent pro-inflammatory effects, CD40L regulates the development and stability of thrombus in ACS. Stability is maintained by the interaction between the lysine-arginine-glutamic acid domain of the CD40L and the platelet $\alpha_{IIb}\beta_3$ receptor.[8]

Whereas inhibition of CD40L results in more stable plaque morphology, CD40L left unchecked engages in destabilizing activities. When anti-CD40L antibody was administered to apoE −/− mice treated with anti-CD40L, a reduction in plaque lipid and inflammatory content was noted, without any effect on the size of the lesion.[9] CD40L is also influential in the production and release of matrix metalloproteinases (MMPs), which are thought to be responsible for degradation of the fibrous cap of the atheromatous plaque. These effects of CD40L support its role in plaque instability and atherothrombosis.

Clinically, the ratio of sCD40L to CD40L provides important prognostic value. In patients presenting with ACS, elevated sCD40L was an independent predictor of death and recurrent myocardial infarction (MI).[10] Data from the Dallas Heart Study noted that sCD40L is not a marker of clinically silent atherosclerotic disease, nor is it associated with traditional risk factors for coronary atherosclerosis, suggesting a separate inflammatory process involved in the genesis

of an ACS.[11] A large, placebo-controlled randomized trial of platelet glycoprotein inhibitors in PCI for ACS showed particular benefit among those patients with elevated sCD40L.[12]

The interaction and communication among platelets and leukocytes is essential to the process of inflammation and its sequelae. Inasmuch as the interaction between platelets is emphasized in this scenario, leukocyte and platelet interactions are also vital to the development of thrombosis in ACS. One of the key intermediaries between platelets and leukocytes is P-selectin and its interaction with the P-selectin glycoprotein ligand (PSGL). In experimental models, P-selectin was shown to be important to the processes of thrombosis and thrombus stability.[13]

P-selectin potentially represents an important target for therapy, given its presence in thrombosis. Clinically, in patients presenting with chest pain, elevated levels of P-selectin were predictive of future troponin I positivity.[14] In apparently healthy women, P-selectin levels were predictive of future cardiovascular events.[15] However, direct measurement of platelet-monocyte aggregates may represent a more sensitive marker than P-selectin, and it remains to be seen whether P-selectin will be of value as a true connection between inflammation and thrombosis.

Leukocytes and Inflammation in Acute Coronary Syndromes and Coronary Atherosclerosis

The inflammatory responses leading to the disruption of plaque in ACS and subsequent events is characterized by a varied cellular presence. The relationship between monocyte-derived macrophages and the pathogenesis of atherosclerotic coronary artery disease has been well studied. The importance of neutrophils, lymphocytes, and mast cells in plaque disruption and thrombosis has become apparent. The value of leukocytosis in acute myocardial infarction may extend beyond simple prognosis and may predict patient response to revascularization strategies.

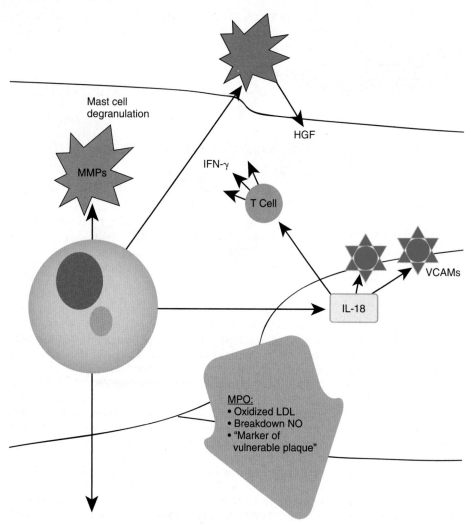

Mast cell
degranulation

MMPs

HGF

IFN-γ

T Cell

VCAMs

IL-18

MPO:
• Oxidized LDL
• Breakdown NO
• "Marker of
vulnerable plaque"

MCP-1: Summons macrophages/monocytes to sites of injury

Figure 1-3. Leukocyte secretory products. HGF, hepatocyte growth factor; IL-18, interleukin-18; INF-γ, interferon-γ; LDL, low-density lipoprotein cholesterol; MCP-1, monocyte chemoattractant protein-1; MMPs, matrix metalloproteinases; MPO, myeloperoxidase; NO, nitric oxide; VCAMs, vascular cell adhesion molecules. (From Anwaruddin S, Askari A, Topol EJ: Redefining risk in acute coronary syndromes using molecular medicine. J Am Coll Cardiol 2007;49:279-289.)

Several studies have assessed the prognostic value of leukocytosis in the setting of ACS, supporting a relationship between leukocytosis and adverse cardiac events during hospitalization for acute MI.[16] In ACS, the presence of neutrophils is being recognized as an important component of acute plaque rupture. Furthermore, elevated neutrophil counts in those with acute MI are associated with suboptimal angiographic results after fibrinolysis.[17] The monocyte-macrophage is central to the events leading to formation of the atherosclerotic plaque and to promoting ongoing inflammation, which may trigger an ACS via an array of leukocyte secretory products. These leukocyte secretory products serve to provide a potential mechanistic link between inflammation and the pathogenesis of atherothrombosis and atherosclerosis (Fig. 1-3).

Myeloperoxidase

Production and release of myeloperoxidase (MPO) from granules is known to occur in both neutrophils and monocytes. MPO is involved in several processes that modulate atherogenesis and coronary inflammation. For example, MPO has the ability to oxidize low-density lipoprotein (LDL) cholesterol, to break down nitric oxide (NO), to regulate endothelial homeostasis, and to modulate NO function in inflammatory processes.[18]

Elevated levels of MPO have been demonstrated in patients with coronary artery disease and have been implicated as having a role in plaque destabilization.[19] An elevated level of MPO at the time of presentation with an ACS was associated with a worse prognosis irrespective of troponin T level,[20] emphasizing the importance of the underlying inflammatory state. It is plausible that the presence of persistent inflammation may contribute to future events. Therefore, the role of MPO as a "marker of the vulnerable plaque" even in the troponin-negative ACS patient has been suggested.[21]

MPO serves to highlight the role of neutrophils in initiation of the events leading to ACS and events occurring immediately after MI. In addition to prognostic value, it provides a direct indication of underlying plaque instability in those with suspected ACS.

Interleukin-18

Interleukin-18 (IL-18) is a cytokine that is capable of inducing production of interferon-γ (IFN-γ) in T lymphocytes and of supporting differentiation of the T_H1 subset of helper T lymphocytes. IL-18 production is increased by stimulation from IL-1β. The resultant increase in IL-18 and the binding to the IL-18 receptor on macrophages and vascular smooth muscle cells results in upregulation of IFN-γ, MMPs, various cytokines, and vascular cell adhesion molecules (VCAMs). Furthermore, IL-18 has been found in atherosclerotic plaques. Increased IL-18 expression results in a "vulnerable plaque morphology," defined by thin cap atheroma and more intraplaque hemorrhage.[22] However, the exact mechanism by which IL-18 contributes to atherosclerotic disease remains controversial.

Although increased IL-18 expression has been noted in patients with ACS as well as in those with known coronary artery disease who are at increased risk of death from cardiovascular causes, the role of IL-18 in ACS is still undetermined and needs to be understood in relation to other factors. The ratio of IL-18, a pro-inflammatory cytokine, to that of IL-10, an anti-inflammatory cytokine, may be more important than the actual quantity of IL-18 itself.[23] Nevertheless, future investigation is necessary before the utility of this cytokine is fully understood.

Matrix Metalloproteinases

MMPs serve to regulate the extracellular environment through breakdown and proteolysis of matrix components, so as to facilitate a favorable environment for cellular development. MMPs are produced in a propeptide form and undergo eventual cleavage in the extracellular environment. MMPs have been implicated in processes such as neointimal hyperplasia, left ventricular remodeling, and formation of vascular aneurysms.

MMP-9, or gelatinase B, and MMP-2, or gelatinase A, are thought to be involved in the development of plaque instability. Local release of these factors is believed to degrade the fibrous cap of the atherosclerotic plaque. Evidence to support the involvement of MMPs in ACS has come from small clinical studies. Higher blood levels of MMP-2 and MMP-9 have been noted in ACS patients compared with healthy controls. Although elevated MMP-9 concentrations were associated with an increased hazard ratio of cardiovascular death after adjusting for clinical confounders,[24] what was not entirely evident was whether MMP-9 provided prognostic information beyond that conveyed by other biomarkers of inflammation typically examined in ACS. Although preliminary work with MMPs is suggestive of their participation in ACS, future translational and clinical investigations need to examine not only MMPs but also their relationship with tissue inhibitors of metalloproteinases (TIMPs). This regulatory association is important, and an improved understanding of it may provide more accurate and more valuable insight as to the significance of MMPs/TIMPs in coronary atherosclerosis and ACS.

Pregnancy-Associated Plasma Protein A

Pregnancy-associated plasma protein A (PAPP-A), a zinc-binding metalloproteinase that is secreted by activated macrophages, fibroblasts, vascular smooth muscle cells, osteoblasts, and placental syncytiotrophoblasts, functions to activate insulin-like growth factor-1 (IGF-1) through actions on IGF-binding protein (IGF-BP). Although the role for PAPP-A as a biomarker for Down syndrome during pregnancy is well established, its potential role with respect to coronary atherosclerosis and ACS has only recently been recognized.

PAPP-A has been found in higher concentrations in unstable plaques from patients dying as a result of ACS. In addition, circulating levels of PAPP-A have been shown to be significantly higher in patients with unstable coronary syndromes versus stable angina.[25] Furthermore, an elevated PAPP-A level was an independent predictor of a 6-month combined primary end point of cardiovascular events, including mortality, in a study of troponin I–negative patients presenting with ACS.[26] Although the findings are quite preliminary, both PAPP-A and the ratio of PAPP-A to proMBP[27] have correlated with extent of coronary atherosclerosis in stable angina.

Although PAPP-A may be present in the unstable plaque in ACS and in peripheral blood of patients with coronary atherosclerosis, its role remains undefined. Some have postulated that, through proteolytic breakdown of IGF-BP activating IGF-1, PAPP-A is able to mediate pro-atherogenic functions and may participate in local inflammatory processes.[28] Conversely, IGF-1 may be protective in coronary and systemic vascular disease, and lower IGF-1 levels may actually predict adverse cardiac events.[29] PAPP-A may simply be a marker of atherosclerotic disease and not directly involved in the pathogenesis.[30] Although these possibilities remain intriguing, it is premature to advocate for the clinical use of PAPP-A in the absence of a proven, pertinent mechanism.

Hepatocyte Growth Factor

Hepatocyte growth factor (HGF), a growth factor originally thought to be important in cellular growth and development, possesses characteristics that underscore a potential purpose in ACS. In the context of acute plaque rupture and thrombosis, there appears to be a relationship between thrombus formation and release of HGF. This appears to be dependent on the presence of mast cells as an intermediary. Perhaps, through activation of the thrombin receptor on mast cells, release of heparin leads to elevated HGF release from the extracellular matrix.

Clinically, significantly higher levels of HGF were demonstrated in patients with chest pain and evidence of acute thrombosis (from ACS, aortic dissection, or acute pulmonary emboli) compared with those without evidence of thrombosis.[31] Similar findings were noted in patients who presented with cerebral infarction and unstable angina. It has been suggested that elevated levels of HGF may be protective in the ACS setting. Although HGF release may be a direct response to acute thrombosis and subsequent myocardial injury, larger studies are needed to validate these findings and to determine whether any relationship exists between levels of HGF and clinical prognosis.

T Cells and Interferon-γ

Supporting the inflammatory basis for atherosclerosis and ACS is the involvement of specific subsets of T lymphocytes. Helper T (T_H) lymphocytes are central mediators of inflammation. T_H1 subsets are pro-inflammatory and express cytokines such as IFN-γ, IL-2, and tumor necrosis factor-β (TNF-β). In contrast, T_H2 cells are responsible for regulating humoral immunity and attenuating inflammation. That T cells are involved in the progression of atherosclerosis has been shown by transfer of CD4+ T cells into B cell– and T cell–deficient apoE$^{-/-/scid/scid}$ mice, which resulted in worsening of atherosclerotic disease and upregulation of IFN-γ secretion.[32]

In ACS, higher levels of T-cell activation have been noted and are thought to be independent of ischemic injury. Significantly higher levels of T_H1 CD4+ cells were observed in patients with unstable angina, compared with controls. Similar findings were noted in patients with acute MIs.[33]

The functional significance of the presence of T_H1 cells in unstable coronary syndromes may be related to expression and release of IFN-γ. Downstream activation of monocyte-macrophages may result from T_H1-mediated IFN-γ release. Upregulation of IFN-γ–inducible genes in monocytes occurs in unstable angina, further supporting T_H1-mediated activation of macrophages in ACS.[34]

A GENETIC BASIS FOR INFLAMMATION

The ability to quantify and eventually treat inflammation as a risk factor for cardiovascular disease may hinge on a proper understanding of the determinants of inflammation. A complex phenotype such as inflammation is strongly influenced by genetics, which may help explain the variation in inflammatory status among those with coronary disease. The discovery of myocyte enhancer factor 2A (MEF2A) and its relationship to MI illustrated the intricate relationship between genetics and clinical cardiology.[35] In addition, specific haplotypes in the gene encoding for the 5-lipoxygenase activating protein (FLAP) have been shown to confer an increased risk of MI and stroke in selected populations.[36] FLAP appears to modulate the production of pro-inflammatory intermediaries such as leukotriene B4 that are believed to be of significance in coronary disease. Furthermore, upregulation of the leukotriene pathway

is also associated with a haplotype of the leukotriene A4 hydrolase (LTA4H) gene, which also confers a risk of MI.[37]

Targeting these pathways based on genetic risk could represent a novel method of identifying and treating inflammation as it relates to MI and coronary atherosclerosis. FLAP inhibitors have been used in a prospective, randomized fashion to demonstrate a reduction in inflammatory biomarkers among those carrying haplotypes associated with increased risk.[38] As the tools used to facilitate discovery of such markers improve, so will both our understanding of the complex nature of inflammation as it relates to coronary disease and our ability to modulate it.

INFLAMMATION AND PERCUTANEOUS CORONARY INTERVENTION

The treatment of stable yet symptomatic coronary atherosclerosis and unstable coronary atherothrombosis has progressed from balloon angioplasty to the modern era of DES and will continue to evolve. Adjunctive medical therapy in the form of statins, glycoprotein inhibitors, and thienopyridines and antithrombin agents has also been a mainstay of treatment aimed at controlling risk factors and progression of disease, both at the time of intervention and afterward. The ultimate success or failure of PCI and management of coronary atherosclerosis varies among individuals. Beyond technical considerations, revascularization has been and will continue to be limited in efficacy by one major variable—inflammation. The focus of treatment must address inflammation to improve outcomes in PCI.

Many of the challenges faced by interventional cardiologists are rooted in problems related to inflammation, a process mediating the response to injury after insult to the endothelial integrity imparted by PCI. The resultant neointima formation has been noted to be a significant problem and occurs as a result of cell death and inflammation. Although DES have been able to temper this process, they are neither a definitive nor a perfect solution.[39,40] Inflammation is a more prominent force, not only in the initiation and propagation of disease, such as in ACS, but also in response to injury after PCI.

Inflammation as a Response to Injury: Pathobiology and Clinical Significance

The pathobiology of the arterial response to injury in the form of PCI with stent deployment has been extensively examined. Stenting leads to an acute inflammatory response, followed by chronic inflammation. Within minutes after stent deployment, an intense reaction to injury consists of platelet activation and accumulation, expression of adhesion molecules, leukocyte recruitment, and thrombus formation. The degree of injury likely determines the resultant inflammatory response and eventual restenosis (Figs. 1-4 and 1-5). In autopsy studies, pathologic data suggest that stent deployment leading to

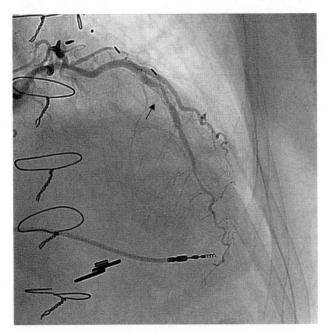

Figure 1-4. Angiogram demonstrating in-stent restenosis of a sirolimus-eluting stent in the middle left anterior descending artery *(arrow)*.

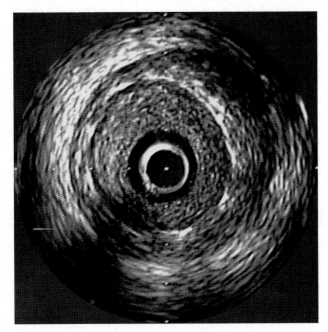

Figure 1-5. Intravascular ultrasound (IVUS) demonstrating severe in-stent restenosis.

arterial medial fracture, particularly deep into lipid-rich plaque, is associated with a higher degree of inflammatory infiltrate, increased neointimal thickness, and neoangiogenesis.[41] Clinical factors associated with restenosis, particularly in diabetics, include longer stent length, active tobacco use, smaller arterial reference diameter, and inflammatory state as determined by CRP level.[42]

Leukocyte infiltration as a response to injury remains an important feature of this inflammatory assault, as does leukocyte adhesion to endothelial cells and to platelets. The expression of neutrophil adhesion molecules, particularly the integrins CD11b/CD18 (now ITGAM/ITGB2) known as the membrane attack complex (MAC-1), increases after PCI with bare metal stents (BMS) in patients with single-vessel coronary atherosclerosis and is strongly correlated with the risk of restenosis. The correlation between MAC-1 expression, as a surrogate marker of leukocyte activation, and neointimal hyperplasia has been examined in MAC-1 −/− mice. After endothelial denudation, a limited leukocyte presence and a reduction in the degree of neointimal hyperplasia were noted.[43]

The response-to-injury hypothesis appears to involve a complex interplay among platelets, leukocytes, fibrin, and other components. The release of a multitude of cytokine mediators, such as MCP-1, IL-6, IL-1, and TNF-α, appears to coordinate this effort. The end result is neointimal hyperplasia leading to restenosis. The potential exists to establish molecular targets, such as MAC-1, with the aim of developing specific therapies to combat inflammation.

The significance of these findings is highlighted by the influence of inflammation on clinical outcomes. Leukocytosis, a nonspecific surrogate marker of inflammatory response across the spectrum of ACS, has been demonstrated to be an ominous sign. In the setting of PCI, peak circulating monocyte count has been shown to be associated with angiographic restenosis at 6 months.[44]

Biomarkers of Inflammation and Percutaneous Coronary Intervention

Inflammatory biomarkers have also been used to quantify systemic inflammation to assess the relation between inflammation and restenosis in PCI. Preprocedural levels of sCD40L were examined prospectively and found to be predictors of restenosis at 6 months in patients undergoing PCI for stable angina.[45] CRP elevation is more commonly used as a measure of inflammatory status after coronary stent implantation. Levels of hsCRP were shown to rise across a translesional gradient, both in patients with angina and in those who had undergone PCI, suggesting local production of CRP or increased local release of CRP-rich thrombus.[46] In patients with stable coronary disease who underwent PCI, elevated postprocedural levels of CRP were noted and supported a robust inflammatory response.

The rationale of predicting outcomes using preprocedural measures of inflammation remains controversial, because pre-PCI levels of CRP and IL-6 have not been shown to correlate with in-stent restenosis after PCI.[47] In 483 patients with stable or unstable angina who underwent coronary intervention with BMS, elevated CRP and lipoprotein(a) predicted adverse cardiac events at 1 year, but the association did not hold for in-stent restenosis.[48] Prospective investigation of 276 patients who had undergone PCI with BMS for both stable angina and unstable

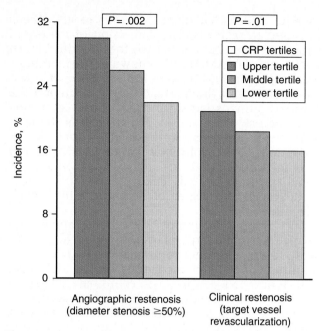

Figure 1-6. Incidence of angiographic and clinical restenosis in three groups defined by the change in C-reactive protein (Δ CRP) after percutaneous coronary interventions. (Redrawn from Dibra A, Mehilli J, Braun S, et al: Inflammatory response after intervention assessed by serial C-reactive protein measurements correlates with restenosis in patients treated with coronary stenting. Am Heart J 2005;150:344-350.)

coronary syndromes demonstrated that preprocedural CRP levels were predictive of increased rates of restenosis and worse clinical outcomes after adjusting for the presence of unstable coronary disease.[49] Given the available data, it is difficult to make definitive conclusions regarding the utility of the preprocedural inflammatory state, particularly in the population of patients with stable angina. In ACS, however, an assessment of the baseline inflammatory state may provide valuable prognostic information.

Clinically, a rise in postprocedural CRP has been shown to correlate with in-stent restenosis at 6 months after PCI. In 1800 patients with either stable or unstable angina undergoing PCI, peak postprocedure CRP level strongly correlated with both angiographic and clinical restenosis (Fig. 1-6). Those patients in the highest tertile of postprocedure increase in CRP level also had higher 30-day rates of stent thrombosis, death, MI, or target vessel revascularization.[50] Alternatively, a return of post-PCI CRP levels to baseline 72 hours after intervention was highly predictive of event-free survival over a 1-year period in a prospective study of 81 consecutive patients with one-vessel stable angina. Therefore, the postprocedural rise in CRP appears to provide a consistent correlation with future risk of restenosis.

GENETICS, INFLAMMATION, AND RESTENOSIS

Inflammation as a response to injury in the post-PCI population is not a universal phenomenon and begs the question of individual genetic susceptibility. The presence of genetic polymorphisms may help define susceptibility and may affect the selection of therapy for certain patients undergoing PCI. The inflammatory response may, in part, be determined by underlying genetic predisposition. The value of such information, beyond traditional risk factors of restenosis (e.g., diabetes), will be determined in studies of large populations. The Genetic Determinants of Restenosis (GENDER) project is one of the studies that have set out to examine possible genetic risk factors.

Although the information generated from these studies is only preliminary, it accomplishes two tasks—the first is to generate hypotheses regarding possible novel mechanisms for restenosis, and the second is to encourage larger-scale studies to validate these ideas. The data from most of these studies is obtained in smaller populations, so the possibility exists that these associations between clinical events and polymorphisms may not exist. Furthermore, most of these studies are of selected populations, and generalization to other ethnic groups or races may not be appropriate. Even where the associations have been proven to be robust in large numbers of subjects, genetic epidemiologic studies do not elucidate pathophysiologic mechanisms.

Polymorphisms have been examined in many different components of the complex array of factors involved in restenosis (Table 1-1). Inflammatory markers such as interleukins, selectins, MMPs, and proteins involved in platelet aggregation and the renin-angiotensin system have been examined, among others. Whether the same polymorphisms are responsible for restenosis in those with DES remains to be seen; however, the idea of a genetic basis for this inflammatory response to injury may allow for both selectively directed therapy and the development of newer therapies directed specifically at known genetic targets.

INFLAMMATION AND DRUG-ELUTING STENTS

Clinical restenosis occurs as a result of both injury to the vessel and the underlying atherosclerotic and inflammatory burden. With the introduction of the sirolimus-eluting (Cypher [Cordis, Johnson and Johnson]) stents and the paclitaxel-eluting (Taxus [Boston Scientific]) stents, potent anti-inflammatory drugs have been applied with the aim of reducing the inflammatory response to injury. Large clinical trials support a reduction in the rate of clinical restenosis with DES compared with BMS.[39,40] The relationship between the inflammatory milieu and the DES is a complex one, at best. Attempting to understand this dynamic may help to define the limitations of these stents and how best to use them.

Defining the inflammatory state through the use of baseline levels of biomarkers or changes in levels is perhaps a simplistic estimation of the events that constitute a complex process. An appreciation of the relationship between DES and inflammation first requires an understanding that the inflammatory

Table 1-1. Genetic Polymorphisms and the Risk of Restenosis

Polymorphism	Study	Follow-up	N and Procedure	Clinical Outcome	Results	Comments
LPL (8p22) polymorphisms: −93/T/G Ser447Ter Asp9Asn Asn291Ser	Monraats et al[86]	9 mo	3104 (PCI)	TVR by either PCI or CABG	Ser447Ter associated with decreased risk of TVR after PCI	BMS used. Ser447Ter SNP codes for a stop codon
Angiotensinogen: 235Met/Thr, T174M, A(−6)G, AT1R: 1166A/C, T810A AT2R: 1675G/A, 2123A HO-1: Polymorphism in promoter region	Wijpkema et al[87]	9.6 mo	2987 (PCI)	1° end point: TVR 2° end point: clinical restenosis	287 with TVR, 327 with 2° endpoint; AT1R 1166CC associated with 1° (P = .007) and 2° (P = .002) end points	Relationship still significant after adjustment for use of ACE inhibitors
48 different polymorphisms in 34 genes associated with inflammatory mediators such as adrenergic receptor, various interleukins, CSF, complement, NOS, SDF-1	Monraats et al[88]	9.6 mo	3104 (PCI)	TVR as defined by PCI or CABG 1 mo after procedure	β_2-adrenergic receptor (ADRB2) Gly16Gly variant associated with increased risk of TVR, even after adjusting for diabetes, age, gender, and smoking status	CD14 (−260T/T), eotaxin gene (−1328A/A), and CSF2 gene (117Thr/Thr) variants were associated with lower risk of TVR
Fractalkine (FKN) receptor polymorphisms: V249I and T280M	Niessner et al[89]	1° End point: 6 mo 2° End point: 2 yr	365 (PCI)	1° end point: Clinical ISR 2° end point: Clinical re-ISR	Restenosis in 25% of patients; I249 allele associated with restenosis	Risk is associated with both ISR and recurrent ISR
Toll-like receptor SNPs: TLR-2 Arg753Gln TLR-4 Asp299Gly	Hamann et al[90]	6 mo	206 (PTCA) and 182 (stent)	Angiographic restenosis at 6 mo	TLR-2 Arg754Gln SNP associated with restenosis after PTCA and stent	Risk of this SNP and restenosis was higher in females than in males
Interferon-γ: IFNG T874A IFN-γ receptor: IFNGR1 C−56T IFNGR2 A839G	Tiroch et al[91]	Variable depending on end point	2591 (stent)	1° end point: Clinical (1 yr) and angiographic (6 mo) ISR 2° end point: Death and nonfatal MI (1 yr)	IFN and IFN receptor genotypes not found to have an association with ISR	No association found; however, authors attributed lack of observed relationship to complexity of molecular processes
SNPs of APOE gene: −219G/T 113G/C, 334T/C, 472T/C	Koch et al[92]	6-mo angiographic follow-up, 1 yr clinical	1850 (stent)	1° end point: angiographic restenosis at 6 mo and TVR at 1 yr 2° end point: death and nonfatal MI (1 yr)	No relationship found between APOE and either end point	

ACE, angiotensin-converting enzyme; APOE, apolipoprotein E; BMS, bare metal stent; CABG, coronary artery bypass grafting; CSF, colony-stimulating factor; DES, drug-eluting stent; IFN, interferon; ISR, in-stent restenosis; MI, myocardial infarction; NOS, nitric oxide synthase; PCI, percutaneous coronary intervention; PTCA, percutaneous transluminal coronary angioplasty; SDF-1, stromal-derived factor-1; SNP, single nucleotide polymorphism; TVR, target vessel revascularization.

state exists at multiple levels. Deployment of DES may have different effects on inflammation in the coronary versus the systemic setting. Clinical studies have examined these relationships (Table 1-2). Most support a local inflammatory milieu that is separate from the systemic inflammatory state and suggest that the use of DES may protect the local environment from outside inflammatory forces. A postprocedural rise in markers of systemic inflammation with the use of BMS, although paralleled with the use of DES, predicts outcome with regard to angiographic restenosis only when using BMS (Fig. 1-7). Other data sets suggest a relationship between the systemic

inflammatory response and the type of stent used. The differences between these data sets may be explained by many factors, including differences in timing of serum measurements, use of adjunctive therapies (e.g., heparin, glycoprotein IIb/IIIa inhibitors), the small size of these studies, and the lack of randomization in some. A substudy of the Randomized Trial to Evaluate Relative PROTECTion Against Post-PCI Microvascular Dysfunction and Post-PCI Ischemia Among Anti-Platelet and Anti-Thrombotic Agents (PROTECT-TIMI 30) noted a significant reduction in CRP and in troponin I rise with DES versus BMS after adjustment for variables

Table 1-2.   Relationship of Stent Type to Inflammation and Restenosis

Study	N	Design	End Points	Results	Comments
Gaspardone et al[93]	160	Nonrandomized; BMS, DES, or DEXs; low risk	Angiographic restenosis at 12.9 mo, CRP rise after procedure	No differences noted in CRP levels after procedure, but lower rate of restenosis in DES group	Although CRP elevation was predictive of restenosis, DES had a much lower rate of restenosis. Suggests that systemic inflammatory state may not be reflective of local environment.
Dibra et al[94]	301	Randomized; SES vs. BMS; low risk	Change in CRP; 6-mo angiographic follow-up for restenosis	Higher restenosis rate in BMS vs. SES	Elevated CRP levels in BMS group predicted restenosis, but restenosis in SES group was independent of rise in CRP
de la Torre-Hernandez et al[95]	300	Nonrandomized; SES vs. BMS; low risk	Change in CRP; 4-6 mo and 12 mo clinical follow-up assessing for MACE (death, MI, TVR)	CRP elevation similar in both groups, but the relation to restenosis was noted in BMS	The relationship between systemic inflammation (CRP) and restenosis holds only for BMS
Gogo et al[96]	75	Nonrandomized; SES vs. BMS; ACS included but no STEMI	Change in IL-6, IL-1Ra, CRP 24 hr after PCI	No difference in rise of inflammatory markers between DES and BMS	Evidence to support the idea that the systemic inflammatory response does not influence restenosis in DES population
Kim et al[97]	67	Nonrandomized; DES vs. BMS; low-risk population	CRP levels at various time points after PCI; 6 mo clinical follow-up, angiogram at 6 mo	Lower CRP levels with DES; greater-diameter stenosis and late lumen loss in BMS, although angiographic follow-up was incomplete	Suggests that the use of DES can alter systemic inflammatory conditions
Gibson et al[51]	665 DES, 139 BMS	Nonrandomized to stent type; NSTEMI patients undergoing PCI	CRP, IL-6, RANTES, sCD40L, TnI, PT F1.2, CK-MB at three time points	No differences noted with regard to sCD40L, RANTES, CK-MB, PT F1.2; rise in CRP and TnI was higher among those with BMS	In high-risk population, the benefit of DES may be in its effects on the microcirculation more so than on systemic inflammation

ACS, acute coronary syndrome; CK-MB, creatine kinase MB fraction; CRP, C-reactive protein; DES, drug-eluting stents; DEXs, dexamethasone eluting stents; IL, interleukin; MACE, major adverse cardiac event; NSTEMI, non-ST-segment elevation myocardial infarction; PCI, percutaneous coronary intervention; PT F1.2, prothrombin fragment 1.2; RANTES, regulated upon activation, normal T cell expressed and secreted; sCD40L, soluble CD40 ligand; SES, sirolimus-eluting stent; STEMI, ST-segment elevation myocardial infarction; TnI, troponin I; TVR, target vessel revascularization.

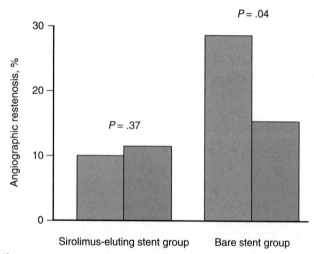

Figure 1-7. Angiographic restenosis (percentage) among patients whose postprocedure change in C-reactive protein levels were higher than the median *(purple bars)* and those whose values were no higher than the median *(blue bars)* in bare metal stent and sirolimus-eluting stent groups. (Redrawn from Dibra A, Ndrepepa G, Mehilli J, et al: Comparison of C-reactive protein levels before and after coronary stenting and restenosis among patients treated with sirolimus-eluting versus bare metal stents. Am J Cardiol 2005;95:1238-1240.)

such as diabetes, randomized treatment assignment to eptifibatide or bivalirudin, myocardial perfusion, epicardial artery perfusion, and duration of clopidogrel pretreatment. No significant differences were noted between the groups in regard to other markers such as sCD40L, RANTES, creatine kinase MB fraction (CK-MB), and prothrombin fragment F1.2.[51] Although this difference is intriguing, it may be more the result of an improved post-PCI microcirculatory status with the use of DES, as well as a reduction in myocardial injury (lower troponin I), and subsequent response to this (lower CRP). Whereas these studies presented varied conclusions with regard to the effects of DES on systemic inflammation, the populations sampled were also quite different in risk and ACS status.

The enthusiasm for the reduction in clinical and angiographic restenosis noted with the advent of DES has been tempered by the real concern for stent thrombosis in patients who have received DES (Fig. 1-8). In a large, prospective, observational study of 2239 patients, stent thrombosis complicated the course of 1.3% of patients receiving either sirolimus-eluting or paclitaxel-eluting stents. Fourteen patients had subacute stent thrombosis (≤30 days), and 15

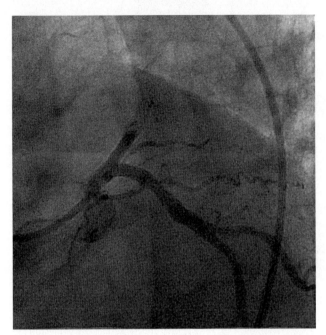

Figure 1-8. Angiogram demonstrating subacute stent thrombosis of a paclitaxel-eluting stent in the proximal left anterior descending artery (left anterior oblique caudal projection).

patients had late stent thrombosis (>30 days); 13 of these 29 patients died.[52] The factors associated with stent thrombosis from this study included premature cessation of antiplatelet therapy, diabetes mellitus, reduced ejection fraction, bifurcation lesions, and renal failure.

The "real world" experience has been replicated in other studies and continues to be slightly higher than noted in larger studies. Although the incidence of stent thrombosis at 30 days appears to be similar between DES and BMS, there is concern about the occurrence of late stent thrombosis in the DES population. The duration of antiplatelet therapy in these patients has come into question as a result. It remains difficult to accurately define the true incidence of stent thrombosis, given the various definitions (both clinical and angiographic) used.

The pathobiology of DES placement is important to understand, because stent thrombosis may limit widespread use of DES. Postmortem studies in late stent thrombosis of BMS have elucidated possible mechanisms, including plaque disruption at stent borders, and stenting across ostia of branch vessels, among others.[53] The drug-release characteristics of the sirolimus-eluting stent and the paclitaxel-eluting stent differ as to the time required for release of the drug, potentially contributing to their safety profiles. Sirolimus is completely released by 6 weeks, whereas paclitaxel-eluting stents are thought to retain drug over a longer period. Although paclitaxel is a useful drug to temper the inflammatory response to injury in the form of restenosis, it has been shown in animal models to delay healing after stent placement, particularly in higher doses.[54] Specifically, fibrin deposition, increased vessel wall inflammation, and

intraintimal hemorrhage were noted with paclitaxel-eluting stents. Delayed endothelial healing and persistent fibrin deposition, as seen with DES use, leave the segment of the artery vulnerable to thrombosis and highlight the need for potent antiplatelet therapy. Autopsy findings of incomplete endothelialization and fibrin deposition in late stent thrombosis with DES and the presence of eosinophil infiltrates suggest that, while preventing neointimal hyperplasia, DES also affect the normal healing process.[55]

The concept of delayed healing is seen again in the context of overlapping placement of stents for longer angiographic lesions. Histologic study of overlapping DES has revealed delayed arterial healing, increased inflammatory cellular infiltrate (notably eosinophils), and fibrin deposition. These observations were made in both types of DES, but were greater in paclitaxel-eluting stents.[56] Delayed healing secondary to higher local content of anti-inflammatory drugs, a hypersensitivity reaction, or both is offered as a possible mechanistic explanation. The decision to cease antiplatelet therapy after DES implantation is problematic, because premature discontinuation may have disastrous consequences. Inflammation complicates the use of stents in the treatment of atherosclerotic coronary disease, as a response to injury in the healing process with the use of BMS and in the context of delayed endothelialization and stent thrombosis with DES. Finding a balance in this complex situation remains a challenge.

ADJUVANT MEDICAL THERAPY: TARGETING INFLAMMATION

The pervasive nature of inflammation in the context of ACS and PCI is hard to dispute. Many of the complications and obstacles faced in treating patients with ACS and those undergoing PCI are undoubtedly related to inflammation. Although current therapies employed to treat atherosclerosis and ACS are directed at reducing platelet aggregation, preventing thrombosis, and controlling lipid levels, their ultimate benefit may lie in their ability to modulate inflammation (Fig. 1-9).

Quantification of inflammatory risk may help improve the ability to determine prognosis and to treat many patients with ACS and with coronary atherosclerosis. Much of the evidence for this statement has come from clinical and translational experimental work with currently available medical therapy. Although these various adjuvant therapies are not specifically directed at treating inflammation, their secondary effects on established markers of inflammation have been assessed in numerous studies.

Statin Therapy (HMG-CoA Reductase Inhibitors)

The use of 3-hydroxy-3-methylglutaryl coenzyme A (HMG-CoA) reductase inhibitors (statins) in ACS and coronary atherosclerosis has illuminated the role of the potential nonlipid effects of these drugs. Statin

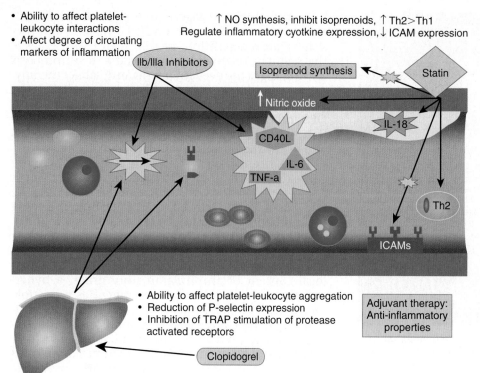

- Ability to affect platelet-leukocyte interactions
- Affect degree of circulating markers of inflammation

IIb/IIIa Inhibitors

↑ NO synthesis, inhibit isoprenoids, ↑ Th2>Th1
Regulate inflammatory cyotkine expression, ↓ ICAM expression

Isoprenoid synthesis

Statin

↑ Nitric oxide

IL-18

CD40L

IL-6

TNF-a

Th2

ICAMs

- Ability to affect platelet-leukocyte aggregation
- Reduction of P-selectin expression
- Inhibition of TRAP stimulation of protease activated receptors

Clopidogrel

Adjuvant therapy: Anti-inflammatory properties

Figure 1-9. Anti-inflammatory effects of adjuvant medical therapy in percutaneous coronary interventions. ICAM, intravascular cell adhesion molecule; IL, interleukin; NO, nitric oxide; Th, helper T cells; TNF-a, tumor necrosis factor-α; TRAP, thrombin receptor agonist peptide.

therapy is thought to affect inflammatory processes contributing to atherosclerosis. Specifically, statins produce "pleiotropic" effects by actions on isoprenoids. By inhibiting the production of isoprenoids, statins interfere with G protein–mediated upregulation of transcription factors responsible for inflammatory signaling.[57]

Statins can affect numerous pathways that contribute to inflammation, including adhesion molecules, cytokines, and a variety of inflammatory cell types. A reduction in the levels of ICAM-1/CD54 and CD18/CD11a by statins has been shown to occur through reduction of messenger RNA (mRNA) transcript.[58] Statins have the ability to downregulate leukocyte mRNA for various cytokines such as IL-6, IL-8, and MCP-1. Statins also affect the balance of helper T lymphocytes by favoring a higher proportion T_H2 versus T_H1 cells.[59] By affecting these pathways, statins may hinder progression of atherosclerotic plaque or avert the onset of an ACS.

Clinically, statins such as atorvastatin and simvastatin reduce recurrent ischemia after ACS[60] and improve mortality in patients with coronary artery disease.[61] Benefits attributed to statin use include lipid-independent effects such as reductions in CRP and serum amyloid A (SAA) with intensive statin therapy over a 16-week period.[62,63] Although intensive statin therapy has been found to improve clinical outcomes, patients with lower CRP levels as a result of intensive treatment have fewer clinical events, independent of LDL levels, supporting the premise that control of inflammation in ACS leads to a reduction in clinical events.

The Reversing Atherosclerosis with Aggressive Lipid Lowering (REVERSAL) study randomly assigned 657 patients to receive intensive statin therapy with either atorvastatin 80 mg or pravastatin 40 mg. Intensive therapy with atorvastatin resulted in a greater reduction in CRP and a corresponding reduction in the progression of atherosclerotic disease as assessed by intravascular ultrasound (IVUS).[64]

In the context of PCI, statin therapy has been proven to reduce periprocedural complications and to improve short- and long-term outcomes (Table 1-3) (Fig. 1-10). Conceptually, the anti-inflammatory properties of statin therapy may reduce the response to injury induced by PCI and periprocedural complications, including microembolization.[65] In contrast to most secondary prevention studies, statin use in the context of PCI has demonstrated a mortality benefit (Fig. 1-11).

Multiple studies have also demonstrated a reduction in the periprocedural CK and CK-MB elevations with statin therapy, which have been shown to predict adverse long-term outcomes. A reduction of myonecrosis resulting from pretreatment with statins before PCI may help to explain the reduction in short- and long-term mortality. In the context of PCI, the benefit of statin therapy appears to be distinct from that observed in the secondary prevention trials. The mechanism of statin-induced reduction in myonecrosis may involve a decrease in the postprocedural inflammatory response, as supported by the Atorvastatin for Reduction of MYocardial Damage during Angioplasty—Cell Adhesion Molecules (ARMYDA-CAMs) substudy.[66]

Table 1-3. Effect of Statin Therapy on Percutaneous Coronary Intervention

Study	N	Study Design	Population	Outcomes	Results	Comments
Chan et al[98]	1552	Prospective, nonrandomized	Elective or urgent PCI	MI or death at 1 yr	Pretreatment with statins was associated with reduced mortality at 1 yr and less periprocedural MI	Statins were especially effective in those with hsCRP in highest quartile
Chan et al[99]	5052	Prospective, nonrandomized; propensity analysis used	Excluded MI or cardiogenic shock	Death at 30 days and at 6 mo after PCI	Statin therapy remained independent predictor of survival at 30 days and 6 mo	No significant differences were noted in incidence of nonfatal MI or rate of repeat revascularization
Hong et al[100]	202	Prospective, randomized	Low EF, PCI for AMI	Death, AMI, CVA, angiographic restenosis, repeat PCI/CABG, LV function	Reduction in 1-yr mortality and restenosis; improvement in LV function	Simvastatin use was not an independent predictor of restenosis after PCI. Small study with incomplete angiographic follow-up
Gaspardone et al[101]	223	Prospective, observational, nonrandomized; three groups (pretreatment, post-treatment, none)	Stable angina, normal LV function, baseline normal CRP level	CRP level at 24 and 48 hr and primary combined end point of death, MI, and TVR at 6 mo	Reduction in primary end point with pretreatment and post-treatment groups driven by TVR	No difference between groups with respect to MI or CV death at 6 mo. By 48 hr, CRP levels in pretreatment and post-treatment groups were not significantly different. Small study size.
Schomig et al[102]	4520	Prospective, observational	Excluded patients >80 yr, cardiogenic shock, in-hospital mortality, and life expectancy <1 yr	All-cause mortality at 1 yr	3585 patients were discharged after PCI on statin and had 49% adjusted risk reduction of primary outcome	Nonrandomized, observational study with potential for bias. No difference noted in TVR rate.
Saia et al[103]	847	Prospective, randomized to fluvastatin or placebo, intention to treat	First PCI, no prior PCI or CABG	Event-free survival at 4 yr; LDL, HDL, total cholesterol	30% reduction in risk of adverse cardiac event at 4 yr after PCI vs. placebo	Significant reduction in non-target vessel revascularization was noted in the statin group
Pasceri et al[104]	153	Prospective, randomized to statin vs. placebo 7 days before PCI	Chronic stable angina without previous statin therapy	Periprocedural MI after elective PCI	Significant reduction in procedural myocardial injury with atorvastatin	Authors postulated the effect may be anti-inflammatory, reduction in microembolization, and platelet adhesion
Chang et al[105]	119	Prospective, nonrandomized, comparing pretreatment vs. no pretreatment	ACS patients undergoing PCI	24-hr CK-MB elevation and 6-mo combined CV event rate	Pretreatment reduced peri-PCI CK-MB rise and risk of combined CV event rate after adjusting for baseline characteristics	Nonrandomized, small sample size, only 64% received GP IIb/IIIa inhibitors
Iwakura et al[65]	293	Prospective, observational, nonrandomized, statin pretreatment vs. no pretreatment	First STEMI	Intracoronary myocardial contrast echocardiographic evidence of no-reflow after PCI	33 Patients with pretreatment had lower incidence of no-reflow	Single-center, observational study could introduce bias. Possible anti-inflammatory effects reduce microembolization during PCI
Lee et al[106]	1658	Prospective, randomized, after first PCI in those with "average" lipid levels	USA, stable angina, or silent ischemia	MACE in the first 6 mo and secondary end point of MACE without TVR	In those with USA and stable angina, statin use reduced the risk of MACE	Authors postulated that the effect is independent of lipid-lowering effects

ACS, acute coronary syndrome; AMI, acute myocardial infarction; CABG, coronary artery bypass grafting; CK-MB, creatine kinase MB fraction; CV, cardiovascular; CRP, C-reactive protein; CVA, cerebrovascular accident; EF, ejection fraction; GP, glycoprotein; HDL, high-density lipoprotein; hsCRP, high-sensitivity C-reactive protein; LDL, low-density lipoprotein; LV, left ventricle; MACE, major adverse cardiac event; MI, myocardial infarction; PCI, percutaneous coronary intervention; STEMI, ST-segment elevation myocardial infarction; TVR, target vessel revascularization; USA, unstable angina.

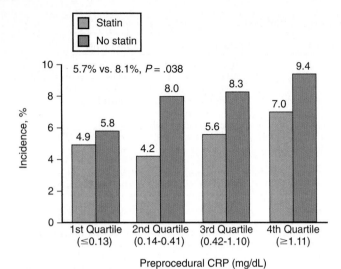

Figure 1-10. Relationship of preprocedural inflammatory state (C-reactive protein [CRP]) and statin use to periprocedural myocardial infarction (MI). (Redrawn from Chan AW, Bhatt DL, Chew DP, et al: Relation of inflammation and benefit of statins after percutaneous coronary interventions. Circulation 2003;107:1750-1756.)

Antiplatelet Therapy (Clopidogrel)

Antiplatelet therapy has also proved to be valuable in the context of ACS and coronary atherosclerosis. In the context of PCI, antiplatelet therapy has become a mainstay for its ability to reduce stent thrombosis and ischemic events. The Clopidogrel for the Reduction of Events During Observation (CREDO) study demonstrated the benefit of using clopidogrel before elective PCI with respect to ischemic events over a 1-year period.[67] In the setting of PCI for ACS (non-ST-elevation myocardial infarction [NSTEMI] or unstable angina), pretreatment with clopidogrel was noted to reduce the risk of MI, cardiovascular death, and need for revascularization.[68] The use of clopidogrel in the setting of rescue PCI led to a significant reduction in MI and death from cardiovascular causes.[69]

Platelets provide a vital link between inflammation and thrombosis, and clopidogrel may have anti-inflammatory actions by way of its effects on platelet function, albeit separate from its inhibition of the adenosine diphosphatase (ADP) receptor. Platelet function has been shown to be highly variable after clopidogrel loading. The fact that clopidogrel can affect platelet activity through other pathways, including via inhibition of thrombin receptor agonist peptide (TRAP) stimulation of the protease-activated receptors (PAR), has important implications for understanding the mechanism of clopidogrel—specifically the potential for clopidogrel to alter TRAP-induced platelet-leukocyte aggregation, suggesting a possible anti-inflammatory effect.[70] Others have noted the ability of clopidogrel to reduce platelet-leukocyte aggregates and P-selectin expression.[71]

The benefits of clopidogrel may extend well beyond its antiplatelet and antithrombotic effects. In 833 patients undergoing PCI, pretreatment with clopidogrel (median duration, 5 days) was associated with a reduction in the postprocedural rise in CRP (Fig. 1-12) and, in some, a postprocedural decline in CRP level.[72] Other makers of inflammation, such as platelet expression of CD40L and P-selectin, were reduced after pretreatment with clopidogrel (median, 5 days).[73] Although these studies were nonrandomized, the data remain provocative regarding the anti-inflammatory effects of clopidogrel when pretreatment is initiated before PCI.

Although the potential benefits of pretreatment with clopidogrel in the setting of PCI are established, the optimal duration of pretreatment remains controversial. The PCI-Clopidogrel in Unstable angina to prevent Recurrent Events (PCI-CURE) study demonstrated benefits of pretreatment given a median of 6 days before PCI in a relatively high-risk NSTEMI population. Among those undergoing elective PCI (Table 1-4), data from CREDO has shown fewer adverse cardiovascular events with greater than 15 hours of pretreatment (Fig. 1-13). However, the Plavix Reduction Of New Thrombus Occurrence (PRONTO) study suggested that the duration of pretreatment before elective PCI has no bearing on platelet function, and that even 3 hours of pretreatment will achieve significant platelet inhibition. In that study, 300 mg of clopidogrel, regardless of the duration of pretreatment, resulted in a peak in platelet activity both at 2 hours and 2 days after PCI. Whereas the PRONTO analysis suggested that duration of pretreatment is of little consequence to platelet inhibition, post-PCI peaks in platelet activity and improved outcomes with longer duration of pretreatment imply an alternative benefit to clopidogrel loading. That benefit may come in the form of anti-inflammatory properties, as described earlier. Anti-inflammatory effects may be responsible for avoiding post-PCI rises in cardiac troponins.[74] Higher loading doses may help achieve a more rapid benefit while improving clinical outcomes, as was noted in the Antiplatelet therapy for Reduction of MYocardial Damage during Angioplasty (ARMYDA-2) study,[75] and in such circumstances the duration of pretreatment may not be relevant.[76] It is unclear whether the benefit of a 600-mg loading dose is related to a more potent anti-inflammatory effect.

Glycoprotein IIb/IIIa Inhibitors

Glycoprotein IIb/IIIa inhibitors have established a niche in the adjuvant treatment of ACS and in elective PCI. The benefits of these medications have been demonstrated in many large-scale clinical trials, both in the context of elective PCI and in PCI for ACS. Their potent antithrombotic actions are most likely responsible for their effects, but the advantages of their use probably involve anti-inflammatory action as well. Although the Intracoronary Stenting and Antithrombotic Regimen: Rapid Early Action for Coronary Treatment (ISAR-REACT) study demonstrated no benefit to the addition of abciximab in patients

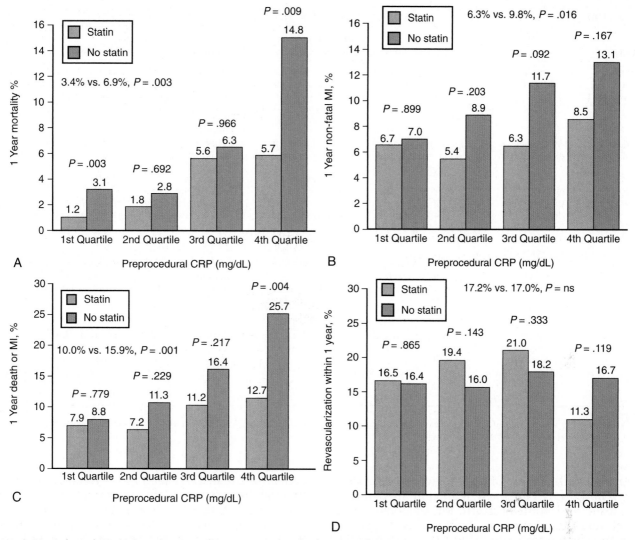

Figure 1-11. A through **D,** Major adverse cardiac events within the first year after percutaneous coronary intervention (PCI), stratified by statin pretreatment before PCI and preprocedural C-reactive protein (CRP) level. MI, myocardial infarction. (Redrawn from Chan AW, Bhatt DL, Chew DP, et al: Relation of inflammation and benefit of statins after percutaneous coronary interventions. Circulation 2003;107:1750-1756.)

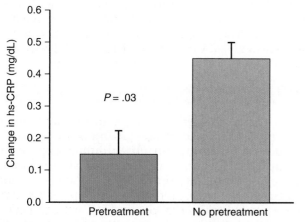

Figure 1-12. Mean change in high-sensitivity CRP (hs-CRP) according to clopidogrel pretreatment. Averaged data are shown as means + standard error of the mean (SEM). (Redrawn from Vivekananthan DP, Bhatt DL, Chew DP, et al: Effect of clopidogrel pretreatment on periprocedural rise in C-reactive protein after percutaneous coronary intervention. Am J Cardiol 2004;94:358-360.)

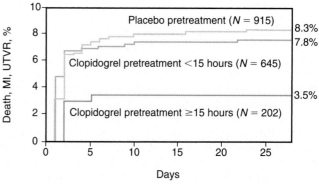

Figure 1-13. Kaplan-Meier curve of the occurrence of the combined end point of death, myocardial infarction (MI), and urgent target vessel revascularization (UTVR) in patients randomly assigned to receive placebo, clopidogrel (300-mg loading dose) less than 15 hours before percutaneous coronary intervention (PCI), or the same dose of clopidogrel 15 hours or longer before PCI. (Redrawn from Steinhubl SR, Berger PB, Brennan DM, Topol EJ: Optimal timing for the initiation of pre-treatment with 300 mg clopidogrel before percutaneous coronary intervention. J Am Coll Cardiol 2006;47:939-943.)

Table 1-4. Duration of Pretreatment with Clopidogrel before Percutaneous Coronary Intervention

Study	N	Primary End Point	Duration of Pretreatment	Outcome	Comments
Steinhubl et al[107]	1762 to undergo elective PCI	28-day combined end point of death, MI, or urgent TVR	Randomized to 300 mg of clopidogrel or placebo at 3 hr (minimum) to 24 hr (maximum) before PCI	Longer duration of pretreatment (>15 hr) was associated with a significant reduction in the primary end point	At least 15 hr of pretreatment is required to see benefit of clopidogrel over placebo before PCI
Kandzari et al[76]	2159 to undergo elective PCI	30-day combined end point of death, MI, or urgent TVR	600 mg of clopidogrel given at 2-3 hr, 3-6 hr, 6-12 hr, or >12 hr before PCI	No benefit of treatment noted beyond 2-3 hr of pretreatment	Authors suggested rapid and maximal platelet inhibition is the result of a higher dose
Hochholzer et al[108]	1001 patients undergoing diagnostic catheterization, 428 of whom underwent PCI	30-day composite of MACE; other end points included platelet aggregation/function	Pretreatment with 600 mg of clopidogrel at intervals from 1 to 6 hr before PCI	For those undergoing PCI, no significant differences in MACE if pretreatment was <2 vs. ≥2 hr	Degree of platelet inhibition was time dependent during first 2 hr
Gurbel et al[109]	100 patients undergoing elective PCI	Multiple markers of platelet function	Pretreatment with 300 mg of clopidogrel at 24, 12, or 3-6 hr before PCI or with 75 mg at the time of PCI	Pretreatment at all time points was associated with platelet inhibition	Authors suggested that platelet inhibition is not time dependent
Patti et al[75]	255 patients undergoing PCI randomized to 600 or 300 mg of clopidogrel (25% had NSTEMI/ACS)	30-day combined end point of death, MI, or TVR	300 mg or 600 mg of clopidogrel 4-8 hr before PCI	End point occurred in 4% of high-dose group vs. 12% of lower-dose group	End point driven primarily by occurrence of periprocedural MI, although end point was measured only out to 30 days

ACS, acute coronary syndrome; MACE, major adverse cardiac event; MI, myocardial infarction; NSTEMI, non-ST-segment elevation myocardial infarction; PCI, percutaneous coronary intervention; TVR, target vessel revascularization.

pretreated with 600 mg of clopidogrel before elective PCI,[77] ISAR-REACT-2 noted reduction in a 30-day composite end point of death, MI, or urgent target vessel revascularization in high-risk ACS patients with an elevated troponin I who were randomized to abciximab versus placebo after pretreatment with clopidogrel.[78]

The use of glycoprotein IIb/IIIa inhibitors, particularly abciximab, appears to affect the degree of circulating markers of inflammation such as sCD40L and platelet-leukocyte aggregates[79] and affects the rise of inflammatory markers such as IL-6, TNF-α, and CRP after angioplasty, suggesting a potent anti-inflammatory effect. The Chimeric c7E3 Fab Anti-Platelet Therapy in Unstable REfractory angina (CAPTURE) investigators noted the importance of inflammation when they stratified an ACS population as high risk defined by a heightened state of inflammation (elevated sCD40L). Abciximab therapy, they observed, was particularly of benefit for those with higher sCD40L.[12] Although abciximab has been shown to be of particular value in those with elevated troponin levels, the benefit may come from preventing distal microembolization and myonecrosis.

Direct Thrombin Inhibitors

The use of direct thrombin inhibitors (DTIs) in the setting of elective PCI has added to the armamentarium of adjunctive therapies in PCI. The potential benefit of use of DTIs such as bivalirudin may lie in their ability to modulate inflammation after PCI. Substudies of the Randomized Evaluation in PCI Linking Angiomax to Reduced Clinical Events 2 (REPLACE-2) study suggested that the use of bivalirudin, compared with unfractionated heparin and eptifibatide, may lead to a reduction in markers of inflammation 1 month out from PCI.[80] Furthermore, it appears that DTIs may affect platelet surface expression of pro-inflammatory markers such as P-selectin.[81] Lower rates of platelet-leukocyte aggregation may be just as significant a factor as the effect on platelet aggregation in the setting of inflammation after PCI.

FUTURE DIRECTIONS

Novel therapeutic strategies are in development or have been examined in the setting of ACS and PCI to address inflammation. The Immunosuppressive Therapy for Prevention of Restenosis after Coronary Artery Stent Implantation (IMPRESS) study demonstrated a benefit to prednisone therapy in patients with elevated CRP after elective PCI with respect to clinical end points at 12 months and angiographic restenosis at 6 months.[82] Although this was one of the only studies demonstrating a benefit to steroid therapy initiated after PCI, the duration of treatment (45 days) was considerably longer than in other studies.

P38 mitogen-activated protein kinase (p38 MAPK) inhibitors have recently garnered attention for potential anti-inflammatory actions in the context of ACS as well. Studies have shown that p38 MAPK inhibitors reduce CRP-mediated inflammatory cytokine production.[83] Preliminary data have demonstrated the ability of p38 MAPK inhibitors to reduce inflammation in patients with ACS. Although large-scale clinical randomized data are not yet available, the promise of targeting inflammation remains exciting.

The issue of late stent thrombosis with DES is an important one, reviewed in Chapter 31, which occurs in low frequency but has serious late sequelae, including sudden death. It is possible that markers of arterial inflammation may be useful in predicting this uncommon event, for the selective use of long-term dual antiplatelet therapy or more aggressive prevention.

The most effective method of treatment will rely heavily on early identification of those at risk for either potent inflammatory underpinnings in ACS or robust inflammatory responses after PCI. Molecular biomarkers representative of inflammation, as discussed, will play a vital role in the diagnosis. Molecular imaging is also likely to become a formidable player in the process of early identification of inflammation. The ability to noninvasively quantify the degree of inflammation at the level of the endothelial cell using VCAM targeting peptides with magnetic resonance imaging[84] may help identify patients at higher risk earlier on and allow for more aggressive medical anti-inflammatory therapy to improve efficacy of standard interventional therapy.

In the setting of both elective PCI and emergent PCI for ACS, modulation of inflammation will affect post-PCI outcomes, in both the short and the long term. In the setting of elective PCI, it is imperative that patients be pretreated with adjuvant medical therapy before the procedure, so as to derive the maximal anti-inflammatory benefit from these drugs to prevent postprocedural complications related to inflammation. In the setting of ACS, rapid action, in terms of "door to balloon" time, is necessary to ensure optimal outcomes. The price of acting quickly is the inability to adequately modulate inflammation in ACS. Often, it is unrealistic to expect longer duration of pretreatment with statins or clopidogrel in this setting, and therefore it is unlikely that patients truly derive the maximum potential benefit from these drugs in this setting. The answer to this problem may lie in other medications with faster onset of action. One such drug on the horizon is cangrelor, a potent, reversible intravenous PY12 inhibitor with a short half-life and a rapid onset of action. Small phase II clinical studies have shown safety and efficacy in the setting of PCI.[85] Although more data are necessary, particularly in the context of PCI for ACS, it remains an attractive alternative to achieve more rapid platelet inhibition and potentially anti-inflammatory benefit in the setting of emergent PCI for ACS.

CONCLUSION

Defining inflammatory status in patients with ACS and in those with coronary atherosclerosis is becoming paramount to the efficient risk assessment and appropriate treatment of patients. As our grasp of molecular and genetic tools improves, the ability to break down the complex pathways and modulate them as potential therapeutic targets in susceptible individuals will take hold. The implications are far reaching and hold the potential to significantly alter the way clinical medicine is practiced. Nowhere is this more relevant than in interventional cardiology. From novel devices and instruments in PCI to adjuvant therapy focused on modulating inflammation, clinical practice will evolve over time. Whether this translates into improved clinical outcomes is yet to be determined. However, what will take place is a more individualized strategy of therapy based on a more complex profile of risk, one that incorporates inflammation as a vital component.

REFERENCES

1. Topol EJ: Simon Dack Lecture: The genomic basis of myocardial infarction. J Am Coll Cardiol 2005;46:1456-1465.
2. Ridker PM, Cushman M, Stampfer MJ, et al: Inflammation, aspirin, and the risk of cardiovascular disease in apparently healthy men. N Engl J Med 1997;336:973-979.
3. Ridker PM, Hennekens CH, Buring JE, Rifai N: C-reactive protein and other markers of inflammation in the prediction of cardiovascular disease in women. N Engl J Med 2000; 342:836-843.
4. Norja S, Nuutila L, Karhunen PJ, Goebeler S: C-reactive protein in vulnerable coronary plaques. J Clin Pathol 2006, Jun 21 Epub ahead of print.
5. Ridker PM: Rosuvastatin in the primary prevention of cardiovascular disease among patients with low levels of low-density lipoprotein cholesterol and elevated high-sensitivity C-reactive protein: Rationale and design of the JUPITER trial. Circulation 2003;108:2292-2297.
6. Henn V, Slupsky JR, Grafe M, et al: CD40 ligand on activated platelets triggers an inflammatory reaction of endothelial cells. Nature 1998;391:591-594.
7. Wagner AH, Guldenzoph B, Lienenluke B, Hecker M: CD154/CD40-mediated expression of CD154 in endothelial cells: Consequences for endothelial cell-monocyte interaction. Arterioscler Thromb Vasc Biol 2004;24:715-720.
8. Andre P, Prasad KS, Denis CV, et al: CD40L stabilizes arterial thrombi by a beta3 integrin–dependent mechanism. Nat Med 2002;8:247-252.
9. Lutgens E, Gorelik L, Daemen MJ, et al: Requirement for CD154 in the progression of atherosclerosis. Nat Med 1999;5:1313-1316.
10. Varo N, de Lemos JA, Libby P, et al: Soluble CD40L: Risk prediction after acute coronary syndromes. Circulation 2003;108:1049-1052.
11. de Lemos JA, Zirlik A, Schonbeck U, et al: Associations between soluble CD40 ligand, atherosclerosis risk factors, and subclinical atherosclerosis: Results from the Dallas Heart Study. Arterioscler Thromb Vasc Biol 2005;25: 2192-2196.
12. Heeschen C, Dimmeler S, Hamm CW, et al: Soluble CD40 ligand in acute coronary syndromes. N Engl J Med 2003; 348:1104-1111.
13. Yokoyama S, Ikeda H, Haramaki N, et al: Platelet P-selectin plays an important role in arterial thrombogenesis by forming large stable platelet-leukocyte aggregates. J Am Coll Cardiol 2005;45:1280-1286.

14. Yazici M, Demircan S, Durna K, et al: Relationship between myocardial injury and soluble P-selectin in non-ST elevation acute coronary syndromes. Circ J 2005;69:530-535.

15. Ridker PM, Buring JE, Rifai N: Soluble P-selectin and the risk of future cardiovascular events. Circulation 2001;103:491-495.

16. Menon V, Lessard D, Yarzebski J, et al: Leukocytosis and adverse hospital outcomes after acute myocardial infarction. Am J Cardiol 2003;92:368-372.

17. Kirtane AJ, Bui A, Murphy SA, et al: Association of peripheral neutrophilia with adverse angiographic outcomes in ST-elevation myocardial infarction. Am J Cardiol 2004;93:532-536.

18. Eiserich JP, Baldus S, Brennan ML, et al: Myeloperoxidase, a leukocyte-derived vascular NO oxidase. Science 2002;296:2391-2394.

19. Fu X, Kassim SY, Parks WC, Heinecke JW: Hypochlorous acid oxygenates the cysteine switch domain of pro-matrilysin (MMP-7): A mechanism for matrix metalloproteinase activation and atherosclerotic plaque rupture by myeloperoxidase. J Biol Chem 2001;276:41279-41287.

20. Baldus S, Heeschen C, Meinertz T, et al: Myeloperoxidase serum levels predict risk in patients with acute coronary syndromes. Circulation 2003;108:1440-1445.

21. Brennan ML, Penn MS, Van Lente F, et al: Prognostic value of myeloperoxidase in patients with chest pain. N Engl J Med 2003;349:1595-1604.

22. de Nooijer R, von der Thusen JH, Verkleij CJ, et al: Overexpression of IL-18 decreases intimal collagen content and promotes a vulnerable plaque phenotype in apolipoprotein-E-deficient mice. Arterioscler Thromb Vasc Biol 2004;24:2313-2319.

23. Chalikias GK, Tziakas DN, Kaski JC, et al: Interleukin-18: Interleukin-10 ratio and in-hospital adverse events in patients with acute coronary syndrome. Atherosclerosis 2005;182:135-143.

24. Blankenberg S, Rupprecht HJ, Poirier O, et al: Plasma concentrations and genetic variation of matrix metalloproteinase 9 and prognosis of patients with cardiovascular disease. Circulation 2003;107:1579-1585.

25. Bayes-Genis A, Conover CA, Overgaard MT, et al: Pregnancy-associated plasma protein A as a marker of acute coronary syndromes. N Engl J Med 2001;345:1022-1029.

26. Lund J, Qin QP, Ilva T, et al: Circulating pregnancy-associated plasma protein A predicts outcome in patients with acute coronary syndrome but no troponin I elevation. Circulation 2003;108:1924-1926.

27. Cosin-Sales J, Christiansen M, Kaminski P, et al: Pregnancy-associated plasma protein A and its endogenous inhibitor, the proform of eosinophil major basic protein (proMBP), are related to complex stenosis morphology in patients with stable angina pectoris. Circulation 2004;109:1724-1728.

28. Cosin-Sales J, Kaski JC, Christiansen M, et al: Relationship among pregnancy associated plasma protein-A levels, clinical characteristics, and coronary artery disease extent in patients with chronic stable angina pectoris. Eur Heart J 2005;26:2093-2098.

29. Conti E, Carrozza C, Capoluongo E, et al: Insulin-like growth factor-1 as a vascular protective factor. Circulation 2004;110:2260-2265.

30. Crea F, Andreotti F: Pregnancy associated plasma protein-A and coronary atherosclerosis: Marker, friend, or foe? Eur Heart J 2005;26:2075-2076.

31. Hata N, Matsumori A, Yokoyama S, et al: Hepatocyte growth factor and cardiovascular thrombosis in patients admitted to the intensive care unit. Circ J 2004;68:645-649.

32. Zhou X, Nicoletti A, Elhage R, Hansson GK: Transfer of CD4(+) T cells aggravates atherosclerosis in immunodeficient apolipoprotein E knockout mice. Circulation 2000;102:2919-2922.

33. Cheng X, Liao YH, Ge H, et al: TH1/TH2 functional imbalance after acute myocardial infarction: Coronary arterial inflammation or myocardial inflammation. J Clin Immunol 2005;25:246-253.

34. Liuzzo G, Vallejo AN, Kopecky SL, et al: Molecular fingerprint of interferon-gamma signaling in unstable angina. Circulation 2001;103:1509-1514.

35. Wang L, Fan C, Topol SE, et al: Mutation of MEF2A in an inherited disorder with features of coronary artery disease. Science 2003;302:1578-1581.

36. Helgadottir A, Manolescu A, Thorleifsson G, et al: The gene encoding 5-lipoxygenase activating protein confers risk of myocardial infarction and stroke. Nat Genet 2004;36:233-239.

37. Helgadottir A, Manolescu A, Helgason A, et al: A variant of the gene encoding leukotriene A4 hydrolase confers ethnicity-specific risk of myocardial infarction. Nat Genet 2006;38:68-74.

38. Hakonarson H, Thorvaldsson S, Helgadottir A, et al: Effects of a 5-lipoxygenase-activating protein inhibitor on biomarkers associated with risk of myocardial infarction: A randomized trial. JAMA 2005;293:2245-2256.

39. Moses JW, Leon MB, Popma JJ, et al: Sirolimus-eluting stents versus standard stents in patients with stenosis in a native coronary artery. N Engl J Med 2003;349:1315-1323.

40. Stone GW, Ellis SG, Cox DA, et al: A polymer-based, paclitaxel-eluting stent in patients with coronary artery disease. N Engl J Med 2004;350:221-231.

41. Farb A, Weber DK, Kolodgie FD, et al: Morphological predictors of restenosis after coronary stenting in humans. Circulation 2002;105:2974-2980.

42. Hong SJ, Kim MH, Ahn TH, et al: Multiple predictors of coronary restenosis after drug-eluting stent implantation in patients with diabetes. Heart 2006;92:1119-1124.

43. Simon DI, Dhen Z, Seifert P, et al: Decreased neointimal formation in Mac-1(−/−) mice reveals a role for inflammation in vascular repair after angioplasty. J Clin Invest 2000;105:293-300.

44. Fukuda D, Shimada K, Tanaka A, et al: Circulating monocytes and in-stent neointima after coronary stent implantation. J Am Coll Cardiol 2004;43:18-23.

45. Turker S, Guneri S, Akdeniz B, et al: Usefulness of preprocedural soluble CD40 ligand for predicting restenosis after percutaneous coronary intervention in patients with stable coronary artery disease. Am J Cardiol 2006;97:198-202.

46. Inoue T, Kato T, Uchida T, et al: Local release of C-reactive protein from vulnerable plaque or coronary arterial wall injured by stenting. J Am Coll Cardiol 2005;46:239-245.

47. Segev A, Kassam S, Buller CE, et al:. Pre-procedural plasma levels of C-reactive protein and interleukin-6 do not predict late coronary angiographic restenosis after elective stenting. Eur Heart J 2004;25:1029-1035.

48. Zairis MN, Ambrose JA, Manousakis SJ, et al: The impact of plasma levels of C-reactive protein, lipoprotein (a) and homocysteine on the long-term prognosis after successful coronary stenting: The Global Evaluation of New Events and Restenosis After Stent Implantation Study. J Am Coll Cardiol 2002;40:1375-1382.

49. Walter DH, Fichtlscherer S, Sellwig M, et al: Preprocedural C-reactive protein levels and cardiovascular events after coronary stent implantation. J Am Coll Cardiol 2001;37:839-846.

50. Dibra A, Mehilli J, Braun S, et al: Inflammatory response after intervention assessed by serial C-reactive protein measurements correlates with restenosis in patients treated with coronary stenting. Am Heart J 2005;150:344-350.

51. Gibson CM, Karmpaliotis D, Kosmidou I, et al: Comparison of effects of bare metal versus drug-eluting stent implantation on biomarker levels following percutaneous coronary intervention for non-ST-elevation acute coronary syndrome. Am J Cardiol 2006;97:1473-1477.

52. Iakovou I, Schmidt T, Bonizzoni E, et al: Incidence, predictors, and outcome of thrombosis after successful implantation of drug-eluting stents. JAMA 2005;293:2126-2130.

53. Farb A, Burke AP, Kolodgie FD, Virmani R: Pathological mechanisms of fatal late coronary stent thrombosis in humans. Circulation 2003;108:1701-1706.

54. Farb A, Heller PF, Shroff S, et al: Pathological analysis of local delivery of paclitaxel via a polymer-coated stent. Circulation 2001;104:473-479.

55. Joner M, Finn AV, Farb A, et al: Pathology of drug-eluting stents in humans: Delayed healing and late thrombotic risk. J Am Coll Cardiol 2006;48:193-202.

56. Finn AV, Kolodgie FD, Harnek J, et al: Differential response of delayed healing and persistent inflammation at sites of overlapping sirolimus- or paclitaxel-eluting stents. Circulation 2005;112:270-278.

57. Ray KK, Cannon CP: Pathological changes in acute coronary syndromes: The role of statin therapy in the modulation of inflammation, endothelial function and coagulation. J Thromb Thrombolysis 2004;18:89-101.

58. Rezaie-Majd A, Prager GW, Bucek RA, et al: Simvastatin reduces the expression of adhesion molecules in circulating monocytes from hypercholesterolemic patients. Arterioscler Thromb Vasc Biol 2003;23:397-403.

59. Hakamada-Taguchi R, Uehara Y, Kuribayashi K, et al: Inhibition of hydroxymethylglutaryl-coenzyme a reductase reduces Th1 development and promotes Th2 development. Circ Res 2003;93:948-956.

60. Schwartz GG, Olsson AG, Ezekowitz MD, et al: Effects of atorvastatin on early recurrent ischemic events in acute coronary syndromes: The MIRACL study—A randomized controlled trial. JAMA 2001;285:1711-1718.

61. Randomised trial of cholesterol lowering in 4444 patients with coronary heart disease: The Scandinavian Simvastatin Survival Study (4S). Lancet 1994;344:1383-1389.

62. Ridker PM, Cannon CP, Morrow D, et al: C-reactive protein levels and outcomes after statin therapy. N Engl J Med 2005; 352:20-28.

63. Kinlay S, Schwartz GG, Olsson AG, et al: High-dose atorvastatin enhances the decline in inflammatory markers in patients with acute coronary syndromes in the MIRACL study. Circulation 2003;108:1560-1566.

64. Nissen SE, Tuzcu EM, Schoenhagen P, et al: Effect of intensive compared with moderate lipid-lowering therapy on progression of coronary atherosclerosis: A randomized controlled trial. JAMA 2004;291:1071-1080.

65. Iwakura K, Ito H, Kawano S, et al: Chronic pre-treatment of statins is associated with the reduction of the no-reflow phenomenon in the patients with reperfused acute myocardial infarction. Eur Heart J 2006;27:534-539.

66. Patti G, Chello M, Pasceri V, et al: Protection from procedural myocardial injury by atorvastatin is associated with lower levels of adhesion molecules after percutaneous coronary intervention: Results from the ARMYDA-CAMs (Atorvastatin for Reduction of MYocardial Damage during Angioplasty-Cell Adhesion Molecules) substudy. J Am Coll Cardiol 2006;48: 1560-1566.

67. Steinhubl SR, Berger PB, Mann JT 3rd, et al: Early and sustained dual oral antiplatelet therapy following percutaneous coronary intervention: A randomized controlled trial. JAMA 2002;288:2411-2420.

68. Mehta SR, Yusuf S, Peters RJ, et al: Effects of pretreatment with clopidogrel and aspirin followed by long-term therapy in patients undergoing percutaneous coronary intervention: The PCI-CURE study. Lancet 2001;358:527-533.

69. Sabatine MS, Cannon CP, Gibson CM, et al: Effect of clopidogrel pretreatment before percutaneous coronary intervention in patients with ST-elevation myocardial infarction treated with fibrinolytics: The PCI-CLARITY study. JAMA 2005;294:1224-1232.

70. Xiao Z, Theroux P: Clopidogrel inhibits platelet-leukocyte interactions and thrombin receptor agonist peptide-induced platelet activation in patients with an acute coronary syndrome. J Am Coll Cardiol 2004;43:1982-1988.

71. Klinkhardt U, Bauersachs R, Adams J, et al: Clopidogrel but not aspirin reduces P-selectin expression and formation of platelet-leukocyte aggregates in patients with atherosclerotic vascular disease. Clin Pharmacol Ther 2003;73:232-241.

72. Vivekananthan DP, Bhatt DL, Chew DP, et al: Effect of clopidogrel pretreatment on periprocedural rise in C-reactive protein after percutaneous coronary intervention. Am J Cardiol 2004;94:358-360.

73. Quinn MJ, Bhatt DL, Zidar F, et al: Effect of clopidogrel pretreatment on inflammatory marker expression in patients undergoing percutaneous coronary intervention. Am J Cardiol 2004;93:679-684.

74. Nienhuis MB, Ottervanger JP, Miedema K, et al: Pre-treatment with clopidogrel and postprocedure troponin elevation after elective percutaneous coronary intervention. Thromb Haemost 2006;95:337-340.

75. Patti G, Colonna G, Pasceri V, et al: Randomized trial of high loading dose of clopidogrel for reduction of periprocedural myocardial infarction in patients undergoing coronary intervention: Results from the ARMYDA-2 (Antiplatelet therapy for Reduction of MYocardial Damage during Angioplasty) study. Circulation 2005;111:2099-2106.

76. Kandzari DE, Berger PB, Kastrati A, et al: Influence of treatment duration with a 600-mg dose of clopidogrel before percutaneous coronary revascularization. J Am Coll Cardiol 2004;44:2133-2136.

77. Kastrati A, Mehilli J, Schuhlen H, et al: A clinical trial of abciximab in elective percutaneous coronary intervention after pretreatment with clopidogrel. N Engl J Med 2004;350: 232-238.

78. Kastrati A, Mehilli J, Neumann FJ, et al: Abciximab in patients with acute coronary syndromes undergoing percutaneous coronary intervention after clopidogrel pretreatment: The ISAR-REACT 2 randomized trial. JAMA 2006;295:1531-1538.

79. Furman MI, Krueger LA, Linden MD, et al: GPIIb-IIIa antagonists reduce thromboinflammatory processes in patients with acute coronary syndromes undergoing percutaneous coronary intervention. J Thromb Haemost 2005;3:312-320.

80. Keating FK, Dauerman HL, Whitaker DA, et al: The effects of bivalirudin compared with those of unfractionated heparin plus eptifibatide on inflammation and thrombin generation and activity during coronary intervention. Coron Artery Dis 2005;16:401-405.

81. Keating FK, Dauerman HL, Whitaker DA, et al: Increased expression of platelet P-selectin and formation of platelet-leukocyte aggregates in blood from patients treated with unfractionated heparin plus eptifibatide compared with bivalirudin. Thromb Res 2006;118:361-369.

82. Versaci F, Gaspardone A, Tomai F, et al: Immunosuppressive Therapy for the Prevention of Restenosis after Coronary Artery Stent Implantation (IMPRESS study). J Am Coll Cardiol 2002;40:1935-1942.

83. Lim MY, Wang H, Kapoun AM, et al: P38 inhibition attenuates the pro-inflammatory response to C-reactive protein by human peripheral blood mononuclear cells. J Mol Cell Cardiol 2004;37:1111-1114.

84. Nahrendorf M, Jaffer FA, Kelly KA, et al: Noninvasive vascular cell adhesion molecule-1 imaging identifies inflammatory activation of cells in atherosclerosis. Circulation 2006;114: 1504-1511.

85. Greenbaum AB, Grines CL, Bittl JA, et al: Initial experience with an intravenous P2Y12 platelet receptor antagonist in patients undergoing percutaneous coronary intervention: Results from a 2-part, phase II, multicenter, randomized, placebo- and active-controlled trial. Am Heart J 2006;151:689 e1-689 e10.

86. Monraats PS, Rana JS, Nierman MC, et al: Lipoprotein lipase gene polymorphisms and the risk of target vessel revascularization after percutaneous coronary intervention. J Am Coll Cardiol 2005;46:1093-1100.

87. Wijpkema JS, van Haelst PL, Monraats PS, et al: Restenosis after percutaneous coronary intervention is associated with the angiotensin-II type-1 receptor 1166A/C polymorphism but not with polymorphisms of angiotensin-converting enzyme, angiotensin-II receptor, angiotensinogen or heme oxygenase-1. Pharmacogenet Genomics 2006;16:331-337.

88. Monraats PS, Pires NM, Agema WR, et al: Genetic inflammatory factors predict restenosis after percutaneous coronary interventions. Circulation 2005;112:2417-2425.

89. Niessner A, Marculescu R, Kvakan H, et al: Fractalkine receptor polymorphisms V2491 and T280M as genetic risk

factors for restenosis. Thromb Haemost 2005;94:1251-1256.

90. Hamann L, Gomma A, Schroder NW, et al: A frequent toll-like receptor (TLR)-2 polymorphism is a risk factor for coronary restenosis. J Mol Med 2005;83:478-485.

91. Tiroch K, von Beckerath N, Koch W, et al: Interferon-gamma and interferon-gamma receptor 1 and 2 gene polymorphisms and restenosis following coronary stenting. Atherosclerosis 2005;182:145-151.

92. Koch W, Mehilli J, Pfeufer A, et al: Apolipoprotein E gene polymorphisms and thrombosis and restenosis after coronary artery stenting. J Lipid Res 2004;45:2221-2226.

93. Gaspardone A, Versaci F, Tomai F, et al: C-reactive protein, clinical outcome, and restenosis rates after implantation of different drug-eluting stents. Am J Cardiol 2006;97:1311-1316.

94. Dibra A, Ndrepepa G, Mehilli J, et al: Comparison of C-reactive protein levels before and after coronary stenting and restenosis among patients treated with sirolimus-eluting versus bare metal stents. Am J Cardiol 2005;95:1238-1240.

95. de la Torre-Hernandez JM, Sainz-Laso F, Burgos V, et al: Comparison of C-reactive protein levels after coronary stenting with bare metal versus sirolimus-eluting stents. Am J Cardiol 2005;95:748-751.

96. Gogo PB Jr, Schneider DJ, Watkins MW, et al: Systemic inflammation after drug-eluting stent placement. J Thromb Thrombolysis 2005;19:87-92.

97. Kim JY, Ko YG, Shim CY, et al: Comparison of effects of drug-eluting stents versus bare metal stents on plasma C-reactive protein levels. Am J Cardiol 2005;96:1384-1388.

98. Chan AW, Bhatt DL, Chew DP, et al: Relation of inflammation and benefit of statins after percutaneous coronary interventions. Circulation 2003;107:1750-1756.

99. Chan AW, Bhatt DL, Chew DP, et al: Early and sustained survival benefit associated with statin therapy at the time of percutaneous coronary intervention. Circulation 2002;105:691-696.

100. Hong YJ, Jeong MH, Hyun DW, et al: Prognostic significance of simvastatin therapy in patients with ischemic heart failure who underwent percutaneous coronary intervention for acute myocardial infarction. Am J Cardiol 2005;95:619-622.

101. Gaspardone A, Versaci F, Proietti I, et al: Effect of atorvastatin (80 mg) initiated at the time of coronary artery stent implantation on C-reactive protein and six-month clinical events. Am J Cardiol 2002;90:786-789.

102. Schomig A, Mehilli J, Holle H, et al: Statin treatment following coronary artery stenting and one-year survival. J Am Coll Cardiol 2002;40:854-861.

103. Saia F, de Feyter P, Serruys PW, et al: Effect of fluvastatin on long-term outcome after coronary revascularization with stent implantation. Am J Cardiol 2004;93:92-95.

104. Pasceri V, Patti G, Nusca A, et al: Randomized trial of atorvastatin for reduction of myocardial damage during coronary intervention: results from the ARMYDA (Atorvastatin for Reduction of MYocardial Damage during Angioplasty) study. Circulation 2004;110:674-678.

105. Chang SM, Yazbek N, Lakkis NM: Use of statins prior to percutaneous coronary intervention reduces myonecrosis and improves clinical outcome. Catheter Cardiovasc Interv 2004;62:193-197.

106. Lee CH, de Feyter P, Serruys PW, et al: Beneficial effects of fluvastatin following percutaneous coronary intervention in patients with unstable and stable angina: Results from the Lescol Intervention Prevention Study (LIPS). Heart 2004;90:1156-1161.

107. Steinhubl SR, Berger PB, Brennan DM, Topol EJ. Optimal timing for the initiation of pre-treatment with 300 mg clopidogrel before percutaneous coronary intervention. J Am Coll Cardiol 2006;47:939-943.

108. Hochholzer W, Trenk D, Frundi D, et al: Time dependence of platelet inhibition after a 600-mg loading dose of clopidogrel in a large, unselected cohort of candidates for percutaneous coronary intervention. Circulation 2005;111:2560-2564.

109. Gurbel PA, Cummings CC, Bell CR, et al: Onset and extent of platelet inhibition by clopidogrel loading in patients undergoing elective coronary stenting: The Plavix Reduction Of New Thrombus Occurrence (PRONTO) trial. Am Heart J 2003;145:239-247.

CHAPTER

2 Diabetes

Marco Roffi and Michael Brandle

KEY POINTS

- Diabetes-associated deaths, more that two thirds of them cardiovascular-related, are rising exponentially, following the diabetes "epidemics" observed in Western countries.
- Diabetes confers a cardiovascular risk equivalent to aging 15 years.
- Coronary artery disease is more prevalent, is more severe, and occurs at younger age in patients with diabetes. Chronic hyperglycemia, dyslipidemia, and insulin resistance have been associated with an accelerated form of atherogenesis, characterized by a prothrombotic state, enhanced inflammation, and endothelial dysfunction.
- Diabetic patients undergoing coronary revascularization have worse outcomes compared with nondiabetic individuals, both in the setting of percutaneous coronary interventions (PCI) and in coronary artery bypass grafting (CABG). Subgroup analyses of randomized trials and registries have suggested that CABG is superior to PCI in diabetic patients with multivessel disease. Ongoing randomized trials that focus for the first time on diabetic patients may settle the controversy.
- Diabetic patients with both non-ST-elevation acute coronary syndromes and ST-elevation myocardial infarction have higher short- and long-term morbidity and mortality rates than their nondiabetic counterparts. This finding is explained partly by a higher baseline risk profile and partly by a lesser degree of adherence to evidence-base therapies in this patient population. At the same time, however, diabetic patients derive a grater benefit than nondiabetic individuals from aggressive management, including early invasive strategy, glycoprotein IIb/IIIa inhibition, and possibly primary angioplasty.
- The association between aggressive glucose-lowering strategies and reduction in diabetes-related adverse outcomes has been established in clinical trials for microvascular but not macrovascular complications. Nevertheless, optimization of the glucose level remains a main goal in diabetes treatment.
- Aggressive modification of additional risk factors, including blood pressure and cholesterol level control, cigarette smoking cessation, weight loss, and exercise, is key cardiovascular prevention.
- Metabolism modulation with thiazolidinediones has been associated in ex vivo studies with anti-inflammatory and thrombus-reducing properties. In addition, rosiglitazone has been shown to prevent diabetes in individuals with impaired glucose metabolism. However, a reduction in cardiovascular events associated with these agents has not yet been convincingly demonstrated.
- The ultimate goal in diabetes care remains the cure of the disease by regeneration of beta-cell mass and/or beta-cell function. The role of pluripotent cells in this setting needs to be defined.

Diabetes mellitus defines a group of metabolic diseases that are characterized by dysfunction in insulin secretion, insulin action, or both. The resulting chronic hyperglycemia may cause failure of various organs, including eyes, kidneys, nerves, heart, and the arterial vasculature. In the last decades, an increase in the prevalence of diabetes of epidemic proportion has been observed in Western countries, and, with a delay, the developing world will follow a similar pattern. Diabetes-associated cardiovascular disease (CVD) involves both the macrovasculature and the microvasculature. The focus of this chapter is the macrovascular complications, specifically coronary artery disease (CAD); microvascular manifestations such as nephropathy, neuropathy, and retinopathy are only marginally addressed. The increased cardiovascular (CV) risk observed in individuals with diabetes is in part a consequence of the associated metabolic disturbances and in part is explained by the clustering of additional CV risk factors, such as hypertension, dyslipidemia, and central obesity. For the purpose of this chapter, "diabetes" refers to type 2 diabetes mellitus, which accounts for 90% to 95% of all diabetes cases in Western countries.

THE BURDEN OF THE DISEASE

Worldwide, the estimated prevalence of diabetes for all age groups was 2.8% in the year 2000 and will be 4.4% in the year 2030.[1] As a consequence, the total number of people affected from this condition is expected to double during the same period, from 171 million to 366 million. Within the United States, according to the American Diabetes Association (ADA), diabetes affected 20.6 million people in 2005, corresponding to 9.6% of all individuals older than 20 years of age.[2] In that same year, 1.5 million new cases of diabetes were diagnosed. Importantly, in approximately one third of affected individuals, the condition remains unrecognized.[2] With respect to gender, half of those affected are women.[3] In 2004, the U.S. Department of Health and Human Services (USDHHS) estimated that approximately 40% of U.S. adults aged 40 to 74 years, or 41 million people, had prediabetes, a glucose metabolic disturbance predisposing to overt diabetes, heart disease, and stroke.[3]

Diabetes was the sixth leading cause of death listed on U.S. death certificates in 2002.[2] Most likely, this number greatly underestimates the impact of this condition, because it has been demonstrated that diabetes is rarely reported as the cause of death. Adults with diabetes have a two- to fourfold higher CV death rate than nondiabetic individuals. With respect to gender, the adjusted risk of CV death among men is three times higher than in nondiabetic individuals, while in diabetic women the risk is up to six times higher.[4] Whereas the U.S. age-adjusted mortality rates of other major multifactorial diseases (e.g., heart disease, stroke, cancer) have declined or remained stable over the last 20 years, the diabetes "epidemic" has led to a 30% increase in diabetes-related deaths in the same time span (Fig. 2-1).[5] The total estimated cost of diabetes in the United States in 2002 was $132 billion, comprising $92 billion for direct medical costs and $40 billion for indirect costs (e.g., disability, work loss, premature mortality). Total health care costs associated with this condition are expected to rise to $192 billion by the year 2020.[6]

DIAGNOSTIC CRITERIA FOR DIABETES, PREDIABETES, AND METABOLIC SYNDROME

The diagnostic criteria for diabetes recommended by the ADA are presented in Table 2-1. In the absence of unequivocal hyperglycemia, one of these criteria must be confirmed on a subsequent day to establish the diagnosis. Although the plasma level of hemoglobin A_{1c} (HbA_{1c}) reflects mean plasma glucose concentrations over the preceding 2 to 3 months, the use of this parameter for the diagnosis of diabetes is currently not recommended.[7] Before the development of diabetes, subjects pass through a stage of impaired glucose metabolism characterized by impaired fasting glucose (IFG) levels or impaired glucose tolerance (IGT) (see Table 2-1). These two metabolic disturbances predispose to diabetes and CVD and were recently grouped in the term *prediabetes*. A cluster of lipid and non-lipid risk factors of metabolic origin mediated by insulin resistance, such as pathologic glucose metabolism, obesity, hypertension, and dyslipidemia, was designated the *metabolic*

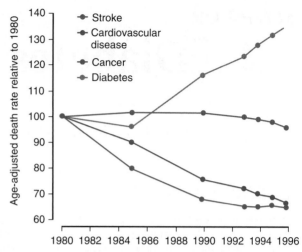

Figure 2-1. Increase in age-adjusted diabetes mellitus–related mortality in the United States between 1980 and 1996. (From McKinlay J, Marceau L: US public health and the 21st century: Diabetes mellitus. Lancet 2000;356:757–761.)

syndrome. Several organizations have proposed definitions of the metabolic syndrome that differ not only in the set of criteria included but also in the cutoff values used to define the presence or absence of an individual component of the syndrome (Table 2-2). However, both the concept and the clinical utility of the metabolic syndrome were recently critically appraised.[8]

PATHOPHYSIOLOGY OF ATHEROSCLEROSIS IN DIABETES

Coronary artery disease is more prevalent, is more severe, and occurs at a younger age in patients with diabetes. Several metabolic abnormalities, including chronic hyperglycemia, dyslipidemia, and insulin

Table 2-1. Diagnostic Criteria for Diabetes Mellitus, Impaired Glucose Tolerance, and Impaired Fasting Glucose According to the American Diabetes Association

Diabetes mellitus
Symptoms of diabetes (e.g., polyuria, polydipsia, unexplained weight loss) and a casual plasma glucose concentration ≥200 mg/dL (11.1 mmol/L)
OR
Fasting plasma glucose ≥126 mg/dL (7.0 mmol/L)
OR
2-hr plasma glucose ≥200 mg/dL (11.1 mmol/L) during an oral glucose tolerance test (OGTT)

Impaired glucose tolerance (IGT)
2-hr plasma glucose ≥140 mg/dL (7.8 mmol/L) but <200 mg/dL (11.1 mmol/L) during OGTT

Impaired fasting glucose (IFG)
2001 definition: Fasting plasma glucose ≥110 mg/dL (6.1 mmol/L) but <126 mg/dL (7 mmol/L)
2004 definition: Fasting plasma glucose ≥100 mg/dL (5.6 mmol/L) but <126 mg/dL (7 mmol/L)

From Diagnosis and classification of diabetes mellitus. Diabetes Care 2006;29(Suppl 1):S43-S48. Copyright American Diabetes Association.

Table 2-2. Definitions of the Metabolic Syndrome

	WHO (1999)	NCEP ATP Iii (2001)	IDF (2004)
	IGT or diabetes and/or insulin resistance* PLUS two or more of the following factors:	Three or more of the following five risk factors:	Central obesity (ethnicity-specific) PLUS any two of the following five factors:
Fasting plasma glucose	—	≥100 mg/dL (5.6 mmol/L)[†]	≥100 mg/dL (5.6 mmol/L) or previously diagnosed diabetes
Blood pressure	≥140/90 mm Hg	≥130/≥85 mm Hg	≥130 or ≥85 mm Hg or treatment of previously diagnosed hypertension
Triglycerides	≥150 mg/dL (1.7 mmol/L) and/or	≥150 mg/dL (1.7 mmol/L)	≥150 mg/dL (1.7 mmol/L) or specific treatment for this abnormality
HDL-cholesterol	Men: <35 mg/dL (0.9 mmol/L) Women: <39 mg/dL (1.0 mmol/L)	Men: <40 mg/dL (1.03 mmol/L) Women: <50 mg/dL (1.29 mmol/L)	Men: <40 mg/dL (1.03 mmol/L) Women: <50 mg/dL (1.29 mmol/L)
Obesity	Men: waist–hip ratio >0.90 Women: waist–hip ratio >0.85 and/or BMI >30 kg/m²	Men: waist circumference >102 cm Women: waist circumference >88 cm	Europid[‡] men: waist circumference ≥94 cm Europid[‡] women: waist circumference ≥80 cm
Microalbuminuria	≥20 µg/min or albumin-creatinine ratio ≥30 mg/g	—	—

BMI, body mass index; HDL, high-density lipoprotein; IDF, International Diabetes Federation; IGT, impaired glucose tolerance; NCEP ATP III, Adult Treatment Panel III of the National Cholesterol Education Program; WHO, World Health Organization.
*Insulin resistance: insulin sensitivity measured under hyperinsulinemic euglycemic conditions, glucose uptake below lowest quartile for background population under investigation.
[†]The 2001 American Diabetes Association (ADA) definition identified fasting plasma glucose of ≥110 mg/dL (6.1 mmol/L) as elevated. This was modified in 2004 to be ≥100 mg/dL (5.6 mmol/L), in accordance with the ADA's updated definition of impaired fasting glucose.
[‡]The values for other ethnic groups are reported in the manuscript.
Adapted from Alberti KG, Zimmet P, Shaw J: Metabolic syndrome: A new world-wide definition. A Consensus Statement from the International Diabetes Federation. Diabet Med 2006;23:469-480.

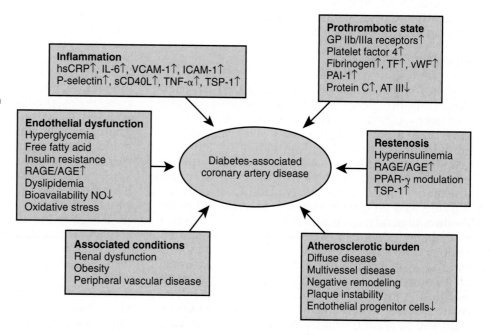

Figure 2-2. Pathophysiology of diabetes mellitus-associated coronary artery disease. AGE, advanced glycation end products; AT, antithrombin; GP, glycoprotein; hsCRP, high-sensitivity C-reactive protein; ICAM-1, intracellular adhesion molecule-1; IL-6, interleukin-6; NO, nitric oxide; PAI-1, plasminogen activator inhibitor-1; PPAR-γ, peroxisome proliferator-activated receptor-γ; RAGE, receptor for AGE; sCD40L, soluble CD40 ligand; TF, tissue factor; TNF-α, tumor necrosis factor-α; TSP-1, thrombospondin-1; VCAM-1, vascular cell adhesion molecule-1; vWF, von Willebrand factor. (Adapted from Roffi M, Topol EJ: Percutaneous coronary intervention in diabetic patients with non-ST-segment elevation acute coronary syndromes. Eur Heart J 2004;25:190-198.)

resistance, have been associated with the accelerated atherogenesis observed in diabetes and may confer vulnerability for CV events, both spontaneous and in the setting of coronary revascularization (Fig. 2-2).[9] In addition to metabolic disturbances, diabetes alters the function of multiple cell lines, including endothelial cells, smooth muscle cells, and platelets. Despite the description of several peculiarities charac-terizing diabetes-associated atherosclerosis, the exact mechanisms underlying the initiation and progres-sion of the atherosclerotic process remain elusive.

Insulin Resistance

Together with dyslipidemia, hypertension, and obesity, insulin resistance is a key feature of the metabolic syndrome. In addition, it is the first measurable metabolic disturbance among individuals who will subsequently develop type 2 diabetes. Insulin resistance describes a reduced sensitivity in body tissues to the action of insulin, which affects both glucose disposal in muscles and fat and insulin suppression of hepatic glucose output. As a consequence, higher concentrations of insulin are needed to stimulate peripheral glucose disposal and to suppress hepatic glucose production in patients with type 2 diabetes than those without diabetes. On a biologic level, insulin resistance has been associated with increased coagulation, pro-inflammation, and endothelial dysfunction, among other conditions.[10] In insulin-resistant subjects, endothelium-dependent vasodilation is reduced, and the severity of the impairment correlates with the degree of insulin resistance. Abnormal endothelium-dependent vasodilation in insulin-resistant states may be explained by alterations in intracellular signaling that reduce the production of nitric oxide (NO). Finally, insulin resistance is associated with elevations in free fatty acid levels, which may also contribute to decreased NO synthase activity and reduced production of NO in insulin-resistant states.[11] With respect to the clinical implications, insulin resistance has been associated with an increased CV risk. Recently, even among nondiabetic patients, high fasting plasma insulin was found to be an independent risk factor of long-term mortality in individuals with acute myocardial infarction (MI) and of new onset of heart failure in elderly patients without known heart disease.[12,13]

Endothelial Dysfunction

Diabetes vascular disease is characterized by endothelial dysfunction, a biologic abnormality that has been related to hyperglycemia, increased free fatty acid production, decreased bioavailability of endothelium-derived NO, formation of advanced glycation end products (AGE), altered lipoproteins, hypertension, and, as previously mentioned, insulin resistance.[11] A decreased bioavailability of endothelium-derived NO, with subsequent impaired endothelium-dependent vasodilation, has been observed in diabetic individuals even before the development of detectable atherosclerosis. NO is a potent vasodilator and a key compound of the endothelium-mediated control mechanisms of vascular relaxation. In addition, it inhibits platelet activation, limits inflammation by reducing leukocyte adhesion to endothelium and migration into the vessel wall, and reduces vascular smooth muscle cell proliferation and migration. As a consequence, an intact NO metabolism in the vessel wall has a protective effect by inhibiting atherogenesis. The impaired vasodilation observed among diabetic individuals may also be caused by an increased production of vasoconstrictors, and particularly endothelin-1. Despite the evidence of increased endothelin-1, angiotensin II, and abnormal sympathetic nervous system activity, the mechanisms of vascular smooth muscle cell dysfunction and hypertension in diabetes remain elusive.[11]

The formation of AGE is the consequence of the oxidation of amino groups by glucose. Additional processes induced by augmented AGE production include subendothelial cellular proliferation and matrix expression, cytokine release, macrophage activation, and expression of adhesion molecules.[14] Although the underlying mechanisms remain incompletely understood, it has been postulated that oxidative stress due to chronic hyperglycemia plays an important role in the etiology of diabetic complications. Hyperglycemia may induce the production of reactive oxygen species in the mitochondria, both directly via glucose metabolism and auto-oxidation and indirectly through the formation of AGE and binding of AGE receptors.

Prothrombotic State

The observation that diabetic patients have a hypercoagulable state is based both on the increased risk of thrombotic events and on laboratory abnormalities. An angioscopic study performed in patients with acute coronary syndromes (ACS) revealed that plaque ulceration and intracoronary thrombus were more frequent among diabetic patients than among their nondiabetic counterparts. Similarly, the incidence of thrombus was found to be higher in atherectomy specimens from patients with diabetes than in those from nondiabetic patients.[15] Diabetic individuals have increased platelet activation and aggregation in response to shear stress and platelet agonists.[16] In addition, an increased platelet-surface expression of the glycoprotein (GP) Ib receptor, which mediates binding to von Willebrand factor, and of the GP IIb/IIIa receptor, which mediates platelet-fibrin interaction, have been described. Moreover, decreased endothelial production of the antiaggregants NO and prostacyclin; increased levels of procoagulant agents such as fibrinogen, tissue factor, von Willebrand factor, platelet factor 4, and factor VII; and decreased concentrations of endogenous anticoagulants such as protein C and antithrombin III have been documented (see Fig. 2-2).[17] Finally, elevated levels of plasminogen activator inhibitor-1 (PAI-1) may impair endogenous tissue plasminogen activator–mediated fibrinolysis.[18] Overall, diabetes is characterized by increased intrinsic platelet activation, decreased endogenous inhibition of platelet activity, and increased blood coagulation in the presence of impaired endogenous fibrinolysis. Ex vivo studies have documented in diabetic patients the association between plasma glucose and level of platelet-dependent thrombosis, as well a reduction of thrombogenicity after improvement in glucose control.

Inflammatory State

Inflammation has been related not only to acute CV events but also to initiation and progression of atherosclerosis. Several CV risk factors, including diabetes, may trigger an inflammatory state. Although white blood cells are commonly considered to be the principal mediators of inflammation, a key role of platelets in the inflammatory process has recently been demonstrated. The interaction between diabetes and inflammation appears complex.[19] Although it is plausible that metabolic disturbances associated with this condition trigger vascular inflammation, the converse may also be true. Accordingly, C-reactive protein (CRP) has been shown to independently predict the risk of developing type 2 diabetes.[20] Inflammatory parameters elevated in diabetes, and in the context of insulin resistance in the absence of overt diabetes, include high-sensitivity C-reactive protein (hsCRP), interleukin-6 (IL-6), tumor necrosis factor-α (TNF-α), and the circulating (soluble) form of CD40 ligand (sCD40L) (see Fig. 2-2). In addition, an increased expression of adhesion molecules, such as endothelial (E)-selectin, vascular cell adhesion molecule-1 (VCAM-1), and intracellular adhesion molecule-1 (ICAM-1) has been detected. The morphologic substrate of increased vascular inflammatory activity can be derived by an analysis of coronary atherectomy specimens of patients with ACS: tissue from diabetic patients exhibits a larger content of lipid-rich atheroma and a more pronounced macrophage infiltration, compared with specimens from nondiabetic individuals.[15] The receptor for AGE (RAGE) may play an important role in inflammatory processes and endothelial activation, most likely accelerating the processes of coronary atherosclerotic development, especially in diabetic patients. Recently, it has been demonstrated that CRP, a key pro-inflammatory cytokine in patients with atherosclerosis, upregulates RAGE expression in endothelial cells. These observations reinforce the mechanistic links in diabetes among inflammation, endothelial dysfunction, atherothrombosis, and, as detailed later, accelerated restenosis.

Plaque Instability and Impaired Vascular Repair

In addition to promoting atherogenesis, diabetes conveys plaque instability.[21] It has been shown that atherosclerotic lesions in diabetic patients have fewer vascular smooth muscle cells compared with those of controls. As the source of collagen, vascular smooth muscle cells strengthen the atheroma, making it less likely to rupture and cause thrombosis. In addition, diabetic endothelial cells may produce an excess of cytokines that decrease the de novo synthesis of collagen by vascular smooth muscle cells. Finally, diabetes enhances the production of matrix metalloproteinases that lead to breakdown of collagen, potentially decreasing the mechanical stability of the plaque's fibrous cap. Overall, diabetes alters vascular smooth muscle function in ways that promote atherosclerotic lesion formation, plaque instability, and clinical events.[21]

It has been demonstrated that diabetic patients have a larger amount of lipid-rich plaques, which may be more prone to rupture.[15] Moreover, recent observations have suggested that, in diabetic patients, human endothelial progenitor cells, which are supposed to be important regulators vascular repair,

exhibit impaired proliferation, adhesion, and incorporation into vascular structures.[22] In addition to the dysfunction described, the number of endothelial progenitor cells obtained from diabetic patients in culture was found to be reduced compared with age- and sex-matched control subjects, and the reduction was inversely related to HbA$_{1c}$ levels.[23] An investigation documented that the level of endothelial progenitor cells was particularly low among diabetic patients with peripheral arterial disease (PAD) and hypothesized that depletion of this cell line may be involved in the pathogenesis of diabetic complications of the peripheral vasculature.[24]

CARDIOVASCULAR DISEASE IN DIABETES

Heart disease and stroke account for more than two thirds of all deaths among diabetic patients.[2] A recent population-based study documented that diabetes confers a CV risk equivalent to aging 15 years.[25] In 2001, the Adult Treatment Panel III of the National Cholesterol Education Program (NCEP ATP III) recommended that diabetes be considered a CAD risk equivalent, thus mandating aggressive CV risk prevention.[26] The notion of diabetes as a CAD risk equivalent came initially from a Finnish population-based study with 7-year follow-up involving 1059 diabetic patients and 1373 nondiabetic patients, which showed that diabetic patients without known CAD had the same likelihood of experiencing an MI as nondiabetic counterparts with a previous history of MI.[27] A similar observation was made in a registry enrolling more than 8000 patients with ACS, which showed that diabetic patients with no previous CVD had the same long-term morbidity and mortality as nondiabetic patients with established CVD before hospital admission.[28] Finally, additional data were provided by the 18-year follow-up of the mentioned Finnish study.[29] Adjusted multivariate Cox hazard models indicated that diabetic subjects without prior MI had mortality rates similar to those of nondiabetic subjects with prior MI (Fig. 2-3). In addition, diabetic subjects without prior evidence of CVD (i.e., MI, angina, or ischemic ECG changes) had a significantly higher risk of death than nondiabetic subjects with prior evidence of CVD (hazard ratio [HR] = 1.5 for men and 3.5 for women).[29]

Anatomic Pattern of Coronary Artery Disease

Autopsy and angiographic studies have shown that patients with diabetes more frequently have left main coronary artery lesions, multivessel disease, and diffuse CAD. A recent angiographic study on 534 patients with angina demonstrated that the greater the impairment of glucose metabolism (i.e., normal, IGT, newly diagnosed diabetes, or known diabetes), the smaller the average vessel diameter and longer the coronary lesions.[30] It is common belief that diabetic patients have an impaired ability to develop coronary collaterals compared with nondiabetic counterparts. However, a recent study measuring coronary collateral flow using intracoronary pressure

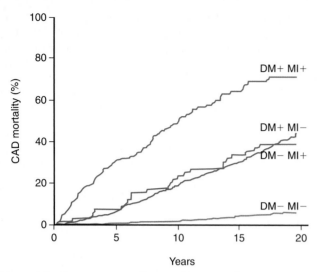

Figure 2-3. Coronary artery disease (CAD) mortality over 18 years according to the status of diabetes (DM) and prior myocardial infarction (MI). (From Juutilainen A, Lehto S, Ronnemaa T, et al: Type 2 diabetes as a "coronary heart disease equivalent": An 18-year prospective population-based study in Finnish subjects. Diabetes Care 2005;28:2901-2907.)

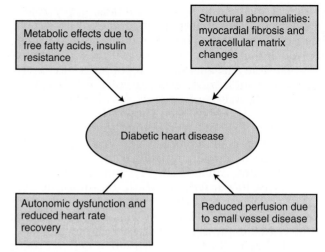

Figure 2-4. Pathogenesis of diabetic heart disease (assuming subclinical coronary artery disease and left ventricular hypertrophy have been excluded). (From Marwick TH: Diabetic heart disease. Heart 2006;92:296-300.)

and Doppler guidewires did not find differences between diabetic and nondiabetic patients in the setting of stable CAD.[31] Finally, intravascular ultrasound (IVUS) studies have shown that coronary arteries of diabetic patients are less likely to undergo favorable remodeling—an early compensatory enlargement at atherosclerotic sites—in response to atherosclerosis.

Heart Failure and Diabetic Cardiomyopathy

Epidemiologic and clinical evidence links diabetes and heart failure. The Framingham study documented increases of 2.5-fold and fivefold in the incidence of heart failure in diabetic men and women, respectively. Diabetes has been shown to promote both systolic and diastolic heart failure. Abnormal echocardiographic findings compatible with diastolic dysfunction were found in approximately one third of diabetic patients after exclusion of left ventricular hypertrophy or ischemia.[32] In the 1970s, the observation that diabetic patients may suffer from congestive heart failure in the absence of hypertension, CAD, or other evident source of cardiac disease led to the concept of diabetic cardiomyopathy, also called diabetic heart disease. Although the exact mechanisms underlying the condition are unknown, the accumulation of extracellular matrix proteins, and in particular of collagen, appears to be a key biologic dysfunction (Fig. 2-4).[33] The deposition may be the result of excess production, reduced degradation, and/or chemical modification of extracellular matrix proteins. These processes are believed to be induced directly or indirectly by hyperglycemia. Fibrosis may be the result of both increased activity of angiotensin II receptors and increased levels of angiotensin II.

At a cellular level, structural changes identified in the myocardium of animal models of diabetes include increases in the extracellular space, extracellular fibrosis, myocyte atrophy, and apoptosis.[34] These changes have been related to an increased vascular permeability caused by microvascular disease. Analogies have been identified between myocardial changes and the involvement of renal glomeruli in diabetic nephropathy, including increased thickness of the basement membrane, reduction of capillary density, and increased permeability with consequent increases of extracellular volume.[34] Clinical and pathologic consequences include myocardial hypertrophy, impaired contraction, diastolic dysfunction, and impaired exercise capacity.[33] The relation between glycemic control and diabetic myocardial abnormalities has been variable and contradictory. Although epidemiologic, clinical, and laboratory evidence supports the notion of diabetic cardiomyopathy, this concept is not universally accepted.

Cardiac Neuropathy

Cardiac neuropathy is characterized by an attenuation of heart rate variability in response to breathing, Valsalva and posture maneuvers, and an impairment of heart rate recovery following exercise. A recent population-based study including more than 2000 individuals demonstrated that diabetes was the primary contributor to reduced heart rate variability.[35] Growing evidence suggests that cardiac neuropathy in diabetes mediates alterations in the regulation of coronary vasodilator function in both epicardial and resistance coronary vessels, causing perfusion abnormalities even in the absence of obstructive epicardial CAD.[36] In addition, the absence of warning anginal symptoms during ischemia in patients with diabetes has been linked to autonomic neuropathy involving afferent sympathetic fibers, a key component of the cardiac pain perception pathway. Clinical studies have confirmed an association of silent infarction and ischemia with autonomic diabetic neuropathy.[36] However, it remains to be determined whether diabetes-associated autonomic dysfunction contributes to the excess CV mortality observed in this patient population.

Peripheral Arterial and Cerebrovascular Disease

Epidemiologic evidence confirms an association between diabetes and PAD, with a twofold to fourfold increased incidence compared with nondiabetic individuals. In the Framingham cohort, the presence of diabetes increased the risk of claudication by fourfold in men and ninefold in women. A study addressing the prevalence of PAD among 631 patients according to the degree of associated metabolic disturbance found that the rate of abnormal ankle-brachial index ranged from 7% in individuals with normal glucose tolerance to 21% in those requiring multiple antidiabetic medications.[37] Diabetes-associated PAD is characterized by extensive vascular calcification and a more frequent infrapopliteal involvement. The lower limb amputation rate among diabetic patients is up to 13 times higher than that of nondiabetic individuals. In 2002, more than 80,000 lower limb amputations were performed in the United States in patients with diabetes, corresponding to more than 60% of all nontraumatic lower limb amputations.[2]

Similarly to what is observed in the coronary and peripheral arterial circulations, diabetes also mediates cerebrovascular disease. Patients with diabetes have higher prevalence and a more advanced stage of extracranial and intracranial atherosclerosis than nondiabetic individuals. Case-control stroke studies and prospective epidemiologic data have correlated poor glycemic control and stroke risk and have identified diabetes as an independent predictor of ischemic stroke, with an increased risk ranging from 1.8-fold to almost sixfold.[38] Particularly ominous appears to be the impact of this condition on individuals younger than 55 years, as documented by a greater than 10-fold increased risk of stroke. In addition, diabetes increases the risk of stroke-related dementia more than threefold, doubles the risk of recurrence, and increases total and stroke-related mortality.

CARDIOVASCULAR DIAGNOSTIC MODALITIES IN DIABETES PATIENTS

Diabetic patients have significantly higher rates of silent ischemia than the general population. It has been estimated that as many as 12.5 million diabetic patients have asymptomatic CAD in the United States.[39] In most of the studies addressing the issue, the prevalence of silent ischemia among diabetic individuals has been greater than among nondiabetic counterparts. As previously mentioned, the absence of warning anginal symptoms during ischemia in patients with diabetes has been linked to autonomic

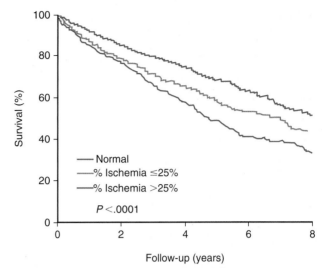

Figure 2-5. Kaplan-Meier survival curves for patients with diabetes mellitus according to dobutamine stress echocardiography results and extent of inducible ischemia. % ischemia, percentage of ischemic segments. (From Chaowalit N, Arruda AL, McCully RB, et al: Dobutamine stress echocardiography in patients with diabetes mellitus: Enhanced prognostic prediction using a simple risk score. J Am Coll Cardiol 2006;47:1029-1036.)

neuropathy. As a consequence of the lack of symptoms associated with ischemia, the diagnosis of CAD may be delayed or missed, which probably contributes to the fact that diabetic patients more frequently present at a later CAD stage than nondiabetic individuals. The diagnostic and prognostic value of stress testing in diabetes has been extensively investigated (Fig. 2-5; Tables 2-3 and 2-4).[40]

Exercise ECG testing is a well established and inexpensive test to guide the clinician in the diagnosis and risk stratification of diabetic patients with suspected CAD. The sensitivity and specificity for diagnosis of CAD in diabetic patients presenting with angina and in nondiabetic patients appear comparable. In asymptomatic patients, a positive exercise ECG test may be helpful to identify a subgroup of patients with advanced CAD. Patients with a negative stress test in the presence of normal exercise capacity are at low risk of CV events, at least in the short run. Stress nuclear imaging has the most extensive literature among the noninvasive modalities for both diagnostic and prognostic purposes in diabetes. With respect to stress echocardiography, several studies have addressed its prognostic accuracy in diabetes, whereas the data on its diagnostic value are scarce (see Tables 2-3 and 2-4).[40]

The ADA consensus guidelines for CAD screening in people with diabetes are listed in Table 2-5.[7] In particular, testing is recommended for patients with an abnormal resting ECG or with evidence of PAD or carotid disease and for those with symptoms possibly related to CAD (i.e., chest pain, dyspnea, fatigue), although the data for this indication are less compelling. In diabetic patients with neither

Table 2-3. Summary of Studies Using Stress Testing in the Diagnosis of Suspected Coronary Artery Disease in Diabetic Patients

Type of Test	Study*	N	Reference Standard	Sensitivity (%)	Specificity (%)	PPV (%)	NPV (%)
ECG	Lee et al	190	Angiography	47	81	85	41
DSE	Hennessy et al	52	Angiography	82	54	84	50
Nuclear	Kang et al	138	Angiography	86	56	NA	NA

*Full references for studies can be found in the source article.
ECG, exercise electrocardiographic stress test; DSE, dobutamine stress echocardiography; NA, not available; NPV, negative predictive value; PPV, positive predictive value.
From Albers AR, Krichavsky MZ, Balady GJ: Stress testing in patients with diabetes mellitus: Diagnostic and prognostic value. Circulation 2006;113:583-592.

Table 2-4. Summary of Studies Using Stress Testing in the Diagnosis of Coronary Artery Disease in Asymptomatic Diabetic Patients

Type of Test	Study*	N	Reference Standard	Sensitivity (%)	Specificity (%)	PPV (%)	NPV (%)
ECG	Blandine et al	98	Angiography	NA	NA	90	NA
ECG	Koistinen et al	136	Angiography	NA	NA	94	NA
ECG	Bacci et al	206	Angiography	NA	NA	79	NA
ECG	Penfornis et al	56	Angiography	NA	NA	60	NA
DSE	Penfornis et al	56	Angiography	NA	NA	69	NA
Nuclear	Blandine et al	103	Angiography	NA	NA	63	NA
Nuclear	Wackers et al	1123	None	NA	NA	NA	NA
Nuclear	Rajagopalan et al	1427	Angiography	92	68	89	60
Nuclear	Penfornis et al	56	Angiography	NA	NA	75	NA

*Full references for studies can be found in the source article.
DSE, dobutamine stress echocardiography; ECG, exercise electrocardiographic stress test; NA, not available; NPV, negative predictive value; PPV, positive predictive value.
From Albers AR, Krichavsky MZ, Balady GJ: Stress testing in patients with diabetes mellitus: Diagnostic and prognostic value. Circulation 2006;113:583-592.

symptoms nor evidence of cardiac or peripheral vascular disease, the ADA guidelines recommend testing for those who have two or more CV risk factors (i.e., dyslipidemia, hypertension, active smoking, family history of premature CAD, or albuminuria). Although the short-term prognosis (i.e., up to 2 years) in diabetic patients after a negative stress imaging test is excellent, multiple studies have found that those patients may suffer high late-event rates. This phe-

nomenon is not seen in the nondiabetic population and is possibly the expression of rapid atherosclerosis progression and increased risk of plaque rupture. This observation has led some investigators to suggest that stress tests should be repeated every 2 years, although the value of such a strategy has not been studied.

REVASCULARIZATION IN DIABETIC PATIENTS WITH STABLE CORONARY DISEASE

Almost 1.5 million coronary revascularization procedures, either coronary artery bypass grafting (CABG) or percutaneous coronary interventions (PCI), are performed each year in the United States, and approximately one quarter of them involve diabetic patients.[41] The randomized data on diabetic patients are scarce and are mainly derived from subgroup analyses of revascularization trials of patients with multivessel disease initiated in the late 1980s and early 1990s. Overall, diabetic patients with multivessel disease seem to have a better prognosis after CABG than after PCI. Although diabetic patients frequently have concurrent risk factors and comorbidities, diabetes has been identified as an independent predictor of CV events during and after revascularization, both percutaneous and surgical. Several pathophysiologic peculiarities of diabetic atherosclerosis previously discussed may negatively affect prognosis and response to coronary revascularization.

Table 2-5. Indications for Cardiac Testing in Diabetic Patients according to the American Diabetes Association

Testing for CAD is warranted in patients with ≥1 of the following characteristics:
Typical or atypical cardiac symptoms
Resting ECG suggestive of ischemia or infarction
Peripheral or carotid occlusive arterial disease
Sedentary lifestyle, age ≥35 years, and plans to begin a vigorous exercise program

Testing is also warranted for patients with ≥2 of the following risk factors in addition to diabetes:
Total cholesterol ≥240 mg/dL (6.2 mmol/L), LDL cholesterol ≥160 mg/dL (4.1 mmol/L), or HDL cholesterol <35 mg/dL (0.9 mmol/L)
Blood pressure >140/90 mm Hg
Smoking
Family history of premature CAD
Positive micro/macroalbuminuria test

CAD, coronary artery disease; ECG, electrocardiogram; HDL, high-density lipoprotein; LDL, low-density lipoprotein.
Adapted from Diagnosis and classification of diabetes mellitus. Diabetes Care 2006;29(Suppl 1):S43-S48.

Percutaneous Coronary Intervention

Whereas in-hospital and 30-day outcomes after PCI in diabetic patients are comparable to those of non-diabetics, large-scale registries have identified diabetes as an independent predictor of long-term mortality and need for repeat revascularization. Putative mechanisms negatively affecting outcomes may include endothelial dysfunction, prothrombotic state, greater propensity for restenosis and adverse vascular remodeling after angioplasty, increased protein glycosylation, and vascular matrix deposition (see Fig. 2-2).[9] All of these processes appear to be exacerbated by hyperglycemia and hyperinsulinemia. In addition, diabetic patients more frequently have noncardiac comorbidities that may also negatively affect outcomes.

Restenosis has been a main challenge in the percutaneous treatment of diabetic patients. Restenosis in the diabetic population is reviewed here, and details about vessel wall response after catheter-induced barotrauma can be found in Chapter 32. The restenotic process in diabetic patients is characterized by excessive proliferative response and increased vascular matrix deposition.[9] Mechanisms that may play a role include the interaction of the RAGE and its ligand, the peroxisome proliferator–activated receptor (PPAR)-γ, and thrombospondin-1 (TSP-1). RAGE is a cell surface molecule that is expressed at low levels in homeostasis but becomes upregulated at the site of vascular injury, particularly within the expanding neointima. In animal studies, blockade of RAGE resulted in significantly decreased neointimal proliferation, migration, and expression of extracellular matrix proteins. Finally, the link between insulin resistance and restenosis after coronary stenting was recently documented in humans. Among 120 patients undergoing coronary stenting who had an oral glucose tolerance test (OGTT), insulin sensitivity independently predicted the minimal lumen diameter at follow-up.[42]

Stents

In the diabetic population, the benefit of stenting was initially demonstrated in a single-center analysis comparing angiographic and clinical outcomes in 314 diabetic patients, matched for baseline characteristics, who underwent either stenting or percutaneous transluminal coronary angioplasty (PTCA).[43] At 6 months, the restenosis rate was significantly lower in the stent group than in the PTCA group (27% versus 62%). At 4 years, the incidence of cardiac death or nonfatal MI was lower in the stent group (14.8% versus 26.0%; P = .02), as was the need for repeat revascularization (35.4% versus 52.1%; P = .001). On a broader scale, a dramatic benefit of stenting in diabetic patients was detected in a study comparing outcomes of the diabetic cohorts of the 1997-2001 National Heart, Lung, and Blood Institute (NHLBI) Dynamic Registry, which was characterized by a large use of stents (87%), and the 1985-1986 NHLBI PTCA registry, in which patients were treated with PTCA only. The most recently performed procedures were characterized by an impressive reduction in in-hospital complications such as abrupt vessel closure (0.9% versus 2.2%), MI (1.0% versus 7.4%), urgent CABG (0.8% versus 6.2%), and death (1.9% versus 4.3%).[44] However, restenosis remains a limitation of stent-based PCI, particularly in diabetic patients. A meta-analysis of six stent trials identified diabetes as an independent predictor of restenosis (odds ratio [OR] = 1.3), and, among the 1166 diabetic patients included, the overall rate of restenosis was 37%.[45] The most important conditions predisposing to in-stent restenosis among diabetic patients have been a small reference vessel diameter and long stented segments.

Within the Do Tirofiban And Reopro Give similar Efficacy outcomes Trial (TARGET), contemporary PCI (i.e., based on third-generation-stents and triple antiplatelet therapy) was associated with similar 30-day event rates among diabetic (n = 1117) and nondiabetic patients (n = 3692).[46] In addition, no significant difference in major adverse cardiac events (MACE) at 6 months was observed, although diabetic patients had greater target vessel revascularization (TVR) than nondiabetic patients (10.3% versus 7.8%, P = .008). At 1 year, there was a trend toward increased mortality in the diabetic group (2.5% versus 1.6%, P = .056), but diabetes was not an independent predictor of mortality. These encouraging results were not replicated in another recent stent study that included a large diabetic population (n = 2694), the Prevention of REStenosis with Tranilast and its Outcomes (PRESTO) trial.[47] Although no difference in in-hospital events was observed between diabetic and nondiabetic patients, after adjustments for baseline characteristics, diabetes was identified as independent predictor of death (relative risk [RR] = 1.9) and of TVR (RR = 1.3) at 9 months.

Within registries, the outcomes of diabetic patients in recent years have remained unfavorable compared with those of nondiabetics, despite a broader use of stents. The NHLBI Dynamic Registry enrolled consecutive patients (1058 with diabetes and 3571 without diabetes) who underwent PCI from July 1997 to June 1999. At 1 year, diabetic patients had significantly higher adjusted risks of mortality (RR = 1.8) and of repeat revascularization (RR = 1.4).[48] Similarly, an analysis of 100,253 PCI patients enrolled in the 1998-2000 American College of Cardiology–National Cardiovascular Data Registry (ACC-NCDR) showed that diabetes was an independent predictor even of in-hospital mortality (OR = 1.4).[49]

Drug-Eluting Stents

Drug-eluting stents (DES) have revolutionized the field of interventional cardiology by dramatically reducing the incidence of restenosis and, as a consequence, the need for TVR (see Chapter 15). The available information on DES in diabetic patients remains scarce and is derived from registries or from subgroup analyses of randomized trials comparing the siroli-mus-eluting stent (SES) Cypher (Cordis, Johnson and Johnson), or the paclitaxel-eluting stent (PES) Taxus (Boston Scientific), with bare metal stents (BMS). Among diabetic patients (n = 279) enrolled in the randomized Sirolimus-Eluting Bx-Velocity Balloon Expandable Stent in the Treatment of Patients with de novo Native Coronary Artery Lesions (SIRIUS) trial, SES implantation was associated with a significant reduction in restenosis compared with BMS implantation (6.9% versus 22.3%; $P < .001$).[50] The relative risk reduction (RRR) was of the same magnitude in diabetic and nondiabetic patients. However, because of higher event rates in the diabetic population, the absolute benefit was greater than among nondiabetic patients (154 versus 111 restenoses prevented per 1000 patients treated). The incidence of MACE was also significantly reduced in diabetic patients, from 25% in those with BMS to 9.2% in those with SES.

With respect to the PES, among the 155 diabetic patients enrolled in the TAXUS IV trial (one third of them on insulin), a significant improvement in outcomes compared with BMS was detected.[51] At 12 months, the TVR rate was reduced from 24.0% to 11.3%, and the MACE rate was reduced from 27.7% to 15.6%. The first study that addressed the efficacy of DES specifically in diabetics randomly assigned 160 patients to SES or BMS.[52] At 9 months, the in-segment late lumen loss was significantly less in the SES group (0.06 mm) than in the BMS group (0.47 mm). As a result, the incidence of target lesion revascularization (7.3% versus 31.3%) and of MACE (11.3% versus 36.3%) were significantly lower in the SES group.

Despite these findings, several observations suggest that diabetic restenosis may be resilient even in the setting of DES. Accordingly, in the SIRIUS trial, diabetes remained an independent predictor of poor angiographic and clinical outcome among patients undergoing SES implantation.[50] In addition, in the same trial, the restenosis rate among diabetic patients with lesions longer than 15 mm in vessels smaller than 2.5 mm was as high as 23.7%. Finally, in the small group of patients treated with insulin (n = 82), the benefit in terms of restenosis with drug elution was modest (35.0% versus 50.0%; $P = .38$). Similarly, in the e-Cypher registry including more than 15,000 patients undergoing SES implantation, both non-insulin-requiring and insulin-requiring diabetes were independent predictors of MACE at 12 months (OR = 1.4 and OR = 2.2, respectively).[53] Although not of all the reports have identified diabetes as an independent predictor of poor DES-based PCI outcome, the results of a recent single-center experience on 260 consecutive diabetic patients undergoing multivessel DES implantation are sobering: the study detected a 9-month MACE rate of 25%.[54] Particularly high were the event rates among patients taking insulin (adjusted OR = 2.7). With respect to subacute or late stent thrombosis,

diabetes was not found to be a predictor of increased events in the BMS era. Conversely, in the e-Cypher registry, insulin treatment at baseline was found to be an independent predictor of late stent thrombosis (OR = 2.8)[53] Similarly, in a prospective cohort of 2229 patients undergoing DES implantation, diabetes was found to be an independent predictor of late stent thrombosis (OR = 3.7).[55] It remains to be determined whether late DES thrombosis will become a clinically relevant problem, particularly in the diabetic population. Potentially, the clopidogrel resistance associated with diabetes could be an underlying link.[56] With respect to whether SES or PES may be the best choice for the diabetic patients, no conclusion can be made at this point, although a randomized angiographic study of 250 diabetic patients favored SES.[57]

Coronary Artery Bypass Surgery

Paralleling what was described for PCI, diabetes also negatively affects outcomes after CABG. The impact of diabetes on morbidity and mortality in patients undergoing surgical coronary revascularization was addressed in a retrospective cohort study, based on the 1997 Society of Thoracic Surgery (STS) database, that included 41,663 diabetic patients among a total population of 146,786 patients.[58] At 30 days, the mortality rate was significantly higher in the diabetes group (3.7% versus 2.7%). The unadjusted and adjusted OR for mortality in these diabetic patients were 1.4 and 1.2, respectively. With respect to diabetes treatments at presentation, the adjusted OR for mortality among patients taking oral hypoglycemic drugs was 1.1, and that for patients taking insulin was 1.4. In addition, the overall morbidity rate and the infection rate were significantly higher in the diabetic patients. With respect to long-term mortality after CABG, a prospective New England cohort study that included 11,186 consecutive diabetic patients and 25,455 nondiabetic patients undergoing CABG from 1992 to 2001 detected a significantly higher annual mortality rate among diabetic patients (5.5%) compared with nondiabetics (3.1%).[59]

In addition to increased periprocedural morbidity and mortality, as well as long-term mortality, diabetes is associated with an increased rate of repeat revascularization after CABG. A prospective analysis on 26,927 patients who were contacted every 5 years up to 25 years after CABG at a single institution in the United States identified diabetes as an independent predictor of subsequent coronary revascularization (Fig. 2-6).[60] As part of the metabolic syndrome, diabetes is frequently associated with obesity, hypertension, and hypertriglyceridemia. The impact of these four factors (the "deadly quartet") on 8-year mortality after CABG was assessed in a single-center database that included 6428 patients.[61] Compared with individuals who had no risk factors, the HR for mortality increased from 1.6 among those with one risk factor to 3.9 for those with four risk factors. The yearly mortality rate ranged from 1% in patients with

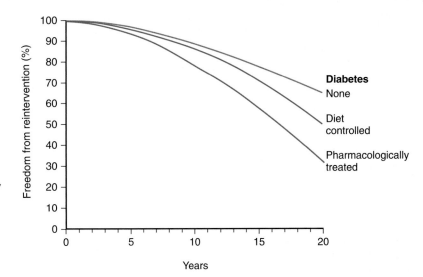

Figure 2-6. Predicted freedom from repeat coronary revascularization after coronary artery bypass surgery stratified by diabetes mellitus and its treatment. (From Sabik JF, Blackstone EH, Gillinov AM, et al: Occurrence and risk factors for reintervention after coronary artery bypass grafting. Circulation 2006;114:I454-460.)

no risk factors to 3.3% in patients with four risk factors. The prevalence and impact of undiagnosed diabetes were addressed in a German retrospective analysis of 7310 patients undergoing CABG between 1996 and 2003.[62] In this cohort, 5.2% of the patients had undiagnosed diabetes, defined as a fasting plasma glucose level of 126 mg/dL or higher. The perioperative mortality rate was significantly higher in the group of patients with undiagnosed diabetes (2.4%), compared with nondiabetic individuals (0.9%) or with patients with known diabetes (1.4%).

The use of multiple arterial conduits, including bilateral internal mammary artery (IMA) grafts, has been shown to improve the long-term results of CABG and reduce the need for repeat revascularization.[60] A recently published observational cohort showed improved 10-year survival and lower rates of recurrent MI and repeat CABG in diabetic patients with preserved left ventricular function who received bilateral IMA grafts.[63] Additionally, and in contrast with previous reports, no significant difference in the incidence of sternal wound infections was detected. With respect to the impact of off-pump surgery, a retrospective analysis compared 346 diabetic patients undergoing off-pump CABG with control subjects and showed reduced complication rates but no survival advantage.[64]

Adjunctive Metabolic Intervention at the Time of Coronary Revascularization

Recent studies have underscored the importance of optimal glycemic control at the time of coronary revascularization, both in the setting of PCI and with CABG. A prospective single-center analysis correlated HbA$_{1c}$ and the 12-month TVR rate in 179 diabetic patients undergoing PCI and demonstrated that diabetic patients with optimal glycemic control (i.e., HbA$_{1c}$ ≤7%) had a TVR rate similar to that of nondiabetic patients ($n = 60$): 15% versus 18%.[65] Those with HbA$_{1c}$ greater than 7% had a significantly higher TVR

rate (34%). In a multiple logistic regression analysis, HbA$_{1c}$ greater than 7% was identified as significant independent predictor of TVR (OR = 2.9). In addition, optimal glycemic control was associated with a significantly lower rate of cardiac rehospitalization and recurrent angina at 12 months. Opposing these results, a single-center retrospective analysis of prospectively acquired registry data addressing outcomes after PCI among 1373 diabetic patients stratified for baseline HbA$_{1c}$ found comparable results in terms of "death" and "death or MI" in various HbA$_{1c}$ strata (HbA$_{1c}$ <8.0%, 8.0% to 10.0%; HbA$_{1c}$ >10%, unknown).[66]

The importance of strict blood glucose control at the time of CABG was underscored in a single-center experience involving 3554 diabetic patients treated either with subcutaneous insulin (1987-1991) or with continuous insulin infusion (1992-2001).[67] The latter group had a lower in-hospital mortality rate (2.5% versus 5.3%). In a multivariate regression model, continuous insulin infusion was identified as an independent protective factor against death (OR = 0.43).[67] Another single-center prospective study randomized 141 diabetic patients undergoing CABG to either tight glycemic control (target serum glucose concentration, 125 to 200 mg/dL) using glucose-insulin-potassium infusion or standard therapy (target, <250 mg/dL) using intermittent subcutaneous insulin beginning before anesthesia and continuing for 12 hours after surgery.[68] Patients allocated to glucose-insulin-potassium achieved lower serum glucose levels, had significantly less perioperative atrial fibrillation, and had a significantly shorter postoperative length of stay. In addition, the active treatment group showed a significant survival advantage over the initial 2 years after surgery and significantly fewer episodes of recurrent ischemia or wound infections at follow-up.

Another concept aimed at improving the outcomes of diabetic and nondiabetic patients undergoing PCI relies on modulation of the PPAR-γ receptor, which is expressed by all major cell lines in the vasculature, including endothelial cells, smooth muscle cells, and monocyte/macrophages. Thiazolidinediones (TZD) bind with high affinity to and activate the PPAR-γ receptor, thereby enhancing the insulin-mediated glucose transport into adipose tissue and skeletal muscle (insulin sensitizers). Troglitazone, rosiglitazone, and pioglitazone inhibit vascular smooth muscle cell proliferation in vitro at drug levels therapeutic for antidiabetic therapy.[69] In a small randomized trial, the administration of troglitazone after coronary stenting was associated with a reduction of restenosis on IVUS follow-up.[70] However, the drug was withdrawn from the market after reports of severe hepatotoxicity. Recently, a positive effect on restenosis was reported with rosiglitazone. Among 95 diabetic patients, randomization to TZD for 6 months after PCI was associated with a significant reduction in restenosis compared with controls (17.6% versus 38.2%; $P = .03$). Baseline and follow-up HbA_{1c} levels did not differ between the two groups.[71]

In a randomized, placebo-controlled, double-blind trial, the effect of 6 months of pioglitazone treatment on neointima volume measured by IVUS was studied in 50 nondiabetic patients undergoing BMS-based PCI.[72] Compared with controls, subjects receiving pioglitazone had significant reductions in both neointima volume within the stented segment and binary restenosis rate. Importantly, in this study population of nondiabetic patients, pioglitazone treatment did not significantly change fasting blood glucose, fasting insulin, HbA_{1c} levels, or lipid parameters. These data bolster the hypothesis that TZD, in addition to their metabolic effects, exhibit direct antirestenotic effects in the vasculature.

The clinical relevance of long-term therapy with insulin sensitizers in association with coronary revascularization in diabetic patients is being tested in the Bypass Angioplasty Revascularization Investigation 2 Diabetes (BARI 2D), an NHLBI-sponsored trial investigating 2368 diabetic patients with mild angina or documented myocardial ischemia and at least 1 significant (>50%) coronary lesion on angiography.[73] Patients were enrolled between 2001 and 2005 and randomly assigned, in a 2 × 2 factorial design, to two glucose management regimens (insulin-sensitizing or insulin-providing) and to either medical therapy or mechanical revascularization (CABG or PCI). The primary end point is 5-year mortality. Aspirin, statins, β-blockers, and angiotensin-converting enzyme (ACE) inhibitors are mandatory if not contraindicated.

CABG VERSUS PCI

It remains a source of discussion what the best revascularization strategy for diabetic patients with multivessel CAD may be. The scarce data available have been accumulated over the years from post-hoc analysis of randomized trials (Table 2-6) and from single-center or multicenter registries.[74] Particular emphasis has been placed on the results of the Bypass Angioplasty Revascularization Investigation (BARI) trial, a

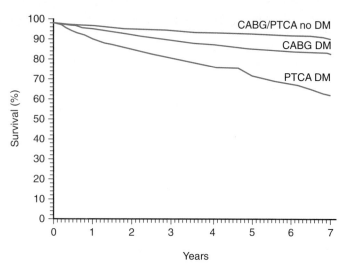

Figure 2-7. Kaplan-Meier estimates of survival for diabetic patients randomized in the BARI trial according to treatment assignment. The survival curves for PTCA and CABG among nondiabetic patients are virtually superimposed and here represented as a single line. CABG, coronary artery bypass surgery; DM, diabetes mellitus; PTCA, percutaneous transluminal coronary angioplasty. (Adapted from BARI investigators: Seven-year outcome in the Bypass Angioplasty Revascularization Investigation [BARI] by treatment and diabetic status. J Am Coll Cardiol 2000;35:1122-1129.)

study that randomized patients with multivessel disease to CABG or PTCA between 1988 and 1991. Among the 353 diabetic patients enrolled, CABG demonstrated a greater survival benefit than PTCA, and this difference persisted to 7 years (76.6% versus 55.7%, respectively; $P = .0011$) (Fig. 2-7).[75] Conversely, the survival curves of nondiabetic patients randomized to CABG or PTCA remained virtually superimposed. Subgroup analyses of the small diabetic group of patients enrolled in the Emory Angioplasty vs. Surgery (EAST) and the Coronary Angioplasty vs. Bypass Revascularization Investigation (CABRI) trials showed a trend for better long-term survival benefit for CABG compared with PTCA (see Table 2-6). In contrast, the Randomized Intervention Treatment of Angina (RITA-1) trial showed a trend toward more deaths among diabetic patients who underwent CABG compared with balloon-only PCI. In a meta-analysis including the subgroup of diabetic patients ($n = 537$) of EAST, CABRI, and BARI, the absolute survival benefit for CABG was 8.6% at 4 years.[76] At 6.5 years, however, the difference was no longer significant. The applicability of these results is limited by the fact that the trials were conducted before the availability of coronary stents and GP IIb/IIIa inhibitors. In addition, there was no systematic use of ACE inhibitors, β-blockers, aspirin, or statins.

With respect to stenting, the only randomized study comparing stent-based PCI with CABG that had a sufficient number of diabetic patients was the Arterial Revascularization Therapy Study (ARTS).[77] At 5 years, comparable results were obtained with PCI and CABG in 208 diabetic patients. The respective

Table 2-6. Diabetic Subgroup Results in Randomized Trials of CABG versus PCI

Study and Year	Patient Profile	Treatment Groups (N)	Repeat Revasc. (%)	Mortality %	P Value	Comments
RITA-1, 1993	One- to three-vessel CAD; angina or ischemia	CABG (33) PTCA (29)		24.2 at 6.5 yr 6.9 at 6.5 yr	.09	32% had single-vessel CAD; stents not used
EAST, 1994	Multivessel CAD; referred for revasc.; LVEF >25%	CABG (30) PTCA (29) CABG PTCA		10.0 at 3 yr 6.9 at 3 yr 24.5 at 8 yr 39.9 at 8 yr	NA .23	Single-center study; stents not used
CABRI, 1995	Multivessel CAD; angina or ischemia; LVEF >35%	CABG (60) PTCA (64)		12.5 at 4 yr 22.6 at 4 yr	NA	Stent use rare
BARI, 1996	Multivessel CAD; angina or ischemia	CABG (180) PTCA (173) CABG PTCA	11.1 at 7 yr 69.9 at 7 yr	19.4 at 5 yr 34.5 at 5 yr 25.6 at 7 yr 44.3 at 7 yr	.003 .001	81% IMA use; stents not used
ARTS, 2001	Multivessel CAD; angina or ischemia; LVEF >30%	CABG (96) Stent (112) CABG Stent CABG Stent	3.1 at 1 yr* 22.3 at 1 yr* 8.4 at 3 yr* 41.1 at 3 yr* 27.5 at 5 yr* 42.9 at 5 yr*	3.1 at 1 yr 6.3 at 1 yr 4.2 at 3 yr 7.1 at 3 yr 8.3 at 5 yr 13.4 at 5 yr	.294 .39 .27	89% IMA use; 3.5% glycoprotein IIb/IIIa inhibitor use
AWESOME, 2001	Medically refractory unstable angina; high CABG risk†	CABG (79) PCI (65) CABG PCI	35 at 1 yr‡ 49 at 1 yr‡ 46 at 5 yr‡ 51 at 5 yr‡	19 at 1 yr 14 at 1 yr 34 at 5 yr 26 at 5 yr	.27 .27	54% stent use; 11% glycoprotein IIb/IIIa inhibitor use

CABG, coronary artery bypass graft surgery; CAD, coronary artery disease; IMA, internal mammary artery; LVEF, left ventricular ejection fraction; NA, not available; PCI, percutaneous coronary interventions; PTCA, percutaneous transluminal coronary angioplasty; revasc., revascularization.
*Combines absolute rates of repeat CABG and PCI.
†Prior heart surgery, myocardial infarction within 7 days, LVEF <35%, age >70 yr, or balloon pump use.
‡Includes revascularization or unstable angina.
Adapted from Flaherty JD, Davidson CJ: Diabetes and coronary revascularization. JAMA 2005;293:1501-1508.

rates of death, stroke, or MI were 25.0% with PCI and 19.8% with CABG. Diabetic patients treated with stenting had a lower event-free survival rate at 5 years (54.5%) compared with those undergoing CABG (25.0%) owing to the difference in the rates of repeat revascularization (42.9% versus 10.4%, respectively). The mortality rates did not differ (see Table 2-6). A comparison of the 1-year mortality rate among diabetic patients enrolled in the BARI (1996) and ARTS (2001) trials suggests an improvement in outcomes over time. The 1-year mortality rates in the two studies were 6.4% and 3.1%, respectively, with CABG and 11.2% and 6.3% with PCI. Such findings may reflect differences in patient selection or may indeed express an improvement in the revascularization and medical management of diabetic patients.

An indirect comparison between PCI and CABG results is also possible using registries. As an example, PCI outcomes of 857 BARI-eligible patients (23% with diabetes) treated within the NHLBI Dynamic Registry were compared with those of 904 patients randomized to PTCA in the BARI trial.[78] Stents and GP IIb/IIIa antagonists were used in 76% and 24% of cases, respectively. A dramatic decrease in both abrupt vessel closure (1.5% versus 9.5%) and need for in-hospital CABG (1.9% versus 10.2%) was observed in the more contemporary patient group. No difference

in in-hospital mortality was observed. Among diabetic patients, the survival at 1 year within the group of BARI-eligible NHLBI Dynamic Registry patients was similar to that observed in the BARI-CABG group (92.1% versus 93.6%). However, such comparisons must be interpreted with caution, because the favorable outcomes of the registry patients may also be the result of improved medical management.

A registry conducted by the Northern New England Cardiovascular Disease Study Group evaluated 5-year mortality rates among patients undergoing revascularization procedures in a large regional database linked to the national death index.[79] A subset of 7159 patients with diabetes treated between 1992 and 1996 was examined. Of those, 2766 patients (736 PCI and 2030 CABG) had similar profiles to diabetic patients randomized in the BARI trial. After adjustment for differences in baseline characteristics, patients treated with PCI had significantly higher mortality than those undergoing CABG (HR = 1.5). When stratified for severity of disease, the difference in mortality remained significantly higher for PCI in the setting of three-vessel but not two-vessel disease.[79] Similarly, a single-center experience of 2319 consecutive diabetic patients (265 PCI, 2054 CABG) undergoing coronary revascularization in the late 1990s detected a significantly higher 5-year mortality rate

Table 2-7. Putative Explanations for the Survival Benefit of CABG over PCI in Diabetic Patients

More complete revascularization
Less myocardium at risk on follow-up
Diabetes predicts restenosis after PTCA but not graft failure on follow-up
Less disease progression in untreated segments
CABG may convey a survival benefit in the setting of subsequent Q-wave MI
Risk associated with repeat revascularization due to restenosis after PCI may negatively impact long-term survival

CABG, coronary artery bypass grafting; MI, myocardial infarction; PCI, percutaneous coronary intervention; PTCA, percutaneous transluminal coronary angioplasty.

with PCI versus CABG (adjusted HR = 1.7 for non-insulin-treated patients and 2.6 for insulin-treated patients).[80]

Further comparative analyses of the outcomes of diabetic patients undergoing CABG or multivessel PCI relied on databases of several New York cardiac registries. A total of 37,212 patients (33% with diabetes) undergoing CABG and 22,102 patients (25% with diabetes) undergoing stent-based PCI between 1997 and 2000 were indentified.[81] At 3 years, a significant mortality reduction was observed among patients undergoing CABG, with the adjusted HR ranging from 0.59 to 0.71, according to the extension of atherosclerotic involvement. The observed reduction missed statistical significance only in the subgroup of diabetic patients with two-vessel CAD and no involvement of the left anterior descending coronary artery.

Explaining the Mortality Benefit of CABG

Several hypotheses have been formulated to explain the mortality benefit associated with CABG over PTCA suggested from the randomized trials (Table 2-7).[74] The survival advantage of CABG among diabetic patients in BARI was limited to those who received at least one IMA graft. In addition, although diabetic patients in the CABG and PTCA groups had a similar mean number of significant lesions (3.5 versus 3.4), 87% of all intended vessels were successfully bypassed with CABG, but only 76% of vessels with significant lesions were successfully revascularized with PTCA.[82] As expression of a less complete revascularization, in the BARI trial diabetic patients had more jeopardized myocardium after PTCA than after CABG.[83] In addition, within the PTCA group, diabetic patients a had significantly higher increase in jeopardized myocardium at 1 year compared with nondiabetic patients. These findings are an expression of both restenosis and disease progression in untreated segments. In contrast, among CABG patients, diabetes was not associated with a percentage increase in jeopardized myocardium at angiographic follow-up.[83]

Furthermore, an analysis of all BARI-eligible diabetic patients (n = 641) revealed that the rate of Q-wave MI in the first 5 years after revascularization was similar after PCI or CABG (approximately 8% to 9%), but at the same time the associated risk of death was substantially reduced in patients who underwent CABG (adjusted RR = 0.09).[84] These results suggest that CABG provided greater protection from death after ischemic events in diabetic patients. Finally, whereas diabetic patients in the BARI trial had markedly greater restenosis after PTCA than nondiabetic individuals, graft patency in the CABG group was not influenced by diabetic status.[85] The long-term survival advantage of CABG over PCI in diabetic patients may therefore, in part, result from having a more durable restoration of flow conveyed by CABG without the risk of a repeat revascularization procedure, as was frequently the case in the PTCA group.

CABG in the Era of Drug-Eluting Stents

So far, no study comparing DES implantation and surgery has been completed. Indirect information on the potential for DES to compete with CABG can be derived from the ARTS II study, a prospective multicenter registry of patients undergoing multivessel PCI with SES implantation, matched to the randomized patients included in the ARTS I trial of CABG versus stenting. In the subgroup of 367 diabetic patients, the 1-year MACE rate in ARTS II was 15.7%, similar to the rate in the CABG group of ARTS I (14.6%).[86] There were no statistically significant differences in the rates of death (2.5% versus 2.1%), cerebrovascular accident (0% versus 5.2%), or MI (0.6% versus 2.1%), but a higher repeat revascularization rate was observed in ARTS II (12.6% versus 4.2%). Because occlusive restenosis occurs more frequently in diabetic patients than in nondiabetics and has been associated with increased long-term mortality among diabetics, DES treatment has theoretically the potential to improve survival in this patient population.[87] It is encouraging that the mortality rate among diabetic patients at 1 year was 11.2% in the PTCA arm of BARI, 6.3% in the stent arm of ARTS I, and only 2.5% in ARTS II.[86]

A study sponsored by the NHLBI, the Future Revascularization Evaluation in patiEnts with Diabetes mellitus: Optimal Management of multivessel disease (FREEDOM) trial, will compare DES-based PCI and CABG in 2400 diabetic patients with multivessel disease. The primary end point will be all-cause mortality, nonfatal MI, and stroke. The study will have a parallel registry of approximately 2000 patients, and the overall study duration will be 5 years. In addition, the Coronary Artery Revascularization in Diabetes (CARDia) trial is currently randomizing 600 diabetic patients in the United Kingdom and Ireland to CABG or PCI (with either BMS or DES).[88] The primary end point will be a composite of death, nonfatal MI, and cerebrovascular accident at 1 year. Additional data on costs, quality of life, and cognitive function are being collected, and follow-up will extend for 3 to 5 years.

NON-ST-ELEVATION ACUTE CORONARY SYNDROMES

The high prevalence of abnormal glucose metabolism in patients with CAD, and in particular among those with acute manifestations of the disease, was recently confirmed in large-scale surveys in both the United States and Europe. Within the U.S. CRUSADE (Can Rapid risk stratification of Unstable angina patients Suppress ADverse outcomes with Early implementation of the ACC/AHA guidelines) registry, among 46,410 patients with non-ST-elevation ACS, the prevalence of diabetes was 33%.[89] Within the National Registry of Myocardial Infarction (NRMI), the prevalence of diabetes among patients presenting with ST-elevation MI (STEMI) and non-ST-elevation MI (NSTEMI) was 27% and 34%, respectively.[90] In the Euro Heart Survey, glucose metabolism was addressed among 2854 patients with stable CAD and 2107 patients with unstable CAD.[91] The overall prevalence of diabetes was approximately 30% in both groups. Among unstable CAD patients without known diabetes, an OGTT detected IGT in 36% and diabetes in 22% of cases. In the stable CAD group those proportions were 37% and 14%, respectively (Fig. 2-8).[91]

Diabetic patients, compared with nondiabetics, more frequently have characteristics and comorbidities that may negatively affect outcomes in the setting of ACS.[92] However, several studies have shown that diabetes remains an independent predictor of short-term morbidity and mortality after accounting for imbalances in baseline characteristics, a notion recently reinforced by an analysis of the CRUSADE registry (Table 2-8).[92] Also, in the lung run, diabetic patients presenting with non-ST-elevation ACS have significantly higher rates of mortality and morbidity, recurrent MI, stroke, and heart failure compared with nondiabetic counterparts.[28] Recent data from the Euro Heart Survey suggest that in this setting the mortality rate is particularly high among diabetic women.[4] Importantly, in ACS, even prediabetes (i.e., fasting glucose levels between 100 and 126 mg/dL) is associated with increased CV risk.[93]

Early Invasive Versus Conservative Strategy

In diabetic patients with non-ST-segment elevation ACS, the positive impact of an early invasive strategy can be derived from subgroup analyses of large-scale randomized studies. The Fragmin and Fast Revascularisation during InStability in Coronary artery disease (FRISC II) study randomized 2457 patients to an invasive or conservative strategy and detected a significant survival benefit associated with the invasive strategy at 1 year.[94] The reduction in 1-year death or MI associated with early coronary angiography followed by revascularization (if needed) was marked among diabetic patients ($n = 299$), in terms of relative and particularly of absolute risk reduction (39% and

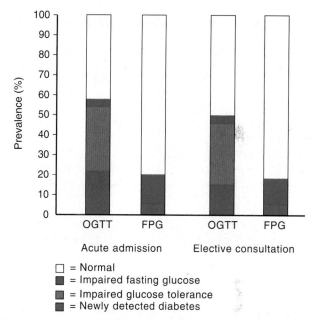

Figure 2-8. Prevalence of abnormal glucose regulation in patients without known diabetes mellitus in the Euro Heart Survey assessed by oral glucose tolerance test (OGTT) or fasting plasma glucose (FPG). (From Bartnik M, Ryden L, Ferrari R, et al: The prevalence of abnormal glucose regulation in patients with coronary artery disease across Europe. Eur Heart J 2004;25:1880-1890.)

Table 2-8. In-Hospital Clinical Outcomes in Diabetic Patients with Non-ST-Elevation Acute Coronary Syndromes in the CRUSADE Registry

Clinical Outcome	Nondiabetic (N = 31,049)	NIDDM (N = 9,773)	IDDM (N = 5,588)	Adjusted Odds Ratio (95% CI)	
				NIDDM*	IDDM†
Death (%)	4.4	5.4	6.8	1.14 (1.02-1.29)	1.29 (1.12-1.49)
Reinfarction(%)	3.2	3.5	3.8	1.07 (0.96-1.19)	1.07 (0.93-1.24)
Congestive heart failure (%)	8.0	12.4	13.7	1.25 (1.16-1.34)	1.19 (1.09-1.31)
Shock (%)	2.5	3.2	3.5	1.22 (1.05-1.41)	1.18 (0.97-1.44)
Red blood cell transfusion (%)	12.9	17.4	20.8	1.31 (1.23-1.40)	1.51 (1.40-1.63)

ACS, acute coronary syndromes; CI, confidence interval; IDDM, insulin-dependent diabetes mellitus; NIDDM, non-insulin-dependent diabetes mellitus.
*Nondiabetic vs. type 2 diabetic patients.
†Nondiabetic vs. IDDM patients.
From Brogan GX, Peterson ED, Mulgund J, et al: Treatment disparities in the care of patients with and without diabetes presenting with non-ST-segment elevation acute coronary syndromes. Diabetes Care 2006;29:9-14.

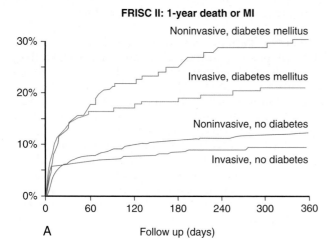

FRISC II: 1-year death or MI

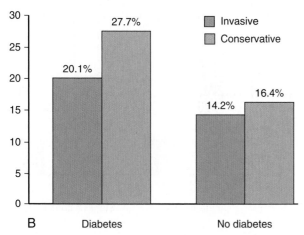

TACTICS: 6-month death, MI, rehospitalization for ACS

Figure 2-9. Outcomes according to diabetic status in the FRISC II **(A)** and TACTICS **(B)** trials of invasive versus conservative strategy in acute coronary syndromes (ACS). MI, myocardial infarction. (**A,** From Norhammar A, Malmberg K, Diderholm E, et al: Diabetes mellitus: The major risk factor in unstable coronary artery disease even after consideration of the extent of coronary artery disease and benefits of revascularization. J Am Coll Cardiol 2004;43:585-591; **B,** Data from Cannon CP, Weintraub WS, Demopoulos LA, et al: Comparison of early invasive and conservative strategies in patients with unstable coronary syndromes treated with the glycoprotein IIb/IIIa inhibitor tirofiban. N Engl J Med 2001;344:1879-1887.)

9.3%, respectively) (Fig. 2-9). Among nondiabetics, the effect was less pronounced (28% and 3.1%, respectively). Because of differences in sample size, the benefit observed barely missed statistical significance in diabetic patients but achieved it in nondiabetic individuals. In addition, diabetic patients undergoing early invasive therapy had a 38% reduction in the relative risk of 1-year death (7.7% versus 12.5%), again not reaching statistical significance owing to the small sample size.[94]

In the Treat Angina with Aggrastat and Determine Cost of Therapy with an Invasive or Conservative Strategy (TACTICS)-TIMI 18 trial, an early invasive strategy was associated with a significant 22% reduc-tion in the relative risk of death, MI, or rehospitaliza-tion for ACS at 6 months, compared with an early conservative strategy.[95] All patients were treated with aspirin, clopidogrel, and tirofiban. Diabetic patients derived a greater benefit than nondiabetics from an early invasive strategy, in terms of both absolute (7.6% versus 1.8%) and relative (27% versus 13%) event reduction at 6 months (see Fig. 2-9).

According to the 2002 Guidelines of the European Society of Cardiology (ESC), diabetes patients with ACS are to be classified automatically as high risk and therefore qualify for an early invasive strategy and for GP IIb/IIIa receptor inhibitors on top of standard treatment.[96] Within the CRUSADE registry, however, diabetic patients had a statistically significant lesser chance to get early coronary angiography compared with nondiabetic individuals.[89]

Coronary Artery Bypass Surgery

The only randomized trial that has compared CABG with PCI in patients with ACS was the AWESOME trial.[97] This study compared the two revascularization strategies in patients who had medically refractory unstable angina and were at high risk for adverse outcomes with CABG. Among 2431 patients identi-fied, 454 were considered acceptable for both PCI and CABG; 1650 patients were not deemed to be candi-date for both therapies and entered a physician-directed registry, and the 327 who were considered candidates for both treatment but refused random-ization entered a patient-choice registry. Overall, dia-betes prevalence was 31%. The respective CABG and PCI 3-year survival rates for diabetic patients were 72% and 81% for those randomized, 85% and 89% for those in the patient-choice registry, and 73% and 71% for those in the physician-directed registry.[97] None of these differences was statistically significant. These results must be interpreted with caution because, from both a surgical perspective (left IMA used in 70% of cases) and an interventional perspec-tive (stents and GP IIb/IIIa antagonists used in 54% and 11% of patients respectively), the way patients were revascularized may not comply with current standards. Nevertheless, CABG and PCI appear to be comparable options for high-risk dia-betic patients with ACS, and the choice of revascu-larization should be made individually based on coronary anatomy, ventricular function, age, and comorbidities.

ST-ELEVATION MYOCARDIAL INFARCTION

Paralleling the observations for non-ST-elevation ACS, diabetes is also an independent predictor of morbidity and mortality in STEMI. A retrospective study evaluating admission glucose of 141,680 patients presenting with acute MI demonstrated a linear correlation between glucose level and mortal-ity (Fig. 2-10).[98] Compared with individuals with admission glucose levels of 110 mg/dL or less, the hazard ratios for mortality for those with glucose

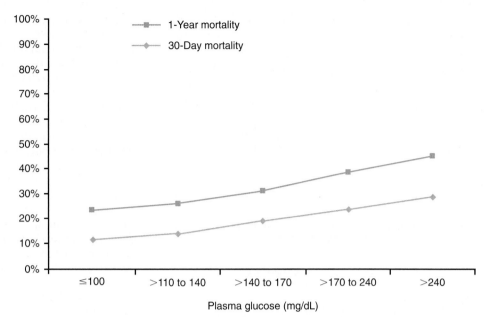

Figure 2-10. Relationship between admission plasma glucose values and 30-day and 1-year mortality rates among patients presenting with acute myocardial infarction. (From Kosiborod M, Rathore SS, Inzucchi SE, et al: Admission glucose and mortality in elderly patients hospitalized with acute myocardial infarction: Implications for patients with and without recognized diabetes. Circulation 2005;111: 3078-3086.)

levels of more than 110 to 140, more than 140 to 170, more than 170 to 240, and more than 240 mg/dL were 1.1, 1.3, 1.5, and 1.8 at 30 days and 1.1, 1.2, 1.3, and 1.5 at 1 year, respectively.

The impact of diabetes on outcomes after the acute MI phase was addressed in a contemporary large-scale study, the VALsartan In Acute myocardial iNfarcTion (VALIANT) trial.[99] The study enrolled 3400 patients with known diabetes, 580 patients with newly diagnosed diabetes, and 10,719 patients with no diabetes. At 1 year, patients with previously known and newly diagnosed diabetes had similar increased risks of mortality (adjusted HR = 1.4 and 1.5, respectively) and of CV events (adjusted HR = 1.4 and 1.3, respectively), compared with nondiabetics. Similarly to what is observed in the setting of non-ST-elevation ACS, diabetic patients are exposed less frequently to evidence-based therapy in the management of acute MI. According to the Swedish Register of Information and Knowledge about Swedish Heart Intensive care Admissions (RIKS-HIA), after adjustments for differences in baseline characteristics, patients with diabetes were significantly less likely than nondiabetics to be treated with reperfusion therapy, heparins, statins, or revascularization but more likely to receive ACE inhibitors[100] (Fig. 2-11). Importantly, the same analysis documented a mortality benefit associated with the administration of several of these therapies in the diabetic population (Fig. 2-12).

Reperfusion Therapy

With respect to fibrinolytic therapy, the meta-analysis of the Fibrinolytic Therapy Trialists' Collaborative Group involving all of the large randomized trials of fibrinolytic therapy versus placebo in STEMI demonstrated a greater than twofold survival benefit at 35 days among diabetic patients (n = 2236), compared with nondiabetics (n = 19,423), corresponding to 3.7

and 1.5 lives saved per 100 patients treated, respectively. Whereas CABG in the setting of STEMI is typically reserved for failed PCI and for MI-related mechanical complications, primary PCI may be preferred over thrombolytic therapy in diabetic patients. However, the data to support this notion are limited. In a pooled analysis on a total of 367 diabetic patients enrolled in 11 randomized trials, allocation to

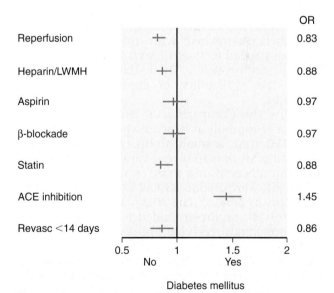

Figure 2-11. Likelihood of receiving various treatments in diabetic and nondiabetic patients with acute myocardial infarction in the RIKS-HIA registry, after adjustment for baseline characteristics. Horizontal lines indicate odds ratio (OR) ±95% confidence interval. ACE, angiotensin-converting enzyme; LMWH, low-molecular-weight heparin; revasc, revascularization. (From Norhammar A, Malmberg K, Ryden L, et al: Underutilisation of evidence-based treatment partially explains for the unfavourable prognosis in diabetic patients with acute myocardial infarction. Eur Heart J 2003;24:838-844.)

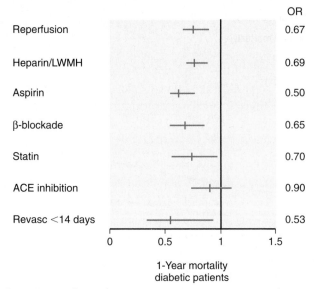

	OR
Reperfusion	0.67
Heparin/LWMH	0.69
Aspirin	0.50
β-blockade	0.65
Statin	0.70
ACE inhibition	0.90
Revasc <14 days	0.53

1-Year mortality
diabetic patients

Figure 2-12. Effects of various treatments on 1-year mortality rate in patients with diabetes mellitus in the RIKS-HIA registry. Horizontal lines indicate odds ratio (OR) ±95% confidence interval. ACE, angiotensin-converting enzyme; LMWH, low-molecular-weight heparin; revasc, revascularization. (From Norhammar A, Malmberg K, Ryden L, et al: Underutilisation of evidence-based treatment partially explains for the unfavourable prognosis in diabetic patients with acute myocardial infarction. Eur Heart J 2003;24:838-844.)

primary PCI led to a reduction in death or nonfatal MI at 30 days compared with fibrinolytic therapy (9.2% versus 19.3%; $P < .05$).[101] Overall, the benefit of primary PCI over thrombolytic therapy was greater in diabetic compared with nondiabetic patients (number needed to treat to save one life [NNT] = 10 and 16, respectively). These data were generated before the availability of stents or GP IIb/IIIa inhibitors.

Within the Comparison of Angioplasty and Prehospital Thrombolysis In acute Myocardial infarction (CAPTIM) trial, a small group of diabetic patients with acute MI ($n = 103$) were randomized to prehospital thrombolysis or a more contemporary primary PCI (stents were used in 83% of cases, and GP IIb/IIIa inhibitors in 27%).[102] The 30-day incidence of death, recurrent MI, or stroke tended to be higher in diabetic individuals receiving fibrinolysis than in those undergoing mechanical reperfusion (21.0% versus 8.8%; $P = .09$). The difference was driven by the higher, although not statistically significant, mortality rate in the fibrinolysis group (13.0% versus 5.3%). A single-center retrospective analysis including a limited number of diabetic patients ($n = 202$) treated with reperfusion therapy for STEMI detected a significantly lower 1-year incidence of death or reinfarction in patients treated with primary PCI ($n = 103$), compared with those undergoing fibrinolysis (19.4% versus 36.4%, respectively).[103] Stents (92%) and GP IIb/IIIa antagonists (63%) were broadly used in the setting of primary PCI.

The Controlled Abciximab and Device Investigation to Lower Late Angioplasty Complications (CADILLAC) trial aimed to determine the benefits of stent implantation over PTCA and abciximab over placebo in patients with STEMI, using a 2×2 factorial design. The study demonstrated that even in the primary PCI era diabetic patients ($n = 346$) had worse outcomes than nondiabetic individuals ($n = 1736$).[104] Accordingly, the incidence of death, disabling stroke, reinfarction, or ischemic TVR at 1 year was 21.9% in diabetics and 16.8% in nondiabetics ($P < .02$). The difference was driven by increased rates of death (6.1% versus 3.9%; $P = .04$) and TVR (16.4% versus 12.7%; $P = .07$) among diabetics. The rates of restenosis and TVR at 1 year were significantly reduced in diabetic patients who underwent routine stenting compared with balloon angioplasty (21.1% versus 47.6% and 10.3% versus 22.4%, respectively).

Aggressive Glucose-Lowering Therapy

The Diabetes mellitus, Insulin Glucose infusion in Acute Myocardial Infarction (DIGAMI) study was designed to test the hypothesis that intensive glucose-lowering therapy in patients with diabetes and acute MI would improve outcomes. A total of 620 patients were randomized to either standard treatment (controls) or standard treatment plus insulin-glucose infusion titrated according to glucose levels for at least 24 hours, followed by subcutaneous insulin treatment for 3 months after discharge. Active treatment was associated with a statistically significant mortality reduction at 3.5 years (33% versus 44%; RRR = 0.72) (Fig. 2-13). This translated into an impressive NNT of 9. Nevertheless, mortality remained elevated, underscoring the high risk of this patient population. In addition, insulin infusion was associated with a reduction in recurrent MI and heart failure rates at follow-up. In the DIGAMI 2 study, three glucose-lowering strategies were compared in 1253 diabetic patients with suspected acute MI: group 1 received an acute insulin-glucose infusion titrated to glucose levels for 24 hours, followed by insulin-based long-term glucose control; group 2 received insulin-glucose infusion for 24 hours followed by standard glucose control; and group 3 received routine metabolic management according to local practice.[105] At 2 years, the mortality rates in the three groups were comparable (23.4%, 22.6%, and 19.3%, respectively) (Fig. 2-14), and no significant differences in nonfatal MI or stroke were detected. Against the expectations, the achieved blood glucose levels during the study period were identical in the three groups. The trial was stopped prematurely because of slow enrollment and lack of funding.

Taken together, the results of the DIGAMI trials may be reconciled by stating that, in diabetic patients with acute MI, aggressive glucose lowering appears to be critical, irrespective of how this goal is achieved. In addition, it is not the metabolic effect on the myocardium of a glucose-insulin-potassium infusion per se that improves outcomes, but the associated

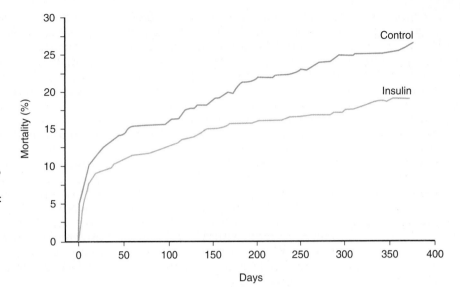

Figure 2-13. One-year mortality curves in diabetic patients with acute myocardial infarction randomized in the DIGAMI trial to either insulin infusion or control therapy. (From Malmberg K, Ryden L, Efendic S, et al: Randomized trial of insulin-glucose infusion followed by subcutaneous insulin treatment in diabetic patients with acute myocardial infarction [DIGAMI study]: Effects on mortality at 1 year. J Am Coll Cardiol 1995;26:57-65.)

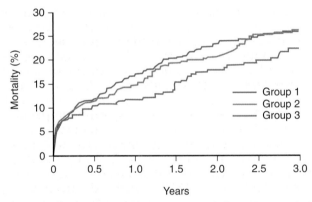

Figure 2-14. Three-year mortality curves in diabetic patients with acute myocardial infarction randomized in the DIGAMI 2 trial according to three different glucose-lowering strategies (for details see the text). (From Malmberg K, Ryden L, Wedel H, et al: Intense metabolic control by means of insulin in patients with diabetes mellitus and acute myocardial infarction [DIGAMI 2]: Effects on mortality and morbidity. Eur Heart J 2005;26:650-661.)

glucose-lowering effect. Accordingly, in a randomized study enrolling 20,201 patients with STEMI primarily treated with thrombolytic therapy, glucose-insulin-potassium infusion for 24 hours did not influence 30-day CV mortality or morbidity among either nondiabetic or diabetic individuals.[106]

ANTITHROMBOTIC THERAPY IN DIABETES

Aspirin and Clopidogrel

Data on the efficacy of antiplatelet therapy for primary prevention in patients with diabetes are limited. The only prospective randomized study has been the Early Treatment Diabetic Retinopathy Study (ETDRS), which enrolled 3711 diabetic patients in the 1980s and randomized them to aspirin 650 mg/day or placebo.[107] The administration of aspirin over 5 years was associated with a nonsignificant reduction in all-cause mortality and in fatal or nonfatal MI (RR = 0.91 and 0.83, respectively). In the secondary prevention setting, the Antiplatelet Trialist Collaboration demonstrated that prolonged use of an antiplatelet agent (mainly aspirin) among 5126 diabetic patients was associated with only a modest, nonsignificant benefit over placebo (RRR = 7%).[108] Information on which oral antiplatelet agent may be best suited for diabetic patients in the prevention setting can be derived from a subgroup analysis of the only large-scale head-to-head comparison, the Clopidogrel versus Aspirin in Patients at Risk of Ischemic Events (CAPRIE) trial. Among 3866 diabetic patients, the adenosine diphosphatase (ADP) (P2Y12) receptor antagonist clopidogrel (75 mg/day) was found to be superior to aspirin (325 mg/day) in the composite of ischemic and bleeding events over 2 years (RRR = 14.5%).[109] Accordingly, the number of ischemic or bleeding events prevented with clopidogrel per year among 1000 treated patients was 9 in the nondiabetic group, 21 in the diabetic group overall, and 38 in the insulin-treated group. These results were not considered to be strong enough, and aspirin remains the first-line antiplatelet agent for CV prevention, even among diabetic patients. The ADA recommends aspirin (72 to 162 mg/day) indefinitely for all diabetic patients with evidence of CVD and in the primary prevention setting for individuals older than 40 years of age with one or more CV risk factors or albuminuria.[110]

The Clopidogrel for High Atherothrombotic Risk and Ischemic Stabilization, Management, and Avoidance (CHARISMA) trial investigated the safety and efficacy of long-term administration of aspirin (75 to 162 mg/day) and clopidogrel (75 mg/day), compared with aspirin alone, in patients with established atherosclerotic disease or with multiple CV risk factors.[111] In the large diabetic population enrolled (n = 6556), no benefit of the combination therapy was observed after a median follow-up of 28 months, whereas the bleeding rate increased. With respect to patients undergoing PCI, the Clopidogrel for the Reduction of Events During Observation (CREDO) study randomized patients either to a 300-mg loading dose followed by 12 months of clopidogrel therapy or to no loading dose and clopidogrel treatment for 1 month on top of aspirin. Among 560 diabetic patients, the benefit of pretreatment and prolonged clopidogrel therapy was modest (RRR = 11.2%) compared with the benefit of this regimen observed among 1556 patients without diabetes (RRR = 32.8%).[112]

In the setting of non-ST-elevation ACS, aspirin remains a cornerstone of therapy, although specific data for diabetic patients are lacking. The Clopidogrel in Unstable angina to prevent Recurrent Events (CURE) trial randomized patients with ACS primarily medically managed to aspirin or aspirin plus clopidogrel for 9 to 12 months. Diabetic patients ($n = 2840$) derived only a modest, nonsignificant benefit from the combined treatment (death, MI, or stroke rate = 14.2% versus 16.7%). Among patients undergoing PCI in the trial, the benefit of the combined antiplatelet therapy was less marked (RR = 0.77) among diabetic patients compared with nondiabetic ones (RR = 0.66).[113] With respect to STEMI, the ClOpidogrel and Metoprolol in Myocardial Infarction Trial (COMMIT) in China randomized 45,852 patients with suspected acute MI to clopidogrel on top of aspirin or aspirin alone for a mean of 15 days.[114] Allocation to clopidogrel led to a modest but statistically significant relative risk reduction (9%) in death, reinfarction, or stroke during the treatment period. Limitations of the study included the lack of reperfusion therapy (approximately 50% received fibrinolysis, but primary PCI was performed only in isolated cases). No information on diabetic patients has so far been reported.

The CLopidogrel as Adjunctive Reperfusion TherapY (CLARITY)-TIMI 28 trial randomized patients receiving fibrinolytic therapy for acute MI to clopidogrel (300-mg loading dose followed by 75 mg/day) or placebo. At 30 days, the incidence of CV death, recurrent MI, or recurrent ischemia leading to urgent revascularization was reduced by 20% in those receiving clopidogrel therapy.[115] No subgroup analysis addressing the diabetic patients enrolled in the main trial ($n = 575$) is currently available. Nevertheless, among the 282 diabetic patients who underwent PCI during their index hospitalization, pretreatment with clopidogrel resulted in a 39% reduction in 30-day events, although this difference was not statistically significant owing to the small sample size.[116] Because of the results of the COMMIT and CLARITY-TIMI 28 trials, the U.S. Food and Drug Administration expanded the indications of clopidogrel for STEMI in August 2006. Overall, clopidogrel treatment for up to 1 year is indicated in diabetic patients presenting with ACS or undergoing PCI. Conversely, its role in the long-term prevention setting still needs to be defined. Although resistance to both aspirin and clopidogrel has been described in diabetic patients, the clinical relevance of these findings remains undetermined. Newer P2Y12 antagonists that have reversible action or are suitable for intravenous administration are currently being tested. Data on the diabetic population are lacking.

Glycoprotein IIb/IIIa Receptor Antagonists

The use of intravenous platelet GP IIb/IIIa receptor inhibitors and stents has markedly reduced the early hazard in diabetic patients undergoing PCI. In the Evaluation of Platelet IIb/IIIa Inhibitor for Stenting (EPISTENT) trial, abciximab halved the risk of death, MI, or urgent revascularization at 30 days among diabetic patients undergoing stenting compared with placebo (12.1% versus 5.6%, respectively). The observed event rate was comparable to that of abciximab-treated nondiabetic patients (5.2%). A pooled analysis of three early abciximab trials demonstrated a significant 1-year mortality rate reduction among diabetic patients randomized to the drug compared with placebo (2.5% versus 4.5%).[117] The Intracoronary Stenting and Antithrombotic Regimen: is abciximab a Superior Way to Eliminate Elevated Thrombotic risk in diabetics (ISAR-SWEET) study demonstrated that, among 701 low-risk diabetic patients, abciximab did not confer additional benefit on top of aspirin and a high clopidogrel loading dose (i.e., 600 mg > 2 hours before PCI).[118] However, the study excluded ACS and insulin-treated diabetic patients. The question whether one GP IIb/IIIa inhibitor rather than another may be preferable in diabetic patients was addressed in a subgroup analysis of the TARGET trial, the only head-to-head comparison thus far performed. Among the 1117 diabetic patients enrolled, randomization to abciximab or tirofiban at the time of PCI led to comparable outcomes for up to 1 year.[46] In particular, no difference was observed in terms of TVR or late mortality, suggesting that the non-GP IIb/IIIa properties of abciximab (such as vitronectin and $\alpha M\beta 2$ [Mac-1] receptor inhibition) do not translate into a long-term clinical benefit among diabetic patients.

In the setting of non-ST-segment elevation ACS, although the overall impact of GP IIb/IIIa receptor inhibitors used in a conservative setting has been modest,[119] a mortality benefit was detected among diabetic patients. Accordingly, the meta-analysis of the diabetic populations ($n = 6458$) enrolled in the six large-scale trials of GP IIb/IIIa inhibitors in ACS detected a highly significant 26% mortality reduction associated with the use of these agents at 30 days, compared with placebo (Fig. 2-15).[120] These findings were reinforced by a statistically significant interaction between treatment and diabetic status. The use of these potent platelet inhibitors was associated with a similar proportionate reduction in mortality for patients treated with insulin and for those treated with diet or with oral hypoglycemic drugs. Even more striking was the mortality reduction (70%) associated with the use of GP IIb/IIIa inhibitors among the diabetic patients who underwent PCI (see Fig. 2-15).

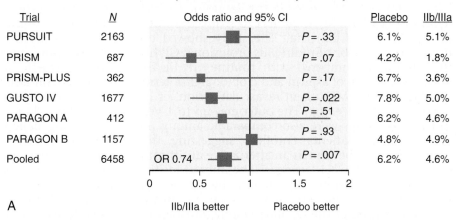

Diabetic patients with ACS: 30 day-mortality

Trial	N	Odds ratio and 95% CI		Placebo	IIb/IIIa
PURSUIT	2163		P = .33	6.1%	5.1%
PRISM	687		P = .07	4.2%	1.8%
PRISM-PLUS	362		P = .17	6.7%	3.6%
GUSTO IV	1677		P = .022	7.8%	5.0%
PARAGON A	412		P = .51	6.2%	4.6%
PARAGON B	1157		P = .93	4.8%	4.9%
Pooled	6458	OR 0.74	P = .007	6.2%	4.6%

A

IIb/IIIa better   Placebo better

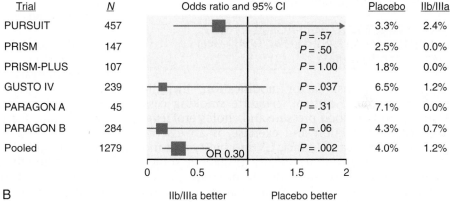

Diabetic patients with ACS undergoing PCI: 30 day-mortality

Trial	N	Odds ratio and 95% CI		Placebo	IIb/IIIa
PURSUIT	457		P = .57	3.3%	2.4%
PRISM	147		P = .50	2.5%	0.0%
PRISM-PLUS	107		P = 1.00	1.8%	0.0%
GUSTO IV	239		P = .037	6.5%	1.2%
PARAGON A	45		P = .31	7.1%	0.0%
PARAGON B	284		P = .06	4.3%	0.7%
Pooled	1279	OR 0.30	P = .002	4.0%	1.2%

B

IIb/IIIa better   Placebo better

Figure 2-15. Meta-analysis of six randomized, placebo-controlled trials demonstrating the effect of platelet glycoprotein IIb/IIIa inhibitors (IIb/IIIa) on 30-day mortality among diabetic patients with acute coronary syndromes (ACS): **A,** overall benefit; **B,** efficacy among patients who underwent in-hospital percutaneous coronary intervention (PCI). The data are reported as odds ratios with 95% confidence intervals (CI) and corresponding probability (P) values. Values lower than 1.0 indicate a survival benefit of IIb/IIIa. (From Roffi M, Chew DP, Mukherjee D, et al: Platelet glycoprotein IIb/IIIa inhibitors reduce mortality in diabetic patients with non-ST-segment-elevation acute coronary syndromes. Circulation 2001;104:2767-2771.)

With respect to putative mechanisms underlying the preferential benefit of GP IIb/IIIa inhibitors observed among diabetic patients, an hypothesis was generated by an in vitro study in which the blood of diabetic (n = 35) and nondiabetic (n = 38) individuals was exposed to pharmacologic concentrations of abciximab, tirofiban, and eptifibatide.[121] The assessment of fibrinogen-binding capacity with flow cytometry after exposure to 1 µmol/L ADP showed that GP IIb-IIIa antagonists inhibited platelet activation to a greater extent in blood from the diabetic patients. The decreased rate of fibrinogen binding after platelet activation was thought to be a consequence of glycation of the GP IIb/IIIa receptor, which may subsequently enhance the inhibitory function of GP IIb-IIIa antagonists.[121] Despite the preferential benefit from GP IIb/IIIa antagonists in the setting of non-ST-elevation ACS, data from the US NRMI registry including more than 60,000 patients with NSTEMI showed that diabetic patients had a significantly lesser chance to be treated with these potent platelet inhibitors than did nondiabetic individuals.[122]

The value of GP IIb/IIIa inhibitors for diabetic patients at the time of mechanical revascularization for STEMI cannot be adequately assessed, because few data are available. In a small, placebo-controlled, randomized trial with abciximab for stent-based primary PCI, the use of the GP IIb/IIIa antagonists among diabetic patients (n = 53) led to a significantly lower mortality rate at 6 months (0% versus 16.7%), as well as a reduced rate of reinfarction.[123] Within the previously mentioned CADILLAC trial, no benefit of abciximab in terms of morbidity or mortality was observed among 346 lower-risk diabetic patients treated with either PTCA or stents for acute MI.[104]

Anticoagulants

The Superior Yield of the New strategy of Enoxaparin, Revascularization, and Glycoprotein IIb/IIIa inhibitors (SYNERGY) trial compared the low-molecular-weight heparin (LMWH) enoxaparin with unfractionated heparin (UFH) in 9978 ACS patients undergoing early invasive strategy and found no difference in outcomes at 30 days and 6 months in the overall study population or in the diabetic cohort (n = 2926).[124] The Aggrastat-to-Zocor (A-to-Z) trial randomized 3987 ACS patients to enoxaparin or UFH on top of aspirin and tirofiban and found no benefit of enoxaparin. Among diabetic patients (n = 751), the composite of death, MI, or refractory ischemia at 30 days was nonsignificantly lowered with enoxaparin (8.4% versus 10.7%).[125] Heparin and LMWH should be seen as equivalent alternatives for diabetic patients in the setting of ACS and PCI.

The value of a bivalirudin-based antithrombotic strategy for PCI was studied in the Randomized Evaluation in PCI Linking Angiomax to reduced Clinical Events 2 (REPLACE-2) trial. The study showed the noninferiority of bivalirudin plus provisional GP IIb/IIIa inhibition compared with routine GP IIb/IIIa inhibition on top of aspirin and clopidogrel in terms of 30-day death, MI, urgent revascularization, or in-hospital major bleeding. The outcomes up to 1 year in the two groups were also comparable among the 1624 diabetic patients enrolled, suggesting that bivalirudin may be seen as an alternative antithrombotic agent in the PCI setting.[126] The interest for this compound has also been reinforced by a recent ex vivo human study showing that both bivalirudin and the combination of the GP IIb/IIIa antagonist eptifibatide plus heparin achieved marked reductions in total thrombus formation and fibrin deposition in diabetic patients undergoing PCI.[127]

PREVALENCE AND MANAGEMENT OF CARDIOVASCULAR RISK FACTORS AND TREATMENT GOALS

Aggressive CV risk factor modification, including optimal glycemic control, cigarette smoking cessation, control of blood pressure and cholesterol levels, and weight reduction and exercise, is an essential part of diabetes care. In fact, CV morbidity and mortality rates increase more steeply in diabetic subjects than in nondiabetic ones in the presence of additional risk factors. Table 2-9 summarizes the recommended treatment goals according to the ADA.[7] Based on the human and financial costs associated with diabetes-related complications, lifestyle and pharmacologic interventions to prevent diabetes are a logical and cost-effective strategy.[128] Dietary intervention, increased physical activity, and moderate weight loss not only improve glycemic control but also lower blood pressure and favorably affect lipid metabolism. Regular physical activity may reduce HbA$_{1c}$ levels by 10% to 20%, both systolic and diastolic blood pressure by 5 to 12 mm Hg, and triglyceride levels by 20% and may increase high-density lipoprotein (HDL)-cholesterol levels. Large cohort

Table 2-9. Treatment Goals for Diabetic Patients According to the American Diabetes Association

Glycemic control	
Hemoglobin A$_{1c}$	<7.0%
Preprandial capillary plasma glucose	90-130 mg/dL (5.0-7.2 mmol/L)
Peak postprandial capillary plasma glucose	<180 mg/dL (<10.0 mmol/L)
Blood pressure	<130/80 mm Hg
Lipids	
Low-density lipoprotein (LDL)	<100 mg/dL (<2.6 mmol/L)
Triglycerides	<150 mg/dL (<1.7 mmol/L)
High-density lipoprotein (HDL)	>40 mg/dL (>1.1 mmol/L)

Adapted from Standards of medical care in diabetes—2006. Diabetes Care 2006;29(Suppl 1):S4-S42.

studies have documented that higher levels of habitual aerobic fitness and/or physical activity are associated with significantly lower cardiovascular and overall mortality rates among diabetic individuals. To achieve and maintain effective lifestyle modifications, diabetic subjects should receive multidisciplinary counseling by dietitians, diabetes educators, exercise trainers, and physicians.

Smoking doubles the CV morbidity and mortality risk among diabetic individuals.[7] In addition, smoking has been associated with premature diabetes-related microvascular complications. Nicotine replacement or bupropion therapy is an effective element to include for smoking cessation in combination with behavioral interventions. Persistent abstinence of tobacco use remains one of the major goals in prevention of CVD in nondiabetic as well in diabetic subjects.[7]

Hyperglycemia

Several studies have demonstrated the link between elevated HbA$_{1c}$ plasma levels and CV risk. A multivariate analysis of the United Kingdom Prospective Diabetes Study (UKPDS) study involving 2693 diabetic patients without known CV disease demonstrated that, for each increment of 1% in HbA$_{1c}$ at baseline, the CV risk increased independently by approximately 10% over a median follow-up of 8 years. Although hyperglycemia has been associated with CVD and epidemiologic evidence links lower blood glucose levels to a decrease in CV events, aggressive blood glucose control in type 2 diabetes within randomized trials has not been shown to significantly reduce macrovascular events,[129] with the exception of patients presenting with acute MI[105] or undergoing CABG.[67] On the other hand, aggressive glucose-lowering therapy was associated with a significant reduction in microvascular complications.[129] A putative explanation for the observed lack of benefit of glucose-lowering therapies on macrovascular complications is that the achieved differences in HbA$_{1c}$ between control and intervention groups within the trials was insufficient. Optimal glycemic control, achieved with diet, exercise, and oral antidiabetic agents or insulin, remains a major goal in treatment of type 2 diabetes.[7]

In type 1 diabetes, optimization of glycemic control is effective in preventing or delaying retinopathy, nephropathy, and neuropathy. Within the Diabetes Control and Complications Trial (DCCT), fewer CV events occurred in the intensive-treatment group than in the conventional-treatment group, but the small number of CV events in the relatively young cohort precluded a determination of whether the use of intensive diabetes therapy affected the risk of CVD. Long-term follow-up data on the DCCT/Epidemiology of Diabetes Interventions and Complications (EDIC) study cohort showed that intensive insulin therapy reduced significantly the risk of nonfatal MI, stroke, or CV death by 57% among 1182 patients monitored for 17 years.[130] Therefore, intensive diabetes therapy has long-term beneficial effects on the risk of CVD in patients with type 1 diabetes.

Hypertension

Hypertension is a major independent CV risk factor in diabetes, and a direct correlation between blood pressure levels and CV risk has been demonstrated. Several recent studies using various antihypertensive drug regimens have demonstrated the benefit of lowering blood pressure to less than 140 mm Hg systolic and 80 mm Hg diastolic in subjects with diabetes. The UKPDS trial showed that tight blood pressure control may be more beneficial than tight glycemic control in terms of CV risk reduction in diabetes. Based on these clinical trials and epidemiologic studies, a target blood pressure goal of less than 130/80 mm Hg for diabetic patients has been recommended (see Table 2-9).[7] Behavioral factors that favorably affect hypertension include weight loss, regular aerobic activity, and limitation of alcohol and sodium intake. These nonpharmacologic strategies may also positively affect glycemic and lipid control. Additional pharmacologic therapy should be initiated early if lifestyle modifications are insufficient or in the presence of moderate to severe hypertension at the time of diagnosis. Among diabetic patients, hypertension can rarely be managed within the target zone with only one agent, and at least one third of patients require three or more medications.

ACE inhibitors or angiotensin receptor blockers (ARB), often in combination with a thiazide diuretic, should be considered as initial therapy (Table 2-10). The use of β-blockers in diabetic patients with CAD is associated with improved survival, even in those without a previous MI. Therefore, in this subgroup of patients, β-blockers and the combination of β-blockers and ACE inhibitors are considered the regimens of choice. It should be emphasized that β-blockers are not contraindicated in diabetic subjects with impaired hypoglycemia awareness, nor in those with PAD, particularly if cardioselective β_1-blockers are used. With respect to calcium channel blockers, dihydropyridines have been shown to decrease cardiac events and stroke, whereas nondihydropyridines reduce the progression of diabetic nephropathy.[131] Because randomized trials have

shown that the efficacy of dihydropyridine calcium channel blockers on CV event reduction is inferior to that observed with ACE inhibitors, calcium antagonists should be used as a second- or third-line regimen. On a broad perspective, optimal blood pressure control is more important than the drug class used to achieve it.

Dyslipidemia

The most common pattern of dyslipidemia among subjects with diabetes is characterized by elevated triglyceride and decreased HDL-cholesterol levels; mean levels of total cholesterol and low-density lipoprotein (LDL)-cholesterol often are not different in diabetic and nondiabetic subjects. With respect to LDL-cholesterol, however, diabetic individuals have a greater proportion of the particularly atherogenic small, dense LDL particles.[132] Lipid management aimed at lowering LDL-cholesterol has been shown to reduce macrovascular disease and mortality in diabetic individuals with and without overt CAD and without respect to baseline cholesterol levels. According to the ADA, the primary goal of therapy is an LDL-cholesterol level lower than 100 mg/dL (<2.6 mmol/L) for all subjects with diabetes (see Table 2-9).[7] The target HDL-cholesterol levels are greater than 40 mg/dL (1.03 mmol/L) in men and >50 mg/dL (1.29 mmol/L) in women. With respect to triglycerides, levels should be lower than 150 mg/dL (1.7 mmol/L).[7] In the secondary CV prevention setting, the use of statins is associated with a significant reduction in total mortality and in major CVD events.[133] The absolute clinical benefit achieved by lipid lowering may be greater in diabetic than in nondiabetic subjects.

With respect to primary prevention, the MRC/BHF Heart Protection Study looked at simvastatin treatment over a 5-year period, and the Collaborative Atorvastatin Diabetes Study (CARDS) used atorvastatin over a 4-year period; both demonstrated that, among diabetic individuals with no history of coronary events, statin treatment reduced major coronary events significantly.[134,135] Because fibrates effectively reduce triglycerides and increase HDL-cholesterol levels, they may be especially useful in diabetes-associated dyslipidemia. In a subgroup analysis of the Fenofibrate Intervention and Event Lowering in Diabetes (FIELD) study, the administration of this agent to patients with no previous CV disease and to younger (<65 years) individuals was associated with significant reductions in total CV events (19% and 20%, respectively).[136] However, within the entire study population of 9795 diabetic patients, fenofibrate did not reduce significantly the primary end point of CAD death and nonfatal MI. Therefore, the use of this drug class should be considered only in the presence of insufficient lipid control with statins. With respect to the combination of statins and ezitimibe, outcome data in the diabetic population are lacking. Treatment of dyslipidemia in diabetic patients should not be limited to prescription of

Table 2-10. Recommended Treatment of Hypertension in Subjects with Diabetes

Hypertension only	ACE-I, ARB, diuretics, or β-blockers
Hypertension with microalbuminuria or nephropathy	ACE-I or ARB (if neither is tolerated, non-dihydropyridine calcium channel blockers)
Hypertension and previous MI	β-Blockers and ACE-I
Hypertension and known CAD but no previous myocardial infarction	ACE-I

ACE-I, angiotensin-converting enzyme inhibitor; ARB, angiotensin receptor blocker; CAD, coronary artery disease.

statins. Regular physical activity and weight loss lead to decreased triglyceride and increased HDL-cholesterol levels. Improved glycemic control mainly lowers triglyceride levels and has only a modest effect on raising HDL. Alcohol consumption should be reduced for triglyceride levels greater than 175 mg/dL (2 mmol/L).

Diabetic Nephropathy

Renal failure is a major independent predictor of cardiovascular events. Diabetes is the leading cause of renal failure in Western countries. In 2002 in the United States, diabetic nephropathy accounted for more than 40% of the new cases of renal failure, and 44,000 diabetic patients began treatment for end-stage renal disease.[2] The condition underlying diabetic nephropathy is microvascular disease. Even in the absence of renal failure, albuminuria is a frequent finding in diabetes. Any degree of albuminuria has been found to be a risk factor for CV events, regardless of the presence or absence of diabetes.[137] In addition, diabetic nephropathy with or without renal failure is a key determinant of risk after both PCI and CABG. A single-center analysis involving 1575 diabetic patients undergoing PCI showed that patients with renal failure had significantly more in-hospital complications than those with normal renal function, including mortality (2.6% versus 0.5%, respectively), neurologic events (3.1% versus 0.6%), and gastrointestinal bleeding (2.9% versus 0.9%).[138] The 1-year mortality rate was strikingly higher in patients with chronic renal insufficiency (16%) than in those with preserved renal function (5%). Similarly, an analysis reviewing more than 480,000 patients undergoing CABG demonstrated that, compared with patients with normal renal function, the adjusted OR for mortality was 1.7 among patients with moderate renal dysfunction, 3.2 among those with severe dysfunction, and 3.6 among patients undergoing dialysis.[139]

Multifactorial Intervention

The Steno-2 study compared the efficacy of a targeted, intensified, multifactorial intervention with that of conventional treatment on modifiable risk factors for CV disease in 160 patients with diabetes and microalbuminuria.[140] The primary end point was a composite of CV death, nonfatal MI, stroke, revascularization, and amputation. Intensive treatment was characterized by a stepwise implementation of behavior modification and pharmacologic therapy that targeted hyperglycemia, hypertension, dyslipidemia, and microalbuminuria, along with secondary CV prevention with aspirin. Conventional treatment was in accordance with national guidelines. After a mean follow-up of 8 years, patients receiving intensive therapy had a significantly lower risk of CVD (HR = 0.47), nephropathy (HR = 0.39), retinopathy (HR = 0.42), and autonomic neuropathy (HR = 0.37). The authors concluded that a target-driven, long-term, intensified intervention aimed at multiple risk

factors in patients with type 2 diabetes and microalbuminuria halves the risk of CV and microvascular events.

Other Pharmacologic Approaches

In addition to the potential beneficial effect on restenosis described previously, TZD have shown anti-inflammatory and anti-thrombotic properties in diabetes. From a clinical perspective, in the PROspective pioglitAzone Clinical Trial In macroVascular Events (PROACTIVE) study, pioglitazone therapy in 5238 diabetic patients was associated with a nonsignificant 10% reduction in the primary end point (composite of all-cause mortality, nonfatal MI, stroke, ACS, endovascular or surgical intervention in the coronary or leg arteries, and amputation above the ankle), compared with placebo. Allocation to pioglitazone led to a significant 16% reduction in the main secondary end point (composite of all-cause mortality, non-fatal MI, and stroke).[141] However, significantly more hospitalizations for heart failure were reported in the active treatment arm. More data will be available from BARI 2D ancillary studies, which will allow insights into the modulation of diabetes-associated inflammation, procoagulation, and progression of CAD mediated by insulin-sensitizing or insulin-providing regimens.[73]

Currently, there are two additional areas of strong interest in research/clinical application in the field of diabetes and cardiovascular disease. The first is optimization of blood glucose control, either by continuous insulin therapy and glycemic monitoring (closed loop) or by new therapeutic agents such as glucagon-like peptide-1 agonists and dipeptyl-peptidase-IV inhibitors. Second, endocannabinoid receptor antagonists have been shown to improve obesity and the overall cardiovascular risk profile. However, it remains to be determined whether these strategies may lead to a reduction in macrovascular or microvascular complications in diabetes.

DIABETES PREVENTION

The best way to prevent CV complications in diabetes is to prevent the disease itself. Several studies performed over the last decade have shown that, in subjects at high risk for development of diabetes, lifestyle modifications and pharmacologic interventions may effectively prevent or delay the onset of the disease. Regular physical activity, diet, and weight reduction in high-risk subjects with IGT were shown to reduce the risk of developing diabetes by 31% to 58%. Several drugs also were able to reduce the progression from IGT to diabetes. The risk of developing diabetes decreased with metformin by 31% over 2.8 years, with acarbose by 25% over 3.5 years, with troglitazone in women with a history of gestational diabetes by 56% over 5 years, and with orlistat in obese subjects with IGT by 45% over 4 years. Finally, the Diabetes REduction Assessment with ramipril and rosiglitazone Medication (DREAM) trial recently showed that rosiglitazone, administered for 3 years, reduced the incidence of diabetes by 62% in middle-aged adults ($N = 5269$) with IFG, IGT, or both.[142]

ACKNOWLEDGMENT

The authors would like to acknowledge Ms. Karin Zambelis for providing assistance with graphics.

REFERENCES

1. Wild S, Roglic G, Green A, et al: Global prevalence of diabetes: Estimates for the year 2000 and projections for 2030. Diabetes Care 2004;27:1047-1053.
2. American Diabetes Association: National Diabetes Fact Sheet, Diabetes Statistics. Available at http://www.diabetes.org/diabetes-statistics.jsp (accessed March 20, 2007).
3. American Heart Association: Heart Disease and Stroke Statistics—2006 Update. Dallas, Texas, 2006.
4. Dotevall A, Hasdai D, Wallentin L, et al: Diabetes mellitus: Clinical presentation and outcome in men and women with acute coronary syndromes. Data from the Euro Heart Survey ACS. Diabet Med 2005;22:1542-1550.
5. McKinlay J, Marceau L: US public health and the 21st century: Diabetes mellitus. Lancet 2000;356:757-761.
6. Hogan P, Dall T, Nikolov P: Economic costs of diabetes in the US in 2002. Diabetes Care 2003;26:917-932.
7. Diagnosis and classification of diabetes mellitus. Diabetes Care 2006;29(Suppl 1):S43-S48.
8. Reaven GM. The metabolic syndrome: Is this diagnosis necessary? Am J Clin Nutr 2006;83:1237-1247.
9. Roffi M, Topol EJ: Percutaneous coronary intervention in diabetic patients with non-ST-segment elevation acute coronary syndromes. Eur Heart J 2004;25:190-198.
10. Kim JA, Montagnani M, Koh KK, et al: Reciprocal relationships between insulin resistance and endothelial dysfunction: Molecular and pathophysiological mechanisms. Circulation 2006;113:1888-1904.
11. Creager MA, Luscher TF, Cosentino F, et al: Diabetes and vascular disease: Pathophysiology, clinical consequences, and medical therapy. Part I. Circulation 2003;108:1527-1532.
12. Kragelund C, Snorgaard O, Kober L, et al: Hyperinsulinaemia is associated with increased long-term mortality following acute myocardial infarction in non-diabetic patients. Eur Heart J 2004;25:1891-1897.
13. Ingelsson E, Sundstrom J, Arnlov J, et al: Insulin resistance and risk of congestive heart failure. JAMA 2005;294:334-341.
14. Bierhaus A, Hofmann MA, Ziegler R, et al: AGEs and their interaction with AGE-receptors in vascular disease and diabetes mellitus: I. The AGE concept. Cardiovasc Res 1998;37:586-600.
15. Moreno PR, Murcia AM, Palacios IF, et al: Coronary composition and macrophage infiltration in atherectomy specimens from patients with diabetes mellitus. Circulation 2000;102:2180-2184.
16. Knobler H, Savion N, Shenkman B, et al: Shear-induced platelet adhesion and aggregation on subendothelium are increased in diabetic patients. Thromb Res 1998;90:181-190.
17. Carr ME: Diabetes mellitus: A hypercoagulable state. J Diabetes Complications 2001;15:44-54.
18. Anand SS, Yi Q, Gerstein H, et al: Relationship of metabolic syndrome and fibrinolytic dysfunction to cardiovascular disease. Circulation 2003;108:420-425.
19. Biondi-Zoccai GG, Abbate A, Liuzzo G, et al: Atherothrombosis, inflammation, and diabetes. J Am Coll Cardiol 2003;41:1071-1077.
20. Freeman DJ, Norrie J, Caslake MJ, et al: C-reactive protein is an independent predictor of risk for the development of diabetes in the West of Scotland Coronary Prevention Study. Diabetes 2002;51:1596-1600.
21. Beckman JA, Creager MA, Libby P:. Diabetes and atherosclerosis: Epidemiology, pathophysiology, and management. JAMA 2002;287:2570-2581.
22. Tepper OM, Galiano RD, Capla JM, et al: Human endothelial progenitor cells from type II diabetics exhibit impaired proliferation, adhesion, and incorporation into vascular structures. Circulation 2002;106:2781-2786.
23. Loomans CJ, de Koning EJ, Staal FJ, et al: Endothelial progenitor cell dysfunction: A novel concept in the pathogenesis of vascular complications of type 1 diabetes. Diabetes 2004;53:195-199.
24. Fadini GP, Miorin M, Facco M, et al: Circulating endothelial progenitor cells are reduced in peripheral vascular complications of type 2 diabetes mellitus. J Am Coll Cardiol 2005;45:1449-1457.
25. Booth GL, Kapral MK, Fung K, et al: Relation between age and cardiovascular disease in men and women with diabetes compared with non-diabetic people: A population-based retrospective cohort study. Lancet 2006;368:29-36.
26. Executive Summary of The Third Report of The National Cholesterol Education Program (NCEP) Expert Panel on Detection, Evaluation, and Treatment of High Blood Cholesterol in Adults (Adult Treatment Panel III). JAMA 2001;285:2486-2497.
27. Haffner SM, Lehto S, Ronnemaa T, et al: Mortality from coronary heart disease in subjects with type 2 diabetes and in nondiabetic subjects with and without prior myocardial infarction. N Engl J Med 1998;339:229-234.
28. Malmberg K, Yusuf S, Gerstein HC, et al: Impact of diabetes on long-term prognosis in patients with unstable angina and non-Q-wave myocardial infarction: Results of the OASIS Registry. Circulation 2000;102:1014-1019.
29. Juutilainen A, Lehto S, Ronnemaa T, et al: Type 2 diabetes as a "coronary heart disease equivalent": An 18-year prospective population-based study in Finnish subjects. Diabetes Care 2005;28:2901-2907.
30. Kataoka Y, Yasuda S, Morii I, et al: Quantitative coronary angiographic studies of patients with angina pectoris and impaired glucose tolerance. Diabetes Care 2005;28:2217-2222.
31. Zbinden R, Zbinden S, Billinger M, et al: Influence of diabetes mellitus on coronary collateral flow: An answer to an old controversy. Heart 2005;91:1289-1293.
32. Fang ZY, Schull-Meade R, Leano R, et al: Screening for heart disease in diabetic subjects. Am Heart J 2005;149:349-354.
33. Asbun J, Villarreal FJ: The pathogenesis of myocardial fibrosis in the setting of diabetic cardiomyopathy. J Am Coll Cardiol 2006;47:693-700.
34. Marwick TH: Diabetic heart disease. Heart 2006;92:296-300.
35. Ziegler D, Zentai C, Perz S, et al: Selective contribution of diabetes and other cardiovascular risk factors to cardiac autonomic dysfunction in the general population. Exp Clin Endocrinol Diabetes 2006;114:153-159.
36. Wackers FJ, Young LH, Inzucchi SE, et al: Detection of silent myocardial ischemia in asymptomatic diabetic subjects: The DIAD study. Diabetes Care 2004;27:1954-1961.
37. Beks PJ, Mackaay AJ, de Neeling JN, et al: Peripheral arterial disease in relation to glycaemic level in an elderly Caucasian population: The Hoorn study. Diabetologia 1995;38:86-96.
38. Goldstein LB, Adams R, Alberts MJ, et al: Primary prevention of ischemic stroke: A guideline from the American Heart Association/American Stroke Association Stroke Council. Circulation 2006;113:e873-e923.
39. Wackers FJ, Zaret BL: Detection of myocardial ischemia in patients with diabetes mellitus. Circulation 2002;105:5-7.
40. Albers AR, Krichavsky MZ, Balady GJ: Stress testing in patients with diabetes mellitus: Diagnostic and prognostic value. Circulation 2006;113:583-592.
41. Smith SC Jr, Faxon D, Cascio W, et al: Prevention Conference VI: Diabetes and Cardiovascular Disease. Writing Group VI: Revascularization in diabetic patients. Circulation 2002;105:e165-e169.
42. Piatti P, Di Mario C, Monti LD, et al: Association of insulin resistance, hyperleptinemia, and impaired nitric oxide release

with in-stent restenosis in patients undergoing coronary stenting. Circulation 2003;108:2074-2081.

43. Van Belle E, Perie M, Braune D, et al: Effects of coronary stenting on vessel patency and long-term clinical outcome after percutaneous coronary revascularization in diabetic patients. J Am Coll Cardiol 2002;40:410-417.

44. Williams DO, Jacobs AK, Vlachos HA, et al: Marked improvements in in-hospital outcomes following contemporary PCI in patients with diabetes. J Am Coll Cardiol 2004;43(Suppl A):56A.

45. Gilbert J, Raboud J, Zinman B: Meta-analysis of the effect of diabetes on restenosis rates among patients receiving coronary angioplasty stenting. Diabetes Care 2004;27:990-994.

46. Roffi M, Moliterno DJ, Meier B, et al: Impact of different platelet glycoprotein IIb/IIIa receptor inhibitors among diabetic patients undergoing percutaneous coronary intervention: TARGET 1-year follow-up. Circulation 2002;105:2730-2736.

47. Mathew V, Gersh BJ, Williams BA, et al: Outcomes in patients with diabetes mellitus undergoing percutaneous coronary intervention in the current era: PRESTO trial. Circulation 2004;109:476-480.

48. Laskey WK, Selzer F, Vlachos HA, et al: Comparison of in-hospital and one-year outcomes in patients with and without diabetes mellitus undergoing percutaneous catheter intervention (from the NHLBI Dynamic Registry). Am J Cardiol 2002;90:1062-1067.

49. Shaw RE, Anderson HV, Brindis RG, et al: Development of a risk adjustment mortality model using the American College of Cardiology–National Cardiovascular Data Registry (ACC-NCDR) experience: 1998-2000. J Am Coll Cardiol 2002;39:1104-1112.

50. Moussa I, Leon MB, Baim DS, et al: Impact of sirolimus-eluting stents on outcome in diabetic patients: A SIRIUS substudy. Circulation 2004;109:2273-2278.

51. Hermiller JB, Raizner A, Cannon L, et al: Outcomes with the polymer-based paclitaxel-eluting TAXUS stent in patients with diabetes mellitus: The TAXUS-IV trial. J Am Coll Cardiol 2005;45:1172-1179.

52. Sabate M, Jimenez-Quevedo P, Angiolillo DJ, et al: Randomized comparison of sirolimus-eluting stent versus standard stent for percutaneous coronary revascularization in diabetic patients: The Diabetes and Sirolimus-Eluting Stent (DIABETES) trial. Circulation 2005;112:2175-2183.

53. Urban P, Gershlick AH, Guagliumi G, et al: Safety of coronary sirolimus-eluting stents in daily clinical practice: One-year follow-up of the e-Cypher registry. Circulation 2006;113:1434-1441.

54. Stankovic G, Cosgrave J, Chieffo A, et al: Impact of sirolimus-eluting and paclitaxel-eluting stents on outcome in patients with diabetes mellitus and stenting in more than one coronary artery. Am J Cardiol 2006;98:362-366.

55. Iakovou I, Schmidt T, Bonizzoni E, et al: Incidence, predictors, and outcome of thrombosis after successful implantation of drug-eluting stents. JAMA 2005;293:2126-2130.

56. Angiolillo DJ, Bernardo E, Ramirez C, et al: Insulin therapy is associated with platelet dysfunction in patients with type 2 diabetes mellitus on dual oral antiplatelet treatment. J Am Coll Cardiol 2006;48:298-304.

57. Dibra A, Kastrati A, Mehilli J, et al: Paclitaxel-eluting or sirolimus-eluting stents to prevent restenosis in diabetic patients. N Engl J Med 2005;353:663-670.

58. Carson JL, Scholz PM, Chen AY, et al: Diabetes mellitus increases short-term mortality and morbidity in patients undergoing coronary artery bypass graft surgery. J Am Coll Cardiol 2002;40:418-423.

59. Leavitt BJ, Sheppard L, Maloney C, et al: Effect of diabetes and associated conditions on long-term survival after coronary artery bypass graft surgery. Circulation 2004;110:II41-II44.

60. Sabik JF, Blackstone EH, Gillinov AM, et al: Occurrence and risk factors for reintervention after coronary artery bypass grafting. Circulation 2006;114:I454-I460.

61. Sprecher DL, Pearce GL: How deadly is the "deadly quartet"? A post-CABG evaluation. J Am Coll Cardiol 2000;36:1159-1165.

62. Lauruschkat AH, Arnrich B, Albert AA, et al: Prevalence and risks of undiagnosed diabetes mellitus in patients undergoing coronary artery bypass grafting. Circulation 2005;112:2397-2402.

63. Endo M, Tomizawa Y, Nishida H: Bilateral versus unilateral internal mammary revascularization in patients with diabetes. Circulation 2003;108:1343-1349.

64. Magee MJ, Dewey TM, Acuff T, et al: Influence of diabetes on mortality and morbidity: Off-pump coronary artery bypass grafting versus coronary artery bypass grafting with cardiopulmonary bypass. Ann Thorac Surg 2001;72:776-780.

65. Corpus RA, George PB, House JA, et al: Optimal glycemic control is associated with a lower rate of target vessel revascularization in treated type II diabetic patients undergoing elective percutaneous coronary intervention. J Am Coll Cardiol 2004;43:8-14.

66. Hasdai D, Rizza RA, Grill DE, et al: Glycemic control and outcome of diabetic patients after successful percutaneous coronary revascularization. Am Heart J 2001;141:117-123.

67. Furnary AP, Gao G, Grunkemeier GL, et al: Continuous insulin infusion reduces mortality in patients with diabetes undergoing coronary artery bypass grafting. J Thorac Cardiovasc Surg 2003;125:1007-1021.

68. Lazar HL, Chipkin SR, Fitzgerald CA, et al: Tight glycemic control in diabetic coronary artery bypass graft patients improves perioperative outcomes and decreases recurrent ischemic events. Circulation 2004;109:1497-1502.

69. Law RE, Goetze S, Xi XP, et al: Expression and function of PPARgamma in rat and human vascular smooth muscle cells. Circulation 2000;101:1311-1318.

70. Takagi T, Akasaka T, Yamamuro A, et al: Troglitazone reduces neointimal tissue proliferation after coronary stent implantation in patients with non-insulin dependent diabetes mellitus: A serial intravascular ultrasound study. J Am Coll Cardiol 2000;36:1529-1535.

71. Choi D, Kim SK, Choi SH, et al: Preventative effects of rosiglitazone on restenosis after coronary stent implantation in patients with type 2 diabetes. Diabetes Care 2004;27:2654-2660.

72. Marx N, Wohrle J, Nusser T, et al: Pioglitazone reduces neointima volume after coronary stent implantation: A randomized, placebo-controlled, double-blind trial in nondiabetic patients. Circulation 2005;112:2792-2798.

73. Brooks MM, Frye RL, Genuth S, et al: Hypotheses, design, and methods for the Bypass Angioplasty Revascularization Investigation 2 Diabetes (BARI 2D) Trial. Am J Cardiol 2006;97:9G-19G.

74. Flaherty JD, Davidson CJ: Diabetes and coronary revascularization. JAMA 2005;293:1501-1508.

75. BARI Investigators: Seven-year outcome in the Bypass Angioplasty Revascularization Investigation (BARI) by treatment and diabetic status. J Am Coll Cardiol 2000;35:1122-1129.

76. Hoffman SN, TenBrook JA, Wolf MP, et al: A meta-analysis of randomized controlled trials comparing coronary artery bypass graft with percutaneous transluminal coronary angioplasty: One- to eight-year outcomes. J Am Coll Cardiol 2003;41:1293-1304.

77. Serruys PW, Ong AT, van Herwerden LA, et al: Five-year outcomes after coronary stenting versus bypass surgery for the treatment of multivessel disease: The final analysis of the Arterial Revascularization Therapies Study (ARTS) randomized trial. J Am Coll Cardiol 2005;46:575-581.

78. Srinivas VS, Brooks MM, Detre KM, et al: Contemporary percutaneous coronary intervention versus balloon angioplasty for multivessel coronary artery disease: A comparison of the NHLBI Dynamic Registry and the BARI study. Circulation 2002;106:1627-1633.

79. Niles NW, McGrath PD, Malenka D, et al: Survival of patients with diabetes and multivessel coronary artery disease after surgical or percutaneous coronary revascularization: Results of a large regional prospective study. J Am Coll Cardiol 2001;37:1008-1015.

80. Brener SJ, Lytle BW, Casserly IP, et al: Propensity analysis of long-term survival after surgical or percutaneous revascular-

ization in patients with multivessel coronary artery disease and high-risk features. Circulation 2004;109:2290-2295.

81. Hannan EL, Racz MJ, Walford G, et al: Long-term outcomes of coronary-artery bypass grafting versus stent implantation. N Engl J Med 2005;352:2174-2183.

82. Detre KM, Guo P, Holubkov R, et al: Coronary revascularization in diabetic patients: A comparison of the randomized and observational components of the Bypass Angioplasty Revascularization Investigation (BARI). Circulation 1999;99:633-640.

83. Kip KE, Alderman EL, Bourassa MG, et al: Differential influence of diabetes mellitus on increased jeopardized myocardium after initial angioplasty or bypass surgery: Bypass Angioplasty Revascularization Investigation. Circulation 2002;105:1914-1920.

84. Detre KM, Lombardero MS, Brooks MM, et al: The effect of previous coronary-artery bypass surgery on the prognosis of patients with diabetes who have acute myocardial infarction. N Engl J Med 2000;342:989-997.

85. Schwartz L, Kip KE, Frye RL, et al: Coronary bypass graft patency in patients with diabetes in the Bypass Angioplasty Revascularization Investigation (BARI). Circulation 2002;106:2652-2658.

86. Macaya C, Garcia H, Serruys PW. Sirolimus-eluting stent versus surgery and bare metal stenting in the treatment of diabetic patients with multivessel disease: A comparison between ARTS II and ARTS I. Circulation 2005;112(Suppl II):II-655.

87. Van Belle E, Ketelers R, Bauters C, et al: Patency of percutaneous transluminal coronary angioplasty sites at 6-month angiographic follow-up: A key determinant of survival in diabetics after coronary balloon angioplasty. Circulation 2001;103:1218-1224.

88. Kapur A, Malik IS, Bagger JP, et al: The Coronary Artery Revascularisation in Diabetes (CARDia) trial: Background, aims, and design. Am Heart J 2005;149:13-19.

89. Bhatt DL, Roe MT, Peterson ED, et al: Utilization of early invasive management strategies for high-risk patients with non-ST-segment elevation acute coronary syndromes: Results from the CRUSADE Quality Improvement Initiative. JAMA 2004;292:2096-2104.

90. Roe MT, Parsons LS, Pollack CV, et al: Quality of care by classification of myocardial infarction: Treatment patterns for ST-segment elevation vs non-ST-segment elevation myocardial infarction. Arch Intern Med 2005;165:1630-1636.

91. Bartnik M, Ryden L, Ferrari R, et al: The prevalence of abnormal glucose regulation in patients with coronary artery disease across Europe. Eur Heart J 2004;25:1880-1890.

92. Brogan GX, Peterson ED, Mulgund J, et al: Treatment disparities in the care of patients with and without diabetes presenting with non-ST-segment elevation acute coronary syndromes. Diabetes Care 2006;29:9-14.

93. Otten R, Kline-Rogers E, Meier DJ, et al: Impact of pre-diabetic state on clinical outcomes in patients with acute coronary syndrome. Heart 2005;91:1466-1468.

94. Wallentin L, Lagerqvist B, Husted S, et al: Outcome at 1 year after an invasive compared with a non-invasive strategy in unstable coronary-artery disease: The FRISC II invasive randomised trial. Lancet 2000;356:9-16.

95. Cannon CP, Weintraub WS, Demopoulos LA, et al: Comparison of early invasive and conservative strategies in patients with unstable coronary syndromes treated with the glycoprotein IIb/IIIa inhibitor tirofiban. N Engl J Med 2001;344:1879-1887.

96. Bertrand ME, Simoons ML, Fox KA, et al: Management of acute coronary syndromes in patients presenting without persistent ST-segment elevation. Eur Heart J 2002;23:1809-1840.

97. Sedlis SP, Morrison DA, Lorin JD, et al: Percutaneous coronary intervention versus coronary bypass graft surgery for diabetic patients with unstable angina and risk factors for adverse outcomes with bypass: Outcome of diabetic patients in the AWESOME randomized trial and registry. J Am Coll Cardiol 2002;40:1555-1566.

98. Kosiborod M, Rathore SS, Inzucchi SE, et al: Admission glucose and mortality in elderly patients hospitalized with acute myocardial infarction: Implications for patients with and without recognized diabetes. Circulation 2005;111:3078-3086.

99. Aguilar D, Solomon SD, Kober L, et al: Newly diagnosed and previously known diabetes mellitus and 1-year outcomes of acute myocardial infarction: The VALIANT trial. Circulation 2004;110:1572-1578.

100. Norhammar A, Malmberg K, Ryden L, et al: Under utilisation of evidence-based treatment partially explains for the unfavourable prognosis in diabetic patients with acute myocardial infarction. Eur Heart J 2003;24:838-844.

101. Grines C, Patel A, Zijlstra F, et al: Primary coronary angioplasty compared with intravenous thrombolytic therapy for acute myocardial infarction: Six-month follow up and analysis of individual patient data from randomized trials. Am Heart J 2003;145:47-57.

102. Bonnefoy E, Steg PG, Chabaud S, et al: Is primary angioplasty more effective than prehospital fibrinolysis in diabetics with acute myocardial infarction? Data from the CAPTIM randomized clinical trial. Eur Heart J 2005;26:1712-1718.

103. Hsu LF, Mak KH, Lau KW, et al: Clinical outcomes of patients with diabetes mellitus and acute myocardial infarction treated with primary angioplasty or fibrinolysis. Heart 2002;88:260-265.

104. Stuckey TD, Stone GW, Cox DA, et al: Impact of stenting and abciximab in patients with diabetes mellitus undergoing primary angioplasty in acute myocardial infarction (the CADILLAC trial). Am J Cardiol 2005;95:1-7.

105. Malmberg K, Ryden L, Wedel H, et al: Intense metabolic control by means of insulin in patients with diabetes mellitus and acute myocardial infarction (DIGAMI 2): effects on mortality and morbidity. Eur Heart J 2005;26:650-661.

106. Mehta SR, Yusuf S, Diaz R, et al: Effect of glucose-insulin-potassium infusion on mortality in patients with acute ST-segment elevation myocardial infarction: The CREATE-ECLA randomized controlled trial. JAMA 2005;293:437-446.

107. ETDRS Investigators: Aspirin effects on mortality and morbidity in patients with diabetes mellitus. JAMA 1992;268:1292-1300.

108. Antiplatelet Trialists Investigators: Collaborative meta-analysis of randomised trials of antiplatelet therapy for prevention of death, myocardial infarction, and stroke in high risk patients. BMJ 2002;324:71-86.

109. Bhatt DL, Marso SP, Hirsch AT, et al: Amplified benefit of clopidogrel versus aspirin in patients with diabetes mellitus. Am J Cardiol 2002;90:625-628.

110. Standards of medical care in diabetes—2006. Diabetes Care 2006;29(Suppl 1):S4-S42.

111. Bhatt DL, Fox KA, Hacke W, et al: Clopidogrel and aspirin versus aspirin alone for the prevention of atherothrombotic events. N Engl J Med 2006;354:1706-1717.

112. Steinhubl SR, Berger PB, Mann JT, et al: Early and sustained dual oral antiplatelet therapy following percutaneous coronary intervention: A randomized controlled trial. JAMA 2002;288:2411-2420.

113. Mehta SR, Yusuf S, Peters RJ, et al: Effects of pretreatment with clopidogrel and aspirin followed by long-term therapy in patients undergoing percutaneous coronary intervention: The PCI-CURE study. Lancet 2001;358:527-533.

114. Chen ZM, Jiang LX, Chen YP, et al: Addition of clopidogrel to aspirin in 45,852 patients with acute myocardial infarction: Randomised placebo-controlled trial. Lancet 2005;366:1607-1621.

115. Sabatine MS, Cannon CP, Gibson CM, et al: Addition of clopidogrel to aspirin and fibrinolytic therapy for myocardial infarction with ST-segment elevation. N Engl J Med 2005;352:1179-1189.

116. Sabatine MS, Cannon CP, Gibson CM, et al: Effect of clopidogrel pretreatment before percutaneous coronary intervention in patients with ST-elevation myocardial infarction treated with fibrinolytics: The PCI-CLARITY study. JAMA 2005;294:1224-1232.

117. Bhatt DL, Marso SP, Lincoff AM, et al: Abciximab reduces mortality in diabetics following percutaneous coronary intervention. J Am Coll Cardiol 2000;35:922-928.

118. Mehilli J, Kastrati A, Schuhlen H, et al: Randomized clinical trial of abciximab in diabetic patients undergoing elective percutaneous coronary interventions after treatment with a high loading dose of clopidogrel. Circulation 2004;110: 3627-3635.

119. Roffi M, Chew D, Mukherjee D, et al: Platelet glycoprotein IIb/IIIa inhibition in acute coronary syndromes: Gradient of benefit related to the revascularization strategy. Eur Heart J 2002;23:1441-1448.

120. Roffi M, Chew DP, Mukherjee D, et al: Platelet glycoprotein IIb/IIIa inhibitors reduce mortality in diabetic patients with non-ST-segment-elevation acute coronary syndromes. Circulation 2001;104:2767-2771.

121. Keating FK, Whitaker DA, Sobel BE, et al: Augmentation of inhibitory effects of glycoprotein IIb-IIIa antagonists in patients with diabetes. Thromb Res 2004;113:27-34.

122. Peterson ED, Pollack CV, Roe MT, et al: Early use of glycoprotein IIb/IIIa inhibitors in non-ST-elevation acute myocardial infarction: Observations from the National Registry of Myocardial Infarction 4. J Am Coll Cardiol 2003;42:45-53.

123. Montalescot G, Barragan P, Wittenberg O, et al: Platelet glycoprotein IIb/IIIa inhibition with coronary stenting for acute myocardial infarction. N Engl J Med 2001;344:1895-1903.

124. Mahaffey KW, Cohen M, Garg J, et al: High-risk patients with acute coronary syndromes treated with low-molecular-weight or unfractionated heparin: Outcomes at 6 months and 1 year in the SYNERGY trial. JAMA 2005;294:2594-2600.

125. Blazing MA, de Lemos JA, White HD, et al: Safety and efficacy of enoxaparin vs unfractionated heparin in patients with non-ST-segment elevation acute coronary syndromes who receive tirofiban and aspirin: A randomized controlled trial. JAMA 2004;292:55-64.

126. Gurm HS, Sarembock IJ, Kereiakes DJ, et al: Use of bivalirudin during percutaneous coronary intervention in patients with diabetes mellitus: An analysis from the REPLACE-2 trial. J Am Coll Cardiol 2005;45:1932-1938.

127. Lev EI, Patel R, Karim A, et al: Anti-thrombotic effect of bivalirudin compared with eptifibatide and unfractionated heparin in diabetic patients: An ex vivo human study. Thromb Haemost 2006;95:441-446.

128. Herman WH, Hoerger TJ, Brandle M, et al: The cost-effectiveness of lifestyle modification or metformin in preventing type 2 diabetes in adults with impaired glucose tolerance. Ann Intern Med 2005;142:323-332.

129. UK Prospective Diabetes Study (UKPDS) Group. Intensive blood-glucose control with sulphonylureas or insulin compared with conventional treatment and risk of complications in patients with type 2 diabetes (UKPDS 33). Lancet 1998; 352:837-853.

130. Nathan DM, Cleary PA, Backlund JY, et al: Intensive diabetes treatment and cardiovascular disease in patients with type 1 diabetes. N Engl J Med 2005;353:2643-2653.

131. Ruggenenti P, Fassi A, Ilieva AP, et al: Preventing microalbuminuria in type 2 diabetes. N Engl J Med 2004;351:1941-1951.

132. Siegel RD, Cupples A, Schaefer EJ, et al: Lipoproteins, apolipoproteins, and low-density lipoprotein size among diabetics in the Framingham offspring study. Metabolism 1996;45: 1267-1272.

133. Pyorala K, Pedersen TR, Kjekshus J, et al: Cholesterol lowering with simvastatin improves prognosis of diabetic patients with coronary heart disease. Diabetes Care 1997;20:614-620.

134. MRC/BHF Heart Protection Study of cholesterol-lowering with simvastatin in 5963 people with diabetes: A randomised placebo-controlled trial. Lancet 2003;361:2005-2016.

135. Colhoun HM, Betteridge DJ, Durrington PN, et al: Primary prevention of cardiovascular disease with atorvastatin in type 2 diabetes in the Collaborative Atorvastatin Diabetes Study (CARDS): Multicentre randomised placebo-controlled trial. Lancet 2004;364:685-696.

136. Keech A, Simes RJ, Barter P, et al: Effects of long-term fenofibrate therapy on cardiovascular events in 9795 people with type 2 diabetes mellitus (the FIELD study): randomised controlled trial. Lancet 2005;366:1849-1861.

137. Gerstein HC, Mann JF, Yi Q, et al: Albuminuria and risk of cardiovascular events, death, and heart failure in diabetic and nondiabetic individuals. JAMA 2001;286:421-426.

138. Nikolsky E, Mehran R, Turcot D, et al: Impact of chronic kidney disease on prognosis of patients with diabetes mellitus treated with percutaneous coronary intervention. Am J Cardiol 2004;94:300-305.

139. Cooper WA, O'Brien SM, Thourani VH, et al: Impact of renal dysfunction on outcomes of coronary artery bypass surgery: Results from the Society of Thoracic Surgeons National Adult Cardiac Database. Circulation 2006;113:1063-1070.

140. Gaede P, Vedel P, Larsen N, et al: Multifactorial intervention and cardiovascular disease in patients with type 2 diabetes. N Engl J Med 2003;348:383-393.

141. Dormandy JA, Charbonnel B, Eckland DJ, et al: Secondary prevention of macrovascular events in patients with type 2 diabetes in the PROactive Study: A randomised controlled trial. Lancet 2005;366:1279-1289.

142. Gerstein HC, Yusuf S, Bosch J, et al: Efect of rosiglitazone on the frequency of diabetes in patients with impaired glucose tolerance or impaired fasting glucose: A randomised controlled trial. Lancet 2006;368:1096-1115.

3 Functional Testing and Multidetector Computed Tomography

Mario J. Garcia

KEY POINTS

- Functional tests such as stress electrocardiography, stress echocardiography, or stress nuclear perfusion imaging have limited accuracy for the detection of anatomical disease but provide important prognostic information.
- Impaired chronotropic response and heart rate recovery are powerful predictors of outcomes. However, it is unknown whether these variables are modifiable by revascularization.
- A normal exercise echocardiogram or myocardial perfusion imaging result is associated with a low risk for cardiac events. The extent of stress-induced segmental wall motion and perfusion abnormalities helps define incremental levels of risk and which populations of patients will benefit most from revascularization.

- Positron emission tomography (PET) is one of the most sensitive methods for the identification of viable myocardium. The detection of gadolinium-delayed enhancement by cardiac magnetic resonance (CMR) is the most sensitive method for identifying scarred, nonviable myocardium.
- A normal multidetector computed tomography (MDCT) coronary angiogram study virtually excludes the presence of coronary artery disease. However, functional testing should be considered after MDCT studies that show moderate anatomical coronary stenosis, given the relative overestimation of stenosis severity by MDCT.

Patients with known or suspected coronary artery disease (CAD) who are asymptomatic or have stable symptoms are often evaluated noninvasively. Functional tests such as stress electrocardiography, stress echocardiography, or stress nuclear perfusion imaging are intended to detect and quantify the presence of ischemia based on electrical, mechanical, or perfusion abnormalities, indirectly establishing the burden of CAD. Functional test results have limited accuracy for the detection of anatomic disease but have been shown to provide important prognostic information, including the prediction of benefit from revascularization. More recently, multidetector computed tomography (MDCT) has emerged as a tool to evaluate the coronary anatomy noninvasively. This test is promising and has clearly established its ability to exclude the presence of significant coronary atherosclerosis. This chapter reviews the current applications of these and other noninvasive modalities for the evaluation of patients with CAD.

STRESS TESTING

For many years, it has been known that the symptoms of CAD depend on the balance of myocardial oxygen supply and oxygen demand. Most patients with CAD have normal resting blood flow, even in the presence of epicardial coronary artery stenosis. Myocardial perfusion pressure and blood flow are maintained by compensatory dilation of the coronary arterioles. During stress, myocardial oxygen demand increases, but myocardial blood flow cannot increase any further, leading to the development of ischemia. Myocardial ischemia results in progressive metabolic and functional alterations, including reduced relative perfusion, abnormal regional diastolic and systolic myocardial function, and electrical repolarization abnormalities. On these principles, various stress testing modalities attempt to indirectly establish the diagnosis of obstructive CAD by identifying one or several of these sequelae.

Stress may be accomplished by a number of methods, including exercise, pharmacologic maneuvers, and even mental tests. The choice depends on the specific patient. Whenever possible, exercise is the preferred modality, because the information obtained may be more easily related to functional limitations. The choice of electrocardiography (ECG), echocardiography, nuclear perfusion imaging, or magnetic resonance imaging (MRI) also depends on specific circumstances and local expertise. There is no clear superiority of any of these modalities. However, specificity appears to be higher with stress echocardiography and sensitivity higher with nuclear perfusion imaging. Accordingly, many clinicians prefer stress echocardiography for individuals with lower pretest probability of having disease, and nuclear perfusion imaging for those with higher risk. Even though exercise ECG is less costly, this modality is less commonly used than imaging stress modalities because of its lower sensitivity and specificity. In addition, exercise ECG cannot localize the ischemic region, rendering it less useful as a guide for targeting revascularization.

Over the last decade, the prognostic utility of stress testing has been increasingly recognized. Exercise capacity, heart rate (HR) response, and the extent of ST depression, wall motion, and perfusion abnormalities are powerful predictors of outcome. Patients with decreased exercise tolerance and chronotropic incompetence during exercise stress testing have been shown to have increased adverse events, independently of other factors.

Chronotropic incompetence may be a marker of impaired autonomic dysfunction, which has been associated with cardiac events. Chronotropic response may be defined as the proportion of age-predicted maximal HR achieved, or the proportion of HR reserve used. The latter is defined as follows:

Proportion of HR Reserve Used =
    (Peak HR − Resting HR)/(220 − Age − Resting HR)

It is the preferred method, because it has been shown to be largely independent of age, functional capacity, or exercise protocol. Chronotropic incompetence is defined as failure to use at least 80% of the HR reserve. Chronotropic incompetence has been shown to be associated with angiographic severity of CAD and increased mortality.

HR recovery is another index that appears to be related to autonomic tone. Most evidence suggests that a rapid reactivation of vagal tone is the major determinant of HR fall during the first 30 seconds to 1 minute after exercise. Unlike chronotropic incompetence, HR recovery is not significantly affected by the administration of β-blockers. HR recovery is calculated as the difference in HR at peak versus HR at 1 minute after exercise. A value of less than 12 beats/min is considered abnormal. Patients evaluated for suspected or known CAD who have an abnormal HR recovery have a markedly increased mortality rate, independent of other risk factors.[1]

Although both impaired chronotropic response and HR recovery are powerful predictors of outcomes, it is unknown whether these factors are modifiable. Moreover, their association with mortality may be independent of the presence or severity of CAD. Therefore, they may have limited value in guiding diagnostic and therapeutic strategies.

Electrocardiographic Stress Testing

From the beginning, the application of exercise stress testing for the diagnosis of obstructive CAD has been focused on the presence and extent of ST-segment deviations during and immediately after exercise. This is obtained by serial recordings of the 12-lead electrocardiograph (ECG), which is often aided by computer analysis.

Exercise ECG testing has modest diagnostic utility, mostly in patients with an intermediate pretest likelihood for having disease. It is now recognized that the early reported sensitivities of exercise ECG testing were affected by a verification bias. In other words, the performance of coronary angiography was influenced by the results of the exercise test. This verification bias leads to overestimation of sensitivity and underestimation of specificity. Recent data suggest that the true sensitivity of exercise testing is only about 50%. Despite this limitation, exercise ECG testing remains a useful prognostic test. An index derived from the exercise ECG test that incorporates exercise time, magnitude of ST-segment deviation, and angina, also known as the Duke Treadmill Score, has proved to be a powerful prognosticator of events. The Duke Treadmill Score is calculated as follows:

Duke Treadmill Score = Exercise time −
    (5 × Max ST deviation) − (4 × Angina index)

where Max ST deviation is the maximum ST-segment deviation (elevation or depression) noted in any of the 12 ECG leads, compared with baseline. The treadmill angina index is defined as having a value of 0 if no angina occurs, 1 if angina occurs during exercise but is not test-limiting, or 2 if test-limiting angina occurs. Exercise time is based on the Bruce Protocol.

Using the Duke Treadmill Score, patients may be divided into categories of low risk (score greater than or equal to +5), intermediate risk (score less than 5 but greater than or equal to −10), and high risk (score less than −10). In the original study, the 5-year survival rates among patients categorized as having low, intermediate, and high risk were 97%, 91%, and 72%, respectively. Of note, the exercise treadmill score provided prognostic information independent of coronary angiography findings. The ability of the score to predict risk has been validated in many different subpopulations, including women. The annual cardiac death rate has been reported to be very low (0.3% to 1.2% per year) in patients with low-risk scores. Recent studies suggest, however, that exercise

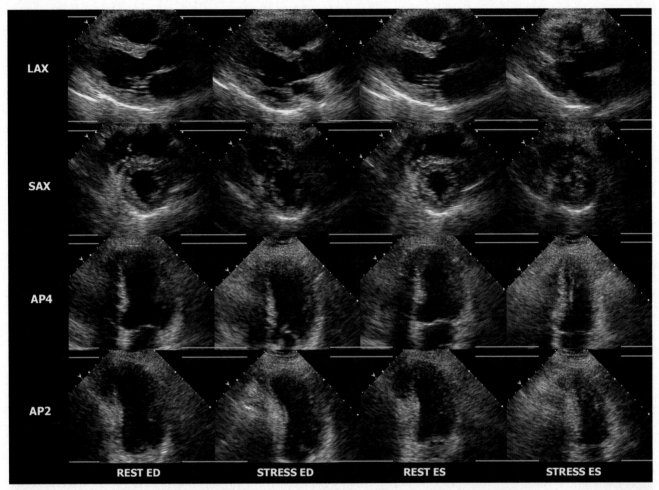

Figure 3-1. Normal stress echocardiographic response. Images obtained at end-diastole (ED) and end-systole (ES) at rest and immediately after exercise stress from the parasternal long axis (LAX), short axis (SAX), and apical four-chamber (AP4) and two-chamber (AP2) windows. Notice the decrease in ES left ventricular cavity size after stress.

capacity is the most important factor in the Duke Treadmill Score.[2]

Stress Echocardiography

Stress echocardiography is based on the identification of regional wall motion abnormalities, which occur as a result of an increase in oxygen demand without a matched increased in oxygen supply in the presence of a coronary stenosis. The test has gained increasing acceptance with the introduction of digital echocardiography, harmonic imaging, and the use of contrast agents, all of which have incrementally contributed to increased image quality, reproducibility, and accuracy. However, the performance and interpretation of stress echocardiography require intensive skills. Therefore, accuracy may vary significantly among echocardiographic laboratories in clinical practice. Recent studies suggest that real-time three-dimensional (3D) echocardiography facilitates faster data acquisition and better image segmentation, and therefore may lead to improved diagnostic accuracy.[3]

Most commonly, regional wall motion is assessed from parasternal long, parasternal short, and apical images, using a 17-segment model of the left ventricle (LV).[4] Each segment is described as normal, hypokinetic, akinetic, or dyskinetic, and the results of the individual segments are averaged to calculate a global wall motion score. Recent studies suggest that new quantitative indices of regional contractility, such as strain imaging, are useful in identifying stress-induced ischemia and/or viable myocardium in dysfunctional segments.[5]

Stress echocardiography is used to establish the diagnosis, determine prognosis, or evaluate the need for revascularization in patients with known or suspected CAD. The test may also be used to evaluate patients with cardiomyopathy or valvular heart disease. The diagnosis of CAD is based on detection of either resting or stress-induced regional wall motion abnormalities (Figs. 3-1 through 3-3). A resting regional wall motion abnormality implies in most cases a prior myocardial infarction. A stress-induced regional wall motion abnormality implies, in most cases, ischemia caused by obstructive CAD.

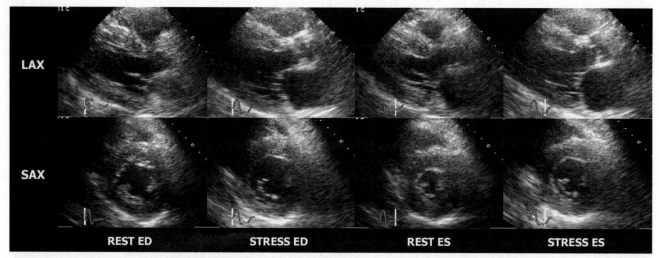

Figure 3-2. Abnormal stress echocardiographic response in a patient with severe multivessel coronary artery disease. Images obtained at end-diastole (ED) and end-systole (ES) at rest and immediately after exercise stress from the parasternal long axis (LAX) and short axis (SAX) windows. Notice the ES dilatation of the left ventricular cavity size.

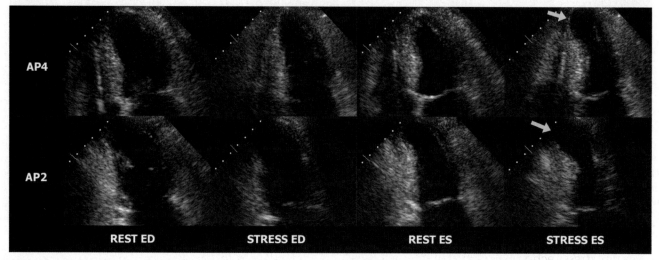

Figure 3-3. Abnormal stress echocardiographic response in a patient with severe stenosis of the middle left anterior descending coronary artery. Images obtained at end-diastole (ED) and end-systole (ES) at rest and immediately after exercise stress from the apical four-chamber (AP4) and two-chamber (AP2) windows. Notice the relative ES dilatation of the left ventricular apical segments *(arrows)*.

Exercise Echocardiography

Exercise stress testing may be performed with treadmill, supine or prone bicycle, or even arm ergometry. Treadmill stress echocardiography is by far the most commonly used modality in the United States. With treadmill exercise, only pre-exercise and post-exercise images are obtained, both with the patient in the supine lateral position. Post-exercise images need to be obtained within 1 minute after termination of exercise. Any delay may result in resolution of regional wall motion abnormalities, reducing the sensitivity of the test for moderate, single-vessel disease. Bicycle ergometry allows the operator to obtain images while the patient is still exercising, so, in theory, it is capable of detecting milder, transient wall motion abnormalities caused by ischemia. Either treadmill or bicycle ergometry allows evaluation of

important functional data such as exercise capacity, blood pressure response, and hemodynamic responses to exercise, including assessment of cardiac output and pulmonary pressures, as well as ECG ST analysis. The final interpretation of the test takes into account all of these variables.

Several studies have reported sensitivities ranging from 71% to 97% and specificities ranging from 64% to more than 90%. The differences in results often relate to the use of different thresholds to define wall motion abnormalities. If hypokinesis or akinesis is defined as a threshold, sensitivity tends to be lower and specificity higher. On the other hand, if tardokinesis (delayed contraction or postsystolic shortening) or lack of hyperkinesis is used as a threshold, sensitivity is higher and specificity tends to be lower. Accuracy parameters also vary according to whether coronary stenosis is defined at a 50% or 70% stenosis

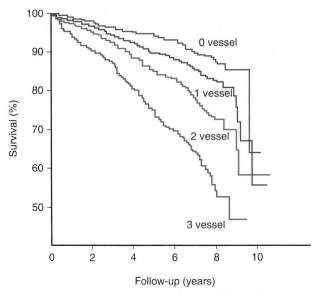

Figure 3-4. Mortality rates of patients according to the total extent of wall motion abnormalities (summed stress score, expressed as vessel territories) at peak stress (N = 5375 patients). (From Marwick TH, Case C, Vasey C, et al: Prediction of mortality by exercise echocardiography: A strategy for combination with the Duke treadmill score. Circulation 2001;29:2566-2571.)

threshold. The sensitivity of exercise echocardiography is lower for the detection of single-vessel disease, particularly that involving the circumflex coronary artery. In patients with multivessel disease, ischemia often is detected only in the territory supplied by the most stenotic vessel, especially if the test is discontinued at submaximal workload.

Resting or exercise-induced wall motion abnormalities may occur in the presence of cardiomyopathy, microvascular disease, severe hypertension (increased afterload), or valvular disease and are often the cause of false-positive interpretations.

Several stress echocardiographic variables have been shown to provide important prognostic value in patients with known or suspected CAD (Fig. 3-4). A low exercise wall motion score index or a fall in exercise ejection fraction is highly predictive of increase risk for adverse cardiac events. This prognostic decision point is similar to that of a radionuclide perfusion defect size of more than 15%. Echocardiographic variables have incremental independent prognostic utility over other variables such as the Duke Treadmill Score.[6] The rate of cardiac events in individuals with a normal exercise echocardiogram has been reported in several studies to be less than 1% per year.

Pharmacologic Stress Echocardiography

The most commonly employed agents for pharmacologic stress echocardiography are dobutamine, dipyridamole, and adenosine. Dobutamine is the most commonly used stressor in the United States. Dobutamine is administered by continuous infusion at incremental rates of 5 to 50 µg/kg/min. It is often complemented with handgrip exercise and/or atro-

pine (0.5 to 2.0 mg) to increase HR. Dobutamine increases myocardial oxygen demand by increasing contractility and HR. The use of adenosine and dipyridamole is more popular in Europe and South America. It is believed that these agents induce ischemia by inducing coronary steal. In order to induce sufficient ischemia to result in regional wall motion abnormalities, the doses are typically higher than those used with pharmacologic myocardial perfusion stress.

Reported sensitivities and specificities of dobutamine echocardiography have been similar to those for exercise echocardiography. The sensitivity is reduced in patients with concentric hypertrophy who experience cavity obliteration early during the test and in those patients who do not reach their target HR.

Echocardiographic variables obtained during pharmacologic stress have also been shown to have significant prognostic value.[7] A normal dobutamine stress echocardiogram is associated to a low cardiac event rate in patients with suspected CAD and in those at clinically determined intermediate or high cardiac risk undergoing noncardiac surgery. The presence of stress-induced regional wall motion abnormalities, particularly when detected at low HRs, is a strong predictor of cardiac events. Dobutamine stress echocardiography allows further risk stratification even in patients receiving perioperative β-blockers with intermediate or high risk.[8]

Dobutamine echocardiography may be performed for risk assessment in patients after myocardial infarction. In this setting, extensive resting regional wall motion abnormalities, stress-induced ischemia, absence of viability, and worsening LV function with stress are associated with increased risk of adverse events. In patients with ischemic heart disease and chronic LV dysfunction, dobutamine echocardiography is useful to identify myocardial viability. Improvement in regional contractility at lower rates of dobutamine (5 to 10 µg/kg/min) in segments that are akinetic or hypokinetic at rest predicts functional recovery after revascularization, particularly if those same segments exhibit reduction in contractility at high dobutamine rates (biphasic response). Patients with ischemic LV dysfunction and viable myocardium who undergo revascularization have better outcomes than those who are not revascularized or those who have no evidence of viability, regardless of revascularization. The sensitivity for prediction of recovery of function with dobutamine echocardiography ranges between 74% and 88%, and the specificity ranges between 73% and 87%. Compared with radionuclide perfusion techniques, dobutamine stress echocardiography has higher specificity, lower sensitivity, but overall similar accuracy for predicting functional recovery (Fig. 3-5).[9]

Contrast Perfusion Imaging

The new echocardiographic contrast agents consist of inert perfluorocarbon gases encapsulated in a biodegradable shell. Contrast microbubbles have a small diameter (<10 μm) that allows them to cross the pulmonary capillary bed. These agents are commercially available and are approved for endocardial border definition in patients with suboptimal echocardiographic images. When exposed to ultrasound,

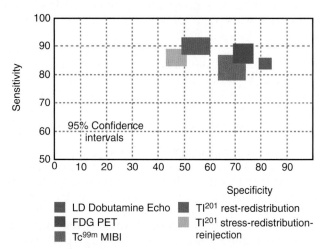

Figure 3-5. Receiver operating characteristic display, indicating 95% confidence intervals for various imaging techniques used for the evaluation of myocardial viability. The most effective modalities are located closer to the upper right corner of the graph. In this display, a smaller square reflects narrower confidence intervals. FDG PET, ^{18}F-fluorodeoxyglucose positron emission tomography; LD, low dose; Tc^{99m} MIBI, technitium-99m sestamibi; Tl^{201}, thallium 201. (From Bax JJ, Wijns W, Cornel JH, et al: Accuracy of currently available techniques for prediction of functional recovery after revascularization in patients with left ventricular dysfunction due to chronic coronary artery disease: Comparison of pooled data. J Am Coll Cardiol 1997;30:1451-1460.)

these microbubbles act as strong reflectors because of their liquid-gas interface. Over the last decade, there has been growing interest in the application of contrast microbubbles for the assessment of myocardial perfusion. Because the LV myocardium has a dense capillary bed, the injection of contrast microbubbles results in myocardial enhancement that is proportional to the myocardial blood volume. During vasodilator stress, in the presence of a flow-limiting stenosis, there is a reduction in capillary blood flow and myocardial blood volume in the segments supplied by the stenotic vessel. This may be detected as either a delay in myocardial enhancement after contrast injection or a relative reduction in enhancement in ischemic compared with normal segments (Figs. 3-6 and 3-7).

Studies have shown relatively good agreement between myocardial contrast echocardiography and single-photon emission computed tomography (SPECT) for the detection of ischemia.[10,11] A study performed in a group of patients determined to be at high risk but without resting wall motion abnormalities reported a sensitivity of 85% by myocardial contrast echocardiography versus 74% by SPECT for the detection of obstructive CAD.[12] The high spatial and temporal resolution of myocardial contrast echocardiography makes it suitable for the detection of nontransmural ischemia and milder ischemia, in which blood flow may be reduced but blood volume is preserved (late enhancement). However, data have been limited to few reports, and, in some studies where the sensitivity has been reported to be high, the specificity has been low. A recently published multicenter trial performed in 123 patients reported a sensitivity of 84% but a specificity of 56%.[13] Moreover, current protocols for image acquisition and interpre-

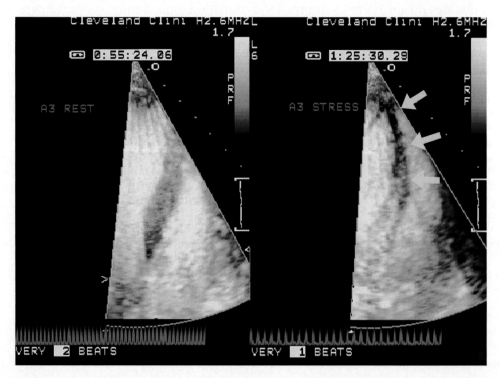

Figure 3-6. Myocardial contrast perfusion study showing a stress-induced (adenosine) perfusion defect not present at rest in the middle and apical anteroseptal region *(arrows)* in a patient with severe stenosis of the middle left anterior descending coronary artery.

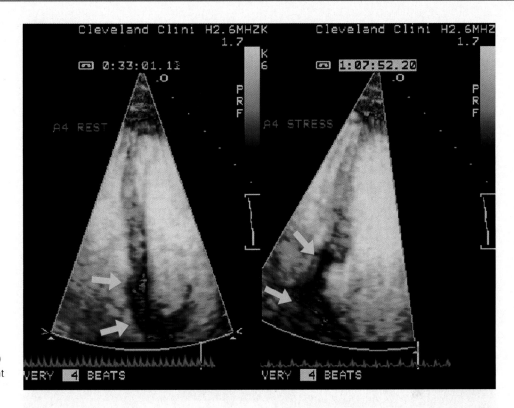

Figure 3-7. Myocardial contrast perfusion study showing a perfusion defect present both at rest and during stress (adenosine) in the basal septal region *(arrows)* in a patient with an occluded right coronary artery.

tation are considerably more technically demanding than those required for SPECT imaging. Therefore, at the present time, the clinical use of myocardial contrast echocardiography for perfusion assessment is limited to a few centers.

Stress Nuclear Perfusion Imaging

The assessment of myocardial perfusion by nuclear scintigraphic methods relies on the administration of a radionuclide isotope that is accumulated by the myocardium in proportion to blood flow. Nuclear perfusion imaging is performed with either single photon–emitting or dual photon–emitting isotopes using SPECT or positron emission tomography (PET) systems.

SPECT is the most common system used for myocardial perfusion imaging. Most SPECT studies are done with thallium 201, technetium-99m sestamibi, and technetium-99m tetrofosmin. Currently, the technetium 99m–labeled tracers are preferred for their higher photon energy, which results in less attenuation artefact. These isotopes emit single photons that travel through tissues and need to be detected on a position-sensitive detector. The direction of the traveling photon is determined by adding a lead collimator that acts as an X-ray filter between the source and the detector. This collimator rejects most of the photons not traveling along certain directions; as a result, only a percentage of the emitted photons are used for imaging. Spatial resolution is given by the space between the bars in the collimator. Increasing spatial resolution requires higher rejection of photons, reducing efficiency and increasing radiation exposure to the patient.

Most dual photon–emitting isotopes are cyclotron produced. These isotopes decay with the emission of a positron, which, after a series of collisions with atomic electrons from the tissues, is annihilated with a nearby electron and produces two high-energy photons emitted in opposite directions. A PET system relies on the simultaneous detection of these photons. These photons travel toward detectors positioned around the subject, where they interact, are absorbed, and produce an electrical signal. The detector signals are processed by specialized coincidence circuitry, and, if the difference in the time of arrival of these photons is smaller than a predetermined value (typically 10 ns), then a signal is recorded. Unlike SPECT imaging, PET does not require collimation, because the position of the emitting target is determined by the simultaneous registration of the two photons at 180 degrees apart. Therefore, the efficiency of PET is several magnitudes greater, providing higher resolution, lower noise, and lower radiation exposure. The signals recorded are used to reconstruct a 3D image. The spatial resolution of PET images is closely related to the physical size of the detector elements.

With either SPECT or PET cardiac perfusion studies, images are obtained after stress and at rest. For segmentation of the LV, a 17-segment model is applied. Images are interpreted visually or with the use of automated quantification based on normalized data. Myocardial scar is determined by the presence of a relative perfusion defect (compared to the segment with highest counts) that persists on both stress and resting images. Ischemia is determined by the presence of a perfusion defect on stress images that improves or resolves on the resting images (Figs. 3-8 through 3-11).

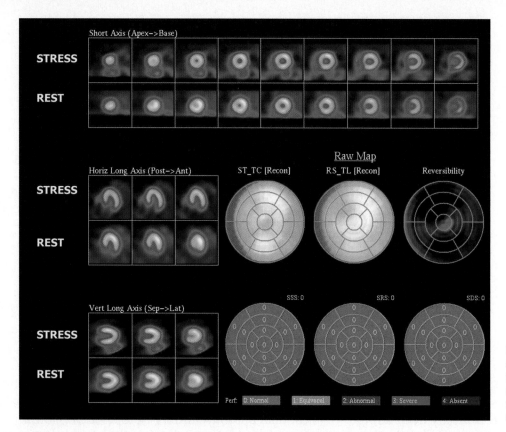

Figure 3-8. Single-photon emission computed tomography (SPECT) technetium-99m sestamibi exercise stress study showing normal myocardial perfusion during stress and at rest.

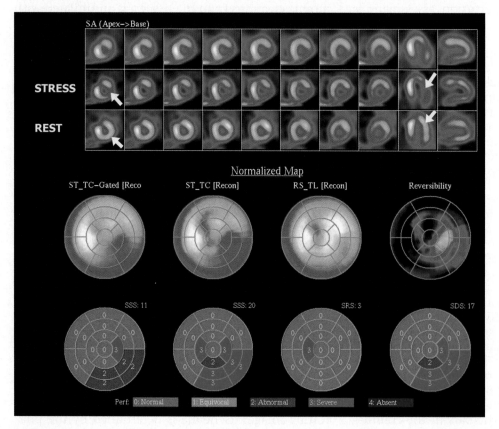

Figure 3-9. Single-photon emission computed tomography (SPECT) technetium-99m sestamibi exercise stress study showing a large myocardial perfusion defect in the posterolateral walls during stress *(white arrows)* with complete reversibility on the resting study, indicating ischemia.

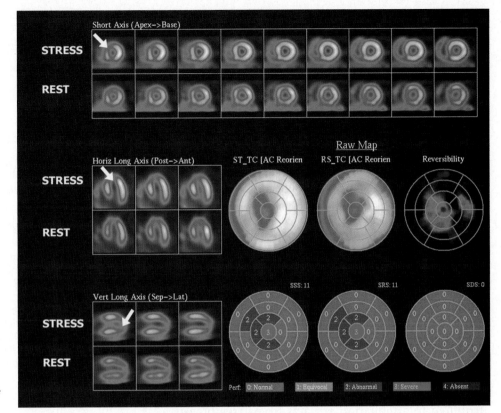

Figure 3-10. Single-photon emission computed tomography (SPECT) technetium-99m sestamibi exercise stress study showing a mid-size myocardial perfusion defect in the anteroseptal and apical walls during stress *(white arrows)* without reversibility on the resting study, indicating scar.

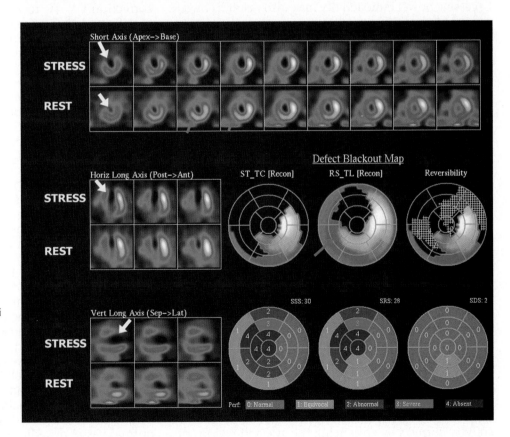

Figure 3-11. Single-photon emission computed tomography (SPECT) technetium-99m sestamibi exercise stress study showing a large myocardial perfusion defect in the anteroseptal, anterior, and inferior walls during stress *(white arrows)* with partial reversibility (inferior and septal walls, *green arrow*) on the resting study, indicating both scar and ischemia.

Exercise Nuclear Perfusion Imaging

Exercise stress is well suited for SPECT imaging. At peak exercise, either on a treadmill or on a bicycle ergometer, patients are injected with the radioisotope. Acquisition of the stress images is performed from a few minutes to 1 hour after exercise, depending on the radioisotope used. Resting images are obtained before or after the exercise images, after the administration of a separate dose of the isotope. Different isotopes may be used for resting and for stress imaging, such as thallium 201 injected at rest and technetium-99m sestamibi injected at peak stress.

The mean reported sensitivity and specificity for exercise SPECT are 86% and 74%, respectively.[14] However, most of the studies reported are potentially subject to verification bias, which means that the sensitivity may be overestimated and the specificity underestimated. To estimate the true specificity of the test, the normalcy rate has been studied in populations at low risk of having CAD, and the mean normalcy rate in these populations was reported to be 89%. Sensitivity and specificity were higher for the detection of multivessel disease, followed by single-vessel disease in the left anterior descending artery distribution, in the right coronary artery, and in the circumflex artery. False-positive results are often attributed to attenuation artifacts from large breasts in women, or to the diaphragm in obese individuals. Excessive bowel radioactivity may also result in negative or false-positive results.

More recently, the introduction of ECG-gated SPECT imaging has allowed assessment of LV function in addition to perfusion. Studies have shown a good correlation for assessment of LV ejection fraction between SPECT and other tomographic modalities.[15] However, LV volumes may be underestimated and ejection fraction overestimated in ventricles with a small LV cavity and hypertrophy of the walls, because of partial volume effects. The accuracy of SPECT determination of LV volumes and ejection fraction is also limited in patients with extensive perfusion defects and LV aneurysm, because the entire geometry of the LV cavity cannot be defined. However, the additional information derived from regional systolic function in gated studies has improved the diagnostic accuracy of the test. Frequently, artefacts caused by soft tissue attenuation may be discriminated from true ischemia or scar by the demonstration of normal regional wall motion.

Another recent advancement in SPECT imaging has been the introduction of attenuation correction. Commercially available SPECT attenuation correction systems measure the nonhomogeneous attenuation distribution, using external collimated radionuclide sources or X-ray computed tomography (hybrid systems). Application of attenuation correction in patients with excessive subdiaphragmatic activity corrects by enhancing the affected regions of the myocardium, such as the inferior and posterior LV walls. Several studies have shown significant improvement in specificity and modest improvements in sensitivity with the use of attenuation

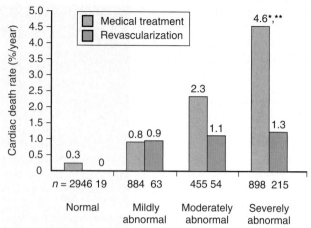

Figure 3-12. Rates of cardiac death per year as a function of scan result and type of treatment. Purple bars represent patients undergoing medical treatment after single-photon emission computed tomography (SPECT); teal bars represent patients undergoing revascularization after SPECT. *$P < .01$ versus patients undergoing revascularization early after SPECT; **$P < .001$ within patients undergoing revascularization early after SPECT. (From Hachamovitch R, Berman DS, Shaw LJ, et al: Incremental prognostic value of myocardial perfusion single photon emission computed tomography for the prediction of cardiac death: Differential stratification for risk of cardiac death and myocardial infarction. Circulation 1998;97:535-543.)

correction.[16,17] A recent study demonstrated that specificity decreases dramatically in obese patients as indexed body mass increases without attenuation correction, but it remains high in all groups with attenuation correction.[18]

Several studies have shown that a normal exercise stress SPECT study predicts a very low likelihood (<1%) of adverse events such as cardiac death or myocardial infarction for at least 12 months, and that this level of risk is independent of gender, age, symptom status, and even presence of anatomic CAD. In those patients with abnormal scans, baseline clinical characteristics such as diabetes, as well as the extent and severity of SPECT perfusion abnormalities, permit definition of incremental levels of risk and which populations of patients will benefit most from revascularization (Fig. 3-12).[19]

Pharmacologic Nuclear Perfusion Imaging

In the United States, many patients who are referred for evaluation of suspected or known CAD are unable to exercise. Both adenosine and dipyridamole are vasodilator agents that, in the absence of epicardial artery stenosis, increase myocardial blood flow three to five times over baseline. In the presence of a stenosis, a relative perfusion defect may be seen; it indicates either failure to increase regional blood flow compared to myocardial segments supplied by a normal vessel or reduced myocardial blood flow due to coronary steal. For this reason, in some patients with multivessel disease and balanced ischemia, the pharmacologic stress SPECT study may appear as normal. The mean reported sensitivity and specificity of adenosine SPECT for the detection of CAD are similar to those of exercise SPECT studies—90% and 75%, respectively. With dipyridamole SPECT, sensitivity is similar (89%), but the specificity is lower (65%). As previously discussed, verification bias may exaggerate true sensitivity and underestimate specificity. The sensitivities and specificities are also higher for multivessel than for single-vessel disease.

Pharmacologic stress SPECT studies may be performed also with dobutamine. The mean reported sensitivity and specificity for this test are 82% and 75%, respectively. In contrast to dobutamine echocardiography, monitoring of ischemia-induced functional abnormalities is difficult with SPECT. For this reason, dobutamine is not a preferred stressor in most clinical instances.

Pharmacologic SPECT is a powerful prognosticator in populations of patients with suspected CAD and in those who at risk and are being evaluated before noncardiac surgery. The risk of death in patients with normal scans has been reported to be low but higher than in patients with negative exercise SPECT (1% to 3% per year). This probably reflects higher comorbidities in selected populations of patients who cannot exercise. In patients undergoing noncardiac surgery, a pharmacologic stress test has a significant negative predictive value but a low positive predictive value.[19a,19b] For that reason, it has been recommended that this test be applied only to populations of patients with moderate clinical risk, such as those with anginal symptoms, prior infarction, and/or diabetes.

Pharmacologic stress imaging may be performed with PET. The higher spatial resolution, higher efficiency, and lower attenuation make PET a superior method in certain patient groups, such as obese patients. Cardiac PET has also been validated for the quantitative assessment of regional myocardial perfusion, LV function, and viability. Current PET stress myocardial perfusion protocols require pharmacologic stress because of the short half-life of rubidium-82. This is the preferred radioisotope for assessment of perfusion in clinical practice, given that it can be produced on site without a cyclotron from a column generator. Two other radioisotopes approved for cardiac PET use in the United States are nitrogen-13 ammonia (perfusion) and ^{18}F-FDG (metabolism-viability). In patients with suboptimal-quality SPECT results, follow-up cardiac PET has demonstrated superior accuracy. A majority of the PET studies obtained in patients with equivocal SPECT results are unequivocally normal or low risk.[20]

PET is one of the most sensitive methods for identifying myocardial viability in patients with ischemic LV dysfunction. PET defines viable myocardium as the presence of a perfusion-metabolism mismatch. Images are obtained with a perfusion isotope such as rubidium-82 and a metabolic agent such as ^{18}F-FDG. Scar myocardium exhibits reduced uptake of both tracers, whereas ischemic viable myocardium shows preserved metabolic activity (Fig. 3-13). The extent of viability by PET has been shown in numerous studies to predict functional myocardial recovery after revascularization. Patients with viable myocardium by PET who undergo revascularization have improved survival compared to those with viable myocardium who receive medical therapy or those without viability regardless of treatment.

Magnetic Resonance Imaging

MRI is an excellent method for the assessment of global and regional systolic LV function. The most widely used steady-state free precession technique (SSFP) allows clear identification of endocardial borders caused by a high blood pool signal. In addition, the tomographic approach allows measurement of volumes without geometric assumptions, resulting in accurate measurements even in those patients with previous myocardial infarction and distorted LV geometry. Image quality is preserved even in obese patients, making it ideal for those patients with technically difficult echocardiographic images. In addition, with the use of intravenous paramagnetic contrast agents, MRI may provide an accurate assessment of myocardial perfusion.

Dobutamine MRI

MRI may be used to obtain global and regional LV function at rest and during bicycle or pharmacologic stress. Dobutamine is the most commonly used stressor for the evaluation of ischemia-induced regional wall motion abnormalities. The mean reported sensitivity and specificity for the detection of obstructive CAD are 89% and 84%, respectively. The protocols used are similar to those used in echocardiography for the evaluation of both ischemia and viability. One of the limitations of dobutamine MRI is the inability to obtain accurate ECG monitoring of ST-segment deviation during the test. For this reason, many centers have favored the use of vasodilator stress and MRI perfusion imaging.

MRI Perfusion Imaging

The intravenous injection of a paramagnetic agent such as gadolinium diethylenetriaminepentaacetic acid (DTPA) may be used to evaluate myocardial perfusion. Gadolinium DTPA is an extracellular agent that, during its first pass, enhances the intravascular compartment. This is followed by extracellular deposition. Areas of fibrosis and scarring in the LV accumulate gadolinium over time, exhibiting "delayed enhancement." With the use of a fast imaging protocol with steady-state precession (FISP)-based sequence, the first-pass enhancement of the myocardium may be imaged by MRI almost in real time. MRI allows identification of areas of myocardial hypoenhancement at rest in the presence of severely reduced myocardial blood flow (Fig. 3-14). In most circumstances, however, resting blood flow is normal in segments supplied by stenotic vessels because of compensatory arteriolar vasodilation. However, adenosine or dipyridamole may induce ischemia in these cases by reducing myocardial perfusion pressure.

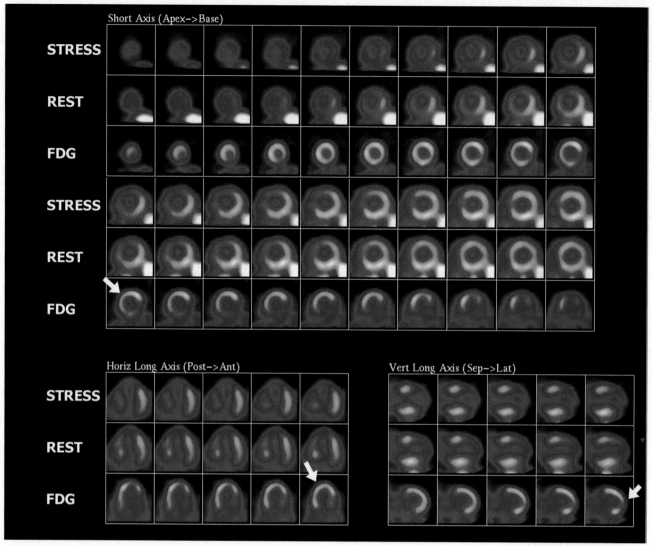

Figure 3-13. Positron emission tomography (PET) myocardial viability study obtained in a patient with ischemic left ventricular dysfunction. Both resting and stress rubidium-82 images show an extensive anteroapical perfusion defect *(arrow)*. The fluorine-18 fluorodeoxyglucose (FDG) images show matched preserved metabolic activity, indicating hypoperfused but viable myocardium *(arrows)*.

The high spatial resolution of cardiac MRI permits visualization of nontransmural ischemia or infarction. A study comparing cardiac MRI and SPECT for the detection of CAD demonstrated similar sensitivities for both techniques for the detection of transmural ischemia or infarction.[21] However, SPECT identified only 28% of subendocardial infarcts, whereas MRI identified 92%. MRI studies have shown abnormal myocardial perfusion also in patients with syndrome X[22] and in others with microvascular disease.

Quantitative analysis of the MRI perfusion images can be performed to determine the ratio of stress to resting blood flow, known as the myocardial perfusion reserve (MPR). Studies have shown that, in patients with obstructive coronary disease, MPR increases after percutaneous intervention.[23]

Delayed gadolinium-enhanced MRI is a powerful technique to evaluate the presence of scar in patients with ischemic LV dysfunction. The extent of infarct transmurality, as determined by MRI, predicts functional recovery in patients referred for revascularization (Figs. 3-15 and 3-16).[24]

COMPUTED TOMOGRAPHY

Computed tomography is rapidly emerging as a non-invasive method to evaluate the coronary anatomy. Technical advances available in modern scanners now permit adequate image quality in most patients. Image acquisition and interpretation can be performed very rapidly, making this technology suitable for the evaluation of ambulatory patients.

MDCT technology has recently overcome many of its previous limitations and now can provide ECG-gated acquisition with short acquisition time, sub-millimeter spatial resolution, and adequate temporal resolution (100 to 220 msec), thus allowing excellent

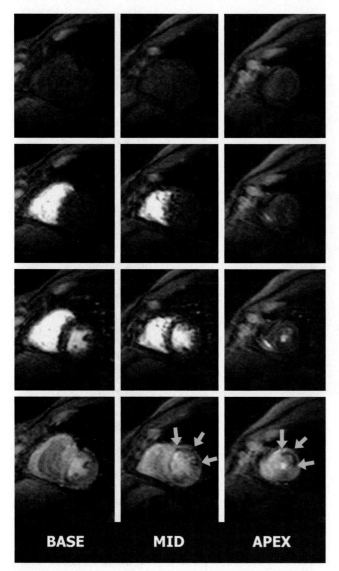

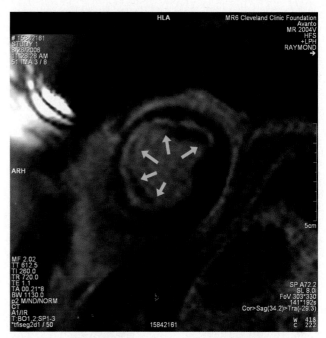

Figure 3-15. Cross-sectional image at the middle of the left ventricle obtained 20 minutes after injection of gadolinium DTPA demonstrates a large area of subendocardial fibrosis (white rim indicated by *arrows*) involving 50% of transmural thickness in the septum and anterior walls.

Figure 3-14. First-pass gadolinium DTPA myocardial perfusion study. From top to bottom, sequential cross-sectional images obtained at the base (*left*), midlevel (*middle*), and apex (*right*) of the heart. The first row of images is acquired before arrival of the contrast agent. The second row demonstrates arrival to the right ventricle. The third row shows arrival to the left ventricular cavity, and the fourth row shows enhancement of the myocardium. The arrows demonstrate an area of subendocardial hypoenhancement in a patient with severe stenosis of a large marginal branch.

Calcium Scoring

With EBCT scanners, the most widely used measure of calcium burden has been the calcium score, based on a radiographic density-weighted volume of plaques with pixel numbers of a least 130 Hounsfield units (HU). More recently, MDCT has been shown to provide comparable and reproducible results. The prognostic value of coronary calcification has been clearly established. Keelan and colleagues[25] demonstrated that a coronary calcium Agatston score greater than 100 was an independent predictor (odds ratio [OR] = 1.88) of cardiovascular outcomes (death and nonfatal myocardial infarction) at 7 years' follow-up. Although very high calcium scores impart an approximate 10-fold increased risk, they do not always imply a tight coronary stenosis. The role of EBCT screening of asymptomatic individuals is controversial, and the incorporation of this type of investigation into a comprehensive risk screening with CRP and cholesterol measurements is ongoing. There is some evidence to support the incorporation of calcium scores into an overall risk stratification of older individuals using clinical algorithms such as the Framingham Risk Score. In the South Bay Heart Watch study,[26] a calcium score of more than 300 was associated with a significant increase in coronary heart disease event risk compared with that determined by clinical score alone. These data support the hypothesis that high coronary calcium scores can modify predicted risk, especially among patients in the intermediate-risk category, for whom clinical

visualization of the coronary arteries. Moreover, the rate of technologic advancement leading to improved coronary angiography with MDCT has rapidly exceeded that of electron-beam computed tomography (EBCT) or MRI. Image quality is undergoing constant refinement, and the number of uninterpretable coronary studies has gradually decreased, from 20% to 40% with the 4-detector system, to 15% to 25% with 16 detectors, and now as low as 3% to 10% with 64-detector systems.

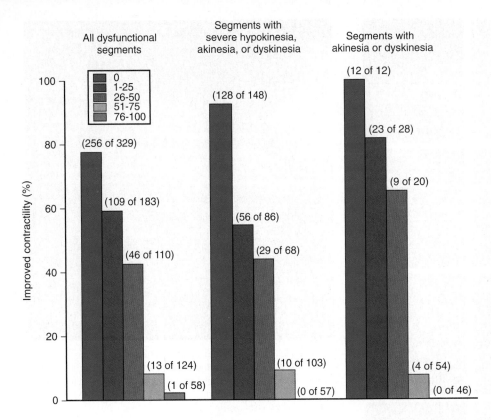

Figure 3-16. Relation between the transmural extent (percentage) of hyperenhancement before revascularization and the likelihood of functional recovery (*N* = 804 dysfunctional segments in 50 patients). (From Kim RJ, Wu E, Rafael A, et al: The use of contrast-enhanced magnetic resonance imaging to identify reversible myocardial dysfunction. N Engl J Med 2000;343:1445-1453.)

decision making is the most difficult. Those at low risk by clinical score derived no additional benefit from calcium scoring. The use of the calcium score scanning to improve cardiovascular risk prediction in people with no cardiac symptoms who are at low absolute risk is very expensive. Some even suggest that its wide clinical implementation can in aggregate have a detrimental effect on the quality of life of screened populations.[27]

Computed Tomographic Coronary Angiography

Although the actual acquisition of MDCT studies takes less than 15 seconds, patient preparation and data interpretation require extensive training and extreme attention to detail. Even in expert hands, the average time required for interpretation exceeds by far the time required for interpretation of nuclear perfusion or echocardiographic studies.

Patient selection is critical when performing MDCT coronary angiography. A stable, low HR is required at the time of the procedure, because motion artifacts can occur, given current limitations in temporal resolution of existing scanners. Oral and/or intravenous β-blockers are administered before the study to obtain, ideally, a resting HR lower than 60 beats/min. β-Blockers reduce HR variability during the scan, and for that reason we recommend their administration almost routinely, unless contraindicated.

MDCT provides complex and detailed 3D data sets, which are reconstructed from the raw data file,

according to specific phases of the cardiac cycles. In most patients with a heart rate lower than 70 beats/min, the best phase free of motion is centered on 75% of the R-R interval, corresponding to the diastasis phase of diastole. At higher rates, diastasis disappears, so image reconstruction at about 50% of the cardiac cycle is preferred. Nevertheless, there is significant patient-to-patient variability, and often several phases reconstructed at 5% to 10% intervals need to be examined.

Once the best phase for analysis is determined, examination of each vessel is performed from 3D multiplanar reconstructed images. Careful adjustment of image windowing parameters is done to differentiate the iodine-enhanced lumen from calcified and noncalcified plaques. This procedure is repeated for each vessel segment and its branches.

Both EBCT and MDCT are very useful in assessing the origin and course of congenitally anomalous coronary arteries and the 3D relationship of such arteries with the aorta and the pulmonary arterial trunk.[28-30] Myocardial bridges and coronary arterial-venous fistulas can also be well visualized by EBCT and MDCT.

Evaluation of Coronary Artery Stenosis by MDCT

Figures 3-17 and 3-18 are MDCT coronary angiograms obtained, respectively, from a patient with normal coronaries and a patient with severe multivessel disease. The corresponding invasive angiogram

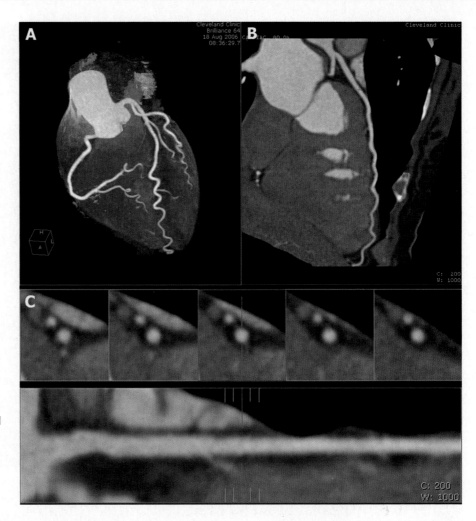

Figure 3-17. Multidetector computed tomographic (MDCT) coronary angiography showing normal coronary arteries. **A,** Volume-rendered maximum-intensity projection of the aortic root and coronary arteries. **B,** Curved multiplanar reconstruction of the left anterior descending coronary artery (LAD). **C,** Series of cross-sectional images obtained from the mid-LAD at 1-mm intervals.

from the latter individual is shown in Figure 3-19. Several single-center studies have investigated the accuracy of MDCT coronary angiography for the detection of coronary artery stenosis in patients with known or suspected CAD referred for invasive coronary angiography.[31-41] In all of these studies, analysis of the MDCT data was performed by investigators blinded to the results of invasive angiography, and in many, it was limited to coronary segments of more than 1.5 or 2 mm in diameter. In most cases, significant coronary artery stenosis was defined as a reduction in diameter of more than 50%, in order to define sensitivity, specificity and positive and negative predictive values. The prevalence of significant CAD in patients enrolled in these studies was 53% to 83%. A few studies have also reported the performance characteristics of MDCT, using each patient as the unit of analysis. Based on these single studies, the sensitivity of MDCT coronary angiography ranged between 72% and 95% per coronary segment, and between 85% and 100% when using each patient as the denominator unit. The specificity per segment has been reported to be between 86% and 98%, and between 78% and 86% per patient. Positive predictive values have ranged from 72% to 90% per segment and from 81% to 97% per patient; negative predictive values were between 97% and 99% per segment and 82% and 100% per patient. As expected, sensitivity was higher in those studies that excluded segments with a diameter smaller than 1.5 mm. Most experts agree that the ability to detect obstructive coronary disease in smaller-caliber vessels is less important, because myocardial revascularization is often not required or cannot be performed.

We recently completed a multicenter trial that studied the accuracy of MDCT coronary angiography performed with 16-slice scanners.[42] We enrolled 238 patients with high or intermediate risk who were clinically referred for diagnostic angiography. Patients first underwent a calcium score scan, followed by MDCT angiography if the Agatston calcium score was less than 600, before invasive angiography. Coronary angiography and MDCT data sets were quantitatively analyzed by blinded independent core laboratories. Among the 187 patients who underwent MDCT, there were 89 segments (5.5%) in 59 patients (32%) with stenosis greater than 50% by conventional angiography. Of 1629 segments larger than 2 mm in diameter, 71% were evaluable on MDCT. All nonevaluable segments were censored "positive," because in clinical practice they would also lead to performance of angiography. Using this

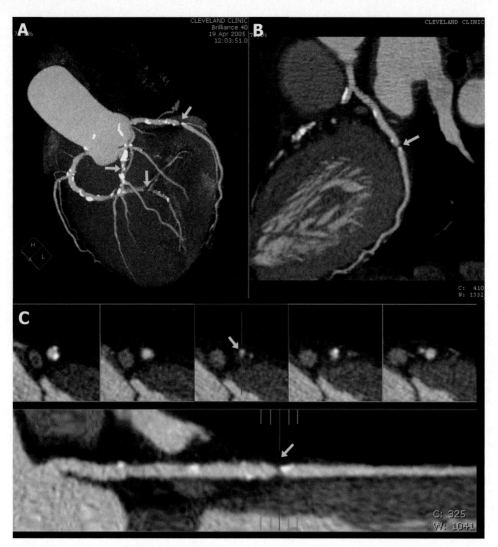

Figure 3-18. Multidetector computed tomographic (MDCT) coronary angiography showing obstructive multivessel disease. **A,** Volume-rendered maximum-intensity projection of the aortic root and coronary arteries. **B,** Curved multiplanar reconstruction of the left circumflex coronary artery (LCX). **C,** Series of cross-sectional images obtained from the mid-LCX at 1-mm intervals. Arrows indicate areas of severe stenosis caused predominantly by noncalcified (dark) atherosclerotic plaques.

approach, the sensitivity, specificity, and positive and negative predictive values for detecting greater than 50% luminal stenoses were 89%, 65%, 13%, and 99%, respectively. In a patient-based analysis, the respective values for detecting subjects with at least one "positive" segment were 98%, 54%, 50%, and 99%. The high number of nonevaluable and false-positive segments in this study indicated that 16-slice MDCT may lead to an excessive number of catheterizations or additional functional testing if applied indiscriminately. Nevertheless, given its high sensitivity and high negative predictive value, 16-slice MDCT may be very useful for excluding coronary disease in selected patients in whom a false-positive or inconclusive stress test result is suspected. It is anticipated that the lower number of nonevaluable segments seen with 64-slice scanners will result in higher specificity and positive predictive values, allowing wider implementation of this test.

It is likely that there always will be a discrepancy between MDCT and invasive coronary angiography for the quantitative assessment of luminal stenosis. Unlike angiography, MDCT highlights both the lumen and the wall vessel plaque. Therefore, MDCT may be more comparable to intravascular ultrasound

(IVUS) than to invasive angiography. In addition, MDCT can provide an infinite number of projections because of its 3D nature. In many cases, a presumed false-positive MDCT finding may actually represent a false-negative coronary angiogram, if adequate projections in the latter test were not obtained (Fig. 3-20).

Accurate assessment of previously stented coronary vessels remains an important limitation to MDCT coronary angiography.[43] A noninvasive, accurate test for in-stent restenosis would be invaluable for patients with postintervention chest pain. This is particularly true because the widespread use of drug-eluting stents reduces the incidence of in-stent restenosis, thereby reducing the yield from repeat invasive coronary angiography. In a study using 16-slice MDCT, only 126 (64%) of 232 stents could be evaluated.[44] Smaller stents, in vessels smaller than 3 mm, were harder to accurately evaluate. Internal luminal diameter is often underestimated. More recently, another study evaluated 13 stented segments using 64-slice MDCT.[39] Two stents with severe stenosis were accurately identified; two other stents with moderate stenosis were called normal by MDCT; and four stents with no angiographic restenosis were thought to be stenotic by MDCT. The ability to evaluate the lumen of stented vessels depends on the type and diameter of the stent. Practical delineation of in-stent stenosis remains difficult in lumens smaller than 3 mm in diameter.

MDCT has been proposed for the evaluation of coronary artery bypass grafts (CABG) (Fig. 3-21). A study using 16-slice MDCT reported successful visualization in all bypass conduits after exclusion of three subjects due to poor overall image quality.[45] The reported sensitivity, specificity, and positive and negative predictive values for detecting total graft occlusion were 96%, 95%, 81%, and 99%, respectively. However, evaluation of the distal anastomosis site was possible only in 75% of the cases. Motion artifacts and interference by surgical clips often limit the assessment of vessel anastomosis. Therefore, determining total vein graft occlusion is straightforward, but quantifying moderate stenoses can be difficult. Analysis of the native vessels is often more difficult in patients with previous CABG, due to poor run-off, more extensive calcification, and smaller lumen size. This can potentially limit the diagnostic utility of MDCT angiography in this setting. MDCT angiography may also help characterize the 3D location of preexisting coronary grafts in relationship to each other and to the chest wall in patients undergoing repeat sternotomy. In patients with previous CABG, MDCT should be considered as complementary to invasive angiography for those in whom direct catheterization carries a risk, such as patients with suspected atheroma or patients in whom a high contrast load should be avoided. MDCT may also be useful in symptomatic patients with recent CABG in whom graft occlusion is suspected.

Evaluation of Atherosclerotic Plaque Morphology by MDCT

Until recently, IVUS was the only diagnostic tool capable of detecting the presence, extent, and composition of atherosclerotic plaques in the coronary

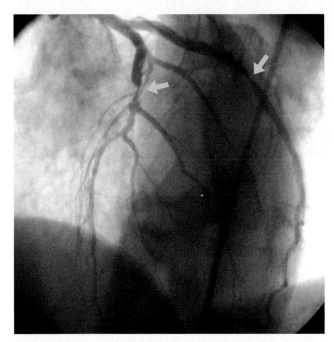

Figure 3-19. Angiographic left anterior projection of the left coronary artery and branches obtained by catheterization in the patient shown in Figure 3-18. Arrows indicate severe stenotic lesions in the left anterior descending coronary artery and the left circumflex coronary artery.

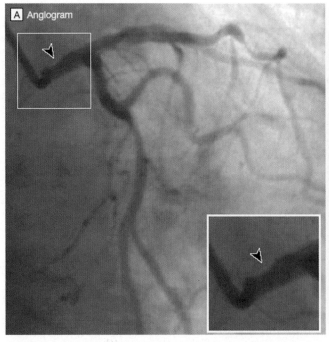

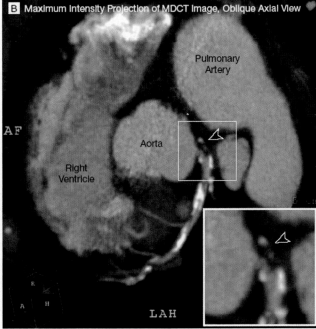

Figure 3-20. A patient with a large mixed atherosclerotic plaque at the left main ostium (*arrowheads*). Quantitative analysis indicated 65% stenosis by multidetector computed tomography (MDCT) coronary angiography (*right*) versus 34% by invasive angiography (*left*), probably owing to difference in angiographic projections. (From Garcia MJ, Lessick J, Hoffmann MHK: Accuracy of 16-row multidetector computed tomography for the assessment of coronary artery stenosis. JAMA 2006;296:403-411.)

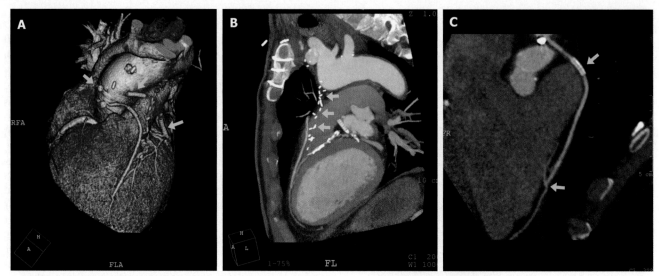

Figure 3-21. Multidetector computed tomographic (MDCT) coronary angiography obtained in a patient with previous coronary artery bypass grafts. **A,** Volume-rendered projection of the heart. Arrows indicate the stump of an occluded bypass to the circumflex and stents previously deployed in this vessel. The graft is not visualized because of the lack of contrast opacification. **B,** Oblique sagittal maximum-intensity projection shows a series of staples, corresponding to an occluded left internal thoracic graft to the left anterior descending coronary artery (LAD). **C,** Curved multiplanar reconstruction of a saphenous vein bypass graft to the LAD. The arrows indicate a stent in the proximal segment and the location of anastomosis to the distal LAD.

arteries in vivo.[46,47] However, the wide application of IVUS as a screening tool for risk assessment is impractical because of the need for and high cost of invasive catheterization. In contrast to invasive coronary angiography, MDCT angiography is also capable of imaging the vessel wall. Recent studies have documented the ability of MDCT to visualize atherosclerotic coronary plaques[48-50] and to differentiate calcified from noncalcified lesions based on Hounsfield unit values.[51] In a series of 22 patients clinically referred for IVUS, MDCT correctly identified the presence of coronary atherosclerotic plaques in 41 of 50 affected segments.[50] Whether MDCT could be used in clinical practice as a screening test remains to be proven, but in selected patients at low-to-intermediate risk, it could potentially help to justify lifelong aggressive preventive intervention. MDCT plaque characterization could also potentially help in devising optimal revascularization strategies.

Cardiac CT, like invasive angiography, involves radiation exposure. The "effective dose," expressed in milli-Sieverts (mSv), depends on multiple factors, including volume of acquisition required, duration of the scan, and radiation energy level used. The volume of acquisition is typically 12 to 16 cm for coronary angiography and 18 to 25 cm for angiography for coronary bypass conduits. The radiation energy level required to obtain adequate image quality also depends on the weight of the patient. Obese individuals require a larger amount of energy owing to scattering and attenuation. Current generation systems with 64 detectors provide a typical dose range in the order of 8 to 14 mSv for MDCT coronary angiography with the use of tube current modulation. This compares to 2 to 6 mSv for invasive angiography, 15 to 25 mSv for nuclear stress myocardial perfusion studies, and 3.6 mSv from yearly background radiation exposure. Therefore, careful analysis of the long-term risk from radiation versus potential benefits derived should be taken into consideration when indicating this study, particularly in younger individuals who are at higher risk.

Guiding Interventions with MDCT

Because of its 3D capabilities, MDCT has a great potential to be used to guide interventions. In electrophysiology, MDCT has already been adopted, because it provides an anatomic roadmap for complex electrophysiologic procedures such as radiofrequency ablation of atrial fibrillation.

Certain properties need to be understood when comparing MDCT and invasive coronary angiography:

1. In MDCT, 3D images of the coronary arteries include atherosclerotic wall plaques. Therefore, in most cases, it is difficult to quantify luminal narrowing from the 3D images. Quantification of luminal stenosis is accomplished by analysis of cross-sectional or curved multiplanar reconstructed images, but these do not provide accurate 3D representation.
2. The contrast agent is not injected as a short bolus; neither is it selectively injected in a coronary vessel. Therefore, one cannot determine the presence of reduced flow or whether opacification of a vessel occurs from anterograde filling or from collaterals. However, this may represent an advantage, such as in visualization of chronic occlusions.
3. The anatomic information obtained in 3D space includes other anatomic structures in the thorax.

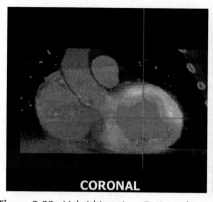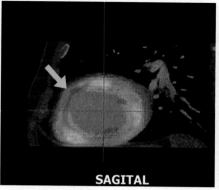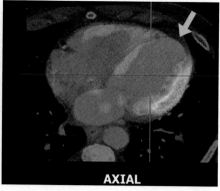

CORONAL SAGITAL AXIAL

Figure 3-22. Hybrid imaging. Fusion of anatomic (multidetector computed tomography) and functional images (rubidium-82 positron emission tomography) in a patient with a large apical myocardial infarction *(arrows)*. Notice the thinning of the myocardium, which matches the lack of perfusion.

Tools exist that allow the display of the coronary images alone, but they often require some user manipulation.

Perhaps one of the most exciting potential applications of MDCT is in the anatomic definition of chronically occluded vessels. MDCT may define patency, anatomic course, caliber of the vessel, length of the stenotic segment, and extent of calcification. In addition, MDCT images may be projected side-by-side with the fluoroscopy images in the catheterization laboratory.

HYBRID IMAGING

Until the advent of coronary CT angiography, non-invasive imaging for the detection of CAD had relied mainly on functional imaging techniques to assess perfusion or wall motion abnormalities as indirect evidence of CAD. Functional imaging proved to be very valuable in determining prognosis and establishing the need for revascularization. However, neither echocardiographic, SPECT, nor MRI stress testing can establish the presence of mild-to-moderate CAD. Moreover, decisions regarding revascularization cannot rely solely on functional imaging without knowledge of the coronary anatomy.

MDCT is now capable of providing detailed information about the coronary anatomy, including luminal stenosis and wall plaque. Because of the latter, it may establish the presence of atherosclerosis even earlier than invasive coronary angiography. However, the technique is limited in spatial and temporal resolution, making difficult the differentiation between moderate and severe luminal stenosis in most cases.

The rationale for the development of PET-CT or SPECT-CT hybrid systems is that, in most symptomatic patients, knowledge of both coronary anatomy and functional data is required. Hybrid systems consist of an MDCT and either a SPECT or a PET camera mounted next to each other, sharing the same patient table. This facilitates the registration of functional and anatomic data in 3D space (Fig. 3-22). In theory, other hybrid combinations, such as PET-

MRI, are also possible. In other medical fields such as oncology, the use of hybrid PET-CT systems has replaced the use of either modality alone. In oncologic applications, the benefit of integrating anatomic and functional data is clear, given the small size and large possible volume of distribution of metastatic tumors. However, in cardiology, the development of the technology has advanced before a clinical need has been clearly established. Several questions need to be answered before the clinical community in cardiology universally adopts hybrid systems: Is the dual information necessary in all patients? Will the cost of implementation be feasible if only a fraction of the patients having studies are using both capabilities? Could both MDCT angiography and nuclear perfusion imaging be performed with limited radiation exposure? Is the information obtained in a hybrid system superior to the information obtained from separate MDCT and PET or SPECT systems reviewed together? We certainly wait for all these questions to be answered. In the meantime, hybrid systems will likely prove to be powerful research tools in basic and clinical studies.

CONCLUSIONS

All noninvasive imaging modalities that were discussed in this chapter are very useful in guiding clinical decisions in the cardiac patient. But in a world with limited resources, one must choose appropriately the test that may be the best to answer a specific clinical dilemma.

Given the recent adoption of MDCT technology, evidence to support improved clinical outcomes or reduced costs is lacking. One must recognize that outcome data will become available over time, with increased clinical utilization. Meanwhile, the high negative predictive value of this test makes it ideal for establishing or excluding CAD in patients with low-to-intermediate risk. When used as a primary test, a normal MDCT study virtually excludes the presence of CAD. MDCT studies that demonstrate the presence of atherosclerotic plaque without significant luminal stenosis may be useful to establish the need for implementing secondary prevention, although outcome data are lacking to support the clinical utility of this strategy. Functional testing should follow MDCT studies that show moderate-to-severe stenosis in most cases, given the high prevalence of false-positive MDCT results. In patients who have nondiagnostic, equivocal, or unexpected functional stress test results, MDCT may also be useful as a confirmatory test, reducing the need for diagnostic coronary angiography. The utility of MDCT is less clear in patients with already established CAD. In them, functional stress testing should be considered as the first choice for evaluation of symptoms.

REFERENCES

1. Cole CR, Blackstone EH, Pashkow FJ, et al: Heart-rate recovery immediately after exercise as a predictor of mortality. N Engl J Med 1999;341:1351-1357.
2. Nishime EO, Cole CR, Blackstone EH, et al: Heart rate recovery and treadmill exercise score as predictors of mortality in patients referred for exercise ECG. JAMA 2000;284:1392-1398.
3. Ahmad M, Xie T, McCulloch M, et al: Real-time three-dimensional dobutamine stress echocardiography in assessment stress echocardiography in assessment of ischemia: Comparison with two-dimensional dobutamine stress echocardiography. J Am Coll Cardiol 2001;37:1303-1309.
4. Quinones MA, Douglas PS, Foster E, et al: ACC/AHA clinical competence statement on echocardiography: A report of the American College of Cardiology/American Heart Association/American College of Physicians/American Society of Internal Medicine Task Force on Clinical Competence. J Am Coll Cardiol 2003;41:687-708.
5. Voigt JU, Exner B, Schmiedehausen K, et al: Strain-rate imaging during dobutamine stress echocardiography provides objective evidence of inducible ischemia. Circulation 2003;107: 2120-2126.
6. Marwick TH, Case C, Vasey C, et al: Prediction of mortality by exercise echocardiography: A strategy for combination with the Duke treadmill score. Circulation 2001;103:2566-2571.
7. Sicari R, Pasanisi E, Venneri L, et al: Stress echo results predict mortality: A large-scale multicenter prospective international study. J Am Coll Cardiol 2003;41:589-595.
8. Boersma E, Poldermans D, Bax JJ, et al: Predictors of cardiac events after major vascular surgery: Role of clinical characteristics, dobutamine echocardiography, and beta-blocker therapy. JAMA 2001;285:1865-1873.
9. Bax JJ, Poldermans D, Elhendy A, et al: Sensitivity, specificity, and predictive accuracies of various noninvasive techniques for detecting hibernating myocardium Curr Probl Cardiol 2001;26:141-186.
10. Heinle SK, Noblin J, Goree-Best P, et al: Assessment of myocardial perfusion by harmonic power Doppler imaging at rest and during adenosine stress: Comparison with (99m)Tc-sestamibi SPECT imaging. Circulation 2000;102:55-60.
11. Wei K., Crouse L, Weiss J, et al: Comparison of usefulness of dipyridamole stress myocardial contrast echocardiography to technetium-99m sestamibi single-photon emission computed tomography for detection of coronary disease (PB127 multicenter phase 2 trial results). Am J Cardiol 2003;91:1293-1298.
12. Peltier M, Vancraeynest D, Pasquet A, et al: Assessment of the physiologic significance of coronary disease with dipyridamole real-time myocardial contrast echocardiography. J Am Coll Cardiol 2004;43:257-264.
13. Jeetley P, Hickman M, Kamp O: Myocardial contrast echocardiography for the detection of coronary artery stenosis: A prospective multicenter study in comparison with single-photon emission computed tomography. J Am Coll Cardiol 2006;47:141-145 (Epub 2005 Dec 15).
14. Underwood SR, Anagnostopoulos C, Cerqueira M, et al: Myocardial perfusion scintigraphy: The evidence. Eur J Nucl Med Mol Imaging 2004;31:261-291.
15. Ioannidis JP, Trikalinos TA, Danias PG: Electrocardiogram-gated single-photon emission computed tomography versus cardiac magnetic resonance imaging for the assessment of left ventricular volumes and ejection fraction: A meta-analysis. J Am Coll Cardiol 2002;39:2059-2068.
16. Hendel RC, Berman DS, Cullom SJ, et al: Multicenter clinical trial to evaluate the efficacy of correction for photon attenuation and scatter in SPECT myocardial perfusion imaging. Circulation 1999; 99:2742-2749.
17. Links JM, Becker LC, Rigo P, et al: Combined corrections for attenuation, depth-dependent blur, and motion in cardiac SPECT: A multicenter trial. J Nucl Cardiol 2000;7:414-425.
18. Bateman TM, Heller GV, Johnson LL, et al: Relative performance of attenuation-corrected and uncorrected ECG-gated SPECT myocardial perfusion imaging in relation to body mass index. Circulation 2003;108:IV-455.
19. Hachamovitch R, Hayes SW, Friedman JD, et al: Identification of a threshold of inducible ischemia associated with a short-term survival benefit with revascularization compared to medical therapy in patients with no prior CAD undergoing stress myocardial perfusion SPECT. Circulation 2003;107: 2899-2906.
19a. Eagle KA, Coley CM, Newell JB, et al: Combining clinical and thallium data optimizes preoperative assessment of cardiac risk before major vascular surgery. Am Intern Med 1989;110:859-866.
19b. Tischler MD, Lee TH, Hirsch AT, et al: Prediction of major cardiac events after peripheral vascular surgery using dipyridamole echocardiography. Am J Cardiol 1991;68:593-597.
20. Bateman TM, McGhie I, O'Keefe JH, et al: High clinical value of follow-up myocardial perfusion PET in patients with a diagnostically indeterminate myocardial perfusion SPECT study. Circulation 2003;108:IV-454.
21. Wagner A, Mahrholdt H, Holly TA, et al: Contrast-enhanced MRI and routine single photon emission computed tomography (SPECT) perfusion imaging for detection of subendocardial myocardial infarcts: An imaging study. Lancet 2003;361: 374-379.
22. Panting JR, Gatehouse PD, Yang GZ, et al: Abnormal subendocardial perfusion in cardiac syndrome X detected by cardiovascular magnetic resonance imaging. N Engl J Med 2002;346: 1948-1953.
23. Al-Saadi N, Nagel E, Gross M, et al: Noninvasive detection of myocardial ischemia from perfusion reserve based on cardiovascular magnetic resonance. Circulation 2000;101:1379-1383.
24. Kim RJ, Wu E, Rafael A, et al: The use of contrast-enhanced magnetic resonance imaging to identify reversible myocardial dysfunction. N Engl J Med 2000;343:1445-1453.
25. Keelan PC, Bielak LF, Ashai K, et al: Long-term prognostic value of coronary calcification detected by electron-beam computed tomography in patients undergoing coronary angiography. Circulation 2001;104:412-417.
26. Greenland P, LaBree L, Azen SP, et al: Coronary artery calcium score combined with Framingham score for risk prediction in asymptomatic individuals. JAMA 2004;291:210-215.
27. O'Malley PG, Greenberg BA, Taylor AJ: Cost-effectiveness of using electron beam computed tomography to identify patients at risk for clinical coronary artery disease. Am Heart J 2004;148:106-113.
28. Taylor AJ, Byers JP, Cheitlin MD, Virmani R: Anomalous right or left coronary artery from the contralateral coronary sinus: "High-risk" abnormalities in the initial coronary artery course and heterogeneous clinical outcomes. Am Heart J 1997;133: 428-435.
29. Shi H, Aschoff AJ, Brambs HJ, et al: Multislice CT imaging of anomalous coronary arteries. Eur Radiol 2004;14:2172-2181.
30. Memisoglu E, Hobikoglu G, Tepe MS, et al: Congenital coronary anomalies in adults: Comparison of anatomic course visualization by catheter angiography and electron beam CT. Catheter Cardiovasc Interv 2005;66:34-42.
31. Nieman K, Cademartiri F, Lemos PA, et al: Reliable noninvasive coronary angiography with fast submillimeter multislice

spiral computed tomography. Circulation 2002;106:2051-2054.

32. Ropers D, Baum U, Pohle K, et al: Detection of coronary artery stenoses with thin-slice multi-detector row spiral computed tomography and multiplanar reconstruction. Circulation 2003;107:664-666.

33. Kuettner A, Beck T, Drosch T, et al: Diagnostic accuracy of noninvasive coronary imaging using 16-detector slice spiral computed tomography with 188 ms temporal resolution. J Am Coll Cardiol 2005;45:123-127.

34. Dewey M, Laule M, Krug L, et al: Multisegment and halfscan reconstruction of 16-slice computed tomography for detection of coronary artery stenoses. Invest Radiol 2004;39:223-229.

35. Kuettner A, Trabold T, Schroeder S, et al: Noninvasive detection of coronary lesions using 16-detector multislice spiral computed tomography technology: Initial clinical results. J Am Coll Cardiol 2004;44:1230-1237.

36. Mollet NR, Cademartiri F, Nieman K, et al: Multislice spiral computed tomography coronary angiography in patients with stable angina pectoris. J Am Coll Cardiol 2004;43:2265-2270.

37. Martuscelli E, Romagnoli A, D'Eliseo A, et al: Accuracy of thin-slice computed tomography in the detection of coronary stenoses. Eur Heart J 2004;25:1043-1048.

38. Raff GL, Gallagher MJ, O'Neill WW, et al:. Diagnostic accuracy of noninvasive coronary angiography using 64-slice spiral computed tomography. J Am Coll Cardiol 2005;46:552-557.

39. Leber AW, Knez A, von Ziegler F, at al: Quantification of obstructive and nonobstructive coronary lesions by 64-slice computed tomography: A comparative study with quantitative coronary angiography and intravascular ultrasound. J Am Coll Cardiol 2005;46:147-154.

40. Mollet NR, Cademartiri F, van Mieghan CA, et al: High-resolution spiral computed tomography coronary angiography in patients referred for diagnostic conventional coronary angiography. Circulation 2005;112:2318-2323.

41. Leschka S, Alkadhi H, Plass A, et al: Accuracy of MSCT coronary angiography with 64-slice technology: First experience. Eur Heart J 2005;26:1482-1487.

42. Garcia MJ, Lessick J, Hoffmann MHK: Accuracy of 16-row multidetector computed tomography for the assessment of coronary artery stenosis. JAMA 2006;296:404-411.

43. Gilard M, Cornily JC, Rioufol G, et al: Noninvasive assessment of left main coronary stent patency with 16-slice computed tomography. Am J Cardiol 2005;95:110-112.

44. Hong C, Chrysant GS, Woodard PK, et al: Coronary artery stent patency assessed with in-stent contrast enhancement measured at multi-detector row CT angiography: Initial experience. Radiology 2004;233:286-291.

45. Schlosser T, Konorza T, Hunold P, et al: Noninvasive visualization of coronary artery bypass grafts using 16-detector row computed tomography. J Am Coll Cardiol 2004;44:1224-1229.

46. Vince D, Dixon K, Cothern R, et al: Comparison of texture analysis methods for the characterization of coronary plaques in intravascular ultrasound images. Comput Med Imag Graph 2000;24:221-229.

47. Kostamaa H, Donoran J, Kasaoka E, et al: Calcified plaque cross-sectional area in human arteries: Correlation between intravascular ultrasound and undercalcified histology. Am Heart J 1999;(3):482-488.

48. Kopp A, Schoroeder S, Baumbach A, et al: Non-invasive characterization of coronary lesion morphology and composition by multislice CT: First results in comparison with intracoronary ultrasound. Eur Radiol 2001;11:1607-1611.

49. Schoenhagen P, Tuzcu EM, Stillman AE, et al: Non-invasive assessment of plaque morphology and remodeling in mildly stenotic coronary segments: Comparison of 16-slice computed tomography and intravascular ultrasound. Coron Artery Dis 2003;14:459-462.

50. Achenbach S, Moselewski F, Ropers D, et al: Detection of calcified and noncalcified coronary atherosclerotic plaque by contrast-enhanced, submillimeter multidetector spiral computed tomography: A segment-based comparison with intravascular ultrasound. Circulation 2004;109:14-17.

51. Carrascosa PM, Capunay CM, Garcia-Merletti P, et al: Characterization of coronary atherosclerotic plaques by multidetector computed tomography. Am J Cardiol 2006;97:598-602.

4 Extent of Atherosclerotic Disease and Left Ventricular Function

Douglass A. Morrison

KEY POINTS

- The relative roles of medical therapy, coronary artery bypass grafting (CABG), and percutaneous coronary intervention (PCI) in the treatment of patients with coronary artery disease (CAD) are evolving.
- Traditionally, CABG has been recommended, largely on anatomic and functional bases, over a broad clinical and/or physiologic spectrum. Anatomic features such as greater than 70% epicardial narrowing of all three major coronary arteries; greater than 50% narrowing of the left main coronary artery; or greater than 70% narrowing of two major coronary arteries, if one of them is the left anterior descending artery, as well as functional criteria such as left ventricular ejection fraction (LVEF) less than .55, have been used to select patients with stable or unstable angina or myocardial infarction (MI) for CABG.
- Although some structural features, such as "diffuse disease" or "small-caliber targets," are used to deny patients CABG on a regular basis, these features are hard to define and therefore have not generally found their way into practice guidelines.
- Reperfusion therapy has revolutionized the care of patient with acute MI; it has spawned several major shifts in the clinical choice between CABG and PCI, all of which are primarily a matter of physiology, not anatomy. Randomized studies of patients with ST-segment elevation myocardial infarction (STEMI), comparing fibrinolytic therapy with emergency PCI, are concordant in showing improved survival, reduced reinfarction, reduced stroke, and reduced late revascularization with PCI. (In part because of the significance of time to complete reperfusion, very few patients in these trials were sent to CABG, regardless of anatomy.) Randomized trials of patients with non-ST-
segment elevation myocardial infarction (NSTEMI), comparing aggressive with conservative treatment, are also concordant in demonstrating advantage to early revascularization. (Again, only a minority of these patients were revascularized by CABG.) Moreover, every CABG registry has demonstrated that operating between day 1 and day 7 after an MI is an extremely high-risk endeavor.
- Almost independent of the extent of anatomic CAD and the resting LVEF, emergent or urgent revascularization in any of the following settings, indicates PCI, rather than CABG, if at all technically achievable:
  - cardiogenic shock,
  - hemodynamic instability,
  - acute pulmonary edema,
  - acute STEMI, and
  - recurrent or refractory NSTEMI.
- Comorbidities, which render CABG high risk for mortality and/or morbidity, can also shift emphasis toward PCI and away from CABG, as in the following examples:
  - chronic obstructive pulmonary disease, which increases the risks of mediastinitis, prolonged mechanical ventilation, and/or atrial fibrillation;
  - ascending aortic disease or carotid vascular disease, either of which increases the risks of postoperative stroke and/or mental impairment; and
  - liver disease, which greatly increases the risk with several anesthetic agents for post-CABG liver failure.
- In the future, the objective, evidence-based choice between CABG and PCI is more a matter of clinical setting and patient physiology than of coronary anatomy and/or resting left ventricular global systolic performance.

The fundamental point of this chapter is to synthesize from four decades of disparate trials and registries a shift in emphasis from anatomic to physiologic thinking about (1) whether to revascularize, (2) how to revascularize, and (3) how to measure success of revascularization.[1,2] An important caveat is that the

physiologic approach emphasizes that the decision whether to revascularize, based on potential clinical benefit, should be answered before trying to answer the question of how to revascularize (i.e., CABG versus PCI).[2] Focusing the decision of whether to revascularize on relief of medically refractory myo-

Table 4-1. Randomized Trials of CABG versus Medical Therapy*

Trial	N	Years	Exclusions	Major Outcome in First Report	Primary Result in First Report
VA Stable Angina	686	1972-1974	Recent MI Heart failure Severe LV dysfunction	Survival at 5 yr	No difference
European Stable Angina	768	1973-1976	LVEF <.50 LMCA disease	Survival at 7 yr	CABG better
CASS Stable Angina	780	1975-1979	LMCA disease	Survival at 5 yr	No difference
NHLBI Unstable Angina	288	1972-1976	LMCA disease	Survival at 30 mo	No difference
VA Unstable Angina	468	1976-1978	LMCA disease	Survival at 5 yr	No difference

*None of these trials enrolled patients with acute MI, hemodynamic instability, severe LV dysfunction, prior CABG, or age >70 years. Medical therapy consisted of antianginals (nitrates, β-blockers, or calcium channel blockers) on an as-needed basis; aspirin was not routine, and statins, ACE inhibitors, and angiotensin receptor blockers were not yet available. The subset of LMCA disease was included only in the first VA study. The world literature of patients with left main stenosis, randomly allocated between the medical therapy of the early 1970s and CABG, consists of 91 U.S. veterans. Percutaneous coronary intervention was not yet available at the time of these studies. Use of the internal mammary artery was not common, and cardioplegia has evolved since these trials.

ACE, angiotensin-converting enzyme; CABG, coronary artery bypass grafting; CASS, Coronary Artery Surgery Study; LMCA, left main coronary artery; LV, left ventricular; LVEF, left ventricular ejection fraction; MI, myocardial infarction; NHLBI, National Heart, Lung and Blood Institute; NIH, National Institutes of Health; PCI, percutaneous coronary intervention; VA, Veterans Administration.

Modified from Morrison DA, Sacks J: Balancing benefit against risk in the choice of therapy for coronary artery disease (CAD): Lessons from prospective, randomized, clinical trials (RCTs) of percutaneous coronary intervention (PCI) and coronary artery bypass graft surgery (CABG). Minerva Cardioangiol 2003;51:585-597, with permission of Minerva Cardioangiologica.

cardial ischemia places optimal medical therapy before any revascularization. It also serves to emphasize the importance of medical management and risk factor modification after revascularization. Focusing on medically refractory ischemia as the primary indication for revascularization also serves to refine the definition of success. A "successful" CABG or PCI would not be a procedure in which the patient only survives and has a patent conduit; rather, it would require relief of the ischemia and/or symptoms for which the patient underwent the procedure in the first place.

THE EVOLUTION OF REVASCULARIZATION FOR THE TREATMENT OF MYOCARDIAL ISCHEMIA AND THE ORIGINS OF THE "ANATOMIC PARADIGM"

The optimal roles of medical therapy and risk factor modification alone, compared with percutaneous coronary intervention (PCI) plus medical therapy, or with coronary artery bypass graft surgery (CABG) plus medical therapy, have not yet been fully defined. With technologic advances and changing operator experience, their relative roles are changing.[1,2]

CABG was introduced in the late 1960s, after the advent of the heart-lung bypass machine made it possible to operate on a still heart. Despite the complexity and significant potential morbidity of the procedure, CABG was shown to be accompanied by relief of acute ischemia and resolution of anginal symptoms in most patients. There was an almost immediate call to develop randomized clinical trials to determine whether the relief of ischemia and symptoms led to even more favorable outcomes, such as prevention of coronary events and improved survival. By the mid-1970s, three trials, of approximately 800 patients each, were completed that compared the medical therapy of that period with CABG (Table 4-1) in relatively low-risk patients with stable

angina. These were the Veterans Affairs (VA) Cooperative Study; the European Cooperative Study; and the National Heart, Lung and Blood Institute (NHLBI) Coronary Artery Surgery Study (CASS).[1-4] They were followed by two trials (VA and NHLBI) of medical therapy versus CABG in patients with unstable angina (myocardial infarction [MI] within 30 days, as defined by the World Health Organization criteria, was one exclusion criteria).

None of these five trials demonstrated any evidence to suggest prevention of subsequent MI by CABG. Four of the five trials failed to demonstrate a survival difference between CABG and medical therapy in their first reports, which included follow-up of from 3 to 5 years.[1-4] Subsequent analyses and reports of longer follow-up demonstrated survival benefits for CABG among selected anatomic subsets: (1) left main coronary artery stenosis greater than 50%; (2) three-vessel stenoses greater than 70% (proximal left anterior descending [LAD], circumflex, and posterior descending, or anterior, lateral, and inferior territories); and (3) two-vessel stenoses greater than 70% (provided that LAD was one of the two), especially if (4) mild to moderately reduced left ventricular function, as measured by the ejection fraction (LVEF) is present. Meta-analysis of long-term results demonstrated an overall survival benefit with initial CABG. It is important to recognize which clinical categories of patients were systematically excluded from these trials, so as to avoid overgeneralizing the results. Another significant limitation of these trials derives from the very limited medical therapy in use at the time they were completed.

Through consecutive versions of the American College of Cardiology/American Heart Association (ACC/AHA) Guidelines for CABG, MI, and angina, the relative role of CABG has continued to be defined primarily in terms of numbers of major epicardial coronary arteries with greater than 50% (left main) or greater than 70% (LAD, circumflex, posterior

Table 4-2. Randomized Clinical Trials of Medical Therapy versus PCI in Patients with Stable Coronary Artery Disease*

Trial	Years	N	Major Outcome	Result	Caveats and Comments
ACME (One-vessel)	1987-1990	212	Exercise tolerance	PCI better	Pre-stent era
ACME (Two-vessel)	1987-1990	101	Exercise tolerance	No difference	Pre-stent era
RITA-2	1992-1996	1018	Death or MI	PCI better	9% with stents
AVERT	1995-1996	341	Any ischemic event	No difference	39% of PCI = stents 25% of PCI = no lipid
ACIP	1991-1993	558	Mortality at 2 yr	No difference	Both CABG or PCI
MASS (LAD)	1994	214	Event-free survival	CABG	Both CABG or PCI
COURAGE†	1999-2004	2287	Death or MI	No difference	PCI with stents

*For the most part, these studies included only low-risk patients and demonstrated relatively little benefit from revascularization. Medical management was not optimal at the time most were conducted. Medical therapy has improved significantly since all of these trials were completed. PCI outcomes have improved since these trials were completed.

†Boden WE, O'Rourke RA, Teo KK, et al; COURAGE Trial Research Group: Optimal medical therapy with or without PCI for stable coronary disease. N Engl J Med 2007;356:1503-1516.

ACIP, Asymptomatic Cardiac Ischemia Pilot Study; ACME, Angioplasty Compared to Medicine; AVERT, Atorvastatin versus Revascularization Treatments; CABG, coronary artery bypass grafting; COURAGE, Clinical Outcomes Utilizing Revascularization and Aggressive Drug Evaluation; LAD, left anterior descending coronary artery; MASS, Medicine, Angioplasty or Surgery Study; MI, myocardial infarction; PCI, percutaneous coronary intervention; RITA-2, Randomized Intervention Treatment of Angina-2.

Modified from Morrison DA, Sacks J: Balancing benefit against risk in the choice of therapy for coronary artery disease (CAD): Lessons from prospective, randomized, clinical trials (RCTs) of percutaneous coronary intervention (PCI) and coronary artery bypass graft surgery (CABG). Minerva Cardioangiol 2003;51:585-597, with permission of Minerva Cardioangiologica. Compare with Table 11 in Smith SC Jr, Feldman TE, Hirshfeld JW Jr, et al: ACC/AHA/SCA&I guideline update for percutaneous coronary intervention: Summary article. Cath Cardiovasc Intervent 2006;67:87-112.

descending) narrowings and LVEF greater than or less than .55—virtually regardless of symptoms, documented ischemia, or medical therapy that the patients are receiving.[3] The trial results and guideline recommendations constitute the core of the "anatomic paradigm" for revascularization decision-making.

PCI, using only a balloon, was introduced in the late 1970s.[1] Because general anesthesia, sternotomy, and heart-lung bypass were not a part of early PCI, the procedure had much less morbidity than CABG but was applied only to stable patients with relatively simple, single-vessel (>70%) disease. An important lesson was that ballooned lesions could suddenly occlude, leading to acute MI and even death. Surgical teams were held on standby so as to emergently perform CABG on patients with acute occlusion from PCI. Only proximal lesions and relatively "simple" lesions could be approached with early wire and balloon technology. The largest part of early PCI courses and textbooks focused on the myriad selection factors, and in those years, most practitioners speculated that PCI would not be applied to more than 5% to 10% of patients with symptomatic coronary artery disease (CAD). Anatomic characteristics of individual lesions (length, diameter of reference or "normal" segment, presence of thrombus, presence of calcification, presence of tortuosities, ostial location, bifurcation, saphenous vein graft lesions) were used to further refine the patient selection process for PCI, in terms of likelihood of success and likelihood of complication.[1,2]

The early randomized comparisons of PCI with medical therapy were even more limited in numbers of patients, categories of patients, and outcomes than the trials of medical therapy versus CABG (Table 4-2).[1,2,5-7] A small VA trial (ACME) and a larger trial from the United Kingdom (RITA-2) documented relief of ischemia and relief of anginal symptoms. A small pilot trial funded by the NHLBI (ACIP) sup-

ported revascularization by either CABG or PCI for patients with documented myocardial ischemia, even in the absence of symptoms. None of these trials, nor any large registry series, supported either prevention of MI or survival benefit with balloon-only PCI. All of these trials were limited to clinically and angiographically "simple" cases.

Despite the lack of evidence supporting a survival benefit, use of PCI grew at an exponential rate during this period, primarily by application to low-risk patients with single-vessel disease, many of whom had neither symptoms nor documented ischemia. There was little emphasis on trying to optimize medical therapy for relief of ischemia or improving outcomes before performing PCI.[1,2,5-7] In essence, PCI staked out a territory that was largely distinct from that of CABG on anatomic grounds; this lent further support to the "anatomic paradigm" of revascularization decision-making.

As technology improved and operator experience widened, PCI was applied to a larger spectrum of the CAD population and began to be considered as an alternative to CABG for patients with single-vessel CAD and for some patients with two-vessel CAD, provided that the anatomic features were favorable. The clinical spectrum approached with PCI remained clinically low risk, and surgical standby remained a routine part of the procedure. Because PCI was being applied to some patients with multivessel disease (mostly two-vessel disease excluding the LAD) who previously had been considered for CABG, there was a call to compare PCI with CABG. Over the 1980s and 1990s, nine trials of balloon-only PCI versus CABG were completed and reported: BARI, EAST, GABI, CABRI, RITA, ERACI I, MASS I, and the studies from Lausanne and Toulouse (Table 4-3).[1-5,8] More than 90% of the screened patients were excluded before enrollment in any of these trials, mostly for clinical or angiographic features that made them unfavorable for balloon-only PCI. As in the previous

Table 4-3. Randomized Trials Comparing Balloon-Only PCI with CABG

Trial	Years	No. Screened	No. Enrolled	Mean Age (Yr)	Mean LVEF	Prior MI (%)	Diabetes (%)	Angina Grade 3/4 (%)	PCI Mortality	CABG Mortality
BARI	1988-1991	12,530	1,829	61	.57	55	25	64	14 at 5 yr	11 at 5 yr
CABRI	1988-1993	23,047	1,054	60	.63	42	12	62	4 at 1 yr	2 at 1 yr
EAST	1987-1990	5,118	392	62	.61	41	23	80	7 at 3 yr	6 at 3 yr
GABI	1986-1991	8,981	359	59	.56	47	13	—	2 at 1 yr	5 at 1 yr
RITA	1989-1991	27,975	1,011	57	—	43	6	59	3 at 2.5 yr	4 at 2.5 yr
ERACI-I	1988-1990	1,409	127	57	.61	50	11	100	5 at 1 yr	5 at 1 yr
MASS	1988-1991		142	56	.75	0	23	—	1 at 3 yr	1 at 3 yr
Lausanne			134	56	—	—	12	78		
Toulouse			152	67	—	38	13	53		

BARI had both the largest enrollment (1829) and the largest proportion of screened patients enrolled (15%). None of these studies had stents, glycoprotein IIb/IIIa inhibitors, or "dual antiplatelet therapy" available. All studies excluded patients with MI within the previous 5 days, those with prior CABG, and those who required emergency revascularization. Some studies excluded patients with total occlusions (GABI), more than two total occlusions (EAST, ERACI-I), or greater than 2-cm length (GABI). Functional exclusions included, in some cases, ">50% of LV potentially involved in the event of abrupt occlusion" (GABI).

BARI, Bypass Angioplasty Revascularization Investigation; CABG, coronary artery bypass grafting; CABRI, Coronary Angioplasty versus Bypass Revascularization Investigation; EAST, Emory Angioplasty versus Surgery; ERACI I, Argentine Randomized Trial of Percutaneous Transluminal Coronary Angioplasty Versus Coronary Artery Bypass Surgery in Multivessel Disease I; GABI, German Angioplasty Bypass Surgery Investigation; LVEF, left ventricular ejection fraction; MASS I, Medicine, Angioplasty or Surgery Study I; MI, myocardial infarction; PCI, percutaneous coronary intervention; RITA, Randomized Intervention Treatment of Angina.

Modified from Morrison DA, Sacks J: Balancing benefit against risk in the choice of therapy for coronary artery disease (CAD): Lessons from prospective, randomized, clinical trials (RCTs) of percutaneous coronary intervention (PCI) and coronary artery bypass graft surgery (CABG). Minerva Cardioangiol 2003;51:585-597, with permission of Minerva Cardioangiologica. Compare with Table 10 in Smith SC Jr, Feldman TE, Hirshfeld JW Jr, et al: ACC/AHA/SCA&I guideline update for percutaneous coronary intervention: Summary article. Cath Cardiovasc Intervent 2006;67:87-112.

trials of medical therapy versus CABG, medical therapy was neither standardized nor mandated.[1,2,8]

None of these trials demonstrated a difference in subsequent MI rate or survival, comparing patients initially treated with PCI versus CABG, on follow-up of 3 to 5 years. Alternatively, even in this low-risk and small subset of CAD patients, relief of angina and need for subsequent revascularization both favored CABG from the beginning. Longer follow-up, meta-analysis of multiple trials, and at least one subset (diabetes) have all allowed for demonstration of a survival advantage with CABG, even among these low-risk patients.[1-4] None of these results challenged the "anatomic paradigm" that CABG is routinely indicated for patients with left main disease and/or three-vessel disease, whereas PCI is indicated for favorable patients with one-vessel disease and patients with two-vessel disease in an area of active conflict between the two revascularization methods.[1,2]

In the ensuing decades, PCI advanced rapidly and a host of moderate to large (>1000 patients) randomized trials documented the objective clinical advances. Specifically. the application of bare metal stents and the use of advanced antiplatelet pharmacologic therapies, including thienopyridines rather than Coumadin anticoagulation for stenting, and glycoprotein IIB/IIIa inhibitors have greatly reduced the problem of acute and subacute occlusive syndromes.[9-19] PCI-associated rates of MI, death, and emergent CABG have all declined as a result of these advances, and these declines have occurred despite a far wider application, in both clinical and angiographic terms.[9-19]

Perhaps the most important broadening of clinical application of PCI has been to include patients with acute coronary syndromes and, more specifically, patients with acute MI. During the past 20 years, more than 20 randomized trials, including more than 8000 patients with acute ST-segment elevation myocardial infarction (STEMI), have compared revascularization with contemporary medical therapy, including fibrinolysis (Table 4-4).[20-24] Taken together, these trials demonstrate a survival benefit, with reduced rates of cardiac events and stroke, for revascularization, predominantly by PCI.[20-24] Similarly, more than 6000 patients with high-risk unstable angina, mostly non-ST-segment elevation myocardial infarction (NSTEMI), have been randomly allocated between a conservative strategy of medical therapy and an aggressive strategy using predominantly PCI (Table 4-5).[25-27] These trials have documented an objective clinical advantage for PCI (FRISC II, TACTICS-TIMI 18, RITA-3).[7,25-27] PCI can be justified for almost all STEMI and most high-risk NSTEMI patients for emergent or urgent relief of medically refractory ischemia.[20-27] The higher the clinical risk of MI patients, the more likely they will also enjoy a survival benefit compared with optimal contemporary medical management ("revascularization paradox").[1,2] It is primarily the application of PCI to high-risk clinical subsets, coupled with randomized trial demonstration of major clinical advantage of PCI relative to contemporary medical therapy, that has allowed for *evidence-based* application of PCI to anatomic subsets (two- and three-vessel disease) previously reserved for CABG. The rationale for this application has been predominantly physiologic (acute MI and/or medically refractory ischemia), and the definition of success has been almost completely physiologic (relief of ischemia, termination of acute infarction, recovery of ventricular function, enhanced survival).

When CABG was introduced, medical therapy consisted of antianginal medications such as nitrates, β-blockers, and calcium channel blockers on an "as

Table 4-4. Trials of PCI versus Thrombolysis in Patients with STEMI

First Author	Number		Lytic	Stent	Gp IIb/IIIa	Death (%)		Total Stroke (%)	
	PCI	Lytic				PCI	Lytic	PCI	Lytic
Zilstra	152	149	SK	No	No	1	7	0.7	2
Riberio	50	50	SK	No	No	6	2	0	0
Grinfeld	54	58	SK	No	No	9	14	—	—
Zilstra	47	53	SK	No	No	2	2	2	4
Akhras	42	45	SK	No	No	0	9	—	—
Widimsky	101	99	SK	Yes	No	7	14	0	1
DeBoer	46	41	SK	Yes	No	7	22	2	7
Widimsky	429	421	SK	Yes	Yes	7	10	—	—
DeWood	46	44	Duteplase	No	No	7	5	—	—
Grines	195	200	TPA 3 hr	No	No	3	7	0	4
Gibbons	47	56	Duteplase	No	No	4	4	0	0
Ribichini	55	55	Acc. tPA	No	No	2	6	0	0
Garcia	95	94	Acc. tPA	No	No	3	11	—	—
GUSTO IIB	565	573	Acc. tPA	No	No	6	7	1	2
LeMay	62	61	Acc. tPA	Yes	Yes	5	3	2	3
Bonnefoy	421	419	Acc. tPA	Yes	Yes	5	4	0	1
Schomig	71	69	Acc. tPA	Yes	Yes	4	7	—	—
Vermeer	75	75	Acc. tPA	Yes	No	7	7	3	3
Andersen	790	782	Acc. tPA	Yes	NA	7	8	1	2
Kastrati	81	81	Acc. tPA	Yes	Yes	3	6	1	1
Aversano	225	226	Acc. tPA	Yes	Yes	5	7	1	4
Grines	71	66	Acc. tPA	Yes	Yes	8	12	0	5
Hochman	152	150	Acc. tPA	Yes	Yes	47	56	3	1

Acc. tPA, accelerated tissue plasminogen activator; GUSTO IIB, Global Use of Strategies to Open Occluded Arteries in Acute Coronary Syndromes IIB; PCI, percutaneous coronary intervention; SK, streptokinase; STEMI, ST-segment elevation myocardial infarction; TPA, tissue plasminogen activator.
Adapted from Keeley EC, Boura JA, Grines CL: Lancet 2003;361:13-20.) Reproduced from Morrison DA, Sacks J: Balancing benefit against risk in the choice of therapy for coronary artery disease (CAD): Lessons from prospective, randomized, clinical trials (RCTs) of percutaneous coronary intervention (PCI) and coronary artery bypass graft surgery (CABG). Minerva Cardioangiol 2003;51:585-597, with permission of Minerva Cardioangiologica.

Table 4-5. NSTEMI/Unstable Angina Strategy Trials*

Trial	Years	N	Strategy (%)		Death or MI At 6-12 Mo (%)		Death At 6-12 Mo (%)	
			Conserv.	Invas.	Conserv.	Invas.	Conserv.	Invas.
TIMI-IIIb (U.S.)	1989-1992	1473	50	63	12	11	—	—
VANQWISH (U.S. VA)	1993-1996	920	33	44	14	23	8	14
FRISC-II (Scandinavia)	1996-1998	2457	9	71	14	10	4	2
TACTICS-TIMI 18 (U.S.)	1997-1999	220	36	61	10	7	4	3
RITA-3 (U.K.)	1997-2001	1810	10	44	8	8	4	5
ICTUS (Netherlands)[†]	2001-2003	1200	40	76	14.4[‡]	19.9[‡]	4.5[‡]	4.4[‡]

*The trials with the biggest differences between invasive and conservative strategies in their primary end points were trials that included more contemporary therapy and had the largest differences in proportions of patients receiving conservative versus invasive pharmacotherapy (FRISC-II, TACTICS-TIMI, and RITA-3). Multivariate analysis of TIMI-IIIb yielded four variables that identified a high-risk subset that did benefit from early invasive strategy; patients in this subset had age >65 yr, ST depression at presentation, "complicated angina," and elevated CK-MB. Both FRISC II and TACTICS-TIMI 18 demonstrated benefit in reduction of death and MI only among patients with elevated troponin on presentation, and the highest reductions occurred among older patients with diabetes, prior MI, and electrocardiographic ST depression as well as troponin elevation. All of these factors are also predictors of adverse outcome; accordingly, the "revascularization paradox" (i.e., patients with the most long-term benefit often also have the highest short-term risk) is supported by these data in aggregate.
†Hirsch A, Windhausen F, Tijssen JG, et al: Long-term outcome after an early invasive versus selective invasive treatment strategy in patients with non-ST-elevation acute coronary syndrome and elevated cardiac troponin T (the ICTUS trial): A follow-up study. Lancet 2007;369:827-835.
‡Two-year, not 12-month results.
Conserv., conservative strategy; FRISC-II, Fragmin and Revascularization during InStability in Coronary Artery Disease II; ICTUS, Invasive versus Conservative Treatment in Unstable Coronary Syndromes; Invas., invasive strategy; MI, myocardial infarction; NSTEMI, non-ST-segment elevation myocardial infarction; RITA-3, Randomized Intervention Trial of unstable Angina-3; TACTICS, Treat Angina with Aggrastat and Determine Cost of Therapy with an Invasive or Conservative Strategy; TIMI, Thrombolysis in Myocardial Infarction; VANQWISH, Veterans Affairs Non-Q-Wave Myocardial Infarction Strategies In-Hospital.
Modified from Morrison DA, Sacks J: Balancing benefit against risk in the choice of therapy for coronary artery disease (CAD): Lessons from prospective, randomized, clinical trials (RCTs) of percutaneous coronary intervention (PCI) and coronary artery bypass graft surgery (CABG). Minerva Cardioangiol 2003;51:585-597, with permission of Minerva Cardioangiologica. Compare with Table 18 in Smith SC Jr, Feldman TE, Hirshfeld JW Jr, et al: ACC/AHA/SCA&I guideline update for percutaneous coronary intervention: Summary article. Cath Cardiovasc Intervent 2006;67:87-112.

needed" basis.[1-4] Not only had there been no documentation of survival benefit with any form of medical therapy (beyond blood pressure control), but the early CABG trials regarded the "need" for medication after CABG as an indication of "failed" CABG.

The mindset developed among clinicians and patients that revascularization "fixed" the problem of atherosclerosis, whereas medical therapy simply "put it off." Patients were encouraged to "get it over with". Many patients continue to be convinced that CABG

Table 4-6. Trials of PCI versus CABG in the Bare Metal Stent Era*

Trial	Years	N	Age (Yr)	LVEF	Prior MI (%)	Diabetes (%)	Two- Or Three- Vessel Disease (%)	Unstable Angina (%)	Exclusions	Death Follow-up	PCI	CABG
ARTS	1997-1998	1205	61	.60	44	17	98	37	LVEF <.30	1 yr	6%	3%
SoS	1996-1999	988	62	.57	45	14	100	24	MI within 48 hr	2 yr	5%	2%
MASS II	2000	611	60	.68	44	30	0	—	Only single-vessel LAD included	1 yr	2%	1%
ERACI II	1996-1998	5619	61		29	17	95	92	—	25 mo	1%	4%
AWESOME	1995-2000	2431	67	.45	71	33	82	100	Only "medically refractory" cases included	3 yr	20%	21%

*All of these trials, except ERACI II, excluded unprotected left main coronary artery disease. All of these trials, except AWESOME, excluded prior CABG. Only AWESOME mandated any definition of "medically refractory." Average time between randomization and treatment in ARTS was 28 days for CABG and 11 days for PCI. Nine of 22 PCI deaths in SoS were cancer-related (statistical aberration).

ARTS, Arterial Revascularization Therapies Study; AWESOME, Angina With Extemely Serious Operative Mortality Evaluation; CABG, coronary artery bypass grafting; ERACI II, Argentine Randomized Trial of Percutaneous Transluminal Coronary Angioplasty Versus Coronary Artery Bypass Surgery in Multivessel Disease (Estudio Randomizado Argentino de Angioplastia vs. Cirugía) II; LAD, left anterior descending coronary artery; LVEF, left ventricular ejection fraction; MASS II, Medicine, Angioplasty or Surgery Study II; MI, myocardial infarction; PCI, percutaneous coronary intervention; SoS, Stent or Surgery Trial.

Modified from Morrison DA, Sacks J: Balancing benefit against risk in the choice of therapy for coronary artery disease (CAD): Lessons from prospective, randomized, clinical trials (RCTs) of percutaneous coronary intervention (PCI) and coronary artery bypass graft surgery (CABG). Minerva Cardioangiol 2003;51:585-597, with permission of Minerva Cardioangiologica. Compare with Table 10 in Smith SC Jr, Feldman TE, Hirshfeld JW Jr, et al: ACC/AHA/SCA&I guideline update for percutaneous coronary intervention: Summary article. Cath Cardiovasc Intervent 2006;67:87-112.

or PCI will "fix" their problem but that medical therapy, which has many side effects and is costly and inconvenient, only temporizes.

In the 3 decades since PCI was introduced, medical therapy and risk factor modification have evolved dramatically.[1,2] Numerous large trials, megatrials, and meta-analyses have provided support for prolonged survival with each of the following medical therapies, among subgroups with both stable and unstable CAD: aspirin,[28,29] statins and other lipid-lowering drugs,[30] β-blockers,[31] and angiotensin-converting enzyme inhibitors (ACE) inhibitors and/or angiotensin receptor blocking agents (ARBs).[32]

A fundamental implication of the advances in medical therapy over the last 3 decades is that the inference that CABG will lead to prolonged survival in purely anatomic subsets is much less likely in 2008 than it was in 1970.[2] In addition, all trials and registries are concordant in suggesting that patients continue to derive multiple objective clinical benefits, including survival benefit, if they continue optimal medical management after either CABG or PCI.[3,5] Patients who continue optimal medical management and risk factor modification will likely go on to more "successful" long-term CABG or PCI outcomes.[2]

Despite the advances in technology and experience, many practitioners and observers have continued to view the choice between CABG and PCI largely in anatomic terms. Some of this tendency derives from the limiting of comparative trials in the bare metal stent era to clinically low-risk patients, and the screening and enrolling of patients starting with a "multivessel" classification (Table 4-6).[33-37] Additionally, many interventionists have seen the failure to demonstrate a survival difference between CABG and PCI in the pre-stent trials (see Table 4-3), not as a function of either low risk/low event rates or modest sample sizes leading to limited power and type I error

(failure to detect a difference where there is truly a difference), but rather reflecting the reality of the situation. (For example, compare the interventional view in Klein[38] with the surgical view in the CABG Guideline.[3]) From the interventionist's perspective, the only task remaining for PCI to supplant CABG for multivessel disease was to reduce the late repeat revascularization difference by reducing restenosis. By this (anatomic) thinking, drug-eluting stents could allow, by inference, the notion that stents "prolong life" in three-vessel disease.[10-14]

THE ANATOMIC (CONVENTIONAL) PARADIGM IN CLINICAL PRACTICE

As outlined in both the 1991 and the 2004 CABG Guidelines, left main coronary artery stenosis of greater than 50% is a class I indication for CABG in stable patients with either asymptomatic, mild angina or moderate angina, regardless of the level of LV function, regardless of whether myocardial ischemia has been documented, and without mention of any form of medical therapy. The same applies for greater than 70% narrowing of all three major vascular territories.

Further extension of the anatomic approach includes application to two-vessel disease, by separating those patients with or without proximal narrowing greater than 70% in the LAD. The complex formulas and figures, especially the control or "medical therapy" arms displayed in the 1991 Guideline, were derived primarily from the VA Cooperative Stable Angina Study, which was completed by the early 1970s and did not routinely include any of the four categories of medications subsequently shown to have survival benefit.

Acute MI was divided into Q and non-Q types in the 1991 CABG Guideline, and, in general, early post-MI CABG was proscribed. Nevertheless, specific direction was not given (beyond coronary anatomy) regarding which, if any, MI patients would be better served with PCI than with CABG.

By the 2004 CABG Guideline Update, clinical patient subgroups were expanded to include asymptomatic or mild angina, stable angina, unstable angina/NSTEMI, STEMI, poor LV function, and life-threatening arrhythmias, to be consistent with both the PCI Guidelines, the MI Guidelines, and the Stable and Unstable Angina Guidelines.

As outlined in the 1988 PCI Guideline, the first major "cut-point" in PCI Guidelines was between single-vessel and multivessel CAD; multivessel disease referred to greater than 70% diameter stenoses in two more major epicardial vessels. Particularly given the possibility of acute occlusion with attendant acute MI and need for emergency CABG, each category of recommendation was accompanied by an estimate of the likelihood of success and the likelihood of acute occlusive syndrome based on an anatomic scheme introduced in that Guideline. The ACC/AHA lesion classification was for balloon-only angioplasty, because stents had not yet become available. Type A lesions were said to be associated with greater than 85% success and a low risk of acute complications. Type A lesions were discrete (<10 mm), concentric, readily accessible, nonangulated, smooth lesions with little or no calcification that were less than totally occlusive, not ostial, not bifurcated, and free of thrombus. Type B anatomic lesions were said to be associated with 60% to 85% success and a moderate risk of complications. Type B lesions included those that were 10 to 20 mm in length, eccentric, of moderate tortuosity, with moderate angulation, irregular contour, moderate to heavy calcification, total occlusion of less than 3 months' duration, ostial location, presence of bifurcation necessitating two guidewires, and containing thrombus. Class C anatomic features were said to be associated with less than 60% acute success and a high risk of acute complications. Class C features included greater than 2 cm length, excessive tortuosities, angulation of greater than 90 degrees, total occlusion of longer than 3 months' duration, inability to protect major side branches, and degenerated saphenous vein graft lesion.

CLINICAL EXAMPLES OF THE ANATOMIC PARADIGM IN PRACTICE

For purposes of illustration, consider two hypothetical 74-year-old patients (male or female; diabetic or not), one stable and the other unstable, in whom coronary angiography was completed and showed 50% left main narrowing and 70% proximal circumflex and right coronary artery stenoses. In the stable patient, the LAD has an additional high-grade, discrete stenosis, whereas in the unstable patient, there is a 100% thrombotic occlusion. The unstable patient is suffering an acute anterior MI with ST elevation and has a blood pressure of 80 mm Hg on high-dose dopamine (>20 μg/kg/min), despite a pulmonary

wedge pressure of 22 mm Hg. In other words, this patient has anterior STEMI with cardiogenic shock. The stable patient has Canadian Cardiovascular Society Class II angina, is receiving no medical therapy, and has not had a provocative test for ischemia. The ACC/AHA CABG Guidelines suggest that both patients should receive CABG as a class I recommendation, based on level of evidence "A" (multiple trials and or meta-analysis).[1-5] Perusal of the reference list shows that the multiple trials are the five CABG versus medical therapy trials alluded to previously, although later publications of longer follow-up are cited (see Table 4-1).[3,4]

Regarding our unstable patient with acute STEMI, this patient would not have been excluded by the more than 20 trials of thrombolytic therapy versus primary PCI that supported revascularization, more than 90% of which was accomplished by PCI (see Table 4-4).[5,28,29] However, all five CABG versus medical therapy trials excluded patients who were hemodynamically unstable, within 30 days of an MI, and older than 70 years of age and therefore would have excluded our patient with STEMI and shock (see Table 4-1).[3,4] The SHould we emergently revascularize Occluded Coronaries in cardiogenic shocK? (SHOCK) trial of cardiogenic shock would provide support for the decision to revascularize our unstable patient, but, because there was no randomization between CABG and PCI in that trial (two thirds of revascularizations were by PCI), it does not help with the choice of revascularization method.[2,5] Given the speed of reperfusion and its importance, many operators and hospitals would use primary PCI to care for this STEMI patient. Facilities without PCI, or operators without sufficient experience and comfort, might use thrombolytics and an intra-aortic balloon pump (IABP), and the SHOCK trial provides support for this approach. The CABG Guidelines' own caveats regarding the timing of surgery relative to MI might be used to declare CABG a "prohibitive risk" in many settings.[3]

For our stable patient, the ACC/AHA Guidelines would give a class I recommendation for CABG, based on class A evidence. Nevertheless, based on the patient's age, he or she would have been excluded from the three CABG versus medical therapy trials (see Table 4-1).[1-4] The patient would likely undergo CABG at most hospitals. In fact, in many communities, radio and television advertisements extol the importance of using calcium scores to guide asymptomatic and untreated subjects to coronary angiography; patients with three-vessel CAD go on to provide testimonials as to having their lives "saved" by CABG.

LIMITATIONS OF RANDOMIZED TRIALS AND HOW THEY AFFECT THE VALIDITY OF THE ANATOMIC PARADIGM

The primary limitation of applying randomized trial results to clinical practice involves generalizability issues, such patient exclusions, and changes in "standard" therapy that render trials "outdated". The results of a randomized trial do not necessarily apply to populations that were systematically excluded from that trial. Because most trials, especially procedural trials, exclude patients with complex and high-risk conditions, their results provide the most guidance for the simplest decisions. Almost all CABG trials have systematically excluded patients within 7 to 30 days of an acute MI, patients with LVEF less than .35, hemodynamically unstable patients, patients with anatomy deemed unfavorable for CABG (no anatomic contraindication is harder to define than "diffuse disease"), patients older than 70 years of age, patients with one or more prior heart surgeries, and patients with severe comorbidities, including but not limited to chronic obstructive pulmonary disease, pulmonary hypertension, prior stroke, cancer, severe liver disease, and severe renal failure.

The results of randomized trials do not necessarily apply in the same way if either the control (standard) therapy or the active therapy has undergone major improvement since completion of the trial. With highly significant improvements in survival resulting from the use of aspirin, statins, β-blockers, and ACE inhibitors/ARBs, the likely long-term mortality of medical therapy arms in 2008 is substantially better than it was in the 1960s, when medical therapy was compared with CABG. Although CABG has also improved since the 1960s, there is no body of large randomized trials showing superiority of current techniques to those of 40 years ago. For example, although it is believed that routine use of the left internal mammary or thoracic artery as a conduit is an important clinical advance, there is not one randomized trial comparing use of the internal mammary artery with saphenous vein graft implantation into the same recipient vessels, under the same conditions, with the same adjuncts and follow-up. This dearth of prospective randomized trials also applies to cardioplegic techniques, and it stands in marked contrast to PCI advances such as bare metal stents, drug-eluting stents, thienopyridines, direct thrombin inhibitors, and glycoprotein IIb/IIIa inhibitors, each of which has been compared with "standard" therapy in thousands of randomized subjects.

Beyond the generic limitations of randomized trials, there are additional limitations on trials of procedures. In revascularization trials, blinding of subjects or caregivers is impossible. Because caregivers provide medications and patients choose whether to use them, undergoing a procedure can bias the subsequent use of medications known to alter survival among patients with CAD. Put another way, it can be said that any good clinician is trying to bias the outcome of his or her patients toward a favorable result. The clinician does this by prescribing and encouraging compliance with evidence-based medical therapy, among many other ways.

Additionally, the sample sizes of revascularization trials are an order of magnitude less than those of the megatrials of pharmacologic agents, and operators tend to select low-risk patients. Low risk means low

event rate, and smaller numbers of subjects with lower event rates translates into significantly less power to detect meaningful differences in trials of procedures. The power of a study to detect differences is also reduced by large numbers of crossovers, which are expected in any trial of a procedure that is effective.

LIMITATIONS OF REGISTRIES AND HOW THEY AFFECT THE VALIDITY OF THE ANATOMIC PARADIGM

To supplement the anatomic conclusions derived from the aforementioned 1960s trials, the practice guidelines and other authoritative sources cite the results of several large prospective registries. The Duke database is a long-term, single-center registry that is often cited, and the State of New York, VA, and Society of Cardiovascular Surgeons all maintain large, multicenter registries. These registries have the advantages of consistent definition of variables. Nevertheless, they all are prone to the epidemiologic triad of alternative explanations for their results; specifically, selection bias, confounding, and/or information bias may be a possible or even a probable alternative explanation for many of their findings.

With regard to the possibility of selection bias, the conventional wisdom, during the entire period that most registries have existed, has been that patients with left main and/or three-vessel disease have better survival with CABG.[3,39-41] This conclusion has been promulgated by the ACC/AHA Guidelines.[3] Under these circumstances, what kinds of patients with left main and/or three-vessel CAD would not be offered CABG at Duke or in the State of New York? Among the categories of patients likely to be denied CABG are the following groups: patients with shock, cancer, "diffuse disease," or life-threatening comorbidities; moribund patients; demented patients; patients with recent cardiac arrest; and so on. At the end of 10 years, the favorable patients with left main and/or three-vessel disease who underwent CABG may have more survivors than the medical therapy group, but this may be as much a function of the inclusion of such high-risk patients only in the medical arm as of a difference between CABG and medical therapy. This sampling problem cannot be adequately dealt with by any multivariable method unless all of the significant groups have been defined and measured during the period of the registry. This limitation also applies to multicenter registries and is not made less important by simply having a larger registry.

Confounding is the mixing of effects. Because of the multiplicity of anatomic and physiologic associations, as well as treatment with clinical associations, it is another extremely common form of systematic bias or alternative explanation for study results. The major advantage of the randomized trial is that an adequately powered randomized study tends to balance both known and unrecognized confounding factors; therefore, the observed results of the trial can be safely inferred to result from differences in treatment rather than differences in the patient groups. A simple example is that most patients who undergo CABG go through some form of postprocedure rehabilitation, during which they are likely to get risk factor and medication reinforcement that they would not get if they were in the medical arm of the registry. Sophisticated attempts to "correct" for inadvertent imbalances between compared groups (e.g., propensity analysis) are dependent on the validity and objectivity of the measurements used to define clinical and angiographic and procedural characteristics. Clearly, one cannot "correct" for undefined and unmeasured variables. Perhaps the most common anatomic factor cited for "turning down" patients for CABG, and a commonly cited reason for procedural MI or other adverse outcome of CABG, is "diffuse disease" or "poor targets." This factor is so subjective that no trial or registry has defined it or attempted to measure it.

The third major alternative is information bias, which means misclassification or systematic differences in the way outcomes are measured. Specific examples include the detection of MI or stroke after PCI versus after CABG versus among medically treated patients. The PCI Guideline recommends highly sensitive troponin measurement for every PCI patient with chest pain and even gives a IIa ("ought to consider") recommendation to routine troponin measurement after PCI. In contrast, CABG patients with chest pain or change in mental status are often assumed to have surgery-related or intensive care unit–related symptoms, and measurement of enzymes or electrocardiographic recording is usually eschewed. Medical patients are probably in the middle, getting electrocardiograms and/or enzyme analysis primarily based on their presentation with new symptoms.

THE VERY DIFFERENT ADVANTAGES AND DISADVANTAGES OF PCI AND CABG

A fundamental result of reviewing randomized trial comparisons of two treatment options is the tendency to see them as "either-or" rather than complementary options.[1,2] In particular, the fact that the major rationale for CABG, historically, has been anatomic has fostered an emphasis on the anatomic differences (advantages/disadvantages) between CABG and PCI. Nevertheless, the physiologic differences between the two revascularization techniques turn out to be every bit as important.

The major advantage for CABG, which has a structural or anatomic basis, is the ability to achieve "complete revascularization," even in the face of one or more chronic total occlusions. This allows for the application of CABG to anatomic subsets that are not approachable with PCI. A second major advantage of CABG, namely the superior durability of its results (at least compared with bare metal stents), is at least partly structural, in that bypass conduits protect territories, whereas stents treat lesions. But another major advantage of CABG has been its near-simultaneous treatment of multiple vessels at the same procedure,

which has been possible because the patient's physiologic state is "controlled" by general anesthesia, intubation/ventilation, heart-lung bypass, sternotomy exposure, cardioplegia, and so on. It is from these control factors that two of the major disadvantages of CABG compared with PCI derive.[2] First, it takes finite time to initiate these control features, and this time can translate into necrosis if the patient is suffering from an acute MI. Second, each of these control features contributes to the overall morbidity of CABG. This morbidity is also enhanced if CABG is undertaken during an MI. Other patient comorbidities, such as severe cerebrovascular disease or severe pulmonary disease, can compound the interaction of MI, time, and the invasive control features of CABG.[2,42]

In contrast, the major advantages of contemporary PCI (which includes stents, thienopyridines, and glycoprotein IIb/IIIa inhibitors, among other adjuncts) are speed of achieving normal or near-normal perfusion and relatively mild morbidity. Because of these factors, patients with an acute MI can often be rapidly stabilized by a single-lesion procedure, with more complete revascularization achieved by either PCI or CABG during subsequent procedures, which they undergo at much lower risk (because their ischemic, hemodynamic, and/or electrical instability has been relieved). All of these advantages apply to acute coronary syndromes (STEMI and NSTEMI), which are purely physiologic subsets.

The major disadvantages of PCI include inability to treat chronic total occlusions and inability to protect territories rather than lesions. These are structural issues that apply primarily to stable patients.

Medical therapy and risk factor modification have been shown to provide clinical benefit for stable and unstable patients.[43-46] Furthermore, stability implies time to document ischemia that is medically refractory, whereas instability implies ischemia that is refractory. Acute coronary syndrome is a reason to consider emergent or urgent revascularization, most often by PCI. Stable coronary syndromes provide time to optimize medical management and document ischemia, before considering either CABG or PCI. Neither PCI nor CABG provides either a "cure" or prevention of future events. Both PCI and CABG (like acute MI) can be viewed as opportunities to help patients change their lifestyles to become more cardioprotective.[43-46]

RELATIVE COSTS OF CABG AND PCI AND THE CHANGE FROM ANATOMIC TO FUNCTIONAL DECISION MAKING

Most of the limited cost effectiveness studies come from randomized trial data.[47] Because the rates of survival, MI, and stroke in most trials of CABG and PCI have not been significantly different and the short-term costs and morbidity of CABG are so much greater, most trials have shown a short-term cost advantage for PCI, which is often made up for over the long term (see Tables 4-3 and 4-6).[47] Additionally, repeat revascularization has consistently favored

Table 4-7. Complex PCI Means Lower Likelihood of Success and/or Higher Likelihood of Complication: How Bare Metal Stents (BMS) and Drug-Eluting Stents (DES) Have Changed PCI for the Better

Feature	BMS More Helpful than Balloon PCI	DES More Helpful than BMS
Anatomic Feature		
2.5-3.5 mm diameter; <20 mm long; without calcium, thrombus, tortuosity, or bifurcation	STRESS, BENESTENT	RAVEL, SIRIUS, TAXUS IV, Babapulle et al* meta-analysis of DES, ISAR-DESIRE
Diffuse	BENESTENT II	RESEARCH registry, C-SIRIUS
Small caliber	ISAR-SMART, SISCA, BESMART, COMPASS, CHIVAS, SVS, SISA, COAST, RAP, LASMAL	RESEARCH registry
Osteal	Cohort	Cohort
Bifurcation	Cohorts using T stent, Y stent, V stent, "kissing" stents, or "culotte"	Cohorts using Crush or "kissing" stents
Heavy calcium	Cohorts including both Rotablator and Excimer laser registries	Cohort
Saphenous vein	SAVED	Cohort
Chronic total	SICCO, GISSOC, TOSCA, SARECCO, SPATCO	RESEARCH registry
Thrombus-containing	EPISTENT	
Clinical Feature		
STEMI	Stent-PAMI, PASTA, GRAMI, FRESCO, CADILLAC	RESEARCH registry
NSTEMI	EPISTENT	RESEARCH registry
Shock	Antonucci et al†	
Left main coronary artery disease		Valgimigli et al‡

*Babapulle MN, Joseph L, Belisle P, et al: A hierarchical Bayesian meta-analysis of randomized clinical trials of drug-eluting stents. Lancet 2004;364:583-591.
†Antonucci D, Valenti R, Migliorini A, et al: Abciximab therapy improves survival in patients with acute myocardial infarction compliated by early cardiogenic shock undergoing coronary artery stent implantation. Am J Cardiol 2002;90:353-357.
‡Valgimigli M, Malagutti P, Aoki J, et al: Sirolimus-eluting versus paclitaxel-eluting stent implantation for the percutaneous treatment of left-main coronary artery disease: A combined RESEARCH and T-SEARCH long-term analysis. J Am Coll Cardiol 2006;47:507-514.
BENESTENT, Belgian Netherlands Stent Study; BESMART, Bestent in Small Arteries; C-SIRIUS, Canadian Study of the Sirolimus-Eluting Stent in the Treatment of Patients with Long De Novo Lesions in Small Native Coronary Arteries; CADILLAC, Controlled Abciximab and Device Investigation to Lower Late Angioplasty Complications; CHIVAS, Coronary Heart Disease Stenting in Small Vessels Versus Balloon Angioplasty Study; COAST, Heparin-COAted STents in small coronary arteries; COMPASS, Cilostazol or Multilink for Percutaneous coronary Angioplasty of Small vessel Study; EPISTENT, Evaluation of Platelet IIb/IIIa Inhibitor for Stenting; FRESCO, Florence Randomized Elective Stenting in Acute Coronary Occlusions; GISSOC, Gruppo Italiano di tudio sullo Stent nelle Occlusioni Coronariche; GRAMI, Gianturco-Roubin in Acute Myocardial Infarction; ISAR-DESIRE, Intracoronary Stenting or Angioplasty for Restenosis Reduction: Drug-Eluting Stents for In-Stent Restenosis; ISAR-SMART, Intracoronary Stenting or Angioplasty for Restenosis Reduction in Small Arteries; LASMAL, Latin American Small Vessels; NSTEMI, non-ST-segment elevation myocardial infarction; PASTA, Primary Angioplasty versus Stent Implantation in Acute Myocardial Infarction; RAP, Restenosis en Arterias Pequenas; RAVEL, Randomized Study with the Sirolimus-Eluting Velocity Balloon Expandable Stent; RESEARCH, Rapamycin-Eluting Stent Evaluated At Rotterdam Cardiology Hospital; SARECCO, Stent or Angioplasty after Recanalization of Chronic Coronary Occlusions; SAVED, Saphenous Vein De Novo; SICCO, Stenting in Chronic Coronary Occlusion; SIRIUS, Sirolimus-Eluting Bx-Velocity Balloon Expandable Stent in the Treatment of Patients with De Novo Native Coronary Artery Lesions; SISA, Stenting in Small Arteries; SISCA, Stenting in Small Coronary Arteries; SPATCO, Stent versus Percutaneous Angioplasty in Chronic Total Occlusion; STEMI, ST-segment elevation myocardial infarction; Stent-PAMI, Stent Primary Angioplasty in Myocardial Infarction; STRESS, Stent Restenosis Study; SVS, Small Vessel Study; T-SEARCH, Taxus-Stent Evaluated At Rotterdam Cardiology Hospital; TOSCA, Total Occlusion Study of Canada.
Revised from Morrison DA: Multivessel percutaneous coronary intervention (PCI): A new paradigm for a new century. Minerva Cardioangiol 2005;53:361-378, with permission of Minerva Cardioangiologica. Compare with Tables 20 and 28 in Smith SC Jr, Feldman TE, Hirshfeld JW Jr, et al: ACC/AHA/SCA&I guideline update for percutaneous coronary intervention: Summary article. Cath Cardiovasc Intervent 2006;67:87-112.

CABG, or at least it did before the completion of any trials incorporating drug-eluting stents.[2,5,47]

A major alternative result is the 2006 cost-effectiveness study from the AWESOME trial.[48] Because that trial focused on patients with medically refractory myocardial ischemia and high-risk factors for CABG outcome, its survival trends have always favored PCI. By 5 years of follow-up, the survival difference for the entire trial population reached a *P* value of .06, which is almost "significant" by conventional standards.[48] In addition, by 5 years, the cost difference was still more than $20,000, in favor of PCI.[48] Accordingly, in this population of high-risk patients with acute coronary syndromes, including acute MI, hemodynamic instability, severe LV dysfunction, and older age, PCI appears to be economically "dominant."[48]

These results resonate with the cost-effectiveness results from the Swiss Trial of Invasive versus Medical therapy in Elderly patients with chronic symptomatic coronary-artery disease (TIME), in which a medically refractory, elderly cohort was randomized between contemporary medical therapy and revascularization (primarily accomplished by PCI).[7,49] The TIME investigators found revascularization to be clinically advantageous, in terms of symptoms and hospitalization, but somewhat more expensive than medical therapy alone.

STENTS AND THE "LEVELING OF THE ANATOMIC PLAYING FIELD"

As summarized in Table 4-7, both bare metal stents and drug-eluting stents have been tested, by randomized trial and/or registry, in a number of the anatomic classifications that the ACC/AHA lesion scheme defined as high-risk.[5] The reductions in both acute and long-term adverse outcomes and improvements in clinical success are major components of the broadening of the anatomic application of PCI to relief of myocardial ischemia. A major test of this "leveling of the anatomic playing field" hypothesis will be whether the proportion of screened patients who are enrolled in the trials of drug-eluting stents versus CABG, such as the National Institutes of Health (NIH)-sponsored Future Revascularization Evaluation in patiEnts with Diabetes mellitus: Optimal Management of multivessel disease (FREEDOM) trial, is not considerably higher than the less than 10% of almost all of the trials of pre-stent PCI versus CABG (see Table 4-3).[2,8]

SUMMARY: FROM STRUCTURE TO FUNCTION

Since the early 1970s, the decision to offer patients with myocardial ischemia CABG surgery has been largely determined by the extent of CAD and left ventricular function. Based on subset analyses and long-term follow-up of the trials listed in Table 4-1, the notion has persisted that patients with left main

Table 4-8. Caring for the Individual Patient with Myocardial Ischemia Secondary to CAD: Changing the Primary Focus for Revascularization Decisions from Coronary Anatomy to Clinical Syndromes and Clinical (Functional) Outcomes—Specific Questions to be Answered

General Concept 1: Every CAD patient benefits from risk factor modification and optimal medical management.
Have the following management approaches been tried or are they appropriate:
    Smoking cessation?
    Diet?
    Exercise program?
    Blood pressure check?
    LDL and HDL check?
    HbA$_{1c}$ check?
    Aspirin?
    Statin?
    ACE inhibitor or ARB?
    β-blocker?

General Concept 2: Begin consideration of revascularization by assessing potential benefit. The primary benefit of any form of revascularization is relief of myocardial ischemia with attendant resolution of ischemic symptoms. A survival benefit is significantly less likely in an individual patient, given the improvements in medical therapy, but it is most likely for the highest-risk patients and most "evidence-based" for those with high clinical risk.
Is this stable or unstable ischemia?
Is there an acute myocardial infarction?
Is this patient hemodynamically unstable?
Is this patient electrically unstable?
Is there a large area of ischemia?
Are there medically refractory symptoms?

General Concept 3: After concluding that this patient is likely to benefit from revascularization performed at this time, begin choosing between CABG and PCI, with a comparison of relative benefits.
Are there one or more chronic total occlusions?
Has this patient had prior CABG with one or more patent conduits?
Has the left internal mammary artery already been used?
Is a conduit available?

General Concept 4: Risk versus benefit is multifactorial.
Is there an acute infarct?
Is this patient hemodynamically unstable?
Is there acute pulmonary edema?
Does this patient have cardiogenic shock?
Are downstream vessels favorable for grafting?
Are lesions favorable for stenting?

General Concept 5: Risk versus benefit is dynamic; that is, there are important individual differences among surgeons/interventionists and among patients.
Is the surgeon comfortable taking on this case?
Is the interventionist comfortable taking on this case?
Is this patient willing to undergo CABG?
Is this patient willing to undergo PCI?

General Concept 6: Costs are both short term and long term; there are also important cost consequences of taking people out of the workforce.
Is this patient at high risk for postoperative pulmonary morbidity?
Is this patient at high risk for postoperative cerebral morbidity?
Is this patient at high risk for postoperative hepatic morbidity?
Is this patient at high risk for postoperative renal morbidity?
Is this patient at high risk for one or multiple restenoses postoperatively?
Is this patient likely to return to work after CABG?
Is this patient likely to return to work after PCI?

ACE, angiotensin-converting enzyme; ARB, angiotensin receptor blocker; CABG, coronary artery bypass grafting; CAD, coronary artery disease; HbA$_{1c}$, glycosylated hemoglobin; HDL, high-density lipoprotein cholesterol; LDL, low-density lipoprotein cholesterol; PCI, percutaneous coronary intervention.

narrowing of greater than 50% or three-vessel stenoses greater than 70%, or even two-vessel stenoses greater than 70% in which one of the vessels is the proximal LAD, derive a survival benefit from CABG relative to medical therapy (anatomic paradigm).

The medical therapy administered in the original trials of CABG versus medical therapy consisted of little more than antianginal medications used on an "as needed" basis. In the ensuing four decades, multiple large, well-done, randomized clinical trials have established a survival benefit for four different forms of medical therapy among a broad spectrum of CAD patients. Aspirin, lipid-lowering therapies (especially statins), β-blockers, and ACE inhibitors and/or ARBs have all been shown to enhance survival, as well as reducing other objective adverse outcomes of CAD.

These advances in medical therapy, coupled with the small but significant rates of mortality and morbidity associated with both CABG and PCI, are among the reasons to skeptically consider a potential "survival benefit" of revascularization. A more common and far more easily justified reason to consider revascularization is to relieve "medically refractory" myocardial ischemia, particularly if the ischemia is accompanied by symptoms. Accordingly, documentation of medically refractory myocardial ischemia provides the answer to the first question of myocardial revascularization: Is this patient likely to derive clinical benefit from revascularization at this time? It is only after this question has been answered that one needs to consider the relative advantages and disadvantages of PCI versus CABG (physiologic paradigm).[1,2]

Two of the relative advantages of PCI, namely speed of reperfusion and relatively low morbidity, are among the reasons that most randomized trial data, and most clinical applications of revascularization to patients with MI (STEMI and NSTEMI) have been by PCI (see Tables 4-4 and 4-5).[1,2,20-27] In contrast, for stable patients with medically refractory ischemia, anatomic considerations continue to be relevant to the choice between CABG and PCI.[2,3,5] Specific advantages of CABG include its potential to revascularize chronically occluded vessels with collaterals supplying viable myocardium, the fact that conduits protect territories rather than simply treating lesions, and the greater durability of conduits compared with bare metal stents (although drug-eluting stents may change the picture).

Based on these principles, physiologic, rather than anatomic, considerations are most useful in determining whether to revascularize and how urgently to revascularize. STEMI is an emergent indication and high-risk NSTEMI is an urgent indication. Coronary anatomy, including both number of vessels and lesion characteristics, continues to aid the decision between CABG and PCI, as well as formulation of patient-specific strategies.

Advantages of using a physiologic frame of reference (i.e., clinical presentations and outcomes) rather than an anatomic one for clinical decision-making include (1) re-emphasis on medical therapy and risk factor modification before and after revascularization; (2) redefining the indications for procedures to be more clearly evidence-based; and (3) redefining clinically successful revascularization procedures.[1,2,43-46] Table 4-8 provides a simple algorithm incorporating the physiologic paradigm (clinical presentations and clinical outcomes) rather than anatomic decision-making.

REFERENCES

1. Morrison DA, Serruys P (eds): Medically Refractory Rest Angina. New York, Marcel Dekker, 1992.
2. Morrison DA, Serruys P (eds): High Risk Cardiac Revascularization and Clinical Trials. London, Martin Dunitz, 2002.
3. Eagle KA, Guyton RA, Davidoff R, et al: ACC/AHA guideline update for coronary artery bypass graft surgery: Summary article. Circulation 2004;110:1168-1176.
4. Yusuf S, Zucker D, Peduzzi P, et al: Effect of coronary artery bypass graft surgery on survival: Overview of 10-year results from randomized trials by the Coronary Artery Bypass Graft Surgery Trialists Collaboration. Lancet 1994;344:563-570.
5. Smith SC Jr, Feldman TE, Hirshfeld JW Jr, et al: ACC/AHA/SCA&I guideline update for percutaneous coronary intervention: Summary article. Cath Cardiovasc Intervent 2006;67:87-112.
6. Bourassa MG, Knatterud GL, Pepine CJ, et al; for the ACIP Investigators: Asymptomatic Cardiac Ischemia Pilot (ACIP) Study: Improvement of cardiac ischemia at 1 year after PTCA and CABG. Circulation 1995;92(Suppl II):II-1-7.
7. The TIME Investigators: Trial of invasive versus medical therapy in elderly patients with chronic symptomatic coronary-artery disease (TIME): A randomized trial. Lancet 2001;358:951-957.
8. Pocock SJ, Henderson RA, Rickards AF, et al: Meta-analysis of randomized trials comparing coronary angioplasty with bypass surgery. Lancet 1995;346:1184-1189.
9. George BS, Voorhees WD, Roubin GDS, et al: Multicenter investigation of coronary stenting to treat acute or threatened closure after percutaneous transluminal coronary angioplasty: clinical and angiographic outcomes. J Am Coll Card 1993;22:135-143.
10. Serruys PW, de Jaegere P, Kiemeneij F, et al; for the BENESTENT Study Group: A comparison of balloon-expandable-stent implantation with balloon angioplasty in patients with coronary artery disease. N Engl J Med 1994;331:489-495.
11. Fischman DI, Leon M, Baim DS, et al: A randomized comparison of coronary stent placement and balloon angioplasty in the treatment of coronary artery disease. N Engl J Med 1994;331:496-501.
12. Moses JW, Leon MB, Popma JJ, et al; for the SIRIUS Investigators: Sirolimus-eluting stents versus standard stents in patients with stenosis in a native coronary artery. N Engl J Med 2003;349:1315-1323.
13. Stone GW, Ellis SG, Cox DA, et al; for the TAXUS-IV investigators: A polymer-based, paclitaxel-eluting stent in patients with coronary artery disease N Engl J Med 2004;350:221-231.
14. Babapulle MN, Joseph L, Belisle P, et al: A hierarchical Bayesian meta-analysis of randomized clinical trials of drug-eluting stents. Lancet 2004;364:583-591.
15. Leon MB, Baim DS, Popma JJ, et al: A clinical trial comparing three antithrombotic-drug regimens after coronary-artery stenting. Stent Anticoagulation Restenosis Study investigators. N Engl J Med 1998;339:1665-1671.
16. Bertrand ME, Legrand V, Boland J, et al: Randomized multicenter comparison of conventional anticoagulation versus antiplatelet therapy in unplanned and elective coronary stenting: The Full Anticoagulation versus Aspirin and Ticlopidine (FANTASTIC) study. Circulation 1998;98:1597-1603.
17. The Direct Thrombin Inhibitor Trialists' Collaborative Group: Direct thrombin inhibitors in acute coronary syndromes: Principal results of a meta-analysis based on individual patients' data. Lancet 2002;359:294-302.

18. Antoniucci D, Valenti R, Migliorini A, et al: Abciximab therapy improves survival in patients with acute myocardial infarction complicated by early cardiogenic shock undergoing coronary artery stent implantation. Am J Cardiol 2002;90: 353-357.

19. The EPISTENT Investigators: Randomized placebo-controlled and balloon-angioplasty controlled trial to assess safety of coronary stenting with use of platelet glycoprotein IIb/IIIa blockade. Lancet 1998;352:87-92.

20. DeWood MA, Spores J, Notske R, et al: Prevalence of total coronary occlusion during the early hours of transmural myocardial infarction. N Engl J Med 1980;303:897-902.

21. DeWood MA, Stifter WF, Simpson CS, et al: Coronary angiographic findings soon after non-Q myocardial infarction. N Engl J Med 1986;315:417-423.

22. Fibrinolytic Therapy Trialists' (FTT) Collaborative Group: Indications for fibrinolytic therapy in suspected acute myocardial infarction: Collaborative overview of early mortality and major morbidity results from all randomized trials of more than 1000 patients. Lancet 1994;343:311-322.

23. Keeley EC, Boura JA, Grines CL: Primary angioplasty versus intravenous thrombolytic therapy for acute myocardial infarction: A quantitative review of 23 randomized trials. Lancet 2003;361:13-20.

24. Weaver WD, Simes J, Betrieu A, et al: Comparison of primary coronary angioplasty and intravenous thrombolytic therapy for acute myocardial infarction: A quantitative review. JAMA 1997;278:2093-2098.

25. Fragmin and Fast Revascularization during InStability in Coronary artery disease investigators: Invasive compared with non-invasive treatment in unstable coronary artery disease. FRISC II prospective randomized multicentre study. Lancet 1999;3554:708-715.

26. Cannon CP, Weintraub WS, Demopoulos LA, et al; for the TACTICS–Thrombolysis in Myocardial Infarction 18 investigators: Comparison of early invasive and conservative strategies in patients with unstable coronary syndromes treated with the glycoprotein IIb/IIIa inhibitor tirofiban. N Engl J Med 2001;344:1879-1887.

27. Fox KAA, Poole-Wilson PA, Henderson RA, et al; for the Randomized Intervention Trial of unstable Angina (RITA) Investigators: Interventional versus conservative treatment for patients with unstable angina or non-ST-elevation myocardial infarction: The British Heart Foundation RITA 3 randomized trial. Lancet 2002;360:743-751.

28. Antiplatelet Trialists Collaboration: Collaborative overview of randomized trials of antiplatelet therapy-I: Prevention of death, myocardial infarction and stroke by prolonged antiplatelet therapy in various categories of patients. BMJ 1995;308:81-106.

29. Yusuf S, Wittes J, Friedman L: Overview of results of randomized clinical trials in heart disease II: Unstable angina, heart failure, primary prevention with aspirin, and risk factor modification. JAMA 1988;260:2259-2263.

30. Larosa JC, Hunninghake D, Bush D, et al: The cholesterol facts: A summary of the evidence relating dietary fats, serum cholesterol, and coronary heart disease. A joint statement by the American Heart Association and the National Heart, Lung, and Blood Institute. The Task Force on Cholesterol Issues, American Heart Association. Circulation 1998;97:946-952.

31. Yusuf S, Peto R, Lewis J, et al: Beta blockade during and after myocardial infarction: An overview of the randomized trials. Prog Cardiovasc Dis 1985;27:335-371.

32. ACE Inhibitor Myocardial Infarction Collaborative Group: Indications for ACE inhibitors in the early treatment of acute myocardial infarction: Systematic overview of individual data from 100,000 patients in randomized trials. Circulation 1998; 97:2202.

33. Rodriguez A, Bernardi V, Navia J, et al: Argentine randomized study: Coronary angioplasty with stenting versus coronary bypass surgery in patients with multiple-vessel disease (ERACI II): 30-day and one-year follow-up results. J Am Coll Cardiol 2001;37:51-58.

34. Serruys PW, Unger F, Sousa JE, et al; for the Arterial Revascularization Therapies Study Group: Comparison of coronary-artery bypass surgery and stenting for the treatment of multivessel disease. N Engl J Med 2001;344:1117-1124.

35. Serruys PW, Unger F, van Hout BA, et al; for the ARTS study group: The ARTS (Arterial Revascularization Therapies Study): Background, goals and methods. Int J Cardiovasc Intervent 1999;2:41-50.

36. Stent or Surgery Investigators: Coronary artery bypass surgery versus percutaneous coronary intervention with stent implantation in patients with multivessel coronary artery disease (the stent or surgery trial): A randomized controlled trial. Lancet 2002;360:965-970.

37. Morrison DA, Sethi G, Sacks J, et al; for the AWESOME co-investigators: Percutaneous coronary intervention versus bypass graft surgery for patients with medically refractory myocardial ischemia and risk factors for adverse outcome with bypass: A multicenter, randomized trial. J Am Coll Cardiol 2001;38:143-149.

38. Klein LW: Are drug-eluting stents the preferred treatment for multivessel coronary artery disease? J Am Coll Cardiol 2006; 47:22-26.

39. Hannan EL, Racz MJ, McCallister BD, et al: A comparison of three-year survival after coronary artery bypass graft surgery and percutaneous transluminal coronary angioplasty. J Am Coll Cardiol 1999;33:63-72.

40. Hannan EL, Racz MJ, Walford G, et al: Long-term outcomes of coronary-artery bypass grafting versus stent implantation. N Engl J Med 2005;152:2174-2183.

41. Jones RH, Hannan EL, Hammermeister KE, et al: Identification of preoperative variables needed for risk adjustment of short-term mortality after coronary artery bypass graft surgery. The Working Group Panel on the Cooperative CABG Database Project. J Am Coll Cardiol 1996;28:1478-1487.

42. Roach GW, Kanchugar M, Mangano CM, et al; for the Multicenter Study of Perioperative Ischemia Research Group and the Ischemia Research and Education Foundation Investigators: Adverse cerebral outcomes after coronary bypass surgery. N Engl J Med 1996;335:1867-1863.

43. Pearson T, Rapaport E, Criqui M, et al: Optimal risk factor management in the patient after coronary revascularization. AHA Medical/Scientific Statement. Circulation 1994;90:3125-3133.

44. Smith SC Jr, Allen J, Blair SP, et al: AHA/ACC guidelines for secondary prevention for patients with coronary and other atherosclerotic vascular disease: 2006 Update. J Am Coll Cardiol 2006;47:2130-2139.

45. LaBresh KA, Ellrodt AG, Gliklich R, et al: Get with the guidelines for cardiovascular secondary prevention pilot results. Arch Intern Med 2004;164:203-209.

46. Mehta RH, Montoye CK, Gallogy M, et al: GAP Steering Committee of the American College of Cardiology: Improving quality of care for acute myocardial infarction. The Guidelines Applied in Practice (GAP) Initiative. JAMA 2002:287:1269-1276.

47. Hlatky MA, Rogers WJ, Johnstone I, et al; BARI Investigators: Medical care costs and quality of life after randomization to coronary angioplasty or coronary bypass surgery. N Engl J Med 1997;336:92-99.

48. Stroupe KT, Morrison DA, Hlatky MA, et al; for the Investigators of Veterans Affairs Cooperative Study No. 385 (AWESOME): Cost-effectiveness of coronary artery bypass grafts versus percutaneous coronary intervention for revascularization of high-risk patients. Circulation 2006;114:1229-1231.

49. Claude J, Schindler C, Kuster GM, et al; for the Trial of Invasive versus Medical therapy in Elderly (TIME) Investigators: Cost-effectiveness of invasive versus medical management of elderly patients with chronic symptomatic coronary artery disease. Eur Heart J 2004;25:2195-2203.

5 Renal Dysfunction

Uptal D. Patel and Brahmajee K. Nallamothu

KEY POINTS

- Renal dysfunction after cardiac catheterization and percutaneous coronary intervention (PCI) is common, is primarily due to exposure to contrast agents, and is associated with worse clinical outcomes.
- The prevalence of chronic kidney disease is rising, and it is a key risk factor for renal dysfunction after cardiac catheterization and PCI.
- The presence of chronic kidney disease and end-stage renal disease is associated with worse short- and long-term outcomes even after successful PCI, including higher rates of restenosis and repeat revascularization. The use of coronary stenting and drug-eluting stents may diminish this risk.

- Calculation of glomerular filtration rates and a simple risk score can help identify high-risk patients before their procedure beyond the use of serum creatinine levels alone.
- Established keys to preventing renal dysfunction after cardiac catheterization and PCI include periprocedural hydration and use of low- or iso-osmolar contrast agents.
- Evidence appears to favor the safety and efficacy of antioxidant agents such as *N*-acetylcysteine in high-risk patients, but not all trials are consistent.
- Intraprocedural strategies should consistently be used to minimize the volume of contrast agent exposure as much as possible.

Renal dysfunction is a widely-recognized complication of cardiac catheterization and percutaneous coronary intervention (PCI). A transient rise in serum creatinine levels, a common marker for the development of mild renal dysfunction, occurs in up to 15% of patients undergoing these procedures. Although many of these rises are unlikely to be clinically significant, even short-term renal dysfunction after cardiac catheterization and PCI has been associated with longer hospital stays and greater inpatient costs, as well as worse short- and long-term mortality.

Renal dysfunction after cardiac catheterization and PCI is believed to be primarily caused by intraprocedural exposure to contrast agents that are nephrotoxic in high doses.[1] The single most important risk factor that has been linked to the development of renal dysfunction after cardiac catheterization and PCI is the presence of preexisting chronic kidney disease (CKD). Other clinical factors such as diabetes mellitus and hemodynamic instability, which are also highly prevalent in this population, may also contribute to and exacerbate its clinical course. In a small proportion of patients, renal dysfunction is related to renal atheroembolic disease from diffuse atherosclerosis of the aorta. In patients without CKD or other risk factors, the development of renal dysfunction after these procedures is rare.

Importantly, recent diagnostic and therapeutic advances have improved our ability to identify those

patients who are at the highest risk for developing renal dysfunction and, further, to minimize its occurrence. In this chapter we provide a summary of these data, with an additional focus on patients with CKD, given its strong association with worsening renal dysfunction as well as subsequent cardiovascular complications. We also briefly comment on patients with end-stage renal disease (ESRD), a group that represents a growing segment of the population undergoing coronary revascularization. Finally, we discuss the role of nonpharmacologic and pharmacologic strategies for reducing the likelihood of developing renal dysfunction in high-risk patients.

PATHOPHYSIOLOGY OF RENAL DYSFUNCTION

The most common reason for renal dysfunction after cardiac catheterization and PCI is related to the use of intravascular contrast agents. Despite their widespread use in imaging studies, the exact mechanisms responsible for the development of contrast-related nephropathy remain unknown.[1] Most studies suggest that both direct toxic injury to the renal tubules and ischemic injury to the renal medulla from vasomotor changes and decreased perfusion are responsible. The latter appears to be mediated partly by the development of reactive oxygen species such as superoxide and has important implications for treatment with scavenging agents.[2] Diabetes mellitus and heart failure also may exacerbate contrast-related nephropathy, specifically through impairment of vasodilatory responses in the renal vasculature.[3]

A much less common but well-recognized cause of renal dysfunction after cardiac catheterization and PCI is renal atheroembolic disease. This disease process is part of the larger cholesterol embolization syndrome that can result from the embolism of minor atheromatous debris from the aorta or other large vessels to small arteries in various vascular beds.[4] The clinical spectrum of renal atheroembolic disease therefore includes blue toe syndrome, livedo reticularis, visual deficits, and abdominal pain from mesenteric ischemia.[4] Laboratory abnormalities include elevated eosinophil counts in the blood and eosinophiluria. Renal dysfunction is believed to be caused by distal and partial occlusion of the small arteries that leads to ischemic atrophy, as opposed to large areas of infarction.[5] Treatment for renal atheroembolic disease is largely supportive.

Finally, additional factors may exacerbate the development of renal dysfunction after cardiac catheterization and PCI. Many medications may directly contribute to renal toxicity or worsen microvasculature changes in the renal medulla, extending areas of ischemic injury. Table 5-1 lists several of these agents, as well as others that should be monitored closely because of their potential interactions with contrast agents.[6] For example, metformin can cause lactic acidosis in the setting of renal dysfunction, which has led the U.S. Food and Drug Administration to recommend withholding it on the day of exposure to contrast agents and for 48 to 72 hours after such exposure. Similarly, volume depletion and hemodynamic changes from heart failure or cardiogenic shock may aggravate contrast-related nephropathy. In case reports, anticoagulants such as warfarin and heparin have been implicated as causative agents in renal atheroembolic disease, given their potential to prevent proper healing of atheroma in the aorta after instrumentation.[5,7]

RENAL DYSFUNCTION, RISK FACTORS, AND PROGNOSIS

The most commonly used definition of renal dysfunction after cardiac catheterization and PCI in the literature (which refers primarily to contrast-related nephropathy) is a rise in serum creatinine levels of 0.5 mg/dL or a 25% increase from baseline. Although its reported incidence ranges from 8% to 15% in the general population,[8] the clinical importance of this change in most cases is uncertain given its transitory nature. In only a few of these patients (<1%) will this abnormality extend beyond a few weeks and require the need for renal replacement therapy with either hemodialysis or peritoneal dialysis. In most cases with long-term complications, patients have preexisting evidence of advanced CKD.

In addition to CKD, several other risk factors for developing renal dysfunction after cardiac catheterization and PCI have been identified (Table 5-2). Most importantly, these appear to be related to demographic factors such as advanced age, comorbidities (e.g., diabetes mellitus), periprocedural factors such as hemodynamic instability or heart failure, and evidence of volume depletion.[9] Additional factors include the use of intra-aortic balloon pumps and nephrotoxic medications such as nonsteroidal anti-inflammatory drugs (NSAIDs). A key and potentially modifiable factor is the use of high volumes of contrast agents. Several investigators have suggested a maximum allowable contrast dose that is dependent on the degree of CKD at baseline (Fig. 5-1).[10,11]

Over the last several years, several risk-prediction models have been developed to predict a patient's risk of developing renal dysfunction (and specifically contrast-related nephropathy) after cardiac catheterization and PCI. A recent model by Mehran and colleagues, developed in 8357 patients undergoing PCI, uses eight readily-available variables to calculate an

---

Table 5-1. Concomitant Drugs to Monitor with Exposure to Contrast Agents

Drugs influencing renal hemodynamics
Nonsteroidal anti-inflammatory drugs (NSAIDs)
Cyclooxygenase-2 inhibitors
Nesiritide
Angiotensin-converting enzyme (ACE) inhibitors
Angiotensin receptor blockers
Dipyridamole

Drugs that cause tubular toxicity
Diuretics, including mannitol
Antibiotics, including aminoglycosides, vancomycin,
   amphotericin B
Immunosuppressants, including tacrolimus and cyclosporine A

Drugs with potentially enhanced toxicity after
contrast-induced nephropathy
Metformin
Statins

Adapted from Erley C: Concomitant drugs with exposure to contrast media. Kidney Int Suppl 2006;(100):S20-S24.

Table 5-2. Risk Factors for the Development of Contrast-Induced Nephropathy

Clinical factors
Advanced age
Female gender
Chronic kidney disease
Diabetes mellitus
Peripheral vascular disease
Hypertension
Ejection fraction <40%

Presenting factors
Acute coronary syndrome
Hypotension
Heart failure
Volume depletion
Concomitant nephrotoxic medications
Anemia

Procedural factors
Intra-aortic balloon pump placement
Multivessel disease
Contrast amount
Contrast type

overall risk score for predicting both contrast-related nephropathy and nephropathy requiring dialysis (Fig. 5-2).[12] Variables in this model are scored from 1 to 6 and then summed to generate risks of contrast-related nephropathy ranging from 7.5% to 57.3% and risks of nephropathy requiring dialysis from 0.04% to 12.6%. Use of models such as these allows clinicians to appropriately discuss the potential benefits and risks of cardiac catheterization with high-risk patients before their procedure. It also may help target potential strategies to minimize the risk of developing renal dysfunction.

In most cases, renal dysfunction after cardiac catheterization and PCI is completely reversible and has no apparent long-term effects. Contrast-related nephropathy typically results in a clinical course consistent with acute tubular necrosis and nonoliguric renal dysfunction. Abnormalities in serum creatinine levels start within 24 to 48 hours after the procedure, peak at 5 days, and then completely resolve within 2 to 4 weeks.[13] The need for renal replacement therapy with hemodialysis or peritoneal dialysis is extremely rare.[11] Among those who do require renal replacement therapy, fewer than 50% require it permanently. The requirement for renal replacement

therapy appears to be more likely in the setting of renal atheroembolic disease, which has a more progressive course than contrast-related nephropathy and a lower likelihood of recovery.

Importantly, both the presence of CKD at baseline and the development of renal dysfunction after cardiac catheterization and PCI have been associated with several clinical outcomes unrelated to renal disease. Several studies have shown that patients with CKD at baseline who undergo PCI are at a higher risk of mortality and major adverse clinical events, both in routine cases and in the setting of ST-elevation myocardial infarction.[14,15] In addition, the development of renal dysfunction after cardiac catheterization and PCI has been shown to result in longer hospital stays and greater inpatient costs.[16] Recent reports also suggest that the development of contrast-related nephropathy predicts short- and long-term mortality.[17-20] What remains unclear from this literature, however, is whether the presence of CKD at baseline or the development of renal dysfunction after PCI is simply a marker of greater disease acuity or represents an additional comorbidity like diabetes mellitus.

CHRONIC KIDNEY DISEASE AND END-STAGE RENAL DISEASE

Chronic Kidney Disease

The population of patients with CKD worldwide is growing at a tremendous rate. Consequently, these high-risk patents are now encountered much more frequently in the cardiac catheterization laboratory. In one recent registry, for example, 25% of patients undergoing PCI had at least mild CKD.[14] For the interventional cardiologist, identifying these patients is important for two reasons. First, this group

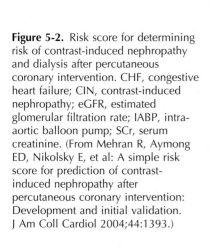

Figure 5-1. Calculation of maximum allowable contrast dose based on degree of chronic kidney disease. (Redrawn from Cigarroa RG, Lange RA, Williams RH, et al: Dosing of contrast material to prevent contrast nephropathy in patients with renal disease. Am J Med 1989;86:649.)

Figure 5-2. Risk score for determining risk of contrast-induced nephropathy and dialysis after percutaneous coronary intervention. CHF, congestive heart failure; CIN, contrast-induced nephropathy; eGFR, estimated glomerular filtration rate; IABP, intra-aortic balloon pump; SCr, serum creatinine. (From Mehran R, Aymong ED, Nikolsky E, et al: A simple risk score for prediction of contrast-induced nephropathy after percutaneous coronary intervention: Development and initial validation. J Am Coll Cardiol 2004;44:1393.)

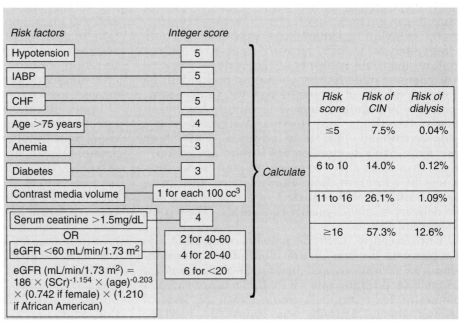

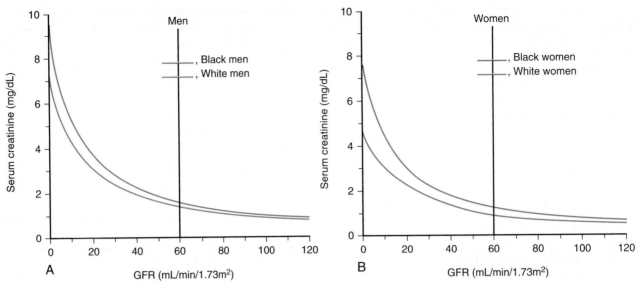

Figure 5-3. Relationship of measured serum creatinine levels to measured glomerular filtration rates in the Modification of Diet in Renal Disease Study in men **(A)** and in women **(B)**. Confidence intervals for serum creatinine levels were wider at lower levels of GFR. (From Levey AS, Bosch JP, Lewis JB, et al: A more accurate method to estimate glomerular filtration rate from serum creatinine: A new prediction equation. Modification of Diet in Renal Disease Study Group [comment]. Ann Intern Med 1999;130:464.)

represents those patients who are at the highest-risk for developing renal dysfunction after PCI and who require specific preventive therapies before their procedure. Second, patients with CKD at baseline are also more likely to have worse cardiovascular outcomes after their procedure. This latter finding results, in part, from the well-established relationship between CKD and cardiovascular disease.

Several clinical factors are useful in identifying individuals at increased risk for CKD. Estimates of the incidence and prevalence of CKD indicate that 20 million people are currently affected in the United States,[21] with diabetes mellitus and hypertension accounting for as much as 70% of the disease burden in this country. Additional clinical factors associated with CKD include autoimmune diseases, systemic infections, urinary stones, lower urinary tract obstruction, reduction in kidney mass, exposure to certain drugs such as NSAIDs, recovery from acute kidney failure, and a family history of kidney disease. Several sociodemographic factors are also useful in identifying individuals at increased risk for CKD. Ethnic minority populations, including African Americans, Native Americans, and Hispanic Americans, bear a disproportionate burden of advanced CKD[22] and are more likely to develop ESRD than are whites.[23] Such disparities also may result, in part, from differences in education, household income, and insurance status.[24,25] Different rates of access to care and to delivery of higher-quality care are also likely to be important factors.[26]

Until recently, defining patients with CKD was problematic because of the multitude of nonstandardized definitions and inaccurate assessments of glomerular filtration rate (GFR). In the cardiovascular literature, for example, a serum creatinine level of greater than 1.5 mg/dL was commonly used to

identify CKD at baseline,[27] whereas levels greater than 2.0 to 2.5 mg/dL have been used to exclude patients from several large cardiovascular randomized clinical trials. Despite its frequent use, the serum creatinine level alone also has several limitations. Most importantly, a normal serum creatinine value does not necessarily reflect normal kidney function, and standard reference ranges for normal often misclassify patients with early disease (Fig. 5-3).[28] Such errors result from the fact that serum creatinine alone does not accurately reflect the level of GFR because of nonlinear relationships that vary according to age, gender, race, and lean body mass. A number of factors other than changes in true GFR account for this relationship (especially in the presence of CKD), including tubular secretion or reabsorption, generation, and extrarenal elimination of the endogenous filtration marker, creatinine. Furthermore, some drugs, such as trimethoprim in Bactrim, can inhibit tubular secretion of creatinine, whereas others, such as noncreatinine chromogens, can interact with common assays used for measurement.

Direct measurements of GFR may be more accurate, but they require either intravenous infusions of exogenous filtration markers such as inulin, iothalamate, iohexol, and ethylenediaminetetraacetic acid (EDTA) or the careful collection of timed urine specimens. However, these methods also have significant measurement errors and are too expensive and difficult to perform in routine practice. Indirect measurements of GFR are obtained by incorporating serum creatinine values into formulas such as the Cockcroft-Gault equation or the Modification of Diet in Renal Disease (MDRD) study equation.[29] Although the MDRD study equation has generally been purported to have less bias, both formulas have limitations in accuracy, especially for patients with normal kidney function.[30] In addition, these formulas do not perform well for many other individuals who were not well represented in the cohorts from which these equations were developed, including those who have very high or very low muscle mass, weight, or age; are severely ill or hospitalized; ingest no meat or large amounts of meat; or are from minority racial and ethnic groups such as Asians or Hispanics.[30] More recently, serum cystatin C has been suggested as a superior alternative to serum creatinine in quantifying GFR in patients with CKD, because cystatin C has a fairly constant rate of production.[30] However, serum levels of cystatin C may also be influenced by age, gender, and muscle mass.[31] In addition, many laboratories are not yet equipped to perform this test.

The National Kidney Foundation now specifically defines CKD as the presence of sustained abnormalities of renal function, manifested by either a reduced GFR or presence of kidney damage. Kidney damage is defined as structural or functional abnormalities of the kidney, in the presence or absence of decreased GFR, that is manifested by either pathologic abnormalities (assessed by renal biopsy) or markers of kidney damage including laboratory abnormalities (in the composition of blood or urine) and radiographic abnormalities (on imaging tests).[29] Once GFR has been assessed, patients with CKD can be stratified into five stages (Table 5-3) in order of increasing impairment: stage 1, GFR $\geq$ 90 mL/min per 1.73 m^2; stage 2, 60-89 mL/min; stage 3, 30-59 mL/min; stage 4, 15-29 mL/min; and stage 5, less than 15 mL/min. Patients with GFRs of 60 mL/min or higher are considered to have CKD if they meet additional criteria, demonstrating evidence of kidney damage based on pathologic, laboratory, or imaging tests. Such markers of kidney damage include proteinuria, abnormalities of the urinary sediment, and abnormal radiologic findings. In all cases, CKD requires that kidney disease has persisted for 3 months or longer.

Patients with advanced CKD are at particularly high risk for complications after interventional procedures, because they are close to requiring initiation of renal replacement therapy but have not yet reached ESRD. They also are far more likely to die or suffer cardiovascular events than to progress to ESRD.[32,33] Even patients with milder forms of CKD are at greater risk for cardiovascular events than for adverse renal outcomes.[34] The risk of adverse outcomes is progressive, with an independent, graded association between reduced GFR and risk of hospitalizations, cardiovascular events, and death.[32,34,35] Consequently, the National Kidney Foundation, the American Heart Association, and the Seventh Joint National Committee on Prevention, Detection, Evaluation, and Treatment of High Blood Pressure have classified the presence of CKD as a cardiovascular risk factor.[29,33,36]

Mechanisms by which renal dysfunction increases cardiovascular risk are unclear and under investigation. The progressive increase in cardiovascular risk associated with declining kidney function is largely explained by a larger burden of traditional risk factors.[37] However, CKD is also associated with many nontraditional risk factors associated with renal decline, including albuminuria, proteinuria, homocysteinemia, elevated uric acid levels, anemia, dysregulation of mineral metabolism and arterial calcification, oxidative stress, inflammation, malnutrition, endothelial dysfunction, insulin resistance, and conditions promoting coagulation, all of which are associated with accelerated atherosclerosis.[27,29,33] Finally, another contributing factor may be the paradox of lower rates of appropriate therapy with risk-factor modification and intervention among CKD patients than in the general population, despite established awareness of their high cardiovascular risk, a concept referred to as "therapeutic nihilism."[38]

End-Stage Renal Disease

Not all patients with CKD go on to develop ESRD; in fact, most die of other, nonrenal causes, especially from cardiovascular disease. However, patients with ESRD who do undergo cardiac catheterization and PCI represent an important group that may be at risk

Table 5-3. Stages of Chronic Kidney Disease (CKD), Action Recommendations, and Prevalence

CKD Stage	Description	GFR (mL/min/1.73 m²)	Action Recommendation	Prevalence (%)
1	Kidney damage with normal or increased GFR	≥90	Diagnosis and treatment Treatment of coexisting conditions Slowing progression CVD risk reduction	2.8
2	Kidney damage with mild decrease in GFR	60-89	Estimation of progression	2.8
3	Moderate decrease in GFR	30-59	Evaluation and treatment of complications	3.7
4	Severe decrease in GFR	15-29	Referral to nephrologist Consideration for renal replacement therapy	0.1
5	Kidney failure	<15 or dialysis	Replacement (if uremia present)	0.2

CVD, cardiovascular disease; GFR, glomerular filtration rate.
Adapted from National Kidney Foundation: K/DOQI clinical practice guidelines for chronic kidney disease: Evaluation, classification, and stratification. Kidney Disease Outcome Quality Initiative. Am J Kidney Dis 2002;39:S1-S266.

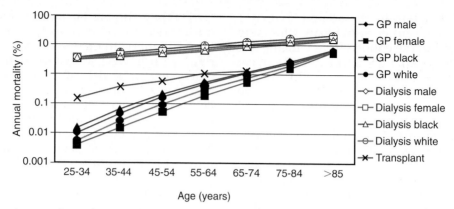

Figure 5-4. Cardiovascular mortality in the general population (GP, data from the National Center for Health Statistics) compared with patients with end-stage renal disease treated by dialysis (data from United States Renal Data System, 1994-1996). (From Sarnak MJ, Levey AS, Schoolwerth AC, et al: Kidney disease as a risk factor for development of cardiovascular disease: A statement from the American Heart Association Councils on Kidney in Cardiovascular Disease, High Blood Pressure Research, Clinical Cardiology, and Epidemiology and Prevention. Circulation 2003;108:2155.)

for intraprocedural as well as short- and long-term complications.

Overall, the epidemiology of ESRD is better understood than that of CKD. In the United States, both the incidence and the prevalence of ESRD have doubled in the past decade and are expected to increase significantly in the future.[23] In 2003, more than 450,000 people required dialysis or transplantation for ESRD in the United States; however, by 2030, estimates suggest that this number will increase to more than 2 million people.[23] The dramatically increased rates of cardiovascular disease and accelerated atherosclerosis have long been recognized in ESRD.[39] More than 50% of deaths among patients with ESRD are caused by cardiovascular events, and more than 20% of cardiac deaths can be attributed to acute myocardial infarction.[40] The 2-year mortality rate after myocardial infarction among patients with ESRD is approximately 50%, twice the mortality rate after myocardial infarction in the general population.[33,40] This excess cardiovascular mortality risk ranges from 500-fold higher in individuals aged 25 to 35 years to fivefold higher in individuals older than 85 years of age (Fig. 5-4).[41]

In most patients who are receiving chronic dialysis, postprocedure dialysis is not routinely needed after exposure to contrast agents.[42,43] But the studies in this area involved only a selected group of patients. So, although it appears that most patients can be maintained on their routine schedule for dialysis, special care and attention may be needed for specific groups, such as those with poor cardiac function or evidence of residual renal function, which is more common among patients treated with peritoneal dialysis.

Relationship of Chronic Kidney Disease and ESRD with Clinical Outcomes

An additional concern regarding patients with advanced CKD and ESRD is the anatomy of their coronary arteries, which are frequently diffusely diseased.[44] These issues can raise technical challenges in the delivery of coronary devices during routine PCI, particularly for those with ESRD caused by extensive coronary calcification. Additional strategies such as rotational atherectomy may be required under these circumstances for plaque modification before coronary stent delivery.

After PCI, the presence of CKD and ESRD is also associated with higher rates of major adverse cardiovascular events, including restenosis and repeat target vessel revascularization. In the era before routine stenting, restenosis was a substantial problem, with rates as high as 80% in patients with ESRD. Although the likelihood of these complications has diminished with the availability of newer devices, there still appears to be an increased risk.[45,46] For example, Rubenstein and colleagues demonstrated that CKD was independently predictive of worse outcomes, including repeat revascularization, in a cohort of 3334 patients undergoing PCI during a period when coronary stenting and atherectomy were being introduced (Fig. 5-5).[46] Within their study population, there also appeared to be no difference between patients with CKD and those with ESRD.[46] Although the data are limited, some reports also have suggested that the development of drug-eluting stents may minimize the risk of restenosis even further in patients with CKD and ESRD.[47,48] This area requires further investigation.

Another critical issue in these patients is determining the risks and benefits of PCI versus surgical revascularization. This is a controversial area, and clinical trials have been unable to directly inform this issue, because most have excluded patients with significant CKD and ESRD. In the absence of adequate clinical trial data, this decision is often individualized and relies on the goals of treatment, the likelihood of technical success with PCI, and the patient's operative risk with bypass surgery.[49,50]

Finally, it is important for the interventional cardiologist to appropriately select and dose adjunctive drug therapy in patients with CKD and ESRD. The

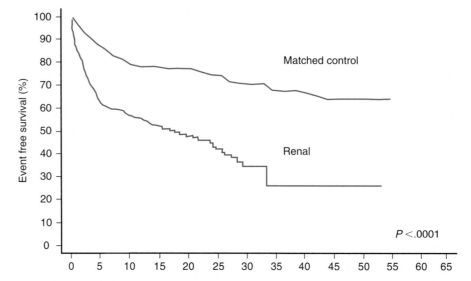

Figure 5-5. Kaplan-Meier event-free survival for major adverse cardiovascular events, including repeat revascularization, in patients with chronic kidney disease including end-stage renal disease (Renal) versus matched control patients undergoing percutaneous coronary intervention. (From Rubenstein MH, Harrell LC, Sheynberg BV, et al: Are patients with renal failure good candidates for percutaneous coronary revascularization in the new device era? Circulation 2000;102:2966.)

risks and benefits of many drugs routinely used as adjunctive therapy in PCI, including glycoprotein IIb/IIIa inhibitors and bivalirudin, need to be carefully weighed in this population because of their diminished renal clearance and potentially increased risk for bleeding.[51,52]

MINIMIZING THE RISK OF RENAL DYSFUNCTION

Patients with CKD often have existing comorbidities that may complicate their procedure and postprocedure management. As always, developing a systematic approach that incorporates the patient's history, physical examination, and laboratory studies is critical. As described earlier, the clinician needs to pay particular attention to accurate assessment of the degree of CKD at baseline, as well as several clinical risk factors that have been consistently associated with poor outcomes in patients with CKD (e.g., diabetes mellitus, hemodynamic instability). Most of the approaches described here are designed to minimize the risk of contrast-related nephropathy, which is the most likely cause of renal dysfunction after

cardiac catheterization and PCI. These approaches are summarized in Table 5-4.

Periprocedural Strategies

Most strategies to reduce the risk of procedural complications in patients with CKD must be considered even before cardiac catheterization and PCI begin. These include measures to carefully prepare the patient with adequate hydration and the use of specific drug therapies.

Hydration

Adequate hydration is a particular concern because most patients are asked to avoid oral intake starting the night before their procedure. They can easily present to the catheterization laboratory in a relatively dehydrated state. It is important to initiate intravenous fluid early in these cases, while carefully monitoring patients with heart failure who may be sensitive to rapid volume changes. The most well-studied fluid regimen in clinical trials has been 0.45%

Table 5-4.   Strategies to Minimize Contrast-Induced Nephropathy in At-Risk Patients

Periprocedural strategies	
Hydration	0.9 NS 1 mL/kg/hr starting 6 to 12 hr before and after procedure or D5W with sodium bicarbonate 154 mEq/L at 3 mL/kg/hr starting 1 hr before procedure and continuing at 1 mL/kg/hr for 6 hr after procedure
N-Acetylcysteine	600-1200 mg orally twice daily starting the day before the procedure for 2 days
Ascorbic acid	3 g orally 2 hr before procedure and 2 g orally two times the next day
Hemofiltration	Starting 4-6 hr before the procedure and continued for 18-24 hr after
Intraprocedural strategies	
Avoid nephrotoxic medications (e.g., NSAIDs)	
Minimize use of contrast agents	Selective left ventriculography, smaller catheters, biplane coronary angiography
Use low- or iso-osmolar contrast agents	

D5W, 5% dextrose in water; NS, normal saline; NSAIDs, nonsteroidal anti-inflammatory drugs.

normal saline infusions at a rate of 1 mL/kg/hour for 6 to 12 hours before the procedure and continuing after the procedure.[53] Data from a large trial suggested that the substitution of isotonic saline for 0.45% normal saline may modestly reduce the incidence of contrast-related nephropathy, particularly among patients with diabetes mellitus and those receiving large doses of contrast agents.[54] In a small clinical trial of 36 patients with serum creatinine levels at baseline equal to or greater than 1.4 mg/dL, it was demonstrated that 1 L orally followed by 6 hours of intravenous hydration starting at the time of contrast agent exposure was equivalent to preprocedural intravenous hydration.[55] This approach may be more realistic for outpatients who come in the day of their procedure.

From a practical standpoint, a quick assessment of the adequacy of hydration is possible before contrast injection by assessing the left ventricular end-diastolic pressure with a pigtail or multipurpose catheter even if a pulmonary capillary wedge pressure is unavailable. If the patient appears to be dehydrated based on hemodynamic parameters, then fluid boluses may be given intermittently before contrast agent exposure.

Recently, there has been great interest in the use of sodium bicarbonate infusions to hydrate patients with CKD during the periprocedural period. Sodium bicarbonate may relieve oxidative stress, which is a possible mechanism of action by which contrast-related nephropathy occurs. In a recently published clinical trial, 119 patients with serum creatinine levels equal to or greater than 1.1 mg/dL who were undergoing diagnostic catheterization were randomly assigned to receive either sodium bicarbonate or sodium chloride boluses and infusions before and after their procedure.[56] Although those who received sodium bicarbonate were significantly less likely to develop contrast-related nephropathy, some have raised methodologic concerns about this study, particularly because of its early unscheduled termination. However, the major benefit of this approach is that it requires no new procedures, but simply replaces one infusion with another.

Medications

Several medications have also been used to reduce the risk of contrast-related nephropathy. The most extensively studied of these agents is N-acetylcysteine, which has been evaluated in at least 20 randomized clinical trials.[57] The premise behind the use of N-acetylcysteine is that it acts as a scavenger of reactive oxygen species and promotes vasodilatory effects in the renal medulla. The first of these trials was reported by Tepel and colleagues, who evaluated its use in 83 patients receiving intravenous contrast agents for computed tomography.[58] They found a relative risk reduction of approximately 90% in contrast-related nephropathy with the use of acetylcysteine, but not all studies have shown a consistent

benefit. In total, the evidence suggests that there is a potential benefit with its use. It is certainly reasonable to consider its use in high-risk patients, given its good safety profile and low cost.

The most commonly studied regimen for N-acetylcysteine has been 600 mg orally, given twice a day starting 1 day before the procedure, but there is evidence that other routes of administration are effective and that higher doses may result in even better clinical outcomes. In one study, intravenous N-acetylcysteine was prepared as 150 mg/kg in 500 mL 0.9% saline and given over 30 minutes starting just before contrast agent exposure.[59] This study demonstrated efficacy with the use of intravenous N-acetylcysteine, and this may be an effective alternate regimen if time constraints prevent its oral use. Most recently, in a provocative trial of 354 patients, the use of N-acetylcysteine routinely in all patients undergoing primary PCI for ST-elevation myocardial infarction, regardless of serum creatinine levels at baseline, also demonstrated benefit.[60] Not only did it prevent the development of contrast-related nephropathy, but, remarkably, its use led to a reduction in in-hospital deaths. In this study, there appeared to be dose-dependent effects, with a higher dose of N-acetylcysteine (1200 mg bolus intravenously, followed by 1200 mg orally twice a day for 2 days) being superior to standard doses.

Another important medication that has been studied extensively in randomized clinical trials is fenoldapem. Fenoldapem works as a dopamine-receptor agonist and is believed to preserve renal blood flow despite insults from contrast agent exposure. A series of small clinical studies had suggested significant benefit in the reduction of contrast-related nephropathy, particularly in high-risk patients.[61,62] However, enthusiasm for fenoldapem has fallen since publication of the large, multicenter CONTRAST trial in 2003.[63] In that study, no benefit was seen with fenoldapem in 315 patients with estimated GFRs of less than 60 mL/min who underwent cardiac catheterization.

Additional agents that have been studied include ascorbic acid, captopril, theophylline (or aminophylline), dopamine, atrial natriuretic peptides, calcium channel blockers, and prostaglandin E_1. Most of these agents have been studied in only a few trials (ascorbic acid[64]) or have produced conflicting results (theophylline[65]). Their routine use cannot be recommended. Medications that should be avoided unless otherwise indicated include mannitol or furosemide for forced diuresis (without hemodynamic monitoring), given their potential to result in volume depletion and to exacerbate renal dysfunction.[53]

Other Strategies

Several other nonpharmacologic strategies have been suggested as approaches for minimizing renal dysfunction after cardiac catheterization and PCI. However, many of these strategies require intense resources, and their use is limited to the highest-risk patients.

The use of forced diuresis with a combination of intravenous hydration, furosemide, dopamine, and mannitol may be valuable, but only if implemented after the measurement of right- and left-sided filling pressures with adjustments made according to baseline pressures.[66] In this setting, with a careful protocol to ensure adequate hydration, one clinical trial suggested that the use of forced diuresis led to higher urine flow rates. However, only modest clinical benefits were noted in regard to serum creatinine levels and the incidence of contrast-related nephropathy.

Another approach that has been suggested is the routine use of hemodialysis or hemofiltration after or during contrast agent exposure. Although contrast agents can be effectively removed from blood by hemodialysis, several studies have suggested that use of hemodialysis is not associated with better clinical outcomes.[43] One explanation for the lack of efficacy is that hemodialysis may result in hemodynamic or inflammatory changes that are nephrotoxic and offset the benefit of removal of contrast agents. To better address this issue, Marenzi and colleagues recently studied the use of hemofiltration in 114 patients with severe CKD undergoing PCI.[67] Hemofiltration has the advantage of avoiding hypovolemia, and it can provide high-volume hydration without concerns of intravascular congestion. In this group, the use of hemofiltration starting at least 4 to 6 hours before PCI was associated with improved clinical outcomes, including lower rates of renal replacement therapy, in-hospital mortality, and 1-year mortality. The intensive resources required for this intervention limit its use to tertiary-care centers and the highest-risk patients.

Finally, another recently proposed mechanism for contrast agent removal after cardiac catheterization is coronary sinus cannulation followed by contrast agent removal with an extracorporeal absorbing column.[68] The feasibility of this system was demonstrated in a swine model and awaits human use.

Intraprocedural Strategies

Intraprocedural strategies for patients with CKD largely depend on (1) the choice of contrast agent, (2) minimizing the volume that is used, and (3) avoiding use of potentially nephrotoxic medications. However, this must be done without sacrificing the operator's ability to adequately and safely perform the procedure, which always requires a careful balance. Appropriate visualization of the lesion and adjacent coronary anatomy is essential for success during PCI and should not be sacrificed.

General strategies to consider include the use of smaller guiding catheters whenever possible, because they are associated with lower volumes of contrast agents. It is also important to minimize the use of contrast agents during the diagnostic portion of the case if ad hoc PCI is performed. This can be done by avoiding left ventriculograms and using noninvasive tests such as echocardiography to evaluate systolic wall motion and function. The use of biplane coronary angiography, which allows the operator to obtain two simultaneous views with one injection during cineangiography, is another commonly used tool.

Choice and Use of Contrast Agent

The choice of contrast agent is an important intraprocedural consideration and has evolved considerably over the last several years with the development of low- and iso-osmolar contrast agents. Traditional iodine-based contrast agents were hypertonic and included ionic compounds such as diatrizoate (Hypaque, Renografin) that frequently caused mild hemodynamic changes in addition to contrast-related nephropathy. Given substantially lower costs in recent years, most laboratories have switched to the routine use of low-osmolar, non-ionic contrast agents for improved hemodynamic effects and patient comfort. An important effect of low-osmolar agents is believed to be reductions in contrast-related nephropathy. In a meta-analysis that included data from 25 trials, the risk of contrast-related nephropathy was 39% lower in patients who received low-osmolar contrast agents, compared with hypertonic contrast agents.[69] This benefit appeared to be even more pronounced in patients with preexisting renal disease, with a 50% risk reduction in that population.

More recently, the introduction of iodixanol (Visipaque), an iso-osmolar contrast agent, has raised the question of whether the incidence of contrast-related nephropathy can be further reduced. In a widely cited study of patients with CKD and diabetes mellitus, the use of iso-osmolar contrast agents reduced the incidence of contrast-related nephropathy by more than 90%, compared with low-osmolar contrast agents.[70] An additional study comparing these two types of contrast agents also suggested a reduction in major adverse cardiovascular events with the use of iso-osmolar contrast in patients undergoing high-risk PCI.[71]

Finally, some investigators have begun to use alternative, non–iodine-based contrast agents such as gadolinium, particularly for peripheral angiography. Although case reports of its use in the coronary circulation do exist, many questions remain regarding the overall safety and feasibility of this approach, particularly given the high serum osmolality of these agents.[72,73]

Regardless of the selection of a contrast agent, it is imperative that the least amount of volume required for adequate visualization of the coronary artery and technical success of the procedure be used. For patients who are at particularly high risk, the maximum allowable contrast dose should be calculated before the procedure, so that the interventional cardiologist and team can be aware of its use during the procedure. Staging of nonurgent procedures is also a possibility in many settings and will minimize the risk of developing contrast-related nephropathy. Unfortunately, there are few data on how long one should wait before staging procedures.

REFERENCES

1. Persson PB, Tepel M: Contrast medium-induced nephropathy: The pathophysiology. Kidney Int Suppl 2006;(100):S8-S10.
2. Katholi RE, Woods WT Jr, Taylor GJ, et al: Oxygen free radicals and contrast nephropathy. Am J Kidney Dis 1998;32:64-71.
3. Toprak O, Cirit M: Risk factors for contrast-induced nephropathy. Kidney Blood Press Res 2006;29:84-93.
4. Fukumoto Y, Tsutsui H, Tsuchihashi M, et al: The incidence and risk factors of cholesterol embolization syndrome, a complication of cardiac catheterization: A prospective study. J Am Coll Cardiol 2003;42:211-216.
5. Mannesse CK, Blankestijn PJ, Man in 't Veld AJ, et al: Renal failure and cholesterol crystal embolization: A report of 4 surviving cases and a review of the literature. Clin Nephrol 1991;36:240-245.
6. Erley C: Concomitant drugs with exposure to contrast media. Kidney Int Suppl 2006;(100):S20-S24.
7. Hyman BT, Landas SK, Ashman RF, et al: Warfarin-related purple toes syndrome and cholesterol microembolization. Am J Med 1987;82:1233-1237.
8. Barrett BJ, Parfrey PS: Clinical practice: Preventing nephropathy induced by contrast medium. N Engl J Med 2006; 354:379-386.
9. Mehran R, Nikolsky E: Contrast-induced nephropathy: Definition, epidemiology, and patients at risk. Kidney Int Suppl 2006;(100):S11-S15.
10. Cigarroa RG, Lange RA, Williams RH, et al: Dosing of contrast material to prevent contrast nephropathy in patients with renal disease. Am J Med 1989;86:649-652.
11. Freeman RV, O'Donnell M, Share D, et al: Nephropathy requiring dialysis after percutaneous coronary intervention and the critical role of an adjusted contrast dose. Am J Cardiol 2002;90:1068-1073.
12. Mehran R, Aymong ED, Nikolsky E, et al: A simple risk score for prediction of contrast-induced nephropathy after percutaneous coronary intervention: Development and initial validation. J Am Coll Cardiol 2004;44:1393-1399.
13. McCullough PA, Sandberg KR: Epidemiology of contrast-induced nephropathy. Rev Cardiovasc Med 2003;4(Suppl 5): S3-S9.
14. Blackman DJ, Pinto R, Ross JR, et al: Impact of renal insufficiency on outcome after contemporary percutaneous coronary intervention. Am Heart J 2006;151:146-152.
15. Sadeghi HM, Stone GW, Grines CL, et al: Impact of renal insufficiency in patients undergoing primary angioplasty for acute myocardial infarction. Circulation 2003;108: 2769-2775.
16. McCullough PA, Wolyn R, Rocher LL, et al: Acute renal failure after coronary intervention: Incidence, risk factors, and relationship to mortality. Am J Med 1997;103:368-375.
17. Rihal CS, Textor SC, Grill DE, et al: Incidence and prognostic importance of acute renal failure after percutaneous coronary intervention. Circulation 2002;105:2259-2264.
18. Marenzi G, Lauri G, Assanelli E, et al: Contrast-induced nephropathy in patients undergoing primary angioplasty for acute myocardial infarction. J Am Coll Cardiol 2004;44: 1780-1785.
19. Bartholomew BA, Harjai KJ, Dukkipati S, et al: Impact of nephropathy after percutaneous coronary intervention and a method for risk stratification. Am J Cardiol 2004;93:1515-1519.
20. Gupta R, Gurm HS, Bhatt DL, et al: Renal failure after percutaneous coronary intervention is associated with high mortality. Catheter Cardiovasc Interv 2005;64:442-448.
21. Coresh J, Astor BC, Greene T, et al: Prevalence of chronic kidney disease and decreased kidney function in the adult US population: Third National Health and Nutrition Examination Survey. Am J Kidney Dis 2003;41:1-12.
22. Hsu CY, Lin F, Vittinghoff E, et al: Racial differences in the progression from chronic renal insufficiency to end-stage renal disease in the United States. J Am Soc Nephrol 2003;14:2902-2907.
23. U.S. Renal Data System, USRDS 2005 Annual Data Report: Atlas of End-Stage Renal Disease in the United States. Bethesda, MD, National Institutes of Health, National Institute of Diabetes and Digestive and Kidney Diseases, 2005.
24. Tarver-Carr ME, Powe NR, Eberhardt MS, et al: Excess risk of chronic kidney disease among African-American versus white subjects in the United States: A population-based study of potential explanatory factors. J Am Soc Nephrol 2002; 13:2363-2370.
25. Kinchen KS, Sadler J, Fink N, et al: The timing of specialist evaluation in chronic kidney disease and mortality. Ann Intern Med 2002;137:479-486.
26. Powe NR, Melamed ML: Racial disparities in the optimal delivery of chronic kidney disease care. Med Clin North Am 2005;89:475-488.
27. Best PJ, Reddan DN, Berger PB, et al: Cardiovascular disease and chronic kidney disease: Insights and an update. Am Heart J 2004;148:230-242.
28. Levey AS, Bosch JP, Lewis JB, et al: A more accurate method to estimate glomerular filtration rate from serum creatinine: A new prediction equation. Modification of Diet in Renal Disease Study Group [comment]. Ann Intern Med 1999;130: 461-470.
29. National Kidney Foundation: K/DOQI clinical practice guidelines for chronic kidney disease: Evaluation, classification, and stratification. Kidney Disease Outcome Quality Initiative. Am J Kidney Dis 2002;39:S1-S266.
30. Stevens LA, Coresh J, Greene T, et al: Assessing kidney function: Measured and estimated glomerular filtration rate. N Engl J Med 2006;354:2473-2483.
31. Knight EL, Verhave JC, Spiegelman D, et al: Factors influencing serum cystatin C levels other than renal function and the impact on renal function measurement. Kidney Int 2004; 65:1416-1421.
32. Go AS, Chertow GM, Fan D, et al: Chronic kidney disease and the risks of death, cardiovascular events, and hospitalization. N Engl J Med 2004;351:1296-1305.
33. Sarnak MJ, Levey AS, Schoolwerth AC, et al: Kidney disease as a risk factor for development of cardiovascular disease: A statement from the American Heart Association Councils on Kidney in Cardiovascular Disease, High Blood Pressure Research, Clinical Cardiology, and Epidemiology and Prevention. Circulation 2003;108:2154-2169.
34. Patel UD, Young EW, Ojo AO, et al: CKD progression and mortality among older patients with diabetes. Am J Kidney Dis 2005;46:406-414.
35. Anavekar NS, Gans DJ, Berl T, et al: Predictors of cardiovascular events in patients with type 2 diabetic nephropathy and hypertension: A case for albuminuria. Kidney Int Suppl 2004;(92):S50-S55.
36. Chobanian AV, Bakris GL, Black HR, et al: The Seventh Report of the Joint National Committee on Prevention, Detection, Evaluation, and Treatment of High Blood Pressure: The JNC 7 report [comment] [erratum appears in JAMA 2003 Jul 9;290(2):197]. JAMA 2003;289:2560-2572.
37. Shlipak MG, Fried LF, Cushman M, et al: Cardiovascular mortality risk in chronic kidney disease: Comparison of traditional and novel risk factors. JAMA 2005;293:1737-1745.
38. Anavekar NS, McMurray JJ, Velazquez EJ, et al: Relation between renal dysfunction and cardiovascular outcomes after myocardial infarction. N Engl J Med 2004;351:1285-1295.
39. Lindner A, Charra B, Sherrard DJ, et al: Accelerated atherosclerosis in prolonged maintenance hemodialysis. N Engl J Med 1974;290:697-701.
40. Herzog CA, Ma JZ, Collins AJ: Poor long-term survival after acute myocardial infarction among patients on long-term dialysis. N Engl J Med 1998;339:799-805.
41. Levey AS, Beto JA, Coronado BE, et al: Controlling the epidemic of cardiovascular disease in chronic renal disease: What do we know? What do we need to learn? Where do we go from here? National Kidney Foundation Task Force on Cardiovascular Disease. Am J Kidney Dis 1998;32:853-906.

42. Hamani A, Petitclerc T, Jacobs C, et al: Is dialysis indicated immediately after administration of iodinated contrast agents in patients on haemodialysis? Nephrol Dial Transplant 1998; 13:1051-1052.

43. Deray G: Dialysis and iodinated contrast media. Kidney Int Suppl 2006;(100):S25-S29.

44. Bocksch W, Fateh-Moghadam S, Mueller E, et al: Percutaneous coronary intervention in patients with end-stage renal disease. Kidney Blood Press Res 2005;28:275-279.

45. Azar RR, Prpic R, Ho KK, et al: Impact of end-stage renal disease on clinical and angiographic outcomes after coronary stenting. Am J Cardiol 2000;86:485-489.

46. Rubenstein MH, Harrell LC, Sheynberg BV, et al: Are patients with renal failure good candidates for percutaneous coronary revascularization in the new device era? Circulation 2000; 102:2966-2972.

47. Daemen J, Lemos P, Aoki J, et al: Treatment of coronary artery disease in dialysis patients with sirolimus-eluting stents: 1-Year clinical follow-up of a consecutive series of cases. J Invasive Cardiol 2004;16:685-687.

48. Halkin A, Mehran R, Casey CW, et al: Impact of moderate renal insufficiency on restenosis and adverse clinical events after paclitaxel-eluting and bare metal stent implantation: Results from the TAXUS-IV Trial. Am Heart J 2005;150: 1163-1170.

49. Reddan DN, Szczech LA, Tuttle RH, et al: Chronic kidney disease, mortality, and treatment strategies among patients with clinically significant coronary artery disease. J Am Soc Nephrol 2003;14:2373-2380.

50. Williams M: Coronary revascularization in diabetic chronic kidney disease/end-stage renal disease: A nephrologist's perspective. Clin J Am Soc Nephrol 2006;1:209-220.

51. Freeman RV, Mehta RH, Al Badr W, et al: Influence of concurrent renal dysfunction on outcomes of patients with acute coronary syndromes and implications of the use of glycoprotein IIb/IIIa inhibitors. J Am Coll Cardiol 2003;41:718-724.

52. Alexander KP, Chen AY, Roe MT, et al: Excess dosing of antiplatelet and antithrombin agents in the treatment of non-ST-segment elevation acute coronary syndromes. JAMA 2005; 294:3108-3116.

53. Solomon R, Werner C, Mann D, et al: Effects of saline, mannitol, and furosemide to prevent acute decreases in renal function induced by radiocontrast agents. N Engl J Med 1994; 331:1416-1420.

54. Mueller C, Buerkle G, Buettner HJ, et al: Prevention of contrast media-associated nephropathy: Randomized comparison of 2 hydration regimens in 1620 patients undergoing coronary angioplasty. Arch Intern Med 2002;162:329-336.

55. Taylor AJ, Hotchkiss D, Morse RW, et al: PREPARED: Preparation for Angiography in Renal Dysfunction: A randomized trial of inpatient vs outpatient hydration protocols for cardiac catheterization in mild-to-moderate renal dysfunction. Chest 1998;114:1570-1574.

56. Merten GJ, Burgess WP, Gray LV, et al: Prevention of contrast-induced nephropathy with sodium bicarbonate: A randomized controlled trial. JAMA 2004;291:2328-2334.

57. Nallamothu BK, Shojania KG, Saint S, et al: Is acetylcysteine effective in preventing contrast-related nephropathy? A meta-analysis. Am J Med 2004;117:938-947.

58. Tepel M, van der Giet M, Schwarzfeld C, et al: Prevention of radiographic-contrast-agent-induced reductions in renal function by acetylcysteine. N Engl J Med 2000;343:180-184.

59. Baker CS, Wragg A, Kumar S, et al: A rapid protocol for the prevention of contrast-induced renal dysfunction: The RAPPID study. J Am Coll Cardiol 2003;41:2114-2118.

60. Marenzi G, Assanelli E, Marana I, et al: N-Acetylcysteine and contrast-induced nephropathy in primary angioplasty. N Engl J Med 2006;354:2773-2782.

61. Madyoon H, Croushore L, Weaver D, et al: Use of fenoldopam to prevent radiocontrast nephropathy in high-risk patients. Catheter Cardiovasc Interv 2001;53:341-345.

62. Kini AS, Mitre CA, Kamran M, et al: Changing trends in incidence and predictors of radiographic contrast nephropathy after percutaneous coronary intervention with use of fenoldopam. Am J Cardiol 2002;89:999-1002.

63. Stone GW, McCullough PA, Tumlin JA, et al: Fenoldopam mesylate for the prevention of contrast-induced nephropathy: A randomized controlled trial. JAMA 2003;290:2284-2291.

64. Spargias K, Alexopoulos E, Kyrzopoulos S, et al: Ascorbic acid prevents contrast-mediated nephropathy in patients with renal dysfunction undergoing coronary angiography or intervention. Circulation 2004;110:2837-2842.

65. Bagshaw SM, Ghali WA: Theophylline for prevention of contrast-induced nephropathy: A systematic review and meta-analysis. Arch Intern Med 2005;165:1087-1093.

66. Stevens MA, McCullough PA, Tobin KJ, et al: A prospective randomized trial of prevention measures in patients at high risk for contrast nephropathy: Results of the P.R.I.N.C.E. Study. Prevention of Radiocontrast Induced Nephropathy Clinical Evaluation. J Am Coll Cardiol 1999;33:403-411.

67. Marenzi G, Bartorelli AL: Hemofiltration in the prevention of radiocontrast agent induced nephropathy. Minerva Anestesiol 2004;70:189-191.

68. Michishita I, Fujii Z: A novel contrast removal system from the coronary sinus using an adsorbing column during coronary angiography in a porcine model. J Am Coll Cardiol 2006;47:1866-1870.

69. Barrett BJ, Carlisle EJ: Metaanalysis of the relative nephrotoxicity of high- and low-osmolality iodinated contrast media. Radiology 1993;188:171-178.

70. Aspelin P, Aubry P, Fransson SG, et al: Nephrotoxic effects in high-risk patients undergoing angiography. N Engl J Med 2003;348:491-499.

71. Davidson CJ, Laskey WK, Hermiller JB, et al: Randomized trial of contrast media utilization in high-risk PTCA: The COURT trial. Circulation 2000;101:2172-2177.

72. Sarkis A, Badaoui G, Azar R, et al: Gadolinium-enhanced coronary angiography in patients with impaired renal function. Am J Cardiol 2003;91:974-975, A4.

73. Bokhari SW, Wen YH, Winters RJ: Gadolinium-based percutaneous coronary intervention in a patient with renal insufficiency. Catheter Cardiovasc Interv 2003;58:358-361.

CHAPTER

6 Evidence-Based Interventional Practice

Franz-Josef Neumann and Heinz Joachim Büttner

KEY POINTS

- When coronary revascularization is considered, prognostic and symptomatic indications need to be distinguished.
- In general, percutaneous coronary intervention (PCI) for single-vessel disease is justified only if improvement of symptoms can be anticipated.
- In patients with multivessel disease without relevant left main coronary artery involvement and without diabetes mellitus, survival after PCI is similar to that after coronary artery bypass grafting (CABG), provided that complete revascularization can be achieved.
- In patients with diabetes mellitus, it is unclear whether multivessel PCI can achieve a prognostic benefit similar

to that of CABG. Depending on the chances for success and the risks for surgery, multivessel PCI may offer a reasonable option in diabetic patients.
- Currently available evidence does not allow proposing PCI for distal left main coronary artery disease in patients who are good candidates for surgery. PCI appears to be an acceptable alternative to CABG in poor surgical candidates.
- In many instances, individualized decisions must be taken jointly by the cardiac surgeon and the interventional cardiologist.

CHANGING PARADIGMS OF CORONARY REVASCULARIZATION

When the era of interventional cardiology began with the pioneering work of Andreas Grüntzig on plain balloon angioplasty, percutaneous coronary intervention (PCI) was a treatment option only for isolated proximal coronary lesions not involving the ostia or the left main stem. In the late 1980s, coronary stents were developed with the goals of reducing the risk of restenosis and achieving a more predictable acute result of angioplasty, thus avoiding the dreaded abrupt closure due to dissection. As shown subsequently, stents were successful in achieving this goal. Nevertheless, they created a new problem: subacute stent thrombosis. After intense research on peri-interventional and postinterventional antithrombotic treatment, the concept of dual or triple antiplatelet therapy emerged, which largely resolved the issue of subacute stent thrombosis. The use of coronary stents in conjunction with optimized antithrombotic treatment extended the spectrum of coronary lesions for which PCI was considered a reasonable treatment option and thereby led to a substantial expansion of interventional techniques. With the large number of patients being treated with coronary stents, restenosis due to neointima formation became a serious problem. Although

various studies demonstrated that stents reduce the need for reintervention compared with plain balloon angioplasty,[1-3] restenosis rates continued to be relevant, ranging from just above 10% in the most simple lesions to more than 50% with diffuse disease in patients with diabetes.

Therefore, it is not surprising that the community of interventional cardiologists celebrated the advent of the new drug-eluting stents as a major breakthrough, given that the initial studies suggested zero restenosis rates. It has become clear that drug-eluting stents reduce the need for target vessel reintervention by about 80% compared with a bare metal stent, thereby largely reducing but not eliminating the problem of restenosis. Subsequently, drug-eluting stents led to another massive expansion of the proportion of patients treated with PCI. With the widespread use of drug-eluting stents for PCI, reports appeared pointing toward a new problem that was not perceived with bare metal stents: late (>30 days to 1 year) and very late (>1 year after stent implantation) stent thrombosis. Thorough reevaluation of the data from randomized trials with uniform application of definitions for definite, probable, and possible stent thrombosis showed no difference in stent thrombosis rates between drug-eluting stents and bare metal stents until 1 year after stent implantation.[4-7] However, there was evidence of a slight, 0.1%

to 0.2% per year increase in the risk of very late stent thrombosis associated with drug-eluting stents until 4 years after stent implantation. Although there were no significant differences in the cumulative rates for death or myocardial infarction at 4 years, as compared to bare metal stents, the impact of drug-eluting stents on serious late complications is a major scientific and clinical challenge, due to their overall low incidence and the long follow-up periods needed. A tradeoff between the marked reduction in target vessel revascularization on one hand and death or myocardial infarction (MI) on the other hand would not be acceptable in the presence of alternative treatment options such as bare metal stents or bypass surgery. (A list of trial abbreviations and acronyms is presented in Table 6-1.)

Despite remaining issues to be addressed, the use of PCI has increased exponentially over the past decades. Initially, this increase came at the expense of lone medical therapy. However, with the advent of drug-eluting stents, there has been a shift of patients with multivessel disease and other complex coronary anatomies from CABG to PCI. In many countries, this has led to a decrease in CABG procedures, sometimes by as much as 20% per year, because the demographically driven increase in numbers of patients needing coronary revascularization could not compensate for the shift from surgery to interventional cardiology. This shift from surgery to PCI has been facilitated by both physician and patient preference to take the supposedly easier approach to coronary revascularization, given the conception that the problem of restenosis has been largely solved. However, there is reasonable concern that this has led to overuse of PCI and that in many patients PCI, as the easier approach, may not yield the same outcome as CABG, which for a number of indications is an established treatment option with a well-documented survival benefit compared with medical therapy.

SCOPE OF THIS CHAPTER

When comparing PCI with lone medical treatment or bypass surgery, it is important to scrutinize the evidence indicating that PCI offers at least equal benefit to CABG on the one hand, or superior benefit to lone medical treatment on the other hand. A number of randomized studies and analyses from large-scale registries have been performed. Despite this large database, currently available evidence is difficult to interpret for two reasons. First, because of rapid technologic and pharmacologic development in both the surgical and the interventional field, the therapeutic approaches often are outdated by the time the results of a study appear. Second, with any of the modern treatments, mortality, the most important benchmark for studies, is so low that huge numbers of patients are needed to assess this end point. Therefore, most studies concentrate either on surrogate end points or composite end points that combine events of diverse clinical importance (e.g.,

Table 6-1. Trial Abbreviations and Acronyms

ACIP	Asymptomatic Cardiac Ischemia Pilot study
ACME	Angioplasty Compared to Medicine
APPROACH	Alberta Provincial Project for Outcome Assessment in Coronary Heart Disease
ARTS	Arterial Revascularization Therapies Study
AVERT	Atorvastatin versus Revascularization Treatments
AWESOME	Angina With Extremely Serious Operative Mortality Evaluation
BARI	Bypass Angioplasty Revascularization Investigation
CABRI	Coronary Angioplasty versus Bypass Revascularization Investigation
CASS	Coronary Artery Surgery Study
COMBAT	Randomized Comparison of Bypass Surgery versus Angioplasty Using Sirolimus-Eluting Stent in Patients With Left Main Coronary Artery Disease
COURAGE	Clinical Outcomes Utilizing Revascularization and Aggressive Drug Evaluation
EAST	Emory Angioplasty versus Surgery Trial
ECSS	European Coronary Surgery Study
ERACI	Argentine Randomized Trial of Percutaneous Transluminal Coronary Angioplasty Versus Coronary Artery Bypass Surgery in Multivessel Disease
FREEDOM	Future Revascularization Evaluation in Patients with Diabetes Mellitus: Optimal Management of Multivessel Disease
FRISC	Fragmin and Revascularization during Instability in Coronary Artery Disease
GABI	German Angioplasty Bypass Surgery Investigation
ICTUS	Invasive versus Conservative Treatment in Unstable Coronary Syndromes
ISAR-SWEET	Intracoronary Stenting and Antithrombotic Regimen: Is Abciximab a Superior Way to Eliminate Elevated Thrombotic Risk in Diabetics?
MASS	Medicine, Angioplasty or Surgery Study
MATE	Medicine versus Angiography in Thrombolytic Exclusion
RESEARCH	Rapamycin-Eluting Stent Evaluated At Rotterdam Cardiology Hospital [registry]
RITA	Randomized Intervention Treatment of Angina
SIMA	Stenting versus Internal Mammary Artery
SoS	Stent or Surgery Trial
SYNTAX	Synergy Between PCI with Taxus Drug-Eluting Stent and Cardiac Surgery
TACTICS	Treat Angina with Aggrastat and Determine Cost of Therapy with an Invasive or Conservative Strategy
TIMI	Thrombolysis in Myocardial Infarction
TRUCS	Treatment of Refractory Unstable Angina without Cardiac Surgery
T-SEARCH	Taxus-Stent Evaluated At Rotterdam Cardiology Hospital registry
VA-Study	Veterans Administration Cooperative Study
VANQWISH	Veterans Affairs Non-Q-Wave Myocardial Infarction Strategies In-Hospital
VINO	Value of First Day Angiography/Angioplasty in Evolving Non-ST Segment Elevation Myocardial Infarction: An Open Multicenter Randomized Trial

death and target vessel revascularization). Despite these difficulties, it is important to make therapeutic decisions on the basis of evidence as much as possible. This review summarizes and discusses the evidence that is currently available to present a rationale for clinical decision-making.

Pharmacologic therapy and coronary revacularization by either CABG or PCI are the mainstays of treatment for coronary artery disease. The prime objective of such treatment is improved survival (prognostic indication); other reasonable treatment goals are relief of symptoms and improved quality of life (symptomatic indication). In pursuing these goals, prevention of MI is a key issue that pertains to both survival and quality of life. When deciding about the optimal revascularization strategy in a patient with coronary artery disease, it is necessary to first determine whether there is a prognostic or symptomatic indication for coronary revascularization and then choose the most appropriate revascularization modality.

This chapter intends to present criteria for both of these elements in clinical decision-making about coronary revascularization. It focuses primarily on the prognostic indication for coronary revascularization. Based on a review of the general criteria for indication of revascularization, the efficacy and safety of PCI compared with CABG are discussed. Thereafter, the role of PCI in symptomatic indications for coronary revascularization is addressed, predominantly in comparison with lone medical therapy. The focus is on stable coronary disease. Acute coronary syndromes, including MI, are touched on only briefly, because they are discussed in depth in other chapters.

CRITERIA FOR PROGNOSTIC INDICATION OF CORONARY REVASCULARIZATION

Role of Clinical Presentation

ST-Segment Elevation Myocardial Infarction

In acute MI, fibrinolysis reduces the mortality rate by 18%, compared with conservative treatment, as was shown by a meta-analysis of the randomized trials in this setting.[8] In addition to this benefit, coronary reperfusion by primary PCI reduces in-hospital mortality by an additional 35%.[9] This risk reduction is consistent with the pooled analysis of registry data of more than 100,000 patients (Fig. 6-1). In addition to its effect on survival, PCI compared with fibrinolysis reduces the risk of reinfarction and of stroke, particularly that of hemorrhagic stroke.[10] The initial benefit is maintained during long-term follow-up.[10] The largest survival benefit with PCI is obtained when the delay conferred by PCI compared with fibrinolysis is shorter than 35 minutes.[9] Nevertheless, even with delays ranging between 35 and 120 minutes, there is a significant survival benefit with PCI, about 18% on average.[9] Beyond 2 hours of delay between PCI and fibrinolysis, however, a benefit from PCI as compared with fibrinolysis cannot be shown with currently available data. Although fibrinolysis is more effective within the first 1 to 3 hours after onset of pain than after longer delays, the benefit from PCI compared with fibrinolysis is largely independent of

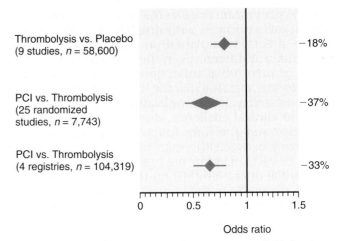

Figure 6-1. Reperfusion strategies in acute myocardial infarction. The diamonds indicate the odds ratio for death with 95% confidence intervals. PCI, percutaneous coronary intervention.

the time from onset of pain to intervention.[9] CABG in the setting of MI, although it can be performed, delays reperfusion compared with PCI and is associated with a high perioperative risk. Hence, CABG has only a niche indication in this setting. In summary, acute MI is an accepted and well-documented prognostic indication for PCI.

Non-ST-Segment Elevation Acute Coronary Syndromes

In acute coronary syndromes without ST-segment elevation, there has been a long-standing debate about two competing treatment strategies.[11] The conservative strategy reserves coronary angiography and revascularization for those patients who continue to have spontaneous or inducible myocardial ischemia despite maximal medical therapy. The invasive strategy, on the other hand, recommends coronary angiography and revascularization regardless of the primary success of medical treatment. Various studies have addressed this issue. A meta-analysis published in 2005 concluded that the invasive strategy, while increasing the risk of in-hospital death and MI (so-called early hazard), significantly reduced death and MI during the entire follow-up period, ranging from 6 months to 2 years in various studies, by 18% (95% confidence interval [CI], 2% to 42%).[12] Supporting this analysis, the 5-year follow-up of RITA-3 revealed that the benefit of the invasive strategy with respect to death and MI continued to increase with time, compared with the conservative strategy.[13] At 5 years after intervention, the incidence of death and MI was 20.0% in the conservative arm but 16.6% in the interventional arm (P = .04). Moreover, there was an increased survival benefit of the invasive strategy during the 5-year follow-up (88% vs. 85%) that almost reached statistical significance (P = .054). The recently reported 5-year follow-up of FRISC-II also demonstrated a significant reduction in the long-term incidence of death and MI by the invasive strategy compared with the conservative strategy (5-year incidence, 19.9% vs. 24.5; P = .009).[14]

The benefit from the invasive strategy compared with the conservative strategy is not uniform across the spectrum of acute coronary syndromes. The major, more recent clinical studies, FRISC-2, TACTICS-TIMI 18, and RITA-3,[15-17] consistently show that the benefit from the invasive strategy is linked to various markers of risk, whereas patients without these risk markers may be treated according to the same principles as patients with stable angina. The risk factors that could be established in previous studies include elevated myocardial marker proteins, dynamic ST-segment changes, ongoing myocardial ischemia, hemodynamic instability, and diabetes mellitus.[18]

This concept of routine invasive strategy was recently challenged by the ICTUS trial.[19] The ICTUS trial accepted the need for coronary revascularization in most patients but challenged troponin levels as the sole criterion for revascularization. The ICTUS trial randomized 1200 patients to a routine invasive versus a selective invasive strategy. To be included, patients had to have unstable angina with elevated cardiac troponin levels. During 1-year follow-up, 54% of the patients in the selective invasive arm and 76% of the patients in the routine invasive arm underwent coronary revascularization. It is noteworthy that the rate of coronary revascularization in the conservative arm of ICTUS was as high as in the invasive arm of RITA-3. During 1-year follow-up, the primary end point of ICTUS (death, MI, and hospital readmission for unplanned coronary revascularization) was not significantly different between the two treatment arms. Secondary analyses, however, revealed a significant increase of MIs in the invasive arm (15% vs. 10%), which could be attributed to an early hazard of the intervention. The ICTUS trial is consistent with other previous trials that suggested that there is a need for revascularization in the majority of patients presenting with high-risk acute coronary syndromes. As a new aspect, ICTUS suggests that there may be an optimal rate of coronary revascularization, above which the potential benefit from revascularization is reversed by peri-interventional complications. It appears that in low-risk patients the long-term benefit from revascularization cannot compensate for the incidence of peri-interventional complications. In this respect, ICTUS challenges the elevation of myocardial marker proteins as the only criterion for recommending revascularization. Using a Bayesian approach to the analysis of all available or published studies on treatment strategies in acute coronary syndromes, including ICTUS, it can be demonstrated that there is a more than 94% probability that the invasive approach will yield a benefit with respect to death and MI and a 75% probability that this benefit will be a least 5% (Fig. 6-2).[11]

In summary, the majority of patients with high-risk acute coronary syndromes benefit from coronary revascularization with respect to death and MI. The results of RITA-3 and FRISC II even suggest a

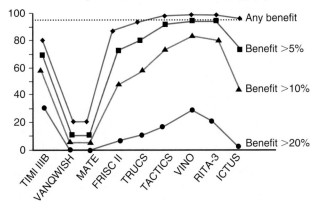

Figure 6-2. Bayesian analysis of trials comparing conservative versus invasive strategy in acute coronary syndromes with respect to death and myocardial infarction during 6- to 12-month follow-up. The curves show the probability of a benefit with the invasive strategy, of the extent specified, based on sequential analysis of the trials in chronologic order. The dotted horizontal line represents the boundary for conventional statistical significance. (From Neumann FJ, Kastrati A, Schwarzer G: New aspects in the treatment of acute coronary syndromes without ST-elevation: ICTUS and ISAR-COOL in perspective. Eur Heart J Suppl 2007;9: A4–A10.)

long-term survival benefit with prudent use of coronary revascularization.

Stable Angina—Severe Angina or Large Ischemic Area

Among patients with chronic stable angina, those with severe angina, large or multiple perfusion defects on functional testing, or a low threshold for induction of ischemia (Table 6-2) have a poor prognosis, with an annual mortality risk greater than 3%. If these high-risk features are associated with double- or triple-vessel disease, patients benefit from revascularization regardless of left ventricular function. In an analysis of 5303 patients of the CASS registry, surgical benefit was greatest in patients who exhibited at least 1 mm of ST-segment depression and who could exercise only into stage 1 or less. In the surgical group with triple-vessel disease and severe exercise-induced ischemia, 7-year survival was 81%, whereas it was

Table 6-2. Conditions Indicating Poor Prognosis* in Stable Angina

High-risk treadmill score
Stress-induced large or moderate size nuclear perfusion defect (particularly if anterior wall)
Stress-induced multiple perfusion defects with left ventricular dilation or increased lung parenchymal uptake of thallium-201 isotope
Echocardiographic wall motion abnormality involving >2 segments developing at a low dose of dobutamine (≤10 µg/kg/min) or at a low heart rate (120 beats/min)
Stress-induced echocardiographic evidence of extensive ischemia

*Average annual mortality risk >3%.

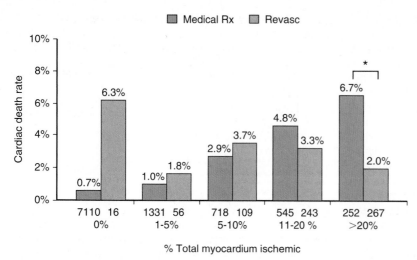

Figure 6-3. Observed cardiac death rates during a mean follow-up of 1.9 years in patients undergoing revascularization (Revasc) versus medical therapy (Medical Rx) as a function of the amount of inducible ischemia. *, $P < .001$. (From Hachamovitch R, Hayes SW, Friedman JD, et al: Comparison of the short-term survival benefit associated with revascularization compared with medical therapy in patients with no prior coronary artery disease undergoing stress myocardial perfusion single photon emission computed tomography. Circulation 2003;107:2900-2907.)

58% in the corresponding medical group.[20] Likewise, in another registry including 2023 patients with severe angina and two-vessel disease, 6-year survival was 76% in patients treated medically and 89% in patients treated surgically ($P < .001$).[21] Cox multivariate analyses showed that surgical treatment was a beneficial independent predictor of survival for patients with two-vessel coronary disease and Canadian Heart Association class III or IV angina.

The ACIP study was a more recent trial that was designed to compare the efficacy of medical therapy versus revascularization.[22] In ACIP, 558 patients with angiographically documented coronary artery disease, mostly multivessel disease, and stable coronary artery disease were randomly assigned to medical therapy, either adjusted to suppress angina or adjusted to suppress both angina and evidence of ischemia during ambulatory electrocardiographic (ECG) monitoring or revascularization with either PCI or CABG. Revascularization was significantly more effective in relieving ischemia than either of the medical strategies. During 1-year follow-up, the ACIP trial appeared to show better outcome in patients treated with revascularization. Mortality was 4.4% and 1.6% in the two conservative groups, whereas none of the patients in the revascularization group died during in the first year. The apparent benefit of revascularization therapy was largely confined to patients with double- or triple-vessel disease.

A recent registry of 10,627 consecutive patients who underwent exercise or adenosine myocardial perfusion single-photon emission computed tomography demonstrated that patients with a large ischemic area on functional testing benefit from revascularization. The patients included in this retrospective analysis had no prior MI or revascularization and were followed up for a mean of 1.9 years. The treatment, received within 60 days after stress testing, was revascularization by either CABG or PCI in 671 patients and medical therapy in 9956 patients. To adjust for nonrandomization of treatment, a propensity score was developed. On the basis of the Cox

proportional hazards model predicting cardiac death, patients undergoing medical therapy demonstrated a survival advantage compared with patients undergoing revascularization in the setting of no or mild ischemia, whereas patients undergoing revascularization had an increasing survival benefit over patients undergoing medical therapy if moderate to severe ischemia was present (Fig. 6-3).[23]

Therefore, although adequately powered randomized trials addressing the impact of severe angina or large perfusion defects on outcome in patients with chronic stable angina are lacking, the bulk of the currently available evidence suggests that these patients benefit from revascularization, particularly if more than one vessel is affected.

Role of Coronary Anatomy

Up to now, understanding of the anatomic conditions that constitute a survival benefit from coronary revascularization versus lone medical therapy has been largely based on milestone studies performed during the 1970s. Soon after CABG was introduced in 1969, three randomized trials compared surgical revascularization with lone medical therapy: the VA-Study, the ECSS, and the CASS. Although these studies are outdated in many aspects, including a low use of arterial conduits and limited means of pharmacologic risk factor modification or of platelet inhibition, it is unlikely that they will ever be replicated. In concert with analyses of large registry databases, the early studies established the conditions in which CABG improves survival compared with medical therapy (Table 6-3).

A meta-analysis of all published randomized trials of CABG versus lone medical treatment for coronary artery disease identified left main disease (diameter stenosis $\geq$ 50%), multivessel disease, and involvement of the proximal left anterior descending coronary artery (LAD) as significant predictors of a survival benefit from CABG.[24] In the cumulative experience of seven studies, the VA-study being the first, surgical

Table 6-3. Conditions in Which CABG Improves Survival Compared with Medical Therapy

Left main coronary artery disease
Triple- or double-vessel disease involving the proximal LAD
Triple- or double-vessel disease in the presence of severe angina or large areas of ischemia on functional testing
Triple-vessel disease associated with impaired left ventricular function

LAD, left anterior descending coronary artery.

revascularization for left main disease was associated with a 65% relative reduction in mortality compared with lone medical therapy.[24] Notably, in left main disease, there was a survival benefit of surgery irrespective of the presence or absence of spontaneous or inducible symptoms or signs of ischemia or reduced left ventricular function. The same is also true for triple- or double-vessel disease involving the proximal LAD.[25]

In all other conditions, the indication for surgical coronary revascularization depends on a combination of anatomic and clinical criteria. If triple-vessel disease is associated with impaired left ventricular function (left ventricular ejection fraction [LVEF] <50%), surgical revascularization improves survival irrespective of LAD involvement.[26,27] In the presence of severe angina or large areas of ischemia on functional testing, surgical revascularization of triple- or double-vessel disease is also indicated for both symptomatic and prognostic reasons, even in the absence of left ventricular dysfunction.[20,21]

Coronary revascularization has never been shown to confer a survival benefit in patients with single-vessel disease. This is also true for isolated proximal LAD stenoses. The meta-analysis by Yusuf showing a survival benefit from surgery in patients with LAD involvement must be interpreted with the notion that this result was obtained in a cohort consisting predominantly of patients with multivessel disease.[24] More recently, the randomized MASS trial compared lone medical treatment with plain balloon angioplasty or CABG in 214 patients with symptomatic, isolated, high-grade stenosis of the LAD.[28] During a 5-year follow-up, there was no appreciable difference among the three treatment arms in either death or MI. Although the power to detect small differences in event rates was low in MASS, the results were consistent with the current judgment that there is no prognostic indication for coronary revascularization in stable single-vessel disease.

No study has ever demonstrated that the risk of subsequent MI can be reduced in patients with stable angina by either bypass surgery or PCI. Concerning PCI, the recently published COURAGE trial confirmed this old notion in the setting of contemporary PCI and medical therapy.[29] The degree of stenosis is a notoriously poor predictor of subsequent events. Although the risk of subsequent MI is higher with high-grade stenoses than with low-grade stenoses, the latter are by far more frequent. Therefore, most infarctions are triggered by low-grade stenoses. The current means of identifying vulnerable plaques are limited. Several techniques for assessing the vulnerability of plaques appear promising, including intravascular ultrasound, optical coherence tomography, intracoronary thermography, and palpography. Nevertheless, the prognostic impact of the findings obtained by these methods has not been established by prospective studies.

Role of Technical Feasibility

Apart from the extent and distribution of coronary artery disease, the probability of achieving complete revascularization is an important criterion in choosing the most appropriate revascularization strategy.

In CABG, a number of studies have demonstrated that patients who achieve complete revascularization have better long-term outcomes than those with incomplete revascularization.[30] The same is also true for PCI. Several studies of the pre-stent era confirmed better long-term outcomes after complete versus incomplete revascularization.[31,32] Reasons for not treating all diseased vessels may include technical obstacles such as heavy calcification, tortuous vessels, or chronic total occlusions; the presence of serious concomitant disease; or the intention to treat only the "culprit lesion" that is thought to be responsible for the patient's symptoms.

A recent analysis of 21,945 stent patients from New York State's Percutaneous Coronary Interventions Reporting System assessed the issue of incomplete revascularization with current practices of coronary revascularization. A follow-up period of 3 years was reported.[33] In this registry, 68.9% of the stented patients were incompletely revascularized. After adjustment for comorbidities and other baseline characteristics associated with increased risk, incompletely revascularized patients were significantly more likely to die at any time than completely revascularized patients (adjusted hazard ratio [HR] = 1.15; 95% CI: 1.01 to 1.30). The risk associated with incomplete revascularization was higher the greater the number of vessels that were not revascularized, and it was higher with nonrevascularized chronic total occlusions than with nonrevascularized subtotal stenoses. Incompletely revascularized patients with total occlusions and two or more nonrevascularized vessels were at the highest risk compared with completely revascularized patients (HR = 1.36; 95% CI: 1.12 to 1.66) (Fig. 6-4).

Given the major impact of the extent of revascularization on long-term survival, consideration must be given to the likelihood of achieving complete revascularization. If PCI is unlikely to achieve complete revascularization, surgery may offer better prospects for revascularization. Yet, this may not always be the case. In some instances, poor target vessels for CABG may be treated by PCI with higher chances of success.

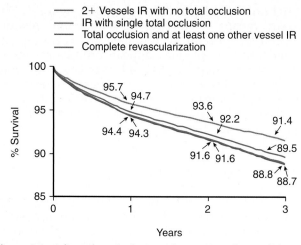

Figure 6-4. Adjusted survival curves for stenting: three subgroups with incomplete revascularization (IR) versus the group with complete revascularization. (From Hannan EL, Racz M, Holmes DR, et al: Impact of completeness of percutaneous coronary intervention revascularization on long-term outcomes in the stent era. Circulation 2006;113:2406-2412.)

PROGNOSTIC INDICATION FOR REVASCULARIZATION: PCI VERSUS CABG

Multivessel Disease

From the late 1980s to the early 1990s, several studies were designed, conducted, and reported that compared plain balloon angioplasty with CABG. Among them there were three larger trials, RITA ($N = 1011$), CABRI ($N = 1154$), and BARI ($N = 1829$), and three smaller trials, GABI ($N = 358$), EAST ($N = 392$), and the Toulouse monocentric study ($N = 152$). In each of these trials, survival was similar after PCI and after CABG, as was the incidence of Q-wave MI, but repeat revascularization was more frequently needed after PCI. In a meta-analysis based on data extracted from the literature, however, Hoffman and colleagues showed a significant survival benefit from surgery compared with PCI: 3% absolute at 5 years and 4% absolute at 8 years.[34]

However, the results of the early studies that antedated the stent era are not reflective of the current practice of coronary revascularization. Since those studies were completed, major advances have been achieved in PCI, CABG surgery, and medical treatment. With respect to PCI, coronary stents, currently implanted in more than 80% of all PCIs, have improved the safety and predictability of PCI, with a dramatic decline in the need for emergency CABG, and have reduced the incidence of restenosis by about 10% absolute, compared with plain balloon angioplasty. Moreover, modern adjunctive antiplatelet therapy has reduced the risk of peri-interventional MI by about one half. As for CABG, several advances such as off-pump surgery, minimally invasive surgical approaches, and, most importantly, the widespread use of arterial conduits up to complete arterial revascularization have been introduced. Moreover, irrespective of the revascularization strategy, patients with coronary artery disease have profited from recognition of the importance of risk factor reduction and of vigorous drug therapy to achieve this goal.

For these reasons, results of randomized trials performed in the pre-stent era cannot be transferred to current practice. This chapter will, therefore, focus on the contemporary studies performed with stents and modern pharmacotherapy.

Lessons from Studies with Bare Metal Stents

Randomized Studies

Five randomized trials have compared stenting with CABG for multivessel disease: ARTS,[35,36] SoS,[37] ERACI-2,[38,39] MASS-2,[40] and AWESOME.[41]

ARTS was the largest trial comparing PCI with CABG for treatment of multivessel disease.[35,36] ARTS included a total of 1205 patients with at least two de novo lesions that were located in different vessels and territories, not including the left main coronary artery. Acute MI, but not unstable angina, was an exclusion criterion. Patients could be included if the cardiac surgeon and interventional cardiologist agreed that the same extent of revascularization could be achieved by either technique. Six hundred patients were randomly assigned to stenting and 605 to bypass surgery; 67% of the patients had a double-vessel disease, and 32% had triple-vessel disease. At 1 year, there was no significant difference between the stent group and the CABG group in terms of the incidence of death (2.5% vs. 2.8%; relative risk [RR] = 0.89; 95% CI: 0.45 to 1.77), cerebrovascular accident (1.5% vs. 2.0%; RR = 0.78; 95% CI: 0.34 to 1.76), or MI (5.3% vs. 4.0%; RR = 1.29; 95% CI: 0.80 to 2.06). The 5-year follow-up of the ARTS trial has now been published.[35] At 5 years, the incidence of death was 8% in the stent group versus 7.6% in the CABG group (RR = 1.05; 95% CI: 0.71 to 1.55; $P = .83$). Likewise, there was no significant difference in cerebrovascular accident (3.8% vs. 3.5%; RR = 1.10; 95% CI: 0.62 to 1.97; $P = .76$), Q-wave MI (6.7% vs. 5.6%; RR = 1.19; 95% CI: 0.76 to 1.85; $P = .47$), non–Q-wave MI (1.8% vs. 0.8%; RR = 2.22; 95% CI: 0.78 to 6.35; $P = .14$), or the composite thereof (18.2% vs. 14.9%; RR = 1.22; 95% CI: 0.95 to 1.58; $P = .14$) (Fig. 6-5). Consistent with the findings at 1 year, however, there was a significant difference in the incidence of repeat revascularization, and this had widened over time (30.3% vs. 8.8%; RR = 3.46; 95% CI: 2.61 to 4.60; $P < .001$). In the stent group, 10.5% of the revascularizations involved CABG, compared with 1.2% in the CABG group. In summary, the 5-year outcome with respect to the serious end points of death, MI, and cerebrovascular accident was similar for both the nonsurgical approach and the surgical approach. With the primarily catheter-based approach, there was a 90% chance of avoiding CABG during the subsequent 5 years, with similar outcome in relation to the end points, but at the

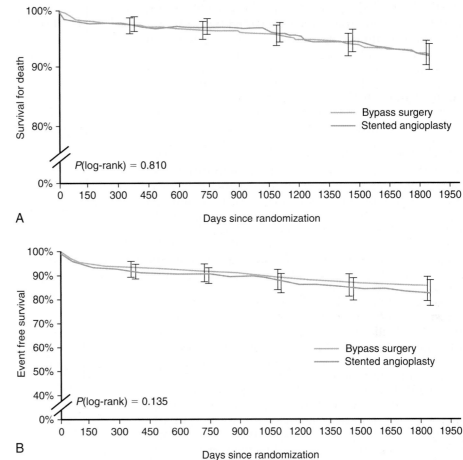

Figure 6-5. Five-year outcome in ARTS. **A,** Kaplan-Meier curves showing freedom from death. **B,** Kaplan-Meier curves showing freedom from death, cerebrovascular accident, or myocardial infarction. (From Serruys PW, Ong AT, van Herwerden LA, et al: Five-year outcomes after coronary stenting versus bypass surgery for the treatment of multivessel disease: The final analysis of the Arterial Revascularization Therapies Study (ARTS) randomized trial. J Am Coll Cardiol 2005;46:575-581.)

expense of a 20% higher incidence of repeat catheter interventions.

The second largest trial comparing stenting with CABG for multivessel disease was the SoS.[37] The multicenter SoS trial included 488 patients randomized to stenting and 500 patients randomized to CABG. Symptomatic patients with multivessel coronary artery disease were considered for inclusion and enrolled if the consensus view of the surgeon and the interventionist was that revascularization was clinically indicated and appropriate by either strategy. All patients were followed up for a minimum of 1 year. In this study, 38% of the PCI group and 47% of the CABG group had three-vessel disease. During a median follow-up of 2 years, 21% of the patients in the PCI group required additional revascularization procedures, compared with 6% of the CABG group (RR = 3.85; 95% CI: 2.59 to 5.79; $P < .001$). The incidence of death and acute MI was similar in both groups (9% vs. 10%; $P = .08$). There were, however, more deaths in the PCI group than in the CABG group (5% vs. 2%; HR = 2.91; 95% CI: 1.29 to 6.53; $P = .01$). Although mortality was not the primary end point of the study, the data suggested that there was a survival benefit from CABG compared with PCI.

ERACI-2 randomly assigned 450 patients with multivessel disease to either PCI or CABG. More than 90% of the patients had unstable angina, and 56%

of the patients had triple-vessel disease. At 900 days, there was a better survival with PCI than with CABG (96.9% vs. 92.5%; $P < .017$). Likewise, there was a better survival free of MI with PCI than with CABG (97.7% vs. 93.7%; $P < .017$). As in the other studies, however, freedom from new revascularization procedures was significantly better with CABG (95.2% vs. 82.2%; $P < .01$). At 5-years' follow-up,[39] patients initially treated with PCI had similar survival and freedom from nonfatal MI than those initially treated with CABG (92.8% vs. 88.4% and 97.3% vs. 94%, respectively; $P = .16$), but freedom from repeat revascularization procedures was significantly lower with PCI (71.5% vs. 92.4%; $P < .001$).

MASS-2 comprised 611 patients with multivessel disease who were randomly assigned to CABG, PCI, or medical therapy; 58% of the patients had triple-vessel disease, and 92% had LAD involvement).[32] At 1 year, the incidence of death was lowest with a medical treatment (1.5%), although the difference was not significantly different among the three treatment arms. Comparing the two revascularization modalities, 1-year mortality was similar with PCI and CABG (4.5% vs. 4.0%; $P = .23$), whereas Q-wave MI was significantly more frequent with PCI (8.3% vs. 2.0%; $P = .01$). Similar to the other studies, repeat intervention was needed more often after PCI than after CABG surgery (12.3% vs. 0.5%; $P < .001$).

The studies described so far compared PCI with CABG in cohorts that were well suited for both procedures. The important question, whether patients at high risk for CABG surgery and refractory myocardial ischemia should undergo PCI as an alternative procedure, was addressed in AWESOME.[41] This multicenter study included patients with myocardial ischemia refractory to medical management and the presence of one or more risk factors for adverse outcome with CABG, including prior open heart surgery, age older than 70 years, LVEF less than 35%, MI within 7 days, or the need for intra-aortic balloon pumping. Over a 5-year period 2431 patients met the entry criteria. By physician consensus, 1650 patients formed a physician-directed registry assigned to CABG (n = 692), PCI (n = 651), or further medical therapy (n = 307), and 781 were angiographically eligible for random allocation. Among the patients who were angiographically acceptable, 454 consented to randomized assignment between CABG and PCI, and the remaining 327 constituted a patient choice registry. At all time points during the 5-year follow-up of the randomized study, there was a nonsignificant survival benefit of PCI over CABG (97% vs. 95% at 30 days, 75% vs. 70% at 5 years).[42] Within the first 3 years after randomization, more patients randomized to PCI received a subsequent revascularization (37% vs. 18%; P < .001), but between 3 and 5 years of follow-up, repeat revascularization was similarly frequent in both the PCI group and the CABG group (6% vs. 4%). In the physician-directed subgroup, the 3-year survival rate was 76% for both CABG and PCI. In the patient choice subgroup, the 3-year survival rate was 80% with CABG but 98% with PCI. The findings of the AWESOME Registry[43] therefore support the findings of the main study. The AWESOME investigators specifically addressed the issue of whether PCI is the preferred option for repeat intervention in patients with previous CABG.[44] In the subgroup with previous CABG, 3-year survival rates were 73% with CABG and 76% with PCI in the randomized patients; 71% and 77%, respectively, in the physician-directed registry; and 65% and 86% (P = .001) in the patient choice registry. The authors concluded that PCI is preferable to CABG for many post-CABG patients.

Recently, four major studies were incorporated in a meta-analysis that was based on individual patient data. This meta-analysis confirmed the results of most of the individual studies.[45] The meta-analysis included ARTS, SoS, ERACI-2, and MASS-2 but excluded AWESOME, because the high-risk characteristics of the patients in AWESOME were clearly different from the patient population of the four other trials. This meta-analysis confirmed that PCI with stent placement was associated with a similar 1-year incidence of death, myocardial infarction, or stroke, compared with CABG (Fig. 6-6). Nevertheless, the need for repeat revascularization was considerably higher after PCI, although the observed gap with CABG surgery was narrowed (from approximately 30% reported in the pre-stent era) to approximately

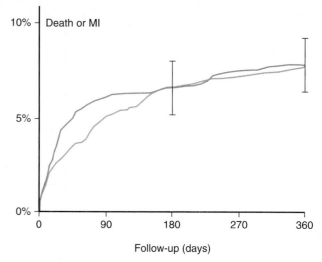

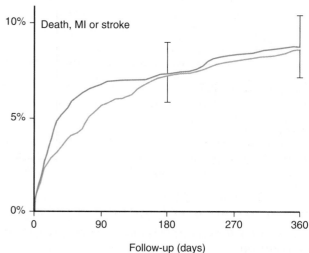

Figure 6-6. Meta-analysis of ARTS, SoS, ERACI-2, and MASS-2. Incidence of adverse cardiovascular events during 1-year follow-up in patients allocated to percutaneous coronary intervention with multiple stenting *(blue line)* or coronary artery bypass grafting *(green line)*. MI, myocardial infarction. (From Mercado N, Wijns W, Serruys PW, et al: One-year outcomes of coronary artery bypass graft surgery versus percutaneous coronary intervention with multiple stenting for multisystem disease: A meta-analysis of individual patient data from randomized clinical trials. J Thorac Cardiovasc Surg 2005;130:512-519.)

14%. Compared with PCI, CABG was associated with a slightly lower frequency of recurrent angina (77% vs. 82%; P = .002).

Another meta-analysis based on aggregate data from ARTS, SoS, ERACI-2 and SIMA, a study on isolated proximal LAD stenosis, extended the analysis to a follow-up of 3 years.[34] The point estimates for the 3-year incidence of death and nonfatal MI were both lower after PCI than after CABG; however, a significant difference was found only for nonfatal MI (Fig. 6-7). Moreover, this meta-analysis confirmed that the 1-year incidence of repeat intervention was higher (by 15% absolute) after PCI than after CABG, but it did not demonstrate any

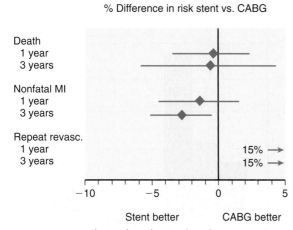

% Difference in risk stent vs. CABG

Figure 6-7. Meta-analysis of randomized studies comparing stenting with coronary artery bypass grafting (CABG), showing risk difference for various events at 1 year and at 3 years. The lines represent 95% confidence interval. MI, myocardial infarction; revasc., revascularization.

significant further changes with 1 to 3 years of follow-up.

Registries

It has been argued that the randomized studies comparing PCI with CABG in multivessel disease comprised only a small proportion of the patients presenting at dedicated high-volume centers.[46] Therefore, the results of these trials may not be applicable to most patients needing coronary revascularization. It is, therefore, an important question whether the absence of a substantial difference in survival between PCI and CABG can also be verified in large registries.

A large registry of the Cleveland Clinic comprised 6033 consecutive patients with multivessel disease undergoing either CABG ($n = 5161$) or PCI ($n = 872$) from 1995 to 1999.[47] A stent was placed in 70% of the patients. The 1- and 5-year unadjusted mortality rates were 5% and 16% for PCI and 4% and 14% for CABG (unadjusted HR = 1.13; 95% CI: 1.0 to 1.4; $P = .07$). In the propensity-adjusted analysis, however, PCI was associated with an increased risk of death (propensity-adjusted HR = 2.3; 95% CI: 1.9 to 2.9; $P < .001$). This difference was observed across all categories of propensity for PCI. When the proportional-hazards model was restricted to patients who had stenting, as compared to those referred for CABG, stenting was associated also with a higher death risk (adjusted HR = 2.2; 95% CI: 1.7 to 2.9; $P < .001$). When interpreting these data, it must be considered that, at an interval of 5 years, the data will favor CABG to a certain extent simply because that time period precedes the development of severe graft disease while capturing most events in the PCI cohort. Moreover, the authors noted that, during the era covered by this registry, the routine use of more potent antiplatelet therapy was not yet established.

More recently, survival data of 59,314 patients with multivessel disease from the New York cardiac registries were published.[48] This analysis comprised 37,212 patients undergoing CABG and 22,102 patients undergoing stenting between 1997 and 2000. The median follow-up was 706 days in the CABG group and 585 days in the stenting group. Patients were stratified into various anatomic groups depending on two-vessel or three-vessel involvement and LAD involvement. The observed (unadjusted) survival rate was significantly higher after stent placement than after CABG among patients with two-vessel disease without involvement of the LAD ($P = .03$), whereas the opposite was true among patients who had three-vessel disease with involvement of the proximal LAD ($P < .01$). There was no significant treatment-related difference in survival in the other anatomic groups. Patients who underwent CABG were significantly older than patients who received stents; they were more likely to be white men and less likely to be Hispanic. Patients who underwent CABG also had a significantly lower LVEF and were less likely than patients who received stents to have had a MI in the week before the procedure. Also, the CABG group had a significantly higher prevalence of coexisting conditions, such as diabetes or renal failure, and was significantly more likely to have three-vessel disease. After adjusting for these differences, the estimated survival curves significantly favored CABG in each of the anatomic subgroups. The largest benefit from CABG was seen in patients with three-vessel disease and involvement of the proximal LAD, with an adjusted HR of 0.64 (95 CI: 0.56 to 0.74).

Despite these statistically clear-cut results, the implications of the findings in this registry must be interpreted cautiously. Not all patients undergoing PCI in the New York area were included in this registry. Moreover, several limitations derive from the nonrandomized nature of this comparison. There may be a risk ascertainment bias, because patients undergoing CABG receive a more thorough clinical workup before the procedure than do patients undergoing PCI. It is also conceivable that there may be differences in follow-up management between the stent group and the CABG group, because CABG may offer a stronger incentive for lifestyle changes and preventive medical treatments. In addition, it must be considered that risk adjustment by proportional-hazard models cannot fully substitute for randomization, because comprehensive inclusion of all confounders is impossible. One important confounder that was not included in risk adjustment, incomplete revascularization, was subsequently published by the same authors. Sixty-nine percent of the patients receiving a stent in this registry had incomplete revascularization. In the same registry, incomplete revascularization after PCI had a statistically significant and clinically relevant impact on outcome, as discussed earlier. Between patients completely revascularized and those incompletely revascularized there was a 2.1% survival disadvantage at 3 years in the absence of a total occlusion and a 2.7% difference in the presence of a nonrecanalized total occlusion.[33] The difference between complete and incomplete revascularization within the stent group of the New York registry was on the same order of magnitude as the difference between the stent group and the CABG group in the entire registry.

The Rotterdam group reported a single-center, matched, propensity-controlled comparison of stenting versus CABG for multivessel disease.[49] This study compared 409 consecutive patients who underwent an elective coronary intervention with stent placement between 1995 and 1999, in whom at least two stents were implanted for multiple vessels, with 409 patients who underwent CABG during the same time period, who were selected from 1723 CABG patients by propensity score matching. The cumulative survival rates after stenting were 93%, 90%, and 82% at 3, 5, and 8 years, respectively; after CABG, these rates were 97%, 93%, and 87%, respectively ($P = .02$). Moreover, among patients treated with a stent, additional revascularization procedures were more common than among patients treated with CABG (30.6% vs. 20.4% at 8 years; $P < .001$). Most of the repeat interventions in the PCI group occurred within the first year: 20% of the patients underwent an additional coronary revascularization (2.2% CABG, 13.9% PCI, 3.7% both procedures). There were no significant differences in the incidences of MI and stroke. It is noteworthy that the survival benefit of CABG was largely driven by the patients with left main stenosis, whereas no significant difference in survival was reported for patients with multivessel disease in the absence of left main involvement.

Recently, a comprehensive analysis from the Duke registry was published.[50] This registry comprised 18,481 patients with significant coronary artery disease between 1986 and 2000 who were assigned by physician preference to medical therapy ($n = 6862$), PCI ($n = 6292$), or CABG ($n = 5327$). Each group was categorized into three subgroups according to baseline severity of coronary artery disease: low severity (predominantly single-vessel disease), intermediate severity (predominantly two-vessel) and high severity (all three-vessel). Mortality was evaluated by Cox models adjusted for cardiac risk, comorbidity, and propensity for selection of a specific treatment. In all three anatomic subgroups, revascularization conferred a significant survival benefit compared with medical therapy (Fig. 6-8). The extent of this survival benefit varied with the degree of coronary artery disease, ranging from an additional 8 months gained during 15 years in the low-severity group to 24 months gained in the high-severity group. In the low- and intermediate-severity groups, the benefit from revascularization was independent of treatment modality, with similar results by CABG or PCI. In the high-severity subgroup, however, CABG was associated with a small but significant survival benefit of 8 months during 15 years. It is noteworthy that the impact of revascularization versus medical treatment was substantially larger

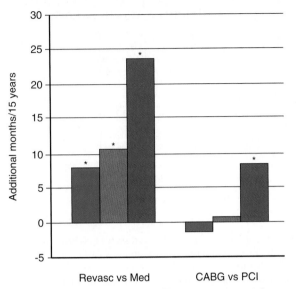

Figure 6-8. Adjusted survival difference versus initial treatment selection. Results are shown according to severity of coronary artery disease: low *(blue bar)*, intermediate *(orange bar)*, and high *(purple bar)*. *, $P < .05$; CABG, coronary artery bypass grafting; PCI, percutaneous coronary intervention; Revasc, revascularization. (From Smith PK, Califf RM, Tuttle RH, et al: Selection of surgical or percutaneous coronary intervention provides differential longevity benefit. Ann Thorac Surg 2006;82:1420-1428.)

than the impact of the choice of revascularization modality. The authors also compared CABG versus PCI in various prespecified time periods: era 1 (pre-stent era), 1986-1990; era 2, 1991-1995; and era 3 (stent era), 1996-2000. In this analysis, the benefit of surgery versus PCI increased with time, reaching a survival benefit of approximately 5 months per 7 years during era 3.

In summary, contemporary registry data suggest a small survival benefit of CABG versus PCI in patients with multivessel disease. A large proportion of this survival benefit appears to be attributed to patients with left main disease and to those patients who do not achieve complete revascularization with PCI. Hence, the registry data are consistent with the results of randomized trials such as ARTS, in which a high probability of complete revascularization with PCI was an entry criterion and left main stenosis was an exclusion criterion. The registry data therefore do not suggest that the key findings of the randomized trials (i.e., comparable survival after PCI or CABG in patients with multivessel disease without left main involvement and with complete revascularization) cannot be transferred to daily practice.

Lessons from Studies with Drug-Eluting Stents

ARTS II, a 45-center, 607-patient registry, intended to compare 1-year outcomes of the sirolimus-eluting stent against the historical results of the two arms of ARTS I.[51] Patients were stratified to ensure that at least one third had three-vessel disease to achieve a number of treatable lesions per patient comparable to ARTS I. Compared with ARTS I, ARTS II comprised a higher-risk cohort: 53.5% had three-vessel disease, and diabetes was present in 26.2%. Mean stented length was 72.5 mm, with 3.7 stents implanted per patient. The 1-year survival rate was 99.0%, the composite of death/stroke and MI-free survival was 96.9%, and freedom from revascularization was 91.5%. In the unadjusted comparison with the historical control arms of ARTS I-CABG and ARTS I-PCI, the respective relative risks and 95% CIs for the end points were (1) freedom from repeat revascularization, 2.03 (1.23-3.34) and 0.44 (0.31-0.61), respectively; and (2) freedom from death, stroke, MI, and revascularization, 0.89 (0.65-1.23) and 0.39 (0.30-0.51), respectively. The authors concluded that surgery still afforded a lower need for repeat revascularization, although overall event rates in ARTS II approached those of the surgical results and were significantly better than bare stenting in ARTS I. The three year clinical outcome of ARTS II (presented at the 56th Annual Scientific Session, American College of Cardiology, New Orleans, 2007) confirmed the favorable results during long-term follow-up. In the unadjusted comparison of ARTS II with ARTS I-CABG and ARTS I-PCI, freedom from death, stroke, and MI until three years was 92.0%, 89.1%, and 87.2%, respectively (for ARTS II versus ARTS I-CABG, log rank P = .07; for ARTS II versus ARTS I-PCI, log rank P = .004), and freedom from death, stroke, MI and repeat revascularization up to three years was 80.6%, 83.8%, and 66.0%, respectively (for ARTS II versus ARTS I-CABG, log rank P = .22; for ARTS II versus ARTS I-PCI, log rank P < .001). So the overall major adverse event rate of ARTS II at three years is noninferior to ARTS I-CABG.

The promising results of ARTS II have to be interpreted cautiously, because ARTS II did not account for advances in surgical technique that may have occurred since the days of ARTS I. Despite this limitation, there is currently no evidence-based reason for withholding the benefit of drug-eluting stents with respect to reintervention from patients with multivessel disease. Randomized studies that clarify the role of drug eluting-stents compared with CABG for multivessel disease are currently underway.

Special Considerations in Diabetic Patients

Compared with nondiabetic patients, patients with diabetes often have a more advanced coronary atherosclerosis with diffuse disease in small-lumen vessels. With any treatment modality for coronary revascularization, diabetic patients have an inferior outcome compared with nondiabetics. This was first shown for CABG. In patients with diabetes mellitus, CABG is associated with a more rapid progression of atherosclerosis of both grafted and nongrafted vessels, as well as an accelerated degeneration of venous bypass grafts, compared with nondiabetics. Nevertheless, CASS demonstrated that in older diabetics

coronary revascularization confers a substantial benefit compared with lone medical therapy.[52] Likewise, PCI in patients with diabetes is associated with a substantially increased risk of adverse short-term and long-term outcome compared with PCI in nondiabetics. In particular, it the risk of restenosis after any type of PCI is substantially increased in diabetics.[53,54] Moreover, whereas restenosis has little impact on survival in patients without diabetes, Bertrand and coworkers demonstrated that restenosis after plain balloon angioplasty in diabetics has a major impact on 10-year mortality, with a 45% relative increase for nonocclusive stenosis and more than a twofold increase with occlusive stenosis.[55] The risk of peri-interventional death and MI is also increased by about twofold after plain balloon angioplasty in diabetics compared with nondiabetics.[56]

Because coronary revascularization in diabetics differs in many aspects from that in nondiabetics, the indications for PCI in diabetics deserve special attention.

Studies on Plain Balloon Angioplasty

Four of the studies comparing CABG with plain balloon angioplasty for multivessel disease reported subgroup analyses for diabetics. The largest of these subgroup analyses was derived from BARI, which included 353 patients with diabetes. During the 5-year follow-up, the mortality rate of diabetics randomized to plain balloon angioplasty was 34.5%, and after seven years it was 44.3%, whereas after CABG the respective mortality rates were 19.4% (P = .03) and 23.6% (P = .01).[57] The difference in mortality in BARI could be attributed to a difference in cardiac mortality (20.6% vs. 5.8% during 5-year follow-up). MIs showed a similar incidence in both treatment groups but were less often lethal in surgically treated patients. This may be attributed, at least in part, to a less complete revascularization in the PCI arm. The findings in BARI led to a clinical alert of the National Heart, Lung and Blood Institute, abandoning plain balloon angioplasty as a treatment option for multivessel coronary artery disease.

There has been considerable debate about the results of BARI, because the meta-analysis of the 5-year follow-up of the three smaller studies reporting subgroup analyses for diabetics, RITA, CABRI, and EAST, did not reveal a significant disadvantage of multivessel PCI versus CABG in diabetics.[58] Nevertheless, the 8-year follow-up results of EAST demonstrated a significant survival benefit of CABG over PCI.[59] In addition, seven registries were reported comparing plain balloon angioplasty with bypass surgery. In each of these registries, adjusted mortality after catheter intervention was higher than after bypass surgery. However, statistical significance was reached only in the largest registry, the Northern New England Cardiovascular Disease Study Group, and in the subgroup of the Emory registry with insulin treatment.[60,61] Except for the Emory registry, adjustment did not include completeness of revascularization, probably because incomplete revascularization was considered an inherent problem of the interventional approach. In the Emory registry, the adjustment for completeness of revascularization abrogated the differences between catheter treatment and bypass surgery. These findings again point to the importance of achieving complete revascularization with PCI.

The studies during the era of plain balloon angioplasty are not transferable to current practice. As first demonstrated by the studies on abciximab, the increased risk of thrombotic complications during early and longer term follow-up can be abrogated by intense antiplatelet therapy.[62,63] More recently, the ISAR-SWEET study suggested that a similar effect can be achieved by effective pretreatment with clopidogrel.[64] In addition, it was shown by various studies that stents compared with plain balloon angioplasty reduce the subsequent incidence of restenosis, although this incidence continues to be higher than in nondiabetics.[54,65,66] Given the major impact of restenosis on survival, it is plausible that stents, compared with plain balloon angioplasty, may improve the long-term outcome of PCI substantially. Finally, the recently improved means of achieving tight metabolic control can further improve outcome after catheter intervention. Independent studies demonstrated that outcome after PCI in diabetic patients with tight metabolic control is similar to that in nondiabetic patients.[67,68]

Studies with Bare Metal Stents

Of the studies comparing bare metal stents with bypass surgery, ARTS, AWESOME, and ERACI-2 reported subgroup analyses for diabetics (Fig. 6-9).

Of the 1205 patients included in ARTS, 112 diabetics were randomly assigned to stent implantation and 69 to bypass surgery.[69] The incidence of major adverse events during hospital stay was similar in both groups except for stroke, which was significantly more frequent in the surgical patients than in the interventional patients (0% vs. 4.2%; $P = .04$). During 1-year follow-up, this trend continued to prevail (1.8% vs. 6.3%; $P = .10$). Mortality during 1-year follow-up, however, was higher in the stent group (6.3%) than in the surgical group (3.1%) although

statistical significance was missed ($P = .294$). The incidence of MI was also higher by trend in the PCI group than in the CABG group (6.3% vs. 3.1%; $P = .294$). As in the entire ARTS cohort, the need for repeat intervention (mostly catheter intervention) was significantly higher in the PCI group than in the CABG group. Overall event-free survival of diabetics during 1-year follow-up after stent implantation was significantly lower than after surgery (63.4% vs. 84.4%; $P < .05$). Notably, in the PCI group, there was a significant difference in event-free survival between diabetics and nondiabetics (63.4% vs. 76.2%) which was not present in the surgical group. In the aggregate, ARTS suggested CABG as the preferred treatment for multivessel disease in diabetics. Nevertheless, the number of diabetics included in ARTS was too low to allow definite conclusions.

ARTS included a patient cohort with low to intermediate risk for CABG. The AWESOME study addressed patients with a high risk for CABG (see earlier discussion). The number of diabetics included in AWESOME was 144 in the randomized study, 89 in the patient choice registry, and 525 in the physician choice registry.[70] In the randomized study, the 4-year mortality rate for diabetics after PCI was not significantly different than after CABG, with the point estimates favoring the former (19% vs. 28%; $P = .27$). Similar results were obtained in the patient choice registry (11% vs. 15%; $P = .73$) and in the physician choice registry (29% vs. 27%; $P = .77$). The results of AWESOME, therefore, suggest that, in diabetic patients with multivessel disease and refractory angina who have an increased risk for CABG, coronary stent implantation is a safe alternative to surgical revascularization.

The combined analysis of the 90 diabetics in ERACI (without stent) and ERACI-2 (with stent) demonstrated no benefit of CABG during 1-year follow-up, compared with PCI. The composite end point of death and MI was somewhat higher in the surgical group than in the stent group (6.5% vs. 4.5% and 13% vs. 4.5%, respectively). Because of the low number of patients included in ERACI and the short follow-up period, these data should be interpreted cautiously.

The only large registry that addressed stent-supported PCI versus bypass surgery in patients with diabetes, APPROACH, did not reveal any benefit of CABG compared with PCI.[71]

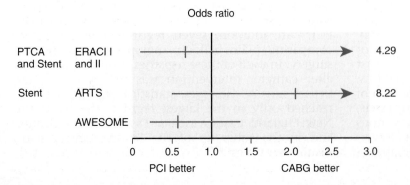

Figure 6-9. Odds ratios for mortality after stenting versus coronary artery bypass grafting (CABG) in the diabetic cohorts of ERACI-1, ERACI-2, ARTS, and AWESOME. The horizontal lines represent 95% confidence intervals. PCI, percutaneous coronary intervention; PTCA, percutaneous transluminal coronary angioplasty.

Studies with Drug-Eluting Stents

Drug-eluting stents are particularly appealing for patients with diabetes mellitus because they offer a solution to the most crucial problem of PCI in this patient subset, restenosis. A recently published meta-analysis of the diabetic patients in randomized studies comparing drug-eluting stents with bare metal stents confirmed that drug-eluting stents confer a similar relative reduction in restenosis in diabetics and in nondiabetics, compared with bare metal stents.[72] The same meta-analysis did not reveal any safety issues with respect to the 1-year incidence of death or the composite of death and nonfatal MI. Based on the older studies for PCI in diabetes, it may be anticipated that the reduction in restenosis conferred by drug-eluting stents compared with bare metal stents may confer a survival benefit during longer-term follow-up.

As of this writing, the role of drug-eluting stents in the treatment of multivessel disease in patients with diabetes cannot be judged by evidence-based criteria. Thus far, data from large registries and randomized trials comparing drug-eluting stents with CABG for multivessel disease in diabetics are lacking. A large trial sponsored by the National Institutes of Health addressing this issue, FREEDOM, is underway.

Left Main Coronary Artery Disease

Since the early days of A. Grüntzig, most interventional cardiologists have considered percutaneous transluminal coronary angiography (PTCA) of unprotected left main stem lesions to be contraindicated because of the almost inevitable fatality when the procedure fails. In a series of 129 patients undergoing PTCA of unprotected left main stenoses, the procedural and 3-year mortality rates were 9.1% and 65%, respectively, with a need for subsequent revascularization in 42%.[73] Because CABG was established as a therapy that reduces mortality compared with lone medical treatment, plain PTCA was completely abandoned.

Lessons from Studies with Bare Metal Stents

Randomized Studies
Thus far, there have been no randomized studies comparing coronary stent placement with CABG for left main disease. It is therefore unknown whether the survival benefit after coronary stenting is similar to that after CABG in patients with left main coronary artery disease.

Registries
Various groups have reported favorable results after stenting of unprotected left main stenoses.[74-79] The efficiency of stents in reducing acute complications and restenosis, particularly in large-diameter vessels,

explains the attractiveness of stenting for percutaneous treatment of left main disease. Moreover, stents overcome the elastic recoil within the aortic wall, which represents a major problem with left main PTCA. Accordingly, reported rates of restenosis at 6-month follow-up have ranged between 7% and 22% for stenting of unprotected left main stenosis,[76,77,80] corresponding to a rate of repeat revascularization between 10% and 17%.[74-77,81-83] The risk of restenosis appears to be the highest in lesions involving the distal part of the left main coronary artery.[80] In patients with elective stenting of unprotected left main disease, mortality varies considerably, depending on the clinical setting, with an early (≤30 days) mortality rate ranging from 0% to 6%[74,76,77] and a late (≥6 months) mortality rate ranging between 2% and 32%.[74-77,81,83] In the Korean experience of 270 consecutive patients with stent treatment of unprotected left main disease, the 3-year cardiac mortality rate was $3.2\% \pm 1.1\%$, and the rate of survival without MI or reintervention was $77.7\% \pm 2.7\%$. The majority of events occurring during the first 3 years were reinterventions within the first 6 months (17.2%).[79] Similar results were obtained at 5-year follow-up.[78]

Strong predictors of late mortality include LVEF less than 40%[74] and increased risk for CABG.[75] Among poor candidates for surgery, stenting of the left main coronary artery carried a 9% mortality risk in the first month and an 11% risk in the first year.[75] On the other hand, stenting of the left main in 93 patients who were good candidates for surgery was associated with a 30-day mortality rate of 0% and a 1-year mortality rate of 2.5% in a single-center series.[75]

The registry data suggest that, similar to CABG, PCI carries a higher long-term and short-term risk in the presence of left main disease, compared with more distal coronary lesions. The findings also indicate that the risk for major complications after PCI, at least during the mid-term up to 5 years, appears to be on the same order of magnitude as that after CABG. Obviously, the registry data cannot establish equivalence to surgery. Nevertheless, the data indicate that stenting of the left main coronary artery may be a reasonable option if there is good reason to avoid surgery, such as severe concomitant disease or advanced age.

Lessons from Studies with Drug-Eluting Stents

Randomized Studies
As with bare metal stents, data from randomized studies comparing drug-eluting stents with CABG for unprotected left main coronary artery disease are not yet available. Several randomized studies addressing this issue are underway.

Registries
Several registries have addressed the efficacy and safety of drug-eluting stents in the treatment of left main coronary artery disease. In 2005, three key studies were published that comprised cohorts of 85 to 102 patients treated with drug-eluting stents for

Table 6-4. Mid-Term Outcome After Implantation of Drug-Eluting Stents (DES) versus Bare Metal Stents (BMS) for Unprotected Left Main Coronary Artery Disease

Parameter	Valgimigli et al[79]		Park et al[77]		Chieffo et al[78]	
	DES	BMS	DES	BMS	DES	BMS
No. patients	95	86	102	121	85	64
Follow-up	503 days	503 days	12 mo	30 mo	6 mo	6 mo
ACS (%)	52	50	59.8	67.8	30.9	42.1
Death (%)	14	16	0	0	3.5*	14.1
Nonfatal MI (%)	4*	12	6.9	8.3	7.1	7.8
TVR (%)	6*	23	2.0*	17.4	20	30.6
Any MACE	24*	45	2.0*	18.6	20.0*	35.9
Stent thrombosis (%)	nr	nr	0	0	1.2	0
Binary restenosis (%)	nr	nr	7.0	30.3	19.0	30.6

*$P < .05$.
ACS, acute coronary syndromes; TVR, target vessel revascularization; MACE, major adverse cardiac event; MI, myocardial infarction; nr, not reported.

unprotected left main disease and historical control groups of 64 to 121 patients receiving bare metal stents.[84-86] As shown in Table 6-4, the historical comparisons suggested that drug-eluting stents, compared with bare metal stents, reduced the risk of major adverse cardiac events during mid-term follow-up (6-12 months), a benefit that can be attributed largely to a reduction in the need for target vessel revascularization. This benefit prevailed after adjustment for differences in baseline characteristics between the respective study cohorts, which in general favored bare metal stents.

It is noteworthy that the incidence of severe complications such as cardiac death and MI was high, particularly in the series of Valgimigli and colleagues.[86] When interpreting these results, it must be taken into account that each of the registries included a large proportion of patients with acute coronary syndromes. The study of Valgimigli also included patients with acute ST-segment elevation MI and cardiogenic shock. In fact, seven of the deaths in the drug-eluting stent group of this study occurred in patients who presented with cardiogenic shock.

In the study of Park and associates, late lumen loss was lowest in the group of patients who could be treated with a single stent and highest in the group treated with the crushing technique.[84] These observations are consistent with the findings of the combined analysis of the RESEARCH and T-SEARCH registries, which demonstrated a significantly elevated risk in patients with distal left main disease.[87,88] In this analysis, the incidence of major adverse cardiac events during a median follow-up of 587 days was 30% in patients with distal left main disease versus 11% in those without. After adjustment for confounders and surgical risk status, distal left main disease remained a significant independent predictor of major adverse cardiac events (HR = 2.79; 95%-CI: 1.17 to 8.9; $P = .032$).

The registry data suggest a substantial benefit of drug-eluting stents versus bare metal stents but cannot assess the long-term risks, nor can they assess the efficacy compared with CABG. While randomized studies such as COMBAT and SYNTAX are underway, two nonrandomized studies comparing implantation of drug-eluting stents for unprotected left main disease with CABG have been published. The study by Lee and associates[89] compared 50 patients who underwent PCI with drug-eluting stents for unprotected left main disease with 123 patients from the same institutions who underwent CABG. High-risk patients (Parsonett score >15) made up 46% of the CABG group and 64% of the PCI group ($P = .04$). Median follow-up was 6.7 months in the CABG group and 5.6 months in the PCI group. Freedom from major adverse cardiac and serious vascular events including death, MI, cerebrovascular events, and target vessel revascularization was 83% after CABG and 89% after PCI ($P = .20$). Freedom from death, MI, and cerebrovascular events at 6 months was significantly higher after PCI (95.6%) than after CABG (82.9%) ($P = .03$) (Fig. 6-10). By multivariable Cox regression analysis, CABG was an independent predictor of major adverse cardiovascular and cerebrovascular events.

Similar results were obtained in the study by Chieffo and colleagues.[90] This study compared 107 patients with unprotected left main disease treated with PCI and drug-eluting stent implantation with 142 patients undergoing CABG. At 1 year, the rate of death, MI, and cerebrovascular events was significantly lower with PCI than with CABG (3.7% vs. 8.5%; $P < .001$). This difference prevailed after adjustment by propensity analysis with respect to baseline differences between the two cohorts (adjusted odds ratio = 0.39; 95% CI: 0.18 to 0.82; $P = .01$). On the other hand, there was a significant increase in target vessel revascularization in the PCI-treated patients (19.6% vs. 3.6%).

Although registry data and nonrandomized studies suggest a favorable outcome of PCI with drug-eluting stents for unprotected left main disease, they are far from being conclusive. Apart from the problems associated with the analysis of nonrandomized comparisons, the duration of follow-up is too short, and the number of patients included is too low to address the efficacy of drug-eluting stents with respect to survival.

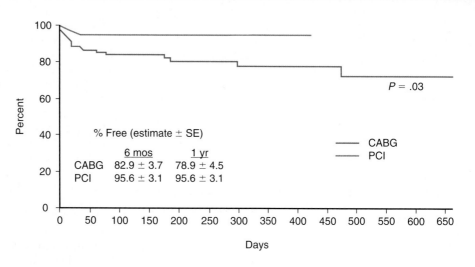

Figure 6-10. Freedom from death, myocardial infarction, and cerebrovascular events in unprotected left main coronary artery disease after treatment with percutaneous coronary intervention (PCI) with drug-eluting stent implantation versus coronary artery bypass grafting (CABG). (From Lee MS, Kapoor N, Jamal F, et al: Comparison of coronary artery bypass surgery with percutaneous coronary intervention with drug-eluting stents for unprotected left main coronary artery disease. J Am Coll Cardiol 2006;47:864-870.)

SYMPTOMATIC INDICATION FOR REVASCULARIZATION: PCI VERSUS MEDICAL THERAPY ALONE

Several studies from the pre-stent era compared PCI with lone medical therapy in patients with single- or double-vessel disease without a prognostic indication for CABG.

The Veterans Affairs ACME trial was the first randomized trial to compare plain balloon angioplasty with medical therapy.[91] In this study, 212 patients with single-vessel disease, stable angina pectoris, and positive results on stress testing or MI within the preceding 3 months were randomized to an initial strategy of plain balloon angioplasty or medical therapy. The primary end points were change in exercise tolerance and change in symptoms at 6 months. Compared with lone medical therapy, balloon angioplasty significantly improved treadmill exercise performance, with an increase in duration of 2.1 ± 3.1 minutes after angioplasty versus 0.5 ± 2.2 minutes without PCI. Moreover, 64% of the patients primarily treated with balloon angioplasty were free of angina pectoris at 6 months, compared with 45% of those in the medical therapy group. Balloon angioplasty was also associated with greater improvement in quality-of-life variables. No significant difference was seen in the frequency of death and MI between the two groups. For the entire cohort, the study demonstrated significant improvement of symptoms with early angioplasty. On the other hand, among patients who become symptom-free on medical therapy, there was no advantage of PCI, because the conservative approach was not associated with any excess MIs or deaths.

Subsequently, the study was extended by including 201 patients with double-vessel coronary disease (ACME-2).[92] At 6 months, patients treated with plain balloon angioplasty and those treated with plain medical therapy had similar degrees of improvement in exercise duration, freedom from angina, and overall quality-of-life score. There was no appreciable increased hazard observed with the conservative approach. This part of the ACME trial suggested that patients with double-vessel disease achieved less benefit from an interventional approach than did patients with single-vessel disease. This may be attributed in part to the limitations that were prevalent in the era of plain balloon angioplasty, which included a relatively high risk of restenosis and inability to achieve full revascularization in a large proportion of patients.

The largest trial comparing balloon angioplasty with medical therapy was RITA-2, which included 1018 patients with single-vessel or multivessel disease.[93] Most of the patients had stable angina and preserved left ventricular function, although unstable angina and left ventricular dysfunction did not constitute an exclusion criterion. Of the patients included, 60% had single-vessel disease, 33% double-vessel disease, and 7% had triple-vessel disease. The primary end point of the trial was the composite of all-cause death and nonfatal MI during a median follow-up of 2.7 years. The incidence of the primary end point was significantly higher in the PTCA arm compared with the conservative arm (6.3% vs. 3.3%; $P = .02$). This difference was largely due to one periprocedural death and seven periprocedural MIs. As in the ACME trial, balloon angioplasty was more efficient in reducing symptoms than the primary medical approach. At 3 months, medical therapy was associated with a 60.5% higher prevalence of grade 2 or worse angina compared with balloon angioplasty ($P < .01$), a difference that attenuated to 7.6% during follow-up. There also was a larger improvement in total exercise time in the balloon angioplasty group compared with the medically treated group. Subgroup analysis revealed that patients with more severe symptoms at study entry obtained a larger symptomatic benefit from balloon angioplasty than did patients with minor symptoms.

A recent study, AVERT, included 341 patients with single- or double-vessel disease who were randomly assigned to either medical treatment including vigorous risk factor modification with state-of-the-art statin therapy or PCI and usual care.[94] The primary study end point was the composite of a variety of

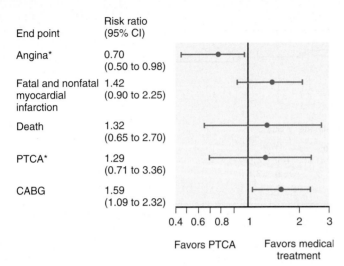

End point	Risk ratio (95% CI)
Angina*	0.70 (0.50 to 0.98)
Fatal and nonfatal myocardial infarction	1.42 (0.90 to 2.25)
Death	1.32 (0.65 to 2.70)
PTCA*	1.29 (0.71 to 3.36)
CABG	1.59 (1.09 to 2.32)

0.4 0.6 0.8 1   2   3

Favors PTCA   Favors medical treatment

Figure 6-11. Pooled risk ratios for various end points from six randomized controlled trials comparing percutaneous transluminal coronary angioplasty (PCTA) with medical treatment in patients with nonacute coronary heart disease. CABG, coronary artery bypass grafting; CI, confidence interval; MI, myocardial infarction. (From Bucher HC, Hengstler P, Schindler C, Guyatt GH: Percutaneous transluminal coronary angioplasty versus medical treatment for non-acute coronary heart disease: Meta-analysis of randomised controlled trials. BMJ 2000;321:73-77.)

events including cardiac death, nonfatal MIs, stroke, CABG, PCI, or hospitalization for unstable angina. One ore more ischemic events occurred in 13% of the medically treated patients and in 21% of the PCI-treated patients during the follow-up period of 18 months. When adjusted for interim analyses that were performed, this difference did not reach statistical significance, although the unadjusted level of significance was $P = .048$. The study did not assess relief of angina. AVERT is difficult to interpret, because state-of-the-art risk factor modification was not instituted in the PCI arm. It is known that patients undergoing PCI obtain particular benefit from high-dose statin treatment. Therefore, the patients who were randomly assigned to balloon angioplasty were penalized by not receiving established treatments for secondary prevention in coronary artery disease. Hence, AVERT cannot answer the key question of whether best-possible medical therapy combined with best-possible PCI will provide superior freedom from death and nonfatal MI as well as better relief of angina, compared with best-possible medical therapy alone. This issue has been addressed in the randomized COURAGE trial.[29] COURAGE included 2287 patients with stable angina who received optimized state-of-the-art medical therapy. Patients were randomly assigned to revascularization by PCI or conservative management alone. Confirming earlier studies, COURAGE did not find a benefit of PCI with respect to death and myocardial infarction during a median follow-up of 4.6 years (19.0% in the PCI group versus 18.5% in the medical-therapy group; HR = 1.05; 95% CI: 0.87 to 1.27; $P = .62$). There was, however, a significant difference in the rates

of freedom from angina throughout most of the follow-up period, favoring PCI. When interpreting the results of COURAGE two aspects need to be considered. First, severe angina (CCS IV) or a markedly positive stress test precluded participation in the study, thus limiting the potential benefit from revascularization. Second, COURAGE pursued the strategy of culprit-lesion treatment. Although seventy percent of the patients had multivessel disease, most of the patients received only one stent. Hence, the revascularization strategy in COURAGE might have fallen short of the full potential of PCI.

A meta-analysis that included ACME (1 and 2), RITA-2, and AVERT as well as MASS and one smaller German trial, demonstrated a significant 30% reduction in angina but a significant increase in the need for CABG with PCI, compared with medical treatment, as well as trends toward increased risk of death, MI, and nonscheduled PCI (Fig. 6-11).[95] This meta-analysis supported the concept that PCI, compared with lone medical therapy in patients with stable angina, reduces symptoms but may be associated with a higher incidence of serious complications such as death and MI. However, none of the studies included in this meta-analysis used contemporary interventional techniques such as the systematic use of stents, vigorous peri-interventional and postinterventional antiplatelet treatment, and strict risk factor modification, in particular with statins, in patients treated with PCI. Modern peri-interventional and postinterventional drug therapy would have reduced the risk of death and MI, and each of the three elements of modern interventional treatment—stents, statins and antiplatelet drugs—would have reduced the need for subsequent unplanned revascularization procedures. Hence, it may be anticipated that with modern interventional approaches the complications of catheter intervention may be substantially lower without corrupting the beneficial effect of this treatment on angina, compared with lone medical therapy.

Although the benefit/risk ratio of PCI versus medical treatment in patients without an established indication for CABG will be superior with modern interventional techniques, there is currently no evidence from randomized studies that in this setting PCI compared with medical therapy reduces the risk of death or nonfatal MI. Therefore, in patients who are free of symptoms under an antianginal medication that is well tolerated, there is no established benefit of PCI. Accordingly, current guidelines suggest that, for patients with stable angina, PCI should be reserved for those who are not free of symptoms with lone medical therapy or who have substantial side effects. This recommendation was challenged recently by a large meta-analysis from the Duke University Medical Center registry that included 18,481 patients (see Fig. 6-8).[50] As detailed earlier, this study demonstrated that, even in patients with low-severity coronary artery disease (one or two vessels = 75%, none = 95%), the initial revascularization by PCI conferred a significant survival benefit (8 months in 7 years, adjusted for pertinent covariables).

SUMMARY

When coronary revascularization is considered, prognostic and symptomatic indications need to be distinguished. With prognostic indications, PCI offers an alternative to CABG; with symptomatic indications, PCI competes with medical treatment.

In general, PCI for single-vessel disease is justified only if improvement of symptoms can be anticipated.

In patients with multivessel disease without relevant left main coronary artery involvement and without diabetes mellitus, survival after PCI is at least not substantially inferior to that after CABG, provided that complete revascularization can be achieved. Patients must be informed that the higher need for repeat procedures after PCI has to be weighed against the discomfort of surgery.

In patients with diabetes mellitus, it is unclear whether multivessel PCI can achieve a prognostic benefit similar to that of CABG. Nevertheless, stents, vigorous antiplatelet treatment, and tight metabolic control have been shown to improve the outcome of PCI in diabetic patients substantially. Depending on the chances for success and the risk for surgery, multivessel PCI may offer a reasonable option even in diabetic patients.

Currently available evidence does not allow proposing PCI for distal left main coronary artery disease in patients who are good candidates for surgery. Promising results from recent registries indicate that PCI is an acceptable alternative to CABG in poor surgical candidates.

In many instances, individualized decisions must be taken that consider the likelihood of complete revascularization and the risk associated with either approach, the patient's life expectancy based on age and comorbidities, and the patient's preference after thorough counseling. Such decisions are best reached jointly by the cardiac surgeon and the interventional cardiologist.

REFERENCES

1. Serruys PW, de Jaegere P, Kiemeneij F, et al: A comparison of balloon-expandable-stent implantation with balloon angioplasty in patients with coronary artery disease. Benestent Study Group. N Engl J Med 1994;331:489-495.
2. Betriu A, Masotti M, Serra A, et al: Randomized comparison of coronary stent implantation and balloon angioplasty in the treatment of de novo coronary artery lesions (START): A four-year follow-up. J Am Coll Cardiol 1999;34:1498-1506.
3. Fischman DL, Leon MB, Baim DS, et al: A randomized comparison of coronary-stent placement and balloon angioplasty in the treatment of coronary artery disease. Stent Restenosis Study Investigators. N Engl J Med 1994;331:496-501.
4. Spaulding C, Daemen J, Boersma E, et al: A pooled analysis of data comparing sirolimus-eluting stents with bare-metal stents. N Engl J Med 2007:356:989–997.
5. Stone GW, Moses JW, Ellis SG, et al: Safety and efficacy of sirolimus- and paclitaxel-eluting coronary stents. N Engl J Med 2007;356:998-1008.
6. Mauri L, Hsieh W, Massaro JM, et al: Stent thrombosis in randomized clinical trials of drug eluting stents. N Engl J Med 2007;356:1020-1029.
7. Kastrati A, Mehilli J, Pache J, et al: Analysis of 14 trials comparing sirolimus-eluting stents with bare-metal stents. N Engl J Med 2007;356:1030-1039.
8. Fibrinolytic Therapy Trialists' (FTT) Collaborative Group: Indications for fibrinolytic therapy in suspected acute myocardial infarction: Collaborative overview of early mortality and major morbidity results from all randomised trials of more than 1000 patients. Lancet 1994;343:311-322.
9. Boersma E: The Primary Coronary Angioplasty vs. Thrombolysis Group. Does time matter? A pooled analysis of randomized clinical trials comparing primary percutaneous coronary intervention and in-hospital fibrinolysis in acute myocardial infarction patients. Eur Heart J 2006;27:779-788.
10. Keeley EC, Boura JA, Grines CL: Primary angioplasty versus intravenous thrombolytic therapy for acute myocardial infarction: A quantitative review of 23 randomised trials. Lancet 2003;361:13-20.
11. Neumann FJ, Kastrati A, Schwarzer G: New aspects in the treatment of acute coronary syndromes without ST-elevation: ICTUS and ISAR-COOL in perspective. Eur Heart J Suppl 2007;9:A4-A10.
12. Mehta SR, Cannon CP, Fox KA, et al: Routine vs selective invasive strategies in patients with acute coronary syndromes: A collaborative meta-analysis of randomized trials. JAMA 2005;293:2908-2917.
13. Fox KA, Poole-Wilson P, Clayton TC, et al: 5-Year outcome of an interventional strategy in non-ST-elevation acute coronary syndrome: The British Heart Foundation RITA 3 randomised trial. Lancet 2005;366:914-920.
14. Lagerqvist B, Husted S, Kontny F, et al: 5-Year outcomes in the FRISC-II randomised trial of an invasive versus a non-invasive strategy in non-ST-elevation acute coronary syndrome: A follow-up study. Lancet 2006;368:998-1004.
15. Cannon CP, Weintraub WS, Demopoulos LA, et al: Comparison of early invasive and conservative strategies in patients with unstable coronary syndromes treated with the glycoprotein IIb/IIIa inhibitor tirofiban. N Engl J Med 2001; 344:1879-1887.
16. Fox KA, Poole-Wilson PA, Henderson RA, et al: Interventional versus conservative treatment for patients with unstable angina or non-ST-elevation myocardial infarction: The British Heart Foundation RITA 3 randomised trial. Randomized Intervention Trial of unstable Angina. Lancet 2002;360:743-751.
17. FRISC II Investigators: Invasive compared with non-invasive treatment in unstable coronary-artery disease: FRISC II prospective randomised multicentre study. Lancet 1999;354: 708-715.
18. Bertrand ME, Simoons ML, Fox KA, et al; Task Force on the Management of Acute Coronary Syndromes of the European Society of Cardiology: Management of acute coronary syndromes in patients presenting without persistent ST-segment elevation. Eur Heart J 2002;23:1809-1840.
19. de Winter RJ, Windhausen F, Cornel JH, et al: Early invasive versus selectively invasive management for acute coronary syndromes. N Engl J Med 2005;353:1095-1104.
20. Weiner DA, Ryan TJ, McCabe CH, et al: The role of exercise testing in identifying patients with improved survival after coronary artery bypass surgery. J Am Coll Cardiol 1986;8: 741-748.
21. Mock MB, Fisher LD, Holmes DR Jr, et al: Comparison of effects of medical and surgical therapy on survival in severe angina pectoris and two-vessel coronary artery disease with and without left ventricular dysfunction: A Coronary Artery Surgery Study Registry Study. Am J Cardiol 1988;61: 1198-1203.
22. Pepine CJ, Geller NL, Knatterud GL, et al: The Asymptomatic Cardiac Ischemia Pilot (ACIP) study: Design of a randomized clinical trial, baseline data and implications for a long-term outcome trial. J Am Coll Cardiol 1994;24:1-10.
23. Hachamovitch R, Hayes SW, Friedman JD, et al: Comparison of the short-term survival benefit associated with revascularization compared with medical therapy in patients with no prior coronary artery disease undergoing stress myocardial perfusion single photon emission computed tomography. Circulation 2003;107:2900-2907.
24. Yusuf S, Zucker D, Peduzzi P, et al: Effect of coronary artery bypass graft surgery on survival: Overview of 10-year results from randomised trials by the Coronary Artery Bypass Graft Surgery Trialists Collaboration. Lancet 1994;344:563-570.

25. ECSS Group: Long-term results of prospective randomised study of coronary artery bypass surgery in stable angina pectoris. European Coronary Surgery Study Group. Lancet 1982;2:1173-1180.

26. Passamani E, Davis KB, Gillespie MJ, Killip T: A randomized trial of coronary artery bypass surgery: Survival of patients with a low ejection fraction. N Engl J Med 1985;312:1665-1671.

27. Peduzzi P, Hultgren HN: Effect of medical vs surgical treatment on symptoms in stable angina pectoris: The Veterans Administration Cooperative Study of surgery for coronary arterial occlusive disease. Circulation 1979;60:888-900.

28. Hueb WA, Bellotti G, de Oliveira SA, et al: The Medicine, Angioplasty or Surgery Study (MASS): A prospective, randomized trial of medical therapy, balloon angioplasty or bypass surgery for single proximal left anterior descending artery stenoses. J Am Coll Cardiol 1995;26:1600-1605.

29. Boden WE, O'Rourke RA, Teo KK, et al: Optimal medical therapy with or without PCI for stable coronary disease. N Engl J Med 2007;356:1503-1516.

30. Bell MR, Gersh BJ, Schaff HV, et al: Effect of completeness of revascularization on long-term outcome of patients with three-vessel disease undergoing coronary artery bypass surgery: A report from the Coronary Artery Surgery Study (CASS) Registry. Circulation 1992;86:446-457.

31. Bourassa MG, Kip KE, Jacobs AK, et al: Is a strategy of intended incomplete percutaneous transluminal coronary angioplasty revascularization acceptable in nondiabetic patients who are candidates for coronary artery bypass graft surgery? The Bypass Angioplasty Revascularization Investigation (BARI). J Am Coll Cardiol 1999;33:1627-1636.

32. Cowley MJ, Vandermael M, Topol EJ, et al: Is traditionally defined complete revascularization needed for patients with multivessel disease treated by elective coronary angioplasty? Multivessel Angioplasty Prognosis Study (MAPS) Group. J Am Coll Cardiol 1993;22:1289-1297.

33. Hannan EL, Racz M, Holmes DR, et al: Impact of completeness of percutaneous coronary intervention revascularization on long-term outcomes in the stent era. Circulation 2006;113:2406-2412.

34. Hoffman SN, TenBrook JA, Wolf MP, et al: A meta-analysis of randomized controlled trials comparing coronary artery bypass graft with percutaneous transluminal coronary angioplasty: One- to eight-year outcomes. J Am Coll Cardiol 2003;41:1293-1304.

35. Serruys PW, Ong AT, van Herwerden LA, et al: Five-year outcomes after coronary stenting versus bypass surgery for the treatment of multivessel disease: The final analysis of the Arterial Revascularization Therapies Study (ARTS) randomized trial. J Am Coll Cardiol 2005;46:575-581.

36. Serruys PW, Unger F, Sousa JE, et al: Comparison of coronary-artery bypass surgery and stenting for the treatment of multivessel disease. N Engl J Med 2001;344:1117-1124.

37. SoS Investigators: Coronary artery bypass surgery versus percutaneous coronary intervention with stent implantation in patients with multivessel coronary artery disease (the Stent or Surgery trial): A randomised controlled trial. Lancet 2002;360:965-970.

38. Rodriguez A, Bernardi V, Navia J, et al: Argentine Randomized Study—Coronary Angioplasty with Stenting versus Coronary Bypass Surgery in patients with Multiple-Vessel Disease (ERACI II): 30-Day and one-year follow-up results. ERACI II Investigators. J Am Coll Cardiol 2001;37:51-58.

39. Rodriguez AE, Baldi J, Fernandez Pereira C, et al: Five-year follow-up of the Argentine randomized trial of coronary angioplasty with stenting versus coronary bypass surgery in patients with multiple vessel disease (ERACI II). J Am Coll Cardiol 2005;46:582-588.

40. Hueb W, Soares PR, Gersh BJ, et al; The Medicine, Angioplasty, or Surgery Study (MASS-II): A randomized, controlled clinical trial of three therapeutic strategies for multivessel coronary artery disease: One-year results. J Am Coll Cardiol 2004;43:1743-1751.

41. Morrison DA, Sethi G, Sacks J, et al: Percutaneous coronary intervention versus coronary artery bypass graft surgery for patients with medically refractory myocardial ischemia and risk factors for adverse outcomes with bypass: A multicenter, randomized trial. J Am Coll Cardiol 2001;38:143-149.

42. Stroupe KT, Morrison DA, Hlatky MA, et al: Cost-effectiveness of coronary artery bypass grafts versus percutaneous coronary intervention for revascularization of high-risk patients. Circulation 2006;114:1251-1257.

43. Morrison DA, Sethi G, Sacks J, et al: Percutaneous coronary intervention versus coronary bypass graft surgery for patients with medically refractory myocardial ischemia and risk factors for adverse outcomes with bypass: The VA AWESOME multicenter registry. Comparison with the randomized clinical trial. J Am Coll Cardiol 2002;39:266-273.

44. Morrison DA, Sethi G, Sacks J, et al: Percutaneous coronary intervention versus repeat bypass surgery for patients with medically refractory myocardial ischemia: AWESOME randomized trial and registry experience with post-CABG patients. J Am Coll Cardiol 2002;40:1951-1954.

45. Mercado N, Wijns W, Serruys PW, et al: One-year outcomes of coronary artery bypass graft surgery versus percutaneous coronary intervention with multiple stenting for multisystem disease: A meta-analysis of individual patient data from randomized clinical trials. J Thorac Cardiovasc Surg 2005;130:512-519.

46. Grapow MT, von Wattenwyl R, Guller U, et al: Randomized controlled trials do not reflect reality: Real-world analyses are critical for treatment guidelines! J Thorac Cardiovasc Surg 2006;132:5-7.

47. Brener SJ, Lytle BW, Casserly IP, et al: Propensity analysis of long-term survival after surgical or percutaneous revascularization in patients with multivessel coronary artery disease and high-risk features. Circulation 2004;109:2290-2295.

48. Hannan EL, Racz MJ, Walford G, et al: Long-term outcomes of coronary-artery bypass grafting versus stent implantation. N Engl J Med 2005;352:2174-2183.

49. van Domburg RT, Takkenberg JJ, Noordzij LJ, et al: Late outcome after stenting or coronary artery bypass surgery for the treatment of multivessel disease: A single-center matched-propensity controlled cohort study. Ann Thorac Surg 2005;79:1563-1569.

50. Smith PK, Califf RM, Tuttle RH, et al: Selection of surgical or percutaneous coronary intervention provides differential longevity benefit. Ann Thorac Surg 2006;82:1420-1428.

51. Serruys PW, Ong ATL, Morice MC, et al: Arterial Revascularisation Therapies Study Part II: Sirolimus-eluting stents for the treatment of patients with multivessel de novo coronary artery lesions. EuroInterv 2005;1:147-156.

52. Barzilay JI, Kronmal RA, Bittner V, et al: Coronary artery disease and coronary artery bypass grafting in diabetic patients aged > or = 65 years: Report from the Coronary Artery Surgery Study (CASS) Registry. Am J Cardiol 1994;74:334-339.

53. Van Belle E, Abolmaali K, Bauters C, et al: Restenosis, late vessel occlusion and left ventricular function six months after balloon angioplasty in diabetic patients. J Am Coll Cardiol 1999;34:476-485.

54. Elezi S, Kastrati A, Pache J, et al: Diabetes mellitus and the clinical and angiographic outcome after coronary stent placement. J Am Coll Cardiol 1998;32:1866-1873.

55. Van Belle E, Ketelers R, Bauters C, et al: Patency of percutaneous transluminal coronary angioplasty sites at 6-month angiographic follow-up: A key determinant of survival in diabetics after coronary balloon angioplasty. Circulation 2001;103:1218-1224.

56. Kip KE, Faxon DP, Detre KM, et al: Coronary angioplasty in diabetic patients: The National Heart, Lung, and Blood Institute Percutaneous Transluminal Coronary Angioplasty Registry. Circulation 1996;94:1818-1825.

57. BARI Investigators: Seven-year outcome in the Bypass Angioplasty Revascularization Investigation (BARI) by treatment and diabetic status. J Am Coll Cardiol 2000;35:1122-1129.

58. Ellis SG, Narins CR: Problem of angioplasty in diabetics. Circulation 1997;96:1707-1710.

59. King SB, Kosinski AS, Guyton RA, et al: Eight-year mortality in the Emory Angioplasty versus Surgery Trial (EAST). J Am Coll Cardiol 2000;35:1116-1121.

60. Weintraub WS, Stein B, Kosinski A, et al: Outcome of coronary bypass surgery versus coronary angioplasty in diabetic patients

with multivessel coronary artery disease. J Am Coll Cardiol 1998;31:10-19.

61. Niles NW, McGrath PD, Malenka D, et al: Survival of patients with diabetes and multivessel coronary artery disease after surgical or percutaneous coronary revascularization: Results of a large regional prospective study. Northern New England Cardiovascular Disease Study Group. J Am Coll Cardiol 2001;37:1008-1015.

62. Marso SP, Lincoff AM, Ellis SG, et al: Optimizing the percutaneous interventional outcomes for patients with diabetes mellitus: Results of the EPISTENT diabetic substudy. Circulation 1999;100:2477-2484.

63. Bhatt DL, Marso SP, Lincoff AM, et al: Abciximab reduces mortality in diabetics following percutaneous coronary intervention. J Am Coll Cardiol 2000;35:922-928.

64. Mehilli J, Kastrati A, Schühlen H, et al: Randomized clinical trial of abciximab in diabetic patients undergoing elective percutaneous coronary interventions after treatment with a high loading dose of clopidogrel. Circulation 2004;110:3627-3635.

65. Van Belle E, Bauters C, Hubert E, et al: Restenosis rates in diabetic patients: A comparison of coronary stenting and balloon angioplasty in native coronary vessels. Circulation 1997;96:1454-1460.

66. Van Belle E, Perie M, Braune D, et al: Effects of coronary stenting on vessel patency and long-term clinical outcome after percutaneous coronary revascularization in diabetic patients. J Am Coll Cardiol 2002;40:410-417.

67. Otsuka Y, Myazaki S, Okumura H: Abnormal glucose tolerance, not small vessel diameter, is a determinant of long-term prognosis in patients treated with balloon coronary angioplasty. Eur Heart J 2000;21:1790-1796.

68. Takagi T, Akasaka T, Yamamuro A, et al: Troglitazone reduces neointimal tissue proliferation after coronary stent implantation in patients with non-insulin dependent diabetes mellitus: A serial intravascular ultrasound study. J Am Coll Cardiol 2000;36:1529-1535.

69. Abizaid A, Costa MA, Centemero M, et al: Clinical and economic impact of diabetes mellitus on percutaneous and surgical treatment of multivessel coronary disease patients: Insights from the Arterial Revascularization Therapy Study (ARTS) trial. Circulation 2001;104:533-538.

70. Sedlis SP, Morrison DA, Lorin JD, et al: Percutaneous coronary intervention versus coronary bypass graft surgery for diabetic patients with unstable angina and risk factors for adverse outcomes with bypass: Outcome of diabetic patients in the AWESOME randomized trial and registry. J Am Coll Cardiol 2002;40:1555-1566.

71. Dzavik V, Ghali WA, Norris C: Long-term survival in 11,661 patients with multivessel coronary artery disease in the era of stenting: A report from the Alberta Provincial Project for Outcome Assessment in Coronary Heart Disease (APPROACH) investigators. Am Heart J 2001;142:119-126.

72. Scheen AJ, Warzee F, Legrand VM: Drug-eluting stents: Meta-analysis in diabetic patients. Eur Heart J 2004;25:2167-2168; author reply 2168-2169.

73. O'Keefe JH, Hartzler GO, Rutherford BD, et al: Left main coronary angioplasty: Early and late results of 127 acute and elective procedures. Am J Cardiol 1989;64:144-147.

74. Ellis SG, Tamai H, Nobuyoshi M, et al: Contemporary percutaneous treatment of unprotected left main coronary stenoses: Initial results from a multicenter registry analysis 1994-1996. Circulation 1997;96:3867-3872.

75. Silvestri M, Barragan P, Sainsous J, et al: Unprotected left main coronary stenting: Immediate and medium-term outcomes of 140 elective procedures. J Am Coll Cardiol 2000;35:1543-1550.

76. Park SJ, Park SW, Hong MK, et al: Stenting of unprotected left main coronary artery stenoses: Immediate and late outcomes. J Am Coll Cardiol 1998;31:37-42.

77. Park SJ, Hong MK, Lee CW, et al: Elective stenting of unprotected left main coronary artery stenosis: Effect of debulking before stenting and intravascular ultrasound guidance. J Am Coll Cardiol 2001;38:1054-1060.

78. Lee BK, Hong MK, Lee CW, et al: Five-year outcomes after stenting of unprotected left main coronary artery stenosis in patients with normal left ventricular function. Int J Cardiol 2006;115:208-213 (Epub 2006 Aug 9).

79. Park SJ, Park SW, Hong MK, et al: Long-term (three-year) outcomes after stenting of unprotected left main coronary artery stenosis in patients with normal left ventricular function. Am J Cardiol 2003;91:12-16.

80. Suarez de Lezo J, Medina A, Romero M, et al: Predictors of restenosis following unprotected left main coronary stenting. Am J Cardiol 2001;88:308-310.

81. Lopez JJ, Ho KK, Stoler RC, et al: Percutaneous treatment of protected and unprotected left main coronary stenoses with new devices: Immediate angiographic results and intermediate-term follow-up. J Am Coll Cardiol 1997;29:345-352.

82. Laruelle CJ, Brueren GB, Ernst SM, et al: Stenting of "unprotected" left main coronary artery stenoses: Early and late results. Heart 1998;79:148-152.

83. Wong P, Wong V, Tse KK, et al: A prospective study of elective stenting in unprotected left main coronary disease. Catheter Cardiovasc Interv 1999;46:153-159.

84. Park SJ, Kim YH, Lee BK, et al: Sirolimus-eluting stent implantation for unprotected left main coronary artery stenosis: Comparison with bare metal stent implantation. J Am Coll Cardiol 2005;45:351-356.

85. Chieffo A, Stankovic G, Bonizzoni E, et al: Early and mid-term results of drug-eluting stent implantation in unprotected left main. Circulation 2005;111:791-795.

86. Valgimigli M, van Mieghem CA, Ong AT, et al: Short- and long-term clinical outcome after drug-eluting stent implantation for the percutaneous treatment of left main coronary artery disease: Insights from the Rapamycin-Eluting and Taxus Stent Evaluated At Rotterdam Cardiology Hospital registries (RESEARCH and T-SEARCH). Circulation 2005;111:1383-1389.

87. Valgimigli M, Malagutti P, Rodriguez-Granillo GA, et al: Distal left main disease is a major predictor of outcome in patients undergoing percutaneous intervention in the drug-eluting stent era: An integrated clinical and angiographic analysis based on the Rapamycin-Eluting Stent Evaluated At Rotterdam Cardiology Hospital (RESEARCH) and Taxus-Stent Evaluated At Rotterdam Cardiology Hospital (T-SEARCH) registries. J Am Coll Cardiol 2006;47:1530-1537.

88. Valgimigli M, Malagutti P, Rodriguez Granillo GA, et al: Single-vessel versus bifurcation stenting for the treatment of distal left main coronary artery disease in the drug-eluting stenting era: Clinical and angiographic insights into the Rapamycin-Eluting Stent Evaluated at Rotterdam Cardiology Hospital (RESEARCH) and Taxus-Stent Evaluated at Rotterdam Cardiology Hospital (T-SEARCH) registries. Am Heart J 2006;152:896-902.

89. Lee MS, Kapoor N, Jamal F, et al: Comparison of coronary artery bypass surgery with percutaneous coronary intervention with drug-eluting stents for unprotected left main coronary artery disease. J Am Coll Cardiol 2006;47:864-870.

90. Chieffo A, Morici N, Maisano F, et al: Percutaneous treatment with drug-eluting stent implantation versus bypass surgery for unprotected left main stenosis: A single-center experience. Circulation 2006;113:2542-2547.

91. Parisi AF, Folland ED, Hartigan P: A comparison of angioplasty with medical therapy in the treatment of single-vessel coronary artery disease. Veterans Affairs ACME Investigators. N Engl J Med 1992;326:10-16.

92. Folland ED, Hartigan PM, Parisi AF: Percutaneous transluminal coronary angioplasty versus medical therapy for stable angina pectoris: Outcomes for patients with double-vessel versus single-vessel coronary artery disease in a Veterans Affairs Cooperative randomized trial. Veterans Affairs ACME Investigators. J Am Coll Cardiol 1997;29:1505-1511.

93. RITA-2 Investigators: Coronary angioplasty versus medical therapy for angina: The second Randomised Intervention Treatment of Angina (RITA-2) trial. Lancet 1997;350:461-468.

94. Pitt B, Waters D, Brown WV, et al: Aggressive lipid-lowering therapy compared with angioplasty in stable coronary artery disease. N Engl J Med 1999;341:70-76.

95. Bucher HC, Hengstler P, Schindler C, Guyatt GH: Percutaneous transluminal coronary angioplasty versus medical treatment for non-acute coronary heart disease: Meta-analysis of randomised controlled trials. BMJ 2000;321:73-77.

7 Preoperative Coronary Intervention

Craig R. Narins

KEY POINTS

- Perioperative myocardial infarction (MI) can result from coronary plaque rupture or from a myocardial oxygen supply-demand mismatch related to a preexisting coronary stenosis.
- Perioperative MI, even if clinically silent, is a powerful predictor of future adverse cardiac events.
- The indications for performing preoperative coronary angiography are typically the same as those in the nonoperative setting.
- Perioperative β-blocker therapy has been associated with reduced cardiac event rates among patients at risk for complications during noncardiac surgery.
- The benefit of using coronary revascularization to "get the patient through" noncardiac surgery is unproven.
- Because no prospective trial to date has demonstrated short- or long-term benefits from a strategy of routine

- preoperative percutaneous coronary intervention (PCI) among patients with coronary disease, the indications for preoperative PCI at this time remain limited and uncertain.
- The procedural risks of PCI are increased among patients with comorbidities requiring impending surgery, especially peripheral vascular disease.
- Noncardiac surgery performed within 6 weeks after coronary stent implantation is associated with very high rates of stent thrombosis and major cardiac events.
- The risk-benefit decision regarding whether to perform preoperative PCI is typically complex and requires multidisciplinary input from the cardiologist, surgeon, and other involved subspecialists.

Of the more than 30 million surgical procedures requiring the use of general anesthesia performed annually in the United States, approximately one third involve patients who are at risk for or have known coronary artery disease. Given the physiologic stresses that accompany surgery, the perioperative period represents a time of substantially heightened risk for adverse cardiac events among these individuals. A variety of algorithms have been developed to assist practitioners in predicting which patients are at elevated risk for perioperative cardiac events, but in clinical practice there remains a great deal of physician-to-physician variability in the approach to preoperative risk assessment. Even more so, among patients documented to have significant coronary disease, controversy persists as to whether and when preoperative coronary revascularization may have a beneficial role in reducing the likelihood of subsequent cardiac events.

Despite these uncertainties, preoperative assessment remains a common indication for coronary angiography in clinical practice. Among individuals who do ultimately undergo percutaneous coronary intervention (PCI) before noncardiac surgery, various

technical issues exist that are unique to the preoperative setting. This chapter provides a clinically oriented review of preoperative PCI, including the indications for coronary angiography before upcoming surgery, the utility of various medical and interventional strategies to reduce perioperative risk among patients with known or suspected coronary disease, and the technical aspects of performing angioplasty and stenting before noncardiac surgery.

PERIOPERATIVE MYOCARDIAL INFARCTION

Pathophysiology

Similar to myocardial infarction (MI) outside the context of surgery, perioperative MI can result either from atherosclerotic plaque rupture, with subsequent thrombotic occlusion of the involved coronary artery, or from a transient stress-induced mismatch of myocardial oxygen supply and demand, often in the setting of a fixed coronary artery stenosis. Among patients with fatal perioperative MI, autopsy series have demonstrated histologic characteristics of recent plaque rupture in approximately 50% of cases. Clinical studies employing routine continuous electrocardiographic (ECG) monitoring during and after noncardiac surgery demonstrate that the most nonfatal perioperative MIs are preceded by ST-segment depression rather than elevation, supporting the concept that most surgically related MIs result from a myocardial oxygen supply-demand mismatch rather than acute thrombotic occlusion. Clinical studies also suggest that most perioperative MIs are nontransmural in nature. For example, in a study of 232 high-risk individuals who had routine myocardial enzyme determinations after noncardiac surgery, 10% of patients were ruled-in for postoperative MI, but only 1% ultimately developed new Q waves on their ECG.

In one large retrospective analysis that examined clinical and angiographic data from 1242 patients who underwent preoperative coronary angiography followed by vascular surgery at a single center from 1984 to 1991, the incidence of perioperative MI or death was 1.7%. In 57% of instances, MI could be attributed to a known occluded collateralized coronary artery, again invoking the development of a myocardial supply-demand mismatch as an important contributor to the development of MI.[1] Within this same cohort, however, several patients did develop a postsurgical MI in a coronary territory without a corresponding obstructive lesion on the presurgical angiogram, corroborating the finding from autopsy series that plaque rupture with subsequent vessel thrombosis serves as a potential mechanism for perioperative MI. From a clinical standpoint, the potential for rupture of a previously nonobstructive plaque highlights a mechanism by which perioperative MI can occur despite the absence of ischemia on presurgical stress testing or of significant coronary stenosis on coronary angiography.

Timing

In most instances, perioperative MI does not occur during the surgical procedure itself, but rather within the first 48 hours after surgery. Among MIs diagnosed in one cohort of 323 patients undergoing noncardiac surgery, 94% occurred by the second postoperative day, with approximately half occurring on the day of surgery. Indeed, the first few hours after surgery, when the patient is emerging from general anesthesia, is the period that poses the greatest risk for myocardial ischemia (Fig. 7-1). This period is associated with multiple hemodynamic stresses and hematologic alterations that can predispose to either plaque rupture or a myocardial oxygen supply-demand mismatch. Spikes in plasma catecholamine levels and increases in sympathetic nervous system tone are observed during withdrawal of general anesthesia. These changes typically result in increased heart rate, blood pressure, and myocardial contractility, leading to greater myocardial oxygen demand. Likewise, these neuroendocrine alterations can favor coronary vasospasm or changes in shear stress within the coronary arteries. In addition, tissue injury inherent in

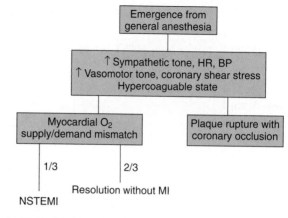

Figure 7-1. Pathophysiologic events contributing to the genesis of perioperative myocardial infarction (MI). BP, blood pressure; HR, heart rate; NSTEMI, non–ST-segment elevation myocardial infarction.

surgical procedures tends to engender a procoagulant state, often associated with generalized platelet activation, reductions in endogenous tissue plasminogen activator levels, and increased plasminogen activator inhibitor levels, all changes that can favor coronary thrombosis. Other factors that may adversely influence the balance of myocardial oxygen delivery and demand in the early postoperative period include anemia resulting from surgical blood loss, tachycardia or hypertension induced by postoperative pain, and fluid shifts frequently seen after surgical procedures.

Incidence

The incidence of myocardial ischemia and infarction in the period surrounding noncardiac surgery is a function of both the type of surgery and the risk profile of the population being studied. The type of surgery influences the likelihood of adverse perioperative cardiac events in two primary ways. First, the specific condition being addressed by the surgical procedure often can serve as an indicator of the patient's likelihood of harboring concomitant coronary artery disease. For example, because of the systemic nature of atherosclerosis, approximately two thirds of patients undergoing vascular surgery also possess significant coronary artery disease, and only 10% of such patients have angiographically normal coronary arteries (Fig. 7-2). Second, the type of surgery being performed can greatly influence the degree of intraoperative hemodynamic stress to which the patient will be exposed, and consequently has a bearing on the likelihood of cardiac complications. Surgical procedures associated with greater amounts of perioperative pain or blood loss, longer periods of recovery and immobility, or greater degrees of intraoperative alterations in blood pressure or heart rate (e.g., cross-clamping of the aorta during abdominal aortic aneurysm repair, manipulation of the carotid

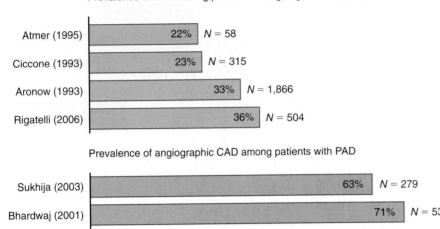

Prevalence of PAD among patients undergoing cardiac catheterization

Atmer (1995) — 22% *N* = 58
Ciccone (1993) — 23% *N* = 315
Aronow (1993) — 33% *N* = 1,866
Rigatelli (2006) — 36% *N* = 504

Prevalence of angiographic CAD among patients with PAD

Sukhija (2003) — 63% *N* = 279
Bhardwaj (2001) — 71% *N* = 53

Figure 7-2. Frequency of concomitant coronary artery disease (CAD) and peripheral arterial disease (PAD) among patients referred for coronary angiography *(top)* and among patients undergoing coronary angiography in the setting of documented PAD *(bottom)*. (Data from Aronow WS, Ahn C: Am J Cardiol 1994;74: 64-65; Atmer B, et al: International Angiol 1995;14:89-93; Bhardwaj R, et al: Indian Heart J 2001;53:189-191; Ciccone M, et al: International Angiol 1993;12:25-28; Rigatelli G, Rigatelli G: Int J Cardiol 2006;106:35-40; Sukhija R, et al: Am J Cardiol 2003;92: 304-305.)

baroreceptor during carotid endarterectomy) typically are associated with greater likelihoods of perioperative cardiac events.

The incidence of myocardial ischemia during vascular surgical procedures has ranged from 10% to 30% in various studies.[2] In one study of 188 individuals who underwent continuous ECG monitoring during and after vascular surgery, ST abnormalities compatible with myocardial ischemia were noted in 20% of patients, 6.5% of whom were ultimately ruled-in for MI. Whereas the duration of ischemia was variable (range, 29 to 625 minutes), in all instances the ST depression was preceded by the onset of tachycardia and marked by eventual resolution of ECG changes without the development of new Q waves.[3] The American College of Cardiology/American Heart Association (ACC/AHA) guidelines for perioperative assessment classify specific operations as high risk (>5% reported cardiac event rate), intermediate risk (1%-5%), or low risk (<1%) (Table 7-1).

Table 7-1. Cardiac Risk* for Noncardiac Surgical Procedures

High (reported cardiac risk often >5%)
Emergent major operations, particularly in the elderly
Aortic and other major vascular surgery
Peripheral vascular surgery
Anticipated prolonged surgical procedures associated with large fluid shifts and/or blood loss

Intermediate (reported cardiac risk usually <5%)
Carotid endarterectomy
Head and neck surgery
Intraperitoneal and intrathoracic surgery
Orthopedic surgery
Prostate surgery

Low (reported cardiac risk usually <1%)
Endoscopic procedures
Superficial procedures
Cataract surgery
Breast surgery

*Death and/or myocardial infarction.
From Eagle KA, Berger PB, Calkins H, et al: ACC/AHA guideline update for perioperative cardiovascular evaluation for noncardiac surgery: Executive summary. A report of the American College of Cardiology/ American Heart Association Task Force on Practice Guidelines. Circulation 2002;105:1257-1267.

Clinical Implications

Perioperative MI, whether clinically apparent or silent, is associated with increased mortality in both the short and long term. Most perioperative infarctions are asymptomatic and detected only by serial ECG and myocardial enzyme monitoring. Likewise, in-hospital mortality is uncommon in the setting of perioperative MI, with hospital survival rates typically greater than 90%, similar to rates for MI in the nonoperative setting. However, in a manner analogous to clinically silent MI detected after PCI, even smaller infarcts detected after noncardiac surgery are associated with striking increases in medium- to late-term mortality. In one series of 229 patients who had routine serial myocardial enzyme determinations performed over a 3-day period after major vascular surgery, elevated serum troponin levels were detected in 12% of the patients. Whereas increased troponin levels were not associated with a greater likelihood of in-hospital mortality, by 6 months those patients with perioperative troponin elevations demonstrated a sixfold increase in mortality and a 27-fold excess rate of subsequent MI compared with patients without a perioperative troponin rise. A dose-response relationship was noted within this cohort, whereby higher postoperative troponin concentrations were associated with progressively greater likelihoods of adverse events during follow-up.[4] In a longer-term surveillance study of 447 patients who underwent vascular surgery, elevations in serum troponin and/or creatine kinase (CK) levels were associated with a highly significant twofold to fourfold increase in mortality during a mean follow-up period of 32 months, independent of other clinical factors such as age or prior cardiac history. Even minor elevations in biomarker levels during the initial 72 hours after surgery were predictive of late mortality (Fig. 7-3).[5] Similarly, in a separate group of 391 patients who underwent vascular surgery, postoperative troponin elevation was associated with significant elevations in death or MI, both at 30 days (hazard ratio [HR] = 5.5; 95% confidence interval [CI]: 3.2 to 9.4) and at 18 months (HR = 4.7; 95% CI:

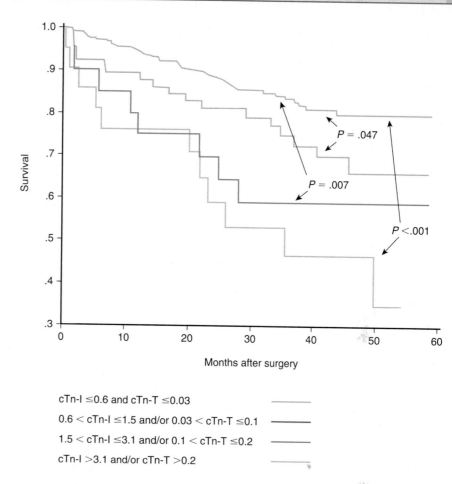

Figure 7-3. Relationship between degree of troponin elevation after vascular surgery and subsequent mortality among 447 patients. cTn-I, cardiac troponin-I; cTn-T, cardiac troponin-T. (From Landesberg G, Shatz V, Akopnik I, et al: Association of cardiac troponin, CK-MB, and postoperative myocardial ischemia with long-term survival after major vascular surgery. J Am Coll Cardiol 2003;42:1547-1554.)

2.9 to 7.6), even after adjustment for other clinical predictors of adverse events.[6]

Determining Operative Risk

Concepts

For the process of preoperative evaluation to be a clinically useful exercise, two goals must be accomplished. First, the evaluation must result in the identification of a subgroup of patients who are at heightened risk of short- or long-term cardiac complications during or after surgery. Second, and equally important, once this higher-risk group is identified, there must exist some intervention that can modify that risk, whether canceling the surgery or intervening to make the surgery safer, such as by prescribing a medication, changing the operative approach or route of anesthesia, or correcting an underlying problem (e.g., through coronary revascularization). Several models have been devised that allow prediction of operative risk based on a patient's clinical history and the results of noninvasive testing. In culling findings from a wealth of studies, the ACC/AHA consensus guidelines for preoperative evaluation before noncardiac surgery have become a widely used clinical tool, not only to identify operative risk but to serve as a guideline for the appropriateness of further testing and intervention.[7] A complete review of preoperative risk stratification is beyond the scope of this chapter, but the key principles, as specifically related to indications for performing coronary angiography and revascularization before planned noncardiac surgery, will be summarized.

The ACC/AHA guidelines recommend a stepwise approach to determining the need for invasive testing before noncardiac surgery. First, patient-specific risk is determined through assessment of clinical risk factors and symptoms, overall functional capacity, and the timing and results of prior coronary evaluation and treatment, if applicable. Second, surgery-specific cardiac risk is determined based on the expected incidence of cardiac events associated with the particular surgery that the patient is scheduled to undergo, as previously discussed. The decision whether to perform noninvasive stress testing is then based on assessment of these patient-specific and surgery-specific risks (Table 7-2; see Table 7-1). For example, a low-risk patient undergoing a low-risk surgery typically does not require further testing, because the results would be unlikely to alter surgical risk or outcome. Likewise, for high-risk individuals, such as patients with unstable angina or recent MI,

Table 7-2. Clinical Predictors of Increased Perioperative Cardiovascular Risk*

Major risk
Unstable coronary syndromes
  Acute or recent MI with evidence of important ischemic risk by
    clinical symptoms or noninvasive study
  Unstable or severe angina (CCS class III or IV)
Decompensated heart failure
Significant arrhythmias
  High-grade atrioventricular block
  Symptomatic ventricular arrhythmias with underlying heart
    disease
  Supraventricular arrhythmias with uncontrolled ventricular rate
Severe valvular disease

Intermediate risk
Mild angina pectoris (CCS class I or II)
Previous MI by history or pathologic Q waves
Compensated or prior heart failure
Diabetes mellitus
Renal insufficiency

Minor risk
Advanced age
Abnormal ECG (left ventricular hypertrophy, left bundle branch
  block, ST-T abnormalities)
Rhythm other than sinus
Low functional capacity
History of stroke
Uncontrolled systemic hypertension

*Death, MI, or heart failure.
CCS, Canadian Cardiovascular Society; ECG, electrocardiogram;
  MI, myocardial infarction.
From Eagle KA, Berger PB, Calkins H, et al: ACC/AHA guideline update
for perioperative cardiovascular evaluation for noncardiac surgery:
Executive summary. A report of the American College of Cardiology/
American Heart Association Task Force on Practice Guidelines.
Circulation 2002;105:1257-1267.

who are scheduled to undergo a high-risk procedure, proceeding directly to coronary angiography is probably the most cost-effective and clinically useful strategy. As a general principle, noninvasive testing tends to be most cost-effective and clinically helpful in determining the need for subsequent angiography among patients with intermediate risk features.[8] One group of investigators, for example, examined both the costs of preoperative cardiac testing and surgical outcomes before and after implementation of the AHA/ACC guidelines at their center; they determined that more selective referral for noninvasive testing, as advocated by the guidelines, was associated with reduced costs without sacrificing the low rate of cardiac events at their institution.[9]

Indications for Coronary Angiography

The indications for performing coronary angiography as part of a preoperative assessment are essentially identical to those used to justify coronary angiography in the nonoperative setting. Typical indications include the following:

1. Noninvasive test results suggesting a high risk of adverse outcomes, such as the presence of extensive (multivessel distribution) myocardial ischemia. For example, among a subgroup of patients with abnormal dobutamine stress echocardiography results before noncardiac surgery, the rate of perioperative cardiac events was found to be still relatively low (2.8%) in patients with a more limited extent of ischemia (1-4 segments) but much higher (36%) in those with more extensive ischemia (≥5 segments), despite the use of β-blocker therapy.[10]
2. An equivocal noninvasive test result in a patient with multiple clinical risk factors facing high-risk surgery
3. The presence of exertional angina not responsive to appropriate medical therapy, especially if the patient is facing a moderate- or high-risk surgical procedure
4. The presence of unstable angina

It is important to emphasize that, given the current absence of prospective data indicating that surgical risk can be favorably influenced by preoperative coronary revascularization, the concept that PCI or coronary artery bypass grafting (CABG) should be undertaken to "get the patient through" a subsequent noncardiac surgery is not supported by evidence-based standards, and these interventions should be used sparingly for this indication. Consequently, the ACC/AHA consensus guidelines assert that preoperative coronary revascularization is most likely "appropriate for only a small subset of patients at very high risk." Despite the published guidelines, a substantial amount of physician-to-physician variability exists in clinical practice regarding the role of preoperative coronary revascularization. In one study, 31 physicians were presented with the clinical scenarios and angiographic findings of 12 patients scheduled for vascular surgery and asked to make recommendations with respect to the appropriateness of coronary revascularization. The physicians' recommendations deviated from published guidelines in 40% of cases, and the likelihood of discordance between two cardiologists was 54%.[11]

PHARMACOLOGIC THERAPY

β-Blockers

By reducing adrenergic stimulation, β-blockers have the potential to ameliorate cardiac stress in the perioperative setting, thereby reducing the likelihood of clinical cardiac events.[12] Potential cardioprotective effects of β-blockers include (1) reduction in myocardial oxygen demand via the negative inotropic and chronotropic effects of these agents; (2) increase in myocardial oxygen supply, brought about by prolongation of coronary diastolic filling time; (3) reduced arrhythmic potential despite perioperative increases in sympathetic tone; (4) decreased coronary shear stress, lowering the likelihood of coronary plaque rupture; and (5) anti-inflammatory effects, also possibly reducing the potential for plaque disruption. With respect to patients undergoing vascular surgery, although the presence of severe peripheral arterial disease previously was viewed as a contraindication to β-blocker therapy, recent studies have shown that

Table 7-3. Results of Randomized Trials of β-Blocker Therapy during Noncardiac Surgery

Study	Drug	N	Follow-up	Composite Cardiac End Point (%)		All-Cause Mortality (%)		Nonfatal Myocardial Infarction (%)	
				β-Blocker	Placebo	β-Blocker	Placebo	β-Blocker	Placebo
McSPI	Atenolol	200	2 yr	17*	32	10*	21	NR	NR
DECREASE	Bisoprolol	112	30 days	3*	34	3*	17	0*	17
DIPOM	Metoprolol XL	921	18 mo	21	20	16	16	NR	NR
MaVS	Metoprolol	497	30 days	10	12	0.4	2.8	7.7	8.4

*P < .05.
NR, not reported.

these agents are well tolerated and are associated with a substantial survival benefit in patients with vascular disease.[13]

Based primarily on the results of two small randomized trials, the ACC/AHA guidelines for perioperative evaluation and management recommend (class I or IIa) the routine use of β-blocker therapy for patients with either established coronary disease, ischemia on preoperative stress testing, or multiple clinical risk factors who are scheduled to undergo an intermediate- or high-risk surgical procedure.[14] In the Dutch Echocardiographic Cardiac Risk Evaluation Applying Stress Echocardiography (DECREASE) trial, 112 patients with evidence of ischemia on stress echocardiography before vascular surgery were randomized to oral bisoprolol or placebo starting at least 7 days before surgery and continuing for 30 days postoperatively.[15] Although the study was limited by its small sample size, nonblinded design, and low number of adverse events, bisoprolol therapy was associated with dramatic reductions in 30-day cardiac death (3.4% vs. 17%) and nonfatal MI (0% vs. 17%). The Multicenter Study of Perioperative Ischemia (McSPI) randomized 200 patients undergoing a variety of noncardiac surgical procedures to either a combination of oral and intravenous atenolol or placebo, initiated before the induction of anesthesia and continued for up to 7 days postoperatively.[16] Although β-blocker therapy was not associated with a reduction in perioperative MI or death, it was associated with a 50% reduction in the number of ischemic episodes on continuous ECG monitoring during the index hospitalization, as well as a 65% relative reduction in cardiac mortality (and a 55% reduction in all-cause mortality) at 2-year follow-up. The reason that a short course of β-blocker therapy during the perioperative period was associated with such a dramatic reduction in late mortality in this cohort is not clear.

Interestingly, two larger and more recently completed randomized studies failed to demonstrate benefit from perioperative β-blocker therapy (Table 7-3).[17,18] In the Diabetic Postoperative Mortality and Morbidity (DIPOM) trial, 921 patients with type 2 diabetes mellitus who were scheduled for noncardiac surgery and not already using β-blocker therapy were randomized to receive either metoprolol or placebo, initiated 2 hours before surgery and continued up to 8 days postoperatively. At 18-month follow-up, there

were no differences based on treatment assignment in the incidence of either the primary composite end point of death, MI, unstable angina, or heart failure (21% vs. 20% for metoprolol vs. placebo) or all-cause mortality (16% vs. 16%). Similarly, in the Metoprolol after Vascular Surgery (MaVS) trial of 497 patients undergoing elective vascular surgery, metoprolol begun 2 hours before the operation and continued for 6 days afterward was not associated with a significant reduction in 30-day cardiac death (0% vs. 0.4% for metoprolol vs. placebo) or nonfatal MI (7.7% vs. 8.4%), although a trend toward reduced all-cause mortality was apparent with β-blocker therapy (0.4% vs. 2.8%).

A large observational study that examined outcomes of more than 100,000 patients who received β-blocker therapy during admission for noncardiac surgery suggests a relationship between a patient's degree of cardiac risk and the likelihood of benefit from perioperative β-blockers.[19] Among individuals at the highest risk for perioperative cardiac events, β-blocker therapy was associated with a 43% relative reduction in the risk of in-hospital death after surgery; however, among patients with the lowest preoperative cardiac risk index, use of β-blockers was associated with a surprising 10% to 43% increased rate of in-hospital mortality (Fig. 7-4).

Based on current data, several important unanswered questions exist regarding the use of β-blockers in the perioperative setting, including (1) the optimal timing of therapy, including the issues of how long before surgery β-blockers should be initiated, and for what duration they should be continued postoperatively; (2) whether a class-effect exists, or whether certain β-blocker agents are superior for preventing perioperative events; (3) whether the β-blocker dose should be individually titrated to effect (e.g., target heart rate), or whether a standard dose is sufficient; and (4) which patients are most likely to derive benefit from perioperative β-blocker therapy.[20]

Two large ongoing trials should help to further clarify the role of β-blockers. Until then, physicians should adhere to the current ACC/AHA guidelines, which advocate the use of β-blockers for higher-risk patients undergoing intermediate- or high-risk surgical procedures. Recent surveys have demonstrated that appropriate perioperative β-blocker therapy remains widely underused in clinical practice.[21] It should also be recognized that potential adverse

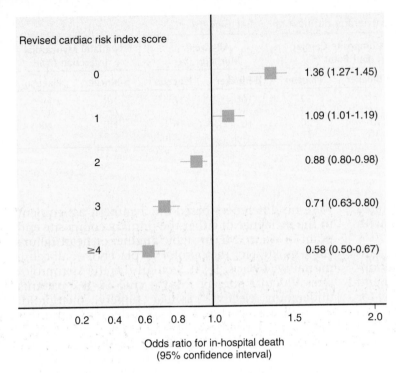

Revised cardiac risk index score

0	1.36 (1.27-1.45)
1	1.09 (1.01-1.19)
2	0.88 (0.80-0.98)
3	0.71 (0.63-0.80)
≥4	0.58 (0.50-0.67)

0.2   0.4   0.6   0.8   1.0   1.5   2.0

Odds ratio for in-hospital death
(95% confidence interval)

Figure 7-4. Odds ratios for in-hospital death among patients receiving β-blocker therapy during hospitalization for noncardiac surgery, based on the patient's Revised Cardiac Risk Index score. Patients with lower scores (0,1) demonstrated increased mortality rates relative to patients not taking β-blockers at the time of surgery. Among patients at higher cardiac risk, however, use of β-blockers was associated with lower perioperative mortality rates. (From Lindenauer PK, Pekow P, Wang K, et al: Perioperative beta-blocker therapy and mortality after major noncardiac surgery. N Engl J Med 2005;353:349-361.)

effects of β-blocker administration can occur. In the MaVS trial, for example, patients randomized to pretreatment with β-blockers were significantly more likely to develop intraoperative hypotension or bradycardia requiring treatment. β-Blocker therapy likewise should be used with caution in low-risk individuals until further data emerge, given the paradoxical increase in mortality among lower-risk patients in the retrospective analysis discussed earlier. In summary, although β-blocker therapy most likely will continue to play an important role in perioperative management, because the antiadrenergic actions of β-blockers counter only one of several possible pathophysiologic mechanisms of perioperative MI, determination of other approaches to MI prevention will remain essential.[22] As evidenced in clinical trials, perioperative cardiac events can still occur in more than 10% of patients receiving β-blocker therapy.

Statins

Several observational studies have suggested that 3-hydroxy-3-methylglutaryl coenzyme A (HMG-CoA) reductase inhibitor therapy administered at the time of noncardiac surgery is associated with a reduction in major adverse events. In a retrospective review of more than 750,000 operations performed at 329 hospitals, Lindenauer and colleagues noted that patients who were receiving lipid-lowering therapy at surgery (which included stains in 91% of cases) demonstrated a 30% relative reduction in all-cause hospital mortality (2.13% vs. 3.05%; P < .001), and the benefits of lipid-lowering therapy appeared to be greatest among higher-risk patients.[23] Likewise, Poldermans and asso-

ciates, in a case-control study involving patients who underwent major vascular surgery at a single center, noted an independent, greater than fourfold reduction in perioperative mortality among patients receiving statins at the time of surgery.[24] In another analysis of patients who underwent open abdominal aortic aneurysm repair, statin use was associated with significant reductions in adjusted 30-day death or MI (3.7% vs. 11.0%), in late (median, 4.7 years) all-cause mortality (18% vs. 50%), and in cardiac mortality (11% vs. 34%).[25]

These provocative findings require confirmation in a randomized controlled trial before firm treatment recommendations are possible. However, most patients undergoing vascular surgery already possess indications for chronic statin therapy for the prevention of cardiac events, and among patients already receiving treatment it seems reasonable to continue statin therapy through the perioperative course. Potential mechanisms by which statins may reduce perioperative cardiac complications relate to the plaque-stabilizing effects of these agents, including their anti-inflammatory and antithrombotic properties, and their beneficial influences on plaque-related endothelial dysfunction. Whereas β-blockers exert their primary cardioprotective effects through their influence on myocardial oxygen supply and demand, the principal effect of statins in the perioperative period may be related to the prevention of atherosclerotic plaque rupture. These two forms of therapy may therefore be especially complementary, a hypothesis that is currently being evaluated in the prospective DECREASE-IV study, in which a combination of fluvastatin and bisoprolol therapy is being examined in the perioperative setting.[26,27]

α_2-Receptor Agonists

α_2-Receptor agonists inhibit central sympathetic nervous system outflow, resulting in a reduction of peripheral norepinephrine release. Clinically, these agents possess anxiolytic, analgesic, and sedative effects; attenuate hemodynamic instability in response to anesthesia and surgery; and serve as coronary vasodilators in the presence of atherosclerotic disease.[28] A meta-analysis of seven randomized placebo-controlled trials involving 1648 patients with known or suspected coronary disease undergoing vascular surgery demonstrated that α_2-receptor agonist therapy was associated with significant reductions in both perioperative mortality (odds ratio [OR] = 0.47; 95% CI: 0.25 to 0.90) and MI (OR = 0.47; 95% CI: 0.46 to 0.94) (Fig. 7-5).[29] Treatment duration among the trials ranged from a single preoperative dose, to treatment continuation for up to 3 days postoperatively. Confirmation of the benefits of α_2-receptor agonist therapy with a large randomized trial seems warranted. The interaction and relative efficacy of α_2-receptor agonists compared with perioperative β-blocker therapy also remains uncertain and warrants clarification in well-designed clinical trials. Currently, the use of α_2-receptor antagonist therapy for the prevention of perioperative events remains a class IIb recommendation in the ACC/AHA perioperative guidelines.

Other Noninterventional Strategies

A variety of other medical and supportive measures have been recommended to reduce the likelihood of ischemic cardiac complications after noncardiac surgery, although randomized controlled trial data evaluating these strategies are typically absent. Among individuals with known or suspected coronary disease, aspirin should be reinitiated as soon as possible after surgery. Perioperative hypertension should be controlled, and patients with left ventricular dysfunction or history of congestive heart failure should receive angiotensin-converting enzyme inhibitor therapy if possible.[30] Postoperative pain should be controlled aggressively to keep catecholamine

levels down, anemia should be corrected to optimize myocardial oxygen delivery, and overall fluid balance should be closely monitored and treated. One large randomized trial demonstrated no benefit for routine use of a pulmonary artery catheter to guide therapy, compared with standard care, among 1994 elderly high-risk patients undergoing major noncardiac surgery.[31]

PREOPERATIVE CORONARY REVASCULARIZATION

Because most episodes of perioperative myocardial ischemia and infarction are related to the presence of one or more preexisting fixed coronary stenoses, the performance of coronary revascularization before surgery traditionally has been looked upon as a potential means to limit the occurrence of ischemic events during and after surgery. Recent data, however, have cast doubts on the utility of routine coronary revascularization before noncardiac surgery, although many clinicians remain convinced that certain higher-risk individuals may benefit from such an approach. Whereas coronary revascularization is typically performed preoperatively with the intention of decreasing the likelihood of subsequent adverse cardiac events, it must be remembered that coronary revascularization itself is associated with risks that are separate from (and additive to) those of surgery. Therefore, for a strategy of PCI or CABG followed by noncardiac surgery to be fruitful, the coronary revascularization procedure must decrease the risks of the subsequent surgery by a degree sufficient to overcome the increased cumulative risk inherent in performing two procedures instead of one.

Coronary Artery Bypass Grafting

Several retrospective and registry-based studies have examined outcomes of patients with prior CABG who subsequently required a major noncardiac surgical procedure. Among patients with remote CABG, noncardiac surgery appears safe. Among 1961 patients monitored in the Coronary Artery Surgery Study (CASS) registry, patients with prior CABG had signifi-

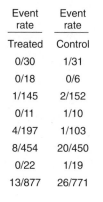

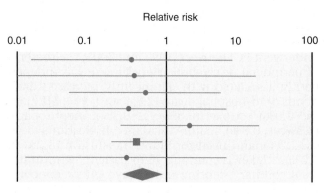

Figure 7-5. Meta-analysis of seven randomized trials of α_2-receptor agonist therapy versus placebo for mortality prevention during noncardiac surgery. (From Wijeysundera DN, Naik JS, Beattie WS: Alpha-2 adrenergic agonists to prevent perioperative cardiovascular complications: A meta-analysis. Am J Med 2003;114:742-752.)

Event rate Treated	Event rate Control
0/30	1/31
0/18	0/6
1/145	2/152
0/11	1/10
4/197	1/103
8/454	20/450
0/22	1/19
13/877	26/771

Relative risk

Favors α-2 agonists   Favors control

cantly reduced postoperative mortality (1.7% vs. 3.3%; *P* = .03) and MI (0.8% vs. 2.7%; *P* = .002) after noncardiac surgery, compared to patients with medically managed coronary disease. The mean duration between CABG and subsequent noncardiac surgery in this study was 4.1 years. Other observational reports have indicated that, for patients with prior CABG, mortality rates associated with noncardiac surgery are comparable to those observed among patients without evidence of coronary disease.

Although a history of remote CABG may be protective during future surgical procedures, the role of CABG undertaken as a preemptive measure among patients discovered to possess severe coronary artery disease during a preoperative risk assessment remains unproven. Performance of CABG can substantially delay subsequent noncardiac surgery, and prophylactic CABG may not be feasible if the required noncardiac surgical procedure is urgent or semiurgent. Attempting to perform noncardiac surgery very shortly after CABG may be associated with further increased operative risks. For example, in one observational report, patients undergoing vascular surgery within 1 month after CABG demonstrated a fivefold increase in operative mortality compared with matched controls who underwent vascular surgery without preceding CABG (20.6% vs. 3.9%; *P* < .005).[32]

Percutaneous Coronary Intervention

Risks of Preoperative PCI

Decision analyses have suggested that coronary angiography and intervention before vascular surgery should be carried out only if the risk of the vascular surgery is relatively high (>5% mortality risk) and the anticipated risk of angiography and revascularization is relatively low (<3% mortality risk). However, many studies have demonstrated that the short- and long-term risks of performing PCI are substantially increased among patients with comorbidities requiring noncardiac surgery, especially if PCI is performed in individuals with concomitant peripheral vascular disease. Among 2340 patients enrolled in the BARI trial or registry, the presence of peripheral vascular disease was associated with a 50% relative increase in major in-hospital cardiovascular events after PCI (11.7% vs. 7.8%) and an almost twofold increased likelihood of adverse events after CABG. Similarly, within another large registry of 25,114 patients who underwent PCI between 1997 and 2001, the presence of peripheral or cerebral artery disease was independently associated with significantly increased likelihoods of in-hospital death (2.8% vs. 1.3%), MI (3.0% vs. 2.0%), stroke (0.8% vs. 0.3%), nephropathy (3.3% vs. 0.8%), major vascular complications (3.4% vs. 2.2%), and need for blood transfusion (8.2% vs. 4.2%).[33] Likewise, among 7696 patients who underwent coronary stenting at the Mayo Clinic, concomitant peripheral arterial disease was associated with an independent, nearly twofold increase in the likelihood of in-hospital death, as well as a significantly increased composite event rate of death, MI, CABG, or target vessel revascularization at 2 years.[34] The significantly elevated risks of performing PCI in the setting of coexisting peripheral vascular disease, as highlighted by these studies, should be considered when deciding whether to undertake PCI in patients with planned vascular surgery.

Clinical Studies of Preoperative PCI

A variety of retrospective analyses extending from the pre-stent era to current practice have addressed the utility of preoperative PCI for reducing the likelihood of adverse cardiac events. The conclusions that can be drawn from these studies are, however, quite limited. Almost all reports suffer from small size, retrospective design, frequent absence of standardized indications to determine which patients were referred for PCI, wide variety of surgical procedures, variable timing between preoperative PCI and subsequent noncardiac surgery (days to years), and, perhaps most importantly, lack of control groups in most studies. Also, in these retrospective trials, because patients who died after PCI would not have gone on to noncardiac surgery and therefore would not be included in follow-up, the true complication rates from a strategy of preoperative PCI are likely to have been underreported.[35] Within studies of preoperative angioplasty performed in pre-stent era, in-hospital mortality after noncardiac surgery ranged from 0% to 2.7% for patients who had undergone either recent (within 2 weeks) or remote (up to 29 months) preoperative balloon angioplasty (Table 7-4). Higher perioperative mortality rates (ranging from 2.9% to 20%) were reported in several more recent studies that examined outcomes of coronary stent implantation shortly before noncardiac surgery, but again none of these observational reports employed a control group (Table 7-5).[36-40]

In one retrospective analysis of 501 patients who underwent a major vascular surgical procedure, pre-

Table 7-4. Complication Rates of Noncardiac Surgery after Balloon Angioplasty

Author (Year)*	N	Myocardial Infarction (%)	Death (%)	Interval Between Angioplasty and Surgery
Allen (1991)	148	0.7	2.7	11 mo
Huber (1992)	50	5.6	1.9	9 days
Elmore (1993)	14	0	0	10 days
Jones (1993)	108	3.7	0.9	14 days
Gottlieb (1998)	194	0.5	0.5	11 days
Posner (1999)	686	2.2	2.6	1 yr
Hassan (2001)	251	0.8	0.8	21 mo

*Complete references for these studies can be found in the source article.
Adapted from Eagle KA, Berger PB, Calkins H, et al: ACC/AHA guideline update for perioperative cardiovascular evaluation for noncardiac surgery: Executive summary. A report of the American College of Cardiology/American Heart Association Task Force on Practice Guidelines. Circulation 2002;105:1257-1267.

Table 7-5. Complication Rates of Noncardiac Surgery after Recent Coronary Bare Metal Stent Placement

Author (Year)	N	Myocardial Infarction (%)	Death (%)	Major Bleeding (%)	Interval Between Stenting and Surgery
Kaluza (2000)	40	17.5	20	27.5	≤42 days
Wilson (2003)	207	1.4	2.9	33	<35 days
Vicenzi (2006)	103	11.7	4.9	3.9	≤42 days
Reddy (2005)	56	10.7	7.1	5.4	≤42 days
Total	**406**	**6.9**	**5.7**	**21.2**	

operative PCI did appear to confer benefit. Within this cohort, the presence of moderate to severe inducible ischemia on preoperative thallium stress testing was associated with an overall 22.4% incidence of perioperative MI. Patients who underwent coronary revascularization before surgery, however, had only a 6.4% incidence of postoperative MI, which was similar to the rate observed among patients without ischemia on preoperative stress testing.[41]

The CARP Trial

To date, only one prospective randomized study, the Coronary Artery Revascularization Prophylaxis (CARP) trial, has examined the strategy of preoperative coronary revascularization for the reduction of early and late perioperative cardiac events after major vascular surgery.[42] The CARP trial included 510 patients scheduled for vascular surgery at 1 of 18 Veterans Affairs medical centers. Patients were eligible for inclusion if angiographically proven coronary artery disease with at least 70% stenosis in at least one major epicardial coronary artery was present. Patients were randomized to undergo either coronary revascularization followed by vascular surgery (n = 258) or vascular surgery without preceding coronary revascularization (n = 252). Among the group randomized to coronary revascularization, 41% of patients underwent CABG and 59% were treated with PCI. The median age of enrolled patients was 66 years; angina was noted in 38%, 42% had a prior MI, and 74% were considered to possess at least an intermediate risk for a perioperative cardiac event based on either clinical risk factors or the results of noninvasive testing. Patients with a left main coronary artery stenosis of 50% or greater, a left ventricular ejection fraction of less than 20%, or severe aortic stenosis were excluded. β-Blocker therapy was employed in approximately 85% of patients in both study arms.

The final results of the CARP trial indicated that preoperative revascularization was not associated with any apparent benefit over conservative therapy. Whereas patients assigned to coronary revascularization had a significantly longer delay between randomization and vascular surgery (54 versus 18 days), coronary revascularization was not associated with a reduction in the occurrence of adverse cardiac events after vascular surgery, either at 30-day or at 2.7-year follow-up (Fig. 7-6). Furthermore, subgroup analysis

indicated that preoperative revascularization was not associated with a survival benefit in any low- or high-risk patient subgroup.

One criticism of the CARP trial was that process of preoperative risk stratification used in the study did not follow the ACC/AHA guidelines, by which coronary angiography is considered only after noninvasive testing has demonstrated moderate or severe inducible ischemia. In the study, noninvasive testing was not mandated, and fewer than 50% of enrolled subjects underwent a stress imaging study in which moderate or severe ischemia was documented before coronary angiography was performed.[43] Nevertheless, it is difficult not to concede that the population studied in the CARP trial represented a high-risk group of patients, as evidenced by the substantial overall 22% mortality rate at 2.7 years. Because the CARP trial included almost exclusively male patients and was limited to vascular surgery, generalization of results is somewhat restricted. Also, because only 9% of patients who were screened for study inclusion were ultimately enrolled, the possibility of selection bias exists; investigators may have excluded some

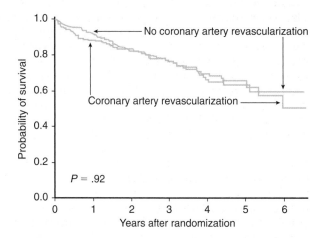

No. at risk

Revascularization	226	175	113	65	18	7
No revascularization	229	172	108	55	17	12

Figure 7-6. Kaplan-Meier survival curve for patients enrolled in the CARP trial. There was no difference in early or late mortality after noncardiac surgery among patients with coronary artery disease who were randomized to undergo preoperative coronary revascularization rather than conservative therapy. (From McFalls EO, Ward HB, Moritz TE, et al: Coronary-artery revascularization before elective major vascular surgery. N Engl J Med 2004;351:2795-2804.)

patients they believed to be at higher risk, simply referring them for revascularization outside the context of the study.

Despite its potential shortcomings, the CARP results lend strong support to the concept that performing prophylactic coronary revascularization for the purpose of "getting a patient through" noncardiac surgery is generally not appropriate. It should be stressed that the majority of patients enrolled in the CARP trial were at intermediate risk for perioperative events, and the results of the study may not apply to higher-risk patients (including those with left main coronary artery disease, poor ejection fraction, severe valvular heart disease, unstable angina or angina not responsive to medical therapy, or recent MI). One retrospective analysis suggested that the subset of patients with three or more clinical risk factors and extensive ischemia on a stress imaging study has increased surgical risk despite β-blocker therapy and may represent an appropriate group in which to consider preoperative coronary revascularization.[10]

In summary, pending the results of further prospective trials, there is not sufficient evidence to suggest that routine preoperative PCI is effective in reducing the risk of noncardiac surgery among patients with documented coronary artery disease who are at moderate clinical risk. In these individuals, preoperative PCI should be performed only for patients who have an indication for coronary revascularization unrelated to the noncardiac surgery. For a limited group of patients at higher risk, data are lacking, and the perceived risks and benefits of preoperative revascularization need to be carefully weighed on an individual basis. Multidisciplinary communication, including the patient's medical specialist, cardiologist, cardiac surgeon, anesthesiologist, and surgeon intending to perform the noncardiac procedure, can be quite helpful in determining a rational preoperative strategy. Such a discussion can allow consideration of issues such as life expectancy; anticipated risks and benefits of PCI, CABG, and the planned noncardiac surgery itself; the urgency of the noncardiac surgery; and the potential risks that medical treatments such as aspirin or thienopyridine therapy may pose during the noncardiac surgery.

Technical Considerations of PCI

When the decision has been made to proceed with preoperative PCI, several important technical considerations exist. Foremost is the length of delay that is permissible between the PCI and the subsequent noncardiac surgical procedure, which often dictates whether stand-alone balloon angioplasty, bare metal stenting, or drug-eluting stent implantation is performed.

Balloon Angioplasty
Because of less reliable short- and long-term results, balloon angioplasty without stent placement has become an infrequently used strategy among most patients undergoing PCI. Stand-alone balloon angioplasty may have a role in the preoperative setting, however, because this approach does not mandate the subsequent use of thienopyridine therapy and therefore allows surgery to be performed with little delay after PCI. Among 350 patients who underwent balloon angioplasty within 2 months before noncardiac surgery at the Mayo Clinic from 1988 to 2001, the incidence of perioperative death or MI was only 0.9%. No perioperative events occurred among the subset of 162 patients in this cohort who underwent their noncardiac surgical procedure more than 2 weeks after coronary angioplasty.[44]

Current ACC/AHA guidelines recommend delaying surgery for at least 1 week after balloon angioplasty to allow for initial healing at the site of vessel injury and to overcome the time frame during which acute vessel closure and recoil typically occurs. Surgery should not be delayed for longer than 8 to 12 weeks after angioplasty, however, because restenosis becomes a potential concern after this interval. Therefore, for a patient in whom PCI is deemed necessary before surgery, delay of surgery for more than 1 to 2 weeks is undesirable, and balloon angioplasty without stenting may represent a reasonable option. It should be kept in mind, however, that abrupt vessel closure or an inadequate angiographic result occurs in approximately 10% of attempts at stand-alone balloon angioplasty, and unplanned stenting may become necessary.

Bare Metal Stents
Among patients undergoing PCI, routine stent implantation is associated with improved immediate and late results compared with balloon angioplasty alone. In the face of noncardiac surgery, however, the presence of a recently placed coronary stent introduces the possibility of stent thrombosis during the perioperative period, an event that is associated with substantial morbidity and mortality. Antiplatelet therapy with acetylsalicylic acid (ASA) and a thienopyridine is typically recommended for at least 2 to 4 weeks after placement of a bare metal stent, to reduce the likelihood of stent thrombosis while stent endothelialization is occurring, which mandates a longer delay between PCI and subsequent noncardiac surgery. If noncardiac surgery is undertaken soon after coronary stent implantation, several retrospective reports have demonstrated an alarmingly high rate of adverse cardiac events (see Table 7-5).

An observational report by Kaluza and colleagues was the first to highlight concerns regarding stent placement before noncardiac surgery.[36] Among 40 patients who underwent bare metal stenting less than 6 weeks before noncardiac surgery, there were 8 deaths, 7 MIs, and 11 major bleeding episodes at the time of surgery. The majority of ischemic cardiac events were the result of stent thrombosis, and all episodes of MI and death occurred among patients who underwent surgery within 2 weeks after stent implantation. In a subsequent report from the Mayo Clinic, among 207 patients who underwent a surgical procedure within 2 months after coronary bare metal stent implantation, the incidence of perioperative death, MI, or stent thrombosis was lower but still of concern at 4.0%. All events occurred among patients who underwent surgery within 6 weeks after stent implantation, with no major cardiac complications reported when surgery was delayed for longer than 6 weeks.[37] In a separate analysis of 56 patients who underwent noncardiac surgery after remote or recent coronary stenting, perioperative major adverse cardiac events or bleeding occurred in 8 (50%) of 16 patients who had surgery within 42 days after stent placement but in no patient whose surgery was performed more than 42 days after the stent procedure.[39]

Vicenzi and colleagues performed a prospective evaluation of 103 patients who required noncardiac surgery within 1 year after coronary stenting.[40] In an attempt to limit thrombotic events, all patients were started on either unfractionated or low-molecular-weight heparin before surgery, and their baseline antiplatelet therapy was continued throughout the perioperative period if feasible or, if necessary, discontinued for as short a duration as possible. Despite these precautions, the incidence of major and minor cardiovascular events was 43%, and the overall surgical mortality rate was 4.9%. The risk of an adverse event was 2.1-fold higher among patients who underwent noncardiac surgery after recent (<35 days) rather than more remote (>90 days) coronary stenting.

In summary, based on the association between stent placement and perioperative stent thrombosis when the interval between PCI and surgery is short, it appears preferable to delay surgery for 6 weeks after bare metal stent implantation. This permits at least partial endothelialization of the stent as well as completion of a full course of thienopyridine therapy, and it also allows for drug discontinuation and return of platelet function before surgery. Of note, the performance of surgery soon after discontinuation of antiplatelet medications may itself predispose to thrombotic events, because withdrawal of oral antiplatelet medications outside the context of surgery has been associated with increased rates of death, MI or bleeding events in the ensuing 30 days.[45]

Drug-Eluting Stents

Drug-eluting stents have reduced the likelihood of restenosis after PCI compared to bare metal stents, yet they may not be well suited for use in the preoperative period. By inhibiting cellular proliferation, not only do drug-eluting stents limit the development of fibrointimal hyperplasia, but they also inhibit the protective process of stent endothelialization. The possibility of stent thrombosis therefore remains a concern for months to years (instead of weeks) after drug-eluting stent implantation and mandates a prolonged course of thienopyridine therapy.[46] According to package labeling, dual antiplatelet therapy is recommended for at least 3 months after sirolimus-eluting stent placement and 6 months after implantation of a paclitaxel-coated stent, although

reports of later thrombosis with both stent types suggest that even longer courses of thienopyridine therapy may be beneficial.[47]

Interruption of antiplatelet therapy to permit the performance of many types of noncardiac surgery even months after drug-eluting stent implantation may be hazardous. Although definitive studies examining the potential consequences of drug eluting stent implantation before noncardiac surgery are lacking, perioperative stent thrombosis has been reported after cessation of antiplatelet therapy up to 21 months after placement of a sirolimus- or paclitaxel-eluting stent.[48-50]

Recommendations

From a technical standpoint, if PCI is believed to be necessary as a prelude to noncardiac surgery, the primary factors that dictate the procedural approach are (1) the amount of time available between PCI and surgery and (2) whether the planned surgical procedure allows for continuation of antiplatelet therapy during the perioperative period (Fig. 7-7). If surgery is urgent, for a life-threatening problem, PCI is typically not performed. Stand-alone balloon angioplasty may be considered in instances in which surgery can be delayed for at least 1 week, because this approach circumvents the need for thienopyridine therapy and the possibility of perioperative stent thrombosis. As noted, however, the possibility that bailout stent placement may become necessary during attempts at balloon angioplasty should be considered. A strategy of simple balloon angioplasty may also be less likely to yield adequate results with certain disease patterns, such as multivessel or left main disease. Bare metal stent placement appears to represent the preferred approach if surgery can be postponed for preferably 6 weeks after stent placement, to permit stent endothelialization and completion and washout of thienopyridine therapy. If the bleeding risks of the

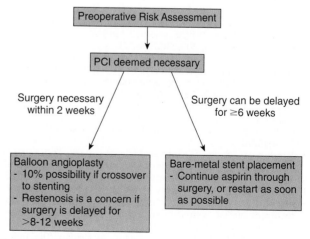

Figure 7-7. Technical considerations of preoperative percutaneous coronary intervention (PCI).

planned surgical procedure are low, such that aspirin and thienopyridine can be continued perioperatively, it may be possible, if necessary, to perform surgery 2 to 4 weeks after stent placement, although the safety of this approach remains uncertain, and postponing surgery for a full 6 weeks is recommended. At present, based almost exclusively on theoretical concerns, the use of drug-eluting stents should be avoided before planned noncardiac surgery. If a patient who has undergone recent drug-eluting stent implantation requires unexpected noncardiac surgery, the surgery should probably be delayed as long as safely possible, and aspirin and thienopyridine therapy should be reinitiated as soon as possible after surgery.

REFERENCES

1. Ellis SG, Hertzer NR, Young JR, Brener S: Angiographic correlates of cardiac death and myocardial infarction complicating major nonthoracic vascular surgery. Am J Cardiol 1996; 77:1126-1128.
2. Mackey WC, Fleisher LA, Haider S, et al: Perioperative myocardial ischemic injury in high-risk vascular surgery patients: Incidence and clinical significance in a prospective clinical trial. J Vasc Surg 2006;43:533-538.
3. Landesberg G, Mosseri M, Zahger D, et al: Myocardial infarction after vascular surgery: The role of prolonged stress-induced, ST depression-type ischemia. J Am Coll Cardiol 2001;37:1839-1845.
4. Kim LJ, Martinez EA, Faraday N, et al: Cardiac troponin I predicts short-term mortality in vascular surgery patients. Circulation 2002;106:2366-2371.
5. Landesberg G, Shatz V, Akopnik I, et al: Association of cardiac troponin, CK-MB, and postoperative myocardial ischemia with long-term survival after major vascular surgery. J Am Coll Cardiol 2003;42:1547-1554.
6. Bursi F, Babuin L, Barbieri A, et al: Vascular surgery patients: Perioperative and long-term risk according to the ACC/AHA guidelines: The additive role of post-operative troponin elevation. Eur Heart J 2005;26:2448-2456.
7. Eagle KA, Berger PB, Calkins H, et al: ACC/AHA guideline update for perioperative cardiovascular evaluation for noncardiac surgery: Executive summary. A report of the American College of Cardiology/American Heart Association Task Force on Practice Guidelines. Circulation 2002;105:1257-1267.
8. Mukherjee D, Eagle KA: Perioperative cardiac assessment for noncardiac surgery: Eight steps to the best possible outcome. Circulation 2003;107:2771-2774.
9. Froehlich JB, Karavite D, Russman PL, et al: American College of Cardiology/American Heart Association preoperative assessment guidelines reduce resource utilization before aortic surgery. J Vasc Surg 2002;36:758-763.
10. Boersma E, Poldermans D, Bax JJ, et al: Predictors of cardiac events after major vascular surgery: Role of clinical characteristics, dobutamine echocardiography, and beta-blocker therapy. JAMA 2001;285:1865-1873.
11. Pierpont GL, Moritz TE, Goldman S, et al: Disparate opinions regarding indications for coronary artery revascularization before elective vascular surgery. Am J Cardiol 2004;94: 1124-1128.
12. London MJ, Zaugg M, Schaub MC, Spahn DR: Perioperative beta-adrenergic receptor blockade: Physiologic foundations and clinical controversies. Anesthesiology 2004;100:170-175.
13. Narins CR, Zareba W, Moss AJ, et al: Relationship between intermittent claudication, inflammation, thrombosis, and recurrent cardiac events among survivors of myocardial infarction. Arch Intern Med 2004;164:440-446.
14. Fleisher LA, Beckman J, Brown K, et al: ACC/AHA 2006 guideline update on perioperative cardiovascular evaluation for noncardiac surgery: Focused update on perioperative beta-blocker therapy. A report of the American College of Cardiology/American Heart Association Task Force on Practice Guidelines. J Am Coll Cardiol 2006;47:2343-2355.
15. Poldermans D, Boersma E, Bax JJ, et al: The effect of bisoprolol on perioperative mortality and myocardial infarction in high-risk patients undergoing vascular surgery. Dutch Echocardiographic Cardiac Risk Evaluation Applying Stress Echocardiography Study Group. N Engl J Med 1999;341: 1789-1794.
16. Mangano DT, Layug EL, Wallace A, Tateo I: Effect of atenolol on mortality and cardiovascular morbidity after noncardiac surgery. Multicenter Study of Perioperative Ischemia Research Group. N Engl J Med 1996;335:1713-1720.
17. Juul AB, Wetterslev J, Kofoed-Enevoldsen A, et al: The Diabetic Postoperative Mortality and Morbidity (DIPOM) trial: Rationale and design of a multicenter, randomized, placebo-controlled, clinical trial of metoprolol for patients with diabetes mellitus who are undergoing major noncardiac surgery. Am Heart J 2004;147:677-683.
18. Yang H, Raymer K, Butler R, et al: Metoprolol After Vascular Surgery (MaVS). [Abstract.] Can J Anaesth 2004;51:A7.
19. Lindenauer PK, Pekow P, Wang K, et al: Perioperative beta-blocker therapy and mortality after major noncardiac surgery. N Engl J Med 2005;353:349-361.
20. Kertai MD, Bax JJ, Klein J, Poldermans D: Is there any reason to withhold beta blockers from high-risk patients with coronary artery disease during surgery? Anesthesiology 2004;100: 4-7.
21. Lindenauer PK, Fitzgerald J, Hoople N, Benjamin EM: The potential preventability of postoperative myocardial infarction: Underuse of perioperative beta-adrenergic blockade. Arch Int Med 2004;164:762-766.
22. Devereaux PJ, Yusuf S, Yang H, et al: Are the recommendations to use perioperative beta-blocker therapy in patients undergoing noncardiac surgery based on reliable evidence? CMAJ 2004;171:245-247.
23. Lindenauer PK, Pekow P, Wang K, et al: Lipid-lowering therapy and in-hospital mortality following major noncardiac surgery. JAMA 2004;291:2092-2099.
24. Poldermans D, Bax JJ, Kertai MD, et al: Statins are associated with a reduced incidence of perioperative mortality in patients undergoing major noncardiac vascular surgery. Circulation 2003;107:1848-1851.
25. Kertai MD, Boersma E, Westerhout CM, et al: Association between long-term statin use and mortality after successful abdominal aortic aneurysm surgery. Am J Med 2004;116: 96-103.
26. Kertai MD, Boersma E, Westerhout CM, et al: A combination of statins and beta-blockers is independently associated with a reduction in the incidence of perioperative mortality and nonfatal myocardial infarction in patients undergoing abdominal aortic aneurysm surgery. Eur J Vasc Endovasc Surg 2004;28: 343-352.
27. Schouten O, Poldermans D, Visser L, et al: Fluvastatin and bisoprolol for the reduction of perioperative cardiac mortality and morbidity in high-risk patients undergoing non-cardiac surgery: Rationale and design of the DECREASE-IV study. Am Heart J 2004;148:1047-1052.
28. Wallace AW, Galindez D, Salahieh A, et al: Effect of clonidine on cardiovascular morbidity and mortality after noncardiac surgery. Anesthesiology 2004;101:284-293.
29. Wijeysundera DN, Naik JS, Beattie WS: Alpha-2 adrenergic agonists to prevent perioperative cardiovascular complications: A meta-analysis. Am J Med 2003;114:742-752.
30. Henke PK, Blackburn S, Proctor MC, et al: Patients undergoing infrainguinal bypass to treat atherosclerotic vascular disease are underprescribed cardioprotective medications: Effect on graft patency, limb salvage, and mortality. J Vasc Surg 2004;39: 357-365.
31. Sandham JD, Hull RD, Brant RF, et al: A randomized, controlled trial of the use of pulmonary-artery catheters in high-risk surgical patients. N Engl J Med 2003;348:5-14.
32. Breen P, Lee JW, Pomposelli F, Park KW: Timing of high-risk vascular surgery following coronary artery bypass surgery: A 10-year experience from an academic medical centre. Anaesthesia 2004;59:422-427.

33. Mukherjee D, Eagle KA, Smith DE, et al: Impact of extracardiac vascular disease on acute prognosis in patients who undergo percutaneous coronary interventions. Am J Cardiol 2003; 92:972-974.

34. Singh M, Lennon RJ, Darbar D, et al: Effect of peripheral arterial disease in patients undergoing percutaneous coronary intervention with intracoronary stents. Mayo Clin Proc 2004;79:1113-1118.

35. Priebe HJ: Perioperative myocardial infarction: Aetiology and prevention. Br J Anaesth 2005;95:3-19.

36. Kaluza GL, Joseph J, Lee JR, et al: Catastrophic outcomes of noncardiac surgery soon after coronary stenting. J Am Coll Cardiol 2000;35:1288-1294.

37. Wilson SH, Fasseas P, Orford JL, et al: Clinical outcome of patients undergoing non-cardiac surgery in the two months following coronary stenting. J Am Coll Cardiol 2003;42: 234-240.

38. Godet G, Riou B, Bertrand M, et al: Does preoperative coronary angioplasty improve perioperative cardiac outcome? Anesthesiology 2005;102:739-746.

39. Reddy PR, Vaitkus PT: Risks of noncardiac surgery after coronary stenting. Am J Cardiol 2005;95:755-757.

40. Vicenzi M, Meislitzer T, Heitzlinger B, et al: Coronary artery stenting and non-cardiac surgery: A prospective outcome study. Br J Anaesth 2006;6:686-693.

41. Landesberg G, Mosseri M, Shatz V, et al: Cardiac troponin after major vascular surgery: The role of perioperative ischemia, preoperative thallium scanning, and coronary revascularization. J Am Coll Cardiol 2004;44:569-575.

42. McFalls EO, Ward HB, Moritz TE, et al: Coronary-artery revascularization before elective major vascular surgery. N Engl J Med 2004;351:2795-2804.

43. Landesberg G, Mosseri M, Fleisher LA: Coronary revascularization before vascular surgery. N Engl J Med 2005;352: 1492-1495.

44. Brilakis ES, Orford JL, Fasseas P, et al: Outcome of patients undergoing balloon angioplasty in the two months prior to noncardiac surgery. Am J Cardiol 2005;96:512-514.

45. Collet JP, Montalescot G, Blanchet B, et al: Impact of prior use or recent withdrawal of oral antiplatelet agents on acute coronary syndromes. Circulation 2004;110:2361-2367.

46. McFadden EP, Stabile E, Regar E, et al: Late thrombosis in drug-eluting coronary stents after discontinuation of antiplatelet therapy. Lancet 2004;364:1519-1521.

47. Ong AT, McFadden EP, Regar E, et al: Late Angiographic Stent Thrombosis (LAST) events with drug-eluting stents. J Am Coll Cardiol 2005;45:2088-2092.

48. Auer J, Berent R, Weber T, Eber B: Risk of noncardiac surgery in the months following placement of a drug-eluting coronary stent. J Am Coll Cardiol 2004;43:713.

49. Nasser M, Kapeliovich M, Markiewicz W: Late thrombosis of sirolimus-eluting stents following noncardiac surgery. Cath Cardiovasc Intervent 2005;65:516-519.

50. Murphy JT, Fahy BG: Thrombosis of sirolimus-eluting coronary stent in the postanesthesia care unit. Anesth Analg 2005;101:971-973.

CHAPTER

8   Gender and Ethnicity Issues in Percutaneous Coronary Intervention

Leslie Cho

KEY POINTS

- Women who present for percutaneous coronary intervention (PCI) are older and have more comorbidities than men. Women and men have similar short- and long-term mortality rate after PCI. However, women have 1.5 to 4 times higher vascular complication and bleeding rates than men.
- The diagnosis of microvessel dysfunction should be considered in women who have abnormal stress test results with perfusion defect but minimal coronary artery disease on angiography.
- Women and men have similar benefit with glycoprotein IIb/IIIa inhibitor, adenosine diphosphate (ADP) receptor inhibitors, and direct thrombin inhibitors. The benefit of

aspirin in secondary prevention is well known in women and men. However, aspirin and primary prevention differ between men and women. Women have fewer ischemic strokes and men have fewer myocardial infarctions with aspirin therapy.
- Race-specific analyses in PCI are still rare. However, African American patients who present for PCI are younger, female, and more likely to have comorbidities and present with acute coronary syndromes (ACS) or ST-segment elevation myocardial infarction (STEMI).
- African American patients have a lower long-term survival rate after PCI than their white counterparts.

Cardiovascular disease (CVD) remains the leading cause of death in the United States, regardless of gender and race.[1] Until recently, information extrapolated from large studies and registries has been applied to all population groups irrespective of gender, race, or ethnicity. However, there is a growing body of literature that has shown differences in CVD manifestation and treatment based on gender and race. This chapter explores gender and racial differences in percutaneous coronary intervention (PCI), acute myocardial infarction (MI), acute coronary syndromes (ACS), stable angina, and adjunctive pharmacotherapy.

GENDER

CVD is the leading cause of mortality and morbidity in women in the United States. It claims the lives of more women then the next five major causes of death in women combined.[1] CVD in women occurs about 10 years later than in men, and in part this has contributed to the misconception that CVD is predominantly a problem of male gender. Many of the

outcome differences reported between women and men may be explained by differences in comorbidities, pathophysiologic differences between genders, and disparities in treatment and outcomes after the cardiovascular event.[1]

Percutaneous Coronary Intervention

More than 1 million PCIs are performed annually in the United States, and an estimated 33% of patients undergoing PCI are women.[1,2] Compared with men, women undergoing PCI are 5 years older and have higher prevalences of hypertension, diabetes, and other comorbidities.[3-5] They are less likely to have had a history of MI, PCI, or coronary artery bypass grafting (CABG). At the time of PCI, they have less multivessel disease and are more likely to present with unstable angina.[3-5] Unlike men, they require more urgent procedures and are more likely to have rotational atherectomy. Paradoxically, given their higher risk profile, women tend to have similar lesion types, less multivessel disease, and more preserved left ventricular (LV) function than men.[3-5] However,

Table 8-1. In-Hospital Death and Myocardial Infarction after PCI by Gender

Study (Year)	No. Women/No. Men	Women (%)	Men (%)	Adjusted OR (95% CI)
Peterson (2001)	35,571/74,137			
Death		1.8	1.0	1.07 (0.9-1.2)
MI		1.5	1.2	1.25 (1.1-1.4)
Jacobs (2002)	895/1,629			
Death		2.2	1.3	1.6 (0.76-3.35)
MI		0.2	0.7	
Lansky (2002)	2,077/5,295			
Death		1.4	0.7	2.28 (1.15-4.55)
Watanabe (2001)	29,227/53,556			
Death		1.2	0.6	1.65 (1.33-2.04)
Malenka (2002)	3,983/8,057			
Death		1.04	0.79	1.24 (0.96-1.60)
MI		1.71	1.36	1.02 (0.85-1.24)

CI, confidence interval; MI, myocardial infarction; OR, odds ratio.

despite better LV function, women tend to have higher incidence of congestive heart failure and more functional impairment after revascularization than men.[2]

Early reports of patients undergoing balloon angioplasty showed lower procedural success rates in women. However, recent studies have reported similar procedural success rates (>90%) in both groups.[3,4,6-8] In addition, earlier registry studies showed that women had higher in-hospital mortality rates after PCI even after adjusting for baseline comorbidites.[3,9] Improved morbidity and mortality outcomes have been reported in more recent studies, despite the older age in women.[3-5,10-13] Table 8-1 shows the recently published data regarding rates of in-hospital death and MI by gender. Table 8-1 includes large published studies since 2000 that reported age and risk factor adjusted odds ratios. Even though there are variations in each of the studies, they show no gender difference in in-hospital mortality and morbidity rates. With the recent advances in PCI with newer-generation stents, balloons, smaller sheath sizes and catheters, and advances in adjunctive pharmacotherapies, adjusted long-term mortality and morbidity rates after PCI are also similar between men and women (Table 8-2;

Fig. 8-1).[3,4,7] There has been much controversy surrounding less frequent utilization of diagnostic catheterization and delays in PCI in women compared with men.[14] These issues are addressed further in the discussions of ACS and MI.

Microvascular Dysfunction

Recently, there has been renewed interest in microvascular dysfunction in women. Of note, women have smaller epicardial arteries than men, independent of body size.[15] Women taking androgens have much larger arteries than control women, and androgen-deprived men have smaller arteries than control men.[16,17] Moreover, male patients who have received transplanted female donor hearts show progressive epicardial vessel enlargement independent of body size.[18] However, there is no change in vessel size for male hearts transplanted into women. These findings suggest that sex hormones have a unique effect on arterial remodeling. Much is still unknown regarding this effect.

Most women undergoing cardiac catheterization for chest pain have minimal coronary artery disease (CAD).[19] However, many of these women have abnormal stress test findings and continue to have

Table 8-2. Long-Term (1-Year) Outcome of PCI by Gender

Study (Year)	No. Women/No. Men	Women (%)	Men (%)	Adjusted OR (95% CI)
Jacobs (2002)	895/1,629			
Death		6.5	4.3	1.26 (0.85-1.87)
Death/MI		11.1	9.0	1.14 (0.86-1.50)
Lansky (2002)	2,077/5,295			
Death		4.4	3.3	—
MACE		29.2	32.7	
Mehili (2000)	1,001/3,263			
Death		4.0	4.1	0.99 (0.54-1.13)
MACE		6.0	5.8	—
Chiu (2004)	5,301/12,738			
Death		7	5	1.14 (0.93-1.41)
MACE		—	—	1.05 (0.97-1.13)

*No difference between genders noted; however, OR was not reported.
CI, confidence interval; MACE, major adverse cardiac events; MI, myocardial infarction; OR, odds ratio; PCI, percutaneous coronary intervention.

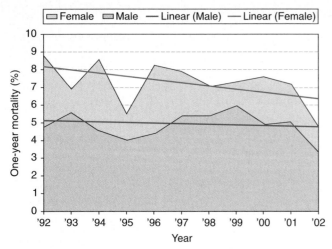

Figure 8-1. One-year unadjusted mortality rates after percutaneous coronary intervention in women and men between 1992 and 2002 at The Cleveland Clinic Foundation. (From Chiu JH, Bhatt DL, Ziada KM, et al: Impact of female sex on outcome after percutaneous coronary intervention. Am Heart J 2004; 148:998-1002.)

symptoms. Innovations in the technique of phosphorus-31 nuclear magnetic resonance (NMR) spectroscopy have shed light on this issue. Phosphorus-31 NMR can monitor myocardial high-energy phosphates, phosphocreatine, and adenosine triphosphate (ATP) after stress. A transient decrease in the ratio of myocardial phosphocreatine to ATP during exercise indicates myocardial ischemia. In the National Institute of Health–National Heart, Lung and Blood Institute (NHLBI)–sponsored Women's Ischemia Syndrome Evaluation (WISE) study, 20% of women with chest pain and minimal CAD had evidence of myocardial ischemia with a decreased phosphocreatine/ATP ratio with exercise.[20] The magnitude of ischemia in these women was equal to or greater than that in patients with 70% stenosis of the left anterior descending coronary artery.[20] Myocardial ischemia in these women is most likely caused by microvascular smooth muscle cell dysfunction and endothelial dysfunction. Vascular testing with adenosine or nitroprusside infusion has shown smooth muscle cell dysfunction, and testing with endothelium-dependent vasodilators such as acetylcholine has shown endothelial dysfunction in these women.[21] Patients with microvessel dysfunction have higher risk for death or MI.[21]

Gender and Devices

No gender-based comparisons were made in the earlier randomized clinical trials comparing bare metal stent (BMS) with balloon angioplasty. Restenosis and revascularization rates were not well defined for women after BMS because of the small sample of women in prospective trials with systematic angiographic follow-up. Even though women tend to have smaller vessel size and higher prevalence of diabetes, initially there were intriguing studies reporting that women had similar or lower rates of target vessel

revascularization (TVR) than their male counterparts after PCI.[22,23] However, with systematic angiographic and clinical follow-up, these reports have not been validated.

In the era of drug-eluting stents (DES), both sirolimus- and taxus-eluting stents have shown favorable outcomes in women. Both the SIRIUS trial and the TAXUS IV trial demonstrated DES superiority, with reduction in restenosis, TVR, and major adverse cardiac events at 1 year follow-up in women and men.[24,25] In TAXUS IV, 1314 patients with severe coronary artery stenosis were randomized to paclitaxel stent versus BMS. Women comprised 27.9% of the study population. Restenosis rates were similar in women and men treated with TAXUS stent (7.6% vs. 8.6%; $P = .80$), as was late loss (0.23 vs. 0.22 mm; $P = .90$).[25] Compared to women receiving BMS stents, those receiving TAXUS stents had a significant reduction in 9-month restenosis (29.2% vs. 8.6%; $P < .001$) and 1-year target lesion revascularization (TLR; 14.9% vs. 7.6%; $P = .02$).[25] Of note, women had a higher unadjusted TLR rate than men at 1 year; however, female gender was not an independent predictor of TLR (odds ratio [OR] = 1.72; 95% CI: 0.68 to 4.37; $P = .25$).[25] In the SIRIUS study, 1058 patients with severe coronary artery stenosis were randomized to sirolimus stent versus BMS. A total of 305 women were enrolled in the trial. The rate of TLR in women randomized to DES was 3.4%, compared with 16.5% in BMS group ($P < .001$).[24] In men, the rate of TLR was 4.4% in the sirolimus group and 16.6% in the BMS group ($P < .001$).[24] In summary, restenosis and revascularization rates are similar between women and men and appear to be directly related to smaller vessel size, body surface area, and incidence of diabetes.

Few gender-based studies exist on the efficacy of directional coronary atherectomy (DCA). However, DCA appears to be associated with lower procedural success and more bleeding complications in women.[26] Likewise, large devices such as Excimer laser angioplasty also appear to be associated with a higher morbidity rate in women, with higher coronary perforation rates.[26] No gender-specific data exist on rotational atherectomy, cutting balloon angioplasty, extraction atherectomy, or gamma brachytherapy.

Vascular Complications

Women have experienced greater vascular complications, such as major hematoma, retroperitoneal bleed, bleeding complications requiring transfusion, and vascular injury requiring surgery, than men after PCI.[6,27-31] Much of this has been postulated to be the result of smaller vessel size and aggressive anticoagulation. With development of weight-adjusted heparin dosing, introduction of smaller sheath sizes, and early sheath removal, vascular complications have decreased.[7,27,29] However, even in the current era, women continue to have a 1.5 to 4 times higher risk of vascular complications compared to men.[7,27-29,32] Table 8-3 shows rates for various vascular complica-

Table 8-3. Vascular Complications by Gender

Study (Year)	No. Women/No. Men	Women (%)	Men (%)	P Value
Chiu (2004)	5,301/12,738			
Blood transfusion		12	4	<.001
Major hematoma		5	2	<.001
Pseudoaneurysm		0.6	0.3	.005
Lansky (2002)	562/1,520			
Major hematoma		2.5	1.5	.005
Retroperitoneal bleed		0.5	0.2	.05
Surgical repair		3.8	2.4	.001
Welty (2001)	2,101/3,888			
Vascular injury		1.6	0.6	.001
Peterson (2001)	35,571/74,137			
Vascular injury		5.4	2.7	.001

tions by gender from recently published large studies. Of note, there have been no gender-specific data regarding arterial vascular puncture closure devices.

Gender Differences by Clinical Syndrome

Acute Coronary Syndromes

Women who present with ACS are older and have higher incidences of diabetes and hypertension compared to men. They also have less severe CAD, with greater absence of critical obstructions and more preserved LV function. In ACS, women were more likely to have elevated C-reactive protein (CRP) and brain natriuretic peptide (BNP), whereas men were more likely to have elevated creatine kinase-MB (CK-MB) and troponin.[33]

There have been four major randomized trials that compared invasive versus conservative strategy for ACS and reported findings in women.[34-37] Whereas these trials consistently showed benefit in men, the results in women were conflicting.

The Treat Angina with Aggrastat and Determine Cost of Therapy with an Invasive or Conservative Strategy (TACTICS-TIMI 18) trial enrolled 2220 patients, 34% women. A significant reduction in the primary end point of death, MI, and rehospitalization at 6 months occurred in the overall group.[12,33,34] Among women subjects, there was a trend toward lower rates of the primary end point at 6 months in the invasive treatment group (17.0% vs. 19.6% in the conservative treatment group; P = not significant [NS]).[34] As in other ACS studies, women enrolled in TACTICS-TIMI 18 were less likely to have elevated CK-MB or troponin. When the results of invasive versus conservative strategies were evaluated by measurement of cardiac biomarkers, benefit from invasive strategy was seen in both genders.[33] For men with at least one positive biomarker, 22.1% of patients receiving conservative treatment had a primary end point of death, MI, or rehospitalization, compared with 14.2% of those assigned to the invasive strategy (OR = 0.58; 95% CI: 0.41 to 0.82).[33] Similarly, among women with positive biomarkers, 25.8% of those assigned to the conservative strategy and 17.5% of those treated invasively reached the primary end

point (OR = 0.61; 95% CI: 0.38 to 0.96).[33] In both groups, this difference was predominantly mediated by troponin elevation, because there was no statistical difference in outcome by treatment strategy for troponin-negative patients who were BNP or CRP positive (for women, OR = 0.54; 95% CI: 0.12 to 16.6; for men, OR = 1.12; 95% CI: 0.36 to 3.5).[33] If all markers were negative, regardless of gender, there was a nonsignificant trend toward increased death or MI in the invasive group.

The Fragmin and Revascularization during Instability in Coronary Artery Disease II (FRISC II) trial enrolled 2457 patients, of whom 30% were women. They found that, unlike men, women did not benefit from early invasive treatment.[37] The incidence of death or MI at 6 months in women was 10.5% in the invasive group and 8.3 % in the conservative group (OR = 1.26; 95% CI: 0.80 to 1.97).[37] In men, there was a significant reduction of events at 6 months in the invasive strategy group (19% vs. 36%; OR = 0.53; 95% CI: 0.45 to 0.65).[37] A similar finding was seen in the Randomized Intervention Treatment of Angina 3 (RITA 3), which enrolled 1810 ACS patients, including 38% women, to receive either invasive or conservative therapy.[35] Men benefited more from an early intervention strategy, with reduction in death or nonfatal MI at 1 year (adjusted OR = 0.63; 95% CI: 0.41 to 0.98), than did women (OR = 1.79; 95% CI: 0.95 to 3.35; interaction P = .007).

It is important to understand the outcomes in TACTICS-TIMI18, FRISC II, and RITA-3. First, RITA-3 and FRISC II included women who were at lower risk than the women in the TACTICS-TIMI 18 study. In TACTICS-TIMI 18, women with negative troponin, CK-MB, BNP, or CRP in the invasive strategy group had an increased risk of death, MI, or hospitalization (OR = 3.1; 95% CI: 1.17 to 8.31).[33] Men without marker elevation had no significant benefit with invasive strategy (OR = 1.2; 95% CI: 0.64 to 2.25). However, both women and men with elevated biomarkers benefited from an invasive strategy. Secondly, FRISC II did not routinely use glycoprotein IIb/IIIa (GP IIb/IIIa) inhibitors and had much higher rates of mortality with CABG. The CABG mortality rate in women was 9.9%, compared with 1.2% in men.[37] Therefore, the benefit of early invasive therapy may have been diluted owing to the high mortality rate associated with CABG. Moreover, FRISC II and RITA 3 used delayed invasive strategies. In summary, in light of current evidence, women with ACS who have high-risk features such as elevated CK-MB and troponin, benefit from an early invasive strategy with adjunctive GP IIb/IIIa inhibitor use.[12,38]

Much has been reported on gender differences in diagnosis and treatment of ACS, ST-segment elevation myocardial infarction (STEMI), and stable angina.[39-44] Studies have shown delays in diagnosis and health care–seeking behavior as well as underutilization of cardiac catheterization and revascularization in women compared to men with ACS.[39-44] In 2005, the Can Rapid Risk Stratification of Unstable Angina Patients Suppress Adverse Outcomes with Early Implementation of the American College of Cardiology/American Heart Association Guidelines (CRUSADE) National Quality Improvement Initiative investigators published their registry data on gender differences in patients with non–ST-elevation myocardial infarction (NSTEMI)/ACS. In this large registry of more than 35,000 patients, of whom 41% were women, they found that women were less likely to receive guideline-recommended therapy such as heparin (adjusted OR = 0.91; 95% CI: 0.86 to 0.97), angiotensin-converting enzyme (ACE) inhibitors (adjusted OR = 0.95; 95% CI: 0.90 to 0.99), and GP IIb/IIIa inhibitors (adjusted OR = 0.87; 95% CI: 0.81 to 0.92) than men during acute hospitalization.[39] Even among troponin-positive patients, women were less likely to receive GP IIb/IIIa inhibitors (adjusted OR = 0.87; 95% CI: 0.81 to 0.92). Moreover, women were less likely to undergo diagnostic catheterization (adjusted OR = 0.86; 95% CI: 0.82 to 0.91) or PCI (adjusted OR = 0.91; 95% CI: 0.86 to 0.96) during hospitalization.[39] Women were also less likely to receive guideline-recommended medical therapies such as aspirin (adjusted OR = 0.91; 95% CI: 0.85 to 0.98), ACE inhibitors (adjusted OR = 0.93; 95% CI: 0.88 to 0.98), and statin therapy (adjusted OR = 0.92; 95% CI: 0.88 to 0.98) at the time of discharge. The CRUSADE registry confirms the unfortunate presence of continued treatment disparities between the groups. These findings call for significant improvements in the care of ACS patients and highlight the importance of continued investigations into barriers that contribute to these differences.

ST-Segment Elevation Myocardial Infarction

Women with MI are older and have more comorbidities than their male counterparts. Moreover, they are likely to present to hospital later then men, with higher Killip class. At the time of presentation, women have less severe CAD and more preserved LV function. In most cases, the initial presentation of CAD in women is sudden cardiac death or acute MI. Surprisingly, there appear to be plaque morphology differences between women and men with acute MI. Autopsy studies have shown more plaque erosion than plaque rupture in young women after fatal MI, compared with men or with older women (Fig. 8-2).[45,46] Also, women appear to have more distal microvascular embolization than men during fatal MI.[47]

The overall superiority of primary PCI over fibrinolytic therapy has been demonstrated for women.[48] Because women have more comorbidities at presentation, the absolute benefit with primary PCI is greater for women than for men. An estimated 56 deaths could be prevented for every 1000 women treated with primary PCI, compared with 42 fewer deaths per 1000 men.[48] One study showed gender-associated differences in the amount of myocardial salvage after primary PCI for STEMI. In this study, myocardial salvage achieved by primary PCI was greater in women than in men.[49] Improved salvage may be due to gender-specific hypoxic tolerance. Female cells have a higher baseline expression of the protein Bcl-2, showing a higher inherited hypoxic tolerance than male cells.[49]

There have been gender-specific data regarding primary stenting versus primary balloon angioplasty in STEMI. Women with STEMI benefitted from primary stenting, with less reinfarction, TVR, and TLR.[23] More recently, the Controlled Abciximab and Device Investigation to Lower Late Angioplasty Complications (CADILLAC) trial, which enrolled 2082 patients including 27% women to receive either bare metal stent or primary balloon angioplasty with or without GP IIb/IIIa inhibitor, found superior efficacy and safety with primary stenting, with or without abciximab, compared to balloon angioplasty (Fig. 8-3).[32] For women, primary stenting resulted in a reduction in the 1-year composite end point of death, reinfarction, ischemia-driven TVR, or disabling stroke, from 28.1% to 19.1% (P = .01), compared with percutaneous transluminal coronary angioplasty (PTCA).[32] The addition of abciximab to primary stenting significantly reduced the 30-day ischemic TVR without increasing bleeding or stroke rates for women.[32]

There has been much controversy surrounding mortality rate differences between women and men after STEMI (Table 8-4). There appears to be a higher in-hospital mortality rate in women undergoing PCI for STEMI compared to men. A large study using Nationwide Inpatient Sample of 11,717 women and 24,028 men found 5.2% in-hospital mortality in women and 2.7% in men. Even after adjusting for age, hypertension, institutional volume, and pulmonary disease, women had a higher mortality rate (OR = 1.47; 95% CI: 1.23 to 1.75).[50] Similarly, the New York State Department of Health database found that women had a significantly higher adjusted in-hospital mortality rate (OR = 2.69; 95% CI: 1.4 to 5.2).[13] However, at 30 days and at 1 year, there was no apparent difference in mortality rate between the two groups.

Of note, female gender is an independent risk factor for the development of cardiogenic shock as complication of acute MI.[51] However, there is no gender difference in the mortality rate of cardiogenic

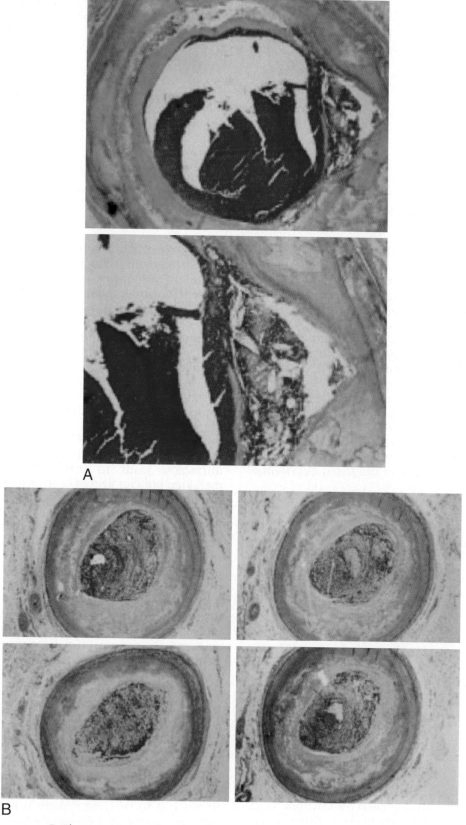

Figure 8-2. A, Plaque rupture. **B,** Plaque erosion. (From Arbustini E, Dal Bello B, Morbini P, et al: Plaque erosion is a major substrate for coronary thrombosis in acute myocardial infarction. Heart 1999;82:269-272.)

Table 8-4. Short- and Long-Term Outcomes in Patients with Myocardial Infarction after PCI by Gender

Study (Year)	No. Women/No. Men	Women (%)	Men (%)	Adjusted OR (95% CI)
Watanabe (2001)	11,717/24,028			1.47 (1.23-1.75)
In-hospital death		5.2	2.7	2.69 (1.4-5.2)
Vakili (2001)	317/727			
In-hospital death		7.9	2.3	
Mehili (2000)	502/1,435			
30-day death		8.4	8.5	—
1-yr death		13.8	12.9	0.65 (0.49-0.87)
Lansky (2005)	562/1,520			
30-day death		4.6	1.1	—
1-yr death		7.6	3.0	1.11 (0.53-2.36)
Antonucci (2001)	230/789			
6-mo death		12	7	1.25 (0.63-2.47)

CI, confidence interval; OR, odds ratio; PCI, percutaneous coronary intervention.

shock once age is adjusted. Therefore, the ACC/AHA guideline for the treatment of STEMI recommends PCI or CABG for patients younger than 75 years of age who are in cardiogenic shock and have lesions amenable to revascularization, regardless of gender.[2]

Many studies have shown delays in time to treatment or time to invasive diagnostic testing and revascularization in women. Women with STEMI are less likely to undergo primary angioplasty within 2 hours or to have accepted pharmacologic treatment on admission. Even at discharge, women are less likely to be receiving accepted medical treatment.[52-54] The older age of women compared to men with STEMI, their symptom differences, and the delay in presentation after acute MI have been suggested as potential explanations. Although these factors may explain initial treatment differences, they do not explain the treatment disparities once the diagnosis has been made. Continued quality improvement in the diagnosis and treatment of women with CAD is needed.

Adjunctive Pharmacotherapy

Antiplatelet Therapy

Aspirin

Aspirin remains the mainstay of antiplatelet therapy in patients with CAD. It acts by irreversibly inactivating cyclooxygenase (COX), which leads to the inhibition of platelet thromboxane A_2 synthesis, which ultimately leads to inhibition of thromboxane-mediated platelet aggregation. Aspirin's effectiveness in secondary prevention is well known. Antithrombotic Trialist Collaboration III demonstrated, in a meta-analysis of 287 randomized trials, the benefit of aspirin after coronary artery revascularization and for the secondary prevention of CVD.[55] Use of aspirin resulted in an estimated 23% to 30% mortality reduction in patients with ACS or MI, although no gender-specific analyses were reported. A study of 2418 women with CAD found a significant 39% relative risk reduction in cardiovascular mortality with aspirin therapy versus no aspirin therapy.[56] However, aspirin's role in primary prevention has been controversial for women.

An early prospective prevention cohort study of 87,678 healthy women aged 34 to 65 years found that 325 mg of aspirin taken one to six times a week was associated with a significant reduction of MI ($P = .005$).[57] However, a recent randomized primary prevention trial of 39,876 women receiving 100 mg aspirin administered every other day found no cardiovascular risk reduction (relative risk [RR] = 0.91; 95% CI: 0.80 to 1.15).[58] Aspirin reduced the risk of ischemic stroke by 24% but had no effect on the risk of MI. Of note, there was a consistent cardiovascular risk reduction with aspirin in women older than 65 years of age. A meta-analysis of six randomized controlled trials of primary prevention in 51,342 women and 44,114 men demonstrated gender-

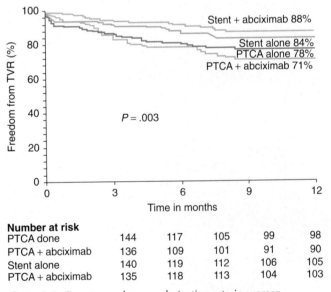

Figure 8-3. Target vessel revascularization rate in women enrolled in the CADILLAC trial. (From Lansky AJ, Pietras C, Costa RA, et al: Gender differences in outcomes after primary angioplasty versus primary stenting with and without abciximab for acute myocardial infarction: Results of the Controlled Abciximab and Device Investigation to Lower Late Angioplasty Complications [CADILLAC] trial. Circulation 2005;111: 1611-1618.)

Number at risk					
PTCA done	144	117	105	99	98
PTCA + abciximab	136	109	101	91	90
Stent alone	140	119	112	106	105
PTCA + abciximab	135	118	113	104	103

Figure labels: Stent + abciximab 88%; Stent alone 84%; PTCA alone 78%; PTCA + abciximab 71%; $P = .003$

specific benefit.[59] In women, aspirin decreased the rate of ischemic stroke (OR = 0.76; 95% CI: 0.63 to 0.93; P = .0008) but had no benefit in reducing MI. In contrast, men had a reduction in MI (OR = 0.68; 95% CI: 0.54 to 0.86; P = .001) but no significant reduction in the incidence of stroke.[59]

The treatment variability has been attributed to baseline clinical differences as well as to unique gender-specific responses to aspirin therapy. Recently, a study assessing platelet reactivity and response to low-dose aspirin therapy in unaffected individuals from families with premature CAD found that women, compared with men, had consistently more reactive platelets to multiple agonists in both whole blood and platelet-rich plasma.[60] After aspirin therapy, men and women showed similar inhibition of platelets in the COX-1 direct pathway. In aggregation assays that were indirectly dependent on the COX-1 pathway, women had modestly more platelet reactivity than men after aspirin therapy.[60] These findings are similar to one in Women's Health Study, which showed similar thromboxane and prostacyclin concentrations between men and women after low-dose aspirin therapy.[58]

Aspirin resistance also appears to be more common in women. A recent study of 326 patients with CVD assessed the prevalence and clinical significance of aspirin resistance by optical platelet aggregation.[61,62] Seventeen of the 326 patients were aspirin resistant. In this study, aspirin resistance was defined as mean platelet aggregation of at least 70% with 10 µmol adenosine diphosphate (ADP) and a mean aggregation of at least 20% with 0.5 mg/mL arachidonic acid. Women were more likely to be aspirin resistant.[61,62] A much larger study from the Heart Outcome Prevention Evaluation (HOPE) trial assessed the relationship between aspirin resistance and the risk of adverse cardiovascular outcomes.[63] Patients in the study had a history of CAD, stroke, peripheral vascular disease, or diabetes, plus at least one other cardiovascular risk factor. Aspirin resistance was determined by measuring urinary levels of 11-dehydrothromboxane B_2, a stable metabolite of thromboxane A_2. Higher baseline urinary levels of 11-dehydrothromboxane B_2 were associated with an increased rate of MI, stroke, or cardiovascular death (P = .01).[63] Female gender was independently associated with higher baseline levels of 11-dehydrothromboxane B_2, indicating that women may be more resistant to aspirin (P = .0004).[63]

Of greater concern is the lack aspirin therapy in women with CAD. In a large secondary prevention trial of women, only 83% of those with established CAD or CVD were receiving aspirin therapy.[64] Even in patients with stable angina, women were less likely to be given aspirin therapy. This dismal rate has been confirmed in other large registries and speaks to the treatment gap that still exists in practice.[64-67] Despite the advances in therapy, proven medical treatments after PCI, such as use of aspirin, ACE inhibitors, β-blockers, and statins, continue to be underutilized in all patients and most specifically in women.[64-67]

Thienopyridines

Clopidogrel and ticlopidine inhibit platelet aggregation by inhibiting ADP receptor binding to platelet. When given in addition to aspirin, these agents reduce the rates of subacute stent thrombosis after stent implantation. The PCI-CURE substudy of the Clopidogrel in Unstable Angina to Prevent Recurrent Events (CURE) investigation enrolled 2658 patients with ACS treated with PCI, of whom 30.2% were women, to either long-term or short-term clopidogrel plus aspirin. The researchers found that clopidogrel for up to 12 months was superior to aspirin alone.[68] There was a trend toward benefit in women (RR = 0.77; 95% CI: 0.52 to 1.15) and a statistically significant benefit in men (RR = 0.65; 95% CI: 0.48 to 0.87). In the Clopidogrel for the Reduction of Events During Observation (CREDO) trial, which enrolled 2116 patients (29% women), long-term treatment with clopidogrel for up to 12 months after elective PCI, compared with short-term clopidogrel, was associated with a 27% relative risk reduction in the primary end point of death, MI, or stroke.[69] In women, there was 32% relative risk reduction in the primary end point, which did not reach statistical significance (OR = 32.1; 95% CI: 58.9 to –12.1).[69] In regard to clopidogrel loading dose, there are no gender-specific data. The optimal timing and loading dose for women at either high or low risk is yet to be determined. The Intracoronary Stenting and Antithrombotic Regimen: Rapid Early Action for Coronary Treatment (ISAR-REACT) trial, which enrolled 2159 low-risk PCI patients pretreated with 600 mg of clopidogrel to receive either abciximab or placebo, found no additional benefit with GP IIb/IIIa inhibitor.[70] In that study, women made up 24% of the population. All patients who had a diagnosis of ACS, insulin-requiring diabetes, or other high-risk criteria were excluded from the trial. The rates of death, MI, and TVR at 30 days did not differ between the abciximab and placebo groups in either the entire population (4.0% vs. 4.0%; P = NS) or the female subset (3.0% vs. 3.0%; P = NS).[70]

Glycoprotein IIb/IIIa Inhibitor

GP IIb/IIIa inhibitors in addition to unfractionated heparin are beneficial for women undergoing PCI and are not associated with an independent risk of major bleeding complications, although the risk of minor bleeding complications is increased in women.[29] In the pooled analysis of abciximab high-risk PCI trials, abciximab conferred equal benefit in men and women.[29] The composite incidence of death, MI, or urgent revascularization was reduced from 16.0% to 9.9% at 6 months in women (P < .001), and at 1 year there was a significant reduction in mortality (4.0% vs. 2.5%; P = .03) in women treated with abciximab. Although women experienced more major bleeding than men (3.0% vs. 1.3%; P < .05), this finding was independent of abciximab treatment. However, abciximab therapy was associated with increased minor bleeding in women (6.7% vs. 4.7% with placebo; P = .01).[29]

A meta-analysis of six large placebo-controlled trials of mostly small-molecule GP IIb/IIIa inhibitors in ACS patients undergoing PCI showed a significant reduction in the combined end point of death or nonfatal MI after PCI.[71] This benefit extended to 6 months after the index PCI. In this meta-analysis, a highly significant interaction was seen between gender and treatment.[71] In men, there was 19% reduction in the rate of death or MI at 30 days with GP IIb/IIIa inhibitor compared with placebo (OR = 0.81; 95% CI: 0.75 to 0.89).[71] By contrast, in women, there was an 11% increased risk of death or MI at 30 days with GP IIb/IIIa inhibitor use (OR = 1.15; 95% CI: 1.01 to 1.30).[71] Even after adjusting for age and comorbidities, there was still a gender difference in treatment effect. However, once patients were stratified according to troponin concentration, there was no differential treatment effect between women and men.[71] A reduction in the rate of death or MI at 30 days with GP IIb/IIIa inhibitor was seen in women (OR = 0.93; 95% CI: 0.68 to 1.28) and in men (OR = 0.82; 95% CI: 0.65 to 1.03) with positive baseline troponin, whereas no risk reduction was seen in patients with negative troponin.[71] Similar findings were also reported in the TACTICS-TIMI 18 study.[33]

Tirofiban and eptifibatide have both been shown to be safe and efficacious in women during PCI.[72,73] However, abciximab has been shown to be superior to tirofiban in preventing periprocedural and 30-day ischemic complications, a finding that was consistent regardless of gender.[74] Abciximab has never been compared directly with double-bolus eptifibatide. In women undergoing PCI for STEMI, use of the GP IIb/IIIa inhibitor resulted in a reduction of short-term ischemic events.[32] However, the use of GP IIb/IIIa inhibitor in rescue PCI after failed thrombolysis was associated with increased bleeding rates, especially in women and the elderly.[75,76]

Antithrombin Agents

Unfractionated Heparin
Unfractionated heparin has been used as the main anticoagulation therapy in PCI. In the early days of PCI, empiric heparin dosing was used. However, activated clotting times (ACT) after a fixed dose of unfractionated heparin vary substantially because of differences in body size, concomitant use of other medications, and the presence of certain disease states that increase heparin resistance (e.g., ACS). This issue is of particular concern in women, because they tend to have higher rates of bleeding. Therefore, weight-based dosing of heparin is essential for women.[26] In those patients who are not receiving a GP IIb/IIIa inhibitor, a weight-adjusted heparin dose of 70 to 100 U/kg should be given to achieve an ACT of 250 to 300 seconds with the HemoTec device or 300 to 350 seconds with the Hemochron device.[77] The unfractionated heparin bolus should be reduced to 50 to 70 U/kg when GP IIb/IIIa inhibitors are given, to achieve a target ACT of 200 seconds with either the HemoTec or the Hemochron device.[77]

Low-Molecular-Weight Heparin
The efficacy and safety of the low-molecular-weight heparin (LMWH) enoxaparin in patients with ACS undergoing PCI was studied in two noninferiority trials.[78,79] The Aggrastat-to Zocor (A-to-Z) study enrolled 3987 patients, of whom 29% were women, and the Superior Yield of the New Strategy of Enoxaparin, Revascularization, and Glycoprotein IIb/IIIa Inhibitors (SYNERGY) study enrolled 9978 patients, of whom 34% were women. Neither study found any statistical benefit of enoxaparin over standard unfractionated heparin in PCI.[78,79] In the A-to-Z trial, 8.6% of women taking enoxaparin reached the primary end point of death, MI, or refractory ischemia at 7 days, compared with 9.3% of the women taking unfractionated heparin; this difference was not statistically significant.[78] In the SYNERGY trial, patients with ACS who were treated to early invasive strategy were given either enoxaparin or unfractionated heparin. At 30 days, death or MI had occurred in 13.5% of the women taking enoxaparin, compared with 12.9% of those taking unfractionated heparin (P = .59).[79] Bleeding rate by gender has not been reported.

Direct Thrombin Inhibitors
The direct thrombin inhibitor bivalirudin has emerged as an alternative antithrombotic therapy during PCI. The Randomized Evaluation in PCI Linking Angiomax to reduced Clinical Events-2 (REPLACE-2) trial demonstrated that the bivalirudin with provisional GP IIb/IIIa inhibitor was not inferior to heparin and GP IIb/IIIa inhibition with regard to major adverse cardiac events and was associated with less bleeding among patients undergoing PCI.[80] This trial enrolled 6010 subjects, of whom 1537 were women. In prospectively defined analysis of gender, there was no difference in individual or composite ischemic end points of death, MI, or urgent revascularization at 30 days or at 6 months between genders with bivalirudin versus heparin and GP IIb/IIIa inhibitor.[27] Among women treated with heparin and GP IIb/IIIa inhibitor, the composite of death, MI, and urgent revascularization at 30 days occurred in 7.5%, compared with 6.7% for women treated with bivalirudin (P = .58). In women, major bleeding occurred in 5.9% of those in the heparin and GP IIb/IIIa inhibitor group, compared with 3.7% of those in the bivalirudin group (P = .04). Likewise, minor bleeding was decreased (28.2% vs. 16.0%; P < .001) and access site bleeding was decreased (4.1% vs. 1.6%; P = .003) with bivalirudin.[27] Thus, for lower-risk female patients undergoing PCI, bivalirudin appears to provide similar protection against ischemic events and fewer bleeding events than heparin and GP IIb/IIIa inhibitor.

Table 8-5. Prevalence of CAD and Mortality by Race (2003)

Parameter	White		African American		Mexican American	
	Men	Women	Men	Women	Men	Women
Prevalence of CAD	8.9%	5.4%	7.4%	7.5%	5.6%	4.3%
Prevalence of MI	5.1%	2.4%	4.5%	2.7%	3.4%	1.6%

ETHNICITY

Currently African Americans, Hispanic Americans, Asian Americans, and Native Americans make up 30% of the U.S. population. By 2050, they will make up 47.5% of the population. Therefore, it is important to understand the dissimilarities among these and other ethnic/racial groups and determine whether they are clinically relevant. Discussion on race or ethnicity in medicine is fraught with difficulties, because "race" is neither a scientific nor a physiologic category. Race can provide information regarding similar environmental factors and some physiologic risk factors such as obesity, diabetes, and hypertension; however, because it is self-reported, it is often prone to inaccuracies. The importance of environment cannot be overemphasized, because the genetic variance between the races is only 0.1%.

Coronary Artery Disease

Heart disease is the leading cause of death for all races in the U.S. population. African Americans experience the highest rates of mortality from heart disease, 1.6 times that of whites.[1] The average annual death rate due to heart disease by race is shown in Table 8-5. The prevalence of CAD is also higher in African Americans compared to their white counterparts, regardless of gender.[1] Furthermore, onset of disease occurs 5 years earlier in African Americans. Death rates from stroke are also higher among African Americans.

Various ethnic minority groups are experiencing increasing rates of ischemic heart disease. Rates for CAD are increasing in Asian Americans, Hispanic Americans, and Native Americans.[1] Despite the increased incidence of CAD in African Americans, the presence of obstructive epicardial CAD on angiography is less than whites.[81] Paradoxically, there is greater extent of atherosclerosis in African Americans despite less obstructive CAD. The increased prevalence of CAD in African Americans is most likely due to increased rates of hypertension, diabetes, and smoking, and not to inherent differences in pathophysiology of CAD.[81] Of note, African Americans tend to have more peripheral arterial disease than their white counterparts (adjusted OR = 2.39; 95% CI: 1.11 to 5.12). This was seen in the National Health and Nutrition Examination Survey in United States.[82] It was confirmed by the NHLBI Genetic Epidemiology Network of Arteriopathy (GENOA) study, which also showed that the difference was not explained by risk factor differences.[83] African American men (adjusted OR = 4.7; 95% CI: 1.4 to 16.0) and women (adjusted OR = 2.2; 95% CI: 1.2 to 4.2) had higher rates of peripheral arterial disease even after adjusting for age and comorbidities than did white Americans.

Percutaneous Coronary Intervention

African American patients undergoing PCI are younger, more likely to be female, and more likely to have hypertension, diabetes, and chronic renal insufficiency than their white counterparts. They are more likely to have urgent PCI rather than elective PCI. Immediate procedural success rates between African Americans and whites appear to be similar.[84-87] Short-term rates of death or MI are also similar between the groups after PCI.[88-90] However, some have reported lower long-term survival rates in African Americans than in their white counterparts[87,91] (Table 8-6). In a large PCI registry, there was an increased adjusted mortality rate among African Americans at 2 years (OR = 1.47; 95% CI: 1.06 to 2.04). In another large single-center PCI registry study, there was an increased 2-year adjusted mortality rate in African Americans (OR = 1.45; 95% CI: 1.14-1.84).[84]

Table 8-6. Short- and Long-Term Outcomes after PCI in African Americans

Study (Year)	No. of Patients (% African American)	Adjusted Event Rate Comparing African American to White (OR [95% CI])
Maynard (2001)	24625 (11%)	
In-hospital death		0.97 (0.83-1.12) Death
2-yr death		1.11 (1.05-1.17) Death
Leborgne (2004)	10561 (12%)	
1-yr death		1.35 (1.06-1.71) Death
Slater (2003)	4618 (9.7%)	
1-yr death		0.65 (0.36-1.14) Death, MI, or CABG
2-yr death		1.47 (1.06-2.04) Death, MI, or CABG
Chen (2005)	8832 (8.0%)	
1-yr death		1.45 (1.14-1.84) Death or MI

CABG, coronary artery bypass grafting; CI, confidence interval; MI, myocardial infarction; OR, odds ratio.

Differences in long-term outcomes after PCI are likely to be multifactorial, potentially due to differences in access and quality of health care for African Americans. African Americans receive fewer preventive health care services and less specialist care, and physicians treating them have been less well trained clinically.[92-94] Another possibility is the excess prevalence of LV hypertrophy together with increased endothelin-1 levels in African Americans.[95] Endothelin-1, a potent vasoconstrictor, is stimulated by transforming growth factor-β (TGF-β), which is increased in African Americans with hypertension. The combination of LV hypertrophy and endothelial dysfunction in conjunction with CAD may contribute to greater rates of mortality.[81] Despite the recent interest in the field, race-specific analyses in PCI are still rare.

Acute Coronary Syndromes

In ACS, African American patients are more likely to be younger and to have hypertension, diabetes, heart failure, and renal insufficiency. They are also less likely to have insurance coverage or specialist care.[96,97] Recently, the investigator of CRUSADE, a large NSTEMI registry, found that African American patients were likely to receive more older ACS treatments, such as aspirin, β-blockers, and ACE inhibitors, but were significantly less likely to receive newer ACS therapies such as GP IIb/IIIa inhibitors, clopidogrel, and statin therapy.[96] Also, African Americans were less likely to receive cardiac catheterization, revascularization, or smoking cessation counseling. The rates of in-hospital death and postadmission MI were similar between African American and Caucasian patients in CRUSADE (adjusted OR = 0.92; 95% CI: 0.81 to 1.05).[96] However, in TACTICS-TIMI 18, African American patients were had an increased risk of death, MI, or rehospitalization (adjusted OR = 1.34; 95%CI: 1.14 to 3.48).[97] There may be several factors explaining the decreased rates of catheterization and revascularization in African Americans. In addition to patient preference and physician recommendations, African American patients with ACS are more likely to be treated in low-volume hospitals.[98,99] Although there are some data regarding race-specific differential responses to antihypertensive medications, to our knowledge there are no race-specific data on adjunctive PCI pharmacotherapy.

ST-Segment Elevation Myocardial Infarction

At the time of presentation with STEMI, African Americans are younger, more likely to be female, have more comorbidities, and present in higher Killip class.[100] Because of their younger age, they are less likely to have disease in two or more vessels. In a large fibrinolytic trial, the 30-day survival rate was similar between African Americans and whites. However, African Americans had a higher rate of in-hospital stroke (OR = 1.75; 95% CI: 1.19 to 2.59) and

more major bleeding events (OR = 1.32; 95% CI: 1.13 to 1.55).[100] At 5 years, there was a significantly higher death rate among African Americans despite their younger age (OR = 1.63; 95% CI: 1.41 to 1.90).[100] In another registry, young African Americans (<65 years) had a higher in-hospital mortality rate compared with whites of the same age, and decreasing age was associated with a higher risk of in-hospital death for African Americans compared to whites.[101]

There have been studies demonstrating different practice patterns according to racial/ethnic group in acute MI.[98,101-103] African Americans are less likely to undergo cardiac catheterization and revascularization after STEMI.[98,101-103] Recently, a study was reported that assessed racial and ethnic differences in the time to acute reperfusion treatment for patients with STEMI, using the National Registry of Myocardial Infarction (NRMI).[98] The researchers found that white patients tended to be older than patients of racial and ethnic minority groups, and insurance status differed significantly between the groups. The types of hospitals to which patients presented also differed markedly by race.[98] They found that the door to drug time and the door to balloon time were significantly longer for patients who were nonwhite. Even after adjusting for age, gender, insurance status, clinical characteristics, time of arrival, time since symptom onset, and hospital characteristics, there was still a difference between white and nonwhite patients. In the fully adjusted model, door to balloon time was 8.7 minutes longer for African Americans compared with whites ($P < .001$) and 3.7 minutes longer for Hispanic American patients compared with whites ($P = .002$).[98] Likewise in the fully adjusted model, door to drug time was 5.1 minutes longer in African Americans ($P < .001$), 1.3 minutes longer in Hispanic Americans ($P = .006$), and 1.7 minutes longer in Asian Americans ($P = .01$) than in their white counterpart.[98] A substantial portion of the racial and ethnic disparity in time to treatment was accounted for by the hospital to which the patient was admitted. Nevertheless, even after adjusting for hospital and clinical factors, there remained racial and ethnic treatment disparities.

Treatment Differences

Owing to complex issues of social, political, physiologic, and genetic variances in population subgroups, there are disparities in health care. African Americans and members of other ethnic minority groups are less likely to undergo cardiovascular procedures such as catheterization and revascularization, either with stent or with CABG.[104,105] Although it is important to note that ethnic minority patients are more likely to be treated in low-volume hospitals and more likely to refuse invasive procedures than their Caucasian counterparts, there still appears to be some amount of treatment disparities.[106-109] In a review of more than 100 studies, The National Institute of Medicine found in 2001 that minority patients were less likely to receive needed services compared to their white counterparts, even after accounting for reduced access to health care.[110] The committee considered three sets of factors associated with treatment differences given the assumption that each group had similar access to health care. The first set of factors were those related to the operation of health care systems, such as lack of interpretative services for non–English-speaking patients or the fact that minority group members are more likely to be enrolled in lower-cost health plans that place greater limits on testing and access to specialists. The second set of factors were from the providers, such as bias against minority patients or greater uncertainty in diagnosis in these patients on the part of health care providers. Lastly, they considered patient preferences.[110] The report concluded that, even though "myriad sources contribute to these [treatment] disparities, some evidence suggests that bias, prejudice, and stereotyping on the part of the healthcare providers may contribute to differences in care."[110] Studies have shown that, regardless of the physicians' race, practitioners use information about patients' ethnicity, age, and lifestyle to make decisions about cardiac intervention.[103] To eliminate disparities in care The National Institute of Medicine recommended a comprehensive, multilevel strategy including training and education of health care providers, as well as policy and regulatory strategies that address health plans and health services, to promote better use of clinical practice guidelines.[110]

CONCLUSION

Much has been learned in the last few years regarding gender and racial differences in CAD. There is much more to be learned regarding differences in pathophysiology, clinical manifestations, treatment responses, and outcomes in these groups. The pervasive and continuing treatment disparities found for women and minority patients should remind all health care providers and researchers of the need to improve understanding and quality of care for these patients.

REFERENCES

1. Thom T, Haase N, Rosamond W, et al: Heart disease and stroke statistics: 2006 Update. A report from the American Heart Association Statistics Committee and Stroke Statistics Subcommittee. Circulation 2006;113:e85-e151.
2. Smith SC Jr, Feldman TE, Hirshfeld JW Jr, et al: ACC/AHA/SCAI 2005 guideline update for percutaneous coronary intervention: A report of the American College of Cardiology/American Heart Association Task Force on Practice Guidelines (ACC/AHA/SCAI Writing Committee to Update 2001 Guidelines for Percutaneous Coronary Intervention). Circulation 2006;113:e166-e286.
3. Jacobs AK, Johnston JM, Haviland A, et al: Improved outcomes for women undergoing contemporary percutaneous coronary intervention: A report from the National Heart, Lung, and Blood Institute Dynamic registry. J Am Coll Cardiol 2002;39:1608-1614.
4. Malenka DJ, Wennberg DE, Quinton HA, et al: Gender-related changes in the practice and outcomes of percutaneous coronary interventions in Northern New England from 1994 to 1999. J Am Coll Cardiol 2002;40:2092-2101.
5. Jacobs AK: Coronary revascularization in women in 2003: Sex revisited. Circulation 2003;107:375-377.
6. Alfonso F, Hernandez R, Banuelos C, et al: Initial results and long-term clinical and angiographic outcome of coronary stenting in women. Am J Cardiol 2000;86:1380-1383, A5.
7. Peterson ED, Lansky AJ, Kramer J, et al: Effect of gender on the outcomes of contemporary percutaneous coronary intervention. Am J Cardiol 2001;88:359-364.
8. Trabattoni D, Bartorelli AL, Montorsi P, et al: Comparison of outcomes in women and men treated with coronary stent implantation. Catheter Cardiovasc Interv 2003;58:20-28.
9. Jacobs AK: Women, ischemic heart disease, revascularization, and the gender gap: What are we missing? J Am Coll Cardiol 2006;47(3 Suppl):S63-S65.
10. Ferguson TB Jr, Hammill BG, Peterson ED, et al: A decade of change: Risk profiles and outcomes for isolated coronary artery bypass grafting procedures, 1990-1999. A report from the STS National Database Committee and the Duke Clinical Research Institute. Society of Thoracic Surgeons. Ann Thorac Surg 2002;73:480-489; discussion 489-490.
11. Wong SC, Sleeper LA, Monrad ES, et al: Absence of gender differences in clinical outcomes in patients with cardiogenic shock complicating acute myocardial infarction: A report from the SHOCK Trial Registry. J Am Coll Cardiol 2001;38:1395-1401.
12. Glaser R, Herrmann HC, Murphy SA, et al: Benefit of an early invasive management strategy in women with acute coronary syndromes. JAMA 2002;288:3124-3129.
13. Vakili BA, Kaplan RC, Brown DL: Sex-based differences in early mortality of patients undergoing primary angioplasty for first acute myocardial infarction. Circulation 2001;104:3034-3038.
14. Schulman KA, Berlin JA, Harless W, et al: The effect of race and sex on physicians' recommendations for cardiac catheterization. N Engl J Med 1999;340:618-626.
15. Sheifer SE, Canos MR, Weinfurt KP, et al: Sex differences in coronary artery size assessed by intravascular ultrasound. Am Heart J 2000;139:649-653.
16. Herman SM, Robinson JT, McCredie RJ, e al: Androgen deprivation is associated with enhanced endothelium-dependent dilatation in adult men. Arterioscler Thromb Vasc Biol 1997;17:2004-2009.
17. McCredie RJ, McCrohon JA, Turner L, et al: Vascular reactivity is impaired in genetic females taking high-dose androgens. J Am Coll Cardiol 1998;32:1331-1335.
18. Herity NA, Lo S, Lee DP, et al: Effect of a change in gender on coronary arterial size: A longitudinal intravascular ultrasound study in transplanted hearts. J Am Coll Cardiol 2003;41:1539-1546.
19. Quyyumi AA: Women and ischemic heart disease: Pathophysiologic implications from the Women's Ischemia Syndrome Evaluation (WISE) study and future research steps. J Am Coll Cardiol 2006;47(3 Suppl):S66-S71.
20. Buchthal SD, den Hollander JA, Merz CN, et al: Abnormal myocardial phosphorus-31 nuclear magnetic resonance spectroscopy in women with chest pain but normal coronary angiograms. N Engl J Med 2000;342:829-835.
21. von Mering GO, Arant CB, Wessel TR, et al: Abnormal coronary vasomotion as a prognostic indicator of cardiovascular events in women: Results from the National Heart, Lung, and Blood Institute-Sponsored Women's Ischemia Syndrome Evaluation (WISE). Circulation 2004;109:722-725.
22. Mehilli J, Kastrati A, Bollwein H, et al: Gender and restenosis after coronary artery stenting. Eur Heart J 2003;24:1523-1530.
23. Antoniucci D, Valenti R, Moschi G, et al: Sex-based differences in clinical and angiographic outcomes after primary angioplasty or stenting for acute myocardial infarction. Am J Cardiol 2001;87:289-293.
24. Moses JW, Leon MB, Popma JJ, et al: Sirolimus-eluting stents versus standard stents in patients with stenosis in a native coronary artery. N Engl J Med 2003;349:1315-1323.
25. Lansky AJ, Costa RA, Mooney M, et al: Gender-based outcomes after paclitaxel-eluting stent implantation in patients with coronary artery disease. J Am Coll Cardiol 2005;45:1180-1185.

26. Lansky AJ, Hochman JS, Ward PA, et al: Percutaneous coronary intervention and adjunctive pharmacotherapy in women: A statement for healthcare professionals from the American Heart Association. Circulation 2005;111:940-953.

27. Chacko M, Lincoff AM, Wolski KE, et al: Ischemic and bleeding outcomes in women treated with bivalirudin during percutaneous coronary intervention: A subgroup analysis of the Randomized Evaluation in PCI Linking Angiomax to Reduced Clinical Events (REPLACE)-2 trial. Am Heart J 2006;151:1032 e1-e7.

28. Chiu JH, Bhatt DL, Ziada KM, et al: Impact of female sex on outcome after percutaneous coronary intervention. Am Heart J 2004;148:998-1002.

29. Cho L, Topol EJ, Balog C, et al: Clinical benefit of glycoprotein IIb/IIIa blockade with abciximab is independent of gender: Pooled analysis from EPIC, EPILOG and EPISTENT trials. Evaluation of 7E3 for the Prevention of Ischemic Complications. Evaluation in Percutaneous Transluminal Coronary Angioplasty to Improve Long-Term Outcome with Abciximab GP IIb/IIIa blockade. Evaluation of Platelet IIb/IIIa Inhibitor for Stent. J Am Coll Cardiol 2000;36:381-386.

30. Lansky AJ, Mehran R, Dangas G, et al: New-device angioplasty in women: Clinical outcome and predictors in a 7,372-patient registry. Epidemiology 2002;13(3 Suppl):S46-S51.

31. Welty FK, Lewis SM, Kowalker W, Shubrooks SJ Jr: Reasons for higher in-hospital mortality >24 hours after percutaneous transluminal coronary angioplasty in women compared with men. Am J Cardiol 2001;88:473-477.

32. Lansky AJ, Pietras C, Costa RA, et al: Gender differences in outcomes after primary angioplasty versus primary stenting with and without abciximab for acute myocardial infarction: Results of the Controlled Abciximab and Device Investigation to Lower Late Angioplasty Complications (CADILLAC) trial. Circulation 2005;111:1611-1618.

33. Wiviott SD, Cannon CP, Morrow DA, et al: Differential expression of cardiac biomarkers by gender in patients with unstable angina/non-ST-elevation myocardial infarction: A TACTICS-TIMI 18 (Treat Angina with Aggrastat and determine Cost of Therapy with an Invasive or Conservative Strategy–Thrombolysis In Myocardial Infarction 18) substudy. Circulation 2004;109:580-586.

34. Cannon CP, Weintraub WS, Demopoulos LA, et al: Comparison of early invasive and conservative strategies in patients with unstable coronary syndromes treated with the glycoprotein IIb/IIIa inhibitor tirofiban. N Engl J Med 2001;344:1879-1887.

35. Clayton TC, Pocock SJ, Henderson RA, et al: Do men benefit more than women from an interventional strategy in patients with unstable angina or non-ST-elevation myocardial infarction? The impact of gender in the RITA 3 trial. Eur Heart J 2004;25:1641-1650.

36. Hochman JS, McCabe CH, Stone PH, et al: Outcome and profile of women and men presenting with acute coronary syndromes: A report from TIMI IIIB. TIMI Investigators. Thrombolysis in Myocardial Infarction. J Am Coll Cardiol 1997;30:141-148.

37. Lagerqvist B, Safstrom K, Stahle E, et al: Is early invasive treatment of unstable coronary artery disease equally effective for both women and men? FRISC II Study Group Investigators. J Am Coll Cardiol 2001;38:41-48.

38. Hochman JS, Tamis-Holland JE: Acute coronary syndromes: Does sex matter? JAMA 2002;288:3161-3164.

39. Blomkalns AL, Chen AY, Hochman JS, et al: Gender disparities in the diagnosis and treatment of non-ST-segment elevation acute coronary syndromes: Large-scale observations from the CRUSADE (Can Rapid Risk Stratification of Unstable Angina Patients Suppress Adverse Outcomes With Early Implementation of the American College of Cardiology/American Heart Association Guidelines) National Quality Improvement Initiative. J Am Coll Cardiol 2005;45:832-837.

40. Canto JG, Allison JJ, Kiefe CI, et al: Relation of race and sex to the use of reperfusion therapy in Medicare beneficiaries with acute myocardial infarction. N Engl J Med 2000;342:1094-1100.

41. Daly C, Clemens F, Lopez Sendon JL, et al: Gender differences in the management and clinical outcome of stable angina. Circulation 2006;113:490-498.

42. Ghali WA, Faris PD, Galbraith PD, et al: Sex differences in access to coronary revascularization after cardiac catheterization: Importance of detailed clinical data. Ann Intern Med 2002;136:723-732.

43. Guru V, Fremes SE, Austin PC, et al: Gender differences in outcomes after hospital discharge from coronary artery bypass grafting. Circulation 2006;113:507-516.

44. Vaccarino V: Angina and cardiac care: Are there gender differences, and if so, why? Circulation 2006;113:467-469.

45. Arbustini E, Dal Bello B, Morbini P, et al: Plaque erosion is a major substrate for coronary thrombosis in acute myocardial infarction. Heart 1999;82:269-272.

46. Burke AP, Farb A, Malcom G, Virmani R: Effect of menopause on plaque morphologic characteristics in coronary atherosclerosis. Am Heart J 2001;141(2 Suppl):S58-S62.

47. Kolodgie FD, Burke AP, Wight TN, Virmani R: The accumulation of specific types of proteoglycans in eroded plaques: A role in coronary thrombosis in the absence of rupture. Curr Opin Lipidol 2004;15:575-582.

48. Tamis-Holland JE, Palazzo A, Stebbins AL, et al: Benefits of direct angioplasty for women and men with acute myocardial infarction: Results of the Global Use of Strategies to Open Occluded Arteries in Acute Coronary Syndromes Angioplasty (GUSTO II-B) Angioplasty Substudy. Am Heart J 2004;147:133-139.

49. Mehilli J, Ndrepepa G, Kastrati A, et al: Gender and myocardial salvage after reperfusion treatment in acute myocardial infarction. J Am Coll Cardiol 2005;45:828-831.

50. Watanabe CT, Maynard C, Ritchie JL: Comparison of short-term outcomes following coronary artery stenting in men versus women. Am J Cardiol 2001;88:848-852.

51. Hasdai D, Califf RM, Thompson TD, et al: Predictors of cardiogenic shock after thrombolytic therapy for acute myocardial infarction. J Am Coll Cardiol 2000;35:136-143.

52. Gan SC, Beaver SK, Houck PM, et al: Treatment of acute myocardial infarction and 30-day mortality among women and men. N Engl J Med 2000;343:8-15.

53. Marrugat J, Sala J, Masia R, et al: Mortality differences between men and women following first myocardial infarction. RESCATE Investigators. Recursos Empleados en el Sindrome Coronario Agudo y Tiempo de Espera. JAMA 1998;280:1405-1409.

54. Vaccarino V, Parsons L, Every NR, et al: Sex-based differences in early mortality after myocardial infarction. National Registry of Myocardial Infarction 2 Participants. N Engl J Med 1999;341:217-225.

55. Collaborative meta-analysis of randomised trials of antiplatelet therapy for prevention of death, myocardial infarction, and stroke in high risk patients. BMJ 2002;324:71-86.

56. Harpaz D, Benderly M, Goldbourt U, et al: Effect of aspirin on mortality in women with symptomatic or silent myocardial ischemia. Israeli BIP Study Group. Am J Cardiol 1996;78:1215-1219.

57. Manson JE, Stampfer MJ, Colditz GA, et al: A prospective study of aspirin use and primary prevention of cardiovascular disease in women. JAMA 1991;266:521-527.

58. Ridker PM, Cook NR, Lee IM, et al:. A randomized trial of low-dose aspirin in the primary prevention of cardiovascular disease in women. N Engl J Med 2005;352:1293-1304.

59. Berger JS, Roncaglioni MC, Avanzini F, et al: Aspirin for the primary prevention of cardiovascular events in women and men: A sex-specific meta-analysis of randomized controlled trials. JAMA 2006;295:306-313.

60. Becker DM, Segal J, Vaidya D, et al: Sex differences in platelet reactivity and response to low-dose aspirin therapy. JAMA 2006;295:1420-1427.

61. Gum PA, Kottke-Marchant K, Poggio ED, et al: Profile and prevalence of aspirin resistance in patients with cardiovascular disease. Am J Cardiol 2001;88:230-235.

62. Gum PA, Kottke-Marchant K, Welsh PA, et al: A prospective, blinded determination of the natural history of aspirin resistance among stable patients with cardiovascular disease. J Am Coll Cardiol 2003;41:961-965.

63. Eikelboom JW, Hirsh J, Weitz JI, et al: Aspirin-resistant thromboxane biosynthesis and the risk of myocardial infarction, stroke, or cardiovascular death in patients at high risk for cardiovascular events. Circulation 2002;105:1650-1655.

64. Vittinghoff E, Shlipak MG, Varosy PD, et al: Risk factors and secondary prevention in women with heart disease: The Heart and Estrogen/progestin Replacement Study. Ann Intern Med 2003;138:81-89.

65. Jani SM, Montoye C, Mehta R, et al: Sex differences in the application of evidence-based therapies for the treatment of acute myocardial infarction: The American College of Cardiology's Guidelines Applied in Practice projects in Michigan. Arch Intern Med 2006;166:1164-1170.

66. Califf RM, DeLong ER, Ostbye T, et al: Underuse of aspirin in a referral population with documented coronary artery disease. Am J Cardiol 2002;89:653-661.

67. Kim C, Beckles GL: Cardiovascular disease risk reduction in the Behavioral Risk Factor Surveillance System. Am J Prev Med 2004;27:1-7.

68. Mehta SR, Yusuf S, Peters RJ, et al: Effects of pretreatment with clopidogrel and aspirin followed by long-term therapy in patients undergoing percutaneous coronary intervention: The PCI-CURE study. Lancet 2001;358:527-533.

69. Steinhubl SR, Berger PB, Mann JT 3rd, et al: Early and sustained dual oral antiplatelet therapy following percutaneous coronary intervention: A randomized controlled trial. JAMA 2002;288:2411-2420.

70. Kastrati A, Mehilli J, Schuhlen H, et al: A clinical trial of abciximab in elective percutaneous coronary intervention after pretreatment with clopidogrel. N Engl J Med 2004;350:232-238.

71. Boersma E, Harrington RA, Moliterno DJ, et al: Platelet glycoprotein IIb/IIIa inhibitors in acute coronary syndromes: A meta-analysis of all major randomised clinical trials. Lancet 2002;359:189-198.

72. Iakovou I, Dangas G, Mehran R, et al: Gender differences in clinical outcome after coronary artery stenting with use of glycoprotein IIb/IIIa inhibitors. Am J Cardiol 2002;89:976-979.

73. Fernandes LS, Tcheng JE, O'Shea JC, et al: Is glycoprotein IIb/IIIa antagonism as effective in women as in men following percutaneous coronary intervention? Lessons from the ESPRIT study. J Am Coll Cardiol 2002;40:1085-1091.

74. Topol EJ, Moliterno DJ, Herrmann HC, et al: Comparison of two platelet glycoprotein IIb/IIIa inhibitors, tirofiban and abciximab, for the prevention of ischemic events with percutaneous coronary revascularization. N Engl J Med 2001;344:1888-1894.

75. Cantor WJ, Kaplan AL, Velianou JL, et al: Effectiveness and safety of abciximab after failed thrombolytic therapy. Am J Cardiol 2001;87:439-442, A4.

76. Jong P, Cohen EA, Batchelor W, et al: Bleeding risks with abciximab after full-dose thrombolysis in rescue or urgent angioplasty for acute myocardial infarction. Am Heart J 2001;141:218-225.

77. Chew DP, Bhatt DL, Lincoff AM, et al: Defining the optimal activated clotting time during percutaneous coronary intervention: Aggregate results from 6 randomized, controlled trials. Circulation 2001;103:961-966.

78. Blazing MA, de Lemos JA, White HD, et al: Safety and efficacy of enoxaparin vs unfractionated heparin in patients with non-ST-segment elevation acute coronary syndromes who receive tirofiban and aspirin: A randomized controlled trial. JAMA 2004;292:55-64.

79. Ferguson JJ, Califf RM, Antman EM, et al: Enoxaparin vs unfractionated heparin in high-risk patients with non-ST-segment elevation acute coronary syndromes managed with an intended early invasive strategy: Primary results of the SYNERGY randomized trial. JAMA 2004;292:45-54.

80. Lincoff AM, Bittl JA, Harrington RA, et al: Bivalirudin and provisional glycoprotein IIb/IIIa blockade compared with heparin and planned glycoprotein IIb/IIIa blockade during percutaneous coronary intervention: REPLACE-2 randomized trial. JAMA 2003;289:853-863.

81. Yancy C: Heart Disease in Varied Populations, 7th ed. Philadelphia, Elsevier Saunders, 2005.

82. Selvin E, Erlinger TP: Prevalence of and risk factors for peripheral arterial disease in the United States: Results from the National Health and Nutrition Examination Survey, 1999-2000. Circulation 2004;110:738-743.

83. Kullo IJ, Bailey KR, Kardia SL, et al: Ethnic differences in peripheral arterial disease in the NHLBI Genetic Epidemiology Network of Arteriopathy (GENOA) study. Vasc Med 2003;8:237-242.

84. Chen MS, Bhatt DL, Chew DP, et al: Outcomes in African Americans and whites after percutaneous coronary intervention. Am J Med 2005;118:1019-1025.

85. Maynard C, Wright SM, Every NR, Ritchie JL: Racial differences in outcomes of veterans undergoing percutaneous coronary interventions. Am Heart J 2001;142:309-313.

86. Minutello RM, Chou ET, Hong MK, Wong SC: Impact of race and ethnicity on inhospital outcomes after percutaneous coronary intervention: Report from the 2000-2001 New York State Angioplasty Registry. Am Heart J 2006;151:164-167.

87. Slater J, Selzer F, Dorbala S, et al: Ethnic differences in the presentation, treatment strategy, and outcomes of percutaneous coronary intervention: A report from the National Heart, Lung, and Blood Institute Dynamic Registry. Am J Cardiol 2003;92:773-778.

88. Marks DS, Mensah GA, Kennard ED, et al: Race, baseline characteristics, and clinical outcomes after coronary intervention: The New Approaches in Coronary Interventions (NACI) registry. Am Heart J 2000;140:162-169.

89. Mastoor M, Iqbal U, Pinnow E, Lindsay J Jr: Ethnicity does not affect outcomes of coronary angioplasty. Clin Cardiol 2000;23:379-382.

90. Iqbal U, Pinnow EE, Lindsay J Jr: Comparison of six-month outcomes after percutaneous coronary intervention for Whites versus African-Americans. Am J Cardiol 2001;88:304-305.

91. Leborgne L, Cheneau E, Wolfram R, et al: Comparison of baseline characteristics and one-year outcomes between African-Americans and Caucasians undergoing percutaneous coronary intervention. Am J Cardiol 2004;93:389-393.

92. Bach PB, Pham HH, Schrag D, et al: Primary care physicians who treat blacks and whites. N Engl J Med 2004;351:575-584.

93. Gornick ME, Eggers PW, Reilly TW, et al: Effects of race and income on mortality and use of services among Medicare beneficiaries. N Engl J Med 1996;335:791-799.

94. Lillie-Blanton M, Maddox TM, Rushing O, Mensah GA: Disparities in cardiac care: Rising to the challenge of Healthy People 2010. J Am Coll Cardiol 2004;44:503-508.

95. Schiffrin EL: Role of endothelin-1 in hypertension and vascular disease. Am J Hypertens 2001;14(6 Pt 2):83S-89S.

96. Sonel AF, Good CB, Mulgund J, et al: Racial variations in treatment and outcomes of black and white patients with high-risk non-ST-elevation acute coronary syndromes: Insights from CRUSADE (Can Rapid Risk Stratification of Unstable Angina Patients Suppress Adverse Outcomes With Early Implementation of the ACC/AHA Guidelines?). Circulation 2005;111:1225-1232.

97. Sabatine MS, Blake GJ, Drazner MH, et al: Influence of race on death and ischemic complications in patients with non-ST-elevation acute coronary syndromes despite modern, protocol-guided treatment. Circulation 2005;111:1217-1224.

98. Bradley EH, Herrin J, Wang Y, et al: Racial and ethnic differences in time to acute reperfusion therapy for patients hospitalized with myocardial infarction. JAMA 2004;292:1563-1572.

99. Trivedi AN, Sequist TD, Ayanian JZ: Impact of hospital volume on racial disparities in cardiovascular procedure mortality. J Am Coll Cardiol 2006;47:417-424.

100. Mehta RH, Marks D, Califf RM, et al: Differences in the clinical features and outcomes in African Americans and whites with myocardial infarction. Am J Med 2006;119:70 e1-e8.

101. Manhapra A, Canto JG, Vaccarino V, et al: Relation of age and race with hospital death after acute myocardial infarction. Am Heart J 2004;148:92-98.

102. Barnhart JM, Fang J, Alderman MH: Differential use of coronary revascularization and hospital mortality following acute myocardial infarction. Arch Intern Med 2003;163:461-466.

103. Chen J, Rathore SS, Radford MJ, et al: Racial differences in the use of cardiac catheterization after acute myocardial infarction. N Engl J Med 2001;344:1443-1449.

104. Lucas FL, DeLorenzo MA, Siewers AE, Wennberg DE: Temporal trends in the utilization of diagnostic testing and treatments for cardiovascular disease in the United States, 1993-2001. Circulation 2006;113:374-379.

105. Werner RM, Asch DA, Polsky D: Racial profiling: The unintended consequences of coronary artery bypass graft report cards. Circulation 2005;111:1257-1263.

106. Hughes D, Griffiths L: "But if you look at the coronary anatomy": Risk and rationing in cardiac surgery. Sociol Health Illn 1996;18:172-197.

107. Whittle J, Conigliaro J, Good CB, Joswiak M: Do patient preferences contribute to racial differences in cardiovascular procedure use? J Gen Intern Med 1997;12:267-273.

108. Rosen AB, Tsai JS, Downs SM: Variations in risk attitude across race, gender, and education. Med Decis Making 2003;23:511-517.

109. Shen JJ, Wan TT, Perlin JB: An exploration of the complex relationship of socioecologic factors in the treatment and outcomes of acute myocardial infarction in disadvantaged populations. Health Serv Res 2001;36:711-732.

110. Unequal Treatment: Confronting Racial and Ethnic Disparities in Healthcare. Washington DC, The Institute of Medicine, 2001.

Pharmacologic Intervention

9 Role of Platelet Inhibitor Agents in Percutaneous Coronary Interventions

Hussam Hamdalla and Steven R. Steinhubl

KEY POINTS

- Platelets are critical to the atherothrombotic process by contributing to the inflammatory response with thrombus formation.
- Aspirin, although frequently referred to as a weak antiplatelet agent, provides clinical benefits that are virtually unmatched in cardiovascular medicine.
- Dual therapy to inhibit platelet activation with a thienopyridine and aspirin provide at least additive antithrombotic protection in specific clinical situations, such as percutaneous coronary intervention (PCI). Adequate pretreatment with 600 mg of clopidogrel more than 2 hours

before the procedure in stable patients with negative troponin levels can inhibit the procedural ischemic complications with no further benefit from adding abciximab at the time of PCI.
- GP IIb/IIIa receptor inhibitors provide the maximum benefit in patients with elevated troponin levels on admission, especially those who are destined to undergo PCI.
- Platelet variability in response to antiplatelet therapy is well recognized, but further understanding about how to better measure it and adjust therapy accordingly is needed.

Antiplatelet therapy has been an important component of adjunctive medical therapy during percutaneous coronary interventions (PCIs) since the inception of this technique almost 30 years ago. Just how critical a role it played was not fully appreciated until early placebo-controlled studies established the importance of aspirin use in decreasing the risk of acute thrombotic complications by roughly 75%. Several hundred thousand patients have been enrolled in randomized trials to establish the optimal antiplatelet regimens to prevent acute and long-term thrombotic complications in patients undergoing a PCI or presenting with an acute coronary syndrome (ACS).

Despite the fact that antiplatelet therapies have been available for more than 100 years, have been studied in more patients than virtually any other pharmacologic class, and are one of our most effective therapeutic interventions, there are a number of basic aspects of platelets and antiplatelet therapy that remain poorly understood. In this chapter, we review the current understanding of the role of platelets in atherothrombosis and the clinical data supporting

antiplatelet agents in various clinical settings, particularly PCI.

PLATELET BIOLOGY

Platelet Cell Biology

The platelet is a small, circulating, anucleate, disk-shaped cell that is formed from the cytoplasm of megakaryocytes and has a life span of 7 to 10 days. Platelets normally circulate in an inactive form, although they do continue to circulate after activation. Activation classically occurs after exposure of subendothelial molecules to the blood after spontaneous plaque rupture or vessel damage during angioplasty (Fig. 9-1). Packaged internally inside the platelets are primarily two types of granules. The α-granule is the larger of the two and stores the adhesive proteins (i.e., fibrinogen, fibronectin, vitronectin, von Willebrand factor [vWF] and thrombospondin) and glycoproteins (GP) (i.e., GP IIb/IIIa, GP Ib-IX-V, and P-selectin). The dense granules are smaller and carry the soluble activating agents (i.e., adenosine

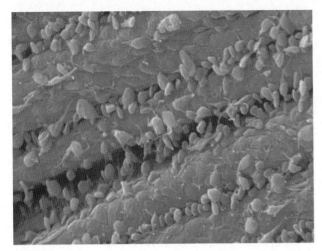

Figure 9-1. Electron microscopic view of platelets adhering to the endothelium.

diphosphate [ADP] and serotonin) and divalent cations.[1]

Platelet Function

Adhesion

Platelets circulating in the blood vessels do not interact with other platelets or other cell types under normal physiologic conditions. Disruption of the endothelial layer and exposure of the subendothelial matrix triggers a cascade of events terminating in thrombus formation. Subendothelial constituents, the most important of which is collagen, provide a surface for the platelets to adhere to. *Initiation* begins with the rolling, arrest, and activation of moving platelets by the collagen/vWF complex to form a platelet monolayer. Collagen serves as a substrate for platelet adhesion and as a potent platelet agonist. Platelets possess two types of collagen receptors: GP Ia/IIa and GP VI. GP Ia/IIa serves as an anchor through which platelets attach directly to the exposed collagen in the subendothelium. Adhesive proteins, including vWF and fibronectin, are present in the platelets, plasma, and subendothelial matrix and play an integral role in the platelet adhesion. The vWF rapidly attaches to platelets to promote adhesion through interaction with GP Ib/IX/V complex and GP IIb/IIIa.

Activation

Circulating platelets are restrained from activation in the blood through the inhibitory action of the prostaglandin (PG) I_2 and nitric oxide (NO). After exposure to collagen or other platelet agonists, intracellular signaling results in the activation and expression of the GP Ia/IIa and GP IIb/IIIa, allowing them to bind to collagen and fibrinogen, respectively. The extension of the platelet plug occurs when additional activated platelets accumulate on top of the platelet monolayer. This is mediated through the local release and accumulation of molecules such as thrombin, ADP, thromboxane A_2 (TxA$_2$), and epinephrine. In contrast to platelet activation by collagen, platelet activation by most of the agonists involved in extension of the platelet plug is very rapid. Platelet agonists typically cause activation by the G protein–coupled receptors (GPCRs) on the platelet surface (Fig. 9-2). Thrombin, the most potent platelet agonist, activates platelets by binding with the protease-activated receptor (PAR), which is a GPCR. There are two PAR receptors on the human platelet: PAR-1 and PAR-4. The PAR receptors are activated when thrombin binds to the receptor N terminus, cleaving it and exposing a new N terminus that serves as a tethered ligand. Thrombin increases the cytosolic Ca^{2+} concentration and inhibits cyclic adenosine monophosphate (cAMP) formation; it also induces cell-surface expression of the adhesion molecule P-selectin and CD40 ligand and activation of the GP IIb/IIIa to mediate platelet aggregation. ADP, a weaker agonist, is stored in the platelet-dense granules and released on platelet activation. ADP activates platelets through two receptors, $P2Y_1$ and $P2Y_{12}$, and activation triggers TxA$_2$ formation, protein phosphorylation, and an increase in cytosolic Ca^{2+} concentration, with a platelet shape change. Although ADP has long been known to be a platelet agonist, the $P2Y_1$ and $P2Y_{12}$ receptors were not identified until recently. When ADP stimulates the $P2Y_{12}$ receptor, it inhibits adenylate cyclase. Adenylyl cyclase generates cAMP, which is a potent inhibitor of platelet activation. TxA$_2$ is produced from arachidonate in platelets by the cyclooxygenase pathway and has a very short half-life (approximately 30 seconds), confining the platelet activation to the site of injury. TxA$_2$ causes shape change, aggregation, secretion, protein phosphorylation, and an increase in cytosolic Ca^{2+}, while having little or no direct effect on cAMP formation. In contrast with ADP and thrombin, epinephrine is a weak activator of human platelets and appears to serve primarily as a potentiator of platelet responses to other agonists.

Aggregation

Platelet aggregation is cell-to-cell adhesion that is mediated by the binding of fibrinogen or vWF to the activated GP IIb/IIIa. This process is a key event in the thrombus formation. The GP IIb/IIIa is a member of the integrin family of heterodimeric receptors that mediate cell adhesion and signaling. It is the most abundant platelet surface glycoprotein, and it is specific to the platelets. In the resting platelet, GP IIb/IIIa maintains a low affinity to ligand binding, allowing platelets to circulate in the blood without forming clots. Conformational changes in the GP IIb/IIIa ensue after platelet activation that increases the affinity of the receptor to the ligand. Ligand binding to the GP IIb/IIIa receptor triggers an outside-in signal that contributes to the adhesive strengthening and to irreversible platelet aggregation.

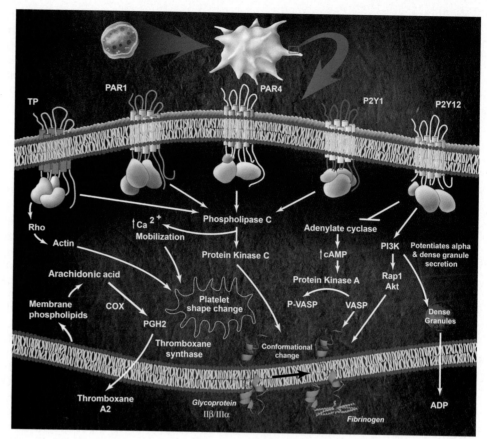

Figure 9-2. Diagram highlighting the platelet receptors' mechanism of action, with their intracellular signaling and interactions leading to the final common changes in platelet shape and receptor expression. ADP, adenosine diphosphate; Akt, serine/threonine protein kinase; cAMP, cyclic adenosine monophosphate; COX, cyclo-oxygenase enzyme; PAR, protease-activated receptor; PGH2, prostaglandin H2; PI3K, phosphoinositide-3 kinase; TP, thromboxane A2 receptor.

Platelets as Inflammatory Cells

An increasing body of evidence links platelets to the inflammatory process of atherosclerosis.[1] Platelets appear to be a primary source for the inflammatory mediators responsible for the vascular endothelial injury that promotes atherosclerosis. Among the more than 300 proteins released by the platelets, CD40 ligand (CD40L), P-selectin, interleukin (IL)-1β, platelet factor-4, and RANTES (regulated on activation, normal T cell expressed and secreted) have an established role in the progression and stability of atherosclerosis. Platelet activation increases the CD40L expression; this is subsequently cleaved to produce the soluble CD40L that is released into the circulation. The release of stored CD40L from activated platelets, which is the source for more than 90% of circulating sCD40L, stimulates endothelial cells to produce cytokines, such as IL-1 and IL-18, and increases thrombotic activity. The P-selectin expressed on the surface of activated platelets binds to P-selectin glycoprotein ligand-1 (PSGL-1) on leukocytes, promoting the formation of platelet-leukocyte complexes.

Platelets, long thought to play only a reactionary role at the time of endothelial disruption, are now recognized as important mediators of the inflammatory process. More evidence from prospective, randomized trials is lacking, and our understanding of the platelet's role as an inflammatory cell needs further refinement to be able to better prevent and treat the atherosclerotic process.

Measuring Platelet Function

Animal Models

Defining and measuring platelet function in vivo remains a considerable challenge.[2] The animal models were developed to function as a bridge between the in vitro findings and in vivo clinical studies.

Folts' Model

This animal model was first described by John Folts more than 15 years ago and continues to be frequently used today in the evaluation of antithrombotic agents. In this model, blood flow is typically measured in the circumflex or left anterior descending artery using a Doppler flow probe. Distal to the flow probe, endothelial or medial injury is induced by a vascular clamp. A plastic cylinder is placed around the vessel at the site of vascular injury producing a critical stenosis. Platelet rich thrombus formation begins to form in the stenosed lumen causing a decline in the coronary flow until it becomes occlusive thrombus. The thrombus is then embolized in the distal circulation, and blood flow is restored to normal, until platelets re-accumulate and again occlude the vessel. These cyclic flow reductions

(CFRs) are repetitive, permitting the testing of different antithrombotic regimens.

Badimon Chamber

Perfusion chambers allow the dynamics of platelet deposition to be extensively studied. The Badimon chamber is a well-recognized perfusion model that allows the study of thrombus formation under controlled hemodynamic conditions after plaque rupture in the vicinity of a stenotic lesion. Arterial blood is drawn from the animal carotid or femoral artery into the tubular perfusion chamber and then returned through the vein. The tubelike perfusion chamber is designed to mimic the cylindrical shape typical of the vasculature, to accept a variety of biologic and prosthetic materials, and to simulate a broad range of physiologic flow conditions. Platelet deposition on the surface is evaluated by ^{111}In-labeled platelets injected into the animal. Perfusion systems have allowed studies using laminar flow; however, new systems to create turbulent flow are being developed.

Ex Vivo Studies

Aggregometry

The historical standard for platelet function testing is light transmittance aggregometry (LTA), although there are multiple theoretical and practical limitations to its clinical applicability. LTA is tedious and requires a fair degree of technical expertise in its performance and interpretation. Platelet aggregation studies are performed using platelet-rich plasma. When platelets are suspended in the plasma unaggregated, they create a turbid solution that absorbs light. On adding an agonist to the solution, platelets are activated, and aggregation is initiated. The aggregated platelets clump together and fall to the bottom of the tube, increasing light transmittance. The spectrophotometry generated is recorded as a function of time. The degree and speed of aggregation depend on the strength and type of agonist used.

Flow Cytometry

Flow cytometry is a powerful tool to study platelet function and includes a variety of assays for multiple purposes. The platelets, with or without activation with an agonist, are labeled with fluorescent monoclonal antibodies specific for the marker of interest, such as P-selectin or the activated confirmation of the GP IIb/IIIa receptor, and are then passed through a flow chamber with a focused beam of laser light. After the laser light activates the fluorophore at the excitation wavelength, detectors process the emitted fluorescence and light-scattering properties of the cells. The intensity of the emitted light is directly proportional to the antigen density. Flow cytometry permits more specific assessment of platelet function in different clinical disorders and in diagnosing specific congenital platelet disorders. It also has the advantage of directly analyzing platelets in their physiologic milieu of whole blood using a small sample, even in patients with thrombocytopenia. The activation state and the reactivity of circulating platelets can be determined through the use of specific platelet activation markers. The disadvantage of flow cytometry is the high cost and complicated sample preparation.

VerifyNow

The VerifyNow (Accumetrics, Inc., San Diego, CA), previously known as the Ultegra-Rapid Platelet Function Assay (RPFA), is a whole-blood, point-of-care assay originally developed to provide simple and rapid functional assessment of GP IIb/IIIa receptor blockade. The test is based on the principle that fibrinogen-coated polystyrene beads will agglutinate in whole blood in proportion to the number of available platelet GP IIb/IIIa receptors. Blood samples are drawn into a standard citrated tube, or PPACK (Phe-Pro-Arg chloromethyl ketone), can be used as an anticoagulant. The blood is then drawn into a disposable plastic cartridge containing fibrinogen-coated beads and a specific agonist, depending on what drug effect is being monitored: thrombin-receptor-activating peptide (TRAP) for GP IIb/IIIa antagonists, arachidonic acid for aspirin, and a combination of ADP and prostacyclin for P2Y$_{12}$ antagonists. As the platelets are activated, they interact with fibrinogen-coated beads and agglutinate, allowing increased light transmittance across the solution. The rate of change in absorbance is plotted against a fixed time interval and reported as platelet aggregation units (PAU=mV/10 sec). The VerifyNow eliminates the need for sample preparation, and it is an automated test. Analysis is duplicated to avoid errors, and it provides a rapid digital readout.

Platelet Function Analyzer-100

The Platelet Function Analyzer (PFA)-100 (Dade Behring, Miami, FL) provides a simple and sensitive test that was developed as an alternative to the bleeding time. This test is based on platelet activation using high shear force by vacuum suction through a capillary stainless steel tube. A small sample of citrated whole blood is drawn into a disposable cartridge and then through the stainless steel tube. The blood is then passed through a small aperture (150 μm in diameter) onto a membrane coated with collagen and epinephrine (CEPI) or collagen and ADP (CADP). Initial adhesion to the membrane is a function of the high shear rates, but subsequent platelet aggregation is the response to the release of the platelet content and the presence of epinephrine or ADP. As the clot forms, the aperture becomes totally occluded, and blood flow completely ceases. This parameter is referred to as the *closure time*. As with the bleeding time, this test is sensitive to the platelet count and hematocrit. Although the test is sensitive for the presence of platelet dysfunction, it is not specific, and it is highly dependent on vWF.

Plateletworks

The Plateletworks (Helena Laboratories, Beaumont, TX) platelet aggregation system is a point-of-care test that provides platelet count, standard complete blood cell count (CBC), and platelet micro-aggregation results rapidly. Plateletworks assesses platelet aggregation by comparing the platelet count before and after exposure with a specific platelet agonist. This assay measures the number of free platelets in an agonist-stimulated blood sample compared with baseline platelet count. The assay uses standard platelet counting equipment and avoids the requirement of centrifugation.

ANTIPLATELET THERAPIES

Aspirin

Salicylates are naturally occurring chemicals found in a wide range of plants, including the bark and leaves of the willow tree. They were used for centuries, and the first published research (1763) on the topic is entitled "An Account of the Success of the Bark of the Willow in the Cure of Agues." Aspirin, or acetylsalicylic acid, was made by the chemical substitution of acetic acid group for the carboxyl group and was launched in 1899 by Bayer. However, its cardioprotective and antithrombotic benefits were not recognized till the mid-20th century. Aspirin confers its clinical benefit through the inhibition of prostaglandin (PG) biosynthesis.

Arachidonic acid is metabolized by the cyclooxygenase (COX) enzyme PGH synthase into PGG_2, which is then converted to TxA_2 by thromboxane synthase. Aspirin acetylates the COX enzyme at the catalytic site, resulting in irreversible inhibition.[3] Because platelets are anucleate structures, they are incapable of reproducing and replacing COX for the life span of the platelet. COX produces TxA_2 in the platelets, which leads to platelet aggregation and vasoconstriction, whereas in the endothelial cells, it produces PGI_2, which inhibits platelet aggregation and causes vasodilation. There are two isoforms of the cyclooxygenase enzyme, COX-1 and COX-2, with aspirin being a 170-fold more selective inhibitor of COX-1. Beyond platelet aggregation, COX-1 regulates other normal cellular processes such as gastric cytoprotection, vascular homeostasis, and kidney function. Although both TxA_2 and PGI_2 are inhibited by aspirin, the inhibition of PGI_2 is temporary because endothelial cells are able to regenerate new COX and despite early concerns has never been found to have prothrombotic consequences.

Aspirin's role in the reduction of nonfatal myocardial infarction (MI) and cardiovascular mortality in the setting of an ACS has been well established through a number of placebo-controlled trials. Findings of early trials, including the Veterans Administration Cooperative Study and the Canadian Multicenter Trial, established the benefit of aspirin therapy in unstable angina patients with a more than 50% relative reduction in nonfatal MI and cardiovascular death compared with placebo. The role of aspirin in the acute treatment of patients with an ST-segment elevation MI was verified in the International Study of Infarct Survival (ISIS) 2 trial.[4] Patients who were randomized to a 7-day treatment with aspirin attained more than 20% reduction in vascular death, similar to that achieved by streptokinase alone, and there was an additive benefit when it was combined with streptokinase.

The role of aspirin in the long-term therapy of patients with established cardiovascular disease is less conclusive. In one of the first placebo-controlled trials of long-term aspirin in secondary prevention, the Aspirin Myocardial Infarction Study (AMIS), patients with a previous history of MI who were randomized to daily aspirin did not have a survival benefit at the end of 3-year follow-up compared with placebo. It was not until the Antiplatelet Trialists' combined the results of all 11 placebo-controlled post-MI trials, including slightly less than 20,000 patients, that a significant benefit of aspirin in terms of recurrent nonfatal MI (4.7% versus 6.5%, $P < .00001$) and vascular death (8.1% versus 9.4%, $P < .005$) was established.

Aspirin for primary prevention has been evaluated in a number of placebo-controlled trials. One of the first to establish its role in cardiovascular disease prevention in low risk, healthy individuals was in the U.S. Health Physicians Study. There was a significant 44% reduction in the risk of first MI but no overall survival benefit. A later trial, including 39,876 U.S. female health care professionals who were 45 years or older, were randomized to aspirin or placebo for primary prevention. Although there was a small but significant reduction in stroke, this was not accompanied with any cardiovascular benefit, except in those older than 65 years.[5]

Thienopyridines

Ticlopidine, the prototype thienopyridine, was introduced more than 30 years ago. Although initially it was developed as an anti-inflammatory agent, it was quickly found to have antiplatelet effects that were subsequently shown to be specific for ADP's platelet-stimulating properties. However, it did not come to the forefront in the treatment and prevention of cardiovascular disease until stents were used in the coronary arteries. Clopidogrel was the second thienopyridine to be developed as a safer, better-tolerated, and more rapid-acting alternative to ticlopidine. Although clopidogrel is roughly 10 times more potent than ticlopidine on a molar basis, chronic dosing was designed to achieve levels of platelet inhibition similar to ticlopidine. Prasugrel has been added to the class of thienopyridines. This medication was developed as a more potent thienopyridine derivative, about 10 times more potent than clopidogrel and therefore about 100 times more potent than ticlopidine.

Thienopyridines are inactive in vitro and require hepatic metabolism for production of their active metabolite, which has a very short half-life. Once metabolized, the thiol active form irreversibly binds to the $P2Y_{12}$ receptor on the platelet surface and inhibits the ADP-induced platelet aggregation.[6] The antiplatelet effect of ticlopidine requires 2 to 3 days to become clinically significant and up to a week to achieve its maximum effect. Likewise, clopidogrel requires 3 to 5 days without a loading dose to achieve a similar level of platelet aggregation inhibition. A more rapid onset of action can be achieved with a loading dose: within almost 24 hours after a 300-mg and within 2 hours after a 600-mg loading dose. Prasugrel is being evaluated with doses that achieve faster onset of action and higher level of inhibition in response to ADP-induced aggregation compared with standard doses of clopidogrel.

Thienopyridines also differ in their safety profile, with ticlopidine having a higher ($\approx 20\%$) discontinuation rate because of gastrointestinal intolerance and rash. Although less common, there is a serious risk of neutropenia, with an absolute neutrophil count of less than $1200/mm^3$ reported in 2.4% of patients and severe neutropenia ($<450/mm^3$) in 0.8%. The life-threatening complication of thrombotic thrombocytopenic purpura (TTP) has also been associated with ticlopidine use. Clopidogrel was reported to have a better safety profile with discontinuation rates about 5% in major trials. Its most common reported side effects were rash and diarrhea, but it also was later found to have an association with TTP, but at a much lower incidence than ticlopidine. There will not be sufficient data on prasugrel's safety profile available until the completion of the current phase III trials.

Ticlopidine was initially evaluated in the long-term therapy of stroke and claudication; however, use was later extended to the prevention of cardiac thrombotic events. Ticlopidine was evaluated in patients with unstable angina in a placebo-controlled trial, and similar to the early placebo-controlled aspirin trials, it was found to provide a 46% reduction in the risk of vascular death or MI at 6 months compared with placebo (7.3% versus 13.6%, $P=.009$). The first large-scale trial of clopidogrel was the Clopidogrel versus Aspirin in Patients at Risk for further Ischemic Events (CAPRIE) trial, in which it was compared with aspirin for the long-term prevention of thrombotic events. CAPRIE randomized more than 19,000 patients with atherosclerotic disease, including ischemic stroke, MI, or symptomatic peripheral arterial disease, to clopidogrel or aspirin daily. After a mean follow-up of 2 years, clopidogrel treated patients had a slightly lower risk of the combined end point of ischemic stroke, myocardial infarction and vascular death compared with aspirin (5.3% versus 5.8%, $P<.048$). These studies established thienopyridines as viable alternatives to aspirin in treating coronary disease.

Thienopyridines and aspirin act synergistically to achieve greater in vitro inhibition of thrombosis and improved reductions in ischemic events. This was best demonstrated in the Clopidogrel in Unstable

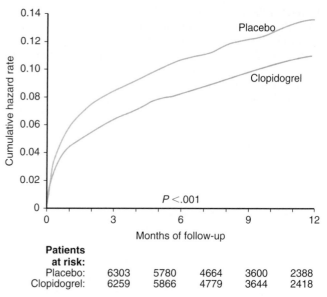

Figure 9-3. Cumulative hazard rates for the first primary outcome (i.e., death from cardiovascular causes, nonfatal myocardial infarction, or stroke) during the 12 months of the Clopidogrel in Unstable Angina to Prevent Recurrent Ischemic Events (CURE) trial. (From The Clopidogrel in Unstable Angina to Prevent Recurrent Events Trial. N Engl J Med 2001;345:494-502.)

Angina to Prevent Recurrent Ischemic Events (CURE) trial.[7] A total of 12,562 patients with non-ST-elevation ACSs were randomized to the combination of clopidogrel and aspirin or to aspirin alone. The combination's superiority was demonstrated with a 20% reduction in the major cardiac events (11.5% versus 9.3%; $P<.001$) at the end of the 9-month follow-up period (Fig. 9-3).

Prasugrel is the latest addition to the thienopyridines and is currently undergoing phase III study in the Trial to Assess Improvement in Therapeutic Outcomes by Optimizing Platelet Inhibition with Prasugrel (TRITON)-TIMI 38. In this trial, about 13,000 patients with an ACS undergoing a PCI are being randomized to clopidogrel or prasugrel for up to 1 year.[8]

Glycoprotein IIb/IIIa Antagonists

Irrespective of the platelet agonist that leads to platelet activation, platelet aggregation always occurs through the binding of fibrinogen and vWF to platelets through the integrin GP IIb/IIIa expressed on the surface of activated platelets. Given the central role of platelets in the pathophysiology of ACSs, as well as the marked benefit of aspirin in this patient population, the GP IIb/IIIa receptor antagonists were extensively studied in this population.[9] Abciximab, developed from a murine monoclonal antibody into a chimeric antibody, was the first GP IIb/IIIa receptor inhibitor to become available. The c7E3 Fab Anti-

Table 9-1. Placebo-Controlled Trials of Intravenous Glycoprotein IIb/IIIa Antagonists in Patients with Non-ST-Segment Elevation Acute Coronary Syndrome

Trial	N	Drug	Follow-up	Heparin	PTCA	Primary End Point	Percentage (%) with End Point Placebo	Percentage (%) with End Point IIb/IIIa Inhibitor	P Value
CAPTURE	1,265	Abciximab	30 days	UFH	98%	Death, MI, or urgent revascularization	15.9	11.3	.012
GUSTO IV-ACS	7,800	Abciximab	30 days	UFH or LMWH	2%	Death or MI	8.0	24-Hour infusion: 8.2% / 48-Hour infusion: 9.1%	NS / NS
PURSUIT	10,948	Eptifibatide	30 days	UFH	≈24%	Death or MI	15.7	14.2	.04
PARAGON	2,282	Lamifiban	30 days	UFH or placebo	≈12%	Death or MI	11.7	Low dose with heparin: 10.3%	NS
PARAGON-B	5,225	Lamifiban	30 days	UFH	28%	Death, MI, or severe, recurrent ischemia	12.8	11.8	.33
PRISM	3,231	Tirofiban	48 hours	UFH control arm only	21%	Death, MI, or refractory ischemia	5.6	3.8	.01
PRISM-PLUS	1,560	Tirofiban	7 days	UFH	≈70%	Death, MI, or refractory ischemia	17.9	12.9	.004

ACS, acute coronary syndrome; CAPTURE, c7E3 Fab Antiplatelet Therapy in Unstable Refractory Angina; GUSTO, Global Use of Strategies To Open Occluded Arteries in Acute Coronary Syndromes; LMWH, low-molecular-weight heparin; MI, myocardial infarction; N, number of patients; NS, not significant; PARAGON, Platelet IIb/IIIa Antagonism for the Reduction of Acute Coronary Syndrome Events In a Global Organization Network; PRISM, Platelet Receptor Inhibition for Ischemic Syndrome Management; PRISM-PLUS, Platelet Receptor Inhibition for Ischemic Syndrome Management in Patients Limited by Unstable Signs and Symptoms; PTCA, percutaneous transluminal coronary angioplasty; PURSUIT, Platelet IIb/IIIa in Unstable Angina: Receptor Suppression Using Integrilin Therapy; UFH, unfractionated heparin.

platelet Therapy in Unstable Refractory Angina (CAPTURE) was the first study to randomize patients with unstable angina to either abciximab or placebo (Table 9-1). This study was terminated before full enrollment because of a clear benefit from the abciximab infusion. Patients had a 29% reduction in the combined risk of death, MI, or urgent revascularization at 30-day follow-up in the abciximab arm (11.3% versus 15.9%; *P*=.012), with a 50% reduction in nonfatal MI (4.1% versus 8.2%, *P*=.002). Further analysis revealed this benefit to be limited to those with elevated troponin levels in whom abciximab reduced the risk of death, MI, or urgent revascularization by 78% at the 6-month follow-up. Because all patients underwent revascularization in this study, this prevented the applicability of these findings to medically managed patients.

The Global Use of Strategies to Open Occluded Arteries in Acute Coronary Syndromes (GUSTO) IV-ACS trial was launched to address the role of abciximab in medically managed, high-risk ACS patients (see Table 9-1). Patients presenting with ST-segment depression or elevated cardiac markers were randomized to placebo or abciximab (a 24- or 48-hour infusion). Surprisingly, not only was there no benefit, but there was a potentially harmful effect associated with abciximab infusion that increased with the duration of the infusion. The reasons for these surprising findings are not yet clear but may be related to paradoxical platelet activation with lower levels of GP IIb/IIIa inhibition, as is suspected to have occurred with prolonged abciximab infusions.

When the findings of CAPTURE and GUSTO-IV, along with the post hoc analysis of the unstable angina patients enrolled in the placebo-controlled abciximab PCI trials, are analyzed together, they provide strong, evidence-based guidance for the use of abciximab in the patient presenting with an ACS. However, it should be reserved for those with elevated troponin levels, with therapy to be initiated at the time of PCI. There is no role for abciximab in medical management of unstable angina, and it should be avoided.

Lamifiban is a low-molecular-weight, synthetic, nonpeptide that is a highly specific GP IIb/IIIa antagonist and that was evaluated in unstable angina. In the Platelet IIb/IIIa Antagonism for the Reduction of Acute Coronary Syndrome Events in a Global Organization Network (PARAGON-A) trial, two doses of lamifiban were evaluated (1-μg/min and 5-μg/min infusion) with and without heparin. Although there was no significant difference between the lamifiban and placebo, the low-dose lamifiban did better than the high dose (see Table 9-1). The curves continued to separate until it reached statistical difference at 6 months between the low-dose lamifiban and placebo arm in death and MI. The PARAGON-B trial was designed to adjust the lamifiban dose according to creatinine clearance with a similar design to the PARAGON-A. Similar to the findings in PARAGON-A, there was no significant reduction in the combined end point of death, MI, or recurrent ischemia (see Table 9-1). However, patients with elevated troponin levels had a significant reduction in death or MI (11%

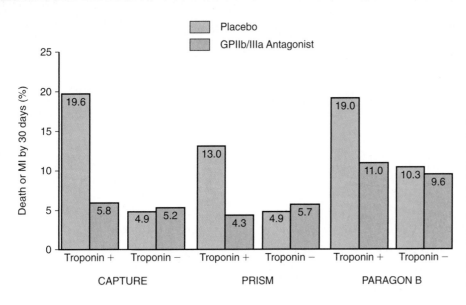

Figure 9-4. Glycoprotein IIb/IIIa effect on the 30-day end point of death and myocardial infarction among patients presenting with elevated troponin levels compared with negative troponin levels. CAPTURE, Chimeric c7E3 Fab AntiPlatelet Therapy in Unstable REfractory angina trial; PARAGON B, Platelet IIb/IIIa Antagonism for the Reduction of Acute Coronary Syndrome Events In a Global Organization Network-B trial; PRISM, Platelet Receptor Inhibition for Ischemic Syndrome Management.

versus 19.4%, *P*=.01), which was not seen in troponin-negative patients. Because of the results of these trials, lamifiban was never marketed commercially.

Tirofiban, a small non–peptide tyrosine derivative, has a rapid onset of action and rapid reversal of effect after drug discontinuation. The Platelet Receptor Inhibition for Ischemic Syndrome Management (PRISM) trial was the first trial to compare tirofiban without heparin against heparin alone in patients with unstable angina. Tirofiban was better than heparin in reducing death, MI, and refractory ischemia at 48 hours (3.8% versus 5.6%, *P*=.01) (see Table 9-1). Similar to all other placebo-controlled GP IIb/IIIa antagonist trials that measured troponins at baseline, tirofiban was beneficial only in those individuals who had elevated troponin levels (Fig. 9-4). The Platelet Receptor Inhibition for Ischemic Syndrome Management in Patients Limited by Unstable Signs and Symptoms (PRISM-PLUS) trial enrolled a higher-risk population compared with PRISM and assigned patients to tirofiban alone, tirofiban with heparin, or heparin alone. The tirofiban-alone arm was discontinued early because of unexpectedly high mortality. The addition of tirofiban to heparin was associated with a reduction in the primary end point of death, MI, or refractory ischemia at 7 days from 17.9% to 12.9% (*P*=.004) (see Table 9-1). The benefit of the tirofiban treatment was found to be greatest in patients who underwent revascularization.

Eptifibatide is a cyclic heptapeptide based on the RGD template, but it substitutes a lysine for an arginine, creating a KGD sequence and increasing its specificity for GP IIb/IIIa. In the Platelet IIb/IIIa in Unstable Angina: Receptor Suppression Using Integrilin Therapy (PURSUIT) trial, almost 11,000 patients with unstable angina were randomized to the eptifibatide or placebo (see Table 9-1). At 30-day follow-up, the primary end point of death or MI was reduced from 15.7% in the placebo group to 14.2% in patients receiving eptifibatide (*P*=.04). Similar to the PRISM-PLUS, those who underwent revascularization had

the maximum benefit derived from the eptifibatide treatment.

A critical review of all of the trials of the parenteral GP IIb/IIIa receptor inhibitors reveals their benefit in selected group of patients.[10] First, patients with ACS who have elevated cardiac markers constitute a high-risk population at increased risk for death, MI, and recurrent ischemia in the ensuing weeks and who derive the greatest benefit from receiving a GP IIb/IIIa antagonist. Second, another consistent finding is that an early revascularization approach seems to be associated with a heightened benefit from the GP IIb/IIIa receptor antagonists.[11] A third group to gain from this therapy are patients with diabetes mellitus presenting with ACS. Diabetes is a well-documented risk factor for atherosclerosis and a marker for worse outcome in patients with established coronary artery disease. A meta-analysis of the 6458 diabetic patients enrolled in the GP IIb/IIIa receptor inhibitors studies was performed to assess the extent of benefit.[12] Diabetics who were randomized to a GP IIb/IIIa receptor inhibitors had a survival benefit at 30 days (4.6% versus 6.2%, *P*=.007), which was more pronounced in those undergoing revascularization (Fig. 9-5).

All of the placebo-controlled trials of the GP IIb/IIIa antagonists have also used unfractionated heparin. Their benefit in addition to or directly compared with other anticoagulants, such as direct thrombin inhibitors, is not established.

Acute MI patients presenting with ST-segment elevation represent a milieu packed with heightened platelet activation. GP IIb/IIIa receptor inhibitors have been used in adjunct with fibrinolytic therapy and mechanical reperfusion. The ReoPro and Primary PTCA Organization and Randomized Trial (RAPPORT) were the first of these trials to use abciximab with primary angioplasty in ST-segment elevation myocardial infarction (STEMI) patients. Patients who received the actual treatment had a significant reduction in combined outcome of death or reinfarction, seen by 7 days (1.4% versus 4.7%, *P*=.047), but there

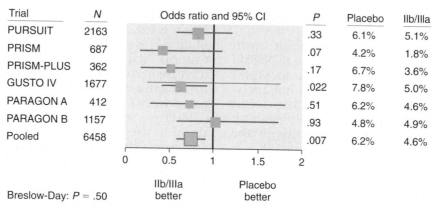

Trial	N	Odds ratio and 95% CI	P	Placebo	IIb/IIIa
PURSUIT	2163		.33	6.1%	5.1%
PRISM	687		.07	4.2%	1.8%
PRISM-PLUS	362		.17	6.7%	3.6%
GUSTO IV	1677		.022	7.8%	5.0%
PARAGON A	412		.51	6.2%	4.6%
PARAGON B	1157		.93	4.8%	4.9%
Pooled	6458		.007	6.2%	4.6%

Breslow-Day: P = .50

IIb/IIIa better — Placebo better

Figure 9-5. Glycoprotein IIb/IIIa effect on 30-day mortality among diabetic patients with acute coronary syndrome. GUSTO, Global Use of Strategies to Open Occluded Arteries in Acute Coronary Syndromes trial; PARAGON, Platelet IIb/IIIa Antagonism for the Reduction of Acute Coronary Syndrome Events In a Global Organization Network trial; PRISM, Platelet Receptor Inhibition for Ischemic Syndrome Management trial; PURSUIT, Platelet IIb/IIIa in Unstable Angina: Receptor Suppression Using Integrilin Therapy trial. (From Roffi M, Chew DP, Mukherjee D, et al: Platelet glycoprotein IIb/IIIa inhibitors reduce mortality in diabetic patients with non-ST-segment-elevation acute coronary syndromes. Circulation 2001;104:2767-2771.)

was attenuation of the benefit by 6 months (6.9% versus 12%, P=.07). Additional placebo-controlled trials of abciximab in the primary PCI population included Abciximab before Direct Angioplasty and Stenting in Myocardial Infarction Regarding Acute and Long-Term Follow-up (ADMIRAL) and the Controlled Abciximab and Device Investigation to Lower Late Angioplasty Complications (CADILLAC) trials. In the ADMIRAL trial, all patients underwent stenting and were randomized to receive either abciximab or placebo. In this trial, there was a pronounced 59% reduction in the combined end point of death, MI, or urgent revascularization at 30 days with abciximab use (6% versus 14.6%, P=.01), and it was maintained at 6 months (7.4% versus 15.9%, P=.02) (Fig. 9-6). In this trial, an increased TIMI grade 3 flow was seen in the abciximab arm before the procedure (16.8% versus 5.4%, P=.01) and immediately afterward (95.1% versus 86.7%, P=.04). This was paralleled by an improvement in the microvascular perfusion when assessed by the Doppler FloWire in the infarct region. The findings of the CADILLAC trial were less consistent, with a strong benefit of GP IIb/IIIa antagonists in primary PCI. This was a larger study that randomized patients to balloon angioplasty or stenting and then to abciximab or placebo. Although stenting lowered the rate of angiographic restenosis at 7 months from 40.8% in the balloon angioplasty arm to 22.2% in the stented arm (P=.01), those who underwent stenting did not achieve the same marked benefit with abciximab compared with stenting with placebo as seen in previous trials.

Despite the partial success of GP IIb/IIIa in conjunction with mechanical reperfusion, the results of the combination with fibrinolytic therapy have not been encouraging. A total of 16,588 patients with STEMI were randomized in the GUSTO V trial to standard-dose reteplase or half-dose reteplase and full-dose abciximab.[13] This study was powered to demonstrate a mortality benefit at 30 days; however, no difference was seen between the reteplase arm

(5.9%) and the half-dose reteplase with abciximab (5.6%). Although there was a significant reduction in the risk of reinfarction, from 3.5% in the reteplase arm to 2.3% in the combination therapy (P<.0001), combination therapy was also associated with an increased risk of severe bleeding and intracranial hemorrhage in those older than 75 years, from 1.1% to 2.1% in the combination therapy (P=.069). Conversely, the Assessment of the Safety and Efficacy of a New Thrombolytic Regimen (ASSENT)-3 study evaluated a combination of half-dose tenecteplase and full-dose abciximab. Patients were randomized to full-dose tenecteplase with unfractionated heparin, tenecteplase and low-molecular-weight heparin, or half-dose tenecteplase and abciximab. The 30-day end point of death, reinfarction, or recurrent ischemia was similar between the tenecteplase and abciximab combination (11.1%) compared with the

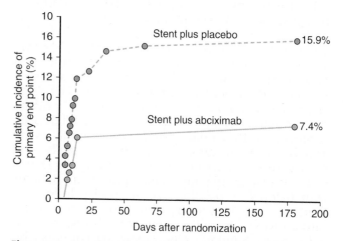

Figure 9-6. Cumulative incidence of composite end point of death, myocardial infarction, or urgent revascularization at 6-months after randomization to abciximab. (From Montalescot G, Barragan P, Wittenberg O, et al, for the ADMIRAL Investigators: Platelet glycoprotein IIb/IIIa inhibition with coronary stenting for acute myocardial infarction. N Engl J Med 2001;344:1895-1903.)

tenecteplase and low-molecular-weight heparin combination (11.4%).

The ongoing, Facilitated Intervention with Enhanced Reperfusion Speed to Stop Events (FINESSE) trial is randomizing 3000 patients with an STEMI receiving mechanical reperfusion to up-front abciximab or abciximab plus half-dose reteplase versus placebo.[14] The results of this trial will help establish the optimal role of GP IIb/IIIa antagonists in the treatment of patients undergoing a planned PCI in the setting of an STEMI.

Phosphodiesterase Inhibitors

Dipyridamole was introduced in 1959 as a coronary vasodilator. It was later found to inhibit platelet aggregation and adhesion and became widely used for stroke prevention, to improve patency of bypass grafts, and to inhibit thrombosis of prosthetic valves. The specific mechanism of action in inhibiting platelet aggregation remains controversial. It is known to inhibit the nucleoside transporter of cell membrane's increasing the plasma concentration of adenosine, which stimulates the A2A receptor, which increases the activity of adenylyl cyclase. It also inhibits the cAMP phosphodiesterase, and these two mechanisms result in increased accumulation of cAMP, which is believed to be responsible for inhibiting platelet aggregation.

The results of early studies suggested that that combination of dipyridamole and aspirin provided no clinical benefit compared with aspirin alone. However, two studies in patients with cerebrovascular disease using an extended-release formulation of dipyridamole with aspirin found a significant reduction in recurrent vascular events compared with aspirin alone. The role of this combination therapy in patients with cardiovascular disease remains poorly understood.

Cilostazol is a selective phosphodiesterase type 3 inhibitor that was introduced in Japan initially for the treatment of symptomatic peripheral arterial occlusion. Through its inhibition of phosphodiesterase type 3, there is increased accumulation of cAMP and cGMP inside the platelet, leading to inhibition of aggregation. However its mechanism of action is not limited to platelet aggregation but extends to arterial vasodilation and inhibition of vascular smooth muscle cell proliferation. Cilostazol has been compared with clopidogrel and ticlopidine as an antiplatelet agent after PCI. In the first study, 490 consecutive patients after elective stenting were given dual antiplatelet therapy using aspirin in all patients with ticlopidine or cilostazol. At 30-day follow-up, there was no significant difference in the major cardiac events, including stent thrombosis, between both groups. Similarly, 689 consecutive patients who underwent elective PCI with stenting were randomized to dual antiplatelet therapy using aspirin with clopidogrel or cilostazol. The rates of major cardiac events, including stent thrombosis, were similar in both groups (2.0% versus 2.6%, $P=.61$). However, the

role of cilostazol in the post–drug-eluting stent population is less well studied, with one very concerning finding from the Asian Paclitaxel-Eluting Stent Clinical Trial (ASPECT) trial, which found a marked increase in stent thrombosis in patients in whom the investigator chose to use cilostazol plus aspirin compared with a thienopyridine plus aspirin.

Multiple studies have evaluated the role of cilostazol in the prevention of neointimal proliferation and reduction of stent restenosis. The largest trial is the Cilostazol for Restenosis Trial (CREST).[15] Patients after elective PCI were randomized to cilostazol (200 mg daily) or placebo for 6 months in addition to aspirin. They all received a bare-metal stent and were treated with clopidogrel for 30 days. At the 6-month follow-up, angiography was performed to determine rate of restenosis. Patients assigned to cilostazol had a significant 36% relative risk reduction in restenosis (22% versus 34.5%, $P=.002$). There was no difference in bleeding, rehospitalization, target-vessel revascularization, MI, or death.

Novel Antiplatelet Agents

The antiplatelet agents available have limitations, and research and development of more practical, efficacious, and better-tolerated antiplatelet regimens remains ongoing. A few of the medications that are being evaluated in phase III trials with the potential for clinical application over the coming years are discussed.

Cangrelor

Thienopyridines have some limitations, including being prodrugs, patient response variability, delay to peak onset, irreversible inhibition, and lack of an intravenous form. Cangrelor is a P2Y$_{12}$ receptor reversible blocker, formerly known as AR-C69931MX, which has an elimination half-life of about 10 minutes and peak onset within less than 2 minutes of an intravenous bolus. Unlike the thienopyridines, this agent acts directly as a reversible, competitive antagonist that does not require metabolic activation. Cangrelor is an ATP analogue that has several-fold selectivity for the P2Y$_{12}$ receptor and competes with ADP in producing anti-aggregatory effects with high potency. Cangrelor was evaluated in phase II trials against the GP IIb/IIIa inhibitor abciximab and was found to achieve rapid and reversible inhibition of platelet aggregation without increased risk of cardiac events and with less bleeding time.[16] A Clinical Trial Comparing Cangrelor to Clopidogrel (CHAMPION) is a phase III trial designed to demonstrate that the efficacy of cangrelor is superior or at least not inferior to clopidogrel in 9000 patients scheduled to undergo an elective or urgent PCI. Patients will be randomized to receive cangrelor or clopidogrel at the time of PCI, with a primary end point of death, MI, or ischemia-driven revascularization at 48 hours. This study will be evaluating the efficacy of cangrelor at reducing the risk of death, MI, or urgent revascularization at 48 hours.

AZD6140

Another agent in a new class of ATP analogues with reversible P2Y$_{12}$ receptor inhibition is AZD6140.[17] Unlike cangrelor, this is an orally active agent without the need for metabolic activation. It has one known active metabolite, and it is as potent as the parent compound in inhibiting the P2Y$_{12}$ receptor. It is believed to contribute to antiplatelet activity. In phase II studies, four doses of the AZD6140 were assessed and compared with a 75-mg dose of clopidogrel over a 30-day period. The 50-mg dose (twice daily) was found to achieve levels of inhibition similar to those of the 75-mg dose of clopidogrel; however, all three of the higher doses (100 mg bid, 200 mg bid, and 400 mg once daily) achieved more robust and complete inhibition of platelet aggregation at 2 hours after initiation of the medication and throughout the follow-up period. There was only one episode of major bleeding that was noticed (with the highest dose), and more importantly, there was increased incidence of dyspnea associated with the escalating dose of the medication. The Can PLATelet Inhibition be Optimized to Prevent Vascular Events (PLATO) trial is planned to enroll about 16,000 patients within 24 hours of an ACS and randomize patients to AZD6140 or clopidogrel, both in addition to aspirin.

PAR-1 Inhibitor

Thrombin is the most potent platelet agonist known and acts on the platelet through the PAR-1 and PAR-4 receptors. PAR-1 is the high-affinity thrombin receptor and the target of SCH 530348, an oral agent that achieves clinically relevant levels of platelet inhibition within 1 hour of a loading dose. SCH 530348 is undergoing clinical testing in a phase II, dose-ranging study involving 800 patients undergoing PCI. In this trial, SCH 530348 is being added to clopidogrel and aspirin.

ANTIPLATELET THERAPIES IN PERCUTANEOUS CORONARY INTERVENTION

Aspirin

Aspirin is an integral part of the antithrombotic regimen in every procedure in interventional cardiology, although it has frequently been described as a weak antiplatelet agent. Although in a test tube that does appear to be the case, there are clinically few individual agents more efficacious. Barnathan and colleagues[17a] observed a remarkable reduction in occlusive thrombus from 10.7% without aspirin to 1.8% with aspirin in their first few balloon angioplasty procedures. Schwartz and colleagues evaluated aspirin-dipyridamole combination in the prevention

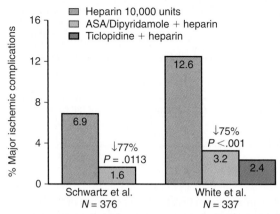

Figure 9-7. Aspirin effect on ischemic complications during percutaneous revascularization compared with placebo. (Data from Schwartz L, Bourassa MG, Lesperance J, et al: Aspirin and dipyridamole in the prevention of restenosis after percutaneous transluminal coronary angioplasty. N Engl J Med 1988;318:1714; White CW, Chaitman B, Knudson ML, et al: Antiplatelet agents are effective in reducing the acute ischemic complications of angioplasty but do not prevent restenosis. Coron Artery Dis 1991;2:757.)

of restenosis after balloon angioplasty. Although there was no reduction in restenosis, the combination therapy was associated with a reduction in the ischemic events to 1.6% from 6.9% in the placebo arm (RR=77%; P=.0113) (Fig. 9-7). Although the adjunctive antithrombotic regimen available to the interventionalist has improved substantially over the past several decades, aspirin remains the cornerstone of therapy in all patients undergoing PCI.

Thienopyridines

The role of thienopyridines in PCI developed from the recognition that aspirin plus aggressive anticoagulation with heparin and warfarin was inadequate in reducing the incidence of acute or subacute thrombosis after coronary stenting. Ticlopidine, which before coronary stenting was limited to primarily patients who had suffered a stroke while taking aspirin, was found to act synergistically with aspirin and therefore was empirically tried as adjunctive therapy after stenting. Subsequent randomized trials confirmed that dual antiplatelet therapy with ticlopidine and aspirin was more effective than aspirin alone or aspirin plus warfarin.

Because of the delay in onset of ticlopidine's full antiplatelet effects for several days, many interventionalists attempted to initiate ticlopidine before the planned intervention when possible. This led to the observation that "pretreatment" with ticlopidine decreased the risk of peri-PCI thrombotic events. The PCI-Clopidogrel in Unstable Angina to Prevent Recurrent Events (PCI-CURE) was one of the first large analyses of blinded dual antiplatelet therapy in the setting of PCI. Of the 12,562 patients enrolled in the CURE trial, 2658 patients underwent PCI. This subset of patients was treated for a median of 10 days before the PCI with clopidogrel or matching placebo, both

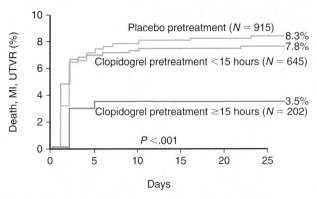

Figure 9-8. Kaplan-Meier curves of the occurrence of the primary combined end point of death, myocardial infarction (MI), and urgent target vessel revascularization (UTVR) in patients randomized to placebo, patients randomized to receive a 300-mg loading dose of clopidogrel that was initiated ≤15 hours before percutaneous coronary intervention, and patients randomized to receive a 300-mg loading dose of clopidogrel that was initiated ≥15 hours before percutaneous coronary intervention. For pretreatment ≥15 hours versus placebo, P=.18; for pretreatment ≥15 hours versus less than 15 hours, P=.033; and for placebo versus pretreatment less than 15 hours, P=.72. (From Steinhubl SR, Berger PB, Brennan DM, Topol EJ: Optimal timing for the initiation of pre-treatment with 300 mg clopidogrel before percutaneous coronary intervention. J Am Coll Cardiol 2006;47:939-943.)

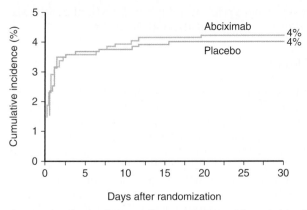

Figure 9-9. The 30-day cumulative incidence of the combined end point of death, myocardial infarction, or urgent-target revascularization in the Intracoronary Stenting and Antithrombotic Regimen-Rapid Early Action for Coronary Treatment (ISAR-REACT) trial. (From Kastrati A, Mehilli J, Schuhlen H, et al: A clinical trial of abciximab in elective percutaneous coronary intervention after pretreatment with clopidogrel. N Engl J Med 2004;350:232-238.)

in addition to aspirin. Patients pretreated with clopidogrel before their PCI experienced a significant reduction in the combined end point of cardiovascular death, recurrent MI, and revascularization (4.5% versus 6.4%; RR=0.70; P=.03) at 30 days.

The Clopidogrel for Reduction of Events During Observation (CREDO) trial was the first placebo-controlled trial designed to address the benefit of clopidogrel pretreatment and long-term 1-year therapy with a clopidogrel in patients undergoing nonurgent PCI.[18] The 28-day end point, which reflected the difference between pretreatment with a 300-mg loading dose compared with no pretreatment and no loading dose, did not demonstrate a significant reduction in the combined end point of death, MI, and urgent target revascularization. However, subsequent analysis found that the timing of pretreatment appeared to influence the clinical benefit of the loading dose, with only those treated more than 15 hours before their PCI achieving a significant reduction in periprocedural ischemic events compared with placebo (Fig. 9-8).[19] The PCI-Clopidogrel as Adjunctive Reperfusion Therapy (PCI-CLARITY) was a prespecified analysis to evaluate the role of clopidogrel pretreatment in STEMI patients.[20] The addition of a 300-mg dose of clopidogrel to thrombolytic therapy in patients with STEMI who underwent PCI a median of 3 days after receiving the study drug was associated with a highly significant reduction in the odds of death, MI, or stroke at 30-days (OR=0.59; 95% CI: 0.43 to 0.81; P=.001).

Although these studies used a 300-mg loading dose, subsequent pharmacodynamic studies found that the maximal antiplatelet effects could be

achieved within 2 hours after a 600-mg loading dose. Clinical data from the ISAR trials support a full clinical benefit of pretreatment within 2 hours of a 600-mg loading dose. Ensuing pharmacodynamic studies have evaluated loading doses up to 900 mg, with conclusions regarding any addition of speed or degree of platelet inhibition compared with 600 mg mixed.

A series of studies started exploring whether the GP IIb/IIIa inhibitors are complementary to the benefit of thienopyridines or if the former can be skipped when adequate pretreatment is given. In the Intracoronary Stenting and Antithrombotic Regimen-Rapid Early Action for Coronary Treatment (ISAR-REACT) study, the addition of abciximab to a 600-mg loading dose more than 2 hours before PCI did not confer any further reduction in the ischemic events (Fig. 9-9).[21] Similarly, in the Intracoronary Stenting and Antithrombotic Regimen: Is Abciximab a Superior Way to Eliminate Elevated Thrombotic Risk in Diabetics (ISAR-SWEET) study, abciximab did not provide any further benefit on top of adequate pretreatment with clopidogrel in diabetic patients.[22] Consistent with the previous findings, patients with small-artery PCI also did not derive any clinical benefit with abciximab if they received a 600-mg clopidogrel loading dose in the Intracoronary Stenting or Angioplasty for Restenosis Reduction in Small Arteries (ISAR-SMART 2) study.[23] However, these studies enrolled only patients with relatively stable coronary artery disease, and the findings should be applied only to similar patient cohorts. Patients presenting with an ACS documented by ST-segment depression or elevated troponin levels were randomized in a similar fashion after a 600-mg loading dose in the ISAR-REACT 2 trial.[24] Contrary to findings of the previous studies, among patients who had elevated troponin levels, further reduction in the relative risk of ischemic events (i.e., combination of

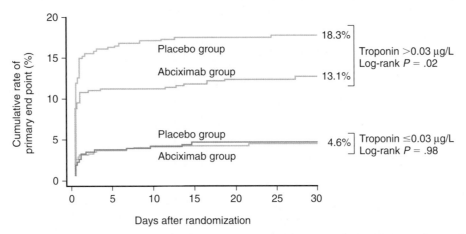

Figure 9-10. Cumulative incidence of death, myocardial infarction, or urgent target revascularization in a subset with or without elevated troponin levels in the Intracoronary Stenting and Antithrombotic Regimen—Rapid Early Action for Coronary Treatment (ISAR-REACT 2) trial. (From Kastrati A, Mehilli J, Neumann FJ, et al: Abciximab in patients with acute coronary syndromes undergoing percutaneous coronary intervention after clopidogrel pretreatment: The ISAR-REACT 2 randomized trial. JAMA 2006;295:1531-1538.)

death, MI, or urgent target revascularization) at 30 days was achieved with abciximab compared with placebo (RR=0.71; 95% CI: 0.54 to 0.95; P=.02) (Fig. 9-10). Consistent with previous findings, patients with no elevation in troponin levels despite having an unstable angina presentation did not benefit from abciximab. A combined analysis of more than 4000 troponin-negative patients from the ISAR trials confirmed the lack of benefit with the addition of abciximab to a 600-mg loading dose of clopidogrel when given more than 2 hours before PCI in this population (Fig. 9-11).

Although dual antiplatelet therapy was embraced in the interventional community for the prevention of stent thrombosis, ticlopidine or clopidogrel was routinely and arbitrarily stopped 2 to 4 weeks after bare-metal stenting. The PCI-CURE analysis evaluated the potential role of prolonged dual antiplatelet therapy up to a mean duration of 8 months after PCI in a subset of patients from the CURE trial. A 21% further reduction between 30 days and the end of

follow-up was identified in the cohort of patients randomized to dual antiplatelet therapy. Likewise, patients enrolled in the CREDO trial and assigned to the 300-mg loading dose were also to continue clopidogrel therapy by protocol out to 1 year, whereas the control arm reverted to aspirin alone after 4 weeks of dual therapy. Overall, the combined benefit of pretreatment and prolonged clopidogrel up to 1 year in CREDO was associated with a 27% (95% CI: 3.9% to 44.4%) relative reduction in the combined primary end point compared with those assigned to routine therapy without pretreatment followed by 4 weeks of dual antiplatelet therapy.[18] Continuation of dual therapy beyond 30 days resulted in further divergence between the two arms, with a 37% reduction in the risk of the combined end point between 29 days and 1 year in the clopidogrel arm compared with the placebo (HR=0.63; 95% CI: 0.4 to 0.98; P=.04) (Fig. 9-12).[25] Collectively, the PCI-CURE and CREDO support the long-term therapy with clopidogrel after PCI to 1 year.

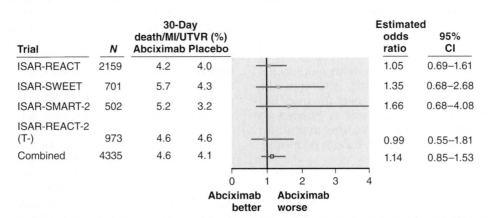

Trial	N	30-Day death/MI/UTVR (%) Abciximab	Placebo		Estimated odds ratio	95% CI
ISAR-REACT	2159	4.2	4.0		1.05	0.69–1.61
ISAR-SWEET	701	5.7	4.3		1.35	0.68–2.68
ISAR-SMART-2	502	5.2	3.2		1.66	0.68–4.08
ISAR-REACT-2 (T-)	973	4.6	4.6		0.99	0.55–1.81
Combined	4335	4.6	4.1		1.14	0.85–1.53

Figure 9-11. A combined analysis of the Intracoronary Stenting and Antithrombotic Regimen—Rapid Early Action for Coronary Treatment (ISAR-REACT), Intracoronary Stenting and Antithrombotic Regimen: Is Abciximab a Superior Way to Eliminate Elevated Thrombotic Risk in Diabetics (ISAR-SWEET), Intracoronary Stenting or Angioplasty for Restenosis Reduction in Small Arteries (ISAR-SMART 2), and the troponin-negative patients in the ISAR-REACT 2 trial. MI, myocardial infarction; (T-), troponin negative; UTVR, urgent target vessel revascularization. (From Hamdalla H, Steinhubl SR: Oral antiplatelet therapy for percutaneous coronary revascularization. Catheter Cardiovasc Interv 2007;69:637-642.)

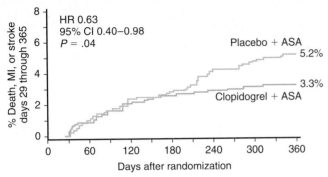

Figure 9-12. Kaplan-Meier estimates of death, myocardial infarction, or stroke from day 29 to 1 year based on randomized treatment assignment in the Clopidogrel for the Reduction of events During Observation (CREDO) trial. (From Steinhubl SR, Topol EJ: Risk reduction with long-term clopidogrel following percutaneous coronary intervention. Eur Heart J 2004;25:2169-2170.)

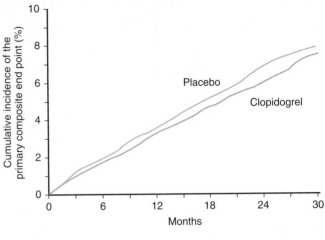

Patients at risk:

Clopidogrel:	7802	7653	7510	7363	5299	2770
Placebo:	7801	7644	7482	7316	5212	2753

Figure 9-13. Cumulative incidence of the combined end point of myocardial infarction, stroke, or cardiovascular death at 30 months in patients randomized to clopidogrel compared with placebo. (From Bhatt DL, Fox KAA, Hacke W, et al: Clopidogrel and aspirin versus aspirin alone for the prevention of atherothrombotic events. N Engl J Med 2006;354:1706-1717.)

With the current use of drug-eluting stents, patients routinely maintain dual antiplatelet therapy for at least 3 to 6 months. However, beyond that point, especially beyond a year, post-PCI therapy remains open for debate. A number of case reports have highlighted that at least some patients treated with drug-eluting stents are at risk for stent thrombosis even beyond 1 year. There is no pathophysiologic basis for assuming that the benefit seen in CURE and CREDO would end at 1 year. The Clopidogrel for High Atherothrombotic Risk and Ischemic Stabilization, Management, and Avoidance (CHARISMA) trial was designed to evaluate long-term treatment with clopidogrel extending beyond 1 year in a wide range of patients with established atherosclerotic disease or multiple risk factors for vascular disease.[26] After randomization, patients were assigned to a 75-mg dose of clopidogrel daily or placebo on top of daily aspirin, and they were followed for a median of 28 months. In the overall population, there was no benefit derived from such a long course of therapy with clopidogrel compared with placebo (6.8% versus 7.3% p 0.22) (Fig. 9-13). However, a prespecified group of symptomatic patients derived a small but significant reduction in the combined end point of cardiovascular death, MI, or stroke with clopidogrel therapy (6.9% versus 7.9% P=.046). Although the CHARISMA trial was designed to answer the question of long-term therapy, more analysis is needed to discern which patients would have the maximum benefit, because such an approach has an economic burden.

Glycoprotein IIb/IIIa Antagonists

Almost 17,000 patients undergoing a PCI have been randomized in placebo-controlled trials in the evaluation of GP IIb/IIIa antagonists (Fig. 9-14). The Evaluation of c7E3 for Prevention of Ischemic Complications (EPIC) trial was the first study and randomized 2099 patients deemed at high risk for thrombotic compli-

cations to abciximab or matching placebo on top of heparin and aspirin.[27] Patients randomized to abciximab derived a 35% (significant) reduction in the combined end point of death, MI, or urgent revascularization at 30 days (12.8 versus 8.3%, P=.008) that was maintained at the 6-month follow-up evaluation (35.1% versus 27.0%; 23% reduction, P=.001) (Fig. 9-15). However, randomization to abciximab was also associated with a significant increase in risk of major bleeding complications compared with placebo (7% versus 14%, P=.001), although as part of the study femoral artery sheaths were left in overnight, and a heparin infusion was also maintained. The management of abciximab-treated patients was better optimized in the 2792 patients randomized in the Evaluation of the PTCA to Improve Long-Term Outcome with Abciximab GP IIb/IIIa Blockade (EPILOG) trial, in which lower-dose, weight-adjusted heparin was used, and femoral sheaths were removed early after the procedure. The results of the EPILOG trial broadened the applicability of the GP IIb/IIIa therapy to include essentially all PCI patients in addition to demonstrating their safety compared with unfractionated heparin alone. By the time the EPILOG was concluded, routine stenting was replacing bailout stenting, and the benefit of routine stenting and the need for a GP IIb/IIIa antagonist in the stented patients were being questioned. Consequently, the Evaluation of Platelet Inhibition in Stenting (EPISTENT) trial was launched, and almost 2400 patients scheduled for a PCI were randomized to abciximab or matching placebo and stent or balloon angioplasty. The study concluded that the benefit of abciximab was independent of stenting

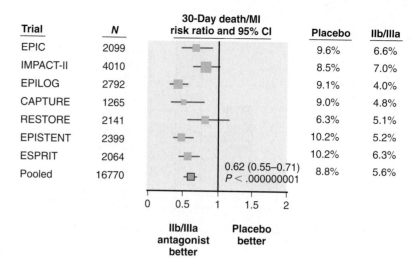

Trial	N	30-Day death/MI risk ratio and 95% CI	Placebo	IIb/IIIa
EPIC	2099		9.6%	6.6%
IMPACT-II	4010		8.5%	7.0%
EPILOG	2792		9.1%	4.0%
CAPTURE	1265		9.0%	4.8%
RESTORE	2141		6.3%	5.1%
EPISTENT	2399		10.2%	5.2%
ESPRIT	2064		10.2%	6.3%
Pooled	16770	0.62 (0.55–0.71) $P < .000000001$	8.8%	5.6%

IIb/IIIa antagonist better   Placebo better

Figure 9-14. A meta-analysis of the glycoprotein IIb/IIIa trials in the patients undergoing revascularization.

and that they are complementary to each other. The incidence of the composite end point of death, MI, or urgent revascularization at 30 days was lower in the group receiving stenting with abciximab (5.3%; OR=0.48; 95% CI: 0.33 to 0.69; P<.001) and the group receiving balloon angioplasty and abciximab (6.9%; OR=0.63; 95% CI: 0.45 to 0.88; P=0.007) compared with those receiving stenting with heparin alone (Fig. 9-16). Overall, the EPIC, EPILOG, and EPISTENT trials showed a robust benefit when using abciximab in PCI that was independent of the device used, without an increased risk of bleeding when heparin dosing is controlled tightly.

As the chimeric antibody abciximab was being clinically evaluated there was early concern regarding its long biologic half-life and potential antigenic effect. This led to the development of the small molecular GP IIb/IIIa inhibitors that are more selective and have a shorter half-life: eptifibatide and tirofiban. The Integrilin to Minimize Platelet aggregation and Coronary Thrombosis-II (IMPACT-II) was the

first trial to evaluate eptifibatide in PCI. The dose that was being evaluated was based on early studies using blood samples collected in sodium citrate, which led to overestimation of platelet aggregation inhibition. This was mirrored with a small, nonsignificant reduction in the ischemic events at 30 days and the 6-month follow-up evaluation. The Enhanced Suppression of the Platelet IIb/IIIa Receptor with Integrilin Therapy (ESPRIT) was designed using a much greater dosing regimen of eptifibatide. Patients randomized to the eptifibatide experienced a 38% reduction in the risk of death, MI, or urgent target vessel revascularization at 30 days (6.4% versus 10.2%, P=.0014). Although the risk of major bleeding was low in the eptifibatide group, it was slightly higher than for heparin alone and depended on the level of anticoagulation achieved.

A similar small GP IIb/IIIa inhibitor, tirofiban, was evaluated in the setting of PCI in the Randomized Efficacy Study of Tirofiban for Outcomes and Restenosis (RESTORE). Patients experienced a reduction in

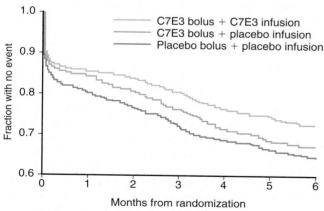

Figure 9-15. Kaplan-Meier survival curves at the 6-month follow-up for patients randomized to abciximab in the Evaluation of c7E3 for Prevention of Ischemic Complications (EPIC) trial. (From Topol EJ, Califf RM, Weisman HF, et al: Randomised trial of coronary intervention with antibody against platelet IIb/IIIa integrin for reduction of clinical restenosis: Results at six months. The EPIC Investigators. Lancet 1994;343:881-886.)

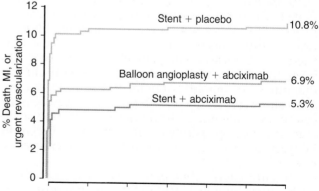

Figure 9-16. Cumulative incidence of the combined end point of myocardial infarction (MI), death, or urgent revascularization for stent with and without abciximab versus balloon angioplasty with abciximab. (From The EPISTENT Investigators: Randomised placebo-controlled and balloon-angioplasty-controlled trial to assess safety of coronary stenting with use of platelet glycoprotein-IIb/IIIa blockade. Evaluation of Platelet IIb/IIIa Inhibitor for Stenting. Lancet 1998;352:87-92.)

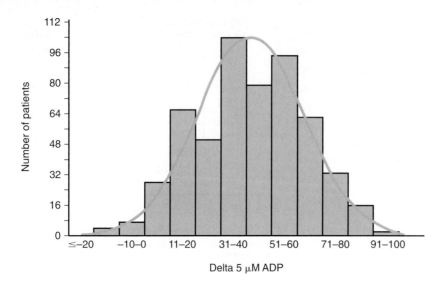

Figure 9-17. Distribution of changes in 5 μmol of adenosine diphosphate (ADP)–induced platelet aggregation in 544 patients after receiving clopidogrel therapy. Negative changes in aggregation values represent aggregation values after the administration of clopidogrel that were higher than the baseline readings. (From Serebruany VL, Steinhubl SR, Berger PB, et al: Variability in platelet responsiveness to clopidogrel among 544 individuals. J Am Coll Cardiol 2005;45:246-251.)

the composite end point of major cardiac events within the first 48 hours; however, at 30-day follow-up, the benefit was lost. Tirofiban was subsequently compared with abciximab in The Do Tirofiban and ReoPro Give Similar Efficacy Trial (TARGET).[28] This was the only trial to compare two different inhibitors of the GP IIb/IIIa receptor directly. Patients randomized to abciximab were found to experience a significantly lower incidence of the 30-day end point of major cardiac events compared with tirofiban (6.0% versus 7.6%; P=.038). The RESTORE and TARGET trials did not support a role for tirofiban at the doses studied in the setting of PCI.

VARIABILITY IN RESPONSE TO ANTIPLATELET THERAPIES

Although the concept of interindividual variability in response to aspirin was recognized as early as 1966, this topic has become of much greater interest to clinicians only recently. The terms *resistance* or *non-responsiveness,* suggesting a dichotomous response, have been used to describe a wide variety of laboratory or clinical entities. There are substantial limitations to this concept. The foremost challenge is that there is no measure of platelet function that has been convincingly shown to correlate with clinical outcomes—thrombotic or hemorrhagic—or evidence that altering therapy based on that measurement improves outcomes. Nonetheless, several small studies have successfully demonstrated a correlation between measured platelet function and thrombotic events.[29]

All antiplatelet therapies have been associated with interindividual variability in response. For aspirin, one of the first studies to evaluate clinical outcome as a measure of platelet responsiveness was a follow-up of 180 aspirin-treated patients with stroke, among whom 33% where described as aspirin nonresponders.[30] A number of studies have followed, with most finding a relationship between platelet function and clinical outcomes. One of the latest,

in patients undergoing PCI, found that patients characterized as aspirin resistant using the VerifyNow device had almost a threefold incidence of post-PCI myonecrosis.[31]

Similar results have been found with clopidogrel. In a heterogeneous group of 544 patients treated with clopidogrel, platelet function studies revealed a bell-shaped normal distribution in which 4.2% of patients were more than two standard deviations above the mean, and 4.8% of patients were at least two standard deviations below the mean, creating categories of hyperresponders and hyporesponders (Fig. 9-17).[32] Although most investigators have found that this variability in response to clopidogrel is associated with the future risk of thrombotic events, the results are inconsistent across all studies.

Because GP IIb/IIIa antagonists are designed to specifically inhibit just one aspect of platelet function, aggregation, and they are dosed to achieve a target level of inhibition, there are more data supporting the importance of achieving a specific level of inhibition with these agents than for aspirin or the thieno-pyridines. Several trials have investigated the role of platelet function monitoring in patients treated with GP IIb/IIIa antagonists. The largest of these, the Assessing Ultegra (AU, or GOLD) trial found that achieving more than 90% inhibition as measured by the VerifyNow device was independently and significantly associated with improved outcomes for patients undergoing a PCI.[33] Similar results in smaller trials established a higher risk of stent thrombosis in patients who have higher platelet reactivity despite clopidogrel therapy.[34,35] Because no studies have yet proved the clinical applicability of altering therapy based on the measured platelet function in patients receiving a GP IIb/IIIa antagonist, variability in response is not routinely measured.

CONCLUSIONS

Antiplatelet therapy is the cornerstone of management of patients with ACS and those undergoing percutaneous revascularization. However, there is much that needs to be learned to optimize this therapy for the individual patient. Over the past 3 decades, antiplatelet therapy has evolved from aspirin monotherapy to triple therapy with GP IIb/IIIa receptor blockers and thienopyridines in addition to aspirin. The importance of upstream inhibition of platelet activation before coronary instrumentation has changed the procedural pharmacologic approach. The benefit of dual antiplatelet therapy regimens has extended beyond the periprocedural period to provide further incremental benefit out to 1 year after the procedure, although longer-term benefit is less well established. The surgical bleeding complications associated with such aggressive regimens has prohibited its wide acceptance and limited the clinical benefit. Ongoing studies to evaluate novel antiplatelet medications that may overcome most of the obstacles that faced the thienopyridines are unending. In recent years, more interest in patients' variability in response to antiplatelet therapy has emerged. Tailoring therapy to individual patients and assessing their inherent risk for ischemic complications is a more appealing approach in managing patients, especially with the growing concern about stent thrombosis in drug-eluting stents.

REFERENCES

1. Gawaz M, Langer H, May AE: Platelets in inflammation and atherogenesis. J Clin Invest 2005;115:3378-3384.
2. Michelson AD: Platelet function testing in cardiovascular diseases. Circulation 2004;110:e489-493.
3. Patrono C, Garcia Rodriguez LA, Landolfi R, Baigent C: Low-dose aspirin for the prevention of atherothrombosis. N Engl J Med 2005;353:2373-2383.
4. ISIS-2 Collaborative Group: Randomised trial of intravenous streptokinase, oral aspirin, both, or neither among 17,187 cases of suspected acute myocardial infarction: ISIS-2. ISIS-2 (Second International Study of Infarct Survival) Collaborative Group. Lancet 1988;2:349-360.
5. Ridker PM, Cook NR, Lee IM, et al: A randomized trial of low-dose aspirin in the primary prevention of cardiovascular disease in women. N Engl J Med 2005;352:1293-1304.
6. Savi PPD, Herbert JMPD: Clopidogrel and ticlopidine: P2Y12 adenosine diphosphate-receptor antagonists for the prevention of atherothrombosis. Semin Thromb Hemost 2005: 174-183.
7. The Clopidogrel in Unstable Angina to Prevent Recurrent Events Trial. I. Effects of clopidogrel in addition to aspirin in patients with acute coronary syndromes without ST-segment elevation. N Engl J Med 2001;345:494-502.
8. Wiviott SD, Antman EM, Winters KJ, et al, for the Randomized Comparison of Prasugrel (CS-747, LY640315), a Novel Thienopyridine P2Y12 Antagonist, with Clopidogrel in Percutaneous Coronary Intervention: Results of the Joint Utilization of Medications to Block Platelets Optimally (JUMBO)-TIMI 26 Trial. Circulation 2005;111:3366-3373.
9. Quinn MJ, Byzova TV, Qin J, et al: Integrin alphaIIbbeta3 and its antagonism. Arterioscler Thromb Vasc Biol 2003;23: 945-952.
10. Boersma E, Harrington RA, Moliterno DJ, et al: Platelet glycoprotein IIb/IIIa inhibitors in acute coronary syndromes: A meta-analysis of all major randomised clinical trials. Lancet 2002;359:189-198.
11. Roffi M, Chew DP, Mukherjee D, et al: Platelet glycoprotein IIb/IIIa inhibition in acute coronary syndromes. Gradient of benefit related to the revascularization strategy. Eur Heart J 2002;23:1441-1448.
12. Roffi M, Chew DP, Mukherjee D, et al: Platelet glycoprotein IIb/IIIa inhibitors reduce mortality in diabetic patients with non-ST-segment-elevation acute coronary syndromes. Circulation 2001;104:2767-2771.
13. Lincoff AM, Califf RM, Van de Werf F, et al: Mortality at 1 year with combination platelet glycoprotein IIb/IIIa inhibition and reduced-dose fibrinolytic therapy vs conventional fibrinolytic therapy for acute myocardial infarction: GUSTO V randomized trial. JAMA 2002;288:2130-2135.
14. Ellis SG, Armstrong P, Betriu A, et al: Facilitated percutaneous coronary intervention versus primary percutaneous coronary intervention: Design and rationale of the Facilitated Intervention with Enhanced Reperfusion Speed to Stop Events (FINESSE) trial. Am Heart J 2004;147:E16.
15. Douglas JS Jr, Holmes DR Jr, Kereiakes DJ, et al, for the Cilostazol for Restenosis Trial: Coronary stent restenosis in patients treated with cilostazol. Circulation 2005;112:2826-2832.
16. Greenbaum AB, Grines CL, Bittl JA, et al: Initial experience with an intravenous P2Y12 platelet receptor antagonist in patients undergoing percutaneous coronary intervention: Results from a 2-part, phase II, multicenter, randomized, placebo- and active-controlled trial. Am Heart J 2006;151:689.
17. Husted S, Emanuelsson H, Heptinstall S, et al: Pharmacodynamics, pharmacokinetics, and safety of the oral reversible P2Y12 antagonist AZD6140 with aspirin in patients with atherosclerosis: A double-blind comparison to clopidogrel with aspirin. Eur Heart J 2006;27:1038-1047.
17a. Barnathan ES, Schwartz JS, Taylor L, et al: Aspirin and dipyridamole in the prevention of acute coronary thrombosis complicating coronary angioplasty. Circulation 1987;76:125-134.
18. Steinhubl SR, Berger PB, Mann JT III, et al, for the CREDO Investigators: Early and sustained dual oral antiplatelet therapy following percutaneous coronary intervention. A randomized controlled trial. JAMA 2002;288:2411-2420.
19. Steinhubl SR, Berger PB, Brennan DM, Topol EJ: Optimal timing for the initiation of pre-treatment with 300 mg clopidogrel before percutaneous coronary intervention. J Am Coll Cardiol 2006;47:939-943.
20. Sabatine MS, Cannon CP, Gibson CM, et al: Effect of clopidogrel pretreatment before percutaneous coronary intervention in patients with ST-elevation myocardial infarction treated with fibrinolytics: The PCI-CLARITY study. JAMA 2005;294: 1224-1232.
21. Kastrati A, Mehilli J, Schuhlen H, et al: A clinical trial of abciximab in elective percutaneous coronary intervention after pretreatment with clopidogrel. N Engl J Med 2004;350:232-238.
22. Mehilli J, Kastrati A, Schuhlen H, et al: Randomized clinical trial of abciximab in diabetic patients undergoing elective percutaneous coronary interventions after treatment with a high loading dose of clopidogrel. Circulation 2004;110: 3627-3635.
23. Hausleiter J, Kastrati A, Mehilli J, et al: A randomized trial comparing phosphorylcholine-coated stenting with balloon angioplasty as well as abciximab with placebo for restenosis reduction in small coronary arteries. J Intern Med 2004;256: 388-397.
24. Kastrati A, Mehilli J, Neumann FJ, et al: Abciximab in patients with acute coronary syndromes undergoing percutaneous coronary intervention after clopidogrel pretreatment: The ISAR-REACT 2 randomized trial. JAMA 2006;295:1531-1538.
25. Steinhubl SR, Topol EJ: Risk reduction with long-term clopidogrel following percutaneous coronary intervention. Eur Heart J 2004;25:2169-2170; author reply 2170-2171.
26. Bhatt DL, Fox KAA, Hacke W, et al: Clopidogrel and aspirin versus aspirin alone for the prevention of atherothrombotic events. N Engl J Med 2006;354:1706-1717.
27. The EPIC Investigation: Use of a monoclonal antibody directed against the platelet glycoprotein IIb/IIIa receptor in high-risk coronary angioplasty. N Engl J Med 1994;330:956-961.
28. Mukherjee D, Topol EJ, Bertrand ME, et al: Mortality at 1 year for the direct comparison of tirofiban and abciximab during percutaneous coronary revascularization: Do tirofiban and ReoPro give similar efficacy outcomes at trial 1-year follow-up. Eur Heart J 2005;26:2524-2528.
29. Gum P, Kottke-Marchant K, Welsh PA, et al: A prospective, blinded determination of the natural history of aspirin resis-

tance among stable patients with cardiovascular disease. J Am Coll Cardiol 2003;41:961-965.

30. Grotemeyer KH, Scharafinski HW, Husstedt LW: Two-year follow-up of aspirin responder and aspirin non-responder. A pilot study including 180 post-stroke patients. Thromb Res 1993;71:397-403.

31. Chen WH, Lee PY, Ng W, et al: Aspirin resistance is associated with a high incidence of myonecrosis after non-urgent percutaneous coronary intervention despite clopidogrel pretreatment. J Am Coll Cardiol 2004;43:1122-1126.

32. Serebruany VL, Steinhubl SR, Berger PB, et al: Variability in platelet responsiveness to clopidogrel among 544 individuals. J Am Coll Cardiol 2005;45:246-251.

33. Steinhubl SR, Talley JD, Braden AJ, et al: Point-of-care measured platelet inhibition correlates with a reduced risk of an adverse cardiac event after percutaneous coronary intervention: Results of the GOLD (AU—Assessing Ultegra) multicenter study. Circulation 2001;103:2572-2578.

34. Gurbel PA, Bliden KP, Samara W, et al: Clopidogrel effect on platelet reactivity in patients with stent thrombosis: Results of the CREST Study. J Am Coll Cardiol 2005;46:1827-1832.

35. Muller I, Besta F, Schulz C, et al: Prevalence of clopidogrel non-responders among patients with stable angina pectoris scheduled for elective coronary stent placement. Thromb Haemost 2003;89:783-787.

CHAPTER

10 Anticoagulation in Percutaneous Coronary Intervention

Derek P. Chew

KEY POINTS

- Although the impact of ischemic events on late mortality is well appreciated, a robust link between bleeding events and late mortality is emerging. These factors bear careful consideration when weighing efficacy and safety considerations among antithrombotic therapies.
- Platelets and coagulation play a synergistic role in the generation of thrombus. Improved antithrombin approaches reduce the dependence on antiplatelet therapy for achieving suppression of ischemic events.
- The activated clotting time (ACT) provides semiquantitative information for guiding heparin therapy in the absence of glycoprotein IIb/IIIa inhibition. The ACT is of limited value in guiding heparin therapy in the context of concurrent glycoprotein IIb/IIIa inhibition or when enoxaparin or bivalirudin is used.
- Although unfractionated heparin remains the main anticoagulant used in PCI worldwide, evidence demonstrates

suboptimal suppression of ischemic events among high-risk patients.
- Clinical trial evidence suggests that enoxaparin can be extended from the up-stream therapy for acute coronary syndrome (ACS) to the anticoagulant used during percutaneous coronary intervention (PCI) without increases in ischemic complications. Small increases in bleeding events are seen among ACS patients undergoing PCI, but not among elective patients.
- Bivalirudin (with provisional glycoprotein IIb/IIIa inhibition) provides comparable suppression of ischemic events while reducing bleeding events compared with heparin and planned glycoprotein IIb/IIIa inhibition. Similar benefits are observed when this agent is used in the up-stream management of ACS patients undergoing invasive management.

Pharmacologic strategies for the prevention of periprocedural ischemic complications during percutaneous coronary intervention (PCI) continue to evolve, with an expanding array of antithrombin therapies now available to the interventional cardiologist. Later clinical trial evidence also supports novel direct and indirect inhibitors of thrombin across the diverse array of patients undergoing PCI. The data have highlighted the importance of suppressing ischemic and bleeding adverse outcomes within modern interventional cardiology practice. Some of the newer agents are associated with greater ease of use, reduced need for monitoring, and less bleeding when used in conjunction with more robust platelet inhibition. This chapter discusses the modern biology of coagulation and its key effector, thrombin; the monitoring of anticoagulants in the catheter laboratory; and the clinical trial evidence supporting the use of indirect and direct inhibitors of the thrombin as anticoagulants in PCI.

THE BIOLOGY OF COAGULATION: THERAPEUTIC TARGETS

Conceptualization of the coagulation cascade continues to evolve, with an increasing appreciation of the complex interplay between the coagulative proteins, platelets, and cellular phospholipid membranes. Although the subsequent discussion will focus on the coagulative factors that serve as targets of modern antithrombotic regimens, additional effects on platelet-mediated thrombosis and vascular tissue function should not be ignored.

The Central Role of Thrombin

Disruption of endothelial integrity and expression of pro-thrombotic molecules such as tissue factor leads to the activation of the soluble coagulative proteins (Fig. 10-1). This amplifying cascade converges on the

165

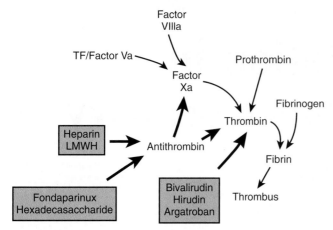

Figure 10-1. The schematic representation of the relationship between coagulation and arterial thrombosis highlights specific targets for therapy.

generation of activated factor X (FXa) and the pro-thrombinase complex, which leads to the conversion of thrombin from its parent molecule, prothrombin. Thrombin generation leads to multiple effects influencing the formation of thrombosis.[1] Specifically, thrombin catalyses the conversion of fibrin from fibrinogen, enabling clot formation while also activating factors V, VIII, and X and thereby promoting its own generation. Through direct effects on the protease activated receptor (PAR)-1, thrombin promotes platelet activation, leading to the expression of CD40 ligand, P-selectin, and the glycoprotein IIb/IIIa receptor, as well as the secretion of vasoactive agents, including adenosine diphosphate, serotonin, and thromboxane A$_2$. Direct effects of thrombin on endothelial cells and smooth muscle cells results in the expression of adhesion molecules, enabling plate-let and leukocyte attachment, whereas its effect on endothelial membrane permeability contributes to the transmigration of the cellular and cytokine-mediated inflammatory response within the vascular wall. Although thrombin promotes vasodilation in the intact endothelium, it contributes to vasoconstriction where the endothelium is damaged or denuded. Thrombin also appears to promote fibroblast cytokine production, and it is mitogenic (Fig. 10-2).[2]

However, thrombin has a short circulating half-life, and in the context of a normal endothelial barrier the effects of thrombin are tightly controlled by a negative-feedback mechanism. Antithrombin is a single-chain plasma glycoprotein produced by the liver. As an inhibitor of coagulation, this molecule has the ability to bind to thrombin, factor Xa, and factor IXa in equimolar concentrations. Antithrombin's action is increased more than 1000-fold by binding of pentasaccharide chains containing heparins. The pentasaccharide sequence enables the binding of heparins to antithrombin and augments the binding affinity for thrombin and the other clotting factors. Antithrombin is also activated by the glycosaminoglycan heparin sulfate, which is found on the surface of endothelial cells. Other pathways for the inhibition of thrombin exist. These include the binding of thrombin to thrombomodulin and protein C, together with protein S. This inactivates the upstream coagulation proteins, factors Va and VIIIa, and promotes the release of tissue plasminogen activator.

Thrombin plays a central effector role in the vascular response to balloon and stent-induced vascular injury and remains an important therapeutic target for the prevention of ischemic complications during PCI. A schematic of the structure of the thrombin molecule is presented in Figure 10-3. Separate

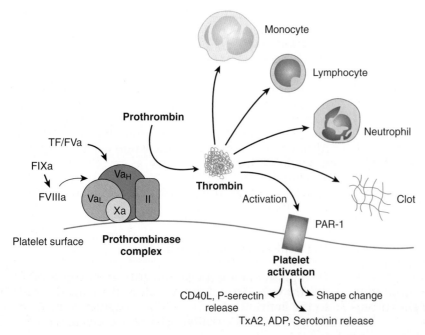

Figure 10-2. The central role of thrombin in thrombosis and inflammation. PAR-1, protease-activating receptor-1; TF, tissue factor.

Table 10-1. Clinical End Point Definitions of Bleeding and Ischemia Used in Clinical Trials of Antithrombotic Agents in Percutaneous Coronary Intervention

End Point	Definition
Myocardial infarction (after PCI)	CK-MB elevation >3 times the upper limit of normal or the development of new Q waves. If CK-MB is unavailable, total CK may be used.
Myocardial infarction (after CABG)	CK-MB elevation >5 times the upper limit of normal and the development of new Q waves, or CK-MB elevation >10 times the upper limit of normal without new Q waves. If CK-MB is unavailable, total CK may be used.
Myocardial infarction (not periprocedural)	CK-MB elevation >2 times the upper limit of normal or the development of new Q waves. If CK-MB is unavailable, total CK may be used.
TIMI major bleeding	Intracerebral hemorrhage, or any bleeding associated with a >5 g/dL fall in hemoglobin or a 15% absolute decrease in hematocrit.*
TIMI minor bleeding	Any bleeding event associated with a >3 g/dL fall in hemoglobin or a 10% absolute decline in hematocrit, or a >4 g/dL fall in hemoglobin or a 12% absolute decline in hematocrit in the absence of overt bleeding.*
Major bleeding (REPLACE-2 definition)	Intracerebral hemorrhage or any bleeding event associated with a >3 g/dL fall in hemoglobin, or a >4 g/dL fall in hemoglobin in the absence of overt bleeding, or any red cell transfusion of 2 or more units*
GUSTO severe or life-threatening bleeding	Intracerebral hemorrhage or bleeding the causes hemodynamic compromise or requires intervention
GUSTO minor bleeding	Bleeding that requires transfusion but does not case hemodynamic compromise

*All calculations of falls in hemoglobin are adjusted for any transfusion by the Landefeld index.
CABG, coronary artery bypass grafting; CK-MB, creatine kinase MB fraction; GUSTO, Global Use of Strategies to Open Occluded Arteries in Acute Coronary Syndromes trial; PCI, percutaneous coronary intervention; REPLACE-2, Randomized Evaluation in PCI Linking Angiomax to reduced Clinical Events 2; TIMI, Thrombolysis in Myocardial Infarction trial.

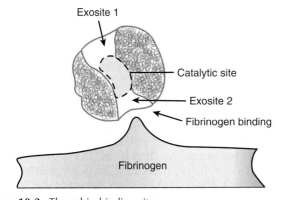

Figure 10-3. Thrombin binding sites.

substrate recognition sites are involved in the binding of heparin, fibrinogen, and thrombomodulin, and the catalytic site is responsible for the serine protease activity and is blocked by the direct thrombin inhibitors.[3]

Adverse Events after Percutaneous Coronary Intervention

Improvements in interventional techniques and refinements in antithrombotic therapies have led to a decline in the incidence of ischemic complications after PCI. Further refinement of antithrombotic strategies can be considered a two-edged sword, with improved prevention of ischemic complications potentially leading to an increase in bleeding complications (Table 10-1). Although the relationship between periprocedural myocardial infarction (MI)

has been widely debated, several studies using data from large-scale clinical trials demonstrate an excess risk of mortality with creatine kinase MB fraction (CK-MB) elevations of greater than three times the upper limit of normal. However, other studies have observed an excess in mortality only at higher degrees of myonecrosis, such as more than five times the upper limit of normal or when there is the development of Q waves. In an analysis of patients enrolled in the Randomized Evaluation in PCI Linking Angiomax to reduced Clinical Events 2 (REPLACE-2) study, a CK-MB elevation greater than or equal to three times the upper limit of normal was associated with a 3.5-fold excess risk of mortality at 12 months and accounted for 13.2% of all mortality seen by 12 months (Fig. 10-4).[4] This forms the threshold definition for periprocedural (within 48 hours) MI within many PCI trials of adjunctive pharmacotherapy. In contrast, weighing the clinical significance of bleeding events reductions in hemoglobin has been less robustly examined. Factors contributing to this uncertainty include a nonstandardized approach to the recognition and reporting of clinical events in clinical trials and the lack of routine assessment of blood loss after PCI. Nevertheless, several studies demonstrate a substantial increase in early and late mortality associated with Thrombolysis In Myocardial Infarction (TIMI) major and minor bleeding after PCI. In an analysis by Kinnaird and colleagues examining 10,974 patients over a 10-year period, major bleeding events were associated with an approximately 10-fold excess in mortality and an approximately threefold excess in non-Q-wave MI.[5] Urgent revascularization and Q-wave MI were also increased. In the analysis of REPLACE-2, TIMI minor or greater bleeding accounted for 3.9% of all the mortality

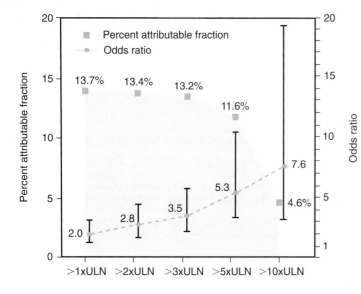

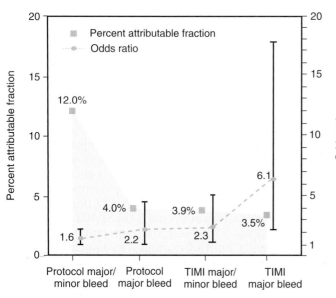

Figure 10-4. Relationships among ischemic events, bleeding events, and late mortality.

observed with a 2.3-fold relative risk, whereas a bleeding event meeting the TIMI major criteria was associated with a 6.1-fold excess mortality risk (see Fig. 10-4).

These observations raise the question of how to weigh bleeding and ischemia relative to each other. From a statistical perspective, combining these end points may increase the likelihood of observing no difference between therapies, and therefore assessment of noninferiority may be better conducted on ischemic and bleeding end points separately. However, from a clinical perspective, bleeding and ischemic events are associated with substantial adverse outcomes and the combined consideration remains a clinical imperative.

Monitoring of Anticoagulation

Various assays, including the activated clotting time (ACT), ecarin clotting time (ECT), and Factor Xa levels, have been used to monitor the therapeutic effect of anticoagulants during PCI. However, the correlation between the levels achieved with these assays with the various agents and clinical events have been studied only retrospectively. The relationship between the assay level achieved and clinical events is also influenced by concomitant antiplatelet therapy. In the context of unfractionated heparin therapy, increasing levels of ACT are associated with a modest reduction in periprocedural ischemic events, but a moderate excess in bleeding events.[6] In contrast, when heparin is given with abciximab, ischemic events are lower, with little further reduction in events at higher ACT levels but a substantial increase in bleeding events (Fig. 10-5).

The ACT assay is not as useful for monitoring the efficacy of enoxaparin and the other low-molecular-weight heparins (LMWHs), with lesser degrees of prolongation in this assay observed.[7] Traditional laboratory-based factor Xa assays also remain impractical for catheter laboratory use. The ENOX assay (Rapidpoint) is a whole-blood, point-of-care assay that correlates with laboratory enoxaparin-induced anti-Xa levels.[8] The Evaluating Enoxaparin Clotting times (ELECT) study explored the relationship between the ENOX assay results and clinical outcomes among 445 patients receiving subcutaneous or intravenous enoxaparin before PCI. There was a nonsignificant and nonlinear association between the ENOX times and ischemic complications, whereas bleeding events increased with greater ENOX times. ENOX times of between 250 and 450 seconds (correlating with anti-FXa levels of between 0.8 and 1.8 IU/mL) for intraprocedural anticoagulation and levels of less than 200 to 250 seconds for sheath removal when enoxaparin is used have been recommended.

In contradistinction to both heparin and LMWH, bivalirudin is generally associated with greater prolongation of ACT. This effect appears to occur in a dose-dependent manner, although no gradient of benefit with respect to ischemic or bleeding events has been observed across the range of ACT values recorded at the doses studied within clinical trials.[9] Despite the higher ACT levels, lower rates of bleeding have been consistently observed, potentially highlighting the limited value of ACT in predicting clinical events with this agent. The ACT provides qualitative but not quantitative information about bivalirudin and is of value only in determining if this agent was effectively administered. As a possible clinical alternative, the monitoring of these agents with the ECT may be more appropriate. Measurements based on this test appear to better correlate with plasma bivalirudin and hirudin levels.[10] Whether levels based on this assay evolve to recommended targets for therapy remains to be established.

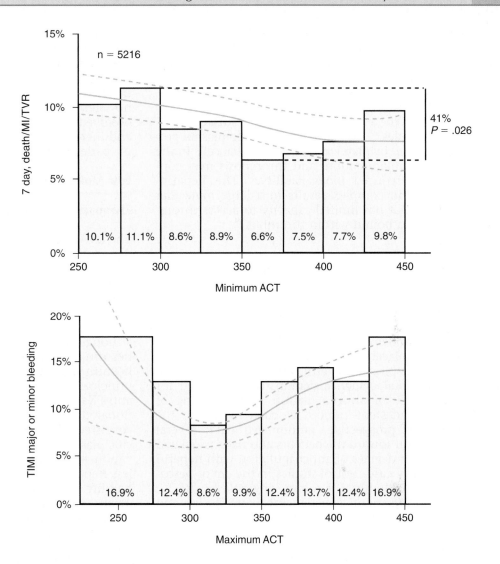

Figure 10-5. Relationship between activated clotting time (ACT) and outcome with heparin.

Unfractionated Heparin

Heparin Pharmacology

Unfractionated heparin is a heterogeneous group of glycosaminoglycans of various lengths (5000 to 30,000 daltons; mean, 15,000 daltons) that exhibits a high-affinity for antithrombin. This binding augments antithrombin's enzymatic inactivation of thrombin, factor Xa, and factor IXa, with its effects on thrombin being the most pronounced.[11] Given heparin's reliance on antithrombin for a therapeutic effect, it is considered as an indirect antithrombin. The antithrombin effect of heparin requires the simultaneous binding of heparin, antithrombin, and thrombin. Consequently, molecules smaller than 18 saccharides lack sufficient length to simultaneously span antithrombin and thrombin and do not exhibit antithrombin activity. These smaller molecules account for up to two thirds of unfractionated heparin preparations. Thrombin inactivation by heparin also oc-curs by heparin-cofactor II, an enzyme with specific activity for thrombin, but it requires much higher heparin levels than the heparin-antithrombin

pathway. However, the anti-factor Xa effects of heparin do not depend on simultaneous binding of antithrombin and factor Xa, and antithrombin effects therefore are observed across a wider range of saccharide chain lengths.

Pharmacokinetic heterogeneity is also observed, because larger heparin molecules are cleared more rapidly, and attenuation of heparin's antithrombin effect is faster relative to its anti-factor Xa effect. The activated partial thromboplastin time (aPTT) and in vivo anticoagulant effect have an imperfect correlation. The elimination of unfractionated heparin is initially through rapid but saturable metabolism within endothelial cells and macrophages (zero-order kinetics), followed by slower renal clearance (first-order kinetics). The plasma half-life depends on the dose administered and is approximately 1 hour at doses of 100 IU/kg. In the context of excessive dosing or perforation/excessive bleeding, unfractionated heparin can be reversed by the administration of protamine. However, the clinical efficacy safety and efficacy of this strategy is not well established.

Increasingly, the limitations of heparin have been appreciated. These limitations include the activation of platelets; a dependence on antithrombin levels; nonspecific binding to plasma protein; an inability to inhibit clot bound thrombin; and direct binding to platelet factor-4 contributing to heparin induced thrombocytopenia in 1% to 3% of treated patients. Platelet activation by heparin is evidenced by an increase in the expression of platelet surface adhesion molecules.[12] Nonspecific binding to plasma proteins secreted by platelets and endothelial cells in the setting of inflammation, and thrombosis may contribute to reduced bioavailability.[13] The heparin-antithrombin complex results in a large molecular structure that has limited capacity to access thrombin and FXa bound within thrombus.[14]

Clinical Data for Unfractionated Heparin

Worldwide, unfractionated heparin remains the mainstay anticoagulant for patients undergoing PCI. Despite this fact, there are no prospective, randomized data to demonstrate the relative efficacy of this agent over placebo, and current dosing recommendations are empirical. Nevertheless, clinical experience and anecdotal evidence demonstrate the need for some degree of anticoagulation in the setting of balloon- and stent-induced vascular injury. In the absence of prospective, randomized data, several studies point toward the benefits and risks associated with greater degrees of anticoagulation with heparin in PCI. Early case-control studies in the era of percutaneous transluminal coronary angioplasty (PTCA) suggest that patients experiencing acute closure and death or urgent revascularization had lower ACT levels than those not experiencing these complications.[15,16] Similarly, among 403 patients randomized to heparin (5000 units IV or 20,000 units IV) before balloon angioplasty, those receiving the higher dose experienced a nonsignificant reduction in the rate of death, MI, acute vessel closure, and repeat intervention (8.0% versus 12.5%, P = NS) but an increased rate of bleeding complications (20% versus 6%, P < .001).[17] Weight-adjusted dosing has been studied as a strategy to reduce the variability in dose response. In a 400-patient, randomized trial assessing weight-adjusted dosing compared with higher fixed dosing, the weight-adjusted strategy was not associated with superior efficacy or safety, although earlier sheath removal was afforded.

Nevertheless, pooled analysis of heparin-only–treated patients enrolled in several randomized clinical trials suggests that there is a gradient of benefit associated with increasing degrees of anticoagulation, with commensurate risk of bleeding events. This analysis suggests that ACT levels in excess of 350 seconds are associated with fewer ischemic events, although bleeding rates also increase at these levels.[6] Such levels of anticoagulation are not required when concomitant glycoprotein (GP) IIb/IIIa inhibition is used, and the relevance of these data in the context of pretreatment with thienopyridines is not known.[18] These observations have also been difficult to demonstrate in smaller studies in which the initial heparin doses, and therefore the ACT levels, achieved were lower.[19] In contrast, the available data do not support the use of prolonged heparin infusions after PCI for the prevention of subacute ischemic events, in which no significant reduction in ischemic events is observed, but there is a clear excess in bleeding events and increased length of stay.[20] This is especially true for patients receiving GP IIb/IIIa inhibition.

Low-Molecular-Weight Heparin

Pharmacology

The LMWHs are produced by chemical or enzymatic depolymerization of unfractionated heparin, resulting in heparin fragments with a mean molecular weight that is approximately 30% of most unfractionated heparin preparations. However, the molecular size of the heparin molecules still varies, and anticoagulant characteristics remain heterogeneous, although more predictable, compared with those of heparin.[21] Although between 25% and 50% of the heparin molecules retain antithrombin activity, the principal effect of the LMWHs is the inhibition of anti-FXa by antithrombin. Compared with unfractionated heparin, the LMWHs demonstrate a more consistent dose response as a result of less nonspecific plasma protein binding, as well less platelet activation and platelet factor-4 interactions leading to less heparin-induced thrombocytopenia. The longer half-life of this agent provides a more convenient means of prolonged anticoagulation before PCI among patients with acute coronary syndrome (ACS). Clearance is achieved by renal excretion, and the biologic half-life is increased in those with renal failure (Table 10-2).

Several small studies have explored the various dosing strategies for the use of enoxaparin in PCI. Adequate levels of anti-FXa were observed in patients 2 to 8 hours after subcutaneous dosing of enoxaparin (1 mg/kg bid), and in those receiving an additional 0.3-mg/kg intravenous dose 8 to 12 hours after subcutaneous dosing at 1.0 mg/kg.[22] Other investigators have suggested that doses as low as 0.5 mg/kg of intravenous enoxaparin may be safe and efficacious, while enabling easier sheath management, although a fourth of the patients in this study also received a GP IIb/IIIa inhibitor.[23] Some evidence suggests that enoxaparin may be reversed by the intravenous administration of protamine, but these data are limited.

Clinical Data on Enoxaparin

For the available LMWHs, most data support the use of enoxaparin in PCI. Interest in the use of enoxaparin in patients undergoing PCI has emerged from its use in patients with ACS. In general, these data suggest at least equal efficacy, if not modest superiority, with respect to ischemic complications compared

Table 10-2. Features of Low-Molecular Weight Heparins

Property	Unfractionated Heparin	Enoxaparin	Bivalirudin
Mean molecular mass (daltons)	15,000	5,000	2,180
Dependence on antithrombin	Yes	Yes	No
Anti-Xa : anti-IIa activity	1	2-4	No anti-Xa activity
Half-life (minutes)	≈60	≈240	25
Bioavailability	+ to +++	++++	++++
Subcutaneous absorption	++	++++	—
Binding to plasma proteins	+++	+	—
Binding to platelets or macrophages	++	+	—
Antigenicity/HITS	++	+	—
Clearance	Renal	Renal	Renal/proteolysis
Protamine neutralization	++++	++	—

HITS, heparin-induced thrombocytopenia syndrome; plus signs represent relative strength.

with heparin, with a modest excess in bleeding events in the context of invasively and conservatively managed patients.

The initial reported experience with enoxaparin specifically in PCI includes a series of studies performed by the National Investigators Collaborating on Enoxaparin (NICE) study group. These studies explored enoxaparin without abciximab (NICE-1) and with abciximab (NICE-4) in patients undergoing PCI and compared these historically with the arms of the Evaluation in Percutaneous Transluminal Coronary Angioplasty to Improve Long-Term Outcome with Abciximab GP IIb/IIIa Blockade (EPILOG) and Evaluation of Platelet IIb/IIIa Inhibitor for Stenting (EPISTENT) trials, respectively (Fig. 10-6).[24] The NICE-3 registry addressed outcomes among ACS patients receiving the various intravenous GP IIb/IIIa inhibitors, with PCI being left to the discretion of the investigator.

The NICE-1 registry assessed enoxaparin (1.0 mg/kg IV) without GP IIb/IIIa inhibition before coronary intervention in 828 patients undergoing elective and urgent PCI. The primary study end point was in-hospital and 30-day major hemorrhage. Minor bleeding,

the need for any transfusion, and the composite ischemic end point of death, MI, and urgent revascularization were also examined. Key exclusion criteria were acute MI within 24 hours, recent fibrinolysis (3 days), prior LMWH within 12 hours, thrombocytopenia less than 100,000/mL, and serum creatinine level higher than 2.5 mg/dL. In this group, at least one stent was placed in 85% of patients, aspirin was administered to all patients, and clopidogrel pretreatment was at the discretion of the treating interventionalist. Arteriotomy closure devices were not permitted and the protocol was prescriptive with respect to the time for sheath removal (4 to 6 hours). In the study without concomitant GP IIb/IIIa inhibition, major hemorrhage occurred in 1.1% of patients, with minor hemorrhage and transfusions occurring in 6.2% and 2.7% of patients, respectively. The composite ischemic end point of death, MI, and urgent revascularization at 30 days was observed in 7.7% of patients, with MI occurring in 5.4% of cases.[24]

In the very similar NICE-4 protocol, 818 patients received enoxaparin (0.75 mg/kg) and abciximab (0.25-mg/kg bolus and 0.125-μg/kg/min infusion).[24] In this study, 88% of patients received a bare-metal

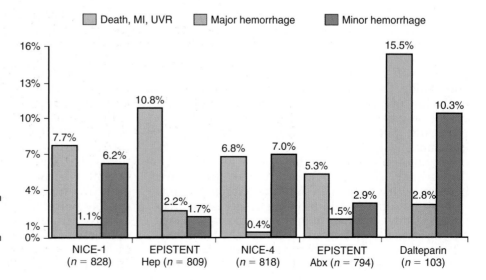

30 Day Outcomes

☐ Death, MI, UVR   ☐ Major hemorrhage   ☐ Minor hemorrhage

Figure 10-6. Observational studies with low-molecular-weight heparins in percutaneous coronary intervention contrasted with events in the Evaluation of Platelet IIb/IIIa Inhibitor for Stenting (EPISTENT) trial.

stent. The use of closure devices was not permitted. Inclusion and exclusion criteria and clinical end point definitions were similar to those used in the NICE-1 study. In NICE-4, major hemorrhage and minor hemorrhage were reported in 0.4% and 7.0% of patients, respectively, with transfusions required in 1.8% of cases. The composite ischemic event of death, MI, or urgent revascularization by 30 days occurred in 6.8% of patients, suggesting that enoxaparin may confer a similar level of efficacy and safety as observed with unfractionated heparin in the context of abciximab therapy.[24]

Employing a noncontrolled observational design, the NICE-3 study reported bleeding and ischemic events among 671 patients presenting with ACS and treated with tirofiban, eptifibatide, or abciximab.[25] Within this population, 43% underwent PCI. By 30 days, death, MI, and urgent revascularization were observed in 1.6%, 5.1%, and 6.8% of patients, respectively. The primary end point of non–CABG-related major bleeding was reported in 1.9% of patients by 30 days. Although numerically higher than the rates observed in other studies, interpretation of these results is hampered by the uncontrolled nature of the study design. Other observational data in the setting of ACS also suggest that enoxaparin is safe and efficacious among ACS patients undergoing PCI. Subgroup analysis of 4676 patients undergoing PCI in the ExTRACT-TIMI 25 study suggests that the incidence of death or MI may be reduced with enoxaparin compared with heparin among patients who have received fibrinolysis for ST-segment elevation myocardial infarction (STEMI) (10.7% for enoxaparin versus 13.8% for heparin, $P = .001$), with no significant excess in bleeding complications. Similarly, the larger subgroup analysis of 4687 unstable angina and non-ST-segment elevation ACS patients undergoing PCI in the Superior Yield of the New Strategy of Enoxaparin, Revascularization and Glycoprotein IIb/IIIa Inhibitors (SYNERGY) study observed comparable rate of 30-day death or MI rates, with a slight excess in bleeding events.[26]

Two randomized studies have been more optimally designed to examine the relative clinical risks and benefits of enoxaparin among patients undergoing PCI. The Coronary Revascularization Using Integrillin and Single bolus Enoxaparin (CRUISE) study randomized 261 elective or urgent PCI patients to enoxaparin (1 mg/kg IV) or heparin, with all patients receiving eptifibatide.[27] This small study reported no difference in the rate of bleeding complications or angiographic complications (6.3% versus 6.2%, $P = NS$) during the procedure. Similarly, there were no differences in ischemic end points at 48 hours or 30 days. Several other randomized studies have been too small to demonstrate clear benefits with enoxaparin over heparin, with a meta-analysis of these studies demonstrating no difference in bleeding or ischemia.[28] The largest study directly addressing enoxaparin use among patients undergoing PCI was the Safety and Efficacy of Intravenous Enoxaparin in Elective Percutaneous Coronary Intervention: an International

Randomized Evaluation (STEEPLE) trial.[29] This study randomized 3528 patients to intravenous enoxaparin (0.5 mg/kg; $n = 1070$), intravenous enoxaparin (0.75 mg/kg; $n = 1228$), or ACT-adjusted unfractionated heparin ($n = 1230$). The primary end point was non–CABG-related, protocol-defined bleeding by 48 hours (but not using the TIMI or Global Use of Strategies to Open Occluded Arteries in Acute Coronary Syndromes [GUSTO] scales), with the ischemic end points at 30 days also reported as secondary end points. In this study, GP IIb/IIIa inhibition and thienopyridines were used in about 40% and 95% of patients, respectively, with drug-eluting stents deployed in 57% of patients; 16% of cases involved multivessel intervention. At 48 hours, enoxaparin was associated with a lower rate of protocol-defined major and minor bleeding (6.0% for enoxaparin at 0.5 mg/kg versus 6.6% for enoxaparin at 0.75 mg/kg versus 8.7% for heparin; $P = .0014$), with most of the benefit driven by reductions in major bleeding (1.2% for enoxaparin at 0.5 mg/kg versus 1.2% for enoxaparin at 0.75 mg/kg versus 2.8% for heparin; $P = .004$ and $P = .007$). However, no difference was seen when the TIMI or GUSTO definitions of bleeding were applied, and there was no difference in the rate of transfusion. The composite end point of death, MI, or urgent revascularization at 30 days favored the unfractionated heparin arm, although these differences did not reach statistical significance and met a broad noninferiority boundary (Fig. 10-7). These results suggest that enoxaparin is a viable alternative to heparin, producing modest reductions in bleeding risk. However, the nonblinded nature of this study is of concern and confirmation of this result with other trials will be required.

Clinical Data for Dalteparin

Data for dalteparin are limited, with disappointing results suggesting that further clinical development of this agent for catheter laboratory use is unlikely.[30] In a dose-ranging study of 107 patients, 4 patients received dalteparin (120 U/kg) less than 8 hours before PCI and received an additional 40 U/kg (1 patient) or no further LMWH (3 patients). The remaining patients were randomized to 40 U/kg given intravenously (27 patients) or 60 U/kg given intravenously (76 patients) at the beginning of the procedure, with all patients receiving aspirin and abciximab. However, three early thrombotic events led to the decision to unblind the study and terminate the 40-U/kg arm. In this trial, death, MI (CK > three times the upper limit of normal), and urgent revascularization were observed in 15.5% of patients overall, whereas major hemorrhage and transfusion each occurred in 2.8% of patients. Although inadequately powered to fully evaluate the clinical utility of this agent among patients undergoing PCI, these event rates are higher than commonly seen in modern PCI trials, and further adequately controlled studies with this agent have not been performed.

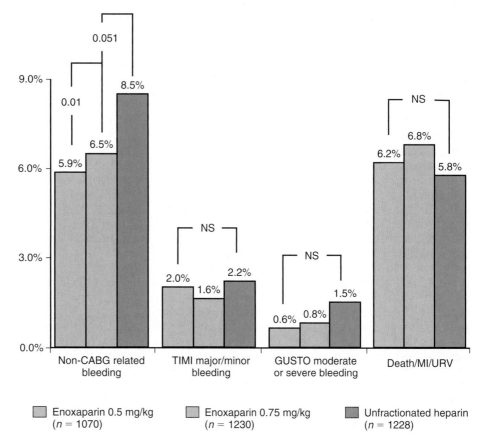

Figure 10-7. Protocol-defined major bleeding and ischemic events in the Safety and Efficacy of Intravenous Enoxaparin in Elective Percutaneous Coronary Intervention: An International Randomized Evaluation (STEEPLE) trial. CABG, coronary artery bypass grafting; GUSTO, Global Use of Strategies To Open Occluded Arteries in Acute Coronary Syndromes trial; MI, myocardial infarction; TIMI, Thrombolysis In Myocardial Infarction trial; URV, urgent revascularization.

Pentasaccharide and Hexadecasaccharide

Two novel indirect thrombin inhibitors have entered phase IIb and phase III clinical development. Fondaparinux, a pentasaccharide, and a hexadecasaccharide are both synthetic molecules that mimic the biologically active sequence of heparin in its interaction with antithrombin. Given that these molecules are short, their principal effect is the inactivation of FXa, as seen with the LMWHs in contradistinction to unfractionated heparin.[31] Similarly, these agents have relatively long half-lives, offering once-daily dosing regimens. These agents are not reversed by protamine and require the administration of factor VII concentrates. Given the pharmacokinetic characteristics, the initial interest with these agents has been for the treatment of patients presenting with acute coronary syndromes. The only large-scale trial evaluating a substantial number of patients undergoing coronary intervention is the Organization to Assess Strategies in Acute Ischemic Syndromes (OASIS)-5 trial. In this trial of 20,078 ACS patients randomized to enoxaparin or fondaparinux, 6207 patients underwent coronary intervention. Among these patients, no differences in ischemic complications were observed, though a benefit with fondaparinux was evident with respect to bleeding events compared with enoxaparin (8.8% for enoxaparin versus 3.3% for fondaparinux; $P < .001$). However, a substantial number of patients undergoing PCI received unfractionated heparin in both arms of the study. The protocol was modified during the study to ensure the use of heparin in the fondaparinux arm owing to a higher rate of catheter-related thrombosis (0.5% for enoxaparin versus 1.3% for fondaparinux; $P = .001$). Dedicated randomized trials of these agents, as stand-alone antithrombotic strategies or in combination with other antithrombins and antiplatelet agents in PCI, are awaited.

Direct Thrombin Inhibitors

Pharmacology

The direct thrombin inhibitor hirudin, found in the saliva of the medicinal leech *Hirudo medicinalis,* is the prototypical molecule of this class. Hirudin is a 65–amino acid protein that forms a stable noncovalent complex with thrombin.[31] With two domains, the NH$_2$ terminal core domain and the COOH terminal tail, the hirudin molecule inhibits the catalytic site and the anion binding exosite in a two-step process. An initial ionic interaction leads to a rearrangement of the thrombin-hirudin complex and the subsequent formation of a tighter, irreversible 1 : 1 bond.[3] This complex and tight binding of hirudin to thrombin helps account for the highly specific effect of hirudin on thrombin. Generally, the direct thrombin inhibitor molecules are smaller than the indirect thrombin inhibitors and consequently demonstrate greater efficacy for the inhibition of clot-bound thrombin, in addition to their effects on fluid-phase thrombin.[31,32] Two forms of recombinant hirudin (r-hirudin) have been developed, one with a sulfated Tyr63 and the other without this change. The non-sulfated tyrosine molecule appears to have a 10-fold lower affinity for thrombin compared with the naturally occurring compound.

The hirudin-thrombin interaction offers a method for categorizing the other direct thrombin inhibitors, which have been divided into univalent and bivalent molecules. The univalent molecules, dabigatran, argatroban, melagatran, and the oral prodrug, ximelagatran, inhibit only the catalytic site and inactivate only fibrin-bound thrombin. The thrombin inhibition provided by these agents is less robust than that observed with hirudin, because dissociation leads to some residual thrombin activity. Argatroban, the only one of these agents approved for use in PCI, binds to the apolar-binding site adjacent to the catalytic site and provides competitive inhibition. The bivalent molecules, recombinant hirudin and bivalirudin, bind to the catalytic site and at least one of the exosites. Although the interaction between hirudin and thrombin is irreversible, the inhibition provided by bivalirudin is more transient. Bivalirudin is a synthetic 20–amino acid molecule with two domains. These are targeted toward the anion-binding exosite and catalytic sites, which are linked by four glycine spacers. Given the shorter amino acid chain length compared with hirudin, bivalirudin exhibits less avid ionic binding. Cleavage of the bivalirudin molecule at the Arg-Pro bond of the amino-terminal extension by thrombin itself enables the release of the thrombin active site for further thrombotic activity. This in part accounts for the shorter half-life of bivalirudin compared with hirudin and may account for some of the reduced bleeding risk seen with this agent.

Several other direct thrombin inhibitors have been developed in addition to those discussed, but they have not yet found a clinical role in the catheterization laboratory.[33] All available agents approved for use in PCI require parenteral administration. With the exception of argatroban, these agents are cleared renally, and clearance is attenuated in the setting of reduced renal function. In the setting of excessive dosing or bleeding, these agents can be removed by hemofiltration. Argatroban is primarily eliminated through hepatic metabolism, and dose reduction in the setting of hepatic dysfunction is required. However, renal function also influences dosing.[34] Bivalirudin also undergoes proteolysis within the plasma, contributing to its shorter half-life and relatively constant elimination characteristics even among patients with mild to moderate renal impairment (see Table 10-2). Nevertheless, dose attenuation is required for patients with creatinine clearance less than 30 mL/min. These agents are not reversed by protamine. Nonspecific measures such as transfusion of blood products, including fresh frozen plasma, and local measures are recommended in the context of active bleeding.

Clinical Evidence of Direct Thrombin Inhibition

This class of agents, particularly bivalirudin, has emerged as a useful alternative to heparin as an anticoagulant among patients undergoing PCI as an adjunct and alternative to GP IIb/IIIa inhibition. Early trials with hirudin focused on the prevention of restenosis in the setting of balloon angioplasty. Although no anti-restenotic effect was evident, reductions in early ischemic events were observed. These agents have found a role in the management of patients with heparin-induced thrombocytopenia (i.e., argatroban and bivalirudin), whereas most recent data suggest that improved thrombin inhibition with bivalirudin enables sparing of GP IIb/IIIa inhibition in most patients undergoing PCI.

Clinical Evidence for Hirudin

The first large-scale, randomized trial of direct thrombin inhibition in PCI was the Hirudin in a European Trial Versus Heparin In the Prevention of Restenosis after PTCA (HELVETICA) trial.[35] In this study, 1141 unstable angina patients undergoing balloon angioplasty received either of two dose regimens of hirudin or unfractionated heparin. Patients receiving intravenous hirudin experienced a reduction in early cardiac events within 96 hours (hirudin arms combined, RR = 0.61; 95% CI: 0.41 to 0.90; P = .023). However, in this study, the primary end point was event-free survival at 7 months, and for this end point, there were no differences between the three treatment arms, whereas similar rates of restenosis were observed. In the angioplasty substudy of STEMI patients of the Global Utilization of Strategies to Open Occluded Coronary Arteries IIb (GUSTO IIb) trial, 503 patients undergoing PTCA were randomized to hirudin or heparin.[36] Hirudin resulted in a 23% (P = NS) reduction in death, MI, or stroke at 30 days.

A benefit with hirudin in the setting of PCI is also evident from other observational studies. Among all patients undergoing PCI in the GUSTO IIb (ST elevation, [randomized] and non-ST elevation ACS [physician discretion]), a reduction in 30-day MI among the hirudin group (n = 672) compared with those receiving heparin (n = 738) was seen (4.9% versus 7.6%, P = .04), and a nonsignificant excess in bleeding was observed.[37] Likewise, analysis of the OASIS-2 trial of unstable angina patients randomized to heparin or hirudin, assessing the outcomes in 172 patients undergoing PCI within 72 hours of randomization, provides similar conclusions.[38] Although the study was observational and relatively small, the rate of death or MI at 96 hours was lower among hirudin-treated patients compared with those receiving heparin (6.4% versus 21.4%; OR = 0.30; 95% CI: 0.10 to 0.88) and 35 days (6.4% versus 22.9%; OR = 0.25; 95% CI: 0.07 to 0.86). Caution should be exercised when interpreting this nonrandomized comparison. Nevertheless, these observations led to a meta-analysis of direct thrombin inhibition drawn from

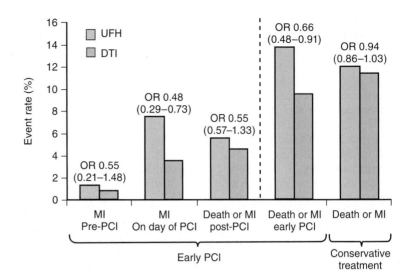

Figure 10-8. The relative impact of direct thrombin inhibition in invasive and conservative management of acute coronary syndromes. DTI, direct thrombin inhibitor; MI, myocardial infarction; PCI, percutaneous coronary intervention; UFH, unfractionated heparin.

two PCI and nine ACS trials (N = 35,970), including data for bivalirudin and the univalent direct thrombin inhibitors, that reported a beneficial effect linked to the timing of PCI.[39] Among patients undergoing PCI within 72 hours of randomization, the direct thrombin inhibitors were associated with lower rates of death or MI (OR = 0.66; 95% CI: 0.48 to 0.91) compared with heparin. In this analysis, a reduction in bleeding was driven by the benefits observed in the PCI trials (Fig. 10-8). In contrast, a more modest effect was documented when PCI was delayed after 72 hours. No benefit with these agents over heparin was observed in the context of conservative management.

Clinical Evidence for Argatroban

For the widespread application to patients undergoing PCI, argatroban has not been studied in large-scale, randomized clinical trials. However, as an alternative to heparin among patients with heparin-induced thrombocytopenia syndrome (HITS), results of a small case series totaling 151 patients suggest that this agent is safe.[40,41] Similarly, a small, non-blinded, uncontrolled study of argatroban administered to patients treated with abciximab (n = 150) and eptifibatide (n = 2) suggests that the combinations of these agents is at least feasible, but evidence defining the absolute benefits and risk associated with argatroban in the context of modern intervention practice is still lacking.[42]

Clinical Evidence for Bivalirudin

Clinical studies with bivalirudin constitute the bulk of evidence supporting the role of direct thrombin inhibition in the context of PCI. The first large-scale study with bivalirudin in the context of balloon angioplasty was with the Bivalirudin Angioplasty Study (BAT).[43,44] Initially published in 1995, the trial was conducted in the era before coronary stenting,

thienopyridine use, and intravenous GP IIb/IIIa inhibition. In context of urgent or elective angioplasty, 4312 patients were randomized to bivalirudin (1 mg/kg bolus and 2.5 mg/kg/hr infusion) or high-dose unfractionated heparin. A subgroup of 741 post-MI patients underwent stratified randomization to the same treatment arms. Randomization to bivalirudin provided a 22% reduction (6.2% versus 7.9%, P = .039) in death, myocardial infarction, or urgent revascularization and a 62% reduction (3.9% versus 9.7%, P < .001) in major bleeding events at 7 days. Among this stratified post-MI subgroup, the triple ischemic end point was reduced by 46% by 90 days (OR = 0.54; 95% CI: 36 to 0.81; P = .009).

The advent of GP IIb/IIIa inhibition required two smaller pilot studies exploring the incremental benefits of bivalirudin among PCI patients receiving modern antiplatelet therapies. The Comparison of Abciximab Complications with Hirulog for Ischemic Events Trial (CACHET) A/B/C studies explored the role of bivalirudin with routine or provisional use of abciximab use in 208 patients undergoing coronary angioplasty and stenting. Within this small study, a promising reduction in bleeding events without excess ischemic events was observed.[45] The Randomized Evaluation of PCI Linking Angiomax to reduced Clinical Events (REPLACE)-1 study employed a less prescriptive design, randomizing 1056 PCI patients to 0.75 mg/kg and 1.75 mg/kg/hr of bivalirudin or 60 to 70 U/kg of heparin with GP IIb/IIIa inhibition (i.e., abciximab, eptifibatide, or tirofiban) provisionally, routinely, or not at all at the discretion of the interventional cardiologist. Stents and GP IIb/IIIa inhibition were used in approximately 85% and 76% of patients, respectively. A nonsignificant benefit favoring the use of bivalirudin was observed at 48 hours in terms of ischemic and bleeding complications, despite the liberal use of GP IIb/IIIa inhibition.[46]

In the largest trial of antithrombotic therapy in PCI performed, the REPLACE-2 study enrolled 6010 patients undergoing elective or urgent coronary intervention. Randomization was to bivalirudin

(0.75 mg/kg and 1.75 mg/kg/hr IV) and provisional abciximab or eptifibatide versus the planned use of these GP IIb/IIIa inhibitors and heparin (65 mg/kg IV), conducted in a double-blind, double-dummy manner.[47] The commonly used "triple ischemic end point" of death, MI or urgent revascularization by 30 days was assessed with a noninferiority design. The major exclusions to this study were patients presenting with STEMI undergoing PCI for reperfusion, patients at significant risk for bleeding, or those requiring dialysis. As a result, approximately 50% of patients underwent PCI for an ACS, multivessel intervention was undertaken in about 15% of cases, and saphenous vein graft intervention occurred in 6% of patients. Provisional use of a GP IIb/IIIa inhibitor was permitted for coronary dissection, thrombus formation, unplanned stenting, slow flow, distal embolization, and ongoing clinical instability in the bivalirudin arm, whereas provisional placebo was used in the arm of patients already receiving GP IIb/IIIa inhibition. Among bivalirudin treated patients, GP IIb/IIIa inhibition was used in 7.5% of procedures. In contrast, 5.2% of heparin and GP IIb/IIIa inhibition-treated patients received provisional placebo (P = .002). Pretreatment with a thienopyridine, mostly clopidogrel, was administered in 86% of patients. Bivalirudin (plus provisional GP IIb/IIIa inhibition) was associated with a nonsignificant excess in ischemic events (7.6% for heparin and GP IIb/IIIa inhibition versus 7.9% for bivalirudin; OR = 1.09; 95% CI: 0.90 to 1.32; P = .40) but met the boundary for noninferiority. In contrast, bleeding events were significantly reduced when evaluated by the TIMI criteria or the slightly broader protocol definition that included blood transfusion (4.1% for heparin and GP IIb/IIIa inhibition versus 2.4% for bivalirudin, P < .001). Reduced vascular access site events accounted for a large proportion of this bleeding benefit. Despite inadequate power to assess the benefit with respect to mortality, assessment of 12-month events demonstrated a lower point estimate for mortality with bivalirudin (1.6% versus 2.5%, P = .16).[48] The nonsignificant excess in early MI was not associated with an excess in late mortality.

These data are further supported by the results of the Acute Catheterization and Urgent Intervention Triage Strategy (ACUITY), a trial of antithrombotic therapy among ACS patients undergoing early invasive management. Among this high-risk patient population, the strategy of bivalirudin with bailout use of GP IIb/IIIa inhibition was associated with a slight but nonsignificant excess in ischemic events, with significant reduction of bleeding events (Fig. 10-9). Overall, when considered in a combined end point of ischemia and bleeding, the use of bivalirudin was "not inferior" to heparin or LMWH and a GP IIb/IIIa inhibitor. However, this was a complex trial, in which the timing of the GP IIb/IIIa inhibitor was also randomized to "upstream use" or "in cath-lab" initiation. As with the bivalirudin versus heparin or LMWH comparison, the in-catheter laboratory initiation of GP IIb/IIIa inhibition was associated with slightly

more ischemic events and fewer bleeding events. Although the noninferiority margin for these comparisons was met, results of longer follow-up of these patients will be needed to evaluate the relative efficacy and safety of these strategies.

Pooled analysis of the randomized clinical trial experience with bivalirudin in PCI, including 11,638 patients (bivalirudin, 5861; heparin, 5777) demonstrates a reduction in the incidence of death, MI, revascularization, and major bleeding (7.8% versus 10.8%, P < .001) with this direct thrombin inhibitor at 48 hours. This large clinical trial experience also suggests a benefit with respect to mortality alone, despite the very low rate of events (0.01% versus 0.02%, P = .049). Consistent with the individual trial data, reductions for major bleeding were substantial (2.7% versus 5.8%, P < .001).[49] The impact of bivalirudin-based strategies compared with eptifibatide-based strategies on measures of coronary flow after intervention have shown mixed results that are difficult to interpret in the context of large-scale clinical data that show no difference between these strategies.[50] Limited, uncontrolled series also report experiences with bivalirudin with other interventional technologies, including drug-eluting stents, brachytherapy, and peripheral intervention. These results suggest an ischemic and bleeding profile that is consistent with the large-scale clinical trials despite their observational nature.[51-53]

TREATMENT OF SPECIAL GROUPS

With the broad array of therapies available, weighing the limitations and benefits of each approach is often difficult. In many patients, the use of unfractionated heparin remains a safe and efficacious choice, especially in the context of pretreatment with a thienopyridine and the planned used of GP IIb/IIIa inhibition. However, in specific high-risk populations, the decision to use an alternative antithrombotic strategy may be considered.

ST-Segment Elevation Myocardial Infarction

Although the efficacy of hirudin has been explored in the context of primary PCI with balloon angioplasty in the GUSTO IIb study (discussed earlier), there are no randomized studies to optimally evaluate the risks and benefits of using enoxaparin or bivalirudin in the context of primary or rescue PCI. Nevertheless, a small, observational series suggests that bivalirudin is a feasible anticoagulant in primary PCI.[36,54] Similar small series have been described for the use of enoxaparin in the context of liberal GP IIb/IIIa use.

Transitioning from Upstream Management to the Catheter Laboratory

Extrapolation of the clinical experience with unfractionated heparin suggests that the degree of anticoagulation required during PCI is greater than that

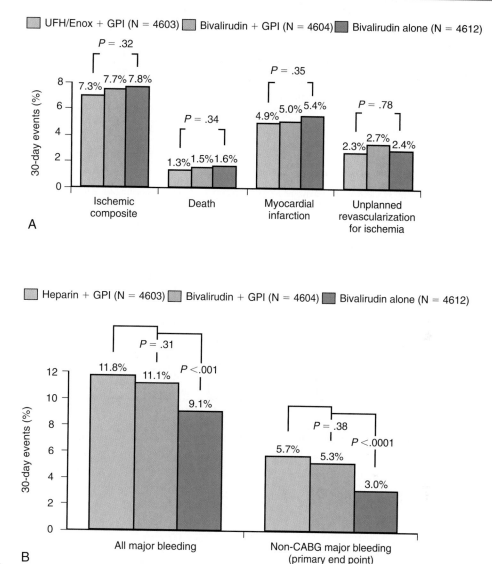

Figure 10-9. Ischemic and bleeding outcomes with bivalirudin versus bivalirudin/glycoprotein IIb/IIIa inhibition versus heparin **(A)** or low-molecular-weight/glycoprotein IIb/IIIa inhibition **(B)** in the Acute Catheterization and Urgent Intervention Triage Strategy (ACUITY) trial. CABG, coronary artery bypass grafting; UFH, unfractionated heparin.

required during the medical management of patients presenting with ACS. As a result, strategies have evolved to optimize the antithrombin therapies for ACS patients proceeding to PCI while already receiving one of these agents. Among patients being treated with heparin, an ACT-guided approach is recommended, with an additional 20 to 50 U/kg administered intravenously to achieve an ACT longer than 200 to 250 seconds when concomitant GP IIb/IIIa inhibition is planned and more than 300 to 350 seconds when heparin is the sole agent. Data on enoxaparin suggest that PCI can proceed without additional dosing when the procedure is occurring within 8 hours of the subcutaneous dose, and an additional intravenous bolus of 0.3 mg/kg is recommended when the delay is 8 to 12 hours. Outside this window, a dose of 0.75 mg/kg given intravenously should be administered regardless of GP IIb/IIIa inhibition use based on results of the SYNERGY study. Among patients receiving infusions of bivalirudin, an additional bolus of 0.5 mg/kg and an increase in the

infusion rate to 1.75 mg/kg were shown to be safe and efficacious in the ACUITY study, regardless of GP IIb/IIIa use (Table 10-3). Whether switching between agents when transitioning to invasive management is safe has not been prospectively evaluated.

Decreased Renal Function

Increased ischemic and bleeding events are observed among patients with renal dysfunction. Analyses of the randomized clinical trial experience with bivalirudin suggests that the relative benefits of this agent in terms of bleeding complications and ischemic complications is preserved.[55,56] In absolute terms, among patients with at least moderate renal dysfunction (creatinine clearance <60 mL/min), bivalirudin is associated with a greater absolute benefit with respect to bleeding without an excess risk of ischemic events (Fig. 10-10). With enoxaparin, and fondaparinux, there are limited data examining the relative risks and benefits in the context of patients

Table 10-3. Dosing of the Available Antithrombin Agents

Status	Unfractionated Heparin	Enoxaparin	Bivalirudin
No prior treatment	60-100 units/kg IV*	0.5-0.75 mg/kg IV	0.75 mg/kg IV with 1.75 mg/kg/hr infusion
Upstream ACS management	60 IU/kg IV and 800-1000 IU/hr infusion	1.0 mg/kg SC bid	0.1 mg/kg IV with 0.25 mg/kg/hr infusion
Additional bolus before PCI	20-50 IU/kg*	<8 hr since last dose: none 8-12 hr since last SC dose: 0.3 mg/kg IV	0.5 mg/kg IV bolus
Infusion during PCI	None	None	1.75 mg/kg/hr infusion

*Targeting and ACT >200 seconds with concomitant glycoprotein IIb/IIIa inhibition or ACT >300-350 seconds without concomitant glycoprotein IIb/IIIa inhibition.
ACS, acute coronary syndrome; ACT, activated clotting time; PCI, percutaneous coronary intervention.

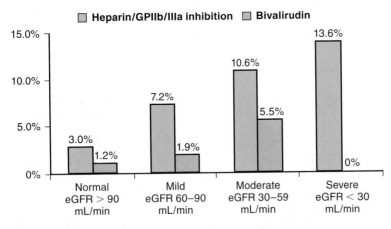

Protocol defined bleeding

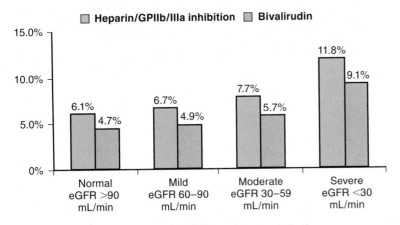

30-day death/MI/urgent revascularisation

Figure 10-10. Relationship between renal function and outcomes with bivalirudin. eGFR, estimated glomerular filtration rate.

with renal impairment. However, given the reliance on renal elimination for these agents, their use is not expected to be an optimal choice.

Diabetes

Subgroup analysis of randomized clinical trials appears to indicate that abciximab provides substantial benefits in terms of reduced repeat revascularization and mortality among diabetic patients, with comparable effects observed with tirofiban. Clinical trial evidence with bivalirudin supports similar con-clusions. In the REPLACE-2 study of bivalirudin and provisional GP IIb/IIIa inhibition compared with heparin and GP IIb/IIIa inhibition, bivalirudin-treated diabetic patients experienced a lower, but nonsignificant rate of mortality at 12 months (2.3% versus 3.9%, P = NS). No difference in the rate of 30-day bleeding and ischemic outcomes was observed.[57] Although the long-term effects of enoxaparin-based strategies in diabetic patients have not been reported, a substantial rate of concomitant GP IIb/IIIa use in these studies will limit the interpretation of these data.

Heparin-Induced Thrombocytopenia

HITS precludes the use of unfractionated heparin during PCI. Although the rate of HITS is less frequent with the LMWHs, cross-reactivity with these agents is observed and may be associated with increased rates of ischemic and bleeding complications. Whether pentasaccharides and hexadecasaccharides are safe and efficacious in this context has yet to be determined. The direct thrombin inhibitors are well suited to the management of HITS patients requiring PCI. Observational data for argatroban suggest that this agent can be safely used as an alternative to heparin in these patients. Case reports with recombinant hirudin (lepirudin) suggest that the use of this agent is also feasible.[58] Similarly, a registry of 52 HITS patients receiving bivalirudin before PCI reported a 96% rate of freedom from death, Q-wave MI, and emergent CABG. Thrombocytopenia (platelet counts $<50 \times 10^9$/L) was not observed among these patients, suggesting that bivalirudin is also an alternative anticoagulation strategy within this uncommon but high-risk subgroup.[59]

Glycoprotein IIb/IIIa–Sparing, Combination Approaches and Economic Considerations

When required, combination antithrombotic strategies, including pretreatment with thienopyridines, intravenous GP IIb/IIIa inhibition, and the direct or indirect thrombin inhibitors, appear to be safe. However, given the cost of GP IIb/IIIa inhibition and the increased risk of bleeding events, efforts to refine antithrombotic approach and define patient subsets that may not derive incremental benefits from these agents have continued. Optimization of anticoagulant therapies may mitigate the dependence on potent platelet inhibition. With respect to antithrombin therapy, the only trial optimally designed to address this question has been the REPLACE-2 study, in which comparable ischemic outcomes were observed, although a slightly greater rate of provisional GP IIb/IIIa inhibition was also seen. Pretreatment with thienopyridines did not appear to influence this relationship.[60] Given reductions in drug costs and cost associated with bleeding, the bivalirudin strategy was economically attractive.[61] Whether such conclusions can be made regarding the LMWHs or the oligosaccharides has not been addressed in adequately designed and powered studies.

Direct thrombin inhibition provides theoretical advantages for combination pharmacotherapies in PCI. Providing potent inhibition of thrombin-induced platelet activation, synergistic effects with agents blocking the activation and aggregation of platelets can be expected, in contrast to the effects of heparin.[62,63] The combination of bivalirudin and GP IIb/IIIa inhibition in a planned and provisional strategy also appears to be safe. Although not a randomized comparison, patients in the REPLACE-1 study receiving both bivalirudin and GP IIb/IIIa inhibition experienced a nonsignificant excess in bleeding events compared with those receiving bivalirudin alone, and ischemic events were not significantly lower than heparin and GP IIb/IIIa inhibition-treated patients in this pilot study.[46] However, the incremental value of this approach in routine PCI is likely to be modest.

CONCLUSIONS

Substantial clinical trial evidence supports the use of the novel coagulants among patients undergoing PCI. These agents demonstrate improved efficacy and safety compared with heparin and enable less use of GP IIb/IIIa inhibition. The optimal antithrombotic strategies for treatment of STEMI are likely to be answered in clinical trials that are ongoing.

REFERENCES

1. Davie EW, Kulman JD: An overview of the structure and function of thrombin. Semin Thromb Hemost 2006;32(Suppl)1: 3-15.
2. Zucker TP, Bonisch D, Muck S, et al: Thrombin-induced mitogenesis in coronary artery smooth muscle cells is potentiated by thromboxane A_2 and involves upregulation of thromboxane receptor mRNA. Circulation 1998;97:589-595.
3. Tulinsky A: Molecular interactions of thrombin. Semin Thromb Hemost 1996;22:117-124.
4. Chew DP, Bhatt DL, Lincoff AM, et al: Clinical end point definitions following percutaneous coronary intervention and their relationship to late mortality: An assessment by attributable risk. Heart 2005;92:945-950.
5. Kinnaird TD, Stabile E, Mintz GS, et al: Incidence, predictors, and prognostic implications of bleeding and blood transfusion following percutaneous coronary interventions. Am J Cardiol 2003;92:930-935.
6. Chew DP, Bhatt DL, Lincoff AM, et al: Defining the optimal activated clotting time during percutaneous coronary intervention: Aggregate results from 6 randomized, controlled trials. Circulation 2001;103:961-966.
7. Cavusoglu E, Lakhani M, Marmur JD: The activated clotting time (ACT) can be used to monitor enoxaparin and dalteparin after intravenous administration. J Invasive Cardiol 2005;17: 416-421.
8. Saw J, Kereiakes DJ, Mahaffey KW, et al: Evaluation of a novel point-of-care enoxaparin monitor with central laboratory anti-Xa levels. Thromb Res 2003;112:301-306.
9. Cheneau E, Canos D, Kuchulakanti PK, et al: Value of monitoring activated clotting time when bivalirudin is used as the sole anticoagulation agent for percutaneous coronary intervention. Am J Cardiol 2004;94:789-792.
10. Casserly IP, Kereiakes DJ, Gray WA, et al: Point-of-care ecarin clotting time versus activated clotting time in correlation with bivalirudin concentration. Thromb Res 2004;113:115-121.
11. Rosenberg RD, Lam L: Correlation between structure and function of heparin. Proc Natl Acad Sci U S A 1979;76:1218-1222.
12. Xiao Z, Theroux P: Platelet activation with unfractionated heparin at therapeutic concentrations and comparisons with a low-molecular-weight heparin and with a direct thrombin inhibitor. Circulation 1998;97:251-256.
13. Young E, Cosmi B, Weitz J, Hirsh J: Comparison of the non-specific binding of unfractionated heparin and low molecular weight heparin (enoxaparin) to plasma proteins. Thromb Haemost 1993;70:625-630.
14. Weitz JI, Hudoba M, Massel D, et al: Clot-bound thrombin is protected from inhibition by heparin-antithrombin III but is susceptible to inactivation by antithrombin III-independent inhibitors. J Clin Invest 1990;86:385-391.

15. Narins CR, Hillegass WB Jr, Nelson CL, et al: Relation between activated clotting time during angioplasty and abrupt closure. Circulation 1996;93:667-671.

16. Ferguson JJ, Barasch E, Wilson JM, et al: The relation of clinical outcome to dissection and thrombus formation during coronary angioplasty. Heparin Registry Investigators. J Invasive Cardiol 1995;7:2-10.

17. Boccara A, Benamer H, Juliard JM, et al: A randomized trial of a fixed high dose vs a weight-adjusted low dose of intravenous heparin during coronary angioplasty. Eur Heart J 1997;18:631-635.

18. Brener SJ, Moliterno DJ, Lincoff AM, et al: Relationship between activated clotting time and ischemic or hemorrhagic complications: Analysis of 4 recent randomized clinical trials of percutaneous coronary intervention. Circulation 2004;110:994-998.

19. Tolleson TR, O'Shea JC, Bittl JA, et al: Relationship between heparin anticoagulation and clinical outcomes in coronary stent intervention: Observations from the ESPRIT trial. J Am Coll Cardiol 2003;41:386-393.

20. Friedman HZ, Cragg DR, Glazier SM, et al: Randomized prospective evaluation of prolonged versus abbreviated intravenous heparin therapy after coronary angioplasty. J Am Coll Cardiol 1994;24:1214-1219.

21. Weitz JI: Low-molecular-weight heparins. N Engl J Med 1997;337:688-698.

22. Martin JL, Fry ET, Sanderink GJ, et al: Reliable anticoagulation with enoxaparin in patients undergoing percutaneous coronary intervention: The pharmacokinetics of enoxaparin in PCI (PEPCI) study. Catheter Cardiovasc Interv 2004;61:163-170.

23. Choussat R, Montalescot G, Collet JP, et al: A unique, low dose of intravenous enoxaparin in elective percutaneous coronary intervention. J Am Coll Cardiol 2002;40:1943-1950.

24. Kereiakes DJ, Grines C, Fry E, et al: Enoxaparin and abciximab adjunctive pharmacotherapy during percutaneous coronary intervention. J Invasive Cardiol 2001;13:272-278.

25. Ferguson JJ, Antman EM, Bates ER, et al: Combining enoxaparin and glycoprotein IIb/IIIa antagonists for the treatment of acute coronary syndromes: Final results of the National Investigators Collaborating on Enoxaparin-3 (NICE-3) study. Am Heart J 2003;146:628-634.

26. Ferguson JJ, Califf RM, Antman EM, et al: Enoxaparin vs unfractionated heparin in high-risk patients with non-ST-segment elevation acute coronary syndromes managed with an intended early invasive strategy: Primary results of the SYNERGY randomized trial. JAMA 2004;292:45-54.

27. Bhatt DL, Lee BI, Casterella PJ, et al: Safety of concomitant therapy with eptifibatide and enoxaparin in patients undergoing percutaneous coronary intervention: Results of the Coronary Revascularization Using Integrilin and Single bolus Enoxaparin Study. J Am Coll Cardiol 2003;41:20-25.

28. Borentain M, Montalescot G, Bouzamondo A, et al: Low-molecular-weight heparin vs. unfractionated heparin in percutaneous coronary intervention: A combined analysis. Catheter Cardiovasc Interv 2005;65:212-221.

29. Montalescot G, White HD, Gallo R, et al: Enoxaparin versus unfractionated heparin in elective percutaneous coronary intervention. N Engl J Med 2006;355:1006-1017.

30. Kereiakes DJ, Kleiman NS, Fry E, et al: Dalteparin in combination with abciximab during percutaneous coronary intervention. Am Heart J 2001;141:348-352.

31. Weitz JI, Bates SM: New anticoagulants. J Thromb Haemost 2005;3:1843-1853.

32. Weitz JI, Leslie B, Hudoba M: Thrombin binds to soluble fibrin degradation products where it is protected from inhibition by heparin-antithrombin but susceptible to inactivation by antithrombin-independent inhibitors. Circulation 1998;97:544-552.

33. Di Nisio M, Middeldorp S, Buller HR: Direct thrombin inhibitors. N Engl J Med 2005;353:1028-1040.

34. Arpino PA, Hallisey RK: Effect of renal function on the pharmacodynamics of argatroban. Ann Pharmacother 2004;38:25-29.

35. Serruys PW, Herrman JP, Simon R, et al: A comparison of hirudin with heparin in the prevention of restenosis after coronary angioplasty. Helvetica Investigators. N Engl J Med 1995;333:757-763.

36. A clinical trial comparing primary coronary angioplasty with tissue plasminogen activator for acute myocardial infarction. The Global Use of Strategies to Open Occluded Coronary Arteries in Acute Coronary Syndromes (GUSTO IIb) Angioplasty Substudy Investigators. N Engl J Med 1997;336:1621-1628.

37. Roe MT, Granger CB, Puma JA, et al: Comparison of benefits and complications of hirudin versus heparin for patients with acute coronary syndromes undergoing early percutaneous coronary intervention. Am J Cardiol 2001;88:1403-1406, A6.

38. Mehta SR, Eikelboom JW, Rupprecht HJ, et al: Efficacy of hirudin in reducing cardiovascular events in patients with acute coronary syndrome undergoing early percutaneous coronary intervention. Eur Heart J 2002;23:117-123.

39. Sinnaeve PR, Simes J, Yusuf S, et al: Direct thrombin inhibitors in acute coronary syndromes: Effect in patients undergoing early percutaneous coronary intervention. Eur Heart J 2005;26:2396-2403.

40. Matthai WH Jr: Use of argatroban during percutaneous coronary interventions in patients with heparin-induced thrombocytopenia. Semin Thromb Hemost 1999;25(Suppl)1:57-60.

41. Lewis BE, Matthai WH Jr, Cohen M, et al: Argatroban anticoagulation during percutaneous coronary intervention in patients with heparin-induced thrombocytopenia. Catheter Cardiovasc Interv 2002;57:177-184.

42. Jang IK, Lewis BE, Matthai WH Jr, Kleiman NS: Argatroban anticoagulation in conjunction with glycoprotein IIb/IIIa inhibition in patients undergoing percutaneous coronary intervention: An open-label, nonrandomized pilot study. J Thromb Thrombolysis 2004;18:31-37.

43. Bittl JA, Strony J, Brinker JA, et al: Treatment with bivalirudin (Hirulog) as compared with heparin during coronary angioplasty for unstable or postinfarction angina. Hirulog Angioplasty Study Investigators. N Engl J Med 1995;333:764-769.

44. Bittl JA, Chaitman BR, Feit F, et al: Bivalirudin versus heparin during coronary angioplasty for unstable or postinfarction angina: Final report reanalysis of the Bivalirudin Angioplasty Study. Am Heart J 2001;142:952-959.

45. Lincoff AM, Kleiman NS, Kottke-Marchant K, et al: Bivalirudin with planned or provisional abciximab versus low-dose heparin and abciximab during percutaneous coronary revascularization: Results of the Comparison of Abciximab Complications with Hirulog for Ischemic Events Trial (CACHET). Am Heart J 2002;143:847-853.

46. Lincoff AM, Bittl JA, Kleiman NS, et al: Comparison of bivalirudin versus heparin during percutaneous coronary intervention (the Randomized Evaluation of PCI Linking Angiomax to Reduced Clinical Events [REPLACE]-1 trial). Am J Cardiol 2004;93:1092-1096.

47. Lincoff AM, Bittl JA, Harrington RA, et al: Bivalirudin and provisional glycoprotein IIb/IIIa blockade compared with heparin and planned glycoprotein IIb/IIIa blockade during percutaneous coronary intervention: REPLACE-2 randomized trial. JAMA 2003;289:853-863.

48. Lincoff AM, Kleiman NS, Kereiakes DJ, et al: Long-term efficacy of bivalirudin and provisional glycoprotein IIb/IIIa blockade vs heparin and planned glycoprotein IIb/IIIa blockade during percutaneous coronary revascularization: REPLACE-2 randomized trial. JAMA 2004;292:696-703.

49. Ebrahimi R, Lincoff AM, Bittl JA, et al: Bivalirudin vs heparin in percutaneous coronary intervention: A pooled analysis. J Cardiovasc Pharmacol Ther 2005;10:209-216.

50. Gibson CM, Morrow DA, Murphy SA, et al: A randomized trial to evaluate the relative protection against post-percutaneous coronary intervention microvascular dysfunction, ischemia, and inflammation among antiplatelet and antithrombotic agents: The PROTECT-TIMI-30 trial. J Am Coll Cardiol 2006;47:2364-2373.

51. Allie DE, Hebert CJ, Lirtzman MD, et al: A safety and feasibility report of combined direct thrombin and GP IIb/IIIa inhibition with bivalirudin and tirofiban in peripheral vascular disease intervention: Treating critical limb ischemia like acute coronary syndrome. J Invasive Cardiol 2005;17:427-432.

52. Dangas G, Lasic Z, Mehran R, et al: Effectiveness of the concomitant use of bivalirudin and drug-eluting stents (from the prospective, multicenter BivAlirudin and Drug-Eluting STents [ADEST] study). Am J Cardiol 2005;96:659-663.

53. Kuchulakanti P, Wolfram R, Torguson R, et al: Bivalirudin compared with IIb/IIIa inhibitors in patients with in-stent restenosis undergoing intracoronary brachytherapy. Cardiovasc Revasc Med 2005;6:154-159.

54. Stella JF, Stella RE, Iaffaldano RA, et al: Anticoagulation with bivalirudin during percutaneous coronary intervention for ST-segment elevation myocardial infarction. J Invasive Cardiol 2004;16:451-454.

55. Chew DP, Bhatt DL, Kimball W, et al: Bivalirudin provides increasing benefit with decreasing renal function: A meta-analysis of randomized trials. Am J Cardiol 2003;92:919-923.

56. Chew DP, Lincoff AM, Gurm H, et al: Bivalirudin versus heparin and glycoprotein IIb/IIIa inhibition among patients with renal impairment undergoing percutaneous coronary intervention (a subanalysis of the REPLACE-2 trial). Am J Cardiol 2005;95:581-585.

57. Gurm HS, Sarembock IJ, Kereiakes DJ, et al: Use of bivalirudin during percutaneous coronary intervention in patients with diabetes mellitus: An analysis from the randomized evaluation in percutaneous coronary intervention linking angiomax to reduced clinical events (REPLACE)-2 trial. J Am Coll Cardiol 2005;45:1932-1938.

58. Manfredi JA, Wall RP, Sane DC, Braden GA: Lepirudin as a safe alternative for effective anticoagulation in patients with known heparin-induced thrombocytopenia undergoing percutaneous coronary intervention: Case reports. Catheter Cardiovasc Interv 2001;52:468-472.

59. Mahaffey KW, Lewis BE, Wildermann NM, et al: The anticoagulant therapy with bivalirudin to assist in the performance of percutaneous coronary intervention in patients with heparin-induced thrombocytopenia (ATBAT) study: Main results. J Invasive Cardiol 2003;15:611-616.

60. Saw J, Lincoff AM, DeSmet W, et al: Lack of clopidogrel pre-treatment effect on the relative efficacy of bivalirudin with provisional glycoprotein IIb/IIIa blockade compared to heparin with routine glycoprotein IIb/IIIa blockade: A REPLACE-2 substudy. J Am Coll Cardiol 2004;44:1194-1199.

61. Cohen DJ, Lincoff AM, Lavelle TA, et al: Economic evaluation of bivalirudin with provisional glycoprotein IIB/IIIA inhibition versus heparin with routine glycoprotein IIB/IIIA inhibition for percutaneous coronary intervention: Results from the REPLACE-2 trial. J Am Coll Cardiol 2004;44:1792-1800.

62. Harding SA, Din JN, Sarma J, et al: Promotion of proinflammatory interactions between platelets and monocytes by unfractionated heparin. Heart 2006;92:1635-1638.

63. Keating FK, Dauerman HL, Whitaker DA, et al: Increased expression of platelet P-selectin and formation of platelet-leukocyte aggregates in blood from patients treated with unfractionated heparin plus eptifibatide compared with bivalirudin. Thromb Res 2005;118:361-369.

11 Lipid Lowering in Coronary Artery Disease

Kausik K. Ray and Christopher P. Cannon

KEY POINTS

- Epidemiologic studies suggest a linear relationship between cholesterol and coronary heart disease risk.
- There is a linear relationship between the magnitude of low-density lipoprotein cholesterol (LDL-C) reduction and clinical benefit.
- Randomized trials have shown that intensive statin therapy reduces major cardiovascular events by 16% and heart failure by 27% compared with moderate statin therapy.

- In patients with coronary artery disease, LDL-C should be less than 70 mg/dL.
- Beyond LDL-C reduction, lowering C-reactive protein levels with statins is associated with greater reductions in coronary artery disease risk.
- Raising high-density lipoprotein levels appears to be beneficial, and many trials are ongoing.

EPIDEMIOLOGY

Coronary artery disease (CAD) is the largest cause of premature death in the Western world (Fig. 11-1). We are born with an LDL cholesterol (LDL-C) level of 0.8 mmol/L, which increases throughout life (Fig. 11-2A). Several epidemiologic studies have demonstrated a relationship between elevated total cholesterol and LDL-C and an increased risk of death or nonfatal myocardial infarction (MI).[1-4] The relationship between cholesterol and risk of coronary heart disease (CHD) is linear, with no apparent threshold below which risk declines (see Fig. 11-2B),[5] suggesting that interventions that reduce cholesterol the most are also likely to have the greatest impact on CHD risk reduction. The central role of cholesterol in the pathophysiology of CAD has pushed lipid-lowering therapy to the forefront of medical management of this condition.

NATIONAL CHOLESTEROL EDUCATION PROGRAM RECOMMENDATIONS

To help reduce the prevalence of elevated blood cholesterol levels in adult Americans, the National Heart, Lung, and Blood Institute (NHLBI) of the National Institutes of Health (NIH) launched the National Cholesterol Education Program (NCEP) in 1985.[6] For the first time, there was a consensus by leading experts in the field on the measurement, detection, and treatment of patients with hypercholesterolemia. The report established criteria that defined candidates with high blood cholesterol levels who should

receive medical intervention and provided guidelines on how to detect, set goals, treat, and monitor these patients over time. The NCEP-1 treatment guidelines recommended that all adults older than 20 years have a blood cholesterol measurement at least once every 5 years. Patients with levels greater than 200 mg/dL (5.2 mmol/L), confirmed by a second blood cholesterol measurement, were advised to adopt a Step 1 fat-controlled diet. Patients with cholesterol exceeding 240 mg/dL (6.2 mmol/L) were candidates for intensive treatment with a Step 2 diet and sometimes with drugs, as were those with cholesterol levels in the range of 5.2 to 6.2 mmol/L (200 to 240 mg/dL) who were at especially high risk because they already had CAD or two other risk factors. It was also recommended that drugs for lowering blood cholesterol should be used only when the indication has been confirmed by measuring LDL-C and as a supplement to the dietary treatment. These guidelines were the first initial steps toward the management of lipids that have become commonplace today.

EARLY NONSTATIN LIPID-LOWERING TRIALS

In the Lipid Research Clinics–Coronary Primary Prevention Trial (LRC-CPPT),[7] cholestyramine therapy resulted in a 13% reduction in LDL-C and a significant 19% reduction in fatal and nonfatal MI at 7 years (Table 11-1). During the first 2 years of the trial, higher event rates occurred in the cholestyramine group versus the placebo group. The Coronary Drug Project evaluated the effects of estrogen,

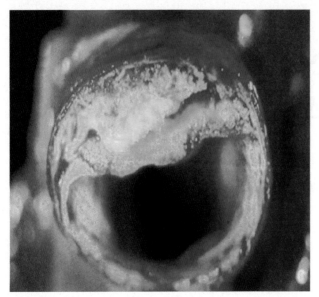

Figure 11-1. Lipid-rich atherosclerotic plaque in a coronary artery.

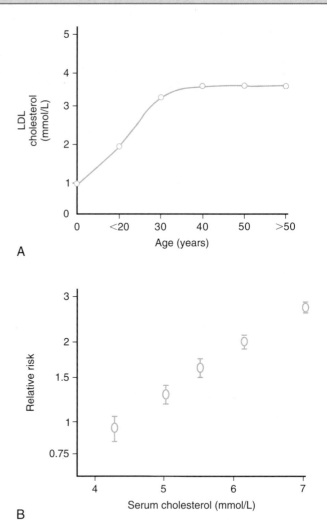

Figure 11-2. A, The change in low-density lipoprotein cholesterol (LDL-C) levels throughout life. **B,** The relationship between cholesterol and long-term risk of congestive heart failure (CHD). (**A,** data from Freedman DS, Srinivasan SE, Cresanta JL, et al: Cardiovascular risk factors from birth to 7 years of age: The Bogalusa Heart Study. Serum lipids and lipoproteins. Pediatrics 1987;80[Pt 2]:789-796 and from Webber LS, Srinivasan SE, Wattigney WA, Berenson GD: Tracking of serum lipids and lipoproteins from childhood to adulthood. The Bogalusa Heart Study. Am J Epidemiol 1991;133:884-899; **B,** data from Law MR, Wald NJ: Risk factor thresholds: Their existence under scrutiny. BMJ 2002;324:1570-1576.)

dextrothyroxine, clofibrate, and niacin on recurrent disease in men. Clofibrate resulted in an 8% reduction in total cholesterol and a 25% reduction in triglycerides but no significant reduction on the combined end point of cardiac death and nonfatal MI at 5 years.[8] Subjects who were assigned to niacin treatment achieved a 10% reduction in total cholesterol and a 25% reduction in triglyceride levels. At 5 years, a dose of niacin (3 g/day) was associated with a significant reduction in CHD death or MI (25.6% versus 30.1%, $P < .005$).[9] Benefit was not evident after the second year of therapy. The Stockholm Ischaemic Heart Disease Prevention study evaluated the combination of niacin (3 g/day) and clofibrate (2 g/day).[10] Total mortality and, notably, CHD mortality were significantly reduced in the lipid-lowering therapy group (16.8% and 21.9% versus the control group rates of 26.4% and 29.7%, $P < .05$ and $P < .01$, respectively). A significant reduction in nonfatal MI was reported at 44 months (6.8% versus 13.6%, $P < .01$). No significant benefit from gemfibrozil therapy was observed in the secondary prevention arm of the Helsinki Heart Study.[11] However, gemfibrozil therapy did reduce the rates of MI and CHD death in men in the secondary prevention Veterans Affairs High-Density Lipoprotein Cholesterol Intervention Trial (VA-HIT) (see Table 11-1).[12]

EARLY SECONDARY PREVENTION STATIN TRIALS

During a decade of clinical research, successive trials using statins have demonstrated the benefit of lowering serum cholesterol in a wide range of clinical conditions compared with diet alone. The first of these trials was the Scandinavian Simvastatin Survival Study (4S) trial, which randomized 4444 patients with angina pectoris or previous MI and serum cholesterol levels of 215 to 312 mg/dL (5.5 to 8.0 mmol/L)

to a lipid-lowering diet or to treatment with simvastatin (average dose of 20 mg/day).[13] Over 5 years, simvastatin produced mean reductions in total cholesterol and LDL-C levels of 25% and 35%, respectively. Statin therapy was associated with an absolute 4% reduction in mortality and a relative risk reduction in all-cause mortality of 30% ($P = .0003$). Significant reductions were also observed for CHD death (42%), major CHD event (34%), and the need for revascularization (37%). This was the first trial in the modern era that provided definitive proof that lipid-lowering therapy was safe and reduced the risk of cardiac death or nonfatal MI. The Cholesterol and Recurrent Events (CARE) trial quickly followed 4S

Table 11-1. Early Trials of Lipid Lowering with Nonstatin Regimens

Trial	Therapy	Lipid Differential	Outcome Treatment vs. Controls	P Value
Lipid Research Clinics-Coronary Primary Prevention Trial (LRC-CPPT)	Cholestyramine	−9% TC −13% LDL-C	CHD death or MI 7% vs. 8.60%	<0.05
Coronary Drug Project	Clofibrate	−8% TC −25% TG	CHD death 14.1% vs. 16.20%	0.06
Coronary Drug Project	Niacin	−10% TC −25% TG	CHD death 15.9% vs. 16.20%	0.5
Stockholm Ischemic Heart Disease	Niacin + clofibrate	−13% TC −19% TG	CHD death 16.8% vs. 26.40%	<0.01
Helsinki Heart	Gemfibrozil	−10% TC −41% TG	CHD death or MI 7.4% vs. 6.3%	0.14
Veterans Affairs High-Density Lipoprotein Cholesterol Intervention Trial (VA-HIT)	Gemfibrozil	−4% TC −31% TG	CHD death 17.3% vs. 21.70%	0.006
Bezafibrate Infarction Prevention (BIP)	Bezafibrate	−4% TC −21% TG	CHD death or MI 13.6% vs. 15%	0.26

LDL-C, low-density-lipoprotein cholesterol; TC, total cholesterol; TG, triglycerides.

with consistent findings, demonstrating a reduction in major coronary events with pravastatin (40 mg) versus placebo, as well as reductions in the rates of revascularization and stroke in patients with normal cholesterol levels.[14]

The Long-Term Intervention with Pravastatin in Ischaemic Disease (LIPID) trial was the largest of the three early secondary prevention trials (N = 9014 patients), and it confirmed the mortality findings of 4S in a population with an overall lower total cholesterol level.[15] LIPID demonstrated that among patients with a history of MI or hospitalization for unstable angina and initial plasma total cholesterol levels of 155 to 271 mg/dL (3.97 to 6.95 mmol/L), pravastatin (40 mg/day) reduced CHD death by 1.9%, resulting in a 24% relative risk reduction ($P < .001$). Similarly, overall mortality was reduced (22%), as were rates for recurrent MI (29%), stroke (19%), and coronary revascularization (20%). These three trials demonstrated the cumulative benefit of statins across a range of baseline cholesterol values.

HEART PROTECTION STUDY AND CHOLESTEROL TREATMENT TRIAL META-ANALYSIS

The large Heart Protection Study (HPS) demonstrated that the magnitude of benefit from statin therapy (40 mg of simvastatin) was similar at each level of baseline LDL-C, including subjects with an LDL-C level below 100 mg/dL (2.56 mmol/L).[16] HPS studied approximately 20,000 patients who were able to tolerate simvastatin (after a run-in phase) for 5 years and assessed the on-treatment (rather than intention to treat) effect of a standard dose of a statin rather than a specific cholesterol or LDL-C target. HPS, however, included a range of patients with CAD; those with prior vascular disease, such as peripheral vascular disease or stroke; and subjects without prior clinical manifestations of vascular disease who were considered at high risk, such as diabetics.[17] The implications of this trial for clinical practice were that physicians did not need to treat to specific targets,

because subjects with vascular disease all derived similar proportional reductions in risk with simvastatin (40 mg).

Preliminary evidence indicated that some overall benefit existed for statin therapy in different circumstances, such as at different ages, in men and women, and at different levels of established risk factors, but additional data involving several thousand more patients were needed to provide large-scale evidence of benefit in individual subgroups. The Cholesterol Treatment Trial (CTT) collaborators set out to undertake a prospective meta-analysis of mortality and morbidity from all relevant large-scale, randomized trials of statin therapy.[18] Data on 90,056 individuals were combined. During a mean follow-up of 5 years, there was a significant 12% reduction in all-cause mortality per 38.6-mg/dL (1-mmol/L) reduction in LDL-C, a 19% reduction in coronary mortality, a 24% reduction in the need for revascularization, and a 17% reduction in stroke. Overall, a 38.6-mg/dL (1-mmol/L) reduction in LDL was associated with a 21% reduction in any major vascular event; an absolute reduction in LDL-C of 1.8 mg/dL (0.05 mmol/L) reduced major cardiovascular events by 1%. Importantly, a similar proportional benefit was observed in different age groups, across genders, at different levels of baseline lipids (including triglycerides and high-density lipoprotein cholesterol [HDL-C]), and equally among those with prior CAD and cardiovascular risk factors and in those without (Fig. 11-3). The CTT meta-analysis collected data on 5103 new cases of cancer, with no evidence that statins increased the overall incidence of any form of cancer (HR = 1.0; $P = .9$).

These data demonstrate that compared with placebo, statin therapy is safe and reduces the 5-year incidence of major coronary events, coronary revascularization, and stroke among those at high risk for vascular disease or with preexisting disease. This magnitude of benefit is related to the magnitude of LDL-C reduction and is independent of the initial lipid profile or other presenting characteristics. The

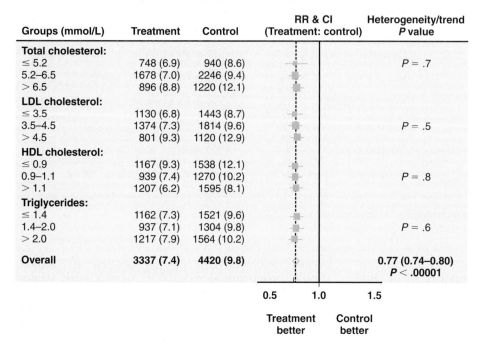

CTT collaboration effects on major coronary events per mmol/L LDL cholesterol reduction subdivided by baseline lipid values

Groups (mmol/L)	Treatment	Control	RR & CI (Treatment: control)	Heterogeneity/trend P value
Total cholesterol:				
≤ 5.2	748 (6.9)	940 (8.6)		P = .7
5.2–6.5	1678 (7.0)	2246 (9.4)		
> 6.5	896 (8.8)	1220 (12.1)		
LDL cholesterol:				
≤ 3.5	1130 (6.8)	1443 (8.7)		
3.5–4.5	1374 (7.3)	1814 (9.6)		P = .5
> 4.5	801 (9.3)	1120 (12.9)		
HDL cholesterol:				
≤ 0.9	1167 (9.3)	1538 (12.1)		
0.9–1.1	939 (7.4)	1270 (10.2)		P = .8
> 1.1	1207 (6.2)	1595 (8.1)		
Triglycerides:				
≤ 1.4	1162 (7.3)	1521 (9.6)		
1.4–2.0	937 (7.1)	1304 (9.8)		P = .6
> 2.0	1217 (7.9)	1564 (10.2)		
Overall	**3337 (7.4)**	**4420 (9.8)**		0.77 (0.74–0.80) P < .00001

0.5   1.0   1.5

Treatment better   Control better

Figure 11-3. The relationship between baseline lipid levels and the benefit of statin therapy was shown in the Cholesterol Treatment Trial (CTT) meta-analysis. The effects of major coronary events per 1 mmol/L of low-density lipoprotein (LDL) cholesterol reduction subdivided by baseline lipid values are shown. (Modified from Baigent C, Keech A, Kearney PM, et al: Efficacy and safety of cholesterol-lowering treatment: Prospective meta-analysis of data from 90,056 participants in 14 randomised trials of statins. Lancet 2005;366:1267-1278.)

absolute benefit correlates chiefly with an individual's absolute risk of cardiovascular events, reinforcing the need to consider long-term statin therapy among all individuals at high risk for any type of major vascular event.

INTENSIVE STATIN THERAPY FOR ACUTE CORONARY SYNDROME

The early trials looking at treatment of acute coronary syndrome (ACS) (i.e., 4S, CARE, and LIPID) excluded patients within the first 4- to 6-month period after ACS. The Myocardial Ischemia Reduction with Acute Cholesterol Lowering (MIRACL) trial provided the first evidence that statin therapy initiated early after ACS reduced adverse clinical events by 16 weeks.[19] However, the higher than usual dose of statin (80 mg of atorvastatin) and lack of an active comparator coupled with an absence of long-term safety data limited the widespread applicability of its findings.

PROVE IT-TIMI 22 Trial

The Pravastatin or Atorvastatin Evaluation and Infection Therapy–Thrombolysis In Myocardial Infarction 22 (PROVE IT-TIMI 22) was the first large-scale study of statin therapy comparing two active comparators. In the PROVE IT-TIMI 22) trial, patients who had been hospitalized for ACS within the preceding 10 days (N = 4162) were randomized to 40 mg of pravastatin (i.e., standard therapy) or 80 mg of atorvastatin daily (i.e., intensive therapy).[20] The primary end point was a composite of death from any cause, MI,

documented unstable angina requiring rehospitalization, revascularization (performed at least 30 days after randomization), and stroke.

In PROVE IT, the median LDL-C level achieved during treatment was 95 mg/dL (2.46 mmol/L) in the standard-therapy group and 62 mg/dL (1.60 mmol/L) in the high-dose group (P < .001). Kaplan-Meier estimates of the rates of the primary end point at 2 years were 26.3% for standard therapy and 22.4% for intensive therapy, reflecting a 16% reduction in the hazard ratio (HR) in favor of intensive therapy (P = .005). Muscle-related side effects were low and not significantly different between groups. There were no cases of rhabdomyolysis.

A to Z Trial

The Aggrastat to Zocor study (A to Z trial) compared an early initiation of an intensive statin regimen with delayed initiation of a less-intensive regimen in patients with ACS.[21] Patients with ACS (N = 4497) received 40 mg of simvastatin for 1 month, followed by 80 mg thereafter, which was compared with placebo for 4 months, followed by 20 mg of simvastatin. The primary end point was a composite of cardiovascular death, nonfatal MI, readmission for ACS, and stroke. The median LDL-C level on placebo was 122 mg/dL (3.16 mmol/L) at 1 month and was 77 mg/dL (1.99 mmol/L) at 8 months on 20 mg of simvastatin. The median LDL-C concentration achieved at 1 month while taking 40 mg of simvastatin was 68 mg/dL (1.76 mmol/L) and was 63 mg/dL (1.63 mmol/L) at 8 months while taking 80 mg of simvastatin. Overall, 16.7% in the placebo plus simvastatin group experienced the primary end point, compared with 14.4% in the simvastatin only group (40 mg/80 mg), reflecting a hazard ratio of 0.89 (P = .14). Myopathy (i.e., creatine kinase >10 times the upper limits of normal with muscle symptoms) occurred in 9 patients (0.4%) receiving 80 mg of simvastatin, in no patients receiving lower doses of simvastatin, and in 1 patient receiving placebo (P = .02).

The PROVE IT-TIMI 22 and A to Z trials compared similar intensive and moderate statin therapy after ACS, with apparently disparate results. An analysis comparing and contrasting the two trials observed differences between the trials in baseline demographic characteristics, geographic location, and use of percutaneous coronary intervention (PCI).[22] The LDL-C level difference was greater early in the A to Z trial than in PROVE IT (≤4 months), but the difference was less late in the trials. Significant C-reactive protein (CRP) reduction also occurred earlier in PROVE IT. With common end points, an early favorable separation of event curves was seen in PROVE IT but not in the A to Z trial. Clinical end point rates and reductions were similar in both trials after 4 months. Factors that may explain this disparity include the statin regimen in the early phase, leading to differences in the magnitude of LDL-C lowering and CRP levels and differences in the early use of PCI. In summary, the results of these trials support a strategy of early, intensive statin therapy coupled with revascularization when appropriate in patients after ACS (Fig. 11-4).[22]

INTENSIVE STATIN THERAPY IN STABLE CORONARY ARTERY DISEASE

Despite the landmark results from PROVE IT, which led to NCEP recommending an optional LDL-C goal of less than 70 mg/dL in high-risk patients,[23] several questions arose, such as whether intensive statin therapy was safe over a longer period and whether intensive statin therapy was as beneficial in subjects with stable CAD as in ACS patients. The Treating to New Targets (TNT)[24] and Incremental Decrease in Endpoints through Aggressive Lipid Lowering (IDEAL)[25] trials addressed these issues and provided approximately 50,000 patient-years of data on the safety and efficacy of intensive statin therapy.

TNT Trial

The TNT trial compared a strategy of intensive lipid lowering using 80 mg of atorvastatin with 10 mg of atorvastatin in patients with stable CHD in 10,001 patients over 5.5 years. The definition of CHD in the study population included patients with previous MI, those with stable angina with objective evidence of atherosclerotic CHD, or patients who had undergone revascularization. After an open-label run-in phase with 10 mg of atorvastatin for 8 weeks, patients were randomized to 10 or 80 mg of atorvastatin (i.e., double-blind period). The primary end point of TNT was the time to occurrence of a major cardiovascular event, defined as CHD death, nonfatal MI, resuscitated cardiac arrest, and fatal or nonfatal stroke. During the open-label phase, LDL-C levels fell from 152 mg/dL (3.9 mmol/L) to a mean of 98 mg/dL (2.6 mmol/L). Among those randomized to 80 mg of atorvastatin after the open-label phase, LDL-C fell further by 21.4% to a mean of 77 mg/dL (2 mmol/L). A significant further reduction in triglycerides was observed with the 80-mg dose, but there was no significant difference in HDL-C levels between doses. The primary end point occurred in 8.7% of the 80-mg atorvastatin group and in 10.9% of the 10-mg atorvastatin group, reflecting a 22% risk reduction (HR = 0.78; P < .001). Clinical benefit appeared within 6 months against a background of aggressive medical therapy. This benefit was largely driven by significant reductions in nonfatal MI (HR = 0.78; range, 0.66 to

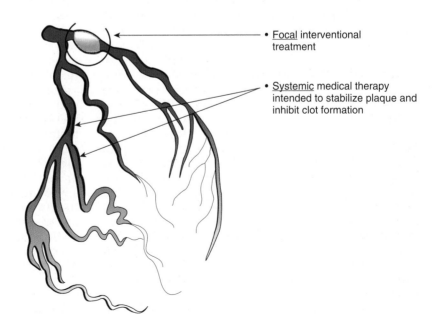

- Focal interventional treatment

- Systemic medical therapy intended to stabilize plaque and inhibit clot formation

Figure 11-4. Complementary benefit of percutaneous coronary intervention and intensive statin therapy in patients with acute coronary syndrome. (Redrawn from Ambrose JA, Martinez EE: A new paradigm for plaque stabilization. Circulation 2002;105:2000-2004.)

0.93; $P = .004$) and fatal or nonfatal stroke (HR = 0.75; $P = .02$). A trend in favor of cardiovascular death was also observed, which was not significant. Overall, intensive therapy was safe, with no excess risk of adverse effects occurring with intensive therapy.

IDEAL Trial

The Incremental Decrease in Endpoints through Aggressive Lipid Lowering (IDEAL) trial was a randomized, open-label trial that compared a strategy of achieving an approximately 35% reduction in LDL-C using the 20/40-mg dose of simvastatin versus a strategy of achieving a 55% reduction in LDL-C using 80 mg of atorvastatin in patients with a history of MI. Patients were recruited months to years after the index MI, making IDEAL comparable in design to the 4S and CARE trials.[13,14] Approximately 70% of patients were on statin therapy before study entry, and about 50% of participants were subjects previously enrolled in the 4S trial. The primary end point was coronary death, nonfatal MI, or resuscitated cardiac arrest. IDEAL enrolled 8888 patients and had a mean follow-up period of 4.8 years. During follow-up, the mean LDL-C level was 104 mg/dL (2.69 mmol/L) in the 20/40-mg simvastatin group and 82 mg/dL (2.12 mmol/L) in the 80-mg atorvastatin group. Major coronary events tended to be lower with intensive therapy (HR 0.89; $P = .07$) but did not achieve statistical significance. Major cardiovascular events and any coronary event were significantly reduced by 13% ($P = .02$) and 16% ($P < .001$), respectively, in the 80-mg atorvastatin group. There was no excess risk of noncardiovascular death with intensive therapy (HR = 0.92; $P = .47$). With the exception of transient elevations in liver transaminase levels, there were no significant differences between treatments.

The results of the TNT and IDEAL trials further establish the important role for intensive statin therapy in the management of patients with stable CAD and extend the observations from PROVE IT-TIMI 22 in ACS patients to patients with stable disease. The IDEAL trial disproved the earlier concerns raised by TNT that intensive statin therapy might be associated with an excess risk of noncardiovascular mortality and provided further safety data on 80 mg of atorvastatin in more than 20,000 patient-years of follow-up. Some observers have questioned the importance of TNT and IDEAL, citing that the benefit of intensive therapy in these trials tends to be driven by the so-called soft end points, such as recurrent MI or revascularization, compared, for instance, with the landmark 4S trial, in which total mortality was reduced in the statin group compared with placebo. However, in the decade since 4S was completed, the management of CAD has improved dramatically with greater use of additional cardioprotective medication and greater use of revascularization. It is therefore unlikely that a significant benefit in all-cause mortality would be observed with intensive compared with standard therapy unless a much larger trial (perhaps requiring about 50,000 patients) with a longer follow-up is conducted.

Atherosclerosis is a chronic disease, and patients who are commenced on statins require this treatment for the remainder of their lives. The benefits of intensive therapy observed in TNT and IDEAL over about 5 years are likely to translate into even greater reductions in the number of events over a longer period, providing significant benefits for individuals and health care systems.

META-ANALYSIS OF INTENSIVE VERSUS STANDARD THERAPY

The four intensive versus standard therapy trials used different end points to assess clinical benefit and were each underpowered to assess the historical end point of CHD death, or nonfatal MI. A literature-based meta-analysis was conducted to obtain consistent large-scale evidence across trials. All eligible trials were required to have at least 1000 participants and a treatment duration of at least 2 years.[26] The four trials discussed previously—PROVE IT-TIMI 22,[20] A to Z,[21] TNT,[24] and IDEAL[25]—were identified, providing information on 27,548 patients and approximately 120,000 patient-years of follow-up data.[20,21,24,25] A separate meta-analysis of the same four trials also assessed the effect of intensive versus standard therapy for reductions in hospitalization with heart failure.[27]

The average, pooled baseline LDL-C level in the four trials was 130 mg/dL (3.3 mmol/L), which was reduced on average to 101 mg/dL (2.59 mmol/L). With intensive therapy, the average LDL-C level was lowered further to 75 mg/dL (1.92 mmol/L).[26] This additional reduction in LDL-C was associated with a 16% reduction in the risk of CHD death or MI (OR -0.84; $P = .00003$) (Fig. 11-5). Similarly, there was a reduction in the risk of any major cardiovascular event by 16% ($P < .0001$). There was a favorable trend toward reduction in CHD death (OR = 0.88; $P = .054$) and no excess risk in non-cardiovascular mortality was observed (OR = 1.03; $P = .73$). Reductions were observed for stroke (OR = 0.82; $P = .012$) and for hospitalization for CHF (OR = 0.73; $P < .001$).[27]

Statin therapy is now recommended for all patients with established atherosclerotic vascular disease. This meta-analysis extends the earlier findings (i.e., CTT meta-analysis) and demonstrates that beyond standard therapy, additional intensive LDL-C reduction provides an additional 16% reduction in risk of CHD or nonfatal MI or any major cardiovascular event, or approximately a 50% reduction versus placebo. Given the improvement in standards of medical care and use of revascularization over the past decade, these additional benefits may seem modest but are achieved over 2 to 5 years. Given the chronic, lifelong nature of these diseases, these benefits throughout an individual's life would be expected to translate into greater absolute benefits by preventing recurrent, multiple events.

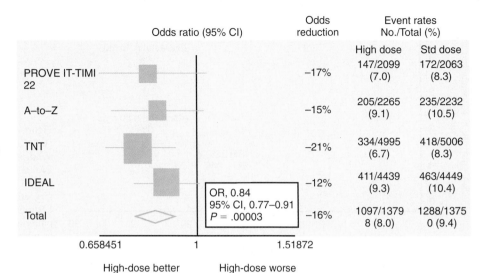

	Odds ratio (95% CI)	Odds reduction	Event rates No./Total (%)	
			High dose	Std dose
PROVE IT-TIMI 22		−17%	147/2099 (7.0)	172/2063 (8.3)
A–to–Z		−15%	205/2265 (9.1)	235/2232 (10.5)
TNT		−21%	334/4995 (6.7)	418/5006 (8.3)
IDEAL		−12%	411/4439 (9.3)	463/4449 (10.4)
Total	OR, 0.84 95% CI, 0.77–0.91 P = .00003	−16%	1097/13798 (8.0)	1288/13750 (9.4)

0.658451   1   1.51872

High-dose better   High-dose worse

Figure 11-5. Meta-analysis of intensive versus standard therapy, showing reductions in coronary heart disease, death, or nonfatal myocardial infarction. (Data from Cannon CP, Steinberg BS, Murphy SA, et al: Meta-analysis of cardiovascular outcomes trials comparing intensive versus moderate statin therapy. J Am Coll Cardiol 2006;48:438-445.)

Observational studies have suggested that among patients with heart failure, a low LDL-C level is associated with an increased risk of adverse events.[28,29] However, it is likely that these observations are confounded given the results of the meta-analysis, which showed reductions in the risk of the development of heart failure with intensive versus standard therapy. Although it is not immediately intuitive what role lowering LDL-C levels plays in reducing the risk of heart failure, results of the latest meta-analysis may reflect the beneficial effects of high-dose statin therapy beyond LDL-C reduction, the so-called pleiotropic effect.

EARLY BENEFITS OF INTENSIVE STATIN THERAPY FOR ACUTE CORONARY SYNDROME

The risk of adverse clinical events is greatest in the first 6 months after the index ACS event. The early trials of statin therapy in patients with stable CAD suggested that the benefits of statin therapy appeared only after 1 to 2 years.[13,14] Although plaque rupture is a feature of ACS (Fig. 11-6), it has become apparent that ACS is a pancoronary process with multiple vulnerable or ruptured plaques (Fig. 11-7). Although angioplasty and stenting treat a culprit lesion effectively, potent systemic therapy is required to passivate other vulnerable sites.[30]

The PROVE IT trial, conducted in patients enrolled within 10 days of experiencing an ACS, demonstrated the superiority of intensive versus standard statin therapy in these patients over a period of 2 years, but it was unclear whether this benefit was related principally to a very early benefit, to a late benefit after patients had stabilized, or to a combination of the two. Using a composite end point of death, MI, or rehospitalization for recurrent ACS (i.e., the common end point in ACS trials), the benefit of intensive statin therapy was assessed in the first 30 days after ACS and in more stable patients from 6 months through end of study.[31] This particular analysis

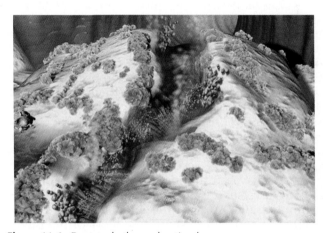

Figure 11-6. Ruptured atherosclerotic plaque.

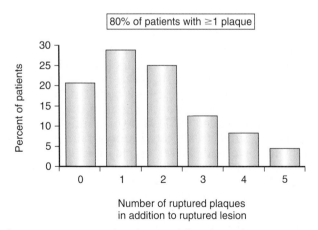

Figure 11-7. Intravascular ultrasound data shows that acute coronary syndrome patients have multiple vulnerable or ruptured plaques. (Data from Rioufol G, Finet G, Ginon I, et al: Multiple atherosclerotic plaque rupture in acute coronary syndrome: A three-vessel intravascular ultrasound study. Circulation 2002;106:804-808.)

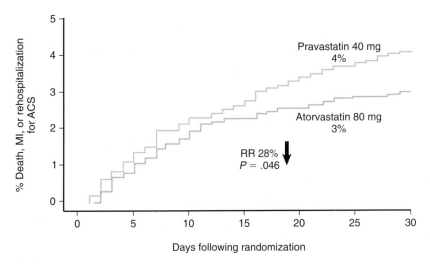

Figure 11-8. Early benefit of intensive standard statin therapy within 30 days after acute coronary syndrome (ACS) in the Pravastatin or Atorvastatin Evaluation and Infection Therapy (PROVE IT) trial. (Data from Ray KK, Cannon CP, McCabe CH, et al, for the PROVE IT-TIMI 22 Investigators: Early and late benefits of high-dose atorvastatin in patients with acute coronary syndromes: Results from the PROVE IT-TIMI 22 trial. J Am Coll Cardiol. 2005;46:1405-1410.)

demonstrated that the composite end point occurred in 15.7% of patients assigned to 80 mg of atorvastatin and in 20.0% of patients assigned to 40 mg of pravastatin, reflecting a risk reduction of 24% ($P = .0002$). Benefit in favor of 80 mg of atorvastatin was observed as early as 15 days after randomization and was significant by day 30. The composite end point occurred in 3.0% of the intensive-therapy group and in 4.2 % of the standard-therapy group at 30 days, reflecting a 28% risk reduction at 30 days ($P = .046$) with 80 mg of atorvastatin (Fig. 11-8). In addition to greater reductions in LDL levels, 80 mg of atorvastatin reduced CRP levels to a greater extent than 40 mg of pravastatin, independent of effects on LDL (1.6 mg/L versus 2.3 mg/L, $P < .0001$). Commencing 6 months after ACS to the end of the study, the composite end point occurred in 9.6% of the intensive-therapy group and 13.1% of the standard-therapy group, representing a 28% further risk reduction ($P = .003$) in favor of high-dose atorvastatin (80 mg). This suggests that among patients who tolerate high-dose statin therapy, continuation of high-dose therapy is beneficial and provides early and late benefits.

PROVE IT demonstrated that high-dose statin therapy lowers LDL-C and CRP concentrations at 30 days and is associated with a reduction in clinical events. In contrast, the A to Z trial showed a greater difference in resulting LDL levels between intensive versus moderate statin regimens but no difference in CRP levels at 30 days and, significantly, no early benefit was observed.[21,22] Despite matching for LDL-C at day 30, subjects allocated atorvastatin were less likely to have had an MI or recurrent ACS in the previous 30 days, suggesting that the early benefit is related to effects beyond the concentration of LDL-C and that lowering CRP levels may reduce inflammation and may be more important than lipid lowering with respect to early benefits.[32]

A meta-analysis of 13 randomized trials of early statin therapy for management of ACS assessed the early benefit of statin therapy using cumulative data on 17,963 patients.[33] Only five of the trials enrolled more than 1000 patients, and of these, only three trials had follow-up periods for more than 4 months, and only two trials followed patients for more than 1 year. This meta-analysis assessed major cardiovascular events, including stroke. In particular, the latter end point requires about 2 years to demonstrate a clinical benefit and might have attenuated any observed early benefits on CHD. In this analysis, early benefit was not observed at 1 month after ACS (HR = 1.02) but appeared by 4 months (HR = 0.84) and was significant by 6 months (HR = 0.76).

INTENSIVE STATIN THERAPY AND ATHEROSCLEROSIS

Given the clinical impact of statin therapy of cardiovascular event reduction in patients with CAD, it is intuitive to expect that statins would reverse atherosclerosis disease burden. Several trials used angiography to assess the impact of standard-dose statin therapy on the extent of angiographic disease. Although standard doses of statins reduced LDL-C levels by 20% to 30%, they failed to demonstrate regression of disease burden, but instead consistently showed that in the presence of CAD, statins reduce the rate of progression of disease.[34]

REVERSAL Trial

The Reversing Atherosclerosis with Aggressive Lipid Lowering (REVERSAL) trial compared the effects of two statin regimens administered for 18 months in 654 patients. Patients were randomized to a moderate-lipid-lowering regimen consisting of 40 mg of pravastatin (licensed in the United States for reducing atherosclerosis progression) or an intensive-lipid-lowering regimen consisting of 80 mg of atorvastatin. The primary efficacy parameter was the percentage of change in atheroma volume (i.e., follow-up value minus baseline). Secondary efficacy parameters included change in total atheroma volume, change in percentage of atheroma volume, and change in atheroma volume in the most severely diseased 10-mm vessel subsegment.

The baseline LDL-C concentration fell from 150.2 mg/dL (3.89 mmol/L) in both treatment groups to 110 mg/dL (2.85 mmol/L) in the pravastatin group and to 79 mg/dL (2.05 mmol/L) in the atorvastatin group (P < .001). CRP levels decreased 5.2% with pravastatin and 36.4% with atorvastatin (P < .001). In subjects receiving standard therapy, the percentage of change in atheroma volume from baseline was 2.7% (P < .001), and in those allocated to intensive therapy, it was –0.4% (P = .98; for difference between groups, P = .02). Similar differences between groups were observed for secondary efficacy parameters, including change in total atheroma volume (P = .02), change in percentage of atheroma volume (P < .001), and change in atheroma volume in the most severely diseased 10-mm vessel subsegment (P < .01).

ASTEROID Trial

A Study to Evaluate the Effect of Rosuvastatin on Intravascular Ultrasound-Derived Coronary Atheroma Burden (ASTEROID) assessed whether intensive statin therapy with 40 mg of rosuvastatin could regress atherosclerosis in patients with CAD assessed by intravascular ultrasound (IVUS). A motorized IVUS pullback was used to assess coronary atheroma burden at baseline and after 24 months of treatment in 507 patients.

The mean (SD) baseline LDL-C level of 130.4 mg/dL declined to 60.8 mg/dL; mean HDL-C level at baseline was 43.1 mg/dL, increasing to 49.0 mg/dL; and the median concentration of triglycerides fell from 135 mg/dL to 109 mg/dL. The mean change in percentage of atheroma volume from baseline for the entire vessel was –0.98 %. The mean change in atheroma volume in the most diseased 10-mm subsegment was –6.1 mm³ (P < .001 versus baseline). Change in total atheroma volume showed a 6.8% median reduction (P < .001 versus baseline).

These two studies using IVUS confirm that standard statin therapy does not arrest the progression of atherosclerosis and that more intensive therapy is required to stop or even regress preexisting disease burden (Fig. 11-9). Although the findings in ASTEROID appear more dramatic than the initial findings in REVERSAL, some key differences should be considered. There was no active comparator arm in ASTEROID, which makes it unclear what effect other statin regimens would have had in the same population. This is particularly important because in REVERSAL, specific subgroups such as nondiabetics and those with lower LDL-C levels appeared to derive greater benefit from 80 mg of atorvastatin. Compared with REVERSAL, there were a greater number of patients in the ASTEROID trial and consequently greater power to demonstrate regression. The ASTEROID population had a lower baseline LDL-C concentration, had a lower baseline level of triglycerides, and had fewer diabetics, which might have favored demonstration of disease regression resulting from intensive therapy. In ASTEROID, there was higher percentage of patients with no IVUS follow-up for clinical end points compared with REVERSAL, highlighting the difficulty of comparing trials. Nevertheless, these trials and similar studies such as the Early Statin Treatment in Patients with Acute Coronary Syndrome: Demonstration of the Beneficial Effect on Atherosclerotic Lesions by Serial Volumetric Intravascular Ultrasound Analysis during Half a Year after Coronary Event (ESTABLISH trial), which studied ACS patients[35,36] cumulatively, demonstrate the need for intensive lipid reduction to arrest disease progression in subjects with established atherosclerosis.

MECHANISMS OF BENEFIT

Intensity of Low-Density Lipoprotein Reduction

Given prior epidemiologic data and clear evidence that a statin is better than placebo and that an intensive statin regimen is better than a standard-dose

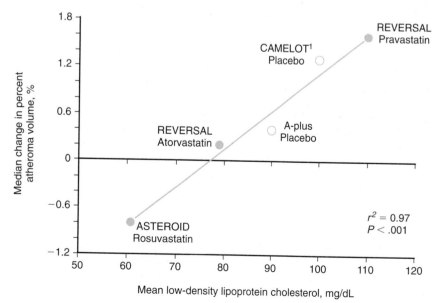

Figure 11-9. Relationship between low-density lipoprotein cholesterol and atherosclerosis progression on intravascular ultrasound in the Reversing Atherosclerosis with Aggressive Lipid Lowering (REVERSAL), Comparison of Amlodipine vs Enalapril to Limit Occurrences of Thrombosis (CAMELOT), Avasimibe and Progression of Coronary Lesions Assessed by Intravascular Ultrasound (A-PLUS), and A Study to Evaluate the Effect of Rosuvastatin on Intravascular Ultrasound-Derived Coronary Atheroma Burden (ASTEROID) trials, (Data from Nissen SE, Nicholls SJ, Sipayhi I, et al: Effect of very high-intensity statin therapy on regression of coronary atherosclerosis: The ASTEROID trial. 2006,;295:1555-1565.)

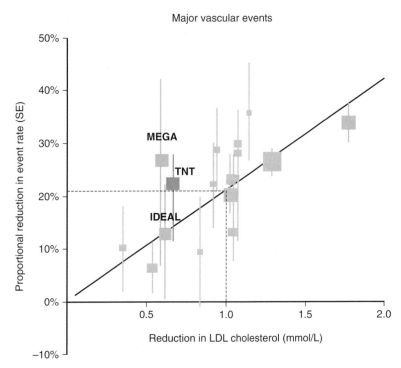

Major vascular events

Figure 11-10. Updated Cholesterol Treatment Trial (CTT) meta-analysis, including the Treating to New Targets (TNT), Individualized Dosing Efficacy versus Flat Dosing to Assess Optimal Pegylated Interferon Therapy (IDEAL), and Management of Elevated Cholesterol in the Primary Prevention Group of Adult Japanese (MEGA) trials, showing the linear relationship between low-density lipoprotein cholesterol (LDL-C) reduction and clinical risk reduction. (Modified from Baigent C, Keech A, Kearney PM, et al: Efficacy and safety of cholesterol-lowering treatment: Prospective meta-analysis of data from 90,056 participants in 14 randomised trials of statins. Lancet. 2005;366:1267-1278.)

statin regimen, subjects with CAD who achieved the lowest levels of LDL-C would be expected to be at lowest risk for recurrent events. In the CTT meta-analysis, when all trials were considered and a regression line forced through zero, a linear relationship between lower LDL-C levels and risk reduction was observed. The current intensive versus moderate statin therapy trials also fit this regression model, suggesting that the greater the LDL-C difference between two strategies, the greater is the clinical benefit (Fig. 11-10).

However, the long-term efficacy of statin therapy in patients achieving very low LDL-C levels (<100 mg/dL) remained poorly assessed until recently. In an analysis from PROVE IT-TIMI 22, the relationship between achieved LDL-C levels and clinical outcomes with 80 mg of atorvastatin was assessed by dividing these patients into subgroups by achieved LDL-C levels at 4 months (>80 to 100, >60 to 80, >40 to 60, ≤40 mg/dL) and correlating this with risk of subsequent adverse events.[37] Among almost 2000 subjects with 4-month LDL-C data available, about 90% had LDL-C levels less than 100 mg/dL (2.59 mmol/L). Compared with the reference group (LDL-C level of 80 to 100 mg/dL), the hazard of death, MI, stroke, recurrent ischemia, and revascularization was lower among patients with LDL-C levels between more than 40 and 60 (HR = 0.76) and lowest among those with LDL-C levels less than or equal to 40 mg/dL (HR = 0.61). There was no excess risk of adverse events at these low levels of LDL-C. It is not necessary to reduce the dose of a statin if the resultant LDL-C levels fall well below guideline recommendations. These results suggest the possibility that further LDL-C lowering beyond the new guideline optimal goal of less than 70 mg/dL (1.8 mmol/L) may translate into additional clinical benefit.

Reduction in C-Reactive Protein Levels

Statins possess pleiotropic effects that are mediated by HMG-CoA reductase but are not dependent on lowering of LDL-C levels (Fig. 11-11). All statins lower CRP levels, in part related to the statin dose. In PROVE IT, the median levels of CRP were similar in the 80-mg atorvastatin and 40-mg pravastatin groups (12.2 and 11.9 mg/L, respectively; $P = .60$) at study entry, but they were significantly lower in the atorvastatin group than in the pravastatin group at 30 days (1.6 versus 2.3 mg/L, $P < .001$), 4 months (1.3 versus 2.1 mg/L, $P < .001$), and the end of the study (1.3 versus 2.1 mg/L, $P < .001$). Although the levels of LDL-C and CRP were reduced by statin therapy at 30 days, the correlation between the achieved values was weak. (r = .16; $P = .001$) (i.e., less than 3% of the variance in achieved CRP levels was explained by the variance in achieved LDL). Because there are other known correlates of CRP in statin-naïve subjects, further assessment from PROVE IT performed a cross-sectional analysis of the relationship between on-treatment uncontrolled risk factors and CRP levels.[38] These factors were defined as body mass index (BMI) greater than 25 kg/m^2 (i.e., World Health Organization's cutoff for overweight), blood pressure higher than 130/85 mm Hg, glucose concentration higher than 110 mg/dL, triglyceride level greater than 150 mg/dL (i.e., Adult Treatment Panel III of the National Cholesterol Education Program's cutoffs), HDL level less than 50 mg/dL, LDL-C level equal to or greater than 70 mg/dL, and smoking. An increase

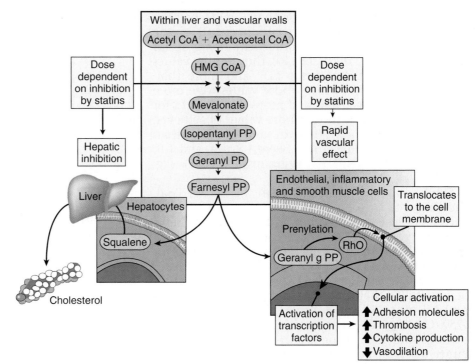

Figure 11-11. Inhibition of HMG-CoA reductase leads to low-density lipoprotein cholesterol (LDL-C)–mediated effects through the liver and nonlipid-related effects in the vessel wall. (From Ray KK, Cannon CP: The potential relevance of the multiple lipid-independent (pleiotropic) effects of statins in the management of acute coronary syndromes. J Am Coll Cardiol 2005;46:1425-1433.)

in incremental risk factor burden (i.e., number of uncontrolled risk factors present) was associated with an increase in CRP values (Fig. 11-12). Among patients allocated to standard therapy, the CRP level was 3.8 mg/L (interquartile range [IQR]: 1.9, 7.8) when seven uncontrolled risk factors were present and 1.0 mg/L (IQR: 0.7, 2.1) when none were present (*P* < .0001 for trend). However, among patients allocated intensive therapy, the corresponding CRP levels were lower and ranged from 2.4 mg/L (IQR: 1.7, 5.7) to 0.8 mg/L (IQR: 0.4, 1.2) (*P* < .0001 for trend). In this population, in which everyone received a statin, prior randomization to 80 mg of atorvastatin was associated with a 27% lower CRP compared with 40 mg of pravastatin (*P* < .0001) independently of LDL-C, triglyceride, and HDL levels and other correlates of CRP, such as age, gender, glycemia, blood pressure, smoking, and BMI.[38]

At 30 days, the median LDL concentration was approximately 70 mg/L, and the median CRP level was approximately 2 mg/L. At 30 days, patients in whom statin therapy resulted in LDL-C levels less than 70 mg/dL had lower age-adjusted rates of recurrent MI or CHD death compared with those who did not achieve this goal (2.7 versus. 4.0 events per 100 person-years, *P* = .008). Despite the minimal correlation between LDL-C and CRP levels, an identical difference in the age-adjusted rates of events was also observed among patients in whom statin therapy resulted in CRP levels of less than 2 mg/L compared with those in whom statin therapy resulted in higher CRP values (2.8 versus 3.9 events per 100 person-years, *P* = .006). Patients who had achieved LDL-C levels less than 70 mg/dL and CRP levels less than 2 mg/L had the lowest risk of recurrent events, whereas those with LDL-C levels more than

Figure 11-12. Relationships among uncontrolled risk factors, statin therapy, and achieved C-reactive protein (CRP) levels. (From Ray KK, Cannon CP: The potential relevance of the multiple lipid-independent (pleiotropic) effects of statins in the management of acute coronary syndromes. J Am Coll Cardiol 2005;46:1425-1433.)

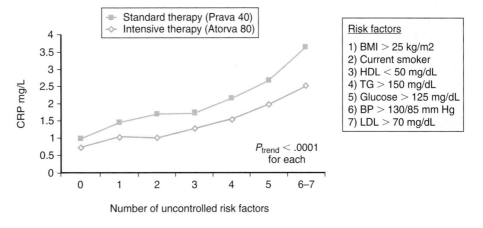

70 mg/dL and CRP levels more than 2 mg/L had the highest risk. Hazard ratios for recurrent events among patients whose values were more than 70 mg/dL for LDL-C and below 2 mg/L for CRP, those whose values were less than 70 mg/dL for LDL and more than 2 mg/L for CRP, and those whose values were more than 70 mg/dL for LDL-C and more than 2 mg/L for CRP, compared with those whose values of achieved LDL-C were less than 70 mg/dL and CRP less than 2 mg/L (i.e., reference group), were 1.3, 1.4, and 1.9, respectively (for trend across groups, P < .001) (Fig. 11-13A).

Similar data have emerged from the A to Z Trial, showing that subjects who achieve a low CRP level with high-dose statin therapy and those who achieve the dual goals of LDL-C levels less than 70 mg/dL and CRP levels less than 2 mg/L are at lower risk for recurrent events (see Fig. 11-13B).[39] Meta-analysis of achieved CRP levels in the PROVE IT and A to Z trials demonstrated that the adjusted risk of death or recurrent MI of a CRP value greater than 2 mg/L is 1.43 (95% CI: 1.2 to 1.7). These secondary prevention data demonstrate that using statin therapy to achieve target levels of both LDL-C and CRP decreases the risk of recurrent MI and CHD death among patients with ACS. Whether CRP is causally related to risk or is a marker remains unclear, but several lines of evidence suggest that it is an important player in mediating cardiovascular risk (Fig. 11-14). These data support the hypothesis that therapies designed to reduce inflammation after ACS may improve cardiovascular outcomes.

Apolipoprotein B

Although the clinical benefits of statins appear to be predominantly related to LDL-C–mediated effects, the LDL-C level incompletely measures atherogenic lipoproteins, and measurement of the concentration of apolipoprotein B (apoB), which is a direct measurement of the concentration of proatherogenic particles (e.g., LDL-C, VLDL, IDL), and measurement of non-HDL-C, which reflects the cholesterol concentration of atherogenic lipoproteins or the total cholesterol to HDL ratio, provide alternative approaches. The debate regarding the choice of the best lipid parameter has further intensified with apparently conflicting evidence between prospective studies.[40-42] In statin trials, conflicting data exists about whether on-treatment lipid values alone explain the totality of the benefits of statin therapy. In the Air Force/Texas Coronary Atherosclerosis Prevention Study (AFCAPS/TexCAPS) trial, on-treatment apoB values appeared to be a superior marker of on-treatment efficacy compared with LDL-C levels, and the on-treatment apoB/A-I ratio appeared to explain the entire benefit of statin therapy in this trial.[43] In contrast, the much larger LIPID trial suggested that the proportion of the treatment effect explained by reductions in LDL-C was 52%, compared with 67% for apoB,[44] suggesting that nonlipid-related effects may also contribute to the long-term benefit of

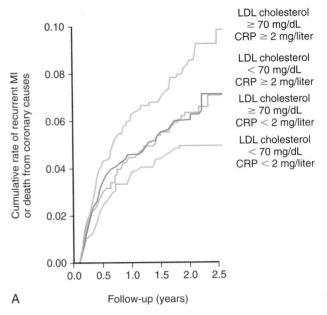

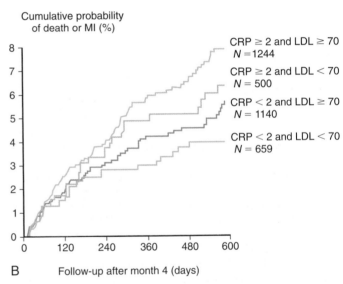

Figure 11-13. Clinical benefit of achieving the dual goals of low-density lipoprotein (LDL) less than 70 mg/dL and C-reactive protein (CRP) levels of less than 2 mg/L with statin therapy in the Pravastatin or Atorvastatin Evaluation and Infection Therapy–Thrombolysis In Myocardial Infarction 22 (PROVE IT-TIMI 22) **(A)** and Aggrastat to Zocor (A to Z) trials **(B),** showing the benefit of achieving dual goals. (**A,** from Ridker PM, Cannon CP, Morrow D, et al, for the Pravastatin or Atorvastatin Evaluation and Infection Therapy–Thrombolysis in Myocardial Infarction 22 (PROVE IT-TIMI 22) Investigators: C-reactive protein levels and outcomes after statin therapy. N Engl J Med 2005;352:20-28; **B,** from Morrow DA, de Lemos JA, Sabatine MS, et al: Clinical relevance of C-reactive protein during follow-up of patients with acute coronary syndromes in the Aggrastat-to-Zocor Trial. Circulation 2006;114:281-288.)

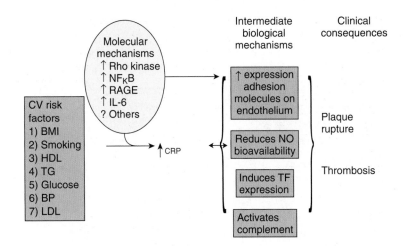

Figure 11-14. Schematic of putative mechanisms by which C-reactive protein (CRP) may mediate cardiovascular (CV) risk. BMI, body mass index; BP, blood pressure; HDL, high-density lipoprotein; IL-6, interleukin-6; LDL, low-density lipoprotein; NO, nitric oxide; TF, tissue factor; TG, triglycerides.

statins. There is little conclusive evidence to suggest that we should measure apoB as an alternative to LDL-C in routine clinical practice.

Oxidized Low-Density Lipoprotein

Oxidized phospholipids (OxPLs) exist within atherosclerotic plaques and are bound by lipoprotein(a) in plasma. Circulating levels of oxidized LDL are strongly associated with angiographically documented CAD and therefore may contribute to the pathogenesis of atherosclerosis.[45] In the MIRACL trial, high-dose atorvastatin reduced the total apoB-containing OxPLs by 29.7%, as well as reducing apoB levels by 30%. When normalized per apoB-100, compared with placebo, atorvastatin increased the OxPL/apoB level (9.5% versus –3.9%, $P < .0001$). These data suggest that atorvastatin treatment results in enrichment of OxPLs on a smaller pool of apoB particles, which may contribute to the reduction in ischemic events after ACS observed in MIRACL.[46]

HDL as a carrier of excess cellular cholesterol in the reverse cholesterol transport pathway is believed to provide protection against atherosclerosis. In reverse cholesterol transport, peripheral tissues (e.g., vessel-wall macrophages) remove their excess cholesterol through the ATP-binding cassette transporter A1 (ABCA1) to poorly lipidated apolipoprotein A-I, forming pre-HDL. HDL consists of a heterogeneous class of lipoproteins containing approximately equal amounts of lipid and protein (Fig. 11-15). The various HDL subclasses vary in quantitative and qualitative content of lipids, apolipoproteins, enzymes, and lipid transfer proteins, resulting in differences in shape, density, size, charge, and antigenicity. Assessment of HDL-C measures the cholesterol content of all these HDL subclasses and is therefore a crude marker of reverse cholesterol transport.

A large number of prospective, observational studies have generally reported inverse associations between HDL-C concentrations and the risk of CHD,[47-52] with the largest study reporting that a 1 mg/dL higher HDL-C concentration is associated with a 2% lower risk of CHD in men and 3% lower risk in women.[47] The association for HDL-C is proportionally about 50% stronger in women than in men.[47] The American National Cholesterol Education Program considers HDL-C to be an optional secondary target of lipid treatment,[23] whereas the European Consensus Panel recommend a minimum target for HDL of 40 mg/dL (1.03 mmol/L) in certain patients, such as diabetics,[53] but the relevance of the latter recommendation is unclear in light of limited data from clinical trials.

Raising High-Density Lipoprotein Cholesterol Levels

Fibrates, which are agonists of the PPAR-α receptor, increase the hepatic production of apolipoprotein A-I, which is the principal lipoprotein contained in the HDL particle and that raises HDL levels by approximately 10% to 15% (although others have shown almost no effect). Niacin reduces the hepatic clearance of the mature HDL particle, raising circulating HDL-C levels by 20% to 30%. Cholesterol ester–transfer protein (CETP) is a plasma glycoprotein that facilitates the transfer of cholesteryl esters from HDL-C to apoB-containing lipoproteins and triglycerides from apoB-containing lipoproteins to HDL. Increasing the triglyceride content of HDL increases its clearance, thereby reducing HDL-C levels.

Cholesterol Ester Transfer Protein Inhibition

Humans with CETP deficiency due to molecular defects in the *CETP* gene have markedly elevated plasma levels of HDL-C and apolipoprotein A-I, suggesting that CETP inhibition may increase HDL-C levels. A phase II trial assessed the relative efficacy of torcetrapib in addition to different doses of atorvastatin at raising HDL.[54] The addition of 60 mg of torcetrapib was associated with an increase in HDL of about 55% when added to 80 mg of atorvastatin, compared with about a 40% increase in HDL when used alone. The addition of 60 mg of torcetrapib to atorvastatin reduced the LDL/HDL ratio significantly,

Reverse cholesterol transport

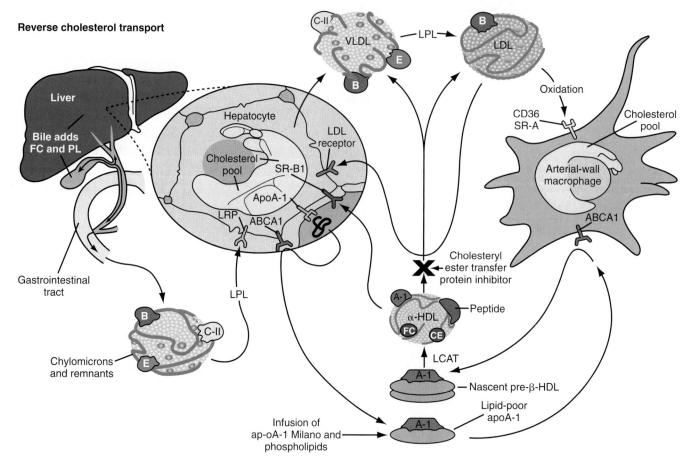

Figure 11-15. The reverse cholesterol transport pathway of high-density lipoprotein (HDL). Lipid-poor pre-β-HDL cholesterol, rich in apolipoprotein A-I (apoA-I), is synthesized by the liver or intestinal mucosa and released into the circulation, where it promotes the transfer of excess cellular-free cholesterol (FC) from macrophages to apoA-I by interacting with the ATP-binding cassette transporter A1 (ABCA1) in arterial wall macrophages. Plasma lecithin-cholesterol acyltransferase (LCAT) converts free cholesterol in pre-β-HDL cholesterol to cholesteryl ester (CE), resulting in the maturation of pre-β-HDL cholesterol to mature α-HDL cholesterol. The α-HDL cholesterol is transported to the liver by a direct or indirect pathway. In the direct pathway, selective uptake of cholesteryl ester by hepatocytes occurs with the scavenger receptor, class B, type 1 (SR-B1). In the indirect pathway, HDL cholesterol cholesteryl ester is exchanged for triglycerides in apolipoprotein B–rich particles (B), LDL cholesterol, and very-low-density lipoprotein (VLDL) cholesterol through cholesteryl ester-transfer protein (CETP), with the uptake of cholesteryl ester by the liver through the low-density lipoprotein (LDL) receptor (LDLR). Cholesterol that is returned to the liver is secreted as bile acids and cholesterol. Acquired triglycerides in the modified HDL cholesterol particle are subjected to hydrolysis by hepatic lipase (HL), thereby regenerating small HDL cholesterol particles and pre-β-HDL cholesterol for participation in reverse cholesterol transport. E, apolipoprotein-E–rich particles; PL, plasma lecithin. (Modified from Brewer HB Jr: Increasing HDL cholesterol levels. N Engl J Med 2004;350:1491-1494. Copyright 2004 Massachusetts Medical Society. All rights reserved.)

and when added to 80 mg of atorvastatin, it resulted in an LDL/HDL ratio of less than 1 (Fig. 11-16). However, in December 2006, Pfizer halted the development of torcetrapib due to a 60% observed increase in deaths in a phase III trial. The relevance of these biologic changes and the role of CETP inhibition remains unproved.

Fibrates and Niacin

A variety of studies have assessed the relative merit of raising HDL-C levels using fibrates or niacin (discussed previously). A meta-analysis of these data suggests that there is a 2.5% reduction in CHD events for every 1% rise in HDL-C levels with fibrates and a 1.7% reduction per 1% rise in HDL-C levels with niacin.[55] Niacin raises HDL-C by levels of approximately 28%, but its use has been limited by side effects, notably flushing mediated by prostaglandins. Using ultrasound and measurements of carotid intima–media thickness, niacin has been shown to attenuate and may reverse atherosclerosis.[56] This concept is being tested in the large-scale 20,000 patient Heart Protection-2 study, combining niacin with an antiflushing agent in a Chinese population with CHD or high-risk equivalent.

Overall, the effects of fibrates on HDL-C levels are modest. This was most recently demonstrated in the Fenofibrate Intervention and Event Lowering in Diabetes (FIELD) trial, in which long-term treatment with fenofibrate to raise HDL-C concentrations and lower triglyceride levels was assessed in subjects

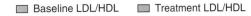

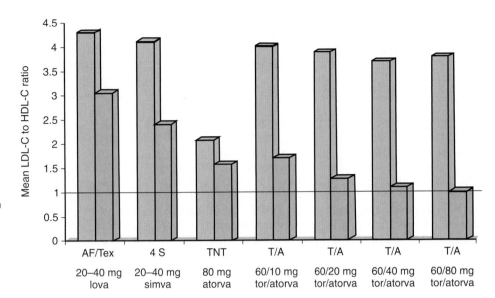

Figure 11-16. Effect of torcetrapib (60 mg) in addition to atorvastatin on the low-density lipoprotein/high-density lipoprotein (LDL/HDL) ratio in subjects with hyperlipidemia compared with earlier statin-only trials. (Data from references 24, 43, 54, 63.)

with type 2 diabetes and total blood cholesterol concentrations of less than 251 mg/dL (6.5 mmol/L).[57] At the end of the trial, LDL-C levels fell from 120 mg/dL (3.07 mmol/L) to 95 mg/dL (2.43 mmol/L) in subjects allocated fenofibrate and to 101 mg/dL (2.60 mmol/L) in the placebo group. Triglyceride levels were also lower in the fenofibrate group— 131 mg/dL (1.47 mmol/L) versus 166 mg/dL (1.87 mmol/L)—but HDL-C levels were not significantly different—44 mg/dL (1.13 mmol/L) versus 44 mg/dL (1.12 mmol/L)—compared with placebo. The differences in lipid levels between treatment groups decreased during the trial, particularly among patients receiving additional lipid-lowering therapy. Overall, 5.9% of patients on placebo and 5.2% of those on fenofibrate experienced the primary end point (P = .16). There was a significant 24% reduction in nonfatal MI but a nonsignificant increase in CAD mortality of 19%. Total cardiovascular events were significantly reduced by 11%, predominantly reflecting a 21% reduction in coronary revascularization. Overall, the FIELD trial failed to demonstrate a significant benefit of an agent that predominantly reduces triglyceride levels and raises HDL levels in a high-risk population. This finding might have resulted from an unequal, excess use of statin therapy in subjects allocated to placebo. Given the benefits of statin therapy among diabetics in the Collaborative Atorvastatin Diabetes Study (CARDS) trial[58] and in subgroups of other trials,[17] there is little evidence to suggest that fibrates are an alternative first-line treatment to statins for the management of dyslipidemia in diabetics. It remains to be seen whether adding a fibrate to statin therapy will reduce cardiovascular risk among diabetics, as is being assessed in the Action to Control Cardiovascular Risk in Diabetes (ACCORD) trial.

Glitazones

Glitazones are a novel class of agents that stimulate the PPAR-γ receptor, improve glycemic control, and have favorable effects on dyslipidemia, in particular reducing triglycerides and raising HDL-C levels. The Prospective Pioglitazone Clinical Trial in Macrovascular Events (PROACTIVE) trial was a placebo-controlled trial that assessed the benefit of a PPAR-γ agonist pioglitazone in stable type 2 diabetic subjects with evidence of macrovascular disease. Patients with evidence of coronary, cerebral, or peripheral arterial disease and an HgbA$_{1c}$ level greater than 6.5% despite treatment were considered eligible for the study (N = 5238).

Compared with placebo, pioglitazone was associated with a 0.8% versus 0.3% reduction in HgbA$_{1c}$ from baseline (P < .0001) and an 11.4% versus 1.8% reduction in triglycerides (P < .0001). Significantly, pioglitazone raised HDL-C levels by 19%, compared with 10.1% in the placebo group (P < .0001), and reduced the LDL/HDL ratio by 9.5%, compared with 4.2% (P < .0001). The primary end point of mortality, nonfatal MI, stroke, ACS, coronary or peripheral arterial revascularization, and above-knee amputation tended to be lower in patients allocated pioglitazone (HR = 0.9; P = .095). The secondary end point of mortality, nonfatal MI, and stroke was reduced by 16% among patients allocated pioglitazone (P = .027). The overall findings of PROACTIVE, which included nonacute end points such as limb amputation, were neutral. However, a significant reduction in the secondary end point of death, nonfatal MI, and stroke was observed, raising the possibility that PPAR-γ agonists may be of value as adjunctive therapy to statins among patients with diabetes and macrovascular disease. However, these findings require validation in further clinical trials. The differences in glycemic control between treatments were modest, but large differences in HDL-C levels were observed with pioglitazone. It is possible that the beneficial effects of pioglitazone may not be due just to effects on glycemia but may also be related to beneficial effects on atherogenic dyslipidemia or systemic inflammation.[55]

Triglycerides

Hypertriglyceridemia is a strong predictor of CHD. Prospective studies such as the Multiple Risk Factor Intervention Trial (MRFIT) show that the adjusted risk of a fatal or nonfatal CHD event is greater among subjects with triglyceride levels of 200 mg/dL or higher. This was the result regardless of whether the subjects were in a fasting or nonfasting state. The Whitehall II study showed the potential relevance of combining triglycerides and cholesterol in risk prediction. There is also an inverse relationship between serum levels of HDL-C and triglycerides, with low serum HDL-C levels representing an independent risk factor for cardiovascular disease and the so-called atherogenic lipid triad, consisting of high serum triglyceride levels, low serum HDL-C levels, and a preponderance of small, dense, LDL-C particles. This feature is particularly common in obesity and insulin-resistant states. More than 2.5 million deaths each year worldwide are weight related, with cardiovascular disease the leading cause. Although modification of nutrition and physical activity is the cornerstone of therapy for obesity, pharmacotherapy focusing on improvement of the metabolic risk profile in patients who are at high risk for diabetes and cardiovascular disease may be required.

Endocannabinoid Blockers

The endocannabinoid system contributes to the physiologic regulation of energy balance, food intake, and lipid and glucose metabolism through central and peripheral effects. This system consists of endogenous ligands and two types of G protein–coupled cannabinoid receptors. The CB1 receptor is located in several brain areas and in a variety of peripheral tissues, including adipose tissue. Compared with wild-type animals, CB1-knockout mice have leaner body composition, but this lean phenotype is not fully explained by changes in food intake. Stimulation of the CB_1 receptors in fat cells promotes lipogenesis and inhibits the production of adiponectin, a cytokine derived from adipose tissue that has potentially important antidiabetic and antiatherosclerotic properties.[59] The system may provide a possible treatment target for high-risk overweight or obese patients.

The RIO Trials

The RIO trials assessed the efficacy and safety of rimonabant (doses of 5 and 20 mg/day) in reducing body weight and improving cardiovascular risk factors in overweight patients (Table 11-2).[60-62] The primary efficacy measure was weight loss, and secondary efficacy measures included changes in metabolic factors. Consistently across these trials, 5 mg of rimonabant had little effect, but 20 mg of rimonabant reduced body weight by about 6 kg (see Table 11-2), reduced triglycerides by approximately 5% to 14%, and increased HDL-C levels by approximately 10% to 21% compared with placebo (Fig. 11-17).

Taken together, the trials of rimonabant suggest that CB1 receptor blockade in patients with adverse cardiovascular risk factors or obesity ameliorates metabolic abnormalities. In view of the residual cardiovascular risk observed among patients despite risk factor modification with statins and control of blood pressure, this novel strategy may be a useful adjunct to current therapeutic regimens. However, the potential cardioprotective effects of rimonabant and similar agents require assessment in clinical trials before definitive conclusions can be made. These potential cardioprotective effects may be offset by a significant excess of side effects, such as nausea and depression, which have led to a high discontinuation rate in the clinical outcome trials conducted. Because these trials are of relatively short duration (1 to 2 years) and it appears that weight gain and adverse cardiometabolic risk recurs after drug cessation, the long-term tolerability of these agents needs to be further assessed. These side effects may limit the widespread use of these agents.

Table 11-2. Trials of Rimonabant in Subjects with Obesity Showing Effects on Weight Loss and Lipids

Trial	Population	N	Study Duration	Change in TG	Change in HDL	Change in Weight with Rimonabant (20 mg)
RIO Europe	BMI >30 or BMI >27 with untreated hypertension or dyslipidemia	1507	1 yr	−14% (P < .001)	+21% (P < .001)	−6.6 kg (P < .001)
RIO Lipids	BMI 27-40 with TG 150-703 mg/dL or TC/HDL ratio >4.5	1036	1 yr	−13% (P < .001)	+10% (P < .001)	−6.7 kg (P < .001)
RIO North America	BMI >30 or BMI >27 with untreated hypertension or dyslipidemia	3045	2 yr	−5% (P < .001)	+11% (P < .001)	−6.3 kg (P < .001)

BMI, body mass index; HDL, high-density lipoprotein; TG, triglycerides.

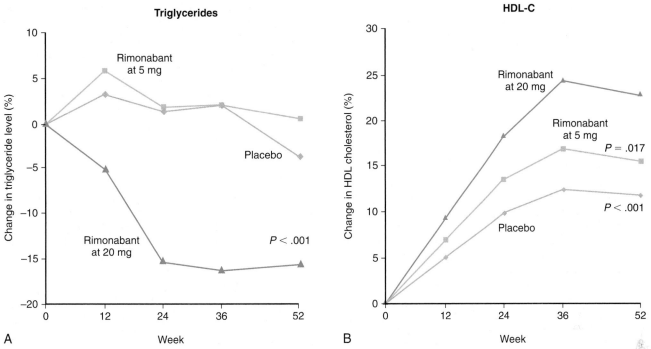

Figure 11-17. Changes in triglyceride **(A)** and high-density lipoprotein cholesterol (HDL-C) **(B)** levels with rimonabant in the Rimonabant In Obesity Lipids (RIO-Lipids) trial. (Modified from Despres JP, Golay A, Sjostrom L, for the Rimonabant in Obesity-Lipids Study Group: Effects of rimonabant on metabolic risk factors in overweight patients with dyslipidemia. N Engl J Med 2005;353:2121-2134.)

Acyl-coenzyme A:Cholesterol Acyltransferase inhibitors

Acyl-coenzyme A:cholesterol acyltransferase (ACAT) is an enzyme that esterifies cholesterol in a variety of tissues. In some animal models, ACAT inhibitors have antiatherosclerotic effects. In an IVUS study of 408 patients with angiographically documented coronary disease, patients assigned the ACAT inhibitor pactimibe (100 mg/day) did not show any significant difference in the progression of atherosclerosis. The change in percent of atheroma volume was similar in the pactimibe and placebo groups (0.69% and 0.59%, respectively; $P = .77$). However, both secondary efficacy variables assessed by means of IVUS showed unfavorable effects of pactimibe treatment. Compared with baseline values, the normalized total atheroma volume showed significant regression in the placebo group (-5.6 mm^3, $P = .001$) but not in the pactimibe group (-1.3 mm^3, $P = .39$; $P = .03$ for the comparison between groups). The atheroma volume in the most diseased 10-mm subsegment regressed by 3.2 mm^3 in the placebo group, compared with a decrease of 1.3 mm^3 in the pactimibe group ($P = .01$). After the preliminary results of the ACAT IntraVascular Atherosclerosis Treatment Evaluation (ACTIVATE) were revealed in October 2005, clinical trials of pactimibe ceased worldwide. In patients with CAD, pactimibe failed to reduce atherosclerosis progression compared with usual care and had some proatherogenic effects. Although the study was not powered for clinical outcomes, ACTIVATE failed to demonstrate any beneficial effect of pactimibe on adverse cardiovascular outcomes.

CONCLUSIONS

All patients with CAD benefit from statin therapy, with no apparent threshold below which benefit is absent. Intensive statin therapy reduces cardiovascular events and atherosclerotic disease progression compared with standard therapy and therefore should be considered the standard of care for patients with CAD. In addition to important reduction of LDL-C levels, intensive statin therapy reduces inflammation, which appears to be particularly important in the early benefits observed in ACS patients, and has important contributions thereafter to long-term risk reduction. Beyond statin therapy, the data for other agents that favorably alter lipid profiles are unclear, but potential benefits of agents that raise HDL-C levels or significantly lower triglyceride levels are being investigated.

REFERENCES

1. Kannel WB, Dawber TR, Friedman GD, et al: Risk factors in coronary heart disease. An evaluation of several serum lipids as predictors of coronary heart disease; the Framingham Study. Ann Intern Med 1964;61:888-899.
2. Kannel WB, Castelli WP, Gordon T, McNamara PM: Serum cholesterol, lipoproteins, and the risk of coronary heart disease. The Framingham Study. Ann Intern Med 1971;74: 1-12.

3. Neaton JD, Wentworth D: Serum cholesterol, blood pressure, cigarette smoking, and death from coronary heart disease. Overall findings and differences by age for 316,099 white men. Multiple Risk Factor Intervention Trial Research Group. Arch Intern Med 1992;152:56-64.

4. Neaton JD, Blackburn H, Jacobs D, et al: Serum cholesterol level and mortality findings for men screened in the Multiple Risk Factor Intervention Trial. Multiple Risk Factor Intervention Trial Research Group. Arch Intern Med 1992;152:1490-500.

5. Law MR, Wald NJ: Risk factor thresholds: Their existence under scrutiny. BMJ 2002;324:1570-1576.

6. Lowering blood cholesterol to prevent heart disease. National Institutes of Health Consensus Development Conference Statement. Natl Inst Health Consens Dev Conf Consens Statement 1985;5:27.

7. The Lipid Research Clinics Coronary Primary Prevention Trial results. I. Reduction in incidence of coronary heart disease. JAMA 1984;251:351-364.

8. Stamler J: The coronary drug project—Findings with regard to estrogen, dextrothyroxine, clofibrate and niacin. Adv Exp Med Biol 1977;82:52-75.

9. Canner P, Berge K, Wenger N, et al: Fifteen year mortality in Coronary Drug Project patients: Long-term benefit with niacin. J Am Coll Cardiol 1986;8:1245-1255.

10. Carlson L, Danielson M, Ekberg I, et al: Reduction of myocardial reinfarction by the combined treatment with clofibrate and nicotinic acid. Atherosclerosis 1977; 28:81-86.

11. Frick M, Heinonen O, Huttunen J, et al: Efficacy of gemfibrozil in dyslipidaemic subjects with suspected heart disease. An ancillary study in the Helsinki Heart Study frame population. Ann Med 1993;25:41-45.

12. Rubins HB, Robins SJ, Collins D, et al: Gemfibrozil for the secondary prevention of coronary heart disease in men with low levels of high-density lipoprotein cholesterol. Veterans Affairs High-Density Lipoprotein Cholesterol Intervention Trial Study Group. N Engl J Med 1999;341:410-418.

13. Randomised trial of cholesterol lowering in 4444 patients with coronary heart disease: The Scandinavian Simvastatin Survival Study (4S). Lancet 1994;344:1383-1389.

14. Sacks FM, Pfeffer MA, Moye LA, et al: The effect of pravastatin on coronary events after myocardial infarction in patients with average cholesterol levels. Cholesterol and Recurrent Events Trial Investigators. N Engl J Med 1996;335:1001-1009.

15. Prevention of cardiovascular events and death with pravastatin in patients with coronary heart disease and a broad range of initial cholesterol levels. The Long-Term Intervention with Pravastatin in Ischaemic Disease (LIPID) Study Group. N Engl J Med 1998;339:1349-1357.

16. MRC/BHF Heart Protection Study of cholesterol lowering with simvastatin in 20,536 high-risk individuals: A randomised placebo-controlled trial. Lancet 2002;360:7-22.

17. Collins R, Armitage J, Parish S, et al: MRC/BHF Heart Protection Study of cholesterol-lowering with simvastatin in 5963 people with diabetes: A randomised placebo-controlled trial. Lancet 2003;361:2005-2016.

18. Baigent CA. Keech PM, Kearney L, et al: Efficacy and safety of cholesterol-lowering treatment: Prospective meta-analysis of data from 90,056 participants in 14 randomised trials of statins. Lancet 2005;366:1267-1278.

19. Schwartz GG, Olsson AG, Ezekowitz MD, et al: Effects of atorvastatin on early recurrent ischemic events in acute coronary syndromes: The MIRACL study: A randomized controlled trial. JAMA 2001;285:1711-1718.

20. Cannon CP, Braunwald E, McCabe CH, et al: Intensive versus moderate lipid lowering with statins after acute coronary syndromes. N Engl J Med 2004;350:1495-1504.

21. De Lemos JA, Blazing MA, Wiviott SD, et al: Early Intensive vs a delayed conservative simvastatin strategy in patients with acute coronary syndromes: Phase Z of the A to Z Trial. JAMA 2004;292:1307-1316.

22. Wiviott SD, de Lemos JA, Cannon CP, et al: A tale of two trials: A comparison of the post-acute coronary syndrome lipid-lowering trials A to Z and PROVE IT-TIMI 22. Circulation 2006;113:1406-1414.

23. Grundy SM, Cleeman JI, Merz CN, et al: Implications of recent clinical trials for the National Cholesterol Education Program Adult Treatment Panel III guidelines. Circulation 2004;110:227-239.

24. LaRosa JC, Grundy SM, Waters DD, et al: Intensive lipid lowering with atorvastatin in patients with stable coronary disease. N Engl J Med 2005;352:1425-1435.

25. Pedersen TR, Faergeman O, Kastelein JJ, et al: High-dose atorvastatin vs usual-dose simvastatin for secondary prevention after myocardial infarction: The IDEAL study: A randomized controlled trial. JAMA 2005;294:2437-2445.

26. Cannon CP, Steinberg BA, Murphy SA, et al: Meta-analysis of cardiovascular outcome trials comparing intensive versus moderate statin therapy. J Am Coll Cardiol 2006;82:438-445.

27. Scirica BM, Morrow DA, Cannon CP, et al: Intensive statin therapy and the risk of hospitalization for heart failure after an acute coronary syndrome in the PROVE IT-TIMI 22 study. J Am Coll Cardiol 2006;47:2326-2331.

28. Horwich TB, Hamilton MA, Maclellan WR, Fonarow GC: Low serum total cholesterol is associated with marked increase in mortality in advanced heart failure. J Card Fail 2002;8:216-224.

29. Rauchhaus M, Clark AL, Doehner W, et al: The relationship between cholesterol and survival in patients with chronic heart failure. J Am Coll Cardiol 2003;42:1933-1940.

30. Ray KK, Cannon CP: The potential relevance of the multiple lipid-independent (pleiotropic) effects of statins in the management of acute coronary syndromes. J Am Coll Cardiol 2005;46:1425-1433.

31. Ray KK, Cannon CP, McCabe CH, et al: Early and late benefits of high-dose atorvastatin in patients with acute coronary syndromes: Results from the PROVE IT-TIMI 22 trial. J Am Coll Cardiol, 2005;46:1405-1410.

32. Cannon CP, Ray KK, Braunwald E: Reply. J Am Coll Cardiol 2006;48:852-853.

33. Hulten E, Jackson JL, Douglas K, et al: The effect of early, intensive statin therapy on acute coronary syndrome: A meta-analysis of randomized controlled trials. Arch Intern Med 2006;166:1814-1821.

34. Ballantyne CM: Clinical trial endpoints: Angiograms, events, and plaque instability. Am J Cardiol 1998;82(6A):5M-11M.

35. Okazaki S, Yokoyama T, Miyauchi K, et al: Early statin treatment in patients with acute coronary syndrome: Demonstration of the beneficial effect on atherosclerotic lesions by serial volumetric intravascular ultrasound analysis during half a year after coronary event. The ESTABLISH Study. Circulation 2004;110:1061-1068.

36. Hong MK, Lee CW, Kim YK, et al: Usefulness of follow-up low-density lipoprotein cholesterol level as an independent predictor of changes of coronary atherosclerotic plaque size as determined by intravascular ultrasound analysis after statin (atorvastatin or simvastatin) therapy. Am J Cardiol 2006;98:866-870.

37. Wiviott SD, Cannon CP, Morrow DA, et al: Can low-density lipoprotein be too low? The safety and efficacy of achieving very low low-density lipoprotein with intensive statin therapy: A PROVE IT-TIMI 22 substudy. J Am Coll Cardiol 2005;46:1411-1416.

38. Ray KK, Cannon CP, Cairns R, et al: Relationship between uncontrolled risk factors and C-reactive protein levels in patients receiving standard or intensive statin therapy for acute coronary syndromes in the PROVE IT-TIMI 22 trial. J Am Coll Cardiol, 2005;46:1417-1424.

39. Morrow DA, de Lemos JA, Sabatine MS, et al: Clinical relevance of C-reactive protein during follow-up of patients with acute coronary syndromes in the Aggrastat-to-Zocor Trial. Circulation 2006;114:281-288.

40. Ridker PM, Rifai N, Cook NR, et al: Non-HDL cholesterol, apolipoproteins A-I and B100, standard lipid measures, lipid ratios, and CRP as risk factors for cardiovascular disease in women. JAMA 2005;294:326-333.

41. Pischon T, Girman CJ, Sacks FM, et al: Non-high-density lipoprotein cholesterol and apolipoprotein B in the prediction of coronary heart disease in men. Circulation 2005;112:3375-3383.

42. Denke MA: Weighing in before the fight: Low-density lipoprotein cholesterol and non-high-density lipoprotein cholesterol versus apolipoprotein B as the best predictor for coronary heart disease and the best measure of therapy. Circulation 2005;112:3368-3370.

43. Gotto AM Jr, Whitney E, Stein EA, et al: Relation between baseline and on-treatment lipid parameters and first acute major coronary events in the Air Force/Texas Coronary Atherosclerosis Prevention Study (AFCAPS/TexCAPS). Circulation 2000;101:477-484.

44. Simes RJ, Marschner IC, Hunt D, et al: Relationship between lipid levels and clinical outcomes in the Long-term Intervention with Pravastatin in Ischemic Disease (LIPID) trial: To what extent is the reduction in coronary events with pravastatin explained by on-study lipid levels? Circulation 2002; 105:1162-1169.

45. Tsimikas S, Brilakis ES, Miller ER, et al: Oxidized phospholipids, Lp(a) lipoprotein, and coronary artery disease. N Engl J Med 2005;353:46-57.

46. Tsimikas S, Witztum JL, Miller ER, et al: High-dose atorvastatin reduces total plasma levels of oxidized phospholipids and immune complexes present on apolipoprotein B-100 in patients with acute coronary syndromes in the MIRACL trial. Circulation 2004;110:1406-1412.

47. Gordon DJ, Probstfield JL, Garrison RJ, et al: High-density lipoprotein cholesterol and cardiovascular disease. Four prospective American studies. Circulation 1989;79:8-15.

48. Gordon T, Castelli WP, Hjortland MC, et al: High density lipoprotein as a protective factor against coronary heart disease. The Framingham Study. Am J Med 1977;62:707-714.

49. Multiple risk factor intervention trial. Risk factor changes and mortality results. Multiple Risk Factor Intervention Trial Research Group. JAMA 1982;248:1465-1477.

50. Assmann G, Schulte H, von Eckardstein A, Huang Y: High-density lipoprotein cholesterol as a predictor of coronary heart disease risk. The PROCAM experience and pathophysiological implications for reverse cholesterol transport. Atherosclerosis 1996;124(Suppl):S11-S20.

51. Jacobs DR Jr, Mebane LL, Bangdiwala SI, et al: High density lipoprotein cholesterol as a predictor of cardiovascular disease mortality in men and women: The follow-up study of the Lipid Research Clinics Prevalence Study. Am J Epidemiol 1990;131:32-47.

52. Gordon DJ, Knoke J, Probstfield JL, et al: High-density lipoprotein cholesterol and coronary heart disease in hypercholesterolemic men: The Lipid Research Clinics Coronary Primary Prevention Trial. Circulation 1986;74:1217-1225.

53. Chapman MJ, Assmann G, Fruchart JC, et al: Raising high-density lipoprotein cholesterol with reduction of cardiovascular risk: The role of nicotinic acid—A position paper developed by the European Consensus Panel on HDL-C. Curr Med Res Opin 2004;20:1253-1268.

54. Thuren T: Torcetrapib Phase 2 Factorial Study A3071026. American Heart Association Scientic Sessions, 2005.

55. Birjmohun RS, Hutten BA, Kastelein JJ, Stroes ES: Efficacy and safety of high-density lipoprotein cholesterol-increasing compounds: A meta-analysis of randomized controlled trials. J Am Coll Cardiol 2005;45:185-197.

56. Taylor AJ, Sullenberger LW, Lee HJ, et al: Arterial Biology for the Investigation of the Treatment Effects of Reducing Cholesterol (ARBITER) 2: A double-blind, placebo-controlled study of extended-release niacin on atherosclerosis progression in secondary prevention patients treated with statins. Circulation 2004;110:3512-3517.

57. Keech A, Simes RJ, Barter P, et al: Effects of long-term fenofibrate therapy on cardiovascular events in 9795 people with type 2 diabetes mellitus (the FIELD study): Randomised controlled trial. Lancet 2005;366:1849-1861.

58. Colhoun HM, Betteridge DJ, Durrington PN, et al: Primary prevention of cardiovascular disease with atorvastatin in type 2 diabetes in the Collaborative Atorvastatin Diabetes Study (CARDS): Multicentre randomised placebo-controlled trial. Lancet 2004;364:685-696.

59. Okamoto Y, Kihara S, Ouchi N, et al: Adiponectin reduces atherosclerosis in apolipoprotein E-deficient mice. Circulation 2002;106:2767-2770.

60. Van Gaal LF, Rissanen AM, Scheen AJ, et al: Effects of the cannabinoid-1 receptor blocker rimonabant on weight reduction and cardiovascular risk factors in overweight patients: 1-year experience from the RIO-Europe study. Lancet 2005;365:1389-1397.

61. Despres JP, Golay A, Sjostrom L, for the Rimonabant in Obesity-Lipids Study Group: Effects of rimonabant on metabolic risk factors in overweight patients with dyslipidemia. N Engl J Med 2005;353:2121-2134.

62. Pi-Sunyer FX, Aronne LJ, Heshmati HM, et al: Effect of rimonabant, a cannabinoid-1 receptor blocker, on weight and cardiometabolic risk factors in overweight or obese patients: RIO-North America: A randomized controlled trial. JAMA 2006;295:761-775.

63. Pedersen TR, Olasson AG, Faergerman O, et al: Lipoprotein changes and reduction in the incidence of major coronary heart disease events in the Scandinavian Simvastatin Survival Study (4S). 1998;97:1453-1460.

CHAPTER

12 Angiotensin-Axis Inhibition

Marc A. Pfeffer

KEY POINTS

■ Pharmacologic inhibition of the renin-angiotensin-aldosterone system has provided important mechanistic insights into cardiovascular disease progression and offers a means to reduce morbidity and mortality in a variety of cardiovascular conditions.

■ Angiotensin-converting enzyme (ACE) inhibitors are one of the extensively studied classes of pharmacologic compounds.

■ ACE inhibitors and angiotensin receptor blockers (ARBs) reduce the risk of progression to end-stage renal disease.

■ ACE inhibitors and ARBs are effective in reducing clinical events in patients with symptomatic heart failure and reduced left ventricular ejection fraction. Concomitant use in one study resulted in incremental benefits.

■ Several ACE inhibitors and one ARB are effective in reducing clinical events in high-risk acute myocardial infarction patients, but their combination did not offer incremental improvements.

■ Aldosterone inhibition has been shown to be effective in treating severe heart failure and in patients with acute heart failure complicating myocardial infarction.

■ In patients with stable coronary artery disease, the addition of an ACE inhibitor to conventional risk factor modification lowers the risk of cardiovascular events.

■ All inhibitors of the renin-angiotensin-aldosterone system, when used in clinically effective doses, can result in significant hyperkalemia.

Clinical use of inhibitors of the renin-angiotensin system (RAS) had relatively modest early expectations attributed to high plasma renin activity with angiotensin-converting enzyme (ACE) inhibitors specifically developed for the treatment of hypertension. From this relatively humble beginning, RAS inhibitors have emerged as major pharmacologic advances based on definitive clinical trial documentation of their benefits in prolonging survival and reducing cardiovascular and renal morbidity (Fig. 12-1). This rise to prominence of ACE inhibitors and angiotensin receptor blockers (ARBs) over the past 3 decades has been based on primary observations from quality mechanistic studies in animals, such as the attenuation of adverse left ventricular remodeling after myocardial infarction (MI) and the slowing of progression of renal dysfunction, leading to major clinical outcome trials and on secondary benefits first observed in the clinical trials stimulating basic investigations to provide the mechanistic underpinnings for the newly discovered clinical benefits. This progress can be attributed to cross-fertilization between data from basic laboratory research and randomized clinical trials, which support each other in the advancement of clinical care methods and in understanding the mechanisms that interrupt disease progression.[1]

APPLICATIONS OF ANGIOTENSIN-CONVERTING ENZYME INHIBITORS AND ANGIOTENSIN RECEPTOR BLOCKERS

Systemic Hypertension

On the basis of its prevalence in the aging population and the direct pathophysiologic links of elevated blood pressure to atherosclerosis, stroke, MI, sudden death, and heart failure, hypertension is the most important population-attributable and modifiable risk factor for cardiovascular events.[2] Sustained lowering of arterial pressure is the major and critical mechanism by which antihypertensive therapies reduce the incidence of adverse cardiovascular events.[3,4] With the establishment of the importance of blood pressure reduction, the field has matured to the point that placebo-controlled trials in hypertension are considered unethical. To attempt to demonstrate the importance of a specific compound, contemporary trials usually compare different classes of antihypertensive agents.

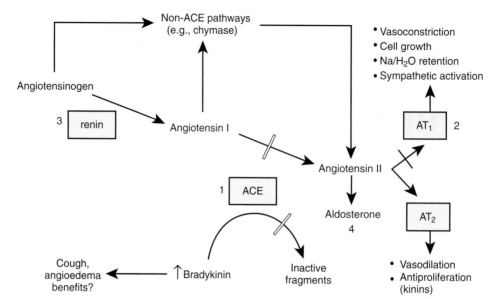

Figure 12-1. Four pharmacologic sites of inhibition of the renin-angiotensin-aldosterone system. 1, Angiotensin-converting enzyme (ACE) inhibitor reduces the conversion of angiotensin I to angiotensin II and also limits the breakdown of bradykinin; 2, angiotensin type 1 receptor blocker or angiotensin receptor blocker (ARB) blocks the action of angiotensin II at the AT1 receptor; 3, renin inhibition blocks the cleavage of angiotensinogen into angiotensin I; 4, aldosterone inhibitor reduces the influence of aldosterone on renal tubules and other tissues. (From McMurray JV, Pfeffer MA, Swedberg K, Dzau V: Which inhibitor of the renin-angiotensin system should be used in chronic heart failure and acute myocardial infarction? Circulation 2004;110:3281-3288.)

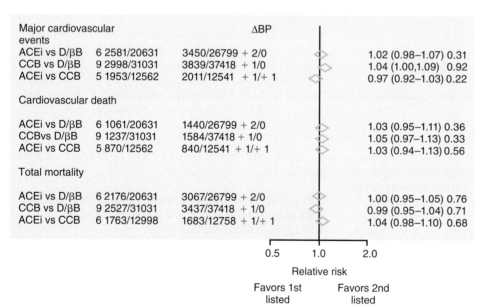

Figure 12-2. Meta-analysis of outcomes of hypertensive patients treated with different antihypertensive agents. Blood pressure (BP)–lowering regimens are based on different drug classes. Mean BP difference between the first and second treatment regimens are shown. ACEi, angiotensin-converting enzyme inhibitor; CCB, calcium channel blocker; D/βB, diuretic-and/or β-blocker–based regimens. (From Williams B: Recent hypertension trials: Implications and controversies. J Am Coll Cardiol 2005;45:813-827.)

In the context of comparator trials of antihypertensive compounds, the clinical mandate of obtaining adequate blood pressure control frequently requires use of multiple agents, which confounds interpretation of the results. Overall, ACE inhibitors have not consistently distinguished themselves as clearly superior to other effective blood pressure–lowering therapies in reducing cardiovascular risk in patients with hypertension (Fig. 12-2).[4,5] The Captopril Prevention Project (CAPPP) reported similar clinical outcomes comparing an ACE inhibitor with a β-blocker–based antihypertensive regimen in more than 10,000 patients with essential hypertension.[6] Similarly, in the smaller U.K. Prospective Diabetes Study, the level of blood pressure control in diabetic patients had more influence on clinical outcomes than whether an ACE inhibitor or β-blocker was used.[7] The Antihypertensive and Lipid Lowering Treatment to Prevent Heart Attack Trial (ALLHAT) compared the cardiovascular event rates of more than 40,000 patients with hypertension plus an additional risk factor, who were randomized to a strategy of an initial antihypertensive therapy based on a diuretic (i.e., chlorthalidone), calcium antagonist (i.e., amlodipine), α-adrenergic blocker (i.e., doxazosin), or ACE inhibitor (i.e., lisinopril).[8] The α-blocker arm was discontinued early by the Data Safety Committee after it became apparent that more cardiovascular events, particularly heart failure, were occurring with this therapy compared with the diuretic group.[9] The other three arms went to completion, and for the primary end point of fatal coronary heart disease or nonfatal MI, no differences were apparent between these three classes of antihypertensive agents when used as initial therapy. However, for several clinically important secondary outcomes, the diuretic-based regimen was thought to be superior.[10] In contrast, in the Second Australian National Blood Pressure Study (ANBP2), fewer cardiovascular events were observed in elderly hypertensive patients randomized to the ACE inhibitor (i.e., enalapril) regimen compared with a diuretic (i.e., hydrochlorothiazide) as initial therapy.[11]

As an even newer class of antihypertensive agents, several ARBs have accepted the challenge of addressing whether their use favorably influences morbidity and mortality in hypertension. In the Losartan Intervention of Endpoint (LIFE) trial, the clinical outcomes of blood pressure control with losartan were compared with those of the β-blocker atenolol in more than 9000 hypertensive patients with electrocardiographic evidence of left ventricular hypertrophy.[12] In this trial, the ARB-based regimen was shown to be even more effective in reducing the primary end point of death, MI, or stroke than the β-blocker. This difference in clinical events occurred predominantly because of lower rates of stroke, despite similar achieved blood pressures and comparable use of diuretics as the second-line agents.[13] Of the many major antihypertensive clinical outcome trials, LIFE is unique in showing a difference in clinical event rates between classes of agents that could not be accounted for by differential blood pressures. Although smaller and not as adequately statistically powered, the Study on Cognition and Prognosis in the Elderly (SCOPE) had similar trends for clinical benefits with the ARB candesartan.[14]

In the Valsartan Antihypertensive Long-term Use Evaluation (VALUE), valsartan was compared with amlodipine in more than 15,000 patients with hypertension plus another risk factor.[15] As opposed to the LIFE trial, in which the ARB was shown to be superior to the β-blocker in reducing clinical events, in VALUE, the picture was mixed for ARB compared with a calcium channel blocker. During the early drug titration phase, blood pressure lowering was initially better with the calcium channel blocker, and overall, this was associated with fewer strokes compared with the ARB arm. However, the primary end point of cardiac events was not different between the two antihypertensive regimens. The results of the Morbidity and Mortality After Stroke (MOSES) study, which compared the effects of the ARB eprosartan with effects of the calcium channel blocker nitrendipine in 1400 stroke survivors requiring antihypertensive therapy, contraindicated the VALUE findings.

Although achieved systolic arterial pressures were comparable (average, 133 mm Hg), the stroke patients randomized to the ARB had fewer cardiovascular events than those randomized to the calcium channel blocker.[16]

Because a high proportion of patients with hypertension require multiple antihypertensive agents for adequate blood pressure control, the traditional focus of clinical trials with administration of a single first agent becomes less clinically relevant than determination of the optimal combination of antihypertensive agents to most safely and effectively lower an individual's cardiovascular risk profile. The Anglo-Scandinavian Cardiac Outcomes Trial (ASCOT) compared a strategy of blood pressure control using a calcium channel blocker (i.e., amlodipine) and adding an ACE inhibitor (i.e., perindopril) as needed for blood pressure control versus a β-blocker (i.e., atenolol) and adding a diuretic (i.e., bendroflumethiazide) as needed for blood pressure control in almost 20,000 patients with hypertension and multiple cardiovascular risks.[17] Randomization to the calcium channel blocker–ACE inhibitor strategy was found to be associated with a lower risk of major cardiovascular events compared with the beta-blocker and diuretic as first- and second-line therapies. Although the blood pressure control was greater in the calcium channel blocker–ACE inhibitor group, the observed difference in cardiovascular events (16% reduction) was greater than what would be anticipated from the blood pressure differential (2.7-mm Hg systolic pressure).

Despite only suggestive and by no means definitive data that indicated unique clinical benefits beyond blood pressure control across classes of antihypertensive therapies, ACE inhibitors and ARBs are an important part of the therapeutic armamentarium for treatment of hypertension to reduce blood pressure and, more importantly, cardiovascular risks. The cardiovascular benefits of inhibiting the RAS that have been demonstrated in certain higher-risk populations are probably the key to their appeal to frontline clinicians for use in individuals with even less overt disease and risks.

Renal Protection

ACE inhibitors and ARBs of the RAS have earned their designation as *renal protective*. Clinical trials have definitely demonstrated that the use of an ACE inhibitor in patients with diabetic nephropathy and nondiabetic nephropathy can slow the progression of renal disease and forestall the need for dialysis. In patients with juvenile diabetes and nephropathy, randomization to captopril reduced the proportion of patients who had a doubling of serum creatinine levels or needed renal transplantation.[18] The African-American Study in Kidney Disease (AASK), comparing an ACE inhibitor (i.e., ramipril) and calcium channel blocker (i.e., amlodipine), was prematurely terminated when it became clear that patients randomized to ramipril had a lower incidence of progression to dialysis.[19] The development of micro-albuminuria was also decreased by the ACE inhibitor trandolapril.[20]

In patients with type 2 diabetes and proteinuria, two separate studies with ARBs demonstrated improved clinical outcomes compared with other antihypertensive strategies. In the Reduction of End-points in NIDDM with the Angiotensin II Antagonist Losartan (RENAAL) study, losartan was associated with fewer patients progressing to a doubling of creatinine levels or needing renal replacement therapy.[21] In the Irbesartan Diabetic Nephropathy Trial (IDNT), despite the similar blood pressure lowering with a regimen based on irbesartan compared with a regimen based on amlodipine or other antihypertensives, fewer renal end points were experienced by those on the ARB than in the two other antihypertensive groups (Fig. 12-3).[22] Together, IDNT and RENAAL provide convincing evidence that an ARB is of particular value in reducing renal failure in patients with diabetic nephropathy. However, it must be acknowledged that the overall balance of cardiovascular events did not favor either class of antihypertensive agents because a reduction in heart failure admissions with the ARBs was offset by fewer atherosclerotic end points in the calcium channel blocker groups. These studies also underscored the difficulties and the importance of blood pressure lowering. In IDNT, achieving systolic blood pressure control approaching 120 mm Hg was associated with the best protection against cardiovascular events.[23] In patients with type 2 diabetes with only microalbuminuria, the ARB irbesartan resulted in a dose-dependent, not blood pressure–dependent, reduction in the risk of developing proteinuria,[24] and valsartan was more effective than amlodipine in reducing albumin excretion.[25]

Taken together, the ACE inhibitors and the ARBs have earned their preferential role in the management of diabetics and others at risk for renal failure. Because there has not been a major head-to-head comparison of ACE inhibitors and ARBs in renal disease, results can only be inferred, but both inhibitors of the RAS can be considered effective in slowing the progression of renal disease and should be used in treating appropriate patients.[26] Although a meta-analysis indicated that there was no specific additional renal protective effect of ACE inhibitors or ARBs compared with other antihypertensive agents,[27] this interpretation is not uniformly accepted.[28] National Kidney Foundation guidelines strongly endorse the use of an ACE inhibitor or ARB to treat diabetics who have hypertension and chronic kidney disease.[29] Their recommendation of a target systolic blood pressure of 130 mm Hg also serves to underscore the practical need for combinations of classes of antihypertensive agents to best limit progression of kidney disease. Although the combination of an ACE inhibitor and an ARB can be effective in reducing proteinuria[30] definitive clinical outcome trials of this combination have not been reported.[31]

Congestive Heart Failure

Angiotensin-Converting Enzyme Inhibitors in Heart Failure

The early clinical trials of ACE inhibitors in heart failure, Cooperative North Scandinavian Enalapril Survival Study (CONSENSUS),[32] Studies of Left Ventricular Dysfunction (SOLVD) Treatment,[33] and Vasodilators in Heart Failure-II (V-HeFT II),[34] have so convincingly demonstrated the importance of inhibiting the RAS with an ACE inhibitor in patients with symptomatic heart failure and depressed ejection fraction that each of the major international society guidelines designate this therapy with its highest endorsement for use in this setting.[35-37] The more contemporary and clinically relevant question is whether the use of an ARB can provide incremental value alone or in combination with more extensively used ACE inhibitors (Fig. 12-4).

Angiotensin Receptor Blockers in Heart Failure

With the proven benefits of ACE inhibitors in the treatment and prevention of heart failure, the clinical value of ARBs had to be demonstrated relative to an ACE inhibitor.[38] In an early head-to-head evaluation in elderly patients with symptomatic heart failure, there was an apparent survival benefit with use of the ARB in a relatively small trial (fewer than 50 deaths) designed to evaluate tolerability.[39] Because this was not a definitive finding and mortality was not the primary prespecified outcome of this study, a much larger trial was undertaken. With more than 3000 patients and more than 500 deaths in the Losartan Heart Failure Survival Study II (ELITE II), losartan (50 mg/day) was not found to be superior to captopril (150 mg/day) because the trend was toward a survival benefit with the ACE inhibitor.[40]

Another approach in ascertaining the clinical value of an ARB in heart failure employed by the Valsartan in Heart Failure Trial (Val-HeFT) tested whether the ARB valsartan provided supplemental benefit in modernly managed patients.[41] Although a survival benefit with the addition of the ARB was not demonstrated, the prespecified co-primary outcome of death, hospitalization for heart failure, treatment for worsening heart failure, or resuscitated sudden death was reduced by 13% in the group randomized to receive valsartan (Fig. 12-5).[41] Small but significant and consistent improvements in left ventricular ejection fraction and functional status supported these observations of reductions in heart failure admissions with the use of valsartan.[42] Because the concurrent medication used by the Val-HeFT cohort was not uniformly distributed, subgroup analyses were performed with respect to other proven therapies for heart failure. In the 7% of the population that at baseline were not receiving an ACE inhibitor, relatively large morbidity and mortality benefits of the ARB were apparent. Although potentially important,

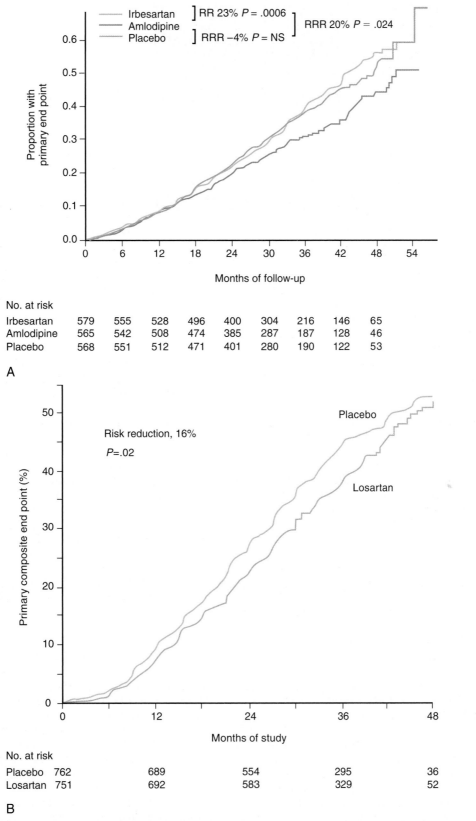

Figure 12-3. Primary end points in the Irbesartan Diabetic Nephropathy Trial (IDNT) **(A)** and Reduction of Endpoints in NIDDM with the Angiotensin II Antagonist Losartan (RENAAL) study **(B)**. (**A,** from Lewis EJ, Hunsicker LG, Clarke WR, et al: Renoprotective effect of the angiotensin-receptor antagonist irbesartan in patients with nephropathy due to type 2 diabetes. N Engl J Med 2001;345:851-860; **B,** from Brenner BM, Cooper ME, de Zeeuw D, et al: Effects of losartan on renal and cardiovascular outcomes in patients with type 2 diabetes and nephropathy. N Engl J Med 2001;345:861-869.)

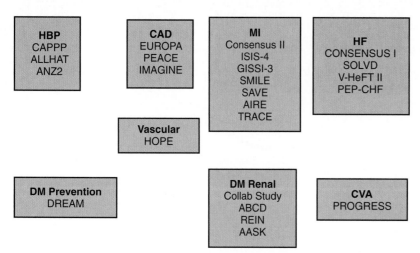

Figure 12-4. Major clinical outcome trials using angiotensin-converting enzyme (ACE) inhibitors. CAD, coronary artery disease; CVA, cerebrovascular accident; DM, diabetes mellitus; HBP, high blood pressure; HF, heart failure; MI, myocardial infarction. (Data from Lewis EJ, Hunsicker, LG, Clarke WR, et al, for the Collaborative Study Group: Renoprotective effect of the angiotensin-receptor antagonist irbesartan in patients with nephropathy due to type 2 diabetes. N Engl J Med. 2001;345:851-860; Brenner BM, Cooper ME, de Zeew D, et al: Effects of losartan on renal and cardiovascular outcomes in patients with type 2 diabetes and nephropathy. N Engl J Med 2001;345:861.)

this observation was from a small subgroup, and the robustness of the finding was questioned. Another subgroup analysis from this study generated an even greater clinical quagmire because it indicated that patients receiving a β-blocker who were randomized to the ARB appeared to have a higher risk of death.[41] With both β-blockers and ACE inhibitors firmly established as lifesaving and current international recommendations for the treatment of symptomatic heart failure with depressed ejection fraction strongly endorsing concurrent use of both, the result of this "triple-therapy" subgroup analysis was of particular concern.[36,37]

The Candesartan in Heart Failure Assessment of Reduction in Mortality and Morbidity (CHARM) program with more than 7000 patients and 3.7 years of follow-up has amassed the largest patient exposure of any randomized, controlled clinical trial in heart failure.[43] The CHARM program is a combination of three integrated protocols evaluating the use of candesartan in heart failure patients with depressed and preserved ejection fractions (see Fig. 12-5). In the depressed ejection fraction (EF) protocols (EF <40%), CHARM-Alternative specifically identified more than 2000 patients that were not being treated with an ACE inhibitor because of previous intolerance.[44] The clear reduction in the primary end point of cardiovascular death or hospitalization for heart failure in those randomized to the ARB was consistent with the results of the no-ACE inhibitor subgroup from Val-HeFT. Together, results of these studies underscore the importance of inhibiting the RAS in patients with depressed ejection fraction heart failure with proven doses of either class of agents.

CHARM-Added randomized approximately 2500 patients, all of whom were on an ACE inhibitor, to address the more vexing question of whether the addition of an ARB to an ACE inhibitor in the presence or absence of a β-blocker could improve clinical outcomes in symptomatic heart failure patients.[45] A 15% reduction in the rates of cardiovascular death or hospitalization for heart failure was obtained by combination therapy, and both of the components of this clinical composite end point achieved statisti-

cal significance. Moreover, these beneficial effects of the ARB were not modified by use of the β-blocker, indicating that in these patients, triple therapy was the most effective strategy. In general, most reconcile the discrepancy of findings of the β-blocker subgroup between Val-HeFT and CHARM as a play of chance and view the CHARM results with a greater number of end points as the more reliable estimates. The lack of a safety signal from the even larger experience of triple therapy in the Valsartan in Myocardial Infarction Trial (VALIANT) provided additional supportive data.[45]

Perhaps the most mechanistically interesting and clinically relevant question concerning the combination use of an ACE inhibitor and ARB in heart failure was posed by the U.S. Food and Drug Administration (FDA) review. Although the CHARM investigators were asked to optimize the dose of ACE inhibitor for their individual patients before randomization, the FDA requested additional analyses to better ascertain whether the observed clinical improvements could be attributed to a relative underdosage of ACE inhibitors. These supplemental analyses indicated that the dose of ACE inhibitor generally used in CHARM-Added was comparable to that achieved in the forced-titration, placebo-controlled ACE inhibitor trials (e.g., SOLVD) and that the beneficial effects observed in CHARM were not modified by the dose of the concomitant ACE inhibitor.[46] The FDA has approved candesartan for the treatment of heart failure (NYHA class II through IV) in patients with left ventricular systolic dysfunction (EF < 40%) to reduce cardiovascular death and to reduce heart failure hospitalizations with the statement that "it [candesartan] also has an added effect on these outcomes when used with an ACE inhibitor."[47]

CHARM-Preserved, the third and perhaps the most specialized protocol of the trio, evaluated the role of the ARB in more than 3000 patients who were selected for signs and symptoms of heart failure but had a quantitative determination of left ventricular ejection fraction of 40% or more.[48] Even though current estimates indicate that 40% to 55% of patients with heart failure have preserved systolic function or

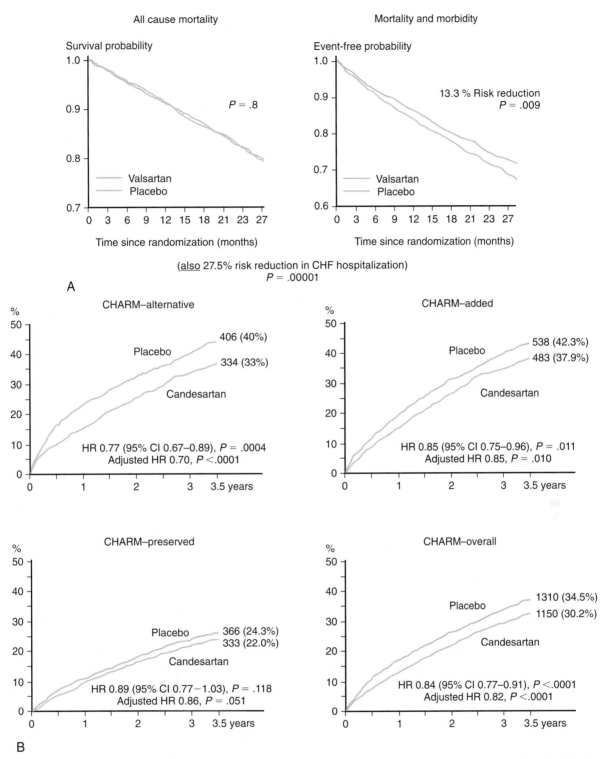

Figure 12-5. Angiotensin receptor blocking (ARB) agents in symptomatic heart failure trials: Valsartan in Heart Failure Trial (Val-HeFT) **(A)** and Candesartan in Heart Failure Assessment of Reduction in Mortality and Morbidity (CHARM) **(B)**.

diastolic dysfunction and that the morbidity and mortality rates are high, this population has been understudied in definitive randomized, controlled clinical trials.[49,50] In these usually elderly patients with frequent comorbidities, neither ACE inhibitors nor β-blockers have been shown to reduce rates of death or hospitalization for heart failure.[51] Although

the use of candesartan in these patients with heart failure and preserved left ventricular function was not associated with a significant improvement in the primary outcome of cardiovascular death or hospitalization for heart failure, there was a borderline trend due to lower rates of hospitalizations for heart failure.[48] Although not definitive, use of ARBs in

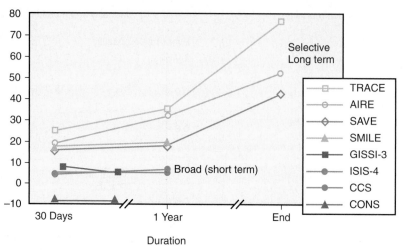

Figure 12-6. Lives saved per 1000 treated patients in all of the major randomized clinical trials of angiotensin-converting enzyme (ACE) inhibition after myocardial infarction (MI). Lives saved per 1000 patients are presented at the initial end point (usually 30 days), at 1 year, and at the end of the respective trials. The *open symbols* represent the selective-inclusion, long-term trials (SAVE, AIRE, and TRACE), and the *filled symbols* represent the broad-inclusion, short-term trials (GISSI-3, ISIS-4, CCS, and CONSENSUS II). The SMILE study represents results after discontinuation of blinded therapy. (Adapted from Solomon SD, Pfeffer MA: Angiotensin-converting enzyme inhibition following myocardial infarction: From left ventricular remodeling to improved survival. In Gersh BJ, Rahimtoola SH [eds]: Acute Myocardial Infarction. New York, Chapman & Hall, 1991, p 704.)

preserved systolic function heart failure remains an open question, with an even larger trial (the Irbesartan in Heart Failure with Preserved Systolic Function [I-PRESERVE]) in progress.[52]

Myocardial Infarction

Angiotensin-Converting Enzyme Inhibitors and Angiotensin Receptor Blockers After Myocardial Infarction

The rationale for the use of an ACE inhibitor after MI was derived from animal experiments that demonstrated that adverse ventricular enlargement and distortion of cavity geometry can be a progressive process after infarction,[53] which can be attenuated by ACE inhibitor therapy.[54,55] It had been demonstrated that even the small increases in ventricular volume after infarction greatly heightened risk of subsequent death and development of heart failure.[56,57] Chronic treatment with ACE inhibitor therapy in animals reduced the extent of remodeling and prolonged survival.[54,58] Early clinical studies confirmed that in selected patients after infarction, progressive enlargement occurred in the months after an infarction and that this process was, as in the animals, modifiable by chronic ACE inhibitor therapy.[59,60]

Clinical Outcome Trials

The cumulative information from eight independent major clinical outcome trials of ACE inhibitors in patients with MI provides the most appropriate quantitation of their benefits and risks in this condition.[61,62] These trials differed in eligibility criteria, time of initiation, and duration of treatment, as well

as the ACE inhibitor employed. A categorization of the trials into selective-inclusion, long-term use or broad-inclusion, short-term use studies has been helpful (Fig. 12-6).

Selective-Inclusion, Long-Term Trials

The Survival and Ventricular Enlargement (SAVE) trial was the first major trial of an ACE inhibitor for MI. SAVE demonstrated that the long-term administration of captopril to survivors of acute MI with baseline left ventricular dysfunction but without overt heart failure would improve survival (i.e., lessen deterioration of cardiac performance) and prevent the development of symptomatic congestive heart failure.[63] The Acute Infarction Ramipril Evaluation (AIRE) investigators identified high-risk patients on clinical grounds by the early development of heart failure complicating the acute MI and found that randomization to the ACE inhibitor ramipril resulted in a 27% reduction in the risk of death.[64] The Trandolapril Cardiac Evaluation (TRACE) study employed a consecutive echocardiographic screening of 6676 patients with acute MI to identify 2606 patients with a wall motion abnormality roughly equivalent to a left ventricular ejection fraction of 35% or less.[65] During the 2 to 4 years of follow-up, there was a 22% reduction in mortality and a 29% reduction in the progression to severe heart failure in the ACE inhibitor group.[65] As in the SAVE and AIRE studies, these reductions were independent of the use of thrombolytics, aspirin, or β-blockers, stressing the additive benefit of ACE inhibitor therapy in the management of patients with MI. The Survival of Myocardial Infarction Long-Term Evaluation (SMILE) also selected a higher-risk population by studying acute anterior infarct patients who did not receive thrombolytic therapy[66] and showed that there was a reduction in the number of patients who died of or developed severe heart failure. When viewed together, the selective-inclusion, long-term trials demonstrated a reduction in the relative risk for death with the use of an ACE inhibitor by about 20%.[62] The lives saved per 1000 treated range from 40 to 70, depending on the mortality rate of the placebo group (see Fig. 12-6).

Broad-Inclusion, Short-Term Trials

Broad-inclusion, short-term trials probed the extent of benefits of ACE inhibitor use in acute MI by evaluating their effectiveness when initiated early in a broader range of patients, including those at lower risk. These trials had a more limited observation period and lower event rates and therefore required much greater sample sizes. The only negative findings for an ACE inhibitor from any major randomized trial in MI patients was from the Cooperative North Scandinavian Enalapril Survival Study II (CONSENSUS II), which evaluated the early use of enalapril, commencing as an intravenous formulation on the first day of the MI.[67] Worrisome increases in hypotension and a trend toward excess mortality with intravenous initiation of an ACE inhibitor led to the early termination of this trial.[68] Fortunately, even larger trials of early use of oral ACE inhibitors in the acute phase of MI did demonstrate a statistically significant survival improvement with the use of this therapy. The Gruppo Italiano per lo Studio della Sopravvivenze nell'Infarto Miocardio (GISSI-3) demonstrated that lisinopril resulted in an 11% reduction in death and severe ventricular dysfunction at 6 weeks.[69] Similarly, with just under 60,000 patients, the International Study of Infarct Survival-4 (ISIS-4) confirmed the early survival benefit of captopril, leading to a 7% reduction in mortality at 1 month.[70] In the Chinese Cardiac Study of approximately 14,000 patients, randomization to captopril was similarly associated with a 6% reduction in early mortality.[71]

These studies of the early use of oral ACE inhibitors provided extensive experience with these agents in the acute myocardial infarct setting. Collectively, this relatively unselected (i.e., minimal systolic pressure above 100 mm Hg) use resulted in 5 lives saved per 1000 patients treated.[72] Angioedema was a rare but worrisome complication. Hypotension and transient renal dysfunction occurred more commonly with the early use of an ACE inhibitor. Although these data support the broad use of ACE inhibitors, a clinical evaluation and selection of higher risk (i.e., anterior location, higher creatinine kinase level, prior infarction, diabetes, Killip class 2 or greater, or cardiac imaging demonstrating depressed ejection fraction) for treatment would concentrate the benefits and reduce the early exposure of low-risk, low-efficacy patients to potential adverse effects of this therapy.[73]

The GISSI-3 and ISIS-4 investigators have stressed that a substantial proportion of the lives saved in their studies of early ACE inhibitor use occurred within the first days and weeks.[61] Their analysis underscores that delaying initiation of therapy is an opportunity lost. In a mechanistic echocardiographic study, the early use of an ACE inhibitor was associated with prompter recovery of ejection fraction and better preservation of left ventricular size.[74] Unlike reperfusion strategies, "early" in the context of ACE inhibitor use in MI is within 1 to 2 days, not minutes to hours.

ACE inhibitors should be considered adjunctive to the other proven beneficial approaches to acute MI.[75] The survival benefits of ACE inhibitors are additive to thrombolytics, β-blockers, and aspirin. Although a theoretical concern has been raised that aspirin use may blunt the benefits of ACE inhibitors,[76] the data support concomitant use.[77] Hospital quality report cards evaluate the number of patients on aspirin, β-blockers, and ACE inhibitors at discharge. Continued long-term use of ACE inhibition in selective high-risk patients will produce the greatest yield (see Fig. 12-6).

Angiotensin Receptor Blockers in Myocardial Infarction

With the demonstrated benefits of an ACE inhibitor after MI, the question of whether more selective blockade of the RAS with an ARB would result in even further improvements in clinical outcomes in this population could be done and interpreted only in the context of a comparator arm of a proven ACE inhibitor. Two major trials tested the relative value of an ARB in high-risk MI patients; both used captopril titrated to 50 mg three times daily as the comparator. The Optimal Therapy in Myocardial Infarction with the Angiotensin II Antagonist Losartan (OPTIMAAL) study of more than 5000 patients showed no benefit of the ARB losartan titrated to 50 mg/day compared with the proven dose of captopril.[78] As in ELITE II, in heart failure patients, there was a strong trend toward better outcomes in the ACE inhibitor group.[79] Together, results of ELITE II and OPTIMAAL indicate that this dose of losartan should not be considered equivalent to the proven dose of captopril in reducing cardiovascular events and raised serious questions about the common clinical practice of substituting an ARB for patients with presumed ACE inhibitor cough.

VALIANT was a three-arm trial with just under 15,000 high-risk patients randomized to an ACE inhibitor (i.e., captopril, target dose of 50 mg three times daily), an ARB (i.e., valsartan, target dose of 160 mg twice daily), or the combination of both the ACE inhibitor and ARB.[80] The patients randomized to the ARB had a morbidity and mortality rate that was very similar to the captopril-assigned patients. Although superiority of the ARB was not demonstrated compared with the ACE inhibitor, the point estimates and narrow confidence intervals for mortality and combined cardiovascular outcomes event were within the predefined noninferiority limits, supporting the conclusion that this dose of valsartan preserves the clinical benefits achieved with the ACE

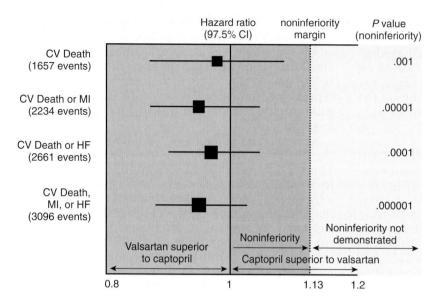

Figure 12-7. Noninferiority analysis in VALIANT demonstrates the preservation of benefits of captopril with the use of valsartan in a high-risk myocardial infarction population.

inhibitor (Fig. 12-7).[80] These data were sufficiently robust to lead to an FDA indication for this regimen of valsartan as an alternative for an ACE inhibitor in these patients.[81] The Joint Commission on Accreditation of Healthcare Organization (JCAHO) also altered its performance to add an ARB as an option for the post-MI regimen.[82]

In VALIANT, the combination of an ARB plus an ACE inhibitor offered no incremental clinical benefit and resulted in more adverse effects attributed to the concurrent use of these two inhibitors of the RAS.[80,83] These findings contrast with those of the CHARM-Added trial, in which reductions in cardiovascular death and hospitalizations for heart failure were achieved with use of dual inhibitors of the RAS.[45,46] Although there are multiple possibilities for this discrepancy, the differences in the stability of these patients (i.e., acute high-risk MI versus stable chronic heart failure), prior existing chronic use of an ACE inhibitor in only the heart failure patients, and the simultaneous introduction of both inhibitors of the RAS in only VALIANT, offer the most likely explanations.[84]

Reducing Aldosterone's Effects

In light of the direct stimulation of aldosterone release by angiotensin II, the RAS is more fully characterized as the renin-angiotensin-aldosterone system (RAAS) (see Fig. 12-1). Reducing local angiotensin II levels or inhibiting receptor binding would also be anticipated to reduce the influence of aldosterone. Beyond its renal actions at the distal tubule to promote sodium resorption in exchange for potassium, aldosterone is an important mediator of interstitial fibrosis.[85,86] The therapeutic importance of directly inhibiting the influence of aldosterone was highlighted in the Randomized Aldactone Evaluation Study (RALES).[87] In this randomized trial of patients with severe heart failure, a reduction in the risk of death was achieved with the addition of

spironolactone in patients who were already being treated with an ACE inhibitor.[87] Because this trial was conducted before the benefits of β-blockers in heart failure were fully demonstrated, only approximately 10% of the patients were concomitantly treated with these agents. Another aldosterone blocker, eplerenone, was also shown to be highly effective in improving survival rates of patients with left ventricular systolic dysfunction and clinical or radiologic evidence of acute heart failure complicating MI.[88] This survival benefit in the Eplerenone Post-AMI Heart Failure Efficacy and Survival Study (EPHESUS) was demonstrated in a more contemporary trial, with 85% of patients on both an ACE inhibitor and a β-blocker.

For high-risk MI patients with reduced left ventricular ejection fraction and acute heart failure, the effectiveness of combining an ACE inhibitor, β-blocker, and aldosterone antagonist appears clear (Fig. 12-8). In patients with heart failure and reduced left ventricular ejection fraction, the combination of an ACE inhibitor and β-blocker is considered the foundation of treatment, and whether the third agent should be an ARB or aldosterone blocker is more subjective.[84,89,90] In all cases, when using combination of RAAS inhibitors, monitoring for hyperkalemia is an important responsibility.[91-93]

Antiatherosclerotic and Vascular Injury

Clinical attention has focused on a more general role for ACE inhibition therapy in management of the broader population of patients with atherosclerotic vascular disease. An important observation from the SAVE and SOLVD studies was that the long-term administration of ACE inhibitor therapy was associated with an important reduction in the incidence of recurrent MI.[94,95] This information about secondary end points from these large trials with long-term follow-up pointed to another potential favorable mechanism of ACE inhibition therapy. Although it

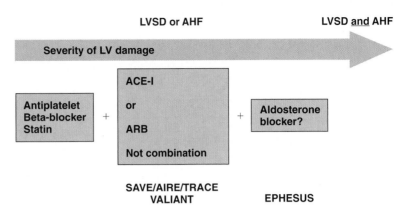

Figure 12-8. Suggested scheme for use of angiotensin-converting enzyme (ACE) inhibitors, angiotensin receptor blocking (ARB) agents, and aldosterone blockers in acute myocardial infarction based on clinical severity. AHF, acute heart failure; LVSD, left ventricular systolic dysfunction. (Adapted from McMurray JV, Pfeffer MA, Swedberg K, Dzau V: Which inhibitor of the renin-angiotensin system should be used in chronic heart failure and acute myocardial infarction? Circulation. 2004;110:3281-3288.)

had been reported that hypertensive individuals with high renin profiles were more likely to experience clinical MIs,[96] an association between the use of ACE inhibitors and a reduction of MI had not been demonstrated until the reports by the SAVE and SOLVD investigators. A meta-analysis of all the major long-term post-MI studies support the observation that ACE inhibitor use results in fewer MIs.[97]

Three major randomized-controlled clinical trials are prospectively evaluating whether the benefits of SAVE and SOLVD can be observed in patients without reduced ejection fraction. The first of these studies, the Heart Outcomes Protection Evaluation (HOPE) has definitively shown that the ACE inhibitor ramipril, when administered to patients with high-risk vascular disease, resulted in clear reductions in the risk of death, MI, and stroke.[98] The study had more than 9000 patients with a sufficient number of events to demonstrate that each of these components of the primary end point were reduced with use of the ACE inhibitor (Fig. 12-9A).[98] The HOPE study added definitive information regarding coronary atherosclerotic events, with clear reductions in the need for angioplasty, bypass surgery, and recurrent MIs. The study was also large enough to demonstrate reductions in stroke with the use of an ACE inhibitor (Table 12-1).

The European Trial on Reduction of Cardiac Events with Perindopril in Stable Coronary Artery Disease (EUROPA) trial randomized more than 12,000 patients with stable coronary disease to conventional therapy plus placebo or the ACE inhibitor perindopril.[99] Although the EUROPA cohort had a better prognosis than the HOPE patients, as manifested by their lower cardiovascular event rates, the ACE inhibitor group still experienced a 20% reduction in the primary end point of cardiovascular death, MI, or cardiac arrest (see Fig. 12-9B). These results provided rather strong confirmation and extension of the clinical importance of inhibiting the RAS with an ACE inhibitor in patients with atherosclerosis.

The Prevention of Events with Angiotensin-Converting Enzyme Inhibition (PEACE) study randomized more than 8000 lower-risk patients with coronary artery disease and documented preserved left ventricular function to continue their contempo-

rary therapy with the addition of either placebo or the ACE inhibitor trandolapril.[100] Neither the primary outcome of cardiovascular death, nonfatal MI, or coronary revascularization procedure or the major secondary end point of cardiovascular death or nonfatal MI was reduced in the ACE inhibitor group (see Fig. 12-9C). As the most contemporary of the three trials, PEACE had the lowest comorbidity as manifested by lower baseline blood pressure, cholesterol, and prevalence of diabetes. These important demographic features were translated into a better prognosis, because the clinical event rates in the placebo group of PEACE were lower than observed in even the ACE inhibitor arms of HOPE or EUROPA. Although appropriate questions have been raised regarding this apparent discrepancy of results, including the lower-risk population and the specific ACE inhibitor tested, other secondary end points, such as development of congestive heart failure and incidence of new diabetes, were reduced in the ACE inhibitor group.[101] The PEACE investigators support their assessment that lower risk may contribute to their negative findings with a retrospective analysis stratifying risk by renal function (i.e., estimated glomerular filtration rate [eGFR]).[102] Although the overall effect of the ACE inhibitor was null in the 16% of patients with chronic kidney disease, as manifested by an eGFR below 60 mL/min/1.73 m^2, there did appear to be a survival benefit in the group randomized to the ACE inhibitor. Moreover, meta-analysis of PEACE, HOPE, and EUROPA for patients with atherosclerosis does show an overall mortality benefit of the ACE inhibitor therapy (Fig. 12-10).[103,104]

The Perindopril Protection Against Recurrent Stroke Study (PROGRESS) demonstrated another vascular disease population that derived clinical benefits from the use of an ACE inhibitor.[105] In this study of more than 6000 patients who had a previous stroke or transient ischemic attack, randomization to active treatment with the ACE inhibitor perindopril with or without the addition of the diuretic indapamide (at the discretion of the treating physician) resulted in a 28% reduction in the risk of subsequent stroke. Moreover, there was a reduction in the risk of nonfatal MI for those on the ACE inhibitor. Although ACE inhibitors have been shown to reduce the need for

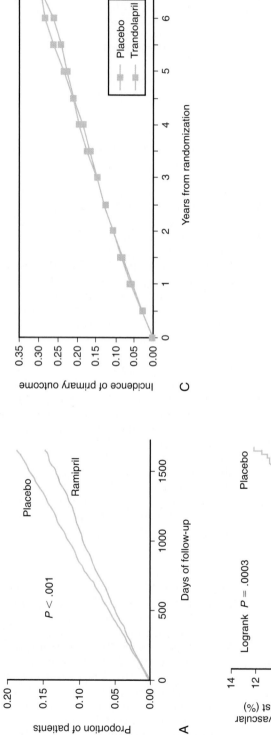

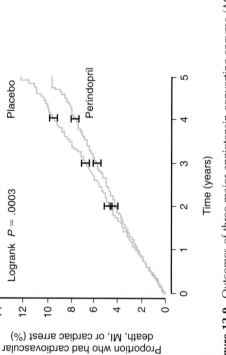

Figure 12-9. Outcomes of three major angiotensin-converting enzyme (ACE) inhibitor–treated vascular or coronary artery disease populations. **A,** HOPE primary outcome of myocardial infarction (MI), stroke, or cardiovascular (CV) death. **B,** EUROPA primary outcome of MI, CV death, or cardiac arrest. **C,** PEACE primary outcome of CV death, coronary artery bypass grafting (CABG), or percutaneous coronary intervention (PCI).

Table 12-1. Incidence of Secondary and Other Outcomes in the Hope Study

Outcome	Ramipril (n = 4645) No. (%)	Placebo (n = 4652) No. (%)	Relative Risk (95% CI)	P Value
Primary Outcomes				
Myocardial infarction, stroke, or death from cardiovascular causes	651 (14.0)	826 (17.8)	0.78 (0.70-0.86)	<.001
Death from cardiovascular causes	282 (6.1)	377 (8.1)	0.74 (0.64-0.87)	<.001
Myocardial infarction	459 (9.9)	570 (12.3)	0.80 (0.70-0.90)	<.001
Stroke	156 (3.4)	226 (4.9)	0.68 (0.56-0.84)	<.001
Death from noncardiovascular causes	200 (4.3)	192 (4.1)	1.03 (0.85-1.26)	.74
Death from any cause	482 (10.4)	569 (12.2)	0.84 (0.75-0.95)	.005
Secondary Outcomes				
Revascularization	742 (16.0)	852 (18.3)	0.85 (0.77-0.94)	.002
Hospitalization for unstable angina	554 (11.9)	565 (12.1)	0.98 (0.87-1.10)	.68
Complications related to diabetes	299 (6.4)	354 (7.6)	0.84 (0.72-0.98)	.03
Hospitalization for heart failure	141 (3.0)	160 (3.4)	0.88 (0.70-1.10)	.25
Other Outcomes				
Heart failure	417 (9.0)	535 (11.5)	0.77 (0.67-0.87)	<.001
Cardiac arrest	37 (0.8)	59 (1.3)	0.62 (0.41-0.94)	.2
Worsening angina	1107 (23.8)	1220 (26.2)	0.89 (0.82-0.96)	.004
New diagnosis of diabetes	102 (3.6)	155 (5.4)	0.66 (0.51-0.85)	<.001
Unstable angina with electrocardiographic changes	175 (3.8)	180 (3.9)	0.97 (0.79-1.19)	.76

From the HOPE Study Investigators: Effects of an angiotensin-converting-enzyme inhibitor, ramipril, on cardiovascular events in high-risk patients. N Engl J Med 2000;342:145.

coronary revascularization procedures, including percutaneous angioplasty,[94,95] two well-done studies have not demonstrated a reduction in coronary restenosis after balloon-only angioplasty.[106,107] The uniqueness of ACE inhibition was also questioned by the Comparison of Amlodipine versus Enalapril to Limit Occurrences of Thrombosis (CAMELOT) study of normotensive patients with known coronary artery disease, in which blood pressure lowering with the calcium channel blocker amlodipine was associated with fewer cardiovascular events than with either placebo or the ACE inhibitor enalapril.[108]

Proposed Mechanisms

In addition to the previously discussed hemodynamic and left ventricular structural benefits, new antiath-erosclerotic mechanisms have been invoked to explain the clinical observations of ACE inhibitors reducing coronary and other vascular events.[109,110] Experimental work has shown that in cholesterol-fed models, ACE inhibitor therapy can lead to reduction in the quantitative extent of atherosclerotic lesions.[111,112] Angiotensin II appears to directly influence the development of atherosclerotic lesions.[113] Another interface between the RAS and vascular events is the balance between thrombolysis and thrombosis. Infusion of angiotensin II in healthy subjects raised levels of plasminogen activator inhibitor-1 (PAI-1), altering fibrinolytic balance toward thrombosis,[114] and in patients with acute infarction, the use of an ACE inhibitor resulted in lower PAI-1 levels.[115] Reduced PAI-1 levels may also be an indicator of a better restoration of endothelial function. In a study of coronary artery nitric oxide–mediated

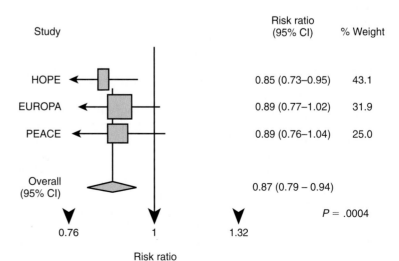

Figure 12-10. Meta-analysis of mortality from three major populations of angiotensin-converting enzyme (ACE) inhibitor–treated vascular or coronary artery disease populations.

vasomotion, less vasoconstriction in response to ace-tylcholine (i.e., improved nitric oxide generation) was observed after 6 months of treatment with an ACE inhibitor.[116] Lowering of local angiotensin II levels may reduce superoxide anions, promote nitric oxide, and limit further vascular damage.[117-119] Involvement of angiotensin II in oxidation and uptake of low-density lipoprotein,[120] in the stimulation of adhesion molecules,[121] and in the destabilization of the atherosclerotic plaque[122] has been invoked to explain some of the observed clinical benefits of ACE inhibitors on vascular events. Although atherosclerosis is considered a chronic inflammatory condition and C-reactive protein (CRP) can be used to assess this risk, the influence of ACE inhibition on this biomarker is unclear. An observational study of 507 patients with a recent ischemic stroke found that ACE inhibitor use was associated with more than a twofold lower CRP level and lower rates of fatal and nonfatal clinical events,[123] but in the randomized experience from the PEACE trial, CRP levels were not lower in the ACE inhibitor group.[124]

Angiotensin Receptor Blockers and Vascular Disease

Because these putative mechanisms link local angiotensin II to the atherosclerotic process, it is theoretically possible that the ARBs will be as effective or even more effective than ACE inhibitors in preventing vascular complications. However, as the clinical trial data unfolded, the question raised was whether the ARBs afforded even equivalent protection from the risk of MI compared with ACE inhibitors.[125] VALIANT provides the largest randomized, head-to-head ACE inhibition and ARB experience in a population at risk for recurrent MI, and no differences were found in rates or total burden of MIs between these two modes of inhibiting the RAS.[126] Similarly, in CHARM, cardiovascular death and nonfatal MIs were reduced by the ARB.[127] In an extensive review of this topic, ARBs were found to be as effective as ACE inhibitors.[128]

A more direct answer to this important question will likely be obtained from the Ongoing Telmisartan Alone and in Combination with Ramipril Global Endpoint Trial (ONTARGET). ONTARGET has randomized more than 25,000 HOPE-type patients to ramipril, the ARB telmisartan, or the combination. An additional 5000 ACE inhibitor–intolerant patients with vascular disease were randomized to telmisartan or placebo.[129] This ambitious research program will provide a quantitative assessment of the relative merits of ACE inhibitor, ARB, and the combination. The progress that has been made with ACE inhibitors has come from a host of definitive, well-conducted clinical trials across the entire spectrum of vascular disease (see Fig. 12-4). The newly developed ARBs also target the widest spectrum of patients with vascular disease in studies that will provide direct comparisons with the ACE inhibitors and that will define the optimal mode of inhibiting the RAS to reduce

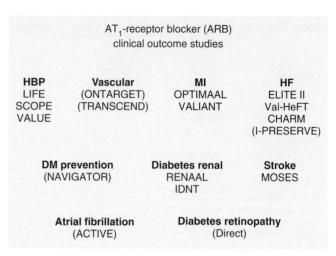

Figure 12-11. Major clinical outcomes trials using AT1-receptor blockers (i.e., angiotensin receptor blockers [ARBs]). DM, diabetes mellitus; HBP, high blood pressure; HF, heart failure; MI, myocardial infarction.

death and the clinical manifestations of vascular disease (Fig. 12-11).[38]

The Jikei Heart Study of more than 3000 Japanese patients with ischemic heart disease, hypertension, or heart failure provides additional support for an important effect of ARBs on atherothrombosis.[130] Subjects were randomized to the ARB valsartan or to conventional therapy. Despite similar blood pressure levels, there were fewer cardiovascular events (predominantly strokes) in the ARB group.

Reduction in the Incidence of Diabetes

The observations that fewer patients randomized to captopril developed diabetes than those randomized to the β-blocker in the CAPPP trial was initially met with skepticism about whether it was a real reduction with the ACE inhibitor or an increase in incidence of diabetes produced by the β-blocker comparator.[6] However, this objection cannot apply to the results of the HOPE trial, which showed a 30% reduction in the new incidence of diabetes in the ramipril arm.[98] There has been a rather consistent reduction in diabetes as assessed as a secondary end point in some of the major trials, including ALLHAT[10] and PEACE.[100] Similarly, major studies in hypertension comparing ARBs with other antihypertensive agents, such as in LIFE[13] and VALUE,[15] and with placebo, such as in the CHARM heart failure program,[43] have indicated that both pharmacologic inhibitors of the RAS reduced the risk of developing new-onset diabetes. A meta-analysis showed an approximately 20% reduction in the risk of developing diabetes in subjects receiving an ACE inhibitor or ARB.[131]

These observations have spurred basic research that has uncovered multiple potential mechanisms, such as reducing potential angiotensin II effect on the pancreatic fibrosis, improving insulin sensitivity in skeletal muscle, improving insulin signaling pathways, and other mechanisms whereby RAS inhibition could influence glucose homeostasis.[132] However, all the consistent and important observations from clinical trials must be considered as nondefinitive because they were derived from secondary end points from studies that were designed to address other questions. As part of a two-by-two factorial design, the Diabetes Reduction Assessment with Ramipril and Rosiglitazone (DREAM) study much more directly and rigorously tested whether an ACE inhibitor could reduce the development of diabetes in an at-risk population.[133] Although the primary end point of incidence of diabetes or death was 9% lower in the ACE inhibitor group, this difference was not statistically significant. A strong suggestion of an effect on glucose metabolism was, however, observed on prespecified secondary outcomes. An accompanying editorial indicated that hospitalization and ascertainment bias could have overestimated the RAS inhibitor influence on the incidence of diabetes in the prior trials and that the 95% confidence interval of DREAM (0.81 to 1.05) still encompassed an important possible benefit.[134] The ongoing Nateglinide And Valsartan in Impaired Glucose Tolerance Outcomes Research (NAVIGATOR), with more than 9000 subjects with impaired glucose tolerance randomized as part of a two-by-two factorial to the ARB valsartan or placebo, should settle this important issue.[135]

Renin Inhibitor Challenge

The cascade that leads to angiotensin II commences with the enzyme renin, which cleaves the peptide angiotensin I from angiotensinogen (see Fig. 12-1). Until recently, this first reaction has not been a clinically available pharmacologic target for inhibiting the RAS.[136,137] Theoretically, inhibition at this site of initiation may provide a unique way to reduce both angiotensin I and II levels while preventing exposure to compensatory escape mechanisms. Renin inhibition would also be anticipated to reduce the influence of other angiotensin peptides[138] more than ACE inhibitors or ARBs. Alternatively, combining a renin inhibitor with an inhibitor of angiotensin II generation (ACE inhibitor) or end receptor blocker (ARB) may provide the most effective means for long-term RAS inhibition. Commercialization of oral renin inhibitors has been severely hampered by a combination of poor bioavailability and a relatively expensive generation and production process. One agent, aliskiren, is emerging as an effective and apparently well-tolerated antihypertensive therapy.[137] The relative merits and clinical usage will undoubtedly depend on clinical outcome studies that go beyond the surrogate of blood pressure reduction. For this agent to be a commercial success, the medical community must be convinced by robust outcomes studies, such as have been conducted with the ACE inhibitors and ARBs, that a renin inhibitor alone or in combination with other proven pharmacologic therapies is safe and effective in reducing cardiovascular risk to justify usage of a new agent.

CONCLUSIONS

The clinical utility of ACE inhibitors has evolved from limited use in severe, refractory hypertension to first-line therapy for essential hypertension. A similar pattern has emerged in the management of patients with ventricular dysfunction. ACE inhibitors were initially administered only to severely compromised patients with heart failure, until further studies (e.g., SOLVD, Pre-SAVE) demonstrated the survival benefits of ACE inhibitors in milder degrees of congestive heart failure and even when used in a preventive manner before the clinical manifestation of overt heart failure in patients with asymptomatic left ventricular dysfunction. With the proven benefits of ACE inhibitors first observed during acute and chronic MI, studies have now extended proof of benefits to high-risk vascular disease and stroke patients. This pattern of testing from severe to milder forms of disease was also used for patients with vascular disease. The development of ARBs offers a unique opportunity to determine whether more complete inhibition of the RAS could produce additional clinical benefits. This is an active area of clinical investigation that will likely determine the relative roles of ACE inhibitors and ARBs alone or in combination. The expanding indications for ACE inhibitor and ARB use have been based on an exciting convergence of basic and clinical investigations that have improved our understanding of pathophysiology, vascular biology, and patient care.

Some of the advancements in the use of these inhibitors of the RAS stemmed from hypotheses derived from basic laboratory research, such as renal nephron protection and the attenuation of adverse left ventricular remodeling after MI, which were translated into clinical benefits by randomized, controlled clinical trials. Other leads for innovative areas of research stemmed from observations of secondary, often not prespecified, end points from the clinical trial experience. These initially unexpected findings, such as reductions in atherosclerotic events and reductions of the incidence of diabetes and atrial fibrillation,[139] provided the impetus for new randomized trials and important mechanistic studies. Inhibiting the angiotensin axis is perhaps one of the best examples of the importance of cross-fertilization between clinical outcomes and basic mechanistic studies.

REFERENCES

1. Pfeffer MA, Frohlich ED: Improvements in clinical outcomes with the use of angiotensin-converting enzyme inhibitors: Cross-fertilization between clinical and basic investigation. Am J Physiol 2006;291:H2021-H2025.
2. Lloyd-Jones DM, Evans JC, Levy D: Hypertension in adults across the age spectrum: Current outcomes and control in the community. JAMA 2005;294:466-472.
3. Turnbull F: Effects of different blood-pressure-lowering regimens on major cardiovascular events: Results of prospectively-designed overviews of randomised trials. Lancet 2003;362:1527-1535.

4. Williams B: Recent hypertension trials: Implications and controversies. J Am Coll Cardiol 2005;45:813-827.

5. Leenen FH, Nwachuku CE, Black HR, et al: Clinical events in high-risk hypertensive patients randomly assigned to calcium channel blocker versus angiotensin-converting enzyme inhibitor in the antihypertensive and lipid-lowering treatment to prevent heart attack trial. Hypertension 2006;48:374-384.

6. Hansson L, Lindholm LH, Niskanen L, et al: Effect of angiotensin-converting-enzyme inhibition compared with conventional therapy on cardiovascular morbidity and mortality in hypertension: The Captopril Prevention Project (CAPPP) randomised trial. Lancet 1999;353:611-616.

7. UK Prospective Diabetes Study Group: Efficacy of atenolol and captopril in reducing risk of macrovascular and microvascular complications in type 2 diabetes: UKPDS 39. BMJ 1998;317:713-720.

8. Davis BR, Cutler JA, Gordon DJ, et al: Rationale and design for the Antihypertensive and Lipid Lowering Treatment to Prevent Heart Attack Trial (ALLHAT). ALLHAT Research Group. Am J Hypertens 1996;9:342-360.

9. The ALLHAT Officers and Coordinators for the ALLHAT Collaborative Research Group: Major cardiovascular events in hypertensive patients randomized to doxazosin vs chlorthalidone: The antihypertensive and lipid-lowering treatment to prevent heart attack trial (ALLHAT). JAMA 2000;283:1967-1975.

10. Major outcomes in high-risk hypertensive patients randomized to angiotensin-converting enzyme inhibitor or calcium channel blocker vs diuretic: The Antihypertensive and Lipid-Lowering Treatment to Prevent Heart Attack Trial (ALLHAT). JAMA 2002;288:2981-2997.

11. Wing LM, Reid CM, Ryan P, et al: A comparison of outcomes with angiotensin-converting–enzyme inhibitors and diuretics for hypertension in the elderly. N Engl J Med 2003;348:583-592.

12. Okin PM, Devereux RB, Jern S, et al: Baseline characteristics in relation to electrocardiographic left ventricular hypertrophy in hypertensive patients: The Losartan intervention for endpoint reduction (LIFE) in hypertension study. The Life Study Investigators. Hypertension 2000;36:766-773.

13. Dahlöf B, Devereux RB, Kjeldsen SE, et al: Cardiovascular morbidity and mortality in the Losartan Intervention For Endpoint reduction in hypertension study (LIFE): A randomised trial against atenolol. Lancet 2002;359:995-1003.

14. Lithell H, Hansson L, Skoog I, et al: The Study on Cognition and Prognosis in the Elderly (SCOPE): Principal results of a randomized double-blind intervention trial. J Hypertens 2003;21:875-886.

15. Kjeldsen SE, Julius S, Brunner H, et al: Characteristics of 15,314 hypertensive patients at high coronary risk. The VALUE trial. The Valsartan Antihypertensive Long-term Use Evaluation. Blood Press 2001;10:83-91.

16. Schrader J, Luders S, Kulschewski A, et al: Morbidity and mortality after stroke, eprosartan compared with nitrendipine for secondary prevention: Principal results of a prospective randomized controlled study (MOSES). Stroke 2005;36:1218-1226.

17. Dahlöf B, Sever PS, Poulter NR, et al: Prevention of cardiovascular events with an antihypertensive regimen of amlodipine adding perindopril as required versus atenolol adding bendroflumethiazide as required, in the Anglo-Scandinavian Cardiac Outcomes Trial-Blood Pressure Lowering Arm (ASCOT-BPLA): A multicentre randomised controlled trial. Lancet 2005;366:895-906.

18. Lewis EJ, Hunsicker LG, Bain RP, Rohde RD: The effect of angiotensin-converting-enzyme inhibition on diabetic nephropathy. The Collaborative Study Group. N Engl J Med 1993;329:1456-1462.

19. Agodoa LY, Appel L, Bakris GL, et al: Effect of ramipril vs amlodipine on renal outcomes in hypertensive nephrosclerosis: A randomized controlled trial. JAMA 2001;285:2719-2728.

20. Ruggenenti P, Fassi A, Ilieva AP, et al: Preventing microalbuminuria in type 2 diabetes. N Engl J Med 2004;351:1941-1951.

21. Brenner BM, Cooper ME, de Zeeuw D, et al: Effects of losartan on renal and cardiovascular outcomes in patients with type 2 diabetes and nephropathy. N Engl J Med 2001;345:861-869.

22. Lewis EJ, Hunsicker LG, Clarke WR, et al: Renoprotective effect of the angiotensin-receptor antagonist irbesartan in patients with nephropathy due to type 2 diabetes. N Engl J Med 2001;345:851-860.

23. Berl T, Hunsicker LG, Lewis JB, et al: Cardiovascular outcomes in the Irbesartan Diabetic Nephropathy Trial of patients with type 2 diabetes and overt nephropathy. Ann Intern Med 2003;138:542-549.

24. Parving HH, Lehnert H, Brochner-Mortensen J, et al: The effect of irbesartan on the development of diabetic nephropathy in patients with type 2 diabetes. N Engl J Med 2001;345:870-878.

25. Viberti G, Wheeldon NM: Microalbuminuria reduction with valsartan in patients with type 2 diabetes mellitus: A blood pressure-independent effect. Circulation 2002;106:672-678.

26. Hostetter TH: Prevention of end-stage renal disease due to type 2 diabetes. N Engl J Med 2001;345:910-912.

27. Casas JP, Chua W, Loukogeorgakis S, et al: Effect of inhibitors of the renin-angiotensin system and other antihypertensive drugs on renal outcomes: Systematic review and meta-analysis. Lancet 2005; 366:2026-2033.

28. Remuzzi G, Ruggenenti P: Overview of randomised trials of ACE inhibitors. Lancet 2006;368:555-556.

29. Levey AS, Coresh J, Balk E, et al: National Kidney Foundation practice guidelines for chronic kidney disease: Evaluation, classification, and stratification. Ann Intern Med 2003;139:137-147.

30. Nakao N, Yoshimura A, Morita H, et al: Combination treatment of angiotensin-II receptor blocker and angiotensin-converting-enzyme inhibitor in non-diabetic renal disease (COOPERATE): A randomised controlled trial. Lancet 2003;361:117-124.

31. MacKinnon M, Shurraw S, Akbari A, et al: Combination therapy with an angiotensin receptor blocker and an ACE inhibitor in proteinuric renal disease: A systematic review of the efficacy and safety data. Am J Kidney Dis 2006;48:8-20.

32. Effects of enalapril on mortality in severe congestive heart failure. Results of the Cooperative North Scandinavian Enalapril Survival Study (CONSENSUS). The CONSENSUS Trial Study Group. N Engl J Med 1987;316:1429-1435.

33. Effect of enalapril on survival in patients with reduced left ventricular ejection fractions and congestive heart failure. The SOLVD Investigators. N Engl J Med 1991;325:293-302.

34. Cohn JN, Johnson G, Ziesche S, et al: A comparison of enalapril with hydralazine-isosorbide dinitrate in the treatment of chronic congestive heart failure. N Engl J Med 1991;325:303-310.

35. Hunt SA, Baker DW, Chin MH, et al: ACC/AHA guidelines for the evaluation and management of chronic heart failure in the adult: Executive summary. A report of the American College of Cardiology/American Heart Association Task Force on Practice Guidelines (Committee to revise the 1995 Guidelines for the Evaluation and Management of Heart Failure). J Am Coll Cardiol 2001;38:2101-2113.

36. Swedberg K, Cleland J, Dargie H, et al: Guidelines for the diagnosis and treatment of chronic heart failure: Executive summary (update 2005): The Task Force for the Diagnosis and Treatment of Chronic Heart Failure of the European Society of Cardiology. Eur Heart J 2005;26:1115-1140.

37. Adams JF, Lindenfeld J, Arnold JMO, et al: HFSA 2006 Comprehensive Heart Failure Practice Guideline. Journal of Cardiac Failure 2006;12:e1-e122.

38. Skali H, Pfeffer MA: Prospects for ARB in the next five years. J Renin Angiotensin Aldosterone Syst 2001;2:215-218.

39. Pitt B, Segal R, Martinez FA, et al: Randomised trial of losartan versus captopril in patients over 65 with heart failure (Evaluation of Losartan in the Elderly Study, ELITE). Lancet 1997;349:747-752.

40. Pitt B, Poole-Wilson PA, Segal R, et al: Effect of losartan compared with captopril on mortality in patients with symptomatic heart failure: Randomised trial—the Losartan Heart Failure Survival Study ELITE II. Lancet 2000;355:1582-1587.

41. Cohn JN, Tognoni G: A randomized trial of the angiotensin-receptor blocker valsartan in chronic heart failure. N Engl J Med 2001;345:1667-1675.
42. Anand IS, Wong M, Latini R, et al: Relation between changes in ejection fraction over time and subsequent mortality and morbidity in Val-HeFT [abstract]. J Am Coll Cardiol 2003;41(Suppl A):212A
43. Pfeffer MA, Swedberg K, Granger CB, et al: Effects of candesartan on mortality and morbidity in patients with chronic heart failure: The CHARM-Overall programme. Lancet 2003;362:759-766.
44. Granger CB, McMurray JJ, Yusuf S, et al: Effects of candesartan in patients with chronic heart failure and reduced left-ventricular systolic function intolerant to angiotensin-converting-enzyme inhibitors: The CHARM-Alternative trial. Lancet 2003;362:772-776.
45. McMurray JJ, Östergren J, Swedberg K, et al: Effects of candesartan in patients with chronic heart failure and reduced left-ventricular systolic function taking angiotensin-converting-enzyme inhibitors: The CHARM-Added trial. Lancet 2003;362:767-771.
46. McMurray JJ, Young JB, Dunlap ME, et al: Relationship of dose of background angiotensin-converting enzyme inhibitor to the benefits of candesartan in the Candesartan in Heart failure: Assessment of Reduction in Mortality and morbidity (CHARM)-Added trial. Am Heart J 2006;151:985-991.
47. http://www.fda.gov/cder/foi/appletter/2005/020838s022ltr.pdf
48. Yusuf S, Pfeffer MA, Swedberg K, et al: Effects of candesartan in patients with chronic heart failure and preserved left-ventricular ejection fraction: The CHARM-Preserved Trial. Lancet 2003;362:777-781.
49. Owan TE, Hodge DO, Herges RM, et al: Trends in prevalence and outcome of heart failure with preserved ejection fraction. N Engl J Med 2006;355:251-259.
50. Bhatia RS, Tu JV, Lee DS, et al: Outcome of heart failure with preserved ejection fraction in a population-based study. N Engl J Med 2006;355:260-269.
51. Cleland JG, Tendera M, Adamus J, et al: The perindopril in elderly people with chronic heart failure (PEP-CHF) study. Eur Heart J 2006;27:2338-2345.
52. Carson P, Massie BM, McKelvie R, et al: The irbesartan in heart failure with preserved systolic function (I-PRESERVE) trial: Rationale and design. J Card Fail 2005;11:576-585.
53. Pfeffer JM, Pfeffer MA, Fletcher PJ, Braunwald E: Progressive ventricular remodeling in rat with myocardial infarction. Am J Physiol 1991;260:H1406-H1414.
54. Pfeffer JM, Pfeffer MA, Braunwald E: Influence of chronic captopril therapy on the infarcted left ventricle of the rat. Circ Res 1985;57:84-95.
55. Pfeffer MA, Braunwald E: Ventricular remodeling after myocardial infarction. Experimental observations and clinical implications. Circulation 1990;81:1161-1172.
56. Hammermeister KE, DeRouen TA, Dodge HT: Variables predictive of survival in patients with coronary disease: Selection by univariate and multivariate analyses from the clinical, electrocardiographic, exercise, arteriographic, and quantitative angiographic evaluations. Circulation 1979;59:421-430.
57. White HD, Norris RM, Brown MA, et al: Left ventricular end-systolic volume as the major determinant of survival after recovery from myocardial infarction. Circulation 1987;76:44-51.
58. Pfeffer MA, Pfeffer JM, Steinberg C, Finn P: Survival after an experimental myocardial infarction: beneficial effects of long-term therapy with captopril. Circulation 1985;72:406-412.
59. Pfeffer MA, Lamas GA, Vaughan DE, et al: Effect of captopril on progressive ventricular dilatation after anterior myocardial infarction. N Engl J Med 1988;319:80-86.
60. Sharpe N, Smith H, Murphy J, Hannan S: Treatment of patients with symptomless left ventricular dysfunction after myocardial infarction. Lancet 1988;1:255-259.
61. Latini R, Maggioni AP, Flather M, et al: ACE inhibitor use in patients with myocardial infarction. Summary of evidence from clinical trials. Circulation 1995;92:3132-3137.
62. Flather MD, Yusuf S, Køber L, et al: Long-term ACE-inhibitor therapy in patients with heart failure or left-ventricular dysfunction: A systematic overview of data from individual patients. ACE-Inhibitor Myocardial Infarction Collaborative Group. Lancet 2000;355:1575-1581.
63. Pfeffer MA, Braunwald E, Moyé LA, et al: Effect of captopril on mortality and morbidity in patients with left ventricular dysfunction after myocardial infarction. Results of the Survival And Ventricular Enlargement trial. N Engl J Med 1992;327:669-677.
64. Acute Infarction Ramipril Efficacy (AIRE) Study Investigators: Effect of ramipril on mortality and morbidity of survivors of acute myocardial infarction with clinical evidence of heart failure. Lancet 1993;342:821-828.
65. Køber L, Torp-Pedersen C, Carlsen JE, et al: A clinical trial of the angiotensin-converting-enzyme inhibitor trandolapril in patients with left ventricular dysfunction after myocardial infarction. Trandolapril Cardiac Evaluation (TRACE) Study Group. N Engl J Med 1995;333:1670-1676.
66. Ambrosioni E, Borghi C, Magnani B: The effect of the angiotensin-converting-enzyme inhibitor zofenopril on mortality and morbidity after anterior myocardial infarction. The Survival of Myocardial Infarction Long-Term Evaluation (SMILE) Study Investigators. N Engl J Med 1995;332:80-85.
67. Swedberg K, Held P, Kjekshus J, et al: Effects of the early administration of enalapril on mortality in patients with acute myocardial infarction. Results of the Cooperative New Scandinavian Enalapril Survival Study II (CONSENSUS II). N Engl J Med 1992;327:678-684.
68. Furberg CD, Campbell RW, Pitt B: ACE inhibitors after myocardial infarction [letter]. N Engl J Med 1993;328:967-968.
69. Gruppo Italiano per lo Studio della Sopravvivenza Nell'Infarto Miocardico (GISSI)-3: Effects of lisinopril and transdermal glyceryl trinitrate singly and together on 6-week mortality and ventricular function after acute myocardial infarction. Lancet 1994;343:1115-1122.
70. Fourth International Study of Infarct Survival (ISIS-4): A randomised factorial trial assessing early oral captopril, oral mononitrate, and intravenous magnesium sulphate in 58,050 patients with suspected acute myocardial infarction. Lancet 1995;345:669-685.
71. Chinese Cardiac Study Collaborative Group: Oral captopril versus placebo among 13,634 patients with suspected acute myocardial infarction: Interim report from the Chinese Cardiac Study (CC-1). Lancet 1995;345:686-687.
72. ACE Inhibitor Myocardial Infarction Collaborative Group. Indications for ACE inhibitors in the early treatment of acute myocardial infarction: Systematic overview of individual data from 100,000 patients in randomized trials. Circulation 1998;97:2202-2212.
73. Pfeffer MA: ACE inhibition in acute myocardial infarction [editorial]. N Engl J Med 1995;332:118-120.
74. Pfeffer MA, Greaves SC, Arnold JM, et al: Early versus delayed angiotensin-converting enzyme inhibition therapy in acute myocardial infarction. The Healing and Early Afterload Reducing Therapy trial. Circulation 1997;95:2643-2651.
75. Antman EM, Anbe DT, Armstrong PW, et al: ACC/AHA guidelines for the management of patients with ST-elevation myocardial infarction—Executive summary: A report of the American College of Cardiology/American Heart Association Task Force on Practice Guidelines (Writing Committee to Revise the 1999 Guidelines for the Management of Patients With Acute Myocardial Infarction). Circulation 2004;110:588-636.
76. Hall D: The aspirin-angiotensin-converting enzyme inhibitor tradeoff: To halve and halve not. J Am Coll Cardiol 2000;35:1808-1812.
77. Pfeffer MA: Clinical accomplishments of ACE inhibition therapy: With and without aspirin. In: Goldhaber SZ, Ridker PM, eds. Thrombosis and Thromboembolism. New York: Marcel Dekker, 2002, pp 145-159.
78. Dickstein K, Kjekshus J: Effects of losartan and captopril on mortality and morbidity in high-risk patients after acute myocardial infarction: The OPTIMAAL randomised trial. Optimal Trial in Myocardial Infarction with Angiotensin II Antagonist Losartan. Lancet 2002;360:752-760.

79. Tokmakova M, Solomon SD: Inhibiting the renin-angiotensin system in myocardial infarction and heart failure: Lessons from SAVE, VALIANT and CHARM, and other clinical trials. Curr Opin Cardiol 2006;21:268-272.

80. Pfeffer MA, McMurray JJ, Velazquez EJ, et al: Valsartan, captopril, or both in myocardial infarction complicated by heart failure, left ventricular dysfunction, or both. N Engl J Med 2003;349:1893-906.

81. http://www.fda.gov/medwatch/safety/2005/aug_PI/Diovan_PI.pdf

82. http://www.jointcommission.org/NR/rdonlyres/A73B9038-87B2-4F92-81EF-9DE408EFB90B/0/ChangeinACEIforLVSD-MeasuresIncorpARBs.pdf

83. Mann DL, Deswal A: Angiotensin-receptor blockade in acute myocardial infarction—A matter of dose. N Engl J Med 2003;349:1963-1965.

84. McMurray JJ, Pfeffer MA, Swedberg K, Dzau VJ: Which inhibitor of the renin-angiotensin system should be used in chronic heart failure and acute myocardial infarction? Circulation 2004;110:3281-3288.

85. Struthers AD: Aldosterone blockade in cardiovascular disease. Heart 2004;90:1229-1234.

86. Cohn JN, Colucci W: Cardiovascular effects of aldosterone and post-acute myocardial infarction pathophysiology. Am J Cardiol 2006;97:4F-12F.

87. Pitt B, Zannad F, Remme WJ, et al: The effect of spironolactone on morbidity and mortality in patients with severe heart failure. Randomized Aldactone Evaluation Study Investigators. N Engl J Med 1999;341:709-717.

88. Pitt B, Williams G, Remme W, et al: The EPHESUS trial: Eplerenone in patients with heart failure due to systolic dysfunction complicating acute myocardial infarction. Eplerenone Post-AMI Heart Failure Efficacy and Survival Study. Cardiovasc Drugs Ther 2001;15:79-87.

89. McMurray JJ, Pfeffer MA: Heart failure. Lancet 2005;365:1877-1889.

90. Mielniczuk L, Stevenson LW: Angiotensin-converting enzyme inhibitors and angiotensin II type I receptor blockers in the management of congestive heart failure patients: What have we learned from recent clinical trials? Curr Opin Cardiol 2005;20:250-255.

91. Juurlink DN, Mamdani MM, Lee DS, et al: Rates of hyperkalemia after publication of the Randomized Aldactone Evaluation Study. N Engl J Med 2004;351:543-551.

92. McMurray JJ, O'Meara E: Treatment of heart failure with spironolactone—trial and tribulations. N Engl J Med 2004;351:526-528.

93. Desai AS, McMurray JJV, Granger CB, et al: Incidence and predictors of hyperkalemia in patients with heart failure—an analysis of the Candesartan in Heart failure—Assessment of Reduction in Mortality and morbidity (CHARM) program [abstract 531]. Eur J Heart Fail Suppl 2006;5:115.

94. Rutherford JD, Pfeffer MA, Moyé LA, et al: Effects of captopril on ischemic events after myocardial infarction. Results of the Survival and Ventricular Enlargement trial. SAVE Investigators. Circulation 1994;90:1731-1738.

95. Yusuf S, Pepine CJ, Garces C, et al: Effect of enalapril on myocardial infarction and unstable angina in patients with low ejection fractions. Lancet 1992;340:1173-1178.

96. Alderman MH, Madhavan S, Ooi WL, et al: Association of the renin-sodium profile with the risk of myocardial infarction in patients with hypertension. N Engl J Med 1991;324:1098-1104.

97. Danchin N, Cucherat M, Thuillez C, et al: Angiotensin-converting enzyme inhibitors in patients with coronary artery disease and absence of heart failure or left ventricular systolic dysfunction: An overview of long-term randomized controlled trials. Arch Intern Med 2006;166:787-796.

98. Yusuf S, Sleight P, Pogue J, et al: Effects of an angiotensin-converting-enzyme inhibitor, ramipril, on cardiovascular events in high-risk patients. N Engl J Med 2000;342:145-153.

99. Fox KM, Henderson JR, Bertrand ME, et al: The European trial on reduction of cardiac events with perindopril in stable coronary artery disease (EUROPA). Eur Heart J 1998;19(Suppl J):J52-J55.

100. Braunwald E, Domanski MJ, Fowler SE, et al: Angiotensin-converting-enzyme inhibition in stable coronary artery disease. N Engl J Med 2004;351:2058-2068.

101. Pitt B: ACE inhibitors for patients with vascular disease without left ventricular dysfunction—May they rest in PEACE? N Engl J Med 2004;351:2115-2117.

102. Solomon SD, Rice MM, Jablonski KA, et al: Renal function and effectiveness of angiotensin-converting enzyme inhibitor therapy in patients with chronic stable coronary disease in the Prevention of Events with ACE inhibition (PEACE) trial. Circulation 2006;114:26-31.

103. Al-Mallah MH, Tleyjeh IM, Abdel-Latif AA, Weaver WD: Angiotensin-converting enzyme inhibitors in coronary artery disease and preserved left ventricular systolic function: A systematic review and meta-analysis of randomized controlled trials. J Am Coll Cardiol 2006;47:1576-1583.

104. Dagenais GR, Pogue J, Fox K, et al: Angiotensin-converting-enzyme inhibitors in stable vascular disease without left ventricular systolic dysfunction or heart failure: A combined analysis of three trials. Lancet 2006;368:581-588.

105. Progress Collaborative Group: Randomised trial of a perindopril-based blood-pressure-lowering regimen among 6,105 individuals with previous stroke or transient ischaemic attack. Lancet 2001;358:1033-1041.

106. The MERCATOR Study Group: Does the new angiotensin converting enzyme inhibitor cilazapril prevent restenosis after percutaneous transluminal coronary angioplasty? Results of the MERCATOR Study: A multicenter, randomized, double-blind placebo-controlled trial. Circulation 1992;86:100-110.

107. Faxon DP: Effect of high dose angiotensin-converting enzyme inhibition on restenosis: Final results of the MARCATOR Study, a multicenter, double-blind, placebo-controlled trial of cilazapril. The Multicenter American Research Trial With Cilazapril After Angioplasty to Prevent Transluminal Coronary Obstruction and Restenosis (MARCATOR) Study Group. J Am Coll Cardiol 1995;25:362-369.

108. Nissen SE, Tuzcu EM, Libby P, et al: Effect of antihypertensive agents on cardiovascular events in patients with coronary disease and normal blood pressure: The CAMELOT study: A randomized controlled trial. JAMA 2004;292:2217-2225.

109. Strawn WB, Ferrario CM: Mechanisms linking angiotensin II and atherogenesis. Curr Opin Lipidol 2002;13:505-512.

110. Pagliaro P, Penna C: Rethinking the renin-angiotensin system and its role in cardiovascular regulation. Cardiovasc Drugs Ther 2005;19:77-87.

111. Teo KK, Burton JR, Buller CE, et al: Long-term effects of cholesterol lowering and angiotensin-converting enzyme inhibition on coronary atherosclerosis: The Simvastatin/Enalapril Coronary Atherosclerosis Trial (SCAT). Circulation 2000;102:1748-1754.

112. Weiss D, Kools JJ, Taylor WR: Angiotensin II-induced hypertension accelerates the development of atherosclerosis in apoE-deficient mice. Circulation 2001;103:448-454.

113. Kon V, Jabs K: Angiotensin in atherosclerosis. Curr Opin Nephrol Hypertens 2004;13:291-297.

114. Ridker PM, Gaboury CL, Conlin PR, et al: Stimulation of plasminogen activator inhibitor in vivo by infusion of angiotensin II. Evidence of a potential interaction between the renin-angiotensin system and fibrinolytic function. Circulation 1993;87:1969-1973.

115. Vaughan DE, Rouleau JL, Ridker PM, et al: Effects of ramipril on plasma fibrinolytic balance in patients with acute anterior myocardial infarction. Circulation 1997;96:442-447.

116. Mancini GB, Henry GC, Macaya C, et al: Angiotensin-converting enzyme inhibition with quinapril improves endothelial vasomotor dysfunction in patients with coronary artery disease. The TREND (Trial on Reversing ENdothelial Dysfunction) Study. Circulation 1996;94:258-265.

117. Munzel T, Keaney JF Jr: Are ACE inhibitors a "magic bullet" against oxidative stress? Circulation 2001;104:1571-1574.

118. Strawn WB, Chappell MC, Dean RH, et al: Inhibition of early atherogenesis by losartan in monkeys with diet-induced hypercholesterolemia. Circulation 2000;101:1586-1593.

119. Chen J, Mehta JL: Angiotensin II-mediated oxidative stress and procollagen-1 expression in cardiac fibroblasts: blockade by pravastatin and pioglitazone. Am J Physiol 2006;291: H1738-H1745.

120. Limor R, Kaplan M, Sawamura T, et al: Angiotensin II increases the expression of lectin-like oxidized low-density lipoprotein receptor-1 in human vascular smooth muscle cells via a lipoxygenase-dependent pathway. Am J Hypertens 2005;18:299-307.

121. Graninger M, Reiter R, Drucker C, et al: Angiotensin receptor blockade decreases markers of vascular inflammation. J Cardiovasc Pharmacol 2004;44:335-339.

122. Browatzki M, Larsen D, Pfeiffer CA, et al: Angiotensin II stimulates matrix metalloproteinase secretion in human vascular smooth muscle cells via nuclear factor-kappaB and activator protein 1 in a redox-sensitive manner. J Vasc Res 2005;42:415-423.

123. Di Napoli M, Papa F: Angiotensin-converting enzyme inhibitor use is associated with reduced plasma concentration of C-reactive protein in patients with first-ever ischemic stroke. Stroke 2003;34:2922-2929.

124. Sabatine MS, Morrow DA, Jablonski KA, et al: Investigation of the relation between the new AHA/CDC C-reactive protein cutpoints and cardiovascular outcomes and incident diabetes in patients with stable coronary disease: A PEACE substudy. J Am Coll Cardiol 2006;47(Suppl A):222A.

125. Strauss MH, Hall AS: Angiotensin receptor blockers may increase risk of myocardial infarction: Unraveling the ARB-MI paradox. Circulation 2006;114:838-854.

126. McMurray J, Solomon S, Pieper K, et al: The effect of valsartan, captopril, or both on atherosclerotic events after acute myocardial infarction: An analysis of the Valsartan in Acute Myocardial Infarction Trial (VALIANT). J Am Coll Cardiol 2006;47:726-733.

127. Demers C, McMurray JJ, Swedberg K, et al: Impact of candesartan on nonfatal myocardial infarction and cardiovascular death in patients with heart failure. JAMA 2005;294: 1794-1798.

128. Tsuyuki RT, McDonald MA: Angiotensin receptor blockers do not increase risk of myocardial infarction. Circulation 2006;114:855-860.

129. Sleight P: The ONTARGET/TRANSCEND Trial Programme: Baseline data. Acta Diabetol 2005;42(Suppl 1):S50-S56.

130. Mochizuki S, Shimizu M, Taniguchi I, et al: JIKEI HEART Study—A morbi-mortality and remodeling study with valsartan in Japanese patients with hypertension and cardiovascular disease. Cardiovasc Drugs Ther 2004;18:305-309.

131. Abuissa H, Jones PG, Marso SP, O'Keefe JH Jr: Angiotensin-converting enzyme inhibitors or angiotensin receptor blockers for prevention of type 2 diabetes: A meta-analysis of randomized clinical trials. J Am Coll Cardiol 2005;46: 821-826.

132. Aguilar D, Solomon SD: ACE inhibitors and angiotensin receptor antagonists and the incidence of new-onset diabetes mellitus: An emerging theme. Drugs 2006;66:1169-1177.

133. Bosch J, Yusuf S, Gerstein HC, et al: Effect of ramipril on the incidence of diabetes. N Engl J Med 2006;355:1551-1562.

134. Ingelfinger JR, Solomon CG: Angiotensin-converting-enzyme inhibitors for impaired glucose tolerance—Is there still hope? N Engl J Med 2006;355:1608-1610.

135. Haffner S, Hotman R, Califf R, et al: Targeting post-prandial hyperglycemia to prevent type 2 diabetes: Rationale and design of the NAVIGATOR trial [abstract]. Diabetologia 2002;45(Suppl 2):319.

136. Staessen JA, Li Y, Richart T: Oral renin inhibitors. Lancet 2006;368:1449-1456.

137. Azizi M, Webb R, Nussberger J, Hollenberg NK: Renin inhibition with aliskiren: Where are we now, and where are we going? J Hypertens 2006;24:243-256.

138. Cesari M, Rossi GP, Pessina AC: Biological properties of the angiotensin peptides other than angiotensin II: Implications for hypertension and cardiovascular diseases. J Hypertens 2002;20:793-799.

139. Anand K, Mooss AN, Hee TT, Mohiuddin SM: Meta-analysis: Inhibition of renin-angiotensin system prevents new-onset atrial fibrillation. Am Heart J 2006;152:217-222.

13 Thrombolytic Intervention

Matthews Chacko and Eric J. Topol

KEY POINTS

- Although percutaneous coronary intervention (PCI) has evolved into the preferred reperfusion strategy for ST-segment elevation myocardial infarction (STEMI), many patients present to hospitals that are not PCI-capable institutions or that have poor door-to-balloon times, rendering thrombolytic therapy an important tool in the reperfusion armamentarium.

- Plasminogen activators are serine proteases that participate in the lysis of fibrin by converting plasminogen to plasmin and include the fibrin-specific agents (e.g., tissue-type plasminogen activator, single-chain urokinase plasminogen activator, tenecteplase, staphylokinase, monteplase, palmiteplase, amediplase), the intermediate fibrin-specific agents (e.g., reteplase, lanoteplase), and the non–fibrin-specific agents (e.g., streptokinase, anistreplase, urokinase).

- The degree of myocardial salvage after acute myocardial infarction is related to timely reperfusion, reinforcing the "time is myocardium" principle, with the 2- to 3-hour mark being critical, regardless of which reperfusion strategy is employed.

- In the 30% to 40% of patients who fail thrombolysis (<70% ST segment resolution at 90 minutes or ongoing chest pain), rescue PCI should be performed. There is accumulating evidence that systematic cardiac catheterization and PCI within 24 hours, regardless of the success of thrombolysis, should also be performed.

- There is no evidence that a strategy of facilitated PCI for STEMI should be undertaken.

- Aspirin, unfractionated heparin, and clopidogrel should be administered to all patients with STEMI treated with thrombolysis in the absence of contraindications. There is no significant survival advantage to using GP IIb/IIIa inhibitors, low-molecular-weight heparin, or bivalirudin in the thrombolytic-treated patient despite reductions in reinfarction with these agents.

- Future thrombolytic intervention strategies will enhance epicardial and microvascular thrombus dissolution and will address preempting additional myocardial damage by neutralizing inflammation, apoptosis, and promoting myocardial regeneration.

Atherosclerotic plaque rupture and subsequent thrombus formation through an intricate series of interactions of the coronary artery endothelium, exposed subendothelium, circulating platelets, and coagulation factors leading to occlusion of an epicardial coronary artery are the pathophysiologic underpinnings of ST-elevation myocardial infarction (STEMI). The open-artery hypothesis, in which early reperfusion of the occluded artery translates into myocardial salvage and ultimately improved survival, is the foundation on which reperfusion therapy rests. The evidence for the benefit of thrombolytic therapy as a reperfusion strategy in STEMI is incontrovertible. Pivotal placebo-controlled, randomized trials of patients with STEMI from the 1980s proved the value of early thrombolysis by reducing mortality by approximately 30%.[1] The acceptance of thrombolysis as standard therapy for reperfusion in patients with acute myocardial infarction (MI) ushered in the *thrombolytic era,* a term that characterized the revolu-

tion in attitude among members of the medical community toward the disease.

Although there has been a shift in favor of primary percutaneous coronary intervention (PCI) as the preferred reperfusion strategy in most instances, the American College of Cardiology/American Heart Association (ACC/AHA) STEMI guidelines[1] favor thrombolytic therapy over PCI as the primary reperfusion strategy in patients who are not in cardiogenic shock and have no contraindications to thrombolytic therapy (Table 13-1), who present early (<3 hours), who have no invasive option (e.g., catheter laboratory is unavailable, vascular access issues), or who have a significant delay in performing PCI (e.g., prolonged transport time, door-to-balloon minus door-to-needle time of more than 60 minutes, door-to-balloon time of more than 90 minutes). However, because of concerns about bleeding complications, incomplete patency, and early re-occlusion rates with thrombolytic therapy, combined with the fact that

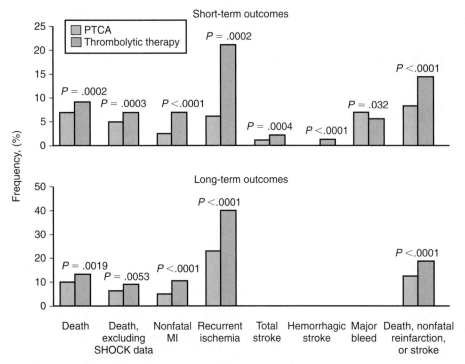

Figure 13-1. Frequency of short-term and long-term outcomes for patients treated with primary percutaneous coronary intervention versus thrombolytic therapy for ST-segment elevation myocardial infarction. (Adapted from Keeley EC, Boura JA, Grines CL: Primary angioplasty versus intravenous thrombolytic therapy for acute myocardial infarction: A quantitative review of 23 randomized trials. Lancet 2003;361:13-20.)

more primary PCI is being performed at smaller hospitals without on-site cardiac surgery back-up,[2] thrombolytic therapy has been superseded by primary PCI for the treatment of STEMI, which has been associated with better clinical outcomes (Fig. 13-1).[3-5] Although PCI has evolved into the preferred reperfusion strategy, particularly at high-volume, experienced centers, approximately 50% of patients with acute MI present to hospitals that are not capable of performing PCI.[6] Moreover, data from the National Registry of Myocardial Infarction (NRMI-4)[7] suggest that door-to-balloon times remain poor, with a median time of 180 minutes for patients transferred from one hospital to another for primary PCI, even within the framework of the current STEMI guidelines, indicating that there are still many patients who experience an inordinate delay in mechanical reperfusion therapy (or even no reperfusion therapy at all) in the real world. Thrombolytic therapy therefore remains an important tool in the pharmacologic armamentarium for treating STEMI, albeit with significant limitations. This chapter reviews the salient issues in thrombolytic intervention, laying the groundwork for a future perspective on the field.

THROMBOLYTIC AGENTS

Thrombolytic therapy was initiated in 1933, when Tillett and Garner[8] described the fibrinolytic activity of β-hemolytic streptococci, leading to the first therapeutic attempt by Tillett and Sherry in 1948 to dissolve a fibrinous pleural effusion.[9] The class of agents known as plasminogen activators are serine proteases that participate in the lysis of fibrin by converting plasminogen to plasmin. They include fibrin-specific agents such as tissue-type plasminogen activator (t-PA), single-chain urokinase plasminogen activator (scu-PA), tenecteplase (TNK), and staphylokinase (SAK), as well as the non–fibrin-specific agents such as streptokinase, anistreplase (anisoylated plasminogen streptokinase activator complex [APSAC]), and urokinase. Reteplase (recombinant plasminogen activator [r-PA]) and lanoteplase (novel plasminogen activator [n-PA]) have intermediate fibrin specificity. Two novel fibrin-specific agents, monteplase (MT-PA) and palmiteplase (YM866), are modified recombi-

Table 13-1. Contraindications to Thrombolytic Therapy in Patients with ST-Segment Elevation Myocardial Infarction

Absolute contraindications	Any prior intracranial bleeding
	Known cerebral AVM or malignancy
	Ischemic stroke (<3 months)
	Aortic dissection
	Active bleeding (nonmenstrual) or bleeding diathesis
	Significant head injury or facial trauma (<3 months)
Relative contraindications	Severe uncontrolled hypertension (>180/110 mm Hg)
	Ischemic stroke (>3 months)
	Traumatic or prolonged CPR (>10 minutes)
	Recent internal bleeding (<2-4 weeks)
	Noncompressible vascular puncture
	Active peptic ulcer disease
	Concurrent anticoagulation with warfarin
	Prior exposure or allergy to streptokinase or anistreplase
	Pregnancy

AVM, arteriovenous malformation; CPR, cardiopulmonary resuscitation.

Table 13-2. Characteristics of Thrombolytic Agents

Feature Source	Streptokinase Group C Streptococci	Tenecteplase Recombinant, Human	Alteplase Recombinant, Human	Anistreplase Group C Streptococci Plasminogen, Anisoylated	Reteplase Recombinant, Human Mutant Tissue-Type Plasminogen Activator
Molecular weight (kd)	47	57*	63-70	131	39
Fibrin specificity	No	Yes	Yes	No	Yes
Metabolism	Hepatic	Hepatic	Hepatic	Hepatic	Renal
Half-life (min)	18-23	20-24	3-4	70-120	14
Mode of action	Activator complex	Direct	Direct	Direct	Direct
Antigenicity	Yes	No	No	Yes	No
Estimated hospital cost/dose ($US)†	$300/1.5 MU	$2200	$2200/100 mg	$1800/30 U	$2200/20 MU

*Data from Tucasso NM, Napi JM: Tenecteplase for treatment of acute myocardial infarction. Ann Pharmacother 2001;35:1233-1240.
†Costs list U.S. prices of usual dose. Data from Granger CB, Califf RM, Topol EJ: Thrombolytic therapy for acute myocardial infarction. Drugs 1992;44:293-325.

nant tissue plasminogen activators with relatively long half-lives that have been tested primarily in Japan but have not been developed for widespread commercial use. Amediplase [K(2) tu-PA] is a fibrin-specific hybrid plasminogen activator with improved clot penetration in animal models, and it is undergoing evaluation in Europe for the treatment of STEMI. The major thrombolytic agents are briefly reviewed with regard to mechanism of action and thrombolytic profile in Table 13-2.

MAJOR HISTORICAL COMPARATIVE THROMBOLYTIC TRIALS

The second Gruppo Italiano per lo Studio della Sopravvivenze nell'Infarcto Miocardio (GISSI-2)/ International trial,[10] with 20,891 patients with STEMI within 6 hours of symptom onset randomly assigned to t-PA or streptokinase, demonstrated no difference in mortality between streptokinase and t-PA with or without subcutaneous heparin (intravenous heparin was rarely used in this trial) but showed a higher rate of ischemic stroke in the t-PA group. The International Study of Infarct Survival-3 (ISIS-3) trial[11] of 41,299 patients randomized to t-PA, streptokinase, or anistreplase demonstrated equivalence of mortality reduction among the three agents but found that streptokinase was associated with the lowest overall rates of stroke (1.1%) and intracerebral hemorrhage (0.3%). Intravenous heparin was not used in this trial, and as has been borne out collectively through other studies of the fibrin-specific plasminogen activators, adjunctive heparin, although not critical to achieve thrombolysis, is important to sustain infarct vessel patency through avoidance of repeat thrombosis. The Global Use of Strategies to Open Occluded Arteries in Acute Coronary Syndromes I (GUSTO I) trial[12] enrolling 41,021 patients promulgated the benefit of "accelerated" t-PA plus intravenous heparin in STEMI, leading to a 15% relative and 1% absolute reduction in mortality (or 10 lives saved per 1000 patients treated) and included an angiographic com-

ponent[13] that led to the major finding that early and complete infarct vessel patency was tightly linked to a reduction in mortality. The GUSTO III trial,[14] enrolling 15,021 patients, failed to show true equivalence of r-PA to accelerated t-PA, but the approximation of the results, especially for death and disabling stroke, combined with the more convenient double-bolus administration of r-PA, made it a viable option for thrombolysis at the time. The Assessment of the Safety of a New Thrombolytic-2 (ASSENT-2) trial,[15] which included 16,949 patients randomized to receive TNK or t-PA, found similar mortality rates but was notable for significantly less bleeding with the highly fibrin-specific TNK compared with t-PA, although this was tempered by a relatively high rate of intracerebral hemorrhage in both groups.

TIMING OF THROMBOLYTIC THERAPY

Early Treatment

The degree of myocardial salvage after acute MI is clearly related to timely reperfusion, reinforcing the "time is myocardium" principle, with the 2- to 3-hour mark being critical (Fig. 13-2).[16] Several randomized trials and registries of prehospital thrombolysis in the United States and Europe have tested the value of very early administration of therapy but have not shown a significant survival benefit with this theoretically advantageous strategy. Based on the current ACC/AHA STEMI guidelines,[1] for patients not in shock who present within 3 hours of symptom onset with a large MI *and* if there is a significant delay anticipated in primary PCI (the preferred reperfusion strategy), in-hospital thrombolytic therapy should be administered. In patients who present after 3 hours, primary PCI appears to be superior to prehospital and in-hospital thrombolysis in terms of myocardial salvage, infarct size, and mortality, possibly owing to time-dependent thrombus resistance to thrombolytic agents[17,18] (Fig. 13-3). There appears to be an early and sustained difference

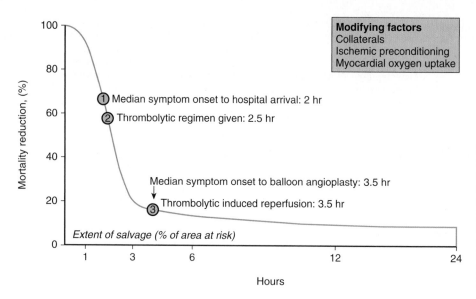

Figure 13-2. Mortality reduction as a function of time, with reperfusion therapy and the potential for myocardial salvage illustrating that unless patients present very early into the course of ST-segment elevation myocardial infarction, thrombolysis before percutaneous coronary intervention can have little benefit. (Adapted from Stone GW, Gersh BJ:. Facilitated angioplasty: Paradise lost. Lancet 2006;367:543-546.)

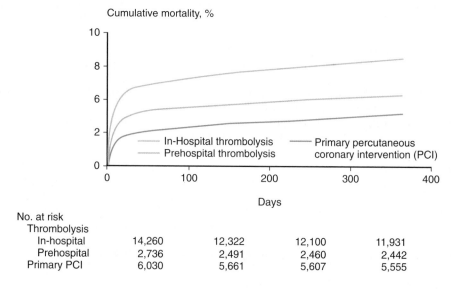

Figure 13-3. Unadjusted cumulative mortality for 26,205 patients with ST-segment elevation myocardial infarction who received reperfusion therapy between 1999 and 2004. (Adapted from Stenestrand U, Lindback J, Wallentin L, for the RIKS-HIA Registry: Long-term outcome of primary percutaneous coronary intervention vs pre-hospital and in-hospital thrombolysis for patients with ST-elevation myocardial infarction. JAMA 2006;296:1749-1756.)

in favor of primary PCI versus thrombolysis as a function of time to reperfusion; it was observed in one large registry study of 26,205 patients that it was not until approximately the 6- to 7-hour mark that the age-adjusted, 1-year mortality rate for primary PCI reached the same level as thrombolysis administered within 2 hours (Fig. 13-4).[18] Even if transfer to another facility is required, the benefit of PCI over thrombolysis in terms of reducing death, reinfarction, and disabling stroke exists for those with STEMI presenting less than 12 hours from symptom onset.[5,19] However, the net benefit of primary PCI over thrombolysis may be neutralized if door-to-balloon time for PCI is 60 minutes longer than door-to-needle time for thrombolysis, given that every 30-minute delay in symptom onset to balloon inflation is associated with a 7.5% increase in death at 1 year.[20] For those who present within 3 to 12 hours of symptom onset and if this delay is anticipated, thrombolysis is considered a viable alternative. Ting and colleagues[21] have developed an evidence-guided approach for

selecting the optimal reperfusion strategy based on incurred ischemia time (or transport time) and fixed ischemia time (or duration of symptoms) (Table 13-3). In the 30% to 40% of patients who fail thrombolysis (<70% ST segment resolution at 90 minutes or ongoing chest pain), rescue PCI should be performed given the benefit of this strategy (Fig. 13-5).[22-24] There is accumulating evidence that systematic cardiac catheterization and PCI within 24 hours, regardless of the success of thrombolysis, should be performed (Fig. 13-6).[24,25]

The facilitated PCI approach with early administration of a thrombolytic agent followed by mechanical revascularization is discussed later in this chapter and in Chapter 19.

Late Treatment

Mega-trials of thrombolytic therapy suggest that most of the benefit is largely confined to the first 12 hours after symptom onset and that many of the

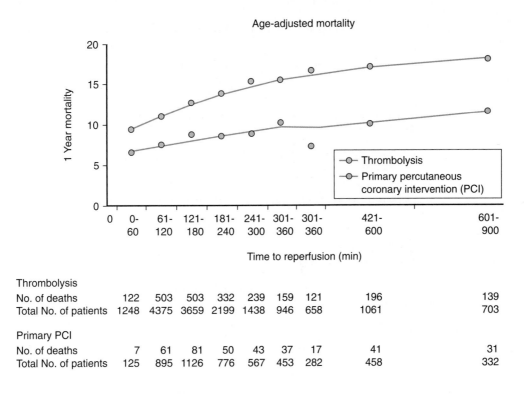

Thrombolysis

	0-60	61-120	121-180	181-240	241-300	301-360	301-360	421-600	601-900
No. of deaths	122	503	503	332	239	159	121	196	139
Total No. of patients	1248	4375	3659	2199	1438	946	658	1061	703

Primary PCI

	0-60	61-120	121-180	181-240	241-300	301-360	301-360	421-600	601-900
No. of deaths	7	61	81	50	43	37	17	41	31
Total No. of patients	125	895	1126	776	567	453	282	458	332

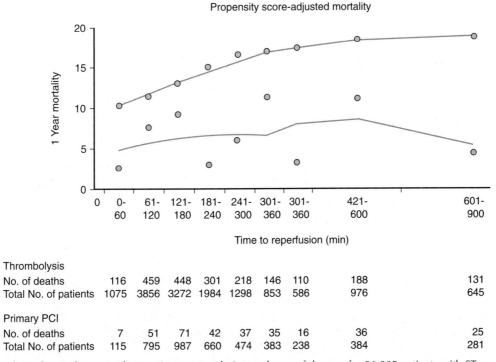

Thrombolysis

	0-60	61-120	121-180	181-240	241-300	301-360	301-360	421-600	601-900
No. of deaths	116	459	448	301	218	146	110	188	131
Total No. of patients	1075	3856	3272	1984	1298	853	586	976	645

Primary PCI

	0-60	61-120	121-180	181-240	241-300	301-360	301-360	421-600	601-900
No. of deaths	7	51	71	42	37	35	16	36	25
Total No. of patients	115	795	987	660	474	383	238	384	281

Figure 13-4. Age-adjusted mortality according to time to reperfusion and type of therapy for 26,205 patients with ST-segment elevation myocardial infarction who received reperfusion therapy between 1999 and 2004. (Adapted from Stenestrand U, Lindback J, Wallentin L, for the RIKS-HIA Registry: Long-term outcome of primary percutaneous coronary intervention vs pre-hospital and in-hospital thrombolysis for patients with ST-elevation myocardial infarction. JAMA 2006;296:1749-1756.)

Table 13-3. 2 × 3 Framework for Selecting a Reperfusion Strategy for Patients with ST-Segment Elevation Myocardial Infarction*

Transport Time (Incurrent Ischemia Time)	Duration of Onset of Symptoms (Fixed Ischemia Time)	
	<3 Hours	**>3 Hours**
<30 min	Primary PCI and GP IIb/IIIa[†]	Primary PCI and GP IIb/IIIa[†]
30-60 min	Thrombolytic agent and clopidogrel[‡]	Primary PCI and GP IIb/IIIa[†]
>60 min	Thrombolytic agent and clopidogrel[‡]	Thrombolytic agent and clopidogrel or primary PCI and GP IIb/IIIa[‡]

*Patients treated with thrombolytic agents should be immediately transferred to a PCI-capable facility in the event of failure to reperfuse.
[†]Based on American Heart Association/American College of Cardiology guidelines.
[‡]Based on clinical trials.
GP IIb/IIIa, platelet glycoprotein IIb/IIIa inhibitor; PCI, percutaneous coronary intervention.
Adapted from Ting HH, Yang EH, Rihal CS: Narrative review: Reperfusion strategies for ST-segment elevation myocardial infarction. Ann Intern Med 2006;145:610-617.

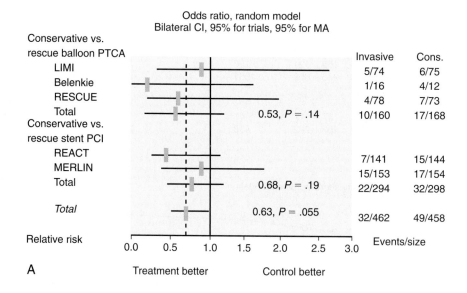

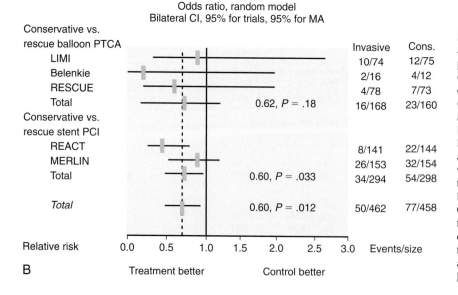

Figure 13-5. Odds ratios for death **(A)** and death or reinfarction **(B)** with rescue percutaneous coronary intervention versus conservative management of ST-segment elevation myocardial infarction at 30 days. (LIMI, LImburg Myocardial Infarction Trial; MA, meta-analysis; MERLIN, Middlesborough Early Revascularization to Limit Infarction; PTCA, percutaneous transluminal coronary angioplasty; REACT, REscue Angioplasty versus Conservative Therapy or repeat thrombolysis trial; RESCUE, Randomized Evaluation of Salvage Angioplasty with Combined Utilization of End points). (Adapted from Collet JP, Montalescot G, Le May M, et al: Percutaneous coronary intervention after failed fibrinolysis: A multiple meta-analysis approach according to the type of strategy. J Am Coll Cardiol 2006;48:1326-1335.)

complications, such as serious bleeding and latent myocardial rupture, occur with late thrombolysis. Two specific trials, the Late Assessment of Thrombolytic Efficacy (LATE) trial[26] and the Estudios Multicentrico Estreptoquinasa Republica Americas Sud (EMERAS)[27] trial, addressed the issue of late thrombolysis and showed no demonstrable survival benefit beyond the 12-hour mark with t-PA or streptokinase, with an excess of serious bleeding complications observed in the latter trial. The Fibrinolytic Therapy Trialists' Collaboration[28] pooled analysis of 52,892 patients enrolled in eight placebo-controlled trials

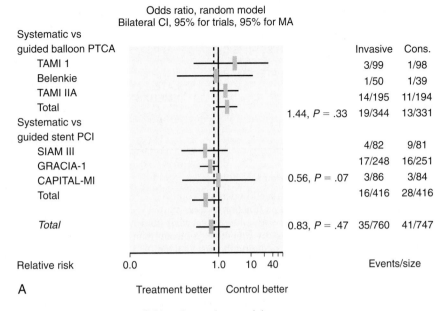

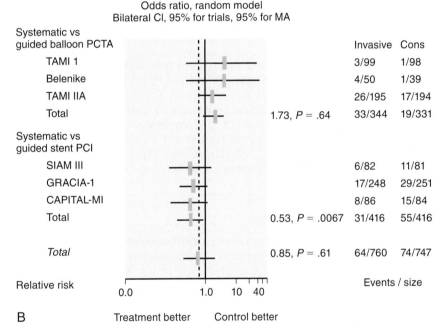

Figure 13-6. Odds ratios for death **(A)** and death or reinfarction **(B)** with systematic versus ischemia-guided percutaneous coronary intervention after ST-segment elevation myocardial infarction. (CAPITAL-MI, Combined Angioplasty and Pharmacologic Intervention versus Thrombolytics Alone in Acute Myocardial Infarction; GRACIA-1, Randomized trial comparing stenting within 24 hours of thrombolysis versus ischemia-guided approach to thrombolyzed acute myocardial infarction with ST-segment elevation; MA, meta-analysis; PTCA, percutaneous transluminal coronary angioplasty; SIAM, Comparison of Invasive and Conservative Strategies After Treatment with Streptokinase in Acute Myocardial Infarction; TAMI, Thrombolysis and Angioplasty in Myocardial Infarction). (Adapted from Collet JP, Montalescot G, Le May M, et al: Percutaneous coronary intervention after failed fibrinolysis: A multiple meta-analysis approach according to the type of strategy. J Am Coll Cardiol 2006;48:1326-1335.)

(excluding LATE) showed significant benefit up to, but not beyond, 12 hours. The available data provide cogent evidence that there is a "golden" first hour and a "dim" 12th hour after symptom onset, illustrating the narrow therapeutic window for thrombolytic therapy (Fig. 13-7), and that health care systems should minimize the delays in patient triage and initiation of reperfusion therapy.

ADJUNCTIVE THERAPIES

One of the remaining challenges of contemporary reperfusion therapy is to achieve tissue-level nutrient flow rather than simply restoring patency of the infarct-related epicardial coronary artery. Microcirculatory reperfusion after thrombolysis is critical, and mechanisms to reduce platelet aggregation, maintain endothelial integrity, and prevent the downstream effects of embolized thrombus and atherosclerotic debris through the use of potent anticoagulant, antithrombotic, and antiplatelet agents have led to several important clinical trials. Adjunctive therapies aimed at improving epicardial and microcirculatory patency while preserving myocardial function are discussed in the following sections.

Aspirin

The standard adjuvant pharmacotherapy for all patients with acute MI undergoing thrombolysis should include 162 to 325 mg/day of aspirin in the absence of a documented allergy to aspirin.[1,29] The benefit of aspirin therapy in ISIS-2 resulted in 25 lives saved per 1000 patients treated, and it prevented

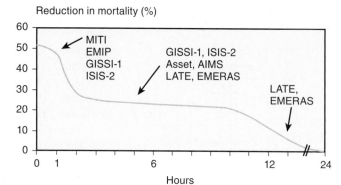

Figure 13-7. Percent mortality reduction derived from thrombolytic therapy is plotted as a function of time from symptom onset to initiation of therapy; the clinical trials from which these data are extrapolated are identified. A greater than 50% reduction in mortality occurs during the first "golden hour," after which the mortality benefit declines to a plateau of approximately 25% reduction until 12 hours, after which there is no apparent survival benefit with thrombolytic therapy. (From Lincoff AM, Topol EJ: The illusion of reperfusion: Does anyone achieve optimal reperfusion during acute myocardial infarction? Circulation 1993;87:1792-1805.)

10 nonfatal reinfarctions and 3 strokes per 1000 patients treated.[30] These findings appear to be durable at 10 years, making the duration of aspirin therapy in this setting indefinite.[31] Aspirin resistance in stable cardiovascular patients occurs at a frequency of approximately 5% and confers a significant risk of death, MI, or stroke compared with those with aspirin sensitivity, although widespread screening is controversial.[32]

Heparin

In the absence of heparin-induced thrombocytopenia or known allergy to heparin, unfractionated heparin should be part of the standard adjuvant pharmacotherapy for patients with acute MI treated with thrombolysis given the thrombin-mediated prothrombotic state that is created. The recommended heparin dose by the AHA/ACC Task Force is a 60-U/kg bolus (maximum, 4000 U) and a continuous intravenous infusion of 12 U/kg/hr (maximum, 1000 U/hr), titrated to keep the activated partial thromboplastin time (aPTT) between 50 and 70 seconds (class I recommendation).[1]

Low-molecular-weight heparin has emerged as an alternative to unfractionated heparin as adjunctive therapy for thrombolysis. The ASSENT-3 trial[33] assessed two different combination strategies: half-dose TNK plus abciximab versus full-dose TNK plus enoxaparin compared with TNK monotherapy (with unfractionated heparin) in 6095 patients, and it demonstrated an impressive reduction in reinfarction for both TNK combination-therapy groups, confirming the potency of the half-dose thrombolytic plus abciximab combination and the efficacy of enoxaparin in this setting. The benefit was tempered by an increased rate of bleeding complications requiring blood trans-

fusions in both of the combination-therapy groups compared with the TNK (plus heparin) monotherapy group. Also disconcerting was the relatively high rate of intracerebral hemorrhage in all three groups of the study (0.8% to 0.9%), particularly in the elderly. The trial did provide encouraging data for the use of TNK plus enoxaparin rather than heparin to reduce the short-term outcome of reinfarction, even though long-term follow-up at 1 year showed no benefit among the treatment groups in terms of mortality.[34] The ENTIRE (Thrombolysis in Myocardial Infarction [TIMI] 23) trial[35] evaluated ST-segment resolution at 180 minutes and early angiographic patency using various combinations of TNK with enoxaparin and abciximab in 461 patients with acute MI and demonstrated a reduction in death or nonfatal MI, as well as increased ST-segment resolution in the combined TNK plus abciximab plus enoxaparin group compared with TNK and either agent, with no increased bleeding complications. Validating the benefit of enoxaparin in reducing reinfarction, the Enoxaparin and Thrombosis Reperfusion for Acute Myocardial Infarction Treatment (ExTRACT)-TIMI 25 trial[36] compared enoxaparin with unfractionated heparin in 20,506 patients with STEMI undergoing fibrinolysis and demonstrated a 17% relative risk reduction in the primary end point of death or nonfatal reinfarction at 30 days (9.9% in enoxaparin group versus 12.0% in unfractionated heparin group, P < .001), driven primarily by a reduction in nonfatal reinfarction.

This benefit was at the cost of a significant increase in major bleeding in those treated with enoxaparin (1.4% in unfractionated heparin group versus 2.1% in enoxaparin group, P < .001), which appears to be problematic with enoxaparin given in conjunction with thrombolytic therapy.

The Cardiovascular Risk Reduction by Early Anemia Treatment with Epoetin-β (CREATE) trial,[37] which enrolled more than 15,000 patients with STEMI treated with thrombolytic therapy randomized to the adjunctive use of the low-molecular-weight heparin, reviparin, or placebo, demonstrated benefit in favor of reviparin regarding the primary composite end point of death, reinfarction, or stroke at 7 days (9.6% versus 11%, P = .005), although this, too, was offset by a small increase in severe bleeding. A meta-analysis by Eikelboom and coworkers[38] of randomized trials of low-molecular-weight heparin versus heparin with thrombolytic therapy in STEMI suggests that the benefit is in favor of low-molecular-weight heparin in terms of preventing reinfarction at 30 days (Fig. 13-8), although this must be weighted against the risk of bleeding, with particular caution in treating elderly patients (>75 years old) and those with significant renal dysfunction, both of which the ACC/AHA Task Force gives a class III recommendation against.[1]

Direct Thrombin Inhibitors

Deficiencies with heparin and low-molecular-weight heparin led to studies of direct thrombin inhibitors,

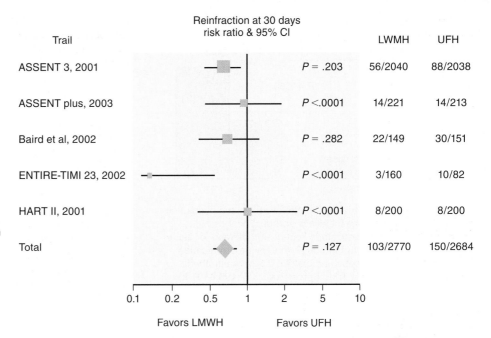

Trail	Reinfraction at 30 days risk ratio & 95% CI		LWMH	UFH
ASSENT 3, 2001		*P* = .203	56/2040	88/2038
ASSENT plus, 2003		*P* <.0001	14/221	14/213
Baird et al, 2002		*P* = .282	22/149	30/151
ENTIRE-TIMI 23, 2002		*P* <.0001	3/160	10/82
HART II, 2001		*P* <.0001	8/200	8/200
Total		*P* = .127	103/2770	150/2684

0.1   0.2   0.5   1   2   5   10

Favors LMWH   Favors UFH

Figure 13-8. Rates of reinfarction in unfractionated heparin (UFH) versus low-molecular-weight heparin (LMWH)–treated patients as adjuncts to thrombolysis in ST-segment elevation myocardial infarction. (Adapted from Eikelboom JW, Quinlan DJ, Mehta SR, et al: Unfractionated and low-molecular-weight heparin as adjuncts to thrombolysis in aspirin-treated patients with ST-elevation acute myocardial infarction: A meta-analysis of the randomized trials. Circulation 2005;112:3855-3867.)

such as hirudin and its synthetic peptide congener bivalirudin, as adjuncts to thrombolytic therapy. Clot-bound thrombin is quarantined from the inhibition of heparin and amplifies its own generation through a positive-feedback loop and activates platelets through thromboxane-independent mechanisms, making it an important effector of thrombus formation. Unlike heparin (or low-molecular-weight heparin), which potentiates the inhibitory effect of antithrombin III on soluble thrombin, which can be highly variable from patient to patient and even within the same patient, direct thrombin inhibitors directly bind soluble and bound thrombin, thereby inactivating it.

Hirudin was tested against unfractionated heparin in two thrombolytic regimens, including streptokinase and t-PA in the GUSTO IIb trial[39] of 4000 STEMI patients, and it demonstrated a favorable interaction with streptokinase (but not t-PA) in terms of 30-day death or reinfarction, illustrating the crucial role of thrombin generation after streptokinase administration and its relation to outcomes.

The largest dedicated trial using a direct thrombin inhibitor was the Hirulog Early Reperfusion Occlusion 2 (HERO-2) study,[40] in which 17,073 patients with STEMI were treated with streptokinase plus heparin or bivalirudin. It demonstrated a relatively high overall mortality rate (10.9% in the streptokinase plus heparin group versus 10.8% in the streptokinase plus bivalirudin group), the reasons for which were unclear, but it might have been related to the use of streptokinase as the thrombolytic agent, the relatively late entry of patients, and the geographic considerations of enrollment. Although it did show a significant reduction in reinfarction (1.6% in streptokinase plus bivalirudin group versus 2.3% in streptokinase plus heparin group, *P* = .001), a trend toward increased intracerebral hemorrhage and blood

transfusions was observed in the streptokinase plus bivalirudin group. Bivalirudin, as an alternative to unfractionated heparin, may be acceptable (class IIa recommendation) in patients with heparin-induced thrombocytopenia and STEMI treated with streptokinase based on the HERO-2 trial.

Glycoprotein IIB/IIIA Inhibitors

The rationale for more potent adjunctive therapies for thrombolysis originated from angiographic studies of thrombolysis monotherapy showing incomplete clot dissolution. Moreover, despite the promise and ease of bolus administration of the second- and third-generation thrombolytic agents, there was no incremental improvement in survival. The combination of a thrombolytic agent at half-dose with full-dose GP IIb/IIIa inhibitor seemed to be particularly attractive in light of a number of studies indicating better infarct vessel patency, more complete angiographic clot dissolution, and more ST-segment resolution. Most of the available data for the use of GP IIb/IIa inhibitors as adjunctive therapy in STEMI involves abciximab and are exemplified by results of the GUSTO V trial,[41] which evaluated the combination of half-dose reteplase plus abciximab compared with full-dose reteplase in 16,588 patients. The main findings of the trial suggested that combination therapy might be particularly useful in younger patients (<75 years old), particularly those with anterior MI. The primary end point of 30-day mortality was slightly better with combination therapy (5.6% versus 5.9%, *P* = .45), which fulfilled noninferiority criteria and represented the first combination reperfusion strategy validated as "at least as good as" full-dose thrombolytic therapy. The trade-off, however, was an increase in bleeding complications requiring blood transfusions in 4% of the

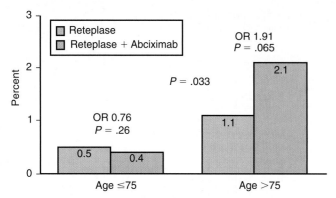

Figure 13-9. GUSTO V trial data plotted to show the interaction of intracranial hemorrhage incidence and treatment by age. (From the GUSTO V Investigators: Reperfusion therapy for acute myocardial infarction with fibrinolytic therapy or combination low dose fibrinolytic therapy and platelet glycoprotein IIb/IIIa inhibition: The GUSTO V Trial. Lancet 2001;357:1905-1914.)

r-PA–treated patients and 5.7% in the combination-treated patients, most of whom were elderly and had a significantly increased risk of intracerebral hemorrhage (Fig. 13-9). Disappointingly, long-term data highlighted that there was no difference in 1-year mortality between the two strategies.[42] A meta-analysis by De Luca and associates[43] summarized the use of abciximab in this context and showed that compared with primary angioplasty for STEMI, abciximab as adjunctive therapy for thrombolysis for STEMI had no mortality benefit at 30 days or long term, and although there were similar reductions in reinfarction at 30 days, the bleeding trade-offs with abciximab were significant.

Regarding the small-molecule GP IIb/IIIa inhibitors, the combination of TNK plus tirofiban versus TNK alone demonstrated more rapid and complete ST-segment resolution in the small, randomized, dose-finding study Fibrinolytics and Aggrastat in ST Elevation Resolution (FASTER)-TIMI 24[44] without an

increase in major bleeding. The SASTRE investigators demonstrated higher rates of TIMI 3 flow and TIMI grade 3 myocardial perfusion (TMP), translating into better clinical outcomes and no increased bleeding risk when tirofiban was used as an adjunct to reperfusion therapy with thrombolysis (i.e., alteplase) and with primary PCI in 144 patients.[45] The Integrilin and Tenecteplase in Acute Myocardial Infarction (INTEGRITI) trial[46] evaluating TNK with combinations of eptifibatide in STEMI showed that double-bolus eptifibatide plus half-dose TNK improved arterial patency and ST-segment resolution over TNK monotherapy, but it was at the expense of increased major bleeding and transfusions, limiting this as a useful strategy. Large-scale trials showing a survival benefit with the adjunctive use of small-molecule GP IIb/IIIa inhibitors with thrombolysis are lacking.

Limited data are available with regard to the role of GP IIb/IIIa inhibitors in rescue PCI after failed full-dose thrombolytic therapy, with particular concern about excess bleeding (despite lower heparin doses), as seen in the GUSTO III subgroup of subjects who underwent rescue angioplasty with abciximab.[47] Small series from the stenting era suggest that short-term clinical outcomes may be improved with this strategy with no significant trade-offs in terms of bleeding complications, although caution is warranted.[48]

Thienopyridines

Clopidogrel was shown in the 45,852 patients in the Clopidogrel and Metoprolol in Myocardial Infarction Trial (COMMIT)[49] to significantly reduce death (7.5% versus 8.1%, P = .03) (Fig. 13-10) and the combined end point of death, reinfarction, or stroke (9.2% versus 10.1%, P = .002) when given to aspirin-treated patients before thrombolytic therapy for STEMI (Fig. 13-11). The Clopidogrel as Adjunctive Reperfusion Therapy (CLARITY)-TIMI 28 trial[50] also supported the

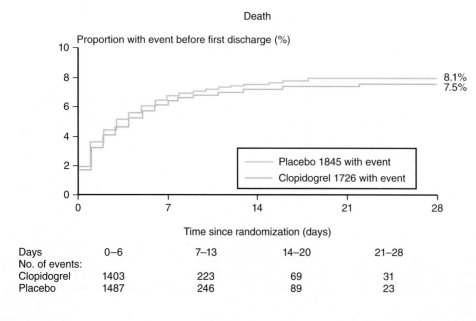

Death

Days	0–6	7–13	14–20	21–28
No. of events:				
Clopidogrel	1403	223	69	31
Placebo	1487	246	89	23

Figure 13-10. Death rates from the COMMIT trial for the addition of clopidogrel to aspirin in 45,852 patients with ST-segment elevation myocardial infarction. (Adapted from Chen ZM, Jiang LX, Chen YP, et al: Addition of clopidogrel to aspirin in 45,852 patients with acute myocardial infarction: Randomized placebo-controlled trial. Lancet 2005;366:1607-1621.)

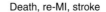

Death, re-MI, stroke

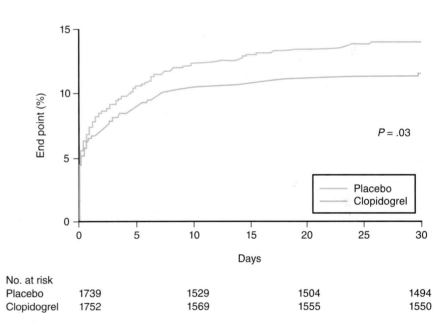

Proportion with event before first discharge (%)

| | Placebo 2310 with event |
| | Clopidogrel 2121 with event |

Time since randomization (days)

Days	0–6	7–13	14–20	21–28
No. of events:				
Clopidogrel	1751	247	91	32
Placebo	1879	301	104	26

Figure 13-11. Combined end point of death, reinfarction, and stroke from COMMIT for the addition of clopidogrel to aspirin in 45,852 patients with ST-segment elevation myocardial infarction. (Adapted from Chen ZM, Jiang LX, Chen YP, et al: Addition of clopidogrel to aspirin in 45,852 patients with acute myocardial infarction: Randomized placebo-controlled trial. Lancet 2005;366:1607-1621.)

P = .03

| | Placebo |
| | Clopidogrel |

Days

No. at risk				
Placebo	1739	1529	1504	1494
Clopidogrel	1752	1569	1555	1550

Figure 13-12. Cumulative incidence of the combined end point of cardiovascular death, recurrent myocardial infarction, or recurrent ischemia leading to the need for urgent revascularization. (Adapted from Sabatine MS, Cannon CP, Gibson CM, et al: Addition of clopidogrel to aspirin and fibrinolytic therapy for myocardial infarction with ST-segment elevation. N Engl J Med 2005;352:1179-1189.)

benefit of clopidogrel pretreatment of thrombolysis in patients who were 75 years or younger with STEMI, and the trial demonstrated reduced rates of death and recurrent MI or ischemia at 30 days (Figs. 13-12 and 13-13), as well as significantly improved coronary blood flow at 48 hours and no excess bleeding with clopidogrel. If aspirin allergy or intolerance precludes the use of aspirin with thrombolysis, clopidogrel is considered an acceptable alternative.[1,51] Prasugrel, a novel thienopyridine P2Y12 receptor antagonist with more potent platelet inhibition and possibly less resistance compared with clopidogrel, is being tested in the moderate- to high-risk acute coronary syndrome population undergoing PCI in the Trial to Assess Improvement in Therapeutic Outcomes by Optimizing Platelet Inhibition with Prasugrel–Thrombolysis in Myocardial Infarction 38 (TRITON-TIMI 38) trial[52] (which will include approximately 3500 STEMI patients), and it remains to be seen whether its application and benefit will be extended to thrombolytic-treated patients. No meaningful studies have compared the thienopyridine ticlopidine with placebo as adjunctive therapy in STEMI patients undergoing thrombolysis. The Study of Ticlopidine versus Aspirin after Myocardial Infarction (STAMI)[53] did address the role of ticlopidine in secondary prevention of cardiovascular events in STEMI patients treated with thrombolysis but found no difference compared with aspirin.

The data in aggregate point to the value of early initiation of clopidogrel in STEMI patients. The optimal loading dose—300 or 600 mg or higher—in the setting of reperfusion has yet to be defined.

Complement Inhibitors

Because complement activation during acute STEMI was thought to mediate ischemia-related and

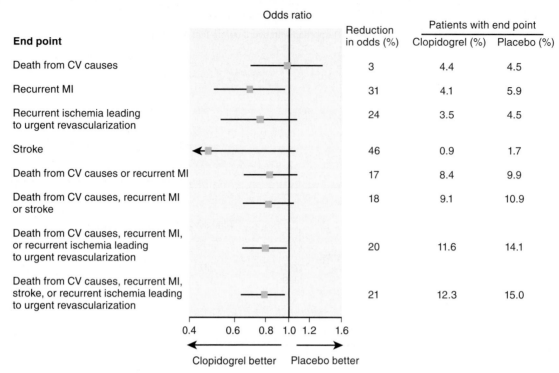

Figure 13-13. Odds ratios for individual and composite clinical end points through 30 days from the CLARITY-TIMI-28 trial. (Adapted from Sabatine MS, Cannon CP, Gibson CM, et al: Addition of clopidogrel to aspirin and fibrinolytic therapy for myocardial infarction with ST-segment elevation. N Engl J Med 2005;352:1179-1189.)

reperfusion myocardial injury, complement inhibition seemed useful in this setting. Disappointingly, the C5 complement monoclonal antibody pexelizumab failed to reduce infarct size or adverse events in patients with STEMI treated with thrombolysis in the Complement Inhibition in Myocardial Infarction Treated with Thrombolytics (COMPLY) trial[54] and cannot be recommended as adjunctive therapy without further study.

Factor XA Inhibitors

The Organization to Assess Strategies for Ischemic Syndromes 6 (OASIS-6) trial[55] evaluated the adjunctive use of the selective factor Xa inhibitor, fondaparinaux, versus unfractionated heparin in 12,092 patients with STEMI and found no benefit in those undergoing primary PCI, but it did show a significant reduction in death and reinfarction at 30 days and at 3 to 6 months for those undergoing thrombolysis treated with fondaparinaux, with no increase in severe bleeding, at least out to 9 days. Among those who underwent PCI, there was an increase in guide catheter thrombosis. Combined with results of the OASIS-5 trial[56] for the non-STEMI population, for whom there was a mortality benefit at 3 and 6 months with less major bleeding with fondaparinaux compared with enoxaparin, there appears to be promise for fondaparinaux across the spectrum of acute coronary syndrome patients, and future trials will determine whether this agent will become the standard of care, at least for those not undergoing PCI, with the realization that the prolonged 9-day administration may limit its widespread adoption.

Facilitated Percutaneous Coronary Intervention

Considerable attention has been given to the concept of facilitated PCI or the use of upstream pharmacologic therapy to serve as a "bridge" to PCI, given that survival is improved if TIMI 3 flow is present before mechanical reperfusion with PCI.[57] The use of full-dose thrombolytic therapy before PCI for STEMI was unhelpful (and even harmful), largely because of the prothrombotic effect of plasminogen activators and the showering of platelet-rich microthrombi into the microvasculature, leading to poorer outcomes in the early major trials that combined thrombolytic therapy with immediate angioplasty.[58] These early trials were conducted before the routine use of intensive antiplatelet therapy (including GP IIb/IIIa inhibitors and thienopyridines) and stents, which have improved outcomes for contemporary PCI for STEMI. The largest facilitated PCI trial was the ASSENT-4 trial,[59] which assessed the role of full-dose TNK and was stopped prematurely because of higher in-hospital mortality in the facilitated compared with the primary PCI group (6% versus 3%, $P = .01$), with ischemic complications such as reinfarction and repeat target vessel revascularization being significantly more frequent in the facilitated group. The strategy of using half-dose thrombolytic therapy plus full-dose GP IIb/IIIa inhibitor before PCI would seem to be a particularly attractive one given the benefit of GP IIb/IIIa inhibitors in those undergoing primary PCI. The prematurely terminated (owing to lack of enrollment) Angioplasty after Combination Therapy or Eptifibatide Monotherapy in Acute Myocardial Infarction (ADVANCE MI) trial[60] tested this strategy and compared eptifibatide plus half-dose TNK with eptifibatide plus placebo before primary PCI for STEMI and found adverse clinical outcomes and higher bleeding rates in the eptifibatide plus half-dose TNK arm despite demonstrating improved pre-PCI coronary flow. The Bavarian Reperfusion Alternatives Evaluation (BRAVE) trial[61] addressed the use of upstream abciximab plus half-dose reteplase versus abciximab monotherapy in 253 patients undergoing PCI for STEMI and found no reduction in infarct size by single-photon emission computed tomography (done between 5 and 10 days after randomization), with nonsignificant trends toward more adverse cardiac events at 6 months and more major bleeding in the abciximab plus Retavase group. A meta-analysis of 17 trials of patients with STEMI by Keeley and colleagues[62] sums up the lack of benefit of the facilitated PCI strategy and demon-

strates that despite achieving initial TIMI 3 flow in a greater number of patients, short-term outcomes (up to 42 days) of target vessel revascularization rates, reinfarction, stroke, and death are significantly increased with the facilitated approach (Fig. 13-14). The data from that analysis were insufficient to make any conclusions about the use of platelet glycoprotein IIb/IIIa inhibitors alone (without lytics) as a viable and potentially preferred facilitative approach to PCI. The ongoing Facilitated Intervention with Enhanced Reperfusion Speed to Stop Events (FINESSE) trial[63] may help to answer unsettled issues regarding facilitated PCI. Facilitated PCI is reviewed in more depth in Chapter 19.

CONCLUSIONS

Despite a deeper molecular, genetic, and pathophysiologic understanding of acute MI and vast improvements in the pharmacologic and mechanical reperfusion tools available, outcomes for STEMI remain suboptimal. Thrombolytic therapy has been the mainstay in the treatment of STEMI for the past

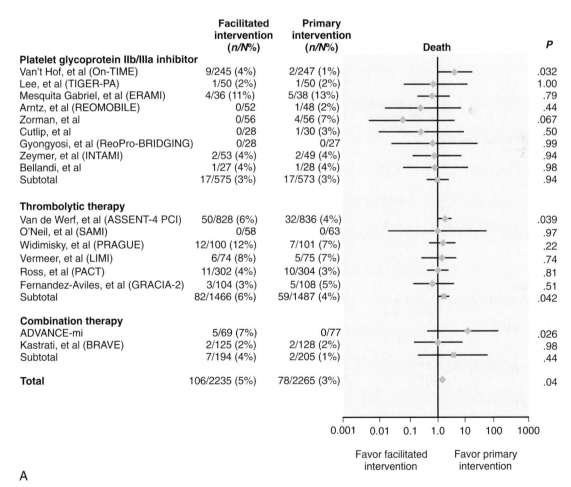

A

Figure 13-14. Odds ratios of short-term death **(A),** nonfatal reinfarction **(B),** and urgent target vessel revascularization **(C)** in patients treated with facilitated or primary percutaneous coronary intervention for ST-segment elevation myocardial infarction. (Adapted from Keeley EC, Boura JA, Grines CL: Comparison of primary and facilitated percutaneous coronary interventions for ST-elevation myocardial infarction: Quantitative review of randomized trials. Lancet 2006;367:579-588.)

Figure continued on next page.

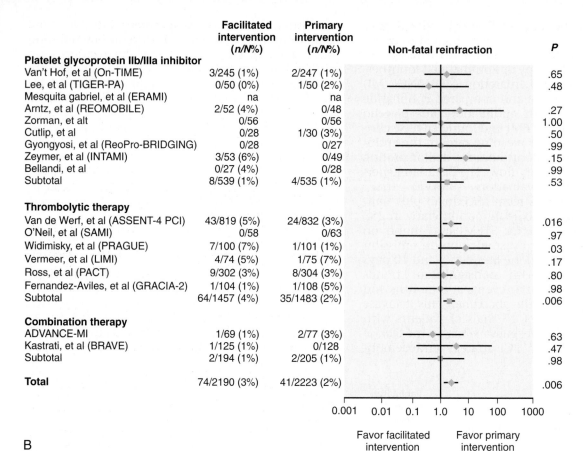

	Facilitated intervention (n/N%)	Primary intervention (n/N%)	Non-fatal reinfraction	P
Platelet glycoprotein IIb/IIIa inhibitor				
Van't Hof, et al (On-TIME)	3/245 (1%)	2/247 (1%)		.65
Lee, et al (TIGER-PA)	0/50 (0%)	1/50 (2%)		.48
Mesquita gabriel, et al (ERAMI)	na	na		
Arntz, et al (REOMOBILE)	2/52 (4%)	0/48		.27
Zorman, et alt	0/56	0/56		1.00
Cutlip, et al	0/28	1/30 (3%)		.50
Gyongyosi, et al (ReoPro-BRIDGING)	0/28	0/27		.99
Zeymer, et al (INTAMI)	3/53 (6%)	0/49		.15
Bellandi, et al	0/27 (4%)	0/28		.99
Subtotal	8/539 (1%)	4/535 (1%)		.53
Thrombolytic therapy				
Van de Werf, et al (ASSENT-4 PCI)	43/819 (5%)	24/832 (3%)		.016
O'Neil, et al (SAMI)	0/58	0/63		.97
Widimisky, et al (PRAGUE)	7/100 (7%)	1/101 (1%)		.03
Vermeer, et al (LIMI)	4/74 (5%)	1/75 (7%)		.17
Ross, et al (PACT)	9/302 (3%)	8/304 (3%)		.80
Fernandez-Aviles, et al (GRACIA-2)	1/104 (1%)	1/108 (5%)		.98
Subtotal	64/1457 (4%)	35/1483 (2%)		.006
Combination therapy				
ADVANCE-MI	1/69 (1%)	2/77 (3%)		.63
Kastrati, et al (BRAVE)	1/125 (1%)	0/128		.47
Subtotal	2/194 (1%)	2/205 (1%)		.98
Total	74/2190 (3%)	41/2223 (2%)		.006

0.001 0.01 0.1 1.0 10 100 1000

Favor facilitated intervention — Favor primary intervention

B

	Facilitated intervention (n/N%)	Primary intervention (n/N%)	Urgent Target vessel revascularization	P
Platelet glycoprotein IIb/IIIa inhibitor				
Van't Hof, et al (On-TIME)	5/245 (2%)	0/247		.039
Lee, et al (TIGER-PA)	0/50	1/50 (2%)		.48
Mesquita gabriel, et al (ERAMI)	na	na		
Arntz, et al (REOMOBILE)	4/52 (8%)	3/48 (6%)		.78
Zorman, et alt	0/56	2/56 (4%)		.24
Cutlip, et al	0/28	1/30 (3%)		.50
Gyongyosi, et al (ReoPro-BRIDGING)	0/28	1/27 (4%)		.46
Zeymer, et al (INTAMI)	2/53 (4%)	1/49 (2%)		.61
Bellandi, et al	0/27	0/28		.99
Subtotal	11/539 (2%)	9/535 (2%)		.99
Thrombolytic therapy				
Van de Werf, et al (ASSENT-4 PCI)	36/825 (4%)	8/836 (1%)		<.0001
O'Neil, et al (SAMI)	8/58 (14%)	1/63 (2%)		.011
Widimisky, et al (PRAGUE)	na	na		
Vermeer, et al (LIMI)	6/74 (8%)	1/75 (1%)		.05
Ross, et al (PACT)	na	na		
Fernandez-Aviles, et al (GRACIA-2)	1/104 (1%)	1/108 (1%)		.98
Subtotal	51/1061 (5%)	11/1082 (2%)		<.0001
Combination therapy				
ADVANCE-MI	na	na		
Kastrati, et al (BRAVE)	4/125 (3%)	1/128 (1%)		.17
Subtotal				
Total	66/1725 (4%)	21/1745 (1%)		.010

0.001 0.01 0.1 1.0 10 100 1000

Favors facilitated intervention — Favors primary intervention

C

Figure 13-14, cont'd

two decades, although primary PCI has evolved into the favored and recommended strategy at most centers. Whichever strategy is used, the timely restoration of epicardial and microvascular flow is crucial to limit myonecrosis, preserve left ventricular function, and improve survival. Thrombolytic agents have improved in terms of ease of administration and will continue to play an important role in the management of STEMI, particularly when primary PCI is not readily available. Future thrombolytic intervention strategies will enhance epicardial and microvascular thrombus dissolution beyond that which is capable today and will address preempting additional myocardial damage by neutralizing inflammation, restraining apoptosis, and promoting myocardial regeneration.

REFERENCES

1. Antman EM, Anbe DT, Armstrong PW, et al: ACC/AHA guidelines for the management of ST-elevation myocardial infarction: A report of the American College of Cardiology/American Heart Association Task Force of Practice Guidelines (Committee to Revise the 1999 Guidelines for the Management of Patients with Acute Myocardial Infarction). Circulation 2004;110:588-636.
2. Aversano T, Aversano LT, Passamani E, et al: Thrombolytic therapy vs primary percutaneous coronary intervention for myocardial infarction in patients presenting to hospitals without on-site cardiac surgery. JAMA 2002;287:1943-1951.
3. Keeley EC, Boura JA, Grines CL: Primary angioplasty versus intravenous thrombolytic therapy for acute myocardial infarction: A quantitative review of 23 randomized trials. Lancet 2003;361:13-20.
4. Boersma E, for the Primary Coronary Angioplasty Versus Thrombolysis-2 (PCAT-2) Trialists' Collaborative Group: Does time matter? A pooled analysis of randomized clinical trials comparing primary percutaneous coronary intervention and in-hospital fibrinolysis in acute myocardial infarction patients. Eur Heart J 2006;27:779-788.
5. Andersen HR, Nielsen TT, Rasmussen K, et al, for the DANAMI-2 Investigators: A comparison of coronary angioplasty with fibrinolytic therapy in acute myocardial infarction. N Engl J Med 2003;349:733-742.
6. Waters RE, Singh KP, Roe MT, et al: Rationale and strategies for implementing community-based transfer protocols for primary percutaneous coronary intervention for acute ST-segment elevation myocardial infarction. J Am Coll Cardiol 2004;43:2153-2159.
7. Nallamothu BK, Bates ER, Herrin J, et al: Times to treatment in transfer patients undergoing primary percutaneous coronary intervention in the United States: National Registry of Myocardial Infarction (NRMI)-3/4 analysis. Circulation 2005;111:761-777.
8. Tillett WS, Garner RI: The fibrinolytic activity of hemolytic streptococci. J Exp Med 1933;58:485-502.
9. Tillett WS, Sherry S: The effect in patients of streptococcal fibrinolysin (streptokinase) and streptococcal desoxyribonuclease on fibrinous, purulent, and sanguineous pleural exudations. J Clin Invest 1949;28:173-190.
10. The International Study Group: In-hospital mortality and clinical course of 20,891 patients with suspected acute myocardial infarction randomized between alteplase and streptokinase with or without heparin. Lancet 1990;336:71-75.
11. ISIS-3 (Third International Study of Infarct Survival) Collaborative Group: ISIS-3: A randomized comparison of streptokinase vs tissue plasminogen activator vs anistreplase and of aspirin plus heparin vs aspirin alone among 41,299 cases of suspected acute myocardial infarction. Lancet 1992;339:753-770.
12. The GUSTO Investigators: An international randomized trial comparing four thrombolytic strategies for acute myocardial infarction. N Engl J Med 1993;329:673-682.
13. The GUSTO Angiographic Investigators: The effects of tissue plasminogen activator, streptokinase, or both on coronary-artery patency, ventricular function, and survival after acute myocardial infarction. N Engl J Med 1993;329:1615-1622.
14. The GUSTO-III Investigators: An international, multicenter, randomized comparison of reteplase with alteplase for acute myocardial infarction. N Engl J Med 1997;337:1118-1123.
15. The Assessment of the Safety and Efficacy of a New Thrombolytic (ASSENT-2) Investigators: Single-bolus tenecteplase compared with front-loaded alteplase in acute myocardial infarction: The ASSENT-2 double-blind randomized trial. Lancet 1999;354:716-722.
16. Stone GW, Gersh BJ: Facilitated angioplasty: Paradise lost. Lancet 2006;367:543-546.
17. Schomig A, Ndrepepa G, Mehilli J, et al: Therapy-dependent influence of time-to-treatment interval on myocardial salvage in patients with acute myocardial infarction treated with coronary artery stenting or thrombolysis. Circulation 2003;108:1084-1088.
18. Stenestrand U, Lindback J, Wallentin L, for the RIKS-HIA Registry: Long-term outcome of primary percutaneous coronary intervention vs pre-hospital and in-hospital thrombolysis for patients with ST-elevation myocardial infarction. JAMA 2006;296:1749-1756.
19. Widimsky P, Budesinsky T, Vorac D, et al: Long distance transport for primary angioplasty vs immediate thrombolysis in acute myocardial infarction. Final results of the randomized national multicentre trial-PRAGUE-2. Eur Heart J 2003;24:94-104.
20. De Luca G, Suryapranata H, Ottervanger JP, Antman EM: Time delay to treatment and mortality in primary angioplasty for acute myocardial infarction: Every minute of delay counts. Circulation 2004;109:1223-1225.
21. Ting HH, Yang EH, Rihal CS: Narrative review: Reperfusion strategies for ST-segment elevation myocardial infarction. Ann Intern Med 2006;145:610-617.
22. Gershlick AH, Stephens-Lloyd A, Hughes S, et al: Rescue angioplasty after failed thrombolytic therapy for acute myocardial infarction. N Engl J Med 2005;353:2758-2768.
23. Patel TN, Bavry AA, Khumbani DJ, Ellis SG: A meta-analysis of randomized trials of rescue percutaneous coronary intervention after failed fibrinolysis. Am J Cardiol 2006;97:1685-1690.
24. Collet JP, Montalescot G, Le May M, et al: Percutaneous coronary intervention after failed fibrinolysis: A multiple meta-analysis approach according to the type of strategy. J Am Coll Cardiol 2006;48:1326-1335.
25. Fernandez-Aviles F, Alonso JJ, Castro-Beiras A, et al: Routine invasive strategy within 24 hours of thrombolysis versus ischaemia-guided conservative approach for acute myocardial infarction with ST-segment elevation (GRACIA-1): A randomized controlled trial. Lancet 2004;364:1045-1053.
26. Wilcox RG, for the LATE Steering Committee: Late assessment of thrombolytic efficacy with alteplase 6-24 hours after onset of acute myocardial infarction. Lancet 1993;342:759-766.
27. Estudio Multicentrico Estreptoquinasa Republicas de America del Sud (EMERAS) Collaborative Group: Randomized trial of late thrombolysis in patients with suspected acute myocardial infarction. Lancet 1993;342:767-772.
28. Fibrinolytic Therapy Trialists' (FTT) Collaborative Group. Indications for fibrinolytic therapy in suspected acute myocardial infarction: Collaborative overview of mortality and major morbidity results from randomized trials of more than 1000 patients. Lancet 1994;343:311-322.
29. Antithrombotic Trialists' Collaboration: Collaborative meta-analysis of randomized trials of antiplatelet therapy for prevention of death, myocardial infarction, and stroke in high-risk patients. BMJ 2002;324:71-86.
30. ISIS-2 (Second International Study of Infarct Survival) Collaborative Group: Randomized trial of intravenous streptokinase, oral aspirin, both or neither among 17,187 cases of

suspected acute myocardial infarction: ISIS-2. Lancet 1988;2: 349-360.

31. Baigent C, Collins R, Appleby P, et al: ISIS-2:10 year survival among patients with suspected acute myocardial infarction in randomised comparison of intravenous streptokinase, oral aspirin, both, or neither. The ISIS-2 (Second International Study of Infarct Survival) Collaborative Group. BMJ 1998; 316:1337-1343.

32. Gum PA, Kottke-Marchant K, Welsh PA, et al: A prospective, blinded determination of the natural history of aspirin resistance among stable patients with cardiovascular disease. J Am Coll Cardiol 2003;41:961-965.

33. The Assessment of the Safety and Efficacy of a New Thrombolytic Regimen (ASSENT)-3 Investigators: Efficacy and safety of tenecteplase in combination with enoxaparin, abciximab, or unfractionated heparin: The ASSENT-3 randomized trial in acute myocardial infarction. Lancet 2001;358:605-613.

34. Sinnaeve PR, Alexander JH, Bogaerts K, et al: Efficacy of tenecteplase in combination with enoxaparin, abciximab, or unfractionated heparin: One-year follow-up results of the Assessment of the Safety of a New Thrombolytic-3 (ASSENT-3) randomized trial in acute myocardial infarction. Am Heart J 2004;147:993-998.

35. Antman EM, Louwerenburg HW, Baars HF, et al, for the ENTIRE-TIMI 23 Investigators: Enoxaparin as adjunctive antithrombin therapy for ST elevation myocardial infarction. Results of the ENTIRE-Thrombolysis In Myocardial Infarction (TIMI) 23 trial. Circulation 2002;105:1642-1649.

36. Antman EM, Morrow DA, McCabe CH, et al, for the ExTRACT-TIMI 25 Investigators: Enoxaparin versus unfractionated heparin with fibrinolysis for ST-segment myocardial infarction. N Engl J Med 2006;354:1477-1488.

37. Yusef S, Mehta SR, Xie C, et al: Effects of reviparin, a low molecular weight heparin, on mortality, re-infarction, and strokes in patients with acute myocardial infarction presenting with ST-segment elevation. JAMA 2005;293:427-435.

38. Eikelboom JW, Quinlan DJ, Mehta SR, et al: Unfractionated and low-molecular-weight heparin as adjuncts to thrombolysis in aspirin-treated patients with ST-elevation acute myocardial infarction: A meta-analysis of the randomized trials. Circulation 2005;112:3855-3867.

39. The Global Utilization of Strategies to Open Occluded Coronary Arteries (GUSTO) IIb Investigators: A comparison of recombinant hirudin versus heparin for the treatment of acute coronary syndromes. N Engl J Med 1996;335:775-782.

40. HERO-2 Trial Investigators: Thrombin-specific anticoagulation with bivalirudin versus heparin in patients receiving fibrinolytic therapy for acute myocardial infarction: The HERO-2 randomised trial. Lancet 2001;358:1855-1863.

41. The GUSTO V Investigators: Reperfusion therapy for acute myocardial infarction with fibrinolytic therapy or combination low dose fibrinolytic therapy and platelet glycoprotein IIb/IIIa inhibition: The GUSTO V Trial. Lancet 2001;357: 1905-1914.

42. Lincoff AM, Califf RM, Van de Werf F, et al: Mortality at 1 year with combination platelet glycoprotein IIb/IIIa inhibition and reduced-dose fibrinolytic therapy vs conventional fibrinolytic therapy for acute myocardial infarction: GUSTO V randomized trial. JAMA 2002;288:2130-2135.

43. De Luca G, Suryapranata H, Stone GW, et al: Abciximab as adjunctive therapy to reperfusion in acute ST-segment elevation myocardial infarction: A meta-analysis of randomized trials. JAMA 2005;293:1759-1765.

44. Ohman EM, Van de Werf F, Antman EM, et al, for the FASTER (TIMI 24) Investigators: Tenecteplase and tirofiban in ST-segment elevation acute myocardial infarction: Results of a randomized trial. Am Heart J 2005;150:79-88.

45. Martinez-Rios MA, Rosas M, Gonzalez H, et al, for the SASTRE Investigators: Comparison of reperfusion regimens with or without tirofiban in ST-elevation acute myocardial infarction. Am J Cardiol 2004;93:280-287.

46. Giugliano RP, Roe MT, Harrington RA, et al, for the INTEGRITI Investigators: Combination reperfusion therapy with eptifibatide and reduced-dose tenecteplase for ST-elevation myocardial infarction: Results of the Integrilin and tenecteplase in acute myocardial infarction (INTEGRITI) Phase II Angiographic Trial. J Am Coll Cardiol 2003;16;41:1251-1260.

47. Miller JM, Smalling R, Ohman EM, et al: Effectiveness of early coronary angioplasty and abciximab for failed thrombolysis (reteplase or alteplase) during acute myocardial infarction (results of the GUSTO-III trial). Global Use of Strategies to Open Occluded Arteries. Am J Cardiol 1999;84:779-784.

48. Gruberg L, Suleiman M, Kapeliovich M, et al: Glycoprotein IIb/IIIa inhibitors during rescue percutaneous coronary intervention in acute myocardial infarction. J Invasive Cardiol 2006;18:63-64.

49. Chen ZM, Jiang LX, Chen YP, et al: Addition of clopidogrel to aspirin in 45,852 patients with acute myocardial infarction: Randomized placebo-controlled trial. Lancet 2005; 366:1607-1621.

50. Sabatine MS, Cannon CP, Gibson CM, et al: Addition of clopidogrel to aspirin and fibrinolytic therapy for myocardial infarction with ST-segment elevation. N Engl J Med 2005; 352:1179-1189.

51. Patrono C, Bachmann F, Baigent C, et al, for the Task Force on the Use of Antiplatelet Agents in Patients with Atherosclerotic Cardiovascular Disease: Expert consensus document on the use of antiplatelet agents. Eur Heart J 2004;25:166-181.

52. Wiviott SD, Antman EM, Gibson CM, et al, for the TRITON-TIMI 38 Investigators: Evaluation of prasugrel compared with clopidogrel in patients with acute coronary syndromes: Design and rationale for the TRial to assess Improvement in Therapeutic Outcomes by optimizing platelet inhibitioN with prasugrel-Thrombolysis In Myocardial Infarction 38 (TRITON-TIMI 38). Am Heart J 2006;152:627-635.

53. Scrutinio D, Cimminiello C, Marubini E, et al, for the STAMI Group: Ticlopidine versus Aspirin after Myocardial Infarction (STAMI) trial. J Am Coll Cardiol 2001;37:1259-1265.

54. Mahaffey KW, Granger CB, Nicolau JC, et al, for the COMPLY Investigators: Effect of pexelizumab, an anti-C5 complement antibody, as adjunctive therapy to fibrinolysis in acute myocardial infarction: The COMPlement inhibition in myocardial infarction treated with thromboLYtics (COMPLY) trial. Circulation 2003;108:1176-1183.

55. Yusuf S, Mehta SR, Chrolavicius S, et al, for the Oasis-6 Trial Group: Effects of fondaparinaux on mortality and reinfarction in patients with acute ST-segment elevation myocardial infarction: The OASIS-6 randomized trial. JAMA 2006;295: 1519-1530.

56. The Fifth Organization to Assess Strategies in Acute Ischemic Syndromes Investigators (OASIS-5): Comparison of fondaparinaux and enoxaparin in acute coronary syndromes. N Engl J Med 2006;354:1464-1476.

57. Stone GW, Cox D, Garcia E, et al: Normal flow (TIMI-3) before mechanical reperfusion therapy is an independent determinant of survival in acute myocardial infarction: Analysis from the Primary Angioplasty in Myocardial Infarction Trials. Circulation 2001;104:636-641.

58. Topol EJ, Califf RM, George BS, et al, for the Thrombolysis and Angioplasty in Myocardial Infarction (TAMI) Study Group: A randomized trial of immediate versus delayed elective angioplasty after intravenous tissue plasminogen activator in acute myocardial infarction. N Engl J Med 1987;317:581-588.

59. ASSENT-4 PCI Investigators: Primary versus tenecteplase-facilitated percutaneous coronary intervention in patients with ST-segment elevation acute myocardial infarction (ASSENT-4 PCI): Randomized trial. Lancet 2006;367:569-578.

60. ADVANCE MI Investigators: Facilitated percutaneous coronary intervention for acute ST-segment elevation myocardial infarction: Results from the prematurely terminated ADdressing the Value of facilitated ANgioplasty after Combination therapy or Eptifibatide monotherapy in acute Myocardial Infarction. Am J Heart 2005;150:116-122.

61. Kastrati A, Mehilli J, Schlotterbeck K, et al, for the Bavarian Reperfusion Alternatives Evaluation (BRAVE) Study Investigators: Early administration of reteplase plus abciximab vs abciximab alone in patients with acute myocardial infarction

referred for percutaneous coronary intervention: A randomized controlled trial. JAMA 2004;291:947-954.

62. Keeley EC, Boura JA, Grines CL: Comparison of primary and facilitated percutaneous coronary interventions for ST-elevation myocardial infarction: quantitative review of randomized trials. Lancet 2006;367:579-588.

63. Ellis SG, Armstrong P, Betriu A, et al: Facilitated percutaneous coronary intervention versus primary percutaneous coronary intervention: Design and rationale of the Facilitated Intervention with Enhanced Reperfusion Speed to Stop Events Investigators. Am Heart J 2004;147:E16.

14 Other Adjunctive Drugs for Coronary Intervention: β-Blockers and Calcium Channel Blockers

Vivek Rajagopal

KEY POINTS

- β-Blockers reduce myocardial oxygen demand and prevent deleterious myocardial remodeling. These properties explain the protective role of β-blockers in the treatment of acute and chronic ischemic coronary syndromes.
- β-Blockers significantly reduce reinfarction and ventricular fibrillation after myocardial infarction.
- In higher-risk myocardial infarction patients, such as those in heart failure or at high risk for developing heart failure, β-blockers increase the risk of cardiogenic shock, counterbalancing the ischemic and arrhythmic benefits.

- As the COMMIT trial demonstrated, intravenous β-blockade provides no overall benefit in patients with acute myocardial infarction. Nevertheless, patients not at high risk for developing cardiogenic shock do benefit from β-blockade.
- Calcium channel blockers are useful agents in chronic treatment of hypertension in coronary artery disease patients.
- In patients with acute myocardial infarction, calcium channel blockers should be used only in β-blocker–intolerant patients who are not at high risk for developing heart failure.

For several decades, β-blockers and calcium channel blockers have been beneficial in a wide spectrum of coronary artery disease, such as stable and unstable angina, non-ST-segment elevation myocardial infarction (NSTEMI), and ST-segment elevation myocardial infarction (STEMI). Many clinical trials since the 1980s have demonstrated benefits of these agents, which work primarily by reducing myocardial oxygen demand.

In this chapter, I discuss the basic pharmacology of these agents, the randomized trials using these agents, and ongoing research. I also provide treatment recommendations.

BETA-BLOCKADE

Beta-Adrenergic Receptors

β-Receptors belong to a well-characterized family of receptors known as G protein–coupled receptors.[1] The pathway involves binding of an agonist (e.g., catecholamines for β-receptors) to an extracellular receptor (Fig. 14-1). Receptor activation causes a coupled G protein to stimulate adenylyl cyclase, which increases intracellular concentrations of cyclic adenosine monophosphate (AMP). Cyclic AMP activates several AMP-dependent protein kinases, which

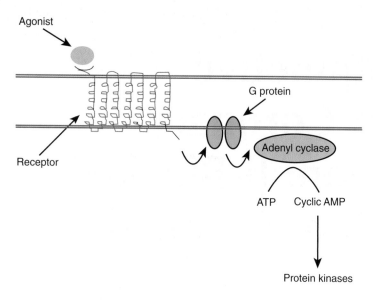

Figure 14-1. β-Receptors belong to the family of G protein–coupled receptors. The pathway involves binding of an agonist, such as a catecholamine, to an extracellular receptor.

phosphorylate other proteins, resulting in a cellular response.

The cellular response for β-receptors differs according to three major subtypes: β_1, β_2, and β_3. Whereas stimulation of β_2-receptors causes bronchodilation and peripheral vasodilation, stimulation of β_1-receptors predominantly affects the heart, increasing contractility and heart rate, as well as increasing lipolysis. The β_3-receptor increases heat production in brown adipose tissue and increases lipolysis in brown and white adipose tissue.[2,3] The β_3-receptor may play a role in obesity and insulin resistance.[3]

Beta-Adrenergic Receptor Blockers

β-Blockers act by directly competing with binding of catecholamines to β-adrenergic receptors. These agents differ in their selectivity, lipid solubility, metabolism, and partial-agonist ability (i.e., intrinsic sympathomimetic ability [ISA]) (Table 14-1). Although some data suggest that these differences may impact efficacy in certain conditions (e.g., chronic conges-

tive heart failure), these differences mainly affect side effects, contraindications, and frequency of dosing. For example, nonselective agents may increase bronchospasm in asthmatic patients. Lipophilic agents may have more central nervous system effects, such as sedation and depression. The type of metabolism affects plasma half-life in patients with renal or hepatic insufficiency. β-Blockers with ISA slow the heart rate less than β-blockers without ISA; β-blockers with ISA are less likely to decrease HDL or increase triglycerides.

Despite these pharmacokinetic differences, efficacy in coronary artery disease arises primarily from β_1-receptor antagonism. In acute myocardial infarction (MI), for example, the catecholamine storm decreases the fibrillation threshold, increases myocardial oxygen consumption, and promotes myocardial necrosis. By decreasing heart rate and contractility, blockade of the β_1-receptor lowers myocardial stress, which decreases necrosis. β-Blockade also raises the fibrillation threshold. By antagonizing lipolysis, β-blockers reduce concentrations of free fatty acids,

Table 14-1.   Beta-Blockers

Drug	Dose (mg)	Frequency	Excretion	Lipid Solubility	ISA
Selective β_1					
Acebutolol	200-600	q 12 hr	Kidney	Moderate	Low
Atenolol	25-200	q 24 hr	Kidney	None	None
Betaxolol	5-20	q 24 hr	Kidney	Moderate	Low
Metoprolol	25-400	q 12 hr	Liver	Moderate	None
Long-acting		q 24 hr			
Nonselective β					
Labetalol (α,β_1,β_2)	100-1200	q 12 hr	Liver	None	None
Nadolol	20-320	q 24 hr	Kidney	Low	None
Pindolol	5-30	q 12 hr	Kidney	Moderate	Moderate
Propranolol	40-320	q 8-12 hr	Liver	High	None
Long-acting		q 12 hr			
Timolol	10-30	q 12 hr	Liver	Moderate	None

ISA, intrinsic sympathomimetic ability.

Ellis K, Kapadia SR: Stable angina. *In* Topol E, Griffin BA (eds): Manual of Cardiovascular Medicine, 2nd ed. Philadelphia, Lippincott Williams & Wilkins, 2004, p 85.

increasing the use of glucose and decreasing the use of oxygen. Although controversial, β-blockers, particularly carvedilol, may also inhibit platelet aggregation, but the mechanism may be membrane interaction instead of β-receptor antagonism.[4]

Given these salubrious effects, it is not surprising that numerous clinical trials have demonstrated the benefits of β-blockers in acute coronary syndromes (ACS). Prudence is still required because β-blockers decrease inotropy and slow atrioventricular conduction, which can be harmful in certain subgroups of patients.

Unstable Angina Pectoris

Because of β-blockers' potent effects in reducing myocardial oxygen demand, treating unstable angina with β-blockers has much intuitive appeal. A few small, randomized trials have supported this approach. Gottlieb and colleagues randomized 81 patients with unstable angina to 4 weeks of propranolol or placebo.[5] All patients received calcium channel blockers or nitrates, or both. Although incidence of death, MI, or need for urgent coronary artery bypass grafting (CABG) did not differ between groups, propranolol significantly reduced frequency and severity of recurrent ischemia. In the Holland Interuniversity Nifedipine and Metoprolol Trial (HINT), 338 patients with unstable angina not pretreated with a β-blocker randomly received nifedipine alone, metoprolol alone, or nifedipine and metoprolol. The odds ratios for recurrent ischemia or MI by 48 hours were 1.15 (95% CI: 0.83 to 1.64) for nifedipine, 0.76 (95% CI: 0.49 to 1.16) for metoprolol, and 0.80 (95% CI: 0.53 to 1.19) for both; not surprisingly, small numbers limited the power of the study, and these differences were not statistically significant. Hohnloser and associates[6] examined the effects of esmolol, a short-acting (half-life of 9 minutes), intravenous β-blocker, in a randomized, placebo-controlled trial of 113 patients. Investigators increased esmolol until they reduced the double product by about 25%; thereafter, the esmolol infusion continued for up to 72 hours.[6] Acute MI or urgent revascularization occurred in 9 patients treated with placebo, compared with 3 patients treated with esmolol (P = .06). In a later randomized trial, Brunner and colleagues[7] randomized 116 patients with unstable angina to placebo or carvedilol at 25 mg twice daily. Patients received 48-hour Holter monitoring to document ischemia. Carvedilol reduced ischemic time by 75% (204 versus 49 minutes, P < .05), with a 66% reduction in the number of ischemic episodes (24 versus 8, P < .05).

Some retrospective data from recent studies demonstrate the benefit of β-blockers in unstable angina. Ellis and associates[8] pooled data from five randomized trials of abciximab during percutaneous coronary intervention (PCI)—EPIC, EPILOG, EPISTENT, CAPTURE, and RAPPORT.[8] Except for RAPPORT, which had STEMI patients, the other four trials included patients with unstable angina or NSTEMI.

The rate of all-cause mortality by 30 days was 0.6% among patients receiving β-blockers, compared with 2.0% for patients not receiving β-blockers. After adjusting for baseline characteristics and propensity score to receive β-blockers, β-blockers remained predictive of lower mortality (HR = 0.25; 95% CI: 0.11 to 0.57; P = .001). This mortality difference persisted at 6 months (1.7% versus 3.7%; adjusted HR = 0.53; 95% CI: 0.29 to 0.94; P = .03). Among patients with unstable angina, β-blockers reduced mortality at 3 months (1.6% to 0.6%, P = .029) and at 6 months (3.1% to 1.4%, P = .009). Curiously, β-blockers did not reduce MI or revascularization rates in the entire group or in the subgroup of patients with unstable angina. Similarly, Ellis[9] demonstrated no effect of β-blockers on postprocedural MI in a large cohort (N = 6700) of patients (most [66%] of whom had unstable angina) undergoing PCI at the Cleveland Clinic from 1997 to 2000. After adjusting for differences in baseline characteristics and propensity to receive preprocedural β-blockers, β-blockers did not independently predict any differences in the postprocedural creatine kinase MB fraction (CK-MB). These retrospective data suggest a mortality benefit not mediated by a lower incidence of MI.

Percutaneous Coronary Intervention

Although trials have evaluated adjunctive β-blockade in patients with unstable angina or MI undergoing PCI, few data exist for the effect of β-blockade as a specific adjunct to PCI. Most data for adjunctive benefit arise from nonrandomized registries.

Sharma and colleagues evaluated 1675 consecutive patients undergoing PCI.[10] None of the patients had MI before PCI. The study authors did not specify how many patients presented with unstable angina. CK-MB level elevation occurred in 13.2% of patients on β-blockers before the procedure, compared with 22.1% of patients not on β-blockers (P < .001). On multivariate analysis, β-blockers remained an independent predictor of lower CK-MB release. Over a mean of 15 months of follow-up, patients on preprocedural β-blockers had a mortality rate of 0.8%, compared with 2.0% for patients not on preprocedural β-blockers (P = .04). Chan and colleagues[11] evaluated 4553 consecutive patients without acute or recent MI who underwent PCI, according to whether they had been treated with β-blockers at the time of the PCI. Of these patients, 2056 (45%) were on β-blockers at the time of the intervention. Mortality rates were lower for patients on β-blockers at 30 days (1.3% versus 0.8%, P = .13) and at 1 year (6.0% versus 3.9%, P = .0014). After adjusting for differences in the baseline characteristics by propensity analysis, β-blocker therapy remained independently predictive of 1-year survival (HR = 0.63; 95% CI: 0.46 to 0.87, P = .0054).

Along with these mortality data, other data suggest a benefit of β-blockers on the rate of restenosis. Jackson and colleagues[12] followed 4840 patients undergoing PCI according to whether they received β-blockers on discharge. Patients treated with β-blockers had a 5-year clinical restenosis rate of 12% compared with 14% for the other group (adjusted OR = 0.83; P = .046). These data, however, are controversial, because a small, randomized trial of adjunctive carvedilol failed to reduce restenosis rates for patients undergoing atherectomy.[13]

In another small, randomized trial, Wang and colleagues[14] examined the effect of intracoronary propranolol during PCI. Although most patients presented with unstable angina or recent MI (28% of propranolol group and 20% of placebo group had stable angina), Wang's trial is most accurately characterized as a β-blocker adjunctive trial, because investigators delivered intracoronary propranolol during the PCI, regardless of whether patients had been started on β-blockers before the PCI (≈65%).

Investigators[14] randomized 150 patients undergoing PCI to placebo or propranolol (15 µg/kg) injected into the distal coronary artery by means of the balloon catheter positioned across the stenosis. CK-MB elevation occurred in 17% of propranolol patients, compared with 36% of placebo patients (P = .01). The incidence of death, MI, or urgent revascularization by 30 days was 18% for the propranolol patients, compared with 40% for the placebo patients (P = .004). The relative risk of MI did not differ between patients on prior β-blocker therapy and patients not on prior therapy.

Acute Myocardial Infarction

Early Trials

The data for β-blockade in acute MI come from 26 small trials and two large trials—the Metoprolol in Acute Myocardial Infarction (MIAMI) trial and the First International Study of Infarct Survival (ISIS-1) trial.[15,16]

The MIAMI Trial
Patients with acute MI within 24 hours of symptom onset (N = 5778) were randomized to receive intravenous metoprolol (15 mg) or placebo, followed by oral metoprolol (200 mg daily) or placebo for 15 days. β-Blockade reduced Q-wave infarction significantly from 53.9% to 50.9% (P = .024), with a nonsignficant reduction in mortality (4.9% to 4.3%, P = .29). The MIAMI trial is significantly limited in its applicability to the modern era. Patients enrolled in MIAMI were low risk (e.g., all Killip class I), and the trial occurred before routine reperfusion, angiotensin-converting enzyme (ACE) inhibition, and statin treatment.

The ISIS-1 Trial
Although ISIS-1 was similarly limited by a lack of reperfusion, its larger size and power are important. ISIS-1 randomized 16,207 patients with suspected acute MI (mean of 5 hours from symptom onset) to the control group or to treatment with intravenous atenolol (5 to 10 mg), followed by 100 mg of oral atenolol daily for 7 days. Treatment with atenolol significantly reduced vascular mortality from 4.57% to 3.89% (P < .04) from days 0 to 7. Atenolol-treated patients also had a significantly lower vascular mortality by 1 year (10.7% versus 12.0%, P < .01), although much of this late difference might have arisen because patients randomized to atenolol were more likely to be discharged on β-blockers compared with controls.

Recent Data—The COMMIT Trial

Given that most data for β-blockade in acute MI are several decades old, benefit for β-blockade in the current era of aggressive use of antiplatelet therapy, thrombolysis or primary angioplasty, statin therapy, and antialdosterone therapy has remained uncertain, and physicians have hoped for trials with modern background therapy to assess the true value of β-blockade. This uncertainty has remained relevant because of persistent fears that β-blockers may exacerbate the condition of some acute MI patients, particularly those with signs and symptoms of congestive heart failure. Fortunately, newer data have come from the large-scale, randomized CLOpidogrel and Metoprolol in Myocardial Infarction Trial (COMMIT). COMMIT was a trial performed in the modern reperfusion era, and it was the largest trial ever investigating β-blockers in acute MI. As such, it is exceptionally important to understand the trial and its implications for patient management.

The COMMIT trial (also known as the Second Chinese Cardiac Study [CCS-2]) was a placebo-controlled, randomized trial with a 2 × 2 factorial design, randomizing acute MI patients to metoprolol or placebo, as well as to clopidogrel or placebo, with a background therapy of aspirin, anticoagulant therapy[16a] (mostly unfractionated heparin), and thrombolysis.

Patient Selection
The scale of the trial was impressive. Between August 1999 and February 2005, COMMIT enrolled 45,852 patients in 1250 Chinese hospitals. Inclusion criteria included left bundle branch block (presumably new), ST-segment elevation, or ST-segment depression within 24 hours of ischemic symptoms. Exclusion criteria included patients scheduled for primary percutaneous intervention (because of combined aspirin and clopidogrel use that would interfere with other study arm) or conditions considered high risk for β-blocker therapy, such as systolic blood pressure less than 100 mm Hg or heart rate less than 50 beats/min, heart block, or cardiogenic shock. Moderate heart failure (Killip class II or III) was not a contraindication, unlike in trials such as MIAMI.[16]

Study Protocol
Patients randomized to metoprolol received a 5-mg intravenous dose, followed by second and third doses as long as systolic blood pressure was higher than 90 mm Hg and the heart rate was higher than

50 beats/min after each dose. Patients then received 50 mg of metoprolol 15 minutes after the last intravenous dose, which was repeated every 6 hours for 24 hours, followed by 200 mg of controlled-release metoprolol once daily up to 4 weeks.

End Points

The COMMIT trial had two primary end points: all-cause mortality until discharge or day 28 and the composite end point of death, reinfarction, or cardiac arrest. Secondary end points included cardiogenic shock, cardiac arrest, and reinfarction. Prespecified subgroup analyses included effects of metoprolol on primary outcomes according to hospital days and the following subgroups: age, sex, time from symptom onset, fibrinolysis, Killip class, heart rate, systolic blood pressure, and shock risk index (absolute risk of shock calculated from Cox regression model using baseline prognostic characteristics).

Results

The large sample size of COMMIT ensured that baseline characteristics between groups were similar (see Fig. 14-3). The mean age was 61 years, with 26% older than 70 years, and 72% of subjects were men. ST-segment elevation occurred in 87%, with left bundle branch block in 6% and ST-segment depression in 7%. Time from symptom onset to treatment was evenly distributed over 24 hours, with approximately one third of patients treated within 6 hours, one third within 6 to 13 hours, and one third within 13 to 24 hours. Although most patients had no signs or symptoms of congestive heart failure, a sizable percentage—24%—had Killip class II or III features on presentation. This contrasts with early β-blocker trials that enrolled lower-risk patients with no evidence of congestive heart failure. In COMMIT, 54% of patients received thrombolysis, with most of these patients receiving urokinase. Of those presenting within 12 hours, 68% received thrombolysis; it is unknown how many of the remaining patients did not receive thrombolytics because of clear contraindications. Slightly fewer metoprolol-treated patients received ACE inhibitors (67.2% versus 69.3%, $P <$ .0001).

The primary composite outcome of death, reinfarction, or cardiac arrest did not differ between metoprolol-treated patients (9.4%) and placebo-treated patients (9.9%) (OR = 0.96%; 95% CI: 0.90 to 1.01; $P =$ .10) (Fig. 14-2). Similarly, the co-primary outcome of death did not differ between metoprolol (7.7%) and placebo (7.8%) patients (Fig. 14-3). Given the prior clinical data supporting early β-blockade in acute MI, reasons for these counterintuitive results require careful dissection; in particular, did β-blockade reduce any particular clinical events, and did β-blockade benefit some patients much more than others?

β-Blockade significantly reduced any reinfarction (2.0% for metoprolol versus 2.5% for placebo, $P =$ .001) and risk of ventricular fibrillation (2.5% versus 3.0%, $P =$ .001). Treatment, however, increased risk

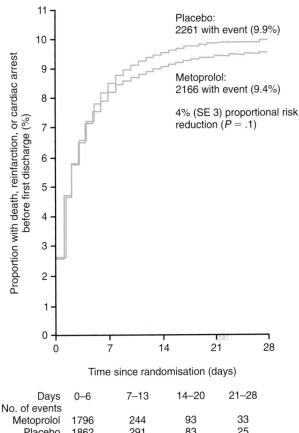

Figure 14-2. Death, reinfarction, or cardiac arrest in COMMIT.

Days	0–6	7–13	14–20	21–28
No. of events				
Metoprolol	1796	244	93	33
Placebo	1862	291	83	25

of cardiogenic shock by 30% (5.0% versus 3.9%, $P <$ .0001). Although β-blockade significantly reduced arrhythmic death by 22% (1.7% for metoprolol versus 2.2% for placebo, $P =$ .0002), β-blockade significantly increased death from cardiogenic shock by 29% (2.2% versus 1.7%, $P =$ .0002). The benefit in reducing arrhythmic death was counteracted by harm in increasing cardiogenic shock. In absolute terms, metoprolol prevented 5 episodes of ventricular fibrillation and 5 episodes of reinfarction per 1000 treated, but it caused 11 episodes of cardiogenic shock per 1000 treated. These effects had differential time courses. In particular, 10 per 1000 excess risk for cardiogenic shock occurred within the first 24 hours. In contrast, reductions in risk of reinfarction and ventricular fibrillation began approximately 48 hours after treatment initiation.

The propensity of metoprolol to cause cardiogenic shock differed according to baseline characteristics. Metoprolol caused a much higher excess of cardiogenic shock in several subgroups: 56.9 per 1000 patients in Killip class III; 34.6 per 1000 patients presenting with heart rates higher than 110 beats/min; 23.3 per 1000 per patients presenting with systolic blood pressure less than 120 mm Hg; and 23.1 per 1000 patients ≥70 years old. Not surprisingly, these differences translated into a much higher risk of cardiogenic shock with metoprolol according to

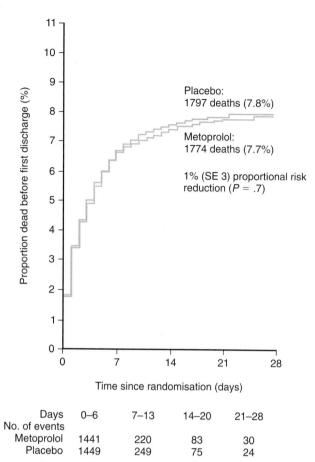

Figure 14-3. Death in COMMIT.

baseline risk of shock: 3.7 per 1000 (low risk) versus 16.2 per 1000 (medium risk) versus 56.9 per 1000 (high risk) ($P < .0001$).

This differential effect on cardiogenic shock translated into a differential effect on mortality according to patients' baseline risk of shock. For patients at high risk for cardiogenic shock, metoprolol caused an absolute *increase* of 24.8 deaths per 1000 treated. Conversely, treatment caused an absolute *decrease* of 4.2 and 4.3 deaths per 1000 treated for medium-risk and low-risk patients, respectively.

Meta-Analysis Using COMMIT Patients
As the COMMIT investigators mentioned, patients in COMMIT had a significantly higher risk of shock and mortality compared with patients enrolled in prior trials. The investigators examined effects of β-blockade on patients in COMMIT, similar to the low-risk patients enrolled in MIAMI (i.e., heart rate >65 beats/min, Killip class I, systolic blood pressure >105 mm Hg). They also pooled these patients with patients from MIAMI, ISIS-1, and 26 small trials (Fig. 14-4). The magnitude of benefit in low-risk COMMIT patients (6.4% to 5.7%) was similar to that of MIAMI patients (4.9% to 4.3%). In the analysis of pooled patients (about 52,000), β-blockade significantly reduced cardiac arrest (3.1% versus 3.6%, $P = .002$),

reinfarction (2.3% versus 2.8%, $P = .0002$), and mortality (4.8% versus 5.5%, $P = .0006$).

Recommendations for Beta-Blockade during Acute Myocardial Infarction

Given COMMIT's applicability to the modern era, and its enormous size (almost twice as many patients as all others combined), the COMMIT data must form the core basis for any recommendations. Accordingly, early intravenous β-blocker therapy for acute MI cannot be recommended for all patients. Nevertheless, the neutrality of the primary end points was driven by excess of cardiogenic shock in patients at increased baseline risk of developing shock. It is rational to consider early β-blockade in patients at low risk for shock (i.e., age <70, heart rate <110 beats/min, systolic blood pressure >120 mm Hg, and Killip class I). This is not supported on a strict scientific basis, because such a group was not prespecified. A stronger recommendation can be made for waiting at least 24 hours to determine clinical stability before beginning β-blockade. Because the cardiogenic shock hazard arises within 24 hours, it is possible that waiting could circumvent this hazard, allowing the "fittest for β-blockade" to emerge, giving these patients the reinfarction and cardiac arrest benefits, which emerge more slowly over the hospital course.

Chronic Therapy after Myocardial Infarction
ISIS-1 demonstrated a sustained benefit of β-blockade for patients with acute MI; 1-year mortality for atenolol-treated patients was 10.7%, compared with 12.0% for placebo patients ($P < .01$). Given that patients randomized to atenolol in this trial were more likely to be discharged on atenolol, the further separation in survival curves at 1 year suggests a beneficial effect of β-blockade given chronically after MI. Pooled data from all long-term trials of β-blockade after MI also show a significant protective effect.[17] Long-term β-blockade reduced sudden death from 5.2% to 3.6% ($P < .0001$), reinfarction from 7.3% to 5.5% ($P < .0001$), and mortality from 9.5% to 7.5% ($P < .0001$) over a follow-up of 1 to 3 years.

The Carvedilol Post-Infarct Survival Control in Left Ventricular Dysfunction (CAPRICORN) trial supported this benefit for patients with recent MI and systolic dysfunction.[18] CAPRICORN randomized 1959 patients with acute MI and a left ventricular ejection fraction of 40 or less to carvedilol (6.25 mg twice daily, starting during hospitalization) or placebo. Carvedilol was titrated up to 25 mg twice daily over 4 to 6 weeks. After a mean follow-up of 15 months, carvedilol treatment reduced all-cause mortality from 15% to 12% (HR = 0.77; 95% CI: 0.60 to 0.98; $P = .03$). The CAPRICORN trial represented modern therapy with aggressive reperfusion, antiplatelet therapy, and anticoagulation; all patients received ACE inhibitors for 48 hours before randomization.

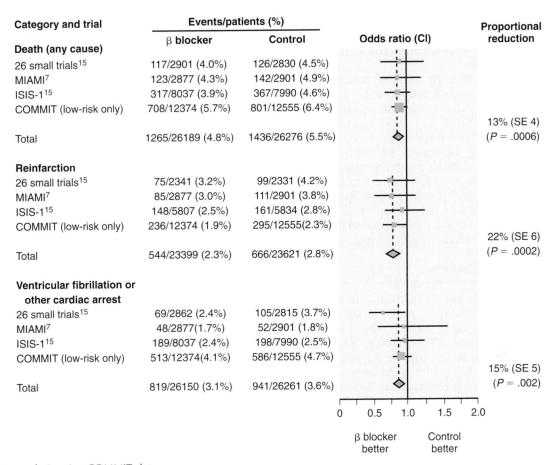

Category and trial	Events/patients (%)		Odds ratio (CI)	Proportional reduction
	β blocker	Control		
Death (any cause)				
26 small trials[15]	117/2901 (4.0%)	126/2830 (4.5%)		
MIAMI[7]	123/2877 (4.3%)	142/2901 (4.9%)		
ISIS-1[15]	317/8037 (3.9%)	367/7990 (4.6%)		
COMMIT (low-risk only)	708/12374 (5.7%)	801/12555 (6.4%)		13% (SE 4)
Total	1265/26189 (4.8%)	1436/26276 (5.5%)		(P = .0006)
Reinfarction				
26 small trials[15]	75/2341 (3.2%)	99/2331 (4.2%)		
MIAMI[7]	85/2877 (3.0%)	111/2901 (3.8%)		
ISIS-1[15]	148/5807 (2.5%)	161/5834 (2.8%)		
COMMIT (low-risk only)	236/12374 (1.9%)	295/12555 (2.3%)		22% (SE 6)
Total	544/23399 (2.3%)	666/23621 (2.8%)		(P = .0002)
Ventricular fibrillation or other cardiac arrest				
26 small trials[15]	69/2862 (2.4%)	105/2815 (3.7%)		
MIAMI[7]	48/2877 (1.7%)	52/2901 (1.8%)		
ISIS-1[15]	189/8037 (2.4%)	198/7990 (2.5%)		
COMMIT (low-risk only)	513/12374 (4.1%)	586/12555 (4.7%)		15% (SE 5)
Total	819/26150 (3.1%)	941/26261 (3.6%)		(P = .002)

0   0.5   1.0   1.5   2.0

β blocker better   Control better

Figure 14-4. Meta-analysis using COMMIT data.

Patient Selection: Role of Genomics

Because β-blockade does not uniformly benefit patients after MI, as the COMMIT trial demonstrated, β-blockers may harm certain subgroups while benefiting others. Clinical trials remain blunt and crude instruments at best.

Suppose, for example, a condition has a 100% mortality rate, and a treatment demonstrates a large absolute reduction in mortality (40%). In that case, 4 of 10 patients given the treatment survive compared with 0 of 10 patients given placebo. That means that 6 treated patients did not receive benefit. This conundrum presented by clinical trials argues for a finer instrument with which to determine benefit.

Given recent advances in pharmacogenomics, characterization of patients' genetic polymorphisms may be a useful instrument to select the best candidates for β-blocker therapy. Lanfear and colleagues studied polymorphisms in the β_1- and β_2-receptors among patients discharged on β-blocker therapy after an ACS.[30] No relationship existed between β_1-receptor polymorphisms and mortality in patients treated or not treated with β-blockers. Polymorphisms in β_2-receptors, however, correlated significantly with mortality among patients discharged on β-blockers. In particular, Kaplan-Meier 3-year mortality rates were 6%, 11%, and 16% for three different polymorphisms (GG, CG, and CC genotypes, respectively, for

polymorphism Gln27Glu; HR = 0.24 [95% CI: 0.09 to 0.68] for GG versus CC, P = .004). Another β_2-receptor polymorphism, Gly16Arg, displayed a correlation between genotypes and mortality. The 3-year Kaplan-Meier mortality rates of 10% for the GG and GA genotypes compared with 20% for the AA genotype (HR = 0.44 [95% CI: 0.22 to 0.85] for GG versus AA and 0.48 [95% CI: 0.27 to 0.86] for GA versus AA (P = .005 for overall comparison). Importantly, these polymorphisms did not correlate with mortality and patients not treated with β-blockers, indicating a specific interaction of the polymorphisms with β-blocker treatment. Although the mechanism of this interaction is unknown, it is possible that these polymorphisms alter left ventricular modeling in response to β-blockade, as has been described for β_1-receptor polymorphisms.[19]

CALCIUM CHANNEL BLOCKADE

Calcium Channels

Intracellular calcium concentrations are tightly regulated by calcium exchangers, ion pumps, and channels. At baseline, cytoplasmic calcium ion concentrations exist at very low levels (<100 nM) compared with extracellular concentrations (>1 mM). When calcium channels open at the plasma membrane or endoplasmic reticular level, intracellular concentrations of calcium rapidly rise; ATP-dependent ion pumps and sodium/calcium exchangers restore equilibrium.

Calcium channels exist as three major subgroups: stretch-operated, receptor-operated, and voltage-dependent forms. The voltage-dependent receptors exist as three subtypes: N, L, and T. The L-type and T-type channels are important to cardiovascular medicine and are inhibited by calcium channel blockers. L-type channels exist throughout the cardiovascular system in cardiac and smooth muscles, and they are responsible for the slow inward current (i.e., plateau phase) of the action potential. T-type channels are found mainly in sinus nodal tissue, with few found in ventricular myocardium.

Calcium Channel Blockers

The three main classes of calcium channel blockers include dihydropyridines, phenylalkylamines, and benzothiazepines (Table 14-2).[20] These classes differ in their vasodilatory and chronotropic effects. In particular, phenylalkylamines (e.g., verapamil) and benzothiazepines (e.g., diltiazem) decrease atrioventricular and sinoatrial conduction, whereas dihydropyridines (e.g., amlodipine) do not. Dihydropyridines are more potent vasodilators. Nifedipine, in particular, can cause profound peripheral vasodilation, resulting in reflex tachycardia. Despite these differences, all classes of calcium channel blockers have been shown to reduce infarct size in animal models. Some authorities have speculated that calcium channel blockers may protect myocardium through coronary vasodilation and decreased ischemic calcium overload.

Calcium Channel Blockade in Acute Myocardial Infarction

Most data for calcium channel blockade after acute MI are more than a decade old. The pivotal trials for early treatment of MI include the Secondary Preven-tion Reinfarction Israeli Nifedipine Trial (SPRINT-II), the first Danish Study Group on Verapamil in Myocardial Infarction Trial (DAVIT), and three small diltiazem trials.[17] None of these trials showed any significant difference in reinfarction or mortality with calcium channel blockade; SPRINT-II was stopped prematurely because of increased mortality in the nifedipine group.

Recent data are limited and hypothesis generating only. In a recent Japanese trial, investigators randomized 1090 patients after acute MI to β-blocker or calcium channel blocker therapy.[21] At a mean follow-up of 455 days, patients treated with calcium channel blockers did not differ in incidence of cardiovascular death (1.1% versus 1.7%), reinfarction (1.3% versus 0.9%), or nonfatal stroke (0.2% versus 0.7%). The calcium channel group had a significantly lower incidence of congestive heart failure (1.1% versus 4.2%, $P = .001$) and coronary spasm (0.2% versus 1.2%, $P = .027$). More data in other populations are required to verify these differences.

Recommendations for Acute Coronary Syndromes

Given the lack of large trials demonstrating benefit in acute MI, calcium channel blockers should not be administered routinely, particularly for patients presenting with STEMI. A prominent exception is the patient who presents with ST-segment elevation after cocaine intoxication. Given the prominent role of coronary vasospasm after cocaine use and the possible exacerbation with β-blockade, it is reasonable to administer calcium channel blockers to these patients.

For patients with unstable angina or NSTEMI, the ACC/AHA guidelines[22] endorse a class I recommendation for some ACS patients: "In patients with continuing or frequently recurring ischemia when β-blockers are contraindicated, a nondihydropyridine calcium antagonist (e.g., verapamil, diltiazem), followed by oral therapy, may be used as initial therapy in the absence of severe left ventricular dysfunction or other contraindications (evidence level B)." These guidelines endorse a class IIa recommendation for other ACS patients with recurrent ischemia already on β-blockers and nitrates: "Oral long-acting calcium antagonists for recurrent ischemia in the absence of contraindications and when β-blockers and nitrates are fully used (evidence level C)." The guidelines also clearly indicate that short-acting dihydropyridines (e.g., short-acting nifedipine) are contraindicated because of their propensity to decrease blood pressure abruptly and worsen ischemia or infarction.

Chronic Therapy after Myocardial Infarction

Early Trials

Like the data for acute treatment, many studies investigating chronic treatment are limited by being more than a decade old. These trials started calcium channel

Table 14-2. Calcium Channel Blockers

Drug	Vasodilatory Effects	Conduction Effects	Negative Inotropy
Phenylalkylamine			
Verapamil	+++	++++	+++
Benzothiazepine			
Diltiazem	++	+++	++
Dihydropyridine			
Amlodipine	+++	+	+
Bepridil	+++	+++	++++
Felodipine	++++	+	0
Isradipine	+++	++	0
Nicardipine	++++	+	0
Nifedipine	++++	+	+
Nisoldipine	+++	+	+

0, No activity; ++++, most potent.

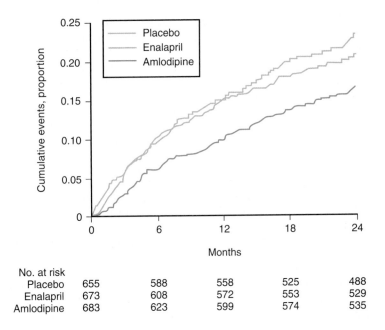

No. at risk

Placebo	655	588	558	525	488
Enalapril	673	608	572	553	529
Amlodipine	683	623	599	574	535

Figure 14-5. Cumulative events in the CAMELOT trial.

blockade weeks to months after MI, continuing these agents long term. Data for nifedipine suggest harm, and trials evaluating verapamil and diltiazem show a nonsignificant reduction in noninfarction, although one large diltiazem trial showed this trend only in patients without congestive heart failure.[17] Taken together, the nifedipine trials demonstrate excess mortality with treatment; however, these trials had small numbers of events and used short-acting nifedipine, not controlled-release nifedipine. When the verapamil and diltiazem data are combined, treatment reduced reinfarction by 22% (95% CI: –33% to 0.8%; $P < .01$).[17]

Later Trials

Several antihypertensive trials of calcium channel blockers have demonstrated similar outcomes with calcium channel blockers compared with other agents. Some of these trials have enrolled patients with a history of MI and provide reassuring data.

The CAMELOT Trial

The Comparison of Amlodipine versus Enalapril to Limit Occurrences of Thrombosis (CAMELOT) study randomized 1991 patients with angiographically documented coronary artery disease (>20%) to amlodipine (10 mg daily), enalapril (20 mg daily), or to placebo.[23] Uniquely, these patients had normal blood pressure at baseline (≈129/77). The primary outcome was incidence of adverse cardiovascular events, including cardiovascular death, resuscitated cardiac arrest, nonfatal MI, coronary revascularization, hospitalization for congestive heart failure, hospitalization for angina pectoris, stroke, or transient ischemic attack (TIA), and any new diagnosis of peripheral vascular disease. The trial had an intravascular ultrasound substudy, with the end point being percent

change in atheroma volume. The mean age of the patients was about 57 years, and 38% of the entire population had a history of MI.

The primary end point occurred in 23.1% of placebo patients, compared with 20.2% of enalapril patients and 16.6% of amlodipine patients, with significant differences between both the enalapril and amlodipine groups compared with placebo (Fig. 14-5). The amlodipine group had a statistical trend for fewer cardiovascular events compared with the enalapril group (HR = 0.81; 95% CI: 0.63 to 1.04; $P = .10$), and amlodipine treatment resulted in significantly fewer hospitalizations for angina (HR = 0.59; 95% CI: 0.42 to 0.84; $P = .003$). Amlodipine also displayed a trend for reduced atheroma progression compared with placebo ($P = .12$); amlodipine-treated patients with baseline blood pressures above mean had significantly reduced atheroma progression compared with placebo ($P < .001$).

The INVEST Trial

The International Verapamil-Trandolapril Study (INVEST) compared a calcium channel blocker strategy to a non–calcium channel blocker strategy for treatment of hypertension in coronary artery disease patients.[24] The trial randomized patients to baseline therapy of long-acting verapamil or atenolol. Patients not meeting the blood pressure goals of the Seventh Report of the Joint National Committee on Prevention, Detection, Evaluation, and Treatment of High Blood Pressure (JNC-7) received trandolapril or hydrochlorothiazide, or both. The primary end point was incidence of death, MI, or stroke.

The 22,576 enrolled patients all had documented coronary artery disease, and about 32% had history of MI. Because secondary hypertensive therapy was not specified, secondary agents differed between the groups. The verapamil arm received more trandolapril than the atenolol arm (62.9% versus 52.4%,

$P < .001$) but received less hydrochlorothiazide (43.7% versus 60.3%, $P < .001$). At a mean follow-up of 2.7 years, results for the the primary end point did not differ between verapamil and atenolol arms (9.93% for verapamil versus 10.17% for atenolol; RR = 0.98; 95% CI: 0.90 to 1.06). Results for the primary end point did not differ according to treatment arm for patients with a history of MI (13.67% for verapamil versus 14.38% for atenolol; RR = 0.95; 95% CI: 0.85 to 1.07).

The INVEST and CAMELOT trials confirm that long-term calcium channel blockade is safe and efficacious in high-risk patients, even those with a history of MI. The JNC-7 guidelines recommend that post-MI patients receive ACE inhibitors and β-blockers; calcium channel blockers have been given a "compelling indication" for patients with diabetes or high coronary artery disease risk. Most patients require multiple medications for blood-pressure control, and these data suggest that calcium channel blockers are a reasonable part of the treatment plan.[25]

Percutaneous Coronary Intervention

As an adjunct to PCI, calcium channel blockers have shown beneficial effects on myocardial perfusion, particularly during a "no-flow" state, and on restenosis. *No-reflow* is slow epicardial flow and inadequate myocardial perfusion despite a patent epicardial vessel. Although mechanisms of no-reflow are incompletely understood, many investigators believe that no-reflow occurs because of widespread microvascular dysfunction from overwhelming thromboembolism and reperfusion injury.

Because calcium channel blockers are potent coronary vasodilators, investigators have used these agents in no-reflow states in hope of opening the plugged microvasculature. Small studies support this idea. In a single-center, nonrandomized study, Hang and colleagues[26] administered intracoronary verapamil to 50 acute MI patients undergoing primary PCI and compared these patients with 50 historical controls. Myocardial perfusion, as measured by the Thrombolysis in Myocardial Infarction Myocardial Perfusion Grade (TMPG), significantly differed with verapamil administration. Specifically, 42% of verapamil-treated patients had TMPG-3, compared with only 14% of control subjects ($P = .004$). Moreover, verapamil treatment was an independent predictor of TMPG (OR = 0.26; 95% CI: 0.12 to 0.58; $P = .001$).

Umemura and colleagues confirmed this benefit of verapamil in patients with acute MI undergoing primary PCI.[31] They performed ^{99m}Tc-tetrofosmin single photon emission computed tomographic (SPECT) imaging before, immediately after, and 1 month after PCI in 101 acute MI patients. No-reflow occurred in 32 (31%) patients. Verapamil administration independently predicted post-PCI TIMI-3 flow (OR 22.4, $P = .002$) and lower infarct size by 1 month according to SPECT imaging.

In addition to improving no-reflow, calcium channel blockers may also lower the incidence of restenosis. Although the most effective agents for reducing neointimal hyperplasia have been sirolimus and paclitaxel, some data exist for a beneficial effect of calcium channel blockers in reducing restenosis. For example, data for benidipine, a dihydropyridine calcium channel blocker, showed that proliferation of vascular smooth muscle cells in culture was significantly reduced by benidipine.[27]

The reduction in vascular smooth muscle cells proliferation leads to less neointimal hyperplasia. Yamazaki and colleagues showed this by randomizing 63 patients after successful coronary stenting to amlodipine (5 mg/day) or quinapril (10 mg/day).[32] Investigators performed quantitative coronary angiography before and immediately after stenting and 3 to 6 months later. Approximately 50% of each group also received intravascular ultrasound examination at follow-up. At follow-up, amlodipine-treated patients had a significantly larger minimal lumen diameter (1.52 ± 0.53 mm versus 1.88 ± 0.64 mm, $P < .01$) and a significantly smaller neointimal area (1.9 ± 0.5 mm^2 versus 2.7 ± 0.8 mm^2, $P < .01$).

This reduction in neointimal proliferation appears to lead to lower rates of clinical events, as demonstrated by the most recent clinical trial of calcium channel blockade after PCI—Verapamil Slow-Release for Prevention of Cardiovascular Events After Angioplasty (VESPA) trial.[28] The VESPA investigators randomized 700 patients after PCI to verapamil (240 mg twice daily for 6 months) or placebo. Most patients (83%) received stents, and follow-up was excellent, with 95% having complete clinical follow-up and 94% receiving angiography at 6 months. The rate of the primary end point, a composite of death, MI, or target vessel revascularization by 1 year, was 19.3% for placebo patients, compared with 29.3% for verapamil patients (RR = 0.66; 95% CI: 0.48 to 0.89; $P = .002$). The end point was driven by a lower risk of target vessel revascularization (26.2% for placebo versus 17.5% for verapamil; RR = 0.67; 95% CI: 0.49 to 0.93; $P = .006$). Verapamil reduced the incidence of restenosis to 75% (13.7% versus 7.8%; RR = 0.57; 95% CI: 0.35 to 0.92; $P = .014$). Despite these promising animal and clinical data, they are limited, and VESPA is a single, small trial. Moreover, the advent of drug-eluting stents has significantly dampened enthusiasm for systemic therapies such as calcium channel blockers.

CONCLUSIONS

Although the COMMIT trial suggests caution for acute intravenous β-blockade after MI, the data are strong for the benefit of β-blockers in the subacute and chronic treatment of patients with MI. Strong recommendations can be made for using β-blockers in all post-MI patients, particularly those with left ventricular dysfunction. Similarly, in stable patients after MI, calcium channel blockers can be a useful adjunct for hypertension and angina treatment.

Despite initial concerns about early, short-acting calcium channel blockers, the data have demonstrated excellent safety and efficacy for these agents. Coupling these therapies with other well-established ones, such as antiplatelet agents, angiotensin receptor blockers, and statins, is important for maximizing benefit for the patient and the public.

REFERENCES

1. Brodde OE, Bruck H, Leineweber K: Cardiac adrenoceptors: Physiological and pathophysiological relevance. J Pharmacol Sci 2006;100:323-337.
2. Emorine LJ, Marullo S, Briend-Sutren MM, et al: Molecular characterization of the human beta 3-adrenergic receptor. Science 1989;245:1118-1121.
3. Collins S, Cao W, Robidoux J: Learning new tricks from old dogs: beta-adrenergic receptors teach new lessons on firing up adipose tissue metabolism. Mol Endocrinol 2004;18: 2123-2131.
4. Petrikova M, Jancinova V, Nosal R, et al: Antiplatelet activity of carvedilol in comparison to propranolol. Platelets 2002; 13:479-485.
5. Gottlieb SO, Weisfeldt ML, Ouyang P, et al: Effect of the addition of propranolol to therapy with nifedipine for unstable angina pectoris: A randomized, double-blind, placebo-controlled trial. Circulation 1986;73:331-337.
6. Hohnloser SH, Meinertz T, Klingenheben T, et al: Usefulness of esmolol in unstable angina pectoris. European Esmolol Study Group. Am J Cardiol 1991;67:1319-1323.
7. Brunner M, Faber TS, Greve B, et al: Usefulness of carvedilol in unstable angina pectoris. Am J Cardiol 2000;85: 1173-1178.
8. Ellis K, Tcheng JE, Sapp S, et al: Mortality benefit of beta blockade in patients with acute coronary syndromes undergoing coronary intervention: Pooled results from the Epic, Epilog, Epistent, Capture and Rapport Trials. J Interv Cardiol 2003;16:299-305.
9. Ellis SG, Brener SJ, Lincoff AM, et al: Beta-blockers before percutaneous coronary intervention do not attenuate postprocedural creatine kinase isoenzyme rise. Circulation 2001;104:2685-2688.
10. Sharma SK, Kini A, Marmur JD, Fuster V: Cardioprotective effect of prior beta-blocker therapy in reducing creatine kinase-MB elevation after coronary intervention: benefit is extended to improvement in intermediate-term survival. Circulation 2000;102:166-172.
11. Chan AW, Quinn MJ, Bhatt DL, et al: Mortality benefit of beta-blockade after successful elective percutaneous coronary intervention. J Am Coll Cardiol 2002;40:669-675.
12. Jackson JD, Muhlestein JB, Bunch TJ, et al: Beta-blockers reduce the incidence of clinical restenosis: Prospective study of 4840 patients undergoing percutaneous coronary revascularization. Am Heart J 2003;145:875-881.
13. Serruys PW, Foley DP, Hofling B, et al: Carvedilol for prevention of restenosis after directional coronary atherectomy: Final results of the European carvedilol atherectomy restenosis (EUROCARE) trial. Circulation 2000;101:1512-1518.
14. Wang FW, Osman A, Otero J, et al: Distal myocardial protection during percutaneous coronary intervention with an intracoronary beta-blocker. Circulation 2003;107:2914-2919.
15. Infarct Survival Collaborative Group: Randomised trial of intravenous atenolol among 16 027 cases of suspected acute myocardial infarction: ISIS-1. First International Study of Infarct Survival Collaborative Group. Lancet 1986;2:57-66.
16. MIAMI Trial Research Group: Metoprolol in acute myocardial infarction (MIAMI). A randomised placebo-controlled international trial. Eur Heart J 1985;6:199-226.
16a. Chen ZM, Pan HC, Chen YP, et al: COMMIT (CLOpidogrel and Metoprolol in Myocardial Infarction Trial) collaborative group: Early intravenous then oral metoprolol in 45,852 patients with acute myocardial infarction: Randomised placebo-controlled trial. Lancet 2005;366:1622-1632.
17. Held P, Teo K, Yusuf S: Effects of medical therapies on acute myocardial infarction and unstable angina pectoris. *In* Topol E (ed): Textbook of Interventional Cardiology, vol 1, 4th ed. Philadelphia, WB Saunders, 2002, 65-78.
18. Dargie HJ: Effect of carvedilol on outcome after myocardial infarction in patients with left-ventricular dysfunction: The CAPRICORN randomised trial. Lancet 2001;357:1385-1390.
19. Terra SG, Hamilton KK, Pauly DF, et al: Beta1-adrenergic receptor polymorphisms and left ventricular remodeling changes in response to beta-blocker therapy. Pharmacogenet Genomics 2005;15:227-234.
20. Sica DA: Pharmacotherapy review: Calcium channel blockers. J Clin Hypertens (Greenwich) 2006;8:53-56.
21. Comparison of the effects of beta blockers and calcium antagonists on cardiovascular events after acute myocardial infarction in Japanese subjects. Am J Cardiol 2004;93:969-973.
22. Braunwald E, Antman EM, Beasley JW, et al: ACC/AHA guidelines for the management of patients with unstable angina and non-ST-segment elevation myocardial infarction: Executive summary and recommendations. A report of the American College of Cardiology/American Heart Association task force on practice guidelines (Committee on the Management of Patients with Unstable Angina). Circulation 2000;102: 1193-1209.
23. Nissen SE, Tuzcu EM, Libby P, et al: Effect of antihypertensive agents on cardiovascular events in patients with coronary disease and normal blood pressure: The CAMELOT study: A randomized controlled trial. JAMA 2004;292:2217-2225.
24. Pepine CJ, Handberg EM, Cooper-DeHoff RM, et al: A calcium antagonist vs a non-calcium antagonist hypertension treatment strategy for patients with coronary artery disease. The International Verapamil-Trandolapril Study (INVEST): A randomized controlled trial. JAMA 2003;290:2805-2816.
25. Chobanian AV, Bakris GL, Black HR, et al: The Seventh Report of the Joint National Committee on Prevention, Detection, Evaluation, and Treatment of High Blood Pressure: The JNC 7 report. JAMA 2003;289:2560-2572.
26. Hang CL, Wang CP, Yip HK, et al: Early administration of intracoronary verapamil improves myocardial perfusion during percutaneous coronary interventions for acute myocardial infarction. Chest 2005;128:2593-2598.
27. Arakawa E, Hasegawa K: Benidipine, a calcium channel blocker, regulates proliferation and phenotype of vascular smooth muscle cells. J Pharmacol Sci 2006;100:149-156.
28. Bestehorn HP, Neumann FJ, Buttner HJ, et al: Evaluation of the effect of oral verapamil on clinical outcome and angiographic restenosis after percutaneous coronary intervention: The randomized, double-blind, placebo-controlled, multicenter Verapamil Slow-Release for Prevention of Cardiovascular Events After Angioplasty (VESPA) Trial. J Am Coll Cardiol 2004;43:2160-2165.
29. Ellis K, Kapadia SR: Stable angina. *In* Topol E, Griffin BA (eds): Manual of Cardiovascular Medicine, 2nd ed. Philadelphia, Lippincott Williams & Wilkins, 2004, p 85.
30. Lanfear DE, Jones PG, Marsh S, et al: Beta 2-adrenergic genotype and survival among patients receiving beta-blocker therapy after an acute coronary syndrome. JAMA 2005;294: 1526-1533.
31. Umemura S, Nakamura S, Sugiura T, et al: The effect of verapamil on the restoration of myocardial perfusion and functional recovery in patients with angiographic no-reflow after primary percutaneous coronary intervention. Nucl Med Commun 2006;27:247-254.
32. Yamazaki T, Taniguchi I, Kurusu T, et al: Effect of amlodipine on vascular responses after coronary stenting compared with an angiotensin-converting enzyme inhibitor. Circ J, 2004;68: 328-333.

Coronary Intervention

CHAPTER

15 Drug-Eluting and Bare Metal Stents

Stephen G. Ellis

KEY POINTS

- Both drug-eluting stents, Cypher and Taxus, reduce clinical restenosis by a relative 50% to 80%, but they have no overall impact on the risk of death or myocardial infarction.
- The principal clinical limitation of drug-eluting stenting is stent thrombosis, which is a multifactorial problem involving failure to adequately expand the stent(s), residual coronary dissection, stent number or length, medication compliance, and possibly genetic factors, such as those predisposing to diminished responsiveness to aspirin and clopidogrel.
- The role of testing for resistance to aspirin and clopidogrel remains poorly defined, with inadequate functional definitions of poor responders, and it represents a major unmet clinical need.

- Thrombosis in drug-eluting stents is often related to withholding antiplatelet therapy before or during noncardiac surgery. The optimal pharmacologic management of such patients remains ill defined. If possible, aspirin should not be stopped; many surgical procedures can be safely performed without stopping aspirin.
- The proper role of drug-eluting stents in patients with complex multivessel disease also eligible for bypass surgery remains to be determined and is the topic of several ongoing randomized trials. The only patient subset with clearly better outcomes with bypass surgery is diabetics with diffuse coronary involvement (i.e., multivessel disease and more than three lesions severe enough to require revascularization).

HISTORICAL BACKGROUND

The introduction of bare metal stents in the late 1980s by Sigwart, Roubin, Palmaz, Schatz, and others dramatically improved the interventionalist's ability to successfully treat balloon or atherectomy device–induced coronary dissections and to minimize post-treatment vessel recoil. The need for emergency surgery was thereby reduced from about 4% to less than 1%, and elective target vessel revascularization (TVR) was reduced by a relative 30% (with the absolute number depending on the nature of the lesion), hastening an era of more aggressive percutaneous revascularization.[1-3]

However, vessel trauma from stent implantation increased late loss (i.e., minimum lumen diameter after the procedure – minimum lumen diameter at follow-up) compared with balloon alone, to about 1.0 mm.[2,3] Given the wide variations in lesion and patient response, clinically relevant restenosis occurred in 20% to 50% of lesions, precipitating a search for a systemic solution and, when that failed, a local, pharmacologic solution to reduce this process, which resulted from neointimal hyperplasia and matrix accumulation.[4]

COMPONENTS OF DRUG-ELUTING STENTS

The drug-eluting stent (DES) consists of three principal components: the stent backbone itself, the pharmacologic agents intended to reduce neointimal hyperplasia and sometimes other adverse effects, and a polymer designed to slow the release of the pharmacologic agent such that it remains at a sufficient concentration for long enough to interdict relevant biologic processes (Fig. 15-1).

Early balloon-expandable stents were made of 316L stainless steel, laser cut from a thin-walled hollow tube. Stainless steel is an alloy predominately composed of relatively inert iron, but it also contains about 5% nickel, and allergy to nickel may be related to restenosis.[5] Some stents have used tantalum, cobalt chromium, or other alloys to allow a reduction in strut size (75 μm compared with 100 to 150 μm) without sacrificing radial strength or radiopacity.[6] First-generation DESs used available bare metal stents to serve as their scaffold or backbone. The original Cypher stent used the BX Velocity backbone, and the Taxus stent used the Express backbone (Fig. 15-2). The ideal scaffold dimensions depend somewhat on the diffusing capability of the pharmacologic agent

Taxus SR and MR

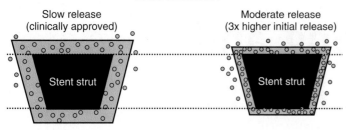

	Slow release (clinically approved)		Moderate release (3x higher initial release)
1 μg/mm²		Dose density	1 μg/mm²
16–18 μm		Coating thickness	6–8 μm
Lower		Paclitaxel/polymer ratio	Higher
Sparser		Drug distribution	Denser
		In vivo release kinetics	
7.5%		Released < 30 days	21.9%
92.5%		Released > 30 days	78.1%

Figure 15-1. Components of drug-eluting stents. The slow-release and moderate-release Taxus stents exemplify the principal components of drug-eluting stents, including the stent backbone, the polymer to which the drug is associated, and the drug itself. Dimensions and release kinetics are provided. (Courtesy of Boston Scientific.)

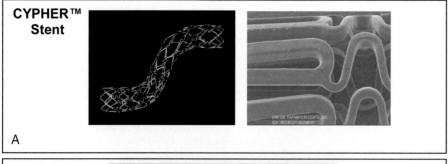

CYPHER™ Stent

A

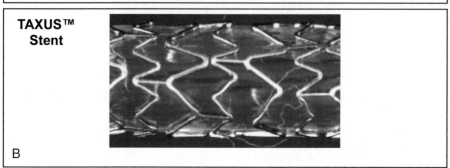

TAXUS™ Stent

B

Figure 15-2. Cypher (**A**) and Taxus (**B**) drug-eluting stents are available in the United States. The drugs released from stents have cytostatic and anti-inflammatory effects. The pharmacologic agents interrupt the cell cycle indirectly (e.g., sirolimus and its cogeners bind to the mammalian target of rapamycin [mTOR] and decrease inflammation by increasing p21 and p27 levels). Alternating macro and micro elements are shown for the Taxus stent. (**A,** Courtesy of Cordis Corporation; **B,** courtesy of Boston Scientific.)

delivered and on design considerations that allow a combination of sufficient radial strength and axial flexibility.[7,8] Newer designs in phase III clinical trials rely on novel, more complex designs (Fig. 15-3). Scaffolds that dissolve over time may be ideal because they allow restoration of physiologic vasomotor tone and access to jailed side branches, and are now being tested.[9-11]

The associations of stent geometry, polymer-drug characteristics, and drug deposition have been difficult to characterize because of the paucity of high-resolution techniques for detecting drug within tissue and for distinguishing it from residual drug adherent to the stent (i.e., radiolabeling and fluorescence labeling of drug are inadequate) and because animal models cannot mimic the effect of complex calcified atheromatous disease on drug deposition. Nonethe-

less, coupled computational fluid dynamics and mass transfer models (Fig. 15-4) provide important and often counterintuitive insights.[8,12]

It appears that abluminal stent-tissue contact may provide considerably less drug to the tissue than does drug eluting off the noncontacting top and distal strut surfaces and that is temporarily "trapped" by stagnant blood in recirculation zones just distal to stent struts.[8] Modeling a drug with modest plasma and tissue binding, Edelman and colleagues[8] found only 11% of total drug delivered was provided directly by the abluminal strut surface itself, and 30% and 43% were provided by the noncontacting stent top and distal strut surfaces, respectively; compare the red (abluminal surface-only coated) with the purple (all surfaces coated) and the green (only adluminal surface coated) curves in Figure 15-4B.

A. ZoMaxx Stent

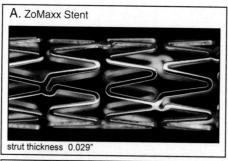

strut thickness 0.029"

B. **Triplex Stent**

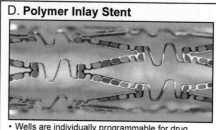

Stainless Steel

Tantalum

25kU   X500   50μm 0000 17 45 SEI

Triplex is a trademark of Uniform Tubing, Inc.

C. **CoStar Stent**

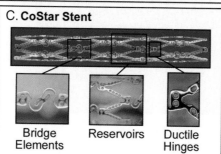

Bridge Elements   Reservoirs   Ductile Hinges

D. **Polymer Inlay Stent**

• Wells are individually programmable for drug concentration enabling controlled spatial drug
• Dose distribution

Figure 15-3. Newer drug-eluting stents are being evaluated. In the ZoMaxx stent (**A**), using Triplex stent material (Uniform Tubing, Inc.) (**B**), the strut thickness is only 0.029 inches. In the Co-Star stent (**C**), using polymer inlay technology (**D**), wells are individually programmable for drug concentration, enabling a controlled spatial drug dose distribution. (**A** and **B**, Courtesy of Abbott Laboratories; **C** and **D**, courtesy of Conor Medsystems.)

If generalizable, these data are important for stent strut geometries, surface coatings (i.e., abluminal may not be better than all-surface coatings), and strut spacing. They explain the distal greater than proximal edge benefit of DES with regard to the late lumen loss seen with TAXUS IV and SIRIUS trials (the former more than the latter owing to drug-binding proteins.[13,14]

Initial coatings were passive and intended principally to decrease stent thrombosis. Covalently bound heparin (i.e., Carmeda coating) and phosphorylcholine gained some acceptance in this regard, although it proved difficult to translate obvious benefit in bench models to the human arena.[15,16] Many polymers carrying antiproliferative agents targeting restenosis have been developed. The ideal polymer coating is biocompatible with blood and tissue. These have not been easy to develop because most induce at least some degree of inflammation and promote local thrombosis.[17] The polymers can be configured to release the biologic payload over the 2 to 4 weeks that most drugs appear to require to minimize the restenosis process, and they minimally adversely affect stent performance. Several concepts have been tested (Fig. 15-5).

The pharmacologic agents used in stents interrupt the cell cycle indirectly (i.e., sirolimus and its cogeners bind to the mammalian target of rapamycin [mTOR], as well as decreasing inflammation by increasing p21 and p27 levels) or principally affect microtubular assembly (i.e., by means of paclitaxel, although this entity affects a number of other restenosis-related pathways) (Figs. 15-6 and 15-7).[18,19] The ideal drug would reduce the smooth muscle cell proliferation and matrix accumulation that characterize restenosis, while minimally inhibiting the endothelial recovery necessary to minimize the risk of thrombosis. Many have been or are being tested (Table 15-1).

Covered stents have been used to treat coronary perforation and applied with less evidence to support their use to treat coronary aneurysms.[20] One or two layers of microporous polytetrafluoroethylene (PTFE) surround or are surrounded by the bare metal stent skeleton. Risk of thrombosis with these devices seems to be somewhat accentuated.

IMPLANTATION TECHNIQUE

Current DES outcomes have improved compared with initial outcomes because of evolution of implantation techniques. This is best exemplified by differences between Cypher stent use in the SIRIUS and New SIRIUS trials.[13,21] Contemporary technique draws on the early experience of Colombo and associates,[22] who observed the importance of high-pressure implantation (i.e., the polymer itself makes the stent somewhat less expanded at a given pressure, such that even at 13 to 15 atm, stents are typically only 75% of nominal diameter),[23] and that from the brachytherapy era and initial Cypher follow-up data, showing a high incidence of edge restenosis, particularly in small vessels[13] (Fig. 15-8), suggesting that minimization of trauma outside the treatment zone was important.

Properly shaped, coaxial guide catheters that provide support sufficient for the clinical and anatomic scenario remain a must. In our laboratory, XB and Amplatz shaped catheters are the workhorses. Guide catheter size ranges from 5 to 8 Fr, depending on the length of the stent to be placed (i.e., its stiffness) and on the tortuosity and elasticity (i.e., calcification) of the vessel to be traversed. After atraumatic placement of an appropriately sized guide catheter,

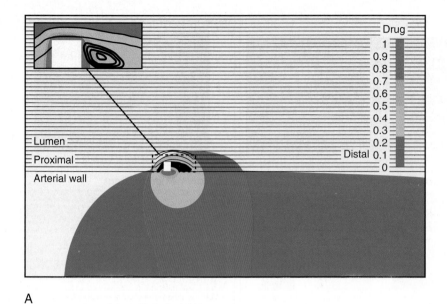

A

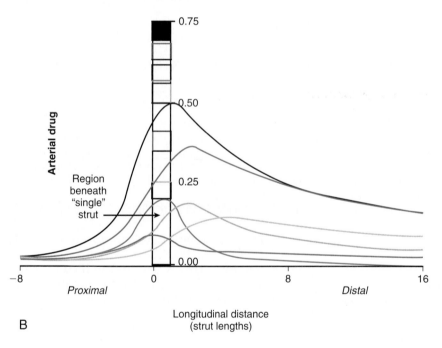

B

Figure 15-4. Modeling drug deposition of a drug-eluting stent (DES). **A,** Single DES strut. Visual representation of drug concentration distribution and blood flow profiles *(black curves).* **Inset,** The high magnification of area is outlined *(dashed line).* **B,** Arterial wall drug concentration profile as function of axial distance along an artery at a depth of 1.5 strut heights into the arterial wall. Each curve represents a case in which 0, 1, or more than 1 surfaces of a single strut were simulated as noneluting *(black line).* (From Balakrishnan SB, Tzafriri AR, Seifert P, et al: Strut position, blood flow, and drug deposition implications for single and overlapping drug-eluting stents. Circulation 2005;111:2958-2965.)

the lesion is predilated with a balloon of sufficient diameter to allow placement of the subsequent stent, with particular attention to prevent trauma to areas that will not be covered by the stent, or it is directly stented if the lesion is neither severely narrowed nor heavily calcified. Direct stenting appears not to adversely affect the anti-restenosis benefit of the Cypher or Taxus stents.[24,25] In 1% to 2% of stenoses, characterized by dense angiographic calcification, debulking to modify vessel compliance with rotational atherectomy or other devices is required to allow safe stent placement and expansion.

The stent diameter should be chosen to approximate a 1.1:1 ratio compared with the angiographically normal adjacent vessel. The stent length should

be chosen to cover the entire length of the lesion ("shoulder to shoulder") if possible. This dictum may occasionally be violated to avoid covering difficult-to-manage side branches, which represent a technical challenge in the absence of a dedicated side-branch stent but usually should be treated with a stent in the side branch and completed with "kissing balloon" inflation only if the side branch is large and diseased at its origin and the interventionalist cannot achieve an adequate result without stenting. Stent overlap at the point of a major side branch should be avoided, especially when using a DES with a thick polymer.[26] The stent itself should be implanted at high pressure (>16 atm) or post-dilated at a similarly high pressure.[23] The latter is preferred, keeping the post-

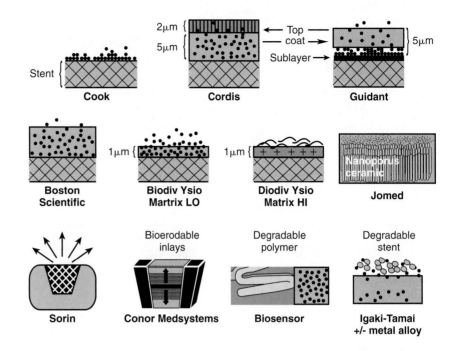

Figure 15-5. Stent and drug delivery systems under evaluation, with a focus on polymer or other drug-deployment systems.

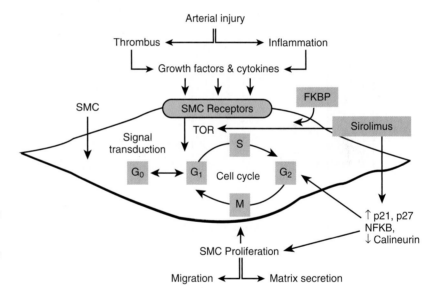

Figure 15-6. The mammalian target of rapamycin (mTOR) pathway and other relevant biologic pathways interdicted by sirolimus in the Cypher drug-eluting stent. FKBP, cytosolic receptor of the macrolide antibiotic rapamycin; NFKB, NF-κB transcription factor; SMC, smooth muscle cell.

dilatation balloon within the confines of the stent, especially when dilating in areas of diffuse disease to minimize the possibility of edge trauma.

TRIALS OF STENTS

Overview of Key Trials

Approval and availability of current DESs rests on results from pivotal randomized trials performed in relatively nonchallenging patient or lesion subsets comparing DESs with bare metal stents. General configuration and patient and lesion entry criteria for the trials of the Cypher, Taxus, and Endeavor stents are shown in Tables 15-2, 15-3, and 15-4.[13,14,27] In general, each DES dramatically reduced TVR relative to its bare metal stent control (Fig. 15-9). The degree

of "neointimal suppression," measured by angiographically confirmed late loss, varied from 0.24 mm (Cypher) to 0.60 mm (Endeavor stent).[13,14,27] Given the relationship between late loss and TVR (Fig. 15-10),[28,29] it was anticipated that the Cypher stent might perform relatively better than the Taxus or Endeavor stents in more challenging lesions, although at least initially it remained uncertain whether the relative potency of these different stent products would remain constant across untested patient and lesion subtypes (e.g., in-stent restenosis, saphenous vein bypass graft stenoses).

After the pivotal trials, the Cypher and Taxus stents have been subjected to studies in more challenging populations and to meta-analyses that allow amalgamation of sufficient clinical results to draw further conclusions.[30] Long-term results for the two products

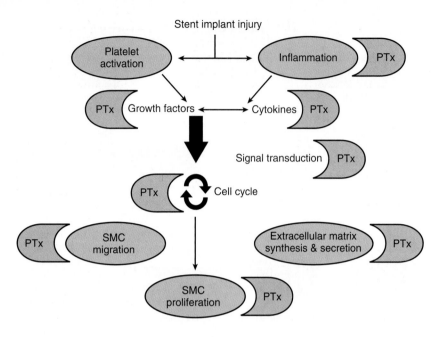

Figure 15-7. Taxus-relevant biologic pathways affected by paclitaxel (PTx). SMC, smooth muscle cell. (Courtesy of Boston Scientific.)

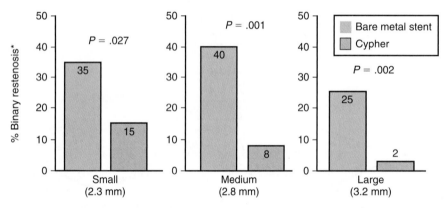

*Overall Cypher = 9.2% (2.0% in-stent)
+ 2.5–3.5 mm ref DM (visual), 15–30 mm length, 28% DM

Figure 15-8. Interim results of the Study of the Sirolimus-Eluting Stent in the Treatment of Patients with Long De Novo Lesions in Small Native Coronary Arteries (SIRIUS) trial presented on European CD mark approval of the stent, highlighting relatively high restenosis rates in small stents, predominantly at the proximal edge.

Table 15-1. Innovation in Next-Generation Drug-Eluting Stents

Manufacturer	Name	Drug	Stent Material	Polymer	Status
Abbott	ZoMaxx	Zotarolimus	Tantalum/stainless steel	Durable	—
Abbott	Zodiac	Zotarolimus, dexamethasone	Tantalum/stainless steel	Durable	—
Biosensors	Axxion	Paclitaxel	Stainless steel	None	CE mark
Biosensors	BioMatrix	Biolimus-A9	Stainless steel	Bioabsorable	—
Boston Scientific	Taxus Liberte	Paclitaxel	Stainless steel	Durable	CE mark
Conor	CoStar	Paclitaxel	Cobalt chromium	Bioabsorable	—
Cordis/J&J	Cypher select	Sirolimus	Stainless steel	Durable	CE mark
Cordis/J&J	Cypher Neo	Sirolimus	Cobalt chromium	Durable	—
Guidant	Champion	Everolimus	Stainless steel	Bioabsorable	—
Guidant	Xience	Everolimus	Cobalt chromium	Durable	CE mark
Medtronic	Endeavor	Zotarolimus	Cobalt chromium	Durable	CE Mark
Orbus	Genous	EPC	Stainless steel	Anti-CD34 antibody	—
Sorin	Janus	Tacrolimus	Stainless steel	None	CE mark
Sahajanand Medical Technologies (SMT)	Infinnium	Paclitaxel	Stainless steel	Bioabsorable	CE mark
Terumo	Nobori	Biolimus-A9	Stainless steel	Bioabsorable	—

CE mark, mandatory declaration by the manufacturer that the medical device meets the appropriate provisions of certain European directives; EPC, endothelial progenitor cells.

Table 15-2. Early Cypher Trials

Characteristic*	C-SIRIUS	SIRIUS	RAVEL	E-SIRIUS
No. of patients (total = 1793)	238	1101	102	352
Randomization (DES or BMS)	1:1	1:1	1:1	1:1
No. of sites	19	53	8	35
Inclusion vessel size (mm)	2.5-3.5	2.5-3.5	2.5-3.0	2.5-3.0
Inclusion lesion length (mm)	≤18	15-30	15-32	15-32
Pre-PCI regimen	100-400 mg of ASA 12 hr before PCI			
	300-375 mg of clopidogrel before or immediately after PCI *or*			
	500 mg ticlopidine ≥24 hr before PCI			
Post-PCI regimen	100-400 mg ASA indefinitely			
	75 mg qd or 250 mg bid of ticlopidine			
Post-discharge thienopyridine (mo)	2	3	2	2
Angiographic follow-up (mo)	6	8	8	8

*Acute myocardial infarction, in-stent restenosis, saphenous vein grafting, and bifurcation not included.
ASA, acetylsalicylic acid; BMS, bare metal stent; C-, Canadian study; DES, drug-eluting stent; E-, European study; PCI, percutaneous coronary intervention; RAVEL, Randomized Study with the Sirolimus-Eluting Velocity Balloon Expandable Stent; SIRIUS, Sirolimus-Eluting Bx-Velocity Balloon Expandable Stent in the Treatment of Patients with De Novo Native Coronary Artery Lesions.

Table 15-3. Early Taxus Trials

Characteristic	Taxus II	Taxus IV	Taxus V	Taxus VI
No. of patients (total = 3445)	529	1314	1156	446
Formulation	SR and MR	SR	SR	MR
Stent platform	NIRx	Express	Express 2	Express
Geography	Global	United States	United States	Europe
Primary end point	6 mo	9 mo	9 mo	9 mo
Angiographic follow-up (%)	97.0	53.9	85.6	93.5
IVUS follow-up (%)	89.6	13.2	25.0	28.3

IVUS, intravascular ultrasound; MR, moderate release rate; SR, slow release rate.

Table 15-4. Endeavor Trials

Characteristic	Endeavor I	Endeavor II	Endeavor III	Endeavor IV
No. of patients (total = 2794)	100	1200	436	1058
Vessel size (mm)	3.0-3.5	2.25-3.5	2.5-3.5	2.5-3.5
Lesion length (mm)	<15	14-27	14-27	<27
Angiographic follow-up (%)	100	50	100	Subset
Clopidogrel (mo)	3	3	≥3	≥6
RCT	No	BMS	Cypher	Taxus
First-degree end point	MACE at 30 days; late loss at 4 mo	TVF	Late loss	TVF

BMS, bare metal stent; MACE, major adverse cardiac event; RCT, randomized, controlled trial; TVF, target vessel failure.

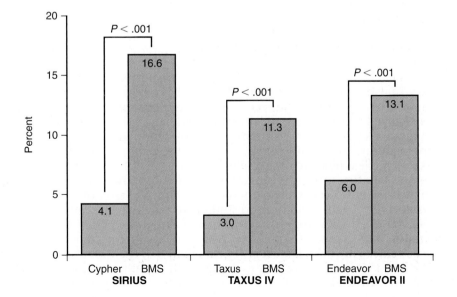

Figure 15-9. Target lesion revascularization in major U.S. randomized trials of drug-eluting stents (DESs). All DESs show significant reduction in restenosis-associated target lesion revascularization. BMS, bare metal stent.

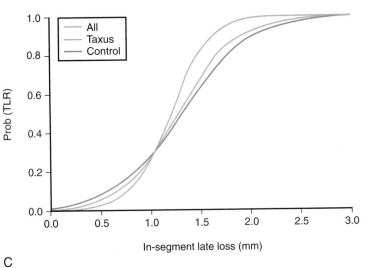

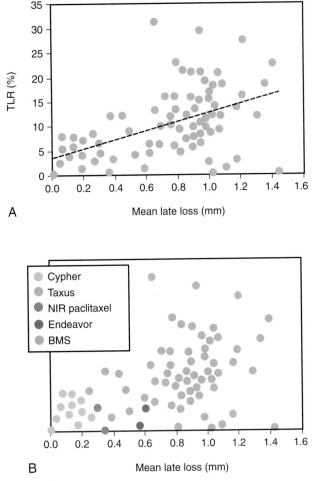

Figure 15-10. A and **B,** Late loss versus target lesion revascularization (TLR) results drawn from a number of key studies. **C,** Late loss and target vessel revascularization modeled on the basis of individual patient data from TAXUS IV. (**A** and **B** from Mauri L, Orav EJ, Candia SC, et al: Robustness of late lumen loss in discriminating drug-eluting stents across variable observational and randomized trials. Circulation 2005;112:2833-2839; **C** from Ellis SG, Popma JJ, Lasala JM, et al: Relationship between angiographic late loss and target lesion revascularization after coronary stent implantation: Analysis from the TAXUS IV trial. J Am Coll Cardiol 2005;45:1193-1200.)

are depicted in Figure 15-11. The long-term follow-up of large numbers of patients in these studies has enabled identification of what appears to be a significant, albeit numerically small, risk of late stent thrombosis for both products.[31] Results also show a dramatic and fairly consistent reduction of clinical events related to restenosis but no reduction in the risk of death or myocardial infarction.[30]

Lessons from Meta-Analyses and Registries

The ideal large, all-comer, head-to-head comparative DES trial has yet to be performed. Trials have been modestly to grossly undersized; they often focus on particular subgroups, minimizing their generalizability; and they are often "contaminated" by required angiographic follow-up, which, owing to the oculostenotic reflex, tends to exaggerate differences in outcomes resulting from differences in late loss. With these caveats, however, meta-analyses combining the results of the eight head-to-head studies are available (Fig. 15-12).[32] They appear to conclusively show the late-loss impact predicted previously, favoring Cypher over Taxus. However, large registry experiences (Figs. 15-13 to 15-15) do not appear to duplicate this result, showing instead overall parity, emphasizing the

possible contaminating effect of protocol-mandated follow-up angiography.[33-35]

USE OF STENTS

Stent Thrombosis: Risk and Management

Several large-scale studies of the carefully selected patients from randomized trials or more general practice[36,37] have attempted to assess the incidence, timing, and risk factors for DES-associated stent thrombosis. Intravascular ultrasound (IVUS) and autopsy studies suggest a correlation with stent underexpansion, dissection, plaque prolapse, and stenting adjacent to vulnerable plaque.[38] The 30-day risk appears to be 0.6% to 1.4%, which is not dissimilar to that with bare metal stents. From 6 months to 2 years, however, some studies suggest numerically small but significant excess risk with DESs. Simolimus- and paclitaxel-eluting stents appear to have similar risks.[30] Consistent findings among the studies are the relation of cessation of clopidogrel therapy, renal failure, and bifurcation lesions to risk of thrombosis, often increasing the risk by more than five times.[36,37] Other studies have found that the thrombosis risk also was related to stent length, in-stent

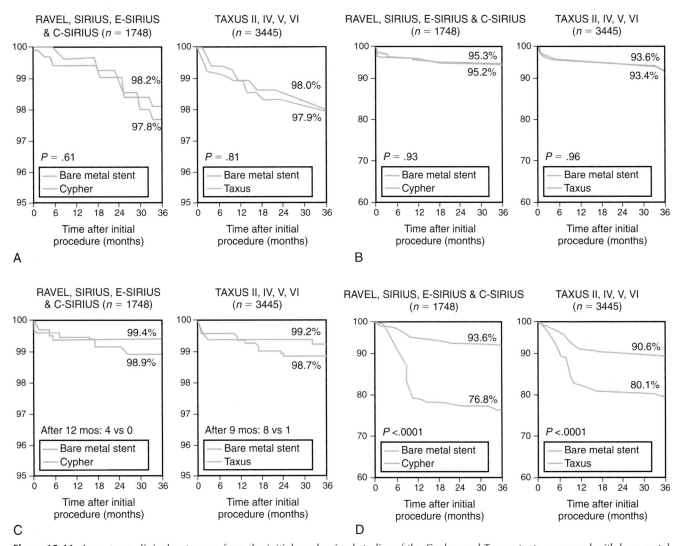

Figure 15-11. Long-term clinical outcomes from the initial randomized studies of the Cypher and Taxus stents compared with bare metal stents. **A,** Freedom from cardiac death. **B,** Freedom from myocardial infarction. **C,** Freedom from stent thrombosis. **D,** Freedom from target lesion revascularization.

restenosis treatment, diabetes, and low ejection fraction, albeit at a lesser magnitude of risk. Stent thrombosis is poorly responsive to fibrinolytic therapy and usually results in myocardial infarction, and because stents are typically placed in large proximal vessels, the result is death in 15% to 48% of cases.[36,37]

Thrombosis should be managed with emergency angioplasty, with aggressive platelet antagonist use, and with IVUS if a mechanical cause is suspected; if there is no obvious mechanical cause and the patient has been taking dual-antiplatelet therapy, further coagulation testing should be performed.[38,39] Late stent thrombosis especially has been related to cessation of dual-antiplatelet therapy in conjunction with hypercoagulative risk of major surgery.[40,41] A DES should be considered contraindicated if surgery that cannot be performed on aspirin is anticipated within approximately 2 years. Although the approach is not yet validated, I suggest aspirin and clopidogrel resistance testing for patients with risk factors before using DESs in the elective setting.[38,39]

Pharmacologic Adjuncts

Periprocedural inhibition of thrombin- and platelet-mediated coagulation is critical. Aspirin, clopidogrel, and thrombin inhibition with bivalirudin or unfractionated heparin provides the basic therapy, with bivalirudin generally favored over heparin owing to less bleeding.[42-44] Glycoprotein IIb/IIIa antagonists such as abciximab add benefit principally in the setting of enzyme-positive acute coronary syndromes (Figs. 15-16 to 15-18).[44] As shown in Figure 15-11C, DESs appear to be prone to late thrombosis, even when used in relatively ideal patients and with "ideal dualantiplatelet therapy."[30,41] The issue of individual patient response or resistance to both aspirin and clopidogrel has also been posited as a contributing factor.[38,39] Current recommendations are for aspirin use indefinitely and clopidogrel use probably for at least 2 years. The optimal aspirin dose remains somewhat conjectural, because the pivotal DES trials required the 325-mg daily dose known to increase

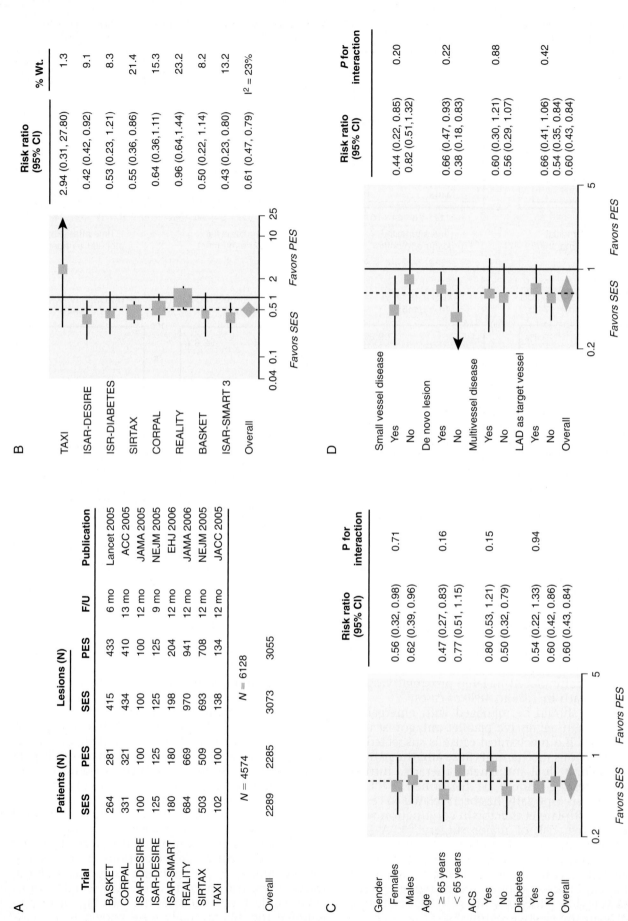

Figure 15-12. A, SIRPACT meta-analysis of the first eight head-to-head randomized trials comparing Cypher and Taxus stents. **B,** Target lesion revascularization in individual studies. **C** and **D,** Target lesion revascularization in selected subgroups. ACS, acute coronary syndrome; F/U, follow-up; LAD, left anterior descending; PES, paclitaxel-eluting stent; SES, sirolimus-eluting stent.

A

Trial	Patients (N) SES	Patients (N) PES	Lesions (N) SES	Lesions (N) PES	F/U	Publication
BASKET	264	281	415	433	6 mo	Lancet 2005
CORPAL	331	321	434	410	13 mo	ACC 2005
ISAR-DESIRE	100	100	100	100	12 mo	JAMA 2005
ISAR-DESIRE	125	125	125	125	9 mo	NEJM 2005
ISAR-SMART	180	180	198	204	12 mo	EHJ 2006
REALITY	684	669	970	941	12 mo	JAMA 2006
SIRTAX	503	509	693	708	12 mo	NEJM 2005
TAXI	102	100	138	134	12 mo	JACC 2005
	N = 4574		*N* = 6128			
Overall	2289	2285	3073	3055		

B

	Risk ratio (95% CI)	% Wt.
TAXI	2.94 (0.31, 27.80)	1.3
ISAR-DESIRE	0.42 (0.42, 0.92)	9.1
ISR-DIABETES	0.53 (0.23, 1.21)	8.3
SIRTAX	0.55 (0.36, 0.86)	21.4
CORPAL	0.64 (0.36,1.11)	15.3
REALITY	0.96 (0.64,1.44)	23.2
BASKET	0.50 (0.22, 1.14)	8.2
ISAR-SMART 3	0.43 (0.23, 0.80)	13.2
Overall	0.61 (0.47, 0.79)	I^2 = 23%

C

	Risk ratio (95% CI)	P for interaction
Gender		
Females	0.56 (0.32, 0.98)	0.71
Males	0.62 (0.39, 0.96)	
Age		
≥ 65 years	0.47 (0.27, 0.83)	0.16
< 65 years	0.77 (0.51, 1.15)	
ACS		
Yes	0.80 (0.53, 1.21)	0.15
No	0.50 (0.32, 0.79)	
Diabetes		
Yes	0.54 (0.22, 1.33)	0.94
No	0.60 (0.42, 0.86)	
Overall	0.60 (0.43, 0.84)	

D

	Risk ratio (95% CI)	P for interaction
Small vessel disease		
Yes	0.44 (0.22, 0.85)	0.20
No	0.82 (0.51, 1.32)	
De novo lesion		
Yes	0.66 (0.47, 0.93)	0.22
No	0.38 (0.18, 0.83)	
Multivessel disease		
Yes	0.60 (0.30, 1.21)	0.88
No	0.56 (0.29, 1.07)	
LAD as target vessel		
Yes	0.66 (0.41, 1.06)	0.42
No	0.54 (0.35, 0.84)	
Overall	0.60 (0.43, 0.84)	

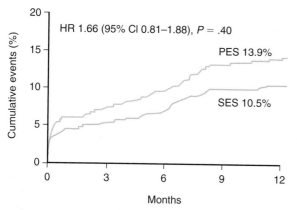

Figure 15-13. Experience of the Thoraxcenter and T-SEARCH registries using Cypher and Taxus stents, showing cumulative adverse cardiac events at 12 months. PES, paclitaxel-eluting stent; SES, sirolimus-eluting stent. (Data from Lemos PA, Serruys PW, van Domburg RT, et al: Unrestricted utilization of sirolimus-eluting stents compared with conventional bare stent implantation in the "real world": The Rapamycin-Eluting Stent Evaluated At Rotterdam Cardiology Hospital (RESEARCH) Registry. Circulation 2004;109:190-195.)

bleeding risk compared with lower doses when used in conjunction with clopidogrel. Because 50% to 60% of the stent thrombosis risk appears in the first month, the higher dose of aspirin should probably be maintained for that period and possibly longer. Whether patients who are relatively resistant to aspirin or clopidogrel should be treated initially with bare metal stents and have DESs used only in the event of restenosis remains to be clarified. Statins, smoking cessation, and proper assessment and treat-

ment of other coronary artery disease risk factors are also imperative.

Role of Coronary Stents in Patient Management

A complete discussion of the role of coronary stents in patient management is beyond the scope of this chapter but is addressed in Chapters 17 to 25. However, certain fundamentals are discussed here.

The balance of benefit and risk must be considered. Benefit beyond improvement of angina-related symptoms (which is important) is largely confined to acute coronary syndrome patients. Death and infarction are clearly prevented only in patients with ST-segment elevation myocardial infarction and moderate- to high-risk patients with non-ST-segment elevation myocardial infarction.[45,46] Whether underpowered "equivalence" trials comparing

	Hazard ratio	(95% CI)	P value
Diabetes	2.34	(1.50, 3.65)	0.001
Stent length (per mm)	1.03	(1.02, 1.05)	0.001
Cypher stent	1.09	(1.04, 1.14)	NS

Figure 15-14. Predictors of target lesion revascularization at 9 months. (Data from Cosgrave J, Agostoni P, Ge L, et al: Clinical outcome following aleatory implantation of paclitaxel-eluting or sirolimus-eluting stents in complex coronary lesions. Am J Cardiol 2005;96:1663-1668.)

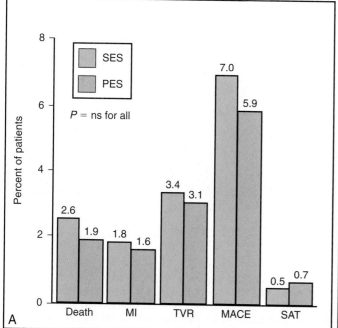

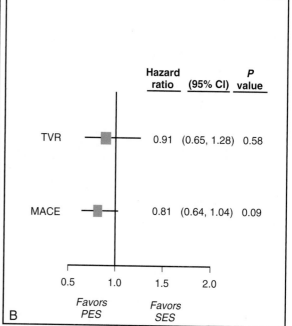

Figure 15-15. The U.S. STENT registry experience for Cypher and Taxus stents. **A,** Clinical outcomes in the STENT registry. **B,** Adjusted hazard ratios for time to event comparing paclitaxel-eluting stent (PES)–only patient with sirolimus-eluting stent (SES)–only patients. MACE, major adverse cardiac event; MI, myocardial infarction; SAT, subaclete thrombosis; TVR, target vessel revascularization.

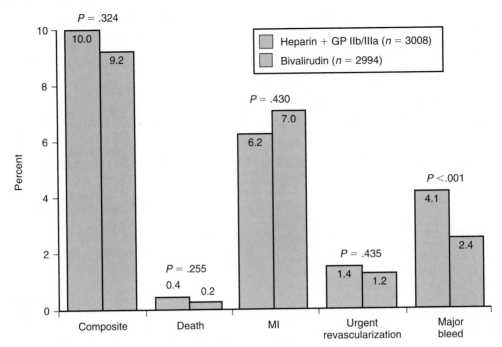

Figure 15-16. Results of REPLACE, the U.S. pivotal trial of bivalirudin for percutaneous coronary intervention, showing the composite quadruple end point and its components. Notice that the benefit is principally a reduction in major bleeding. (Redrawn from Lincoff AM, Bittl JA, Harrington RA, et al, for the REPLACE-2 Investigators. Bivalirudin and provision glycoprotein IIb/IIIa blockade compared with heparin and planned glycoprotein IIb/IIIa blockade during percutaneous coronary intervention. REPLACE-2 randomized trial. JAMA 2003;289:853-863.)

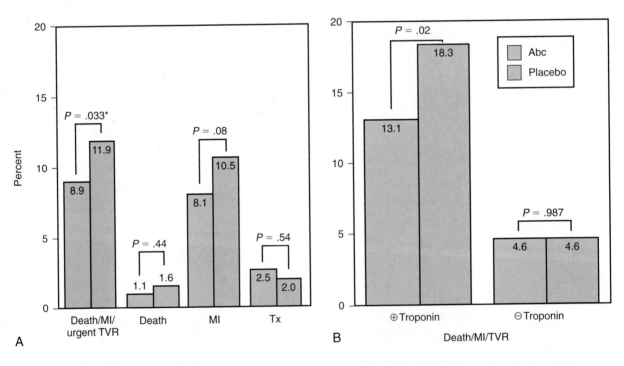

*Benefit confined to troponin ⊕ patients

Figure 15-17. Role of abciximab (Abc) in percutaneous coronary intervention for 2022 patients with acute coronary syndrome (ACS) in the ISAR-REACT II trial. All patients received aspirin, clopidogrel (600-mg loading dose), and heparin. **A,** Overall results. **B,** Triple composite end point for patients with and without elevated troponin levels, showing the benefit of abciximab limited to those with elevated troponin levels. MI, myocardial infarction; TVR, target vessel revascularization; Tx, therapy; asterisk, benefit confined to the troponin-positive patients. (Redrawn from Kastrati A, Mehilli J, Neumann FJ, et al, for the Intracoronary Stenting and Antithrombotic Regimen: Rapid Early Action for Coronary Treatment 2 (ISAR-REACT 2) Trial Investigators: Abciximab in patients with acute coronary syndromes undergoing percutaneous coronary intervention after clopidogrel pretreatment: the ISAR-REACT 2 randomized trial. 2006;295:1531-1538.)

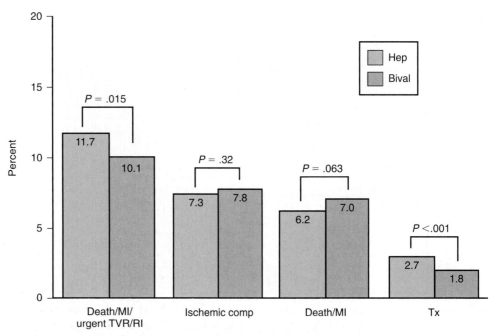

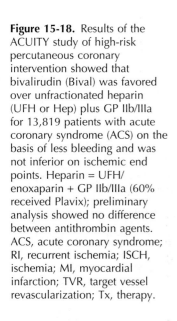

Figure 15-18. Results of the ACUITY study of high-risk percutaneous coronary intervention showed that bivalirudin (Bival) was favored over unfractionated heparin (UFH or Hep) plus GP IIb/IIIa for 13,819 patients with acute coronary syndrome (ACS) on the basis of less bleeding and was not inferior on ischemic end points. Heparin = UFH/ enoxaparin + GP IIb/IIIa (60% received Plavix); preliminary analysis showed no difference between antithrombin agents. ACS, acute coronary syndrome; RI, recurrent ischemia; ISCH, ischemia; MI, myocardial infarction; TVR, target vessel revascularization; Tx, therapy.

Hep = UFH/Enox* + GPIIb/IIIa (60% received plavix) N = 13,819 ACS patients
*Preliminary analysis-no difference between antithrombin agents

percutaneous coronary intervention (PCI) with bypass surgery[47,48] can reasonably extrapolate the benefits of coronary artery bypass grafting on survival compared with medical therapy to PCI is debatable for high-risk patients or perhaps even those with silent ischemia.[49,50]

Against benefit should be assessed the risk of adverse outcomes. Compared with the prestent era, when most severe complications were periprocedural in nature, unplanned bypass surgery has become distinctly uncommon,[51] and most fatal outcomes are related to baseline patient morbidity. Several schemas allow the operator to assess risk (Fig. 15-19).[52,53]

Choosing Stents and Identifying Difficult Subsets

For the interventionalist, the first choice to be made after deciding that PCI is superior to other options is whether to implant a high-priced DES or a more modestly priced bare metal stent. The utility of a DES depends on the resources a medical system or society are willing to spend to improve quality of life corresponding to a lower risk of clinical restenosis. DESs do not impact the risk of death or myocardial infarction compared with bare metal stenting.[30] The risk of clinically meaningful restenosis using bare metal stents can be anticipated based on clinical and anatomic parameters (i.e., longer lesions, smaller vessels, diabetes, saphenous vein graft or ostial location, and lesions with prior restenosis all are at higher risk),[54] although even for a low-risk patient, assurance of an event-free outcome is challenging.[55] It is difficult to be sanguine about placing a $2000 device that will not alter fatal outcome or risk of myocardial infarction and that may only modestly reduce other non-

fatal events, but normative value in this country expects their placement. Formal cost-effectiveness analyses can be performed (Fig. 15-20).[56] The physician must also consider the risk of stent thrombosis in the event antiplatelet therapy must be withdrawn. Patients with expected noncardiac surgery should have bare metal stents placed preferentially.[41]

If the cardiologist has decided to place a DES, the next choice is which one to implant. There is a disparity in outcomes between results of randomized trials often requiring angiography (i.e., generally favoring Cypher over Taxus, with Endeavor not yet directly studied) and large-scale clinical registries (i.e., generally no difference between Cypher and Taxus).[32-35] The impact of greater late loss inhibition is most likely to be evident in long lesions and perhaps in small vessels (although due to stent design, the less potent Taxus stent has a greater drug density with the 2.5-mm stent than with the 3.0- to 3.5-mm stent). Apparent differences between DESs in diabetics and patients with bare metal stent in-stent restenosis have been inconsistent.[13,32] With newer iterations of these stent platforms, differences in deliverability have been minimized. The choice between Cypher and Taxus stents is often made on the basis of subjective issues.

The impact of widespread DES availability on the choice of PCI versus bypass surgery for patients with complex or advanced disease has been considerable, but it is not based on a substantial evidence base. Important large-scale, randomized trials such as FREEDOM (Future Revascularization Evaluation in patiEnts with Diabetes mellitus: Optimal Management of multivessel disease), SYNTAX (Synergy Between PCI with Taxus Drug-Eluting Stent and

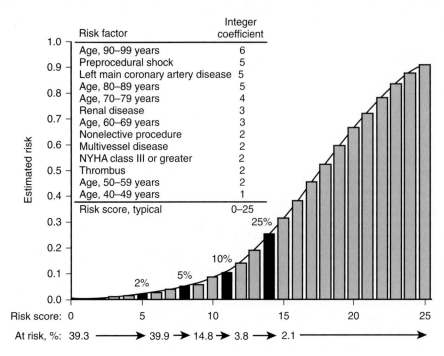

Figure 15-19. Estimating the risk of percutaneous coronary intervention in the contemporary era—the Mayo Clinic model. (Redrawn from Singh M, Lennon RJ, Holmes DR, et al: Correlates of procedural complications and a simple integer risk score for percutaneous coronary intervention. J Am Coll Cardiol 2002;40:387-393.)

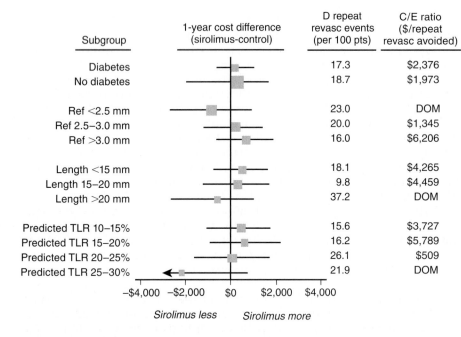

Figure 15-20. Cost effectiveness of the Cypher stent determined in the SIRIUS trial. DOM, subgroups for whom sirolimus stenting was economically dominant; TLR, target lesion revascularization. (Redrawn from Cohen DJ, Bakhai A, Shi C, et al, for the SIRIUS Investigators: Cost-effectiveness of sirolimus-eluting stents for treatment of complex coronary stenoses: Results from the Sirolimus-Eluting Balloon Expandable Stent in the Treatment of Patients with De Novo Native Coronary Artery Lesions (SIRIUS) trial. Circulation 2004;110:508-514.)

Cardiac Surgery), COMBAT (Comparison of Bypass Surgery versus Angioplasty Using Sirolimus-Eluting Stent in Patients with Left Main Coronary Artery Disease), and CARDIA (Coronary Artery Revascularisation in Diabetes) (Fig. 15-21) are ongoing.[57] Data from the ARTS I and II (Arterial Revascularization Therapies Study I and II) trials are often cited to support PCI (Fig. 15-22),[58,59] but the number of patients studied and the duration of follow-up are inadequate to draw anything but general conclusions. The adage that the more diffuse the disease, the more the relative advantage of bypass surgery, still appears to be valid.

SUMMARY

The availability of DESs allows the interventionalist to offer the patient therapy with a much lower risk for necessary repeat treatment, albeit with no difference in the risk of death or myocardial infarction and with the need to take protracted antiplatelet therapy to minimize the added risk of stent thrombosis compared with previously available percutaneous therapies. To be truly transformational, DESs must be developed that better suppress clinical restenosis in high-risk patient subsets and that do not increase the

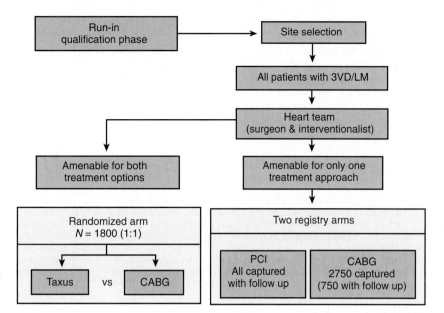

Figure 15-21. The SYNTAX trial configuration for comparing drug-eluting stents with coronary artery bypass grafting (CABG) for high-risk multivessel disease. LM, left main coronary artery. PCI, percutaneous coronary intervention ; 3VD, three-vessel disease. (Courtesy of Boston Scientific.)

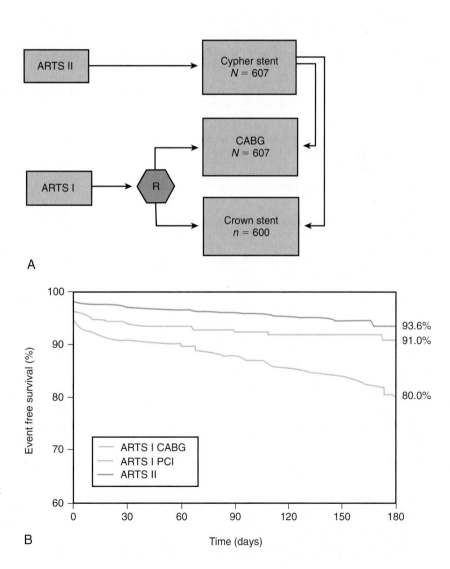

Figure 15-22. A, ARTS I and II study designs for assessing bare metal stents, coronary artery bypass grafting (CABG), drug-eluting stents. **B,** Major adverse cardiac event (MACE)–free survival in ARTS I and II studies. PCI, percutaneous coronary intervention. (Redrawn from Serruys PW, Ong ATL, Morice MC, et al: Arterial Revascularization Therapies Study. Part II. Sirolimus-eluting stents for the treatment of patients with multivessel de novo coronary artery lesions. Eurointervention 2005;2:147-156.)

risk of subsequent thrombotic events. Such devices are already being evaluated, but given the regulatory constraints on approval pathways for drug and device combinations, especially if they involve a new molecular entity, availability in the United States will be unlikely until the next decade. Nonetheless, the interventionalist cardiologists must stay abreast of this rapidly developing field to provide optimal patient care.

REFERENCES

1. George BS, Voorhees WD, Roubin GS, et al: Multicenter investigation of coronary stenting to treat acute or threatened closure after percutaneous transluminal coronary angioplasty: Clinical and angiographic outcomes. J Am Coll Cardiol 1993; 22:135-143.
2. Fischman DL, Leon MB, Baim DS, et al: A randomized comparison of coronary-stent placement and balloon angioplasty in the treatment of coronary artery disease. N Engl J Med 1994; 331:496-501.
3. Serruys PW, de Jaegere P, Kiemeneij F, et al: A comparison of balloon-expandable-stent implantation with balloon angioplasty in patients with coronary artery disease. N Engl J Med 1994;331:489-495.
4. Schwartz RS: Pathophysiology of restenosis: Interaction of thrombosis, hyperplasia, and/or remodeling. Am J Cardiol 1998;81:14E-17E.
5. Koster R, Vieluf D, Kiehn M, et al: Nickel and molybdenum contact allergies in patients with coronary in-stent restenosis. Lancet 2000;356:1895-1897.
6. Kereiakes DJ, Cox DA, Hermiller JB, et al, for the Guidant Multi-Link Vision Stent Registry Investigators: Usefulness of a cobalt chromium coronary stent alloy. Am J Cardiol 2003;92: 463-466.
7. Hwang C, Wu D, Edelman ER: Physiological transport forces govern drug distribution for stent-based delivery. Circulation 2001;104:600-605.
8. Balakrishnan B, Tzafriri AR, Seifert P, et al: Strut position, blood flow, and drug deposition: Implications for single and overlapping drug-eluting stents. Circulation 2005;111: 2958-2965.
9. Tamai H, Igaki K, Kyo E, et al: Initial and 6-month results of biodegradable poly-L-lactic acid coronary stents in humans. Circulation 2000;102:399-404.
10. Vogt F, Stein A, Rettemeier G, et al: Long-term assessment of a novel biodegradable paclitaxel-eluting coronary polylactide stent. Eur Heart J 2004;25:1330-1340.
11. Heublein B, Rohde R, Kaese V, et al: Biocorrosion of magnesium alloys: A new principle in cardiovascular implant technology? Heart 2003;89:651-656.
12. Hwang CE, Wu D, Edelman ER: Physiological transport forces govern drug distribution for stent-based delivery. Circulation 2001;104:600-606.
13. Moses JW, Leon MB, Popma JJ, et al: Sirolimus-eluting stents versus standard stents in patients with stenosis in a native coronary artery. N Engl J Med 2003;349:1315-1323.
14. Stone GW, Ellis SG, Cos DA, et al: A polymer-based, paclitaxel-eluting stent in patients with coronary artery disease. N Engl J Med 2004;350:221-231.
15. Hardhammar PA, van Beusekom HMM, Emanuelsson HU, et al: Reduction in thrombotic events with heparin-coated Palmaz-Schatz stents in normal porcine coronary arteries. Circulation 1996;93:423-430.
16. Moses JW, Buller CEH, Nukta ED: The first clinical trial comparing a coated versus a non-coated coronary stent: The Biocompatibles BiodivYsio Stent in Randomized Controlled Trial. Circulation 2000;102(Suppl II):664.
17. van der Giessen WJ, Lincoff MA, Schwartz RS, et al: Marked inflammatory sequelae to implantation of biodegradable and nonbiodegradable polymers in porcine coronary arteries. Circulation 1996;94:1690-1697.
18. Marx SO, Jayaraman T, Go LO, Marks AR: Rapamycin-FKBP inhibits cell cycle regulators of proliferation in vascular smooth muscle cells. Circ Res 1995;76:412-417.
19. Rowinsky EK, Donehower RC: Paclitaxel (Taxol). N Engl J Med 1995;332:1004-1015.
20. Briguori C, Nishida T, Anzuini A, et al: Emergency polytetrafluoroethylene-covered stent implantation to treat coronary ruptures. Circulation 2000;102:3028-3031.
21. Schofer J, Schluter M, Gershlick AH, et al, for the E-SIRIUS Investigators: Sirolimus-eluting stents for treatment of patients with long atherosclerotic lesions in small coronary arteries: Double-blind, randomized controlled trial (E-SIRIUS). Lancet 2003;362:1093-1099.
22. Colombo A, Hall P, Nakamura S, et al: Intracoronary stenting without anticoagulation accomplished with intravascular ultrasound guidance. Circulation 1995;91:1676-1688.
23. Costa J, Mintz G, Carlier SG, et al: Intravascular ultrasonic assessment of stent diameters derived from manufacturer's compliance charts. Am J Cardiol 2005;96:74-78.
24. Silber S, Hamburger J, Grube E, et al: Direct stenting with Taxus stents seems to be as safe and effective as with predilatation: A post hoc analysis of Taxus II. Herz 2004;29:171-180.
25. Schluter M, Schoefer J, Gershlick AH, et al, for the E- and C-SIRIUS Investigators: Direct stenting of native de novo coronary artery lesions with the sirolimus-eluting stent: A post hoc subanalysis of the pooled E- and C-SIRIUS trials. J Am Coll Cardiol 2005;45:10-13.
26. Stone GW, Ellis SG, Cannon L, et al, for the TAXUS V Investigators: Comparison of a polymer-based paclitaxel-eluting stent with a bare metal stent in patients with complex coronary artery disease. JAMA 2005;294:1215-1223.
27. Kandzari DE: ENDEAVOR III: A prospective, randomized comparison of Zotarolimus-eluting and sirolimus-eluting stents in patients with coronary artery disease. Transcatheter Cardiovascular Therapeutics meeting, 2005, Washington, DC.
28. Mauri L, Orav EJ, Candia SC, et al: Robustness of late lumen loss in discriminating drug-eluting stents across variable observational and randomized trials. Circulation 2005;112: 2833-2839.
29. Ellis SG, Popma JJ, Lasala JM, et al: Relationship between angiographic late loss and target lesion revascularization after coronary stent implantation: Analysis from the TAXUS IV trial. J Am Coll Cardiol 2005;45:1193-1200.
30. Leon MB: Synthesizing the evidence-based medicine DES clinical data: What every practicing interventionalist should know. Available at http://www.tctmd.com/csportal/appmanager/tctmd/main?nfpb=true@pageLabel=TCTMD Content&hdCon=1340410
31. Ellis SG, Colombo A, Grube E, et al: Stent thrombosis with the polymeric paclitaxel drug-eluting stent-incidence, timing and correlates—a TAXUS II, IV, V, and VI meta-analysis of 3445 patients followed up to three years. J Am Coll Cardiol 2007;49:1043-1051.
32. Windecker S, Remondino A, Eberli FR, et al: Sirolimus-eluting and paclitaxel-eluting stents for coronary revascularization. N Engl J Med 2005;353:653-663.
33. Lemos PA, Serruys PW, van Domburg RT, et al: Unrestricted utilization of sirolimus-eluting stents compared with conventional bare stent implantation in the "real world": The Rapamycin-Eluting Stent Evaluated At Rotterdam Cardiology Hospital (RESEARCH) Registry. Circulation 2004;109: 190-195.
34. Cosgrave J, Agostoni P, Ge L, et al: Clinical outcome following aleatory implantation of paclitaxel-eluting or sirolimus-eluting stents in complex coronary lesions. Am J Cardiol 2005;96: 1663-1668.
35. Simonton C, Brodie B, Cheek B, et al: Clinical outcomes of drug-eluting stents in the first year since US approval: Results from the Strategic Transcatheter Evaluation of New Therapies (STENT) group. Am J Cardiol 2004;94(Suppl 6A):207S.
36. Moreno R, Fernandez C, Hernandez R, et al: Drug-eluting stent thrombosis. J Am Coll Cardiol 2005;45:954-960.
37. Iakovou I, Schmidt T, Boizzoni E, et al: Incidence, predictors, and outcome of thrombosis after successful implantation of drug-eluting stents. JAMA 2005;293:2126-2130.

38. Fuji K, Carlier SG, Mintz GS, et al: Stent underexpansion and residual reference segment stenosis are related to stent thrombosis after sirolimus-eluting stent implantation: an intravascular ultrasound study. J Am Coll Cardiol 2005;45: 995-998.

39. Hoffman S, Klamroth R, Landgraf H, et al: Clopidogrel resistance, ASA resistance and coronary stent thrombosis: A causal relation? J Am Coll Cardiol 2005;45:87A.

40. Wenaweser P, Hess O: Stent thrombosis is associated with an impaired response to antiplatelet therapy. J Am Coll Cardiol 2005;45:1748-1752.

41. Ong AT, McFadden EP, Regar E, et al: Late angiographic stent thrombosis (LAST) events with drug-eluting stents. J Am Coll Cardiol 2005;45:2088-2093.

42. Leon MB, Baim DS, Popma JJ, et al: A Clinical trial comparing three antithrombotic-drug regimens after coronary-artery stenting. N Engl J Med 1998;339:1665-1671.

43. Lincoff AM, Bittl JA, Harrington RA, et al, for the REPLACE-2 Investigators: Bivalirudin and provision glycoprotein IIb/IIIa blockade compared with heparin and planned glycoprotein IIb/IIIa blockade during percutaneous coronary intervention. REPLACE-2 randomized trial. JAMA 2003;289:853-863.

44. Kastrati A, Mehilli J, Neumann FJ, et al, for the Intracoronary Stenting and Antithrombotic Regimen: Rapid Early Action for Coronary Treatment 2 (ISAR-REACT 2) Trial Investigators: Abciximab in patients with acute coronary syndromes undergoing percutaneous coronary intervention after clopidogrel pretreatment: the ISAR-REACT 2 randomized trial. JAMA 2006;295:1531-1538.

45. Keeley EC, Boura JA, Grines CL: Comparison of primary and facilitated percutaneous coronary interventions for ST-elevation myocardial infarction: Quantitative review of randomised trials. Lancet 2006;367:579-588.

46. Mehta SR, Cannon CP, Fox KA, et al: Routine vs. selective invasive strategies in patients with acute coronary syndromes: A collaborative meta-analysis of randomized trials. JAMA 2005;293:2908-2917.

47. Serruys PW, Unger F, Sousa JE, et al: Comparison of coronary-artery bypass surgery and stenting for the treatment of multivessel disease. N Engl J Med 2001;344:1117-1125.

48. SOS Investigators: Coronary artery bypass surgery versus percutaneous coronary intervention with stent implantation in patients with multivessel coronary artery disease (the Stent or Surgery trial): A randomized controlled trial. Lancet 2002;360: 965-970.

49. Alderman EL, Bourassa MG, Cohen LS: Ten-year follow-up of survival and myocardial infarction in the randomized Coronary Artery Surgery Study. Circulation 1990;82:1629-1646.

50. Davies RF, Goldberg D, Forman S, et al: Asymptomatic Cardiac Ischemia Pilot (ACIP) study two-year follow-up. Circulation 1997; 95:2037-2048.

51. Seshadri N, Whitlow PL, Acharya N, et al: Emergency coronary artery bypass surgery in the contemporary percutaneous coronary intervention era. Circulation 2002;106:2346-2350.

52. Krone RJ, Shaw RE, Klein LW, et al: Evaluation of the American College of Cardiology/American Heart Association and the Society of Coronary Angiography and Interventions lesion classification system in the current "stent era" of coronary interventions (from the ACC-National Cardiovascular Data Registry). Am J Cardiol 2003;92:389-394.

53. Singh M, Lennon RJ, Holmes DR, et al: Correlates of procedural complications and a simple integer risk score for percutaneous coronary intervention. J Am Coll Cardiol 2002;40: 387-393.

54. Kastrati A, Schoming A, Elezi S: Predictive factors of restenosis after coronary stent placement. J Am Coll Cardiol 1997;30:1428-1436.

55. Ellis SG, Bajzer CT, Bhatt DL, et al: Real-world bare metal stenting: Identification of patients at low and very low risk of 9-month coronary revascularization. Catheter Cardiovasc Interv 2004;63,135-140.

56. Cohen DJ, Bakhai A, Shi C, et al, for the SIRIUS Investigators: Cost-effectiveness of sirolimus-eluting stents for treatment of complex coronary stenoses: Results from the Sirolimus-Eluting Balloon Expandable Stent in the Treatment of Patients with De Novo Native Coronary Artery Lesions (SIRIUS) trial. Circulation 2004;110:508-514.

57. Serruys PW: SYNTAX: Taxus versus CABG in multivessel and left main disease. Available at http://www.tctmd.com/csportal/appmanager/tctmd/main?_nfpb=true&_pageLabel=TCTMDContent&hd Con=1418038

58. Legrand VM, Serruys PW, Unger F, et al, for the Arterial Revascularization Therapy Study (ARTS) Investigators: Three-year outcome after coronary stenting versus bypass surgery for the treatment of multivessel disease. Circulation 2004;109: 1114-1120.

59. Serruys PW, Ong ATL, Morice MC, et al: Arterial Revascularization Therapies Study. Part II. Sirolimus-eluting stents for the treatment of patients with multivessel de novo coronary artery lesions. Eurointervention 2005;2:147-156.

16 Balloon Angioplasty: Is It Still a Viable Intervention?

Jorge R. Alegria and David R. Holmes, Jr.

We shall not cease from exploration and the end of all our exploring will be to arrive where we started and know the place for the first time.

—*T.S. Elliot, Four Quartets*

KEY POINTS

- Percutaneous transluminal coronary angioplasty (PTCA) alone is an option in selected cases.
- Indications for single PTCA include failure to cross the lesion with a stent; treatment of a culprit lesion in an acute coronary syndrome in the setting of coronary anatomy amenable to surgical treatment only, particu-

larly in high-risk patients when complete percutaneous revascularization is not feasible; stenosis at the site of a bypass graft to the native vessel; when prolonged antiplatelet therapy is not feasible or contraindicated; appropriate side branch of a bifurcation lesion; and hypersensitivity to metals used in stents.

Percutaneous transluminal coronary angioplasty (PTCA) was conceived, developed, and refined with the goals of alleviating symptoms, averting cardiomyocyte injury, and restoring epicardial blood flow impaired by acute or chronic effects of coronary atherosclerosis, with the ultimate aim of reducing morbidity and mortality. This tremendous achievement was the result of the application of hydraulic principles to the treatment of coronary artery disease thanks to the creativity and courage of visionary individuals such as Andreas Gruentzig (Fig. 16-1) and technologic advances in the late 1970s and later. The result was treatment of a coronary artery lesion with a balloon that is inflated intraluminally to produce barotrauma that expands the intracoronary lumen, and the new specialty of interventional cardiology revolutionized the way we approach and treat patients with coronary artery disease.

Along with early enthusiasm about PTCA, challenges were identified: coronary artery dissection, abrupt closure, and restenosis. The response to these problems was an enormous and protracted effort of basic, translational, and clinical sciences that produced the contemporary era of drug-eluting stents, when "simple" PTCA appears to have vanished. In the past, treatment with plain PTCA of a tortuous middle left anterior descending coronary artery (LAD)

lesion was a daunting task. Today, the same lesion is comfortably treated with a drug-eluting stent.

A major challenge in an evidence-based interventional cardiology practice, when stenting is the dominant approach, is deciding when to perform PTCA alone. In which patients, in which clinical context, and how should it be done? This chapter provides a synopsis of PTCA and describes the selected cases in which PTCA is a viable intervention. We think that PTCA should continue to be studied and refined; otherwise, we will never know whether we fully perfected the tool that Andreas Gruentzig gave us.

HISTORICAL BACKGROUND

The treatment of coronary artery disease has greatly changed during the past decades. Selective coronary angiography, the procedure necessary to appraise and understand the pathophysiology of coronary artery disease, was developed in 1958 by Mason Sones. While performing an aortogram, he noticed that the catheter engaged the right coronary artery and opacified the lumen.[1] This serendipitous incident prompted the development of the invasive diagnosis and treatment of coronary artery disease, bestowing a device to bring about coronary artery

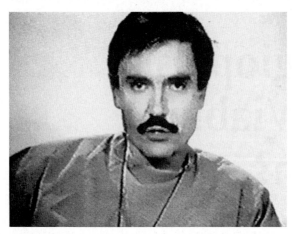

Figure 16-1. Andreas Gruentzig, circa 1978, in Zurich. (Courtesy of A. Gruentzig.)

bypass surgery, thrombolytic therapies, and percutaneous coronary interventions.

The next step occurred in 1964 when Charles Dotter, while performing a vascular diagnostic procedure, noticed the increase in luminal diameter of an iliac occlusion after the passage of the diagnostic catheter through the lesion. Using this observation, Dotter and Judkins successfully developed transluminal angioplasty in the peripheral circulation.[2]

These two groundbreaking events paved the way for the development of PTCA by Andreas Gruentzig, who revolutionized the treatment of coronary artery disease. Gruentzig modified the caged latex balloon catheter previously developed by Porstmann,[3] creating a double-lumen catheter with a distal end having a low-compliance polyvinylchloride (PVC) balloon that he used initially in the peripheral circulation. He first tested in dogs the concept that coronary arteries could be dilated with a diminutive form of the double-lumen catheter balloon. Subsequent tests were performed in human cadavers, followed by performing PTCA in patients undergoing saphenous vein bypass grafting, proving that coronary artery stenosis could be dilated in humans. On September 16, 1977, the first PTCA was performed. A 38-year-old man who had a symptomatic, high-grade stenosis of the proximal LAD underwent successful balloon dilatation, resulting in long-lasting relief of angina and avoidance of single-vessel bypass surgery.[4] Twenty-three years later, the proximal segment of the LAD treated by Gruentzig in that patient revealed no evidence of stenosis (Fig. 16-2),[5] demonstrating the long-lasting beneficial effects of successful PTCA, even when performed with rudimentary equipment.

In 1979, the National Heart, Lung, and Blood Institute (NHLBI) created a registry that ultimately included data from many places worldwide. This registry was fundamental for the widespread appreciation of PTCA as a viable and safe option for patients with coronary artery disease.

During subsequent years, there was a significant improvement in the technique and its results. For example, in the beginning, 65% to 70% of PTCAs were successful, and by 1982, success rates increased to between 80% and 85%, prompted by increased experience with the procedure and the refinement of angioplasty hardware. The large guiding catheters (9 to 10 Fr) were made of solid Teflon and were very challenging to use. Later, a three-layer catheter was developed. The inner surface was composed of Teflon, the middle portion was a woven mesh for torque control, and the outer layer was made of polyurethane for memory. The initial catheter did not allow the use of a wire. It had a double-lumen design, with one lumen used for perfusion and pressure measurements and the second lumen used for the balloon. Simpson and colleagues[6] developed a movable, flexible-tipped guidewire within the balloon dilation catheter that facilitated navigation in the coronary arteries and allowed easier access to complex lesions.

Long-term follow-up of the initial Zurich experience of Gruentzig in treating 133 patients with initially successful PTCA demonstrated a cardiac survival rate of 96% at 6 years and enduring improvement in symptoms in 67% of the patients. The 10-year follow-up of the early Zurich series revealed an overall survival rate of 90% and a survival rate of 95% for patients with single-vessel disease.[7,8]

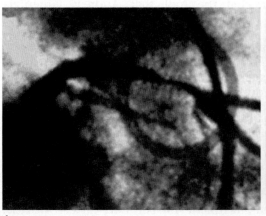

A

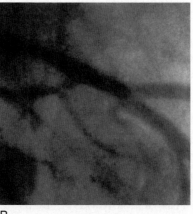

B

Figure 16-2. A, First percutaneous transluminal coronary angioplasty. **B,** The 23-year follow-up angiogram. (From Meier B: The first patient to undergo coronary angioplasty—23-year follow-up. N Engl J Med 2001;344:144-145.)

Initially, the procedure was employed in symptomatic low-risk patients with inducible ischemia and with proximal, nonbifurcated, noncalcified lesions and a normal left ventricular ejection fraction. Later, the NHLBI Registry provided relevant information regarding the evolution of patient selection and outcomes. When the first registry of PTCA for the period between 1977 and 1981 was compared with the registry for the period between 1985 and 1986,[9] the in-hospital mortality rate (1%) and the rate of nonfatal myocardial infarction (MI) (4.3%) were found to be similar, despite a higher-risk population of patients with older age, more multivessel disease, worse left ventricular function, and more frequent history of a previous MI and previous coronary artery bypass grafting.[10]

Two fundamental changes were developed in the technique. Prolonged balloon inflations were used because of the availability of perfusion balloon catheters that decreased coronary artery dissection and acute closure.[11] The use of the monorail catheters and easily extendable guidewires permitted quick and easy withdrawal of the balloon catheter to allow better contrast delivery for angiography, and there was no need to evaluate transstenotic gradients as previously done.

A critical issue to address before the procedure is the use of aspirin. It became clear that pretreatment with aspirin diminished the risk of coronary occlusion at the time of PTCA and afterward.[12]

MECHANISMS

Although the mechanisms of PTCA are not fully defined, they appear to include a complex interplay between physical and biologic factors, such as the balloon behavior (i.e., dilatation), the vessel wall (i.e., plaque characteristics), and the extent of and host response to injury.

The basic physical principles of PTCA are an extension of Laplace's law and were elegantly described by Abele in 1980.[13] Inflation of the balloon creates a "dilating force" that determines the "hoop stress." This dilating force is the consequence of balloon size (i.e., diameter and length) and pressures (Fig. 16-3). The rate and time of total inflation also influence the end result.

The goal of the dilating force created by the balloon in the coronary artery is to create an enduring and healthy larger vessel lumen, thereby augmenting epicardial coronary blood flow. Plain PTCA can achieve this when the balloon is properly inflated, increasing the hydraulic pressure applied to the vessel wall and injuring the artery through a contained barotrauma that produces intimal damage, with fissuring or disruption of the plaque (generally most marked at the plaque shoulder, where an eccentric plaque meets the disease-free wall), partial dehiscence of the intimal plaque from its underlying media, occasional intramedial dissection, stretching of the media and adventitia, and aneurysmal dilatation of the vessel.[14,15]

Plaque fissuring, medial and adventitial stretching, and separation of the atheroma from the underlying media account for an increase in luminal size, intraluminal haziness, and intimal flap or dissection, as identified by angiography or intravascular ultrasound (IVUS).[16,17] These morphologic changes result in irregularly shaped microchannels for blood flow, leading to increased coronary perfusion and to the imaging appearances described previously. Nevertheless, PTCA has the potential to induce severe and life-threatening acute coronary vessel obstruction due to dissection (Fig. 16-4), intraplaque hemorrhage, and luminal thrombosis (Fig. 16-5).

Certain characteristics of the plaque, particularly calcification and eccentricity, can influence the final degree of luminal gain.[17] For instance, when coronary artery rupture occurs in eccentric and heavily calcified lesions, the site of rupture is at the weakest place: the plaque shoulder (Fig. 16-6).[18] The final luminal size results from a complex interplay among distortion of the atherosclerotic plaque or thrombus, disruption of the plaque, expansion of all layers of the vessel, and the local thrombotic and inflammatory responses to the mechanical injury.

Waller and colleagues[19-21] reported their observations in autopsy specimens obtained between 4 hours and 30 days after PTCA. In each specimen, there was

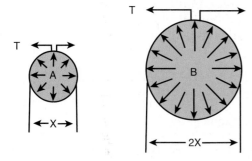

Figure 16-3. Hoop stress (T) is twice as great at an equal pressure in the larger balloon.

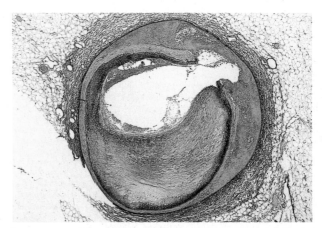

Figure 16-4. Percutaneous transluminal coronary angioplasty with small dissection (Verhoeff-Van Gieson [VVG] stain). (Courtesy W. D. Edwards, MD, Mayo Clinic, Rochester, MN.)

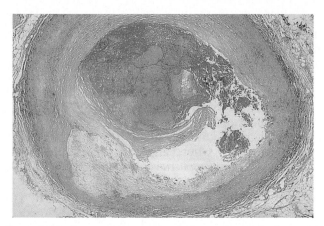

Figure 16-5. Percutaneous transluminal coronary angioplasty with acute thrombosis (hematoxylin and eosin stain). (Courtesy W. D. Edwards, MD, Mayo Clinic, Rochester, MN.)

an intimal crack, tear, fracture, or break associated with various degrees of medial penetration, ranging from localized medial involvement to extensive dissection. No adventitial compromise was observed.

The degree of eccentricity also influences how luminal gain is achieved. For eccentric plaques, luminal enlargement results from stretching the thinner, disease-free portion of the arterial wall.[22] Plaque rupture most commonly occurs at the junction between the plaque and the disease-free portion (see Fig. 16-4).[23] In contrast, soft, concentric plaques may be stretched circumferentially, and firm, fibrocalcific concentric plaques may resist any dilatation.

The mechanisms of PTCA classified by Waller[22] included plaque compression, plaque fracture, plaque fracture with intimal flaps and localized medial dissection, stretching of the disease-free segment, and stretching with compression:

1. *Plaque compression.* Initially, it was hypothesized that the balloon compressed the plaque against the vessel wall to produce a larger lumen. This mechanism only partially explains the results of balloon angioplasty because it assumes that exclusively soft plaque is present, although many atherosclerotic plaques have prominent fibrous components and various amounts of calcium. Although plaque compression may represent an important mechanism in experimental animal models, its effect in humans is overshadowed by intrinsic plaque characteristics.[22]

2. *Plaque fracture.* Likely a major mechanism in humans for sustained luminal expansion after successful PTCA, plaque fracture has been supported by experimental animal models[14,24] and human postmortem studies.[16,25-28] Numerous other terms have been used to describe plaque fracture, such as *splitting, breaking, cracking,* or *fracturing.* Plaque fracture creates multiple new channels by splitting the plaque and producing dissection clefts or breaks of various lengths within the plaque and by partially detaching the intimal plaque from the subjacent media.

3. *Plaque fracture, intimal atherosclerotic flaps, and localized medial dissection.* With this mechanism, significant and persistent luminal cross-sectional area expansion generally requires deep intimal fractures and localized medial dissection.[22]

4. *Stretching of the plaque-free wall segment.* In eccentric lesions, there is a potential for stretching the segments free of atherosclerotic plaque.[29,30] Because of the physical properties of the vessel wall, the balloon overstretches the thinner normal vessel wall segment with no or minimal injury to the thicker atherosclerotic plaque, thereby augmenting the luminal diameter. Weeks later, an appreciable decrease in the lumen may occur because of medial recoil and produce apparent restenosis.[30] This is likely a common occurrence because of the high frequency of eccentric lesions in severe coronary artery disease.[31]

5. *Stretching and minimal or mild compression.* In this situation, an oversized balloon may stretch the entire coronary segment that is concentrically narrowed by a fibrous or fibrocalcific plaque. However, even if the media is ruptured transmurally, the adventitia will often buttress the vessel and prevent the development of a large, epicardial hematoma or a hemopericardium.

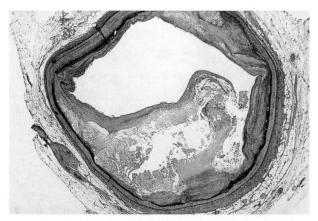

Figure 16-6. Percutaneous transluminal coronary angioplasty with a fracture of the plaque shoulder (VVG stain). (Courtesy W. D. Edwards, MD, Mayo Clinic, Rochester, MN.)

PERCUTANEOUS TRANSLUMINAL CORONARY ANGIOPLASTY

The Technique

Percutaneous transluminal coronary angioplasty is performed in the cardiac catheterization laboratory by an operator with the aim of a potential benefit for a patient who has clinical indications for the procedure. A balloon-tipped catheter is advanced to an area of coronary artery stenosis, the balloon is inflated, and the balloon is then deflated and the catheter removed. The patient must be pretreated with aspirin, and the procedure is performed in serial, logical steps to minimize risks and anticipate complications, demanding focused attention by the operator and the whole team.

It was necessary to gain a significant amount of knowledge about the balloon catheters, size of the original syringes, and pressures to ensure that the dilating force applied to the vessel was the correct amount.[13] In the beginning, the balloon catheters were large, not steerable, and inflexible, limited to accessing the coronaries, but these barriers were overcome in the mid-1980s with a diversification of the balloon angioplasty catheters.

Three types of guidewire interactions were developed. The earlier work was done with an on-the-wire (fixed wire) system,[32,33] which was limited by an inability to exchange balloons and by difficulty navigating the coronary artery. The over-the-wire system developed by Simpson and colleagues[6] in 1982 consisted of a guidewire passed through the balloon catheter lumen and independently guided down through the lesion. This system had good steerability, with the advantage that the balloon could be removed, but it was limited by needing an extension wire. Later, the monorail system[34] consisted of a short segment of catheter that slides over the guidewire, allowing introduction of the balloon after the lesion has been crossed without the need of an extension wire.

Another relevant aspect of PTCA is balloon compliance. The earlier balloons used by Gruentzig were made of PVC and were compliant. Subsequent balloons were compliant or noncompliant.

Longer balloons were developed to intervene in diffuse disease, serial lesions, lesions on a bend, or "tacking-up" dissections. The balloon to be delivered needs several favorable characteristics, including an appropriate profile, trackability, pushability, and lubricity. With experience, problems with the balloons, such as rupture, poor inflation or deflation, breakage, entrapment, or entanglement, became evident.

Because of expanded use of PTCA in higher-risk patients, such as those with multivessel disease, low ejection fraction, hypotension, or cardiogenic shock, the use of the intra-aortic balloon pump emerged as an important adjunctive device.[35]

Guiding Catheters

The guide catheter used for PTCA significantly differs from the diagnostic catheter. To perform PTCA, the guiding catheter should be larger and have lubrication, allowing smooth passage of the balloon catheter. The guide catheter also provides the platform to deliver a balloon in tortuous and often calcified coronary arteries.

Former guiding catheters were large (9.4 Fr) because the balloons were larger than their modern counterparts. Initially, the balloon catheters were made of polytetrafluoroethylene (Teflon, DuPont Co., Wilmington, DE) and were characterized by increased stiffness.[36] Significant improvements in the performance of guiding catheters have been possible with the use of stainless steel braiding that was implanted in the material of the shaft, improving torque control, and very thin Teflon liners were added to the internal lumen of the guiding catheter, enhancing lubricity.

Radiopaque soft catheter tips have reduced injury to the coronary ostium, allowing more manipulation of the guide catheter. Guide catheters provide outstanding backup for balloon transit.

Guide catheter selection is important. When faced with complex lesions and heavily calcified and tortuous vessels, the support that a guide catheter is able to provide can make the difference between a success and failure. If only balloon angioplasty is performed, the need for guide support is less compared with that required for stent implantation.

CLINICAL TRIALS OF PERCUTANEOUS TRANSLUMINAL CORONARY ANGIOPLASTY IN CORONARY ARTERY DISEASE

Overall, the objectives of coronary revascularization are the treatment of symptoms (e.g., angina), improvement in long-term survival, and prevention of nonfatal events (e.g., acute coronary syndromes, heart failure, arrhythmias). Although the risks of serious complications are small, careful patient selection must be undertaken before proceeding with PTCA. For instance, in the multicenter NHLBI Registry of PTCA experience from 1985 to 1986 of intervention in patients with single-vessel disease, the incidences of procedure-related death, nonfatal MI, and coronary artery bypass grafting (CABG) were 0.2%, 3.5%, and 2.9% respectively.[9]

Initially, clinical and angiographic criteria for candidates for PTCA were very restrictive. Patients had to have significant angina and considerable evidence of myocardial ischemia, and be suitable candidates for coronary artery bypass surgery, with preserved left ventricular function; single-vessel disease; and discrete, noncalcified, proximal stenosis. With these criteria in the Coronary Artery Surgery Study (CASS), only 3.7% of patients were eligible for PTCA.[37]

The original indication for PTCA was for chronic stable angina due to single-vessel disease with preserved ventricular function,[38] producing high success rates (>90%) for the treatment of simple lesions.[9] This indication evolved, and the use of PTCA expanded to many patients with coronary artery disease; initially, it was applied empirically, but later randomized trials confirmed its efficacy in stable coronary artery disease.[39] The ultimate success of PTCA is determined by patient characteristics, lesion characteristics, technique and devices, and the physicians' experience, underscoring the idea that PTCA is in some ways an art to be mastered.

Lesion features such as number, severity, length, calcification, eccentricity, ostial involvement, and presence or absence of thrombus can increase the potential for immediate and delayed complications. Other relevant factors are vessel tortuosity, collateral supply, and degree of ventricular dysfunction. Chronic coronary occlusion unfavorably influences the chances of success with PTCA. For instance, if the occlusion has been present for more than 3 months, the success rate is only 50%; however, if it is of recent onset (<3 months) and short, the chance of successful PTCA is approximately 70%.[40-42]

For single-vessel disease, the success rates have been good. In the 1985-1986 NHLBI Registry of a total of 1802 patients without acute MI, single-vessel disease was present in 839 subjects, and the success rate of PTCA was 89% (with success defined as at least a 20% reduction of the narrowing of the vessel diameter).[9] Among patients with single-vessel disease, 84% had clinical success, and all lesions were dilated without in-hospital death, infarction, or need of emergency bypass surgery. These data demonstrated significant progress compared with the PTCA Registry population of 1977 to 1981.

The Angioplasty Compared to Medicine (ACME)[43] study randomly compared PTCA with medical therapy in 212 patients with stable angina coronary, single-vessel disease, a positive exercise test result or MI within the prior 3 months, and evidence of 70% to 99% stenosis of a proximal vessel. Subjects with multivessel disease, women, and patients with decreased left ventricular function were excluded. There was a higher rate of complications in the PTCA-treated group (including emergency bypass surgery), and the PTCA arm had a higher cost but a greater decrease in angina burden, with decreased use of antianginal medications and improvement in exercise tolerance. The rate of repeat PTCA was similar in both groups, but CABG surgery was performed in seven patients from the PTCA group and none in the medically treated subjects. There was no difference in death or rate of MI in both groups. These data suggested that an initial medical approach to single-vessel coronary artery disease was probably better and that the use of PTCA and restenosis created the need for more procedures. Patients were treated with some combination of aspirin, nitroglycerin, β-blockers, and calcium channel blockers, with no use of contemporary therapies such as statins or angiotensin-converting enzyme (ACE) inhibitors.

Another prospective study assessed patients with proximal LAD stenosis, demonstrable ischemia, and preserved ventricular function with an initial approach of PTCA or CABG.[44] Within a 2.5-year follow-up period, 86% of the CABG-treated patients and 43% of the patients treated with PTCA did not have adverse events (P < .01; RR = 2.0; 95% CI: 1.7 to 2.3). The single adverse event that explained this difference was restenosis in the PTCA group.

The subsequent ACME -2 trial[45] tested angioplasty versus medical therapy in 101 men with stable, symptomatic, two-vessel coronary artery disease, evidence of ischemia on nuclear treadmill testing, and a left ventricular ejection fraction greater than 30%. At 6 months of follow-up, both groups had comparable improvement in exercise duration, freedom from angina, and quality of life. There was no evidence of increased hazard with the conservative approach, but because of the small number of subjects, the study was underpowered to detect small differences in outcomes for both strategies.

The Argentine Randomized Trial of Percutaneous Transluminal Coronary Angioplasty versus Coronary Artery Bypass Surgery in Multivessel Disease (ERACI) trial[46] was a single-center trial that randomized 127 patients to PTCA or CABG between 1988 and 1990. Fifty-five percent of patients had double-vessel coronary disease, and 45% had triple-vessel disease. Complete revascularization was accomplished in 51% of PTCA and 88% of CABG patients (P < .001). PTCA and CABG patients did not have different rates of death or nonfatal MI for up to 3 years. Patients in the CABG group were more likely to have event-free survival at 1 year (84% versus 64%; P < .005) due to differences in the occurrence of angina and the need for further revascularization (32% after PTCA, 3% after CABG; P < .001).

The Emory Angioplasty versus Surgery Trial (EAST)[47] was a single-center trial that randomized 392 patients to PTCA or CABG. Sixty percent of patients had double-vessel coronary disease, and the remainder had triple-vessel disease; almost three fourths of patients had involvement of the proximal LAD. In the PTCA group, 88% of targeted lesions were treated successfully. An internal mammary artery graft was used in 90% of CABG patients. The primary end point was the composite of death, Q-wave MI, and a large ischemic thallium defect at 3 years. There was no difference between treatment strategies in the primary end point (27.3% for PTCA versus 26.8% for CABG). The 3-year mortality rate was 7.1% after PTCA and 6.2% after CABG. More than one half of the PTCA group required additional revascularization procedures in 3 years, compared with 13% in the surgical group. Quality-of-life assessments, including overall health, continued employment, and economic status, were similar for the two treatment strategies. All patients who survived to 3 years' follow-up were contacted by telephone after 8 years, and the medical records of nonsurvivors were examined. No difference was observed in late mortality between the two groups (79.3% after PTCA versus 82.7% after CABG, P = .40), although a trend toward better survival was observed in the CABG-treated patients who had diabetes mellitus or proximal LAD disease. No additional difference in revascularization rates after 3 years was seen in these two patient groups.

In the randomized German Angioplasty Bypass Surgery Investigation (GABI) trial,[48] plain angioplasty was compared with CABG in 359 symptomatic patients with multivessel disease. Patients had at least two territories that were clinically and technically possible to intervene in. At 1-year follow-up for

CABG and PTCA demonstrated similar improvements in symptoms (74% versus 71%, respectively). The need of interventions (PTCA or CABG, or both) was greater in the PTCA arm compared with CABG (44% versus 6%, $P < .001$). The follow-up at 13 years showed that both approaches produced similar long-term survival and symptomatic improvement.[49]

The Coronary Angioplasty versus Bypass Revascularization Investigation (CABRI) trial[50] was a multicenter study that randomized 1154 patients to PCI or CABG. Double-vessel disease was present in almost 57% of patients and triple-vessel disease in 42%. This study allowed the use of atherectomy devices and coronary stents. The primary end point of the trial was the combination of death, nonfatal MI, symptom status, and functional capacity. One-year follow-up in the CABRI trial showed no difference in death or nonfatal MI among treatments. PTCA-treated subjects demonstrated a tendency toward more angina and repeat revascularization.

In the landmark Bypass Angioplasty Revascularization Investigation (BARI) trial,[51] subjects with multivessel disease were randomly assigned to an initial treatment strategy of CABG ($n = 914$) or PTCA ($n = 915$), with a mean follow-up of 5.4 years. The 5-year survival rate was 89.3% for CABG patients and 86.3% for PTCA patients ($P = .19$). The in-hospital event rates for CABG and PTCA were 1.3% and 1.1 %, 4.6% and 2.1% for mortality for Q-wave MI ($P < .01$), and 0.8% and 0.2% for stroke, respectively. The 5-year survival rates free from Q-wave MI were 80.4 % and 78%, respectively. At 5 years, 8% of the patients assigned to CABG had undergone additional revascularization procedures compared with 54% of those assigned to PTCA; 69% of those assigned to PTCA did not subsequently undergo CABG. A key observation was that diabetics, who were treated with insulin or oral hypoglycemic agents at baseline, had a 5-year survival rate of 80.6% when treated with CABG, compared with a significantly lower survival rate of 65% for the PTCA group ($P = .003$).

The Medicine, Angioplasty, or Surgery Study (MASS) trial[52] assessed 214 patients with stable angina, normal ventricular function, and high-grade proximal LAD lesions. The subjects were randomized to internal mammary bypass surgery, plain balloon angioplasty, or medical treatment. The primary end point was the combined occurrence of death, MI, and refractory angina requiring revascularization. At the 3-year follow-up, a primary end point had occurred in 3% of CABG patients, 24% of angioplasty patients, and 17% of patients treated medically (by log-rank testing: $P = .0002$ for PTCA versus CABG; $P = .006$ for CABG versus medical therapy; $P = .28$ for PTCA versus medical therapy). Significantly fewer surgical patients reached an end point than PTCA-treated or medically treated patients, and no difference was observed between the medical and PTCA strategies. Differences between treatment strategies were related primarily to the need for subsequent revascularization, and no differences in mortality or infarction rates were seen between groups. Both revascularization techniques

resulted in greater symptomatic relief and decreased exercise-induced ischemia compared with medical therapy alone. At 5 years' follow-up, bypass surgery persisted as offering the best relief of symptoms and freedom from further procedures; angioplasty was superior to medical therapies in relieving angina, and there was no difference between treatments with respect to MI or death. Result of this trial suggested that medical therapy and revascularization (with PTCA or CABG) are equivalent with regard to the end points of death and MI in patients with stable angina and isolated proximal LAD disease. Angina relief was greater with revascularization, and CABG provided superior angina relief and greater freedom from additional procedures (particularly the need for subsequent CABG) than PTCA.

The Randomized Intervention Treatment of Angina (RITA) trial[53] was a large, multicenter study that included stable and unstable angina patients; 58% had Canadian class III or IV angina. Those randomized to PCI were treated with PTCA only. Forty-five percent of randomized patients had single-vessel disease, 43% had double-vessel disease, and 12% had triple-vessel disease. Patients who had previous revascularization with PTCA or CABG or who required urgent revascularization were excluded. The primary end point was the composite of death and nonfatal MI at 5 years. Despite the declared intent of equivalent treatment, achievement of complete revascularization was better in the CABG arm. An internal mammary graft was placed in 76% of CABG patients. At 2.5 years, there were no major differences observed in mortality or MI among patients in the two treatment strategies (8.6% for CABG and 9.8% for PTCA). Rates of death and MI remained comparable for an average of 6.5 years of follow-up.

The RITA-2 trial[54] included a total of 1018 subjects who were randomized to PTCA or medical management, with a mean follow-up of 2.7 years. Patients with single-vessel or multivessel disease, unstable angina, and left ventricular dysfunction were included, but most had stable angina, normal left ventricular function, and single-vessel disease. The primary end point, a composite of all-cause death and nonfatal MI, occurred in 6.3% of patients treated with PTCA and 3.3% of patients medically treated ($P = .02$). This difference was driven by one death and seven nonfatal infarctions related to PTCA. Forty patients (7.9%) in the PTCA group required CABG, including seven for failed PTCA; an additional 11% of patients required further PTCA. In the medical therapy group, 23% required revascularization during follow-up. Angina and total exercise time improved with both strategies, but more so with PTCA. Advantageous effects of PTCA on angina and exercise time at 6 months were limited to patients with grade 2 or worse angina or a baseline exercise time of 9 minutes or less.

The early experience with PTCA in the treatment of patients with acute MI demonstrated that compared with thrombolytic therapy, immediate PTCA reduced the rates of nonfatal reinfarction, was associated with lower serious bleeding, and resulted in at least similar or better left ventricular function, a higher rate of patency of the infarct-related artery, less severe residual stenotic lesion, and less recurrent myocardial ischemia and infarction than thrombolytic therapy.[55,56] When infarct size was assessed by technetium 99m sestamibi scintigraphy, immediate angioplasty did not appear to produce greater myocardial salvage compared with thrombolysis.[57] By early and effective mechanical restoration of epicardial flow, PTCA revolutionized the way acute coronary syndromes were treated.

INDICATIONS FOR PLAIN PERCUTANEOUS TRANSLUMINAL CORONARY ANGIOPLASTY

With the advent of bare metal stents and drug-eluting stents, there was an important decrease in restenosis, and the number of plain PTCA procedures decreased substantially. We believe that there are still indications for PTCA in carefully selected lesions and patients.

Bifurcation Lesions

The bifurcation lesion is particularly challenging because of unpredictable results. The plaque composition (i.e., soft or fibrous) of both branches and the interaction during intervention are critical elements that influence the end result, along with the recognized limitations of coronary angiography to fully characterize the lesions. Each lesion is unique, and the decision to perform PTCA alone, stent the main branch with PTCA of the side branch, or only stent both branches should be based on the anatomic and functional features of the side branch plus the supplied territory, angulation, and amount of disease. Side branches longer than 2.5 mm usually are treated with stenting.

Available data demonstrate that PTCA alone is suboptimal for the treatment of bifurcation lesions. PTCA alone produces high rates of suboptimal angiographic results and higher restenosis rates.

The role of PTCA in bifurcations is mainly in side branches with good anatomic characteristics (e.g., no significant angulation, not calcified), and the exact criteria for single PTCA of a side branch as a first approach remain to be determined. Adjunctive imaging such as coronary computed tomography or magnetic resonance imaging may guide these decisions. Stenting a bifurcation lesion can be performed with success, but there is no advantage to stenting both branches compared with stenting one branch and performing PTCA in the other one.[58]

Small-Vessel Disease

Historically, PCI in small coronary vessels has been a challenging task, with a rate of acute or chronic complications inversely proportional to vessel size. Smaller vessel size is an independent predictor of poor outcomes after PTCA, and the restenosis rates often are high (25% to 50%). Some data on stenting of small vessels suggest higher rates of stent thrombosis, although these findings have not been replicated by others. The benefit of stenting over PTCA is more evident when a larger postprocedural-diameter stenosis is attained. Diabetic patients with small-vessel disease pose even greater challenges to performing PCI.

Predilatation with Balloon and Stenting

PTCA primarily is used for predilatation before stenting to facilitate stent delivery and prevent stent damage. Originally, all patients undergoing stenting were treated with predilatation, which was essential because the earlier stents were bulky with higher profile and stiffness.

PTCA before stenting should be performed when there is significant vessel calcification, tortuosity, and failure to evaluate the correct stent size due to distal vessel underfilling produced by severe stenosis and in ostial lesions. Predilatation has the potential to produce distal embolization and injury beyond the edges of the stent, and it increases the procedural time, x-ray exposure, and costs.

Provisional Stenting

PTCA has been the main treatment of coronary artery disease, but the seriousness of acute complications (mainly acute vessel closure) and the long-term complications of restenosis paved the way for the development of new strategies that resulted in the use of drug-eluting stents. The use of stents has decreased acute complications after failed balloon angioplasty, and they are the best option to decrease the restenosis. However, the technique of balloon angioplasty has improved with increased operator experience, better antiplatelet agents, and the use of backup coronary artery stenting (i.e., use of stenting when PTCA does not accomplish optimal results), or "bailout" stenting (i.e., for definite or threatened abrupt closure), allowing cardiologists to use provisional stenting. This strategy was proposed to reduce costs and rates of in-stent restenosis.[59-61] For example, in the Doppler Endpoint Stenting International Investigation (DESTINI),[60] 370 subjects were randomized to elective stent implantation and 365 to guided PTCA. For 218 lesions (43%), the PTCA result was considered satisfactory (i.e., residual-diameter stenosis ≤35%), coronary flow reserve was more than 2.0 by Doppler ultrasound, and no evidence of threatening dissections was found. The remaining 218 lesions underwent stent implantation. Final residual-diameter stenosis was less in the elective and provisional stent groups (9.3% and 10.2%) than in the optimal PTCA group (24.8%, $P < .00001$). The likelihood of one or more major adverse cardiac events at 12 months was 17.8% in the elective stenting group and 18.9% in the guided-PTCA group (20.1% for optimal PTCA and 18.0% for the provisional stenting subgroup, P = NS). There was no difference for repeat revascularization at 1 year between the elective stenting group and the guided-PTCA group (*P* = NS).

Provisional stenting has been proposed with the use of IVUS. For instance, the Strategy for IVUS-Guided PTCA and Stenting (SIPS) trial reported that IVUS-guided provisional stenting improved 2-year clinical outcomes.[59]

Bailout coronary stent implantation is supported by observational studies that uniformly consider its use a possible option (Table 16-1). In current practice, threatened abrupt closure is treated with the placement of a stent.

Available stents allow higher balloon inflation pressures with PTCA, and stents can be used when potential complications are assessed, such as threatened closure or abrupt closure. The equipment for PTCA has improved considerably, and the use of glycoprotein (GP) IIb/IIIa inhibitors reduces the thrombotic complications associated with angioplasty.[70] Randomized studies have provided valuable information of increased efficacy of balloon angioplasty in control groups of patients who underwent plain balloon angioplasty only. These studies are the Balloon vs Optimal Atherectomy Trial (BOAT),[71] Belgian Netherlands Stent Study-2 (BENESTENT-2),[72] and Evaluation in Percutaneous Transluminal Coronary Angioplasty to Improve Long-Term Outcome with Abciximab GP IIb/IIIa Blockade (EPILOG).[73] The three trials included a total of 4608 patients, and different treatments, such as stenting or directional atherectomy, were used. In the experimental arm, 15.4% required target lesion revascularization (TVR), and 17.5% of the control group (plain PTCA) required TVR. This rate of TVR in the PTCA group (17.5%) represented a considerable advance compared with the previous data for restenosis after PTCA (>20%). This information suggests that a more aggressive approach with balloon dilation using provisional stenting may have a clinical role. Based on the data from EPILOG, BENESTENT, and BOAT, there is a need for a randomized, controlled trial to compare the strategy of using drug-eluting stents with using aggressive angioplasty followed by provisional stenting for suboptimal balloon angioplasty results.[74]

PLAQUE SEALING BY PERCUTANEOUS TRANSLUMINAL CORONARY ANGIOPLASTY: A HYPOTHESIS

Sealing an unpredictable, vulnerable plaque for asymptomatic, angiographically and hemodynamically nonsignificant lesions has been proposed. The rationale is that the vessel that undergoes angioplasty has the potential for "protective" intimal proliferation due to an increase in smooth muscle cells, with a collagen-rich layer creating a fibrous cap that stabilizes a vulnerable plaque.[75,76] This controversial but provocative approach must be carefully tested after the challenge of identification of the unstable plaque are overcome, allowing targeting of sealing angioplasty or stenting.[77,78]

This approach is supported by the long-term prognosis for patients who do not develop restenosis.[79-82] Clinical data suggest that the target site after successful plain PTCA remains stable and is rarely the culprit in subsequent acute coronary events. For instance, the potential for infarction in the segment treated with PTCA was evaluated by Saito and associates[82] in more than 300 patients who experienced an acute MI after PTCA. In 99.3% of cases, the culprit lesion was located in another coronary segment, suggesting that the coronary lesions that undergo angioplasty became stable. A large, retrospective analysis of 4000 patients from different clinical trials evaluated the 1-year mortality and nonfatal MI rates for different diameters of coronary artery stenosis, including a group of subjects with stenotic lesions that were less than 50% of the vessel's diameter stenosis that were treated. Almost two thirds of the patients had a coronary artery stent placed, making it difficult to extrapolate these results to plain PTCA. There was no significant difference in the 1-year mortality and MI rates across the different groups of coronary artery stenosis.

To test the clinical hypothesis of plaque sealing with plain PTCA or stenting, a better understanding of the physical and biologic mechanisms and techniques is needed, and assessment of the vulnerable plaque with imaging, biomarkers, and adequate clinical trials with long-term follow-up should be performed. If plaque sealing is demonstrated to be a

Table 16-1. Outcomes of Bailout Coronary Stenting

Study	N	Study Interval	Follow-up	Stent Type	Successful Deployment (%)	Emergency CABG (%)	Late MI (Q/Non-Q) (%)	Late Death (%)
Herrmann et al.[62]	56	1988-91	30 d	Palmaz-Schatz	98	7	19 (14/5)	4
George et al.[63]	494	1988-91	6 mo	Gianturco-Roubin	95.4	4.3	7.1 (3.8/3.3)	3.6
Lincoff et al.[64]	61	1989-91	6 mo	Gianturco-Roubin	97	4.9	43 (32/11)	3.3
Maiello et al.[65]	32	1990-92	11 mo	Palmaz-Schatz	94	6	12 (9/3)	3
Hearn et al.[66]	116	1987-90	14 mo	Gianturco-Roubin	89	11	34.5 (6.8/27.7)	4
Sutton et al.[67]	415	1989-91	90 d	Gianturco-Roubin	NR	12*	5 (NR)	3
Schömig et al.[68]	339	1989-93	2 yr	Palmaz-Schatz	96.5	1	8.9 (NR)	3
Metz et al.[69]	88	1988-93	In hospital	Several	94	8	26 (8/18)	4.6

*Includes emergency and nonemergency CABG in the first 90 days after stent implantation.
CABG, coronary artery bypass grafting; MI, myocardial infarction; non-Q, non-Q-wave myocardial infarction; NR, not reported; Q, Q-wave myocardial infarction.
From Narins CR, Holmes DR, Topol EJ: A call for provisional stenting: The balloon is back! Circulation 1998;97:1298-1305.

viable option, a new era in cardiology will be established, perhaps creating a preventive interventional practice.

COMPLICATIONS

PCIs have a low rate of serious acute major complications, such as death, MI, perforation, or need for emergency bypass surgery,[83] but the rate of serious acute complications in the early PTCA experience was higher. In the 1977-1983 NHLBI Registry, the mortality rate was 0.9%, rate of emergency CABG was 6.6%, rate of MI was 5.5%, and total rate was 13.6% for major complications among 3079 patients from 105 contributing centers.[84] Complications occurred more frequently in women and patients with unstable angina. The rate of MI decreased with procedural experience, but the rate of coronary dissection or abrupt closure remained unchanged. The second NHLBI Registry (1985-1986)[9] reported that in 1802 consecutive patients, despite being at higher procedural risk than patients in the earlier registry (i.e., older, more multivessel disease, worse left ventricular function, and more frequent history of MI or history of previous CABG), the angiographically determined success rates according to lesion status increased from 67% to 88% ($P < .001$), with similar mortality (1%) and periprocedural MI rates.

Coronary Artery Dissection

Coronary artery dissection is a common complication of PTCA, although most dissections do not result in acute ischemic complications. When coronary artery dissections are small or moderate, a conservative approach can be used.[85] A higher rate of complications was identified for longer dissections, greater degree of stenosis, smaller cross-sectional area, and the use of extraluminal contrast.[86] Other predictors of ischemic complications related to coronary artery dissection and abrupt closure were transient occlusion, residual stenosis of more than 70% of the lumen, and dissections longer than 6 mm.[87]

Anatomic factors play an important role in the development of coronary artery dissection and abrupt closure. For example, PTCA in angulated stenosis resulted in higher initial failure rates and complications.[88] The presence of coronary artery calcium detected by IVUS contributes to dissection after angioplasty.[89]

Abrupt Closure

Among acute complications, abrupt closure is a major hazard, and the complexity is difficult to predict in individual patients. Proposed predictors have included proximal vessel tortuosity, eccentricity, length, and angulation, but in individual patients these measurements proved to be inefficient. The rate of abrupt closure was 4.5% among 1155 patients studied in the first NHLBI Registry between 1979 and 1981.[84] There was a 4.9% rate of overall mortality, 41% rate of MI,

and 72% required emergency bypass surgery. In the late 1980s and early 1990s, the rates of abrupt closure fluctuated between 4% and 8%, with more than one fifth of the patients requiring emergency bypass surgery despite using perfusion devices and longer inflations.[90,91]

Distal Embolization

Distal embolization of some degree is almost universal, and all PCIs in animal experimental models and in humans[26,92] are associated with increased risks of periprocedural MI. The distal embolization of debris during PTCA results in different degrees of obstruction in the distal macrocirculation and microcirculation; the extreme manifestation of "no flow" results in periprocedural MI.

Restenosis after Percutaneous Transluminal Coronary Angioplasty

Restenosis after successful PTCA usually occurs within the first 6 months. It is characterized by lesion complexity and represents a major limitation of the procedure (Fig. 16-7). Data from randomized trials demonstrated rates of angiographically confirmed restenosis of 30% to almost 60% after a successful PTCA.[93-96] For example, for 557 patients who underwent successful PTCA, the NHLBI Registry documented a 33.6% rate of restenosis.[40] Much work needs to be done to clarify the different components of restenosis, but the general consensus is that there are four events: acute elastic recoil, chronic negative remodeling, neointimal hyperplasia, and excessive matrix formation. It is likely that a restenosis is a manifestation of a wound healing response in the vasculature. The combination of inflammation, granulation, and extracellular matrix remodeling influences the degree of restenosis.

Restenosis can be defined angiographically or clinically. The clinical outcome is the most relevant end point. The NHLBI Registry defined restenosis after

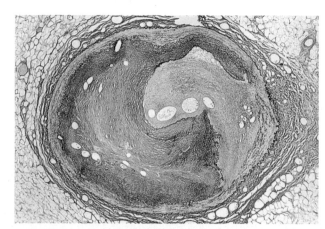

Figure 16-7. Percutaneous transluminal coronary angioplasty with an old occlusive restenosis (VVG stain). (Courtesy W. D. Edwards, MD, Mayo Clinic, Rochester, MN.)

angioplasty by using different percentages of the stenotic diameter at follow-up angiography.[40] The absolute change in minimal lumen diameter determined angiographically at follow-up also has been proposed. The definition could be a binary end point, but restenosis could also be approached as a continuous variable.

Much effort in basic and clinical research has been undertaken to address restenosis. Methods such as directional coronary atherectomy (DCA) and excisional atherectomy were used to prevent restenosis, but they proved to be ineffective. The advent of stents opened a new door for the treatment of coronary artery disease, with a significant reduction in restenosis rates that was demonstrated in randomized trials such as the Stent Restenosis Study (STRESS)[95] and the BENESTENT.[96]

The ability to predict restenosis was important. Multiple clinical, procedural, and angiographic variables were related to restenosis, but their predictive value remained low. Some plausible angiographic variables for predicting restenosis included angulation, length, and proximal location of the lesion; LAD lesions; bifurcation lesions; and lesions that receive collaterals. The final minimal lumen diameter had an inverse relationship to the likelihood of developing restenosis.

Death

In large registry of 8052 PTCA procedures, the incidence of death was 0.4% ($n = 32$), and coronary artery closure was the main cause of death. Decreased left ventricular function and the territory at risk (i.e., jeopardy score) were also important predictors.[97] Other complications of PTCA include vascular injury, coronary perforation, equipment failure, embolization, and air embolism.

PERCUTANEOUS TRANSLUMINAL CORONARY ANGIOPLASTY AS AN OPTION FOR PATIENTS WITH CORONARY ARTERY DISEASE

Histopathologic and clinical data show that after successful dilatation, the area that undergoes balloon angioplasty does not develop instability, avoiding the consequences of acute thrombosis and acute MI. This contrasts with the complication of late thrombosis that is associated with stents and that is associated with high morbidity and mortality rates. The concept that endothelial function may return to normal after PTCA may have larger implications than realized.[98] When a drug-eluting stent is placed, there is endothelial dysfunction in the segment adjacent to the stent.[99,100] In-stent restenosis is difficult to treat, whereas restenosis after PTCA is easier to treat. Balloon angioplasty has a role in the challenging treatment of bifurcation disease, and most trials have demonstrated that stenting one branch and using only balloon angioplasty in the other branch is better than stenting both branches or using PTCA in both branches. In patients with severe, diffuse disease and

small vessels, PTCA alone may be better over time than using several small stents.

Some patients who require revascularization may need to undergo surgery without delay. In that clinical setting, PTCA has a fundamental role in avoiding the need for prolonged therapy with dual antiplatelet agents. If a bare metal stent or a drug-eluting stent is placed with coverage of graft touchdown sites by the metallic platform, the patient will not be a candidate for CABG in the future.

PTCA may be more affordable than other therapies, especially in developing countries or because of reimbursement issues making plain PTCA inexpensive and its use widespread in the population. In selected cases, we need to avoid the hypersensitivity reaction to the polymer or metal in the stents, and we do not know the long-term consequences of this type of foreign material in the coronary artery.

The use of single PTCA (<30%) is declining dramatically owing to the success of novel coronary devices compared with a use greater than 70% in the late 1990s. However, the American College of Cardiology, American Heart Association, and Society for Cardiac Angiography and Interventions (ACC/AHA/SCAI) Task Force's 2005 Guideline Update for Percutaneous Coronary Intervention reminds us that firm evidence (level A data from various randomized clinical trials) is mainly available for stenting over PTCA in selected patients undergoing single-vessel PCI.[101]

SUMMARY

The treatment of coronary artery disease was revolutionized by PTCA, and millions of patients have benefited worldwide. Since the late 1970s, the technique has undergone many improvements and testing in randomized trials, allowing the practice of evidence-based interventional cardiology. Acute (i.e., coronary dissection and abrupt closure) and chronic (i.e., restenosis) complications prompted the development of multiple pharmacologic agents and devices to make the practice safe and efficient. With the abundance of new devices, we are losing sight of the fact that plain PTCA remains a viable option for the treatment of coronary artery disease. We know that successful PTCA can have long-lasting results for more than 2 decades, exemplified by the first lesion treated by the pioneer of the technique, Andreas Gruentzig.

A challenge in interventional cardiology is deciding when to perform plain balloon angioplasty. Individual clinical variables and overall cardiovascular risk should be carefully evaluated. More refined definition of the indications requires a better understanding of the physical and cellular mechanisms of plain balloon angioplasty and randomized trials of simple PTCA with a provisional stenting approach compared with stents. Noninvasive and invasive techniques may help us characterize lesions that should be treated with plain PTCA as initial approach. In the future, treatment of an asymptomatic patient with coronary artery disease and an unpredictable risk may be novel pharmaceutical interventions and inflation of a balloon that will carry cells capable of restoring vessel homeostasis by sealing vulnerable plaques.

Perhaps part of the answer to whether balloon angioplasty is still a viable option resides in the first patient with a proximal LAD stenosis that was dilated by Gruentzig more than 2 decades ago. The enduring result makes us think that plain balloon angioplasty will survive and reach new horizons.

REFERENCES

1. Sheldon WC: F. Mason Sones, Jr.—Stormy petrel of cardiology. Clin Cardiol 1994;17:405-407.
2. Dotter CT, Judkins MP: Transluminal treatment of arteriosclerotic obstruction: Description of a new technic and a preliminary report of its application. Circulation 1964;30:654-670.
3. Porstmann W: A new corset balloon catheter for Dotter's transluminal recanilization with special reference to obliterations of the pelvic arteries [in German]. Radiol Diagn (Berl) 1973;14:239-244.
4. Hurst JW: The first coronary angioplasty as described by Andreas Gruentzig. Am J Cardiol 1986;57:185-186.
5. Meier B: The first patient to undergo coronary angioplasty—23-year follow-up. N Engl J Med 2001;344:144-145.
6. Simpson JB, Baim DS, Robert EW, Harrison DC: A new catheter system for coronary angioplasty. Am J Cardiol 1982;49:1216-1222.
7. King SB 3rd, Schlumpf M: Ten-year completed follow-up of percutaneous transluminal coronary angioplasty: The early Zurich experience. J Am Coll Cardiol 1993;22:353-360.
8. Gruentzig A, King SB 3rd, Schlumpf M, Siegenthaler W: Long-term follow-up after percutaneous transluminal coronary angioplasty. The early Zurich experience. N Engl J Med 1987;316:1127-1132.
9. Detre K, Holubkov R, Kelsey S, et al: Percutaneous transluminal coronary angioplasty in 1985-1986 and 1977-1981. The National Heart, Lung, and Blood Institute Registry. N Engl J Med 1988;318:265-270.
10. Faxon DP, Ruocco N, Jacobs AK: Long-term outcome of patients after percutaneous transluminal coronary angioplasty. Circulation 1990;81(Suppl):IV9-IV13.
11. Jackman JD Jr, Zidar JP, Tcheng JE, et al: Outcome after prolonged balloon inflations of greater than 20 minutes for initially unsuccessful percutaneous transluminal coronary angioplasty. Am J Cardiol 1992;69:1417-1421.
12. Schwartz L, Bourassa MD, Lesperance J, et al: Aspirin and dipyridamole in the prevention of restenosis after percutaneous transluminal coronary angioplasty. N Engl J Med 1988;318:1714-1719.
13. Abele J: Balloon catheters and transluminal dilatation: Technical considerations. AJR Am J Roentgenol 1980;135:901-906.
14. Faxon D, Weber VJ, Haudenschild C, et al: Acute effects of transluminal angioplasty in three experimental models of atherosclerosis. Arterioscler Thromb Vasc Biol 1982;2:125-133.
15. Steele P, Chesebro JH, Stanson AW, et al: Balloon angioplasty. Natural history of the pathophysiological response to injury in a pig model. Circ Res 1985;57:105-112.
16. Soward AL, Essed CE, Serruys PW: Coronary arterial findings after accidental death immediately after successful percutaneous transluminal coronary angioplasty. Am J Cardiol 1985;56:794-795.
17. Farb A, Virmani R, Atkinson JB, Kolodgie FD: Plaque morphology and pathologic changes in arteries from patients dying after coronary balloon angioplasty. J Am Coll Cardiol 1990;16:1421-1429.
18. Saffitz JE, Rose TE, Oaks JB, Roberts WC: Coronary arterial rupture during coronary angioplasty. Am J Cardiol 1983;51:902-904.
19. Waller BF: Early and late morphologic changes in human coronary arteries after percutaneous transluminal coronary angioplasty. Clin Cardiol 1983;6:363-372.
20. Waller BF, Gorfinkel HJ, Rogers FJ, et al: Early and late morphologic changes in major epicardial coronary arteries after percutaneous transluminal coronary angioplasty. Am J Cardiol 1984;53:42C-47C.
21. Waller BF, Rothbaum DA, Pinkerton CA, et al: Status of the myocardium and infarct-related coronary artery in 19 necropsy patients with acute recanalization using pharmacologic (streptokinase, r-tissue plasminogen activator), mechanical (percutaneous transluminal coronary angioplasty) or combined types of reperfusion therapy. J Am Coll Cardiol 1987;9:785-801.
22. Waller BF: Pathology of transluminal balloon angioplasty used in the treatment of coronary heart disease. Cardiol Clin 1989;7:749-770.
23. Sanborn TA, Faxon DP, Haudenschild C, et al: The mechanism of transluminal angioplasty: evidence for formation of aneurysms in experimental atherosclerosis. Circulation 1983;68:1136-1140.
24. Block PC, Fallon JT, Elmer D: Experimental angioplasty: Lessons from the laboratory. AJR Am J Roentgenol 1980;135:907-912.
25. Baughman KL, Pasternak RC, Fallon JT, Block PC: Transluminal coronary angioplasty of postmortem human hearts. Am J Cardiol 1981;48:1044-1047.
26. Block PC, Elmer D, Fallon JT: Release of atherosclerotic debris after transluminal angioplasty. Circulation 1982;65:950-952.
27. Castaneda-Zuniga WR, Formanek A, Tadavarthy M, et al: The mechanism of balloon angioplasty. Radiology 1980;135:565-571.
28. Mizuno K, Kurita A, Imazeki N: Pathological findings after percutaneous transluminal coronary angioplasty. Br Heart J 1984;52:588-590.
29. Saner HE, Gobel FL, Salomonwitz E, et al: The disease-free wall in coronary atherosclerosis: Its relation to degree of obstruction. J Am Coll Cardiol 1985;6:1096-1099.
30. Waller BF: Coronary luminal shape and the arc of disease-free wall: Morphologic observations and clinical relevance. J Am Coll Cardiol 1985;6:1100-1101.
31. Vlodaver Z, Edwards JE: Pathology of coronary atherosclerosis. Prog Cardiovasc Dis 1971;14:256-274.
32. Feldman R, Glemser E, Kaizer J, Standley M: Coronary angioplasty using new 6 French guiding catheters. Cathet Cardiovasc Diagn 1991;23:93-99.
33. Talley JD, Joseph A, Killeavy ES, et al: Multicenter evaluation of a new fixed-wire coronary angioplasty catheter system: Clinical and angiographic characteristics and results. Cathet Cardiovasc Diagn 1991;22:310-316.
34. Pande AK, Meier B, Urban P, et al: Coronary angioplasty with second generation monorail catheters. Int J Cardiol 1991;32:23-27.
35. Alcan KE, Stertzer SH, Wallsh E, et al: The role of intra-aortic balloon counterpulsation in patients undergoing percutaneous transluminal coronary angioplasty. Am Heart J 1983;105:527-530.
36. Williams DO, Riley RS, Singh AK, Most A: Restoration of normal coronary hemodynamics and myocardial metabolism after percutaneous transluminal coronary angioplasty. Circulation 1980;62:653-656.
37. Holmes DR Jr, Vlietstra RE, Fisher LD, et al: Follow-up of patients from the coronary artery surgery study (CASS) potentially suitable for percutaneous transluminal coronary angioplasty. Am Heart J 1983;106(Pt 1):981-988.
38. Ellis SG, Fisher L, Dushman-Ellis S, et al: Comparison of coronary angioplasty with medical treatment for single- and double-vessel coronary disease with left anterior descending coronary involvement: Long-term outcome based on an Emory-CASS registry study. Am Heart J 1989;118:208-220.
39. Holmes DR Jr, Vlietstra RE: Balloon angioplasty in acute and chronic coronary artery disease. JAMA 1989;261:2109-2115.

40. Holmes DR Jr, Vlietstra RE, Smith HC, et al: Restenosis after percutaneous transluminal coronary angioplasty (PTCA): A report from the PTCA Registry of the National Heart, Lung, and Blood Institute. Am J Cardiol 1984;53:77C-81C.

41. Kereiakes DJ, Selmon MR, McAuley BJ, et al: Angioplasty in total coronary artery occlusion: Experience in 76 consecutive patients. J Am Coll Cardiol 1985;6:526-533.

42. Melchior JP, Meier B, Urban P, et al: Percutaneous transluminal coronary angioplasty for chronic total coronary arterial occlusion. Am J Cardiol 1987;59:535-538.

43. Parisi A, Folland E, Hartigan P: A comparison of angioplasty with medical therapy in the treatment of single-vessel coronary artery disease. Veterans Affairs ACME Investigators. N Engl J Med 1992;326:10-16.

44. Goy JJ, Eeckhout E, Burnand B, et al: Coronary angioplasty versus left internal mammary artery grafting for isolated proximal left anterior descending artery stenosis. Lancet 1994;343(8911):1449-1453.

45. Folland ED, Hartigan PM, Parisi AF: Percutaneous transluminal coronary angioplasty versus medical therapy for stable angina pectoris: Outcomes for patients with double-vessel versus single-vessel coronary artery disease in a Veterans Affairs Cooperative randomized trial. Veterans Affairs ACME Investigators. J Am Coll Cardiol 1997;29:1505-1511.

46. Rodriguez A, Boullon F, Perez-Calino N, et al: Argentine randomized trial of percutaneous transluminal coronary angioplasty versus coronary artery bypass surgery in multivessel disease (ERACI): In-hospital results and 1-year follow-up. ERACI Group. J Am Coll Cardiol 1993;22:1060-1067.

47. King SB 3rd, Lembo NJ, Weintraub WS, et al: A randomized trial comparing coronary angioplasty with coronary bypass surgery. Emory Angioplasty versus Surgery Trial (EAST). N Engl J Med 1994;331:1044-1050.

48. Hamm CW, Reimers J, Ischinger T, et al: A randomized study of coronary angioplasty compared with bypass surgery in patients with symptomatic multivessel coronary disease. German Angioplasty Bypass Surgery Investigation (GABI). N Engl J Med 1994;331:1037-1043.

49. Kaehler J, Koester R, Billmann W, et al: 13-Year follow-up of the German angioplasty bypass surgery investigation. Eur Heart J 2005;26:2148-2153.

50. First-year results of CABRI (Coronary Angioplasty versus Bypass Revascularisation Investigation). CABRI Trial Participants. Lancet 1995;346:1179-1184.

51. Five-year clinical and functional outcome comparing bypass surgery and angioplasty in patients with multivessel coronary disease. A multicenter randomized trial. Writing Group for the Bypass Angioplasty Revascularization Investigation (BARI) Investigators. JAMA 1997;277:715-721.

52. Hueb WA, Belotti G, de Oliveire SA, et al: The Medicine, Angioplasty or Surgery Study (MASS): A prospective, randomized trial of medical therapy, balloon angioplasty or bypass surgery for single proximal left anterior descending artery stenoses. J Am Coll Cardiol 1995;26:1600-1605.

53. Coronary angioplasty versus coronary artery bypass surgery: The Randomized Intervention Treatment of Angina (RITA) trial. Lancet 1993;341:573-580.

54. Coronary angioplasty versus medical therapy for angina: the second Randomised Intervention Treatment of Angina (RITA-2) trial. Lancet 1997;350:461-468.

55. Zijlstra F, de Boer MJ, Hoorntje JC, et al: A comparison of immediate coronary angioplasty with intravenous streptokinase in acute myocardial infarction. N Engl J Med 1993;328:680-684.

56. Grines CL, Browne KF, Marco J, et al: A comparison of immediate angioplasty with thrombolytic therapy for acute myocardial infarction. The Primary Angioplasty in Myocardial Infarction Study Group. N Engl J Med 1993;328:673-679.

57. Gibbons RJ, Holmes DR, Reeder GS, et al: Immediate angioplasty compared with the administration of a thrombolytic agent followed by conservative treatment for myocardial infarction. N Engl J Med 1993;328:685-691.

58. Al Suwaidi J, Berger PB, Rihal CS, et al: Immediate and long-term outcome of intracoronary stent implantation for true bifurcation lesions. J Am Coll Cardiol 2000;35:929-936.

59. Cantor WJ, Peterson ED, Popma JJ, et al: Provisional stenting strategies: Systematic overview and implications for clinical decision-making. J Am Coll Cardiol 2000;36:1142-1151.

60. Di Mario C, Moses JW, Anderson TJ, et al: Randomized comparison of elective stent implantation and coronary balloon angioplasty guided by online quantitative angiography and intracoronary Doppler. DESTINI Study Group (Doppler Endpoint STenting INternational Investigation). Circulation 2000;102:2938-2944.

61. Fluck DS, Chenu P, Mills P, et al: Is provisional stenting the effective option? The WIDEST study (Wiktor Stent in De Novo Stenosis). Heart 2000;84:522-528.

62. Herrmann H, Buchbinder M, Clemen MW, et al: Emergent use of balloon-expandable coronary artery stenting for failed percutaneous transluminal coronary angioplasty. Circulation 1992;86:812-819.

63. George B, Voorhees WD 3rd, Roubin GS, et al: Multicenter investigation of coronary stenting to treat acute or threatened closure after percutaneous transluminal coronary angioplasty: clinical and angiographic outcomes. J Am Coll Cardiol 1993;22:135-143.

64. Lincoff A, Topol EJ, Chapekis AT, et al: Intracoronary stenting compared with conventional therapy for abrupt vessel closure complicating coronary angioplasty: A matched case-control study. J Am Coll Cardiol 1993;21:866-875.

65. Maiello L, Colombo A, Gianrossi R, et al: Coronary stenting for treatment of acute or threatened closure following dissection after coronary balloon angioplasty. Am Heart J 1993;125:1570-1575.

66. Hearn J, King SB 3rd, Douglas JS Jr, et al: Clinical and angiographic outcomes after coronary artery stenting for acute or threatened closure after percutaneous transluminal coronary angioplasty. Initial results with a balloon-expandable, stainless steel design. Circulation 1993;88:2086-2096.

67. Sutton J, Ellis SG, Roubin GS, et al: Major clinical events after coronary stenting. The multicenter registry of acute and elective Gianturco-Roubin stent placement. The Gianturco-Roubin Intracoronary Stent Investigator Group. Circulation 1994;89:1126-1137.

68. Schomig A, Kastrati A, Mudra H, et al: Four-year experience with Palmaz-Schatz stenting in coronary angioplasty complicated by dissection with threatened or present vessel closure. Circulation 1994;90:2716-2724.

69. Metz D, Urban P, Camenzind E, et al: Improving results of bailout coronary stenting after failed balloon angioplasty. Cathet Cardiovasc Diagn 1994;32:117-124.

70. Lincoff MA: Platelet glycoprotein IIb/IIIa receptor blockade and low-dose heparin during percutaneous coronary revascularization. N Engl J Med 1997;336:1689-1696.

71. Baim DS, Popma JJ, Sharma SK: Final results in the Balloon vs Optimal Atherectomy Trial (BOAT): 6 month angiography and 1 year clinical follow-up [abstract]. Circulation 1996;94(Suppl I):436.

72. Serruys PW, Emanuelsson H, van der Giessen W, et al: Heparin-coated Palmaz-Schatz stents in human coronary arteries: Early outcome of the BENESTENT-II pilot study. Circulation 1996;93:412-422.

73. The EPILOG Investigators: Platelet glycoprotein IIb/IIIa receptor blockade and low-dose heparin during percutaneous coronary revascularization. N Engl J Med 1997;336:1689-1697.

74. Narins CR, Holmes DR, Topol EJ: A call for provisional stenting: The balloon is back! Circulation 1998;97:1298-1305.

75. Weissberg PL, Clesham GJ, Bennett MR: Is vascular smooth muscle cell proliferation beneficial? Lancet 1996;347:305-307.

76. Meier B: Plaque sealing by coronary angioplasty. Heart 2004;90:1395-1398.

77. Buffon A, Biasucci LM, Liuzzo G, et al: Widespread coronary inflammation in unstable angina. N Engl J Med 2002;347:5-12.

78. Goldstein JA, Demetriou D, Grines CL, et al: Multiple complex coronary plaques in patients with acute myocardial infarction. N Engl J Med 2000;343:915-922.

79. Talley JD, Hurst JW, King SB 3rd, et al: Clinical outcome 5 years after attempted percutaneous transluminal coronary angioplasty in 427 patients. Circulation 1988;77: 820-829.

80. Kadel C, Vallbracht C, Buss F, et al: Long-term follow-up after percutaneous transluminal coronary angioplasty in patients with single-vessel disease. Am Heart J 1992;124:1159-1169.

81. Vandormael M, Deligonul U, Taussig S, Kern MJ: Predictors of long-term cardiac survival in patients with multivessel coronary artery disease undergoing percutaneous transluminal coronary angioplasty. Am J Cardiol 1991;67:1-6.

82. Saito T, Date H, Taniguchi I, et al: Outcome of target sites escaping high-grade (>70%) restenosis after percutaneous transluminal coronary angioplasty. The Am J Cardiol 1999; 83:857-861.

83. Yang EH, Gumina RJ, Lennon RJ, et al: Emergency coronary artery bypass surgery for percutaneous coronary interventions: changes in the incidence, clinical characteristics, and indications from 1979 to 2003. J Am Coll Cardiol 2005;46: 2004-2009.

84. Cowley MJ, Dorros G, Kelsey SF: Acute coronary events associated with percutaneous transluminal coronary angioplasty. Am J Cardiol 1984;53:22C-26C.

85. Albertal M, Regar E, Van Langenhove G, et al: Value of coronary stenotic flow velocity acceleration on the prediction of long-term improvement in functional status after angioplasty. Am Heart J 2001;142:81-86.

86. Black AJ, Namay DL, Niederman AL, et al: Tear or dissection after coronary angioplasty. Morphologic correlates of an ischemic complication. Circulation 1989;79:1035-1042.

87. Bell MR, Reeder GS, Garratt KN, et al: Predictors of major ischemic complications after coronary dissection following angioplasty. Am J Cardiol 1993;71:1402-1407.

88. Ellis SG, Topol EJ: Results of percutaneous transluminal coronary angioplasty of high-risk angulated stenoses. Am J Cardiol 1990;66:932-937.

89. Fitzgerald PJ, Ports TA, Yock PG: Contribution of localized calcium deposits to dissection after angioplasty. An observational study using intravascular ultrasound. Circulation 1992;86:64-70.

90. Lincoff AM, Popma JJ, Ellis SG, et al: Abrupt vessel closure complicating coronary angioplasty: Clinical, angiographic and therapeutic profile. J Am Coll Cardiol 1992;19: 926-935.

91. Kuntz RE, Piana R, Pomerantz RM, et al: Changing incidence and management of abrupt closure following coronary intervention in the new device era. Cathet Cardiovascr Diagn 1992;27:183-190.

92. Adgey AA, Mathew TP, Harbinson MT: Periprocedural creatine kinase-MB elevations: Long-term impact and clinical implications. Clin Cardiol 1999;22:257-265.

93. Topol EJ, Leya F, Pinkerton CA, et al: A comparison of directional atherectomy with coronary angioplasty in patients with coronary artery disease. N Engl J Med 1993;329: 221-227.

94. Adelman AG, Cohen EA, Kimball BP, et al: A comparison of directional atherectomy with balloon angioplasty for lesions of the left anterior descending coronary artery. N Engl J Med 1993;329:228-233.

95. Fischman DL, Leon MB, Baim DS, et al: A randomized comparison of coronary-stent placement and balloon angioplasty in the treatment of coronary artery disease. N Engl J Med 1994;331:496-501.

96. Serruys PW, de Jaegere P, Kiemeniej F, et al: A comparison of balloon-expandable-stent implantation with balloon angioplasty in patients with coronary artery disease. Benestent Study Group. N Engl J Med 1994;331:489-495.

97. Ellis SG, Myler RK, King SB 3rd, et al: Causes and correlates of death after unsupported coronary angioplasty: Implications for use of angioplasty and advanced support techniques in high-risk settings. Am J Cardiol 1991;68:1447-1451.

98. Frielingsdorf J, Kaufmann P, Suter T, et al: Percutaneous transluminal coronary angioplasty reverses vasoconstriction of stenotic coronary arteries in hypertensive patients. Circulation 1998;98:1192-1197.

99. Hofma SH, van der Giessen WJ, van Dalen BM, et al: Indication of long-term endothelial dysfunction after sirolimus-eluting stent implantation. Eur Heart J 2006;27:166-170.

100. Togni M, Windecker S, Cocchia R, et al: Sirolimus-eluting stents associated with paradoxic coronary vasoconstriction. J Am Coll Cardiol 2005;46:231-236.

101. Smith SC Jr, Feldman TE, Hirschfeld JW Jr, et al: ACC/AHA/ SCAI 2005 Guideline Update for Percutaneous Coronary Intervention—Summary article: A report of the American College of Cardiology/American Heart Association Task Force on Practice Guidelines (ACC/AHA/SCAI Writing Committee to Update the 2001 Guidelines for Percutaneous Coronary Intervention). Circulation 2006;113:156-175.

17 Elective Intervention for Chronic Coronary Syndromes: Stable Angina and Silent Ischemia

B. Clay Sizemore, Matheen A. Khuddus, R. David Anderson, and Carl J. Pepine

KEY POINTS

- Event rates for patients with chronic coronary syndromes are relatively low overall.
- Many patients with chronic coronary syndromes have very poor quality of life, mainly because of recurrent angina.
- Revascularization, usually coronary artery bypass grafting is preferred for patients with left main coronary artery or proximal two- or three-vessel obstruction.
- For those without these features who remain limited by angina, percutaneous coronary intervention is usually preferred.
- Therapy must include medication to limit abrupt increases in myocardial oxygen demand, with selected use of interventional procedures to improve the limitation in blood supply.
- Secondary atherosclerosis prevention (e.g., smoking cessation, diet, exercise, aspirin, statins) is required in all patients with chronic coronary syndromes.

INTRODUCTION

Definitions

Despite, and possibly the direct result of, advances in the management of acute coronary syndromes (ACSs), left ventricular dysfunction, and arrhythmias, the number of patients with chronic stable coronary syndromes is increasing. Although most of our efforts have focused on the acute syndromes, our understanding of the pathophysiology of chronic syndromes has lagged.[1]

In this chapter on elective intervention for chronic ischemic syndromes, we use the following terminology. Chronic coronary syndromes (CCS) include the chronic ischemic syndromes of stable angina pectoris, isolated angina pectoris, coronary artery spasm, and silent myocardial ischemia. Acute coronary syndromes (ACS) include unstable angina, non-ST-segment elevation myocardial infarction (NSTEMI), and ST-segment elevation myocardial infarction (STEMI). Coronary artery disease (CAD) includes obstructive coronary atherosclerotic disease, and coronary intervention or coronary revascularization includes all percutaneous coronary interventions (PCIs) and surgical coronary artery bypass grafting (CABG).

Background

In the United States, more than 13 million people have a diagnosis of CAD, and the prevalence of angina pectoris is estimated to be 6.5 million.[2] Determining which patients with these CCS are likely to benefit from elective coronary intervention is difficult, and decision-making requires an understanding of the natural course of this illness, the costs of care, and most importantly, consideration of the patient's symptoms associated with and the pathophysiology of cardiac ischemia.

Prognosis in Chronic Coronary Syndromes

A reasonable body of evidence exists regarding the long-term prognosis of patients with CCS and the effect of revascularization. Although most of these data are from an older era in cardiovascular care,[3-6] the later data also confirm low rates of death, myocardial infarction (MI), stroke, and heart failure.[7-9] Multiple prevention trials performed in this population have established an approximate annual event rate of about 2% to 3% for the composite outcome of death or nonfatal MI.[7,10,11] A validated risk score for predicting near-term events in CCS patients could help decision-making. Several have been proposed from randomized clinical trials in patients with stable angina that were not designed for this purpose.[12,13] These emphasize prior MI and depressed left ventricular systolic function in addition to the electrocardiographic markers and usual cardiac risk factors. They have, however, been derived from relatively small numbers, with follow-up less than 5 years, and none has been replicated in an independent cohort.

Cost Considerations

Decision-making becomes particularly important when considering revascularization, because it must be weighed against the risk of infrequent but potentially serious complications and the costs for intervention. The latter has important implications in terms of rising health care costs, particularly if revascularization can be delayed without increased risk of death or MI by waiting for unacceptable symptom control that significantly impacts quality of life (QOL). With the CCS, health-related QOL often becomes the critical consideration in the choice of an interventional approach versus continued conservative medical care alone. One report estimated that the direct societal costs for "chronic angina" management were in the range of $1.9 to $8.9 billion.[14] For a woman with chest discomfort and CAD at angiography, the estimated lifetime costs of cardiovascular care (i.e., drugs and hospitalizations) are in excess of $1 million.[15]

Symptom Status and Pathophysiology

The pathophysiologic mechanism responsible for symptoms related to cardiac ischemia is poorly understood, and there are wide variations among patients and within a given patient over time. The evidence indicates that women and elderly patients often have symptoms and clinical presentations that are unrecognized as being caused by ischemia because they are truly silent or atypical (e.g., fatigue, back discomfort).[16] Sedentary individuals frequently are not active enough to elicit ischemia-related symptoms. Unfortunately, the converse is also true. Gastrointestinal, pulmonary, musculoskeletal, and even neuropsychiatric pathology can manifest in ways that may be considered typical for angina. For these reasons, evaluation and classification of a patient's symptomatic status must be a detailed process and go beyond the presence or absence of chest discomfort.

Patients with symptoms related to objectively documented myocardial ischemia can be divided into two main groups: those with and those without flow-limiting stenosis in a conduit artery at angiography. Stenosis is often considered to be a diameter reduction of more than 50%, but there is not general agreement until the stenosis reaches more than 70%. Those without such obstructive conduit vessel disease and who manifest objective evidence for myocardial ischemia represent a heterogeneous mix. Some have coronary spasm, severe endothelial dysfunction, microvascular dysfunction, or other disorders creating oxygen supply-demand mismatch (e.g., left ventricular hypertrophy, cardiomyopathy, severe anemia, thyrotoxicosis) (Table 17-1).[17] We comment on the conditions that have interventional aspects, particularly when objective data are available.

In light of these considerations, we examine the evidence from clinical trials, registries, and observational studies relevant to the epidemiology, prognosis, and therapeutic strategies in patients with CCS. This chapter is written with the understanding that aggressive secondary prevention, including optimal lifestyle and pharmacologic risk factor modification, is imperative in all patients at high risk for CCS or with documented CCS, regardless of whether they are candidates for revascularization. If they undergo revascularization, continuation of these secondary prevention measures over their lifetime is essential.

SPECIFIC CONSIDERATIONS

Chronic Stable Angina

Revascularization and Outcomes in the Symptomatic Patient

The two main reasons to consider revascularization in any patient with CAD are improvement of prognosis and alleviation of symptoms to improve the QOL. The risk of major adverse events in patients with CCS is low, but the costs are significant. Methods by which the clinician can identify patient subsets at higher risk are numerous.

Despite the high prevalence of chronic stable angina, relatively little is known about the impact on outcomes of modern coronary revascularization in contemporary patients receiving optimal medical therapy. In the second Medicine, Angioplasty or Surgery Study (MASS-II), 611 patients with chronic stable angina, multivessel CAD, and preserved left ventricular function were randomized to CABG, PCI, or medical therapy.[18] The 1-year survival rates were similar, but the highest frequencies of MI and need for additional revascularization procedures were found in patients assigned to PCI. Medical therapy resulted in much more residual angina than in either intervention group. These are results from a single

Table 17-1. Conditions That Provoke or Exacerbate Ischemia

Increased Oxygen Demand	Decreased Oxygen Supply
Noncardiac Conditions	
Hyperthermia	
Hyperthyroidism	Anemia
Sympathomimetic toxicity (e.g., cocaine use)	Hypoxemia
Hypertension	Pneumonia
Anxiety	Asthma
Arteriovenous fistulas	Chronic obstructive pulmonary disease
	Pulmonary hypertension
	Interstitial pulmonary fibrosis
	Obstructive sleep apnea
	Sickle cell disease
	Sympathomimetic toxicity (e.g., cocaine use)
	Hyperviscosity
	Polycythemia
	Leukemia
	Thrombocytosis
	Hypergammaglobulinemia
Cardiac Conditions	
Hypertrophic cardiomyopathy	Hypertrophic cardiomyopathy
Aortic stenosis	Aortic stenosis
Dilated cardiomyopathy	
Tachycardia	
Ventricular	
Supraventricular	

center trial done in Brazil that are not contemporary. There has been continuing improvement in all three treatment options. The results of the Clinical Outcomes Utilizing Revascularization and Aggressive Drug Evaluation (COURAGE) trial enrolling 2287 patients confirm that PCI did not reduce risk of death, MI, or other major CV events when added to optimal medical therapy. The rates of angina were consistently lower in the PCI group, which translates to improved QOL.[19]

Much of the work on CCS predates advances in medical and surgical approaches. It is nonetheless worth reviewing briefly because it still serves as a cornerstone of management of CAD patients, with the unproven assumption that contemporary medical therapy similarly influences medical and revascularization groups. Three landmark trials addressed these issues: Veterans Administration Cooperative Study, European Coronary Surgery Study (ECSS), and Coronary Artery Surgery Study (CASS).[20-22] All of these studies enrolled patients in the 1970s and published results in the mid-1980s. The first two enrolled only men with stable angina and excluded those with left main coronary artery (LMCA) stenosis from their primary analyses (it was widely accepted by then that revascularization was preferred in these cases).[20-22] The European study also excluded patients with left ventricular dysfunction.[21] The CASS was limited to patients with stable ischemic heart disease, with CCS class I or II angina, and with or without a prior MI.[22] Yusuf and colleagues[23] provided a meta-analysis of the results at 10 years from these three studies plus four smaller, randomized trials and concluded that CABG clearly reduced angina compared with medical therapy. They also found that early revascularization significantly reduced mortality compared with initial medical therapy (Fig. 17-1).

There are important limitations in extrapolating these results to modern practice. Medical therapy was inconsistent and limited to β-blockers, digoxin, diuretics, and aspirin (used in only 20% of the medical arm). There were no statins or angiotensin-converting enzyme (ACE) inhibitors, and calcium antagonists were largely absent. There was a 30% crossover rate to bypass and very limited use of arterial conduits. Although 2649 patients with stable angina were included, only 85 were women, and few were older than 65 years.[23] Despite these limitations, these data serve as a basis for the following discussion.

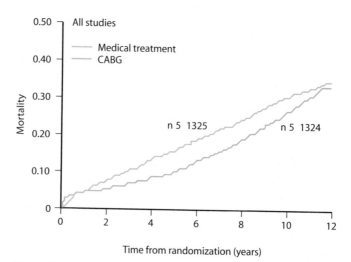

Figure 17-1. Survival curves from meta-analysis of coronary artery bypass grafting (CABG) versus medical therapy trials. (From Yusuf S, Zucker D, Peduzzi P, et al: Effect of coronary artery bypass graft surgery on survival: Overview of 10-year results from randomised trials by the Coronary Artery Bypass Graft Surgery Trialists Collaboration. Lancet 1994;344:563-570.)

Although we have focused on the CABG trials, there are also limited data from trials comparing medical therapy with revascularization by means of PCI confirming the benefits of revascularization. In the multicenter Angioplasty Compared to Medical Therapy Evaluation (ACME), 212 patients with at least one 70% to 99% diameter stenosis and exercise-induced ischemia were randomly assigned to receive conventional medical therapy for angina or percutaneous transluminal coronary angioplasty (PTCA). At 6 months, 64% of PTCA-assigned patients, compared with 46% of medically assigned patients, were free of angina. Patients in the PTCA group also had a greater increase in total exercise duration (2.1 minutes) than the medical group (0.5 minute) and had longer angina-free time on the treadmill.[24] In the second Randomized Intervention Treatment of Angina (RITA-2) trial, 1018 patients with stable angina were randomized to PTCA or medical therapy. Most had at least class 2 angina, and 40% had multivessel disease. Patients assigned to PTCA demonstrated improved treadmill performance, relief of angina, and a greater improvement in perceived QOL (Fig. 17-2). However, the PTCA group had an increased incidence of death or MI after 2.7 years (6.3% versus 3.3%, $P = .02$), largely due to early nonfatal MI related to PCI.[25] Unfortunately, no separate subgroup analysis was done on the patients with multivessel disease. Data from the Duke University database suggest that when single-vessel CAD involves the proximal left anterior descending artery, PCI results in improved survival at 5 years compared with medical therapy.[26] However, there has not been a randomized trial that has demonstrated a clear survival advantage or reduction in MI with PCI compared with medical therapy.

Recently the SWISSI II trial reported the 10-year results in 201 patients of PCI versus medical therapy for silent ischemia following MI. Patients treated with PCI for 1- or 2-vessel disease had lower rates of adverse events (cardiac death, recurrent MI, repeat revascularizations; hazard ratio 0.33, 95% CI, 0.20-0.55, $P < 0.001$) than those treated with medical therapy. Neither the PCI nor the anti-ischemic arms of the trial used contemporary treatments, limiting its broader applicability. Patients undergoing PCI received only balloon angioplasty while medical therapy consisted of only β-blockers, calcium antagonists, and nitrates.[26a]

Refractory Angina

There is general agreement that coronary revascularization is of proven value in patients with disabling symptoms due to transient myocardial ischemia, especially those that recur despite optimal medical therapy.[27] Optimal medical therapy is expected to be individualized for each patient, but it generally includes lifestyle modification and modification of aggravating factors such as obesity, hypertension, anemia, and smoking, in addition to dose titration of anti-ischemic medications (e.g., long-acting nitrates, calcium antagonists, β-blockers). Failure of optimal therapy implies that symptoms due to myocardial ischemia or side effects of medications result in a lifestyle that is unacceptable to the patient. After this definition has been met, the decision for revascularization is usually not difficult, assuming there are not overwhelming comorbidities or other contraindications suggesting an increased risk for complications or that the comorbidity is more likely responsible for the unacceptable lifestyle than the CAD. The comorbidities that most often limit lifestyle more than CAD are chronic pulmonary disease, peripheral vascular disease, and neurologic (e.g., dementia) or muscular (e.g., Parkinson's disease) disorders. Most patients with chronic stable symptoms have multivessel CAD and relatively well-preserved left ventricular function. Only about 3% to 5% of CCS patients have important LMCA obstruction, compared with twice this rate in patients with ACS. When properly selected, about 85% to 90% of these patients have symptoms markedly reduced with successful coronary revascularization.

High-Risk Subsets

The second group likely to benefit from revascularization is patients with findings indicating a high risk of future adverse cardiovascular outcomes. These findings can be categorized as anatomic, functional, and demographic.

Anatomic Considerations

Anatomic findings, including angiographic severity of coronary disease and left ventricular dysfunction,

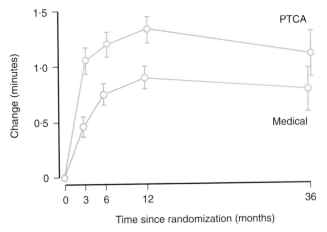

Number of patients

PTCA	469	418	425	369		154
Medical	485	446	436	399		177

Figure 17-2. Changes in Bruce exercise times (mean and standard error) for RITA-2 trial participants. (From Coronary angioplasty versus medical therapy for angina: The second Randomised Intervention Treatment of Angina (RITA-2) trial. RITA-2 trial participants. Lancet 1997;350:461-468.)

are well-established, powerful clinical predictors of long-term outcomes of patients with chronic stable angina.[3,28] The Veterans Administration Cooperative Study demonstrated improved survival in the subgroup of patients with LMCA obstruction randomized to initial surgery.[20] The ECSS Group confirmed these results.[29] As a result, the CASS and subsequent trials excluded patients with LMCA obstruction from randomization. Data from observational studies also support the beneficial effect of surgical revascularization on survival of patients with LMCA obstruction.[30] Surgery is the preferred revascularization approach in patients with LMCA obstruction. However, patients with "protected" LMCA, in which at least one patent bypass graft supplies a left coronary branch, are being treated by percutaneous revascularization with increased frequency. Data from several centers, including recent work involving drug-eluting stents and newer adjunctive pharmacotherapies, suggest that "unprotected" LMCA intervention can be performed with very low mortality and excellent procedural success in selected patients, but restenosis and late sudden death remain concerns.[31-36] Surgical revascularization for more complex bifurcation and distal LMCA anatomy continues to represent the most reliable option.

The extent of CAD was similarly associated with poor outcome in medical management arms of many of the studies evaluating revascularization in patients with stable angina. Although the results of the Veterans Administration Cooperative Study, ECSS, and CASS study were not entirely consistent with regard to the benefit of revascularization in patients with extensive disease, the meta-analysis by Yusuf and colleagues[23] demonstrated that patients with three-vessel disease and those with one- or two-vessel disease, when the proximal left anterior descending artery is involved, derive benefit from CABG. This finding appeared to be independent of LMCA stenosis or left ventricular dysfunction, although analysis of the latter subsets was limited by variable enrollment criteria. Patients deemed to be high risk based on the severity of angina, history of hypertension, MI, or ST-segment depression at rest obtained the greatest benefit in reduction of mortality (Table 17-2). Patients with one- or two-vessel disease and "low-risk profiles" appeared to do better with initial medical therapy.[23]

Left ventricular dysfunction is one of the strongest independent predictors of mortality in patients with CCS.[23] Patients with left ventricular dysfunction are more likely be of advanced age and have other comorbidities such as diabetes and multivessel disease, further affecting their prognosis. There are no randomized trials evaluating optimal therapy for patients with CCS and left ventricular dysfunction. However, limited data from smaller studies and the CASS registry suggest that revascularization in patients with left ventricular dysfunction can result in improved left ventricular function and survival.[20,37-39] The role of myocardial viability testing in daily practice is the subject of intense ongoing investigation, including the Surgical Treatment for Ischemic Heart Failure (STICH) trial. These data will provide insight into the role of intensive medical therapy compared with revascularization with or without ventricular reduction surgery in patients with left ventricular dysfunction.

Table 17-2. Effect of Extent of Coronary Disease on Outcome

Disease Extent	Mean (SE) Survival Time (mo)			P Value	P Value for Interaction
	CABG	Medical Treatment	Difference (1.96 SE)		
Overall	105.51 (0.86)	100.65 (0.97)	4.26 (2.35)	.003	
Vessel disease					
One or two vessels	107.3 (1.2)	106.2 (1.4)	1.8 (3.0)	.25	.02
Three vessels	104.7 (1.2)	98.2 (1.4)	5.7 (3.6)	.001	
Left main	99.6 (4.1)	79.8 (5.7)	19.3 (13.7)	.005	
LV function					
Normal	107.4 (0.9)	103.9 (1.0)	2.3 (2.4)	.06	.01
Abnormal	98.4 (2.2)	88.8 (2.4)	10.6 (6.1)	<.001	
Exercise test					
Missing	101.7 (2.0)	99.1 (2.0)	2.9 (5.2)	.27	.71
Normal	107.5 (1.6)	104.1 (1.8)	3.3 (4.4)	.14	
Abnormal	106.4 (1.2)	100.0 (1.4)	5.1 (3.3)	.002	
Severity of angina					
Class 0, I, II	108.1 (1.0)	104.5 (1.1)	3.3 (2.7)	.02	.16
Class III, IV	100.7 (1.6)	93.0 (1.9)	7.3 (4.8)	.002	
VA-type risk score (clinical data only)					
Low	111.6 (1.7)	112.1 (1.7)	−1.3 (4.1)	.55	.02
Moderate	108.1 (1.3)	106.6 (1.4)	2.1 (3.6)	.25	
High	101.6 (1.7)	92.8 (1.9)	7.8 (4.8)	.001	
Stepwise risk score (clinical and angiographic data)					
Low	110.0 (1.4)	111.7 (1.2)	−1.1 (3.1)	.28	.003
Moderate	108.0 (1.4)	103.1 (1.7)	5.0 (4.2)	.02	
High	98.9 (1.8)	90.0 (2.1)	8.8 (5.4)	.001	

CABG, coronary artery bypass grafting; VA, VA Cooperative Study.

Functional Considerations

Standard coronary angiography and left ventriculography provide anatomic data. However, functional data defining the severity of CAD are also important. In the Asymptomatic Cardiac Ischemia Pilot (ACIP) study, we found the presence of ischemia during stress testing and daily life identified a subgroup with a 2-year risk of death or nonfatal MI that exceeded 8%, which could be reduced with optimal revascularization (i.e., PCI or CABG).[40] A number of exercise stress test findings may be used to identify patients at high risk for adverse outcomes. Data from the CASS Registry on 5302 patients who underwent treadmill testing suggested that revascularization might be more beneficial in patients exhibiting 1 mm of ischemic-type ST-segment depression than in those without this level of ST-segment depression. Revascularization also appeared to be more beneficial in those who could exercise only to stage I or less of the Bruce protocol than in those who exercised longer.[37] The 7-year survival rate of patients in this subgroup was 58% when treated medically, compared with 81% when treated surgically. Exercise testing is valuable in patients with chronic stable angina and may even be done after coronary angiography has defined the anatomic pattern of disease. Stress radionuclide perfusion imaging and pharmacologic stress echo assessment are also useful for selected patients.[41] These tests can be performed when physical limitation, electrocardiographic abnormality that interferes with ST segments, or similar factors preclude other forms of stress testing. Stress radionuclide perfusion imaging provides important information regarding the presence of inducible ischemia, and it provides important prognostic information that is superior to the exercise stress testing or clinical data alone. Stress echocardiography provides prognostic information by examination of left ventricular wall motion and function at rest and in response to exercise.

Demographic Considerations

Other factors that interact with the severity of CAD, such as age, gender, hypertension, and diabetes, are important determinants of morbidity and mortality among patients with various anatomic and functional patterns of CAD. Unfortunately, many important issues, including the health status of the elderly and women, have not been well studied. In trials comparing CABG with medical therapy, the elderly were often excluded, and less than 5% of patients were female.[23] Because age, gender, and comorbidities such as diabetes influence revascularization risks, these considerations are important in decisions about elective intervention.[42]

Although it was previously thought that women undergoing PCI were at higher risk of death compared with men, later studies suggest that it is possible to select women who have similar long-term outcomes compared with men after PCI.[43] This has not been the case with CABG surgery; women continue to have impaired outcomes compared with men after CABG.[44] Data from our institution suggest that the cohort of women seen with chronic stable angina is typically characterized by elderly patients, most of whom have a high frequency of associated illnesses, such as diabetes, hypertension, obesity, and heart failure. Almost one half of this cohort considered to have chronic stable angina also reported angina occurring at rest, and the angina frequency was closely linked with QOL. These considerations suggest that women with chronic stable angina are more likely to be at higher risk for adverse outcomes than patients from previously reported studies who were predominantly men and younger. However, women with CCS have been shown to have a greater incidence of nonobstructive CAD, suggesting that other mechanisms may contribute to their risk.

The elderly are more likely to present with left ventricular dysfunction, multivessel CAD, and associated comorbidities such as diabetes and chronic kidney disease, placing them at higher risk for PCI and often making CABG a more desirable option. Previous studies have demonstrated an increased risk of adverse cardiovascular events in the elderly after PCI. In a prospective registry (Routine versus Selective Exercise Treadmill Testing after Angioplasty [ROSETTA] Registry) designed to evaluate the use of functional testing after PCI, patients 75 years or older were compared with those younger than 75 years old. The older cohort was found to have a higher incidence of death, cardiac death, unstable angina, MI, and the composite end point of all of these outcomes at 6 months after successful PCI. Prior CABG correlated with a higher incidence of events. These elderly patients had a much higher incidence of comorbidities at baseline, which might have explained the differences found.[45] With the advancements in interventional techniques, there has been a substantial reduction in this risk despite the presence of these comorbidities. The Alberta Provincial Project for Outcome Assessment in Coronary Heart Disease (APPROACH) provided observational data on more than 6000 patients older than 70 years, many of whom had stable angina, and it revealed a survival benefit for revascularization in the elderly. The Trial of Invasive versus Medical Therapy in Elderly Patients with Chronic Coronary Artery Disease (TIME) randomized patients older than 75 years to treatment with invasive or medical management. At 6 months, there appeared to be an improvement in the frequency of angina and in QOL and a decrease in major adverse cardiac events (MACEs).[46] By 1 year, in patients who survived the first 6 months, differences in angina and QOL were no longer significant. However, PCI was superior to medical management in reducing MACEs, specifically subsequent rehospitalization or use of revascularization (Fig. 17-3).[47]

Patients with diabetes mellitus have a worse outcome and increased risk for death from cardiovascular causes compared with nondiabetic patients. Many factors are responsible, including a higher prevalence of silent ischemia, heart failure, and mul-

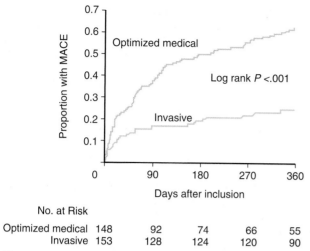

Figure 17-3. Rates of major adverse events (MACE) in the TIME trial over 1 year. (From Pfisterer M, Buser P, Osswald S, et al: Outcome of elderly patients with chronic symptomatic coronary artery disease with an invasive vs optimized medical treatment strategy: One-year results of the randomized TIME trial. JAMA 2003;289:1117-1123.)

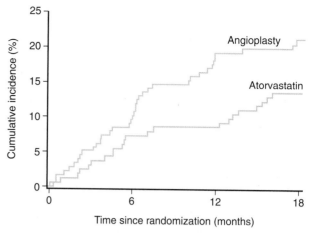

Figure 17-4. Cumulative incidence of first ischemic events in AVERT patients. (From Pitt B, Waters D, Brown WV, et al: Aggressive lipid-lowering therapy compared with angioplasty in stable coronary artery disease. Atorvastatin versus Revascularization Treatment Investigators. N Engl J Med 1999;341:70-76.)

tivessel disease. By some estimates, diabetic patients may comprise 20% to 30% of patients undergoing revascularization. Although the treatment and indications for revascularization in diabetic patients are similar to those in nondiabetic patients, the preferred method of revascularization may be different. Initially, complication rates and angiographic success were similar for diabetic and nondiabetic patients. However, PCI and CABG are associated with higher long-term event rates among diabetic patients. The Bypass Angioplasty Revascularization Investigation (BARI) and the Coronary Angioplasty vs. Bypass Revascularization Investigation (CABRI) demonstrated that CABG improved survival compared with PCI in diabetic patients.[42,48] The advantage seen with CABG was thought to reflect the higher prevalence of multivessel disease and the increased frequency of restenosis in patients undergoing PCI. The major trials of drug-eluting stents have demonstrated that the stents result in a marked reduction of restenosis in diabetic patients, suggesting that PCI may now be an acceptable option.[49,50] However, this option must be further examined in studies evaluating modern revascularization techniques in diabetic patients before any conclusions can be made.

Low-Risk Patients

Concordant with the findings of the surgical revascularization versus medical therapy trials, very-low-risk patients with coronary artery disease without ACS or demonstrable ischemia need to be triaged carefully to an invasive strategy. Results from the early stent era 341-patient Atorvastatin versus Revascularization Treatments (AVERT) trial suggested that aggressive lipid lowering with 80 mg of atorvastatin

might be as effective as PCI and usual care in reducing ischemic events during follow-up. There was a nonsignificant trend toward lower number of events and a longer time to the first ischemic event in the aggressive lipid-lowering arm (Fig. 17-4).[51] In a separate study, a small number of patients with stable coronary disease (mostly CCS class I and II angina) was randomized to PCI or to exercise training. A cohort of 101 patients younger than 70 years who had undergone a coronary angiogram were randomly assigned to PCI or to a daily 20-minute bicycle routine. After 12 months, there were fewer events and the costs for improvement in a single CCS class were less in the exercise group compared with the PCI patients.[52]

Anatomic data should interact with functional and demographic data and with clinical information (specifically symptoms) to yield information important for management. After the data are obtained, the following subgroups should be expected to have improved survival with revascularization: LMCA stenosis, triple-vessel obstruction, double-vessel obstruction involving the proximal left anterior descending artery or when a large amount of myocardium is threatened, single-vessel obstruction involving the proximal left anterior descending artery, and patients who appear to be at high risk based on risk stratification by means of noninvasive tests, such as those with ischemia provokable at low work loads or of severe magnitude. Although more contemporary trials with drug-eluting stent technology and newer adjunctive pharmacotherapies in similar patient cohorts have yet to be completed, some issues surrounding a possible increase in late stent thrombosis reinforce the need for careful patient selection and adherence to published guidelines, especially for low-risk patients.[53-56]

Percutaneous Intervention versus Coronary Artery Bypass Grafting for Stable Angina

Having established that revascularization in general is advantageous to patients with unacceptable symptoms or long-term risk, the next step is choosing a revascularization strategy. Recall from the bypass trials that surgery offered little or no benefit over medical therapy in patients with one- or two-vessel disease and otherwise low-risk profiles. However, many studies reveal that as an initial treatment for single-vessel obstruction, percutaneous revascularization offers earlier and more complete relief of angina than medical therapy, and it is associated with early improved exercise performance (6 months) at a cost of slightly more days in the hospital.

Because of vast differences in patient populations and major discrepancies in the technologies and practices employed, these trials cannot be reliably used for cross-comparison of revascularization strategies. For example, medications and indications have drastically changed. Many trials used only balloon angioplasty without intracoronary stent implantation, a technology that has revolutionized coronary intervention with respect to repeat revascularization. Only in the most recent trials have internal mammary arteries been routinely used for bypass conduits. These issues emphasize the importance of direct head-to-head comparisons, which are largely lacking because of the extreme difficulty in performing them. As a result of the relatively low event rates, these trials have to be very large and prolonged to detect differences. This represents a significant challenge because recent experience suggests that significant advances occur roughly every several years.

For historical reference, it is worth mentioning several of the key trials that directly compared bypass with balloon angioplasty (without stenting). BARI was the largest trial comparing bypass with balloon angioplasty and the only one with a primary outcome of all-cause mortality.[42] The other large trials often cited include RITA and CABRI, both of which were multicenter European trials.[25,48] The two smaller trials that merit limited attention are the German Angioplasty Bypass Surgery Investigation (GABI) and the Emory Angioplasty versus Surgery Trial (EAST).[57,58] All of these trials have enrollment criteria of significant angina or "indication for revascularization," which most commonly consisted of evidence of inducible ischemia. With the exception of BARI and GABI, all trials employed composite primary end points. GABI evaluated only "freedom from angina," and although there was a trend toward less angina after angioplasty, this trial was terminated prematurely and is not discussed further. All the remaining trials used a stenosis value of more than 50% and defined PTCA as successful if the residual stenosis was less than 50%. These definitions would no longer be acceptable end points in contemporary interventional trials. LMCA stenosis and left ventricular systolic dysfunction were exclusion criteria, but BARI and RITA did enroll unstable angina patients (approximately 50%). BARI also enrolled the patients with the highest angiographic complexity, including almost 40% type C lesions or chronic total occlusions. In-hospital events were higher among the surgical groups for effectively all the trials. Although these were modest differences, they were statistically significant and included death, MI, and stroke. The acute crossover to CABG of patients randomized to PTCA was particularly excessive by modern standards. This was later balanced by equivalent long-term outcomes, with the exception of dramatically higher rates of recurrent angina and repeat revascularization in the percutaneously treated groups. BARI was the only trial with a sample that was adequate to support subset analysis. This revealed evidence for a benefit in the form of reduced mortality associated with surgery over PTCA for patients with treated diabetes.

The next major development was the introduction of the intracoronary stent. Two of the more reliable head-to-head comparisons of PCI with CABG reported were the Arterial Revascularization Therapies Study (ARTS), a 1205-patient European randomized trial, and the 454-patient Angina With Extremely Serious Operative Mortality Evaluation (AWESOME) trial, which involved patients deemed at increased risk for perioperative complications. Both studies demonstrated that PCI was an acceptable alternative to CABG, with no difference in mortality. In ARTS, after 5 years, there was no difference in stroke or MI rates, but there was an increase in MACEs for PCI patients, which reflected repeat revascularization procedures (Fig. 17-5).[59] The AWESOME study revealed no difference in 5-year mortality or unstable angina rates between medically refractory patients treated with PCI versus CABG (Fig. 17-6). As seen in other trials, an increased rate of repeat revascularization was seen in the PCI group. At 5 years, there appeared to be a cost advantage for PCI patients.[60,61] The Surgery or Stent (SOS) trial and a second Argentine study (Argentine Randomized Trial of Percutaneous Transluminal Coronary Angioplasty versus Coronary Artery Bypass Surgery in Multivessel Disease [ERACI-2]) are worth mentioning because their findings oppose the otherwise fairly consistent findings outlined for other studies. The SOS suggested a possible mortality benefit with the use of CABG. On further analysis, it becomes apparent that the mortality rate in that arm is exceptionally low at 1% at 1-year of follow-up. Although there was still an increased rate of revascularization, the ERACI-2 suggested a mortality benefit with the use of PCI. In this study, the mortality rate for the surgical group was disproportionately high at 7.6% at 3 years, compared with 3.6% in RITA at 2.5 years.

These trials have notable limitations, mostly related to pharmacologic and technical advances. The critical nature of acute and extended antiplatelet therapy has only recently been appreciated as it relates to PCI. Stents have undergone several generations of improvement, and our understanding of technically appropriate implantation of them continues to evolve.

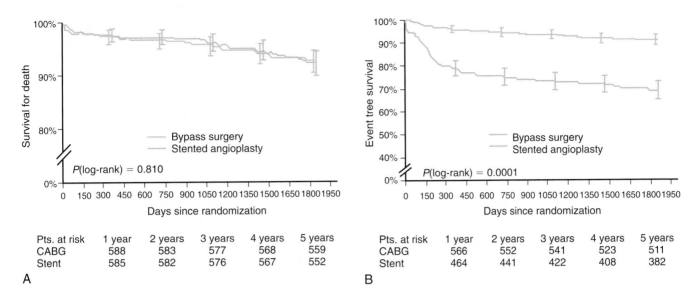

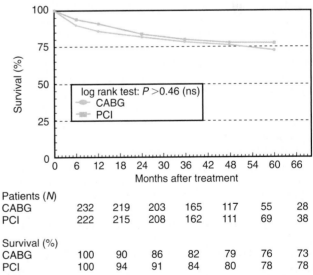

Figure 17-5. A, Kaplan-Meier curves showing freedom from death. **B,** Kaplan-Meier curves showing freedom from revascularization. CABG, coronary artery bypass grafting. (From Serruys PW, Ong AT, van Herwerden LA, et al: Five-year outcomes after coronary stenting versus bypass surgery for the treatment of multivessel disease: The final analysis of the Arterial Revascularization Therapies Study (ARTS) randomized trial. J Am Coll Cardiol 2005;46:575-581.)

Ongoing Trials and Future Directions

Stable obstructive CAD is a problem we have not yet conquered. Many ongoing studies are designed to further elucidate which patients can and should be treated with elective PCI. With the advent of drug-eluting stents, which are discussed in detail elsewhere, the latest series of trials comparing PCI with CABG are well underway. Newer and creative techniques are also being explored for previously less approachable lesions, such as bifurcations, LMCA stenosis, and chronic total occlusions, all of which are also addressed in other chapters.

Coronary Spasm

Coronary spasm as a concept began receiving significant attention in the 1950s with Prinzmetal's work on "variant angina."[62,63] His and others' suspicion that this syndrome was the result of transient increases in "tonus of the vessel wall" has been subsequently well established. Based on the early reports, the term *variant angina* has come to refer to a specific clinical syndrome consisting of recurrent episodes of chest pain (primarily at rest) and associated with ST-segment elevation. With widespread application of coronary angiography, it was recognized that spasm often does occur in the setting of chronic or intermittent ischemia, in which case ST- and T-wave changes on electrocardiography are widely variable. It is generally accepted that the syndrome is also widely variable in terms of clinical manifestations and coronary findings. The earliest reports, appearing in the late 1970s, suggested a high percentage of positive provocation study results related to clinical presentation (e.g., more than 30% in those with rest-only angina and more than 15% for all patients

studied).[64] Data from the same centers in the early 1980s and our subsequent experience suggest that coronary spasm is provoked by ergonovine at a rate of only 2% to 3% among all patients referred for coronary angiography. The most likely explanation

Figure 17-6. Kaplan-Meier survival plot of coronary artery bypass surgery (CABG) versus percutaneous coronary intervention (PCI) in the AWESOME trial. The CABG and PCI number of patients *(N)* and the percentage surviving for each time period are shown at the bottom of the plot. (From Morrison DA, Sethi G, Sacks J, et al: Percutaneous coronary intervention versus coronary artery bypass graft surgery for patients with medically refractory myocardial ischemia and risk factors for adverse outcomes with bypass: A multicenter, randomized trial. Investigators of the Department of Veterans Affairs Cooperative study no. 385, the Angina With Extremely Serious Operative Mortality Evaluation (AWESOME). J Am Coll Cardiol 2001;38:143-149.)

for this reduction in the prevalence of provocable spasm over time is the introduction of calcium antagonists and the rapid proliferation of their use. There also appears to be less well understood differences between white and Japanese populations, which could explain some variability in results from center to center.[65,66]

Most patients with spontaneous or provoked coronary spasm have objective evidence of atherosclerosis, and it is frequently obstructive. These patients merit attempts at intense modification of traditional risk factors. Cigarette smoking has been strongly associated with variant angina.[67] There may be associations with other vasospastic disorders, including migraine headaches and Raynaud's phenomenon.[68,69] Substance abuse, particularly of amphetamines and cocaine, may induce spasm and even MI in the absence of obstructive disease.[70,71] Although noninvasive tests can document transient myocardial ischemia and are useful for formulating a working diagnosis and following the response to therapy, visualization of spasm during coronary angiography is the reference standard. It is critical that true coronary spasm be differentiated from catheter-related spasm. Angiographic evidence for spasm must be associated with objective evidence for myocardial ischemia. Catheter-related spasm typically occurs at or within a centimeter of the catheter tip, and it usually does not cause transient ischemia.

The management of coronary spasm begins with lifestyle interventions such as discontinuation of substance abuse, specifically cocaine. Smoking cessation is critical, as is modification of the traditional risk factors for CAD. Long-acting nitrates and calcium antagonists have been the mainstay of medical thrapy.[72-74] Our typical practice is to start with calcium antagonists at sufficiently high dose and to add a nitrate preparation or calcium antagonist from a different class. It is unusual that we have to resort to second-line drugs, but these have been studied.[75]

Data supporting a role for mechanical revascularization in variant angina are scant at best. There are several very small case series from the PTCA era that were primarily restricted to patients with spasm superimposed on organic lesions.[76-78] Even in these select groups, recurrence of symptoms was unacceptably high. Similarly, there are scattered reports of stenting as a means to treat recalcitrant foci of spasm.[79-81] This practice has not been widely accepted or demonstrated as beneficial, which is not unexpected considering the presumed pathophysiology. Focused, local therapy would have little likelihood for success in a process that seems most consistent with a diffuse abnormality in endothelial or vascular smooth muscle function, whether it is from underlying atherosclerosis or environmental exposure. In a small series of patients with provocable vasospasm who underwent successful stenting, the 6-month follow-up provocation studies suggested a high incidence (almost 40%) of stent-edge spasm. This is additional evidence of the diffuse nature of this dis-

order, suggesting that local therapy is ineffective.[82] There is also evidence to suggest that some patients labeled as vasospastic by testing with acetylcholine actually have microvascular spasm. In these patients, there were signs of ischemia when provoked by acetylcholine in the absence of epicardial vasospasm or fixed obstructive coronary disease.[83] Based on this reasoning and the lack of compelling evidence, we do not include PCI with stenting or CABG in the routine management of coronary spasm in our institution.

Long-term results of drug-eluting stents with regard to vascular function are largely unknown, but investigations indicate that sirolimus- and paclitaxel-eluting stents suppress smooth muscle and endothelial cell replication.[84-86] Concern has been raised that drug-eluting stents have increased the incidence of late thrombosis resulting from deficient or delayed re-endothelialization.[54] Life-threatening refractory coronary spasm has been reported after the use of bare metal stents and drug-eluting stents.[84] Brachytherapy may be a useful adjunctive technique with PCI in selected refractory cases.[87] Against a background of intense antispasm therapy, revascularization may be required when severe proximal atheroma produces coronary stenosis. However, we cannot emphasize too strongly that it is essential to identify the site and extent of spasm, because we and others have observed cases with very diffuse distal coronary spasm that result in recurrent ischemia-related symptoms or occlusion of the graft or native vessel.

The prognosis associated with recognized and treated coronary spasm is generally very good when it is not associated with severe organic stenosis. Yasue and colleagues[88] described a population of 245 patients with variant angina followed for 3 to 10 years. Treatment with calcium antagonists and the extent and severity of CAD were independent predictors of survival without MI. The survival rate at 10 years was 93%.[88] Malignant arrhythmias also may complicate coronary spasm, but data regarding the impact of therapy on future events are limited to a few very small trials and case series, with conflicting results. One series of patients with spasm on medical therapy, in seven of whom implantable cardioverter-defibrillators were placed, revealed that four went on to have appropriate shocks.[89]

Silent Ischemia

Epidemiology

The initial manifestation of CAD can be exceedingly diverse. The incidence of MI manifesting with symptoms other than chest pain has been estimated at 20% to 30%, and at least one report suggested that these patients may have even worse outcomes than those with more typical symptoms.[90] Similarly, Kannel and colleagues[91] estimated that 18% of coronary events have an initial manifestation of sudden death and that women are particularly prone to this presentation. There is a growing body of literature documenting the often subtle or atypical presentation of CAD, particularly in women. Nevertheless, truly silent ischemia has been recognized for decades. Froelicher and coworkers[92] found positive exercise test results for 111 of 1390 healthy male U.S. Air Force members screened. Angiographic stenoses of 50% or greater severity were found in 34 ($\approx$2.5%).[92] The prevalence of silent ischemia appeared to increase with age in the Baltimore Longitudinal Aging Study, in which 2.5% of those younger than 60 years had positive exercise electrocardiographic or thallium studies, whereas in the population older than 70 years, the prevalence was more than 10%.[93]

Silent ischemia affects patients with no prior history of heart disease and those with documented CAD (i.e., concomitant stable angina, unstable angina, and MI). In stable postinfarction and chronic angina patients, silent myocardial ischemia has been estimated to be found on testing in at least 30% to 40%, and we and others have reported data suggesting that it is the most common manifestation of CAD in the chronic disease population, with more than 75% of ischemic episodes during daily life occurring in the absence of symptoms.[94-98]

Diagnostic Methods

There are several methods by which silent ischemia can be identified and quantified. The most accessible and therefore most commonly used modalities are exercise treadmill testing and ambulatory electrocardiographic monitoring. The electrocardiographic diagnosis of ischemia in asymptomatic patients, particularly women and patients with abnormal resting electrocardiograms (e.g., conduction disease, repolarization abnormalities), is plagued by poor specificity.[99,100] For this reason, concomitant imaging, such as echocardiography or nuclear scintigraphy, is recommended by most guidelines. Pharmacologic stress induced by an inotrope or chronotrope such as dobutamine or vasodilators such as adenosine and dipyridamole can be employed in subjects physically unable to exercise. Several other noninvasive modalities for assessing coronary anatomy and perfusion are in various levels of testing and implementation into clinical practice, including computed tomography, magnetic resonance imaging, and positron emission tomography.

Prognosis

In contrast to patients with angina, in whom palliation of symptoms is a primary objective, improving prognosis becomes the management strategy in silent myocardial ischemia. In Multiple Risk Factor Intervention Trial (MRFIT), a large, primary prevention trial that enrolled men without evidence of overt CAD, there was a 3.4-fold increase in CAD mortality among subjects with exercise electrocardiographic criteria for ischemia (Fig. 17-7).[101] The Lipid Research

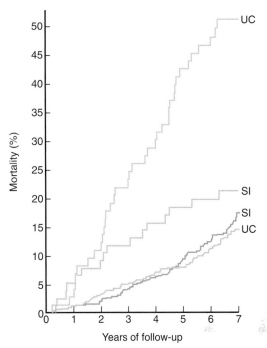

Figure 17-7. Cumulative coronary heart disease (CAD) mortality rates for participants in the Multiple Risk Factor Intervention Trial according to the presence or absence of an abnormal exercise electrocardiographic response. The *teal and purple lines* indicate men with an abnormal baseline exercise electrocardiographic response, and the *blue and pink lines* represent men with a normal exercise electrocardiographic response. SI, special-intervention group; UC, usual-care group. (From Exercise electrocardiogram and coronary heart disease mortality in the Multiple Risk Factor Intervention Trial. Multiple Risk Factor Intervention Trial Research Group. Am J Cardiol 1985;55:16-24.)

Clinics Primary Prevention Trial also revealed a relative risk of CAD mortality of 6.7 in a population of asymptomatic men with silent ischemia and hypercholesterolemia (Fig. 17-8).[102] The ACIP was a multicenter study in which we randomized 558 patients with silent myocardial ischemia and obstructive CAD to one of three treatment strategies: angina-guided medical therapy, ischemia-guided medical therapy, or revascularization. Our results are discussed throughout the remainder of this chapter, but as they relate to prognosis, we did report an association between the baseline number of ischemic episodes at enrollment and cardiac events at 1 year (Fig. 17-9).[103]

Many studies have produced similar results in asymptomatic patients with recent unstable angina or MI. Ambulatory electrocardiographic monitoring– or exercise testing–confirmed silent ischemia before discharge and at follow-up has been associated with significant increases in subsequent cardiovascular events.[96,97,104] One of the few prospectively designed studies with an adequately large sample size, the Multicenter Study of Myocardial Ischemia (MSMI), followed a cohort of 936 patients starting 1 to 6 months after hospitalization for documented MI or unstable angina. At the time of enrollment, each patient underwent exercise treadmill testing or stress

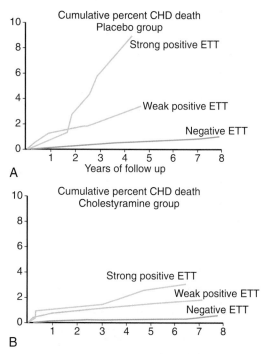

Figure 17-8. Cumulative percentage of death from coronary heart disease in men with strong, weak, and negative exercise treadmill testing (ETT) results in the placebo **(A)** and cholestyramine groups **(B)**. (From Ekelund LG, Suchindran CM, McMahon RP, et al: Coronary heart disease morbidity and mortality in hypercholesterolemic men predicted from an exercise test: The Lipid Research Clinics Coronary Primary Prevention Trial. J Am Coll Cardiol 1989;14:556-563.)

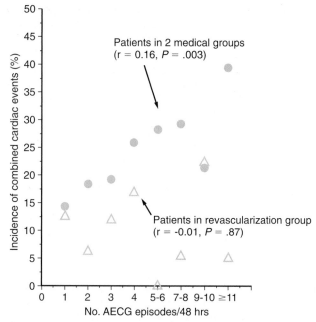

Figure 17-9. Relation between ambulatory electrocardiographic (AECG) ischemic episodes at qualifying visits and incidence of combined cardiac events between week 12 and 1 year. Patients in the two medical groups are indicated by *closed circles,* and patients in the revascularization group are indicated by *open triangles.* The *r* values represent the correlation between the number of AECG ischemic episodes and the incidence of combined cardiac events in the respective groups. (From Stone PH, Chaitman BR, Forman S, et al: Prognostic significance of myocardial ischemia detected by ambulatory electrocardiography, exercise treadmill testing, and electrocardiogram at rest to predict cardiac events by one year (the Asymptomatic Cardiac Ischemia Pilot [ACIP] study). Am J Cardiol 1997;80:1395-1401.)

thallium scintigraphy. Results of this trial contradicted the suggestion of a reduced prognosis for patients with silent ischemia. The study authors offered the possible explanation of a relatively low- to moderate-risk population.

Whether the prognosis for patients with documented ischemia further varies as a function of the presence or absence of symptoms is controversial. An early, retrospective study by Cole and Ellestad[105] analyzed 1402 patients with positive treadmill testing results. They found a doubling of the composite outcome of cardiac death, MI, or progression of angina for the subjects with symptomatic ischemia compared with those with silent ischemia.[105] Mark and associates[106] confirmed these findings in a review of 1698 consecutive patients with symptomatic CAD who had undergone exercise testing and catheterization. Although the group with painless ST-segment deviations did have an increased average annual mortality rate (2.8%) compared with the group with angina and positive exercise test results, CAD was less severe, and the overall prognosis was improved.[106] An additional confirming analysis from the MSMI trial revealed that those with silent ischemia had significantly less severe and extensive ischemia and decreased risk of cardiac events and death than those with overt symptoms.[95,107] Many reports, however,

have not found statistically significant differences in outcomes related to angina versus painless ischemia.[108-114] Despite this apparent and only relatively more benign prognosis compared with overtly symptomatic ischemia, the accumulation of these data and others confirms that silent ischemia is an indicator of increased risk.

Considering the inconvenience and side effects of medical therapy, the rare but occasionally severe complications associated with revascularization, and the absence of a palliative benefit, identifying the silently ischemic patients at the highest risk is a worthy endeavor. Laukkanen and coworkers[115] elegantly described the interactions between silent ischemia and traditional risk factors in a large population of men from eastern Finland in the Kuopio Ischemic Heart Disease (KIHD) risk factor study. Results confirmed that silent ischemia was demonstrably more predictive of acute coronary events and CAD mortality when it occurs in the setting of smoking, hypercholesterolemia, and hypertension (Fig. 17-10 and Table 17-3). Similarly, in patients who have undergone cardiac catheterization, angiographic and hemodynamic findings are presumed to be a crucial part of overall risk assess-

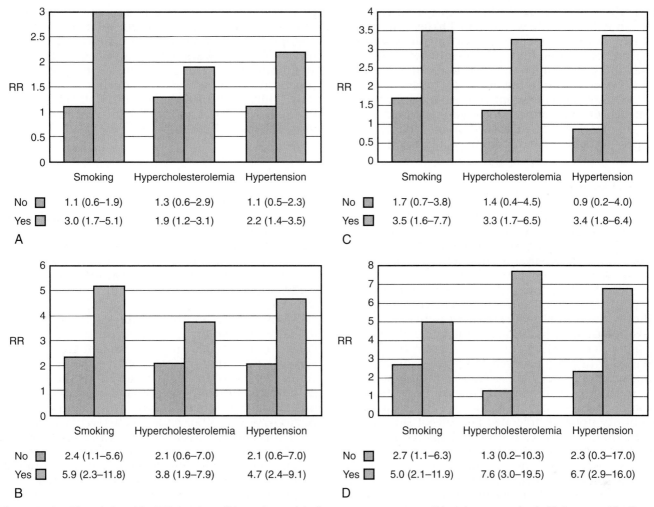

Figure 17-10. The relative risks (RR) (95% confidence intervals) of acute coronary events **(A)** and coronary death **(B)** in men with silent myocardial ischemia during exercise and the RRs of acute coronary events **(C)** and coronary death **(D)** in men with silent ischemia after exercise according to conventional risk factor levels. Men without myocardial ischemia were a reference group. The cutoff for systolic blood pressure was 132 mm Hg, and for serum low-density-lipoprotein cholesterol, it was 3.9 mmol/L. Values were adjusted for age, examination years, alcohol consumption, body mass index, maximal oxygen uptake, diabetes, cigarette smoking, systolic blood pressure, and serum low-density-lipoprotein and high-density-lipoprotein cholesterol, except the risk factor of interest. (From Laukkanen JA, Kurl S, Lakka TA, et al: Exercise-induced silent myocardial ischemia and coronary morbidity and mortality in middle-aged men. J Am Coll Cardiol 2001;38:72-79.)

Table 17-3. Interactions between Silent Ischemia and Traditional Risk Factors

Risk Factor	Acute Coronary Events*		Coronary Death		CVD Death	
	RR (95% CI)	P Value	RR (95% CI)	P Value	RR (95% CI)	P Value
Silent myocardial ischemia during exercise[†]	1.71 (1.14-2.56)	.009	3.51 (1.90-6.50)	<.001	3.26 (1.93-5.52)	<.001
Silent myocardial ischemia during recovery[†]	2.34 (1.31-4.19)	.005	4.71 (2.09-10.6)	<.001	3.67 (1.81-7.46)	<.001

*Included 91 definite and 54 possible episodes of acute myocardial infarction and 29 typical chest pain episodes (angina pectoris) lasting more than 20 minutes and leading to hospitalization.
[†]Each variable was entered separately into a Cox model with age, examination years, cigarette smoking, systolic blood pressure, alcohol consumption, body mass index, maximal oxygen uptake, diabetes, and serum low-density-lipoprotein and high-density-lipoprotein cholesterol.
CI, confidence interval; CVD, cardiovascular disease; RR, relative risk.

ment, but data, specifically in asymptomatic patients, are limited. The ACIP was designed to be a pilot study and was therefore not powered for outcomes or subset analysis, but we did find relationships between event rates and proximal left anterior descending artery or multivessel disease in the medically treated groups.[40] These results are consistent with what can be extrapolated from the data on angiographic determinants of prognosis described earlier in the chapter with respect to patients with chronic stable angina.

Medical Management

After a significantly poor prognosis has been established, therapeutic options must be addressed. As in most discussions of CAD treatment, the initial step is determining whether an invasive treatment strategy is indicated. All patients with known CAD or significant risk factors merit aggressive preventative medical therapy. In terms of pharmacotherapy specifically directed at reducing silent ischemia, studies have focused on traditional antianginal drugs such as β-blockers, calcium antagonists, and nitrates, with all used with the goal of reducing myocardial oxygen consumption. They have been used as monotherapy or in various combinations. This can be particularly helpful in cases in which higher doses of a single agent are not well tolerated because of side effects. Some questions arise. Do these drugs reduce ischemia? Does this reduction translate into reduction in adverse outcomes? The first has been addressed in several studies involving all major classes of drugs mentioned, with clear establishment that the signs of ischemia, particularly those established by ambulatory electrocardiographic monitoring, can be effectively reduced.[116-119]

The data supporting the notion that aggressive suppression of silent ischemia reduces adverse outcomes is far less robust. Comparatively, the β-blockers are the most well studied and effective class. In the Atenolol Silent Ischemia Trial (ASIST), the first randomized and placebo-controlled study to address this issue, we reported a reduction in the number of ischemic episodes and in the accumulative duration of ischemia with atenolol compared with placebo; the latter observation has not been clearly reproduced with other drug classes. We also reported an increase in event-free survival in the atenolol group (120 versus 79 days, $P = .006$).[117] However, the primary outcome in this study was a predefined composite of adverse events, including death, resuscitation from ventricular tachycardia or fibrillation, MI, unstable angina, and revascularization.[117] In a subset analysis from the Angina and Silent Ischemia Study (ASIS), amlodipine appeared particularly useful in cases not associated with increases in heart rate.[120] We found similar reductions in ischemia with β-blockers and calcium antagonists, alone and in combination, in the medical arms of the ACIP study, but we did not find statistically significant differences in outcomes between angina-guided treatment and the more aggressive ischemia-guided treatment.[121] The Angina Prognosis Study in Stockholm (APSIS) compared metoprolol with verapamil, and the Total Ischemic Burden Bisoprolol Study (TIBBS) investigators evaluated bisoprolol versus nifedipine. Both revealed the superiority of β-blockers in reducing ischemia, but only TIBBS confirmed the reduced outcomes finding of ASIST, which was an increase in event-free survival in the bisoprolol group.[122,123]

Revascularization

The data available to guide the decision about when and in whom to perform coronary revascularization on the basis of silent ischemia are scant at best. The National Institutes of Health–sponsored ACIP trial is the only randomized study performed in this specific patient population. Because it was intended as pilot study, the sample size and number of events were somewhat small. Nevertheless, we did find a statistically lower total mortality rate for those assigned to revascularization compared with the angina-guided and ischemia-guided treatment groups (1.1% versus 6.6% and 4.4%, respectively) (Fig. 17-11). Similar relationships were observed for the composite outcome of death, MI, or cardiac hospitalization (including revascularization), with rates of 23% versus 42% and 39%, respectively (Fig. 17-12).[40]

Of the patients assigned to revascularization, 92 underwent PTCA, and 78 were referred for bypass surgery. These strategies were chosen as the optimal revascularization method for the individual cases randomized to revascularization. There were four MIs and one death in the PTCA group, compared with no deaths and two MIs in the bypass group. The composite end point of death, MI, or cardiac hospitaliza-

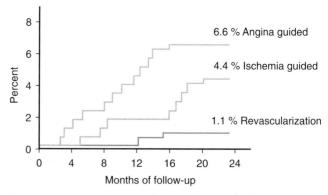

Figure 17-11. Two-year cumulative mortality rates for three treatment strategies. Significant differences were seen between revascularization and angina-guided strategies ($P < .005$) and between revascularization and ischemia-guided strategies ($P < .05$). Angina-guided and ischemia-guided strategies were not significantly different from each other ($P = .34$). (From Davies RF, Goldberg AD, Forman S, et al: Asymptomatic Cardiac Ischemia Pilot (ACIP) study two-year follow-up: Outcomes of patients randomized to initial strategies of medical therapy versus revascularization. Circulation 1997;95:2037-2043.)

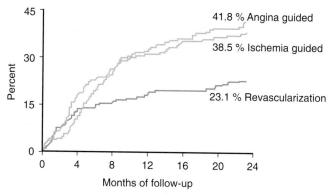

Figure 17-12. Two-year cumulative rates of death, myocardial infarction, or cardiac hospitalization. Differences were significant between revascularization strategy and both angina-guided and ischemia-guided strategies ($P < .003$). The latter were not significantly different from each other ($P = .48$). (From Davies RF, Goldberg AD, Forman S, et al: Asymptomatic Cardiac Ischemia Pilot (ACIP) study two-year follow-up: Outcomes of patients randomized to initial strategies of medical therapy versus revascularization. Circulation 1997;95:2037-2043.)

tion was 32% for PTCA and 13% for bypass. The only statistically significant difference was in the combined outcome ($P = .005$).[40] As in many other trials comparing percutaneous coronary intervention with bypass, this difference was presumably driven largely by subsequent or repeat revascularization in the angioplasty group.

Other than what we can derive from ACIP, which has unfortunately not been followed up by a larger study to confirm its results, the practicing cardiologist is left to extrapolate from the findings of the trials discussed earlier. ACIP did provide a limited analysis of some of the angiographic subgroups. In the medically treated arms, patients who had proximal left anterior descending artery or three-vessel disease had higher event rates at 2 years than those who did not; these differences were not observed in the revascularization group. The results are consistent with those of the previously described studies and with current guidelines for revascularization in stable angina.

SUMMARY

Throughout this textbook the evolving nature of PCI is evident, and pharmacotherapeutic and surgical techniques continue to improve at rapid rates. This is exciting and extremely challenging in that the recommended indications for coronary intervention must also continue to evolve. Patients with CCS, with and without symptoms, continue to represent a significant majority among the overall population of patients with cardiovascular disease. They require continued, aggressive, and specific investigation with regard to PCI. In the societal context of rising health care expenditures, it is equally as important to identify subpopulations that are least likely to derive

benefit. In this regard, it is clear that much more investigation must be done.

REFERENCES

1. Pepine CJ, Nichols WW: The pathophysiology of chronic ischemic heart disease. Clin Cardiol 2007;30:I-4-I-9.
2. Thom T, Haase N, Rosamond W, et al: Heart disease and stroke statistics—2006 Update. A report from the American Heart Association Statistics Committee and Stroke Statistics Subcommittee. Circulation 2006;113:e85-e151.
3. Silverman KJ, Grossman W: Angina pectoris. Natural history and strategies for evaluation and management. N Engl J Med 1984;310:1712-1717.
4. Kamp O, Beatt KJ, De Feyter PJ, et al: Short-, medium-, and long-term follow-up after percutaneous transluminal coronary angioplasty for stable and unstable angina pectoris. Am Heart J 1989;117:991-996.
5. Rupprecht HJ, Brennecke R, Kottmeyer M, et al: Short- and long-term outcome after PTCA in patients with stable and unstable angina. Eur Heart J 1990;11:964-973.
6. Rosengren A, Wilhelmsen L, Hagman M, Wedel H: Natural history of myocardial infarction and angina pectoris in a general population sample of middle-aged men: A 16-year follow-up of the Primary Prevention Study, Goteborg, Sweden. J Intern Med 1998;244:495-505.
7. Fox KM: Efficacy of perindopril in reduction of cardiovascular events among patients with stable coronary artery disease: Randomised, double-blind, placebo-controlled, multicentre trial (the EUROPA study). Lancet 2003;362:782-788.
8. Hjemdahl P, Eriksson SV, Held C, et al: Favourable long term prognosis in stable angina pectoris: An extended follow up of the angina prognosis study in Stockholm (APSIS). Heart 2006;92:177-182.
9. Poole-Wilson PA, Lubsen J, Kirwan BA, et al: Effect of long-acting nifedipine on mortality and cardiovascular morbidity in patients with stable angina requiring treatment (ACTION trial): Randomised controlled trial. Lancet 2004;364:849-857.
10. Braunwald E, Domanski MJ, Fowler SE, et al: Angiotensin-converting-enzyme inhibition in stable coronary artery disease. N Engl J Med 2004;351:2058-2068.
11. Daly CA, de Stavola B, Sendon JL, et al: Predicting prognosis in stable angina—Results from the Euro heart survey of stable angina: Prospective observational study. BMJ 2006;332:262-267.
12. Clayton TC, Lubsen J, Pocock SJ, et al: Risk score for predicting death, myocardial infarction, and stroke in patients with stable angina, based on a large randomised trial cohort of patients. BMJ 2005;331:869.
13. Daly C, Norrie J, Murdoch DL, et al: The value of routine non-invasive tests to predict clinical outcome in stable angina. Eur Heart J 2003;24:532-540.
14. Javitz HS, Ward MM, Watson JB, Jaana M: Cost of illness of chronic angina. Am J Manag Care 2004;10:S358-S369.
15. Shaw LJ, Merz CN, Pepine CJ, et al: The economic burden of angina in women with suspected ischemic heart disease: Results from the National Institutes of Health—National Heart, Lung, and Blood Institute–sponsored Women's Ischemia Syndrome Evaluation. Circulation 2006;114:894-904.
16. Shaw LJ, Bairey Merz CN, Pepine CJ, et al: Insights from the NHLBI-sponsored Women's Ischemia Syndrome Evaluation (WISE) study. Part I. gender differences in traditional and novel risk factors, symptom evaluation, and gender-optimized diagnostic strategies. J Am Coll Cardiol 2006;47:S4-S20.
17. Gibbons RJ, Abrams J, Chatterjee K, et al: ACC/AHA 2002 guideline update for the management of patients with chronic stable angina—Summary article: A report of the American College of Cardiology/American Heart Association Task Force on Practice Guidelines (Committee on the Management of Patients With Chronic Stable Angina). Circulation 2003;107:149-158.

18. Hueb W, Soares PR, Gersh BJ, et al: The Medicine, Angioplasty, or Surgery Study (MASS-II): A randomized, controlled clinical trial of three therapeutic strategies for multivessel coronary artery disease: One-year results. J Am Coll Cardiol 2004;43:1743-1751.

19. Boden WE, O'Rourke RA, Teo KK, et al, for the COURAGE trial Co-Principal Investigators and Study Coordinators: The evolving pattern of symptomatic coronary artery disease in the United States and Canada: baseline characteristics of the Clinical Outcomes Utilizing Revascularization and Aggressive Drug Evaluation (COURAGE) trial. J Am Coll Cardiol 2007;99:208-212.

20. Murphy ML, Hultgren HN, Detre K, et al: Treatment of chronic stable angina. A preliminary report of survival data of the randomized Veterans Administration cooperative study. N Engl J Med 1977;297:621-627.

21. Prospective randomized study of coronary artery bypass surgery in stable angina pectoris: A progress report on survival. Circulation 1982;65:67-71.

22. Coronary Artery Surgery Study (CASS): A randomized trial of coronary artery bypass surgery. Survival data. Circulation 1983;68:939-950.

23. Yusuf S, Zucker D, Peduzzi P, et al: Effect of coronary artery bypass graft surgery on survival: Overview of 10-year results from randomised trials by the Coronary Artery Bypass Graft Surgery Trialists Collaboration. Lancet 1994;344:563-570.

24. Folland ED, Hartigan PM, Parisi AF: Percutaneous transluminal coronary angioplasty versus medical therapy for stable angina pectoris: Outcomes for patients with double-vessel versus single-vessel coronary artery disease in a Veterans Affairs Cooperative randomized trial. Veterans Affairs ACME Investigators. J Am Coll Cardiol 1997;29:1505-1511.

25. Coronary angioplasty versus medical therapy for angina: The second Randomised Intervention Treatment of Angina (RITA-2) trial. RITA-2 trial participants. Lancet 1997;350:461-468.

26. Mark DB, Nelson CL, Califf RM, et al: Continuing evolution of therapy for coronary artery disease. Initial results from the era of coronary angioplasty. Circulation 1994;89: 2015-2025.

26a. Erne P, Schoenenberger AW, Burckhardt D, et al: Effects of percutaneous coronary interventions in silent ischemia after myocardial infarction: The SWISSI II randomized controlled trial. JAMA 2007;297:1985-1991.

27. Braunwald E, Antman EM, Beasley JW, et al: ACC/AHA 2002 guideline update for the management of patients with unstable angina and non-ST-segment elevation myocardial infarction—Summary article: A report of the American College of Cardiology/American Heart Association task force on practice guidelines (Committee on the Management of Patients With Unstable Angina). J Am Coll Cardiol 2002;40: 1366-1374.

28. Burggraf GW, Parker JO: Prognosis in coronary artery disease. Angiographic, hemodynamic, and clinical factors. Circulation 1975;51:146-156.

29. Varnauskas E: Twelve-year follow-up of survival in the randomized European Coronary Surgery Study. N Engl J Med 1988;319:332-337.

30. Conti CR, Selby JH, Christie LG, et al: Left main coronary artery stenosis: Clinical spectrum, pathophysiology, and management. Prog Cardiovasc Dis 1979;22:73-106.

31. Wong P, Wong V, Tse KK, et al: A prospective study of elective stenting in unprotected left main coronary disease. Catheter Cardiovasc Interv 1999;46:153-159.

32. Park SJ, Park SW, Hong MK, et al: Stenting of unprotected left main coronary artery stenoses: Immediate and late outcomes. J Am Coll Cardiol 1998;31:37-42.

33. Ellis SG, Tamai H, Nobuyoshi M, et al: Contemporary percutaneous treatment of unprotected left main coronary stenoses: Initial results from a multicenter registry analysis 1994-1996. Circulation 1997;96:3867-3872.

34. Tan WA, Tamai H, Park SJ, et al: Long-term clinical outcomes after unprotected left main trunk percutaneous revascularization in 279 patients. Circulation 2001;104:1609-1614.

35. Chieffo A, Morici N, Maisano F, et al: Percutaneous treatment with drug-eluting stent implantation versus bypass surgery for unprotected left main stenosis: A single-center experience. Circulation 2006;113:2542-2547.

36. Chieffo A, Stankovic G, Bonizzoni E, et al: Early and mid-term results of drug-eluting stent implantation in unprotected left main. Circulation 2005;111:791-795.

37. Weiner DA, Ryan TJ, McCabe CH, et al: The role of exercise testing in identifying patients with improved survival after coronary artery bypass surgery. J Am Coll Cardiol 1986;8: 741-748.

38. Passamani E, Davis KB, Gillespie MJ, Killip T: A randomized trial of coronary artery bypass surgery. Survival of patients with a low ejection fraction. N Engl J Med 1985;312: 1665-1671.

39. Alderman EL, Bourassa MG, Cohen LS, et al: Ten-year follow-up of survival and myocardial infarction in the randomized Coronary Artery Surgery Study. Circulation 1990;82: 1629-1646.

40. Davies RF, Goldberg AD, Forman S, et al: Asymptomatic Cardiac Ischemia Pilot (ACIP) study two-year follow-up: Outcomes of patients randomized to initial strategies of medical therapy versus revascularization. Circulation 1997;95: 2037-2043.

41. Ritchie JL, Bateman TM, Bonow RO, et al: Guidelines for clinical use of cardiac radionuclide imaging. Report of the American College of Cardiology/American Heart Association Task Force on Assessment of Diagnostic and Therapeutic Cardiovascular Procedures (Committee on Radionuclide Imaging), developed in collaboration with the American Society of Nuclear Cardiology. J Am Coll Cardiol 1995;25:521-547.

42. Five-year clinical and functional outcome comparing bypass surgery and angioplasty in patients with multivessel coronary disease. A multicenter randomized trial. Writing Group for the Bypass Angioplasty Revascularization Investigation (BARI) Investigators. JAMA 1997;277:715-721.

43. Malenka DJ, Wennberg DE, Quinton HA, et al: Gender-related changes in the practice and outcomes of percutaneous coronary interventions in Northern New England from 1994 to 1999. J Am Coll Cardiol 2002;40:2092-2101.

44. Humphries K, Gao M, Pu A, et al: Mortality in women after coronary artery bypass surgery really is higher. Circulation 2005;111:E42-E43.

45. Abenhaim HA, Eisenberg MJ, Schechter D, et al: Comparison of six-month outcomes of percutaneous transluminal coronary angioplasty in patients > or = 75 with those <75 years of age (the ROSETTA registry). Am J Cardiol 2001;87: 1392-1395.

46. Trial of invasive versus medical therapy in elderly patients with chronic symptomatic coronary-artery disease (TIME): A randomised trial. Lancet 2001;358:951-957.

47. Pfisterer M, Buser P, Osswald S, et al: Outcome of elderly patients with chronic symptomatic coronary artery disease with an invasive vs optimized medical treatment strategy: One-year results of the randomized TIME trial. JAMA 2003;289:1117-1123.

48. First-year results of CABRI (Coronary Angioplasty versus Bypass Revascularisation Investigation). CABRI Trial Participants. Lancet 1995;346:1179-1184.

49. Moussa I, Leon MB, Baim DS, et al: Impact of sirolimus-eluting stents on outcome in diabetic patients: A SIRIUS (SIRolImUS-coated Bx Velocity balloon-expandable stent in the treatment of patients with de novo coronary artery lesions) substudy. Circulation 2004;109:2273-2278.

50. Colombo A, Drzewiecki J, Banning A, et al: Randomized study to assess the effectiveness of slow- and moderate-release polymer-based paclitaxel-eluting stents for coronary artery lesions. Circulation 2003;108:788-794.

51. Pitt B, Waters D, Brown WV, et al: Aggressive lipid-lowering therapy compared with angioplasty in stable coronary artery disease. Atorvastatin versus Revascularization Treatment Investigators. N Engl J Med 1999;341:70-76.

52. Hambrecht R, Walther C, Mobius-Winkler S, et al: Percutaneous coronary angioplasty compared with exercise training in patients with stable coronary artery disease: A randomized trial. Circulation 2004;109:1371-1378.

53. McFadden EP, Stabile E, Regar E, et al: Late thrombosis in drug-eluting coronary stents after discontinuation of antiplatelet therapy. Lancet 2004;364:1519-1521.

54. Nordmann AJ, Briel M, Bucher HC: Mortality in randomized controlled trials comparing drug-eluting vs. bare metal stents in coronary artery disease: A meta-analysis. Eur Heart J 2006;27:2784-2814.

55. Joner M, Finn AV, Farb A, et al: Pathology of drug-eluting stents in humans: Delayed healing and late thrombotic risk. J Am Coll Cardiol 2006;48:193-202.

56. Smith SC Jr, Feldman TE, Hirshfeld JW Jr, et al: ACC/AHA/SCAI 2005 Guideline Update for Percutaneous Coronary Intervention—Summary article: A report of the American College of Cardiology/American Heart Association Task Force on Practice Guidelines (ACC/AHA/SCAI Writing Committee to Update the 2001 Guidelines for Percutaneous Coronary Intervention). Circulation 2006;113:156-175.

57. Hamm CW, Reimers J, Ischinger T, et al: A randomized study of coronary angioplasty compared with bypass surgery in patients with symptomatic multivessel coronary disease. German Angioplasty Bypass Surgery Investigation (GABI). N Engl J Med 1994;331:1037-1043.

58. King SB 3rd, Kosinski AS, Guyton RA, et al: Eight-year mortality in the Emory Angioplasty versus Surgery Trial (EAST). J Am Coll Cardiol 2000;35:1116-1121.

59. Serruys PW, Ong AT, van Herwerden LA, et al: Five-year outcomes after coronary stenting versus bypass surgery for the treatment of multivessel disease: The final analysis of the Arterial Revascularization Therapies Study (ARTS) randomized trial. J Am Coll Cardiol 2005;46:575-581.

60. Morrison DA, Sethi G, Sacks J, et al: Percutaneous coronary intervention versus coronary artery bypass graft surgery for patients with medically refractory myocardial ischemia and risk factors for adverse outcomes with bypass: A multicenter, randomized trial. Investigators of the Department of Veterans Affairs Cooperative study no. 385, the Angina With Extremely Serious Operative Mortality Evaluation (AWESOME). J Am Coll Cardiol 2001;38:143-149.

61. Stroupe KT, Morrison DA, Hlatky MA, et al: Cost-effectiveness of coronary artery bypass grafts versus percutaneous coronary intervention for revascularization of high-risk patients. Circulation 2006;114:1251-1257.

62. Prinzmetal M, Kennamer R, Merliss R, et al: Angina pectoris. I. A variant form of angina pectoris; preliminary report. Am J Med 1959;27:375-388.

63. Prinzmetal M, Ekmecki A, Toyoshima H, Kwoczynski JK: Angina pectoris. III. Demonstration of a chemical origin of ST deviation in classic angina pectoris, its variant form, early myocardial infarction, and some noncardiac conditions. Am J Cardiol 1959;3:276-293.

64. Glazier JJ, Faxon DP, Melidossian C, Ryan TJ: The changing face of coronary artery spasm: A decade of experience. Am Heart J 1988;116:572-576.

65. Sueda S, Kohno H, Fukuda H, et al: Frequency of provoked coronary spasms in patients undergoing coronary arteriography using a spasm provocation test via intracoronary administration of ergonovine. Angiology 2004;55:403-411.

66. Sueda S, Ochi N, Kawada H, et al: Frequency of provoked coronary vasospasm in patients undergoing coronary arteriography with spasm provocation test of acetylcholine. Am J Cardiol 1999;83:1186-1190.

67. Sugiishi M, Takatsu F: Cigarette smoking is a major risk factor for coronary spasm. Circulation 1993;87:76-79.

68. Nakamura Y, Shinozaki N, Hirasawa M, et al: Prevalence of migraine and Raynaud's phenomenon in Japanese patients with vasospastic angina. Jpn Circ J 2000;64:239-242.

69. Rosamond W: Are migraine and coronary heart disease associated? An epidemiologic review. Headache 2004;44(Suppl 1):S5-S12.

70. Hung MJ, Kuo LT, Cherng WJ: Amphetamine-related acute myocardial infarction due to coronary artery spasm. Int J Clin Pract 2003;57:62-64.

71. Lange RA, Cigarroa RG, Yancy CW Jr, et al: Cocaine-induced coronary-artery vasoconstriction. N Engl J Med 1989;321:1557-1562.

72. Opie LH: Calcium channel antagonists in the management of anginal syndromes: Changing concepts in relation to the role of coronary vasospasm. Prog Cardiovasc Dis 1996;38:291-314.

73. Lombardi M, Morales MA, Michelassi C, et al: Efficacy of isosorbide-5-mononitrate versus nifedipine in preventing spontaneous and ergonovine-induced myocardial ischaemia. A double-blind, placebo-controlled study. Eur Heart J 1993;14:845-851.

74. Chahine RA, Feldman RL, Giles TD, et al: Randomized placebo-controlled trial of amlodipine in vasospastic angina. Amlodipine Study 160 Group. J Am Coll Cardiol 1993;21:1365-1370.

75. Yasue H, Touyama M, Kato H, et al: Prinzmetal's variant form of angina as a manifestation of alpha-adrenergic receptor-mediated coronary artery spasm: Documentation by coronary arteriography. Am Heart J 1976;91:148-155.

76. Corcos T, David PR, Bourassa MG, et al: Percutaneous transluminal coronary angioplasty for the treatment of variant angina. J Am Coll Cardiol 1985;5:1046-1054.

77. David PR, Waters DD, Scholl JM, et al: Percutaneous transluminal coronary angioplasty in patients with variant angina. Circulation 1982;66:695-702.

78. Leisch F, Herbinger W, Brucke P: Role of percutaneous transluminal coronary angioplasty in patients with variant angina and coexistent coronary stenosis refractory to maximal medical therapy. Clin Cardiol 1984;7:654-659.

79. Jeong MH, Park JC, Rhew JY, et al: Successful management of intractable coronary spasm with a coronary stent. Jpn Circ J 2000;64:897-900.

80. Khatri S, Webb JG, Carere RG, Dodek A: Stenting for coronary artery spasm. Catheter Cardiovasc Interv 2002;56:16-20.

81. Kultursay H, Can L, Payzin S, et al: A rare indication for stenting: Persistent coronary artery spasm. Heart Vessels 1996;11:165-168.

82. Kaku B, Honin IK, Horita Y, et al: The incidence of stent-edge spasm after stent implantation in patients with or without vasospastic angina pectoris. Int Heart J 2005;46:23-33.

83. Sun H, Mohri M, Shimokawa H, et al: Coronary microvascular spasm causes myocardial ischemia in patients with vasospastic angina. J Am Coll Cardiol 2002;39:847-851.

84. Togni M, Windecker S, Cocchia R, et al: Sirolimus-eluting stents associated with paradoxic coronary vasoconstriction. J Am Coll Cardiol 2005;46:231-236.

85. Virmani R, Liistro F, Stankovic G, et al: Mechanism of late in-stent restenosis after implantation of a paclitaxel derivate-eluting polymer stent system in humans. Circulation 2002;106:2649-2651.

86. Wheatcroft S, Byrne J, Thomas M, MacCarthy P: Life-threatening coronary artery spasm following sirolimus-eluting stent deployment. J Am Coll Cardiol 2006;47:1911-1912; author reply 1912-1913.

87. Erne P, Jamshidi P, Juelke P, et al: Brachytherapy: Potential therapy for refractory coronary spasm. J Am Coll Cardiol 2004;44:1415-1419.

88. Yasue H, Takizawa A, Nagao M, et al: Long-term prognosis for patients with variant angina and influential factors. Circulation 1988;78:1-9.

89. Meisel SR, Mazur A, Chetboun I, et al: Usefulness of implantable cardioverter-defibrillators in refractory variant angina pectoris complicated by ventricular fibrillation in patients with angiographically normal coronary arteries. Am J Cardiol 2002;89:1114-1116.

90. Dorsch MF, Lawrance RA, Sapsford RJ, et al: Poor prognosis of patients presenting with symptomatic myocardial infarction but without chest pain. Heart 2001;86:494-498.

91. Kannel WB: Prevalence and clinical aspects of unrecognized myocardial infarction and sudden unexpected death. Circulation 1987;75:II4-II5.

92. Froelicher VF, Thompson AJ, Longo MR Jr, et al: Value of exercise testing for screening asymptomatic men for latent coronary artery disease. Prog Cardiovasc Dis 1976;18:265-276.

93. Fleg JL, Gerstenblith G, Zonderman AB, et al: Prevalence and prognostic significance of exercise-induced silent myocardial

ischemia detected by thallium scintigraphy and electrocardiography in asymptomatic volunteers. Circulation 1990; 81:428-436.

94. Schang SJ Jr, Pepine CJ: Transient asymptomatic S-T segment depression during daily activity. Am J Cardiol 1977;39: 396-402.

95. Narins CR, Zareba W, Moss AJ, et al: Clinical implications of silent versus symptomatic exercise-induced myocardial ischemia in patients with stable coronary disease. J Am Coll Cardiol 1997;29:756-763.

96. Gottlieb SO, Gottlieb SH, Achuff SC, et al: Silent ischemia on Holter monitoring predicts mortality in high-risk postinfarction patients. JAMA 1988;259:1030-1035.

97. Tzivoni D, Gavish A, Zin D, et al: Prognostic significance of ischemic episodes in patients with previous myocardial infarction. Am J Cardiol 1988;62:661-664.

98. Deedwania PC, Carbajal EV: Prevalence and patterns of silent myocardial ischemia during daily life in stable angina patients receiving conventional antianginal drug therapy. Am J Cardiol 1990;65:1090-1096.

99. Morise AP, Diamond GA: Comparison of the sensitivity and specificity of exercise electrocardiography in biased and unbiased populations of men and women. Am Heart J 1995;130:741-747.

100. Orzan F, Garcia E, Mathur VS, Hall RJ: Is the treadmill exercise test useful for evaluating coronary artery disease in patients with complete left bundle branch block? Am J Cardiol 1978;42:36-40.

101. Exercise electrocardiogram and coronary heart disease mortality in the Multiple Risk Factor Intervention Trial. Multiple Risk Factor Intervention Trial Research Group. Am J Cardiol 1985;55:16-24.

102. Ekelund LG, Suchindran CM, McMahon RP, et al: Coronary heart disease morbidity and mortality in hypercholesterolemic men predicted from an exercise test: The Lipid Research Clinics Coronary Primary Prevention Trial. J Am Coll Cardiol 1989;14:556-563.

103. Stone PH, Chaitman BR, Forman S, et al: Prognostic significance of myocardial ischemia detected by ambulatory electrocardiography, exercise treadmill testing, and electrocardiogram at rest to predict cardiac events by one year (the Asymptomatic Cardiac Ischemia Pilot [ACIP] study). Am J Cardiol 1997;80:1395-1401.

104. Deedwania PC: Asymptomatic ischemia during predischarge Holter monitoring predicts poor prognosis in the postinfarction period. Am J Cardiol 1993;71:859-861.

105. Cole JP, Ellestad MH: Significance of chest pain during treadmill exercise: Correlation with coronary events. Am J Cardiol 1978;41:227-232.

106. Mark DB, Hlatky MA, Califf RM, et al: Painless exercise ST deviation on the treadmill: long-term prognosis. J Am Coll Cardiol 1989;14:885-892.

107. Moss AJ, Goldstein RE, Hall WJ, et al: Detection and significance of myocardial ischemia in stable patients after recovery from an acute coronary event. Multicenter Myocardial Ischemia Research Group. JAMA 1993;269:2379-2385.

108. Heller LI, Tresgallo M, Sciacca RR, et al: Prognostic significance of silent myocardial ischemia on a thallium stress test. Am J Cardiol 1990;65:718-721.

109. Travin MI, Flores AR, Boucher CA, et al: Silent versus symptomatic ischemia during a thallium-201 exercise test. Am J Cardiol 1991;68:1600-1608.

110. Bonow RO, Bacharach SL, Green MV, et al: Prognostic implications of symptomatic versus asymptomatic (silent) myocardial ischemia induced by exercise in mildly symptomatic and in asymptomatic patients with angiographically documented coronary artery disease. Am J Cardiol 1987;60: 778-783.

111. Falcone C, de Servi S, Poma E, et al: Clinical significance of exercise-induced silent myocardial ischemia in patients with coronary artery disease. J Am Coll Cardiol 1987;9:295-299.

112. Dagenais GR, Rouleau JR, Hochart P, et al: Survival with painless strongly positive exercise electrocardiogram. Am J Cardiol 1988;62:892-895.

113. Callaham PR, Froelicher VF, Klein J, et al: Exercise-induced silent ischemia: Age, diabetes mellitus, previous myocardial infarction and prognosis. J Am Coll Cardiol 1989;14: 1175-1180.

114. Breitenbucher A, Pfisterer M, Hoffmann A, Burckhardt D: Long-term follow-up of patients with silent ischemia during exercise radionuclide angiography. J Am Coll Cardiol 1990;15:999-1003.

115. Laukkanen JA, Kurl S, Lakka TA, et al: Exercise-induced silent myocardial ischemia and coronary morbidity and mortality in middle-aged men. J Am Coll Cardiol 2001;38:72-79.

116. Knatterud GL, Bourassa MG, Pepine CJ, et al: Effects of treatment strategies to suppress ischemia in patients with coronary artery disease: 12-week results of the Asymptomatic Cardiac Ischemia Pilot (ACIP) study. J Am Coll Cardiol 1994;24:11-20.

117. Pepine CJ, Cohn PF, Deedwania PC, et al: Effects of treatment on outcome in mildly symptomatic patients with ischemia during daily life. The Atenolol Silent Ischemia Study (ASIST). Circulation 1994;90:762-768.

118. Deedwania PC, Carbajal EV, Nelson JR, Hait H: Anti-ischemic effects of atenolol versus nifedipine in patients with coronary artery disease and ambulatory silent ischemia. J Am Coll Cardiol 1991;17:963-969.

119. Stone PH, Gibson RS, Glasser SP, et al: Comparison of propranolol, diltiazem, and nifedipine in the treatment of ambulatory ischemia in patients with stable angina. Differential effects on ambulatory ischemia, exercise performance, and anginal symptoms. The ASIS Study Group. Circulation 1990;82:1962-1972.

120. Andrews TC, Fenton T, Toyosaki N, et al: Subsets of ambulatory myocardial ischemia based on heart rate activity. Circadian distribution and response to anti-ischemic medication. The Angina and Silent Ischemia Study Group (ASIS). Circulation 1993;88:92-100.

121. Pratt CM, McMahon RP, Goldstein S, et al: Comparison of subgroups assigned to medical regimens used to suppress cardiac ischemia (the Asymptomatic Cardiac Ischemia Pilot [ACIP] Study). Am J Cardiol 1996;77:1302-1309.

122. Forslund L, Hjemdahl P, Held C, et al: Prognostic implications of ambulatory myocardial ischemia and arrhythmias and relations to ischemia on exercise in chronic stable angina pectoris (the Angina Prognosis Study in Stockholm [APSIS]). Am J Cardiol 1999;84:1151-1157.

123. Von Arnim T: Prognostic significance of transient ischemic episodes: Response to treatment shows improved prognosis. Results of the Total Ischemic Burden Bisoprolol Study (TIBBS) follow-up. J Am Coll Cardiol 1996;28:20-24.

18 Percutaneous Intervention for Non-ST-Segment Elevation Acute Coronary Syndromes

P. J. de Feyter

KEY POINTS

- Risk assessment at admission and repeated during hospital stay is essential.
- High-risk indicators for progression to acute myocardial infarction (MI) or death are recurrent chest pain, dynamic ST-segment changes, elevated troponin I or T levels, hemodynamic and electrical instability, early post-MI angina, and diabetes mellitus.
- Markers of severe underlying disease important for long-term prognosis are age older than 65 years, history of known coronary artery disease, congestive heart failure, pulmonary edema, new mitral regurgitation, elevated

  levels of inflammatory markers (e.g., C-reactive protein, fibrinogen, interleukin-6), levels of brain natriuretic peptide (BNP) or N-terminal proBNP in upper quartiles, and renal insufficiency.
- High-risk patients are recommended for an early invasive strategy, including coronary angiography and revascularization.
- Low- or intermediate-risk patients are recommended for an initial conservative strategy and ischemia-guided revascularization.

The continuing evolution of the technique of percutaneous coronary intervention (PCI) from balloon to stent implantation to drug-eluting stents combined with adjunctive pharmacologic treatment has broadened the clinical indications for intervention to include patients with stable angina pectoris or acute coronary syndrome (ACS).[1-3]

An ACS is classified as a non-ST-segment elevation ACS (NSTE-ACS) or as an ST-segment elevation ACS (STE-ACS). NSTE-ACS includes patients with unstable angina or non-ST-segment elevation myocardial infarction (NSTEMI), and STE-ACS includes patients with ST-segment elevation myocardial infarction (STEMI). The most appropriate strategy to treat NSTE-ACS patients is still contentious. The European Society of Cardiology (ESC) guidelines[4] and the American College of Cardiology/American Heart Association (ACC/AHA) guidelines[5] recommend an invasive strategy for patients at high-risk, whereas the AHA/ACC guidelines[5] recommend that an interventional strategy or a conservative medical strategy is appropriate for patients at intermediate risk, and

both guidelines recommend an initially conservative approach for patients at low risk.[4,5] Clinical practice differs from the guideline recommendations, and in large-scale international registries, only 25% to 28% of patients with NSTEMI and 18% with unstable angina underwent PCI during hospitalization.[6,7]

In this chapter, we discuss PCI for patients with NSTE-ACS and focus on the pathophysiology and consequences for PCI, risk stratification, adjunctive treatment during PCI, early invasive versus conservative strategy, and the ESC and AHA/ACC guidelines for management of patients with NSTE-ACS.

RATIONALE FOR PERCUTANEOUS CORONARY INTERVENTION IN PATIENTS WITH NON-ST-SEGMENT ELEVATION ACUTE CORONARY SYNDROME

Atherothrombosis is a chronic disease in which cholesterol deposition, inflammation, and intracoronary thrombosis play major roles.[8] Over the years, coronary atherosclerosis silently evolves clinically, which

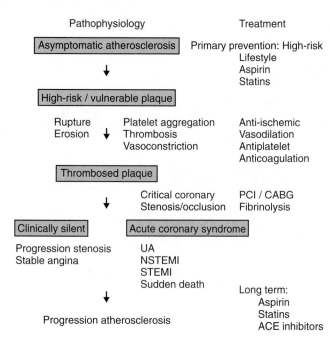

Figure 18-1. Physiopathologic mechanisms underlying acute coronary syndromes. ACE, angiotensin-converting enzyme; CABG, coronary artery bypass grafting; NSTEMI, non-ST-segment elevation myocardial infarction; PCI, percutaneous coronary intervention; STEMI, ST-segment elevation myocardial infarction; UA, unstable angina.

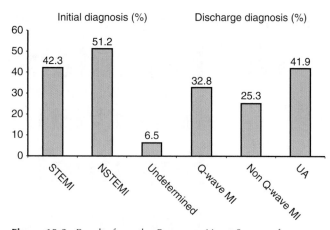

Figure 18-2. Results from the European Heart Survey of acute coronary syndromes in 10.484 patients. MI, myocardial infarction; NSTEMI, non-ST-segment elevation myocardial infarction; STEMI, ST-segment elevation myocardial infarction; UA, unstable angina.

Scope of the Problem

ACS is a major health care problem worldwide. A prospective survey conducted in 103 hospitals and 25 countries in Europe, the European Heart Survey ACS Registry, collected data from 10,484 patients with ACS enrolled during an 8-month period.[7] The initial diagnosis and hospital discharge diagnosis are shown in Figure 18-2. Most patients presented with an initial diagnosis of NSTEMI, and at discharge, most had had unstable angina. The Global Registry of Acute Coronary Events (GRACE Registry) obtained data from 11,543 patients from 18 population-based clusters in 14 countries worldwide and demonstrated that unstable angina was the most frequent presentation at admission and at discharge (Fig. 18-3).[6]

The frequency of invasive procedures in patients with ACS collected in the European Heart Survey-Acute Coronary Syndrome (EHS-ACS) survey is presented in Table 18-1. Approximately one half of these patients underwent coronary angiography, and revas-

eventually may result in the development of a high-risk (i.e., vulnerable) plaque (Fig. 18-1). Rupture or erosion of this high-risk plaque triggers the formation of intracoronary thrombosis and turns the high-risk plaque into a thrombosed plaque, causing a critical stenosis or occlusion of the coronary artery. Although the stenosis may evolve silently, healing may lead to progression of the stenosis, which may occur asymptomatically or may cause angina pectoris. This may cause an ACS with different clinical presentations: unstable angina, NSTEMI, STEMI, and sudden death. All ACS clinical manifestations share a common pathophysiologic pathway, but the duration (i.e., transient or permanent) and severity (i.e., subtotal or total coronary occlusion) are different, not leading to myocardial necrosis (i.e., no troponin or CK-MB release) and clinically manifested as unstable angina or causing myocardial necrosis manifested as NSTEMI or STEMI.

In the first few months after an initial episode of clinical coronary instability, there is a strong tendency for repeat instability caused by progression of the severity of the culprit stenosis or by progression of remote lesions.

The optimal management of unstable angina or NSTEMI has the twin goals of the immediate relief of ischemia and the prevention of progression to acute MI or cardiac death. This can be achieved by a combination of anti-ischemic, antiplatelet, and antithrombotic therapy and invasive procedures (see Fig. 18-1).

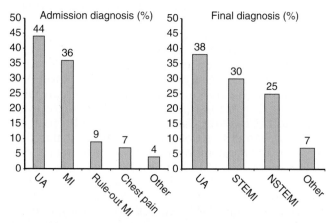

Figure 18-3. Global Registration of Acute Coronary Events (GRACE: 11.543 patients). MI, myocardial infarction; NSTEMI, non-ST-segment elevation myocardial infarction; STEMI, ST-segment elevation myocardial infarction; UA, unstable angina.

Table 18-1. Invasive Procedures Performed in 10,484 Patients in the European Heart Survey of Acute Coronary Syndromes

Type of Disease	Coronary Angiography (%)	Percutaneous Coronary Intervention (%)	Coronary Artery Bypass Grafting (%)
ST-segment elevation myocardial infarction (STEMI)	56.3	40.4	3.4
Non-ST-segment elevation myocardial infarction (NSTEMI)	52.0	25.4	5.4

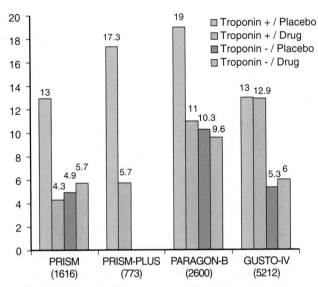

Figure 18-4. The 30-day incidence of death or myocardial infarction (%) in several trials.

Table 18-2. In-Hospital Death or Recurrent Myocardial Infarction

Type of Disease	In-Hospital Death		Reinfarction	
	GRACE (%)	EHS-ACS (%)	GRACE (%)	EHS-ACS (%)
STEMI	7	7	3	2.7
NSTEMI	6	2.4	2	1.4
UA	3	—	—	—
Undetermined ECG	—	11.8	—	1.7

ECG, electrocardiogram; EHS-ACS, European Heart Survey of Acute Coronary Syndromes; GRACE, Global Registry of Acute Coronary Events; NSTEMI, non-ST-segment elevation myocardial infarction; STEMI, ST-segment elevation myocardial infarction; UA, unstable angina.

cularization was performed in a relatively small proportion of NSTEMI patients.

Prognostic data from the EHS-ACS survey and the GRACE survey indicated that the in-hospital mortality and reinfarction rates varied among the various ACS clinical manifestations (Table 18-2)[6,7] but were higher among patients with STEMI. The 30-day mortality rate reported in the EHS-ACS survey was 8.4% for patients with STEMI, 3.5% for those with NSTEMI, and 13.3% for patients with undetermined electrocardiograms.[7]

Prognostic data from some large trials indicated that the 30-day incidence of death and MI varied considerably between control patients at high risk (i.e., troponin positive) and those at low risk (i.e., troponin negative) (Fig. 18-4).[9-12]

Risk Stratification

The risks for patients with NSTE-ACS vary greatly. Various practical risk scores have been developed. The Thrombolysis in Myocardial Infarction (TIMI) risk score, which predicts the risk of 14-day all-cause mortality and new or recurrent MI, is useful for the identification of patients at high risk who may benefit from early revascularization (Fig. 18-5).[13]

The GRACE Registry developed a risk calculator for bedside risk estimation of 6-month mortality for patients after hospitalization for ACS.[14] The overall 6-month mortality rate was 4.8%. Nine predictive variables were identified: older age, previous MI, history of heart failure, increased heart rate, lower systolic blood pressure, serum creatinine level, elevated levels of cardiac biomarkers, ST-segment depression, and no PCI (Fig. 18-6). The estimation of risk at admission is essential, but during hospital admission, the risk may change, and it should be repeatedly assessed.

- Age ≥65 yr
- ≥Anginal events
- ST-segment deviation
- Elevated serum cardiac markers
- ≥3 factors CAD
- Aspirin use (prior 7 days)
- Prior coronary stenosis (>50%)

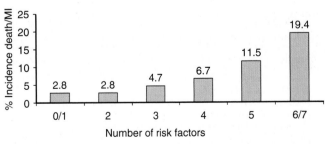

Figure 18-5. The TIMI trial risk score for death or myocardial infarction at 14 days. CAD, coronary artery disease. Score is derived by assigning a value of 0 when a factor is absent and 1 when a factor is present.

1 Age in years   Points
  30 - 39 0
  40 - 49 18
  50 - 59 36
  60 - 69 55
  70 - 79 73
  80 - 89 91
  ≥90 100

2 History of congestive
  heart failure 24

3 History of myocardial
  infarction 12

4 Resting heart rate   Points
  beats / min
  50 - 70 3
  70 - 90 9
  90 - 110 14
  110 - 150 23
  150 - 200 35
  ≥200 43

5 Systolic blood pressure
  mm Hg
  ≤79.9 24
  80 - 99.9 22
  100 - 120 18
  120 - 140 14
  140 - 160 10
  160 - 200 4
  ≥200 0

6 St-segment
  Depression 11

7 Initial serum creatine   Points
  mg/dL
  0 - 0.39 1
  0.4 - 0.79 3
  0.8 - 1.19 5
  1.2 - 1.59 7
  1.6 - 1.99 9
  2.3 - 3.99 15
  ≥4 20

8 Elevated cardiac
  enzymes 15

9 No in-hospital percutaneous
  coronary intervention 14

A

Points
  1............
  2............
  3............
  4............
  5............
  6............
  7............
  8............
  9............

Total risk score_____(Sum of points)
Mortality risk_____(from plot)

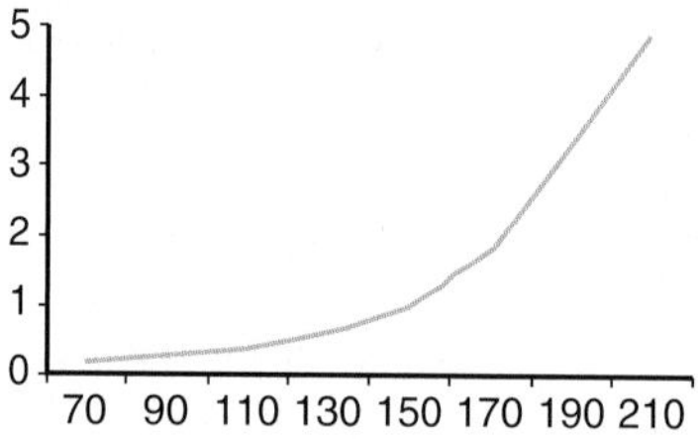

B

Figure 18-6. A, The GRACE Registry developed a risk calculator for bedside risk estimation of 6-month mortality in patients after hospitalization for acute coronary syndrome. **B,** Plot of predicted all-cause mortality.

Predicting a Late Positive Serum Troponin Level in Initially Troponin-Negative Patients with Non-ST-Segment Elevation Acute Coronary Syndrome

It would be valuable to predict which initially troponin-negative patients may have the highest likelihood for a rise in serum troponin levels at 12 hours. Of 1342 patients who were enrolled in the TIMI-IIIB trial, 200 (14.9%) were troponin negative at baseline but developed an elevated troponin I level (≥0.4 ng/mL) at 12 hours.[15] Six independent predictors were identified (Table 18-3), and a score was derived to identify patients with the highest likelihood to become troponin positive later during hospital admis-

sion (Fig. 18-7). The derived score was tested in 855 patients in the Global Use of Strategies To Open Occluded Arteries in Acute Coronary Syndromes IIA (GUSTO IIA) study and similarly predicted a late rise in troponin T levels. This score should help in triage and treatment decision-making for patients presenting with NSTE-ACS who have initially negative values for troponin levels.

ADJUNCTIVE TREATMENT DURING PERCUTANEOUS CORONARY INTERVENTION FOR NON-ST-SEGMENT ELEVATION ACUTE CORONARY SYNDROME

Antiplatelet Treatment

Double-antiplatelet therapy with acetylsalicylic acid (ASA) and clopidogrel is considered standard pretreatment of patients with NSTE-ACS undergoing PCI with or without stent implantation. The optimal timing for initiating clopidogrel is still a matter of debate. The frequency of adverse events is reduced within the first hours of treatment with clopidogrel, but if the patient is referred for surgery, this approach may be associated with more perioperative blood loss.[16] However, given the fact that the need for coronary artery bypass grafting (CABG) is less likely to be necessary even for high-risk NSTE-ACS patients, early

Table 18-3. Predictors of Late Troponin Level Rise in Initially Troponin-Negative Patients

Predictor*	OR	95% CI	P Value
ST-segment deviation	3.52	2.38 to 5.23	<.001
Presentation <8 hr from symptom onset	2.91	1.92 to 4.40	<.001
No prior percutaneous coronary intervention	2.88	1.54 to 5.39	.001
No prior beta blockade	1.74	1.15 to 2.63	.008
Unheralded angina	1.65	1.12 to 2.42	.01
History of myocardial infarction	1.59	1.06 to 2.37	.02

*Late is defined as 12 hours or more.

Table 18-4. ACUITY Trial Results

End Point (30 days)	UFH/Enox + GPI (n = 4603)	Bivalirudin + GPI (n = 4604)	Bivalirduin Alone (n = 4612)	P Value
Net outcome (%)	11.7	11.8	10.1	.0014
Ischemic composite (%)	7.3	7.7	7.8	NS
Major bleeding (%)	5.7	5.3	3.0	<.0001

Enox, enoxaprin; GPI, GP IIb/IIIa inhibitor; NS, not significant; UFH, unfractionated heparin.

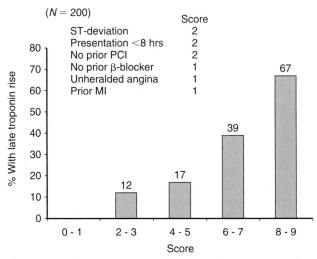

Figure 18-7. The TIMI-III B score used to identify patients who become troponin positive later during hospital admission. MI, myocardial infarction; PCI, percutaneous coronary intervention.

clopidogrel treatment is recommended unless the need for urgent CABG is more likely.

The recommended loading dose of ASA is 500 mg given orally more than 6 hours before the procedure or at least 300 mg administered intravenously directly before the procedure.[4] The recommended loading dose of clopidogrel is 300 mg given at least 6 hours before the procedure or a loading dose of 600 mg administered at least 2 hours before PCI. After the acute phase, the combination of 100 mg/day of ASA and 75 mg/day of clopidogrel during the next 6 to 12 months is recommended. Lifelong ASA treatment may be beneficial.

Anticoagulant Treatment

Since the beginning of PCI, unfractionated heparin (UFH) has been given to prevent thrombosis during intracoronary instrumentation and to minimize thrombosis at the site of the plaque, which is damaged by balloon angioplasty or stent implantation. Treatment with UFH in addition to ASA usually is given based on the data from a meta-analysis demonstrating a reduction of the combined death and MI rate of 7.9% for those treated with UFH compared with 10.3% for those treated with ASA alone.[17] UFH is given as an initial intravenous bolus, usually as 100 IU/kg and guided by the activating clotting time (ACT) in the range of 250 to 300 seconds. If combined with a GP IIb/IIIa inhibitor, the dose of UFH

should be lower: initial intravenous bolus of 50 to 60 IU/kg and ACT in the range of 200 to 250 seconds to prevent excessive bleeding complications. The place of low-molecular-weight heparin (LMWH) in the setting of PCI for NSTE-ACS is controversial. The ESC guidelines prefer to use UFH in high-risk NSTE-ACS patients with planned invasive strategy because of the easy reversibility of UFH by the administration of protamine. However, the AHA/ACC guidelines consider enoxaparin (a LMWH) to be a reliable alternative to UFH.

The role of a direct thrombin inhibitor, bivalirudin, is evolving. The Randomized Evaluation in PCI Linking Angiomax to Reduced Clinical Events II (REPLACE II) trial demonstrated that bivalirudin could be used as an alternative to UFH plus GP IIb/IIIa blockade in patients at low risk who undergo PCI. The efficacy of bivalirudin was further evaluated in the Acute Catheterization and Urgent Intervention Triage Strategy (ACUITY) trial. The ACUITY trial randomized 13,800 patients with moderate- to high-risk unstable angina or NSTEMI undergoing an invasive strategy. There were three treatment groups. Group I received UFH or enoxaparin plus GPI, group II received bivalirudin plus a GP IIb/IIIa inhibitor, and group III received bivalirudin alone. The primary end point at 30 days was a net clinical outcome based on an ischemic composite (i.e., death any cause, MI, or unplanned revascularization for ischemia) or major bleeding. The net outcome was lower with the bivalirudin-alone strategy, which could be ascribed to a significant reduction in major bleeding in the bivalirudin group (Table 18-4).

Glycoprotein IIb/IIIa Inhibitors

In general, the use of GP IIb/IIIa inhibitors (e.g., abciximab, eptifibatide, tirofiban) is recommended in patients undergoing PCI who are at high risk for acute thrombotic complications,[4,5] based on information extracted from GP IIb/IIIa inhibitor studies with planned PCI for NSTE-ACS (Tables 18-5 and 18-6).[18-24] However, in the Evaluation of Platelet IIb/IIIa Inhibitor for Stenting (EPISTENT) and Enhanced Suppression of the Platelet IIb/IIIa Receptor with Integrilin Therapy (ESPRIT) trials, respectively, 43% and 49% of the patients had stable angina. It has been shown that troponin release is associated with an increased risk of major adverse events and that the beneficial effects of GP IIb/IIIa inhibitors are significant in patients with troponin release, whereas the efficacy of GP IIb/IIIa inhibitors is small or non-

Table 18-5. Abciximab with Planned Percutaneous Coronary Intervention in Four Trials

Characteristic	CAPTURE	EPIC	EPILOG	EPISTENT
No. of patients	1265	2099	2792	2399
Primary end point	Death, MI, reintervention	Death, MI, reintervention	Death, MI, urgent revascularization	Death, MI, unplanned revascularization
Time (days)	30	30	30	30
Placebo/drug (%)	15.9/11.3 $P < .05$	12.8/11.4/8.3* $P < .05$	11.7/5.2/5.4* $P < .05$	10.8/5.3/6.9[†] $P < .05$

*Placebo/bolus/bolus + infusion.
[†]Stent + placebo/stent + drug/balloon + drug.
CAPTURE, c7E3 Fab Antiplatelet Therapy in Unstable Refractory Angina; EPIC, Evaluation of 7E3 for the Prevention of Ischemic Complications; EPILOG, Evaluation in Percutaneous Transluminal Coronary Angioplasty to Improve Long-Term Outcome with Abciximab GP IIb/IIIa Blockade; EPISTENT, Evaluation of Platelet IIb/IIIa Inhibitor for Stenting; MI, myocardial infarction.

existent in patients without troponin release (see Fig. 18-4).

Abciximab has been most frequently tested in the setting of NSTEMI ACS and planned PCI. Abciximab has been the preferred GP IIb/IIIa inhibitor by many interventionists. This position was re-enforced by the outcome of the Do Tirofiban and Reopro Give Similar Efficacy Outcomes Trial? (TARGET). The TARGET, a direct comparison of the efficacy of abciximab with that of tirofiban, demonstrated that the primary end point (i.e., composite of death, nonfatal MI, or urgent revascularization at 30 days) was significantly higher in the tirofiban group compared with those receiving abciximab (7.6% versus 6.0%), but at 6 months, this difference was no longer statistically significant.[25]

The high costs of abciximab treatment compared with the costs of tirofiban and eptifibatide has been as issue, particularly in many European countries. The choice is important in case of a bleeding complication or the necessity for urgent bypass surgery. The return of platelet function toward a physiologic state (≤50% inhibition) occurs 12 hours after cessation of abciximab, in contrast to 4 hours with the use of tirofiban and eptifibatide. These factors have favored the use tirofiban or eptifibatide.

Which GP IIb/IIIa inhibitor may be used at upstream management when a patient with NSTE-ACS presents to the hospital, and which GP IIb/IIIa inhibitor should be used during the PCI procedure? There is evidence that tirofiban and eptifibatide show benefit in the upstream management[26,27] and that either abciximab or eptifibatide may be initiated in the catheterization laboratory.

Abciximab in Patients Pretreated Clopidogrel

It was believed that the efficacy of GP IIb/IIIa inhibitors was reduced in patients pretreated with clopidogrel. The Intracoronary Stenting and Antithrombotic Regimen: Rapid Early Action for Coronary Treatment-2 (ISAR-REACT-2) trial addressed this issue. ISAR-REACT-2 was a randomized, double-blind trial of a treatment with abciximab ($n = 1012$) or placebo ($n = 1010$) of patients with NSTE-ACS[28] who were treated with a 600-mg loading dose of clopidogrel. The primary end point was a composite of death, MI, and urgent target vessel revascularization due to myocardial ischemia at 30 days. There was a significant reduction in the primary end point in favor of abciximab in all patients with NSTE-ACS, and this was achieved with no difference in TIMI-defined major bleeding (1.4% versus 1.4%) (Fig. 18-8). Abciximab was highly effective in high-risk NSTE-ACS patients (i.e., troponin positive) but not effective in troponin-negative patients.

EARLY INVASIVE STRATEGY VERSUS CONSERVATIVE STRATEGY FOR PATIENTS WITH NON-ST-SEGMENT ELEVATION ACUTE CORONARY SYNDROME

Two approaches—an early invasive strategy or a conservative strategy—are used for the management of NSTE-ACS. An early invasive strategy involves the use of early coronary angiography and revascularization with PCI or CABG. A conservative strategy involves initial treatment with aggressive pharmacologic treat-

Table 18-6. Eptifibatide and Tirofiban with Planned Percutaneous Coronary Intervention in Three Trials

Characteristic	ESPRIT (Eptifibatide)	IMPACT-II (Eptifibatide)	RESTORE (Tirofiban)
No. of patients	2064	4010	2212
Primary end point	Death, MI, urgent TVR, bailout GP IIb/IIIa	Death, MI, unplanned revascularization, bailout stenting	Death, MI, reintervention, bailout stenting
Time (days)	1	30	30
Placebo/drug (%)	10.5/6.6 $P < .05$	11.4/9.2/9.9*	12.2/10.3

*Placebo/bolus + low dose/bolus + high dose.
GP, glycoprotein; ESPRIT, Enhanced Suppression of the Platelet IIb/IIIa Receptor with Integrilin Therapy; IMPACT-II, Integrilin to Minimise Platelet Aggregation and Coronary Thrombosis-II; MI, myocardial infarction; RESTORE, Randomized Efficacy Study of Tirofiban for Outcomes and REstenosis; TVR, target vessel revascularization.

Table 18-7. Outcomes of Percutaneous Coronary Intervention in Five Trials

Characteristic	FRISC II (N = 2457) (1222/1235)*	TACTICS (N = 2220) (1114/1106)	VINO (N = 131) (64/67)	RITA-3 (N = 1810) (895/915)	ICTUS (N = 1200) (604/596)
Mean age (yr)	65	62	66	63	62
Men (%)	70	66	61	62	62
Diabetes (%)	12	28	25	13	14
Previous MI (%)	22	39	26	39	23
Mean follow-up (mo)	24	6	6	24	12
Invasive/selective revascularization					
At end FU	78/43	61/44	73/39	57/28	79/54
PCI at FU	44/21	42/29	52/13	36/16	61/40
CABG at FU	38/23	22/16	35/30	22/12	18/14

*Early invasive versus conservative strategy.
CABG, coronary artery bypass grafting; FRISC-II, Fast Revascularization during Instability of Coronary Artery Disease-II; FU, follow-up; ICTUS, Invasive Conservative Treatment in Unstable Coronary Syndromes; MI, myocardial infarction; PCI, percutaneous coronary intervention; RITA-3, Randomized Intervention Trial of Unstable Angina; TACTICS, Treat Angina with Aggrastat and Determine Cost of Therapy with an Invasive or Conservative Strategy; VINO, Value of First Day Angiography/Angioplasty In Evolving Non-ST-segment Elevation Myocardial Infarction: an Open Multicenter Randomized Trial.

ment, and coronary angiography with revascularization is used if there is evidence of ischemia spontaneously recurring or provoked during stress testing.

The efficacy of each strategy was tested in the earlier days of PCI, before the use of coronary stents and adjunctive treatment with GP IIb/IIIa inhibition. These studies—TIMI-IIIB, Veterans Affairs Non-Q-Wave Myocardial Infarction Strategies In Hospital (VANQWISH), and Medicine versus Angiography in Thrombolytic Exclusion (MATE)—showed no superiority for either strategy.[29-31] After these trials, the outcome of PCI was improved by the use of stents and adjunctive treatment with thienopyridines and GP IIb/IIIa inhibitors. This prompted the initiation of additional randomized trials: The Fast Revascularization during Instability of Coronary Artery Disease-II (FRISC-II) trial, the Treat Angina with Aggrastat and Determine Cost of Therapy with an Invasive or Conservative Strategy–Thrombolysis in Myocardial Infarction (TACTICS-TIMI 18) trial, the Value of First-Day Angiography/Angioplasty in Evolving Non-ST-Segment Elevation Myocardial Infarction: An Open Multicenter Randomized Trial (VINO), the Random-

ized Intervention Trial of Unstable Angina-3 (RITA-3), and the Invasive versus Conservative Treatment in Unstable Coronary Syndromes (ICTUS) trial. The characteristics of these trials are presented in Table 18-7.[32-36]

With the early invasive strategy approach, early revascularization (in hospital) was achieved in 44% to 76% of the patients, whereas with the conservative strategy, an early revascularization was deemed necessary in 9% to 40% of the patients (Fig. 18-9). The contrast in the frequencies of early revascularization between the early invasive strategy and conservative strategy varied from as low as 24% (TACTICS) to as high as 62% (FRISC-II). Revascularization after hospital discharge was predominantly performed in the patients randomized to an early conservative strategy. The rate of the primary end point of the various trials, defined as a composite of death and MI with or without rehospitalization, was statistically significant in favor of an early invasive strategy in all trials except the RITA-3 and ICTUS trials (Table 18-8). The in-hospital mortality rate and combined in-hospital mortality or nonfatal MI rates are shown in Figures 18-10 and 18-11. The mortality and the combined mortality or nonfatal MI rates at the end of follow-up are presented in Figures 18-12 and 18-13. The RITA-3 trial reported the outcome at a median follow-up of 5 years (Table 18-9).[37] At 1 year, the death and non-

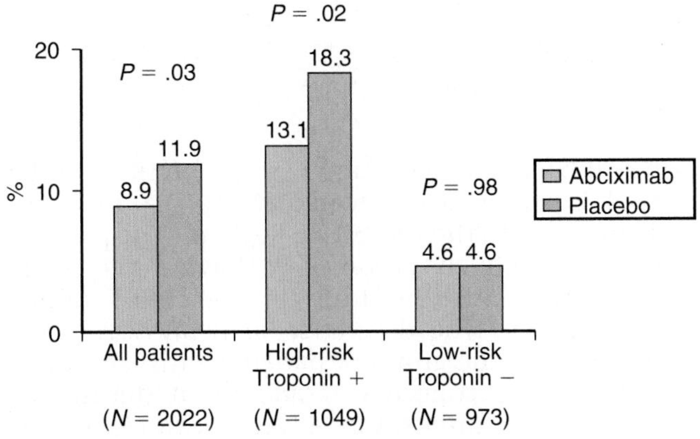

Figure 18-8. Results of the ISAR-REACT 2 trial, comparing abciximab with placebo.

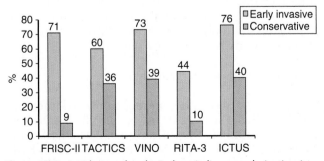

Figure 18-9. Incidence of early (in-hospital) revascularization in several trials.

Table 18-8. Early Invasive versus Conservative Strategies in Five Trials

Trial	Primary End Point	Early Invasive	Conservative	RR or OR	CI 95%, *P* Value
FRISC-II	Death/MI at 1 yr	10.4%	14.1%	RR = 0.74	CI: 0.60 to 0.92 P = .005
TACTICS	Death/MI/rehosp. for ACS at 6 mo	15.9%	19.4%	OR = 0.78	CI: 0.62 to 0.97 P = .025
VINO	Death/MI at 6 mo	6.2%	22.3%		P < .001
RITA-3	Death/MI at 1 yr	7.6%	8.3%	RR = 0.91	CI: 0.67 to 1.25 P = .58
ICTUS	Death/MI/rehosp. <1 yr	22.7%	21.2%	RR = 1.07	CI: 0.87 to 0.133 P = .33

ACS, acute coronary syndrome; FRISC-II, Fast Revascularization during Instability of Coronary Artery Disease-II; ICTUS, Invasive Conservative Treatment in Unstable Coronary Syndromes; MI, myocardial infarction; PCI, percutaneous coronary intervention; RITA-3, Randomized Intervention Trial of Unstable Angina; TACTICS, Treat Angina with Aggrastat and Determine Cost of Therapy with an Invasive or Conservative Strategy; VINO, Value of First Day Angiography/Angioplasty In Evolving Non-ST-segment Elevation Myocardial Infarction: an Open Multicenter Randomized Trial.

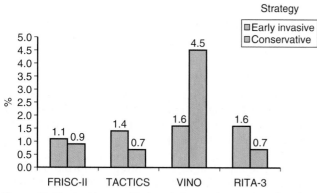

Figure 18-10. Incidence of in-hospital mortality in several trials.

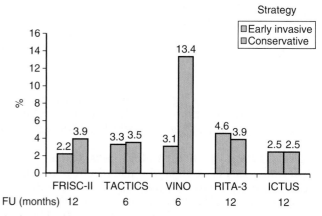

Figure 18-12. Incidence of mortality at the end of follow-up (FU) in several trials.

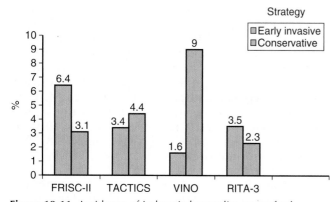

Figure 18-11. Incidence of in-hospital mortality or nonfatal myocardial infarction in several trials.

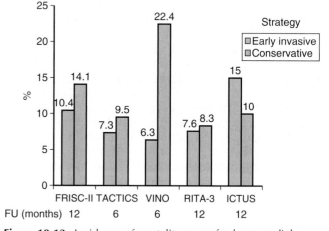

Figure 18-13. Incidence of mortality or nonfatal myocardial infarction at the end follow-up (FU) in several trials.

fatal MI rates were not different between the early invasive strategy and the conservative strategy, but at 5 years, there was a significant difference in favor of the early invasive strategy (Fig. 18-14).

Optimal Timing of Intervention

Few data exist about the optimal timing of intervention in patients with NSTE-ACS. The CRUSADE Registry (Can Rapid Risk Stratification of Unstable Angina Patients Suppress Adverse Outcomes with Early Implementation of the ACC/AHA Guidelines?) investigated whether the outcomes of early catheteriza-

tion and later catheterization were different.[38] A total of 56,352 patients were treated at 310 U.S. hospitals and entered into the CRUSADE Registry. The patients were retrospectively classified as having very early (23.4 hours) catheterization or later (46.3 hours) catheterization. The difference in delay was introduced because the group of patients with later catheterization was collected at admission during the weekend. The in-hospital adverse cardiac events occurring in the two groups are presented in Table 18-10. There was no difference between the two

Table 18-9. RITA-3 Trial Outcomes at a Median Follow-up of 5 Years

Outcome	Early Intervention (*n* = 895)	Conservative Strategy (*n* = 915)	RR, 95% CI, and *P* Value
Follow-up years			
1 yr death/MI	7.6%	8.3%	0.91 (0.67 to 1.25)
5 yr death/MI	16.6%	20.0%	0.78 (0.61 to 0.99), *P* = .044
Death	12.1%	15.1%	0.76 (0.58 to 1.0), *P* = .054
Cardiovasc. death	7.3%	10.6%	0.68 (0.49 to 0.95) *P* = .026
Cardiovasc. death or MI	12.2%	15.9%	0.74 (0.56 to 0.97) *P* = .030

*The benefit is mainly in the high-risk subgroup.
MI, mycoardial infarction.
From Fox KA, Poole-Wilson P, Clayton TC, et al: 5-Year outcome of an interventional strategy in non-ST-elevation acute coronary syndrome: The British Heart Foundation RITA 3 randomised trial. Lancet 2005;366:914-920.

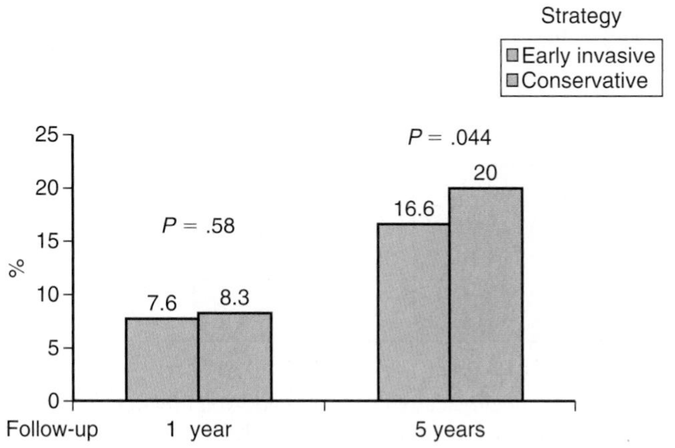

Figure 18-14. Incidence of death or nonfatal myocardial infarction at 5 years' follow-up from the RITA-3 trial.

Table 18-10. Timing of Intervention in Patients with NSTEMI Acute Coronary Syndrome in the CRUSADE Registry

	Timing of Catheterization		
In-Hospital Events	46.3 Hours (*n* = 10,804)	23.4 Hours (*n* = 45,548)	*P* Value
Death (%)	4.4	4.1	.23
Recurrent MI (%)	2.9	3.0	.36
Death/MI (%)	6.6	6.6	.86

CRUSADE, Can Rapid Risk Stratification of Unstable Angina Patients Suppress Adverse Outcomes with Early Implementation of the ACC/AHA guidelines [National Quality Improvement Initiative and Registry]; MI, myocardial infarction, NSTEMI, non-ST-segment elevation myocardial infarction.

groups, but the investigators warned cautiously that they could not exclude an important risk reduction, particularly for early catheterization within 12 hours of presentation.

This issue was addressed in the Intracoronary Stenting with Antithrombotic Regimen COOLing-off (ISAR-COOL) trial.[39] This trial randomized 410 patients who had symptoms of unstable angina plus ST-segment depression or elevation of cardiac troponin T levels. Patients were randomized to antithrombotic pretreatment for 3 to 5 days (the cooling-off

strategy) or very early intervention after pretreatment for less than 6 hours. Antithrombotic pretreatment consisted of heparin, aspirin, clopidogrel, and tirofiban. The outcome is presented in Table 18-11. There was a significant reduction in the combined death and MI rate in favor of the very early intervention strategy. This favorable outcome was predominantly attributable to adverse events occurring before catheterization.

The Early or Late Intervention in Unstable Angina (ELISA) pilot study investigated whether pretreat-

Table 18-11. Outcomes of the ISAR-COOL Trial

Outcome Characteristic	Prolonged Antithrombotic Pretreatment (%) (*n* = 207)	Early Intervention (%) (*n* = 203)	*P* Value
Definitive treatment			
Conservative	28.0	21.7	
CABG	7.7	7.9	
PCI (stents)	64.3	70.4	
30 Days			
Death/MI	11.6	5.9	.04
Death	1.4	0	.25
Non-fatal MI	10.1	5.9	.12
Q-wave	3.4	2.0	
Non-Q-wave	6.8	3.9	
Major bleeding event	3.9	3.0	.61

CABG, coronary artery bypass grafting; ISAR-COOL, Intracoronary Stenting with Antithrombotic Regimen COOLing-off; MI, myocardial infarction; PCI, percutaneous intervention.

ment with a GP IIb/IIIa inhibitor, tirofiban, was beneficial compared with no pretreatment.[40] Two hundred twenty patients with NSTE-ACS were randomized to an early strategy (i.e., early angiography without tirofiban pretreatment) or to a late strategy (i.e., delayed angiography after pretreatment with tirofiban). The primary end point was enzymatic infarct size (LDHQ48) as assessed by the area under the lactate dehydrogenase release curve up to 48 hours after symptom onset. The infarct size and clinical outcome at 30 days are presented (Table 18-12). The study showed that delayed angiography with pretreatment with tirofiban was associated with a smaller enzymatic infarct size. There were no differences in clinical outcome at 30 days.

The CRUSADE quality improvement initiative investigated the use of an early invasive management within 48 hours in 17,926 high-risk NSTEMI patients (Table 18-13).[41] A total of 8037 patients (44.8%) underwent early cardiac catheterization, and of these, 75% were revascularized: 4733 (58.9%) underwent PCI, and 1296 (16.1%) underwent CABG. The unadjusted incidence of in-hospital mortality and postadmission MI was significantly lower for patients who underwent early invasive management than for those not undergoing early invasive management. Patients who underwent early invasive management were younger and had less comorbidity. The adjusted risks for death and MI were lower for patients who underwent early invasive management. In a propensity-

matched pair analysis, the mortality rate remained lower for patients who underwent early invasive management (2.5% versus 3.7%, $P < .01$).

Benefits from Early Invasive Treatment

The FRISC-II and TACTICS trials demonstrated that almost all benefits from an invasive strategy were achieved for the patients with elevated levels of troponin (Figs. 18-15 and 18-16), whereas patients without elevated troponin levels gain little from an

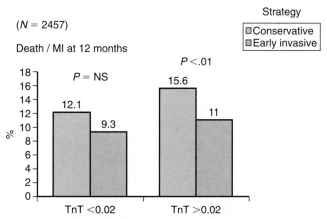

Figure 18-15. Incidence of death or myocardial infarction (MI) in high-risk and low-risk groups from the FRISC II trial ($N = 2457$). TnT, troponin levels.

Table 18-12. Outcomes of the ELISA Pilot Study

Outcome Characteristic	Early Strategy* (n = 109)	Delayed Strategy† (n = 111)
Median time to angiography	6 hr	50 hr
Treatment		
PCI (%)	61	58
CABG (%)	14	19
Conservative (%)	25	23
30-Day clinical outcome of death/MI (%)	9.2	9.0
Enzymatic infarct size (LDHQ48)	629 ± 503	432 ± 441 (P = .02)

*Early angiography and no pretreatment.
†Delayed angiography (24-48 hr) and pretreatment with tirofiban.
CABG, coronary artery bypass grafting; ELISA, Early or Late Intervention in unStable Angina; LDHQ48, cumulative enzyme release up to 48 hours after symptom onset as assessed by the area under the lactate dehydrogenase release curve; MI, myocardial infarction; PCI, percutaneous intervention.

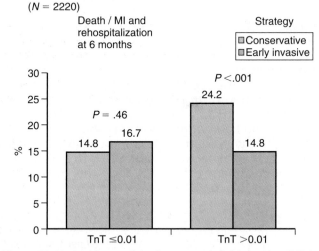

Figure 18-16. Incidence of death or myocardial infarction (MI) in high-risk and low-risk groups from the TACTICS-18 trial.

Table 18-13. Outcomes of the CRUSADE Trial: In-Hospital Death or Myocardial Infarction

Outcome	No Early Invasive Management (n = 9889)	Early Invasive Management (n = 8037)	Adjusted Odds Ratio (95% CI)
Mortality (%)	6.2	2.0	0.63 (0.52 to 0.77)
Post-admission MI (%)	3.7	3.1	0.95 (0.79 to 1.14)
Death or MI (%)	8.9	4.7	0.79 (0.69 to 0.90)

CRUSADE, Can Rapid Risk Stratification of Unstable Angina Patients Suppress Adverse Outcomes with Early Implementation of the ACC/AHA Guidelines; MI, myocardial infarction.

Table 18-14. Rates of Death, Myocardial Infarction, or Rehospitalization for Acute Coronary Syndrome Stratified by TIMI Risk Score

TIMI Risk Score	Event Rate (%)		OR	95% CI
	Invasive	Conservative		
Low (0-2)	19.8	15.1	1.39	1.02 to 1.88
Intermediate (3-4)	18.2	21.8	0.80	0.64 to 0.99
High (5-7)	22.7	34	0.57	0.38 to 0.87

TIMI, Thrombolysis in Myocardial Infarction trial; MI, myocardial infarction; TACTICS, Treat Angina with Aggrastat and Determine Cost of Therapy with an Invasive or Conservative Strategy trial.
Data from TIMI IIIb[15] and TACTICS-TIMI 18[33] trials.

early invasive approach.[32,33] In the TACTICS trial, it was shown that an early invasive strategy had relatively little benefit in patients with an intermediate risk, but for patients with a high TIMI risk score, this strategy was highly effective (Table 18-14).

Based on the evidence, it appears that using an early invasive strategy for high-risk patients with NSTE-ACS is superior to reduce major adverse cardiac events than using a conservative strategy. The overall mortality or combined mortality and MI rates at the end of follow-up of the pooled data from the FRISC, TACTICS, VINO, RITA-3 (1-year follow-up), and ICTUS trials were 3.6% for the early invasive strategy versus 4.7% for the conservative strategy and 10.6% versus 12.4%, respectively. In particular, patients with elevated troponin levels or with high-risk indicators benefit from an early invasive approach in combination with adjunctive treatment with a platelet GP IIb/IIIa inhibitor before, during, and after PCI. Lower-risk patients have almost similar outcomes with either strategy.

Early Invasive Strategy in Women

The benefit of using an early invasive strategy for treating women is achieved primarily in women with high-risk features such as ST-segment changes or elevated troponin levels. Women who were managed with very early aggressive revascularization had a better long-term outcome than men.[42] The combined end point of death and nonfatal MI was significantly reduced at a follow-up of 20 months for women compared with men (OR = 0.65; 95% CI: 0.28 to 0.92).

DRUG-ELUTING STENTS FOR PATIENTS WITH NON-ST-SEGMENT ELEVATION ACUTE CORONARY SYNDROME

No study has exclusively investigated the safety and efficacy of drug-eluting stent (DES) implantation in patients with NSTE-ACS. In various randomized trials comparing the efficacy of DES with that of bare stents to reduce the restenosis and target vessel revascularization rates, the reported proportions of patients with unstable coronary artery disease were between 30% and 50%.[43-46] Although many variables were studied that predicted early in-hospital complications or target vessel revascularization, the presence of unstable coronary artery disease was not reported as a predictive factor. In a subanalysis of the Rapamycin-Eluting Stent Evaluated At Rotterdam Cardiology Hospital (RESEARCH) Registry investigating the safety and efficacy of sirolimus-eluting stents, it was shown that sirolimus stenting in patients with unstable angina and those with stable angina was associated with an almost similar risk reduction in the need for target vessel revascularization compared with bare metal stenting.[47] The hazard ratio at 1 year of clinically driven target vessel revascularization for DES was 0.30 (95% CI: 0.13 to 0.71; $P < .0006$) compared with bare metal stenting. The Basel Stent Kosten Effektivitäts Trial (BASKET) demonstrated that there were fewer adverse cardiac events for patients ($n = 301$) with NSTE-ACS receiving a DES than for those with a bare metal stent.[48]

It may be concluded that the safety and efficacy of DES implantation is similar in patients presenting with stable or unstable coronary artery disease. However, because of delayed healing after DES and the effects of stent implantation in a highly unstable thrombotic milieu, the use of thienopyridines should be continued for at least 6 months (probably 1 year) after DES implantation.

STATINS AND PERCUTANEOUS CORONARY INTERVENTION FOR NON-ST-SEGMENT ELEVATION ACUTE CORONARY SYNDROME

The Myocardial Ischemia Reduction with Aggressive Cholesterol Lowering (MIRACL) trial randomized 3086 patients with unstable coronary artery disease to early treatment with 80 mg of atorvastatin ($n = 1355$) or placebo ($n = 1384$).[49] At 16 weeks, the primary end point (i.e., composite of death, nonfatal MI, cardiac arrest, and recurrent ischemia) occurred in 14.8% in the atorvastatin group and 17.4% in the placebo group ($P = .048$). Only 16% of these patients underwent revascularization.

In the Pravastatin or Atorvastatin Evaluation and Infection Therapy–Thrombolysis In Myocardial Infarction-22 (PROVE IT-TIMI-22) trial, intensive statin treatment in patients hospitalized for an acute coronary syndrome was compared with standard statin therapy.[50] The combined primary end point was death of any cause, MI, documented unstable angina rehospitalization, revascularization (performed at least 30 days after randomization), and stroke. The trial randomized 4162 patients to intensive statin treatment (80 mg of atorvastatin daily, $n = 2099$) or to pravastatin (40 mg, $n = 2063$). Sixty-nine percent of these patients underwent PCI for the treatment of their index acute coronary syndrome before randomization. Three fourths of these patients underwent an early invasive strategy. The low-density-lipoprotein (LDL) cholesterol levels were 106 mg/dL before treatment in each group. The primary end point at the end of follow-up (mean, 24 months) was reached in 22.4% the intensive atorvastatin group and 26.3% in the standard-dose pravastatin group ($P = .005$). The difference in treatment effect started at 30 days, which confirmed the results with statin treatment in the MIRACL trial.

In the Lescol Intervention Prevention Study (LIPS), 1669 patients were randomized to receive 80 mg of fluvastatin or placebo, with treatment starting 2 days after successful PCI.[51] The LIPS study showed that the statin-treated group had a significantly lower incidence of adverse clinical events (24.1%) than the placebo group (26.7%, $P = .01$).

Early and post-PCI statin therapy is beneficial to reduce the adverse coronary event rate. According to the ACC/AHA guidelines, LDL cholesterol reduction is recommended when the level is higher than 130 mg/dL or when, after diet, the LDL level is higher than 100 mg/dL for all patients with an ACS, with or without undergoing revascularization.

MANAGEMENT OF PATIENTS WITH NON-ST-SEGMENT ELEVATION ACUTE CORONARY SYNDROME

American College of Cardiology/American Heart Association Guidelines

NSTE-ACS patients have a wide spectrum of clinical presentations and risks for mortality and morbidity. Risk is considered the most important driver of management decisions, and early risk assessment and repeated risk assessment are based on age, history, character of pain, clinical and electrocardiographic findings, and cardiac markers. The risk level is classified as high, intermediate, or low (Table 18-15), and further management is guided by risk classification. Anti-ischemic treatment together with antiplatelet and anticoagulant treatment forms the cornerstone of management of patients with NSTE-ACS. Antiplatelet treatment consisting of aspirin, clopidogrel, and a platelet GP IIb/IIIa inhibitor is recommended for patients with planned coronary angiography and PCI, and combined treatment with aspirin and clopidogrel is recommended for patients with an early noninterventional approach. Anticoagulation using LMWH (e.g., enoxaparin) or UFH should be added to antiplatelet treatment. An early invasive strategy that includes coronary angiography and revascularization is recommended for patients with high-risk features (Table 18-16). A conservative strategy is recommended for patients without high-risk features. Patients with remaining ischemia or stress test–induced ischemia should be referred for coronary angiography and revascularization.

Coronary revascularization is performed to relieve symptoms and improve prognosis. Depending on the extent and severity of coronary artery disease, suitability of lesions for PCI, and presence of treated diabetes mellitus, patients are referred for CABG or PCI (Table 18-17). Arterial grafting should be performed when possible, and GP IIb/IIIa treatment is recommended during PCI.

Table 18-15. ACC/AHA Risk Stratification: Short-Term Risk Stratification of Death or Nonfatal Myocardial Infarction in Patients with NSTEMI Acute Coronary Syndrome

Feature	High Risk: At Least One of the Following Must Be Present	Intermediate Risk: No High-Risk Feature but Must Have One of the Following	Low Risk: No High- or Intermediate-Risk Feature but May Have Any of the Following
History	Accelerating tempo of ischemic symptoms in preceding 48 hr	Prior MI, peripheral or cerebrovascular disease, or CABG; prior aspirin use	
Character of pain	Prolonged ongoing rest pain (>20 min)	Prolonged (>20 min) rest angina, now resolved, with moderate or high likelihood of CAD Rest angina (<20 min or relieved with rest or sublingual nitroglycerin)	New-onset or progressive CCS class III or IV angina in the past 2 weeks with moderate or high likelihood of CAD
Clinical findings	Pulmonary edema, most likely related to ischemia New or worsening MR murmur S_3 or new or worsening rale Hypotension, bradycardia, tachycardia Age >75 yr	Age >70 yr	
ECG findings	Angina at rest with transient ST-segment changes >0.05 mV Bundle branch block, new or presumed new Sustained ventricular tachycardia	T-wave inversions >0.2 mV Pathologic Q waves	Normal or unchanged ECG pattern during an episode of chest discomfort
Cardiac markers	Elevated (e.g., TnT or TnI >0.1 ng/mL)	Slightly elevated (e.g., TnT >0.01 but <0.1 ng/mL)	Normal

ACC/AHA, American College of Cardiology/American Heart Association; CABG, coronary artery bypass grafting; CAD, coronary artery disease; CSS, Canadian Cardiovascular Society; ECG, electrocardiographic; MI, myocardial infarction; MR, mitral regurgitation; NSTEMI, non-ST-segment elevation myocardial infarction; Tn, troponin (I and T forms).

Table 18-16. American College of Cardiology and American Heart Association High-Risk Indicators for Non-ST-Segment Elevation Acute Coronary Syndrome

- Recurrent angina or ischemia at rest or with low-level activities despite intensive anti-ischemic treatment
- Elevated troponin levels
- New or presumably new ST-segment depression
- Recurrent angina or ischemia with congestive heart failure symptoms, S_3 gallop, pulmonary edema, worsening rales, or new or worsening mitral regurgitation
- High-risk findings on noninvasive stress testing
- Depressed left ventricular systolic function
- Hemodynamic instability
- Sustained ventricular tachycardia
- Percutaneous coronary intervention within 6 months
- Prior coronary artery bypass grafting

Table 18-17. Revascularization of Patients with NSTEMI Acute Coronary Syndrome

CABG	PCI
Left main	One-vessel disease or
Three-vessel disease	Multivessel disease and
Two-vessel disease with LAD	Suitable lesions
Unsuitable lesions PCI	
Patients with diabetes (treated)	

CABG, coronary artery bypass grafting; LAD, left anterior descending coronary artery; NSTEMI, non-ST-segment elevation myocardial infarction; PCI, percutaneous intervention.

European Society of Cardiology Guidelines

The ESC guidelines are slightly different from the ACC/AHA guidelines. Risk stratification determined at admission and repeated during hospitalization is recommended and is a determinant for further management. Patients are classified according to high-risk and low-risk categories based on the presence of high-risk indicators of death or nonfatal MI (Table 18-18).

Treatment consists of anti-ischemic therapy (nitrates and β-blockers), antiplatelet therapy (aspirin and clopidogrel), and anticoagulant therapy (first choice of UFH). A conservative strategy is recommended for low-risk patients, and an early invasive strategy is recommended for high-risk patients.

Comparison of the European Society of Cardiology Guidelines and American College of Cardiology/ American Heart Association Guidelines

The ESC and ACC/AHA guidelines are very similar, but there is a difference in risk assessment. The ACC/AHA guidelines classify three risk categories: high, intermediate, and low. The ESC guidelines classify two risk categories: high and low. The ESC guidelines include diabetes mellitus in the high-risk category. The guidelines' recommendations are not much dif-

Table 18-18. European Society of Cardiology Guidelines for Risk

High-Risk Indicators	Low-Risk Indicators
Elevated troponin levels	Normal troponin levels
Recurrent ischemia	No recurrent ischemia
ST-segment depression	No release of creatine kinase MB
Early unstable angina after	fraction (CK-MB)
myocardial infarction	Presence of negative or flat T
Diabetes mellitus	waves
Hemodynamic instability	Normal electrocardiogram
Major arrhythmias:	
ventricular fibrillation,	
ventricular tachycardia	

ferent for an early invasive strategy or a conservative strategy.

There is a difference in the recommendation for anticoagulant treatment. The ESC guidelines recommend UFH as first-line treatment and acknowledge the advantages of LMWH compared with UFH (i.e., greater bioavailability, convenient administration, decreased risk of thrombocytopenia, and lack of special monitoring) but do not recommend a special compound. The ACC/AHA guidelines recommend enoxaparin as first-line treatment.

Pragmatic Management Approach

We propose a pragmatic approach based on the ACC/AHA and ESC guidelines (Fig. 18-17). The main issues in both guidelines are the importance of early and continuous risk stratification, assessment of troponin levels, high-risk indicators to guide management, reduction of adverse peri-PCI coronary events with platelet GP IIb/IIIa inhibitors, benefits of the addition of clopidogrel to aspirin in patients with a non-interventional approach or planned PCI, and the necessity of postdischarge measures to improve lifestyle and reduction of adverse short- and long-term clinical events with the use of aspirin, β-blockers, statins, and angiotensin-converting enzyme (ACE) inhibitors.

Patients with NSTE-ACS should receive anti-ischemic, antiplatelet, and anticoagulant treatment. An early risk assessment should be performed based on clinical presentation, age, electrocardiographic changes, cardiac enzymes and biomarkers, and clinical course. Patients are at low risk as defined in Tables 18-15 and 18-18 or by having a TIMI risk score of 2 or less. Patients are at intermediate risk as defined in Table 18-15 or by having a TIMI risk score of 3 or 4 with no abnormal biomarkers. Patients are at high risk as defined in Tables 18-15 and 18-18 or by having a TIMI risk score of 5 or higher. An early invasive strategy is recommended for patients with high-risk indicators (see Tables 18-16 and 18-18).

The findings of coronary angiography largely determine whether patients should be referred for PCI or CABG. In general, CABG is indicated for patients with left main coronary artery disease or multivessel disease with compromised left ventricular function, patients with diabetes, and those with

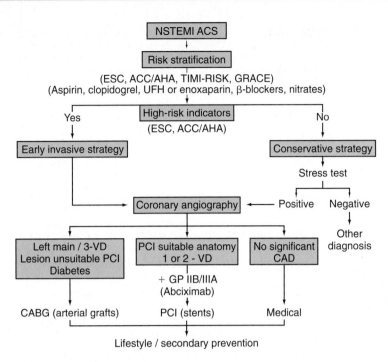

Figure 18-17. Pragmatic approach to manage patients with non-ST-segment elevation myocardial infarction (NSTEMI) acute coronary syndrome (ACS). ACC/AHA, American College of Cardiology/American Heart Association; CABG, coronary artery bypass grafting; CAD, coronary artery disease; ESC, European Society of Cardiology; GRACE, Global Registry of Acute Coronary Events; left main; left main coronary artery; PCI, percutaneous coronary intervention; TIMI-RISK, Thrombolysis in Myocardial Infarction trial risk score; 1- or 2-VD, one- or two-vessel disease; 3-VD, three-vessel disease.

coronary anatomy not suitable for PCI. An attempt should be made to use arterial grafts. PCI is indicated in single-vessel and multivessel disease with lesions suitable for PCI. PCI should preferably include stent implantation, and studies suggest that DESs are safe and reduce in-stent restenosis in patients with NSTE-ACS. Patients undergoing PCI should receive adjunctive treatment with aspirin, clopidogrel, heparin (UFH or LMWH), and a GP IIb/IIIa antagonist. PCI is an alternative to high-risk CABG in patients with refractory myocardial ischemia and severe comorbidity. A conservative approach is recommended for low-risk patients. They should undergo a stress test, and in case of stress-induced ischemia, they should be referred for coronary angiography and revascularization. PCI may also be a reasonable alternative in elderly patients with severe comorbidity. Lifestyle changes and secondary prevention using aspirin β-blockers, statins, and ACE inhibitors should be offered to all survivors of NSTE-ACS.

REFERENCES

1. Gruentzig AR, Senning A, Siegenthaler WE: Non-operative dilatation of coronary artery stenosis: Percutaneous transluminal coronary angioplasty. N Engl J Med 1979;301:61-68.
2. de Feyter PJ, Serruys PW, van den Brand M, et al: Emergency coronary angioplasty in refractory unstable angina. N Engl J Med 1985;313:342-346.
3. Sigwart U, Puel J, Mirkovitch V, et al: Intravascular stents to prevent occlusion and restenosis after transluminal angioplasty. N Engl J Med 1987;316:701-706.
4. Bertrand ME, Simoons ML, Fox KA, et al, for the Task Force on the Management of Acute Coronary Syndromes of the European Society of Cardiology: Management of acute coronary syndromes in patients presenting without persistent ST-segment elevation. Eur Heart J 2002;23:1809-1840.
5. Braunwald E, Antman EM, Beasley JW, et al: American College of Cardiology; American Heart Association. Committee on the Management of Patients With Unstable Angina. ACC/AHA 2002 guideline update for the management of patients with unstable angina and non-ST-segment elevation myocardial infarction—Summary article: A report of the American College of Cardiology/American Heart Association Task Force on Practice Guidelines (Committee on the Management of Patients With Unstable Angina). J Am Coll Cardiol 2002;40:1366-1374.
6. Fox KA, Goodman SG, Klein W, et al, for the GRACE Investigators: Management of acute coronary syndromes. Variations in practice and outcome. Findings from the Global Registry of Acute Coronary Events (GRACE). Eur Heart J 2002;23:1179-1189.
7. Hasdai D, Behar S, Wallentin L, et al: A prospective survey of the characteristics, treatments and outcomes of patients with acute coronary syndromes in Europe and the Mediterranean basin; the Euro Heart Survey of Acute Coronary Syndromes (Euro Heart Survey ACS). Eur Heart J 2002;23:1190-1201.
8. Fuster V, Moreno PR, Fayad ZA, et al: Atherothrombosis and high-risk plaque. Part I. Evolving concepts. J Am Coll Cardiol 2005;46:937-954.
9. A comparison of aspirin plus tirofiban with aspirin plus heparin for unstable angina. Platelet Receptor Inhibition in Ischemic Syndrome Management (PRISM) Study Investigators. N Engl J Med 1998;338:1498-1505.
10. The Platelet Receptor Inhibition in Ischemic Syndrome Management in Patients Limited by Unstable Signs and Symptoms (PRISM-PLUS) Study Investigators: Inhibition of the platelet glycoprotein IIb/IIIa receptor with tirofiban in unstable angina and non-Q-wave myocardial infarction. N Engl J Med 1998;338:1488-1497.
11. Global Organization Network (PARAGON)-B Investigators: Randomized, placebo-controlled trial of titrated intravenous lamifiban for acute coronary syndromes. Circulation 2002;105:316-321.
12. Simoons ML, for the GUSTO IV-ACS Investigators: Effect of glycoprotein IIb/IIIa receptor blocker abciximab on outcome in patients with acute coronary syndromes without early coronary revascularisation: The GUSTO IV-ACS randomised trial. Lancet 2001;357:1915-1924.
13. Antman EM, Cohen M, Bernink PJ, et al: The TIMI risk score for unstable angina/non-ST elevation MI: A method for prognostication and therapeutic decision making. JAMA 2000;284:835-842.
14. Eagle KA, Lim MJ, Dabbous OH, et al: A validated prediction model for all forms of acute coronary syndrome: Estimating

the risk of 6-month postdischarge death in an international registry. JAMA 2004;291:2727-2733.

15. Januzzi JL Jr, Newby LK, Murphy SA, et al: Predicting a late positive serum troponin in initially troponin-negative patients with non-ST-elevation acute coronary syndrome: Clinical predictors and validated risk score results from the TIMI IIIB and GUSTO IIA studies. Am Heart J 2006;151:360-366.

16. Yusuf S, Zhao F, Mehta SR, et al, for the Clopidogrel in Unstable Angina to Prevent Recurrent Events Trial Investigators: Effects of clopidogrel in addition to aspirin in patients with acute coronary syndromes without ST-segment elevation. N Engl J Med 2001;345:494-502.

17. Oler A, Whooley MA, Oler J, Grady D: Adding heparin to aspirin reduces the incidence of myocardial infarction and death in patients with unstable angina. A meta-analysis. JAMA 1996;276:811-815.

18. Hamm CW, Heeschen C, Goldmann B, et al: Benefit of abciximab in patients with refractory unstable angina in relation to serum troponin T levels. c7E3 Fab Antiplatelet Therapy in Unstable Refractory Angina (CAPTURE) Study Investigators. N Engl J Med 1999;340:1623-1629.

19. Use of a monoclonal antibody directed against the platelet glycoprotein IIb/IIIa receptor in high-risk coronary angioplasty. The EPIC Investigation. N Engl J Med 1994;330: 956-961.

20. Platelet glycoprotein IIb/IIIa receptor blockade and low-dose heparin during percutaneous coronary revascularization. The EPILOG Investigators. N Engl J Med 1997;336:1689-1696.

21. Randomised placebo-controlled and balloon-angioplasty-controlled trial to assess safety of coronary stenting with use of platelet glycoprotein-IIb/IIIa blockade. The EPISTENT Investigators. Evaluation of Platelet IIb/IIIa Inhibitor for Stenting. Lancet 1998;352:87-92.

22. Novel dosing regimen of eptifibatide in planned coronary stent implantation (ESPRIT): A randomised, placebo-controlled trial. Lancet 2000;356:2037-2044.

23. Randomised placebo-controlled trial of effect of eptifibatide on complications of percutaneous coronary intervention: IMPACT-II. Integrilin to Minimise Platelet Aggregation and Coronary Thrombosis-II. Lancet 1997;349:1422-1428.

24. The RESTORE Investigators: GP IIb/IIIa blockade with tirofiban during PCI for acute coronary syndromes. RESTORE trial. Circulation 1997;96:1445-1453.

25. Moliterno DJ, Yakubov SJ, DiBattiste PM, et al, for the TARGET investigators: Outcomes at 6 months for the direct comparison of tirofiban and abciximab during percutaneous coronary revascularisation with stent placement: The TARGET follow-up study. Lancet 2002;360:355-360.

26. Theroux P, Alexander J Jr, Dupuis J, et al, for the PRISM-PLUS Investigators: Upstream use of tirofiban in patients admitted for an acute coronary syndrome in hospitals with or without facilities for invasive management. PRISM-PLUS Investigators. Am J Cardiol 2001;87:375-380.

27. Greenbaum AB, Harrington RA, Hudson MP, et al: Therapeutic value of eptifibatide at community hospitals transferring patients to tertiary referral centers early after admission for acute coronary syndromes. PURSUIT Investigators. J Am Coll Cardiol 2001;37:492-498.

28. Kastrati A, Mehilli J, Neumann FJ, et al, for the Intracoronary Stenting and Antithrombotic Regimen Rapid Early Action for Coronary Treatment 2 (ISAR-REACT 2) Trial Investigators: Abciximab in patients with acute coronary syndromes undergoing percutaneous coronary intervention after clopidogrel pretreatment: The ISAR-REACT 2 randomized trial. JAMA 2006;295:1531-1538.

29. Effects of tissue plasminogen activator and a comparison of early invasive and conservative strategies in unstable angina and non-Q-wave myocardial infarction. Results of the TIMI IIIB Trial. Thrombolysis in Myocardial Ischemia. Circulation 1994;89:1545-1556.

30. Boden WE, O'Rourke RA, Crawford MH, et al: Outcomes in patients with acute non-Q-wave myocardial infarction randomly assigned to an invasive as compared with a conservative management strategy. Veterans Affairs Non-Q-Wave Infarction Strategies in Hospital (VANQWISH) Trial Investigators. N Engl J Med 1998;338:1785-1792.

31. McCullough PA, O'Neill WW, Graham M, et al: A prospective randomized trial of triage angiography in acute coronary syndromes ineligible for thrombolytic therapy. Results of the medicine versus angiography in thrombolytic exclusion (MATE) trial. J Am Coll Cardiol 1998;32:596-605.

32. Wallentin L, Lagerqvist B, Husted S, et al: Outcome at 1 year after an invasive compared with a non-invasive strategy in unstable coronary-artery disease: The FRISC II invasive randomised trial. FRISC II Investigators. Fast Revascularisation during Instability in Coronary artery disease. Lancet 2000;356: 9-16.

33. Cannon CP, Weintraub WS, Demopoulos LA, et al: Comparison of early invasive and conservative strategies in patients with unstable coronary syndromes treated with the glycoprotein IIb/IIIa inhibitor tirofiban. N Engl J Med 2001;344: 1879-1887.

34. Spacek R, Widimsky P, Straka Z, et al: Value of first day angiography/angioplasty in evolving Non-ST segment elevation myocardial infarction: An open multicenter randomized trial. The VINO Study. Eur Heart J 2002;23:230-238.

35. Fox KA, Poole-Wilson PA, Henderson RA, et al: Randomized Intervention Trial of unstable Angina Investigators. Interventional versus conservative treatment for patients with unstable angina or non-ST-elevation myocardial infarction: The British Heart Foundation RITA 3 randomised trial. Randomized Intervention Trial of unstable Angina. Lancet 2002;360: 743-751.

36. de Winter RJ, Windhausen F, Cornel JH, et al, for the Invasive versus Conservative Treatment in Unstable Coronary Syndromes (ICTUS) Investigators: Early invasive versus selectively invasive management for acute coronary syndromes. N Engl J Med 2005;353:1095-1104.

37. Fox KA, Poole-Wilson P, Clayton TC, et al: 5-Year outcome of an interventional strategy in non-ST-elevation acute coronary syndrome: The British Heart Foundation RITA 3 randomised trial. Lancet 2005;366:914-920.

38. Ryan JW, Peterson ED, Chen AY, et al, for the CRUSADE Investigators: Optimal timing of intervention in non-ST-segment elevation acute coronary syndromes: Insights from the CRUSADE (Can Rapid risk stratification of Unstable angina patients Suppress ADverse outcomes with Early implementation of the ACC/AHA guidelines) Registry. Circulation 2005;112:3049-3057.

39. Neumann FJ, Kastrati A, Pogatsa-Murray G, et al: Evaluation of prolonged antithrombotic pretreatment ("cooling-off" strategy) before intervention in patients with unstable coronary syndromes: A randomized controlled trial. JAMA 2003;290:1593-1599.

40. van't Hof AW, de Vries ST, Dambrink JH, et al: A comparison of two invasive strategies in patients with non-ST elevation acute coronary syndromes: Results of the Early or Late Intervention in unStable Angina (ELISA) pilot study: 2b/3a upstream therapy and acute coronary syndromes. Eur Heart J 2003;24: 1401-1405.

41. Bhatt DL, Roe MT, Peterson ED, et al: Utilization of early invasive management strategies for high-risk patients with non-ST-segment elevation acute coronary syndromes: Results from the CRUSADE Quality Improvement Initiative. JAMA 2004;292:2096-2104.

42. Mueller C, Neumann FJ, Roskamm H, et al: Women do have an improved long-term outcome after non-ST-elevation acute coronary syndromes treated very early and predominantly with percutaneous coronary intervention: A prospective study in 1,450 consecutive patients. J Am Coll Cardiol 2002;40: 245-250.

43. Morice MC, Serruys PW, Sousa JE, et al: A randomized comparison of a sirolimus-eluting stent with a standard stent for coronary revascularization. N Engl J Med 2002;346: 1773-1780.

44. Moses JW, Leon MB, Popma JJ, et al: Sirolimus-eluting stents versus standard stents in patients with stenosis in a native coronary artery. N Engl J Med 2003;349:1315-1323.

45. Colombo A, Drzewiecki J, Banning A, et al: Randomized study to assess the effectiveness of slow- and moderate-release polymer-based paclitaxel-eluting stents for coronary artery lesions. Circulation 2003;108:788-794.

46. Stone GW, Ellis SG, Cox DA, et al, for the TAXUS-IV Investigators: A polymer-based, paclitaxel-eluting stent in patients with coronary artery disease. N Engl J Med 2004;350:221-231.

47. Lemos PA, Serruys PW, van Domburg RT, et al: Unrestricted utilization of sirolimus-eluting stents compared with conventional bare stent implantation in the "real world": The Rapamycin-Eluting Stent Evaluated At Rotterdam Cardiology Hospital (RESEARCH) registry. Circulation 2004;109: 190-195.

48. Kaiser C, Brunner-La Rocca HP, Buser PT, et al, for the BASKET Investigators: Incremental cost-effectiveness of drug-eluting stents compared with a third-generation bare-metal stent in a real-world setting: Randomised Basel Stent Kosten Effektivitäts Trial (BASKET). Lancet 2005;366:921-929.

49. Schwartz GG, Olsson AG, Ezekowitz MD, et al, for the Myocardial Ischemia Reduction with Aggressive Cholesterol Lowering (MIRACL) Study Investigators: Effects of atorvastatin on early recurrent ischemic events in acute coronary syndromes: The MIRACL study: A randomized controlled trial. JAMA 2001;285:1711-1718.

50. Pravastatin or Atorvastatin Evaluation and Infection Therapy-Thrombolysis in Myocardial Infarction 22 Investigators: Intensive versus moderate lipid lowering with statins after acute coronary syndromes. N Engl J Med 2004;350:1495-504.

51. Lescol Intervention Prevention Study (LIPS) Investigators: Fluvastatin for prevention of cardiac events following successful first percutaneous coronary intervention: A randomized controlled trial. JAMA 2002;287:3215-3222.

19 Percutaneous Coronary Interventions in Acute ST-Segment Elevation Myocardial Infarction

Albert Schömig, Gjin Ndrepepa, and Adnan Kastrati

KEY POINTS

- An estimated 1.2 million Americans have an acute myocardial infarction (MI) annually, and ST-segment elevation MI (STEMI) accounts for about 50% of acute MIs.
- Catheter-based primary percutaneous coronary intervention (PCI) is the mainstay of reperfusion therapy, equaling or surpassing thrombolytic therapy as reperfusion treatment for patients with STEMI in United States.
- PCI is superior to thrombolytic therapy in reducing death, reinfarction, intracranial bleeding, and re-occlusion of infarct-related artery and myocardial ischemia in patients with STEMI, irrespective of the patient's risk and whether interhospital transfer for PCI is required.
- PCI retains its myocardial salvaging capacity and ability to improve clinical outcome over a longer period after symptom onset than thrombolysis and is the therapy of choice for patients presenting early or late after symptom onset.
- Primary stenting is the preferred PCI approach for patients with STEMI. The role of drug-eluting stents needs further evaluation.

- Use of thrombolysis for facilitated PCI as a strategy to promote reperfusion within the time interval from patient presentation to performance of PCI is associated with worse clinical outcome than PCI alone and cannot be recommended for STEMI patients.
- Available evidence supports the use of clopidogrel before treatment and the use of glycoprotein IIb/IIIa receptor inhibitors in patients with STEMI undergoing primary PCI.
- Rescue PCI salvages ischemic myocardium and improves clinical outcome. It is recommended for patients with STEMI after failed thrombolysis.
- Rheolytic therapy or distal protection devices do not improve the results of conventional PCI in STEMI patients and cannot be recommended based on current evidence.
- The adjunctive role of cell-based myocardial repair in the management of patients with STEMI needs further investigation.

It is estimated that 1.2 million Americans have an acute myocardial infarction (MI) annually.[1] Acute MI results mostly from acute thrombotic occlusion of an epicardial coronary artery, typically after disruption or erosion of an atherosclerotic plaque and exposure of thrombogenic material (i.e., plaque lipid content, collagen, and subendothelial extracellular matrix) to circulating blood. Interruption of coronary blood flow results in myocardial ischemia in a blood-deprived myocardial area, which succumbs to myocardial necrosis if the deprivation is severe enough and of sufficient duration. Based on the data of the National Registry of Myocardial Infarction (NRMI) 1,

2, and 3, ST-segment elevation MI (STEMI) accounts for about 50% of acute MIs. Acute coronary thrombosis, apart from serving as pathophysiologic basis for STEMI, forms the rationale for reperfusion therapy aiming at salvaging ischemic myocardium, improving left ventricular function and remodeling, increasing electrical stability, and reducing fatal ventricular arrhythmias. Abundant evidence in the past 25 years testifies to the lifesaving effect and improvement in the quality of life of reperfusion therapy—primary percutaneous coronary intervention (PCI) or thrombolysis—in patients with STEMI. Acute STEMI represents the pathology in which PCI achieves its most impressive lifesaving effect.

A historical perspective of catheter-based reperfusion therapy in patients with STEMI can be found in Chapter 14 of the fourth edition of this textbook.[2] This chapter focuses on the recent achievements in the field of catheter-based reperfusion therapy for patients with STEMI.

SUPERIORITY OF PRIMARY PERCUTANEOUS CORONARY INTERVENTION OVER THROMBOLYSIS

Primary PCI refers to a strategy of emergent coronary angiography followed by coronary angioplasty with or without stenting of the infarct-related artery without prior administration of thrombolytic therapy. Mechanical reperfusion has jumped from the field of clinical research to become the mainstay reperfusion therapy for patients with STEMI. The fourth National Registry of Myocardial Infarction (NRMI-4) has demonstrated that in the United States, PCI has equaled and surpassed thrombolytic therapy as reperfusion treatment for patients with STEMI. It seems that the era of studies comparing mechanical reperfusion (i.e., primary angioplasty or stenting) with pharmacologic thrombolytic therapy is over, and the available data have been reviewed in a couple of meta-analyses. Multiple lines of evidence from randomized studies firmly suggest that catheter-based mechanical reperfusion in patients with STEMI is superior to pharmacologic thrombolytic therapy alone in reducing the composite end point of death, reinfarction, intracranial bleeding, re-occlusion of the infarct-related artery, and recurrent myocardial ischemia.[3,4]

Although thrombolytic therapy has been lifesaving, it has serious limitations. Many patients have relative or absolute contraindications to this therapy, the incidence of intracranial hemorrhage is disproportionately high among elderly patients, the ability to restore normal blood flow in the affected artery is limited, and re-occlusion of the treated artery can result in reinfarction within months of initial treatment.[5] In addition to avoiding these limitations of thrombolytic therapy, PCI has other advantages over thrombolytic therapy, such as restoration of normal coronary blood flow in the infarcted artery in a higher proportion of patients that is durable and relatively independent of time from symptom onset, greater amount of salvaged myocardium, and assessment of coronary anatomy and hemodynamic status, resulting in risk stratification and facilitation of patient care and earlier hospital discharge.[5] A typical example of the efficacy of PCI in patients with STEMI is shown in Figure 19-1.

The lack of availability of medical centers that can offer timely catheter-based invasive treatment for patients with STEMI, rather than clinical effectiveness, is perceived as the most important factor that impedes a wider application of this lifesaving treatment to patients with STEMI. An update of the American College of Cardiology/American Heart Association guidelines defines PCI as a class 1 indication (level of evidence: A) in patients with STEMI (including true posterior MI and MI with new or presumably new left bundle branch block) presenting within 12 hours from symptom onset if performed within 90 minutes of presentation by experienced personnel (i.e., individuals performing more than 75 PCI procedures per year) and in a qualified laboratory staff (i.e., a laboratory that performs more than 200 PCI procedures per year, of which 36 are primary PCI for STEMI, and has a cardiac surgery facility).[6] Even for patients with STEMI who have contraindications to thrombolytic therapy, an analysis of the NRMI has demonstrated that primary PCI significantly improves survival.[7] Similarly, the Stent or Percutaneous Transluminal Coronary Angioplasty for Occluded Coronary Arteries in Patients with Acute Myocardial Infarction Ineligible for Thrombolysis-3 (STOPAMI-3) trial demonstrated that a considerable amount of myocardial salvage is achieved by coronary stenting or balloon angioplasty in patients with STEMI who are considered ineligible for thrombolysis (i.e., presenting later than 12 hours from symptom onset or having contraindications to thrombolysis), as illustrated in Figure 19-2.[8]

Available evidence suggests that primary PCI is superior to thrombolysis in all studied time intervals. A report from the second Primary Coronary Angioplasty vs. Thrombolysis (PCAT-2) Trialists' Collaborative Group demonstrated that primary PCI was superior to thrombolysis in terms of reduction of the 30-day incidence of major adverse cardiac events and that the absolute reduction in mortality by PCI widened over time, from 1.3% within the first hour to 4.2% after more than 6 hours after symptom onset.[9]

The superiority of primary PCI over thrombolysis has been confirmed, particularly for high-risk patients[10] and in centers without on-site cardiac surgery.[11] A report from the Danish Trial in Acute Myocardial Infarction-2 (DANAMI-2) demonstrated that the benefits of PCI are greatest for high-risk patients.[10] For high-risk patients (i.e., those with a Thrombolysis in Myocardial Infarction [TIMI] risk score ≥5), there was a significant reduction in mortality with primary PCI (25.3% versus 36.2% with thrombolysis, $P = .02$), which was not observed for the low-risk group (TIMI risk score of 0 to 4).[10] The Atlantic Cardiovascular Patient Outcomes Research Team (C-PORT) study showed that in centers not providing cardiac surgery, primary PCI is superior to thrombolysis in reducing the composite end point of death, reinfarction, and stroke at 6 weeks (10.7% versus 17.7%, $P = .03$) and at 6 months (12.4% versus 19.9%, $P = .03$).[11]

In aggregate, these studies demonstrate that primary PCI is superior to thrombolysis and should be the preferred strategy of reperfusion in patients with STEMI in all clinical situations and patient subsets. Primary PCI is particularly superior to thrombolysis in patients who present late after symptom onset and those who are considered at high risk.

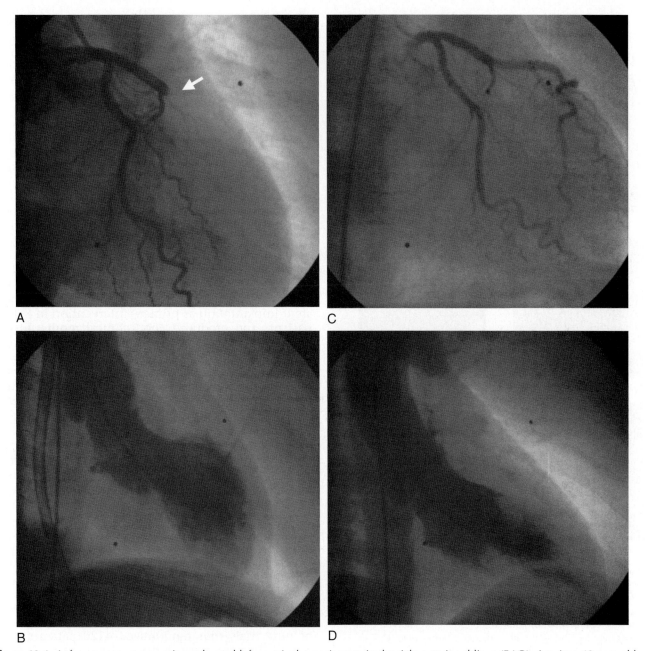

Figure 19-1. Left coronary artery angiography and left ventricular angiogram in the right anterior oblique (RAO) view in a 49-year-old male patient with acute ST-segment elevation anterior myocardial infarction. **A,** Complete thrombotic occlusion *(arrow)* of the left anterior descending coronary artery before coronary stenting. **B,** Left ventricular angiogram before coronary stenting. End-systolic frame of the left ventricular angiogram shows an extensive zone of akinesia in the anterior wall of the left ventricle. **C,** Left coronary artery angiogram performed 6 months after successful stenting. **D,** End-systolic frame of the left ventricular angiogram performed 6 months after stenting shows a marked regional improvement in the left ventricular function.

Because most hospitals do not have PCI capabilities, physicians and hospitals are faced with the challenge of providing timely primary PCI to patients with STEMI.[12] Recognizing the importance of the problem, several regions in the United States have proposed or established triage and transfer protocols to direct without delay patients with STEMI to hospitals with PCI capabilities.[12,13]

APPLICATION OF PRIMARY PERCUTANEOUS CORONARY INTERVENTION

Technical Aspects

From the technical aspect, primary PCI is similar to elective PCI. However, PCI in the early phase of STEMI can be more difficult and requires more

Before intervention   10 days after intervention

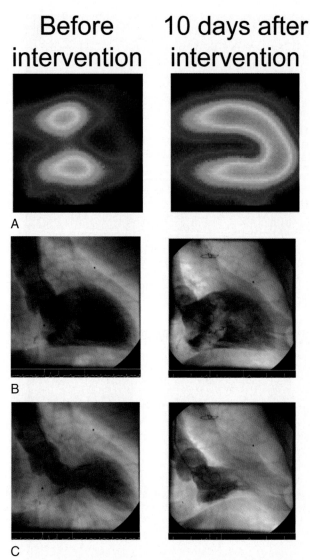

A

B

C

Figure 19-2. Scintigraphic and left ventricular (LV) angiographic images in a 69-year-old patient with acute myocardial infarction treated with coronary artery stenting 16 hours after onset of symptoms. **A,** Vertical long-axis view of technetium 99m sestamibi scintigraphy. **B,** End-diastolic frame of left ventricular angiography in 30-degree, right anterior oblique view. **C,** End-systolic frame of left ventricular angiography in 30-degree, right anterior oblique view. (From Kastrati A, Mehilli J, Nekolla S, et al: A randomized trial comparing myocardial salvage achieved by coronary stenting versus balloon angioplasty in patients with acute myocardial infarction considered ineligible for reperfusion therapy. J Am Coll Cardiol 2004;43:734-741. Copyright Elsevier 2004.)

experience than routine PCI in a stable patient. The goal of primary PCI is to open occluded coronary arteries and restore normal blood flow to the ischemic region. Primary PCI is performed in conditions of increased risk due to hemodynamic and electrical instability, increased thrombogenicity associated with STEMI, and complete thrombotic occlusion of stenotic coronary arteries. Complete occlusion impedes visualization of the coronary artery, makes guidewire or balloon passage through occluded site more difficult, and predisposes to distal embolization of thrombotic material with the potential for further

worsening of the microcirculation. Operators performing primary PCI in STEMI must act rapidly to restore coronary blood flow in the occluded artery as early as possible to stop evolving ischemia and progression to necrosis and to increase the chances of myocardial salvage and infarct size reduction. Vascular access usually is achieved by means of the femoral artery; however, the radial artery is being used increasingly for vascular access. Adjunct antithrombotic therapy is used periprocedurally (see "Periprocedural Antithrombotic Therapy"), and patients are usually anticoagulated with heparin, which is administered during and after procedure (up to 24 hours). The patient is continuously monitored after the procedure and is discharged from the hospital in a few days.

After the initial hesitation to use primary stenting in patients with STEMI because of fears generated by the highly thrombogenic milieu in the infarcted artery, advances in the antiplatelet therapy enabled stent implantation as primary intervention in STEMI patients and produced good clinical results. In the meta-analysis by Keeley and colleagues,[3] 22 randomized trials compared primary PCI with thrombolytic therapy. In 12 trials that compared primary PCI plus stenting with thrombolytic therapy, primary PCI was superior to thrombolytic therapy in terms of lower overall short-term mortality (7% versus 9%, $P = .0002$), nonfatal reinfarction (3% versus 7%, $P < .0001$), stroke (1% versus 2%, $P = .0004$), and the combined end point of death, nonfatal reinfarction, and stroke (8% versus 14%, $P < .0001$). An updated meta-analysis including 24 randomized trials is shown in Table 19-1 and Figure 19-3. The results of primary PCI remained better than the results of thrombolytic therapy during long-term follow-up and were independent of the type of thrombolytic agent used and whether the patient was transferred for primary PCI, which included an average of 38 minutes' delay to initiation of treatment.

Primary stenting has been compared with primary angioplasty alone. A meta-analysis compared results of nine trials that randomized 4120 patients with acute MI to coronary stenting (2050 patients) or to balloon angioplasty alone (2070 patients).[14] In this meta-analysis, there was no difference between patients treated by primary stenting and those treated by balloon angioplasty alone in mortality (3% versus 2.8%) or reinfarction (1.8% versus 2.1%) rates. Major adverse cardiac events were reduced, primarily because of a significant reduction in target vessel revascularization with stenting (9.2% versus 18.7% with primary angioplasty).[14] An analysis of the Primary Angioplasty in Myocardial Infarction (PAMI) trial showed better angiographic results with primary stenting and a sustained benefit in mortality rates for stenting versus balloon angioplasty alone for up to 5 years after STEMI.[15] Compared with balloon angioplasty, stents achieve a better immediate angiographic result because of the larger arterial lumen, less restenosis and re-occlusion, and fewer subsequent ischemic events. Primary stenting has become the

Table 19-1. Randomized Trials Comparing Percutaneous Coronary Intervention with Thrombolysis in Patients with Acute Myocardial Infarction

Trial or First Author	No. of Patients	Type of PCI	Type of Thrombolysis	Source
Akhras	87	PTCA	Streptokinase	J Am Coll Cardiol 1997;29:A235
Andersen	1572	PTCA/stent	t-PA	Clin Cardiol 2002;25:301
Aversano	451	PTCA/stent	t-PA	JAMA 2002;287:1943
Bonnefoy	840	PTCA/stent	t-PA	Lancet 2002;360:825
de Boer	87	PTCA/stent	Streptokinase	J Am Coll Cardiol 2002;39:1723
DeWood	90	PTCA	t-PA	Proceedings of the Thrombolysis and Interventional Therapy in Acute Myocardial Infarction Symposium VI. Washington, DC, George Washington University, 1990, p 28
Garcia	189	PTCA	t-PA	J Am Coll Cardiol 1999;33:605
Gibbons	103	PTCA	t-PA	N Engl J Med 1993;328:685
Grines	395	PTCA	t-PA	N Engl J Med 1993;328:673
Grines	137	PTCA/stent	t-PA	J Am Coll Cardiol 2002;39:1713
Grinfeld	112	PTCA	Streptokinase	J Am Coll Cardiol 1996;27:A222
GUSTO IIb	1138	PTCA	t-PA	N Engl J Med 1997;336:1621
Hochman	302	PTCA/stent	t-PA	N Engl J Med 1999;341:645
Kastrati	162	PTCA/stent	t-PA	Lancet 2002;359:920
Le May	123	PTCA/stent	t-PA	J Am Coll Cardiol 2001;37:985
Ribeiro	100	PTCA	Streptokinase	J Am Coll Cardiol 1993;22:376
Ribichini	110	PTCA/stent	t-PA	J Am Coll Cardiol 1999;32:1687
Schömig	140	PTCA/stent	t-PA	N Engl J Med 2000;343:385
Svensson	205	PTCA/stent	t-PA	Am Heart J 2006;151:798e
Vermeer	150	PTCA/stent	t-PA	Heart 1999;82:426
Widimsky	200	PTCA/stent	Streptokinase	Eur Heart J 2000;21:823
Widimsky	850	PTCA/stent	Streptokinase	Eur Heart J 2003;24:94
Zijlstra	301	PTCA	Streptokinase	N Engl J Med 1993;328:680
Zijlstra	100	PTCA	Streptokinase	J Am Coll Cardiol 1997;29:908

PCI, percutaneous coronary intervention; PTCA, percutaneous transluminal coronary angioplasty; t-PA, tissue-type plasminogen activator.

preferred strategy for primary PCI in STEMI patients.

Drug-eluting stents (DESs), which have significantly reduced restenosis, are being used increasingly in STEMI patients. Results of randomized trials show that implantation of DESs is feasible, safe, and effective in patients with acute STEMI, as shown in Table 19-2 and Figure 19-4.[16-18] The results of the Trial to Assess the Use of the Cypher Stent in Acute Myocardial Infarction Treated with Balloon Angioplasty (TYPHOON) have been published.[17] TYPHOON was a prospective, randomized, single-blind study that compared sirolimus-eluting stents (Cypher, Cordis/ Johnson & Johnson) with conventional bare metal stents in 712 patients with STEMI.[17] The rate of the primary end point, defined as target vessel–related death, recurrent MI, or target vessel revascularization at 1 year, was significantly lower in the sirolimus-eluting stent group than in the bare metal stent group (7.3% versus 14.3%, P = .004).[17] This reduction was driven by a decrease in the rate of target vessel revascularization (5.6% and 13.4%, respectively; P < .001).[17] There was no significant difference between the two groups in the rate of death (2.3% and 2.2%, respectively), reinfarction (1.1% and 1.4%, respectively), or stent thrombosis (3.4% and 3.6%, respectively).[17]

The Paclitaxel-Eluting Stent versus Conventional Stent in Myocardial Infarction with ST-Segment Elevation (PASSION) trial was a prospective, randomized, single-blind study that compared pacli-

taxel-eluting stents (Taxus, Boston Scientific) with conventional bare metal stents in 619 patients with STEMI.[16] The rate of the primary end point, defined as cardiac death, recurrent MI, or target vessel revascularization at 1 year, was not significantly lower in the paclitaxel-eluting stent group than in the bare metal stent group (8.8% versus 12.8%, P = .09).[16] A nonsignificant trend was detected in favor of the paclitaxel-eluting stent group, compared with the bare metal stent group, in the rate of death from cardiac causes or recurrent MI (5.5% versus 7.2%, P = .40) and in the rate of target lesion revascularization (5.3% versus 7.8%, P = .23).[16] The incidence of stent thrombosis during 1 year of follow-up was the same in both groups (1.0%).[16]

Studies of DESs in STEMI patients have shown that the benefit provided by the stents is produced by a reduction in the rate of restenosis.[16-18] However, long-term follow-up studies after implantation of DESs in patients with acute STEMI are lacking. Some reports have raised concerns about the safety of DESs beyond the first year after implantation in patients with stable or unstable angina.[19] While we are waiting for evidence to confirm or refute these preliminary disquieting findings, we still do not know whether the thrombogenic milieu present in acute STEMI makes these patients more prone to thrombotic events in the long term. Considering these circumstances, patients with STEMI who receive DESs are good candidates for long-term, dual-antiplatelet therapy with aspirin plus clopidogrel beyond 1 year. Newer DES

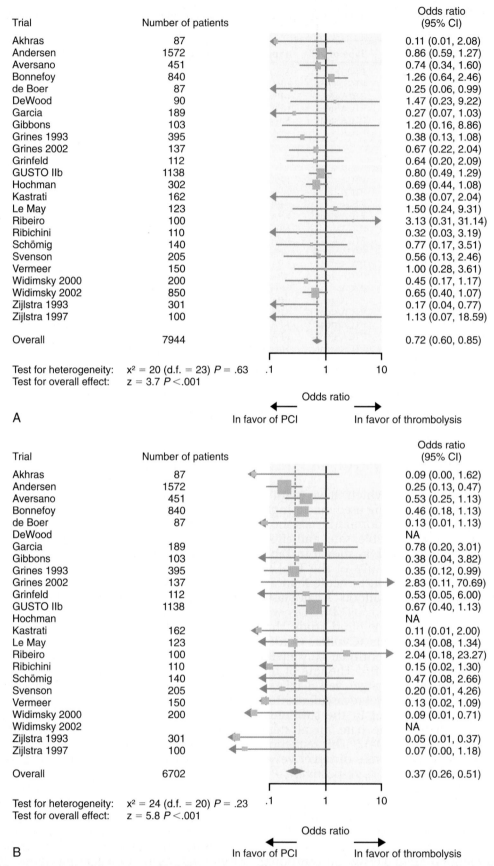

Figure 19-3. Odds ratios (95% confidence interval) of short-term mortality (**A**), recurrent myocardial infarction (**B**), and stroke (**C**) generated by a meta-analysis (random effect model) of 24 randomized trials that have compared primary percutaneous coronary intervention (PCI) with thrombolysis. The first author or the acronym of the trial is shown. (Data sources are provided in Table 19-1.)

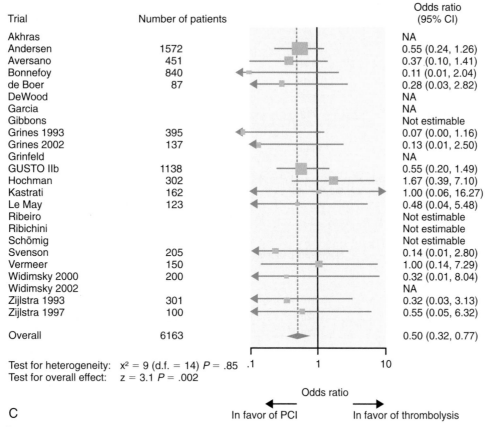

Trial	Number of patients		Odds ratio (95% CI)
Akhras			NA
Andersen	1572		0.55 (0.24, 1.26)
Aversano	451		0.37 (0.10, 1.41)
Bonnefoy	840		0.11 (0.01, 2.04)
de Boer	87		0.28 (0.03, 2.82)
DeWood			NA
Garcia			NA
Gibbons			Not estimable
Grines 1993	395		0.07 (0.00, 1.16)
Grines 2002	137		0.13 (0.01, 2.50)
Grinfeld			NA
GUSTO IIb	1138		0.55 (0.20, 1.49)
Hochman	302		1.67 (0.39, 7.10)
Kastrati	162		1.00 (0.06, 16.27)
Le May	123		0.48 (0.04, 5.48)
Ribeiro			Not estimable
Ribichini			Not estimable
Schömig			Not estimable
Svenson	205		0.14 (0.01, 2.80)
Vermeer	150		1.00 (0.14, 7.29)
Widimsky 2000	200		0.32 (0.01, 8.04)
Widimsky 2002			NA
Zijlstra 1993	301		0.32 (0.03, 3.13)
Zijlstra 1997	100		0.55 (0.05, 6.32)
Overall	6163		0.50 (0.32, 0.77)

Test for heterogeneity: $x^2 = 9$ (d.f. = 14) $P = .85$
Test for overall effect: $z = 3.1$ $P = .002$

.1   1   10

Odds ratio

In favor of PCI   In favor of thrombolysis

C

Figure 19-3, cont'd

Table 19-2. Randomized Trials Comparing Drug-Eluting Stents with Bare Metal Stents in Patients with Acute Myocardial Infarction

Trial (First Author)	No. of Patients	Type of DES	Follow-up (mo)	Source
HAAMU-STENT	164	Taxus	12	Transcatheter Cardiovascular Therapeutics (TCT) Convention, Washington, DC, October 2006
PASSION (Laarman)	619	Taxus	12	N Engl J Med 2006;355:1105
SESAMI	320	Cypher	12	European Paris Course on Revascularization (EuroPCR), Paris, May 2006
STRATEGY (Valgimigli)	175	Cypher	8	JAMA 2005;293:2109
TYPHOON (Spaulding)	712	Cypher	8	N Engl J Med 2006;355:1093

DES, drug-eluting stent; HAAMU-STENT, Helsinki Area Acute Myocardial Infarction Treatment Reevaluation; PASSION, Paclitaxel-Eluting Stent versus Conventional Stent in Myocardial Infarction with ST-Segment Elevation; SESAMI, Sirolimus-Eluting Stent versus Bare Metal Stent in Acute Myocardial Infarction; STRATEGY, Single High Dose Bolus TiRofibAn and Sirolimus Eluting STEnt versus Abiciximab and Bare Metal Stent in Acute MYocardial Infarction; TYPHOON, Trial to Assess the Use of the Cypher Stent in Acute Myocardial Infarction Treated with Balloon Angioplasty.

technologies that avoid the use of permanent polymers, which often are considered responsible for late events, may be particularly useful in patients with STEMI.[20]

In summary, stents with or without drug coatings should be considered the preferred approach for patients with STEMI undergoing primary PCI.

INTERHOSPITAL TRANSFER

The superiority of primary PCI over thrombolysis and the fact that most hospitals have no PCI facility led to the concept of emergency interhospital transfer for primary PCI instead of initial thrombolysis in

the initial hospital for patients with STEMI. Two studies published in 2003—the Danish Trial in Acute Myocardial Infarction-2 (DANAMI-2)[21] and Primary Angioplasty in Patients Transferred from General Community Hospitals to Specialized PTCA Units with or without Emergency Thrombolysis-2 (PRAGUE-2)[22]—compared the outcome of primary PCI in STEMI patients subjected to interhospital transfer from hospitals without PCI to hospitals with PCI capability versus thrombolysis in the initial hospital. The thrombolytic arms received tissue-type plasminogen activator (t-PA) in the DANAMI-2 trial and streptokinase in the PRAGUE-2 trial. Intracoronary bare metal stents were implanted in 93% of interventions in the

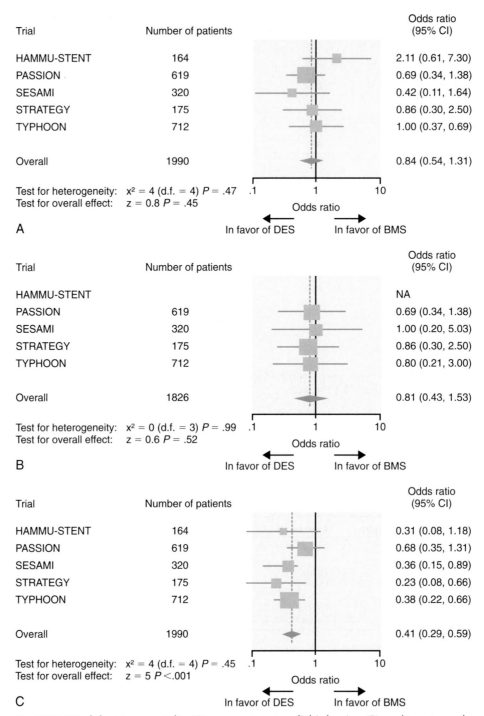

Figure 19-4. Odds ratios (95% CI) of short-term mortality **(A)**, recurrent myocardial infarction **(B)**, and target vessel revascularization **(C)** generated by a meta-analysis (random effect model) of five randomized trials that have compared drug-eluting stents (DES) with bare metal stents (BMS) in patients with acute myocardial infarction. (Data sources are provided in Table 19-2.)

DANAMI-2 trial and in 63% of interventions in the PRAGUE-2 trial. In the DANAMI-2 trial, the rate of the primary composite end point of death, reinfarction, and disabling stroke at 30 days was lower in the PCI group than in thrombolysis group (8.5% versus 14.2%, $P = .002$). Better outcome after PCI was primarily accounted for by a reduction in the rate of reinfarction (1.6% versus 6.3% in the thrombolysis arm, $P < .001$), but also by nonsignificant trends toward lower mortality (6.6% in PCI group versus 7.8% in thrombolysis group, $P = .35$) and stroke (1.1% in the PCI group versus 2% in the thrombolysis group, $P = .15$). The DANAMI-2 trial was halted early by the Data Safety and Monitoring Board after observation of a marked improvement in the clinical outcome of patients in the group with interhospital transfer plus primary PCI.

In the PRAGUE-2 trial, the rate of the primary end point of 30-day mortality was 10% for patients treated by thrombolysis and 6.8% for patients treated by primary PCI (P = .12), whereas the rate of the combined end point of 30-day incidence of death, reinfarction, and stroke was significantly lower for the group with interhospital transfer plus primary PCI than for patients treated with thrombolysis in the initial hospital (8.4% versus 15.2%, P < .003).[22]

Complications during transportations occurred rarely in both studies. Two deaths and three cases of successfully resuscitated ventricular fibrillation were reported during transportation in the PRAGUE-2 trial. No deaths and eight cases of successfully resuscitated ventricular fibrillation during transportation were reported in the DANAMI-2 trial.

A meta-analysis of six randomized trials showed that a strategy of patient transfer plus primary PCI was associated with a 42% reduction in the incidence of the combined end point of death, reinfarction, and stroke compared with a strategy of on-site thrombolysis.[23] An updated meta-analysis including seven randomized trials is provided in Table 19-3 and Figure 19-5. Evidence suggests that patient transfer for PCI is also beneficial for patients with acute MI who receive full-dose thrombolytic therapy in a community hospital. In the third Streptokinase in Acute Myocardial Infarction (SIAM-III) trial, patients presenting within 12 hours of acute MI were randomized to receive immediate stenting within 6 hours (n = 82) or delayed stenting at 2 weeks (n = 81) after full-dose reteplase therapy.[24] Immediate stenting was associated with a significant reduction in the rate of the combined end point of death, reinfarction, ischemic events, and target vessel revascularization at 6 months (25.6% versus 50.6%, P = .001). Quantitative review of studies that have involved the transfer of patients for PCI have suggested that for every 100 patients treated, primary PCI after interhospital transfer instead of on-site thrombolysis prevented seven major adverse cardiac events, defined as death, nonfatal reinfarction, or nonfatal stroke.[25] In aggregate, the results of these trials have expanded the benefits of mechanical reperfusion in patients with STEMI and have had an important impact on clinical practice.

The DANAMI-2 and PRAGUE-2 studies were performed in relatively small countries with highly experienced laboratories and teams committed to the delivery of reperfusion therapy. The time for transportation from community hospital to invasive therapy center was 32 minutes in the DANAMI-2 trial and 48 minutes in the PRAGUE-2 trial. The door-to-balloon interval averaged 26 minutes in both studies. In contrast, a report of the NRMI data showed that in the United States, patients with STEMI who undergo transfer for PCI had a median time interval from initial presentation at the initial hospital to balloon inflation in the invasive therapy center of 180 minutes, which was composed of a median of 120 minutes for decision-making in the initial hospital, transport, and arrival to invasive therapy center and an interval of 53 minutes between arrival and balloon inflation.[26]

The PCI-related time delay has become an integral part of treatment algorithms for patients with STEMI, although the evidence in support of this choice is poor, and the assessment of this issue is difficult. Primary PCI has been found to be superior to thrombolysis despite the inevitable time delay associated with this option[3]; however, several post hoc analyses of randomized trials have aimed at defining a time point in the PCI-related delay beyond which PCI may be inferior to thrombolysis.[27,28] According to current guidelines, thrombolysis should be the preferred treatment option in patients presenting with STEMI

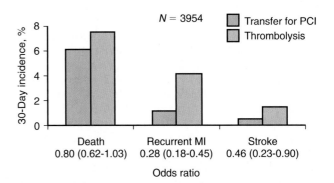

Figure 19-5. Thirty-day incidence of death, recurrent myocardial infarction, and stroke in seven trials that have compared a strategy of patient transfer plus primary percutaneous coronary intervention (PCI) with a strategy of on-site thrombolysis. Odds ratios (OR) and 95% confidence intervals associated with transfer for PCI are shown. (Data sources are provided in Table 19-3.)

Table 19-3. Randomized Trials Comparing Transfer for Percutaneous Coronary Intervention with Immediate Thrombolysis in Patients with Acute Myocardial Infarction

First Author of Trial	No. of Patients	Type of PCI	Type of Thrombolysis	PCI Delay (min)*	Source
Andersen	1572	PTCA/stent	t-PA	62	Clin Cardiol 2002;25:301
Bonnefoy	840	PTCA/stent	t-PA	59	Lancet 2002;360:825
Grines	137	PTCA/stent	t-PA	103	J Am Coll Cardiol 2002;39:1713
Svensson	205	PTCA/stent	t-PA	89	Am Heart J 2006;151:798e
Vermeer	150	PTCA/stent	t-PA	75	Heart 1999;82:426
Widimsky	200	PTCA/stent	Streptokinase	70	Eur Heart J 2000;21:823
Widimsky	850	PTCA/stent	Streptokinase	80	Eur Heart J 2003;24:94

*PCI delay is calculated as the difference in time to treatment between PCI and thrombolysis.
PCI, percutaneous coronary intervention; PTCA, percutaneous transluminal coronary angioplasty; t-PA, tissue-type plasminogen activator.

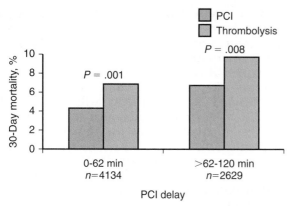

Figure 19-6. Thirty-day mortality in patients treated with percutaneous coronary intervention (PCI) or thrombolysis according to a PCI-related delay of less than 62 minutes or between 62 and 120 minutes. PCI-related delay was calculated as the difference between randomization-to-balloon inflation interval and randomization-to-injection of the fibrinolytic agent interval for each of the hospitals participating in the trials. (Data from Boersma E: Does time matter? A pooled analysis of randomized clinical trials comparing primary percutaneous coronary intervention and in-hospital fibrinolysis in acute myocardial infarction patients. Eur Heart J 2006;27:779-788.)

if a PCI-related delay of more than 60 minutes is assumed.[6] This 60-minute limit was reported by one study,[28] and it was criticized and adjusted to 110 minutes in a later study,[27] until the most thorough time-based meta-analysis was able to show that PCI was superior to thrombolysis, irrespective of the PCI-related time delay characteristic for each participating hospital (Fig. 19-6).[9] A longer PCI-related delay is often associated with less experience and inadequate infrastructure at the primary PCI center,[29] introducing an inevitable bias that is difficult to adjust for in this kind of analysis. Assessment of the relationship between PCI-related time delay and outcome provides helpful information for optimization of the primary PCI network, but it contributes little to the discussion about which reperfusion option to choose in which setting.

In an attempt to shorten PCI-related time delay, direct transportation of patients to hospitals capable of performing primary PCI has been suggested rather than transporting them to the nearest hospital without a PCI facility.[13,30] The data suggest that two thirds of patients with STEMI in the United States present to hospitals without a PCI facility.[13] Almost 80% of the adult population in the United States live within 60 minutes of a hospital with PCI facility, and even among those living closer to hospitals without PCI facilities, almost three fourths would experience less than 30 minutes of additional delay related to direct referral to a hospital with a PCI facility.[31] These data demonstrate that a strategy of patient transfer to hospitals with PCI facilities is feasible and applicable for most patients with STEMI.

In summary, undelayed referral of patients with acute MI to centers with PCI facilities should be the primary objective of the first-contact emergency medical system, even when interhospital transfer is required. This is feasible for most patients with STEMI and should be achieved in the future for all patients with STEMI seeking medical aid.

Percutaneous Coronary Intervention Immediately after Thrombolysis

Previous randomized, prospective trials did not show a benefit for immediate PCI after thrombolysis in terms of increased myocardial salvage, improved left ventricular function, and reduced incidence of reinfarction or mortality.[32] However, advances in mechanical reperfusion devices and adjunctive pharmacologic therapy have had a positive impact on the outcome of PCI immediately after thrombolysis. In the Grupo de Análisis de la Cardiopatía Isquémica Aguda-1 (GRACIA-1) trial, 500 thrombolyzed STEMI patients were randomized to receive coronary stenting within 24 hours or an ischemia-guided conservative approach.[33] At 30 days, both groups had a similar incidence of adverse cardiac events. However, patients randomized to the invasive approach had a reduction in the in-hospital ischemia-driven revascularization (2% versus 12%, $P < .0001$), a shorter hospital stay, and no increase in bleeding compared with patients treated with the conservative approach. By 1 year, patients in the invasive group had a lower frequency of the combined rate of death, reinfarction, or revascularization (9% versus 21%, $P = .0008$), and they showed a trend toward reduced rate of death or reinfarction (7% versus 12%, $P = .07$) compared with patients in the conservative group.

In the Combined Angioplasty and Pharmacological Intervention versus Thrombolysis Alone in Acute Myocardial Infarction (CAPITAL-AMI) trial, 170 patients with high-risk STEMI were randomized within 6 hours to receive tenecteplase plus immediate angioplasty or tenecteplase alone.[34] At 6 months, there was a significant reduction in the incidence of the primary end point (i.e., death, reinfarction, unstable ischemia, or stroke) in the tenecteplase plus PCI group compared with the group receiving tenecteplase alone (11.6% versus 24.4%, $P = .04$). The difference was primarily driven by a significant reduction in the incidence of recurrent unstable ischemia (8.1% versus 20.7%, $P = .03$). There was a trend toward lower incidence of reinfarction in the tenecteplase plus angioplasty group, whereas there were no differences in the rates of death or stroke or bleeding complications among patients who received tenecteplase plus angioplasty compared with those who received tenecteplase alone.[34] Although these studies show that patients with STEMI fare better after thrombolysis followed by PCI compared with thrombolysis alone, they do not address the question of whether thrombolysis is needed at all before PCI.

Facilitated Percutaneous Coronary Intervention

Facilitated PCI refers to a deliberate strategy of PCI preceded by pharmacologic therapy aimed at restoring anterograde flow in the infarct-related artery within the time interval required for performing the PCI in patients with STEMI. It is conceived as an option for filling the time gap between patient presentation and performance of PCI. The pharmacologic regimen consists of drugs known for their ability to restore flow, such as full-dose thrombolysis, half-dose thrombolysis, or a combination of half-dose thrombolysis with glycoprotein IIb/IIIa (GP IIb/IIIa) antagonists. Because of the controversial data about the ability of GP IIb/IIIa antagonists to reopen an affected artery, the isolated use of these drugs may or may not be part of the strategy of facilitated PCI.

There has been a resurgence of interest in combining pharmacologic and mechanical reperfusion strategies, expecting their synergistic action to improve reperfusion and outcome in patients with STEMI.[35] Two factors seem to have served as a rationale for the concept of facilitated PCI. First, ventricular function and prognosis have been better for patients with STEMI who present at the time of primary PCI with spontaneous TIMI flow grade 2 and 3 compared with those who have a TIMI flow grade of 0 and 1 in the infarcted artery. Second, many patients with STEMI cannot undergo mechanical reperfusion without a certain delay owing to a variety of reasons. Facilitated PCI was considered to be advantageous in the reperfusion of patients with STEMI, resulting in a reduction of ischemia time and earlier reperfusion; higher TIMI flow rates in the occluded artery, with facilitation of guidewire or balloon passage; decreased clot burden, and a lower incidence of distal embolization.

Several studies have investigated facilitated PCI in STEMI patients.[36-39] The GRACIA-2 trial randomized 212 patients with acute MI within 12 hours to a strategy of primary PCI with abciximab or to tenecteplase plus enoxaparin, followed by angiography within 2 to 12 hours and intervention if indicated.[36] The study showed no difference in the infarct size or left ventricular function at 6 weeks among patients treated by either approach. No differences in the incidence of major bleeding were observed. A higher proportion of patients assigned to the facilitated PCI group showed complete ST-segment resolution at 6 hours.[36]

The Bavarian Reperfusion Alternatives Evaluation (BRAVE) trial randomized 253 patients with STEMI within 12 hours from symptom onset to facilitated PCI with half-dose reteplase plus abciximab or to abciximab alone. Infarct size estimated by single-photon emission computed tomography (SPECT) 5 to 10 days after randomization was the primary end point of the study. The study reported a higher incidence of TIMI flow grade 3 in the infarct-occluded artery in the reteplase plus abciximab group than in the abciximab-alone group (40% versus 18%, $P <$ .001) but found no difference in the post-PCI TIMI flow grade 3 (87.2% versus 86.7%, $P = .91$) or infarct size (13% versus 11.5%, $P = .81$). The incidence of major bleeding was 5.6% in the reteplase plus abcix-

imab group and 1.6% in the abciximab group ($P = .16$). Within 6 months after randomization, the composite end point of death, recurrent MI, or stroke occurred in 6.4% patients in the reteplase plus abciximab group and 4.7% of patients in the abciximab group ($P = .56$).

The ongoing Facilitated Intervention with Enhanced Reperfusion to Stop Events (FINESSE) trial, a three-arm study with a clinical primary end point, plans to enroll 3000 patients. It will be able to provide evidence on the value of facilitated PCI by half-dose reteplase plus abciximab or abciximab alone versus conventional PCI with abciximab given in the catheterization laboratory.[40]

The Tirofiban Given in the Emergency Room before Primary Angioplasty (TIGER-PA) pilot study included 100 acute MI patients within 12 hours of symptom onset who were randomized to early administration of tirofiban in the emergency department or later administration in the catheterization laboratory.[38] Early administration of tirofiban was associated with an improvement in the initial TIMI flow grade, corrected TIMI frame counts, and TIMI grade myocardial perfusion. The study concluded that early administration of tirofiban is feasible and safe and that it improves angiographic outcome in patients with acute MI undergoing PCI. The 30-day incidence of major adverse cardiac events suggested that early administration of tirofiban might be beneficial.

The Ongoing Tirofiban in Myocardial Infarction Evaluation (On-TIME) trial included 507 patients with acute MI, who were transferred to a PCI center and randomized to early, prehospitalization initiation of tirofiban or to late initiation in the catheterization laboratory.[39] The primary end point was TIMI flow grade 3 in the infarct-related artery at initial angiography. The incidence of TIMI flow grade 3 in the infarct-related artery did not differ significantly among patients with early initiation of tirofiban or those with late initiation of tirofiban (19% versus 15%, $P = .22$). Thrombus or fresh occlusion was present in 60% and 73% in the groups with early and late initiation of tirofiban, respectively ($P = .002$). No differences between groups regarding post-PCI TIMI flow grade in the infarct-related artery or bleeding complications were observed. Thirty-day incidence of death was 3.7% in the group with early initiation of tirofiban and 0.8% in the group with late initiation of tirofiban ($P = .03$). At 1 year, however, mortality was no longer different between the early or late tirofiban groups (4.5% versus 3.7%, $P = .66$). The 1-year combined incidence of death and recurrent MI was not different between groups (7% versus 7%, $P = .99$). The study showed that despite lower prevalence of thrombus or fresh occlusion, early initiation of tirofiban was not associated with beneficial effects in the post-PCI angiographic or 1-year clinical outcome.

The findings of two studies will affect the use of facilitated PCI in patients with STEMI.[41,42] The Assessment of the Safety and Efficacy of a New Treatment Strategy for Acute Myocardial Infarction-4 (ASSENT-

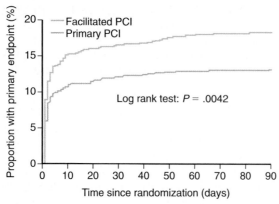

Number at risk

Facilitated PCI 829 703 696 691 685 678 675 673 673 672
Primary PCI   838 747 741 736 730 726 725 724 724 722

Figure 19-7. Kaplan-Meier curves showing a higher incidence of the primary end point (i.e., combination of death, congestive heart failure, or shock within 90 days) with facilitated percutaneous coronary intervention (PCI). (From Primary versus tenecteplase-facilitated percutaneous coronary intervention in patients with ST-segment elevation acute myocardial infarction (ASSENT-4 PCI): Randomised trial. Lancet 2006;367:569-578.)

4) study was a randomized trial of patients with STEMI presenting within 6 hours from the symptom onset, who were scheduled to undergo PCI after an anticipated delay of 1 to 3 hours and who were assigned to standard PCI (n = 838) or PCI preceded by administration of full-dose tenecteplase (n = 829). All patients received aspirin and a bolus without an infusion of unfractionated heparin. The investigators of ASSENT-4 planned to enroll 4000 patients, but the Data and Safety Monitoring Board recommended early cessation because of higher in-hospital mortality in the facilitated PCI group than in the group with standard PCI. The primary end point of ASSENT-4 was death, congestive heart failure, or shock within 90 days from randomization. The primary end point was achieved in 19% of patients in the facilitated PCI group and 13% in the group with standard PCI (RR = 1.39; 95% CI: 1.11 to 1.74; P = .0045) (Fig. 19-7). There were more in-hospital strokes (1.8% versus 0%, P < .001) and a higher incidence of ischemic complications such as reinfarction (6% versus 4%, P = .0279) or repeat target vessel revascularization (7% versus 3%, P = .0041) among patients treated with facilitated PCI than among those treated with standard PCI. The ASSENT-4 trial concluded that a strategy of facilitated PCI consisting of full-dose thrombolysis (i.e., tenecteplase) plus antithrombotic co-therapy and preceding PCI by 1 to 3 hours was associated with worse clinical outcome than a strategy of primary PCI alone and cannot be recommended.[41] Although the reasons for the worse outcome with facilitated PCI remain unclear, the investigators speculated that suboptimal antithrombotic therapy (i.e., absence of infusion of heparin, the absence of up-front loading of clopidogrel, and prohibition of the routine use of GP IIb/IIIa antagonists) and treatment delays in applying thrombolytic therapy (i.e., most patients received thrombolysis later than 2 hours after symptom onset) might have contributed to the failure of facilitated PCI.[41]

The meta-analysis by Keeley and coworkers,[42] which included 17 trials of STEMI patients assigned to facilitated PCI (n = 2237) or primary PCI (n = 2267), showed that facilitated PCI was associated with significantly worse short-term outcomes (up to 42 days) than primary PCI alone: death (5% versus 3%), nonfatal reinfarction (3% versus 2%), urgent target vessel revascularization (4% versus 1%), major bleeding (7% versus 5%), hemorrhagic stroke (0.7% versus 0.1%), and total stroke (1.1% versus 0.3%). The increased rates of adverse events were observed mainly when thrombolytic therapy was used to facilitate PCI.

The evidence offered by the ASSENT-4 PCI trial[41] and the meta-analysis by Keeley and colleagues[42] discourages the use of thrombolytics as pharmacologic facilitation of PCI. The use of thrombolysis for PCI facilitation is not associated with any clinical benefit, although it more than doubles the rate of full restoration of anterograde flow in the infarct-occluded artery before PCI. In the PCI Clopidogrel as Adjunctive Reperfusion Therapy (CLARITY) study, pretreatment with clopidogrel resulted in a highly significant reduction in cardiovascular death, reinfarction, or stroke from randomization through 30 days (7.5% versus 12.0% with placebo, P = .001), although only a slight improvement in TIMI flow was achieved with this pretreatment.[43] This result shows that antithrombotic drugs used in the interval until PCI is performed should not be evaluated only on the basis of their ability to restore the anterograde flow. The failure of thrombolysis to improve the results of subsequent PCI represents a further significant reduction of the role that this treatment deserves in the current reperfusion therapy of patients with STEMI.

In summary, although facilitation of PCI in the sense of promoting reperfusion as the patient is directed to the catheterization laboratory should remain a goal to strive for, available evidence demonstrates that it cannot be achieved with thrombolysis.

Rescue Percutaneous Coronary Intervention

Rescue PCI is defined as PCI performed within 12 hours after failure of thrombolysis in patients with continuing or recurrent myocardial ischemia. In many patients with STEMI, thrombolysis fails to fully restore optimal blood flow in the infarct-occluded artery or after initial restoration of blood flow becomes associated with instability of blood flow, resulting in continuing or recurrent ischemia. In the absence of coronary angiography, partial ST-segment resolution on the surface electrocardiogram or continuation of chest discomfort, even though they are known to be imprecise, can be used as putative markers of failed thrombolysis. Earlier studies have suggested that rescue PCI offers advantages over deferred PCI or conservative therapy after failed thrombolysis, resulting in higher rates of infarct-related artery recanalization, better regional ventricular function, and fewer in-hospital adverse events, including in-hospital death, and better 1-year incidence of death or congestive heart failure.

Some studies have provided confirmation of the beneficial effects of rescue PCI after failed thrombolysis in STEMI patients. The Middlesbrough Early Revascularization to Limit Infarction (MERLIN) trial randomized 307 patients with STEMI and failed thrombolysis (i.e., failure of ST-segment elevation in the lead with maximal elevation to resolve by 50%) who were randomized to emergency coronary angiography with or without rescue PCI or to conservative therapy.[44] The primary end point was all-cause mortality at 30 days. Thirty-day all-cause mortality was similar in the rescue and conservative groups (9.8% versus 11%, $P = .7$). The combined incidence of major adverse cardiac events was reduced in the rescue PCI group (37.3% versus 50.0%, $P = .02$), a result that was driven by less subsequent revascularization (6.5% versus 20.1%; $P = .01$). Reinfarction (7.2% versus 10.4%, $P = .03$) and congestive heart failure (24.2% versus 29.2%, $P = .3$) were less common among patients undergoing rescue PCI. There was an increased incidence of strokes (4.6% versus 0.6%, $P = .03$) and blood transfusions (11.1% versus 1.3%, $P = .001$) among patients treated by rescue PCI compared with those treated by conservative therapy.[44]

The Rescue Angioplasty versus Conservative Treatment or Repeat Thrombolysis (REACT) trial was a multicenter, randomized trial that enrolled 427 patients with STEMI after failed thrombolysis (i.e., less than 50% ST-segment elevation resolution 90 minutes after thrombolysis), who were assigned to repeat thrombolysis (142 patients), conservative treatment (141 patients), or rescue PCI (144 patients).[45] The rate of the composite end point of death, reinfarction, stroke, and severe heart failure within 6 months (primary end point) was significantly reduced in the group with rescue PCI (15.3%) compared with the group with repeated thrombolysis (31%) and the group with conservative therapy (29.8%; $P = .003$). All-cause mortality did not differ significantly among patients in the three groups, but there was significantly less ischemia-driven revascularization in the group with rescue PCI than in patients treated by repeat thrombolysis or conservative therapy (revascularization-free survival rates of 86.2%, 77.6%, and 74.4%, respectively; $P = .05$).

The STOPAMI-4 trial randomized 181 patients with STEMI after failed thrombolysis within 24 hours (i.e., TIMI flow grade of ≤2 during coronary angiography of the infarct related artery) to coronary stenting (90 patients) or to coronary balloon angioplasty (91 patients).[46] The salvage index (i.e., proportion of initial perfusion defect salvaged by rescue intervention), obtained by paired scintigraphic studies performed 7 to 10 days apart, was the primary end point of the trial. The study demonstrated that rescue

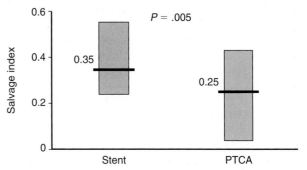

Figure 19-8. Salvage index (median and interquartile range) or the proportion of the initial area at risk salvaged by rescue coronary stenting or percutaneous transluminal coronary angioplasty (PTCA) in patients with failed thrombolysis. (Data from Schömig A, Ndrepepa G, Mehilli J, et al: A randomized trial of coronary stenting versus balloon angioplasty as a rescue intervention after failed thrombolysis in patients with acute myocardial infarction. J Am Coll Cardiol 2004;44:2073-2079.)

angioplasty was associated with a considerable myocardial salvage rate, which was significantly greater with coronary stenting than with angioplasty alone (median [25th, 75th percentiles] salvage index of 0.35 [0.24, 0.56] versus 0.25 [0.04, 0.43]; $P = .005$) (Fig. 19-8). The 1-year mortality rate was 8% for the stent group and 12% for the angioplasty group ($P = .35$). The study was important because it offered a mechanistic explanation of the benefits of rescue PCI after failed thrombolysis. It showed that a large proportion of ischemic myocardium can be salvaged by rescue PCI, although this proportion might be smaller than that reported after primary stenting.[47]

A meta-analysis of five randomized trials of rescue PCI after failed thrombolysis demonstrated a 36% decrease in the risk of death ($P = .048$) and a 28% decrease in the risk of heart failure ($P = .06$) compared with the conservative approach.[48] In summary, rescue PCI (preferentially rescue stenting) improves clinical outcome and should be recommended for patients with STEMI after failed thrombolysis.

Time-to-Treatment Interval and Outcome of Percutaneous Coronary Intervention for ST-Segment Elevation Myocardial Infarction

The time-to-treatment interval is an estimate of overall duration of myocardial ischemia that encompasses the time from the onset of symptoms of coronary occlusion to the initiation of reperfusion therapy (i.e., thrombolysis or primary PCI). Time-to-treatment interval has two components: the interval from the symptom onset to the patient's arrival at the hospital and the time from the patient's arrival to the initiation of reperfusion. Apart from disclosing the duration of myocardial ischemia, the time-to-treatment interval is an index of quality and readiness of the health care system to provide reperfusion therapy in timely fashion. The time-to-treatment and door-to-balloon intervals have been subject of intense research and great efforts are under way to shorten them.[12,49]

Knowledge about the biology of myocardial ischemia and the speed with which it succumbs to necrosis is important to understand the time dependency of efficacy of various reperfusion regimens and the degree of benefit of the reperfusion therapy in general. Experimental studies in dogs by Reimer and associates[50] offer the most complete picture of developments after coronary artery occlusion. Abrupt coronary occlusion results in drastic reduction in the coronary blood flow and myocardial necrosis that progresses gradually and that usually is complete about 6 hours after the onset of occlusion. A rapid phase of cell death, mostly in the subendocardial region, follows the coronary occlusion, and about one half of the ischemic myocardium that is necrotic at 24 hours has already died by 40 minutes of coronary occlusion.[50] A second phase of cell death occurs more slowly in the mid-epicardial and subepicardial myocardium. This phase of myocardial necrosis is completed within 6 hours of coronary occlusion, and about one third of ischemic myocardium is salvageable at 3 hours.[50]

There are considerable differences between coronary occlusion and acute MI in experimental setting and spontaneously occurring coronary occlusion and STEMI in clinical setting. Factors such as a stuttering course of coronary occlusion, spontaneous recanalization, and persistence of anterograde blood flow in the infarct-related artery, collateral circulation, preconditioning, and effects of initial anti-ischemic (antithrombotic) therapy may modify the course of myocardial ischemia progression to necrosis and may extend the time during which ischemic myocardium remains viable. Scintigraphic data have identified viable myocardium in patients with STEMI presenting late (>6 hours) after symptom onset, and this viable myocardium is salvageable when PCI is used as a reperfusion means.

These data suggest the existence of two phases of myocardial salvage: an early phase of myocardial salvage enabled by early reperfusion (within the first hour) and a late phase of myocardial salvage enabled by later reperfusion. During the early phase, reperfusion is associated with substantial and time-dependent myocardial salvage. However, reperfusion therapy within the first hour after coronary occlusion, which is expected to lead to large amounts of myocardial salvage, is hardly achievable. Data from the ASSENT-3 trial have shown that the time-to-treatment interval was less than 2 hours for only 27% of the patients and less than 1 hour for only 3.2%.[51] Reperfusion in the second phase results in a smaller degree of and less time-dependent myocardial salvage. Analysis of time-to-treatment intervals in various studies suggests that most reperfusion studies are performed in the late phase of myocardial salvage, in which primary PCI is clearly superior to thrombolysis in restoring epicardial blood flow in the infarct-related artery. In this phase, a much slower progression of ischemic myocardium to necrosis takes place

owing to residual blood flow or other factors, and myocardial salvage is less time dependent. This may explain the relative independence of myocardial salvage or clinical outcome from time-to-treatment interval when PCI is used as a reperfusion approach (Fig. 19-9).[52]

Time from the onset of symptoms to initiation of reperfusion is an important predictor of myocardial salvage or clinical outcome, particularly with thrombolytic reperfusion. It is widely accepted that the ability of thrombolytic reperfusion to dissolve coronary thrombi and re-canalize occluded coronary arteries and its clinical benefit are heavily time dependent and drastically reduced with the increase in the time-to-treatment interval. The dependence of myocardial salvage or clinical outcome on the time-to-treatment interval in patients with STEMI undergoing PCI is less evident, and the issue is still controversial. A progressive increase in the 1-year mortality rate with every 15-minute increase in the symptom onset-to-balloon time has been reported.[53] However, patients who presented later were older, more often were women, were diabetics, and had a history of coronary bypass surgery.[53] These characteristics are known to have a negative impact on mortality. After adjustment for these factors, the highly significant univariate association ($P < .001$) between time to treatment and mortality was considerably weakened to a borderline significance level ($P = .041$).[53] Patients with a greater delay in admission are also expected to present more frequently with additional adverse characteristics, such as impaired renal function, peripheral arterial disease, or greater inflammatory burden, which were not accounted for in the multivariate model. The lack of adjustment for similar characteristics further widens the gap between statistical and biologic adjustments regarding prognosis. It is highly probable that the more adverse baseline risk profile of patients with longer delay to presentation is the determinant mechanism underlying the apparent association between mortality and time to treatment. Associated comorbidities and the less favorable cardiovascular risk profile may mask the benefits of mechanical reperfusion due to myocardial salvage, and the unfavorable outcome after coronary intervention may erroneously be attributed solely to the longer time-to-reperfusion interval. These considerations are important because the apparent reduction of benefit from PCI with increased time to presentation may be interpreted as a poor incentive for prompt intervention in patients with delayed presentation who are badly in need of this treatment.

Scintigraphic studies provide valuable information on infarct size (Fig. 19-10) and allow assessment of the efficacy of reperfusion in terms of myocardial salvage with a high prognostic value (Fig. 19-11).[54] Several studies have suggested an independence of myocardial salvage or clinical outcome from the time-to-treatment interval in STEMI patients undergoing PCI. In an analysis of the STOPAMI trials that included patients up to 12 hours from symptom

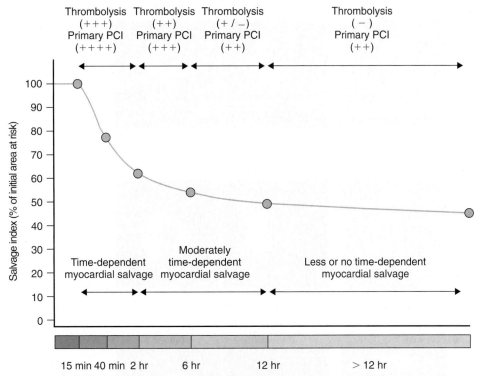

Figure 19-9. Time dependency of myocardial salvage expressed as percentage of initial area at risk and the time dependency of efficacy of thrombolysis or primary percutaneous coronary intervention (PCI). The initial parts of the curve up to 2 hours were reconstructed based on the experimental studies. For the first 15 minutes (15 min) after coronary occlusion, myocardial necrosis is not observed. At 40 minutes (40 min) after coronary occlusion, myocardial cell death develops rapidly, and the myocardial necrosis is confluent. After this point, progression to necrosis is slowed considerably. The other part of the curve showing myocardial salvage from 2 to more than 12 hours from the symptom onset is reconstructed on the basis of data from scintigraphic studies in patients with acute myocardial infarction. Efficacy of reperfusion is expressed as follows: (++++), very effective; (+++), effective; (++), moderately effective; (±), uncertainly effective; (–), not effective. (From Schömig A, Ndrepepa G, Kastrati A: Late myocardial salvage: Time to recognize its reality in the reperfusion therapy of acute myocardial infarction. Eur Heart J 2006;27:1900-1907.)

onset, it was demonstrated that a longer symptom onset-to-treatment interval is associated with less myocardial salvage in patients treated with thrombolysis but not in those treated with coronary stenting. The myocardial salvage index, an estimate of the amount of myocardium salvaged by reperfusion therapy, was reduced markedly with longer time-to-treatment intervals only for patients treated with thrombolysis, but it remained high and relatively constant for those treated with coronary stenting.[47] The Beyond 12 hours Reperfusion AlternatiVe Evaluation-2 (BRAVE-2) trial demonstrated the potential of primary PCI to salvage myocardium and reduce infarct size, even in patients with STEMI presenting 12 to 48 hours from the symptom onset.[55] The median infarct size was 8% in patients with STEMI who were assigned to primary PCI and 13% in patients assigned to conservative treatment ($P < .001$).[55] Data from the NRMI showed that there is no association between symptom onset-to-balloon time and survival in a cohort of 27,080 consecutive patients with acute MI treated with primary angioplasty.[56] Similarly, an analysis of 2635 patients enrolled in 10 randomized trials of primary angioplasty versus thrombolytic therapy demonstrated that with increasing time-to-

presentation interval, major adverse cardiac event rates increased after thrombolysis but remained relatively stable after angioplasty.[57]

One study deserves comment, although it did not deal with patients with acute STEMI. In a selected cohort of patients, the Occluded Artery Trial (OAT) investigators assessed whether opening the occluded artery by PCI 3 to 28 days (median, 8 days) after STEMI could improve the clinical outcome up to 5 years after randomization.[58] The study showed no benefit with this strategy, thereby failing to offer support for the *open artery hypothesis*.[58]

Although the superiority of primary PCI over thrombolysis for longer time-to-presentation intervals is undeniable, there exists controversy about whether primary PCI is superior to thrombolysis when applied early after symptom onset (≤2 hours). Most of this controversy was generated after the publication of a subset analysis from the Comparison of Angioplasty and Prehospital Thrombolysis in Acute Myocardial Infarction (CAPTIM) trial, which enrolled 460 patients and showed that patients with STEMI randomized less than 2 hours after symptom onset had a trend toward lower 30-day mortality with thrombolysis compared with primary PCI (2.2%

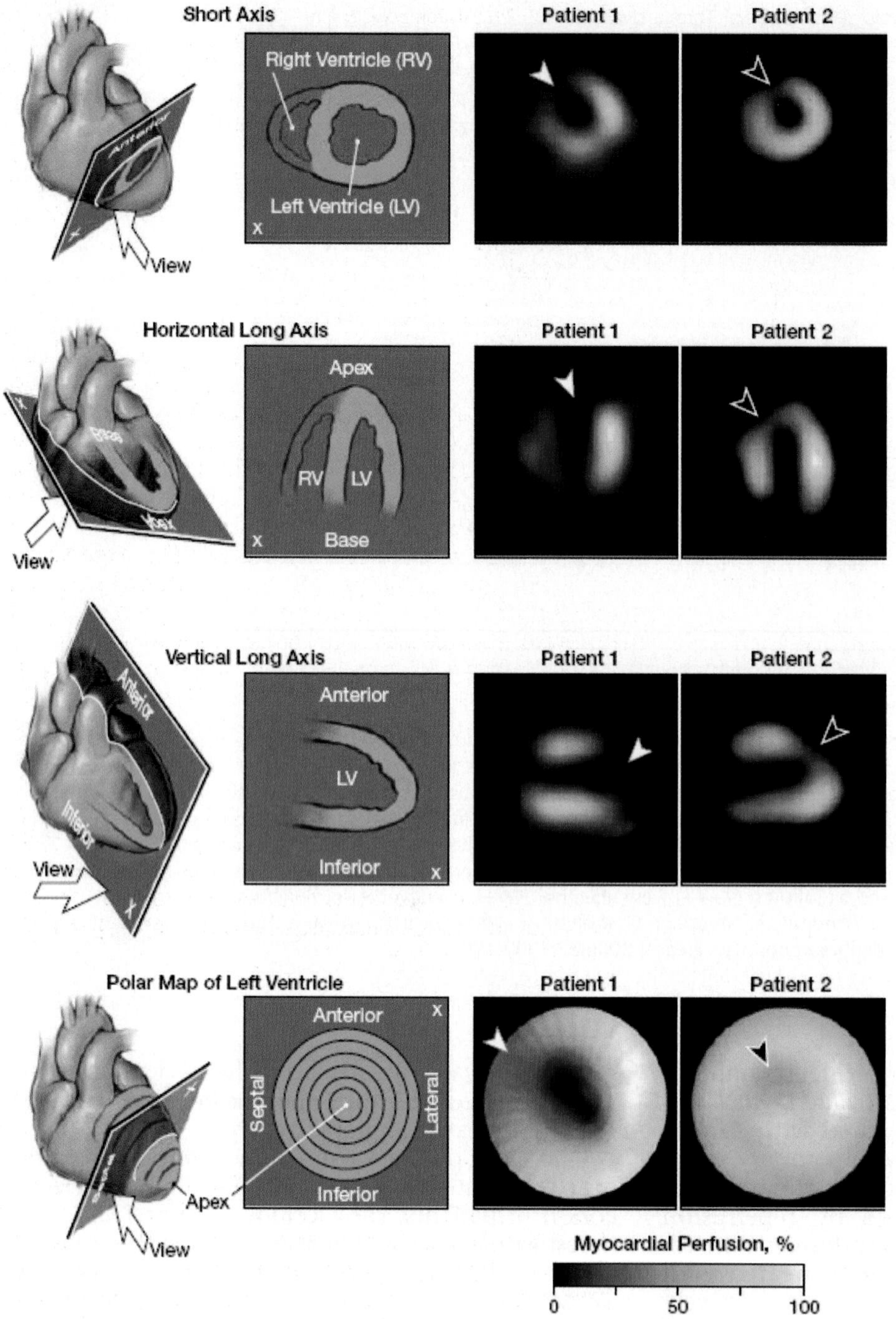

Figure 19-10. Technetium Tc 99m single-photon emission computed tomography images recorded in two patients 1 week after acute myocardial infarction of anterior wall. Patient 1 represents an example of a large myocardial infarction (i.e., perfusion defect involving 38% of the left ventricle; *white arrows*). Patient 2 represents an example of small myocardial infarction of the anterior wall (i.e., perfusion defect of 6% of the left ventricle; *black arrows*). (From Kastrati A, Mehilli J, Schlotterbeck K, et al: Early administration of reteplase plus abciximab vs abciximab alone in patients with acute myocardial infarction referred for percutaneous coronary intervention: A randomized controlled trial. JAMA 2004;291:947-954. Copyright 2004 American Medical Association. All rights reserved.)

versus 5.7%, $P = .058$).[59] The reliability of these results is strongly compromised by the fact that they were produced by a subset analysis of a prematurely terminated trial.

A meta-analysis by the Primary Coronary Angioplasty vs. Thrombolysis-2 (PCAT-2) Trialists' Collaborative Group that was based on individual patient data has demonstrated that primary PCI is superior to thrombolysis in reduction of the 30-day mortality rate, even for a presentation delay of less than 2 hours, as was the case for 2747 patients (4.3% with PCI versus 6.2% with thrombolysis, $P = .03$) (Fig. 19-12).[9] The analysis of a large registry of 26,205 patients with STEMI clearly showed that PCI was superior to prehospital thrombolysis in terms of reduced 30-day and 1-year mortality rates.[60] Based on these data and on the negative findings of the studies on early thrombolysis in the settings of the facilitated PCI strategy despite earlier restoration of flow in a considerable number of patients (see "Facilitated Percutaneous Coronary Intervention"), it is unlikely that the occasionally propagated therapy of prehospital (in ambulance) thrombolysis will be able to compete with a primary PCI strategy. Prehospital thrombolysis carries the risk of exposing many misdiagnosed patients to the hazards of thrombolysis. As

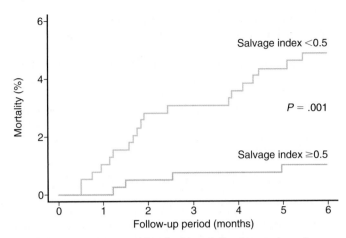

Figure 19-11. Prognostic role of salvage index (proportion of initial area at risk salvaged by reperfusion therapy) illustrated by 6-month mortality curves in two groups of patients with acute myocardial infarction defined by a cutoff median value of 0.5. (Data from Ndrepepa G, Mehilli J, Schwaiger M, et al: Prognostic value of myocardial salvage achieved by reperfusion therapy in patients with acute myocardial infarction. J Nucl Med 2004;45:725-729.)

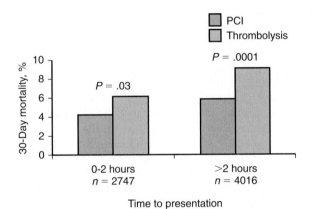

Figure 19-12. Differences in 30-day mortality among patients treated with primary percutaneous coronary intervention (PCI) or thrombolysis according to time to presentation interval dichotomized at the 2-hour interval. (Data from Boersma E: Does time matter? A pooled analysis of randomized clinical trials comparing primary percutaneous coronary intervention and in-hospital fibrinolysis in acute myocardial infarction patients. Eur Heart J 2006;27:779-788.)

long as no specifically designed studies have provided evidence in support of prehospital thrombolysis versus routine PCI in patients calling for medical assistance within 2 to 3 hours from symptom onset, the application of prehospital thrombolysis strategy should be discouraged.

Studies have demonstrated an association between the door-to-balloon interval and survival of patients with STEMI. In a report from NRMI that included data on a cohort of 29,222 patients with STEMI treated with PCI within 6 hours of presentation, longer door-to-balloon intervals were associated with increased in-hospital mortality rates.[61] In-hospital mortality rates were 3%, 4.2%, 5.7%, and 7.4% for

door-to-balloon intervals of 90 minutes or less, 91 to 120 minutes, 121 to 150 minutes, and more than 150 minutes, respectively ($P < .001$).[61] It seems that a high-risk profile and a shorter presentation delay may accentuate this association.[62,63] Despite these data, door-to-treatment times have not decreased significantly in recent years,[64] and greater efforts should be made to improve this parameter. The door-to-balloon time is an indicator of patients' characteristics[26] and experience of the institution providing the primary PCI.[29] Comorbid conditions, absence of chest pain, delayed presentation after symptom onset, less specific electrocardiographic findings, and hospital presentation during off hours were associated with longer total door-to-balloon times.[26] Longer door-to-balloon times were associated with older patients, female sex, nonwhite race, and complex medical histories.[65] Door-to-balloon delay also depended heavily on the hospital characteristics. Presentation at night and treatment at lower-volume facilities were strong independent predictors of longer door-to-balloon intervals.[65,66] Greater experience with primary PCI is associated with shorter door-to-balloon times and lower in-hospital mortality rates for patients with STEMI treated with primary PCI.[29] Primary PCI was superior to thrombolysis, regardless of the door-to-balloon time the treating institution was able to achieve.[9]

In summary, PCI is an invaluable reperfusion treatment option for patients presenting early or late after onset of symptoms. Although prehospital care is critical for successful STEMI management, no evidence supports the use of prehospital thrombolysis.

ASSOCIATED THERAPEUTIC APPROACHES

Rheolytic Therapy and Distal Protection Devices

Although primary PCI is a highly effective therapy in patients with STEMI, there has been great concern that conventional PCI using balloons and stents may dislodge thrombotic material or atherosclerotic plaque debris into the distal circulation, resulting in distal embolization and poor myocardial perfusion after balloon angioplasty or stenting. Distal embolization does occur during PCI for STEMI, and visible debris has been aspirated in 73% of patients.[67] There has been increased interest in developing thrombectomy and distal protection systems to limit distal embolization and improve myocardial perfusion and clinical outcome. Earlier studies including limited numbers of patients tested the safety, feasibility, and efficacy of various devices, demonstrating that embolic protection can be safely performed during PCI in STEMI and that it has positive effects on myocardial reperfusion and outcome.[68] This was also observed in initial, small-scale, randomized studies.[69,70]

Larger studies that evaluated different devices (e.g., Guardwire, Medtronic; Angiojet, Possis Medical; FilterWire, Boston Scientific) with various operational mechanisms failed to demonstrate any positive effect of embolic distal protection on myocardial reperfusion or clinical outcome. The Enhanced Myocardial Efficacy and Recovery by Aspiration of Liberated Debris (EMERALD) trial enrolled 501 patients with STEMI presenting within 6 hours and undergoing primary or rescue PCI to receive angioplasty with balloon occlusion and aspiration distal microcirculatory protection system (GuardWire Plus, Medtronic) versus angioplasty without distal protection. Although the distal balloon occlusion and aspiration system effectively retrieved embolic debris in most patients (73%) undergoing PCI, distal embolic protection did not result in improved microvascular flow, greater reperfusion success, reduced infarct size, or enhanced event-free survival.[67]

In the Protection Devices in PCI Treatment of Myocardial Infarction for Salvage of Endangered Myocardium (PROMISE) trial, which included 200 patients with acute MI, distal protection with Filter-Wire-EX device (Boston Scientific) failed to improve maximal adenosine-induced Doppler flow velocity in the infarct-related artery after PCI or to reduce infarct size as measured by resonance magnetic imaging.[71]

The AngioJet Rheolytic Thrombectomy in Patients Undergoing Primary Angioplasty for Acute Myocardial Infarction (AIMI) study randomized 480 patients with STEMI presenting within 12 hours from symptom onset to treatment with rheolytic thrombectomy (AngioJet catheter, Possis Medical) as an adjunct to primary PCI or PCI alone.[72] Despite effective thrombus removal, greater infarct size was observed in patients with rheolytic thrombectomy compared with patients treated by PCI alone (12.5% versus 9.8% of the left ventricle, $P = .03$). The 30-day incidence of major adverse cardiac events was higher for the group with rheolytic thrombectomy than for the group with PCI alone (6.7% versus 1.7%, $P = .01$), including mortality (4.6% versus 0.8%, $P = .02$).[72] In a later randomized study that enrolled 215 patients with STEMI, thrombectomy pretreatment was associated with an increase in the infarct size as measured by sestamibi SPECT at 30 days (median infarct size of 15% in the group with thrombectomy pretreatment versus 8% in the group with standard PCI, $P = .004$).

Mechanisms of failure of these devices to improve myocardial reperfusion or outcome in patients with STEMI have been revised.[73] In light of the results of these studies, there is no place for thrombectomy or distal embolic protection devices to be used during PCI in patients with STEMI.[74] Whether there is any subgroup of patients with STEMI, such as patients with a large thrombotic burden, who may benefit from this approach remains to be determined in future studies.

Periprocedural Antithrombotic Therapy

Pretreatment with aspirin and clopidogrel and periprocedural heparinization represent the most common forms of adjunct antithrombotic management in patients with STEMI undergoing PCI. Platelet inhibition by various antithrombotic agents used before, during, and after PCI procedures is an integral part of PCI in patients with STEMI.

The use of antithrombotic agents, especially GP IIb/IIIa inhibitors in the setting of facilitated PCI, was described earlier in this chapter (see "Facilitated Percutaneous Coronary Intervention"). However, the short-term and long-term impact of GP IIb/IIIa inhibitors used as adjunctive therapy to primary PCI in STEMI patients remains unclear despite abundant evidence, especially in the case of abciximab. A meta-analysis was able to show a reduction of the 30-day mortality rate from 3.4% to 2.4% when abciximab was used during primary PCI.[75] The results of an updated meta-analysis on the 6- to 12-month outcomes from seven randomized trials are shown in Table 19-4 and Figure 19-13. The discrepancies in the reported effect of abciximab may reflect differences in the risk profiles of patients included in the trials, with higher-risk patients seeming to benefit more from abciximab (Fig. 19-14).

The influence of the timing of administration of GP IIb/IIIa inhibitors relative to PCI has been evaluated. A meta-analysis of six randomized trials (three trials with abciximab and three trials with tirofiban) concluded that early (upfront) administration of these agents is associated with improved coronary patency and favorable trends for clinical outcome.[76]

Table 19-4. Randomized Trials on the Value of Abciximab as an Adjunct to Percutaneous Coronary Intervention in Patients with Acute Myocardial Infarction

Trial (Authors)	No. of Patients	Type of PCI	Blinded Design	Follow-up (mo)	Source
ACE (Antoniucci et al.)	400	Stent	No	12	Circulation 2004;109:1704
ADMIRAL (Montalescot et al.)	300	Stent	Yes	6	N Engl J Med 2001;344:1895
CADILLAC (Stone et al.)	2082	PTCA/stent	No	6	N Engl J Med 2002;346:957
ISAR-2 (Neumann et al.)	401	Stent	No	12	J Am Coll Cardiol 2000;35:915
Petronio et al.	89	PTCA/stent	Yes	6	Am Heart J 2002;143:334
RAPPORT (Brener et al.)	483	PTCA	Yes	6	Circulation 1998;98:734
Zorman et al.	163	PTCA/stent	No	6	Am J Cardiol 2002;90:533

ACE, Abciximab and Carbostent Evaluation; ADMIRAL, Abciximab before Direct Angioplasty and Stenting in Myocardial Infarction Regarding Acute and Long-term Follow-up; CADILLAC: Controlled Abciximab and Device Investigation to Lower Late Angioplasty Complications; ISAR-2, Intracoronary Stenting and Antithrombotic Regimen-2; PCI, percutaneous coronary intervention; PTCA, percutaneous transluminal coronary angioplasty; RAPPORT, ReoPro and Primary PTCA Organization and Randomized Trial.

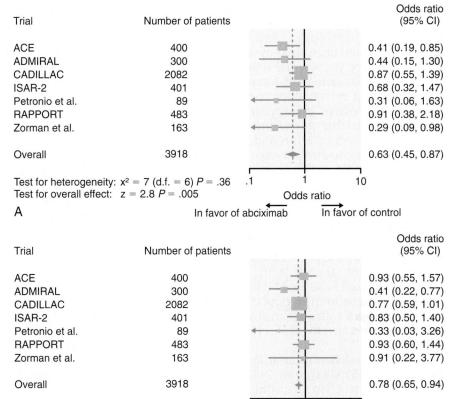

Figure 19-13. Odds ratios (95% confidence interval) of 6- to 12-month mortality **(A)** and target vessel revascularization **(B)** generated by a meta-analysis (random effect model) of seven randomized trials evaluating the platelet glycoprotein IIb/IIIa receptor inhibitor abciximab as an adjunctive therapy to primary percutaneous coronary intervention in patients with acute myocardial infarction. (Data sources are provided in Table 19-4.)

Whether the early benefits achieved with abciximab are sustained over time remains controversial.[77,78] In summary, the evidence supports the use of GP IIb/IIIa inhibitors, abciximab in particular, in many patients with STEMI. Use of these agents requires a reduction of the heparin dose given during the procedure.

The use of a loading dose of clopidogrel before PCI has become a standard after the positive results reported for elective and primary PCI.[43,79] Especially when given in a high loading dose of 600 mg, clopidogrel may attenuate the need of GP IIb/IIIa inhibitors during primary PCI. This hypothesis is being tested in the randomized Bavarian Reperfusion Alternatives Evaluation-3 (BRAVE-3) trial, which is planned to include 800 patients with STEMI. Clopi-dogrel pretreatment may also enable replacement of GP IIb/IIIa inhibitors plus heparin with the direct thrombin inhibitor bivalirudin; this hypothesis is being assessed in the ongoing Harmonizing Outcomes with Revascularization and Stents (HORIZONS) trial.

P2Y12 platelet receptor antagonists (e.g., prasugrel, cangrelor) with a more rapid onset of action than clopidogrel are being assessed in ongoing clinical trials. There are no properly designed studies on the value of low-molecular-weight heparins and factor Xa inhibitors in patients with STEMI treated with PCI. A PCI subset analysis from the Organization for the Assessment of Strategies for Ischemic Syndromes-6 (OASIS-6) trial could not show any benefits with the use of fondaparinux.[80]

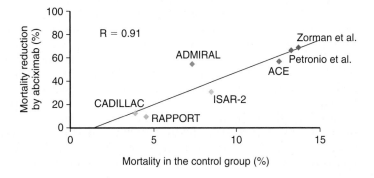

Figure 19-14. Graph showing the dependence of the effect of abciximab (relative reduction of 6- to 12-month mortality) on the baseline risk of the patients (6- to 12-month mortality in the control group). (Data sources are provided in Table 19-4.)

Adjunct Therapies to Enhance Myocardial Salvage

Various pharmacologic and nonpharmacologic approaches have been used as adjunct therapy with PCI to enhance myocardial reperfusion and salvage and to improve outcomes for patients with STEMI. Adenosine and novel adenosine agonists have been tested as adjunctive therapy in these patients. The hypothesis was that adenosine through its salutary effects on microcirculation and its consistently confirmed property to protect myocardium from ischemic injury would promote myocardial salvage and improve clinical outcome. However, the results of research proved to be disappointing regarding the use of adenosine (or adenosine agonists) as adjunctive therapy to PCI in patients with STEMI. The AmP579 Delivery for Myocardial Infarction Reduction (ADMIRE) study tested the AMP579 (i.e., adenosine receptor agonist with A1 and A2 effects) on a randomized basis in 311 STEMI patients undergoing primary balloon angioplasty.[81] The agent failed to reduce infarct size as measured with sestamibi scintigraphy 120 to 216 hours after balloon angioplasty.

In the Acute Myocardial Infarction Study of Adenosine-II (AMISTAD-II) trial, 2118 patients with anterior STEMI receiving thrombolysis or primary angioplasty were randomized to a 3-hour infusion of adenosine (50 or 70 µg/kg/min) or to placebo.[82] Adenosine did not reduce the combined end point of death, new heart failure, and first hospitalization for heart failure within 6 months (16.3% with adenosine versus 17.9% with placebo, P = NS). Infarct size as measured with sestamibi scintigraphy was reduced with high-dose adenosine (70 µg/kg/min) but not with low-dose adenosine (50 µg/kg/min). Based on the results of these studies, there is no place for adenosine as adjunctive therapy with primary PCI in patients with STEMI.

The effects of glucose-insulin-potassium (GIK) therapy in patients with STEMI undergoing PCI have been evaluated. In the Reevaluation of Intensified Venous Metabolic Support for Acute Infarct Size Limitation (REVIVAL) randomized trial conducted among 312 patients with acute MI, GIK therapy did not lead to a reduction of scintigraphically measured infarct size (median salvage index of 0.50 [25th, 75th percentiles: 0.18, 0.87] in the GIK group and 0.48 [25th, 75th percentiles: 0.27, 0.78] in the control group; P = .96) or 6-month mortality rates (5.8% in the GIK group and 6.4% in the control group; P = .85).[83] In the Glucose-Insulin-Potassium Study (GIPS), a randomized trial enrolling 940 patients, the 30-day mortality rate was 4.8% for patients receiving GIK and 5.8% for the control group (P = .50).[84] These results demonstrate that there is no role for GIK as adjunct therapy to primary PCI in patients with STEMI.

Based on the experimental evidence that complement system activation may be involved in the ischemic injury after reperfusion, the effects a C5 complement inhibitor, pexelizumab, on infarct size

in patients with STEMI undergoing primary PCI have been evaluated.[85] The Complement inhibition in Myocardial Infarction Treated with Angioplasty (COMMA) trial randomized 960 patients with STEMI to receive placebo, pexelizumab (2.0-mg/kg bolus), or pexelizumab (2.0-mg/kg bolus and 0.05 mg/kg/hr infusion for 20 hours). The infarct size (measured by creatine kinase-MB area under the curve) or 90-day composite of death, new or worsening heart failure, shock, and stroke (11.1% with placebo, 10.7% with pexelizumab as bolus, and 8.5% with pexelizumab as bolus plus infusion) were unaffected by pexelizumab. However, 90-day mortality was significantly lower with pexelizumab plus bolus infusion (1.8% with pexelizumab versus 5.9% with placebo, P = .014). The reduction in mortality could not be explained by an effect on infarct size but through putatively novel mechanisms.[85] Not enough is known about the impact of complement system inhibitors on the myocardial reperfusion to allow firm recommendations on their use in patients with STEMI as adjunctive therapy to primary PCI.

Nicorandil, a hybrid compound of an ATP-sensitive potassium channel opener and a nitric oxide donor, has been tested as adjunctive therapy in patients with STEMI undergoing PCI.[86] In this study, 368 patients with first STEMI were randomized to receive 12 mg of nicorandil or placebo immediately before PCI. Postprocedural TIMI flow grade 3 (89.7% with nicorandil versus 81.4% with placebo, P = .025), corrected TIMI frame count (21.0 ± 9.1 with nicorandil versus 25.1 ± 14.1 with placebo, P = .0009), and ST-segment elevation resolution greater than 50% (79.5% with nicorandil versus 61.2% with placebo, P = .0002) were improved by nicorandil. During a mean follow-up of 2.4 years, 6.5% of patients assigned to nicorandil and 16.4% of patients assigned to placebo died of cardiovascular causes or had hospital admissions for congestive heart failure (P = .0058). This study showed that nicorandil improved angiographic and myocardial reperfusion markers and long-term clinical outcome.[86] However, further confirmation of the beneficial effects of ATP-sensitive potassium channel openers as adjunctive to primary PCI in patients with STEMI is needed.

In the Caldaret in Patients Undergoing Primary Percutaneous Coronary Intervention for ST-Elevation Myocardial Infarction (CASTEMI) trial, 387 patients with STEMI within 6 hours were randomized to caldaret (an agent supposed to reduce intracellular calcium by inhibiting Na/Ca exchange and enhancing calcium reuptake by the sarcoplasmic reticulum) or to placebo. Caldaret was not associated with a reduction in infarct size or improvement in left ventricular function as assessed by gated SPECT imaging.[87]

Limited information (i.e., trials reported but not published yet) exists for other agents or approaches used as adjunctive to primary PCI in patients with STEMI. The Acute Myocardial Infarction with Hyperoxemic Therapy (AMIHOT) trial randomized patients with acute MI within 24 hours after primary stenting to intracoronary hyperoxemic reperfusion with aqueous oxygen or to the control group.[88] Although the hyperoxemic reperfusion was safe and well tolerated, it did not result in a significant improvement in ST-segment elevation resolution, regional wall motion assessed by serial echocardiography, or infarct size reduction assessed by SPECT.

Active cooling as a means of cardioprotection has been evaluated. The COOLing as an Adjunctive Therapy to Percutaneous Intervention in Patients with Acute Myocardial Infarction (COOL-MI) trial evaluated the effect of systemic hyperthermia by randomizing 395 patients with STEMI presenting within 6 hours to primary PCI with mild hyperthermia or to primary PCI alone.[89] The procedure was well tolerated. There was no effect of cooling in final infarct size as measured by SPECT imaging at 30 days. There was no difference in the infarct size at 7 days.

In summary, there is not sufficient evidence for any of these approaches to have fulfilled expectations regarding enhancement of myocardial salvage and secured a place as an adjunct therapy to PCI in patients with STEMI.

Cell-Based Cardiac Regeneration after ST-Segment Elevation Myocardial Infarction

Intuitively, patients with STEMI may be considered prime candidates for application of cell-based cardiac repair techniques to enhance myocardial recovery after myocardial necrosis by replacing lost myocytes. Animal studies of MI have reported that stem cell and progenitor cell transplantation has resulted in neo-angiogenesis and myogenesis and improved contractile function. Several studies, mostly involving limited numbers of patients, have evaluated the use of stem cell–based techniques for myocardial regeneration in patients with STEMI after PCI. The latest studies in this field are summarized in the form of two meta-analyses of changes in left ventricular function associated with cell-based therapies (Table 19-5 and Fig. 19-15).

The Reinfusion of Enriched Progenitor Cells And Infarct Remodeling in Acute Myocardial Infarction (REPAIR-AMI) trial was a randomized trial that recruited 204 patients with STEMI treated by primary stenting. They were assigned to receive an intracoronary infusion of progenitor cells derived from bone marrow (BMCs) or placebo medium into the infarct artery 3 to 7 days after successful PCI therapy. At 4 months, the absolute improvement in the global left ventricular ejection fraction was significantly greater in the BMC group than in the placebo group (delta of 5.5% ± 7.3% versus 3.0% ± 6.5%; $P = .01$).[90] In another randomized study carried out in 67 patients, intracoronary transfer of BMC 1 day after successful

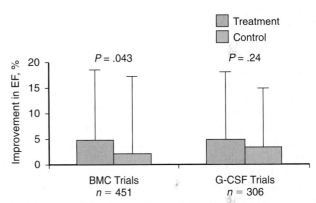

Figure 19-15. Meta-analysis of the randomized cell-based regeneration trials using injection of bone marrow cells (BMC) or granulocyte colony-stimulating factor (G-CSF) in patients with acute myocardial infarction treated with mechanical reperfusion. Modest but significant improvement in the left ventricular ejection fraction (EF) was observed only with BMC therapy. (Data sources are provided in Table 19-5.)

Table 19-5. Randomized Trials on the Value of Stem Cell–Based Therapies after Successful Reperfusion in Patients with Acute Myocardial Infarction

Trial (Authors)	No. of Patients	Started after AMI (days)	Blinded Design	Follow-up (mo)	Source
BMC Trials					
BOOST (Wollert et al.)	60	6	No	6	Lancet 2004;364:141
ASTAMI (Lunde et al.)	100	6	No	6	N Engl J Med 2006;355:1199
REPAIR-AMI (Schächinger et al.)	204	4	Yes	4	N Engl J Med 2006;355:1210
Ruan et al.	20	NA	NA	6	Chin Med J 2005;118:1175
Janssens et al.	67	Few days	Yes	4	Lancet 2006;367:113
G-CSF Trials					
REVIVAL-2 (Zohlnhöfer et al.)	114	5	Yes	6	JAMA 2006;295:1003
Valgimigli et al.	20	1-2	Yes	6	Eur Heart J 2005;26:1838
STEMMI (Ripa et al.)	78	1-2	Yes	6	Circulation 2006;113:1983
FIRSTLINE-AMI (Ince et al.)	50	Same day	No	4	Circulation 2006;112:3097
G-CSF-STEMI (Engelmann et al.)	44	1-7	No	3	J Am Coll Cardiol 2006;48:1712

AMI, acute myocardial infarction; ASTAMI, Autologous Stem Cell Transplantation in Acute Myocardial Infarction; BMC, bone marrow cells; BOOST, BOne MarrOw Transfer to Enhance ST-Elevation Infarct Regeneration; FIRSTLINE-AMI, Front-Integrated Revascularization and Stem Cell Liberation in Evolving Acute Myocardial Infarction by Use of Granulocyte-Colony-Stimulating Factor (FIRSTLINE-AMI); G-CSF, granulocyte colony-stimulating factor; G-CSF-STEMI, Granulocyte Colony-Stimulating Factor ST-Segment Elevation Myocardial Infarction; NA, not applicable; REVIVAL-2, Regenerate Vital Myocardium by Vigorous Activation of Bone Marrow Stem Cells-2; STEMMI, Stem Cells in Myocardial Infarction.

PCI was not associated with greater improvement of left ventricular ejection fraction from 4 days to 4 months after PCI compared with controls, although there was a significant reduction in infarct size with this therapy.[91] In the randomized Autologous Stem Cell Transplantation in Acute Myocardial Infarction (ASTAMI) trial (i.e., effects on left ventricular function by intracoronary injections of autologous mononuclear bone marrow cells in acute anterior wall MI) involving 101 patients with STEMI of anterior wall location, intracoronary BMC injection 5 to 8 days after successful PCI did not improve left ventricular ejection fraction at 6 months.[92] Another study of 35 patients with STEMI treated with coronary stenting raised the possibility that intracoronary stem cell therapy (CD133[+] progenitor cells) could increase the incidence of adverse coronary events, including in-stent re-occlusion, in-stent restenosis, and de novo lesions.[93]

The property of granulocyte colony-stimulating factor (G-CSF) to mobilize stem cells from bone marrow (CD34[+] mononuclear blood stem cells) and increase their circulating levels has been used for stem cell mobilization (G-CSF injection) in patients with STEMI and for harvesting stem cells for intracoronary delivery. Research with this agent has produced conflicting results. The Front-Integrated Revascularization and Stem Cell Liberation in Evolving Acute Myocardial Infarction by Use of Granulocyte Colony-Stimulating Factor (FIRSTLINE-AMI) assessed the effect of G-CSF integrated into primary PCI management of 50 patients with STEMI.[94] Twenty-five of these patients were randomized to receive subcutaneous G-CSF at 10 µg/kg body weight for 6 days in addition to standard care. G-CSF therapy positively affected left ventricular remodeling at 4 months, as evidenced by improved wall motion, left ventricular end-diastolic diameter, and ejection fraction.[94]

In the Stem Cells in Myocardial Infarction (STEMMI) trial, 78 patients with STEMI were randomly assigned to receive G-CSF or placebo for 6 days, starting 1 to 2 days after PCI.[95] The primary end point of systolic wall thickening assessed by magnetic resonance imaging improved 17% in the infarct area in the G-CSF group and 17% in the placebo group ($P = 1.0$). Left ventricular ejection fraction improved similarly in the two groups (8.5% versus 8.0%, $P = .9$).[95]

In the Regenerate Vital Myocardium by Vigorous Activation of Bone Marrow Stem Cells-2 (REVIVAL-2) trial, which was the largest G-CSF trial, 114 patients with STEMI were randomly assigned to G-CSF or placebo for 5 days starting on day 5 after successful PCI.[96] Between baseline and follow-up, left ventricular infarct size according to scintigraphy was reduced by 6.2% ± 9.1% in the G-CSF group and by 4.9% ± 8.9% in the placebo group ($P = .56$), and left ventricular ejection fraction assessed by magnetic resonance imaging was improved by 0.5% ± 3.8% in the G-CSF group and 2.0% ± 4.9% in the placebo group ($P = .14$). Angiographic restenosis occurred in 35.2% of

patients in the G-CSF group and in 30.9% of patients in the placebo group ($P = .79$).[96] Overall, the REVIVAL-2 trial showed that this therapy neither improves left ventricular function nor exerts any negative impact on restenosis as previously reported in a small number of patients.

In summary, although there is sufficient evidence to believe that G-CSF does not represent a useful therapy in patients with STEMI undergoing PCI, further investigations are needed to clarify the role of intracoronary injection of BMCs in these patients.

SPECIAL ISSUES OF PRIMARY PERCUTANEOUS CORONARY INTERVENTION

Risk Factors for Poor Percutaneous Coronary Intervention Outcome

Various studies have identified factors that were associated with poor outcome after primary PCI. They include cardiogenic shock, older age, reduced baseline left ventricular function, triple-vessel disease, diabetes, and comorbidities such as anemia and renal insufficiency. Although ventricular tachycardia and ventricular fibrillation have been reported to occur in 4.3% of primary PCI procedures, they do not seem to affect the outcome.

Cardiogenic Shock

Cardiogenic shock is a serious complication and remains the major cause of death for patients with STEMI. Primary PCI is a class 1 recommendation for patients with STEMI who are younger than 75 years of age and who develop cardiogenic shock within 36 hours of acute MI.[6] Despite advances in the primary PCI technique and adjunctive care, the prognosis of patients with cardiogenic shock that complicates STEMI remains grave. A report involving 483 patients with cardiogenic shock from the American College of Cardiology–National Cardiovascular Data Registry demonstrated that primary PCI was successful in 79% of these patients and that the in-hospital mortality rate was 59.4%.[97] A survey from the NRMI that analyzed the outcome of cardiogenic shock in 293,633 patients demonstrated an increase in PCI rates for patients with shock from 27.4% to 54.4% from 1995 to 2004.[98] The study showed that the increase in PCI rates was associated with a reduction in the overall in-hospital mortality rate from 60.3% to 47.9%.

The Should We Emergently Revascularize Occluded Coronaries for Cardiogenic Shock? (SHOCK) trial randomized 302 patients with acute MI complicated by cardiogenic shock to receive early revascularization (mostly PCI, $n = 152$) or initial medical stabilization ($n = 150$) treatment.[99] At 1 year of follow-up, there was an absolute 13% difference in survival rates favoring patients assigned to early revascularization approach. This benefit in survival remained almost unchanged (13.1% and 13.2%, respectively) at 3 and

6 years of follow-up. The 6-year survival rates for hospital survivors were 62.4% for those assigned to early revascularization and 44.4% for those assigned to initial medical stabilization, with annual rates of death of 8.3% versus 14.3%, respectively. For 1-year survivors, the annual rates of death were 8.0% versus 10.7%, favoring patients assigned to early revascularization. The SHOCK trial demonstrated that almost two thirds of hospital survivors with cardiogenic shock complicating acute MI who were treated with early revascularization survived a 6-year follow-up.[99] The trial strongly recommended early revascularization in patients with acute MI complicated by cardiogenic shock. An analysis of 56 patients with cardiogenic shock who were 75 years old or older and included in the SHOCK trial demonstrated that patients assigned to early revascularization had a higher 30-day mortality rate (75.0% versus 53.1%) than patients 75 years old or older assigned to initial medical stabilization.[100] However, patients 75 years old or older who underwent early revascularization had a lower left ventricular ejection fraction (27.5% versus 35.6%) and higher rate of anterior infarction (62.5% versus 40.6%). These factors may have contributed to the worse result with early revascularization in older patients.

In another report from the SHOCK trial, which enrolled 128 patients with predominantly left ventricular failure who underwent emergency revascularization, PCI (81 patients) was compared with coronary artery bypass graft surgery (47 patients).[101] Although diabetes, the proportion of patients with three-vessel disease, and left main coronary artery involvement were more common in patients undergoing surgery, the 30-day survival rates (55.6% in the PCI group versus 57.4% in the surgery group, P = .86) and the 1-year survival rates (51.9 % in the PCI group versus 46.8% in the surgery group, P = .71) were similar.[101]

Primary Percutaneous Coronary Intervention during Off Hours

The relationship between the time of day when patients with STEMI present to the hospital and the yield of primary PCI or in-hospital mortality has been addressed. In the CADILLAC trial, which included 2082 patients undergoing primary PCI, 49% of patients presented during off hours or weekends.[102] Although there was a 21-minute delay in the time-to-treatment interval for those presenting during off hours, this delay did not impact procedural success, myocardial recovery, or survival after primary PCI. An analysis of 102,086 patients with STEMI who underwent reperfusion (68,439 patients underwent thrombolysis and 33,647 patients underwent PCI) showed that in 67.9% of patients treated with thrombolysis and in 54.2% of patients treated with PCI, reperfusion was performed during off hours.[66] For patients treated by PCI, the door-to-balloon time was 21.3 minutes longer for patients presenting during off hours than those presenting during regular hours

(116.1 minutes versus 94.8 minutes). Patients presenting during off hours and undergoing PCI had a trend to higher in-hospital mortality than patients presenting during regular hours (OR = 1.05; 95% CI: 0.95 to 1.16; P = .30).[66]

Primary Percutaneous Coronary Intervention in the Elderly

Advanced age is an important associate of poor outcome after PCI and thrombolysis. In the Senior Primary Angioplasty in Myocardial Infarction (SENIOR PAMI) trial, 481 patients 70 years old or older were randomized between PCI and thrombolysis.[103] Although it showed trends in favor of PCI regarding the 30-day combined end point of death and disabling stroke (11.3% versus 13%, P = .57), mortality (10% versus 13%, P = .48), disabling stroke (0.8% versus 2.2%, P = .26), or reinfarction (1.6% versus 5.4%, P = .39), the trial was largely underpowered for evaluation of clinical end points.[103]

Primary Percutaneous Coronary Intervention in Women

Numerous studies have demonstrated that mortality rates after acute MI are higher for women than men. Several factors have been linked with the poorer prognosis for women: older age; more comorbidity; higher prevalence of cardiovascular risk factors, including arterial hypertension; diabetes and prior congestive heart failure; longer time-to-hospitalization interval; and undertreatment in the early phase of acute MI, with women less likely than men to undergo coronary angiography, primary PCI, or coronary artery bypass surgery. Despite a less favorable cardiovascular risk profile for women, studies investigating the influence of gender on the outcome after primary PCI have reported no differences in the short- or long-term mortality rates between genders[104,105] and even a higher adjusted survival probability for women (Fig. 19-16).[105] A report from the Global Use of Strategies to Open Occluded Arteries in Acute Coronary Syndromes (GUSTO IIb) Angioplasty Substudy, which randomized patients with acute MI to primary PCI or accelerated tissue plasminogen activator, showed that after adjusting for baseline variables, the 30-day combined end point of death, nonfatal MI, and nonfatal disabling stroke was similar for men and women.[104] However, the absolute number of major events prevented by primary PCI was higher in women than in men (56 events/1000 women treated with primary PCI versus 42 events/1000 men treated with primary PCI).[104] The exact mechanisms of greater benefit from primary PCI in women with acute MI compared with men are not known. A study that included 202 women and 561 men with acute MI who underwent primary PCI showed that the salvaging capacity of primary PCI is greater in women than in men. Median scintigraphically measured salvage index was 0.64 (25th, 75th percentiles: 0.35, 0.95) for women and 0.50 (25th, 75th percen-

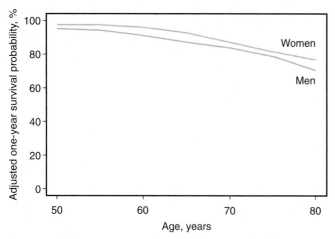

Figure 19-16. Adjusted 1-year probability of survival for women and men with acute myocardial infarction treated with a reperfusion strategy based on percutaneous coronary intervention. (Data from Mehilli J, Kastrati A, Dirschinger J, et al: Sex-based analysis of outcome in patients with acute myocardial infarction treated predominantly with percutaneous coronary intervention. JAMA 2002;287:210-215.)

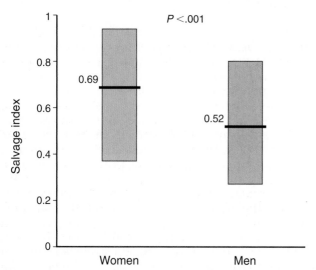

Figure 19-17. Myocardial salvage index (median with interquartile range) for women and men with acute myocardial infarction treated with primary percutaneous coronary intervention. (Data from Mehilli J, Ndrepepa G, Kastrati A, et al: Gender and myocardial salvage after reperfusion treatment in acute myocardial infarction. J Am Coll Cardiol 2005;45:828-831.)

tiles: 0.26, 0.77) for men ($P < .001$) (Fig. 19-17).[106] This study may offer one explanation why women with acute MI may derive a larger absolute benefit from direct PTCA. Based on these studies, primary PCI is strongly recommended in women with STEMI.

CONCLUSIONS

Reperfusion therapies have dramatically improved the prognosis for patients with acute STEMI. Advances in interventional techniques, devices, and antithrom-

botic therapies have enhanced the effectiveness of PCI in patients with STEMI.

More than a decade of randomized clinical trials have shown that primary PCI is superior to thrombolysis as a reperfusion therapy. Its advantages consist of the extremely low number of contraindications, high efficacy in patients presenting early or late after onset of symptoms, and a low number of complications. PCI is also very helpful after failed thrombolysis. Although the proportion of patients with STEMI treated with PCI has been increasing in the past years, major efforts are required to make this therapy available to all patients within a short time from symptom onset.

Patients with STEMI who undergo PCI benefit from pretreatment with effective antiplatelet therapies. In contrast, thrombolysis does not help before PCI and may even be harmful. Additional work is needed to develop effective adjunct therapies that can further promote myocardial salvage after PCI. Intensive experimental and clinical research aiming at myocardial cell regeneration is opening prospects for the improvement of prognosis and quality of life of patients with STEMI.

REFERENCES

1. Thom T, Haase N, Rosamond W, et al: Heart disease and stroke statistics—2006 update: A report from the American Heart Association Statistics Committee and Stroke Statistics Subcommittee. Circulation 2006;113:e85-e151.
2. Brener SJ, Topol EJ: Catheter-Based Reperfusion for Acute Myocardial Infarction, 4th ed. Philadelphia, Elsevier, 2003.
3. Keeley EC, Boura JA, Grines CL: Primary angioplasty versus intravenous thrombolytic therapy for acute myocardial infarction: A quantitative review of 23 randomised trials. Lancet 2003;361:13-20.
4. Grines C, Patel A, Zijlstra F, et al: Primary coronary angioplasty compared with intravenous thrombolytic therapy for acute myocardial infarction: Six-month follow up and analysis of individual patient data from randomized trials. Am Heart J 2003;145:47-57.
5. Keeley EC, Grines CL: Primary coronary intervention for acute myocardial infarction. JAMA 2004;291:736-739.
6. Antman EM, Anbe DT, Armstrong PW, et al: ACC/AHA guidelines for the management of patients with ST-elevation myocardial infarction: A report of the American College of Cardiology/American Heart Association Task Force on Practice Guidelines (Committee to Revise the 1999 Guidelines for the Management of Patients with Acute Myocardial Infarction). Circulation 2004;110:e82-e292.
7. Grzybowski M, Clements EA, Parsons L, et al: Mortality benefit of immediate revascularization of acute ST-segment elevation myocardial infarction in patients with contraindications to thrombolytic therapy: A propensity analysis. JAMA 2003;290:1891-1898.
8. Kastrati A, Mehilli J, Nekolla S, et al: A randomized trial comparing myocardial salvage achieved by coronary stenting versus balloon angioplasty in patients with acute myocardial infarction considered ineligible for reperfusion therapy. J Am Coll Cardiol 2004;43:734-741.
9. Boersma E: Does time matter? A pooled analysis of randomized clinical trials comparing primary percutaneous coronary intervention and in-hospital fibrinolysis in acute myocardial infarction patients. Eur Heart J 2006;27:779-788.
10. Thune JJ, Hoefsten DE, Lindholm MG, et al: Simple risk stratification at admission to identify patients with reduced mortality from primary angioplasty. Circulation 2005;112:2017-2021.

11. Aversano T, Aversano LT, Passamani E, et al: Thrombolytic therapy vs primary percutaneous coronary intervention for myocardial infarction in patients presenting to hospitals without on-site cardiac surgery: A randomized controlled trial. JAMA 2002;287:1943-1951.

12. Jacobs AK, Antman EM, Ellrodt G, et al: Recommendation to develop strategies to increase the number of ST-segment-elevation myocardial infarction patients with timely access to primary percutaneous coronary intervention. Circulation 2006;113:2152-2163.

13. Henry TD, Atkins JM, Cunningham MS, et al: ST-segment elevation myocardial infarction: Recommendations on triage of patients to heart attack centers: Is it time for a national policy for the treatment of ST-segment elevation myocardial infarction? J Am Coll Cardiol 2006;47:1339-1345.

14. Zhu MM, Feit A, Chadow H, et al: Primary stent implantation compared with primary balloon angioplasty for acute myocardial infarction: A meta-analysis of randomized clinical trials. Am J Cardiol 2001;88:297-301.

15. Mehta RH, Harjai KJ, Cox DA, et al: Comparison of coronary stenting versus conventional balloon angioplasty on five-year mortality in patients with acute myocardial infarction undergoing primary percutaneous coronary intervention. Am J Cardiol 2005;96:901-906.

16. Laarman GJ, Suttorp MJ, Dirksen MT, et al: Paclitaxel-eluting versus uncoated stents in primary percutaneous coronary intervention. N Engl J Med 2006;355:1105-1113.

17. Spaulding C, Henry P, Teiger E, et al: Sirolimus-eluting versus uncoated stents in acute myocardial infarction. N Engl J Med 2006;355:1093-1104.

18. Valgimigli M, Percoco G, Malagutti P, et al: Tirofiban and sirolimus-eluting stent vs abciximab and bare-metal stent for acute myocardial infarction: A randomized trial. JAMA 2005;293:2109-2117.

19. Nordmann AJ, Briel M, Bucher HC: Mortality in randomized controlled trials comparing drug-eluting vs. bare metal stents in coronary artery disease: A meta-analysis. Eur Heart J 2006;27:2784-2814.

20. Mehilli J, Kastrati A, Wessely R, et al: Randomized trial of a nonpolymer-based rapamycin-eluting stent versus a polymer-based paclitaxel-eluting stent for the reduction of late lumen loss. Circulation 2006;113:273-279.

21. Andersen HR, Nielsen TT, Rasmussen K, et al: A comparison of coronary angioplasty with fibrinolytic therapy in acute myocardial infarction. N Engl J Med 2003;349:733-742.

22. Widimsky P, Budesinsky T, Vorac D, et al: Long distance transport for primary angioplasty vs immediate thrombolysis in acute myocardial infarction. Final results of the randomized national multicentre trial—PRAGUE-2. Eur Heart J 2003;24:94-104.

23. Dalby M, Bouzamondo A, Lechat P, et al: Transfer for primary angioplasty versus immediate thrombolysis in acute myocardial infarction: A meta-analysis. Circulation 2003;108:1809-1814.

24. Scheller B, Hennen B, Hammer B, et al: Beneficial effects of immediate stenting after thrombolysis in acute myocardial infarction. J Am Coll Cardiol 2003;42:634-641.

25. Zijlstra F: Angioplasty vs thrombolysis for acute myocardial infarction: A quantitative overview of the effects of interhospital transportation. Eur Heart J 2003;24:21-23.

26. Nallamothu BK, Bates ER, Herrin J, et al: Times to treatment in transfer patients undergoing primary percutaneous coronary intervention in the United States: National Registry of Myocardial Infarction (NRMI)-3/4 analysis. Circulation 2005;111:761-767.

27. Betriu A, Masotti M: Comparison of mortality rates in acute myocardial infarction treated by percutaneous coronary intervention versus fibrinolysis. Am J Cardiol 2005;95:100-101.

28. Nallamothu BK, Bates ER: Percutaneous coronary intervention versus fibrinolytic therapy in acute myocardial infarction: Is timing (almost) everything? Am J Cardiol 2003;92:824-826.

29. Nallamothu BK, Wang Y, Magid DJ, et al: Relation between hospital specialization with primary percutaneous coronary intervention and clinical outcomes in ST-segment elevation myocardial infarction: National Registry of Myocardial Infarction-4 analysis. Circulation 2006;113:222-229.

30. Moyer P, Feldman J, Levine J, et al: Implications of the mechanical (PCI) vs thrombolytic controversy for ST segment elevation myocardial infarction on the organization of emergency medical services: The Boston EMS experience. Crit Pathol Cardiol 2004;3:53-61.

31. Nallamothu BK, Bates ER, Wang Y, et al: Driving times and distances to hospitals with percutaneous coronary intervention in the United States: Implications for prehospital triage of patients with ST-elevation myocardial infarction. Circulation 2006;113:1189-1195.

32. Topol EJ, Califf RM, George BS, et al: A randomized trial of immediate versus delayed elective angioplasty after intravenous tissue plasminogen activator in acute myocardial infarction. N Engl J Med 1987;317:581-588.

33. Fernandez-Aviles F, Alonso JJ, Castro-Beiras A, et al: Routine invasive strategy within 24 hours of thrombolysis versus ischaemia-guided conservative approach for acute myocardial infarction with ST-segment elevation (GRACIA-1): A randomised controlled trial. Lancet 2004;364:1045-1053.

34. Le May MR, Wells GA, Labinaz M, et al: Combined angioplasty and pharmacological intervention versus thrombolysis alone in acute myocardial infarction (CAPITAL AMI study). J Am Coll Cardiol 2005;46:417-424.

35. Gersh BJ, Stone GW, White HD, et al: Pharmacological facilitation of primary percutaneous coronary intervention for acute myocardial infarction: Is the slope of the curve the shape of the future? JAMA 2005;293:979-986.

36. Fernandez-Aviles F: Primary optimal percutaneous coronary intervention versus facilitated intervention (tenecteplase plus stenting) in patients with ST-elevated acute myocardial infarction (GRACIA-2). Paper presented at European Society of Cardiology Congress, 2003, Vienna, Austria.

37. Kastrati A, Mehilli J, Schlotterbeck K, et al: Early administration of reteplase plus abciximab vs abciximab alone in patients with acute myocardial infarction referred for percutaneous coronary intervention: A randomized controlled trial. JAMA 2004;291:947-954.

38. Lee DP, Herity NA, Hiatt BL, et al: Adjunctive platelet glycoprotein IIb/IIIa receptor inhibition with tirofiban before primary angioplasty improves angiographic outcomes: Results of the TIrofiban Given in the Emergency Room before Primary Angioplasty (TIGER-PA) pilot trial. Circulation 2003;107:1497-1501.

39. van't Hof AW, Ernst N, de Boer MJ, et al: Facilitation of primary coronary angioplasty by early start of a glycoprotein 2b/3a inhibitor: Results of the ongoing tirofiban in myocardial infarction evaluation (On-TIME) trial. Eur Heart J 2004;25:837-846.

40. Ellis SG, Armstrong P, Betriu A, et al: Facilitated percutaneous coronary intervention versus primary percutaneous coronary intervention: Design and rationale of the Facilitated Intervention with Enhanced Reperfusion Speed to Stop Events (FINESSE) trial. Am Heart J 2004;147:e16-e23.

41. Primary versus tenecteplase-facilitated percutaneous coronary intervention in patients with ST-segment elevation acute myocardial infarction (ASSENT-4 PCI): Randomised trial. Lancet 2006;367:569-578.

42. Keeley EC, Boura JA, Grines CL: Comparison of primary and facilitated percutaneous coronary interventions for ST-elevation myocardial infarction: quantitative review of randomised trials. Lancet 2006;367:579-588.

43. Sabatine MS, Cannon CP, Gibson CM, et al: Effect of clopidogrel pretreatment before percutaneous coronary intervention in patients with ST-elevation myocardial infarction treated with fibrinolytics: The PCI-CLARITY study. JAMA 2005;294:1224-1232.

44. Sutton AG, Campbell PG, Graham R, et al: A randomized trial of rescue angioplasty versus a conservative approach for failed fibrinolysis in ST-segment elevation myocardial infarction: The Middlesbrough Early Revascularization to Limit INfarction (MERLIN) trial. J Am Coll Cardiol 2004;44:287-296.

45. Gershlick AH, Stephens-Lloyd A, Hughes S, et al: Rescue angioplasty after failed thrombolytic therapy for acute myocardial infarction. N Engl J Med 2005;353:2758-2768.

46. Schömig A, Ndrepepa G, Mehilli J, et al: A randomized trial of coronary stenting versus balloon angioplasty as a rescue intervention after failed thrombolysis in patients with acute myocardial infarction. J Am Coll Cardiol 2004;44: 2073-2079.

47. Schömig A, Ndrepepa G, Mehilli J, et al: Therapy-dependent influence of time-to-treatment interval on myocardial salvage in patients with acute myocardial infarction treated with coronary artery stenting or thrombolysis. Circulation 2003;108:1084-1088.

48. Patel TN, Bavry AA, Kumbhani DJ, et al: A meta-analysis of randomized trials of rescue percutaneous coronary intervention after failed fibrinolysis. Am J Cardiol 2006;97: 1685-1690.

49. Bradley EH, Herrin J, Wang Y, et al: Strategies for reducing the door-to-balloon time in acute myocardial infarction. N Engl J Med 2006;355:2308-2320.

50. Reimer KA, Lowe JE, Rasmussen MM, et al: The wavefront phenomenon of ischemic cell death. 1. Myocardial infarct size vs duration of coronary occlusion in dogs. Circulation 1977;56:786-794.

51. Taher T, Fu Y, Wagner GS, et al: Aborted myocardial infarction in patients with ST-segment elevation: Insights from the Assessment of the Safety and Efficacy of a New Thrombolytic Regimen-3 Trial Electrocardiographic Substudy. J Am Coll Cardiol 2004;44:38-43.

52. Schömig A, Ndrepepa G, Kastrati A: Late myocardial salvage: Time to recognize its reality in the reperfusion therapy of acute myocardial infarction. Eur Heart J 2006;27: 1900-1907.

53. De Luca G, Suryapranata H, Ottervanger JP, et al: Time delay to treatment and mortality in primary angioplasty for acute myocardial infarction: Every minute of delay counts. Circulation 2004;109:1223-1225.

54. Ndrepepa G, Mehilli J, Schwaiger M, et al: Prognostic value of myocardial salvage achieved by reperfusion therapy in patients with acute myocardial infarction. J Nucl Med 2004;45:725-729.

55. Schömig A, Mehilli J, Antoniucci D, et al: Mechanical reperfusion in patients with acute myocardial infarction presenting more than 12 hours from symptom onset: A randomized controlled trial. JAMA 2005;293:2865-2872.

56. Cannon CP, Gibson CM, Lambrew CT, et al: Relationship of symptom-onset-to-balloon time and door-to-balloon time with mortality in patients undergoing angioplasty for acute myocardial infarction. JAMA 2000;283:2941-2947.

57. Zijlstra F, Patel A, Jones M, et al: Clinical characteristics and outcome of patients with early (<2 h), intermediate (2-4 h) and late (>4 h) presentation treated by primary coronary angioplasty or thrombolytic therapy for acute myocardial infarction. Eur Heart J 2002;23:550-557.

58. Hochman JS, Lamas GA, Buller CE, et al: Coronary intervention for persistent occlusion after myocardial infarction. N Engl J Med 2006;355:2395-2407.

59. Steg PG, Bonnefoy E, Chabaud S, et al: Impact of time to treatment on mortality after prehospital fibrinolysis or primary angioplasty: Data from the CAPTIM randomized clinical trial. Circulation 2003;108:2851-2856.

60. Stenestrand U, Lindback J, Wallentin L: Long-term outcome of primary percutaneous coronary intervention vs prehospital and in-hospital thrombolysis for patients with ST-elevation myocardial infarction. JAMA 2006;296:1749-1756.

61. McNamara RL, Wang Y, Herrin J, et al: Effect of door-to-balloon time on mortality in patients with ST-segment elevation myocardial infarction. J Am Coll Cardiol 2006;47: 2180-2186.

62. Brodie BR, Hansen C, Stuckey TD, et al: Door-to-balloon time with primary percutaneous coronary intervention for acute myocardial infarction impacts late cardiac mortality in high-risk patients and patients presenting early after the onset of symptoms. J Am Coll Cardiol 2006;47:289-295.

63. Brodie BR, Stone GW, Cox DA, et al: Impact of treatment delays on outcomes of primary percutaneous coronary intervention for acute myocardial infarction: Analysis from the CADILLAC trial. Am Heart J 2006;151:1231-1238.

64. McNamara RL, Herrin J, Bradley EH, et al: Hospital improvement in time to reperfusion in patients with acute myocardial infarction, 1999 to 2002. J Am Coll Cardiol 2006;47: 45-51.

65. Angeja BG, Gibson CM, Chin R, et al: Predictors of door-to-balloon delay in primary angioplasty. Am J Cardiol 2002;89: 1156-1161.

66. Magid DJ, Wang Y, Herrin J, et al: Relationship between time of day, day of week, timeliness of reperfusion, and in-hospital mortality for patients with acute ST-segment elevation myocardial infarction. JAMA 2005;294:803-812.

67. Stone GW, Webb J, Cox DA, et al: Distal microcirculatory protection during percutaneous coronary intervention in acute ST-segment elevation myocardial infarction: A randomized controlled trial. JAMA 2005;293:1063-1072.

68. Limbruno U, Micheli A, De Carlo M, et al: Mechanical prevention of distal embolization during primary angioplasty: Safety, feasibility, and impact on myocardial reperfusion. Circulation 2003;108:171-176.

69. Burzotta F, Trani C, Romagnoli E, et al: Manual thrombus-aspiration improves myocardial reperfusion: The randomized evaluation of the effect of mechanical reduction of distal embolization by thrombus-aspiration in primary and rescue angioplasty (REMEDIA) trial. J Am Coll Cardiol 2005;46: 371-376.

70. Napodano M, Pasquetto G, Sacca S, et al: Intracoronary thrombectomy improves myocardial reperfusion in patients undergoing direct angioplasty for acute myocardial infarction. J Am Coll Cardiol 2003;42:1395-1402.

71. Gick M, Jander N, Bestehorn HP, et al: Randomized evaluation of the effects of filter-based distal protection on myocardial perfusion and infarct size after primary percutaneous catheter intervention in myocardial infarction with and without ST-segment elevation. Circulation 2005;112: 1462-1469.

72. Ali A, Cox D, Dib N, et al: Rheolytic thrombectomy with percutaneous coronary intervention for infarct size reduction in acute myocardial infarction: 30-Day results from a multicenter randomized study. J Am Coll Cardiol 2006;48: 244-252.

73. Limbruno U, De Caterina R, for EMERALD, AIMI, and PROMISE: Is there still a potential for embolic protection in primary PCI? Eur Heart J 2006;27:1139-1145.

74. Schömig A, Kastrati A: Distal embolic protection in patients with acute myocardial infarction: Attractive concept but no evidence of benefit. JAMA 2005;293:1116-1118.

75. De Luca G, Suryapranata H, Stone GW, et al: Abciximab as adjunctive therapy to reperfusion in acute ST-segment elevation myocardial infarction: A meta-analysis of randomized trials. JAMA 2005;293:1759-1765.

76. Montalescot G, Borentain M, Payot L, et al: Early vs late administration of glycoprotein IIb/IIIa inhibitors in primary percutaneous coronary intervention of acute ST-segment elevation myocardial infarction: A meta-analysis. JAMA 2004;292:362-366.

77. ADMIRAL Investigators: Three-year duration of benefit from abciximab in patients receiving stents for acute myocardial infarction in the randomized double-blind ADMIRAL study. Eur Heart J 2005;26:2520-2523.

78. Ndrepepa G, Kastrati A, Neumann FJ, et al: Five-year outcome of patients with acute myocardial infarction enrolled in a randomised trial assessing the value of abciximab during coronary artery stenting. Eur Heart J 2004;25:1635-1640.

79. Kastrati A, Mehilli J, Schuhlen H, et al: A clinical trial of abciximab in elective percutaneous coronary intervention after pretreatment with clopidogrel. N Engl J Med 2004; 350:232-238.

80. Yusuf S, Mehta SR, Chrolavicius S, et al: Effects of fondaparinux on mortality and reinfarction in patients with acute ST-segment elevation myocardial infarction: The OASIS-6 randomized trial. JAMA 2006;295:1519-1530.

81. Kopecky SL, Aviles RJ, Bell MR, et al: A randomized, double-blinded, placebo-controlled, dose-ranging study measuring the effect of an adenosine agonist on infarct size reduction

in patients undergoing primary percutaneous transluminal coronary angioplasty: The ADMIRE (AmP579 Delivery for Myocardial Infarction REduction) study. Am Heart J 2003;146:146-152.

82. Ross AM, Gibbons RJ, Stone GW, et al: A randomized, double-blinded, placebo-controlled multicenter trial of adenosine as an adjunct to reperfusion in the treatment of acute myocardial infarction (AMISTAD-II). J Am Coll Cardiol 2005;45:1775-1780.

83. Pache J, Kastrati A, Mehilli J, et al: A randomized evaluation of the effects of glucose-insulin-potassium infusion on myocardial salvage in patients with acute myocardial infarction treated with reperfusion therapy. Am Heart J 2004;148:e3-e8.

84. van der Horst IC, Zijlstra F, van't Hof AW, et al: Glucose-insulin-potassium infusion inpatients treated with primary angioplasty for acute myocardial infarction: The glucose-insulin-potassium study: A randomized trial. J Am Coll Cardiol 2003;42:784-791.

85. Granger CB, Mahaffey KW, Weaver WD, et al: Pexelizumab, an anti-C5 complement antibody, as adjunctive therapy to primary percutaneous coronary intervention in acute myocardial infarction: The COMplement inhibition in Myocardial infarction treated with Angioplasty (COMMA) trial. Circulation 2003;108:1184-1190.

86. Ishii H, Ichimiya S, Kanashiro M, et al: Impact of a single intravenous administration of nicorandil before reperfusion in patients with ST-segment-elevation myocardial infarction. Circulation 2005;112:1284-1288.

87. Bar FW, Tzivoni D, Dirksen MT, et al: Results of the first clinical study of adjunctive CAldaret (MCC-135) in patients undergoing primary percutaneous coronary intervention for ST-Elevation Myocardial Infarction: The randomized multicentre CASTEMI study. Eur Heart J 2006;27:2516-2523.

88. O'Neill WW: Acute Myocardial Infarction with Hyperoxemic Therapy (AMIHOT): A prospective, randomized, multicenter trial. Paper presented at the Annual Scientific Session of the American College of Cardiology, 2004, New Orleans, LA.

89. O'Neill WW: A prospective, randomized trial of mild systemic hypothermia during PCI treatment of ST elevation MI. Paper presented at Transcatheter Cardiovascular Therapeutics, 2003, Washington, DC.

90. Schachinger V, Erbs S, Elsasser A, et al: Intracoronary bone marrow-derived progenitor cells in acute myocardial infarction. N Engl J Med 2006;355:1210-1221.

91. Janssens S, Dubois C, Bogaert J, et al: Autologous bone marrow-derived stem-cell transfer in patients with ST-segment elevation myocardial infarction: Double-blind, randomised controlled trial. Lancet 2006;367:113-121.

92. Lunde K, Solheim S, Aakhus S, et al: Intracoronary injection of mononuclear bone marrow cells in acute myocardial infarction. N Engl J Med 2006;355:1199-1209.

93. Bartunek J, Vanderheyden M, Vandekerckhove B, et al: Intracoronary injection of CD133-positive enriched bone marrow progenitor cells promotes cardiac recovery after recent myocardial infarction: feasibility and safety. Circulation 2005;112:I178-I183.

94. Ince H, Petzsch M, Kleine HD, et al: Preservation from left ventricular remodeling by front-integrated revascularization and stem cell liberation in evolving acute myocardial infarction by use of granulocyte-colony-stimulating factor (FIRST-LINE-AMI). Circulation 2005;112:3097-3106.

95. Ripa RS, Jorgensen E, Wang Y, et al: Stem cell mobilization induced by subcutaneous granulocyte-colony stimulating factor to improve cardiac regeneration after acute ST-elevation myocardial infarction: Result of the double-blind, randomized, placebo-controlled stem cells in myocardial infarction (STEMMI) trial. Circulation 2006;113:1983-1992.

96. Zohlnhofer D, Ott I, Mehilli J, et al: Stem cell mobilization by granulocyte colony-stimulating factor in patients with acute myocardial infarction: A randomized controlled trial. JAMA 2006;295:1003-1010.

97. Klein LW, Shaw RE, Krone RJ, et al: Mortality after emergent percutaneous coronary intervention in cardiogenic shock secondary to acute myocardial infarction and usefulness of a mortality prediction model. Am J Cardiol 2005;96:35-41.

98. Babaev A, Frederick PD, Pasta DJ, et al: Trends in management and outcomes of patients with acute myocardial infarction complicated by cardiogenic shock. JAMA 2005;294:448-454.

99. Hochman JS, Sleeper LA, Webb JG, et al: Early revascularization and long-term survival in cardiogenic shock complicating acute myocardial infarction. JAMA 2006;295:2511-2515.

100. Dzavik V, Sleeper LA, Picard MH, et al: Outcome of patients aged > or = 75 years in the SHould we emergently revascularize Occluded Coronaries in cardiogenic shocK (SHOCK) trial: Do elderly patients with acute myocardial infarction complicated by cardiogenic shock respond differently to emergent revascularization? Am Heart J 2005;149:1128-1134.

101. White HD, Assmann SF, Sanborn TA, et al: Comparison of percutaneous coronary intervention and coronary artery bypass grafting after acute myocardial infarction complicated by cardiogenic shock: Results from the Should We Emergently Revascularize Occluded Coronaries for Cardiogenic Shock (SHOCK) trial. Circulation 2005;112:1992-2001.

102. Sadeghi HM, Grines CL, Chandra HR, et al: Magnitude and impact of treatment delays on weeknights and weekends in patients undergoing primary angioplasty for acute myocardial infarction (the CADILLAC trial). Am J Cardiol 2004;94:637-640, A639.

103. Grines CL: A prospective randomized trial of primary angioplasty and thrombolytic therapy in elderly patients with acute myocardial infarction (SENIOR-PAMI) Paper presented at Transcatheter Cardiovascular Therapeutics, 2005. Washington, DC.

104. Tamis-Holland JE, Palazzo A, Stebbins AL, et al: Benefits of direct angioplasty for women and men with acute myocardial infarction: Results of the Global Use of Strategies to Open Occluded Arteries in Acute Coronary Syndromes Substudy. Am Heart J 2004;147:133-139.

105. Mehilli J, Kastrati A, Dirschinger J, et al: Sex-based analysis of outcome in patients with acute myocardial infarction treated predominantly with percutaneous coronary intervention. JAMA 2002;287:210-215.

106. Mehilli J, Ndrepepa G, Kastrati A, et al: Gender and myocardial salvage after reperfusion treatment in acute myocardial infarction. J Am Coll Cardiol 2005;45:828-831.

20 Ostial and Bifurcation Lesions

Antonio Colombo and Goran Stankovic

KEY POINTS

- Always consider an ostial lesion as a possible bifurcation lesion except if it is in an aorto-ostial location.
- A 6-Fr guiding catheter is appropriate in most cases. If there is any doubt, a 7- or 8-Fr catheter may be used.
- Do not risk the side branch. If in doubt, protect it with a wire. If there are difficulties in wiring the side branch, consider dilating the main branch first.
- Provisional stenting does not mean accepting a poor final result for an important side branch.

- Treatment of a bifurcation lesion with two stents for the main and side branches as intention to treat is an acceptable approach.
- Liberally use pharmacologic protection with glycoprotein IIb/IIIa inhibitors or bivalirudin.
- Final kissing inflation is preceded by high-pressure inflation on the side branch when implanting two stents.
- When a dedicated drug-eluting stent becomes available for bifurcation lesions, many concepts may change, including more liberal use of a two-stent strategy.

Ostial and bifurcation lesions are discussed in the same chapter because differences between these lesions are relatively minor. A bifurcation lesion is more complex than an ostial lesion because two ostial lesions or one ostial lesion and another blocked vessel are close to each other.

When we refer to *stenting* in this chapter, we mean drug-eluting stent (DES) implantation. Any other stent, such as bare metal stents (BMSs), dedicated bifurcational stents, or other devices are specifically described.

OSTIAL LESIONS

Ostial lesions can be classified as aorto-ostial or as non–aorto-ostial (branch-ostial) lesions.

Aorto-Ostial Lesions

Aorto-ostial lesions are located in the ostium of the right coronary artery, the ostium of the left main coronary artery (LMCA), and the ostium of a saphenous vein graft (SVG). For all of these lesions, the other branch, the aorta, is never pinched by plaque shift.

In this discussion, we assume that the final treatment for all of these lesions will be DES or BMS implantation after different types of lesion preparation.[1-3] DES implantation usually is the preferred approach because of the historically high restenosis rate after BMS implantation, which is reserved for very large vessels (>5 mm) or when there are potential problems with 1 year of dual-antiplatelet therapy.

The aorto-ostial origins of native coronary arteries and SVGs are exposed to nonlaminar turbulent shear forces that may contribute to specific histopathologic characteristics, such as the increased fibrous cellularity, calcification, and sclerosis observed at this location.[4]

The most common risk the operator may face when treating an aorto-ostial lesion is incomplete stent expansion due to fibrosis or calcifications at the lesion site. This specific concern dictates the need to perform adequate lesion preparation. Unfortunately, all our suggestions and guidelines are based only on a C level of evidence, because almost all trials exclude aorto-ostial lesions.[5] An important caveat is that these lesions have been associated with a high incidence of restenosis and the need for reintervention with any approach; an optimal final result is probably the best way to start.

Contemporary Studies

Percutaneous treatment of native coronary and SVG aorto-ostial stenosis has been associated with lower procedural success rates (70% to 97%), frequent in-hospital complications (5% to 12%), and a greater

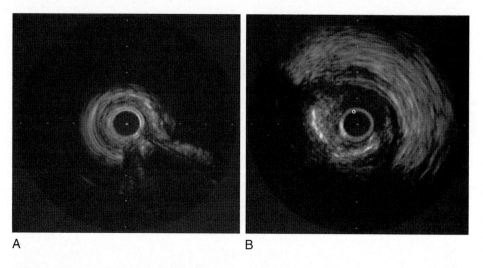

A   B

Figure 20-1. Severely calcified lesion (circumferential calcium ring) before **(A)** (lumen cross-sectional area = 1.3 mm^2) and after lesion preparation with rotational atherectomy **(B)** (lumen cross-sectional area = 4.1 mm^2).

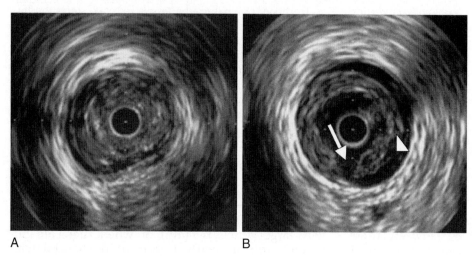

A   B

Figure 20-2. Fibrous plaque before **(A)** (lumen cross-sectional area = 2.2 mm^2) and after lesion preparation with cutting balloon angioplasty **(B)** (lumen cross-sectional area = 8.1 mm^2). The *arrow* points the incision site, and the *arrowhead* identifies dissection plane.

likelihood of late restenosis (28% to 52%) compared with the treatment of nonostial lesions.[4,6-8] An important shift in the outcome after treatment of aorto-ostial lesions came with the introduction of the DES.

In an observational study, Iakovou and colleagues[1] evaluated the clinical and angiographic outcomes of 30 patients with aorto-ostial coronary artery disease treated with sirolimus-eluting stents (SESs) (Cypher, Cordis/Johnson & Johnson, Miami Lakes, FL) and 52 patients treated with BMSs. At the 10-month follow-up assessment, two (6.3%) patients in the SES group and 14 (28%) patients in the BMS group underwent target lesion revascularization (TLR) (*p* = .01). Major adverse cardiac events (MACEs) were less common in the SES group compared with the BMS group (19% versus 44%, *P* = .02). Angiographic follow-up showed lower binary restenosis rates (11% versus 51%, *P* = .001) for the SES group.

Although the results with stents are encouraging, there is no doubt that treating aorto-ostial lesions remain technically challenging, even for experienced operators. This fact must be kept in mind when planning an appropriate treatment strategy.

Proposed Approach

Ideally, intravascular ultrasound (IVUS) should be the first step in deciding whether lesion preparation is needed. If the IVUS catheter is not able to cross the lesion, we usually perform rotational atherectomy with a 1.25- or 1.5-mm burr.

If the IVUS catheter crosses the lesion, we use the information to decide on one of the following approaches. First, superficial calcium extending more than 180 degrees may demand lesion preparation with rotational atherectomy (Rotablator, Boston Scientific, Natick, MA) (Fig. 20-1). Second, severe fibrosis or moderate calcifications may demand the use of a cutting balloon (Cutting Balloon Ultra and Flextome, Boston Scientific) or noncompliant balloon sized to the media-to-media diameter (Fig. 20-2). Third, the presence of soft plaque may permit direct stenting.

When there is the need to perform rotational atherectomy, the procedure is performed with the intent to modify the plaque to allow better stent expansion, not with the goal of debulking the lesion, which means that a single, small burr is the most frequently used device.

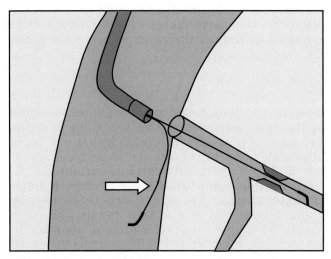

Figure 20-3. A second guidewire is inserted from the guiding catheter into the aorta *(arrow)* to allow advancement of the guiding catheter up to the ostium of the vessel, preventing deep penetration.

When we use the cutting balloon, appropriate sizing is done, with the caution to slightly undersize it to limit the risk of dissecting the aorta. In laboratories in which an excimer laser is available, this device may be a reasonable alternative to the cutting balloon.

Before proceeding with the stent delivery, the best view is selected to fully visualize the ostium of the vessel. Other than the unique value of the anteroposterior or right oblique cranial views to visualize the ostium of the LMCA, most of the projections need to be tailored to the specific anatomy. In difficult situations, the operator should not be reluctant to place a second guidewire that exits from the guiding catheter into the aorta (Fig. 20-3) to allow advancement of the guide catheter to the vessel ostium without penetration.

Stent Placement

When the operator is confident about the optimal view to use to fully cover the ostium, the next step is stent placement. The stent diameter is selected according to the reference vessel size distal to the lesion or according to the diameter of the vessel measured by IVUS. The stent length should fully cover the lesion; stents that are too short may be unstable in their location (i.e., rejection of the stent from the ostium), and stents that are too long may cover the LMCA bifurcation. Most operators use DESs because of their optimal performance in these types of lesions.[1] Only the Taxus stent (Boston Scientific) is available in sizes up to 5 mm, which are sometimes needed for aorto-ostial lesions. When the reference vessel size is large, some operators may consider using BMSs with the assumption that such large vessels are associated with a low-risk of restenosis. Considering the high recurrence rate reported after interventions

in aorto-ostial lesions, we are not confident that the data regarding restenosis and reference vessel size can be applied to this lesion subset.

If the procedure has been conducted with IVUS guidance, the need for postdilatation is determined after an IVUS evaluation performed after stenting. Because the proximal end of the balloon can lie in the aorta, there is no need to select a specific balloon length. Many operators like to inflate the balloon while it protrudes into the aorta at pressures higher than 20 atm, pushing and pulling the inflated balloon cranially and caudally to cause stent flaring.

An Alternative Scenario

In practice, many operators do not perform IVUS, and even if not fully supported by us, we describe an alternative scenario to suite these circumstances. If the aorto-ostial lesion is not severe, many operators perform direct stenting followed by postdilatation as described for other conditions. Otherwise, they perform predilatation with a relatively small balloon. Rotational atherectomy or use of a cutting balloon is reserved for lesions in which calcium is evident on fluoroscopy or in conditions in which the predilating balloon fails to cross the lesion or does not fully expand.

There is a potential problem with these practical approaches: the risk of failing to fully dilate the stent, even with a high-pressure noncompliant balloon. A possible solution is to state that direct stenting should never be performed in aorto-ostial lesions unless we have determined the lesion characteristics by IVUS before intervention. Lesion predilatation should always be done with a balloon sized to the reference vessel diameter. These safeguards allow using an alternative solution in case the predilating balloon does not expand without leaving the problem to be corrected after the stent has been positioned.

When treating SVG aorto-ostial lesions, we prefer to use a filter or a distal occlusive device, despite the low risk for distal embolization.[9] Use of polytetrafluoroethylene (PTFE)–covered stents, which were proposed in the past, has no role in treating these types of lesions, except to treat specific complications.[10]

Branch-Ostial Lesions

Non–aorto-ostial or branch-ostial lesions are a subset of ostial lesions, but they can be included as a subtype of bifurcation lesions if disease is present only at the ostium of a branch.

Contemporary Studies

Treatment of branch-ostial lesions with balloon angioplasty, a BMS, or any other device has been quite problematic and is associated with a high clinical recurrence rate.[11,12] It is not a surprise that these lesions have been excluded from most trials.

The use of DESs has decreased restenotic rates compared with the use of conventional BMSs.[13,14] However, the ostial location of left anterior descending coronary artery (LAD) lesions has been excluded from all randomized trials that have tested the efficacy of DES implantation. The location of the ostial LAD lesion was shown to be an independent predictor of restenosis, even after DES implantation.[15] The implantation of an SES in the LAD has been shown to result in low TLR rates (6% to 9%), comparable to single-vessel bypass surgery revascularization, but ostial LAD lesions were excluded from those studies.[16,17] Reports from single-center registries regarding the use of DESs for ostial LAD lesions are encouraging, with low rates of adverse events at mid-term follow-up.

Vijayakumar and coworkers[18] evaluated clinical outcomes after SES implantation for ostial lesions in 50 patients. The event-free survival rate was 90% at 1 year. There were 5 (10%) target vessel revascularizations (TVRs), 3 (6%) myocardial infarctions (MIs), and 1 (2%) death during a mean follow-up of 414 days. TLR was required in 4 (8%) patients.

Seung and associates[19] evaluated the effectiveness of SES implantation for ostial LAD lesions in 68 consecutive patients. The control group was composed of 77 patients treated with BMSs during the preceding 2 years. In the SES group, stent positioning was intentionally extended into the distal LMCA in 23 patients (34%) with intermediate LMCA narrowing. The procedural success rate was 100% in both groups. The 6-month angiographic restenosis rate was significantly lower in the SES group than in the BMS group (5.1% versus 32.3%, $P < .001$). During the 1-year follow-up period, neither death nor MI occurred in either group, but TLR was less common in the SES group than in the BMS group (0% versus 17%, $P < .001$). In the SES group, there were no restenoses in cases with LMCA coverage, compared with three restenoses (7.9%) in cases with precise stent positioning ($P = NS$). The investigators concluded that SES implantation in ostial LAD lesions achieved excellent results in terms of restenosis and clinical outcomes compared with BMS implantation.

Tsagalou and colleagues[20] investigated early and mid-term clinical and angiographic outcomes of patients with de novo ostial LAD lesions treated with DES (43 patients) or BMS (43 patients) implantation. There were no significant differences with respect to major in-hospital complications between the two groups. Non-Q-wave MIs occurred in 2 patients (4.7%) in the DES group and in 1 patient (2.3%) in the BMS group. At the 9-month follow-up evaluation, 3 patients (7%) in the DES group and 11 patients (25.6%) in the BMS group underwent TLR ($P = .038$). MACEs were less common in the DES group than in the BMS group (9.3% versus 32.6%, $P = .015$). Angiographic follow-up was available for 82% of patients in the DES group and 75% of those in the BMS group and showed lower binary restenotic rates (5.7% versus 31.3%, $P = .01$) and late loss (0.30 versus 1.23 mm, $P = .0001$) in the DES group. The investigators concluded that DES implantation in de novo ostial LAD

lesions appears safe and effective and that it is associated with a significant decrease in the restenosis rate compared with the historical experience with BMSs.

Proposed Approach

Many of the therapeutic considerations expressed for the aorto-ostial lesions are also valid for non–aorto-ostial lesions. The exception is that the risk of incomplete stent expansion due to severe calcification or fibrosis exists, although it is uncommon.

When we are ready for stent placement, two interrelated topics need to be addressed: optimal coverage of the ostium and plaque shift toward the other branch. Many operators prefer a radical approach to this problem, which means stenting across the proximal vessel to ensure full coverage of the ostium. When stenting an ostial LAD lesion, this approach requires placing the stent from the distal LMCA into the LAD and then, if needed, crossing into the left circumflex coronary artery (LCX) and performing a final kissing balloon inflation. Other than occasional case reports, we are not aware of a specific study reporting the long-term results of this strategy or comparisons with other techniques. This approach appears to be quite practical, but it should selectively be used only when there is concern about not being able to fully cover the ostium of the vessel or when the disease extends proximally.

Another approach is to accurately place the stent at the ostium of the diseased branch with a wire or a balloon positioned in the other branch. This sentinel wire or balloon has two functions: to allow better identification of the location of the ostium of the lesion to be treated and to offer the possibility of immediately treating the other branch in case a plaque shift occurs. We usually inflate the sentinel balloon only if a plaque shift has occurred after stenting the ostial lesion. In case we see a reduction of the lumen at the ostium of the other branch, we first administer intracoronary nitroglycerine, and if the lumen reduction is still present, we perform kissing balloon inflation at a low pressure of 5 to 8 atm. This procedure can be done using a 6-Fr guiding catheter, provided that the operator always advances the stent before advancing the sentinel balloon. Figure 20-4 provides an example of this approach. When implanting the two most often used DESs (i.e., Cypher or Taxus stents), our results in the treatment of ostial LAD lesions have been quite rewarding, with a low incidence of adverse events during hospitalization and follow-up, with a significant advantage demonstrated for DESs regarding the need for repeat revascularization compared with the historical experience with BMSs, and with a lack of compromise of the circumflex at follow-up even for patients who required additional treatment of the LCX at the time of the index procedure.[20]

Some operators routinely perform inflation of the sentinel balloon at a low pressure while deploying the stent with the goal of "treating without seeing."

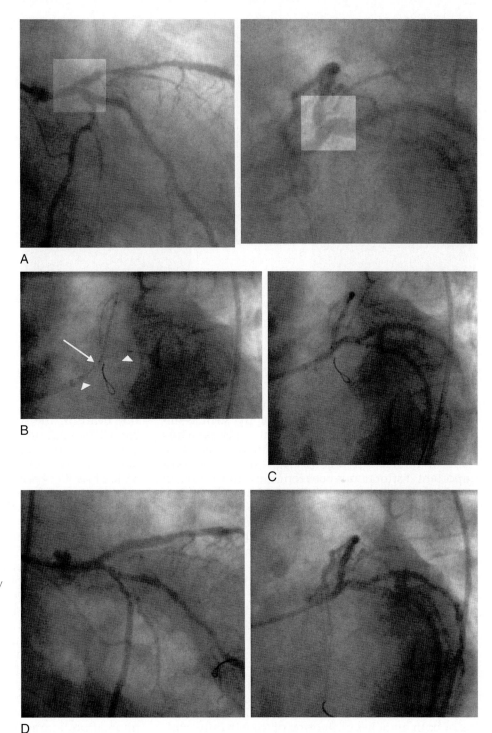

Figure 20-4. An ostial lesion of the left anterior descending coronary artery (LAD) in two projections **(A).** Stent placement at the ostium of the LAD without left main coronary artery (LMCA) coverage *(arrow)* and with a sentinel balloon positioned in the left circumflex coronary artery (LCX) *(arrowheads)* **(B).** The sentinel balloon is not inflated unless plaque shift occurs. The result after stent deployment in the LAD is shown **(C).** In this case, it was not necessary to inflate the sentinel balloon, and the final result is shown in two projections **(D).**

Although this approach may appear simple and practical, there is always a risk of dissecting the nonstented branch, with the need to implant an additional stent.

Lesions at the Ostium of a Diagonal Branch

Lesions at the ostium of a diagonal branch may, in some unlucky conditions, become the origin of a new lesion in the LAD. Operators should be aware that overly aggressive treatment of these lesions might lead to trauma to the LAD, causing a new stenosis in this vessel. Unfortunately, we cannot propose an easy solution to this conundrum other than alerting the operator about the possible risk. Occasionally, a simple cutting balloon dilatation at the ostium of a diagonal branch lesion can provide an acceptable solution (Fig. 20-5).

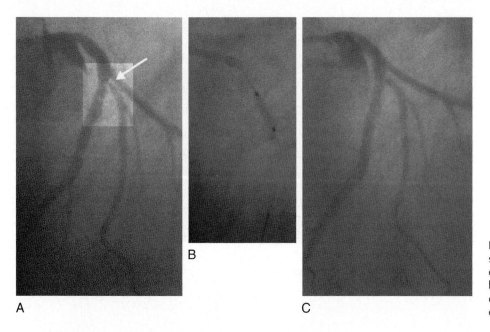

Figure 20-5. Baseline angiogram shows a lesion *(arrow)* at the ostium of a diagonal branch **(A).** Cutting balloon produces 3.0 × 10 mm dilatation at 10 atm **(B),** with the optimal final result **(C).**

BIFURCATION LESIONS

Attempts to classify bifurcation lesions[21-25] suffer all the limitations of coronary angiography, such as different plaque distribution and extent of disease when evaluated by IVUS.[26] There are six different classifications of bifurcation lesions (Fig. 20-6). The most important distinction is between true bifurcations, in which the main branch (MB) and the side branch (SB) are both significantly narrowed (>50% diameter stenosis), and nontrue bifurcations, which include all the other lesions involving a bifurcation. We think that this distinction is a key element in properly planning treatment.

Despite an array of available devices, stenting using DESs remains the default approach to treating bifurcation lesions. Implantation of a single stent in the MB is the most widely used approach.

Contemporary Studies

An SES bifurcation study was the first attempt to provide specific information in this subset of lesions.[27] Eighty-five patients were randomly assigned to stenting of both branches or stenting of the MB only, with provisional stenting of the SB. Data were analyzed by actual treatment received, not by intention to treat. The crossover rate was very high: 22 patients crossed over from stent/percutaneous transluminal coronary angioplasty (PTCA) to stent/stent (51.2%), and two patients crossed from stent/stent to stent/PTCA (4.7%) groups. Angiographic success was ascertained in 59 cases in the stent/stent group (93.6%) and in 17 cases in the stent/PTCA group (77.3%).

The rate of restenosis at 6 months did not differ significantly between the stent/stent (28.0%) and the stent/PTCA (18.7%) groups ($P = .53$). In-stent late luminal loss was also similar in the stent/stent group and the stent/PTCA group for the MB (0.28 versus 0.14 mm, $P = .19$) and for the SB (0.50 versus 0.37 mm, $P = .41$). During the 6-month follow-up, there was one death in the stent/stent group and none in the stent/PTCA group. There was no significant difference between groups in rates of Q-wave MI (1.6% versus 4.5%), non-Q-wave MI (9.5% versus 4.5%), TVR (11.1% versus 9.0%), or target vessel failure (19.0% versus 13.6%). There were three cases of stent thrombosis, all of which occurred in the stent/stent group.

The study had several conclusions:
- Compared with historical studies using BMSs,[21,28,29] clear improvement was achieved in the treatment of bifurcation lesions when one or two stents were implanted.
- The incidence of restenosis in the SB still reaches more than 20%, representing an area where improvement is needed.
- Two other randomized studies confirm that implantation of a stent only in the MB remains the preferred strategy.

Pan and coworkers[30] compared in their randomized study the two strategies for the SES treatment of bifurcation lesions in 91 patients with true coronary bifurcation lesions. All patients received an SES in the main vessel, covering the SB. Patients from group A (47 patients) were randomized to balloon dilation of the involved SB; patients in group B (44 patients) were randomized to receive a second stent at the SB origin. There were no differences between groups regarding baseline clinical and angiographic data. MACEs occurred in three patients from group A (two non-Q-wave MIs and one TLR) and in three patients in group B (one subacute stent thrombosis with subsequent death and two TLRs). Six-month angiographic reevaluation was obtained in 80 patients (88%). Restenosis of the main vessel was observed in

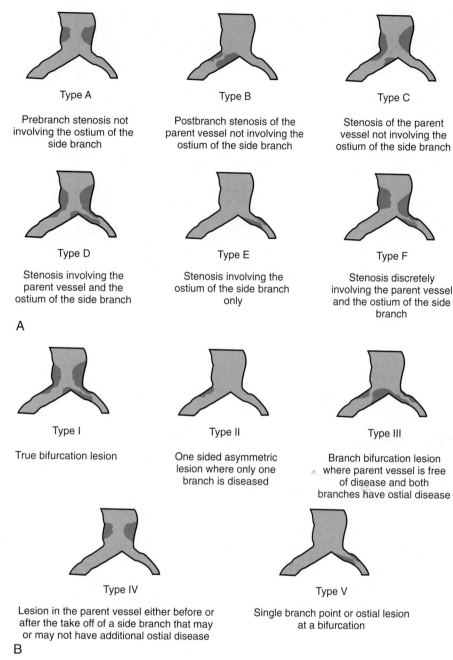

Figure 20-6. Classifications of bifurcations according to plaque distribution: Duke (**A**),[51] Sanborn (**B**).[52]

Continued

one patient (2%) from group A and in four (10%) from group B (*P* = NS). Restenosis of the SB occurred in two patients (5%) from group A and in six patients (15%) from group B (*P* = NS). Both strategies proved to be similarly effective in decreasing restenosis rates, with no differences in terms of clinical outcome.

Steigen and coworkers[31] presented the 6-month results of the Nordic Bifurcation Study at the American College of Cardiology Meeting in Atlanta in 2006. In this study, 413 patients were randomized to stenting of both branches (*n* = 206) with crush, culotte, Y, or other techniques or to provisional stenting (*n* = 207) with SES implantation. The crossover from provisional stenting to stenting two

branches was allowed only if the Thrombolysis in Myocardial Infarction (TIMI)–defined flow after SB dilation was 0. Procedural success was achieved in 97% of cases in the provisional stenting group and in 95% of the both branches stenting group. The SB was stented in only 4.3% of the patients in the provisional stenting group. Final kissing balloon inflation was performed in 32% and 74% of the patients, respectively, (*P* < .001). At 6 months, there was no difference between the two groups regarding cardiac death, MI, index lesion MI, TVR, TLR, and stent thrombosis. Tables 20-1 and 20-2 summarize the most important studies regarding stenting of bifurcation lesions with DES.

Type I
Parent vessel stenosis proximal
and distal to bifurcation

A   B

Type II
Parent vessel stenosis
proximal to bifurcation

A   B

Type III
Parent vessel stenosis
distal to bifurcation

A   B

Type IV
Parent vessel normal, ostial
side branch stenosis

C

Type 1
Lesions located in the main branch, proximal and
distal, and the ostium of side branch

Type 2
Lesions located only in the main branch, proximal
and distal, and not in the ostium of side branch

Type 3
Lesions located in the main branch proximal to
the bifurcation

Type 4
Only the ostium of each branch of the bifurcation
involved with no proximal disease

Type 4a
Lesion located only in
the ostium of main branch

Type 4b
Lesion located only in
the ostium of side branch

D

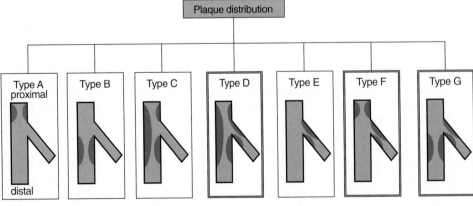

Plaque distribution

Type A
proximal

Type B   Type C   Type D   Type E   Type F   Type G

distal

☐   True bifurcation lesion

E

Figure 20-6, cont'd. Safian (C),[22]
Lefevre (D),[21] SYNTAX study (E).[53]

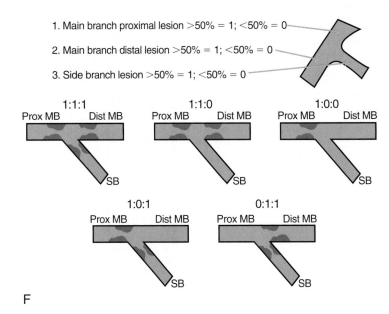

1. Main branch proximal lesion >50% = 1; <50% = 0
2. Main branch distal lesion >50% = 1; <50% = 0
3. Side branch lesion >50% = 1; <50% = 0

Figure 20-6, cont'd. Medina (F).[25]   F

Treatment of Bifurcation Lesions

Guiding Catheter Selection

Most bifurcation lesions can be approached with a 6-Fr guiding catheter because a provisional strategy is used in most cases. The exception is when, owing to lesions characteristics, the operator decides from the very beginning to implant two stents (requiring a 8-Fr guiding catheter, even if technically a 7-Fr guiding catheter can be used with some new DESs).

With the use of very-low-profile balloons (Maverick, Boston Scientific-Scimed, Minneapolis, MN, or any other balloon with similar size features), it is possible to insert two balloons inside a large-lumen, 6-Fr guiding catheter. When using the Endeavor stent (Medtronic, Minneapolis, MN), the insertion of a second balloon to perform kissing inflations requires at least a 7-Fr guiding catheter.

If two stents are needed and a 6-Fr guiding catheter is employed, some limitations must be recognized. The two stents must be inserted and deployed sequentially. The standard crush technique and the V or kissing stents techniques cannot be performed unless an 8-Fr guiding catheter is used. The Taxus Libertè (Boston Scientific) or a second-generation DES may allow the use of a 7-Fr guiding catheter. When the operator knows a priori that two stents will be implanted, an 8-Fr guiding catheter is the best choice.

General Approach to Treating a Bifurcation Lesion

Figure 20-7 summarizes a proposed approach to bifurcation lesions, with an attempt to give directions regarding SB stenting as intention to treat. The most common approach is provisional SB stenting, and it is outlined as follows:

1. Placement of two wires (MB and SB)
2. Predilatation, when needed
3. Stenting of the MB
4. Recrossing with a wire into the SB
5. Crossing with a balloon into the SB
6. Performance of kissing balloon inflation with moderate pressure (8 atm) in the SB, until the balloon is fully expanded
7. Placement of a second stent in the SB only if the result is inadequate

When stenting bifurcations, it is important to protect the SB by inserting a wire to be left in place until the stenting procedure in the MB has been completed, including high-pressure stent deployment or postdilatation. These temporary jailed wires can be retrieved provided that attention is paid to avoid any trauma to the ostium of the proximal coronary with the guiding catheter, which tends to be pulled in.

Difficult Access to the Side Branch

After having attempted different types of wires with all sorts of curves and using all personal tricks, the operator may be left with the impossibility of advancing a wire in the SB. At this point, few options are available: to abort the procedure because the risk of losing the SB is too high considering the size and distribution of the branch (typically an angulated circumflex artery); to perform directional atherectomy on the MB with the intent of removing the plaque, which prevents entry into the SB; or to dilate the MB with a balloon, with the rationale that the plaque modification and a favorable plaque shift can facilitate access of the SB.

Each of the three options has its indication, and the specific anatomic condition, the operator's experience, and the clinical scenario may direct the

Table 20-1. Main Studies with Drug-Eluting Stents Evaluating Provisional Stenting compared with Implantation of Two Stents in Coronary Bifurcations

Author	Study Design	Aim	Number of Patients	Follow-up	1-Stent Group					2-Stent Group			
					Restenosis %					Restenosis %			
					MB	SB	TLR %	ST %		MB	SB	TLR %	ST%
Colombo et al (2004)[27]	Randomized	Both branches vs. provisional stenting	85	6 mos	4.8	14.2	4.5	0		5.7	21.8	9.5	4.7
Pan et al (2005)[30]	Radnomized	Both branches vs. provisional stenting	91	6 mos	2	5	2	0		10	15	5	2.2
Steigen et al (2006)[31]	Randomized	Crush, culotte, Y vs. provisional stenting	413	6 mos	4.6	19.2	1.9	0.5		5.1	11.5	1	0
Tsuchida et al (2007)[54]	Observational	Different subgroup analyses: bifurcations vs. nonbifurcations	607 patients with 324 bifurcations	1 yr	N/A	N/A	9.9	1.5		N/A	N/A	4.9	1.6

1-Stent Group, bifurcation lesions treated with provisional stenting technique; 2-Stent Group, bifurcation lesions treated with both-branch stenting technique; MB, main branch of the bifurcation; N/A, not available; SB, side branch of the bifurcation; ST, stent thrombosis; TLR, target lesion revascularization.

Table 20-2. Main Observational Studies Evaluating Drug-Eluting Stents in Coronary Bifurcations with Main Branch and Side Branch Stenting

Author	Aim	Number of Patients	Follow-up	Final Kissing Inflation Restenosis % MB	SB	TLR %	ST %*	No Final Kissing Inflation Restenosis % MB	SB	TLR %	ST %*
Ge et al (2005)[38]	Crush with FKB vs. without	181	9 mos	8.9	11.1	9.5	2.6	15.5	37.9	24.6	3.0
Hoye et al (2005)[55]	Crush	241	9 mos	6.4	9.6	N/A (9.7 overall)	4	10	41.3	N/A (9.7 overall)	4.2
Moussa et al (2006)[56]	Crush	120	6 mos	N/A	N/A	11.3 overall	1.7 overall	N/A	N/A	11.3 overall	1.7 overall
Sharma et al (2005)[57]	Simultaneous kissing stent	200	9 ± 2 mos	N/A	N/A	4	1	N/A	N/A	N/A	N/A
				Crush				T-Stenting			
Ge et al (2005)[58]	Crush vs. T	182	1 yr	16.2	19.2	14	1.6	13	26.1	31.1	0

*Stent thrombosis defined as per definition in study and does not include intraprocedural stent thrombosis.
FKB, final kissing balloon inflation; MB, main branch of the bifurcation; N/A, not available; SB, side branch of the bifurcation; ST, stent thrombosis; TLR, target lesion revascularization.

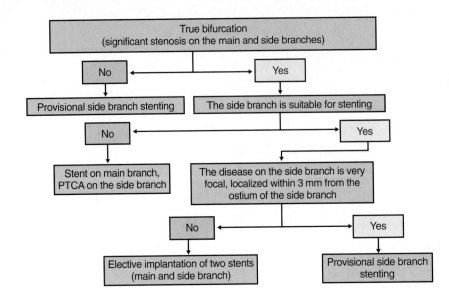

Figure 20-7. Our proposed algorithm for stenting bifurcation lesions. PTCA, percutaneous transluminal coronary angioplasty.

selection of the best strategy. Dilating the MB with a balloon is the option usually employed, and it is most often effective.

Second Stent in the Side Branch after a Provisional Approach

When we are not satisfied with the result obtained with balloon dilatation of the SB and we need to implant a second stent, several other strategies can be used.

T Technique

The T technique (Fig. 20-8) is the one most frequently used to shift from provisional stenting to stenting the SB.[32,33] The T technique consists of advancing a second stent into the SB (after adequate dilation of the MB stent struts). The stent is positioned at the ostium of the SB, trying to minimize any possible gap. A second kissing balloon inflation is performed. The T technique is associated with the risk of leaving a small gap between the stent implanted in the MB and the one implanted in the SB. This gap may contribute to an uneven distribution of the drug and lead to ostial restenosis at the SB. We think this contributed to the restenosis we noticed at the ostium of the SB when two stents were implanted in the sirolimus bifurcation study; the T technique was always used when two stents were implanted.[27] When the angle between the MB and the SB is near 90 degrees and two stents need to be implanted as intention to treat, the T technique is slightly modified by advancement of the two stents at the same time and deployment of the SB stent first (i.e., modified T technique).

Reverse Crush

The reverse crush technique (Fig. 20-9) is performed primarily to allow an opportunity for provisional SB stenting. This technique was developed with the intent to minimize any possible stent gap between the MB and SB stents. The reverse crush technique can be performed using a 6-Fr guiding catheter according to the following steps:

1. A second stent is advanced into the SB and left in position without being deployed.
2. A balloon sized according to the diameter of the MB and shorter than the stent already deployed is advanced in the MB and positioned at the level of the bifurcation, with the operator paying attention to staying inside the stent previously deployed in the MB.
3. The stent in the SB is retracted about 3 mm or less into the MB and deployed. The deploying balloon is removed, and an angiogram is obtained to verify the absence of any distal dissection or the need for an additional stent. If such is the case, the wire from the SB is removed, and the balloon in the MB is inflated at high pressure ($\geq$12 atm).
4. The SB struts are recrossed with a wire and a balloon (a 1.5-mm balloon is sometimes needed). The balloon is sized to the SB reference diameter and inflated at high pressure (12 to 20 atm).
5. Final kissing balloon inflation is performed.

T Stenting and Small Protrusion

T stenting and small protrusion (TAP) can be performed. The reverse crush can be simplified with the TAP technique, which combines some features of the T technique and the crush technique (Fig. 20-10). This technique can be performed as follows:

1. A second stent is advanced in the SB in a way to minimally protrude (1 or 2 mm) into the MB.
2. A balloon is advanced in the MB.
3. The SB stent is deployed as usual ($\geq$12 atm), and the MB balloon is simultaneously inflated at 12 atm or higher pressure.
4. Both balloons are deflated and removed.

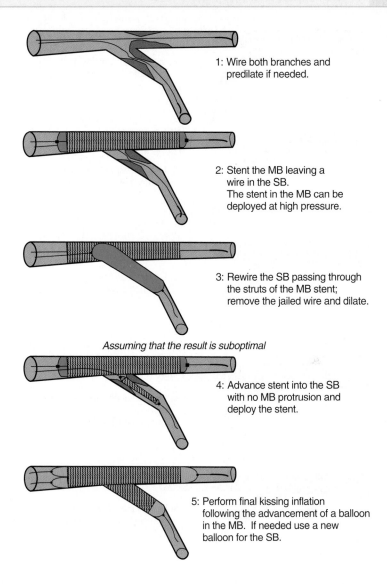

1: Wire both branches and predilate if needed.

2: Stent the MB leaving a wire in the SB. The stent in the MB can be deployed at high pressure.

3: Rewire the SB passing through the struts of the MB stent; remove the jailed wire and dilate.

Assuming that the result is suboptimal

4: Advance stent into the SB with no MB protrusion and deploy the stent.

5: Perform final kissing inflation following the advancement of a balloon in the MB. If needed use a new balloon for the SB.

Figure 20-8. A schematic representation of the T stenting technique. MB, main branch; SB, side branch.

The TAP technique is similar to the V-stenting technique; the only difference is that one of the components of the system is a balloon that is inflated inside a stent previously deployed in the MB. Despite some concerns about stent protrusion into the MB, we have been able to perform IVUS in the MB and SB and, when needed, to advance additional stents distally in the MB and the SB.

Two Stents as Intention to Treat

If the operator estimates that a particular bifurcation will need implantation of two stents (one in the MB and the other in the SB), the techniques we consider suitable in the era of DES implantation are described subsequently. The two-stent approach is reserved for selected true bifurcations after evaluation of additional parameters.

Size and the Territory of Distribution of the Side Branch

The term *side branch* is sometimes associated with a misleading connotation. The terminology may suggest a vessel of less importance compared with the MB. There are various anatomic conditions in which the SB is as important as the MB in terms of the size and territory of distribution. The LMCA, which bifurcates into the LAD and LCX; a right coronary artery that bifurcates in a posterior descending artery and a number of posterolateral branches; and a dominant LCX, which bifurcates into a distal circumflex and a large obtuse marginal branch, are all examples in which the SBs are important vessels that may generate a large ischemic area if left with critical narrowing. The size of the territory supplied by the SB becomes a valuable element to guide the decision to accept a mediocre result at the SB ostium (after balloon angioplasty) compared with the need to have almost 0% residual stenosis (after additional SB stenting).

Angle between the Main and the Side Branch and the Narrowing at the Ostium of the Side Branch

The angle of origin of the SB from the MB can be acute, close to 90 degrees, or obtuse. The narrower the angle between the two branches, the higher is

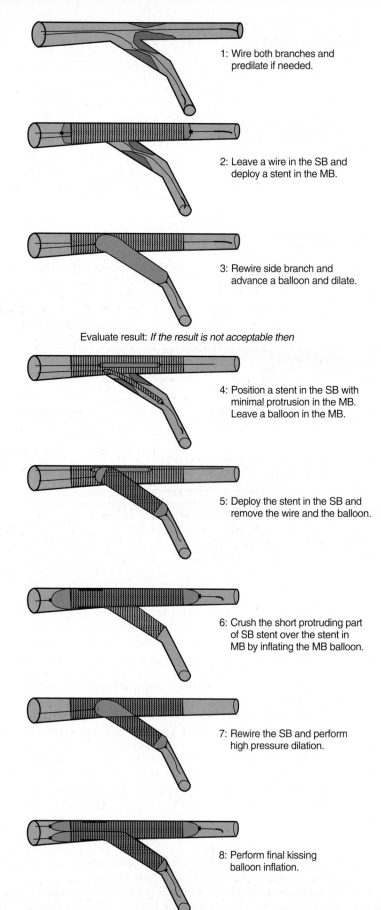

1: Wire both branches and predilate if needed.

2: Leave a wire in the SB and deploy a stent in the MB.

3: Rewire side branch and advance a balloon and dilate.

Evaluate result: *If the result is not acceptable then*

4: Position a stent in the SB with minimal protrusion in the MB. Leave a balloon in the MB.

5: Deploy the stent in the SB and remove the wire and the balloon.

6: Crush the short protruding part of SB stent over the stent in MB by inflating the MB balloon.

7: Rewire the SB and perform high pressure dilation.

8: Perform final kissing balloon inflation.

Figure 20-9. A schematic representation of the reverse crush technique. MB, main branch; SB, side branch.

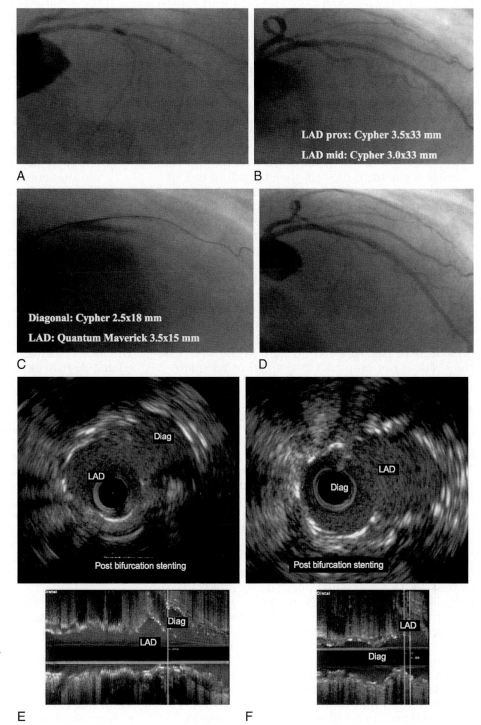

Figure 20-10. T stenting and small protrusion (TAP) technique. The baseline angiogram identifies diffuse disease of the left anterior descending coronary artery (LAD) and ostial or proximal segment of diagonal branch **(A).** After stent implantation in the proximal and middle segments of the LAD and balloon angioplasty at the diagonal branch, the result appears unsatisfactory **(B).** A second stent is advanced in the diagonal branch to minimally protrude (1 or 2 mm) into the LAD, and the balloon is positioned in the LAD. The stent in the diagonal branch is deployed, and the balloon in the LAD is simultaneously inflated **(C).** Angiographic view of the final result **(D).** Transverse and longitudinal views of the final intravascular ultrasound assessment of the LAD **(E)** and the diagonal branch **(F)** confirm optimal stent position in the diagonal branch, with minimal protrusion in the LAD.

the risk of plaque prolapse and compromise of the ostium of the SB.[34] Another element to consider when looking at the angle between the two branches is the difficulty to recross into the SB after stenting of the MB. The severity of the narrowing at the ostium of the SB is another factor influencing the placement of two stents. An additional variable to be considered is the result obtained after balloon dilatation of the SB. All of these elements mean that the selection to implant a second stent may be made at

an intermediate time, occurring after predilatation of the MB and of the SB.

Despite these considerations, the decision to use one, two, or sometimes even three stents (in case of a trifurcation) should be made as early as possible. A timely action affects the result, helps to save time and money, and lowers the risks of complications.

Louvard and associates[24] proposed the use of different strategies according to the morphology of the bifurcation. Their study findings are supported by the results of a large personal experience. Four treatment options are proposed:

Type A treatment: A stent is placed at the SB ostium, followed by placement of another stent in the MB, covering the ostium of the SB.

Type B treatment: MB stenting is followed by stenting of the SB at the ostium level through the struts of the MB stent.

Type C treatment: This technique is known as the culotte or trousers technique or, in some instances, as the Y technique. It consists of implanting a first stent from the proximal to the distal segment of the MB, thereby jailing the SB ostium. A second stent is placed from the proximal MB toward the SB while jailing the distal MB. This approach results in a double layer of stent struts in the proximal part of the MB.

Type D treatment: This strategy consists of placing two stents at the level of the ostia, followed by implantation of another stent in the proximal segment if necessary. This technique is also known as the Y implantation technique.

It is important to know that if we make the decision to use one stent (in the MB), there is usually the possibility of placing a second stent in the SB in case the result is not evaluated as optimal or adequate.

Two-Stent Techniques

The V and the Simultaneous Kissing Stent Techniques

The V and the simultaneous kissing stent (SKS) techniques (Fig. 20-11) are performed by delivering and implanting two stents together.[35,36] When the two stents protrude into the MB with the creation of a double barrel and a very proximal carina, the technique is called SKS.[36] One stent is advanced in the SB, and the other one is advanced in the MB. Both stents are pulled back to create a new carina as close as possible to the original one. The main advantage of the V technique is that the operator can never lose access to any of the two branches. When a final kissing inflation is performed, there is no need to recross any stent. Figure 20-12 shows an example of the V technique performed on the LMCA. The techniques can be performed as follows:

1. Both branches are wired and fully predilated. It is important to perform adequate predilatation to allow full stent expansion.
2. The two stents are positioned into the branches with a slight protrusion of both stents in the main proximal branch. Different operators allow various degrees of protrusion, sometimes creating a rather long (≥5 mm) double barrel in the proximal MB (i.e., SKS). Although we recognize that it is impossible to position the stent exactly at the ostium of each branch, we usually try to limit the length of the new carina to less than 5 mm. Sometimes, it is necessary to advance the first stent more distally into the vessel to facilitate the advancement of the second stent. This maneuver is essential when the kissing stent technique is used to stent a trifurcation using three kissing stents (requiring a 9-Fr guiding catheter). After accurate stent positioning, it is important to verify their correct placement in two projections before deploying the stents. In our experience, each balloon is first inflated individually at a high pressure of 12 atm or more, but other operators inflate the balloons simultaneously.

3. The next step is to inflate both balloons simultaneously at a pressure of about 8 atm. The sizes of the balloon and of the stents are chosen according to the diameter of the vessels to be stented. In the event that the reference vessel size proximal to the bifurcation is relatively small and the operator fears that the two balloons inflated simultaneously may be oversized, the kissing balloon inflation is performed at low pressure (4 atm).

Using the V technique, a metallic neocarina is created within the vessel proximal to the bifurcation. Theoretical concerns about the risk of thrombosis related to this new carina have not been confirmed in our and other operators' experience. The technique has been successfully applied with BMSs and with DESs (Cypher and Taxus). The types of lesions we consider most suitable for this technique are very proximal lesions such as bifurcation of a short LMCA free of disease. Ideally, the angle between the two branches should be less than 90 degrees. The V technique is also suitable for other bifurcations, provided that the portion of the vessel proximal to the bifurcation is free of disease, and there is no need to deploy a stent more proximally. Problems may result in positioning a stent proximal to the double barrel, with the risk of leaving a gap.

Crush Technique: Side Branch Stent Crushed by the Main Branch Stent

The crush technique (Fig. 20-13) was developed with the DES.[37] The sirolimus bifurcation study focused attention on the emerging problem of SB focal restenosis despite use of two Cypher stents (one in the MB and the other in the SB).[27] At that time, the T technique was the default approach when two stents were implanted. The need to obtain full coverage of the ostium of the SB prompted the idea of allowing some protrusion of the SB stent into the MB. The next step was to flatten the SB stent against the MB stent. The angiographic results after the initial application of this technique, which was used only with the Cypher stent, were optimal, and we felt no need for recrossing into the SB to perform a final kissing balloon inflation. Despite favorable short-term clinical outcomes without stent thrombosis, there was a 25% incidence of focal restenosis at the ostium of the SB. Since then, routine recrossing into the SB, inflation of a balloon in the SB, and kissing balloon

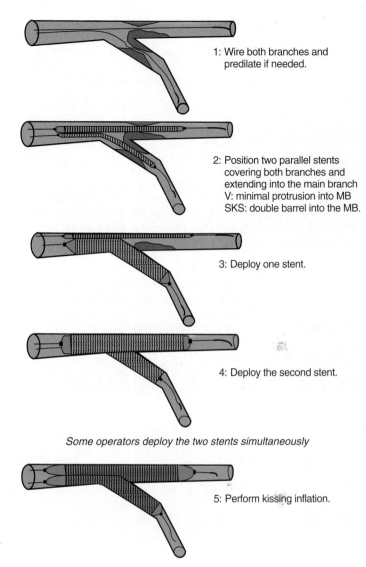

1: Wire both branches and predilate if needed.

2: Position two parallel stents covering both branches and extending into the main branch
V: minimal protrusion into MB
SKS: double barrel into the MB.

3: Deploy one stent.

4: Deploy the second stent.

Some operators deploy the two stents simultaneously

5: Perform kissing inflation.

Figure 20-11. A schematic representation of the simultaneous kissing stents (SKS) technique.

inflation have been performed.[38] Implementation of final kissing balloon inflation was done to enable better strut contact against the ostium of the SB and therefore better drug delivery. The crush technique became a type of simplified culottes technique.[41] Since routine performance of the final kissing balloon inflation, restenosis at the ostium of the SB seems to be declining.[38] The positive aspect is that restenosis usually is focal (<5 mm long) and frequently is not associated with symptoms of ischemia.

The main advantage of the crush technique is that immediate patency of both branches is ensured. This objective is important when the SB is functionally relevant or when wiring is difficult. The main disadvantage is that the performance of the final kissing balloon inflation makes the procedure more laborious because of the need to recross multiple struts with a wire and a balloon.

Ormiston and colleagues[39] reported bench testing with three stent platforms (i.e., BX Velocity, Cordis/Johnson & Johnson; Express II, Boston Scientific; and Driver, Medtronic, Minneapolis, MN) using the crush technique. The investigators stressed the importance of final kissing balloon inflation and concluded that appropriate SB and MB postdilatation is needed to fully expand the stent at the SB ostium, to widen gaps between stent struts overlying the SB (facilitating subsequent access), and to prevent stent distortion.

Performance of the crush technique requires a 7- or 8-Fr guiding catheter, and the technique commits the operator to implant two stents. We subsequently describe a modification of the crush technique that allows provisional SB stenting and permits performing the same or similar approach using a 6-Fr guiding catheter. An angiographic example of the crush technique is presented in Figure 20-14. When the angle between the MB and SB is close to 90 degrees, it is possible to minimize the gap without crushing the SB stent and using the modified T technique. The crush technique can be performed as follows:

1. Both branches are wired and fully dilated. Particular attention is paid to dilating the SB, and we may use a 6-mm-long cutting balloon

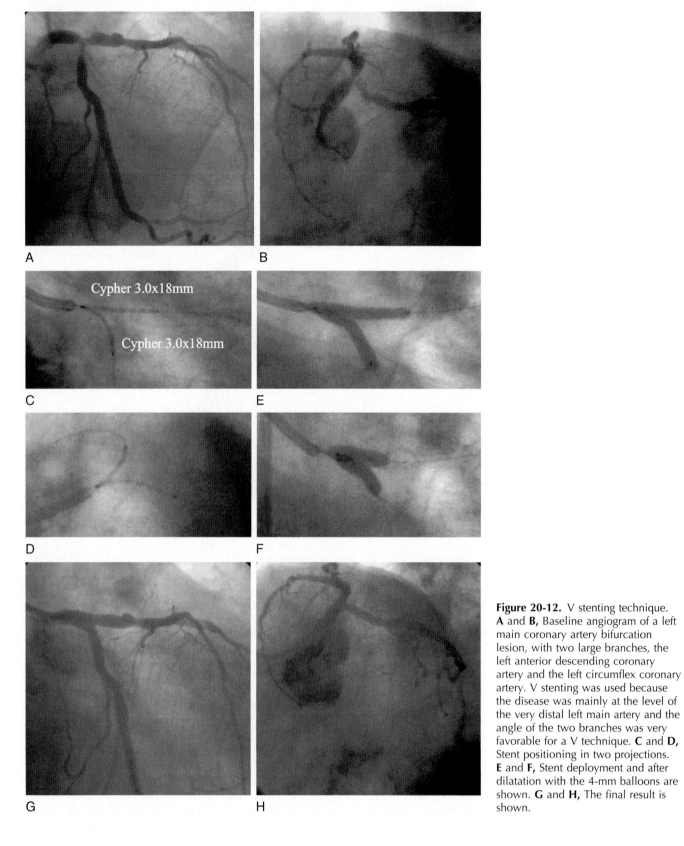

Cypher 3.0x18mm

Cypher 3.0x18mm

A

B

C

E

D

F

G

H

Figure 20-12. V stenting technique. **A** and **B,** Baseline angiogram of a left main coronary artery bifurcation lesion, with two large branches, the left anterior descending coronary artery and the left circumflex coronary artery. V stenting was used because the disease was mainly at the level of the very distal left main artery and the angle of the two branches was very favorable for a V technique. **C** and **D,** Stent positioning in two projections. **E** and **F,** Stent deployment and after dilatation with the 4-mm balloons are shown. **G** and **H,** The final result is shown.

if there is evidence that the predilating balloon does not fully expand at the ostium of the SB.

2. The stent for the SB is positioned in the SB, and the MB stent is advanced.

3. The SB stent is pulled back into the MB by about 2 to 3 mm. This step is verified in at least two projections.

4. The stent in the SB is deployed with at least 12 atm. The balloon is deflated and removed

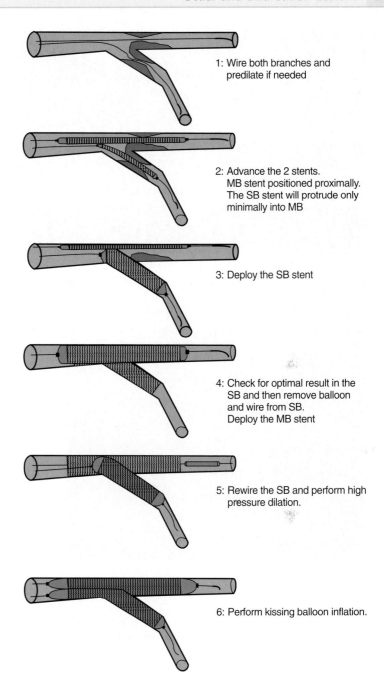

1: Wire both branches and predilate if needed

2: Advance the 2 stents. MB stent positioned proximally. The SB stent will protrude only minimally into MB

3: Deploy the SB stent

4: Check for optimal result in the SB and then remove balloon and wire from SB. Deploy the MB stent

5: Rewire the SB and perform high pressure dilation.

6: Perform kissing balloon inflation.

Figure 20-13. A schematic representation of the crush technique.

from the guiding catheter. An angiogram is obtained to verify that the SB has an appropriate lumen and normal flow and that no distal dissection or residual lesions are present. If an additional stent is needed in the SB, this is the time to perform the implantation. After this check, the wire is removed from the SB, and the stent in the MB is fully deployed at high pressure, usually above 12 atm. An angiogram is obtained after removal of the balloon from the MB.

5. A wire is advanced in the SB. This maneuver may be time consuming in the initial experience with this technique. An average of 2 minutes of fluoroscopy is used to complete

wire advancement in the SB. Besides trying with the initial floppy wire (Balance Universal, Abbott Vascular Devices, Redwood City, CA/ Guidant, Santa Clara, CA), other choices are Rinato-Prowater (Asahi Intec, Japan/Abbott Vascular Devices), Crossit 100 (Abbott Vascular Devices/Guidant), Pilot 50 and Pilot 150 (Abbott Vascular Devices/Guidant). We frequently try first to cross through the stent struts into the SB with the smallest balloon we have on the catheter table; if this balloon fails, we use a Maverick 1.5-mm-diameter balloon. If the 1.5-mm-balloon cannot cross, we consider repositioning the wire and traversing the stent struts in another spot. If

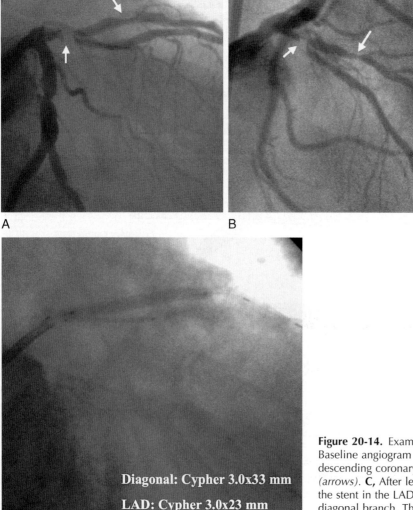

A

B

Diagonal: Cypher 3.0x33 mm

LAD: Cypher 3.0x23 mm

C

Figure 20-14. Example of the crush stenting technique. **A** and **B,** Baseline angiogram of a bifurcation lesion, involving the left anterior descending coronary artery (LAD) and a large diagonal branch *(arrows).* **C,** After lesion predilatation, two stents are positioned with the stent in the LAD placed more proximally than the stent in the diagonal branch. The side-branch stent (diagonal branch) is inflated first. Notice that a long stent was chosen for the diagonal branch to cover a lesion distal to bifurcation site.

the problem remains, we then try a fixed wire balloon, such as an ACE (Boston Scientific). It is important to perform a final dilatation on the stent toward the SB with a balloon appropriately sized to the diameter of this branch and inflated at a high pressure (≥12 atm).

6. A second balloon is advanced over the wire that was left in place in the MB, and kissing balloon inflation is performed at 8 atm or more.

Step Crush
When there is the need to perform a two-stent technique as intention to treat and a 6-Fr guiding catheter is the only available approach (i.e., radial approach), the step crush or modified balloon crush technique can be used.[40] The final result is similar to that obtained with the standard crush technique, with the difference that each stent is advanced and deployed separately. The need for a 6-Fr guiding catheter is the only reason to use this technique. The technique can be performed as follows:

1. Both branches are wired and fully dilated. Particular attention is paid to dilating the SB, and we may use a 6-mm-long cutting balloon if there is evidence that the predilating balloon does not fully expand at the ostium of the SB.
2. A stent is advanced in the SB and protrudes a few millimeters into the MB. A balloon (Maverick balloon or any other balloon with similar size features) is advanced in the MB over the bifurcation.
3. The stent in the SB is deployed, the balloon is removed, an angiogram is performed, and if the result is adequate, the wire is removed. The MB balloon is then inflated (to crush the protruding SB stent) and removed.
4. A second stent is advanced in the MB and deployed (usually at 12 atm or more).

The next steps are similar to those of the crush technique and involve recrossing into the SB, SB stent dilatation, and final kissing balloon inflation.

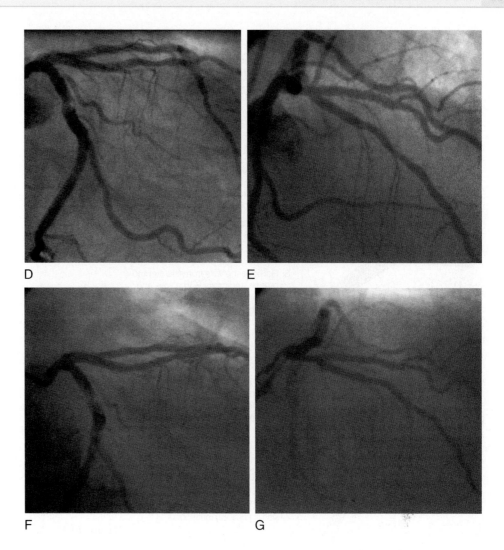

D and E

F and G

Figure 20-14, cont'd D and **E,** Optimal final result. **F** and **G,** The result was maintained at 10-month angiographic follow-up.

Culotte Technique

The culotte technique (Fig. 20-15) uses two stents and leads to full coverage of the bifurcation at the expense of an excess of metal covering of the proximal end.[41]

The culotte technique probably gives the best coverage of the carina. Important caveats about this approach are that with some closed-cell stents such as the Cypher stent, the opening of the struts toward the branches may reach a maximum diameter of only 3 mm. For this reason, the culotte technique should be used only with stents that have a design (i.e., open-cell stents) allowing full opening of the struts toward both branches. The technique can be performed as follows:

1. Both branches are predilated.
2. A stent is deployed across the most angulated branch, usually the SB.
3. The nonstented branch is rewired through the stent struts and dilated.
4. A second stent is advanced and expanded into the nonstented branch, usually the MB.
5. Kissing balloon inflation is performed.

This technique is suitable for all angles of bifurcations and provides near-perfect coverage of the SB ostium. A disadvantage is that like the crush technique, the culotte technique leads to a high concentration of metal with a double-stent layer at the carina and in the proximal part of the bifurcation. Other disadvantages of the technique include rewiring both branches through the stent struts, which can be difficult and time consuming, and a limitation in the maximum opening achievable when a stent with a closed-cell design such as the Cypher is implanted.

Y and Skirt Techniques

The Y technique has historical value because it was the first bifurcation stenting technique demonstrated in a live case course.[42] This technique involves an initial predilatation, followed by stent deployment in each branch. If the results are not adequate, a third stent may also be deployed in the MB.[43] To approximate the proximal stent to the already deployed stents, it is necessary to modify the stent delivery system by placing one stent over two balloons (i.e., skirt stenting).[44] This technique is employed as a last resort for treating very demanding bifurcations in which there is a need to maintain uninterrupted wire access to both branches.

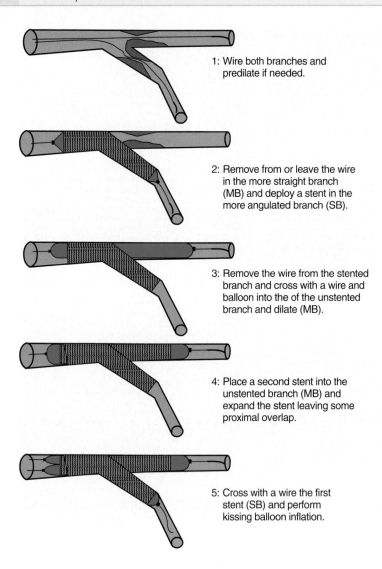

1: Wire both branches and predilate if needed.

2: Remove from or leave the wire in the more straight branch (MB) and deploy a stent in the more angulated branch (SB).

3: Remove the wire from the stented branch and cross with a wire and balloon into the of the unstented branch and dilate (MB).

4: Place a second stent into the unstented branch (MB) and expand the stent leaving some proximal overlap.

5: Cross with a wire the first stent (SB) and perform kissing balloon inflation.

Figure 20-15. A schematic representation of the culotte technique.

Although no definitive statement can be made regarding the best strategy to be used when implantation of two stents is required in a bifurcation, Figure 20-16 provides a schematic approach based on the anatomy of the lesion.

Bifurcation Stents

Dedicated Bifurcation Stents

Several stents have been specifically designed for bifurcation lesions, with particular emphasis on maintaining ease of access to the SB. Initial attempts to develop a specific stent design for bifurcation lesions involved stents with one (NIR side, Medinol, Jerusalem, Israel; AST SLK, Advanced Stent Technologies, Pleasanton, CA) or several (Jomed, Abbott Vascular Devices) larger struts to enhance access to SB ostium. The main drawbacks were poor scaffolding of the SB ostium and difficulties in accurate positioning of a stent at the SB ostium level.

Newer bifurcation stent designs include dedicated bifurcation stents with "intention to stent" the MB and the SB and SB access stents (i.e., provisional SB stenting), in which case the MB is always stented and there is an option to stent the SB.

Other Dedicated Bifurcation Stents

There are several stents specifically designed for bifurcational lesions that have already been used in humans, and some of them already have the CE mark (i.e., European marketing approval) or have been evaluated in animal studies but without any drug-eluting feature.

The Tryton side branch stent (Tryton Medical, Boston, MA) is a single wire stent that requires stenting of the MB and SB branches. In its current design using cobalt chromium, there are no drug-delivery features, but it is likely to incorporate a drug-delivery system for early clinical trials.

The ML Frontier stent (Abbott Vascular Devices/ Guidant) consists of a balloon-expandable stainless steel stent mounted on a delivery system with two

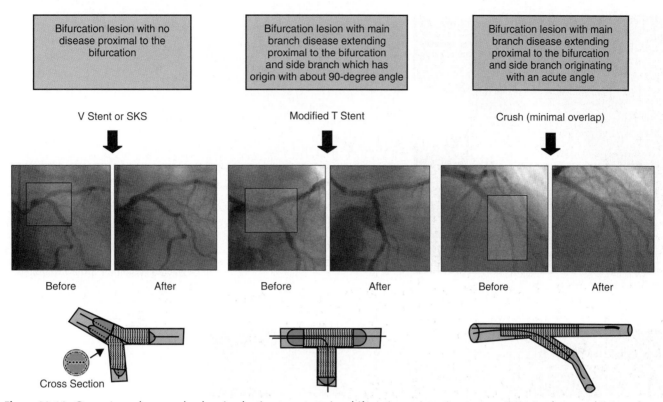

| Bifurcation lesion with no disease proximal to the bifurcation | Bifurcation lesion with main branch disease extending proximal to the bifurcation and side branch which has origin with about 90-degree angle | Bifurcation lesion with main branch disease extending proximal to the bifurcation and side branch originating with an acute angle |

V Stent or SKS   Modified T Stent   Crush (minimal overlap)

Before   After   Before   After   Before   After

Cross Section

Figure 20-16. Our proposed approach when implanting two stents in a bifurcation as intention to treat. SKS, simultaneous kissing stents.

balloons and two guidewires (SB over the wire balloon and MB monorail balloon) designed to maintain wire access to the SB vessel during stent deployment. The advantages of this design are that guidewire crisscross is avoided and SB access is maintained during the whole procedure. This two-balloon, two-wire system requires a 7-Fr guiding catheter.[45] Potential developments are a cobalt chromium platform with polymer-based everolimus-eluting capabilities.

The Twin-Rail bifurcation stent (Invatec, Roncadelle, Italy) has a double-balloon stent delivery system compatible with a 6-Fr guiding catheter. The stent is also available with a single-balloon, two-wire delivery system.

The Nile stent (Minvasis, Gennevilliers, France) is a chromium cobalt stent with dual-balloon delivery system compatible with a 6-Fr guiding catheter. Like all the other provisional SB stents, the Nile stent offers the possibility of adding an SB stent in case of plaque shifting.

The Sideguard stent (Cappella, Auburndale, MA) is a self-expanding stent with a unique delivery system for accurate positioning at the ostium of the SB. The Sideguard stent may need an additional stent to be implanted in the MB. The Sideguard stent tracks over one wire and allows protection of the MB with a wire, a balloon, or a stent. The operator may deploy a stent of her or his choice in the MB after the release of the Sideguard stent. This second balloon-expandable

stent in the MB helps to better flail the proximal segment of the self-expanding SB stent.

Dedicated Drug-Eluting Bifurcation Stents

The Axxess stent (Devax, Irvine, CA) and the Petal stent (Boston Scientific) are the only bifurcation stents likely to reach the market soon. The Axxess stent is modular with three components, with MB proximal stent delivery and distal MB and ostial SB stenting (Fig. 20-17). The stent is made of nitinol, it is self-expanding, and has biolimus A9 drug-delivery feature (Axxess Plus). The current model requires an 8-Fr guiding catheter, and complete coverage of the bifurcation requires the implantation of three stents. The Axxess stent can also be used as an MB or as an SB stent if the lesion is suitable for this approach.

The Petal stent (Boston Scientific) represents the evolution of the AST SLK-View stent, a technology acquired by Boston Scientific (Fig. 20-18). The current Petal stent is a platinum stainless steel stent with a 0.032-inch strut thickness, a dual-wire and dual-balloon delivery system, and a polymer-based paclitaxel-eluting system. The stent has an aperture in the middle segment with struts that protrude into the SB to allow optimal coverage of the ostium. This stent will soon be evaluated in human trials, and it is the

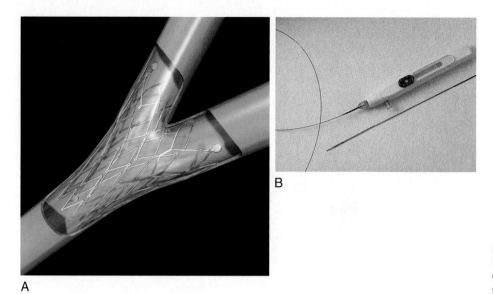

Figure 20-17. The Axxess stent (Devax Inc., Irvine, CA) **(A)** with a dedicated delivery system for a self-expanding stent **(B)**.

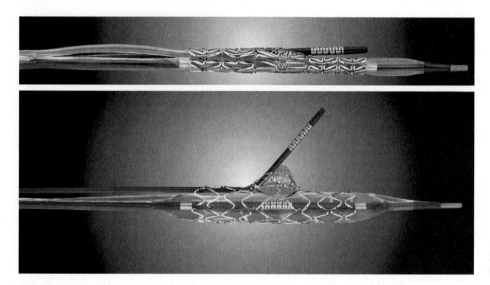

Figure 20-18. The Petal stent (Boston Scientific, Natick, MA) with a dual-balloon system.

most likely competitor to the Axxess stent in the field of dedicated DES bifurcation stents.

Adjunctive Procedures

Rotational Atherectomy

Rotablation allows optimal stent expansion in lesions with severe superficial calcifications. Even if no data are available regarding the role of this technology with DES, we think it is intuitive to aim for optimal stent expansion and symmetry. In the setting of a very calcific lesion, this goal can be achieved only with adequate lesion preparation.

How frequently should a calcific lesion be pretreated with rotational atherectomy, and when is a high-pressure balloon sufficient? Except for information obtained with IVUS or in circumstances in which no balloon would cross the lesion, we cannot provide additional objective guidelines to make a scientific

decision. The operator's judgment remains the most frequent tool dictating the choice of rotational atherectomy. Burr size is typically small (1.25 or 1.5 mm), with the intent to modify the plaque, minimizing the risk of embolization. In our experience, SB stent underdeployment due to inadequate preparation remains the most important cause of restenosis at the ostium of the SB.[46]

Cutting Balloon

Bifurcation lesions with a fibrotic plaque at the SB ostium are an ideal setting for the use of a cutting balloon. The Restenosis Reduction by Cutting balloon Evaluation (REDUCE III) randomized trial evaluated the role of cutting balloon dilatation before stenting compared with standard balloon dilatation in a variety of lesions.[47] This trial reported a lower restenosis rate (11.8% versus 18.8%, $P = .04$) when lesions were predilated with the cutting balloon. The final postprocedural lumen diameter was larger in the cutting balloon arm, and the late loss was 0.74 mm for both strategies, indicating that the main advantage was in enabling better stent expansion.

As discussed in the context of rotational atherectomy, it is difficult to demonstrate that a niche device has an advantage in every lesion. We suggest the use of a cutting balloon in selected, moderately calcific and fibrotic lesions, especially the ones that involve the origin of the SB.

Directional Atherectomy

Directional coronary atherectomy has been considered ideal for bifurcational lesions. There are various indications for plaque removal in this setting, and there are a number of positive anecdotal experiences. Unfortunately, the Atherectomy before Multi-Link Improves Lumen Gain and Clinical Outcomes (AMIGO) trial failed to support the original findings and hypothesis, even in the subgroup of lesions involving a bifurcation.[48] The main problem of directional atherectomy, which might have affected the results of the AMIGO trial, is that the technique is operator dependent. Except for the recent introduction of the Silverhawk device (Fox Hollow Technologies, Redwood City, CA), no further developments in devices were made for a long period.[49] Despite these concerns and despite the lack of scientific evidence supporting the advantage of plaque debulking in bifurcation lesions, our experience in this setting has been favorable, and we still occasionally combine atherectomy and DES when the anatomic setting is appropriate, such as an LMCA stenosis with a large plaque burden demonstrated by IVUS.

Associated Pharmacologic Treatment

When performing bifurcation stenting with one or two stents, we do not usually change our protocol of periprocedural heparin administration (100 U/kg without elective glycoprotein IIb/IIIa inhibitors and 70U/kg with elective glycoprotein IIb/IIIa inhibitors). Use of glycoprotein IIb/IIIa inhibitors is reserved for thrombus-containing lesions, for patients with acute coronary syndromes, or when two stents will be implanted as intention to treat. Glycoprotein IIb/IIIa inhibitors are sometimes administered when the final result at the SB appears suboptimal, but the operator decides not to implant another stent. An alternative to glycoprotein IIb/IIIa inhibitors and heparin is the use of bivalirudin.

We pay close attention to preprocedural preparation with thienopyridines, and when in doubt, we administer a 600-mg loading dose of clopidogrel in the catheterization laboratory.[50] In the sirolimus bifurcation study, clopidogrel was continued for 3 months, and no late episodes of thrombosis were observed.[27] A few thromboses occurred during treatment with clopidogrel, and some of them were associated with an angiographically suboptimal result. The only case of sudden death (4.5 months after the procedure) occurred while the patient was still consuming clopidogrel and aspirin. Unfortunately, the small number of patients enrolled in this trial does not allow us to draw any conclusions regarding the safety of 3-month clopidogrel administration in patients with bifurcation lesions, especially when two stents are used. In our current practice, the duration of combined thienopyridine and aspirin treatment after stent implantation is usually for a minimum of 6 months, and it is usually extended to 1 year.

CONCLUSIONS

The introduction of DESs has made a remarkable improvement in the treatment of bifurcation lesions. The sirolimus bifurcation study, despite the limitations of a small number of patients and the high crossover rate, demonstrated almost full suppression of restenosis in the MB. Restenosis in the SB occurred in about one of five lesions treated, but the restenosis was usually focal and therefore simple to treat. There has been some concern regarding the numerically high thrombosis rate (3 of 85 patients). We think that the learning curve for implanting two stents and the relatively low number of patients enrolled in this study could have magnified the incidence of thrombosis.

The appropriate application of provisional stenting and refinement of stent techniques when implanting two stents will further improve the immediate and long-term follow-up results. The introduction of DESs dedicated for different types of bifurcations may further facilitate the conquest of one of the most challenging areas in interventional cardiology.

REFERENCES

1. Iakovou I, Ge L, Michev I, et al: Clinical and angiographic outcome after sirolimus-eluting stent implantation in aorto-ostial lesions. J Am Coll Cardiol 2004;44:967-971.
2. Kurbaan AS, Kelly PA, Sigwart U: Cutting balloon angioplasty and stenting for aorto-ostial lesions. Heart 1997;77:350-352.
3. Ahmed JM, Hong MK, Mehran R, et al: Comparison of debulking followed by stenting versus stenting alone for saphenous vein graft aortoostial lesions: Immediate and one-year clinical outcomes. J Am Coll Cardiol 2000;35:1560-1568.
4. Kereiakes DJ: Percutaneous transcatheter therapy of aorto-ostial stenoses. Cathet Cardiovasc Diagn 1996;38:292-300.
5. Smith SC Jr, Feldman TE, Hirshfeld JW Jr, et al: ACC/AHA/SCAI 2005 Guideline Update for Percutaneous Coronary Intervention—Summary article: A report of the American College of Cardiology/American Heart Association Task Force on Practice Guidelines (ACC/AHA/SCAI Writing Committee to Update the 2001 Guidelines for Percutaneous Coronary Intervention). Circulation 2006;113:156-175.
6. Heidland UE, Heintzen MP, Michel CJ, Strauer BE: Risk factors for the development of restenosis following stent implantation of venous bypass grafts. Heart 2001;85:312-317.
7. Rocha-Singh K, Morris N, Wong SC, Schatz RA, et al: Coronary stenting for treatment of ostial stenoses of native coronary

arteries or aortocoronary saphenous venous grafts. Am J Cardiol 1995;75:26-29.

8. Jain SP, Liu MW, Dean LS, et al: Comparison of balloon angioplasty versus debulking devices versus stenting in right coronary ostial lesions. Am J Cardiol 1997;79:1334-1338.

9. Shaia N, Heuser RR: Distal embolic protection for SVG interventions: Can we afford not to use it? J Interv Cardiol 2005;18:481-484.

10. Toutouzas K, Stankovic G, Takagi T, et al: Outcome of treatment of aorto-ostial lesions involving the right coronary artery or a saphenous vein graft with a polytetrafluoroethylene-covered stent. Am J Cardiol 2002;90:63-66.

11. Mavromatis K, Ghazzal Z, Veledar E, et al: Comparison of outcomes of percutaneous coronary intervention of ostial versus nonostial narrowing of the major epicardial coronary arteries. Am J Cardiol 2004;94:583-587.

12. Park SJ, Lee CW, Hong MK, et al: Stent placement for ostial left anterior descending coronary artery stenosis: Acute and long-term (2-year) results. Catheter Cardiovasc Interv 2000;49:267-271.

13. Moses JW, Leon MB, Popma JJ, et al: Sirolimus-eluting stents versus standard stents in patients with stenosis in a native coronary artery. N Engl J Med 2003;349:1315-1323.

14. Stone GW, Ellis SG, Cox DA, et al: A polymer-based, paclitaxel-eluting stent in patients with coronary artery disease. N Engl J Med 2004;350:221-231.

15. Lemos PA, Hoye A, Goedhart D, et al: Clinical, angiographic, and procedural predictors of angiographic restenosis after sirolimus-eluting stent implantation in complex patients: An evaluation from the Rapamycin-Eluting Stent Evaluated At Rotterdam Cardiology Hospital (RESEARCH) study. Circulation 2004;109:1366-1370.

16. Sawhney N, Moses JW, Leon MB, et al: Treatment of left anterior descending coronary artery disease with sirolimus-eluting stents. Circulation 2004;110:374-379.

17. Khattab AA, Otto A, Toelg R, et al: Sirolimus-eluting stent treatment for complex proximal left anterior descending artery stenoses: 7-month clinical and angiographic results. J Invasive Cardiol 2005;17:582-586.

18. Vijayakumar M, Rodriguez Granillo GA, Lemos PA, et al: Sirolimus-eluting stents for the treatment of atherosclerotic ostial lesions. J Invasive Cardiol 2005;17:10-12.

19. Seung KB, Kim YH, Park DW, et al: Effectiveness of sirolimus-eluting stent implantation for the treatment of ostial left anterior descending artery stenosis with intravascular ultrasound guidance. J Am Coll Cardiol 2005;46:787-792.

20. Tsagalou E, Stankovic G, Iakovou I, et al: Early outcome of treatment of ostial de novo left anterior descending coronary artery lesions with drug-eluting stents. Am J Cardiol 2006;97:187-191.

21. Lefevre T, Louvard Y, Morice MC, et al: Stenting of bifurcation lesions: Classification, treatments, and results. Catheter Cardiovasc Interv 2000;49:274-283.

22. Safian RD: Bifurcation Lesions. In Safian RD, Freed M (Eds): Manual of Interventional Cardiology. Royal Oak, MI, Physicians' Press, 2001, pp 221-236.

23. Aliabadi D, Tilli FV, Bowers TR, et al: Incidence and angiographic predictors of side branch occlusion following high-pressure intracoronary stenting. Am J Cardiol 1997;80:994-997.

24. Louvard Y, Lefevre T, Morice MC: Percutaneous coronary intervention for bifurcation coronary disease. Heart 2004;90:713-722.

25. Medina A, Suarez de Lezo J, Pan M: A new classification of coronary bifurcation lesions [in Spanish]. Rev Esp Cardiol 2006;59:183.

26. Fujii K, Kobayashi Y, Mintz GS, et al: Dominant contribution of negative remodeling to development of significant coronary bifurcation narrowing. Am J Cardiol 2003;92:59-61.

27. Colombo A, Moses JW, Morice MC, et al: Randomized study to evaluate sirolimus-eluting stents implanted at coronary bifurcation lesions. Circulation 2004;109:1244-1249.

28. Al Suwaidi J, Berger PB, Rihal CS, et al: Immediate and long-term outcome of intracoronary stent implantation for true bifurcation lesions. J Am Coll Cardiol 2000;35:929-936.

29. Yamashita T, Nishida T, Adamian MG, et al: Bifurcation lesions: Two stents versus one stent: Immediate and follow-up results. J Am Coll Cardiol 2000;35:1145-1151.

30. Pan M, de Lezo JS, Medina A, et al: Rapamycin-eluting stents for the treatment of bifurcated coronary lesions: A randomized comparison of a simple versus complex strategy. Am Heart J 2004;148:857-864.

31. Steigen TK, Maeng M, Wiseth R, et al: Randomized study on simple versus complex stenting of coronary bifurcation lesions: The Nordic bifurcation study. Circulation 2006;114:1955-1961.

32. Carrie D, Karouny E, Chouairi S, Puel J: "T"-shaped stent placement: A technique for the treatment of dissected bifurcation lesions. Cathet Cardiovasc Diagn 1996;37:311-313.

33. Nakamura S, Hall P, Maiello L, Colombo A: Techniques for Palmaz-Schatz stent deployment in lesions with a large side branch. Cathet Cardiovasc Diagn 1995;34:353-361.

34. Brunel P, Lefevre T, Darremont O, Louvard Y: Provisional T-stenting and kissing balloon in the treatment of coronary bifurcation lesions: Results of the French multicenter "TULIPE" study. Catheter Cardiovasc Interv 2006;68:67-73.

35. Schampaert E, Fort S, Adelman AG, Schwartz L: The V-stent: A novel technique for coronary bifurcation stenting. Cathet Cardiovasc Diagn 1996;39:320-326.

36. Sharma SK: Simultaneous kissing drug-eluting stent technique for percutaneous treatment of bifurcation lesions in large-size vessels. Catheter Cardiovasc Interv 2005;65:10-16.

37. Colombo A, Stankovic G, Orlic D, et al: Modified T-stenting technique with crushing for bifurcation lesions: Immediate results and 30-day outcome. Catheter Cardiovasc Interv 2003;60:145-151.

38. Ge L, Airoldi F, Iakovou I, et al: Clinical and angiographic outcome after implantation of drug-eluting stents in bifurcation lesions with the crush stent technique: Importance of final kissing balloon post-dilation. J Am Coll Cardiol 2005;46:613-620.

39. Ormiston JA, Currie E, Webster MW, et al: Drug-eluting stents for coronary bifurcations: Insights into the crush technique. Catheter Cardiovasc Interv 2004;63:332-336.

40. Collins N, Dzavik V: A modified balloon crush approach improves side branch access and side branch stent apposition during crush stenting of coronary bifurcation lesions. Catheter Cardiovasc Interv 2006;68:365-371.

41. Chevalier B, Glatt B, Royer T, Guyon P: Placement of coronary stents in bifurcation lesions by the "culotte" technique. Am J Cardiol 1998;82:943-949.

42. Baim DS: Is bifurcation stenting the answer? Cathet Cardiovasc Diagn 1996;37:314-316.

43. Helqvist S, Jorgensen E, Kelbaek H, et al: Percutaneous treatment of coronary bifurcation lesions: A novel "extended Y" technique with complete lesion stent coverage. Heart 2006;92:981-982.

44. Kobayashi Y, Colombo A, Adamian M, et al: The skirt technique: A stenting technique to treat a lesion immediately proximal to the bifurcation (pseudobifurcation). Catheter Cardiovasc Interv 2000;51:347-351.

45. Lefevre T, Ormiston J, Guagliumi G, et al: The Frontier stent registry: Safety and feasibility of a novel dedicated stent for the treatment of bifurcation coronary artery lesions. J Am Coll Cardiol 2005;46:592-598.

46. Costa RA, Mintz GS, Carlier SG, et al: Bifurcation coronary lesions treated with the "crush" technique: An intravascular ultrasound analysis. J Am Coll Cardiol 2005;46:599-605.

47. Ozaki Y, Suzuki T, Yamaguchi T, et al: Can intravascular ultrasound guided cutting balloon angioplasty before stenting be a substitute for drug eluting stent? Final results of the prospective randomized multicenter trial comparing cutting balloon with balloon angioplasty before stenting (REDUCE III) [abstract]. J Am Coll Cardiol 2004;43(Suppl A):1138.

48. Stankovic G, Colombo A, Bersin R, et al: Comparison of directional coronary atherectomy and stenting versus stenting alone for the treatment of de novo and restenotic coronary artery narrowing. Am J Cardiol 2004;93:953-958.

49. Ikeno F, Hinohara T, Robertson GC, et al: Early experience with a novel plaque excision system for the treatment of

complex coronary lesions. Catheter Cardiovasc Interv 2004;61: 35-43.

50. Patti G, Colonna G, Pasceri V, et al: Randomized trial of high loading dose of clopidogrel for reduction of periprocedural myocardial infarction in patients undergoing coronary intervention: Results from the ARMYDA-2 (Antiplatelet therapy for Reduction of MYocardial Damage during Angioplasty) study. Circulation 2005;111:2099-106.

51. Popma J, Leon M, Topol EJ: Atlas of Interventional Cardiology. Philadelphia, PA, WB Saunders, 1994.

52. Spokojny AM, Sanborn TM: The bifurcation lesion. *In* Ellis SG, Holmes DR (Eds): Strategic Approaches in Coronary Intervention. Baltimore, MD, Williams & Wilkins, 1996, p 288.

53. Sianos G, Morel MA, Kappetein AP, et al: The SYNTAX score: An angiographic tool grading the complexity of coronary artery disease. Eurointervention 2005;1:219-227.

54. Tsuchida K, Colombo A, Lefevre T, et al: The clinical outcome of percutaneous treatment of bifurcation lesions in multivessel coronary artery disease with the sirolimus-eluting stent: Insights from the Arterial Revascularization Therapies Study part 11 (ARTS 11). Eur Heart J 2007;4:433-442

55. Hoye A, Iakovou I, Ge L et al: Long term outcomes after stenting of bifurcation lesions with the "crush" technique. J Am Coll Cardiol 2006;47:1949-1958.

56. Moussa I, Costa RA, Leon MB, et al: A prospective registry to evaluate sirolimus-eluting stents implanted at coronary bifurcation lesions using the "crush technique." Am J Cardiol 2006;97:1317-1321.

57. Sharma SK: Simultaneous kissing drug-eluting stent technique for percutaneous treatment of bifurcation lesions in large-size vessels. Catheter Cardiovasc Interv 2005;65:10-16.

58. Ge L, Iakovou I, Cosgrave J, et al: Treatment of bifurcation lesions with two stents: One year angiographic and clinical follow up of crush versus T stenting. Heart 2006;92: 371-376.

CHAPTER

21 Small-Vessel and Diffuse Disease

Masakiyo Nobuyoshi and Hiroyoshi Yokoi

KEY POINTS

■ In light of the paucity of randomized trial data demonstrating the superiority of any particular device in the treatment of small vessel and diffuse disease, treatment needs to be individualized.

■ Rotational atherectomy may provide a rational approach to long-calcified stenoses by rendering them responsive to balloon dilation.

■ Given the substantial incidence of restenosis despite stent placement in the setting of long lesions, until the problem of in-stent restenosis can be ameliorated, the

routine use of stents should be undertaken with extreme caution.

■ Although drug-eluting stents are associated with a lower rate of in-stent restenosis compared with bare metal stents, until the problem of very late stent thrombosis can be ameliorated, the decision to implant a drug-eluting stent or use an alternative revascularization strategy (including a bare metal stent or surgical revascularization) must be made for each patient after consideration of the relative risks and benefits of each therapy.

Small-vessel disease and diffuse coronary disease present considerable challenges to the interventional cardiologist. Compared with treatment of discrete stenoses, percutaneous revascularization of small vessel and diffuse disease is associated with decreased rates of procedural success and a greater incidence of acute complications and restenosis. Patients with diffuse coronary disease often possess other features (e.g., diabetes, multivessel disease) that are associated with adverse procedural outcomes. Patients with diffuse disease may not be suitable candidates for conventional bypass grafting because the disease involves the distal vascular territories.

Despite enthusiastic and favorable observational reports during the preliminary experience with a variety of newer-generation devices, the superiority of ablative and debulking techniques over balloon angioplasty in the treatment of small vessel and diffuse disease has not been confirmed in later randomized trials. Although there have been significant improvements in the short- and long-term outcomes of coronary stenting of discrete stenoses, the data suggest that restenosis rates remain substantial when long or multiple overlapping stents are used to treat small vessel and diffuse disease. This chapter examines potential approaches to the long lesion and emerging concepts regarding treatment of small-vessel and diffuse coronary disease by considering the first-hand experience of treating long lesions at Kokura Memorial Hospital and by reviewing the worldwide literature.

PATHOPHYSIOLOGIC CONSIDERATIONS

The length of a coronary stenosis is an important determinant of its hemodynamic significance, which may affect the decision about whether a particular lesion merits revascularization. Whereas a discrete stenosis of moderate severity may not be flow limiting, a longer stenosis of similar severity may impair distal blood flow. The relationships among stenosis severity, lesion length, and translesional flow in an idealized system are governed by Poiseuille's law, which dictates that flow varies directly as a function of luminal diameter and inversely as a function of lesion length:

$$Flow = \P(\Delta P)(r^4)8/(\eta)(l)$$

In the equation, ΔP is the pressure difference across the stenosis, r is the minimal lumen radius of the stenotic segment, η is blood viscosity, and l is the length of the lesion.[2]

Because flow across the lesion varies in proportion to the fourth power of radius but only as a first power of length, lesion length is expected to exert relatively little effect on translesional flow for discrete (e.g., <5 mm long) stenoses. However, as the length of a stenosis increases, such as from 5 to 25 mm, a fivefold drop in blood flow across the stenosis can occur. Physicians performing coronary angiography or angioplasty must understand this basic concept.[1]

Poiseuille's law describes the flow of fluids through cylindrical tubes in well-controlled experimental settings. It does not take into consideration the complexities of human coronary artery disease, such as plaque irregularity and eccentricity, nonlaminar and pulsatile flow, vasoactive properties of the arterial wall, and the potential for compensatory dilation. There is experimental evidence that lesion length has an important physiologic significance. Short, 40% to 60% coronary narrowings in a canine model with no major resting hemodynamic effects significantly reduced flows when stenosis length was increased to 10 and 15 mm. The hemodynamic effects of a 15-mm-long, 40% to 60% stenosis were similar to those of a discrete 90% narrowing.[3]

BALLOON ANGIOPLASTY FOR SMALL VESSELS AND DIFFUSE DISEASE

Acute Procedural Success and Complications

From the earliest experience with coronary angioplasty, most investigators identified lesion length as a predictor of decreased procedural success and increased periprocedural complications. A twofold increase in adverse procedural sequelae with eccentric lesions longer than 5 mm (24%) compared with dilation of short concentric stenoses (12%) was reported by Meier and colleagues in 1983.[4] Ellis and colleagues[5] identified lesion length twice the reference vessel luminal diameter or longer as an independent predictor of abrupt vessel closure after balloon angioplasty procedures. Data from the 1985-1986 National Heart, Lung, and Blood Institute (NHLBI) Percutaneous Transluminal Coronary Angioplasty (PTCA) Registry support that view.[6] Among 1801 patients who underwent balloon angioplasty, the incidence of abrupt closure was 6.8%, and diffuse lesion morphology predicted abrupt closure with an odds ratio of 2.5. An angiographic success rate of 85.8% but a substantial incidence of major complications was reported by Ghazzal and colleagues; of 184 patients with long (9.1 to 26 mm) lesions who underwent balloon angioplasty, 7.7% needed emergency coronary bypass surgery.[7] Based on these disappointing early reports, the American College of Cardiology/American Heart Association (ACC/AHA) Angioplasty Task Force identified lesion length as an adverse morphologic characteristic for angioplasty and incorporated stenosis length into its widely employed A, B, C lesion classification scheme in 1988.[8]

However several authors have questioned the above relationship. Ellis and colleagues[9] reviewed 350 patients with multivessel coronary disease retrospectively, and lesion length did not emerge as a univariate predictor of procedural success. In the Multi-Hospital Eastern Atlantic Restenosis Trial (M-HEART) enrolling 826 patients, lesion calcification, presence of thrombus, and right coronary artery location affected procedural outcome adversely, but lesion length had no effects.[10] Among 1447 patients enrolled in Coronary Artery Restenosis Prevention on Repeated Thromboxane Antagonism (CARPORT) trial and the Multicenter American Research Trial with Cilazapril after Angioplasty to Prevent Transluminal Coronary Obstruction and Restenosis (MARCATOR) studies, lesion length was not identified as a predictor of major adverse cardiac events following balloon angioplasty.[11]

The inclusion of relatively few patients with nondiscrete stenoses might have biased the results of these studies. For example, in the M-HEART population, 88% of the lesions treated were shorter than 10 mm, and only 1.2% of the lesions were longer than 20 mm.

Data collected in the immediate present era appear to support earlier observations that longer lesions respond less favorably to balloon dilation than shorter stenoses do. Among 533 patients with 1000 treated lesions reported by Myler and colleagues,[12] the procedural success rate decreased from 95% for lesions less than 10 mm long to 91.4% for 10- to 20-mm long lesions and to 88.9% for those longer than 20 mm. Similarly, in a large, retrospective series reported by Tan and colleagues,[13] lesion length was a powerful predictor of procedural success and complications (Fig. 21-1).

The underlying mechanism for the association between lesion length and angioplasty complications is multifactorial. By virtue of their length, diffuse lesions are more likely to be associated with other adverse morphologic characteristics (e.g., overlapping a bifurcation point, an angulated segment of the vessel). The plaque composition of long lesions also may tend to be less uniform, which can predispose to uneven distribution of shear stresses during balloon dilation and consequent dissection. In support of this concept, two reports described a relationship between lesion length and the risk of dissection.[14,15] Proper balloon sizing also may be difficult in the presence of diffuse disease, which often renders the angiographic determination of normal vessel reference diameter impossible.[16]

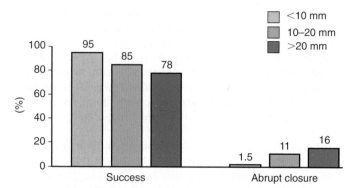

Figure 21-1. Rates of procedural success and abrupt closure after balloon angioplasty as a function of lesion length. (Modified from Tan K, Sulke N, Taub N, Sowton E: Clinical and lesion morphologic determinants of coronary angioplasty success and complications: Current experience. J Am Coll Cardiol 1995;25: 855-865.)

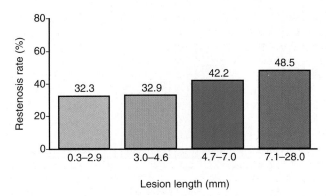

Figure 21-2. Relationship between lesion length and restenosis after balloon angioplasty. (Modified from Hirschfeld JW Jr, Schwartz JS, Jugo R, et al: Restenosis after coronary angioplasty: A multivariate statistical model to relate lesion and procedure variables to restenosis. The M-HEART Investigators. J Am Coll Cardiol 1991;18:647-656.)

Restenosis

Longer lesions carry a heightened risk of restenosis compared with discrete stenoses after balloon angioplasty. Of 510 patients with 598 successfully dilated lesions enrolled in M-HEART and who underwent late follow-up angiography, restenosis occurred in 48.5% of lesions longer than 7 mm compared with 33% of lesions less than 4.6 mm long (Fig. 21-2).[17] Similarly, serial quantitative coronary angiography was performed on 666 lesions immediately and 6 months after successful PTCA in the CARPORT study. Among various clinical and angiographic variables examined, lesion length greater than 6.8 mm was independently associated with subsequent restenosis: 60% greater late loss compared with lesions less than 5.25 mm long.[18]

The Kokura Experience

A retrospective analysis of patients treated at the Kokura Memorial Hospital before the advent of new devices was undertaken. Among all patients undergoing initial PTCA (excluding those in the setting of acute myocardial infarction) between June 1989 and May 1990, 512 patients with 797 lesions could be analyzed by quantitative angiography, of whom 319 patients with 615 lesions had late angiographic follow-up. No significant correlation was found between the lesion length and baseline patient characteristics; however, as shown in Table 21-1, lesions longer than 20 mm were more likely to involve the left anterior descending artery (LAD), possess calcifications, contain thrombus, or represent total occlusions.

As Table 21-2 indicates, the initial results of balloon angioplasty for long lesions in terms of acute luminal gain did not differ significantly from the results achieved in shorter lesions. Consistent with reports from other institutions, however, long (>20 mm) lesions were associated with reduced initial success (74%) and higher restenosis (63%) rates compared with discrete lesions. Restenosis among this group of patients with longer lesions appeared to be related to significantly greater late loss rather than to inadequate initial luminal gain.

Long Balloons

Covering the entire length of a lesion as well as normal proximal and distal vessel segments simultaneously should theoretically distribute pressure more evenly during dilation and produce less shear stress at the transition points between diseased and normal vessel, and the chances of dissection would be reduced.[24] Long lesions often involve angulated segments that respond more favorably to the use of a single, long balloon.[25] Long balloons (30 to 80 mm) hypothetically may enhance the safety and efficacy of dilating long lesions.[19-23]

A few retrospective series seem to confirm these ideas. Brymer and colleagues[19] assigned 44 patients with long (15 to 25 mm) or tandem (<25 mm) lesions to undergo PTCA with standard (20 mm) or long (30 mm) balloons. Lesions treated with long balloons required fewer inflations and were significantly less likely to develop moderate or severe dissections.[19] In a retrospective analysis of 86 long lesions (mean

Table 21-1. Lesion Characteristics

Lesion Type	Short Lesion (n = 817)	Long Lesion* (n = 100)	P Value
Left anterior descending artery (%)	37	56	.002
Irregular (%)	39	47	NS
Calcification (%)	23	36	.002
Thrombus (%)	6	17	.0001
Ostial (%)	13	19	NS
Chronic and occlusion (%)	5	14	.0006

*A long lesion is more than 20 mm long.
NS, not significant.

Table 21-2. Initial and Follow-up Outcomes of Balloon Angioplasty for Long Lesions

| Outcomes | Lesion Length | | | P Value |
	<10 mm	10-20 mm	>20 mm	
Procedure success rate (%)	95	85	74	.0001
Restenosis rate (%)	27	47	63	.0001
Acute gain (mm)	1.50 ± 0.54	1.61 ± 0.60	1.50 ± 0.40	NS
Late loss (mm)	0.53 ± 0.83	0.96 ± 0.91	1.05 ± 0.79	.0001

NS, not significant.

length of 22 ± 11 mm) treated with 30- or 40-mm balloons, Cannon and colleagues[20] reported a clinical success rate of 97%. There was a 35% incidence of dissection, and 12% of patients required adjunctive stent implantation.

Eighty-nine patients with long (mean length of 18 ± 6 mm) stenoses were treated with 30- or 40-mm balloons at Duke University Medical Center over a 12-month period. The procedural success rate of 97%, which compared favorably with historical controls treated with standard-length balloons,[21] and the observed rates of abrupt closure (6%) and major dissection (11%), which were similar to those of patients with discrete stenoses treated concomitantly during the same period,[26] support the safety and efficacy of these balloons. However, angiographically determined restenosis occurred in 55% of patients who returned for follow-up angiography.

At Kokura Memorial Hospital, 1310 lesions longer than 20 mm were treated with balloon angioplasty from 1994 to 1997, and 674 of the lesions were treated with long balloons. The procedural success rate of long balloon angioplasty (87%) was significantly higher than the rate observed with the standard balloon (74%). Acute complications and dissection rates (12% versus 18%) were also less common with long balloons. In concordance with the Duke data, however, restenosis rates remained substantial and were not significantly different (52%) from angioplasty using conventional balloons (63%).

Tapered Balloons

As coronary arteries course distally, there is a natural progressive decline in luminal diameter. In the presence of long stenoses, this natural tapering can present difficulties in terms of proper balloon sizing, especially when longer balloons are used. Sizing a long balloon to match the proximal reference diameter may result in overdilation of the distal side of the lesion with increased potential for dissection, whereas sizing the balloon to the distal reference diameter results in inadequate dilation of the proximal portion of the stenosis. Banka and colleagues[27] measured proximal and distal reference diameters in 100 consecutive coronary stenoses before PTCA; 50% of the arteries examined tapered by more than 0.5 mm between the reference segments, and 23% tapered by 1 mm or more (Fig. 21-3).

In an attempt to overcome the dilemma of balloon sizing in such lesions, tapered balloon catheters were developed. Two uncontrolled series have examined the performance of 25-mm-long balloons that gradually tapered by 0.5 mm over their length (e.g., from 3.5 to 3.0 mm). Banka and colleagues[27] reported an overall success rate of 98%, with a 2.1% incidence of significant dissection after tapered balloon angioplasty of 102 stenotic segments. In a multicenter registry of 115 patients with 129 lesions, a tapered balloon was used as the primary mode of therapy or as secondary treatment after standard balloon or

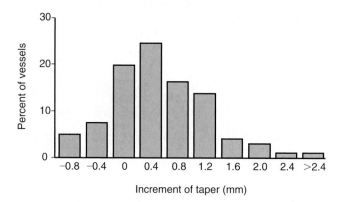

Figure 21-3. Frequency distribution curve for tapering of coronary arteries in 100 stenotic coronary segments. (Modified from Banka VA, Baker HAD, Vemuri DN, et al: Effectiveness of decremental diameter balloon catheters [tapered balloon]. Am J Cardiol 1992; 69:188-193.)

new-device angioplasty. Laird and colleagues[28] reported a procedural success rate of 96%, with severe dissection occurring in 4% and abrupt closure in 4.3%. Although these initial reports of treatment of highly selected patients appear encouraging, randomized trials are necessary to document the superiority of tapered balloon catheters (and perhaps tapered coronary stents) relative to fixed-diameter balloons.

DEBULKING AND ABLATIVE DEVICES

Rotational Atherectomy

From a technical standpoint, rotational atherectomy possesses intrinsic appeal for the treatment of long lesions. This device has the potential to efficiently débride large amounts of plaque material from diffusely diseased vessels. Theoretically, rotational atherectomy may enable the operator to differentially alter the calcific contents of a plaque, converting the target lesion into one with a more homogeneous consistency. After rotational atherectomy, the lesion may be more amenable to balloon angioplasty at lower inflation pressures, potentially resulting in fewer acute complications and better chronic results. Although rotational atherectomy has a favorable impact on procedural success, the data are insufficient to proclaim the superiority of the routine use of rotational atherectomy over that of standard balloon angioplasty in the treatment of long stenoses.

The initial experience with rotational atherectomy by Teirstein and colleagues[29] included a series of 42 patients with high-risk angiographic features (71% having lesions >10 mm long). Lesion length was a predictor of decreased procedural success (92% for discrete lesions versus 70% for lesions >10 mm long) and increased procedural complications. A striking relationship was found between stenosis length and restenosis. Restenosis occurred in 75% of lesions longer than 10 mm, compared with 22% of short lesions. However, these rates might have been

Table 21-3. Procedures and Clinical Events in the ERBAC Study

Outcomes	Balloon Angioplasty (*n* = 222)	Excimer Laser (*n* = 232)	Rotational Atherectomy (*n* = 231)	*P* Value
Procedural success (%)	79.7	77.2	59.2	.019
In-hospital events (%)	3.1	4.3	3.2	.71
Six-month target vessel revascularization (%)	31.9	46.0	42.4	.013
Six-month events* (%)	36.6	47.9	45.9	.057

*Death, myocardial infarction, or repeat revascularization procedure.
ERBAC, Eximer Laser-Rotational Atherectomy-Balloon Angioplasty Comparison.
From Reifart N, Vandormael M, Krajcar M, et al: Randomized comparison of angioplasty of complex coronary lesions at a single center: Excimer Laser,
  Rotational Artherectomy, and Balloon Angioplasty Comparison (ERBAC) study. Circulation 1997;96:91-98.

adversely affected by the failure to employ adjunctive balloon angioplasty after rotational atherectomy in this small series.

As operator experience improved, reports on rotational atherectomy have yielded somewhat more encouraging results. Ellis and colleagues[30] described a procedural success rate of 90% among 316 patients with 400 lesions who underwent rotational atherectomy (followed by adjunctive balloon angioplasty in 82%). Although lesion length was not a determinant of procedural success, lesions longer than 4 mm were associated with an increased risk of major ischemic complications (OR = 3.6), especially non-Q-wave MI (OR = 7.4). In an industry-sponsored registry of 709 patients who underwent rotational atherectomy Warth and colleagues reached similar conclusions.[31] Among patients enrolled in this registry, lesion length was not a predictor of restenosis (37.7% overall); however, lesions longer than 25 mm were excluded. In a subsequent series of 228 patients reported by Leguizamon and colleagues,[32] restenosis was more frequent in long (>20 mm), noncalcified areas (37.7%) than in discrete, calcified lesions (6.3%) treated with rotational atherectomy.

From January 1998 to June 1999, 538 patients with 538 lesions were treated by rotational atherectomy, and quantitative coronary angiography (QCA) parameters were analyzed with a Coronary Artery Surgery Study II (CASS II) system at Kokura Memorial Hospital. Among this cohort, the mean age was 69 years, 41% had diabetes, 38% had previous MI, 62% of the lesions were located in the LAD, 89% were calcified, 11% were ostial lesions, and 7% could not be dilated with a balloon only. Vessel size was 2.35 ± 0.61 mm, and lesion length was 23.4 ± 12.6 mm. Rotational atherectomy was performed with a burr-to-artery ratio of 0.79, and adjunctive balloon angioplasty was used in all treated lesions with a balloon-to-artery ratio of 1.22; stenting was used in 16%. Procedural success, defined as less than 50% diameter stenosis, was 98%, and 96% of procedures were free from major complications. Among patients with procedural complications, angiographically discernible no reflow occurred in 2.7% and perforation in 1.0%. Six-month QCA was available in all cases. Mean minimal lumen diameter (MLD) was 0.93 mm before treatment, 1.82 mm immediately after treatment, and 1.34 mm at 6 months, corresponding to a binary restenosis rate of 52%. Lesions were divided into four subgroups defined by the combination of vessel size and lesion length. A lesion was defined as long if it was more than 15 mm and as focal lesion if it was less than 15 mm long. A vessel was defined as small if it was less than 2.75 mm and large if it was more than 2.75 mm in diameter. Acute and late outcomes were evaluated for each subgroup. The binary restenosis rate significantly increased when long lesions occurred in small vessels (Fig. 21-4).

Although these retrospective analyses have identified lesion length as a significant predictor of periprocedural events and restenosis after rotational atherectomy, these adverse events also increase in frequency when standard balloon angioplasty is used to treat long lesions. One prospective, randomized trial, the Excimer Laser-Rotational Atherectomy-Balloon Angioplasty Comparison (ERBAC), compared the immediate and 6-month results of patients treated with rotational atherectomy versus balloon angioplasty (Table 21-3).[33] In this single-center trial, 685 patients with complex lesion morphology (ACC/AHA type B or C) were randomized to rotational atherectomy, balloon angioplasty, or excimer laser coronary angioplasty (ELCA). Forty-six percent of lesions were longer than 10 mm. Compared with the other two strategies, rotational atherectomy was associated with a significantly higher rate of initial procedural success (89% versus 80% for PTCA versus 77% for ELCA). The incidence of major periprocedural ischemic events did not correlate with any particular device used. Despite the improved procedural success achieved with rotational atherectomy, clinical restenosis, as judged by the need for repeat target lesion

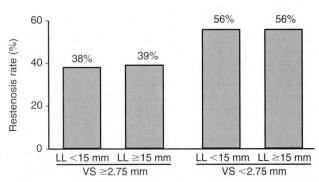

Figure 21-4. Restenosis after rotational atherectomy (*N* = 538): relationship to lesion length and vessel size. LL, lesion length; VS, vessel size.

revascularization at 6 months, was significantly greater among patients assigned to rotational atherectomy (42.4%) and ELCA (46.0%) than among those treated with balloon angioplasty (31.9%).

Despite its failure to favorably influence the rate of restenosis, rotational atherectomy continues to play a role in the initial treatment of heavily calcified lesions that respond poorly to balloon dilation. Meticulous attention to technique (i.e., proper burr sizing, shorter runs, allowance of adequate time between runs for washout of debris, and avoiding drops of greater than 5000 rpm) is particularly important when using rotational atherectomy to treat long lesions.

Excimer Laser Coronary Angioplasty

As with rotational atherectomy, enthusiasm for the use of ELCA in the treatment of long lesions was initially engendered by a series of observational reports during the early experience with the device, only to be lost following the performance of two well-designed randomized, prospective trials. Seven case series, which collectively added more than 5000 patients who underwent ELCA, were published between 1991 and 1994. Overall procedural success was consistently greater than 90%; increasing lesion length did not affect the incidence of adverse effects.[34-40] Restenosis rates after ELCA were 47.6% and 50% in two groups of patients reported by Bittl and colleagues,[35,41] and lesion length did not emerge as a significant risk factor.

Two randomized trials of ELCA versus balloon angioplasty, however, have yielded disappointing results. In the ERBAC trial, the ELCA arm procedural success rate was only 77%, and repeat target lesion revascularization was required significantly more often after ELCA than balloon angioplasty (46.0% versus 31.9%).[33] These results are concordant with those of the prospective Amsterdam-Rotterdam (AMRO) trial, which enrolled only patients with long lesions and stable angina. In this trial, 308 patients with lesions more than 10 mm long were randomized to treatment with ELCA or balloon angioplasty.[42] Adjunctive PTCA was performed in 98% of patients undergoing ELCA. Angiographic success was similar among ELCA- and balloon angioplasty-treated patients (80% versus 79%), as was the incidence of adverse periprocedural events. At the 6-month follow-up, however, late luminal loss as determined by QCA was significantly greater among patients treated with ELCA (0.52 versus 0.34 mm, P = .04), which correlated with a nonsignificant trend toward a greater incidence of angiographic restenosis in the ELCA group (51.6% versus 41.3%, P = .13). Long lesions were associated with a higher late loss index as determined by multivariate analysis.[43] The need for repeat target vessel revascularization was similar among the two groups (21.2% versus 18.5%). However, ELCA was associated with an incremental cost of $4476 per treated lesion compared with balloon angioplasty.[44] In summary, based on the results of the ERBAC and AMRO trials, ELCA appears to provide no immediate or long-term advantages over standard balloon angioplasty in the treatment of long lesions.

Directional Coronary Atherectomy

Popma and colleagues identified lesion length as an independent predictor of smaller residual luminal diameter and abrupt closure after directional coronary atherectomy (DCA).[45-47] Although no randomized trials have directly compared the relative efficacy of DCA and balloon angioplasty for the treatment of long obstructions, several observational investigations suggest the utility of DCA in the treatment of long lesions to be real. Long lesions have been associated with greater residual plaque burden, as assessed by intravascular ultrasound after DCA.[48] For 97 lesions 10 mm or longer treated with DCA, Hinohara and colleagues[49] reported a major complication rate of 6.3%, which increased to 12.5% when only de novo lesions were considered.[49] Selmon and coworkers[50] described an association between increased lesion length and the need for emergency coronary artery bypass grafting after DCA.

Two major randomized studies compared DCA and balloon angioplasty: Coronary Angioplasty vs. Excisional Atherectomy Trial (CAVEAT) and the Canadian Coronary Atherectomy Trial (CCAT) that excluded lesions longer than 12 mm by study protocol. Data from CAVEAT identified increased lesion length as a significant predictor of diminished procedural success.[52-54] Although the acute closure rate of 4.6% during DCA of long lesions did not differ significantly from the rate observed after balloon angioplasty, less than 3% of the lesions treated by DCA were longer than 19 mm at Mooney and colleagues' institution.[51]

Long lesions are associated with a heightened incidence of restenosis when treated with DCA. Hinohara and colleagues[47] reported a restenosis rate of 43% after DCA of long (>10 mm) lesions compared with 26% for lesions less than 10 mm, and Popma and coworkers[55] found lesion length to be a powerful independent predictor of restenosis, with an odds ratio of 4.5.

The efficacy of combining debulking by DCA before stent implantation must be determined. The pivotal randomized Atherectomy before Multilink Stent Improves Lumen Gain and Clinical Outcome Study[56] is currently testing debulking strategies.

CORONARY STENT IMPLANTATION

Coronary stent implantation has become the preferred treatment for discrete de novo stenoses in large-caliber (>3 mm) vessels since 1994. The results of the Stent Restenosis Study (STRESS-1) and the Belgium Netherlands Stent (BENESTENT-1) study laid the foundations for such an approach.[57,58] As reported in these landmark trials, stent implantation was associated with improved procedural success and a reduction in angiographic restenosis relative to balloon angioplasty. In the BENESTENT-2 trial, which used modern techniques of optimal stent deployment in conjunction with heparin-coated stents, angiographically confirmed restenosis occurred in only 16% of patients undergoing stent implantation, compared with 30% in the balloon angioplasty arm.[59] Unfortunately, long lesions (>15 mm) have routinely been excluded from these randomized comparisons of stenting and balloon angioplasty, and uncertainty prevails about whether the benefits of stent placement observed in discrete lesions also apply to long stenoses in which multiple stents or a single long stent is required.

Although many reports have examined the sequelae of stent implantation for long periods, most data exist only in abstract format, are observational in nature, often represent the experience at a single center, and are associated with various angiographic follow-up rates. Despite these limitations, the conclusions of these preliminary studies are remarkably concordant and indicate that the use of long or multiple overlapping stents is associated with restenosis rates that are clearly in excess of those observed when single stents are used to treat discrete stenoses (Table 21-4).[60-69]

The incidence of delivery failure increases when long or multiple stents are used.[64] Implantation of multiple stents was associated with excessive rates of subacute thrombosis compared with rates observed with single stent placement in early reports.[70] However, multiple-stent implantation with complication rates similar to conventional single-stent implantation has been reported with modern stents and deployment techniques and with current antiplatelet agents.[67,71] A procedural success rate of 98%, with a subacute thrombosis rate of only 0.3%, was obtained in 294 consecutive cases of stent implantation in lesions longer than 20 mm at Kokura Memorial Hospital.

The restenosis rate after long- or multiple-stent implantation is higher than with short or single stents. The ten-study (see Table 21-4) composite restenosis rate of 34% is approximately twice that of the 16% rate reported for placement of a single stent in the BENESTENT-2 trial. The need for repeat target vessel revascularization increased with the number of required stents, from 11% for one stent to 23% for two stents and to 29% for three stents, as reported by Aliabadi and colleagues.[72] The presence of diabetes and the need for multiple stents were found to have a marked compounding effect on restenosis by Gaxiola and colleagues.[74] The restenosis rate increased from 10.3% for single-stent implantation to 18% when multiple stents were used in nondiabetic patients and to 37% when multiple stents were required in patients with diabetes.[63]

Kornowski and colleagues[75] were able to implant more than three contiguous stents. Although the acute outcome and the rate of repeat target lesion revascularization were similar to those with one or two short stents, the incidence of MI during follow-up was higher. The investigators[76] also showed that long stents (>25 mm) resulted in similar late clinical outcomes and similar rates of repeat target lesion revascularization, but they produced a higher incidence of major procedural complications compared with short stents (<20 mm).

Figure 21-5 depicts the relative restenosis and repeat target lesion revascularization rates observed at Kokura Memorial Hospital for stented segments meeting the inclusion criteria for the STRESS and BENESTENT trials compared with those observed when stents were used to treat lesions with more complex morphology. Figure 21-6 details the influence of lesion length and vessel size on recurrence rates after coronary stenting. Lesion length and vessel size were significantly related to the binary restenosis rates. The observed difference in binary restenosis of various lesion lengths was primarily related to the difference in relative gain, and that of various vessel sizes was primarily related to the difference in relative loss (Fig. 21-7).

Comparison of Stent Designs for Treatment of Long Lesions

Data are lacking regarding the short- and long-term efficacy of multiple overlapping stents compared with placement of a single long stent, although the latter approach provides potential advantages from the standpoint of procedure duration. The relationship between stent design and restenosis rates also remains incompletely defined.

Table 21-4. Composite Reports of Stent Implantation for Long Lesions

Study	Year	Patients/Lesions	Inclusion	Stent Design	Restenosis Rate (%)
Ellis et al[60]	1992	31/31	Multiple stents	PS	64
Maiello et al[61]	1995	89/108	Lesion length ≥20 mm	PS, GR, Wiktor	35
Yokoi et al[62]	1996	131/136	Lesion length >20 mm	PS, GR, Wallstent	44.1
Gaxiota et al[63]	1997	163/163	Multiple stents	PS	22
Kobayashi and Di Mario[64]	1997	185/234	Long stent (>20 mm)	Multiple	48
Pulsipher et al[65]	1997	73/—	≥3 stents	Unspecified	27.4
Hamasaki et al[66]	1997	—/451	Lesion length ≥15 mm	PS, Cordis	31
Moussa et al[67]	1997	—/258	≥2 stents	PS	29
Williams et al[69]	1999	—/182	Lesion length ≥20 mm	Wallstent	41
Nayeh et al[68]	2001	82/85	Lesion length ≥20 mm	Wallstent, NIR	46, 26

GR, Gianturco-Rubin stent; PS, Palmaz-Schatz.

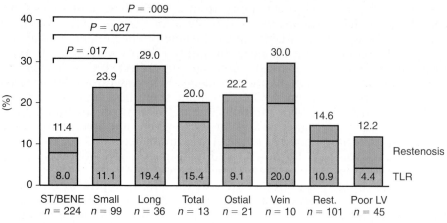

Figure 21-5. Comparison between restenosis and repeat target lesion revascularization rates observed at the Kokura Memorial Hospital.

In an attempt to address these issues, the acute and chronic outcomes for the use of various stents (i.e., Palmaz-Schatz, Gianturco-Roubin, and Wallstent) implanted in 148 lesions longer than 20 mm at Kokura Memorial Hospital between June 1990 and December 1995 were analyzed. Cases involving bypass grafts and acute MI were excluded; only lesions that could be fully covered by the stents were considered.

Because the conventional Palmaz-Schatz stent is available only in short lengths, all Palmaz-Schatz stent cases included in this analysis involved the use of multiple stents. Palmaz-Schatz stents were used to treat 70 lesions, the Gianturco-Roubin stent was used for 38 lesions, and the Wallstent was used for 40 lesions. Although the average lesion length was more than 30 mm for all stents, the Wallstent was typically used for lesions longer than 40 mm. In this nonrandomized comparison, reference diameter was significantly greater in the Wallstent group, and Gianturco-Roubin stents were used most frequently for failed PTCA. The use of multiple stents was undertaken in 100% of the Palmaz-Schatz group, 44% of the Gianturco-Roubin group, and 40% of the Wallstent group.

Procedural success (>50% improvement in vessel narrowing) and freedom from in-hospital complications were independent of stent design. Stent thrombosis occurred in 4.3% of the Palmaz-Schatz group but was not observed in the Gianturco-Roubin or the Wallstent group. QCA demonstrated a significantly larger immediate postprocedural MLD in the Wallstent group, consistent with the larger reference vessel diameter in these patients. Six-month angiography, conducted in 97% of patients, demonstrated no significant differences in MLD among the groups. Binary restenosis rates were high in all groups: 48% for the Palmaz-Schatz stent, 37% for the Gianturco-Roubin stent, and 59% for the Wallstent groups. Repeat target lesion revascularization was required in 31%, 20%, and 40%, respectively. Analysis of MLD demonstrated that late loss indices for the Palmaz-Schatz stent and the Wallstent were uniformly high, even though the initial acute gain was large. In contrast, the smaller acute gain in the Gianturco-Roubin group was compensated for by a more moderate degree of late loss (Table 21-5). In summary, although acute results with all stents in the treatment of lesions longer than 20 mm in length were acceptable, the incidence of late renarrowing was substantial regardless of the type of stent examined. Several newer stent designs are undergoing clinical testing. Follow-up studies are needed to determine whether these new designs afford restenosis benefits over those of the first-generation stents.

Newer-Generation Long Stents

Several newer-generation, flexible, long stents (>20 mm) of various designs have been approved. In an attempt to address the anti-restenotic effect of these stents, the late outcomes were analyzed for various long stents (i.e., GFX, ACS Multi-Link, and Terumo) implanted in 211 lesions longer than 20 mm at Kokura Memorial Hospital between January 1997 and December 2000. GFX long stents (30 mm) were

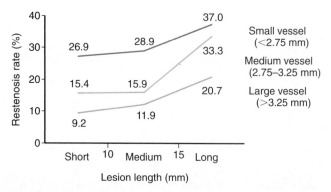

Figure 21-6. Restenosis after coronary stenting ($N = 1048$): relationship to lesion length and vessel size.

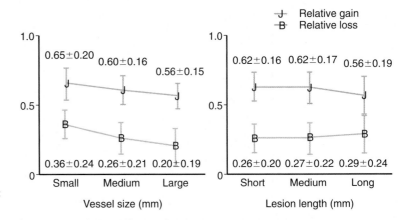

Figure 21-7. Relative gain and relative loss ($N = 1048$): relationship to vessel size and lesion length.

Table 21-5. Kokura Memorial Hospital Series of Long Lesions: Immediate and Follow-up Outcomes

Outcomes	Palmaz-Schatz	Gianturco-Roubin	Wallstent	P Value
Procedural success (%)	100	92	93	NS
Clinical success (%)	91	92	85	NS
MLD before treatment (mm)	0.80 ± 0.45	0.72 ± 0.47	0.89 ± 0.44	NS
MLD after treatment (mm)	2.56 ± 0.40	2.30 ± 0.37	2.82 ± 0.63	.0001
MLD at follow-up (mm)	1.43 ± 0.85	1.61 ± 0.53	1.32 ± 0.60	NS
Restenosis rate (%)	48	37	59	NS

MLD, minimal lumen diameter; NS, not significant.

used to treat 76 lesions, the ACS Multi-Link long stent (35 mm) was used for 42 lesions, and the Terumo long stent was used for 93 lesions (30 mm for 65 lesions and 40 mm for 28 lesions). Binary restenosis rates remained high compared with short lesions in all groups: 40.6% for the GFX long stent, 37.5% for the ACS Multi-Link long stent, and 33.3% for the Terumo long stent.

Full-coverage stenting of long lesions is likely to produce diffuse in-stent restenosis. Treatment of diffuse in-stent restenosis remains exceedingly problematic. Recurrent rates of 42% to 80%[77,78] frequently necessitate multiple additional PTCA procedures and often bypass surgery. The diffuse in-stent restenosis was an independent predictor of long-term outcome after coronary stenting. Angiographically discernible diffuse in-stent restenosis was observed in 44% of multiple Palmaz-Schatz stent, 50% of Gianturco-Roubin stent, 59% of Wallstent, 64% of GFX long stent, 39% of ACS long stent, and 38% of Terumo long stent. Repeat target lesion revascularization was required in 44%, 63%, 70%, 46%, 34%, and 22%, respectively (Fig. 21-8). Newer-generation flexible tube–type long stents such as the ACS Multi-Link long or Terumo long stents are recommended for diffuse disease if stenting is required for their relatively low incidence of diffuse in-stent restenosis.

Full-Coverage Stenting versus Spot Stenting for the Treatment of Long Lesions

Colombo and colleagues[79] described a strategy to treat discrete, high-grade disease within moderately

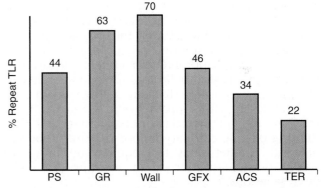

Figure 21-8. Comparison of stent designs to repeat target lesion revascularization (TLR) for in-stent restenosis. ACS, ACS Multi-Link long stent; GFX, GFX long stent; GR, Gianturco-Roubin stent; PS, Palmaz-Schatz stent; TER, Terumo stent.

diseased vessels called *spot stenting,* which consists of short stent implantation only in discrete segments of a long lesion for which intracoronary ultrasound criteria were not satisfied (cross-sectional area >5.5 mm²). With this technique, a 96% procedural success rate and a restenosis rate of 17% were obtained.[79] The long-term outcomes for lesions longer than 20 mm undergoing single (spot stenting) or multiple stent (full-coverage stenting) therapy at Kokura Memorial Hospital were analyzed. Of 95 consecutive patients treated with the Palmaz-Schatz stent, multiple stents were used in 62 and single stents in 33. Although there were no significant differences among the two groups with regard to patient and lesion

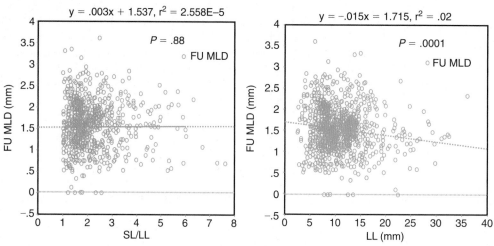

Figure 21-9. Late angiographic outcome: relationship to stent length and lesion length. FU, follow-up; LL, lesion length; MLD, minimal lumen diameter; SL, stent length.

characteristics, the single-stent group contained significantly more emergency cases, and final dilation pressures were also significantly lower. Postprocedural MLD for the multiple- and single-stent groups did not differ significantly, and late angiography also showed no significant differences. Neither restenosis rates (44% and 36%) nor need of repeat target lesion revascularization rates (17% and 17%) were significantly different (Table 21-6).

Reports showed that long stent length was associated with an increased frequency of late in-stent restenosis.[80] If stent length was the only determinant of restenosis, spot stenting might be advantageous and would be an appropriate treatment. However, if lesion length is also a factor, using long stents to completely cover the diseased segment might be preferable. The New Approaches in Coronary Interventions (NACI) investigators have suggested that stenting of long coronary lesions (>20 mm) has significantly higher rates for required repeat target lesion revascularization than stenting of more discrete lesions.[81]

In the series of Kastrati and colleagues,[82] multivariate analysis for both binary restenosis and late lumen loss demonstrated that lesion length was an independent risk factor of restenosis. The risk was further increased by the multiplicity of implanted stents.[82]

To evaluate the impact of stent length on late angiographic outcome with coronary stent implantation, the 6-month follow-up QCA of all consecutive 926 lesions disregarding length treated with a single coronary stent in native arteries between September 1999 and March 2000 at Kokura Memorial Hospital was analyzed. There was no significant relationship between the stent length/lesion length ratio and late angiographic outcome; the late angiographic outcome did correlate significantly with lesion length rather than stent length (Fig. 21-9). It appears that covering the lesion with the least number of nonoverlapping stents may reduce the risks of restenosis.

Overview of the Treatment of Long Stenoses

From the available observational data, stent implantation in long stenoses is associated with restenosis rates twice as high as those seen when single stents are used to treat discrete lesions. This fact may be the cause of the lower rate of event-free survival of patients receiving multiple stents.[73,74] Long lesions are also significantly more prone to restenosis than short lesions after balloon angioplasty, and when restenosis occurs within stents, the prospects for successful long-term control are poorer. Although still incompletely defined, recurrent restenosis rates as high as 80% have been reported after balloon angioplasty for diffuse in-stent restenosis.

Despite these concerns, the use of multiple stents to treat long lesions is a commonplace occurrence in current interventional practice, and several long (>15 mm) stents of various designs have been approved for use in the United States. Randomized clinical trials are needed to document the superiority of this untested approach to traditional long-balloon angioplasty.

EMERGING APPROACHES

Despite the various mechanical approaches discussed earlier, percutaneous revascularization of long lesions

Table 21-6. Kokura Memorial Hospital Series of Long Lesions: Quantitative Coronary Angiographic Data

Outcomes	Full-Coverage Stenting	Spot Stenting	P Value
MLD before treatment (mm)	0.57 ± 0.43	0.63 ± 0.30	NS
MLD after treatment (mm)	2.78 ± 0.63	2.62 ± 0.378	NS
MLD at follow-up (mm)	1.72 ± 1.01	1.76 ± 0.95	NS
Restenosis rate (%)	44	36	NS

MLD, minimal lumen diameter; NS, not significant.

continues to be associated with increased risks of periprocedural complications and late recurrence. It stands to reason that potential benefits afforded by a variety of novel and emerging strategies aimed at increasing the safety and long-term efficacy of angioplasty may be especially evident in the setting of more complex lesion morphologies such as the long lesion.

A series of prospective clinical trials has demonstrated the efficacy of potent antagonists of platelet IIb/IIIa receptor for patients undergoing percutaneous revascularization. Administration of abciximab has significantly reduced occurrence of acute ischemic events in the setting of high- and low-risk PTCA, and benefits have persisted for 3 years of follow-up.[84-87] Results of the IIb/IIIa Platelet Receptor Antagonist 7E3 in Preventing Ischemic Complications (EPIC) trial have been analyzed partially. The benefits of abciximab during angioplasty are not diminished by the presence of adverse lesion characteristics, including lesion length. Because of the propensity for increased late luminal loss, long lesions may be especially responsive to locally delivered ionizing radiation therapy. According to preliminary clinical data, it appears to be especially effective in reducing neointimal hyperplasia after arterial wall injury.[88] Gene-based therapy, currently in the preclinical phase of testing, may ultimately be of benefit in lesion types that are at the highest risk of restenosis.[89] Deploying drug-eluting stents is feasible; the sirolimus-coated stent elicits minimal neointimal proliferation. Additional placebo-controlled trials are necessary to confirm the promising outcomes.[90]

Drug-Eluting Stents

The SIRIUS trial enrolled patients with longer coronary lesions of 15 to 30 mm and allowed long sirolimus-eluting stent (SES) placement (maximum of two overlapping 18-mm SESs). The trial found a 9.2% restenosis rate.[91]

The Rapamycin-Eluting Stent Evaluated At Rotterdam Cardiology Hospital (RESEARCH) registry evaluated the efficacy of SES in 96 consecutive patients (102 lesions) with lesion lengths of more than 36 mm (mean stented length of 61.2 ± 21.4 mm; range, 41 to 134 mm). The binary restenosis rate was 11.9% and in-stent late loss was 0.13 ± 0.47 mm. At long-term follow-up (mean, 320 days), there were two deaths (2.1%), and the overall incidence of major cardiac events was 8.3%.[92]

Clinical trials using a paclitaxel-eluting stent (PES), such as the TAXUS V[93] and TAXUS VI[94] studies, evaluated the efficacy of PES for complex lesions. Both studies included more complex and longer lesion subsets compared with the previous TAXUS trials. In the TAXUS V study using a slow-release PES system, the average lengths of the lesion and total stented segment were 17.3 mm and 28.7 mm, respectively, in the Taxus stent group; 33% of lesions required multiple stents. In this study, the Taxus stent reduced the 9-month target lesion revascularization rate from 15.7% to 8.6% (P < .001) and target vessel revascularization from 17.3% to 12.1% (P = .02) compared with the control group. The angiographic restenosis rate was also lower in the Taxus group than in the control group (18.9% versus 33.9%, P < .001). However, incidence of cardiac death and stent thrombosis did not differ between the two groups.

Tsagalou and colleagues[95] reported the results of multiple DES implantations for 66 patients with diffuse LAD stenosis. In this study, 39 patients were treated with SES (average length of 84 ± 22 mm), and 27 patients were treated with PES (average length of 74 ± 14 mm). The number of stents implanted per patient was 2.8 ± 0.7, and the mean total stent length for the LAD treatment was 80 ± 20 mm. Procedural success was achieved in 95% of cases. Eleven (16.6%) patients had in-hospital non-Q-wave MIs (five SES and six PES), and one patient developed intraprocedural stent thrombosis. All patients had clinical follow-up, and 52 patients (79%) had angiographic follow-up at 6 months. The major adverse cardiac events rate was 15% (7.5% for SES and 7.5% for PES). No patient died, one patient had non-Q-wave MI, and 10 patients (15%) underwent target vessel revascularization.[95]

Aoki and associates[96] reported the results of multiple DES implantations for 122 consecutive patients with de novo coronary lesions. In this study, 81 patients were treated with SES (average length of 77 mm), and 42 patients were treated with PES (average length of 84 mm). The number of stents implanted per patient was 3.3 ± 1.1, and the mean total stent length was 79 mm. Procedural success was achieved in 96% of cases. Seven (5.8%) patients had MIs within 30 days, and one patient developed subacute stent thrombosis. All patients had 1-year clinical follow-up. The major adverse cardiac events rate was 18% (18.5% for SES and 17.1% for PES). Five patients (4.1%) died, 12 patients (10%) had myocardial infarction, and 9 patients (7.5%) underwent target vessel revascularization.[96]

The Multicenter Prospective Nonrandomized Registry Study for Drug-Eluting Stents in Very Long Coronary Lesions (Cypher versus Taxus) (Long-DES Trial) was a nonrandomized registry comparing angiographic and clinical outcomes for 637 patients undergoing stent placement with a bare metal stent (BMS) (n = 177), SES (n = 294), or PES (n = 166) in long coronary lesions. Baseline characteristics were similar in the three arms, including the number of high-risk and diabetic patients enrolled. Average stent length was similar (42.8 mm for SES versus 43.1 mm for PES; P = NS). DES patients received more stents with longer lengths compared with BMS patients. Patients in the SES group had smaller reference vessel diameters (2.80 mm for SES versus 2.9 mm for PES). At the 6-month angiographic follow-up evaluation, completed for approximately 80% of all patients, there was 65% less in-stent late loss in the SES patients compared with the PES patients (0.27 versus 0.78 mm, P < .0001) and 65% less in-segment restenosis in SES patients compared with the PES patients (7.4% versus 21.3%, P < .001). The rate of

Table 21-7. Angiographic and Clinical Outcomes for Implantation of Three Types of Stents

Outcomes	BMS	PES	SES	P Value
Lesions	201	194	223	
Lesion length (mm)	32.0 ± 12.3	36.3 ± 14.5	36.0 ± 14.9	.002
MLD before treatment (mm)	0.78 ± 0.54	0.77 ± 0.49	0.76 ± 0.48	NS
MLD after treatment (mm)	2.60 ± 0.50	2.50 ± 0.45	2.35 ± 0.43	<.001
MLD at follow-up (mm)	1.56 ± 0.69	1.90 ± 0.71	2.21 ± 0.60	<.001
Acute gain (mm)	2.12 ± 0.67	2.01 ± 0.57	1.88 ± 0.59	<.001
Late loss (mm)	1.02 ± 0.67	0.56 ± 0.62	0.14 ± 0.53	<.001
Restenosis rate (%)	42.2	21.3	9.3	<.001

BMS, bare metal stent; NS, not significant; MLD, minimal lesion diameter; PES, paclitaxel-elating stent; SES, serolimus-eluting stent.

target lesion revascularization was significantly lower with DES compared with BMS (2.7% for SES, 5.4% for PES, and 18.6% for BMS; $P < .001$), but the difference between SES and PES was not statistically significant ($P = 0.14$) (Table 21-7).[97]

Recent analyses have suggested that implantation of DES is associated with a higher rate of very late stent thrombosis compared with BMS implantation.[98-100] This complication is evident with SES and PES, but the precise magnitude of this risk and whether this applies to all patients or only to a subset of those who have received DES is incompletely characterized. The presumed mechanism of late susceptibility to stent thrombosis is delayed or incomplete re-endothelialization and possibly an inflammatory response to the stent polymer, although other factors such as fractures and stent malapposition may contribute.[101] The decision to implant a DES rather than use an alternative revascularization strategy (including BMS or surgical revascularization) must be made on an individual patient basis after consideration of the relative risks and benefits of each therapy.

Therapeutic Angiogenesis

Promoting neovascularization by the administration of specific growth factors or genetic material encoding the specific endothelial cell mitogen of soluble basic fibroblast growth factor (i.e., vascular endothelial growth factor [VEGF]) represents another intriguing potential therapeutic approach for patients with diffuse coronary disease.[102] Animal studies have demonstrated angiographically and histologically the feasibility of forming collateral channels in ischemic vascular territories and improved blood flow to ischemic limbs by local or systemic application of such DNA encoding material.[103-105] Isner and colleagues administered naked plasmid DNA to the diseased territory of patients suffering from severe distal lower extremity peripheral vascular disease and rest pain by hydrogel-coated balloons inflated upstream to the disease. Rapid development of collateral vessels associated with augmented blood flow to the limb was observed by intra-arterial Doppler imaging.[106] Similar results have been achieved in animal models with systemic (intramuscular or intra-arterial) administration of DNA encoding VEGF, which possesses tropism for ischemic tissue.[105]

Although therapeutic angiogenesis holds great promise in the treatment of severe, diffuse coronary disease, several issues need to be addressed as these techniques enter phase I clinical testing:

1. Determination of the optimal growth factor or combination thereof to promote neovascularization
2. Development (if necessary) of effective transfecting DNA vectors
3. Determination of the relative efficacy of systemic delivery compared with the more invasive and technically cumbersome local delivery techniques
4. Determination of optimal dosing and the need for and timing of repeat applications
5. Development of methods to ensure delivery of these potent agents only to appropriate target areas
6. Determination of the potential for short- and long-term adverse sequelae related to the administration of these mitogenic, pro-proliferative agents

SUMMARY

In light of the paucity of randomized trial data demonstrating the superiority of any particular device in the treatment of small-vessel and diffuse disease, treatment needs to be individualized. The treatment algorithm used in approaching long lesions at Kokura Memorial Hospital, based on the presence or absence of various ancillary morphologic features, is presented in Figure 21-10. No technique has proven superiority to prevent restenosis over that of standard angioplasty using long balloon catheters. In the ERBAC trial, rotational atherectomy was associated with a modest but statistically significant improvement in acute procedural success compared with balloon angioplasty; it may be a rational approach to long, calcified stenoses by rendering them responsive to balloon dilation. The role of coronary stent placement in the treatment of nondiscrete stenoses has not been defined. Given the substantial incidence of restenosis despite stent placement in the setting of long lesions, until the problem of in-stent restenosis can be ameliorated, the routine use of stents should be undertaken with extreme caution. Perhaps spot stenting the areas failing to respond adequately

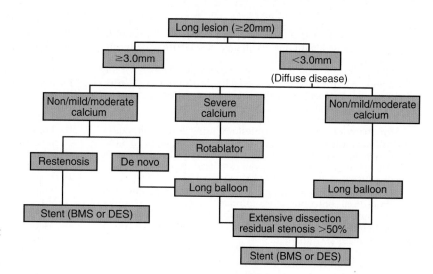

Figure 21-10. Potential approach to the treatment of long lesions and diffuse disease. BMS, bare metal stent; DES, drug-eluting stent.

within a long diseased segment or developing large dissection flaps after balloon dilation may limit the problem of in-stent restenosis. Despite the advent of new devices during the past decade, long lesions continue to present a difficult challenge. The ultimate solution may depend on the development of novel adjunct strategies such as radiation, gene-based therapy, and DESs, which may substantially reduce the potential for neointimal proliferation and thereby stenosis recurrence.

REFERENCES

1. Marcus M, Harrison D, White C, et al: Assessing the physiologic significance of coronary obstructions in patients: Importance of diffuse undetected atherosclerosis. Prog Cardiovasc Dis 1988;31:39-56.
2. Berne R, Levy M: Cardiovascular Physiology. St. Louis, CV Mosby, 1986, pp 109-115.
3. Feldman R, Nichols W, Pepine C, Conti C: Hemodynamic significance of the length of a coronary arterial narrowing. Am J Cardiol 1978;41:865-871.
4. Meier B, Gruentzig AR, Hollman J, et al: Does length or eccentricity of coronary stenoses influence the outcome of transluminal dilatation? Circulation 1983;67:497-499.
5. Ellis SG, Roubin GS, King SBD, et al: Angiographic and clinical predictors of acute closure after native vessel coronary angioplasty. Circulation 1988;77:372-379.
6. Detre KM, Holmes DR Jr, Holubkov R, et al: Incidence and consequences of periprocedural occlusion. The 1985-1986 National Heart, Lung, and Blood Institute Percutaneous Transluminal Coronary Angioplasty Registry. Circulation 1990;82:739-750.
7. Ghazzal Z, Weintraub W, Ba'albaki H, et al: PTCA of lesions longer than 20 mm: Initial outcome and restenosis. Circulation 1990;82:III-509.
8. Ryan TJ, Faxon DP, Gunnar RM, et al: Guidelines for percutaneous transluminal coronary angioplasty. A report of the American College of Cardiology/American Heart Association Task Force on Assessment of Diagnostic and Therapeutic Cardiovascular Procedures (Subcommittee on Percutaneous Transluminal Coronary Angioplasty). Circulation 1988;78:486-502.
9. Ellis SG, Vandormael MG, Cowley MJ, et al: Coronary morphologic and clinical determinants of procedural outcome with angioplasty for multivessel coronary disease. Implications for patient selection. Multivessel Angioplasty Prognosis Study Group. Circulation 1990;82:1193-1202.
10. Savage MP, Goldberg S, Hirshfeld JW, et al: Clinical and angiographic determinants of primary coronary angioplasty success. M-HEART investigators. J Am Coll Cardiol 1991;17:22-28.
11. Hermans WR, Foley DP, Rensing BJ, et al: Usefulness of quantitative and qualitative angiographic lesion morphology, and clinical characteristics in predicting major adverse cardiac events during and after native coronary balloon angioplasty. CARPORT and MERCATOR study groups. Am J Cardiol 1993;72:14-20.
12. Myler RK, Shaw RE, Stertzer SH, et al: Lesion morphology and coronary angioplasty: Current experience and analysis. J Am Coll Cardiol 1992;19:1641-1652.
13. Tan K, Sulke N, Taub N, Sowton E: Clinical and lesion morphologic determinants of coronary angioplasty success and complications: Current experience. J Am Coll Cardiol 1995;25:855-865.
14. Sharma SK, Israel DH, Kamean JL, et al: Clinical, angiographic, and procedural determinants of major and minor coronary dissection during angioplasty. Am Heart J 1993;126:39-47.
15. Reisman M, Cohen B, Warth D, et al: Outcome of long lesions treated with high speed rotational atherectomy. J Am Coll Cardiol 1993;21(Suppl A):443A.
16. Dietz WA, Tobis JM, Isner JM: Failure of angiography to accurately depict the extent of coronary artery narrowing in three fatal cases of percutaneous transluminal coronary angioplasty. J Am Coll Cardiol 1992;19:1261-1270.
17. Hirshfeld JW Jr, Schwartz JS, Jugo R, et al: Restenosis after coronary angioplasty: A multivariate statistical model to relate lesion and procedure variables to restenosis. The M-HEART investigators. J Am Coll Cardiol 1991;18:647-656.
18. Rensing BJ, Hermans WR, Vos J, et al: Luminal narrowing after percutaneous transluminal coronary angioplasty. A study of clinical, procedural, and lesional factors related to long-term angiographic outcome. Coronary Artery Restenosis Prevention on Repeated Thromboxane Antagonism (CARPORT) study group. Circulation 1993;88:975-985.
19. Brymer JF, Khaja F, Kraft PL: Angioplasty of long or tandem coronary artery lesions using a new longer balloon dilatation catheter: A comparative study. Cathet Cardiovasc Diagn 1991;23:84-88.
20. Cannon AD, Roubin GS, Hearn JA, et al: Acute angiographic and clinical results of long balloon percutaneous transluminal coronary angioplasty and adjuvant stenting for long narrowings. Am J Cardiol 1994;73:635-641.
21. Tenaglia AN, Zidar JP, Jackman JD Jr, et al: Treatment of long coronary artery narrowings with long angioplasty balloon catheters. Am J Cardiol 1993;71:1274-1277.
22. Harris WO, Holmes DR Jr: Treatment of diffuse coronary artery and vein graft disease with a 60-mm-long balloon: Early clinical experience. Mayo Clin Proc 1995;70:1061-1067.
23. Cates C, Knopf W, Lembo N, et al: The 80 mm balloon: The first 95 vessel cumulative experience [abstract]. J Am Coll Cardiol 1994;23(Suppl A):58A.

24. Shapiro J, Eigler N, Litvack F: The long lesion. *In* Ellis S, Holmes D Jr (eds): Strategic Approaches in Coronary Intervention. Baltimore, Williams & Wilkins, 1996, pp 260-263.

25. Ellis S: Current approaches to percutaneous treatment of the angulated coronary stenosis. *In* Ellis S, Holmes D Jr (eds): Strategic Approaches in Coronary Intervention. Baltimore, Williams & Wilkins, 1996, pp 281-284.

26. Zidar J, Tenaglia A, Jackman J Jr, et al: Improved acute results for PTCA of long coronary lesions using long angioplasty balloon catheters. J Am Coll Cardiol 1992;19(Suppl A):34A.

27. Banka VS, Baker HAD, Vemuri DN, et al: Effectiveness of decremental diameter balloon catheters (tapered balloon). Am J Cardiol 1992;69:188-193.

28. Laird JR, Popma JJ, Knopf WD, et al: Angiographic and procedural outcome after coronary angioplasty in high-risk subsets using a decremental diameter (tapered) balloon catheter. Tapered Balloon Registry Investigators. Am J Cardiol 1996;77:561-568.

29. Teirstein PS, Warth DC, Haq N, et al: High-speed rotational coronary atherectomy for patients with diffuse coronary artery disease. J Am Coll Cardiol 1991;18:1694-1701.

30. Ellis SG, Popma JJ, Buchbinder M, et al: Relation of clinical presentation, stenosis morphology, and operator technique to the procedural results of rotational atherectomy and rotational atherectomy-facilitated angioplasty. Circulation 1994;89:882-892.

31. Warth D, Leon M, O'Neill W, et al: Rotational Atherectomy Multicenter Registry: Acute results, complications, and 6-month angiographic follow-up in 709 patients. J Am Coll Cardiol 1994;24:641-648.

32. Leguizamon J, Chambre D, Torresani E, et al: High-speed coronary rotational atherectomy. Are angiographic factors predictive of failure, major complications, or restenosis? A multivariate analysis [abstract]. J Am Coll Cardiol 1995; 25(Suppl A):95A.

33. Reifart N, Vandormael M, Krajcar M, et al: Randomized comparison of angioplasty of complex coronary lesions at a single center: Excimer Laser, Rotational Atherectomy, and Balloon Comparison (ERBAC) study. Circulation 1997;96:91-98.

34. Cook SL, Eigler NL, Shefer A, et al: Percutaneous excimer laser coronary angioplasty of lesions not ideal for balloon angioplasty. Circulation 1991;84:632-643.

35. Bittl JA, Sanborn TA: Excimer laser-facilitated coronary angioplasty: Relative risk analysis of acute and follow-up results in 200 patients. Circulation 1992;86:71-80.

36. Hartzler G, Litvack F, Marlolis J, et al: Adjunctive excimer laser coronary angioplasty improves primary PTCA results for lesions >20 mm length. J Am Coll Cardiol 1992;19:48A.

37. Litvack F, Eigler N, Margolis J, et al: Percutaneous excimer laser coronary angioplasty: Results in the first consecutive 3,000 patients. The ELCA investigators. J Am Coll Cardiol 1994;23:323-329.

38. Holmes D, Bresnahan J, Bell M, Litvack FL: Lesion morphology and outcome after laser angioplasty, a prospective evaluation: Excimer Laser Coronary Angioplasty Registry. J Am Coll Cardiol 1993;21(Suppl A):288A.

39. Ghazzal ZM, Hearn JA, Litvack F, et al: Morphological predictors of acute complications after percutaneous excimer laser coronary angioplasty. Results of a comprehensive angiographic analysis: Importance of the eccentricity index. Circulation 1992;86:820-827.

40. Baumbach A, Bittl JA, Fleck E, et al: Acute complications of excimer laser coronary angioplasty: A detailed analysis of multicenter results. Coinvestigators of the U.S. and European Percutaneous Excimer Laser Coronary Angioplasty (PELCA) registries. J Am Coll Cardiol 1994;23:1305-1313.

41. Bittl JA, Kuntz RE, Estella P, et al: Analysis of late lumen narrowing after excimer laser-facilitated coronary angioplasty. J Am Coll Cardiol 1994;23:1314-1320.

42. Appelman YE, Piek JJ, Strikwerda S, et al: Randomized trial of excimer laser angioplasty versus balloon angioplasty for treatment of obstructive coronary artery disease. Lancet 1996;347:79-84.

43. Foley D, Appelman Y, Piek J: Comparison of angiographic restenosis propensity of excimer laser coronary angioplasty and balloon angioplasty in the Amsterdam Rotterdam (AMRO) trial. Circulation 1995;92(Suppl I):I-477.

44. Appelman Y, Birnie E, Piek J, et al: Excimer laser angioplasty versus balloon angioplasty in longer coronary lesions: A cost-effectiveness analysis. Circulation 1995;92(Suppl I):I-512.

45. Popma JJ, De Cesare NB, Ellis SG, et al: Clinical, angiographic and procedural correlates of quantitative coronary dimensions after directional coronary atherectomy. J Am Coll Cardiol 1991;18:1183-1189.

46. Popma JJ, Topol EJ, Hinohara T, et al: Abrupt vessel closure after directional coronary atherectomy. The U.S. Directional Atherectomy Investigator Group. J Am Coll Cardiol 1992;19:1372-1379.

47. Popma JJ, De Cesare NB, Pinkerton CA, et al: Quantitative analysis of factors influencing late lumen loss and restenosis after directional coronary atherectomy. Am J Cardiol 1993;71:552-557.

48. Matar F, Mintz G, Kent K, et al: Predictors of intravascular ultrasound endpoints after directional coronary atherectomy in 170 patients. J Am Coll Cardiol 1994;23(Suppl A):302A.

49. Hinohara T, Rowe MH, Robertson GC, et al: Effect of lesion characteristics on outcome of directional coronary atherectomy. J Am Coll Cardiol 1991;17:1112-1120.

50. Selmon M, Hinohara T, Vetter J, et al: Experience of directional coronary atherectomy: 848 procedures over 4 years. Circulation 1991;84:80A.

51. Mooney MR, Mooney JF, Madison JD, et al: Directional atherectomy for long lesions: Improved results. Cathet Cardiovasc Diagn Suppl 1993;1:26-30.

52. Topol E, Leya F, Pinkerton C, et al: A comparison of directional atherectomy with coronary angioplasty in patients with coronary artery disease: The CAVEAT study group. N Engl J Med 1993;329:221-227.

53. Adelman A, Cohen E, Kimball B, et al: A comparison of directional atherectomy with balloon angioplasty for lesions of the left anterior descending coronary artery. N Engl J Med 1993;329:228-233.

54. Lincoff A, Ellis S, Leya F, et al: Are clinical and angiographic correlates of success the same during coronary atherectomy and balloon angioplasty? The CAVEAT experience. Circulation 1993;88(Suppl I):I-601.

55. Hinohara T, Robertson GC, Selmon MR, et al: Restenosis after directional coronary atherectomy. J Am Coll Cardiol 1992;20:623-632.

56. Simonton CA: Directional coronary atherectomy: optimal atherectomy trials and new combined strategies with coronary stents. Semin Interv Cardiol 2000;5:193-198.

57. Fischman D, Leon M, Baim D, et al: A randomized comparison of coronary-stent placement and balloon angioplasty in the treatment of coronary artery disease. N Engl J Med 1994;331:496-501.

58. Serruys P, De Jaegere P, Kiemeneij F, et al: A comparison of balloon-expandable-stent implantation with balloon angioplasty in patients with coronary artery disease. N Engl J Med 1994;331:489-495.

59. Serruys P, Emanuelsson H, van der Giessen W, et al: Heparin-coated Palmaz Schatz stents in human coronary arteries: Early outcome of the BENESTENT-II pilot study. Circulation 1996;93:412-422.

60. Ellis SG, Savage M, Fischman D, et al: Restenosis after placement of Palmaz-Schatz stents in native coronary arteries. Initial results of a multicenter experience. Circulation 1992;86:1836-1844.

61. Maiello L, Hall P, Nakamura S, et al: Results of stent implantation for diffuse coronary disease assisted by intravascular ultrasound. J Am Coll Cardiol 1995;259(Suppl A):156A.

62. Yokoi H, Nobuyoshi M, Nosaka H, et al: Coronary stenting for long lesions (lesion length >20 mm) in native coronary arteries: Comparison of three different types of stent. Circulation 1996;94(Suppl I):I-685.

63. Gaxiola E, Vlietstra R, Brenner A, et al: Diabetes and multiple stents independently double the risk of short-term revascularization. Circulation 1997;96(Suppl):I-649.

64. Kobayashi Y, Di Mario C: Immediate and follow-up results following single long coronary stent implantation. Circulation 1997;96(Suppl):I-472.

65. Pulsipher M, Baker W, Sawchak S, et al: Outcomes in patients treated with multiple stents. Circulation 1996;94(Suppl): I-332.
66. Hamasaki N, Nosaka H, Kimura T, et al: Influence of lesion length on late angiographic outcome and restenotic process after successful stent implantation. J Am Coll Cardiol 1997; 299(Suppl A):239A.
67. Moussa I, Di Mario C, Moses J, et al: Single versus multiple Palmaz-Schatz stent implantation: Immediate and follow-up results. J Am Coll Cardiol 1997;29(Suppl A):276A.
68. Nageh T, De Belder AJ, Thomas MR, et al: A randomised trial of endoluminal reconstruction comparing the NIR stent and the Wallstent in angioplasty of long segment coronary disease: Results of the RENEWAL Study. Am Heart J 141:971-976, 2001.
69. Williams IL, Thomas MR, Robinson NM, et al: Angiographic and clinical restenosis following the use of long coronary Walstents. Catheter Cardiovasc Diagn 48:287-293, 1999.
70. Doucet S, Fajadet J, Caillard J, et al: Predictors of thrombotic occlusion following coronary Palmaz-Schatz stent implantation. Circulation 1992;86(Suppl I):I-113.
71. Chevalier B, Glatt B, Royer T, Guyon P: Comparative results of short versus long stenting. J Am Coll Cardiol 1997;29(Suppl A):415A.
72. Aliabadi D, Bowers T, Tilli F, et al: Multiple stents increase target vessel revascularization rates. J Am Coll Cardiol 1997;29(Suppl A):276A.
73. Eccleston D, Belli G, Penn I, Ellis S: Are multiple stents associated with multiplicative risk in the optimal stent era? Circulation 1996;94(Suppl I):I-454.
74. Gaxiola E, Vlietstra R, Browne K, et al: Six-month follow-up of patients with multiple stents in a single coronary artery. J Am Coll Cardiol 1997;29(Suppl A):276A.
75. Kornowski R, Mehran R, Hong MK, et al: Procedural results an late clinical outcomes after placement of three or more stents in single coronary lesions. Circulation 2001;103: 192-195.
76. Kornowski R, Bhargava B, Fuchs S, et al: Procedural results and late clinical outcomes after percutaneous interventions using long (> or = 25 mm) versus short (<20 mm) stents. J Am Coll Cardiol 2000;35:612-618.
77. Kimura T, Tamura T, Yokoi H, et al: Long-term clinical and angiographic follow-up after placement of Palmaz-Schatz coronary stent: A single-center experience. J Interv Cardiol 1994;7:129-139.
78. Bauters C, Banos JL, Van Belle E, et al: Six-month angiographic outcome after successful repeat percutaneous intervention for in-stent restenosis. Circulation 1998;97: 318-321.
79. De Gregorio J, Colombo A, et al: Treatment strategies for long and calcified lesions. J Interv Cardiol 1998;11:557-564.
80. Kobayashi Y, De Gregorio J, Kobayashi N, et al: Stented segment length as an independent predictor of restenosis. J Am Coll Cardiol 1999;34:651-659.
81. Saucedo JF, Kennard ED, Popma JJ, et al: Importance of Lesion Length on New Device Angioplasty of Native Coronary Arteries. Catheter Cardiovasc Interv 2000;50:19-25.
82. Kastrati A, Elezi S, Dirschinger J, et al: Influence of lesion length on restenosis after coronary stent placement. J Am Coll Cardiol 1999;83:1617-1622.
83. Narins C, Holmes D Jr, Topol E: The balloon is back: A call for provisional stenting. Circulation 1998;97:1298-1305.
84. The EPIC Investigators: Use of a monoclonal antibody directed against the platelet glycoprotein IIb/IIIa receptor in high-risk coronary angioplasty. N Engl J Med 1994;330: 956-961.
85. The EPILOG Investigators: Platelet glycoprotein IIb/IIIa receptor inhibition with abciximab with lower heparin dosages during percutaneous coronary revascularization. N Engl J Med 1997;336:1689-1696.
86. Brener S, Barr L, Burchenal J, et al: A randomized, placebo-controlled trial of abciximab with primary angioplasty for acute MI. The RAPPORT trial. Circulation 1997;96(Suppl I): I-473.
87. Topol EJ, Ferguson JJ, Weisman HF, et al: Long-term protection from myocardial ischemic events in a randomized trial of brief integrin beta$_3$ blockade with percutaneous coronary intervention. EPIC Investigator Group. Evaluation of Platelet IIb/IIIa Inhibition for Prevention of Ischemic Complications. JAMA 1997;278:479-484.
88. Teirstein P, Massullo V, Jani S, et al: Catheter-based radiotherapy to inhibit restenosis after coronary stenting. N Engl J Med 1997;336:1697-1703.
89. Bennett M, Schwartz S: Antisense therapy for angioplasty restenosis: Some critical considerations. Circulation 1995;92:1981-1993.
90. Sousa JE, Costa MA, Abizaid A, et al: Lack of neointimal proliferation after implantation of sirolimus-coated stents in human coronary arteries. Circulation 2001;103:192-195.
91. Moses JW, Leon MB, Popma JJ, et al: Sirolimus-eluting stents versus standard stents in patients with coronary artery disease. N Engl J Med 2003;349:1315-1323.
92. Degertekin M, Arampatzis CA, Lemons PA, et al: Very long sirolimus-eluting stent implantation for de novo coronary lesions. Am J Cardiol 2005;93:826-829.
93. Stone GW, Ellis SG, Cannon L, et al: Comparison of a polymer-based paclitaxel-eluting stent with a bare metal stent in patients with complex coronary artery disease: A randomized controlled trial. JAMA 2005;294:1215-1223.
94. Dawkins KD, Grube E, Guagliumi G, et al: Clinical efficacy of polymer-based paclitaxel-eluting stents in the treatment of complex, long coronary artery lesions from a multicenter, randomized trial: Support for the use of drug-eluting stents in contemporary clinical practice. Circulation 112:3306-3313, 2005
95. Tsagalou E, Chieffo A, Iakovou I, et al: Multiple overlapping drug-eluting stents to treat diffuse disease of the left anterior decending coronary artery. J Am Coll Cardiol 2005; 45:1570-1573.
96. Aoki J, Ong AT, Rodriguez-Granillo GA, et al: Full metal jacket (stented length >64 mm) using drug-eluting stent for de novo coronary artery lesions. Am Heart J 2005;150: 994-994.
97. Kim YH, Park SW, Lee SW, et al: Comparison of sirolimus-eluting stent, paclitaxel-eluting stent, and bare metal stent in the treatment of long coronary lesions. Catheter Cardiovasc Interv 2006;67:181-187.
98. Pfisterer M, Brunner-La Rocca HP, Buser PT, et al: Late clinical events after clopidogrel discontinuation may limit the benefit of drug-eluting stents. J Am Coll Cardiol 2006;48: 2584-2591.
99. Nordmann AJ, Briel M, Bucher HC: Mortality in randomized controlled clinical trials comparing drug-eluting vs. bare metal stents in coronary artery disease: A meta-analysis. Eur Heart J 2006;27:2784-2814.
100. Bavry AA, Kumbhant DJ, Helton TJ, et al: Late thrombosis of drug-eluting stents: A meta-analysis of randomized clinical trials. Am J Med 2006;119:1056-1061.
101. Joner M, Finn AV, Farb A, et al: Pathology of drug-eluting stents in humans: Delayed healing and late thrombotic risk. J Am Coll Cardiol 2006; 48:193-202.
102. Isner J: Angiogenesis for revascularization of ischemic tissues. Eur Heart J 1997;18:1-2.
103. Takeshita S, Zheng L, Brogi E, et al: Therapeutic angiogenesis: A single intraarterial bolus of vascular endothelial growth factor augments revascularization in a rabbit ischemic hind limb model. J Clin Invest 1994;93:662-670.
104. Shou M, Thirumurti V, Rajanayagam S, et al: Effect of basic fibroblast growth factor on myocardial angiogenesis in dogs with mature collateral vessels. J Am Coll Cardiol 1997;29: 1102-1106.
105. Tsurumi Y, Takeshita S, Chen D, et al: Direct intramuscular gene transfer of naked DNA encoding vascular endothelial growth factor augments collateral development and tissue perfusion. Circulation 1996;94:3281-3290.
106. Isner J, Pieczek A, Schainfeld R, et al: Clinical evidence of angiogenesis after arterial gene transfer of phVEGF165 in a patient with ischemic limb. Lancet 1996;248:370-374.

22 Percutaneous Intervention for Left Main Coronary Artery Stenosis

Seung-Jung Park and Young-Hak Kim

KEY POINTS

- Coronary stents are widely used to overcome the limitations of balloon angioplasty and may be useful for treating unprotected left main coronary artery (LMCA) stenosis.
- Stenting in distal LMCA bifurcation disease is technically more complex than in ostial or shaft lesions.
- With drug-eluting stents, simple (i.e., extending the stent across the circumflex artery) or complex stenting techniques (i.e., multiple stent placement, such as kissing stenting, T stenting, or crush technique) can be used for the treatment of bifurcation LMCA lesions according to vascular size and lesion morphology.
- In bifurcation LMCA lesions with a normal circumflex artery, simple stenting strategy using a crossover technique may be a more effective strategy for reducing the restenosis rate than complex stenting techniques.
- Intravascular ultrasound is a useful adjunct in unprotected LMCA intervention to assess actual vessel size, disease extent of the main vessel and the side branch, and final stent optimization.

- Routine use of debulking atherectomy is not recommended in drug-eluting stent implantation for unprotected LMCA stenosis. However, its selective role is being studied.
- Although an intra-aortic balloon pump is not routinely recommended during the procedure, it should be considered for prevention of hemodynamic collapse in patients with severely depressed left ventricular function.
- When patients with LMCA stenosis had well-preserved left ventricular systolic function and were good candidates for coronary bypass graft surgery, the procedural success rates and in-hospital outcomes after the use of bare metal stents were favorable.
- Use of drug-eluting stents significantly decreased in-stent restenosis when stenting was done for unprotected LMCA stenosis compared with the use of bare metal stents.
- Ongoing randomized studies comparing the safety and efficacy of drug-eluting stents with bypass surgery will determine whether stenting can be an alternative to bypass surgery in patients with unprotected LMCA stenosis.

Left main coronary artery (LMCA) stenosis has several causes (Table 22-1). LMCA stenosis is considered an attractive target for balloon angioplasty because of the vessel's large caliber, the lack of tortuosity, and the short lesion length. Histologically, the LMCA has the most elastic tissue of the coronary vessels, accounting for the poor response of the LMCA to simple balloon angioplasty.[1-3] However, coronary stents have been shown to reduce the immediate need for coronary artery bypass surgery (CABG) for abrupt vessel closure and the likelihood of restenosis after balloon angioplasty. Newer devices are widely used to overcome the limitations of balloon angioplasty and may also be useful for treating unprotected LMCA stenosis in some patients. Stenting of

unprotected LMCA stenosis is therefore considered a therapeutic option in selected patients.[4-23]

TECHNICAL CONSIDERATIONS IN UNPROTECTED LEFT MAIN CORONARY ARTERY STENTING

Ostial Lesions

The ostial LMCA lesion is dilated and stented with the guide tip positioned in the aortic sinus. The proximal end of the stent protrudes slightly to the left (1 to 2 mm) outside the ostium and is expanded against the aortic wall as in stenting of any aorto-ostial lesion (Fig. 22-1). Predilatation before stenting is necessary

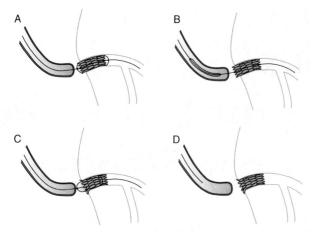

Figure 22-1. Appropriate stenting technique in ostial left main coronary artery (LMCA) intervention. **A,** Stenting at the ostial LMCA with slight protrusion of the stent to the aorta. **B,** Removal of the balloon. **C,** High pressure after dilation for optimal stent expansion and apposition. **D,** Final result.

Table 22-1. Causes of Left Main Coronary Artery Disease

Atherosclerosis
Nonatherosclerotic causes
 Irradiation
 Takayasu's arteritis
 Syphilitic aortitis
 Rheumatoid arthritis
 Aortic valve disease
 Kawasaki disease
 Injury after left main coronary intervention or cardiac surgery
 Idiopathic causes

and is usually performed with undersized, conventional angioplasty balloons. The stent is then deployed by inflating the stent delivery balloon at a nominal or high pressure. After deployment of the stent, the stented segment is often dilated again using high-pressure for the balloon inflation to achieve angiographically confirmed optimal results (Fig. 22-2). Stent size is selected based on the reference artery size and lesion length. Slotted-tube stents, rather than coil stents, are preferable for treatment of LMCA ostial disease because of their strong radial force. Balloon inflations should be brief (<30 seconds) and multiple (>3) to avoid prolonged global ischemia and ischemia-related complications.

Shaft Lesions

The lesion in the midshaft of the LMCA can be predilated and then stented as done for any discrete lesion in other branches (Fig. 22-3). As for ostial LMCA lesions, debulking is recommended in suitable lesion.

Distal Bifurcation Lesions

Approximately two thirds of all significant lesions in the LMCA involve the distal bifurcation. Stenting of distal LMCA bifurcation disease is the most technically complex and potentially high-risk anatomic variant of LMCA intervention. Distal LMCA bifurcation stenting should therefore be performed only by highly skilled interventionists. Patients must also be informed and must fully comprehend the risks and benefits of the percutaneous approach compared with surgical alternatives.

Balloon angioplasty of the distal LMCA bifurcation has been associated with a high rate of complications and restenosis.[24,25] In contrast, numerous reports suggest that stenting in the bifurcation lesion may result in predictable short-term outcomes with durable effects.[26-34] Side branch occlusion due to plaque shifting during balloon angioplasty of a parent vessel is common, and in LMCA bifurcation stenosis, intervention may result in occlusion of the ostium of the left anterior descending artery (LAD) or left circumflex artery (LCX), with disastrous clinical consequences. Various interventional techniques have been tested to reduce or eliminate the risk of side branch occlusion in bifurcating coronary lesions. Plaque debulking with directional and rotational atherectomy has been proposed for bifurcation lesions to reduce plaque shift and side branch compromise.[35] Many bifurcation stent techniques have been explored to prevent side branch occlusion, including T stenting,[27] reverse-Y stenting,[26] trouser-leg stenting,[31] V stenting,[31] culotte stenting,[28] and crush stenting.[34] No single interventional technique has been found to guarantee preserved patency of the parent vessel and side branch. Bifurcation stenting (with or without debulking) is technically demanding, requiring considerable expertise. The complexity of these techniques depends on the specific anatomy of the bifurcation, the approach used, and the stents employed. There is no single optimal technical approach to LMCA bifurcation disease. Moreover, because of the serious clinical consequences of major side branch occlusion during LMCA bifurcation stenting, not all interventionists agree that percutaneous intervention for LMCA bifurcation stenosis is warranted.

At the Asan Medical Center, stenting for LMCA bifurcation stenoses was performed in selected patients.[14] Between November 1995 and March 2002, 80 consecutive patients with unprotected LMCA bifurcation lesions underwent stent placement. Stenting was performed with or without debulking atherectomy at the operator's discretion. If the artery was larger than 3.0 mm in diameter and had no calcification, directional coronary atherectomy (DCA) was usually performed using a 7-Fr catheter. Rotational atherectomy using a step burr approach was performed for calcified lesions. Four major stenting strategies were used, determined by the specific lesion characteristics and anatomy of the distal LMCA bifurcation, including crossover stenting of the

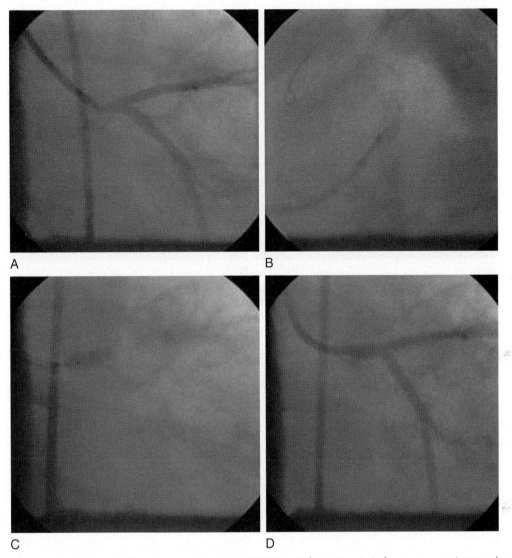

Figure 22-2. An example of unprotected left main coronary artery (LMCA) ostial stenting. **A,** Left coronary angiogram showed a critical narrowing at the ostium of the LMCA. **B,** Directional atherectomy was performed. **C,** The stent was deployed with approximately 1 to 2 mm of proximal struts hanging out into the aorta. **D,** The final angiogram showed no residual stenosis.

LCX, T (Y) stenting, kissing stenting, and bifurcation stenting.

Methods of Stenting

Crossover Technique

Tube stents may be deployed from the LMCA to the proximal portion of LAD if the LCX is diminutive (<2.5 mm) or normal (diameter of stenosis <50%). After stent placement, the LCX is dilated through the first implanted stent strut, as necessary (Figs. 22-4 and 22-5). In the study of Park and colleagues,[14] the LCX ostium was typically covered by a stent without risk of occlusion if it was diminutive or normal. Fifty-four percent of patients were successfully treated with stent placement across the LCX ostium, suggesting that this technique may be widely used for treatment of LMCA bifurcation lesions. However, progression of disease in the side branch lesion

spanned by a stent may be difficult to treat, and a possible risk of side branch occlusion remains an important limitation of this strategy.

T or Y Stenting with or without Simultaneous Kissing Stenting

T or Y stenting with or without simultaneous kissing stenting is performed if the LCX is large and has significant ostial disease. In the bare metal stent (BMS) era, in the T technique (or Y technique, depending on the angle of the bifurcation), after coil stenting (or open-cell design) from the LMCA to the LCX, a slotted-tube stent was sequentially implanted into the LAD through the struts of the coil stent (Figs. 22-6 and 22-7).

The efficacy of T stenting was challenged in the era of the drug-eluting stent (DES). The Study of the Sirolimus-Eluting Stent in the Treatment of Patients

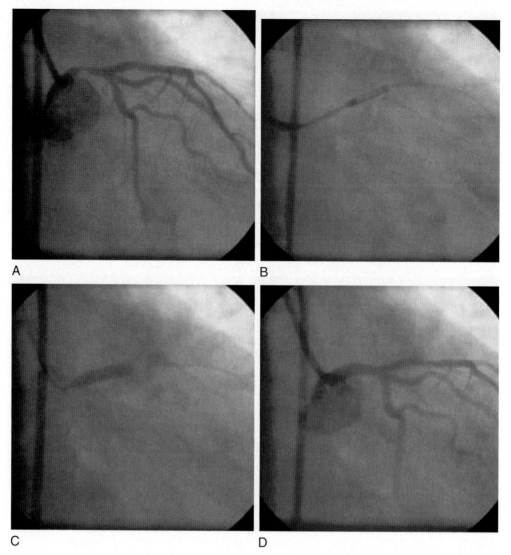

Figure 22-3. An example of unprotected left main coronary artery (LMCA) shaft stenting. **A,** Left coronary angiogram showed a critical eccentric narrowing confined to the midportion of the LMCA. **B,** Directional atherectomy was performed. **C,** The stent was deployed in the body of LMCA. **D,** Final angiogram showed no residual stenosis.

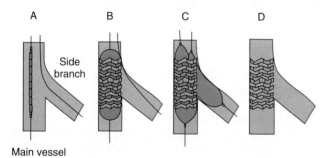

Figure 22-4. Single-stent implantation using the crossover technique in the left circumflex artery. **A,** Wire insertion with optional two-wire technique. **B,** Stent implantation in the main vessel. **C,** Optional kissing balloon dilatation in case of significant stent jail in the side branch after wire insertion into the circumflex artery. **D,** Final result.

with Long De Novo Lesions in Small Native Coronary Arteries (SIRIUS bifurcation study) was a multicenter, randomized trial to assess the feasibility and safety of sirolimus-eluting stent (SES) implantation for bifurcation lesions.[35] In this study, 22 of 43 patients assigned to single SES implantation in the main vessel (group B) were crossed over to T stenting with two SESs, implanted in the main vessel and the side branch (group A) because of flow impairment or residual stenosis of more than 50% of the diameter of the side branch after stent implantation in the main vessel. Sixty-three patients were treated with two stents, and 22 patients were treated with single-stent implantation. Although the high number of crossover patients has made direct comparison of the two groups difficult, the restenosis rates for the two treatment groups were comparably very low (2.3% in group A versus 5.0% in group B). The use of a second stent did not improve the restenosis rate of the side

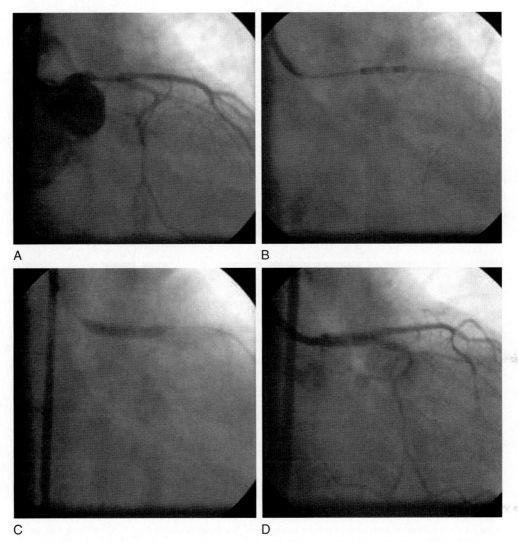

Figure 22-5. An example of unprotected left main coronary artery (LMCA) bifurcation stenting: crossover stenting in the left circumflex artery. **A,** The left coronary angiogram shows a critical eccentric narrowing at the bifurcation site of the LMCA with a normal ostium of the left circumflex artery. **B,** Directional atherectomy was performed from the LMCA toward the left anterior descending artery. **C,** A coronary stent was implanted from LMCA to the left anterior descending artery. **D,** The final angiogram shows no residual stenosis.

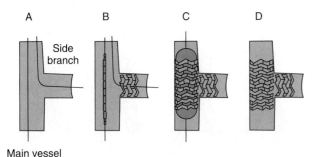

Figure 22-6. T-stenting technique. **A,** The first stent is advanced into the side branch but not expanded, and a second stent is advanced into the main vessel covering the ostium of the side branch. **B,** The first stent is carefully positioned right at the ostium of the side branch or slightly within the main vessel and dilated. **C,** The balloon and wire are removed from the side branch, and then the stent in the main vessel is deployed. **D,** The side branch is rewired, and kissing balloon dilatation of both branches is performed.

branch (19.2% in group A versus 21.1% in group B, P=NS). Overall, the restenosis rate for group A was higher than for group B (25.0% versus 10.0%, P=.20), but it did not achieve statistical significance. The investigators of this study postulated that the relatively high restenosis rate at the side branch in the two-stent implantation group was caused by incomplete coverage of the bifurcation using the T stenting technique. They suggested that T stenting might leave a gap between the two stents at the bifurcation. Other techniques, such as the crush technique or kissing stenting, have been introduced to overcome the problem of T stenting.

Kissing Stenting

Kissing stenting is also a two-stent implantation technique similar to kissing balloon inflation

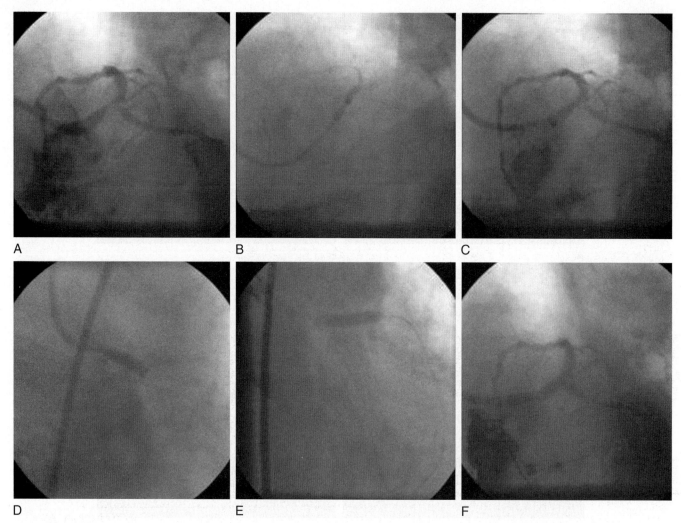

Figure 22-7. An example of unprotected left main coronary artery (LMCA) bifurcation stenting: T (Y) stenting technique. **A,** The left coronary angiogram shows a critical eccentric narrowing at the bifurcation site of the LMCA with ostial narrowing of left circumflex artery. **B,** Directional atherectomy from the LMCA toward the left anterior descending artery was performed. **C,** Another angiogram showed critical narrowing at the ostium of left circumflex artery. **D,** A coronary stent was implanted from the LMCA into the left circumflex artery. **E,** A second coronary stent was implanted from the LMCA to the left anterior descending artery. **F,** Final angiogram shows no residual stenosis.

(Figs. 22-8 and 22-9). A minimum 8-Fr guiding catheter is needed for this technique. The two stents are deployed simultaneously, which creates a double lumen in the main vessel proximal to the bifurcation site. Adjunctive sequential alternative balloon dilatation with final kissing balloon dilatation may be required for optimal stent expansion, especially in the distal part of the bifurcation.[36] This technique is useful for bifurcation lesions with two large side branches with a large diameter of the LMCA trunk. Park[14] suggested that this technique would be appropriate in treating large LMCA lesions (≥4.5 mm). A practical concern of this technique is the difficulty of re-accessing both branches in case of restenosis. However, in the era of DES implantation, this technique was again introduced as one of the appropriate stenting techniques for LMCA bifurcation lesions with a very large proximal vessel.[23] This technique is

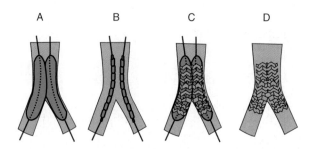

Figure 22-8. Kissing stenting technique. **A,** Both branches are wired and dilated. **B,** The two unexpanded stents are positioned in the bifurcation with parallel proximal stent edges. **C,** The two stents deployed simultaneously. **D,** Final result.

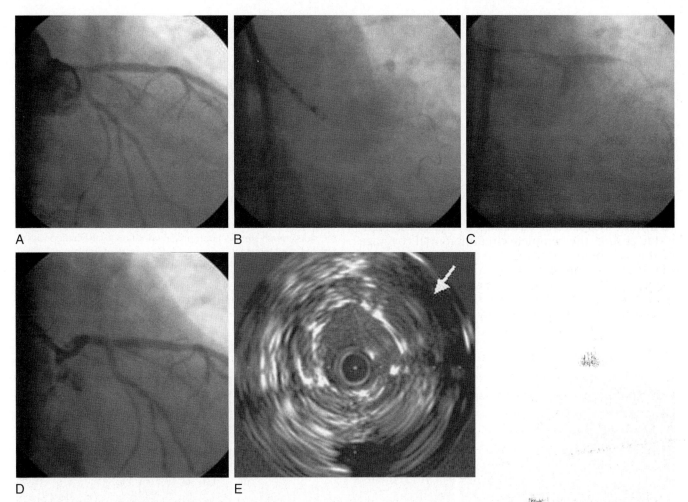

A   B   C

D   E

Figure 22-9. An example of unprotected left main coronary artery (LMCA) bifurcation stenting: kissing stenting technique. **A,** The left coronary angiogram shows critical eccentric narrowing at the bifurcation site of the LMCA and ostial narrowing of the left circumflex artery. **B,** Directional atherectomy was performed. **C,** Simultaneous kissing stenting was performed from the LMCA to the left anterior descending artery and the left circumflex artery. **D,** The final angiogram shows no residual stenosis. **E,** Intravascular ultrasound shows the formation of a new carina at the distal site of the LMCA. The *arrow* indicates the stented ostium of the left circumflex artery.

very safe because access to both branches is always maintained, and it allows complete lesion coverage. Quick performance and easy execution are the major advantages for this technique.

Bifurcation Stenting with Side Branch Access Stenting

The AST SLK-View bifurcation stent (Advanced Stent Technologies, San Francisco, CA) was designed to preserve side branch access and complete the bifurcation stent procedure (Fig. 22-10). The AST SLK-View stent consists of a stainless steel stent with a widened section in the struts located between the proximal and distal ends. A side branch wire exit port passes through this hole, allowing access to the side branch after stenting the main branch. The AST SLK-View stent represents an attractive new approach for treatment of bifurcation lesions. However, further studies are needed to compare this stent with conventional

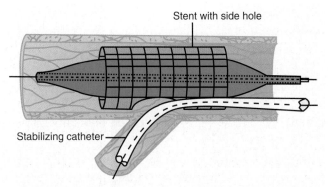

Stent with side hole

Stabilizing catheter

Figure 22-10. SLK-View bifurcation stent system. The main catheter system comprises a main stent with a side hole and a stabilizing catheter. This stent has and expandable side opening with a radiopaque marker. The illustration shows the expanded stent advanced on the two wires in both branches.

stents for treatment of LMCA bifurcation lesions. Preliminary efficacy of this stent system, including outcomes for 11 cases of LMCA bifurcation stenosis, has been presented.[37] In this study, the binary restenosis rates at the 6-month follow-up evaluation were 28.3% and 37.7% for the main vessel and the side branch, respectively.

Crush Technique

The crush technique was introduced by Colombo and colleagues.[38] The procedural steps are shown in Figures 22-11 and 22-12. With the use of DESs, this technique has several advantages. The crush technique ensures the complete circumferential coverage of the side branch ostium. A practical advantage is that the technique is quite safe and relatively simple to execute. This approach gives an immediately successful result with patency of both branches without special technical maneuvers. An important concern

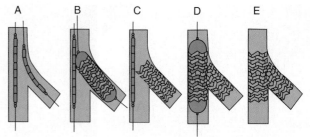

Figure 22-11. Modified T stenting with crushing. **A,** A first stent is advanced into the side branch but not expanded, and a second stent is advanced into the main branch to cover fully the bifurcation. At this point, the proximal marker of the stent in the main vessel is always more proximal in the coronary tree than the proximal marker of the stent for the side branch. **B,** When the side-branch stent is appropriately positioned, the balloon is inflated, and the stent is deployed. **C,** After stent implantation in the side branch, the delivery balloon and the wire are removed from the side branch. **D,** The stent in the main branch is then expanded, and the protruding struts of the stent implanted in the side branch are crushed against the wall of the main vessel.

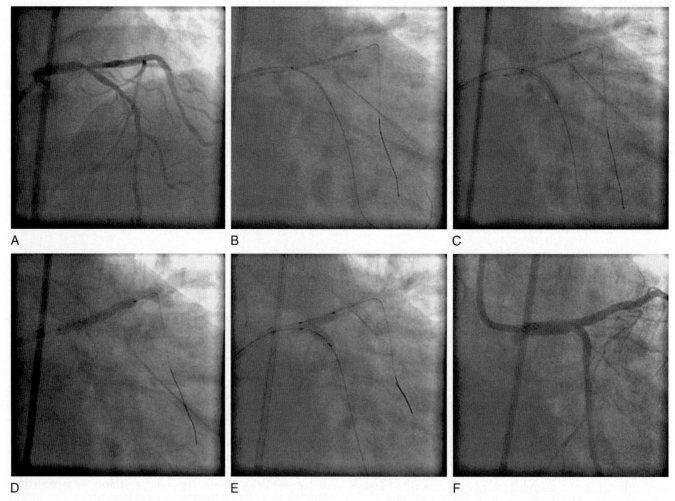

Figure 22-12. An example of unprotected left main coronary artery (LMCA) bifurcation stenting: crushing stent technique. **A,** The left coronary angiogram shows critical eccentric narrowing at the bifurcation site of the LMCA with ostial narrowing of the left circumflex artery (LCX). **B,** Stent positioning. **C,** Stenting was performed in the LCX. **D,** LMCA stenting was performed. **E,** The kissing balloon technique was performed. **F,** The final angiogram shows no residual stenosis.

about this technique is whether the traditional final kissing balloon dilatation is required. Colombo and colleagues[39] suggested that final kissing balloon inflation is very important to achieve long-term patency. Ormiston and coworkers[40] supported the idea with the use of a phantom model. This study demonstrated that it is important to postdilate both stents with appropriately sized balloons.[40] One study achieved a 49% relative reduction in the restenosis rate in the side branch by routine use of final kissing balloon dilation compared with the results of the SIRIUS bifurcation study.[35] The significant reduction of late lumen loss in the side branch after kissing balloon dilation can be explained by better strut contact with the vessel wall and better drug delivery. Kissing balloon dilation may also correct stent deformation and ensure optimal stent scaffolding.

ADJUNCTIVE DEVICES IN UNPROTECTED LEFT MAIN CORONARY ARTERY STENTING

Intravascular Ultrasound

Although intravascular ultrasound (IVUS) provides unique quantitative and qualitative information on coronary artery lesions, the impact of IVUS on long-term clinical outcomes after stent implantation has been controversial. The Can Routine Ultrasound Influence Stent Expansion (CRUISE) study demonstrated that IVUS-guided stent implantation in non-LMCA lesions ensures more effective stent expansion and a larger minimal stent area, resulting in less frequent target vessel revascularization.[41] These results may apply to LMCA intervention as well for several reasons. It is often difficult to evaluate the actual size of the LMCA by angiography.[42] The left main trunk often is short and lacks a normal segment for comparison. Contrast blowback in the aortic cusp may obscure the ostium, and streaming of contrast may result in a false impression of luminal narrowing. Angiography may underestimate stenosis severity, because diffuse disease in the proximal and distal reference segments adjacent to a focal stenosis may be interpreted as normal dimensions, leading to stent undersizing. Preinterventional IVUS examination also provides important information about the underlying lesion morphology and may guide treatment strategy, especially in helping to decide when debulking is necessary or is complete. Angiographically unapparent severe calcification may be seen by IVUS, leading to the decision to performed high-speed rotational atherectomy before stenting to maximize stent expansion. Moreover, negative remodeling (defined as an external elastic membrane cross-sectional area at the lesion site that is smaller than that of the distal reference segment) may be documented in 91% of patients undergoing IVUS-guided stenting of ostial LMCA lesions.[10] In such cases, in which plaque volume is actually reduced compared with non-remodeled or positively remodeled vessels, debulking is unnecessary, and stenting alone should be performed.

Table 22-2. Advantages to Intravascular Ultrasound before and during Left Main Coronary Artery Intervention

Provides precise quantitative measurement
  Reference vessel diameter
  Minimal luminal diameter (before and after)
  Lesion cross-sectional area (before and after)
  Lesion length (automatic pullback)
Characterization of plaque
  Arterial remodeling (positive, negative)
  Plaque stability vs. rupture
  Plaque distribution (eccentric, concentric)
  Plaque composition (soft, fibrous, calcified, mixed; depth of calcium)
  Dissection after predilatation and stenting (length, severity of lumen compromise)
Accurate guidance of procedure
  Decision about additional ballooning
  Decision about treatment strategy in intermediate lesion by quantitative coronary angiography
  Decision about debulking procedure
  Evaluation of stent expansion
  Evaluation of apposition

Performance of IVUS before and during stenting in LMCA stenoses may provide useful information for the selection of the appropriate diameter of balloons and stents, as well as the accurate amount and extent of calcification and need to debulk (Table 22-2). Such information has resulted in changes in the planned procedure and treatment modalities for approximately 40% of non-LMCA lesions.[43] IVUS may also help differentiate which borderline lesions require intervention (with stenting or surgery). However, there are no absolute ultrasound criteria for intervening in a "critical" LMCA stenosis. Important considerations include the patient's symptom status, the presence of other lesions, and the amount of myocardium in jeopardy. Nevertheless, suggested IVUS criteria for significant LMCA disease are stenosis of more than 50% of the vessel diameter, stenosis of more than 60% of the area, and an absolute cross-sectional area less than 7 mm^2 in symptomatic patients or less than 6 mm^2 in asymptomatic patients.

One study evaluated 122 patients with intermediate LMCA disease ($\approx$42% diameter stenosis assessed by quantitative coronary angiography).[44] The 1-year event rate was 14% when LMCA revascularization was deferred based on IVUS findings. When patients with an event were compared with patients without an event, there were no significant differences in left ventricular function or the angiographic diameter stenosis, but the group with events had greater cross-sectional narrowing (70%$\pm$14% versus 53%$\pm$18%, P=.04), smaller minimum LMCA lumen area (6.8$\pm$4.4 versus 10.0$\pm$5.3 mm^2, P=.01), and smaller minimal lumen diameter (MLD) (2.30$\pm$0.69 versus 2.94$\pm$0.81 mm, P=.001). Predictors of cardiac events at 1 year were diabetes mellitus (OR=6.32; 95% CI: 1.82 to 22.04; P=.004), any epicardial vessel with an angiographic stenosis of 50% or more as assessed by quantitative analysis (3.80 [1.08 to 13.39]; P=.037), and the LMCA MLD as assessed by IVUS

Table 22-3. Comparison of Intravascular Ultrasound–Guided Stenting and Angiographically-Guided Stenting in Unprotected Left Main Coronary Artery Stenosis

Characteristic	Intravascular Ultrasound Guidance (n=77)	Angiographic Guidance (n=50)	P Value
Lesion site			.10
Ostium	40 (52%)	19 (38%)	
Body	13 (17%)	6 (12%)	
Bifurcation	24 (31%)	25 (50%)	
Debulking before stenting	30 (39%)	10 (20%)	.02
Reference vessel diameter (mm)	4.0±0.7	4.0±0.6	.46
Minimal luminal diameter			
Before intervention (mm)	1.2±0.5	1.0±0.5	.02
After intervention (mm)	4.2±0.6	4.0±0.6	.003
Follow-up (mm)	2.7±1.0	2.7±1.0	.98
Pressure (atm)	15.1±2.6	15.3±2.8	.33
Angiographic follow-up	59/63 (94%)	41/43 (95%)	.53
Angiographic restenosis rate	11/59 (18.6%)	8/41 (19.5%)	.56

(OR=0.17 [CI: 0.05 to 0.59]; P=.005). When IVUS is used to assess the severity of intermediate LMCA stenoses, decisions to defer to revascularization must consider absolute IVUS dimensions, the presence of diabetes, and the presence of significant lesions in other major epicardial vessels.

The Asan Medical Center reported their experience in stenting 127 unprotected LMCA lesions with (n=77) or without (n=50) IVUS guidance.[10] Debulking procedures before stenting were more frequently performed in the IVUS-guided group (39% versus 20%, P=.02), primarily because of identification of severe calcification with a circumferential arc of more than 90 degrees after IVUS evaluation. According to the IVUS criteria of stent optimization, additional high-pressure balloon angioplasty was performed in 15 (19.5%) of the 77 lesions. As a consequence, the postintervention minimal stent cross-sectional area increased from 10.7±2.8 mm² to 13.0±4.0 mm² after additional balloon angioplasty. The final lumen diameter after stenting was significantly larger in the IVUS-guided group as assessed by quantitative coronary analysis (4.2±0.6 versus 4.0±0.6 mm, P=.003) (Table 22-3). However, the angiographic restenosis and target lesion revascularization rates were not different between the IVUS-guided and angiography-guided procedures in this study. This finding may be explained partly by the fact that the reference vessel size in the current series was large (>4.0 mm) and that the post-stent MLD was also large (>4.0 mm), even in the angiography-guided group. A post-stent MLD of more than 4.0 mm should be large enough to prevent binary restenosis at follow-up. However, we continue to believe that IVUS guidance of unprotected LMCA lesion stenting should be considered, because optimal stent expansion and apposition (which can be verified only by IVUS) may prevent stent thrombosis in the LMCA, a complication with a potentially fatal outcome. In a single center, a small study evaluating the impact of IVUS on unprotected LMCA intervention showed that the incidence of major adverse events was similar: 2 (8%) of 24 in the IVUS group and 7 (20%) of 34 in the non-IVUS group

(P=.18).[45] However, IVUS evaluation may be more crucial in unprotected LMCA intervention for precise lesion assessment, which facilitates selecting and performing optimal stenting strategy.[46]

Debulking Atherectomy

Debulking with directional or rotational atherectomy does not completely eliminate acute recoil and negative vessel remodeling after intervention. The angiographic restenosis rate after directional atherectomy was found to be similar to that of balloon angioplasty alone despite a smaller postprocedural MLD.[47] However, optimally deployed coronary stents reduce the rate of restenosis compared with balloon angioplasty (or directional atherectomy) alone by preventing acute elastic recoil and negative chronic vessel remodeling (although neointimal hyperplasia is increased). Debulking combined with stenting, compared with stenting alone, may result in a larger postprocedural lumen gain and subsequently less angiographic restenosis. Studies have shown that the residual plaque burden is an important predictor of intimal hyperplasia in stented lesions[48] and that aggressive debulking with directional atherectomy before stenting might reduce the residual plaque burden and subsequently reduce the extent of restenosis.[49] This combined approach therefore may be an optimal approach for the management of unprotected LMCA stenoses with a large plaque burden. At the Asan Medical Center, debulking, especially DCA, is performed before stenting if the lesion is suitable. Rotational atherectomy before stenting is also performed if the plaque has diffuse superficial calcification. At the Asan Medical Center, the degree of debulking using directional atherectomy was 30%,[10] compatible with that of other reports (e.g., Stenting after Optimal Lesion Debulking [SOLD] Registry[49]).[50,51] Compared with stent implantation without atherectomy, debulking before stenting in unprotected LMCA lesions was associated with a significant reduction of angiographically confirmed restenosis and target lesion revascularization as assessed by univari-

Table 22-4. Comparison of Angiographic Characteristics and Outcomes in Patients with Unprotected Left Main Coronary Artery Stenoses Undergoing Stenting with Debulking plus Stenting Compared with Stenting Only

Characteristic	Debulking plus Stenting (n=40)	Stenting Only (n=87)	P Value
Lesion site			.003
Ostium	11 (28%)	48 (55%)	
Body	5 (12%)	14 (16%)	
Bifurcation	24 (60%)	25 (29%)	
Debulking before stenting	30 (75%)	47 (54%)	.02
Reference vessel diameter (mm)	4.0±0.6	4.0±0.7	.55
Minimal luminal diameter			
Before intervention (mm)	1.1±0.4	1.1±0.5	.90
After intervention (mm)	4.2±0.7	4.0±0.6	.18
Follow-up (mm)	2.8±1.0	2.7±1.1	.70
Pressure (atm)	15.0±3.1	15.4±2.5	.28
Angiographic follow-up	36/37 (97%)	64/69 (93%)	.31
Angiographic restenosis rate	3/36 (8.3%)	16/64 (25%)	.03
Target lesion revascularization	2/37 (5.4%)	13/69 (18.8%)	.049

ate analysis (Table 22-4).[10] The reduction in the rate of restenosis was most striking in LMCA ostial stenosis. However, debulking atherectomy was not an independent predictor of freedom from restenosis as assessed by multivariate analysis. The most likely explanation is that because of the limited atherectomy device size, the degree of debulking achieved may be insufficient in large LMCA vessels (i.e., mean reference vessel diameter of 4.0 mm). In the non-debulking group, it was possible to achieve just as large an MLD by high-pressure balloon inflations.

DCA may facilitate successful stent placement by removing the plaque and may reduce restenosis rate by improving acute results. A nonrandomized study using BMSs showed that debulking before stenting resulted in significant reduction of angiographic restenosis (P=.034) and target lesion revascularization (P=.049) as assessed by univariate analysis.[52] Hu and associates[53] found similar results for 67 low- to high-risk patients with unprotected LMCA stenosis with distal bifurcation involvement treated with IVUS-guided directional atherectomy. The all-cause mortality, angiographic restenosis, and target lesion revascularization rates at 6 months were 7%, 24%, and 20%, respectively. However, it is unknown whether debulking atherectomy would be advantageous in the era of DES implantation. In practice, the use of debulking has been decreased by the remarkable reduction of restenosis by DESs. Additional research on the effects of DCA and DES implantation is warranted.

Intra-aortic Balloon Pump

Patients with normal left ventricular function are tolerant of global ischemia during balloon occlusion. Although the intra-aortic balloon pump is not routinely recommended during the procedure, it should be considered for prevention of hemodynamic collapse in patients with severely depressed left ventricular function.

BARE METAL STENT IMPLANTATION FOR UNPROTECTED LEFT MAIN CORONARY ARTERY STENOSIS

With the explosive growth of coronary stenting in the 1990s, intervention in the diseased LMCA was again attempted (Table 22-5). The results of these series demonstrated that when patients with LMCA stenosis had well-preserved left ventricular systolic function and were good candidates for bypass graft surgery, the procedural success rates and in-hospital outcomes after stenting were favorable.

Unprotected Left Main Trunk Intervention

A multicenter registry of 107 patients from 25 centers was used to examine the procedural safety and the midterm outcomes of patients who may be considered for percutaneous intervention of unprotected LMCA stenosis.[7] Stents were used in 50%, directional atherectomy in 24%, balloon angioplasty in 20%, and rotational atherectomy in 6% of patients. Technical success was achieved in 96.4% of cases, but 20.6% of patients died while in the hospital, and 10% had nonfatal Q-wave myocardial infarctions (MIs). After post–hospital discharge, outcomes were also unfavorable. Left ventricular function was the most important determinant of survival after LMCA intervention. The Unprotected Left Main Trunk Intervention Multicenter Assessment (ULTIMA) Registry data are difficult to interpret because of inclusion of a very heterogeneous group of patients, including those with poor or good left ventricular function, various degrees of severity of coronary artery disease, and different types of intervention used.[12]

The ULTIMA registry was extended to 279 patients undergoing percutaneous intervention of unprotected LMCA stenosis between July 1993 and July 1998 to examine which patients might have favorable outcomes.[12] Forty-six percent of these patients were deemed inoperable or high-risk surgical candidates. Thirty-eight patients (13.7%) died in the

Table 22-5. Initial and Long-Term Outcomes of Unprotected Left Main Coronary Artery Stenting with Bare Metal Stents

Characteristic	Study Results			
Low-Risk Patients	**Silvestri et al**[11]	**Black et al**[13]	**Park et al**[10]	**Tan et al**[12]
Number	93	53	127	89
Technical success (%)	100	100	99.2	NA
In-hospital outcomes				
Cardiac death (%)	0	1.8	0	0
MI (%)	0	0	1	2.3
Emergent CABG (%)	0	0	1	0
Long-term outcomes				
Duration (mo)	6	7.3±5.8	25.5±16.7	24
Cardiac death (%)	0	1.9	0.8	3.4
MI (%)	0.8	0	0	2.3
TLR (%)	21	15.4	11.8	31.8
High-Risk Patients	**Silvestri et al**[11]	**Black et al**[13]	**Tagaki et al**[15]	**Tan et al**[12]
Number	93	39	67	144
Technical success (%)	100	100	100	NA
In-hospital outcomes				
Cardiac death (%)	9	7.6	0	10.2
MI (%)	4	0	3.0	NA
Emergent CABG (%)	0	0	3.0	NA
Long-term outcomes				
Duration (mo)	6	7.3±5.8	31±23	24
Cardiac death (%)	2	13.8	10.3	29.8
MI (%)	0	0	0	18.8
TLR (%)	10.5	19.4	19.4	50.0

CABG, coronary artery bypass surgery; MI, myocardial infarction; NA, not available; TLR, target lesion revascularization.

hospital, and the remaining patients were followed for a mean of 19 months. The 1-year incidence of all-cause mortality was 24.2% (with 20.2% cardiac mortality), with a 9.8% rate of MI and 9.4% rate of bypass surgery. By multivariate analysis, the independent correlates of death during and after hospitalization were left ventricular ejection fraction of 30% or less, grade 3 or 4 mitral regurgitation, clinical presentation of MI with cardiogenic shock, serum creatinine level of 2.0 mg/dL or higher, and severe lesion calcification (Table 22-6). Decreasing left ventricular ejection fraction was inversely related to events in a nonlinear fashion, with an apparent inflection point at 30%. Except for lesion calcification, the predictors of cardiac death were similar, although different in magnitude: mitral regurgitation grade 3 or 4 (hazard ratio [HR]=5.0); left ventricular ejection fraction of 30% or lower (HR=4.9); MI with cardiogenic shock (HR=4.8; and serum creatinine level of 2.0 mg/dL or higher (HR=3.2). On the basis of this analysis, 32% of the patients could be identi-

fied with three clinical features: age younger than 65 years, left ventricular ejection fraction of 30% or more, and absence of cardiogenic shock from acute MI; they comprised a low-risk group with a 3.4% 1-year mortality rate after LMCA intervention and a 2.3% risk of MI (Table 22-7). There were no periprocedural deaths in this subgroup, and there were no additional deaths or MIs beyond 4 months after discharge (up to 35 months). During the 1-year follow-up of this low-risk group, 24.5% of patients required additional revascularization procedures, including repeat percutaneous intervention in 20.4% and bypass surgery in 11.4% (see Table 22-7).

Similar data were reported by Silvestri and colleagues,[11] who defined a low-risk group as younger than 75 years with no prior bypass great surgery, with a left ventricular ejection fraction of 35% or higher, and with the absence of renal failure, poor coronary runoff, or severe respiratory failure. For these patients, the 1-year mortality rate after unprotected LMCA stenting was 7%, and the need for revascularization

Table 22-6. Correlates of All-Cause Mortality after Unprotected Left Main Coronary Artery Intervention in the ULTIMA Registry

Event	Percent of Study Population	Hazard Ratio	95% CI	P Value
Left ventricular ejection fraction ≤30%	14.3	4.21	2.27 to 7.81	.001
Mitral regurgitation grade 3 or 4	4.1	3.66	1.61 to 8.30	.001
Cardiogenic shock	13.7	3.56	1.73 to 7.34	.001
Serum creatinine ≥2 mg/dL	5.8	3.10	1.30 to 7.39	.011
Severe lesion calcification	8.9	2.32	1.13 to 4.76	.022

All-cause mortality, in-hospital deaths and deaths during follow-up; ULTIMA, Unprotected Left Main Trunk Intervention Multicenter Assessment.

Table 22-7.   One-Year Actuarial Outcomes in the Entire Group and Selected Subgroups of Unprotected Left Main Coronary Artery Intervention from the ULTIMA Registry

Population	Death (%)	Cardiac Death (%)	MI (%)	CABG (%)	Repeat PCI (%)	Death or CABG (%)
All patients (n=278)	24.2	20.2	9.8	9.4	24.2	34.6
LVEF≤30% (n=26)	78.7	73.7	40.1	0.0	67.7	83.7
MR grade 3 or 4 (n=10)	80.0	80.0	0.0	46.7	0.0	90.0
Cardiogenic shock (n=37)	67.6	65.3	0.0	45.8	14.1	78.4
Serum creatinine ≥2 mg/dL (n=16)	68.4	68.4	22.1	0.0	52.8	68.4
Severe calcification (n=21)	56.2	56.2	8.3	10.1	46.0	57.2
Intermediate risk (n=118)	24.4	20.4	14.2	7.8	27.1	33.9
Low risk* (n=89)	3.4	3.4	2.3	11.4	20.4	16.9

*Age <65 years, LVEF>30%, and not in cardiogenic shock.
CABG, coronary artery bypass grafting; PCI, percutaneous coronary intervention; LVEF, left ventricular ejection fraction; MI, myocardial infarction; MR, mitral regurgitation; ULTIMA, Unprotected Left Main Trunk Intervention Multicenter Assessment.

was 28%.[11] To put these data in perspective, the in-hospital mortality rate for patients with LMCA disease undergoing bypass graft surgery was 3.9% as reported by the Society of Thoracic Surgery and 2.3% as reported by The Cleveland Clinic Foundation, with a 1-year mortality rate of 11.3%.[55] In the latter report, the 1-year mortality rate after bypass surgery for a low-risk group similar to that defined in ULTIMA (age <65 years with New York Heart Association congestive heart failure class ≤2) was 5.7%.[12] Patients with LMCA stenosis and poor left ventricular function are recommended for CABG, although patients with well-preserved systolic ventricular performance may have acceptable outcomes after LMCA stenting.

Experience of the Asan Medical Center

The initial report from the ULTIMA Registry demonstrated a relatively high short-term cardiac mortality rate for a heterogenous group of patients.[7] Many of these patients were high risk or ineligible for bypass surgery, and left ventricular ejection fraction was directly related to early and late survival. In the Asan Medical Center experience as reported by Park and associates,[16] only patients with a left ventricular function of 40% or higher were considered for LMCA intervention.

Until January 2001, unprotected LMCA stenting was performed in 156 consecutive patients with normal left ventricular function. The procedural success rate was 99.1%, and 13% underwent multivessel angioplasty during the intervention. There were no procedure-related deaths. However, one patient developed a coronary perforation after DCA, which was successfully treated with a stent graft. During the hospital stay, angiographically documented stent thrombosis occurred in one patient (0.6%) at 3 days after intervention and was complicated by a Q-wave acute MI and the need for elective bypass graft surgery 30 days later. For the remaining patients, the in-hospital clinical outcome was uneventful. Angiographic follow-up data were obtained for 100 of 104 eligible patients (96%). Restenosis was angiographically documented in 19 patients (19%). In the Asan Medical Center study, when

restenosis developed after stenting, it required repeat revascularization, typically within 6 months, and thereafter, most patients were free of symptoms without major adverse cardiac events.

As expected, a smaller reference vessel size was related to a greater likelihood of restenosis, because late lumen loss may be greater in stents implanted into small vessels compared with those implanted in large vessels.[56] As in previous studies of non-LMCA lesions[57] and protected LMCA stenting,[58] the post-stent MLD and minimal lumen cross-sectional area as assessed by IVUS were the most powerful predictors of angiographic restenosis.[59] Target lesion revascularization at the 2-year follow-up was independent of lesion location within the LMCA (Fig. 22-13). As assessed by univariate analysis, there were trends for lower restenosis rates in patients undergoing debulking and in those achieving a large post-stent angiographic MLD, but by multivariate analysis, the reference vessel diameter was the only independent predictor of angiographically observed restenosis in the study.[10] The angiographically confirmed restenosis rate was statistically higher in vessels with

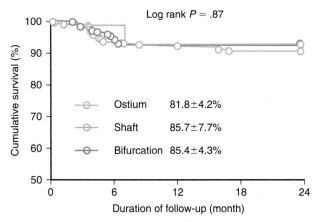

Figure 22-13. Two-year freedom from target lesion revascularization according to the location of the left main coronary artery (LMCA) stenosis in the study by the Asan Medical Center. There were no statistical differences in the 2-year rates of freedom from target lesion revascularization according to location of LMCA stenosis.

Table 22-8. Univariate Determinates of Restenosis in the Parent Vessel after Left Main Coronary Artery Bifurcation Lesion Stenting in the Asan Medical Center Study

Characteristic	Restenosis (*n*=8)	No Restenosis (*n*=35)	*P* Value
Reference artery diameter (mm)	3.4±0.6	3.9±0.6	.03
Minimal lumen diameter (mm)			
Baseline	1.0±0.8	1.1±0.5	.96
Final	3.9±0.7	4.3±0.7	.23
Procedural types			.70
Stenting across the theft circumflex artery ostium	4 (17%)	20 (83%)	
T (Y) or kissing stenting	4 (21%)	15 (79%)	
Debulking performed			.02
Yes	1 (5%)	21 (95%)	
No	7 (33%)	14 (67%)	

a reference diameter of less than 3.6 mm. This cutoff level of 3.6 mm is an arbitrary lower threshold. Although the 31% restenosis rate for these vessels may be slightly higher than that expected in non-LMCA stenting for similar sized arteries, it still is acceptable.

The results of LMCA bifurcation stenting from the Asan Medical Center were published in 2002.[14] Sixty-three consecutive patients were included. DCA was performed in 32 patients (51%). The procedure was successful in all patients, and a prophylactic intra-aortic balloon pump was used in only two patients. In-hospital events did not occur for any patient. Angiographic follow-up was performed for 43 (86%) of the 50 eligible patients reaching the 6-month follow-up point. The angiographic restenosis rate was 28% (including the parent vessel only [LMCA to LAD], 14%; LCX only, 9%; and both, 5%). Restenosis in the parent vessel occurred less frequently in the debulking group than in the non-debulking group (5% versus 33%, *P*=.02). Smaller reference vessel diameter and not having performed debulking were significant univariate predictors of restenosis in the parent vessel (Table 22-8), but debulking was the only independent predictive factor for freedom from restenosis (OR=0.10; 95% CI: 0.01 to 0.90;, *P*=.04). No factors were predictive of restenosis at the side branch. Mean follow-up duration was 19.9±13.7 months (range, 0.23 to 64.6 months). There were two noncardiac deaths but no instances of MI during follow-up. Target lesion revascularization was performed in 6 patients (10%), including repeated percutaneous intervention (*n*=5) and bypass surgery (*n*=1). The event-free survival rate was 86%±6%. In this study, DCA might have been useful for treatment of LMCA bifurcation lesions because a large plaque burden was usually present, and debulking might have prevented plaque shift.

Experience of the ULTRA Registry

The Unprotected Left Main Trunk Angioplasty (ULTRA) study was a multicenter, prospective registry of patients undergoing emergent or elective percutaneous coronary intervention (PCI) for unprotected LMCA stenoses (*n*=284), which was performed in Japan, and the results were presented at the Complex

Catheter Technique meeting in Japan in 2002.[60] This study included very-high-risk patients, including those with acute MI (17%) and patients undergoing emergent intervention for acute coronary syndromes (35%). Coronary stenting, DCA, and other techniques (including conventional balloon angioplasty, cutting balloon angioplasty, and rotablation) were performed in 49%, 37%, and 14% of patients, respectively. The acute result of intervention for 50 patients undergoing LMCA angioplasty in acute MI were very poor, as expected, with a clinical success rate of 64% and an in-hospital mortality rate of 34%. Patients without acute MI, however, had excellent initial and long-term outcomes. In these patients, procedural success was achieved in 99.6% of patients, and major in-hospital complications (i.e., death, Q-wave MI, and emergent bypass surgery) occurred in only 6% of patients. In patients undergoing elective intervention for LMCA disease (*n*=183), the major in-hospital complication rate was only 1%. During 30±11 months of follow-up, the restenosis rate was 22%, and the 1-year event-free survival rate was 89%. These very good initial and long-term outcomes are similar to those of other studies of stenting for low-risk patients with unprotected LMCA stenosis.

Experience of the Multicenter European Study

Black and associates[13] reported the results of stenting unprotected LMCA stenoses in 92 patients from Australia and France. Angiographic success was achieved in 100% of patients, and the mean final stent diameter was 3.9±0.51 mm. Four (4.3%) procedure-related deaths occurred. Neither MI nor emergency bypass surgery occurred during the index hospitalization. During follow-up (7.3±5.8 months; median, 239 days; range, 49 to 1477 days), there were six additional deaths (6.5%): one sudden death was presumed to have a cardiac cause, one was caused by ventricular arrhythmia, three patients died of congestive heart failure, and there was one noncardiac death from lung cancer. The Kaplan-Meier survival estimates found 500- and 1000-day survival estimates of 89% and 85%, respectively. Of the 82 (89%) patients surviving at 6 months, 4 had symptomatic LMCA restenosis and were treated by repeat balloon angioplasty within the stent. Nine other patients had

Table 22-9. In-Hospital and 6-Month Outcomes According to the Risk Group in a European Study of Left Main Coronary Artery Stenting

Complications	Overall (*n*=92)	High Risk* (*n*=39)	Low Risk* (*n*=53)	P Value
In-Hospital Outcomes				
Non Q-wave MI	0	0	0	
Q-wave MI	0	0	0	
Repeat PCI	0	0	0	
CABG	0	0	0	
Death	4 (4.3%)	3 (7.6%)	1 (1.8%)	NS
Noncardiac	1	1	0	
Cardiac	3	2	1	
VF/Arrhythmia		1	1	
Sudden death		0	0	
CHF		1	0	
6-Month Follow-up	**(*n*=88)**	**(*n*=36)**	**(*n*=52)**	
Nonfatal MI	0	0	0	
Re-PCI LMCA	4	1	3	
Re-PCI (other)	9	5	4	
CABG	2	1	1	
Death	6 (6.8%)	5 (13.8%)	1 (1.9%)	NS
Noncardiac	1	1	0	
Cardiac	5	4	1	
VF/arrhythmia		1	1	
Sudden death		1	0	
CHF		2	0	
Total Mortality	10 (10.8%)	8 (20.5%)	2 (3.8%)	<.02

*For high risk patients, bypass surgery was contraindicated; for low-risk patients, bypass surgery was not contraindicated.
CABG, coronary artery bypass graft; CHF, congestive heart failure; LMCA, left main coronary artery; MI, myocardial infarction; NS, not significant; PCI, percutaneous coronary intervention; VF, ventricular fibrillation.

repeat percutaneous intervention in other vessels, and two patients had bypass surgery for restenosis (one for LMCA disease, one for LAD disease). The results differed dramatically, depending on whether LMCA stenting was performed in patients in whom bypass surgery was or was not contraindicated (i.e., high- and low-risk groups, respectively) (Table 22-9). The total mortality rate at 6 months was significantly higher for patients who were not candidates for bypass graft surgery (20.5% versus 3.8%, P<.02). The final stent MLDs and diameters of stenoses were predictive of mortality by univariate analysis (Table 22-10). Lower left ventricular ejection fraction and the presence of three-vessel coronary artery disease

also tended to be more common in patients who died of cardiac causes.

Silvestri and coworkers[11] also examined the outcomes of low-risk patients (*n*=93) and high-risk patients (*n*=47) after LMCA stenting. The high-risk group was composed of patients who were older than 75 years, had history of heart surgery, had a left ventricular ejection fraction less than 35%, had renal failure, had inadequate distal coronary runoff, or had severe respiratory failure. The mortality rate at 1 month was 7% for the high-risk group of patients and 0% for the low-risk group. However, the rate of freedom from major adverse cardiac events at 1 year was similar for the two groups

Table 22-10. Predictors of Cardiac Death in the European Left Main Study Univariate Analysis

Predictors	Cardiac Death (*n*=8)	No Cardiac Death (*n*=84)	P Value
Age (yr)	75±4	74±8	NS
Male gender (%)	63	82	NS
Unstable angina (%)	88	68	NS
Left ventricular ejection fraction (%)	50±14	58±15	<.1
Three-vessel disease (%)	100	71	<.1
Right coronary artery stenosis (%)	75	39	NS
Reference vessel diameter (mm)	3.7±0.6	3.8±0.6	NS
Mean LMCA stenosis (%)	77±11	72±13	NS
Bifurcation stenosis (%)	13	6	NS
Final diameter of stenosis (%)	3.7 (0-20)	1.3 (0-10)	<.05
Final stent diameter (mm)	3.5±0.2	3.9±0.5	<.03
Angioplasty in other vessel (%)	88	63	NS

LMCA, left main coronary artery; NS, not significant.

(66% in high-risk group versus 72% in low-risk group, *P*=NS).

Experience of the French Multicenter Registry

Lefevre presented the French data comparing coronary intervention (*n*=193), bypass surgery (*n*=233), and medical treatment (*n*=57) for LMCA stenoses at the Complex Catheter Technique meeting in Japan in 2002.[61] Eleven centers in France enrolled 483 patients from May 2001 to June 2002 in this study. Thirty-two percent of patients constituted a high-risk group of patients older than 75 years, with pulmonary failure, renal failure, severe peripheral disease, previous bypass graft surgery, previous stroke, and left ventricular ejection fraction less than 30%. Coronary intervention, bypass surgery, or medical therapy was selected for 40%, 48%, and 12% of the cases, respectively, at the operator's or the patient's discretion. High-risk patients were more common in the coronary intervention group than in the bypass surgery group (45% versus 14%), although triple-vessel disease was more common in the surgery group than in the angioplasty group (52% versus 28%). The rates of distal LMCA involvement were similar in the coronary intervention and bypass surgery groups (53% versus 68%). The in-hospital mortality rate was higher after surgery than after coronary intervention (3.8% versus 0%, *P*<.001). At the 6-month follow-up evaluation, the rates of mortality (6.4% with coronary intervention versus 8.1% after surgery) and MI (1.6% versus 1.6%) were similar in the two groups. However, the rate of repeat revascularization of the LMCA was higher in the angioplasty group than the surgery group (15.2% versus 2.7%, *P*=.04). Although these data were not from a randomized, controlled study, the results suggest that LMCA stenting may have comparable long-term results in terms of freedom from death or MI compared with bypass surgery. These favorable initial and intermediate-term outcomes of LMCA stenting for low-risk patients (who would otherwise be candidates for bypass graft surgery) suggested the feasibility of unprotected LMCA stenting.

APPROACH TO IN-STENT RESTENOSIS OF THE UNPROTECTED LEFT MAIN CORONARY ARTERY

In-stent restenosis of the LMCA remains a challenging problem. Because unrecognized LMCA restenosis can manifest as cardiac death, most groups who perform unprotected LMCA stenting recommend elective angiographic restudy at 4 to 6 months after stenting. Elective bypass graft surgery is usually recommended for the treatment of in-stent restenosis of the LMCA. Prior stenting in the LMCA does not interfere with subsequent CABG, and it is the gold standard for the treatment of LMCA stenosis. Alternatively, repeated percutaneous interventions using rotational atherectomy or radiation therapy, or both, in selected patients who refuse surgery have been performed successfully. Further studies and follow-up are needed. The role of drug-eluting stents for treating LMCA in-stent restenosis after bare metal stenting has not been reported.

ELECTIVE INTERVENTION FOR PROTECTED LEFT MAIN CORONARY ARTERY STENOSES

Over the past 25 years, bypass surgery has provided excellent short-term and long-term clinical results for patients with LMCA disease, and the treatment of this lesion has therefore largely remained in the province of the cardiovascular surgeon. However, LMCA stenoses often require treatment after bypass surgery because of progression of native coronary artery disease or bypass graft failure.[62-64] In most cases, a bypass graft is patent to the LAD or to the LCX (or one of their respective branches), resulting in intervention being required for a protected LMCA lesion; the implication is that such a procedure is lower risk than in an unprotected LMCA lesion because ischemia due to LMCA occlusion does not compromise a large portion of the left ventricular myocardium. Conventional balloon angioplasty is often ineffective for a heavy plaque burden and calcification in the unprotected (or protected) LMCA lesion. However, several studies have shown that stenting a protected LMCA stenosis can be safely performed with a high success rate and favorable clinical outcomes (Tables 22-11 and 22-12).[62-71] Kornowski and coworkers[71] reported that stents reduce major in-hospital complications but might not significantly reduce repeat revascularization or major cardiac events at 1 year compared with nonstent LMCA procedures. In their study, diabetes mellitus (OR=3.2, *P*=.04) independently predicted target lesion revascularization, and the final lumen diameter (OR=0.3, *P*=.017) was negatively associated with target lesion revascularization. Nevertheless, the use of stents, alone or after

Table 22-11. In-Hospital Outcomes of Protected Left Main Coronary Artery Intervention

Study	N	Technical Success (%)	Death (%)	Nonfatal Myocardial Infarction (%)	Nonfatal Bypass Surgery (%)
Stertzer et al[65]	8	87	0	0	0
O'Keefe et al[66]	84	—	2.4	0	—
Eldar et al[67]	8	100	0	0	0
Crowley et al[68]	12	100	0	0	0
Lopez et al[69]	46	100	0	0	0
Chauhan et al[70]	14	100	0	0	0
Kornowski et al[71]	124	98	1	1	1

Table 22-12. Long-Term Outcomes of Protected Left Main Coronary Artery Intervention

Study	N	Mean Follow-up (mo)	Deaths after Hospital Discharge (%)	Event-Free Survival* (%)	Restenosis or Bypass Surgery(%)
Stertzer et al[65]	8	46	0	75	—
O'Keefe et al[66]	67	20	10	78	—
Eldar et al[67]	8	24	0	88	38
Crowley et al[68]	12	17	8	92	33
Lopez et al[69]	46	9	2	93	13
Chauhan et al[70]	14	16	14	64	43
Kornowski et al[71]	124	12	0	77	17

* Events include death, myocardial infarction, and revascularization from index intervention.

initial rotational atherectomy, produces the best immediate angiographic results. Technical considerations are similar to those for unprotected LMCA intervention, and precise positioning of the stent is critical, as described previously. Although not proved, pretreatment of heavily calcified LMCA lesions with rotational atherectomy may permit optimal stent expansion with a lower residual stenosis and better long-term clinical outcomes. No comparative data are available examining the outcomes of protected LMCA stenting with repeat bypass surgery. Most experts believe, however, that protected LMCA stenting is preferable to repeat surgery, especially when a left internal mammary artery graft to the LAD is patent.

EMERGENCY INTERVENTION FOR UNPROTECTED LEFT MAIN CORONARY ARTERY STENOSIS

Procedure-Related Complications

LMCA dissection after coronary angiography or an interventional procedure is a rare but serious complication. Careful observation or elective CABG may be a reasonable approach for a non–flow-limiting dissection.[72,73] Emergent CABG or bailout stenting should be performed for a flow-limiting dissection of the LMCA. A retrospective, observational study showed that bailout stenting for LMCA dissection was successful in all cases (n=10) and had very favorable long-term outcomes.[74]

Acute Myocardial Infarction

Because there is paucity of data reporting outcomes of acute MI patients with acute closure of the LMCA, the role of primary angioplasty remains uncertain. Most patients initially presented with cardiogenic shock that required aggressive mechanical support. These patients, unlike those with other forms of acute MI, have high in-hospital mortality and morbidity rates because of left ventricular pump failure. In the ULTIMA registry, the in-hospital cardiac death rate was very high, occurring in more than 50% of patients undergoing primary angioplasty because it cannot prevent acute left ventricular

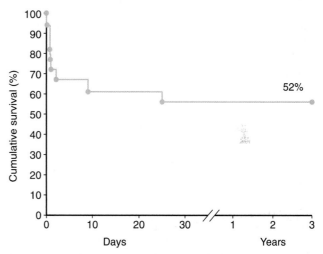

Figure 22-14. Three-year cumulative actuarial survival curve for primary stenting for acute left main coronary artery infarction in 18 patients from the Asan Medical Center.

failure.[75] However, one study showed that 10 surviving patients of 18 patents with LMCA infarction at discharge lived well during the next 39±22 months, except for one patient who required target lesion revascularization (Fig. 22-14).[76] Newer approaches, such as early catheter-based reperfusion therapy plus left ventricular assisted device insertion, may be a good alternative to emergent bypass surgery.

UNPROTECTED LEFT MAIN CORONARY ARTERY STENTING WITH DRUG-ELUTING STENTS

Although, there was a favorable initial outcome after unprotected LMCA intervention using BMSs in low-risk patients, in-stent restenosis is the most important reason for bypass surgery as the first choice for treating unprotected LMCA stenosis. In-stent restenosis in these patients influences long-term survival and may make repeat intervention so difficult that surgery is required. DES implantation remarkably decreases in-stent restenosis in elective patients with relatively simple coronary lesions.[77-79] Along with these results, some studies reported early clinical experience within unprotected LMCA stenting with DESs.

Table 22-13. Comparison of Lesion Characteristics and Procedural Techniques before and after the Era of Drug-Eluting Stents

Characteristic	Chieffo et al[18] DES	Pre-DES	Valgimigli et al[19] DES	Pre-DES	Park et al[17] DES	Pre-DES
Patients (n)	85	64	95	86	102	121
Age	63.2±11.7	65.6±11.7	64±12	66±10	60.3±11.1	57.6±11.9
Male	84.3%	82.3%	66%	62%	71.9%	74.5%
Diabetes mellitus	21.2%	10.9%	30%	22%	84.4%	21.5%
Ejection fraction (%)	51.1±11*	57.4±12.7	41±14	42±13	60.4±8.4	61.8±6.8
Acute MI	NA	NA	17%	20%*	9.8%	6.6%
Cardiogenic shock at entry	NA	NA	9%	12%	0	0
LM plus multivessel involvement (≥2)	NA	NA	80%	69%	58.4%	10.7%
Distal location	81.2%†	57.8%	65%	66%	70.6%†	42.5%
Reference diameter (mm)	3.73±0.6†	4.01±0.7	3.25±0.5	3.37±0.6	3.46±0.65†	3.98±0.69
MLD, before (mm)	1.34±0.5*	1.53±0.6	1.09±0.44	1.05±0.59	1.31±0.57	1.35±0.58
Treated lesions	2.9±1.6†	2.3±1.3	NA	NA	42.2%	34.7%
Stent length (mm)	24.3±12†	15.8±8.6	24±13	20±9	26.6±18.1†	13.3±5.5
DCA (mm)	2.3%†	20.3%	0†	6%	2.9%†	33.1%
MLD, after (mm)	3.3±0.6†	3.8±0.7	2.83±0.49	2.97±0.6	3.36±0.47	4.08±0.57
Bifurcation stenting‡	51 (74%)	NA	40%*	15%	29 (41%)†	9 (18%)
Culotte	10%	NA	36%	11%	0%	0
T technique	8%	NA	44%	88%	3%	89%
Crush	59%	NA	12%	0%	38%	0%
Kissing	24%	NA	8%	0%	59%	11%

*P<.05.
†P<.01.
‡Percentage in patients with bifurcation lesions.
DCA, directional coronary atherectomy; LM, left main; MLD, minimal luminal diameter; MI, myocardial infarction; NA, not available.

Table 22-14. Comparison of Initial and Long-Term Clinical Outcomes before and after the Era of Drug-Eluting Stents

Characteristic	Chieffo et al[18] DES	Pre-DES	Valgimigli et al[19] DES	Pre-DES	Park et al[17] DES	Pre-DES
Patients (n)	85	64	95	86	102	121
Angiographic outcome						
Follow-up rate	NA	NA	NA	NA	84%	82%
MLD, follow-up (mm)	NA	NA	NA	NA	3.25±0.5†	2.78±1.11
Late loss (mm)	0.58†	1.08	NA	NA	0.05±0.57†	1.27±0.90
Restenosis	12 (19%)	15 (30.6%)	NA	NA	6 (7.0%)†	30 (30.3%)
Clinical outcome						
Initial						
Time	In-hospital	In-hospital	30 days	30 days	In-hospital	In-hospital
Death	0	0	10 (11%)	6 (7%)	0	0
MI	5 (5.9%)	5 (7.8%)	4 (4%)	8 (9%)	7 (6.9%)	10 (8.3%)
Stent thrombosis	0	0	0	0	0	0
TVR	0	2 (2.3%)	0	2 (2%)	0	0
Any events	NA	NA	14 (15%)	19 (19%)	7 (6.9%)	10 (8.3%)
Long-term outcomes						
Duration (mo)	6	6	503 (median)		11.7±3.4	30.3±13.7
Death	3 (3.5%)	9 (14.1%)	14%	16%	0	0
MI	NA	NA	4%†	12%	7 (6.9%)	10 (8.3%)
Stent thrombosis	1 (0.1%)	0	NA	NA	0	0
TVR	16 (18.8%)	19 (30.6%)	6%†	12%	2 (2.0%)†	21 (17.4%)
Any events	NA	NA	24%†	45%	9 (7.9%)†	31 (25.6%)

*P<.05.
†p<0.01.
DES, drug-eluting stent; MI, myocardial infarction; MLD, minimal luminal diameter; NA, not available; TVR, target vessel revascularization.

Outcomes of Drug-Eluting Stent Implantation

Three reports have described the mid-term outcomes of unprotected LMCA interventions with DES compared with the pre-DES era. Results are shown in Tables 22-13 and 22-14.

The study of Park and colleagues[17] represents a prospective, ongoing registry of patients with de novo unprotected LMCA stenosis and preserved left ventricular function undergoing elective PCI using SESs. The outcomes of the first 102 patients treated with SESs have been analyzed and compared with

121 patients treated with BMSs, who served as historical controls. The antithrombotic regimen of the patients treated with SESs included aspirin (200 mg/day indefinitely), clopidogrel (300-mg loading dose, followed by 75 mg/day for 6 months), and cilostazol (200-mg loading dose, followed by 100 mg twice daily for 1 month).

The procedural success rate was 100% in the SES and BMS groups. Periprocedural creatine kinase MB fraction (CK-MB) level elevation of three or more times normal developed in 7 SES patients (6.9%) and in 10 BMS patients (8.3%) (P=.69). There were no incidents of death, stent thrombosis, Q-wave MI, or emergent bypass surgery during hospitalization in either group. Quantitative angiographic and IVUS results after the procedures showed that the MLD (4.08±0.57 versus 3.36±0.47 mm, P<.001) and IVUS lesion lumen area (12.41±3.20 versus 9.62±2.57 mm^2, P<.001) after the procedure were larger because of greater acute lumen gain (2.73±0.73 versus 2.06±0.56 mm, P<.001) in the BMS group compared with the SES group. However, at follow-up angiography, lumen loss (0.05±0.57 versus 1.27±0.90 mm, P<.001) and the overall angiographic restenosis rate (7.0% versus 30.3%, P<.001) were significantly lower in the SES group than the BMS group. At 1 year, there were no deaths or acute MIs in either group. Target lesion revascularization at 1 year was performed in 2 SES patients (2.0%) and 21 BMS patients (17.4%) (P<.001). At 12 months, the major adverse cardiac event–free survival rate was 98.0%±1.4% in the SES group and 81.4%±3.7% in the BMS group (P=.0003) (Fig. 22-15).

Chieffo and coworkers[18] reported the outcomes of 85 patients treated with a DES (41 with an SES and 44 with a paclitaxel-eluting stent [PES]), who were compared with 64 patients who received a BMS. During hospitalization, two patients in BMS group had CABG, compared with no patients in the DES group (P=.18); in the BMS group, three had non-Q-wave MI, and two had Q-wave MI, compared with five with non-Q-wave MI in the DES group. One patient had repeat PCI in the BMS group, compared with none in the DES group. No patient in either group died. Procedural success was significantly higher for the DES group than for the BMS group (100% versus 93%, P=.03).

At the 6-month clinical follow-up assessment reported by Chieffo and colleagues,[18] the incidence of major adverse cardiac events was significantly lower in the DES group (17 of 85) than in the BMS group (23 of 64) (20.0% versus 35.9%, P=.039). The all-cause mortality rate is lower for the DES group (3 patients, 3.5%) than the BMS group (9 patients, 14.1%, P=.03). Cardiac deaths were also lower in the DES group (3 patients, 3.5%) than in the BMS group (6 patients, 9.3%), without statistical significance (P=.17). The target lesion revascularization rate did not decrease significantly with DES implantation (14.1%) compared with the BMS implantation (24.2%, P=.13). In the multivariate analysis, only final maximum pressure (atm) (OR=0.85; 95% CI: 0.75 to 0.96; P=.007) correlated to the occurrence of target lesion revascularization. At follow-up angiography, late lumen loss was significantly lower in the DES group than in the BMS group (0.58 versus 1.08 mm, P=.01). However, restenosis occurred in 12 DES patients (19%) and in 15 BMS patients (30.6%, P=.18). the investigators suggested further studies to evaluate the effect of DES in unprotected LMCA intervention.

Valgimigli and colleagues[19] included 95 patients with DES implantation and 86 patients with BMS implantation. There were no significant differences between the DES and the pre-DES groups in the incidence of major adverse cardiovascular events during the first 30 days. After a median follow-up of 503 days (range, 331 to 873 days), the cumulative incidence of major adverse cardiovascular events (i.e., death, MI, or target vessel revascularization) was significantly lower for the DES patients than the pre-DES patients (24% versus 45%; hazard ratio [HR]=0.52; 95% CI: 0.31 to 0.88; P=.01). The mortality rate was similar for the DES (14%) and pre-DES cohort (16%; HR=0.79; 95% CI: 0.38 to 1.66; P=.54), whereas there was a significant reduction in the rate of MI (4% versus 12%; HR=0.22; 95% CI: 0.07 to 0.65; P=.006) and composite death plus MI and in the need for target vessel revascularization (6% versus 23%; HR=0.26; 95% CI: 0.10 to 0.65; P=.004) in the DES group. In the univariate analysis, Parsonnet classification, use of intra-aortic balloon pump, presence of shock at entry, lesion located in the distal LMCA, nonelective intervention, troponin elevation at entry, Thrombolysis in Myocardial Infarction (TIMI) flow grade before and after the procedure, reference vessel diameter, left ventricular ejection fraction, and the use of a DES were identified as significant predictors

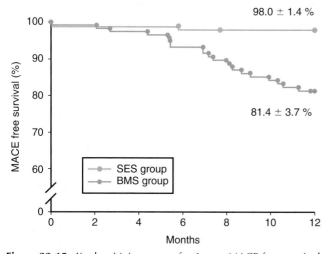

Figure 22-15. Kaplan-Meier curves for 1-year MACE-free survival in patients treated with sirolimus-eluting stents (SES group) and bare metal stents (BMS group). A statistically significant difference was observed between the two groups (P=.0003). MACE, major adverse cardiac events, including death, myocardial infarction, and target lesion revascularization.

of adverse events. In the multivariate analysis, Parsonnet classification, troponin elevation at entry, lesions located at distal site, reference vessel diameter, and the use of a DES were independent predictors of major adverse cardiovascular events.

In the series by De Lezo[20] of 52 patients with unprotected LMCA lesions treated with SESs, primary success was obtained in 50 patients (96%), and 2 patients (4%) developed non-Q-wave MI during the index hospitalization. At a mean follow-up of 12 months, 50 patients (96%) remained asymptomatic, and there were no cases of death or stent thrombosis. Target lesion revascularization was required in one patient (2%).

For the large, Internet-based, postmarketing surveillance e-Cypher registry of 15,169 patients treated in 281 centers, 173 patients were treated for unprotected LMCA stenosis with SESs.[21] The right coronary artery was stenosed or occluded in 54% of patients. A distal bifurcation lesion was present in 62% of the patients. The mean LMCA lesion length was 13.1 ± 7.1 mm, and the mean reference coronary vessel diameter was 3.1 ± 0.4 mm. Overall, 1.01 ± 0.28 SESs per lesion were implanted in native (83%) or restenotic (17%) stenoses. Direct stenting was performed in 33% of patients. The reported in-hospital major adverse cardiac event rate was 0%. At the 6-month clinical follow-up, the incidence of any event was 3.7%, including a 1.8% rate of death, 0.6% rate of MI, and 1.8% rate of target lesion revascularization.

The Korean Multicenter Angioplasty Registry Team (KOMATE) registry, based on the data from five Korean centers, compared outcomes of patients with LMCA stenosis treated with SES versus PES implantation (35 and 19 patients, respectively).[22] Procedural success rates were 100% for both groups. Despite the fact that high-risk patients were included (7.4% of the patients were in cardiogenic shock at study entry), there was only one case of in-hospital death (PES group), a patient with intractable heart failure. At the 6-month clinical follow-up, the overall events rate was 0% for the SES group and 12% for the PES group (all target lesion revascularization) ($P=.07$). Binary restenosis was documented in 1 (8%) of 13 patients treated with SES and 1 (9%) of 11 patients treated with PES.

Technical Considerations

Compared with the pre-DES era, the patients and lesions treated with DESs had higher-risk profiles and disease complexity, such as more multivessel involvement, longer lesions, and more bifurcations (see Table 22-14). Complex stenting procedures were preferred for complete reconstruction of unprotected LMCA bifurcation. In these studies, the crush technique was a new but widely accepted technique for bifurcation lesion stenting. Nevertheless, DES implantation in unprotected LMCA bifurcation lesions showed more favorable long-term outcomes compared with the pre-DES era.

In the study by Park and colleagues,[17] compared with the BMS group, the SES group received more direct stenting, had fewer debulking atherectomies, had more stents implanted, and had more segments stented. IVUS guidance and additional high-pressure balloons were used more frequently in the SES group compared with the BMS group. Extreme overdilation with a balloon at least 1 mm larger than the nominal stent size was performed in 18 SES patients and 4 BMS patients ($P<.001$). Bifurcation stenting, including kissing stenting, T stenting, or crush stenting, of LMCA bifurcation lesions was performed in 40.3% of the SES group and in 17.6% of the BMS group ($P=.010$).

Chieffo and colleagues[18] had a similar pattern of DES implantation. Compared with BMS patients, those treated with a DES had a lower ejection fraction ($51.1\%\pm11\%$ versus $57.4\%\pm13\%$, $P=.002$) and were more often diabetic (21.2% versus 10.9%, $P=.12$) with more frequent distal LMCA involvement (81.2% versus 57.8%, $P=.003$). Moreover, in the DES group, smaller vessels (3.33 ± 0.6 versus 3.7 ± 0.7 mm, $P=.0001$) with more lesions (2.94 ± 1.6 versus 2.25 ± 1.3, $P=.004$) and vessels (2.03 ± 0.69 versus 1.8 ± 0.72, $P=.05$) were treated during the index procedure with longer stents (24.3 ± 12 versus 15.8 ± 8.6 mm, $P=.0001$). In the DES group, an intra-aortic balloon pump was used less frequently (21.2% versus 57.8%, $P=.001$), whereas a trend toward a greater use of inhibitors of glycoprotein IIb/IIIa was observed (28.5% versus 15.6%, $P=.07$). The use of atherectomy devices before stenting was significantly higher in the BMS group than in the DES group.

Two thirds of the patients in Valgimigli and coworkers' two groups had distal LMCA.[19] Patients treated with DESs had significantly more three-vessel disease, more bifurcation stenting, a higher number of stents, and greater total stent length. The nominal stent diameter was on average smaller in the DES group, as judged by the limited availability of DES size.

Drug-Eluting Stent Implantation at Left Main Coronary Artery Bifurcation Stenosis

The location of bifurcation lesions remained a challenge in unprotected LMCA intervention, even in the DES era. All the cases with target vessel failure in the three reports examined in Table 22-14 were caused by restenosis at the unprotected LMCA bifurcation. The report by Chieffo and coworkers[18] did not show a statistically significant benefit of DES over BMS regarding target vessel revascularization. The findings suggested further study focusing on the evaluation of the optimal strategy for improving outcomes of unprotected LMCA bifurcation intervention with DES.

Kim and colleagues[23] reported the results of 116 consecutive patients with de novo unprotected LMCA bifurcation stenoses who underwent elective SES implantation at the Asan Medical Center. Lesions were treated using one of two stenting strategies

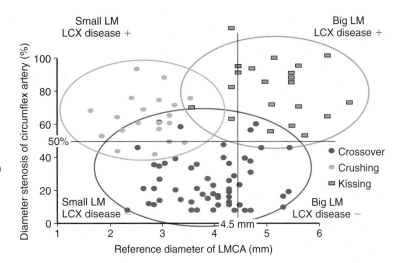

Figure 22-16. Selection of stenting strategy in bifurcation left main stenosis. The presence of ostial left circumflex artery (LCX) disease (diameter stenosis ≥50%) and the reference size of the bifurcation left main (LM) coronary artery stenosis by angiographic and intravenous ultrasound examinations are two important considerations in selecting the stenting strategy.

according to the quantitative angiographic and IVUS measurements (Fig. 22-16). The presence of ostial LCX disease (≥50% diameter stenosis) and the unprotected LMCA bifurcation reference size according to angiographic and IVUS examinations were important considerations in selecting the stenting strategy. In 67 patients (57.8%) with a normal (<50% diameter stenosis) or diminutive (≤2.0 mm) LCX, a simple stenting technique across the ostial LCX was used (i.e., simple group). Final kissing balloon inflation was performed in lesions with significant compromise (≥50% diameter stenosis) of LCX after simple stenting. Alternatively, a complex technique such as a kissing stenting or the crush technique was preferred in 49 (42.2%) patients with a diseased LCX (i.e., complex group). In the complex group, 24 patients who had a relatively large unprotected LMCA that could accommodate two stents proximal to the bifurcation received the kissing stenting technique in an attempt to ensure optimal stent expansion and

sufficient drug release using SESs with diameters of 3.5 mm or less. The crush technique was used in 25 patients with moderately sized, unprotected LMCA lesions. After the crush technique, final kissing balloon dilatation was routinely attempted and was successful in 20 (80%) patients to ensure optimal stent apposition of the two stents at the bifurcation.

In the study of Kim and colleagues,[23] the baseline clinical characteristics did not differ between the two groups, except for more multivessel involvement in the complex group (85.7% versus 68.7%, P=.047). All procedures were successfully performed without any occurrences of death, Q-wave MI, stent thrombosis, or emergent bypass surgery during hospitalization. Procedure-related CK-MB elevation at least three times the normal level occurred in 4 (6.0%) simple group and 3 (6.1%) complex group patients (P=1.0). The results of quantitative angiographic analyses are shown in Table 22-15. The complex group had more

Table 22-15. Angiographic Difference between Simple and Complex Stenting

Characteristic	Simple Group (*n*=69)	Complex Group (*n*=49)	P Value
Patients with follow-up angiogram	57 (85.1%)	41 (83.7%)	.837
Left main coronary artery			
Proximal reference diameter (mm)	3.61±0.72	3.77±0.74	.240
Distal reference diameter (mm)	2.81±0.60	2.75±0.45	.557
Minimal lumen diameter (mm)			
Before procedure	1.11±0.47	1.01±0.47	.269
After procedure	2.97±0.52	2.98±0.36	.931
At follow-up	2.91±0.53	2.56±0.67	.006
Lesion length (mm)	25.8±17.1	26.2±14.5	.918
Acute gain (mm)	1.86±0.58	1.96±0.45	.295
Late loss (mm)	0.13±0.40	0.42±0.63	.009
Restenosis	0	4 (9.8%)	.028
Left circumflex coronary artery			
Distal reference diameter (mm)	2.78±0.66	2.64±0.49	.209
Minimal lumen diameter (mm)			
Before procedure	2.25±0.76	1.39±0.64	<.001
After procedure	2.21±0.77	2.65±0.40	<.001
At follow-up	1.98±0.80	1.97±0.81	.958
Acute gain (mm)	−0.04±0.66	1.26±0.60	<.001
Late loss (mm)	0.20±0.59	0.69±0.72	<.001
Restenosis	3 (5.3%)	7 (17.7%)	.089
Overall restenosis	3 (5.3%)	10 (24.4%)	.024

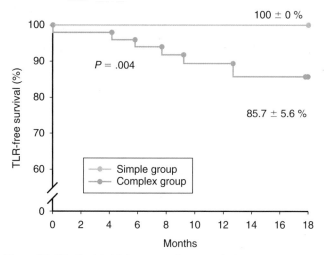

Figure 22-17. Kaplan-Meier curves for target lesion revascularization (TLR)–free survival at 18 months for the simple and complex stenting techniques in the treatment of unprotected left main bifurcation stenosis. A statistically significant difference was observed between the two groups (P=.004).

diseased LCX before the procedure and achieved a more expanded LCX after the procedure. Angiographic follow-up at 6 months was performed for 57 (85.1%) patients in the simple group and 41 (83.7%) patients in the complex group (P=.837). At the main vessel, the late lumen loss (0.13±0.40 versus 0.42±0.63 mm, P=.009) and the angiographic restenosis rate (0% versus 9.8%, P=.028) were lower in the simple group than the complex group. Likewise, late lumen loss at the LCX was also lower in the simple group than in the complex group (0.20±0.59 versus 0.69±0.72 mm, P<.001). Less late lumen loss in the simple group, despite worse postprocedural angiographic outcomes, contributed to the suggestion of a lower LCX restenosis rate than in the complex group (5.3% versus 17.7%, P=.089), although the difference did not reach statistical significance. The simple group had a lower overall angiographic restenosis rate than the complex group (5.3% versus 24.4%, P=.024). For the follow-up period of 18.0±5.3 months in the simple group and 18.0±5.6 months in the complex group (P=.83), no cases of death, stent thrombosis, or MI occurred. Target lesion revascularization was performed in none of the simple group and six (12.2%) patients in the complex group (P=.005). At 18 months, the target lesion revascularization–free survival rate was 100%±0% in the simple group and 85.7%±5.6% in the complex group (P=.004) (Fig. 22-17).

Kim and coworkers[23] suggested that simple crossover stenting of the LCX should be recommended for unprotected LMCA stenosis with a normal LCX. To prevent LCX compromise during and after the procedure, complex stenting techniques were used in true unprotected LMCA bifurcation lesions with a diseased LCX. They further recommended two complex stenting strategies with technical tips to achieve optimal stent expansion at the distal to

bifurcation: kissing stenting after sequential high-pressure dilatation and a crush technique followed by final kissing balloon inflation.

FUTURE PERSPECTIVES

The ultimate proof of the relative value of unprotected LMCA intervention and CABG will depend on the results of randomized clinical trials comparing PCI using DES with the use of CABG. These trials will involve a number of technical considerations that may significantly alter angioplasty outcome.

Two large, randomized studies comparing DES with bypass surgery for unprotected LMCA stenosis are being conducted. The Synergy between Percutaneous Coronary Intervention with Taxus and Cardiac Surgery (SYNTAX) trial is randomizing 1700 patients with de novo triple-vessel disease or LMCA disease (i.e., isolated or with single-, double-, or triple-vessel disease) to PCI with Taxus stents or to CABG. At least 810 patients with unprotected LMCA disease will be enrolled. The trial is powered for noninferiority, with the primary end point being the composite incidence of major adverse cardiac events at 1 year consisting of all-cause death, MI, cerebrovascular events, and repeat revascularization. The Comparison of Bypass Surgery versus Angioplasty using Sirolimus-Eluting Stents in Patients with Left Main Coronary Artery Disease (COMBAT) trial is planning to randomize 1730 patients with unprotected LMCA stenoses with or without disease in other epicardial vessels to revascularization using sirolimus-eluting Cypher stents or to CABG. The primary noninferiority end point is the composite incidence of adverse cardiac events defined as death, MI, and stroke at 2 years.

CONCLUSIONS

Previous studies have shown that the use of coronary stents for the treatment of LMCA stenosis is feasible and is associated with a high rate of procedural success and low rates of early and late complications, such as death, MI, or stent thrombosis, in an otherwise low-risk patient population. However, patients at high risk for CABG have reduced event-free survival after stenting. Compared with historical controls receiving BMSs for LMCA disease, the subsequent rate of target lesion revascularization appears to be diminished by the use of DESs, with similar or enhanced rates of survival and freedom from MI. IVUS guidance during the procedure is strongly encouraged to assess the lesion, select an appropriate stenting technique, and achieve optimal stent placement. DES has been suggested as a reasonable alternative for treating patients with LMCA stenosis. However, for the immediate future CABG must remain the standard of care for most patients with unprotected LMCA disease, pending the results of ongoing and planned, large-scale, prospective, randomized trials comparing DES implantation with CABG.

REFERENCES

1. O'Keefe JH, Hartzler GO, Rutherford BD, et al: Left main coronary angioplasty: Early and late results of 127 acute and elective procedures. Am J Cardiol 1989;64:144-147.
2. Hartzler GO, Rutherford BD, McConohay DR, et al: High-risk percutaneous transluminal coronary angioplasty. Am J Cardiol 1988;61:33G-37G.
3. Eldar M, Schulhoff RN, Hertz I, et al: Results of percutaneous transluminal coronary angioplasty of the left main coronary artery. Am J Cardiol 1991;68:255-256.
4. Macaya C, Alfonso F, Iniguez A, et al: Stenting for elastic recoil during coronary angioplasty of the left main coronary artery. Am J Cardiol 1992;70:105-107.
5. Laham RJ, Carrozza JP, Baim DS: Treatment of unprotected left main stenoses with Palmaz-Schatz stenting. Cathet Cardiovasc Diagn 1996;37:77-80.
6. Lopez JJ, Ho KK, Stoler RC, et al: Percutaneous treatment of protected and unprotected left main coronary stenosis with new devices: Immediate angiographic results and intermediate-term follow-up. J Am Coll Cardiol 1997;29:345-352.
7. Ellis SG, Tamai H, Nobuyoshi M, et al: Contemporary percutaneous treatment of unprotected left main stenoses : Initial results from a multicenter registry analysis 1994-1996. Circulation 1997;96:3867-3872.
8. Park SJ, Park SW, Hong MK, et al: Stenting of unprotected left main coronary artery stenoses: Immediate and late outcome. J Am Coll Cardiol 1998;31:37-42.
9. Kosuga K, Tamai H, Ueda K, et al: Initial and long-term results of angioplasty in unprotected left main coronary artery. Am J Cardiol 1999;83:32-37.
10. Park SJ, Hong MK, Lee CW, et al: Elective stenting of unprotected left main coronary artery stenosis: Effect of debulking before stenting and intravascular ultrasound guidance. J Am Coll Cardiol 2001;38:1054-1060.
11. Silvestri M, Barragan P, Sainsous J, et al: Unprotected left main coronary artery stenting: Immediate and medium-term outcomes of 140 elective procedures. J Am Coll Cardiol 2000;35:1543-1550.
12. Tan WA, Tamai H, Park SJ, et al, for the ULTIMA Investigators: Long-term clinical outcomes after unprotected left main trunk percutaneous revascularization in 279 patients. Circulation 2001;104:1609-1614.
13. Black A, Cortina R, Bossi I, et al: Unprotected left main coronary artery stenting: Correlates of midterm survival and impact of patient selection. J Am Coll Cardiol 2001;37:832-838.
14. Park SJ, Lee CW, Kim YH, et al: Technical feasibility, safety and clinical outcome of stenting of unprotected left main coronary artery bifurcation narrowing Am J Cardiol 2002;104:1609-1614.
15. Takagi T, Stankovic G, Finci L, et al: Results and long-term predictors of adverse clinical events after elective percutaneous interventions on unprotected left main coronary artery. Circulation 2002;106:698-702.
16. Park SJ, Park SW, Hong MK, et al: Long-term (3 years) outcomes after stenting of unprotected left main coronary artery stenosis in patients with normal left ventricular function. Am J Cardiol 2003;91:12-16.
17. Park SJ, Kim YH, Lee BK, et al: Sirolimus-eluting stent implantation for unprotected left main coronary artery stenosis: Comparison with bare metal stent implantation. J Am Coll Cardiol 2005;45:351-356.
18. Chieffo A, Stankovic G, Bonizzoni E, et al: Early and mid-term results of drug-eluting stent implantation in unprotected left main. Circulation 2005;111:791-795.
19. Valgimigli M, van Mieghem CA, Ong AT, et al: Short- and long-term clinical outcome after drug-eluting stent implantation for the percutaneous treatment of left main coronary artery disease: Insights from the Rapamycin-Eluting and Taxus Stent Evaluated At Rotterdam Cardiology Hospital registries (RESEARCH and T-SEARCH). Circulation 2005;111:1383-1389.
20. de Lezo JS, Medina A, Pan M, et al: Rapamycin-eluting stents for the treatment of unprotected left main coronary disease. Am Heart J 2004;148:481-485.
21. Gershlick A, Guagliumi G, Guyon P, et al: Sirolimus-eluting stent and unprotected left main stenosis: The multicenter e-Cypher registry [abstract]. Heart 2005;91:a5-i72.
22. Lee SH, Ko YG, Jang YS, et al: For the Korean Multicenter Angioplasty Team (KOMATE) Investigators: Sirolimus- versus paclitaxel-eluting stent implantation for unprotected left main coronary artery stenosis. Cardiology 2005;104:181-185.
23. Kim YH, Park SW, Hong MK, et al: Comparison of simple and complex stenting techniques in the treatment of unprotected left main coronary artery bifurcation stenosis. Am J Cardiol 2006;97:1597-1601.
24. Lewis B, Leya F, Johnson S, et al: Outcome of angioplasty (PTCA) and atherectomy (DCA) for bifurcation and non-bifurcation lesion in CAVEAT. Circulation 1993;88(Suppl 1):I-601.
25. Mathias DW, Fishman-Mooney J, et al: Frequency of success and complication of coronary angioplasty of a stenosis at the ostium of a branch vessel. Am J Cardiol 1991;67:491-495.
26. Suwaidi JA, Berger PB, Rihal CS, et al: Immediate and long-term outcome of intracoronary stent implantation for true bifurcation lesions. J Am Coll Cardiol 2000;35:929-936.
27. Sheiban I, Albiero R, Marsico F, et al: Immediate and long-term results of "T" stenting for bifurcation coronary lesions. Am J Cardiol 2000;85:1141-1144.
28. Chevalier B, Glatt B, Royer T, Guyon P: Placement of coronary stents in bifurcation lesions by the "culotte" technique. Am J Cardiol 1998;82:943-949.
29. Pan M, Lezo JS, Meding A, et al: Simple and complex stent strategies for bifurcated coronary arterial stenosis involving the side branch origin. Am J Cardiol 1999;83:1320-1325.
30. Cervinka P, Foley DP, Sabaté M, et al: Coronary bifurcation stenting using dedicated bifurcation stents. Catheter Cardiovasc Interv 2000;49:105-111.
31. Lefèvre T, Louvard Y, Morice MC, et al: Stenting of bifurcation lesions: Classification, treatments, and results. Catheter Cardiovasc Interv 2000;49:274-283.
32. Yamashita T, Nishida T, Adamian MG, et al: Bifurcation lesions: Two stents versus one stent—immediate and follow-up results. J Am Coll Cardiol 2000;35:1145-1151.
33. Carlier SG, Giessen WJ, Foley DP, et al: Stenting with a true bifurcated stent: Acute and mid-term follow-up results. Catheter Cardiovasc Interv 1999;47:361-369.
34. Colombo A: Bifurcational lesions and the "crush" technique: Understanding why it works and why it doesn't—a kiss is not just a kiss. Catheter Cardiovasc Interv 2004;63:337-338.
35. Colombo A, Moses JW, Morice MC, et al: Randomized study to evaluate sirolimus-eluting stents implanted at coronary bifurcation lesions. Circulation 2004;109:1244-1249.
36. Sharma SK, Choudhury A, Lee J, et al: Simultaneous kissing stents (SKS) technique for treating bifurcation lesions in medium-to-large size coronary arteries. Am J Cardiol 2004;94:913-917.
37. Ikeno F, Kim YH, Luna J, et al: Acute and long-term outcomes of the novel side access (SLK-View) stent for bifurcation coronary lesions: A multicenter nonrandomized feasibility study. Catheter Cardiovasc Interv 2006;67:198-206.
38. Colombo A, Stankovic G, Orlic D, et al: Modified T-stenting technique with crushing for bifurcation lesions: Immediate results and 30-day outcome. Catheter Cardiovasc Interv 2003;60:145-151.
39. Ge L, Airoldi F, Iakovou I, et al: Clinical and angiographic outcome after implantation of drug-eluting stents in bifurcation lesions with the crush stent technique: Importance of final kissing balloon post-dilation. J Am Coll Cardiol 2005;46:613-620.
40. Ormiston JA, Currie E, Webster MW, et al: Drug-eluting stents for coronary bifurcations: Insights into the crush technique. Catheter Cardiovasc Interv 2004;63:332-336.
41. Fitzgerald PJ, Oshima A, Hayase M, et al: Final results of the Can Routine Ultrasound Influence Stent Expansion (CRUISE) study. Circulation 2000;102:523-530.
42. Hermiller JB, Buller CE, Tenaglia AN, et al: Unrecognized left main coronary artery disease in patients undergoing interventional procedures. Am J Cardiol 1993;71:173-176.

43. Mintz GS, Pichard AD, Kovach JA, et al: Impact of preintervention intravascular ultrasound imaging on transcatheter treatment strategies in coronary artery disease. Am J Cardiol 1994;73:423-430.

44. Abizaid AS, Mintz GS, Abizaid A, et al: One-year follow-up after intravascular ultrasound assessment of moderate left main coronary artery disease in patients with ambiguous angiograms. J Am Coll Cardiol 1999;34:707-715.

45. Agostoni P, Valgimigli M, Van Mieghem CAG, et al: Comparison of early outcome of percutaneous coronary intervention for unprotected left main coronary artery disease in the drug-eluting stent era with versus without intravascular ultrasonic guidance. Am J Cardiol 2005;95:644-647.

46. Hong MK, Park SW, Lee CW, et al: Intravascular ultrasound findings in stenting of unprotected left main coronary artery stenosis. Am J Cardiol 1998;82:670-673.

47. Boehrer JD, Ellis SG, Pieper K, et al: The CAVEAT-I investigators. Directional atherectomy versus balloon angioplasty for coronary ostial and nonostial left anterior descending coronary artery lesions: Results from a randomized multicenter trial. J Am Coll Cardiol 1995;25:1380-1386.

48. Prati F, Di Mario C, Moussa I, et al: In-stent neointimal proliferation correlates with the amount of residual plaque burden outside the stent: An intravascular ultrasound study. Circulation 1999;99:1011-1014.

49. Moussa I, Moses J, Mario CD, et al, for the Stenting after Optimal Lesion Debulking (SOLD) Registry: Angiographic and clinical outcome. Circulation 1998;98:1604-1609.

50. Tsuchikane E, Sumitsuji S, Awata N, et al: Final results of the Stent versus Directional Coronary Atherectomy Randomized Trial (START). J Am Coll Cardiol 1999;34:1050-1057.

51. Simonton CA, Leon MB, Baim DS, et al: Optimal directional coronary atherectomy: Final results of the Optimal Atherectomy Restenosis Study (OARS). Circulation 1998;97:332-339.

52. Cohen MV, Gorlin R: Main left coronary artery disease. Clinical experience from 1964-1974. Circulation 1975;52:275-285.

53. Hu FB, Tamai H, Kosuga K, et al: Intravascular ultrasound-guided directional coronary atherectomy for unprotected left main coronary stenoses with distal bifurcation involvement. Am J Cardiol 2003;92:936-940.

54. Pan M, Lezo JS, Meding A, et al: Simple and complex stent strategies for bifurcated coronary arterial stenosis involving the side branch origin. Am J Cardiol 1999;83:1320-1325.

55. Society of Thoracic Surgery National Database: Available at ctsnet.org/doc/3037

56. Laham RJ, Carrozza JP, Berger C, et al: Long-term outcome of Palmaz-Schatz stenting: Paucity of late clinical stent-related problems. J Am Coll Cardiol 1996;28:820-826.

57. Hoffmann R, Mintz GS, Pichard AD, et al: Intimal hyperplasia thickness at follow-up is independent of stent size: A serial intravascular ultrasound study. Am J Cardiol 1998;82:1168-1172.

58. Kasaoka S, Tobis JM, Akiyama T, et al: Angiographic and intravascular ultrasound predictors of in-stent restenosis. J Am Coll Cardiol 1998;32:1630-1635.

59. Hong MK, Mintz GS, Hong MK, et al: Intravascular ultrasound predictors of target lesion revascularization after stenting of protected left main coronary artery stenoses. Am J Cardiol 1999;83:175-179.

60. Nishikawa H, Nakajima K, Tamai H, et al: ULTRA experiences. Paper presented at the Complex Catheter Therapeutics meeting, 2002, Osaka, Japan.

61. Lefevre T: Left main stenting. Presented at the Complex Catheter Technique 2002 meeting in Japan.

62. Loop FD, Lytle BW, Cosgrove DM, et al: Atherosclerosis of the left main coronary artery: 5 year results of surgical management. Am J Cardiol 1979;44:195-201.

63. Campeau L, Corbara F, Crochet D, Petitclerc R: Left main coronary artery stenosis: The influence of aortocoronary bypass surgery on survival. Circulation 1978;27:1111-1115.

64. Bourassa MG, Fisher LD, Campeau L, et al: Long-term fate of bypass grafts: The Coronary Artery Surgery Study (CASS) and Montreal Heart Institute experiences. Circulation 1985;72(Suppl V):V71-V78.

65. Stertzer SH, Myler RK, Insel H, et al: Percutaneous transluminal coronary angioplasty in left main stem coronary stenosis: A five-year appraisal. Int J Cardiol 1985;9:149-159.

66. O'Keefe JH, Hartzler GO, Rutherford BD, et al: Left main coronary angioplasty: Early and late results of 127 acute and elective procedures. Am J Cardiol 1989;64:144-147.

67. Eldar M, Schulhoff RN, Hertz I, et al: Results of percutaneous transluminal coronary angioplasty of the left main coronary artery. Am J Cardiol 1991;68:255-256.

68. Crowley ST, Morrison DA: Percutaneous transluminal coronary angioplasty of the left main coronary artery in patients with rest angina. Cathet Cardiovasc Diagn 1994;33:103-107.

69. Lopez JJ, Ho KK, Stoler RC, et al: Percutaneous treatment of protected and unprotected left main coronary stenosis with new devices; immediate angiographic results and intermediate-term follow-up. J Am Coll Cardiol 1997;29:345-352.

70. Chauhan A, Zubaid M, Ricci DR, et al: Left main intervention revisited: Early and late outcome of PTCA and stenting. Cathet Cardiovasc Diagn 1997;41:21-29.

71. Kornowski R, Klutstein M, Satler LF, et al: Impact of stents on clinical outcomes in percutaneous left main coronary artery revascularization. Am J Cardiol 1998;82:32-37.

72. Macaya C, Alfonso F, Iniguez A, et al: Stenting for elastic recoil during coronary angioplasty of the left main coronary artery. Am J Cardiol 1992;70:105-107.

73. Garcia-Robles JA, Garcia E, Rico M, et al: Emergency coronary stenting for acute occlusive dissection of the left main coronary artery. Cathet Cardiovasc Diagn 1993;30:227-229.

74. Lee SW, Hong MK, Kim YH, et al: Bail-out stenting for left main coronary artery dissection during catheter-based procedure: Acute and long-term results. Clin Cardiol 2004;27:393-395.

75. Marso SP, Steg G, Plokka T, et al: Catheter-based reperfusion of unprotected left main stenosis during an acute myocardial infarction (the ULTIMA experience). Am J Cardiol 1999;83:1513-1517.

76. Lee SW, Hong MK, Lee CW, et al: Early and late clinical outcomes after primary stenting of the unprotected left main coronary artery stenosis in the setting of acute myocardial infarction. Int J Cardiol 2004;97:73-76.

77. Morice MC, Serruys PW, Sousa JE, et al: A Randomized comparison of a sirolimus-eluting stent with a standard stent for coronary revascularization. N Engl J Med 2002;346:1773-1780.

78. Moses JW, Leon MB, Popma JJ, et al: Sirolimus-eluting stents versus standard stents in patients with stenosis in a native coronary artery. N Engl J Med 2003;349:1315-1323.

79. Stone GW, Ellis SG, Cox DA, et al: A polymer-based, paclitaxel-eluting stent in patients with coronary artery disease. N Engl J Med 2004;350:221-231.

CHAPTER

23 Intervention in Complex Lesions and Multivessel Disease

Peter B. Berger

KEY POINTS

- Percutaneous coronary intervention is associated with the same frequency of death and myocardial infarction as coronary artery bypass grafting in patients with multivessel disease.
- Stents enormously reduce the risk of early coronary artery bypass grafting in patients undergoing multivessel percutaneous coronary intervention.

- The frequency of repeat procedures is reduced with bare metal stents by more than 50% compared with balloon angioplasty.
- There are concerns about late outcomes with drug-eluting stents in patients with complex lesions and multivessel disease.

As initially described, coronary angioplasty was limited to patients with single-vessel disease with a single, discrete, proximal, subtotal, concentric stenosis; well-preserved left ventricular function; and stable angina pectoris refractory to medical therapy. Most patients currently undergoing percutaneous coronary artery intervention have an acute coronary syndrome. Many have had a recent or prior myocardial infarction (MI), and adverse lesion morphology is the rule rather than the exception. More patients than ever have multivessel disease and undergo multilesion or multivessel percutaneous coronary intervention (PCI). Despite the treatment of sicker patients with more complex pathologic anatomy, the short- and long-term outcomes associated with PCI have dramatically improved.

MULTIVESSEL DISEASE

The definition of multivessel disease[1-3] varies greatly from study to study. Depending on which definition is used, the frequency of multivessel disease varies substantially, as do the short- and long-term outcomes of patients with multivessel disease. The different definitions of multivessel disease are one reason that it is difficult to compare PCI with coronary artery bypass grafting (CABG) in nonrandomized trials. However, when similar definitions of multivessel disease are used, most PCI patients with

multivessel disease have two-vessel disease, whereas most patients undergoing CABG with multivessel disease have three-vessel involvement, and they usually have more severe left ventricular dysfunction.

Multilesion PCI should not be confused with multivessel PCI. Although the term *multilesion PCI* refers to PCI of lesions in multiple arterial segments, it does not specify whether the lesions are in a single vessel or multiple vessels. For example, multiple lesions may be dilated in a patient with single-vessel disease or in a patient with multivessel disease. The presence of multivessel disease usually increases the complexity of PCI, even when the lesions are all in the same vessel (or in one vessel and its major branches, which is considered to be single-vessel disease). PCI may be much less complex in a patient with ideal lesions in each of three proximal coronary arteries than in a patient with a single bifurcation lesion or a long, diffuse, calcified lesion in a single, tortuous vessel. For patients with multiple lesions and particularly for those with multivessel disease, each lesion being considered for PCI should be evaluated separately with regard to the risks and benefits of the procedure.

COMPLETE REVASCULARIZATION

The concept of complete revascularization[4-10] initially received attention in the surgical literature when the clinical outcome was found to be related to whether patients had been completely or incompletely revascularized. The results of early series indicated that patients in whom revascularization was complete had a greater reduction of symptoms and improved survival. In three surgical series in which the duration of follow-up ranged from 1 to 5 years, 68% to 87% of patients in whom complete revascularization was achieved were asymptomatic, whereas only 42% to 58% of patients with incomplete revascularization were asymptomatic. Tyras and associates[7] found that patients with complete revascularization also had improved survival.

The importance of complete revascularization, however, may depend in part on the duration of follow-up, because there are some data to suggest that the apparent beneficial effect diminishes with time. Schaff and colleagues[8] evaluated the 10- to 12-year clinical outcomes of 500 consecutive patients who underwent isolated CABG from 1969 to 1972. Preoperative and postoperative variables were tested to identify associations with poor outcome. Only the presence of diseased but ungrafted arteries significantly affected intermediate-term event-free survival. These investigators, however, found that the survival differences between those with complete revascularization and those with incomplete revascularization had disappeared at 10 years. Whether this resulted from progression of disease in the native coronary arteries, late graft failure, or other factors is unknown.

Assessment of the completeness of revascularization is complex, particularly when different revascularization techniques such as PCI and CABG are compared. In some patients, achieving complete revascularization may not be important, because an occluded artery that is not revascularized may supply an area of infarcted myocardium (discussed later). Another confounding variable is that patients in whom complete revascularization can be achieved generally have less severe coronary disease and better left ventricular function; their improved outcome may be the result of better baseline characteristics and less severe disease rather than the revascularization strategy itself. In a study of patients undergoing CABG, Tyras and associates[7] analyzed the actuarial survival corrected for the presence of normal or abnormal left ventricular function. Patients with normal left ventricular function and multivessel disease in whom revascularization was incomplete had a 5-year survival similar to that of patients with complete revascularization, whereas patients with abnormal left ventricular function in whom revascularization was incomplete had a worse clinical outcome than those with complete revascularization. These findings indicate that differences in baseline characteristics may account for the survival differences seen in patients with different degrees of revascularization achieved.

Since these surgical series, the issue of completeness of revascularization has been of great interest with regard to PCI in patients with multivessel disease. However, the impact of different definitions of completeness of revascularization cannot be overemphasized. The frequency with which complete revascularization is achieved with PCI or CABG depends in large part on the definition of complete revascularization. Several series have defined *complete revascularization* as the absence of any lesions with 50% or more stenosis after the procedure. However, given that stenoses less than 70% in native coronary arteries usually do not cause ischemia and may not progress for many years, if ever, such lesions are usually not treated with PCI. It is therefore probably most appropriate to define complete revascularization among patients undergoing PCI as the successful treatment of all lesions with 70% or more stenosis.

The ability to achieve complete revascularization also depends on the selection of patients, because the frequency with which complete revascularization can be achieved is largely a function of the extent of coronary artery disease. In patients with single-vessel disease, complete revascularization is achieved in virtually all patients with just one lesion. In patients with single-vessel disease and incomplete revascularization, usually only a branch vessel with a significant residual stenosis remains, although a distal lesion in an arterial segment too small to treat may account for incomplete revascularization having been achieved. In patients with extensive disease, PCI has been less likely to achieve complete revascularization than CABG; it has generally been achieved in approximately 50% of patients with two-vessel disease but achieved in only 20% to 30% of patients with three-vessel disease (Fig. 23-1).

Several issues must be kept in mind when considering these data. The definition of complete revascularization applied in many surgical series has allowed revascularization to be considered to have been complete if, for example, a lesion in the left anterior descending artery (LAD) was bypassed with a graft to the LAD, even if a lesion in a diagonal branch or in the distal LAD was not bypassed. Dilation of the proximal lesion in the main branch during a PCI procedure usually is not regarded as complete revascularization.

In other surgical series, revascularization has been considered to be complete if a patient with two- or three-vessel disease received two or three grafts, respectively, even if a severe lesion in a major branch remained ungrafted. For example, a patient with a severe LAD and circumflex lesion might have received one graft to the LAD and a second graft to a large diagonal branch, and the patient would be considered to have been completely revascularized, even though the circumflex lesion was not bypassed. Definitions such as these are not generally used for patients undergoing PCI, and their use biases comparisons of the frequency of completeness of revascularization toward surgery over PCI.

The most common reason for failure to achieve complete revascularization with PCI is the presence of one or more chronic occlusions. Success rates with PCI in patients with chronic occlusions remain lower

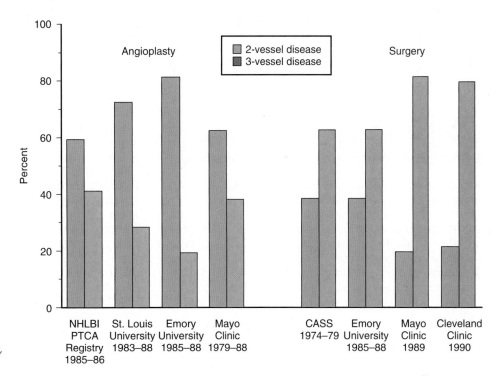

Figure 23-1. Differences in patient populations undergoing percutaneous transluminal coronary angioplasty (PTCA) or surgery. Patients undergoing PTCA have a higher incidence of two-vessel disease compared with patients undergoing surgery, in whom three-vessel disease is more common. (Modified from Berger PB, Holmes DR Jr: Dilatation strategies in patients with multivessel disease. *In* Faxon DP [ed]: Practical Angioplasty. New York, Raven Press, 1993.)

than those in patients with subtotal stenoses, in the 65% to 75% range, particularly when the occlusion is old and when it is long. The presence of an occlusion is not an issue for the surgeon as long as the distal vessel can be well visualized and is of an adequate size.

Other than the presence of a chronic occlusion, the most common reason for incomplete revascularization in patients undergoing PCI is the physician's judgment. A strategy of dilating only the lesion thought to be principally responsible for a patient's ischemia and leaving other lesions untreated has been called a *culprit lesion strategy.* The strategy is generally associated with a good clinical outcome. As a result, the importance of complete revascularization in patients undergoing PCI has been controversial. Some studies have found that the event-free survival is improved for patients with complete revascularization in that the incidences of death, MI, and recurrent angina are decreased. Improved outcome, if real, may be the result of differences in baseline characteristics (discussed earlier). Other studies have not found such an association.

Another complicating factor influencing the completeness of revascularization and its association with improved outcome is the occurrence of restenosis after PCI and graft occlusion after CABG. Complete revascularization at the time of the procedure may be incomplete 3 to 6 months later because of restenosis or graft closure. With PCI, this is less of an issue than before the use of drug-eluting stents, which reduces restenosis by 70% to 90%, but the issue remains relevant, especially for CABG. Most patients undergoing CABG receive at least one vein graft in

addition to an internal mammary artery graft; the likelihood of a vein graft occluding within 18 months was greater than 30% in a the Prevention of Recurrent Venous Thromboembolism-4 (PREVENT-4) trial, the largest randomized trial ever performed with CABG patients.[11] The frequency of occlusion of a vein graft is at least 50% at 10 years.[12] It may be appropriate to consider the concept of transient rather than persistent complete revascularization (i.e., a patient who is completely revascularized who does not develop restenosis or graft occlusion). Given the enormous reduction in restenosis achieved with drug-eluting stents, many believe that such a concept may favor PCI if persistent completeness of revascularization is considered, and that longer-term clinical follow-up of PCI and CABG patients may favor PCI as a result. This is a subject of continuing debate and one that influences the choice of revascularization that physicians must daily consider for their patients.

Differences in clinical outcome related to the completeness of revascularization achieved depend on the viability of myocardium beyond an unrevascularized artery. If the myocardium is not viable, it may not be beneficial to revascularize the region. This approach has been called *incomplete but adequate revascularization,* and it is more common after PCI than CABG.

Improvements in technology have greatly increased the ability to achieve complete revascularization with PCI in patients with multivessel disease. It is fair to conclude that the frequency with which complete revascularization can be achieved in the modern era with PCI and its relation to clinical outcome are unclear. Whether it remains true that CABG leads to more complete revascularization when similar definitions are used, that the difference persists over time, and that it leads to a superior clinical outcome is unknown.

RANDOMIZED TRIALS COMPARING PERCUTANEOUS CORONARY INTERVENTION AND CORONARY ARTERY BYPASS GRAFTING

Any assessment of multivessel PCI among patients requiring revascularization must take into consideration the risks and benefits of the alternative revascularization strategy, CABG. Differences in the baseline clinical and angiographic characteristics of patients undergoing the two procedures and of the definition of success and ascertainment of complications (e.g., procedural MI, restenosis versus late graft closure) make comparisons of observational studies difficult.

Fortunately, since the late 1980s, 11 randomized trials comparing PCI and bypass surgery in patients with predominantly or exclusively multivessel diseases have been performed. They are, in the order in which they were first reported, the Randomised Intervention Treatment of Angina (RITA); the German Angioplasty Bypass Investigation (GABI); the first Argentine Randomized Trial of Percutaneous Transluminal Coronary Angioplasty versus Coronary Artery Bypass Surgery in Multivessel Disease (Estudio Randomizado Argentino de Angioplastia vs. Cirugía [ERACI]); the Coronary Angioplasty versus Bypass Revascularization Investigation (CABRI); the Emory Angioplasty versus Surgery Trial (EAST); BARI; the Arterial Revascularization Therapies Study (ARTS); the second ERACI (ERACI II); the Stent or Surgery (SoS) trial; the second Medicine, Angioplasty, or Surgery (MASS-II) trial; and the Angina With Extremely Serious Operative Mortality Evaluation (AWESOME) study. The first six trials predominantly or exclusively used balloon angioplasty alone in the PCI arms; the subsequent five trials predominantly used bare metal stents. No randomized trials have compared drug-eluting stents and CABG in patients with multivessel disease, although several are ongoing. The following sections review the 11 randomized trials comparing PCI and CABG in patients with multivessel disease.

Balloon Angioplasty versus Coronary Bypass Surgery Trials

RITA

RITA, performed at 16 medical centers throughout Britain, included 1011 patients in whom it was estimated that at least 20% of myocardial mass was supplied by stenotic arteries.[12] RITA was the one of the two trials (along with AWESOME, which is discussed later) that included a minority of patients with single-vessel disease; such patients accounted for approximately one third of those enrolled in the trial. Equivalent degrees of revascularization were required to be achievable by percutaneous transluminal coronary angioplasty (PTCA) and CABG for enrollment. The frequency of primary combined end point of death or nonfatal MI was assessed at 5 years; initially, clinical outcome after a mean follow-up period of 2.5 years was reported. At 2.5 years, there was no significant difference between the PTCA and CABG groups in the primary end point. Death occurred in 3.1% of PTCA and 3.6% of CABG patients. Nonfatal MI occurred in 6.7% of PTCA and in 5.2% of CABG patients. There was no evidence of a treatment difference based on the number of diseased vessels (interaction test $P = .35$). Among the 555 multivessel-disease patients, 26 were PTCA patients, and 27 were CABG patients. When repeat revascularization was included as an end point, 11% of CABG patients died, had a nonfatal MI, or had subsequent PTCA or CABG, compared with 38% of PTCA patients ($P < .001$). Although there was a significant reduction in angina in both treatment groups, angina was significantly more common during follow-up among PTCA patients (31% versus 21% in CABG patients 2 years after enrollment, $P = .007$). The difference reflected more frequent episodes of mild angina among PTCA patients; severe angina occurred in only 6% of patients in both groups. There was no difference between the two groups in exercise capacity at 1 or 2 years after enrollment.

After a median of 6.5 years, there was no significant difference between the PTCA and CABG groups in the primary end point of the trial.[12] Death occurred in 7.6% of PTCA and 9.0% of CABG patients ($P = .51$). Nonfatal MI occurred in 10.8% of PTCA and in 7.4% of CABG patients ($P = .08$). Five years after enrollment, death or nonfatal MI had occurred in 14.1% of PCI patients and 11.1% of the CABG group (not significant [NS]). The rate of death or MI was more than five times higher in the first year than in subsequent years (6.4% versus 1.0%). Similarly, the rate of repeat revascularization procedures declined from 28% and 10% in the first and second years to 3% per year thereafter. The rate of repeat revascularization among CABG patients was 2% per year. Despite the far greater number of repeat procedures required in the PTCA group, the total duration of hospitalization from enrollment through year 5 was greater among CABG patients (20.5 days in the hospital versus 15.9 days in the PCI group). However, angina occurred frequently in PCI patients through the study period, with an average of 10% greater frequency than among CABG patients, and the higher rate was driven by more frequent episodes of mild angina. Class 3 or 4 angina remained rare in both groups. The frequency of events in the small group of diabetic patients ($n = 62$) differed from that in some of the larger studies discussed later in the chapter. Only 2 of 29 diabetic patients undergoing PCI died, compared with 8 of 33 CABG patients ($P = .09$). Death or MI occurred in 5 diabetic PCI patients and 12 diabetic CABG patients ($P = .055$).

ERACI

The single-center ERACI trial was the smallest of the randomized trials, enrolling 127 patients.[13] Significant stenoses had to be amenable to both PTCA and CABG for enrollment. The study had only 70% power to detect a difference in the primary combined end point of survival, freedom from MI, and freedom from any angina during 5 years' follow-up. The small number of patients in this study and the inclusion of any angina during follow-up as a component of the primary end point are limitations. Another limitation is that 13% of patients crossed over from one treatment arm to the other after randomization but before revascularization.

Angioplasty was successful in 92% of attempted lesions, with complete revascularization in 51% of patients, and in 89% of patients when occluded arteries supplying nonviable myocardium were excluded. An internal mammary artery was used in 77% of the surgery patients, and complete revascularization was achieved in 88% of surgery patients.

There were no significant differences in the frequency of death or nonfatal Q-wave MI in the PTCA and CABG groups during the initial hospitalization or the next year (death: 3.2% versus 0%, P = NS; nonfatal Q-wave MI: 9.5% versus 7.8%, P = NS). There was, as expected, more recurrent angina requiring repeat revascularization in the PTCA group. A second revascularization procedure was performed within 1 year in 32% of PTCA patients and in 3.2% of CABG patients. As a result of these repeat procedures, a similar percentage of patients were asymptomatic in both groups at 6 months' follow-up.

After 3 years' follow-up, mortality rates remained similar (4.7% for PTCA versus 9.5% for CABG, P = .5); mortality from cardiovascular causes was 4.7% in both groups (P = 1.0). Q-wave MI rates were also similar (7.8% in both groups).[14] However, 57% of PTCA patients remained free from angina, compared with 79% of CABG patients (P < .001), and 37% of PTCA patients underwent a repeat revascularization procedure, compared with 6.3% of CABG patients (P < .001). Although an economic analysis revealed that the total charges in U.S. dollars, including during hospitalization and the following year, were almost 50% less for the PTCA group at 1 and 3 years, this analysis was limited in that the charges for PTCA and CABG were set by the Argentinean government and do not reflect the true costs.

GABI

The primary end point of the multicenter GABI trial was freedom from class II, III, or IV angina 1 year after study entry.[15] Secondary end points included death, MI, procedure-related complications, repeat interventions, the degree of revascularization, left ventricular function, and an economic comparison. Although the study originally planned to enroll 400 patients to be able to detect a 15% difference in the

prevalence of angina at 1 year, enrollment was terminated after 359 patients when an interim analysis showed that it was highly unlikely that there would be a difference between PTCA and CABG in terms of the primary end point. Of 8981 patients with multivessel disease screened for GABI, 359 patients (4%) were randomized to PTCA (n = 182) or to CABG (n = 177). Of the randomized patients, 337 patients (94%) underwent their assigned procedure. Only patients who underwent their assigned treatment were included in the analysis. Angioplasty was performed on 1.9 ± 0.5 vessels in the PTCA group and was successful in 92% of lesions. Emergency bypass surgery was required in 2.8% of PTCA patients, and elective CABG was required after unsuccessful but uncomplicated PTCA in another 5.7% of patients. Five patients (2.8%) underwent repeat PTCA during the initial hospitalization. CABG patients received 2.2 ± 0.6 grafts; an internal mammary artery was used in only 37% of patients. Two CABG patients required repeat surgical revascularization procedure, and one required PTCA during the initial hospitalization.

In-hospital mortality rates were similar (1.1% for PTCA versus 2.5% for CABG, P = NS). Q-wave MI occurred in fewer PTCA patients (2.3% versus 8.1%, P = .05). At 1 year, the mortality rates were similar in the PTCA and CABG groups (2.6% versus 6.5%, P = NS). MI had occurred in 4.5% of PTCA patients and 9.4% of CABG patients (NS). The cumulative risk of the combined end point of death or nonfatal Q-wave MI was less in PTCA patients (6.0% versus 13.6%, P = .017). Although 44% of PTCA patients required a repeat revascularization procedure compared with 6% of CABG patients, both PTCA and CABG were highly effective at relieving angina. At 3 months, freedom from angina of class II or higher was reported by 60% of PTCA patients and 80% of CABG patients (P = .01). One year after enrollment, 71% of PTCA patients and 74% of CABG patients were free of angina (NS), although more PTCA patients were receiving antianginal medications (12% versus 22%, P = .05).

GABI included an angiographic substudy in which 219 patients (102 PTCA patients and 117 CABG patients) underwent angiography 6 months after the initial procedure.[16] The results of angiography revealed that a severe stenosis (>70%) was present in 19% of PTCA patients. Among the CABG patients, 13% of vein grafts and 7% of internal mammary grafts were occluded.

CABRI

The primary end points of CABRI were mortality, nonfatal infarction, symptomatic status, and functional capacity at 5 to 10 years.[17] In contrast to the other six randomized trials comparing balloon angioplasty and CABG, the use of atherectomy and stents was permitted, although they were infrequently used. Equivalent degrees of revascularization were not required for entry. Among the 1054 patients enrolled, almost two thirds had severe angina (i.e., class III, class IV, or unstable angina), and 41% had a prior MI.

The interim results were initially reported after 1 year of follow-up.[17] The frequency of death and infarction after the two procedures was similar; the percentages of PTCA and CABG patients who died within 30 days were 1.6% and 1.2%, respectively (NS), and the percentages between 30 days and 1 year were 1.8% and 1.0%, respectively (NS). The percentage of patients in the two groups who developed MI in the year after enrollment was also similar (3.7% of PTCA patients versus 3.7% of CABG patients, P = NS). A second revascularization procedure was performed more frequently in patients assigned to PTCA; 1 year after enrollment in the trial, 33% of PTCA patients versus 1.9% of CABG patients had undergone a second revascularization. There was no difference, however, between PTCA and CABG patients in the frequency and severity of angina.

A multivariate analysis of correlates of adverse cardiovascular events in CABRI examined 150 clinical and angiographic variables. Only four were significantly associated with adverse events in the year after enrollment in the trial: a history of peripheral vascular disease (odds ratio [OR] = 3.72; P = .0036), left ventricular ejection fraction (LVEF) (OR = 0.97; P = 0.0305), a history of a cerebral vascular accident (OR = 3.07; P = .0317), and age (OR = 1.05; P = .0416). The assigned revascularization strategy was not a predictor of adverse cardiovascular events in the trial.

The 3-year outcome in the CABRI trial was subsequently reported.[18] Mortality was higher (although not significantly) in the PTCA group (10.9% versus 7.4%; relative risk [RR] = 1.47; 95% CI: 0.99 to 21.9). As in BARI and EAST (discussed later), diabetic patients had considerably better survival with CABG (12.5% versus 22.6%; RR = 1.81; 95% CI: 0.80 to 4.08).

EAST

EAST was a single-center trial for which 5118 patients were screened; 842 patients met the eligibility requirements, and 392 patients (7.7% of screened patients) were enrolled.[19] The primary end point of EAST was a composite of death, infarction, or a large defect on thallium imaging 3 years after enrollment. For patients assigned to PTCA or CABG, the 30-day mortality rate (1.0% versus 1.0%, P = NS) and the frequency of MI (3.5% for PTCA versus 10.0 for CABG, P = NS) were similar. The 3-year mortality rates for PTCA and CABG (7.1% versus 6.2%, P = NS) were also similar. Q-wave MI occurred in 14.1% of PTCA patients and in 19.1% of CABG patients in the 3 years after enrollment (NS). An abnormal thallium scan result was found for a similar number of PTCA and CABG patients (9.6% versus 5.7%, P = NS). At the end of the 3-year follow-up, the combined end point of death, MI, and an abnormal thallium exercise test result was reached by 28.8% of PTCA patients and 27.3% of CABG patients (NS), but repeat revascular-

ization was performed in 56.7% of PTCA patients but only 13.8% of CABG patients (P = .001). Angina was significantly more common in PTCA than CABG patients (19.6% versus 11.7%, P = .05). Protocol angiography 1 and 3 years after the initial revascularization procedure revealed that 59% of the treated segments in the PTCA group and 88% of the grafted segments in the CABG group remained revascularized at 1 year (P < .001). At 3 years, 70% of the treated segments in the PTCA group and 87% of the grafted segments in the CABG group remained widely patent (P < .001).

Eight-year survival rates have been reported for EAST.[20] Survival was similar in the two treatment groups (79.3% in the PTCA group versus 82.7% in the CABG group). Although there were only 59 patients with treated diabetes mellitus in the trial, they tended to have much better survival with CABG (75.5% versus 60.1%, P = .23). There was no interaction between left ventricular function and survival with the different treatment strategies. Repeat revascularization with PTCA or CABG had been performed in 655 of PTCA patients versus 65% of CABG patients (P = .001).

BARI

BARI was the largest randomized trial of PTCA versus CABG, enrolling 1829 patients.[21,22] It was sized to be able to detect a clinically meaningful difference between the two strategies in 5-year mortality by excluding a mortality rate with PTCA of 2.5% or greater than the mortality rate associated with CABG. Follow-up angiography was performed in a subgroup.

Of 12,530 patients who were screened and underwent a detailed angiographic analysis, only 40% of patients were believed by BARI interventional cardiologists to be anatomically suitable for PTCA.[23] The anatomic reasons that patients were judged unsuitable for PTCA (and these were not mutually exclusive) included a nondilatable chronic occlusion (68%), diffuse disease (32%), excessive lesion length (26%), excessive danger (10%), excessive calcification (5%), excessive angulation (5%), excessive tortuosity (3%), and inability to protect a major side branch (3%); miscellaneous other reasons accounted for 3% of exclusions. By comparison, 97% of patients were judged by the participating cardiovascular surgeons to be suitable for CABG. The debate about whether PTCA or CABG is preferable for patients with multivessel coronary disease therefore refers only to the 30% to 50% of patients with multivessel disease suitable for both procedures; most of the remaining patients are clearly better suited for CABG than balloon angioplasty.

A total of 1829 patients were assigned to PTCA (915) or CABG (914); 2435 eligible patients who were not enrolled by physician or patient preference agreed to participate in a registry. In-hospital MIs were more frequent in the CABG group, but the PTCA group required more emergent CABG and repeat PTCA procedures. Survival rates at 5 years were similar for the two groups (89.3% for CABG versus 86.3% for PTCA, $P = .19$). As in all the trials comparing PTCA and CABG, there was a greater need for repeat revascularization with PTCA at 5 years (54% versus 8%). At 7 years, a survival benefit was evident for CABG (84.4% versus 80.9%, $P = .043$), entirely explained by greater survival among patients with treated diabetes (76.4% for CABG versus 55.7% for PTCA, $P = .0011$).[22] There was no difference in survival rates between PTCA and CABG arms for nondiabetics (86.8% versus 86.4%, $P = .72$).

A substudy of BARI aimed to determine whether an initial strategy of PCI was equivalent to CABG in terms of 7-year survival rates for high-risk patients shown to have a survival advantage with CABG over medical therapy.[24] In view of the greater survival among diabetic patients assigned to CABG in BARI, separate analyses of nondiabetic patients were performed. The survival rates at 7 years for patients with three-vessel disease and reduced left ventricular function (ejection fraction <50%) were 70% and 74% ($P = .6$) for all PTCA and CABG patients, respectively ($n = 176$), and 82% and 73% ($P = .29$) when only nondiabetic patients ($n = 124$) were analyzed. The 7-year survival rates were 78% and 71% ($P = .7$), respectively, for patients with two-vessel disease involving the proximal LAD in whom ventricular function was reduced ($n = 72$). The 7-year survival rates for nondiabetic patients with two-vessel disease including the proximal LAD and reduced ventricular function tended to be greater among patients treated with PTCA (90% versus 67%, $P = .13$), although only 46 such patients were enrolled in BARI. In BARI, there was no interaction between left ventricular function and method of revascularization.

The 10-year survival rates have been reported for BARI.[25] Approximately the same absolute difference in survival favoring CABG remains, although the statistical significance has been lost (74% for CABG versus 70.7% for PTCA, $P = .12$). The trend toward greater survival with CABG continues to be explained by greater survival among patients with treated diabetes (57.1% for CABG versus 44.1% for PTCA, $P = .12$).[25] There remains no difference between survival rates with CABG or PTCA for patients without diabetes (78.2% versus 76.8%, $P = .50$).

Coronary Stenting versus Coronary Bypass Surgery Trials

The previous trials assessed the results of primarily balloon angioplasty versus CABG. After the performance of these trials, several randomized trials revealed that the outcome of PCI is superior when stents rather than balloon angioplasty alone are used for a wide variety of clinical presentations and lesion characteristics. Accordingly, more relevant trials were performed.

ERACI II

ERACI II enrolled 450 patients with symptomatic, multivessel disease, including 21 patients with left main coronary artery disease in whom the left main stenosis was believed to be appropriate for stenting.[26] Even though the results of BARI indicated that CABG was preferred for diabetic patients, 17% of patients in ERACI II were diabetics. Abciximab was administered to 28% of the PCI group. The Gianturco-Roubin II stent, shown in randomized trials to be inferior to other stents in terms of clinical outcome, was the primary stent used. At 30 days, the combined frequency of death, Q-wave MI, need for repeat revascularization procedures, and stroke occurred in 3.6% of patients in the PCI group and in 12.3% of patients in the CABG group ($P = .002$). When mortality was analyzed alone, the rate was also lower with PCI (0.9% versus 5.7%, $P < .013$), although the mortality in the CABG group was higher than expected. Using the Kaplan-Meier method of analysis, the PCI group had a greater estimated survival at 900 days than the CABG group (96.9% versus 92.5%, $P < .017$). Although the PCI group had a greater frequency of repeat revascularization (16.8% versus 4.8%, $P < .001$), this frequency of repeat procedures was much lower than had been required in the balloon angioplasty arm of the PTCA versus CABG trials.

The ERACI II investigators have reported the results of their trial with the duration of follow-up extended to 5 years.[27] After 5 years of follow-up, patients initially treated with PCI had similar survival and similar freedom from nonfatal acute MI than those initially treated with CABG (92.8% versus 88.4% and 97.3% versus 94% respectively, $P = .16$). Freedom from repeat revascularization procedures (PCI or CABG) was significantly lower (i.e., worse) among patients initially randomized to PCI than CABG (71.5% versus 92.4%, $P = .0002$). However, with the greater number of repeat procedures performed in patients randomized to PCI, a similar number of patients randomized to each revascularization procedure was asymptomatic or had only class I angina at 5 years (86% for PCI versus 82% for CABG, $P = .916$).

ARTS

ARTS was a multinational study enrolling 1205 patients with multivessel disease (without left main disease).[28] Very-high-risk patients were excluded, and approximately two thirds of the 1205 patients enrolled in the trial had two-vessel disease. At 1 year, there was no difference between the groups in the combined frequency of death, stroke, or MI (91.2% for CABG versus 90.5% for PCI, $P = .69$). The frequency of adverse events considered separately were similar in the CABG and PCI patients: death, 2.8% versus 2.5%; stroke, 2.0 versus 1.5%; infarction, 5.3% versus 4.0%; repeat CABG, 0.5% versus 4.7%; and repeat PCI, 3.0% versus 12.2%. As in all prior studies, repeat revascularization was more frequent in the PCI than in CABG arm, although the difference is narrowing.

An interesting finding in ARTS is the frequency of procedural infarctions with the two revascularization strategies. Serial levels of creatine kinase-myocardial band isoenzyme (CK-MB) were routinely measured in ARTS, and as in most studies in which that was done, it was found that PCI patients more often had elevated levels, usually subclinical, of CK-MB than anticipated. Fully 20% of PCI patients had a CK-MB elevation one to three times the upper limits of normal (ULN) in ARTS, 4% had a peak elevation of three to five times the ULN, and 6% had an elevation greater than five times the ULN; the frequency corresponds in part to the lack of use of glycoprotein IIb/IIIa inhibitors in almost all patients in the trial. However, systematic measurement of CK-MB among the surgery patients revealed elevations of one to three times the ULN in 38%, three to five times the ULN in 7%, and greater than five times the ULN in 12% of CABG patients ($P = .001$). Although there has been much controversy surrounding the frequency and possible long-term clinical significance of such procedural infarctions among patients undergoing PCI in recent years, it should be remembered that such infarctions occur far more commonly and are larger in patients undergoing CABG than those undergoing PCI, even when glycoprotein IIb/IIIa inhibitors are not used during the PCI procedure.

The final secondary end point in ARTS, freedom from major adverse cardiac and cerebrovascular events after 5 years of follow-up, has been reported.[29] At 5 years, there were 48 and 46 deaths in the stent and CABG groups, respectively (8.0% versus 7.6%, $P = .83$; RR = 1.05; 95% CI: 0.71 to 1.55). Among the 208 patients with diabetes, the mortality rate was 13.4% for the stent group and 8.3% for the CABG group ($P = 0.27$; RR = 1.61; 95% CI: 0.71 to 3.63). The rate for overall freedom from death, stroke, or MI was similar for the two groups (18.2% in the stent group versus 14.9% in the surgical group, $P = .14$; RR = 1.22; 95% CI: 0.95 to 1.58). The incidence of repeat revascularization was significantly higher for the stent than for the CABG group (30.3 versus 8.8%, $P = .001$; RR = 3.46; 95% CI: 2.61 to 4.60), which drove the composite event-free survival rate (58.3% for the stent group and 78.2% for the CABG group, $P = .0001$, RR = 1.91; 95% CI: 1.60 to 2.28) in favor of the CABG group.

SoS Trial

In the SoS study, 967 patients were enrolled in 53 European and Canadian centers.[30] There were few restrictions on case selection, few rules about how the procedures were to be performed, and few requirements regarding adjunctive therapy. The median duration of follow-up was 2 years; 1-year follow-up was completed for all patients. The mortality rate at 1 year was lower for CABG than stent patients (0.5% versus 2.5%, $P = .05$), and the difference at 2 years

was even greater (1.2% versus 4.1%, $P = .007$). This result was attributed in large part to a difference in noncardiovascular death; there were eight cancer deaths among the PCI patients and one among the CABG patients, a difference that can only be explained by chance. However, the remarkably low mortality rate for the CABG group (0.5% at 1 year) compared with all previous randomized studies and registry reports further contributed to the significant difference in mortality between the two groups. At 2 years, the frequency of the combined end point of death or Q-wave MI was similar in the two groups (9.3% with CABG versus 9.6% with PCI, $P = NS$). The primary end point of SoS, repeat revascularization at 1 year, was, as in all trials, more frequent among stent patients (13% versus 4.8%) and it remained higher in PCI patients after a median of 2 years (20.3% versus 5.8%; hazard ratio = 3.90; 95% CI: 2.58 to 5.91). The proportions of patients free of angina at that time were 79% with CABG and 66% with PCI.

MASS-II

MASS-II is different from all the other randomized trials comparing PCI with CABG in patients with multivessel disease, because in addition to PCI and CABG arms, a medical therapy arm was included.[31] In MASS-II, 611 patients were randomized to medical therapy ($n = 203$), PCI ($n = 205$), or CABG ($n = 203$). The primary end point was the combined frequency of cardiac death, MI, or unstable angina at 1 year. In the PCI patients, an average of 2.0 vessels were dilated, and angiographic success was achieved in 92% of patients. There were 3.1 vessels grafted in the surgery group. Stents were placed in 70% of PCI patients. The results of MASS-II indicate that after 1 year of follow-up, the mortality rates were not significantly different between the three arms: eight deaths (4.0%) with CABG, nine (4.5%) with PCI, and three (1.5%) with medical therapy. However, the frequency of Q-wave MI was 2% among CABG patients, 5% among medical therapy patients, and 8.3%, among PCI patients ($P = .01$). The frequency of stroke was 1.5%, 1%, and 1.5% in the CABG, PCI, and medical arms, respectively (P-NS). The rate of freedom from any angina at 1 year was 59% among surgery patients, 52% among PCI patients, and 36% among medical therapy patients ($P = .16$ for the CABG versus PCI group). A repeat revascularization procedure was not required in any CABG patient, but repeat revascularization was performed in 14% of PCI patients, and a revascularization procedure was performed in 8% of medical therapy patients.

The reasons that the results of MASS-II differ from all of the other, far larger studies comparing balloon angioplasty and stent placement with CABG are not entirely clear, but several concerns have surfaced about the trial. For example, the frequency of procedural death (2.4%) or Q-wave MI (1.0%) in the PCI arm of MASS-II was 3.4%, higher than in most other studies in the recent era. The timing of the revascularization procedures in patients who were so randomized was unusually slow; for example, only 70% of PCI patients had undergone a PCI procedure within 3 weeks of randomization, by which time two patients had already died (both of noncardiac causes). Repeat angiography was performed by protocol in the PCI arm at 6 months but not in the other two treatment arms; this adds considerable bias and has been conclusively demonstrated to increase the frequency of repeat revascularization procedures, which was the main difference between the treatment arms in MASS-II. The medical therapy received by patients in MASS-II was unusual in that only 77% of patients in the trial received aspirin, 58% of patients received a β-blocker, and 63% of patients received a statin at any point during follow-up period. The ways in which this may have influenced the results of the trial are not known.

AWESOME

The AWESOME study is unique in that it only included patients who had been excluded from prior randomized trials comparing PCI and CABG.[32] In this multicenter trial performed at Veterans Administration hospitals, only patients with medically refractory unstable angina and clinical characteristics known to be associated with an increased risk for CABG, who were amenable to both CABG and PCI, were included. Such characteristics included age older than 70 years, prior bypass surgery, LVEF less than 35%, MI within the prior 7 days, and the need for an intra-aortic balloon pump. The 4554 patients enrolled in AWESOME were older than those in the other trials (mean age, 67 years) and more frequently had diabetes mellitus (32%), triple-vessel disease (45%), prior CABG (31%), and a lower mean LVEF (45%); 21% had an LVEF less than 35%. A total of 19% of AWESOME patients had single-vessel native coronary disease. The early procedural outcome was good, with 30-day survival in these high-risk patients of 95% in patients undergoing CABG and 97% in patients undergoing PCI. Six-month survival was also good (90% versus 94%; *P* = NS for both comparisons).

The results of the AWESOME trial reveal no difference in survival between PCI and CABG patients at 3 years (80% versus 79%, *P* = .46). The frequency of survival free of severe angina was also similar between CABG and PCI patients (65% versus 59%, *P* = NS). MI was not an end point in the trial because serial enzyme measurements were not performed in either group. Because, as in all the randomized comparisons of PCI and CABG, repeat procedures were required more frequently for patients initially undergoing PCI, survival free of both severe angina and repeat revascularization was less common among CABG than PCI patients (61% versus 48%, *P* = .001). Although relatively few women were included in the trial, the inclusion of important subgroups that had been previously been excluded from all the other

trials makes the AWESOME trial a unique and valuable addition to the randomized trials comparing PCI and CABG.

ANALYSIS OF DATA FROM RANDOMIZED TRIALS

Pooled analysis of the 11 PCI versus CABG trials reveals a similar frequency of death (Fig. 23-2) and MI (Fig. 23-3) for the two treatment strategies. Perhaps the most remarkable finding from the stent versus CABG trials is the reduction in the repeat revascularization rates with stenting compared with prior PTCA studies. Despite a greater number of more complex lesions having been treated in the stent trials, the frequency of repeat revascularization was less than

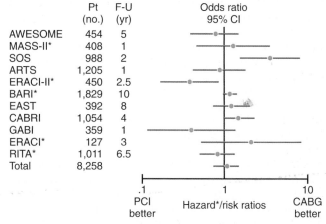

Figure 23-2. Frequency of death (from any cause or only vascular causes when that was all that was reported) in the randomized trials comparing percutaneous coronary intervention (PCI) and coronary artery bypass grafting (CABG). The longest available follow-up is reported, which in some cases is longer than the prespecified time of analysis of the primary end point. *Asterisks* indicate trials that reported hazard ratios rather than risk ratios.

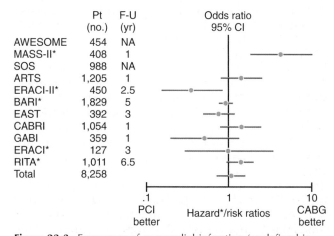

Figure 23-3. Frequency of myocardial infarction (as defined in each of the trials) in the randomized trials comparing percutaneous coronary intervention (PCI) and coronary artery bypass grafting (CABG). The longest available follow-up is reported, which in some cases is longer than the prespecified end point. *Asterisks* indicate trials that reported hazard ratios rather than risk ratios.

one half of that seen in the earlier trials. This is primarily because stents reduce the frequency of restenosis to approximately one half of that seen after balloon angioplasty. However, it also reflects the fact that repeat angiography and follow-up functional tests were not being routinely performed as part of the study protocol of the stent versus CABG trials. The routine performance of functional tests and follow-up angiography in asymptomatic patients increases the frequency of repeat revascularization procedures, and it does so more among patients initially treated with PCI than among those initially treated with CABG.

Several aspects of the performance of PCI in these trials should be carefully considered in clinical decision-making. Few patients in these trials undergoing PCI received a GP IIb/IIIa inhibitor, which improves the clinical outcomes of patients undergoing PCI over the administration of heparin alone. Bivalirudin with bailout GP IIb/IIIa inhibitors was not used, and such therapy improves outcomes over heparin alone, the anticoagulation regimen used most frequently for PCI patients in these trials. Periprocedural infarction was infrequently sought in these trials; when it was, as in the ARTS trial, it was clearly more common among patients undergoing CABG than PCI; the significance of such periprocedural infarctions remains controversial. Pretreatment with a thienopyridine was rarely accomplished; this also reduces procedural complications during PCI and is much more commonly accomplished currently.

Stoke was not included as a component of the primary end point in all of these trials, although many authorities argue that it should be; many patients believe that a significant stroke is a worse outcome than death. If the frequency of stroke were included, it would have favored PCI, because stroke and other neurologic abnormalities are generally more common after CABG than PCI.

The duration of follow-up in all 11 trials was too short to extend into the period when graft occlusion becomes very common. The impact of late graft occlusion on the clinical outcome of patients enrolled in these trials is not clear.

Another important issue to consider is the impact that aggressive risk factor modification might have had in these trials. In BARI, for example, the low-density lipoprotein (LDL) cholesterol level was 143 mg/dL at the time of enrollment and 141 mg/dL 5 years later. It is now clear that intensive secondary prevention is required for all patients with coronary disease, especially those who undergo PCI and CABG. However, it may be particularly critical for PCI patients. Inadequate lipid lowering may favor CABG in that the left internal mammary artery (LIMA) is relatively immune from atherosclerosis for reasons that remain unclear; bypassing the LAD protects a patient from progressive disease and acute occlusion that occurs anywhere in the LAD proximal to the anastomosis of the LIMA, whereas PCI is effective only at the treatment site. If the clinical outcome of PCI is to be optimized in randomized trials comparing it with CABG, particularly in diabetic patients, lipid lowering will be critical.

There are important differences between the 11 prospective, randomized studies comparing coronary angioplasty and bypass surgery. These differences include whether patients with single-vessel disease were included, whether equivalent degrees of revascularization had to be achievable with the different revascularization strategies, whether patients with occluded coronary arteries were eligible, the percentage of internal mammary artery grafts used in the CABG arms, whether stents and other newer interventional devices were permitted, and the planned duration of follow-up.

The length of the follow-up period in most of these studies of 1 to 5 years may favor surgical revascularization over PTCA, because most patients who develop restenosis after coronary angioplasty do so within the first year after the procedure. In contrast, the need for repeat procedures among CABG patients accelerates during the 5 to 10 years after surgery. Follow-up of 1 to 5 years after enrollment in these trials captures virtually all patients who develop restenosis after PCI but captures few patients who require repeat revascularization after CABG. Longer durations of follow-up will be helpful in clarifying these issues, but these trials provide important insights and information into the relative risks and benefits of PTCA and CABG.

Based on the available data from these 11 trials, the following conclusions can be reached:

1. Most patients with multivessel disease being considered for revascularization do not meet the enrollment criteria for these randomized trials (Table 23-1). The results of these trials apply directly only to the minority of patients similar to those enrolled in the trials.

2. Most patients with multivessel disease who require revascularization are better suited for bypass surgery than PCI. The debate about whether PCI or CABG is the most appropriate initial revascularization strategy applies only to the 30% to 50% of patients with multivessel disease suitable for both PCI and bypass surgery. Bare metal stents and drug-eluting stents have increased the appropriateness for PCI in many patients with multivessel disease, but there remain many patients with multivessel disease who are better suited for CABG. These patients include those with left main coronary artery and particularly left main bifurcation lesions; patients with multivessel disease, including undilatable chronic coronary occlusions proximal to viable territory; and possibly patients with two or more bifurcation lesions in major branches not involving the left main coronary artery.

3. In patients with anatomy suitable for both PCI and bypass surgery, the risk of death or MI appears to be similar for the 1 to 10 years

Table 23-1. Comparison of Enrollment, Disease Status, and Left Ventricular Function in 11 Randomized Trials Comparing Percutaneous Coronary Intervention and Coronary Artery Bypass Grafting in Patients with Multivessel Disease

Characteristic	RITA	ERACI	GABI	CABRI	EAST	BARI	ERACI II	ARTS	SOS	MASS-II	AWESOME
Screened*	17,237	1,409	8,981	42,000[†]	5,118	25,200	2,759	Unknown	998	20,769	22,662
Randomizable	Unknown	302	NA	3,000[†]	842	4,110	1,076	Unknown		2,077	781
Randomized	1,011	127	358	1,052	392	1,829	450	1,205	998	611	454
Two-vessel disease (%)	43	55	82	58	60	56	39	68	57	42	37
Triple-vessel disease (%)	12[†]	45	18	40	40	43	57[‡]	32	63	58	45[‡]
Ejection fraction, mean (%)	Unknown	61	56	63	62	58	Unknown	45	57	67	45
Ejection fraction <50%	Unknown	Unknown	21	Unknown	19	23	Unknown	Unknown	Unknown	0	Unknown[§]

*Because most patients screened were not eligible for inclusion, the trials represent a select group of patients, and caution must be used in applying the results of these trials to an individual patient.
[†]Patients with single-vessel disease were permitted in the trial.
[‡]Five percent had left main lesions.
[§]Twenty-one percent had a left ventricular ejection fraction less than 35%.
ARTS, Arterial Revascularization Therapies Study; AWESOME, Angina With Extremely Serious Operative Mortality Evaluation; BARI, Bypass Angioplasty Revascularization Investigation; CABRI, Coronary Angioplasty versus Bypass Revascularization Investigation; EAST, Emory Angioplasty versus Surgery Trial; ERACI, Evaluation of Ranolazine in Chronic Angina; GABI. German Angioplasty Bypass Surgery Investigation; MASS-II, second Medicine, Angioplasty or Surgery Study; RITA, Randomized Intervention Treatment of Angina; SOS, Surgery or Stent.

after the two procedures, whether balloon angioplasty or stents are used in the PCI arm (Table 23-2; see also Figs. 23-2 and 23-3).

4. Among diabetic patients with multivessel disease suitable for either CABG or PCI, balloon angioplasty appears to be associated with a worse outcome than CABG. Diabetic patients with more diffuse and severe triple-vessel disease generally should be treated with CABG rather than balloon angioplasty; this may be true even if stents are used, although it is not certain, especially if drug-eluting stents are used. A large National Institutes of Health (NIH)–funded trial, the Future Revascularization Evaluation in Patients with Diabetes Mellitus: Optimal Management of Multivessel Disease (FREEDOM) trial, is comparing PCI using drug-eluting stents with CABG in diabetic patients with multivessel disease; the results will not be known for several years. Until then, it seems clear that diabetic patients with only a few lesions well suited for both procedures have a good outcome whether PCI or CABG is performed.

5. Approximately 30% to 40% of patients with multivessel disease undergoing balloon angioplasty and perhaps 15% to 20% of patients undergoing bare metal stent placement will need an additional revascularization procedure in the year after the procedure. Patients who are unwilling to risk the likelihood of a second revascularization procedure in the next year may best be treated with CABG.

DRUG-ELUTING STENTS

Although no randomized trials comparing drug-eluting stents and CABG have been performed in patients with multivessel disease, nonrandomized trials have been performed. Perhaps the best are the ARTS II and ERACI III trials. The ARTS investigators enrolled 607 patients in ARTS II who met the inclusion criteria for the ARTS trial and treated them without randomization with drug-eluting Cypher stents. The main goal of ARTS II was to demonstrate noninferiority of PCI using Cypher stents compared with CABG in ARTS I. Patients enrolled in the ARTS II registry were different in some important ways from those enrolled in ARTS I. They were not reviewed by a surgeon and determined to be suitable for CABG. However, approximately 95% of patients with multivessel disease suitable for PCI are suitable for CABG, so whether or to what degree this added bias that favored the PCI arms is not clear. ARTS II patients also had a greater number of high-risk features than the patents in ARTS I, which may have biased the study toward the CABG arm. ARTS II patients had a greater frequency of diabetes, hypertension, diffuse disease, type C lesions, and a greater number of lesions treated than ARTS I patients. Notwithstanding the issues raised by the lack of randomization, patients treated with drug-eluting stents in ARTS II had excellent clinical outcomes. The frequency of death, cardiovascular accident, MI, repeat CABG, and repeat PCI and any of these factors were rare and compared favorably to the frequencies of these events among patients receiving bare metal stents in ARTS I and among CABG patients in ARTS I, the prespecified primary comparator group (Table 23-3).

Table 23-2. Comparison of the Available End Point Data from 11 Randomized Trials

Characteristic	RITA	ERACI	GABI	CABRI	EAST	BARI	ERACI II	ARTS	SoS	MASS-II	AWESOME
Patients enrolled	1011	127	359	1052	392	1829	450	1205	988	611	454
Duration of follow-up (yr)	2.5	3	1	1	3	10	3	1	2	1	3
Mortality rate	ND	ND	ND	ND	ND	ND	ND	ND	Lower with CABG	ND	ND
Myocardial infarction rate	ND	ND	PCI better	ND	ND	ND	PCI better	ND	NA	CABG better	Unknown
Severe angina	ND	ND	ND	ND	Unknown	ND	Unknown	Unknown	Unknown	Unknown	Unknown
Any angina	CABG better at 2.5 yr	ND at 3 yr	ND at 1 yr	ND at 1 yr	CABG better at 3 yr	CABG better at 5 yr	CABG better at 900 days	Unknown	CABG better at 2 yr	CABG better at 1 yr	No difference at 3 yr
Repeat revascularization	PCI 38%, CABG 4%	PCI 37%, CABG 3%	PCI 44%, CABG 4%	PCI 33%, CABG 3%	PCI 57%, CABG 14%	PCI 54%, CABG 8% at 5 yr	PCI 17%, CABG 5% at 900 days	PCI 17%, CABG 4% at 1 yr	PCI 13%, CABG 4.8% at 1 yr	PCI 14%, CABG 0% at 1 yr	Unknown

ARTS, Arterial Revascularization Therapies Study; AWESOME, Angina With Extremely Serious Operative Mortality Evaluation; BARI, Bypass Angioplasty Revascularization Investigation; CABG, coronary artery bypass graft surgery; CABRI, Coronary Angioplasty versus Bypass Revascularization Investigation; EAST, Emory Angioplasty versus Surgery Trial; ERACI, Evaluation of Ranolazine in Chronic Angina; GABI, German Angioplasty Bypass Surgery Investigation; MASS-II, second Medicine, Angioplasty or Surgery Study; NA, not available; ND, no difference; PCI, percutaneous coronary intervention; PTCA, percutaneous transluminal coronary angioplasty; RITA, Randomized Intervention Treatment of Angina; SoS, Surgery or Stent.

Table 23-3. Frequency of Major Adverse Cardiac and Cerebrovascular Events at 1 Year in the ARTS I and ARTS II Trials

Hierarchic MACCE	ARTS II (N = 607)	ARTS I CABG (N = 602)	ARTS I PCI (N = 600)
Death (%)	1.0	2.7	2.7
CVA (%)	0.8	1.8	1.8
MI (%)	1.0	3.5	5.0
Repeat CABG (%)	2.0	0.7	4.7
Repeat PCI (%)	5.4	3.0	12.3
Any MACCE (%)	10.2	11.6	26.5

ARTS, Arterial Revascularization Therapies Study; CABG, coronary artery bypass graft surgery; CVA, cerebrovascular accident; MACCE, major adverse cardiac and cerebrovascular events; MI, myocardial infarction; PCI, percutaneous coronary intervention.

The ERACI investigators enrolled 225 patients in the ERACI III trial who met the criteria for the ERACI II trial and treated them all, without randomization, with drug-eluting stents. They compared the results of these patients with those of patient undergoing CABG in ERACI II. The results of the analysis, which is subject to the same criticisms as those for the ARTS II analysis, suggests (like ARTS II) that drug-eluting stents are a safe and effective means of treating patients with multivessel disease. The results are presented in Table 23-4.

Neither the ARTS II nor ERACI III nonrandomized comparisons should be regarded as definitive. In addition to the limitations of these analyses mentioned, neither analysis could account for the improvements in surgical technique and adjunctive therapies that have occurred since the ARTS and ERACI II trials were performed. Four large, randomized trials are being conducted or are about to be launched in which patients are being randomized to CABG or to drug-eluting stents. They will provide much stronger data about whether, among patients suitable for both CABG and PCI, the use of drug-eluting stents is associated with a similar freedom from death, MI, and the need for repeat revascularization procedures such as CABG.

In the FREEDOM trial, 2400 patients with diabetes mellitus and multivessel disease are being enrolled.

In the Coronary Artery Revascularisation in Diabetes (CARDIA) study, 600 patients with diabetes and either multivessel disease or complex single-vessel disease are being randomized. In Synergy between Percutaneous Coronary Intervention with Taxus and Cardiac Surgery (SYNTAX) trial, 1800 patients with multivessel disease with or without diabetes are being enrolled. SYNTAX also will enroll approximately 900 patients with unprotected left main coronary artery disease. All of these studies will enroll patients who generally meet the clinical and angiographic criteria but do not undergo randomization for one reason or another. These three randomized trials with their registries will provide much greater evidence about whether drug-eluting stents are as safe and effective as CABG in the treatment of patients with multivessel disease, with or without diabetes and with or without left main coronary artery involvement. More information about the true risk of late stent thrombosis of drug-eluting stents placed in off-label situations, including in the treatment of complex anatomy and in patients with multivessel disease, is needed before the most appropriate role of drug-eluting stents in patients with multivessel disease is known.

SUMMARY

PCI is an appropriate therapeutic option for patients with complex or multivessel disease. It is associated with a greater success rate and lower complication rate than achieved before. Whether PCI ought to be preferred in such patients who require revascularization depends on the detailed characteristics of the patient's anatomy and the overall clinical condition, as well as the skill and experience of the operator and of the surgeon who may perform CABG if PCI is not performed. In the past, an important consideration was the patient's willingness to undergo repeat revascularization procedures for restenosis, but that is less of an issue with modern techniques and may no longer be an issue at all since the advent of drug-eluting stents. The risk-benefit ratio of PCI, along with alternative options and their likely outcomes, should be examined and discussed by the primary cardiologist, the patient, and the patient's family.

Table 23-4. Frequency of Major Adverse Events at 1 Year in the ERACI II and ERACI III Trials

MACCE	ERACI II BMS (N = 225)	ERACI II CABG (N = 225)	ERACI III DES (N = 225)	P Value for ERACI III DES vs. ERACI II CABG
Death (%)	3.1	7.6	3.1	.034
MI (%)	2.3	6.2	2.6	.048
Death and MI (%)	5.4	13.8	5.7	.001
Stroke (%)	1.3	0.9	2.2	.56
Repeat PCI/CABG	17	4.9	8.8	.0001
Any MACCE (%)	22.3	19.5	12.0	.047

BMS, bare metal stent; CABG, coronary artery bypass graft surgery; DES, drug-eluting stent; ERACI, Evaluation of Ranolazine in Chronic Angina; MACCE, major adverse cardiac and cerebrovascular events; MI, myocardial infarction; PCI, percutaneous coronary intervention.

REFERENCES

1. Reeder GS, Holmes DR Jr, Detre K, et al: Degree of revascularization in patients with multivessel coronary disease: A report from the National Heart, Lung, and Blood Institute Percutaneous Transluminal Coronary Angioplasty Registry. Circulation 1988;77:638-644.
2. Bell MR, Bailey KR, Reeder GS, et al: Percutaneous transluminal angioplasty in patients with multivessel coronary disease: How important is complete revascularization for cardiac event-free survival? J Am Coll Cardiol 1990;16:553-562.
3. Ellis SG, Cowley MJ, DiSciascio G, et al: Determinants of 2-year outcome after coronary angioplasty in patients with multivessel disease on the basis of comprehensive preprocedural evaluation: Implications for patient selection. The Multivessel Angioplasty Prognosis Study Group. Circulation 1991;83:1905-1914.
4. Cukingnan RA, Carey JS, Wittig JH, et al: Influence of complete coronary revascularization on relief of angina. J Thorac Cardiovasc Surg 1980;79:188-193.
5. Jones EL, Craver JM, Guyton RA, et al: Importance of complete revascularization in performance of the coronary bypass operation. Am J Cardiol 1983;51:7-12.
6. Lavee J, Rath S, Tran-Quang-Hoa, et al: Does complete revascularization by the conventional method truly provide the best possible results? Analysis of results and comparison with revascularization of infarct-prone segments (systematic segmental myocardial revascularization): The Sheba study. J Thorac Cardiovasc Surg 1986;92:279-290.
7. Tyras DH, Barner HB, Kaiser GC, et al: Long-term results of myocardial revascularization. Am J Cardiol 1979;44:1290-1296.
8. Schaff HV, Gersh BJ, Pluth JR, et al: Survival and functional status after coronary artery bypass grafting: Results 10 to 12 years after surgery in 500 patients. Circulation 1983;68(Suppl II):II-200.
9. Lawrie GM, Morris GC Jr, Silvers A, et al: The influence of residual disease after coronary bypass on the 5-year survival rate of 1274 men with coronary artery disease. Circulation 1982;66:717-723.
10. Gohlke H, Gohlke-Barwolf C, Samek L, et al: Serial exercise testing up to 6 years after coronary bypass surgery: Behavior of exercise parameters in groups with different degrees of revascularization determined by postoperative angiography. Am J Cardiol 1983;51:1301-1306.
11. The PREVENT IV Investigators: Efficacy and safety of edifoligide, an E2F transcription factor decoy, for prevention of vein graft failure following coronary artery bypass graft surgery: PREVENT IV: A randomized controlled trial. JAMA 2005;294:2446-2454.
12. RITA Trial Participants: Coronary angioplasty versus coronary artery bypass surgery: The Randomised Intervention Treatment of Angina (RITA) trial. Lancet 1993;341:573-580.
13. Rodriguez A, Boullon F, Perez-Balino N, et al, for the ERACI Group: Argentine Randomized Trial of Percutaneous Transluminal Coronary Angioplasty versus Coronary Artery Bypass Surgery in Multivessel Disease (ERACI): In-hospital results and 1-year follow-up. J Am Coll Cardiol 1993;22:1060-1067.
14. Rodriguez A, Mele E, Peyregne E, et al: Three-year follow-up of the Argentine Randomized Trial of Percutaneous Transluminal Coronary Angioplasty versus Coronary Artery Bypass Surgery in Multivessel Disease (ERACI). J Am Coll Cardiol 1996;27:1178-1184.
15. Hamm CW, Reimers J, Ischinger T, et al: A randomized study of coronary angioplasty compared with bypass surgery in patients with symptomatic multivessel coronary disease. N Engl J Med 1994;331:1037-1043.
16. Rupprecht HJ, Hamm C, Ischinger T, et al: Angiographic follow-up results of a randomized study on angioplasty versus bypass surgery (GABI trial). GABI Study Group. Eur Heart J 1996;17:1192-1198.
17. CABRI trial participants: First-year results of CABRI (Coronary Angioplasty vs. Bypass Revascularization Investigation). Lancet 1995;346:1179-1184.
18. Kurbaan AS, Bowker TJ, Ilsley CD, et al, for the CABRI Investigators (Coronary Angioplasty Versus Bypass Revascularization Investigation): Difference in the mortality of the CABRI diabetic and nondiabetic populations and its relation to coronary artery disease and the revascularization mode. Am J Cardiol 2001;87:947-950.
19. King SB 3rd, Lembo NJ, Weintraub WS: A randomised trial comparing coronary angioplasty with coronary bypass surgery. N Engl J Med 1994;331:1044-1050.
20. King SB 3rd, Kosinski AS, Guyton RA, et al: Eight-year mortality in the Emory Angioplasty versus Surgery Trial (EAST). J Am Coll Cardiol 2000;35:1116-1121.
21. The BARI Protocol: Protocol for the Bypass Angioplasty Revascularization Investigation. Circulation 1991;84(Suppl V):V1-V27.
22. The Bypass Angioplasty Revascularization Investigation (BARI) Investigators: Comparison of coronary bypass surgery with angioplasty in patients with multivessel disease. N Engl J Med 1996;335:217-225.
23. Bourassa MG, Roubin GS, Detre KM, et al: Bypass Angioplasty Revascularization Investigation: Patient screening, selection, and recruitment. Am J Cardiol 1995;75:3C-8C.
24. Berger PB, Velianou JL, Feit F, et al, for the BARI Investigators: Survival following coronary angioplasty versus coronary artery bypass surgery in anatomic subsets in which coronary artery bypass surgery improves survival compared with medical therapy. Results from the Bypass Angioplasty Revascularization Investigation (BARI). J Am Coll Cardiol 2001;38:1440-1449.
25. Detre K, Holubkov R: Coronary revascularization on balance. The Robert L. Frye Lecture. Mayo Clinic Proc 2002;77:72-82.
26. Rodriguez A, Bernardi V, Navia J, et al: Argentine randomized study: Coronary Angioplasty with Stenting versus Coronary Bypass Surgery in Patients with Multiple-Vessel Disease (ERACI II): 30 day and one-year follow-up results. J Am Coll Cardiol 2001;37:51-58.
27. Rodriguez AE, Baldi J, Pereira CF, et al, for the ERACI II Investigators: Five-Year Follow-Up of the Argentine Randomized Trial of Coronary Angioplasty with Stenting versus Coronary Bypass Surgery in Patients with Multiple Vessel Disease (ERACI II). J Am Coll Cardiol 2005;46:582-588.
28. Serruys PW, Unger F, Sousa JE, et al, for the Arterial Revascularization Therapies Study Group: Comparison of coronary artery bypass surgery and stenting for the treatment of multivessel disease. N Engl J Med 2001;344:1117-1124.
29. Serruys PW, Ong ATL, van Herwerden LA, et al: Five-year outcomes after coronary stenting versus bypass surgery for the treatment of multivessel disease: The final analysis of the Arterial Revascularization Therapies Study (ARTS) randomized trial. J Am Coll Cardiol 2005;46:575-581.
30. SoS Investigators: Coronary artery bypass surgery versus percutaneous coronary intervention with stent implantation in patients with multivessel coronary artery disease (the Stent or Surgery trial): A randomised controlled trial. Lancet 2002;360:965-970.
31. Hueb W, Soares PR, Gersh BJ, et al: The Medicine, Angioplasty, or Surgery Study (MASS-II): A randomized, controlled clinical trial of three therapeutic strategies for multivessel coronary artery disease: One-year results. J Am Coll Cardiol 2004;43:1743-1751.
32. Morrison DA, Sethi G, Sacks J, et al, for the Investigators of the Department of Veterans Affairs Cooperative Study no. 385, the Angina With Extremely Serious Operative Mortality Evaluation (AWESOME): Percutaneous coronary intervention versus coronary artery bypass graft surgery for patients with medically refractory myocardial ischemia and risk factors for adverse outcomes with bypass: A multicenter, randomized trial. J Am Coll Cardiol 2001;38:143-149.

CHAPTER
24 Chronic Total Occlusion

Bernhard Meier

KEY POINTS

- Chronic total coronary occlusion is present in almost one third of patients with coronary artery disease, and it is the most common reason not to attempt percutaneous intervention.
- Clinically, a chronic total coronary occlusion imitates a 90% stenosis without its risk of causing infarction.
- The success rate for percutaneous recanalization depends on age, length, and anatomic variables of the occlusion.
- Complications are comparable to those of nontotal lesion angioplasty but usually not related to the occlusion itself.
- Stiff and hydrophilic-coated coronary guidewires yield the highest chance of successfully crossing a chronic total occlusion.

- The technical success rate after accomplished wire passage is more than 90%.
- The common approach to chronic total occlusions after the wire has passed is balloon predilatation with complete coverage with a drug-eluting stent.
- Sophisticated gadgets and techniques may enhance the success rate in selected cases. However, they are not free of complications and should be reserved for experienced specialists.
- The effect of using additional diagnostic tools (e.g., intracoronary ultrasound, computed tomography) on the success rate has not been examined, but it is assumed to be small.

ROLE OF PERCUTANEOUS CORONARY INTERVENTION IN TREATING CHRONIC TOTAL OCCLUSIONS

The initial "chronic" total occlusions tackled by Andreas Gruentzig, the pioneer of percutaneous coronary intervention (PCI), were those that had silently progressed from stenoses while the patients had been on the rather long waiting list for PCI typical for the late 1970s. The primary success rate was 62%.[1]

In contrast to interventional cardiologists, cardiac surgeons may prefer chronic occlusions to stenoses. Both require the same surgical technique, but the occluded coronary artery provides no competitive flow for the graft that may enhance its potential for attrition. Moreover, an occluded native artery will not cause a major clinical problem if the graft closes. The reduced risk aspect of dealing with chronic occlusions pertains also to PCI. However, the heightened intricacy of recanalizing a chronic occlusion rather than dilating a stenosis affects the indications for PCI. Chronically occluded lesions account for 20% to 40% of patients with angiographically documented coronary artery disease, but they represent only 10% of targets for PCI. Chronic occlusions remain the single most important reason not to attempt PCI in

favor of bypass surgery or medical treatment. It appears that better surgical program development means that less time is invested in recanalization of chronic occlusions by PCI operators.

HISTOLOGY AND PATHOPHYSIOLOGY OF CHRONIC TOTAL OCCLUSION

Histology

A chronic total coronary occlusion has several anatomic components.[2,3] An atherosclerotic plaque is invariably present as a major or a minor part of the luminal obstruction. Thrombus is the complementary element. There may be a single clot of uniform structure and age or layers of clots of disparate structures and ages associated with fibrointimal proliferation. The latter situation signifies the occurrence of prior thrombi from previous plaque fissures that might or might not have been totally occlusive. In cases in which they had been totally occlusive, these fissures were partially recanalized before subsequently re-occluding (Fig. 24-1). The most recent thrombus is assumed to obstruct the last lumen that had been patent up to the final complete occlusion of the particular coronary segment. The recanalization

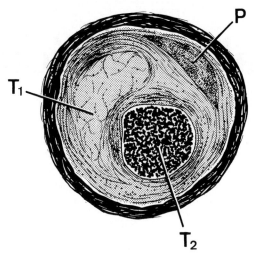

Figure 24-1. Schematic diagram of a cross section of a totally occluded coronary artery segment. There are thrombotic foci (T_1 and T_2) of different ages, indicating a first plaque (P) fissure with an organized and heavily fibrosed thrombus (T_1) and a more recent one causing complete occlusion (T_2). The extent of fibrosis of the most recent thrombus is the decisive factor in determining the chance of successful balloon recanalization.

equipment should be passed through this thrombus. The texture of the thrombus is crucial for success or failure of coronary angioplasty. The older and the more fibrosed a clot is, the smaller the chance to cross it safely.

Spontaneous recanalization of a totally occluded segment may occur by lysis of a clot, development of several new channels through the thrombus (intra-arterial arteries), dilatation of the vasa vasorum, or a combination of these mechanisms. Angiographically, such a recanalization can be readily distinguished from a total occlusion by the presence of antegrade flow, which may coexist with retrograde filling of the distal part of the vessel (demonstrable by angiography in case of ipsilateral collaterals). However, it cannot be discerned which of the aforementioned mechanisms is active for antegrade flow, and the situation is difficult to differentiate from a subtotal stenosis. Tackling a subtotal stenosis that had never been completely occluded before and that shows no collateralization creates the risk of an acute infarction resulting from abrupt vessel closure; tackling a recanalized segment does not. Conversely, it is usually easy to pass a subtotal stenosis with a coronary guidewire, but it may be tedious or impossible even with sophisticated equipment to pass a recanalized segment because the recanalization may consist of several tortuous microchannels in densely fibrosed tissue or be simulated by copious vasa vasorum.

Pathophysiology

Collaterals and Preservation of Myocardial Function

Well-developed collaterals at the time of the acute occlusion of the coronary artery avoid cell death of the subtended myocardium. Poor collaterals may still limit necrosis to the least perfused layers, usually the subendocardium. The performance of collaterals correlates well with duration of occlusion and initial lesion severity. In other words, collaterals are quite common in patients with long-standing coronary astery disease and subtotal stenoses of the vessel in question but are rare in young patients with mild coronary artery disease suffering an acute thrombotic coronary occlusion from a ruptured plaque rather than a significant stenosis. There is a greater propensity for spontaneous recanalization in the young patient with an occlusion based on an insignificant stenosis. They often present with a recanalized vessel but completely lost myocardial function. The typical chronic occlusion to be tackled is therefore one in an elderly patient with established coronary artery disease, complex anatomy in and around the occlusion, and a fairly well-preserved distal myocardium.

Collaterals and Ischemic Symptoms

A total occlusion that is well collateralized is functionally equivalent to a 90% stenosis.[4] It sustains myocardial viability but produces clinically apparent ischemia during periods of increased oxygen demand. Patients with a chronic total coronary occlusion, which was collateralized well enough at the time of the acute event to preserve part or all of the dependent myocardium, are likely to have exertional angina. They may also have chest pain at rest because of increased oxygen demand caused by spells of hypertension or tachycardia, but they lack the major risk of unstable angina (i.e., progression of a lesion to a total occlusion with ensuing myocardial infarction).

PERCUTANEOUS CORONARY INTERVENTION FOR CHRONIC TOTAL OCCLUSION

Rationale

Improvement of clinical symptoms or normalization of a positive exercise test together with a reasonable chance of technical success provide the rationale and ethical basis for PCI in chronic total occlusion.[5] Reduced left ventricular remodeling and improved survival have been observed after successful catheter-based recanalization. The most conspicuous benefit is a significantly lower need for later bypass surgery. Overall, the average left ventricular functional improvement after recanalization of chronic total coronary occlusions is not overwhelming and may escape detection by crude assessment. It is more likely to be found after recanalizing fairly recent occlusions.

Open-Artery Hypothesis

The debate continues about whether an open artery per se provides clinical benefit. The case depicted in

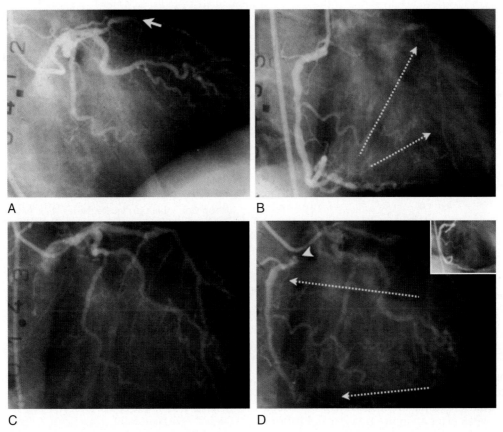

Figure 24-2. Lifesaving recruitment of reverse collaterals after 6 years of dormancy. **A,** Chronic total occlusion of the left anterior descending coronary artery *(arrow)* in a 58-year-old woman with preserved left ventricular function and stable angina pectoris. **B,** Copious collaterals *(dashed arrows)* from the mildly diseased right coronary artery. **C,** Successfully recanalized left anterior descending coronary artery. **D,** Complete occlusion of the orifice of the right coronary artery *(arrowhead)* 6 years later, with resurgence of stable angina after several years without symptoms. The collaterals *(dashed arrows)* had apparently been immediately recruitable because the left ventricular function was still normal. This time, they functioned in a reverse direction from the left anterior descending coronary artery that had stayed patent to the now occluded right coronary artery. Had the left anterior descending coronary artery not been recanalized 6 years earlier, the occlusion of the right coronary artery would have caused an infarction in the inferior and the anterior wall; the left anterior descending coronary artery would still have depended on the collaterals from the right coronary artery. This would not have been compatible with life. **Insert,** The recanalized right coronary artery.

Figure 24-2 may be anecdotal but provides compelling evidence in favor of recanalization. In an individual case, a recanalized artery may provide reverse collaterals to its former donor artery years later, thereby saving the patient's life.

The data available from registries and randomized trials are ambiguous, however.[3,6-9] Figure 24-3 shows the influence of success in a recanalization attempt in three large registries with various follow-up periods. Success has been most instrumental for the survival of patients with attempted revascularization of a chronic total occlusion in two independent registries (Table 24-1).

A first randomized trial from Japan showing a trend for improved survival pertained to recanalization of the left anterior descending coronary artery with a 5-year follow-up (Fig. 24-4).[10] Comparable trials, some not focused on the left anterior descending coronary artery, showed mixed results.[3] None of them unequivocally confirmed the positive results of the Japanese trial.[10]

The Thrombolysis and Angioplasty in Myocardial Infarction (TAMI-6) trial[11] randomized 71 patients within 24 hours of an infarction and had an 81% success rate and a 6-month follow-up period. There was improvement in left ventricular function, but the clinical end points were not influenced.

The Total Occlusion post Myocardial Infarction Intervention Study (TOMIIS)[12] randomized 44 patients 3 to 5 years after an infarction and had a primary success rate of 72% and a follow-up duration of 4 months. The left ventricular ejection fraction was improved by revascularization, but clinical end points were not altered.

The Open Artery Trial (TOAT)[13] randomized 66 patients with an occluded left anterior descending coronary artery about a month after myocardial infarction and had a 94% success rate and a 12-month follow-up. Although left ventricular volumes were increased more in the revascularized group, it showed a benefit in exercise duration and well-being.

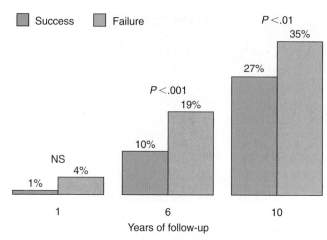

Figure 24-3. Mortality from three different registries with average follow-up periods of 1 year (Total Occlusion Angioplasty Study of the Italian Society of Cardiology [TOAST-GISE] with 286 successful and 83 failed recanalization attempts)[6]; 6 years (British Columbia Cardiac Registry with 1118 successful and 340 failed recanalization attempts)[7,8]; and 10 years (Mid-American Heart Institute, Kansas City, Kansas, with 1491 successful and 514 failed recanalization attempts).[9] NS, not significant.

The Desobstruction Coronaire en Post Infarctus (DECOPI) trial[14] randomized 212 patients (only 17% with an occluded left anterior descending coronary artery) about a week after an acute myocardial infarction to PCI or conservative therapy. The success rate was 96%, and the follow-up period was 34 months. The 6-month patency rates were 83% and 34%, respectively, and the left ventricular ejection fraction was slightly better in the revascularization arm. However, there was no difference in terms of death, reinfarction, or significant arrhythmias (9% or 7%, respectively), but a significant cost saving of 1000 Euros was calculated in favor of the conservative arm.

The Occluded Artery Trial (OAT trial) randomized 2166 patients to recanalization of a chronically *occluded* coronary artery (3-28 days) or to conservative treatment.[15] The outcome was not different

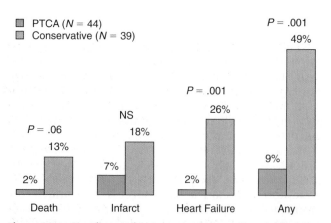

Figure 24-4. Significant adverse events during a 5-year follow-up after a randomized trial with percutaneous transluminal coronary angioplasty (PTCA) or a conservative recanalization attempt for a chronically occluded left anterior descending coronary artery.[10]

Table 24-1. Predictors of Long-Term Mortality after Attempted Revascularization of a Chronic Total Occlusion

Predictors	Hazard Ratio	95% CI
American Heart Institute (2013 patients)*		
Success	0.7	0.5 to 0.8
Age >70 years	1.9	1.5 to 2.4
Ejection fraction <40%	2.1	1.7 to 2.7
Double-vessel disease	1.5	1.1 to 2.2
Triple-vessel disease	1.9	1.4 to 2.7
Diabetes	1.4	1.1 to 1.8
Creatinine >2.0 mg/dL	2.2	1.3 to 3.9
Unstable angina	1.3	1.0 to 1.6
British Columbia Cardiac Registries (1458 patients)†		
Univariate Analysis		
Success	0.44	0.30 to 0.64
Age (per decade)	1.33	1.12 to 1.58
Ejection fraction <50%	2.33	1.58 to 3.43
Multivessel disease	1.62	1.09 to 2.40
Diabetes	1.50	0.99 to 2.27
End-stage renal disease	2.77	1.36 to 5.66
Prior chronic heart failure	1.73	1.10 to 2.76
Cerebral vascular disease	1.92	1.04 to 3.55
Multivariate Analysis		
Failure	2.27	1.56 to 3.30
Age (per decade)	1.33	1.12 to 1.58
Ejection fraction <50%	2.33	1.58 to 3.43
Multivessel disease	1.62	1.09 to 2.40
Prior chronic heart failure	1.73	1.10 to 2.76
End-stage renal disease	2.77	1.36 to 5.66
Cerebral vascular disease	1.92	1.04 to 3.55
Chronic obstructive pulmonary disease	1.64	1.01 to 2.67
Diabetes	1.50	0.99 to 2.27

*Data from Suero JA, Marso SP, Jones PG, et al: Procedural outcomes and long-term survival among patients undergoing percutaneous coronary intervention of a chronic total occlusion in native coronary arteries: A 20-year experience. J Am Coll Cardiol 2001;38:409-414.
†Data from Stone GW, Rutherford BD, McConahay DR, et al: Procedural outcome of angioplasty for total coronary artery occlusion: An analysis of 971 lesions in 905 patients. J Am Coll Cardiol 1990;15:849-856.

regarding death or heat failure but there was a trend toward more infarctions in the revascularization group up to 4 years. A substudy of this trial, the Total Occlusion Study Canada (TOSCA-2), focused on left ventricular function and also found no benefit from revascularization.[16]

An analysis of 11,228 patients treated with thrombolytic therapy showed that the mortality at 30 days was 1.5% if the artery was open and 6.3% if not, and this difference was maintained with an additional 2% mortality rate for both groups from month 2 to 12.[17] A reduced ejection fraction, on the contrary, was a significant harbinger of mortality in the first month (4.3% versus 0.9%) and during months 2 to 12 (additional 4.0% versus 1.2%).

It is important to recanalize an artery early after a myocardial infarction because most of the survival benefit is limited to the first month. Similarly, the vessel also needs to stay patent for a mortality benefit. In a respective study on 528 infarct patients, the long-term mortality rate was 20% if the recanalized artery re-occluded and only 8% if it did not (*P*=.002).[18] This difference was almost exclusively based on cardiovascular mortality (18% versus 5%, *P*=.0001). A

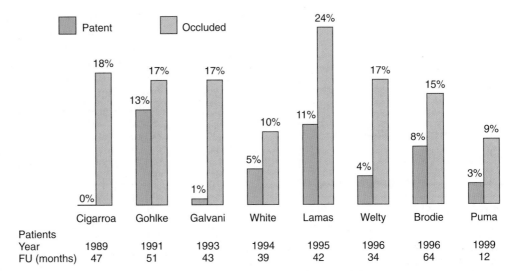

Figure 24-5. Mortality relative to the patency of the infarct-related artery in trials with various follow-up (FU) durations. (Modified from Sadanandan S, Buller C, Menon V, et al: The late open artery hypothesis—A decade later. Am Heart J 2001;142:411-421.)

	Cigarroa	Gohlke	Galvani	White	Lamas	Welty	Brodie	Puma
Patients Year	1989	1991	1993	1994	1995	1996	1996	1999
FU (months)	47	51	43	39	42	34	64	12

mortality benefit of an open infarct artery had been predicted by analyzing the mortality of patients included in the Survival And Ventricular Enlargement (SAVE trial), in which 12% had a patent artery and 23% had an occluded artery ($P<.001$).[19] Figure 24-5 summarizes the influence of a patent artery in a variety of trials.[20] These data are not applicable to a well-collateralized chronic occlusion that had not caused an infarction at the time it shut down.

Indications

Attempts at balloon recanalization of chronic total coronary occlusions are reasonable only if a vessel stump is visible. With an occlusion that is flush at the orifice of the vessel or tapering nicely into a small side branch, there is nowhere to probe for the occluded lumen. The indications for a recanalization attempt are based on a projection of difficulties (particularly duration and length of the occlusion) balanced against the potential benefit for the patient (current symptoms and limitation of activity) and the amount of viable myocardium at stake. The fact that a patient with a coronary occlusion is suffering to an extent to opt for bypass surgery if angioplasty is not offered is a strong argument in favor of a PCI recanalization attempt. Because an angioplasty attempt is less costly and less invasive than coronary artery bypass surgery, the indications need not be restricted to patients selected and ready for surgery if angioplasty proves impossible. Indications may be broad if the recanalization attempt is part of the diagnostic coronary angiogram, because a failure is less costly and imposes on the patient only a somewhat longer procedure. Indications are intermediate if the patient is still hospitalized. Indications should be restrictive if the patient has to travel or interrupt gainful activity to undergo the procedure.

In multivessel disease, the intricacy of recanalizing a chronic occlusion should be taken into consideration. Two or more chronic occlusions are too time consuming, with few exceptions. One or two additional nontotal lesions appear to be reasonable for a single session. If the vessel with the additional lesion provides collaterals to the occluded vessel, recanalization of the occluded vessel should be done first. PCI in the second vessel should be subject to a good result of the recanalization of the first. Occasionally, patients with a chronic occlusion of the right coronary artery are accepted for angioplasty of the left anterior descending or the left circumflex coronary arteries (or vice versa), disregarding the occluded vessel. Although published results of pertinent series have improved with judicious use of stents, the increased risk of interventions on the left anterior descending coronary artery when the dominant right coronary artery is occluded (or vice versa) must be underscored.

Indications for recanalization attempts of chronic total occlusions correlate reciprocally with the local development of coronary artery bypass surgery. The most aggressive country is Japan, where ratios of PCI to coronary artery bypass grafting (CABG) are overall very high. Even in Japan, they vary from more than 200 to less than 1 in individual centers, which invariably have different indication patterns for attempting chronic total occlusions.

Routine Techniques

Knowledge about the length of the occlusion and the course of the vessel at and distal to the occlusion is of paramount importance for a transluminal recanalization. A pre-occlusion film, if available, should be scrutinized before and, in case of problems, during the recanalization attempt. If the distal segment of the artery is filled by ipsilateral or contralateral collaterals, a late freeze-frame of a contrast medium injection into the donor artery showing the distal part of the occluded vessel can be helpful for guidance in conjunction with a freeze-frame of the proximal part of the occluded vessel showing the stump. Injections of contrast medium into the donor vessel during the recanalization attempt may be useful, but they require a second arterial access in case of contralateral collaterals.

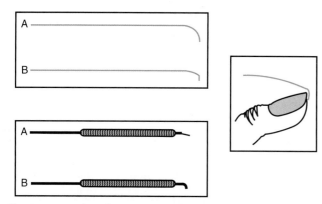

Figure 24-6. When the conventional J at the tip of the guidewire (A) becomes straightened out, it is useless. For difficult lesions (particularly chronic total occlusions), it is beneficial to add an additional sharp bend 1 to 2 mm from the tip of the guidewire (B). This can be achieved by using the thumbnail. It affords steerability even in tight lesions or with a support catheter far advanced.

Attempts to recanalize chronic total coronary occlusions call for adapted techniques and materials. Stiffer wires are commonly recommended and have succeeded in cases in which floppy wires failed. Advancement of the balloon catheter (or any support catheter) close to the tip of the guidewire for further stiffness is common practice. Inflation of the balloon in the stump for optimal support of the penetrating guidewire is a valid option in selected situations.

A simple but often crucial trick consists of custom shaping an additional bend 1 to 2 mm from the guidewire's tip (Fig. 24-6). Once inside the occlusion or with the support catheter far advanced, the conventional J at the tip becomes straightened out and is useless. Steerability is maintained exclusively by this additional bend. If a false lumen is entered, it may help to introduce a second wire and keep it away form the false lumen marked by the first wire (i.e., buddy wire technique).

It is recommended that the integral disappearance of collaterals be ascertained at the end of the procedure. In some cases, the final check for collaterals by an injection of contrast into the contralateral vessel uncovers a silent reclosure or a poor result, which may be amendable. Disappearance of collaterals that had been predominantly ipsilateral is more difficult to access. The watershed phenomenon typically seen in functionally occluded arteries with remaining minimal flow (i.e., contrast medium arriving antegradely and retrogradely and meeting somewhere in the vessel distal to the functional occlusion) should no longer be present.

Dedicated Techniques

Table 24-2 lists techniques developed for chronic total occlusion angioplasty. Some of them existed in the 1980s, and most were first used in peripheral arteries before being adapted to the coronary vasculature.

Conceptually, two approaches are most appealing. The first one, the laser wire, has been abandoned because of an unfavorable cost, intricacy, and risk-benefit record. The second one is the Frontrunner. It consists of a catheter similar to a myocardial bioptome that is advanced into the stump, where the front-end forceps is opened to spread the occluded segment apart. The idea is that the walls separate where they are softest (i.e., at the occluded thrombus), not unlike a butter sandwich being pulled apart (Fig. 24-7). The bulkiness of this equipment and the possibility of not finding the true lumen with this blunt dissection are major limitations that relegate this device to the niche gadgets. Some amendments, such as a bend at the tip and an option to regain the true lumen with a needle tip guided by intravascular ultrasound, have yet to boost its popularity.

Hydrophilic-coated guidewires have emerged as the most successful approach to chronic total occlusions. Equally important is a certain stiffness of the tip, which is often graded by the minimally required deflection force in grams. Hydrophilic-coated guidewires yield a significantly higher success rate than uncoated wires. Once across the occlusion, however, they harbor the risk of perforation of a thin-walled peripheral coronary artery while balloon and stents are manipulated over them. The operator has to painstakingly keep the tip of these wires within a large epicardial artery, never letting it out of sight. This risk of hydrophilic-coated guidewires represents their major drawback, which is not restricted to the realm of chronic total occlusion angioplasty.

Highly seasoned operators may employ the controlled antegrade and retrograde tracking (CART) technique for a particularly difficult recanalization with a clinically compelling indication.[21,22] It implies a retrograde passage of the occluded segment with a hydrophilic-coated guidewire advanced through a particularly well-developed collateral vessel from the collateral donor artery. The wire is subsequently shielded by a flexible vascular sheath. Although this

Table 24-2. Techniques Designed for Chronic Total Occlusion Angioplasty

Technique*	Principal Innovator
High-speed rotational smooth burr†	Kensey
Magnum ball tip wire	Meier
Low-speed rotational smooth burr†	Kaltenbach
High-frequency vibrating wire	Rees
Laser wire†	Several
Ultrasound recanalization	Rosenschein
SafeSteer/SafeCross small wire with optical coherence reflectometry/radiofrequency energy	Hartzler
Frontrunner spreading forceps	Simpson
Buddy wire technique	Katoh
CART retrograde pathfinder technique	Katoh
Crosser wire with relatively low-frequency vibration	Grube
Tornus crossing catheter	Suzuki

*In chronologic order.
†No longer in use.
CART, controlled antegrade and retrograde subintimal tracking.

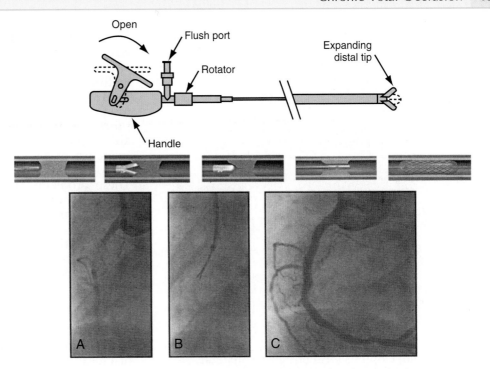

Figure 24-7. Frontrunner is a dedicated tool for chronic occlusion angioplasty. **Top,** Schematic diagram of the device. **Middle,** Schematic diagram of a recanalization, finished with balloon dilation and stenting. **Bottom,** Chronic total occlusion of a right coronary artery (A), recanalized with the Frontrunner (B), and an excellent result achieved by successful passage with the forceps device and adjunctive conventional coronary angioplasty (C). (Courtesy of M. Selmon, Palo Alto, CA.)

wire can often be passed back into the aorta, it is not recommended to grab it with a snare to produce a wire loop. There is a risk of damaging the collaterals or even producing a leak by such wire manipulations despite the protective sheath. The technique is recommended for transseptal but not for epicardial collaterals, even by its protagonists, and the retrogradely passed wire is used solely as a pathfinder. The final recanalization is done antegradely, with the retrograde wire providing a handy optical guide for staying in the true lumen or finding it back after a subintimal passage. The retrograde wire may also create an entry hole for the antegrade wire at the site where it emerges from the occluded segment into the proximal stump.

The "intelligent" recanalization system called SafeSteer or SafeCross is based on optical coherence reflectometry and is designed to distinguish the impenetrable vessel wall from soft occlusion material, thereby guiding progress. After years of poor acceptance, it has been upgraded with a radiofrequency penetration facilitator, and the name was changed from SafeSteer to SafeCross. Reports have been limited to its use in the peripheral circulation.[23]

The Crosser system features 20-MHz vibration generated at the outside end and transmitted to the tip of a coronary guidewire. This fairly simple concept has been successfully used in small clinical series.[24,25] Technical success was achieved in 63%, in cases conventional means had previously failed. These figures should be viewed in light of similar records of other new devices for chronic total occlusion angioplasty when first published and compared in a serial rather than randomized fashion with more conventional approaches.

The Tornus exchange catheter is a fairly straightforward idea.[26] Rarely, successful wire passage may be undermined by the impossibility of crossing the occlusion with a balloon. For this, a flexible metallic catheter with a spiral outer surface structure has been developed. It allows advancement through the occlusion with a screwing motion guided by the correctly placed coronary guidewire. Once across the lesion, the channel should prove to be sufficiently enlarged for passage of a balloon catheter in addition to the option for exchanging the coronary guidewire for a stiffer version before withdrawing the Tornus exchange catheter.

Intracoronary ultrasound has been advocated to help regain the true lumen in the case of a subintimal passage winding up in a dead-end.[27] This technique must be reserved for the few operators with a high volume of chronic total occlusion angioplasty and use of intracoronary ultrasound.

Factors for Success and Failure

Figure 24-8 depicts some of the major factors influencing the technical success of chronic total occlusion recanalization. The absolute figures are likely to vary considerably from operator to operator, depending on his or her determination and use of aggressive devices. However, the significance of the variables on success persists. Duration of occlusion is the key factor for success. The most rapid decline in the chance for success occurs during the first weeks after the occlusion. For nonspecialized operators, it is wise to accept only angiographically ideal occlusions (i.e., short, straight segment in a large vessel with a tapered stump) with a sound clinical indication in the case of an occlusion that is known to be more than a few

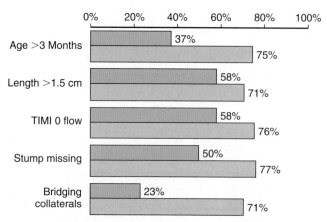

Figure 24-8. Success rates of recanalization attempts for chronic total coronary occlusions with *(green bars)* or without *(purple bars)* the most important risk factors. Depending on indications and revascularization techniques, the absolute figures may be higher or lower. However, the relative differences persist.

months old. Copious local bridging collaterals are an infallible sign of chronicity. The same holds true for the length of the occluded segment or the absence of a proximal stump. Venous bypass grafts with old occlusions should not be tackled.

Complications and Outcomes

The overall risk of angioplasty of occluded vessels lies somewhere between that of diagnostic coronary angiography and that of PCI of nonoccluded vessels. Statistically, it has been shown to be equal to general PCI.[5] This is reflected in Figure 24-9. However, the chronic occlusion usually is not directly responsible

for a dismal outcome but rather reflects the more advanced disease state of the average patient with a chronic occlusion. Many of these patients undergo additional treatment for nonoccluded vessels, or the occlusion has to be approached through significantly diseased coronary arteries. The longer duration of the procedure (implying considerably higher radiation and contrast doses) and the accidental closure of side branches or peripheral coronary arteries by distal embolization are at the base of most complications. These problems are multiplied several-fold by the default use of stents. Whether the risk of distal embolization can be reduced by filter devices has not been elucidated in the setting of chronic total occlusion. However, the negative outcomes of trials in acutely occluded coronary arteries is not promising.[28,29] The same holds true for aspiration devices.[30]

Mortality

Not a single death had been reported in the context of a recanalization attempt of chronic total occlusion until 1990, 13 years after the introduction of coronary angioplasty. Since then, fatal outcomes due to left main coronary artery dissections by the guiding catheter, retracted occlusion material by the balloon, inadvertent air injection during device exchanges, or coronary perforation or rupture have been reported.

Need for Emergency Bypass Surgery

The only conceivable indication for emergency bypass surgery is the occlusion of a not previously occluded coronary artery by inadvertent trauma or

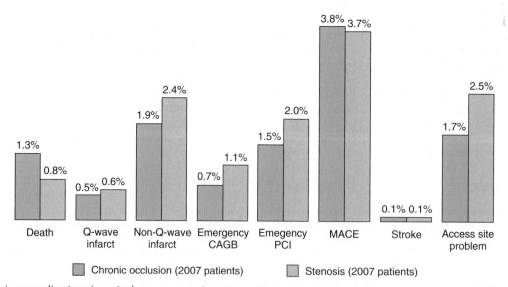

Figure 24-9. Major complications in a single-center experience over 20 years comparing patients who had an angioplasty attempt at treating a chronic total occlusion with patients who had an attempt at treating stenoses only (i.e., matched patient cohorts). None of the differences is significant. CABG, coronary bypass grafting; PCI, percutaneous coronary intervention; MACE, major acute coronary events. (Modified from Suero JA, Marso SP, Jones PG, et al: Procedural outcomes and long-term survival among patients undergoing percutaneous coronary intervention of a chronic total occlusion in native coronary arteries: A 20-year experience. J Am Coll Cardiol 2001;38:409-414.)

by an additional PCI attempt. The failure to pass a chronic total occlusion or its abrupt reclosure cannot create significant ischemia unless a collateral is destroyed in the process. In contrast to some anecdotal reports, this is also a prerequisite for significant ischemia in case of a reclosure of the recanalized segment during follow-up. Collaterals (unless secluded from the recanalized artery by a stent) remain reliably on standby for years, capable to work in both directions (see Fig. 24-1).

Infarction

The most likely explanations for an infarction in the wake of a recanalization of a chronically occluded coronary artery are the occlusion of a hitherto patent side branch or distal embolization of occlusion material. Both complications are compounded by stent implantation, which is routinely done today. It is unlikely that the use of sophisticated protection devices[28-30] is able to significantly prevent such problems.

Perforation or Rupture

Guidewire perforation of the occluded segment is usually harmless because the diseased, thick vessel walls seal spontaneously. Peripheral perforation with hydrophilic-coated guidewires in thin-walled, normal coronary artery segments may lead to tamponade, particularly if there are multiple segments. Rupture of the occluded segment due to balloon inflation or stent placement in a subintimal position or oversizing of the balloon because of overestimation of the nonvisible size of the vessel or inadvertent entry into a small side branch is fortunately rare, but ruptures are often difficult to treat. The use of bulky atherectomy devices increases the risk of rupture. However, these devices are rarely used in chronic total occlusions because they further complicate the technique of an already intricate procedure. Some of the ruptures drain into a ventricle and are clinically innocuous. Some close spontaneously or are contained in the muscle. Some can be remedied percutaneously by implantation of a covered stent to close the hole or to disconnect the leaking artery from the inflow. A noncovered stent may tack back a flap over the hole, but it may also increase the leak. Some leaks require emergency surgery.

Extensive Dissection

Extensive dissection is almost invariably seen after recanalization of a chronic total occlusion, particularly if the occluded segment was rather long. The entire segment is usually fitted with one or several stents to the end of a perfect final aspect. Randomized studies condone this approach because re-occlusion and restenosis are significantly reduced by

elective stenting of the recanalized chronic total occlusion (Fig. 24-10).

The high recurrence rates are a bane but should not be overestimated because many restenoses and occlusions are clinically silent and do not necessarily require reintervention. Nonetheless, there are high hopes for drug-eluting stents to improve on this picture. A first randomized trial (Primary Intracoronary Stent Placement after Successfully Crossing Chronic Total Occlusions [PRISON II]) (Fig. 24-11), comparing the sirolimus-eluting Cypher stent with its passive sibling in total chronic occlusions of 200 patients showed a significant reduction of the restenosis rate from 40% to 10% and of major adverse cardiac events from 20% to 4% with the Cypher stent.[31,32]

An even greater reduction in favor of an inactive stent (i.e., paclitaxel-eluting Taxus stent) was seen in 48 patients compared with matched controls, with a reduction of restenoses from 50% to 10% and of re-occlusion from 20% to 2%.[33] No dedicated head-to-head trials between the Cypher and Taxus stents have been conducted. In the all-comer Sirolimus Taxus (SirTax) trial, which included chronic total occlusions, there was no difference in the outcomes for this small subgroup.[34] In light of the relative innocuousness of a stent thrombosis in a previously chronically occluded lesion and the high relative restenosis rate of bare metal stents in this situation, it is foreseeable that drug-eluting stents may be used exclusively in the near future.

FUTURE PERSPECTIVES

Chronically occluded coronary arteries are a frequent finding in patients needing revascularization. However, the risk posed by the occluded artery itself with conservative treatment is low. Future cardiac events may be more common than in a population without significant coronary disease, but they are caused by progression of other lesions against a background of an extant occlusion rather than by the chronic occlusion itself. The yearly mortality rate is about 4% in the natural course of patients with a chronic total occlusion of the left circumflex or the right coronary artery. It is about 10% if the occlusion is in the left anterior descending coronary artery. Successful recanalization reduces this risk by one half.

The low primary success rate and the moderate clinical improvement to be expected with recanalization of chronic total coronary occlusions warrant moderation on the part of interventional cardiologists when accepting and treating these patients. Even if primary success can be improved by new technologies and skills, the clinical yield will never match that of coronary angioplasty of stenoses. As a comparatively low-yield intervention, percutaneous recanalization of chronic total coronary occlusions should remain low risk and low cost. This sets limits on how sophisticated, complicated, risky, and expensive tools and techniques for percutaneous coronary

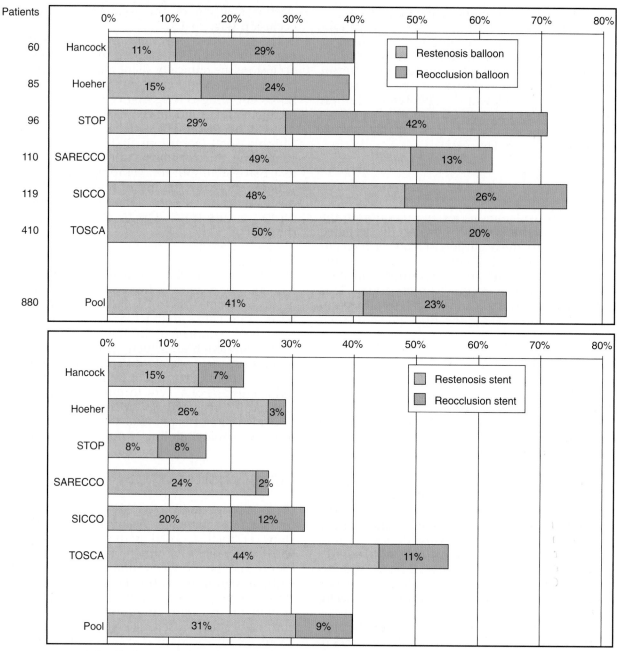

Figure 24-10. Angiographically determined recurrence after balloon angiography (*top*) or stenting (*bottom*) for chronic total coronary occlusions in randomized trials. The occlusion rates varied considerably in relation to the restenosis rates and accounted for more than one half of the recurrences in several studies. All studies demonstrated significant advantages for stenting.

recanalizations can become. Simple mechanical means have a fairly high potential for revascularization, are user friendly, and are associated with relatively little risk, and they are affordable.

The stiff or hydrophilic-coated wires have been the most successful tools for routine recanalization of totally occluded coronary arteries. They are the first choice at most centers. However, neither stiff nor hydrophilic-coated wires should be used by inexperienced operators unaware of their potential for proximal or peripheral dissection (stiff wires) and peripheral perforation (hydrophilic-coated wires), with subsequent severe ischemia or acute or

delayed tamponade. Niche devices such as the Frontrunner, the SafeCross, the Crosser, and the Tornus catheter will continue to be used at highly specialized institutions, flabbergasting delegates of live courses. The same holds true for techniques employing multiple guidewires, retrograde path-finding, or intravascular ultrasound guidance. The endeavors to improve equipment for recanalization of chronic total occlusions are likely to enhance the ease and efficacy of routine coronary angioplasty, just as the development of racecars favorably influences the performance of cars we drive to work.

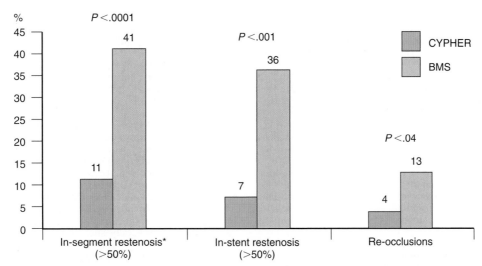

Figure 24-11. Randomized trial comparing the sirolimus-eluting Cypher stent with its bare metal platform (BMS) in 200 patients with chronic total occlusion. There is a marked advantage for the Cypher stent. In-segment restenosis *(asterisk)* is equal to the stented segment plus the proximal and distal 5 mm. (Data from Suttorp MJ, Laarman GJ, Rahel BM, et al: Primary Stenting of Totally Occluded Native Coronary Arteries II [PRISON II]: A randomized comparison of bare metal stent implantation for the treatment of total coronary occlusions. Circulation 2006;114:921-928.)

Uncritically stenting all recanalized occlusions and extending the stents from healthy margin to healthy margin are not warranted. Many ugly-looking recanalized segments were beautifully cleaned out during follow-up in the presrent era. Nevertheless, covering recanalized segments from beginning to end with drug-eluting stents has become the default procedure at most centers and will probably remain so.[35]

Some advocate the use of computed tomography to predefine an occluded segment before making an attempt at chronic total occlusion PCI.[36] A three-dimensional reconstruction picture of the occluded segments may be helpful, but the advantage of attempting PCI ad hoc during the diagnostic coronary angiogram and the quest to contain irradiation (already a problem with chronic occlusion PCI) will confine this technique to patients undergoing coronary computed tomography for reasons other than a previously detected chronic total occlusion planned for a PCI procedure.

The clinical benefit of recanalizing a chronic total occlusions may not always be immediately apparent. However, there is always a possibility that a recanalized vessel can save a patient's life when the prior collateral donor occludes and the myocardium is salvaged thanks to reversed collaterals (see Fig. 24-1). This may sanction (albeit late) a recanalization attempt that was frowned on at the time because of a questionable indication.

REFERENCES

1. Meier B: Chronic total coronary occlusion angioplasty. Cathet Cardiovasc Diagn 1989;17:212-217.
2. Aziz S, Ramsdale DR: Chronic total occlusions—A stiff challenge requiring a major breakthrough: Is there light at the end of the tunnel? Heart 2005;91(Suppl 3):iii42-iii48.
3. Stone GW, Kandzari DE, Mehran R, et al: Percutaneous recanalization of chronically occluded coronary arteries: A consensus document. Part I. Circulation 2005;112:2364-2372.
4. Flameng W, Schwartz F, Hehrlein FW: Intraoperative evaluation of the functional significance of coronary collateral vessels in patients with coronary artery disease. Am J Cardiol 1978;42:187-192.
5. Stone GW, Reifart NJ, Moussa I, et al: Percutaneous recanalization of chronically occluded coronary arteries: A consensus document. Part II. Circulation 2005;112:2530-2537.
6. Olivari Z, Rubartelli P, Piscione F, et al: Immediate results and one-year clinical outcome after percutaneous coronary interventions in chronic total occlusions: Data from a multicenter, prospective, observational study (TOAST-GISE). J Am Coll Cardiol 2003;41:1672-1678.
7. Ramanathan K, Gao M, Nogareda GJ, et al: Successful percutaneous recanalization of a non-acute occluded coronary artery predicts clinical outcomes and survival. Circulation 2001;104:II-415.
8. Stone GW, Rutherford BD, McConahay DR, et al: Procedural outcome of angioplasty for total coronary artery occlusion: An analysis of 971 lesions in 905 patients. J Am Coll Cardiol 1990;15:849-856.
9. Suero JA, Marso SP, Jones PG, et al: Procedural outcomes and long-term survival among patients undergoing percutaneous coronary intervention of a chronic total occlusion in native coronary arteries: A 20-year experience. J Am Coll Cardiol 2001;38:409-414.
10. Horie H, Takahashi M, Minai K, et al: Long-term beneficial effect of late reperfusion for acute anterior myocardial infarction with percutaneous transluminal coronary angioplasty. Circulation 1998;98:2377-2382.
11. Topol EJ, Califf RM, Vandormael M, et al: A randomized trial of late reperfusion therapy for acute myocardial infarction. Thrombolysis and Angioplasty in Myocardial Infarction-6 Study Group. Circulation 1992;85:2090-2099.
12. Dzavik V, Beanlands DS, Davies RF, et al: Effects of late percutaneous transluminal coronary angioplasty of an occluded infarct-related coronary artery on left ventricular function in patients with a recent (6 weeks) Q-wave acute myocardial infarction (Total Occlusion Post-Myocardial Infarction Intervention Study [TOMIIS]—A pilot study). Am J Cardiol 1994;73:856-861.

13. Yousef ZR, Redwood SR, Bucknall CA, et al: Late intervention after anterior myocardial infarction: Effects on left ventricular size, function, quality of life, and exercise tolerance: Results of the Open Artery Trial (TOAT study). J Am Coll Cardiol 2002;40:869-876.

14. Steg PG, Thuaire C, Himbert D, et al: DECOPI (DEsobstruction COronaire en Post-Infarctus): A randomized multi-centre trial of occluded artery angioplasty after acute myocardial infarction. Eur Heart J 2004;25:2187-2194.

15. Hochman JS, Lamas GA, Buller CE, et al: Occluded Artery Trial Investigators: Coronary intervention for persistent occlusion after myocardial infarction. N Engl J Med 2006;355:2395-2407.

16. Dzavik V, Buller CE, Lamas GA, et al: TOSCA-2 Investigators: Randomized trial of percutaneous coronary intervention for subacute infarct-related coronary artery occlusion to achieve long-term patency and improve ventricular function: The Total Occlusion Study of Canada (TOSCA)-2 trial. Circulation 2006;114:2449-2457.

17. Puma JA, Sketch MH Jr, Thompson TD, et al: Support for the open-artery hypothesis in survivors of acute myocardial infarction: Analysis of 11,228 patients treated with thrombolytic therapy. Am J Cardiol 1999;83:482-487.

18. Bauters C, Delomez M, Van Belle E, et al: Angiographically documented late reocclusion after successful coronary angioplasty of an infarct-related lesion is a powerful predictor of long-term mortality. Circulation 1999;99:2243-2250.

19. Lamas GA, Flaker GC, Mitchell G, et al: Effect of infarct artery patency on prognosis after acute myocardial infarction. The Survival and Ventricular Enlargement Investigators. Circulation 1995;92:1101-1109.

20. Sadanandan S, Buller C, Menon V, et al: The late open artery hypothesis—A decade later. Am Heart J 2001;142:411-421.

21. Surmely JF, Tsuchikane E, Katoh O, et al: New concept for CTO recanalization using controlled antegrade and retrograde subintimal tracking: The CART technique. J Invasive Cardiol 2006;18:334-338.

22. Rosenmann D, Meerkin D, Almagor Y: Retrograde dilatation of chronic total occlusions via collateral vessel in three patients. Catheter Cardiovasc Interv 2006;67:250-253.

23. Das T: Optimal therapeutic approaches to femoropopliteal artery intervention. Catheter Cardiovasc Interv 2004;63:21-30.

24. Melzi G, Cosgrave J, Biondi-Zoccai GL, et al: A novel approach to chronic total occlusions: The crosser system. Catheter Cardiovasc Interv 2006;68:29-35.

25. Grube E, Sutsch G, Lim VY, et al: High-frequency mechanical vibration to recanalize chronic total occlusions after failure to cross with conventional guidewires. J Invasive Cardiol 2006;18:85-91.

26. Tsuchikane E, Katoh O, Shimogami M, et al: First clinical experience of a novel penetration catheter for patients with severe coronary artery stenosis. Catheter Cardiovasc Interv 2005;65:368-373.

27. Kimura BJ, Tsimikas S, Bhargava V, et al: Subintimal wire position during angioplasty of a chronic total coronary occlusion: Detection and subsequent procedural guidance by intravascular ultrasound. Cathet Cardiovasc Diagn 1995;35:262-265.

28. Stone GW, Webb J, Cox DA, et al: Distal microcirculatory protection during percutaneous coronary intervention in acute ST-segment elevation myocardial infarction: A randomized controlled trial. JAMA 2005;293:1063-1072.

29. Gick M, Jander N, Bestehorn HP, et al: Randomized evaluation of the effects of filter-based distal protection on myocardial perfusion and infarct size after primary percutaneous catheter intervention in myocardial infarction with and without ST-segment elevation. Circulation 2005;112:1462-1469.

30. Beran G, Lang I, Schreiber W, et al: Intracoronary thrombectomy with the X-sizer catheter system improves epicardial flow and accelerates ST-segment resolution in patients with acute coronary syndrome: A prospective, randomized, controlled study. Circulation 2002;105:2355-2360.

31. Rahel BM, Laarman GJ, Suttorp MJ: Primary stenting of occluded native coronary arteries II—rationale and design of the PRISON II study: A randomized comparison of bare metal stent implantation with sirolimus-eluting stent implantation for the treatment of chronic total coronary occlusions. Am Heart J 2005;149:e1-e3.

32. Suttorp MJ, Laarman GJ, Rahel BM, et al: Primary Stenting of Totally Occluded Native Coronary Arteries II (PRISON II): A randomized comparison of bare metal stent implantation for the treatment of total coronary occlusions. Circulation 2006;114:921-928.

33. Werner GS, Krack A, Schwarz G, et al: Prevention of lesion recurrence in chronic total coronary occlusions by paclitaxel-eluting stents. J Am Coll Cardiol 2004;44:2301-2306.

34. Windecker S, Remondino A, Eberli FR, et al: Sirolimus-eluting and paclitaxel-eluting stents for coronary revascularization. N Engl J Med 2005;353:653-662.

35. Werner GS, Schwarz G, Prochnau D, et al: Paclitaxel-eluting stents for the treatment of chronic total coronary occlusions: A strategy of extensive lesion coverage with drug-eluting stents. Catheter Cardiovasc Interv 2006;67:1-9.

36. Mollet NR, Hoye A, Lemos PA, et al: Value of preprocedure multislice computed tomographic coronary angiography to predict the outcome of percutaneous recanalization of chronic total occlusions. Am J Cardiol 2005;95:240-243.

25 Percutaneous Intervention in Patients with Prior Coronary Bypass Surgery

John S. Douglas, Jr.

KEY POINTS

- Early postoperative ischemia (<30 days) is often caused by graft occlusion or stenosis, and percutaneous coronary intervention (PCI) is frequently feasible.
- Unstable angina or ST-segment elevation myocardial infarction (STEMI) years after coronary artery bypass grafting is most often caused by a saphenous vein graft (SVG) lesion, and native vessel PCI is preferred when possible.
- Intravenous thrombolytic therapy is ineffective in patients with SVG occlusion and STEMI; angiographic evaluation and primary PCI is preferred for STEMI after coronary artery bypass grafting.

- Embolic protection halves the risk of atheroembolic myocardial infarction during SVG PCI and should be used routinely in SVG PCI for de novo lesions.
- Multiple diseased or occluded SVGs, reduced left ventricular function, and available arterial conduits favor repeat coronary artery bypass grafting; patent left internal mammary artery to the left anterior descending coronary artery favors PCI.
- Drug-eluting stents reduce restenosis in SVGs and native coronary arteries and have become the default strategy.

SCOPE OF THE PROBLEM

Although the efficacy of coronary bypass surgery has been enhanced in this fourth decade of application, by the widespread use of arterial grafts, off-bypass and minimally invasive surgical techniques and although attempts have been made to improve graft longevity with antiplatelet agents, lipid-lowering drugs, and gene therapy, the temporary nature of the palliative effect remains a significant health care problem.[1-9] Severe myocardial ischemic syndromes occur in 3% to 5% of patients immediately after surgery,[10-12] and thereafter, recurrent ischemic symptoms appear in 4% to 8% of patients annually.[1-3] Progression of disease in native coronary arteries occurs in approximately 5% of patients annually during the first 10 years. Saphenous vein graft (SVG) attrition is approximately 7% during the first week, even with aspirin therapy; 15% to 20% during the first year; 1% to 2% per year from 1 to 6 years; and 4% per year from 6 to 10 years after surgery; at 10

years, only 40% of patent grafts are free of significant stenosis.[6-19] Although it is clear that arterial grafts are superior,[13,19-24] the limited number of arterial anastomoses that are possible mandates continued heavy reliance on venous conduits. Deterioration of native vessel and graft lumina after surgery results in an increasing need for repeated revascularization procedures.

At Emory University and at the Cleveland Clinic, reoperation was required in 2% to 3% of patients by 5 years, 12% to 15% by 10 years, and 30% by 12 to 15 years after an initial coronary bypass operation.[25,26] At Emory University, reoperative surgery represented 5.4% of coronary surgical procedures in 1982 through 1984 but 15% in 1991 through 2000. Regrettably, the results of reoperative surgery are not as good as those of the first procedure. Even in the most experienced centers, the risk of in-hospital death and nonfatal Q-wave myocardial infarction (MI) is triple that of the initial operation.[25,27] At Emory University, the in-hospital mortality rate for more than 2000 patients undergoing coronary reoperation was 7.0%; it was 4.6% for those younger than 60 years, 8.2% for patients 60 to 69 years old, and 10% for those 70 years or older.[27] In experience confined to the 1990s, the in-hospital mortality rate for reoperative surgery remained more than 7%, and Q-wave infarction, costs, and length of stay were higher than for initial operations.[28] Despite increasing age and complexity postoperative stay after repeat coronary artery bypass grafting (CABG) at Emory decreased significantly from 1985 to 2001, but in-hospital mortality remained constant.[29] In a report from the Cleveland Clinic, the mortality rate was 2.8% at 30 days.[24] In New York state, the in-hospital mortality rate was 4.1% for initial operations but 10.6%, 24.5%, and 38.5% for the first, second, and third reoperations, respectively.[30] At the Mayo Clinic, it was 12% for the second or later reoperations.[31] In addition to being more risky, reoperation was associated with less complete angina relief[31-35] and a reduced graft patency at 5 years of 65% for SVGs and 88% for internal mammary artery (IMA) grafts in patients undergoing recatheterization.[25] Reoperation exhausts the limited supply of graft conduits, restricting future surgical options.

These factors have promoted a conservative approach to reoperation[36] and favored use of percutaneous coronary intervention (PCI).[37-82] There are many symptomatic patients who are candidates for percutaneous methods who would not be considered for reoperation because of limited myocardium now in jeopardy, risk to patent grafts, lack of suitable conduits, poor left ventricular function, advanced age, or coexisting medical problems. Among 3481 patients undergoing their first CABG between 1978 and 1981 at Emory University Hospital, the 5-, 10-, and 12-year freedom from PCI was 0.98, 0.88, and 0.78, respectively.[26] In 1996 through 2000 at Emory University Hospital, approximately 15% of the patients who underwent PCI were patients who had prior coronary bypass surgery. It is in this complex group of patients, those with prior bypass surgery, that percutaneous interventional strategies have the broadest application.

INDICATIONS FOR INTERVENTION

Patients who experience recurrence of ischemia after coronary bypass surgery have diverse anatomic problems (SVG ± native coronary artery ± internal mammary, radial, or gastroepiploic artery graft lesions or subclavian artery stenosis) (Fig. 25-1), and selection for percutaneous intervention must be based on careful analysis of the probabilities for initial success and complications and for long-term safety and efficacy compared with competing strategies.[19,24,25,36,39,83-85] The status of the left anterior descending coronary artery and its graft significantly influences revascularization choices because of its impact on long-term outcome[20-24] and lack of survival benefit of reoperative surgery to treat non–left anterior descending coronary artery ischemia.[24,32-34] Factors favoring surgical revascularization include

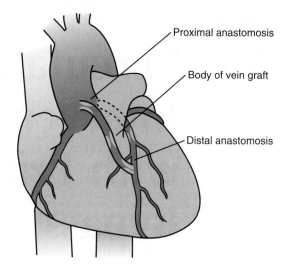

Figure 25-1. Sites of saphenous vein graft stenoses. All lesions between the proximal and distal anastomoses are considered midgraft lesions.

multiple vessel involvement, severe vein graft disease, poor left ventricular function, more total occlusions of native coronary arteries, and available arterial conduits (Table 25-1).[24] Because the choice of percutaneous methods and the relative effectiveness of each are often influenced by the time that has elapsed since surgery, indications are considered in relation to this factor.

Early Postoperative Ischemia

Recurrent ischemia within days of surgery is usually caused by acute vein graft thrombosis. However, stenosis may exist at proximal or distal anastomoses (see Fig. 25-1); the wrong vessel might have been bypassed; or the revascularization might have been rendered incomplete as a result of diffuse disease, stenoses distal to graft insertion, or inaccessible intramyocardial position of a recipient artery. To determine the cause of severe postoperative myocardial ischemia and define therapeutic options, coronary arteriography has been carried out within a few hours of surgery in 3% to 4% of patients in some centers,[10-12] and this strategy is recommended. PCI in patients with early ischemia (usually within 30 days) after CABG is a class I indication in the American College of Cardiology/American Heart Association/Society for Cardiac Angiography and Interventions (ACC/AHA/SCAI) PCI guidelines.[84] Although 44 (29%) of 145 patients catheterized early after surgery had no apparent cause for ischemia, most patients had correctable problems; 30 patients had emergency reoperation, and 44 underwent PCI.[10-12] Graft occlusion or stenosis was present in about 60% and incomplete revascularization in 10% of catheterized patients. In seven patients, focal stenosis was present in a venous or arterial graft distal anastomosis, and although balloon dilation across suture lines was safe in these patients, in our experience (Fig. 25-2) and in that of

Table 25-1. Significant Predictors of Method of Revascularization

Variable*	Chi-square	Odds Ratio†	95% CI
Number of diseased grafts (2 vs. 0)‡	133	0.01	0.01 to 0.03
Number of occluded grafts (2 vs. 0)‡	103	0.05	0.03 to 0.09
Prior infarct	98	37	18 to 75
Chronic obstructive pulmonary disease	82	0.02	0.01 to 0.04
Hyperlipidemia	70	0.11	0.06 to 0.18
Patent LIMA to LAD	57	6.6	4 to 11
Ejection fraction (50% vs. 40%)‡	46	1.3	1.1 to 1.7
Years from 1995 (4.4 vs. 1.5)‡	40	3.0	1.9 to 4.6
Native artery occlusion (2 vs. 1)‡	24	0.41	0.229 to 0.58
Years from CABG (15 vs. 6)‡	23	0.44	0.33 to 0.63
Maximum LAD stenosis (100% vs. 80%)‡	13	0.73	0.61 to 0.86
Maximum LMT stenosis (60% vs. 0%)‡	12	0.47	0.31 to 0.72
Age (73 vs. 60 years)‡	12	1.8	1.3 to 2.6
Unstable angina	8	2.0	1.2 to 3.1
Number of diseased vessels (3 vs. 2)‡	5	2.1	1.1 to 4.1

*Listed in decreasing order of importance.
†Odds ratio >1 denotes higher likelihood of percutaneous coronary intervention.
‡Odds ratio calculated for the 75th vs. 25th percentile for the respective variable in the cohort.
CABG, coronary artery bypass grafting; LAD, left anterior descending coronary artery; LIMA, left internal mammary artery; LMT, left main trunk.
From Loop FD, Lytle BW, Cosgrove DM, et al: Reoperation for coronary atherosclerosis. Ann Surg 1990;212:378-386.

others,[86-88] even a few hours after surgery, extreme care is warranted to ensure an intracoronary position of the steerable guidewire. Balloon sizing should be conservative because we are aware of unreported cases of suture-line disruption and severe hemorrhagic complications. Patients at increased risk for early postoperative ischemia include those undergoing minimally invasive and off-bypass techniques (e.g., surgery on the beating heart)[89,90] (see Fig. 25-2) and perhaps those receiving non-IMA arterial grafts.[6,90]

If a graft is thrombosed, the native vessel is often the best target (see Fig. 25-2A and B), even if it is an old total occlusion. If the native vessel is not a reasonable target, percutaneous intervention on the graft may be effective if thrombus formation is not extensive.[86] Thrombectomy with routine PCI equipment is sometimes effective.[91] The AngioJet thrombectomy device is a valuable adjunctive strategy, and there are a number of simple aspiration catheters.[92] Intracoronary thrombolytic therapy, although technically feasible and effective, has been reported in only a few patients within a week of surgery,[12,93-95] and significant mediastinal bleeding requiring drainage occurred in approximately one third of patients, warranting a cautionary note.[95,96] Whether the risk of bleeding with thrombolytic therapy is significantly reduced at 1 to 4 weeks after surgery, as has been suggested,[97,98] remains to be seen. Native vessel PCI with intracoronary stenting has been reported to be lifesaving in the setting of cardiogenic shock caused by perioperative graft occlusion, and the availability of drug-eluting stents (DESs) enhances this approach.[10,99]

When ischemia recurs 1 to 12 months after surgery, perianastomotic stenoses are one of the most common problems (Fig. 25-3). Stenotic lesions of the distal anastomosis of saphenous vein or arterial grafts can be dilated successfully at this time with little morbid-

ity and good long-term patency in 80% to 90% of patients.[39,53-75] Stenoses in the proximal IMA are rare.[54-56] Stenoses, or in some cases total occlusions, of the middle or distal portions of IMA grafts, radial artery grafts, and gastroepiploic artery grafts may be dilated successfully (Fig. 25-4), especially when a short occlusion can be documented. Stenotic lesions of mid-SVGs occurring within a year of surgery are usually caused by intimal hyperplasia, and these lesions can be dilated with balloon angioplasty or stented with little risk of distal embolization, but recurrence in about 50% of cases in our experience and periprocedural graft perforations have been observed.[79] Although lesions of the proximal vein graft anastomosis (i.e., aorta-SVG junction) have a high restenosis rate, long-term success for up to a decade has been obtained in some patients. Stents, directional atherectomy, and excimer laser angioplasty have all been tried for treatment of proximal anastomotic lesions, with excellent initial results but significant restenosis rates.[100-103] Few data are available regarding use of DESs at this site.

Ischemia 1 to 3 Years after Surgery

Patients with recurrent ischemia 1 to 3 years after surgery frequently have new stenoses in graft conduits and native coronary arteries that are amenable to percutaneous intervention. Whenever possible, native coronary lesions are targeted. Lesions in proximal and middle SVG sites can be instrumented with little risk of distal embolization within this time frame,[39,43,104] unless patients have diabetes or hypercholesterolemia, in which case atherosclerotic lesions may develop in vein grafts in place for 3 years or less. The ACC/AHA/SCAI PCI guidelines consider focal ischemia-producing graft lesions in patients 1 to 3 years after CABG with preserved left ventricular function to be a class IIa indication (i.e., "conflicting

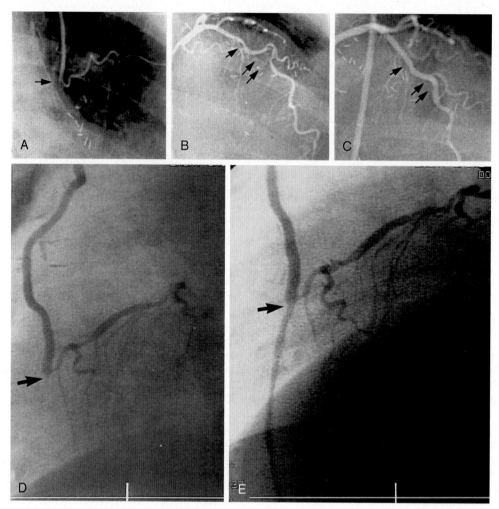

Figure 25-2. Two cases of failure of minimally invasive coronary artery bypass grafting treated with percutaneous catheter-based intervention. *Patient 1:* A 78-year-old woman who underwent intervention in the left internal mammary artery (LIMA) to left anterior descending coronary artery (LAD) through a left fourth intercostal incision without cardiopulmonary bypass because of refractory angina and a long stenosis of a tortuous LAD. Angina at rest recurred within a few hours after surgery, and angiography on the second postoperative day revealed occlusion of the LIMA graft about 4 cm from its insertion into the LAD (**A,** *arrow*). The LAD was tortuous, with multiple, severe stenoses (**B,** *arrows*), and left ventricular function was normal. Angioplasty and stent implantation in the native vessel yielded an excellent angiographic result (**C,** *arrows*) and favorable short-term follow-up. *Patient 2:* Because of disabling angina and a long proximal LAD stenosis, a 60-year-old man underwent minimally invasive LIMA to LAD intervention. About 2 hours after surgery, an electrocardiogram showed anterior ST-segment elevation, and emergency coronary arteriography revealed occlusion of the distal LAD at the graft insertion (**D,** left lateral view, *arrow*). Balloon angioplasty through the LIMA graft was successful (**E,** *arrow*), and the patient remained asymptomatic at the 6-month follow-up assessment.

evidence, weight of evidence/opinion in favor of usefulness").[84]

Recurrent Ischemia More Than 3 Years after Surgery

Beginning about 3 years after implantation, atherosclerotic lesions appear in vein grafts with increasing frequency.[105-107] Unstable ischemic syndromes are common, and aggressive invasive evaluation and therapy are indicated.[108,109] In 70% to 80% of post-CABG patients presenting with acute coronary syndrome, the culprit lesion is located in an SVG.[109,110] Atherosclerotic plaques in vein grafts are morphologically similar to those in native coronary arteries. They contain foam cells, cholesterol crystals, blood elements, and necrotic debris, with less fibrocollage-

nous tissue and calcification than is present in native coronary arteries.[107,110,111] Consequently, the plaques in older vein grafts may be softer and more friable, as well as being larger than those observed in native coronary arteries, and they frequently have associated thrombus formation.[106,112] Angioscopy may be more sensitive than angiography for identification of thrombus and plaque friability. Walts and colleagues[112] reported ruptured plaques with superimposed thrombus in 44% of SVGs removed at reoperation because of graft occlusion. Among 791 preintevention SVGs studied with intravascular ultrasound, 76 (9.6%) had ruptured plaques, and almost one third had more than one.[113] Atheroembolism related to graft intervention may have catastrophic consequences. Consequently, bulky vein graft lesions

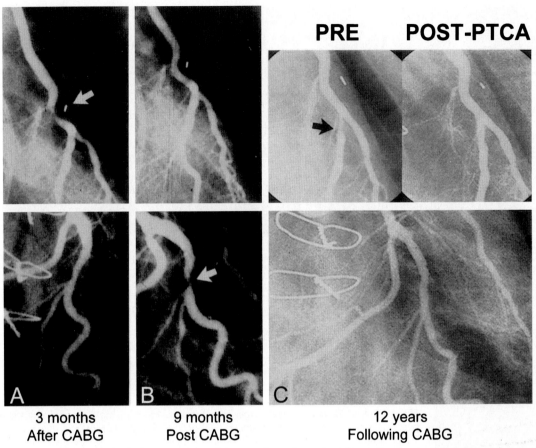

Figure 25-3. A 37-year-old woman had placement of saphenous vein grafts to the left anterior descending (LAD) and posterior descending coronary arteries. Unstable angina recurred 3 months later, and high-grade stenosis was present at the junction of the saphenous vein graft to the LAD (**A,** *top, arrow*). The circumflex coronary artery had minimal disease (**A,** *bottom*). The saphenous vein graft to the posterior descending coronary artery was patent. Balloon angioplasty of the distal anastomosis was successful. Disabling angina recurred 9 months after coronary artery bypass grafting (CABG). Coronary arteriography (**B,** *top*) showed a widely patent distal anastomosis but high-grade stenosis of the circumflex coronary artery (**B,** *bottom, arrow*) that was unresponsive to nitroglycerin. Balloon angioplasty of the circumflex stenosis was successful (residual stenosis of 5%). Twelve years after CABG, angina recurred, and recatheterization showed a high-grade stenosis of the mid-LAD just beyond takeoff of a large diagonal vessel (**C,** *top left, arrow*); the vein graft to the posterior descending coronary artery was occluded. Previous percutaneous transluminal coronary angioplasty (PTCA) sites at the distal anastomosis of the vein graft to the LAD and the circumflex artery (**C,** *bottom*) were widely patent. Balloon angioplasty of the mid-LAD was successful. The patient remained asymptomatic for 4.5 years, when a new thrombotic stenosis in the midportion of the saphenous vein graft to the LAD led to replacement of this graft with a left internal mammary artery. All prior PTCA sites were patent. Surgical benefit was extended over 16 years with three percutaneous procedures.

(i.e., those with a large potential atheroma mass) should be avoided unless one of the newer distal protection strategies appears anatomically suitable, and even then, the outcome is not predictable.

Although the mechanism of balloon angioplasty and stent implantation in older SVGs is similar to that in native coronary arteries,[111,114] elastic recoil of vein grafts may be a more prominent feature. Improved initial luminal outcome has been reported with stent placement and ablative techniques compared with balloon dilation in SVGs, and this has been attributed to reduced recoil.[115-120] However, long-term results in SVGs, even with stents, have been disappointing. Long-term outcomes with DESs in SVGs are not available.

At Emory University Hospital, reoperation is frequently recommended for severe disease of vein grafts to the left anterior descending coronary artery.

In contrast, the presence of a patent IMA graft to this artery may tip the scales toward percutaneous intervention in the right or circumflex coronary artery distributions.[24,39] This is a class IIa indication in the most recent ACC/AHA/SCAI PCI guidelines.[84] Percutaneous intervention is usually not preferred for multiple graft lesions, bulky graft atheromas, or thrombus-laden grafts, which represent a class III indication for PCI.[84] However, intervention may be indicated in highly selected patients (Fig. 25-5). Good intermediate-term outcome favors percutaneous intervention in focal disease of vein grafts supplying small to medium-sized myocardial segments, a class IIa indication[48,80,84,104,121] (see "Results of Intervention").

The role of percutaneous techniques in totally occluded SVGs is controversial.[97,122-140] Balloon angioplasty alone has resulted in high complication rates

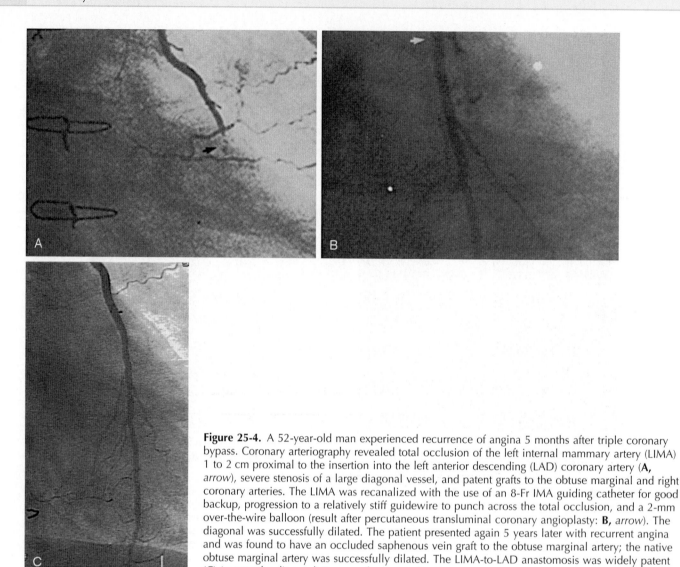

Figure 25-4. A 52-year-old man experienced recurrence of angina 5 months after triple coronary bypass. Coronary arteriography revealed total occlusion of the left internal mammary artery (LIMA) 1 to 2 cm proximal to the insertion into the left anterior descending (LAD) coronary artery (**A,** *arrow*), severe stenosis of a large diagonal vessel, and patent grafts to the obtuse marginal and right coronary arteries. The LIMA was recanalized with the use of an 8-Fr IMA guiding catheter for good backup, progression to a relatively stiff guidewire to punch across the total occlusion, and a 2-mm over-the-wire balloon (result after percutaneous transluminal coronary angioplasty: **B,** *arrow*). The diagonal was successfully dilated. The patient presented again 5 years later with recurrent angina and was found to have an occluded saphenous vein graft to the obtuse marginal artery; the native obtuse marginal artery was successfully dilated. The LIMA-to-LAD anastomosis was widely patent (**C**) (as was the diagonal) 5 years after recanalization.

and low patency in most reports.[133] Unfortunately, prolonged intracoronary thrombolytic therapy has been associated with thromboembolic MI,[122,124-130] hemorrhagic complications,[131,132,134] and relatively low long-term patency. The ACC/AHA/SCAI guidelines consider chronically occluded SVG to be a class III indication (i.e., "procedure not useful, may be harmful").[84] Somewhat more favorable results were obtained in nonocclusive thrombus treated with prolonged thrombolytic therapy,[141] with extractional atherectomy, and with rheolytic thrombectomy.

Although IMA graft lesions are rare at 3 years or more after surgery, graft conduits are frequently used to reach new native coronary artery lesions. Very old native coronary stenoses may present unique challenges because of fibrocalcific disease. Ostial lesions of the right coronary artery or left main coronary lesions may require rotational or directional atherectomy or stent implantation, or both. Subclavian stenoses are an under-recognized, treatable cause of post-CABG ischemia.

Acute Myocardial Infarction

After coronary bypass surgery, approximately 3% of patients experience acute MI annually.[142] Because these patients were excluded from early reperfusion trials, therapy has been based on clinical experience and remains controversial. Reports from the Myocardial Infarction Triage and the Intervention Registry and the National Registry of Myocardial Infarction-2 indicate that patients with prior bypass surgery have a high in-hospital mortality rate with reperfusion strategies,[143,144] probably attributable to the presence of multivessel disease, prior MI, advanced age, and comorbidity.[144,145] In 50% to 70% of patients, the culprit vessel has been found to be a vein graft, and considerable lesion-associated thrombus was a common accompaniment.[146-151] Intravenous thrombolytic therapy was reported to be effective in a small series of patients.[152] However, Grines and colleagues[147] reported a 25% successful reperfusion rate with intravenous therapy, and in the Global Utilization of

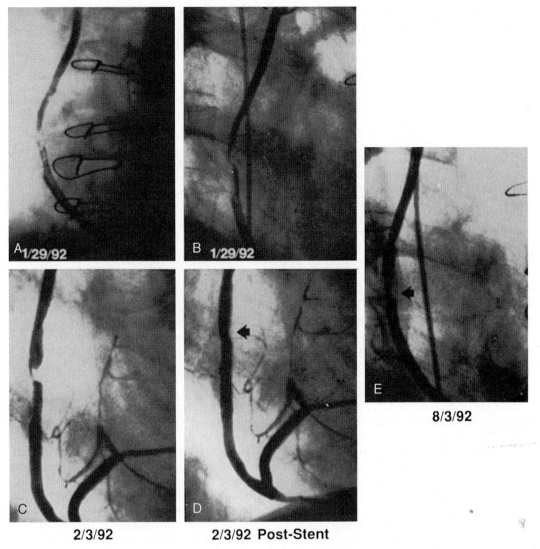

Figure 25-5. A 59-year-old man developed unstable angina 10 years after coronary bypass surgery. **A,** Coronary arteriography revealed a high-grade stenosis with thrombus and poor flow in a sequential saphenous vein graft (SVG) to the posterior descending and circumflex coronary arteries. No narrowing was present in the left anterior descending coronary artery, diagonal, and large anterior marginal systems. The inferior left ventricular wall was moderately hypokinetic. **B,** After infusion of 250,000 units of urokinase into the graft during approximately 1 hour, flow improved, and thrombus was diminished. The patient was maintained on intravenous heparin for 5 days. **C,** Coronary arteriography showed that an eccentric, high-grade focal stenosis was present in the proximal SVG to the right coronary artery without thrombus. **D,** After placement of a 4.0-mm Palmaz-Schatz stent *(arrow)*, the patient became asymptomatic. **E,** Protocol-mandated recatheterization 6 months later revealed excellent patency of the SVG with mild narrowing of approximately 40% at the stent site *(arrow)*. At last follow-up, 10 months after intervention, the patient remained asymptomatic. Although the outcome of this patient was favorable, the availability of AngioJet thrombectomy and methods of distal protection make a more direct approach appealing in some patients with extensive SVG thrombus.

Streptokinase and Tissue Plasminogen Activator for Occluded Coronary Arteries (GUSTO-I) trial, angiography at 90 to 180 minutes after thrombolytic therapy showed that Thrombolysis in Myocardial Infarction (TIMI) grade 2 or 3 flow was achieved in only 48% of SVGs.[148]

Many investigators favor emergency coronary arteriography if it is feasible and the option of more specific intervention, including subselective thrombolytic agents, thrombectomy, and mechanical recanalization.[147,151,153,154] Kahn and associates[153] reported their experience with 72 post-bypass patients who underwent direct PCI without antecedent

thrombolytic therapy at 5.1±4.0 hours from symptom onset. The angiographic success rate was 85% for SVGs and 100% for native coronary arteries. There were no urgent bypass operations, strokes, or transfusions. In-hospital survival was 90% (95% without cardiogenic shock versus 64% with shock). One- and 3-year survival rates were 89% and 87%, respectively. In the Primary Angioplasty in Myocardial Infarction (PAMI) trial of primary angioplasty for initial treatment of acute infarction, the infarct vessel was a venous graft in 45% of post-CABG patients, and the results were similar to those obtained in patients without prior CABG. TIMI grade 3 flow was achieved in 88%.[149] However, in a later and more complete report of 58 post-CABG patients treated with primary PCI for acute MI in PAMI II, the infarct vessel was a bypass graft in 55%, and outcomes were less favorable than for 1042 patients without prior CABG (in-hospital mortality: 9.4% versus 2.6%, $P = .02$; TIMI grade 3 flow: 70% versus 94%, $P < .0001$; 6-month mortality: 14% versus 4%, $P = .001$).[150] Stents, GP IIb/IIIa platelet receptor inhibitors, thrombectomy devices, and distal protection strategies were not used in this study. At the Mayo Clinic, worse outcomes were also reported in 128 post-CABG patients, about one third of whom were treated with stents and 12% with abciximab.[155] Watson and coworkers,[156] reporting outcomes for 21 patients who underwent PCI of SVGs, found high rates of mortality (19%), distal embolization (57%), and no reflow (71%), and the event-free survival rate at 6 months was 55%. The ACC/AHA Task Force Report on Early Management of Acute Myocardial Infarction classified primary percutaneous transluminal coronary angioplasty (PTCA) for vein graft recanalization to be a class IIa intervention that is "acceptable, of uncertain efficacy and may be controversial; weight of evidence in favor of usefulness/efficacy."[157,158]

TECHNICAL STRATEGY

The postoperative patient offers unique challenges to the PCI operator. Catheters are commonly threaded through conduits with unusual origins and courses to reach distal sites, and the targets are frequently rigid lesions known to be present for many years or bulky, friable SVG lesions. Selection of a guiding catheter to achieve coaxial alignment and provide adequate backup support is often the key to success. Figure 25-6 illustrates guide catheter shapes commonly used for vein graft interventions; 7-Fr catheters are favored for many vein graft procedures for optimal visualization, to facilitate stenting, and to accommodate large balloons and distal protection devices. In the presence of severe ostial lesions, when the guide catheter seating may be difficult or impossible, a diagnostic catheter and balloon-on-a-wire dilation catheter may be required. In this setting, predilation with a small balloon may permit subsequent entry of a large balloon, stent, and other devices.

Although some have recommended routine use of oversized balloons and stents for vein graft procedures, it is prudent to size balloons and stents as close to the normal reference segment as possible. This is especially true in older vein grafts, in which vein graft rupture has been reported with modest oversizing (see "Perforation"). Iakovau and coworkers[159] reported no benefit of oversizing with respect to target vessel revascularization (TVR) (31% versus 26%, $P = .3$), and the rate of MI was increased in SVGs (29% versus 17%, $P < .05$).[159] Many vein graft lesions are fibrotic, necessitating high-pressure balloon capacity (>15 atm); rotational atherectomy or a cutting balloon should be considered for undilatable

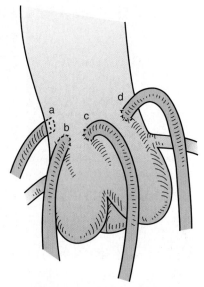

Figure 25-6. Selection of guide catheters for vein graft angioplasty. Obtaining adequate backup becomes more difficult in positions c and d. Selections include a multipurpose shape (a); a multipurpose, right Judkins (b); a hockey stick, left Amplatz, right Judkins (c); and a hockey stick, left Amplatz (d).

lesions.[160] In general, most experienced operators stent from "normal to normal" given the reduced restenosis of DESs and the observation by Ellis and associates[161] that nontarget lesion progression was an important cause of late myocardial ischemic events. When vein grafts are encountered that encircle the heart or in the case of IMA grafts to far distal locations, balloon catheters with extra-long (145-cm) shafts (or shorter guide catheters) may be needed, or the guide catheter can be shortened and a flared, short sheath one size smaller used to close the cut end of the catheter.[162,163] Directional atherectomy usually is not considered for SVG interventions because of the lack of benefit demonstrated in the Coronary Angioplasty Versus Excisional Atherectomy Trial (CAVEAT-II) (see "Results of Intervention"). Coronary stents are commonly used in aorto-ostial sites and in the shaft portions of vein grafts. Debulking before stenting aorto-ostial SVG lesions is probably unnecessary based on the results of observational studies. In vein grafts larger than 4 mm, peripheral or biliary stents have been implanted.[164] In SVGs that are 2.5 to 4.0 mm in diameter, DESs have become the default strategy because of reduced restenosis and target lesion revascularization (TLR) (see "Results of Intervention"), but long-term data are not yet available. Embolic protection strategies, a class I indication in PCI Guidelines for de novo SVG lesions, have been shown to reduce atheroembolic MIs by approximately 50% and should be used routinely in PCI of de novo SVG lesions.[84] However, PCI of restenotic SVG lesions usually does not require embolic protection.

The optimal treatment of complex and thrombus-associated vein graft lesions is controversial. Catheter aspiration of thrombus is sometimes feasible and should be considered.[91,165] The AngioJet, transluminal extraction catheter, ultrasound catheter, X-SIZER device, and excimer laser have been applied to reduce the thrombus and plaque burden before balloon angioplasty or stent implantation.[166-187] Some operators have administered intragraft infusions of a thrombolytic agent for up to 24 hours[141,180-183] or delivered thrombolytic agents locally with a special catheter,[184,185] and reduced thrombus burden has been reported with local administration of abciximab and by administration of a GP IIb/IIIa inhibitor plus an antithrombin for several days or Coumadin anticoagulation for 4 to 6 weeks.[186] Prevention and treatment of slow or no reflow in SVG interventions have been effective with calcium channel blocking drugs (i.e., verapamil or diltiazem or nicardipine in 100-µg increments),[187-190] adenosine,[191] and nitroprusside.[192] When no flow occurs after PCI of an SVG, catheter aspiration of the static column of contrast is sometimes effective in restoring flow (by removing atheromatous gruel), as has been reported in native coronary arteries.[193] In complex SVG lesions, systemic administration of a GP IIb/IIIa platelet receptor inhibitor is common,[194] but there are no convincing data to support this use (discussed later).

When it is necessary to pass a balloon catheter or stent from the graft insertion retrograde into proximal native coronary artery sites (Fig. 25-7), high-performance balloon and stent properties are essential, and changing to a stiffer guidewire after the balloon has passed the initial turn into the artery may be helpful.[195] Virtually all left and right IMA grafts can be approached successfully from the femoral artery. However, an ipsilateral brachial or radial artery approach may be easier in the presence of subclavian tortuosity or disease, or if there is difficulty seating a 6- to 8-Fr IMA guide catheter and especially if considerable IMA graft tortuosity or a distal lesion indicates the need for optimal backup support. A guide catheter specifically designed for right IMA graft angioplasty from the right brachial artery has been reported.[196] An over-the-wire dilation catheter is recommended for most IMA procedures and is strongly favored if a total occlusion must be recanalized or if retrograde passage into the proximal native coronary artery is required (see Fig. 25-7) or extreme graft tortuosity is present. Hydrophilic guidewire coatings are especially helpful in tortuous grafts, in which straightening artifacts and complete graft occlusion can occur with the use of stiff coronary guidewires. Spasm of the IMA can usually be prevented by prophylactic intra-arterial nitroglycerin, but refractory spasm responsive only to balloon inflations is occasionally encountered. After angioplasty, the operator must ensure that withdrawal of a dilation catheter does not cause the guide catheter to be pulled into the origin of the IMA, causing traumatic dissection. Use of balloon-mounted stents has been reported in left and right IMA grafts.[197,198]

In patients with significant subclavian artery stenosis (or occlusion), balloon dilation and stent

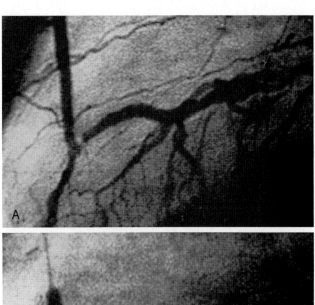
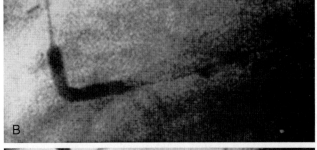
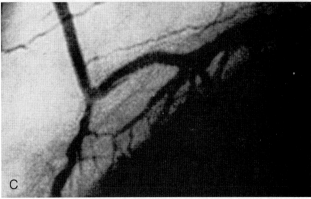

Figure 25-7. Four months after placement of the left internal mammary artery (LIMA) to the distal anterior descending coronary artery, angina recurred in this patient. Coronary arteriography showed a high-grade stenosis of the left anterior descending coronary artery (LAD) at a site just proximal to insertion of the LIMA graft (**A,** left lateral view). The LAD was occluded at its origin. With use of an over-the-wire system, it was possible to pass the steerable guidewire and balloon retrograde in the LAD (**B**) and to dilate the site successfully (**C**), resulting in relief of the angina. (From Douglas JS Jr: Balloon angioplasty: Matching technology to lesions. *In* Vogel JHK, King SB [eds]: Interventional Cardiology: Future Directions, 2nd ed. St. Louis, Mosby–Year Book, 1993, pp 79-88.)

implantation have been reported before and after coronary bypass surgery with a high success rate and infrequent complications, enabling the surgeon to use the left IMA for coronary bypass and improving symptoms in a patient with such a graft already in place[199-201] (Fig. 25-8). To enhance the patient's comfort during IMA graft or subclavian artery interventions, nonionic contrast media have been recom-

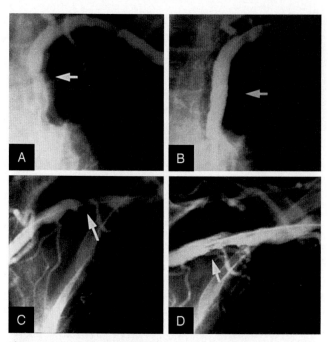

Figure 25-8. A 71-year-old woman with progressive effort fatigue and angina, a markedly positive dobutamine stress echocardiogram (i.e., drop in estimated ejection fraction from 60% to 35%), and a history of two prior coronary artery bypass grafting procedures (12 and 23 years earlier) was found to have a patent left IMA–to–left anterior descending coronary artery graft and a saphenous vein graft to the obtuse marginal artery. The right coronary artery and its graft were occluded. A 45-mm pressure gradient was present across the proximal subclavian artery, and angiography revealed severe stenosis (**A,** arrow). Blood pressure values in the arms were equal, and angiography of the right axillary artery revealed severe focal stenosis (**C,** arrow). Both lesions were treated with placement of 20-mm Palmaz-Schatz stents mounted on a 7-mm balloon catheter (**B** and **D** show post-stent results [arrows]). At follow-up, the patient was dramatically better, with no angina, improved exercise tolerance, and resumption of full household duties with none of the arm fatigue that had limited her previously. This patient illustrates that subclavian artery stenosis can be easily overlooked and that measuring bilateral arm blood pressures may not be sufficient to exclude this diagnosis.

mended; however, a blinded study indicated that ioxaglate, a low-osmolar ionic dimer, was better tolerated than the nonionic monomer iopamidol. Whether this improved tolerance resulted from a lower osmolality (580 versus 616 mOsm/kg of water) or other physical or chemical properties is uncertain.[202]

In patients with protected left main coronary artery disease, the fibrocalcific lesions encountered respond poorly to conventional balloon angioplasty, and although directional atherectomy has been used effectively, the most common strategy is stent implantation with or without prior rotational atherectomy. In patients with poor left ventricular function or a potential for ischemic hemodynamic collapse during intervention, intra-aortic balloon pumping may be used or kept on standby. Use of

in-laboratory cardiopulmonary bypass has been advocated for some particularly high-risk patients.

RESULTS OF INTERVENTION

Percutaneous Coronary Intervention versus Reoperation

Although early results from the National Heart, Lung, and Blood Institute (NHLBI) Registry indicated that an increased risk was associated with PTCA in the post-CABG patient, many subsequent reports, including one from the more recent NHLBI Registry, have failed to confirm this finding.[39-49,203,204] Procedural success rates of approximately 90% were reported even in the early 1980s, when 129 consecutive procedures were performed, with Q-wave MI in one patient and non-Q-wave infarction in four patients, with no procedural mortality.[39] At Emory University between 1980 and 1994, 2613 post-bypass patients underwent catheter-based myocardial revascularization. Compared with 1561 patients treated with reoperative surgery, in-hospital outcomes were more favorable for mortality (1.1% versus 6.9%, $P<.001$), Q-wave infarction (1.4% versus 5.4%, $P<.001$), stroke (0% versus 2.8%, $P=.27$), length of stay (3.0 versus 10.5 days, $P<.001$), and costs ($8500 versus $24,200, $P<.01$); in-hospital CABG was required in 2.9% of angioplasty patients.[205,206] The 10-year survival rate was better in the angioplasty group (62% versus 51%, $P<.0001$), in part related to large differences in baseline variables. Correlates of long-term mortality after angioplasty included ejection fraction, heart failure, age, graft intervention, diabetes, and time from surgery. By 5 years, approximately one half of angioplasty patients required repeated PTCA or CABG, and survival was better for patients who underwent native vessel compared with graft interventions (77% versus 68%, $P<.0001$), an observation not confirmed in the Mayo Clinic experience after correction for baseline differences.[85] Among 632 post-bypass patients revascularized at the Mid-America Heart Institute from 1987 to 1988 and observed for 4 years, patients who underwent angioplasty had a lower in-hospital mortality rates than did those who had reoperation (0.3% versus 7.3%, $P<.0001$), fewer Q-wave MIs (0.9% versus 61%, $P<.0001$), but more repeated interventions (64% versus 8%, $P<.0001$) and equivalent angina relief and 6-year actuarial survival rates (74% and 73%).[207] Improving initial and long-term outcomes were reported for post-CABG patients who underwent PCI at the Mayo Clinic over a 20-year period, perhaps related to improving technology and increased stent use.[85]

In 2191 post-CABG patients who underwent multivessel revascularization at the Cleveland Clinic between 1995 and 2000, 1487 had reoperation and 704 PCI.[24] Initial outcomes were more favorable with PCI for completeness of revascularization (89% versus 71%, $P<.001$), 30-day mortality (1.7% versus 2.8%, $P=.34$), periprocedural Q-wave MI (0.3% versus 1.4%, $P=.01$), and stroke (0.14% versus 1.69%, $P<.001$). In the PCI cohort, 30% underwent PCI of the left main coronary artery, 38% had at least one graft treated, 77% received at least one stent, and 7.7% experienced a non-Q MI (creatine kinase–myocardial band isoenzyme [CK-MB] level four times the upper limit of normal). At 5 years, unadjusted survival was 79.5% for CABG and 75.3% for PCI (P=.008). At 5 years, after adjustment for propensity score, PCI was associated with a hazard ratio for death of 1.47 (P=.09). The interpretation of excess mortality with PCI was hampered by the marked difference in baseline characteristics and small number of patients who could be matched. The only randomized comparison of PCI and CABG in patients after bypass surgery was reported by Morrison and colleagues,[208] who randomized 143 patients (67 to PCI and 75 to CABG). At 3 years, the survival rate was approximately 75%, comparable to the 5-year survival rate in the Cleveland Clinic study; there was no significant advantage of one procedure over the other.

An Emory University experience with 1712 diabetic patients who required repeat revascularization between 1985 and 1999 (1123 with PCI, 589 with reoperation) indicated relatively poor long-term outcomes. Survival rates at 5 years with PCA and reoperation were 62% and 61%, respectively (P=NS).[209] Advanced age and poor left ventricular function were predictors of mortality.

Vein Graft Angioplasty

Although PCI for native vessel stenoses has been firmly established and enhanced with DESs, conduit lesion interventions have been more controversial.

Many centers have reported favorable initial results with balloon angioplasty of vein graft stenoses (Table 25-2). In reports of more than 2000 patients, emergency coronary bypass surgery was needed in 0.3% to 5%, Q-wave MI occurred in 0% to 2.5%, and the overall mortality rate was 0.8%. The most common complication encountered was non-Q-wave MI, which occurred in 13% of 599 patients undergoing 672 vein graft dilations at Emory University.[79] Many of the patients in these early series had relatively ideal lesions that were discrete and free of thrombus. Subsequent cardiac events, however, were common. Even when balloon angioplasty of mid-SVG sites was deemed optimal in one trial, about one half required reintervention within a year.[210] In 599 consecutive patients who underwent balloon dilation of SVGs at Emory University, the 5-year survival rate was 81%, the MI-free survival rate was 62%, and the MI-free, repeat revascularization–free survival rate was 31%.[79] Restenosis occurred in 32% of vein graft lesions dilated within 6 months of surgery and in 43% of those dilated from 6 months to 1 year, 61% from 1 to 5 years, and 64% more than 5 years after surgery (P<.02). Restenosis occurred in 68% of proximal lesions, 61% of midvein graft lesions, and 45% of distal anastomotic lesions (P<.06). Survival at 5 years was 92% for distal lesions, 72% for midvein lesions, and 67% for proximal lesions (P<.0001). The best long-term results with vein graft interventions occurred with stenoses at the distal implantation site within 1 year of surgery; restenosis occurred in only 22% of patients, and late events were rare. The least favorable clinical outcome has been determined for PTCA of totally occluded SVGs. Kahn and associates[133] reported 3-year survival rate of 81%, and only

Table 25-2. Original Reports of Coronary Balloon Angioplasty of Saphenous Vein Grafts

Study	Year	Successful PTCA	Coronary Emboli	Emergency CABG	Death	Acute MI Q-Wave	Acute MI Non-Q Wave
Gruentzig et al[37]	1979	3/5 (60%)	—	0	0	—	—
Ford et al[38]	1980	6/7 (86%)	—	0	0	0	0
Douglas et al[39]	1983	58/62 (94%)	0	0	0	1	0
El Gamal et al[40]	1984	41/44 (93%)	0	1	0	0	2
Block et al[41]	1984	31/40 (78%)	0	0	0	0	0
Dorros et al[42]	1984	26/33 (79%)	0	1	0	—	—
Corbelli et al[43]	1985	43/47 (92%)	0	—	0	—	—
Reeder et al[44]	1986	16/19 (84%)	0	—	1*	0	1
Douglas et al[45]	1986	216/235 (92%)	7 (3%)	0	0	1	15 (7%)
Cote et al[46]	1987	86/101 (85%)	2 (2%)	3 (1.3%)	0	1	—
Pinkerton et al[49]	1988	93/100 (93%)	—	1	—	—	—
Dorros et al[50]	1988	44/53 (83%)	3 (6%)	—	1	1	—
Reed et al[51]	1989	47/52 (90%)	0	—	0	0	0
Cooper et al[52]	1989	18/24 (75%)	—	—	1*	—	—
Platko et al[77]	1989	92/101 (92%)	—	0	1 (1%)	—	—
Plokker et al[78]	1991	409/454 (90%)	—	4 (4%)	3 (0.7%)	—	—
Douglas et al[79]	1991	539/599 (90%)	—	6 (1.3%)	7 (1.2%)	15 (2.5%)	79 (13%)
Miranda et al[104]	1992	410/440 (93%)	—	21 (3.5%)	5 (1.1%)	†	†
Morrison et al[105]	1994	70/75 (93%)	0	†	3%	3%‡	—

*Both patients had intractable congestive heart failure after PTCA of occluded vein grafts.
†A total of 19 patients (5%) had acute MI or urgent CABG or died.
‡Myocardial infarction was not defined.
CABG, coronary artery bypass grafting; MI, myocardial infarction; PTCA, percutaneous transluminal coronary angioplasty.

33% of these patients were free of repeated PTCA or surgery.

Vein Graft Atheroablation

In an attempt to improve outcome of interventions in SVGs, directional atherectomy was performed initially in observational trials with encouraging results.[117,118] However, in the Emory experience treating mostly bulky lesions, 48% experienced non-Q-wave MI.[189] In a randomized multicenter trial of coronary angioplasty versus directional atherectomy for SVG lesions (CAVEAT-II) involving approximately 300 patients, atherectomy was associated with more complications, higher cost, and similar restenosis at 6 months (45% for directional atherectomy versus 50% for PTCA, $P=.49$).[211,212] These factors resulted in a decreased use of directional atherectomy for de novo and restenotic lesions of mid-saphenous vein lesions, for which restenosis rates of 80% have been reported.[118,120]

Excimer laser angioplasty of SVGs has been reported in several large, multicenter trials. In more than 500 lesions, Bittl and colleagues[213] had clinical success in 92%, with in-hospital deaths of 1%, CABG in 1.6%, Q-wave MI in 2.4%, and non-Q-wave infarction in 2.2% of patients. Adjunctive balloon angioplasty was used in 91%, and none of the patients received stents. Predictors of complication-free success were aorto-ostial location, short lesions, and SVG diameter less than 3 mm.[214-216] In 106 consecutive patients subjected to quantitative analysis of procedural and follow-up angiograms, restenosis was identified in 52%, with approximately one half having total occlusion, and the 1-year mortality rate was 9%.[217] These observational results have not supported widespread applications of excimer laser angioplasty in SVG lesions. However, this technology has been used with favorable results to debulk complex lesions before stent implantation. Using this strategy, Hong and coworkers[218] reported 100% procedural success, a 9% rate of non-Q-wave MI, and zero instances of no reflow in 81 patients with degenerated and thrombotic graft lesions.

The extraction atherectomy catheter has been used in a somewhat similar fashion to treat complex vein graft lesions. Application of the this device in 58 thrombotic SVG lesions resulted in less favorable in-hospital outcome than in 125 thrombus-free lesions (clinical success: 69% versus 88%, $P=.01$; higher no reflow: 19% versus 5%) and more complications but comparable restenosis rates of 65%.[171] In the New Approaches to Coronary Intervention (NACI) Registry, experience with 127 extraction atherectomy catheter procedures, distal coronary embolization occurred in 15% of patients, and more than a third of these patients died.[168] Although it has been observed by angioscopy that thrombus removal from the treatment site was relatively complete with use of the this device,[177,178] distal embolization was common, as evidenced by the development of non-Q-wave MI in a significant number of patients. Using

this device to pretreat complex vein graft lesions in 36 patients before stent implantation, Hong and colleagues[218] reported 100% procedural success, 15% rate of non-Q-wave MI, 2.2% rate of no reflow, and 2.9% rate of abrupt closure. Khan and associates[173] reported short-term outcomes for 84 patients with high-risk SVG lesions, noting CK-MB elevations in 50% and no apparent benefit of abciximab in an observational study. The use of this device has been associated with significant complications and cost without proven benefit.

Stone and coworkers[174] reported outcomes of the use of the X-SIZER (ev3, Plymouth, MN) in a randomized trial in 839 diseased SVGs or thrombus-containing native coronary lesions. Major adverse cardiac events (MACEs) were not reduced (16.8% versus 17.1%, $P=.92$), but the occurrence of large MI was reduced from 9.6% to 5.5% ($P=.002$). This device has been approved by the U.S. Food and Drug Administration (FDA) for peripheral vascular intervention.

Bare Metal Stents

Many different stent designs have been used in SVGs (Table 25-3), and newer stents are being evaluated. The self-expanding Wallstent in early experience resulted in successful deployment in more than 95% of patients, but stent thrombosis was reported in up to 10% of patients and restenosis in up to 50%.[226-229] In 62 patients with 93 stent implantations, de Jaegere and colleagues[228] determined an initial clinical success rate of 89% and complication rate of 11%, including an MI rate of 3%, CABG rate of 5%, and in-hospital death rate of 3%. Follow-up of these patients revealed an event-free survival rate of 46% at 1 year and only 30% at 5 years. Safian and associates[232] reported an initial success rate of 95% for 114 patients and, in a randomized format, outcomes similar to those obtained with slotted tubular stent design. In an experience with the Wallstent in 440 patients with degenerated SVGs, Choussat and coworkers[229] reported a 3% initial mortality rate; 9% experienced MI, and the 3-year event-free survival rate was 42%.

Use of the Palmaz-Schatz coronary stent in SVGs has been reported in observational registries,[222,238-241] in nonrandomized comparative studies,[208,223,242] and in a randomized trial comparing balloon angioplasty with stents[224] (Fig. 25-9). The multicenter registry of the use of the Palmaz-Schatz stent in the United States enrolled 589 patients and reported procedural success in 97%, stent thrombosis in 1.4%, in-hospital mortality in 1.7%, Q-wave MI in 0.3%, and urgent bypass surgery in 0.9%.[223] The restenosis rate at 6 months was 18% for de novo lesions and 46% for those with prior procedures, and the 12-month event-free survival rate was 76%. These results were somewhat more favorable than in the subsequent randomized trial and those reported with the Wiktor stent.[230,231] For 290 diabetic patients who underwent SVG stenting with the Palmaz-Schatz stent, in-hospital and late mortality rates were higher than for

Table 25-3. Results of Stenting of Aortocoronary Saphenous Vein Grafts: Selected Reports of 50 or More Patients without the Use of Drug-Eluting Stents

Study	Year	Implantation Success	Early Thromb. (%)	CABG (%)	Death (%)	Acute MI (%)	Restenosis (%)
Palmaz-Schatz stent							
Pomerantz et al[117]	1992	83/84 (99%)	0	0	0	10	36
Carrozza et al[220]	1992	84/84 (100%)	0	0	8	—	—
Fenton et al[221]	1994	196/198 (99%)	0.5	—	—	—	34
Piana et al[222]	1994	147/150 (98%)	1	0	1	7.3	17
Wong et al[223]	1995	571/589 (97%)	1.4	0.9	1.7	0.3	30
Savage et al[224]	1997	105/108 (97%)	1	2	2	4	36
Ahmed et al[225]	2000						
Diabetic		276/290 (95%)	1.2	1.3	2.2	16	TVR: 17
Nondiabetic		604/618 (98%)	1.6	0.6	0.3	20	TVR: 23
Wallstent							
de Scheerder et al[226]	1992	69/69 (100%)	10	0	1.5	7	47
Strauss et al[227]	1992	145/145 (100%)	8	—	—	—	34
de Jaegere et al[228]*	1996	92/93 (99%)	4	5	3	3	—
Choussat et al[229]	2000	126/126 (100%)	0	0	3	9	TVR: 22
Wiktor Stent							
Fortuna et al[230]	1993	101/101 (100%)	2	1	1	3	—
Hanekamp et al[231]	2000	77/78 (99%)	—	—	—	—	22
Various Stents							
Safian et al[232]	1998						
Palmaz-Schatz		101/101 (100%)	—	—	—	—	32
Wallstent		109/114 (95%)	—	—	—	—	13
Wallstent (SVG>4 mm)		197/207 (95%)	—	—	—	—	39
Le May et al[233]	1999	103/106 (98%)	0	0	0	—	—
Dharmadhikari et al[234]	2000						
Covered stents		30	—	3	0	0	Revasc: 20
Noncovered stents		125	—	0	0	8.8	Revasc: 28
Baldus et al[235]†	2000	108/109 (99%)	0.9	0	0	1	26
Nishida et al[236]	2000	97/101 (96%)	—	2	1	10.9	TVR: 21
Bhargava et al[237]	2000	711/719 (99%)	0.7	0.9	1.3	23	TVR: 19
Ashfaq et al[247]	2006	993/1045 (95%)	—	—	0.8	0.7	—
Hong et al[243]‡	2001	925/964 (96%)	—	0.8	2.2	19	TVR: 16
Keeley et al[244]§	2001	—/1062	—	3.0	8	11	Stent: 29 Nonstent: 42

*Ninety percent were Wallstents.
†All were covered stents.
‡In the 1995-1998 experience, 65% of patients received stents.
§Forty-two percent of patients received stents.
CABG, coronary artery bypass grafting; MI, myocardial infarction; Revasc, revascularization; SVG, saphenous vein graft; Thromb., thrombosis; TVR, target vessel revascularization.

nondiabetics, and at 1 year, the rate for TLR was higher and that for event-free survival lower.[225]

Optimal balloon angioplasty of mid-SVG lesions (<20% residual narrowing) in 48 patients was compared with stent implantation in 41 contemporaneously treated but not randomized patients, showing more favorable late outcomes with stenting: mortality in 2.4% versus 8.3% ($P=NS$) and repeated revascularization in 4.9% versus 35% ($P<.01$).[210] Treatment of aorto-ostial SVG lesions with Palmaz-Schatz stenting in 20 patients resulted in restenosis in 7 (35%),[240] and the event-free survival rate at approximately 1 year was 82% for 29 patients with unstable myocardial ischemic presentations.[239] Ahmed and colleagues,[241] who reported outcomes for 320 consecutive patients who underwent stenting of SVG aorto-ostial lesion, 43% of whom had debulking (laser or atherectomy) before stent implantation, found that debulking before stenting afforded no benefit regarding complications (2.2% versus 2.6%), 1-year TLR (19% versus 18%), or cardiac event–free survival (69% versus 68%).[241]

A total of 220 patients with new SVG lesions and angina pectoris or objective evidence of myocardial ischemia were randomly assigned to implantation of Palmaz-Schatz stents or to standard balloon angioplasty in the Saphenous Vein De Novo (SAVED) trial.[224] Patients with a lesion length greater than two stents, MI within 7 days, or evidence of intragraft thrombus were excluded. Patients stented primarily or as a bailout procedure received warfarin anticoagulation. Characteristics of the patients and lesions in the two groups were similar, except the angioplasty group had more diabetes (36% versus 23%, $P=.05$). Patients assigned to stenting had a higher rate of procedural efficacy, defined as a reduction of stenosis to less than 50% of the vessel diameter with the assigned therapy, than did those assigned to angioplasty (92% versus 69%, $P<.001$) (see Fig. 25-9) but experienced more hemorrhagic complications result-

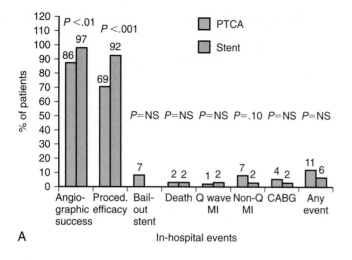

A In-hospital events

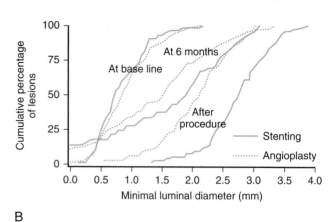

B

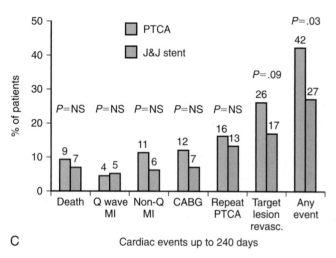

C Cardiac events up to 240 days

Figure 25-9. Results from the Saphenous Vein De Novo (SAVED) trial, a randomized comparison of Palmaz-Schatz stenting and standard balloon angioplasty. **A,** Stents were associated with a higher procedural success rate, whereas other in-hospital events were similar. **B,** The minimal luminal diameter at 6 months was larger in the stent group (1.73 versus 1.49 mm, P=.01). **C,** Late cardiac events were significantly more common in patients in the percutaneous transluminal coronary angioplasty group. (**B,** From Savage MP, Douglas JS Jr, Fischman DL, et al: Stent placement compared with balloon angioplasty for obstructed coronary bypass grafts. Saphenous Vein De novo Trial Investigators. N Engl J Med 1997;337:740-747.)

ing from warfarin anticoagulation. In-hospital complications were otherwise similar in the two groups, although there was a trend toward fewer non-Q-wave infarctions in the stent group. Whether stents have a significant effect in reducing particulate matter embolization is not certain, but it is a possible explanation for this trend. Patients randomized to stents had a larger increase in lumen diameter immediately (1.92 versus 1.21 mm, P<.001) and a greater net gain in lumen diameter at 6 months (0.85 versus 0.54 mm, P=.002). Restenosis occurred in 37% of the stented patients and in 46% of the angioplasty group (P=.24). Late lumen loss was significantly greater in patients who received high-pressure (≥16 atm) stent expansion, suggesting that routine high pressure may be undesirable in SVG stenting. The higher than expected restenosis rate observed in the SAVED stent patients compared with approximately 20% in registry experience is similar to results from the Stent Restenosis Study (STRESS) and U.S. multicenter stent registry in native coronary arteries, for which there also was a discordance between registry and randomized outcomes, including restenosis, suggesting a

bias toward favorable outcomes in observational registries.

The outcome in the SAVED trial with respect to freedom from death, MI, repeated bypass surgery, or revascularization was significantly better in the stent group (73% versus 58%, P=.03).[224] The lack of a significant difference in restenosis rates in the treatment groups was caused by the greater late lumen loss in the stent group (1.1 versus 0.66 mm, P<.01) and the small sample size. The 9% difference in restenosis rates in the SAVED trial approaches that observed in the STRESS and Belgium Netherlands Stent (BENESTENT) trials of stenting in native coronary arteries. The larger late lumen loss with stents emphasized the need for effective antiproliferative strategies. Using the Palmaz-Schatz biliary stent, Wong and coworkers[223] treated 124 patients with 163 SVG lesions with 94% clinical success, one bypass operation, and no Q-wave infarctions or deaths, results comparable to those obtained with the coronary stent in smaller vein grafts.

Several centers have reported outcomes of more contemporary SVG interventions but performed before embolic protection. Comparing the outcomes of 1990-1994 patients with those of the 1995-1998 patients, Hong and colleagues[243] reported similar initial success rates but improved 1-year event-free survival in the more recent experience (71% versus 59%, $P<.0001$) and a lower late mortality rate (6.1% versus 11.3%, $P<.0001$) and a protective effect of stent implantation in both time periods. However, in 1062 patients treated at William Beaumont Hospital from 1993 to 1997, the results were sobering; 89 died in the hospital (8%), and at 3 ± 1 years, another 92 patients had died (9%), and event-free survival was 47%.[244] At a median follow-up of 18 months at the Ottawa Heart Institute, only 44% of patients experienced event-free survival.[233] In a pooled analysis of 627 patients who underwent graft PCI in five large, randomized trials (Evaluation of Platelet IIb/IIIa Inhibition for Prevention of Ischemic Complications [EPIC], Evaluation in PTCA to Improve Long-Term Outcome with Abciximab Glycoprotein IIb/IIIa Blockade [EPILOG], Evaluation of Platelet IIb/IIIa Inhibitor for Stenting [EPISTENT], second Integrelin to Minimize Platelet Aggregation and Coronary Thrombosis [IMPACT II], and Platelet IIb/IIIa in Unstable Angina: Receptor Suppression Using Inte-

grelin Therapy [PURSUIT]), 30-day mortality and MI rates were twice that for native vessel PCI.[245] Factors reported to have the strongest predictive value for late events after SVG stenting included unstable angina, diabetes, previous PTCA, and number of stents.[246] Five-year outcome data from Emory University for 2556 patients who underwent PCI of SVGs emphasized the poorer outcome of diabetics ($n=776$) compared with nondiabetics ($n=1780$) with respect to survival (62.9% versus 78.5%, $P<.0001$) and event-free survival (23% versus 31%, $P=.0001$) (see Fig. 25-10A and B).[247] When only the patients receiving bare metal stents (BMSs) were considered ($n=1045$), in-hospital outcomes of diabetics and nondiabetics were not significantly different, but survival was worse for diabetics at 1 year (89.5% versus 95.5%, $P=.008$) and at 5 years (78.2% versus 87.1%, $P=.009$). Kaplan-Meier survival curves demonstrating survival free of death are shown in Figure 25-10C.

Drug-Eluting Stents

Although BMSs improve initial and long-term outcomes of SVG PCI, the impact is modest because of restenosis and disease progression. DESs have been

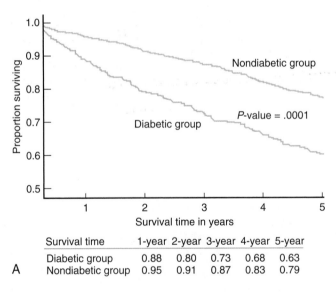

Survival time	1-year	2-year	3-year	4-year	5-year
Diabetic group	0.88	0.80	0.73	0.68	0.63
Nondiabetic group	0.95	0.91	0.87	0.83	0.79

A

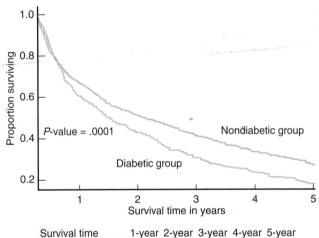

Survival time	1-year	2-year	3-year	4-year	5-year
Diabetic group	0.58	0.45	0.33	0.28	0.23
Nondiabetic group	0.64	0.53	0.43	0.37	0.31

B

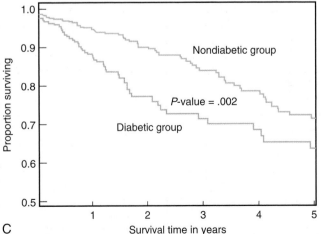

C

Figure 25-10. A, Kaplan-Meier curves show survival free of death for 2556 patients who underwent percutaneous coronary intervention at Emory University Hospital. The 5-year outcomes of nondiabetics are compared with those of treated diabetes. **B,** Kaplan-Meier curves show survival free of death, myocardial infarction, or repeat revascularization. **C,** Kaplan-Meier curves show survival free of death for 1045 patients who underwent bare metal stent implantation in saphenous vein grafts. (From Ashfaq S, Ghazzal Z, Douglas JS, et al: Impact of diabetes on five-year outcomes after vein graft intervention performed prior to the drug-eluting stent era. J Invasive Cardiol 2006;18:100-105.)

shown to significantly reduce restenosis in SVGs. Costa and colleagues[248] implanted sirolimus-eluting stents (SESs) in 76 no-option patients, most of whom had had multiple prior procedures, and found TVR in 16.7% at 6 months. In 19 consecutive patients treated with SES, only one SVG required TLR at 1 year.[249] Ge and associates[250] compared outcomes of 89 patients with BMSs with 61 consecutively treated patients receiving SESs (57%) or paclitaxel-eluting stents (PESs, 43%), reporting lower 6-month restenosis (10% versus 26.7%, P=.03) and TLR (3.3% versus 19.8%, P=.003). In two registry experiences, 6-month outcomes after SVG stenting were favorable with SESs (TLR in 2.5% of 248 patients)[251] and PESs (repeat intervention in 3.9% of 258 patients).[252] Lee and coworkers[253] analyzed outcomes of 139 patients who received DESs for treatment of SVG lesions of a total of 223 consecutive SVG stent procedures reporting that DES implantation was associated with significantly lower rates of mortality, MI, TVR, and MACE. In the only randomized comparison of DESs with BMSs in SVGs, Vermeersch and colleagues[254] implanted SESs in 38 patients with 47 SVG lesions and BMSs in 37 patients with 49 SVG lesions. At 6 months, patients receiving SESs had lower restenosis (13.6% versus 32.6%, P=.03), and TLR rates (5.3% versus 21.6%, P=.047) and lower median neointimal volume (1 versus 24 mm³, P<.001), but they had similar rates of death and MI. Longer-term follow-up studies are needed to determine optimal strategies for the use of DESs in SVGs.

Embolic Protection

Attention has been refocused on the importance of periprocedural elevations of CK-MB and troponin, which indicate myocardial necrosis most often due to atheroembolism,[255,256] because even minor eleva-

tions were shown to have prognostic implications.[257] Even when mostly straightforward single-lesion, single-stent SVG PCI procedures were carried out before the availability of embolic protection, significant creatine kinase elevations were observed in 20% of patients.[258,259] The rate of MI and procedural risk were shown to increase with lesion complexity, length, and estimated plaque volume,[260] and when MI occurred, there was an increased 30-day mortality rate approaching 15%.[261] In more than 1000 patients who underwent SVG stenting, CK-MB elevation was the most powerful predictor of late mortality.[262] Potential approaches to reduce embolic myocardial infarction occurring during SVG PCI include strategies to remove thrombus before PCI, capturing debris that is liberated by filters or occlusion-aspiration techniques, or exclusion of debris by use of a covered stent (discussed later).

The key role played by atheroembolization and confirmation of effective protection strategies were the products of several observational and randomized studies.[261-281] The PercuSurge GuardWire system used a hollow, 0.014-inch wire incorporating a compliant, inflatable distal occlusion balloon (Fig. 25-11). During inflation of the distally placed balloon, flow in the graft was interrupted; the stent was then implanted, followed by aspiration of the graft using a special monorail catheter and deflation of the balloon restoring flow. Webb and associates[264] reported that in 24 older SVGs stented using this system, only one patient had CK elevation more than three times normal and that 95% of the aspirates had typical atherosclerotic debris, including necrotic core, foam cells, cholesterol clefts, and fibrin matrix. The effectiveness of this strategy in a broad range of patients was confirmed in the Saphenous Vein Graft Angioplasty Free of Emboli Randomized (SAFER) trial, in which 801 patients were randomly assigned

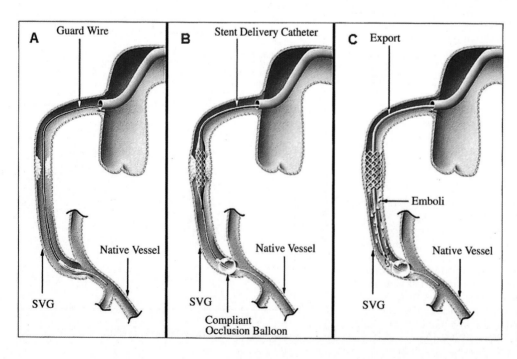

Figure 25-11. The PercuSurge Guardwire device for distal embolic protection. **A,** The lesion is crossed, and the balloon is positioned distally. **B,** After balloon occlusion, the stent is deployed. **C,** The occluded saphenous vein graft (SVG) is aspirated, followed by deflation of the distal occlusion balloon, which restores flow.

to stent implantation with or without use of the GuardWire distal protection.[265] Thirty-day MACEs were reduced by 42% with use of the GuardWire (16.5% to 9.6%, $P=.004$) primarily due to lower rates of MI (8.6% versus 14.7%, $P=.008$).

The PercuSurge system, frequently applicable even in the presence of severe stenosis due to the relatively low profile of the GuardWire, captures small particles and soluble vasoactive agents such as endothelin and serotonin and a variety of coagulation components that have been shown to be liberated during SVG PCI.[266,267] Removal of these vasoactive substances may contribute to improved immediate post-PCI coronary flow and myocardial perfusion as suggested in one study comparing PercuSurge with filter-based distal protection.[268] Analysis of the benefit of PercuSurge in relation to lesion length in SAFER showed that even with lesions less than 10 mm long, a 77% reduction in 30-day MACEs was experienced (2.2% versus 8.1%).[269] In the presence of baseline thrombus, use of the PercuSurge GuardWire was associated with fewer complications (OR=0.624; $P=.02$).[270]

Cohen and coworkers[271] reported that use of the GuardWire balloon occlusion device increased costs at 30 days by less than $650 per patient, with a cost-effectiveness ratio of $3700 per year of life making it highly cost effective. Senter and associates[272] per-

formed a cost analysis of "selective" versus routine use of distal protection, finding that the selective approach cost $42,127 per death prevented, compared with $72,461 using routine distal protection. Patients selected for distal protection had a graft for 8 years or more or had preprocedural thrombus; these were the only independent multivariate predictors of complications in the American College of Cardiology–National Cardiovascular Data Registry (ACC-NCDR) database.[273] Disadvantages of the PercuSurge GuardWire system include the need to completely occlude the target SVG during stent deployment and aspiration (not always well tolerated), a requirement for a relatively long "parking" segment distal to the lesion, inability to protect side branches, and the complexity of the system.

A variety of filters have been applied to SVG interventions (Fig. 25-12). In a 651-patient, randomized, multicenter trial, the FilterWire (Boston Scientific, Natick, MA) was compared with the PercuSurge GuardWire system. The 30-day rates of MACEs, the primary end point, were similar (9.9% with FilterWire compared with 11.6% with the PercuSurge GuardWire system), and there was no difference in death or MI.[274] Analysis of the first 48 patients compared with the next 261 demonstrated trends toward higher MI in the initial patients (19% versus 10%)

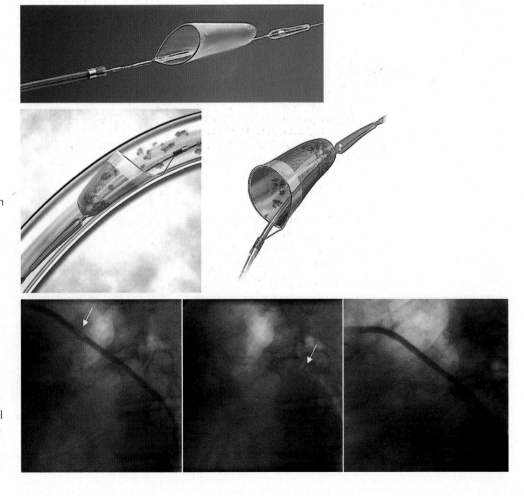

Figure 25-12. The FilterWire. **Top,** The polyurethane nonocclusive filter with 110-μm pore size is mounted on a nitinol loop fixed to a guidewire. **Middle,** The filter is deployed *(left)* distal to the lesion, and the nitinol loop is expanded to the size of the vessel (3.0 to 5.5 mm). The filter is removed *(right)* with a large embolic load. **Bottom,** The saphenous vein graft contains a thrombus *(left, arrow).* The filter is deployed *(center, arrow).* After stenting, the result is excellent *(right).* (From Gorog DA, Foale RA, Malik I, et al: Distal myocardial protection during percutaneous coronary intervention. When and where? J Am Coll Cardiol 2005;46:1434-1445.)

due to failure to obtain good apposition of the filter to the SVG wall, positioning the filter too distal, use of the filter in Y grafts, and carrying out additional interventions after filter removal. Some of the advantages of filters include ease of use, avoidance of ischemia due to preserved coronary flow, and good visualization. Disadvantages include the need to cross the lesion with a somewhat bulky filter, which may cause embolization or require predilation and which has been shown to increase the occurrence of Q wave MI (4.9% versus 0.5%, $P=.04$).[275] Small particles, less than the 100-μm pore size, and soluble agents may not be captured. The former may not be relevant based on a study by Rogers and colleagues[276] reporting that filtering was just as efficient as balloon occlusion in particle capture despite pore sizes larger than the majority of embolic particles. Other problems with filters include the long distal parking segment required and the potential for overwhelming the filter resulting in diminished antegrade flow mimicking no reflow.[277] The optimal strategy if this occurs is to aspirate the stagnant dye column, which may contain suspended debris, followed by filter removal and replacement if more interventional work is needed.

When the TriActiv distal occlusion balloon device (Kensey Nash, Exton, PA) (Fig. 25-13), which incorporates active flush and aspiration, was compared with the GuardWire or FilterWire, the rate of MACEs was similar (8.7% versus 9.2%, $P=NS$), indicating noninferiority.[278] The system is FDA approved and available in the United States. Each of the filters and the two FDA-approved occlusion-aspiration systems discussed earlier require space beyond the lesion for placement of the filter or occlusion balloon. Proximal protection with the Proxis system (St. Jude, St. Paul, MN) is applicable when there is insufficient room beyond the lesion for distal protection. Proxis involves placement of a hydrophilic-coated sheath into the proximal SVG (Fig. 25-14). Inflation of a compliant balloon surrounding this sheath occludes the vein graft, and stent implantation can be carried out, followed by flow-reversal aspiration of the SVG and subsequent balloon deflation restoring flow. When Proxis was compared with the FilterWire or GuardWire in a randomized trial, the rate of MACEs was comparable (9.2% versus 10%, $P=NS$).[279] Advantages of the Proxis device include the ability to insti-

tute embolic protection before the lesion is crossed with a guidewire, to protect side branches, and to handle large embolic loads and use of the guidewire of choice, but the most proximal SVG segment must be disease free, and the graft must be occluded during the procedure for several minutes.

Other filters that have undergone evaluation include the Spider (eV3, Plymouth, MN), which was tested in a 732-patient, randomized trial with 30-day MACEs, the primary end point, occurring in 9.2% of the Spider arm and 8.7% of the approved control device arm, indicating noninferiority.[280] A filter known as the TRAP was compared with unprotected stenting in SVGs in an abbreviated and consequently underpowered 360-patient trial in which there was no difference in the rates of 30-day MACEs between the two groups, but there was a tend toward benefit with the TRAP.[281]

In a meta-analysis of 3430 patients who underwent SVG PCI, 9.4% of those who received embolic protection had a CK-MB level of three or more times normal compared with 22.2% of patients who had unprotected SVG PCI. In multivariate meta-regression, the use of embolic protection and the presence of good left ventricular function were associated with less myonecrosis, but use of GP IIb/IIIa antagonists (discussed later) was not.[282] The reduction of myonecrosis from about 20% to 10% in the meta-analysis parallels closely the results from SAFER[265] and strongly supports use of embolic protection. Patients who benefit the most are those with thrombus, large plaque volume, and degenerated, older grafts.[260,261,270,273] In an unpublished industry survey of approximately 1000 SVG procedures performed in calendar year 2003, 62% were performed without embolic protection, 27% used a filter, 7% used distal occlusion and aspiration, and 4% involved the use of thrombectomy. Occasionally, it is helpful to use both thrombectomy and embolic protection.[283] The type of embolic protection chosen depends on

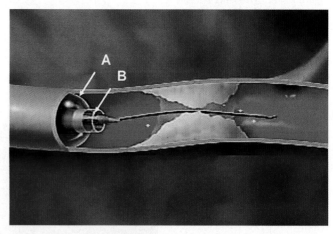

Figure 25-14. The Proxis device consists of a hydrophilic sheath that is placed into the proximal saphenous vein graft (SVG), followed by inflation of the sealing balloon (A), which occludes the SVG. The lesion is crossed with a guidewire; the lesion is then stented, and debris is aspirated by reversing flow in the SVG (B).

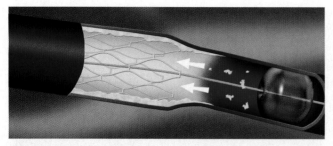

Figure 25-13. The TriActiv system has three components: a distal occlusion balloon, active flushing, and aspiration of debris (*arrows* indicate direction of flow during aspiration).

the anatomy and the patient's ability to tolerate occlusion of the graft for several minutes. In an analysis of 626 patients by Webb and colleagues,[264] 39% of patients were candidates for proximal or distal protection, 18% for distal only, 20% for proximal only, and 23% for neither.

Covered Stents

There have been three randomized trials evaluating the use of the Jomed polytetrafluoroethylene (PTFE)–covered balloon-expandable stent (Fig. 25-15) and one randomized trial of the Boston Scientific PTFE-covered nitinol self-expanding stent in SVGs; all results were negative. In the Randomised Evaluation of Polytetrafluoroethylene-Covered Stent in Saphenous Vein Grafts (RECOVERS) trial, 301 patients undergoing SVG stenting were randomized to Jomed stents or BMSs; the primary end point of in-stent restenosis did not differ (24% versus 24.8%), and the rate of 30-day MACEs was higher in the PTFE group (10.9% versus 4.1%, $P=.049$).[284] In the Stents in Grafts (STING) trial, 211 patients undergoing SVG stenting were randomized to Jomed stents or BMSs, with less favorable outcomes reported for the Jomed-treated patients with respect to restenosis (29% versus 20%), death (8.8% versus 5.8%), and MI (9.8% versus 7.7%).[285]

The Barrier Approach to Restenosis: Restrict Intima and Curtail Adverse Events (BARRICADE) trial was interrupted after 243 of 500 planned patients were enrolled because the primary end point of restenosis with the Jomed stent was trending higher than that with the BMS (39% versus 28%, $P=.14$), as was the

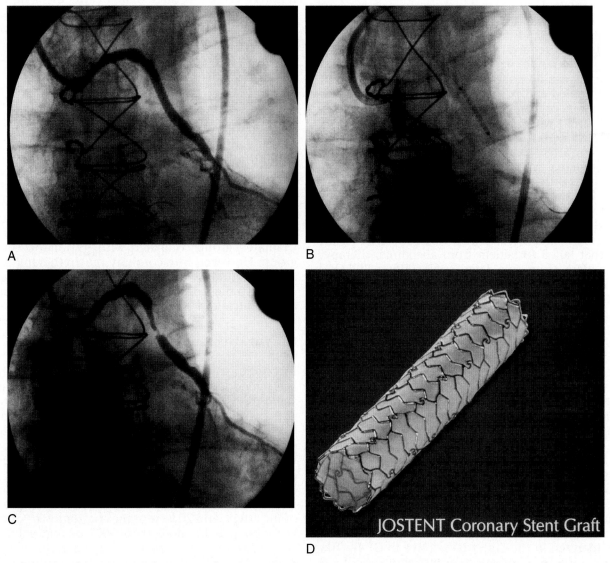

Figure 25-15. Use of a PTFE-covered stent in saphenous vein graft (SVG) percutaneous coronary intervention. The bulky lesion in the SVG to the left coronary artery (**A**) is crossed with a 4.0×19 mm Jostent coronary stent graft (Jomed, Helsingborg, Sweden) (**B**). After balloon inflation to more than 12 atm, an excellent angiographic result was obtained (**C**). This stent design (**D**) is characterized by an expandable PTFE membrane between two layers of stent struts. (Courtesy of Fausto Feres, MD, Sao Paulo, Brazil).

occurrence of total occlusion (20% versus 10% in the BMS group, $P=.09$).[286]

The only randomized trial of the Symbiot PTFE-covered, self-expanding stent (Boston Scientific, Natick, MA) involved 400 patients who received the Symbiot or a BMS. The primary end point, the diameter of stenosis at 8 months, was not different in the two groups, but there was a trend toward increased TVR with the Symbiot (23.5% versus 15.6%, $P=.055$) and nonsignificantly higher rates of MACEs (30.6% versus 26.5%).[287,288] Covered stents are not approved by the FDA for routine use in SVGs, except in the case of perforation.[289,290]

Adjunctive Pharmacotherapy

Accepted adjunctive therapy during PCI of native and SVG PCI includes antithrombotic measures (e.g., aspirin, antithrombin, other antiplatelet agents) and vascular dilators as needed for the treatment of slow or no reflow. Unfractionated heparin was used in most of the SVG studies reported. For the 403 SVG patients in the Randomized Evaluation in PCI Linking Angiomax to reduced Clinical Events (REPLACE) 1 and 2 trials randomized to heparin or bivalirudin, logistic regression analysis revealed no difference in the combined end point (i.e., death, MI, urgent vascularization, or major bleeding), but less minor bleeding occurred with bivalirudin (14.8% versus 22.7%, $P=.037$).[291] Optimal clopidogrel dosing and duration of therapy after SVG PCI have not been studied. The relatively large embolic burden encountered in SVG procedures provides some explanation of the failure of GP IIb/IIIa platelet receptor inhibitors to prevent periprocedural MI in these patients. In an analysis of pooled data from EPIC and EPILOG, Ellis and associates[292] found degenerated SVG to be the only lesion type that failed to benefit from abciximab therapy. When data from five large trials (EPIC, EPILOG, EPISTENT, IMPACT II, and PURSUIT) with a total of more than 600 SVG PCI patients and data from the Cleveland Clinic registry (278 SVG PCI patients) were analyzed, there was no apparent benefit from GP IIb/IIIa inhibitors.[293]

In the meta-analysis of more than 3000 patients undergoing PCI of SVG, use of a GP IIb/IIIa antagonist was a univariate but not multivariate predictor of reduced myonecrosis.[282] In these observational studies, it is difficult to control for the selection bias for use of GP IIb/IIIa inhibitors in sicker patients. In SAFER, patients treated with GP IIb/IIIa inhibitors had a higher incidence of MACEs than patients not treated with these agents.[265] In FIRE, patients chosen for GP IIb/IIIa inhibitor therapy had higher baseline risk and increased rates of 30-day MACEs (13.0% versus 8.0%, $P=.03$). However, when outcomes of GuardWire-treated and FilterWire-treated patients were analyzed in the FIRE trial relative to GP IIb/IIIa inhibitor use in a propensity adjustment, use of GP IIb/IIIa inhibitors with FilterWire was associated with fewer MACEs (i.e., abrupt closure, no reflow, and distal embolization, $P=.023$), whereas there was no

advantage of using GP IIb/IIIa agents with the Guard-Wire.[294] The potential benefit implied by this secondary analysis was offset by a higher requirement for blood transfusion in patients receiving GP IIb/IIIa inhibitors in the study. Possible mechanisms to explain the possible benefit of GP IIb/IIIa antagonists with FilterWire include enhanced filter patency and reduced no-reflow, both favoring capture of debris. The use of microvascular dilators to treat no or slow reflow after PCI or prophylactically before the procedure has not been well studied, but it is an important strategy in SVG PCI.[295]

Restenosis Lesions in Saphenous Vein Grafts

The management of patients with restenosis of SVG stent sites is a topic of considerable interest and a significant clinical problem. As is true in native coronary intervention, treatment of in-stent restenotic lesions in SVGs is safer than treatment of de novo SVG lesions, primarily because of reductions in "slow, no reflow" and periprocedural MI (0% versus 20%, $P=.02$).[296] Recurrences, however, are common; at 1 year, Dangas and coworkers[297] reported TLR in 32% and death of 11% of patients. Better results were obtained in in-stent restenosis lesions in SVGs using intravascular radiation for prevention of recurrence of restenosis. In the Washington Radiation for In-Stent Restenosis Trial for Saphenous Vein Grafts, a double-blind, randomized trial enrolling 120 patients with diffuse in-stent restenosis receiving gamma radiation with ^{192}Ir or placebo, Waksman reported a 65% lower restenosis in the irradiated group at 6 months compared with the control group, but by 36 months target vessel revascularization was not significantly different.[298] Late thrombosis occurred in 8% of the irradiated group compared with 9% of the control group. However, intracoronary brachytherapy is not available in most centers, and DESs have become the default strategy despite the paucity of data to support this application.

Internal Mammary Artery Grafts

In contrast to SVGs, favorable results have been reported with balloon dilation of IMA graft stenoses.[39-74] Lesions at the anastomosis of arterial grafts with the native coronary artery behave much like distal anastomotic lesions of SVGs. They usually occur within a few months of surgery and respond to low-pressure balloon inflations. Successful dilation of ostial or extremely proximal IMA graft lesions has been reported in only a few patients.[53-56] In a report of PCI of 32 IMA graft lesions, 12 were in the midportion of the artery, and 20 were at the anastomosis.[68] Success was obtained in more than 90% of approximately 1000 patients in more than 20 reports in the literature (Table 25-4). Complications occurred infrequently; the most common were IMA dissection and spasm. In a report of 68 patients, 78% had follow-up angiography at a mean of 8 months; restenosis occurred in

Table 25-4. Results of Internal Mammary Artery Graft Intervention

Study	Year	No. of Patients	Success	Complications	Follow-up
Douglas et al[39]	1983	1	0	Nonocclusive dissection	Elective CABG
Kereiakes et al[67]	1984	1	1	0	Asymptomatic at 6 mo
Zaidi and Hollman[57]	1985	1	1	0	Patent at 8 mo
Crean et al[58]	1986	1	1	0	Normal thallium at 4 mo
Dorros and Lewin[59]	1986	7	6	LIMA dissection	No clinical recurrence at 7.7 mo
Steffenino et al[60]	1986	2	2	0	1 asymptomatic at 9 mo, 1 patent at 6 mo
Salinger et al[61]	1986	1	1	IMA spasm	—
Cote et al[46]	1987	5	5	0	—
Stullman and Hilliard[54]	1987	1	1	0	Re-PTCA at 3 mo
Singh[62]	1987	1	1	0	Patent at 6 mo
Pinkerton et al[65]	1987	7	7	0	All asymptomatic
Shimshak et al[68]	1988	26	24	Spasm, 3 dissections	1 of 8 restenosis
Hill et al[63]	1989	11	9	0	2 re-PTCA, 8 of 9 patients asymptomatic
Bell et al[64]	1989	7	7	0	—
Dimas et al[87]	1991	31	28	2 dissections	1 of 7 restenosis
Shimshak et al[88]	1991	86	81	1 QMI	4 late deaths
Sketch et al[53]	1992	14	13	—	1 of 12 restenosis
Hearne et al[69]	1995	68	60	2 dissections	9 restenosis (19%)
Najm et al[70]	1995	34	31	—	4 (14%) of 14 restenosis
Ishizaka et al[71]	1995	46	34	1 spasm	30% restenosis
Gruberg et al[72]	2000	174	168	1 death, 1 CABG 15 non-QMI	7.4% TVR Revascularization at 1 yr
Sharma et al[73]	2001	280	258	30-day mortality: 1.3%	Mortality at 1 yr: 5.7% TVR: 8.3%
Roffi et al[74]	2001	225	196	In-hospital MACE: 8%	MACE at 1 yr: 18% for LIMA, 22% for RIMA

CABG, coronary artery bypass grafting; LIMA, left internal mammary artery; MACE: major adverse cardiac event; PTCA, percutaneous transluminal coronary angioplasty; QMI, Q-wave myocardial infarction; RIMA, right internal mammary artery; TVR, target vessel revascularization.

15% (6 of 40) at the anastomosis of the graft with the coronary artery and in 43% (3 of 7) at midgraft. At a mean interval of 14 months, 76% were in class I or II, and the event-free survival rate was 86%.[69] Sharma and colleagues[73] analyzed outcomes after IMA intervention based on lesion location and the use of a stent versus a balloon alone, finding TLR at 1 year to be lower with balloon angioplasty at the anastomosis (5% versus 30%, *P*=.002). TLR after balloon angioplasty was comparable to stenting in the shaft portion (4.7% versus 4.0%; *P*=1.0) and at the ostium (12% versus 33%, *P*=.59). There are no large series or long-term data regarding stenting in IMA grafts or PCI in gastroepiploic or radial artery grafts.[74,75]

COMPLICATIONS

Given the known increased risk of coronary bypass reoperation, there has been concern that emergency reoperation for failed percutaneous intervention would be associated with marked increased risk (Table 25-5). At Emory University from 1980 to 1989, 1263 patients with prior coronary bypass surgery underwent elective percutaneous intervention; of these patients, 46 (3.6%) underwent reoperation for failed PCI.[299] Three patients (6.5%) died, and 11 (24%) had nonfatal Q-wave MIs. The actuarial 3-year survival rate for the 46 patients was 91%. All early and late deaths occurred in patients with ongoing ischemia at

the time of emergency reoperation. Kahn and associates[300] reported three deaths among 19 patients who had emergency reoperation for failed PCI; two of these had left main coronary artery closure after intervention. Twenty-five percent of survivors had Q-wave MIs. Considering these factors and the high recurrence rate after PCI, some investigators have concluded that percutaneous intervention in patients with prior CABG should be restricted to focal lesions in four angiographic situations: unbypassed native coronary artery, distal anastomoses that are less than 3 years old, SVGs less than 3 years old, and distal native coronary artery lesions reached through fully patent grafts.[80] The ACC/AHA/SCAI PCI guidelines are more permissive, however, extending indications for intervention to include older SVGs, especially when reoperation is not an excellent option.[84]

Abrupt Closure

Because rapid surgical rescue is not possible in patients with prior bypass surgery, abrupt closure of the target vessel in these patients is associated with increased risk. Abrupt closure occurs in 3% to 5% of patients undergoing native vessel angioplasty, is more frequent in the presence of certain angiographic features (i.e., thrombus, long lesion, bifurcation, right coronary artery site, and bend point) and in the presence of unstable angina, but has been ameliorated by stenting.[301] Abrupt closure appears to be less

Table 25-5. Probability of Success, Complications, and Restenosis with Percutaneous Coronary Intervention in Patients after Coronary Artery Bypass Grafting

Lesion Site	Success	Complications	Restenosis (%)	Most Promising Strategy
Internal mammary artery				
Shaft	Good	Dissection	Unknown	DES
DA	Excellent	Rare	10-25	PTCA or DES
Saphenous vein graft				
PA	Good	Embolization >3 yr	20-50	DES
Midvein	Good	Embolization >3 yr	15-25	DES
DA				
≤1 yr after surgery	Excellent	Rare	<20	Balloon or DES
>1 yr after surgery	Good	Embolization >3 yr	15-25	DES
Left main	Good	Dissection	5-40	DES
Subclavian	Excellent	Rare	Infrequent	Stent
Gastroepiploic	Excellent	Rare	Unknown	Unknown
Radial artery	Excellent	Rare	Unknown	DES

DA, distal anastomosis; DCA, directional coronary atherectomy; DES, drug-eluting stent; PA, proximal anastomosis; PTCA, percutaneous transluminal coronary angioplasty; RA, rotational atherectomy.

common in angioplasty of SVGs. In five reports of 448 SVG PCI procedures, abrupt closure occurred in 1.5%.[40,41,43,45,46] A systematic analysis of predictors of this complication in SVG interventions has not been published, but in our experience, thrombus, bulky and eccentric lesions, and infarct-related lesions have an increased risk. Stents and GP IIb/IIIa receptor blockers have also proved to be effective measures in the treatment of threatened and abrupt closure after native vessel and graft angioplasty.

Perforation

Coronary artery perforation is a potential complication of all coronary interventions. Coronary artery perforation has been attributed to vessel wall penetration with guidewires, inflation of a balloon in a subintimal location, or overexpansion of a coronary artery; atheroablative techniques (i.e., atherectomy and laser); and stent implantation. SVG perforation is a rare complication of balloon angioplasty. It was first reported to occur during the performance of 1 (0.5%) of 235 vein graft dilations in 203 patients at Emory University.[45] This patient, as was true of most subsequently described patients, was treated conservatively.[302-304] Prolonged balloon inflation and reversal of anticoagulation were effective in stabilizing most patients. Placement of a second stent has been reported to successfully seal an SVG perforation.[305] Despite the scarring that is present after bypass surgery, vessel perforation may result in extensive hemorrhage, vessel occlusion,[304] and cardiac tamponade,[303] necessitating emergency surgery. The use of covered stents has had an increasing role in the treatment of perforation. In 35 perforations, a PTFE-covered stent was successful in sealing 100%.[306] Because of their large diameter, SVGs are favorable conduits for use of this strategy for sealing perforations (Fig. 25-16).[307,308] Although the use of oversized

balloons has been advocated for vein graft dilations, older vein grafts may rupture with only modest oversizing; rupture occurred in one patient with a balloon-to-SVG ratio of 1.12 to 1.[304] Because of this potential risk, it seems wise to size balloons and stents to the normal adjacent vessel.

No Reflow

The cause of slow or no reflow after native or SVG PCI is multifactorial and probably includes vasospasm and embolization of thrombus and plaque with the latter dominating especially in SVGs. The importance of microvascular spasm is suggested by the observation that vasoconstrictors are released during SVG stent procedures,[266,266a] by the reduction in no reflow when a calcium channel blocker is administered before SVG PCI,[190] by the apparent treatment effect of small-vessel dilators (e.g., calcium channel blockers, adenosine, nitroprusside),[187-192] and by the lack of benefit of nitroglycerin. The dominant role of atheroembolism is apparent from the studies of embolic protection and pathologic studies (Fig. 25-17). Although the use of GP IIb/IIIa inhibitors has been suggested to prevent and treat no flow, this strategy has not been properly tested.

THE FUTURE OF PERCUTANEOUS INTERVENTION

The thorny issues in patients with prior bypass surgery remain vein graft atheroembolism and restenosis and progressive vein graft disease. Major expansion of indications in this subgroup of patients awaits solutions to these problems. To avoid embolization, vein graft atheroma must be removed, excluded from the circulation, fragmented and removed, or ablated. Even with the permissively large lumen of many

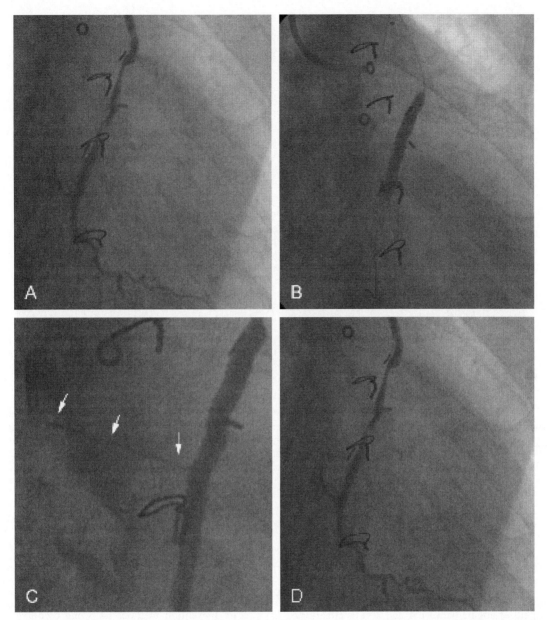

Figure 25-16. A, An 80-year-old man with unstable angina was found to have a long stenosis of an 18-year-old saphenous vein graft to the posterior obtuse marginal coronary artery. **B,** A 4.0×38 mm stent was deployed at 15 atm using the PercuSurge GuardWire system for distal protection (notice the inflated balloon distally). **C,** After balloon deflation, angiography revealed a focal perforation with a jet of contrast *(arrows)*. The patient developed hypotension requiring vasopressor support. Balloon inflation at the site of the perforation failed to seal the hole. **D,** A Jomed stent graft mounted on a 4.0-mm balloon was deployed. It sealed the perforation and provided an excellent angiographic result. The patient's subsequent in-hospital course was uneventful, and at last follow-up, he was doing well. (Courtesy of Ziyad Ghazzal, MD, Atlanta, Georgia).

vein grafts, it is difficult to achieve complete atheroma particle removal reliably, and this accounts for the 10% rate of myonecrosis even with embolic protection. However, a combination of strategies is now available that may permit some cases to be attempted that would previously have been unsuitable for PCI. Competing technologies are continuing to evolve, and it is probable that they will successfully address this important problem of atherembolization.

Restenosis remains a major limiting factor in PCI of SVGs. Although restenosis after placement of DESs occurs less frequently than with other strategies, morbidity and costs related to restenosis continue. How effectively the use of DESs will address this problem of restenosis and treatment of the restenosis lesion remains to be determined, but initial reports are encouraging. An additional overriding issue is the need for strategies to retard disease progression in nontarget sites.

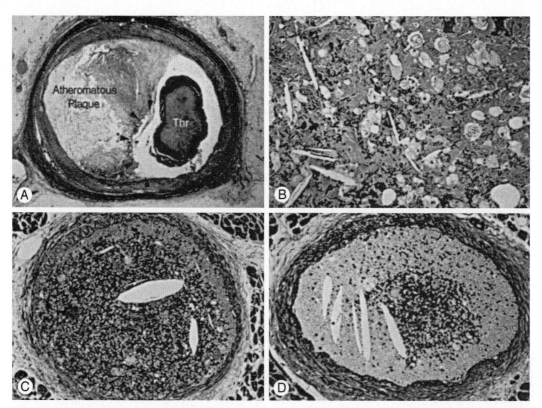

Figure 25-17. Vein graft. **A,** Low-power photomicrograph shows rupture *(arrowheads)* of atheromatous plaque caused by balloon angioplasty and secondary thrombosis (Thr). Sections taken at adjacent sites were involved by such extensive disruption that luminal boundaries were obliterated. **B,** High-power photomicrograph demonstrates the nature of the plaque, with foam cells, cholesterol clefts, blood elements, and necrotic debris. **C** and **D,** Intramural coronary artery branches. Atheromatous emboli obstruct vessels in the anterolateral (**C**) and inferoseptal (**D**) walls of the left ventricle (compare with **B**). (From Saber RS, Edwards WD, Holmes DR Jr, et al: Balloon angioplasty of aortocoronary saphenous vein bypass grafts: A histopathologic study of six grafts from five patients, with emphasis on restenosis and embolic complications. J Am Coll Cardiol 1988;12:1501-1509.)

REFERENCES

1. Campeau L, Lesperance J, Hermann J, et al: Loss of the improvement of angina between 1 and 7 years after aorto-coronary bypass surgery. Circulation 1979;60(Suppl I): I-1-I-5.
2. Johnson WD, Kayser KL, Pedraza PM: Angina pectoris and coronary bypass surgery. Am Heart J 1984;108:1190-1197.
3. Frick MH, Valle M, Harjola PT: Progression of coronary artery disease in randomized medical and surgical patients over a 5-year angiographic follow-up. Am J Cardiol 1983;52:681.
4. Hwang MH, Meadows WR, Palac RT, et al: Progression of native coronary artery disease at 10 years: Insights from a randomized study of medical versus surgical therapy for angina. J Am Coll Cardiol 1990;16:1066-1070.
5. The VA Coronary Artery Bypass Surgery Cooperative Study Group: Eighteen-year follow-up in the Veterans Affairs Cooperative Study of coronary artery bypass surgery for stable angina. Circulation 1992;86:121-130.
6. Khot UN, Friedman DT, Pettersson G, et al: Radial artery bypass grafts have an increased occurrence of angiographically severe stenosis and occlusion compared with left internal mammary arteries and saphenous vein grafts. Circulation 2004;109:2086-2091.
7. Okrainec K, Platt R, Pilote L, et al: Cardiac medical therapy in patients after undergoing coronary artery bypass graft surgery. J Am Coll Cardiol 2005;45:177-184.
8. Alexander JH, Hafley G, Harrington RA, et al: Efficacy and safety of edifoligide, an E2F transcription factor decoy, for prevention of vein graft failure following coronary artery bypass graft surgery: PREVENT IV: A randomized controlled trial. JAMA 2005;294:2446-2454.
9. Goyal A, Alexander JH, Hafley G, et al: Greater use of secondary prevention methods following coronary artery bypass surgery is associated with improved two-year outcomes. Circulation 2006;114(Suppl II):II-796.
10. Reifart N, Haase J, Storger H, et al: Interventional standby for cardiac surgery. Circulation 1996;94(Suppl I):I-86.
11. Rasmussen C, Thiis JJ, Clemmensen P, et al: Management of suspected graft failure in coronary artery bypass grafting. Circulation 1996;94(Suppl I):I-413.
12. Cutlip DE, Dauerman HL, Carrozza JP: Recurrent ischemia within thirty days of coronary artery bypass surgery: Angiographic findings and outcome of percutaneous revascularization. Circulation 1996;94(Suppl I):I-249.
13. Goldman S, Copeland J, Moritz T, et al: Starting aspirin therapy after operation: Effects on early graft patency. Circulation 1991;84:520-525.
14. Fitzgibbon GM, Burton JR, Leach AJ: Coronary bypass graft fate: Angiographic grading of 1400 consecutive grafts early after operation and of 1132 after one year. Circulation 1978;57:1070.
15. Hamby RI, Aintablian A, Handler M, et al: Aortocoronary saphenous vein bypass grafts: Long-term patency, morphology and blood flow in patients with patent grafts early after surgery. Circulation 1979;60:901.
16. Bourassa MG, Enjalbert M, Campeau L, et al: Progression of atherosclerosis in coronary arteries and bypass grafts: Ten years later. Am J Cardiol 1984;53:102C.

17. Bourassa MG, Fisher LD, Campeau L, et al: Long-term fate of bypass grafts: The Coronary Artery Surgery Study (CASS) and Montreal Heart Institute experiences. Circulation 1985;72(Suppl V):V-71-V-78.

18. Fitzgibbon GM, Leach AJ, Kafka HP, et al: Coronary bypass graft fate: Long-term angiographic study. J Am Coll Cardiol 1991;17:1075-1080.

19. Eagle KA, Guyton RA, Davidoff R, et al: ACC/AHA guidelines for coronary artery bypass graft surgery: Executive summary and recommendations. A report of the American College of Cardiology/American Heart Association Task Force on Practice Guidelines (Committee to Revise the 1991 Guidelines for Coronary Artery Bypass Graft Surgery). Circulation 1999;100:1464-1480.

20. Cameron A, Davis KB, Green G, Schaff HV: Coronary bypass surgery with internal-thoracic-artery grafts—effects on survival over a 15-year period. N Engl J Med 1996;334:216-219.

21. Loop FD: Internal-thoracic-artery grafts. N Engl J Med 1996;334:263-265.

22. Cameron AAC, Green GE, Brogno DA, Thornton J: Internal thoracic artery grafts: 20-year clinical follow-up. J Am Coll Cardiol 1995;25:188-192.

23. Mehta R, Honeycutt E, Peterson ED, et al: Impact of internal mammary artery conduit on long-term outcomes after percutaneous intervention of saphenous vein graft. Circulation 2006;114(Suppl I):I-396-I-401.

24. Brener SJ, Lytle BW, Casserly IP, et al: Predictors of revascularization method and long-term outcome of percutaneous coronary intervention or repeat coronary bypass surgery in patients with multivessel coronary disease and previous coronary bypass surgery. Eur Heart J 2006;27:413-418.

25. Loop FD, Lytle BW, Cosgrove DM, et al: Reoperation for coronary atherosclerosis. Ann Surg 1990;212:378-386.

26. Weintraub WS, Jones EL, Craver JM, et al: Incidence of repeat revascularization after coronary bypass surgery. J Am Coll Cardiol 1992;19(Suppl A):98A.

27. Weintraub WS, Jone EL, Craver JM, et al: In-hospital and long-term outcome after reoperative coronary artery bypass graft surgery. Circulation 1995;92(Suppl II):II-50-II-57.

28. Jurkovitz C, Jones EL, Craver JM, et al: Update on reoperative coronary bypass surgery: Results from the 1990's. Circulation 2000;102(Suppl II):II-55.

29. Zhang Z, Weintraub WS, Valedor E, et al: The changing profile of first reoperative coronary artery bypass surgery: Trends over 17 years in 2,770 patients [abstract]. J Am Coll Cardiol 2004;43:267A.

30. Hannan EL, Kilburn H, O'Donnell JF, et al: Adult open heart surgery in New York State. JAMA 1990;264:2768-2774.

31. Pick AW, Mullany CJ, Orszulak TA, et al: Third and fourth operations for myocardial ischemia: Short-term results and long-term survival. Circulation 1996;94(Suppl I):I-413.

32. Lytle BW, Loop FD, Cosgrove DM: Fifteen hundred coronary reoperations: Results and determinants of early and late survival. J Thorac Cardiovasc Surg 1987;93:847-859.

33. Lytle BW, Loop FD, Taylor PT, et al: The effect of coronary reoperation on the survival of patients with stenoses in saphenous vein to coronary bypass grafts. J Thorac Cardiovasc Surg 1993;105:605-614.

34. Lytle BW: The clinical impact of the atherosclerotic saphenous vein to coronary artery bypass grafts. Semin Thorac Cardiovasc Surg 1994;6:81-86.

35. Cameron A, Kemp HG Jr, Green GE: Reoperation for coronary artery disease: 10 years of clinical follow-up. Circulation 1988;78(Suppl I):I-158-I-162.

36. Mills RM, Kalan JM: Developing a rational management strategy for angina pectoris after coronary bypass surgery: A clinical decision analysis. Clin Cardiol 1991;14:191-197.

37. Gruentzig AR, Senning A, Siegenthaler WE: Nonoperative dilatation of coronary-artery stenosis: Percutaneous transluminal coronary angioplasty. N Engl J Med 1979;301:61-68.

38. Ford WB, Wholey MH, Zikria EA, et al: Percutaneous transluminal angioplasty in the management of occlusive disease involving the coronary arteries and saphenous vein bypass grafts. J Thorac Cardiovasc Surg 1980;79:1-11.

39. Douglas JS Jr, Gruentzig AR, King SB III, et al: Percutaneous transluminal coronary angioplasty in patients with prior coronary bypass surgery. J Am Coll Cardiol 1983;2:745-754.

40. El Gamal M, Bonnier H, Michels R, et al: Percutaneous transluminal angioplasty of stenosed aortocoronary bypass grafts. Br Heart J 1984;52:617-620.

41. Block PC, Cowley MJ, Kaltenback M, et al: Percutaneous angioplasty of stenoses of bypass grafts or by bypass graft anastomotic sites. Am J Cardiol 1984;53:666-668.

42. Dorros G, Johnson WD, Tector AJ, et al: Percutaneous transluminal coronary angioplasty in patients with prior coronary artery bypass surgery. J Thorac Cardiovasc Surg 1984;87:17-26.

43. Corbelli J, Franco I, Hollman J, et al: Percutaneous transluminal coronary angioplasty after previous coronary artery bypass surgery. Am J Cardiol 1985;56:398-403.

44. Reeder GS, Bresnahan JF, Holmes DR Jr, et al: Angioplasty for aortocoronary bypass graft stenosis. Mayo Clin Proc 1986;61:14-19.

45. Douglas J, Robinson K, Schlumpf M: Percutaneous transluminal angioplasty in aortocoronary venous graft stenoses: Immediate results and complications. Circulation 1986;74(Suppl II):II-281.

46. Cote G, Myler RK, Stertzer SH, et al: Percutaneous transluminal angioplasty of stenotic coronary artery bypass grafts: 5 years' experience. J Am Coll Cardiol 1987;9:8-17.

47. Ernst JMPG, van der Feltz TA, Ascoop CAPL, et al: Percutaneous transluminal coronary angioplasty in patients with prior coronary artery bypass grafting. J Thorac Cardiovasc Surg 1987;93:268-275.

48. Douglas JS Jr, King SB III, Roubin GS: Percutaneous transluminal coronary angioplasty in patients with prior coronary artery bypass grafting. J Thorac Cardiovasc Surg 1987;93:272-275.

49. Pinkerton CA, Slack JD, Orr CM, et al: Percutaneous transluminal angioplasty in patients with prior myocardial revascularization surgery. Am J Cardiol 1988;61:15G-22G.

50. Dorros G, Lewin RF, Mathiak LM, et al: Percutaneous transluminal coronary angioplasty in patients with two or more previous coronary artery bypass grafting operations. Am J Cardiol 1988;61:1243-1247.

51. Reed DC, Beller GA, Nygaard TW, et al: The clinical efficacy and scintigraphic evaluation of post-coronary bypass patients undergoing percutaneous transluminal coronary angioplasty for recurrent angina pectoris. Am Heart J 1989;117:60-71.

52. Cooper I, Ineson N, Demirtas E, et al: Role of angioplasty in patients with previous coronary artery bypass surgery. Cathet Cardiovasc Diagn 1989;16:81-86.

53. Sketch MH, Quigley PJ, Perez JA, et al: Angiographic follow-up after internal mammary artery graft angioplasty. Am J Cardiol 1992;70:401-403.

54. Stullman WS, Hilliard K: Unrecognized internal mammary artery stenosis treated by percutaneous angioplasty after coronary bypass surgery. Am Heart J 1987;113:393-395.

55. Vivekaphirat V, Yellen SF, Foschi A: Percutaneous transluminal angioplasty of a stenosis at the origin of the left internal mammary artery graft: A case report. Cathet Cardiovasc Diagn 1988;15:176-178.

56. Jacq L, Lancelin B, Brenot P, et al: Percutaneous transluminal angioplasty of ostial lesions of internal mammary artery grafts. Catheter Cardiovasc Interv 2001;52:368-372.

57. Zaidi AR, Hollman JL: Percutaneous angioplasty of internal mammary artery graft stenosis: Case report and discussion. Cathet Cardiovasc Diagn 1985;11:603-608.

58. Crean PA, Mathieson PW, Richards AF: Transluminal angioplasty of a stenosis of an internal mammary artery graft. Br Heart J 1986;56:473-475.

59. Dorros G, Lewin RF: The brachial artery method of transluminal internal mammary artery angioplasty. Cathet Cardiovasc Diagn 1986;12:341-346.

60. Steffenino G, Meier B, Finci L, et al: Percutaneous transluminal angioplasty of right and left internal mammary artery grafts. Chest 1986;90:849-851.

61. Salinger M, Drummer E, Furey K, et al: Percutaneous angioplasty of internal mammary artery grafts stenosis using the

brachial approach: A case report. Cathet Cardiovasc Diagn 1986;12:261-265.

62. Singh S: Coronary angioplasty of internal mammary artery graft. Am J Med 1987;82:361-362.

63. Hill DM, McAuley BJ, Sheehan DJ, et al: Percutaneous transluminal angioplasty of internal mammary artery bypass grafts [abstract]. J Am Coll Cardiol 1989;13:221A.

64. Bell MR, Holmes DR Jr, Vlietstra RE, et al: Percutaneous transluminal angioplasty of left internal mammary artery grafts: Two years' experience with a femoral approach. Br Heart J 1989;61:417-420.

65. Pinkerton CA, Slack JD, Orr CM, et al: Percutaneous transluminal angioplasty involving internal mammary artery bypass grafts: A femoral approach. Cathet Cardiovasc Diagn 1987; 13:414-418.

66. Douglas J, King S, Roubin G, et al: Percutaneous angioplasty of venous aortocoronary graft stenosis: Late angiographic and clinical outcome. Circulation 1986;74(Suppl II):II-281.

67. Kereiakes DJ, George B, Stertzer SH, et al: Percutaneous transluminal angioplasty of left internal mammary artery grafts. Am J Cardiol 1984;55:1215-1216.

68. Shimshak TM, Giorgi LV, Johnson WL, et al: Application of percutaneous transluminal coronary angioplasty to the internal mammary artery graft. J Am Coll Cardiol 1988;12: 1205-1214.

69. Hearne SE, Wilson JS, Harrington J, et al: Angiographic and clinical follow-up after internal mammary artery graft angioplasty: A 9-year experience. J Am Coll Cardiol 1995;25(Suppl A):139A.

70. Najm HK, Leddy D, Hendry PJ, et al: Postoperative symptomatic internal thoracic artery stenosis and successful treatment with PTCA. Ann Thorac Surg 1995;59:323-327.

71. Ishizaka N, Ishizaka Y, Ikari Y, et al: Initial and subsequent angiographic outcome of percutaneous transluminal angioplasty performed on internal mammary artery grafts. Br Heart J 1995;74:615-619.

72. Gruberg L, Dangaas G, Mehran R, et al: Percutaneous revascularization of the internal mammary artery graft: Short- and long-term outcomes. J Am Coll Cardiol 2000;35:944-948.

73. Sharma A, McGlynn S, Pinnow E, et al: Internal mammary artery intervention: To stent or not to stent? A study of 280 patients. Circulation 2001;104(Suppl II):II-705.

74. Roffi M, Mukherjee D, Chew DP, et al: Procedural success and outcomes of percutaneous coronary intervention on arterial bypass grafts. Circulation 2001;104(Suppl II):II-776.

75. Isshiki T, Yamaguchi T, Tamura T, et al: Percutaneous angioplasty of stenosed gastroepiploic artery grafts. J Am Coll Cardiol 1993;22:727-732.

76. Kussmaul WG: Percutaneous angioplasty of coronary bypass grafts: An emerging consensus. Cathet Cardiovasc Diagn 1988;15:1-4.

77. Platko WP, Hollman J, Whitlow PL, et al: Percutaneous transluminal angioplasty of saphenous vein graft stenosis: Long-term follow-up. J Am Coll Cardiol 1989;7:1645-1650.

78. Plokker HW, Meester BH, Serruys PW: The Dutch experience in percutaneous transluminal angioplasty of narrowed saphenous veins used for aortocoronary arterial bypass. Am J Cardiol 1991;67:361-366.

79. Douglas JS Jr, Weintraub WS, Liberman HA, et al: Update of saphenous graft (SVG) angioplasty: Restenosis and long term outcome. Circulation 1991;84(Suppl II):II-249.

80. Loop FD, Whitlow PL: Coronary angioplasty in patients with previous bypass surgery. J Am Coll Cardiol 1990;16: 1348-1350.

81. Webb JG, Myler RK, Shaw RE, et al: Coronary angioplasty after coronary bypass surgery: Initial results and late outcome in 422 patients. J Am Coll Cardiol 1990;16:812-820.

82. Reeves F, Bonan R, Cote G, et al: Long-term angiographic follow-up after angioplasty of venous coronary bypass grafts. Am Heart J 1991;122:620-627.

83. Ryan TJ, Faxon DP, Gunnar RM, et al: Guidelines for percutaneous transluminal coronary angioplasty. J Am Coll Cardiol 1988;12:529-545.

84. Smith SC Jr, Feldman TE, Hirschfeld JW, et al: ACC/AHA/SCAI 2005 guideline update for percutaneous intervention: A report of the American College of Cardiology/American Heart Association Task Force on the Guidelines (ACC/AHA/SCAI Writing Committee to Update the 2001 Guidelines for Percutaneous Coronary Intervention). J Am Coll Cardiol 2006;47:1-121.

85. Mathew V, Clavell AL, Lennon RJ, et al: Percutaneous coronary interventions in patients with prior coronary bypass surgery: Changes in patient characteristics and outcome during two decades. Am J Med 2000;108:127-135.

86. Kahn JK, Rutherford BD, McConahay DR, et al: Early postoperative balloon coronary angioplasty for failed coronary artery bypass grafting. Am J Cardiol 1990;66:943-946.

87. Dimas AP, Arora RR, Whitlow PL, et al: Percutaneous transluminal angioplasty involving internal mammary artery grafts. Am Heart J 1991;122:423-429.

88. Shimshak TM, Rutherford BD, McConahay DR, et al: PTCA of internal mammary artery (IMA) grafts: Procedural results and late follow-up. Circulation 1991;84(Suppl II):II-590.

89. Kim KB, Lim C, Lee C, et al: Off-pump coronary artery bypass may decrease the patency of saphenous vein grafts. Ann Thorac Surg 2001;72:S1033-S1037.

90. Apostolidou IA, Skubas NJ, Depotis GJ, et al: Occurrence of myocardial ischemia immediately after coronary revascularization using radial arterial conduits. Cardiothorac Vasc Anesth 2001;15:433-438.

91. Reeder GS, Lapeyre AC, Edwards WD, et al: Aspiration thrombectomy for removal of coronary thrombus. Am J Cardiol 1992;70:107-110.

92. Whisenant BK, Baim DS, Kuntz RE, et al: Rheolytic thrombectomy with the Possis AngioJet: Technical considerations and initial clinical experience. J Invasive Cardiol 1999;11:421-426.

93. Rentrop P, Blanke H, Karsch KR, et al: Recanalization of an acutely occluded aortocoronary bypass by intragraft fibrinolysis. Circulation 1980;62:1123-1126.

94. Hartzler GO, Johnson WL, McConahay DR, et al: Dissolution of coronary artery bypass graft thrombi by streptokinase infusion. Am J Cardiol 1981;47:493.

95. Rentrop KP, Driesman M, Blanke H, et al: Non-surgical recanalization of early and late bypass occlusion. Circulation 1981;64(Suppl IV):IV-246.

96. Holmes DR, Chesebro JH, Vlietstra RE, et al: Streptokinase for vein graft thrombosis—A caveat. Circulation 1981;63: 729.

97. Frumin H, Goldberg MJ, Rubenfire M, et al: Late thrombolysis of an occluded aortocoronary saphenous vein graft. Am Heart J 1983;106:401-403.

98. Slysh S, Goldberg S, Dervan JP, et al: Unstable angina and evolving myocardial infarction following coronary bypass surgery: Pathogenesis and treatment with interventional catheterization. Am Heart J 1985;109:744-752.

99. Macaya C, Alfonso F, Iniguez A, et al: Stenting for elastic recoil during coronary angioplasty of the left main coronary artery. Am J Cardiol 1992;70:105-107.

100. Kuntz RE, Piana R, Schnitt SJ, et al: Early ostial vein graft stenosis: Management by atherectomy. Cathet Cardiovasc Diagn 1991;24:41-44.

101. Robertson GC, Simpson JB, Vetter JW, et al: Directional coronary atherectomy for ostial lesions. Circulation 1991;84(Suppl II):II-251.

102. Eigler NL, Weinstock B, Douglas JS Jr, et al: Excimer laser coronary angioplasty of aorto-ostial stenoses: Results of the Excimer Laser Coronary Angioplasty (ELCA) Registry in the first 200 patients. Circulation 1993;88:2049-2057.

103. Tierstein P, Stratienko AA, Schatz RA: Coronary stenting for ostial stenoses: Initial results and six month follow-up. Circulation 1991;84(Suppl II):II-250.

104. Miranda CP, Rutherford BD, McConahay DR, et al: Angioplasty of older saphenous vein grafts continues to be a sound therapeutic option. J Am Coll Cardiol 1992;19(Suppl A):350A.

105. Morrison DA, Crowley ST, Veerakul G, et al: Percutaneous transluminal angioplasty of saphenous vein grafts for medically refractory unstable angina. J Am Coll Cardiol 1994;23:1066-1070.

106. Neitzel GF, Barboriak JJ, Pintar K, et al: Atherosclerosis in aortocoronary bypass grafts: Morphologic study and risk

factor analysis 6 to 12 years after surgery. Arteriosclerosis 1986;6:594-600.

107. Smith SH, Greer JC: Morphology of saphenous vein-coronary artery bypass grafts: Seven to 116 months after surgery. Arch Pathol Lab Med 1983;107:13-18.

108. Kugelmass AD, Sadanandan S, Cannon CP, et al: Early invasive strategy improves outcomes in acute coronary syndrome patients with prior CABG: Results from TACTICS-TIMI 18. Circulation 2001;104(Suppl II):II-548.

109. Mathew V, Berger PB, Lennon RJ, et al: Comparison of percutaneous interventions for unstable angina pectoris in patients with and without previous coronary artery bypass grafting. Am J Cardiol 2000;86:931-937.

110. Motwani JG, Topol EJ: Aortocoronary saphenous vein graft disease. Pathogenesis, predisposition, and prevention. Circulation 1998;97:916-931.

111. Waller BF, Rothbaum DA, Gorfinkel HJ, et al: Morphologic observations after percutaneous transluminal balloon angioplasty of early and late aortocoronary saphenous vein bypass grafts. J Am Coll Cardiol 1984;4:784-792.

112. Walts AE, Fishbein MC, Sustaita H, et al: Ruptured atheromatous plaques in saphenous vein coronary artery bypass grafts: A mechanism of acute, thrombotic, late graft occlusion. Circulation 1982;65:197-201.

113. Pregowski J, Tyczyski P, Mintz GS, et al: Incidence and clinical correlates of ruptured plaques in saphenous vein grafts. An intravascular ultrasound study. J Am Coll Cardiol 2005;45:1974-1979.

114. Saber RS, Edwards WD, Holmes DR Jr, et al: Balloon angioplasty of aortocoronary saphenous vein bypass grafts: A histopathologic study of six grafts from five patients, with emphasis on restenosis and embolic complications. J Am Coll Cardiol 1988;12:1501-1509.

115. Hong MK, Popma JJ, Leon MB, et al: Vascular recoil in saphenous vein graft stenoses after investigational angioplasty. J Am Coll Cardiol 1992;19(Suppl A):263A.

116. Leon MB, Ellis SG, Pichard AD, et al: Stents may be the preferred treatment for focal aortocoronary vein graft disease. Circulation 1991;84(Suppl II):II-249.

117. Pomerantz RM, Kuntz RE, Carrozza JP, et al: Acute and long-term outcome of narrowed saphenous venous grafts treated by endoluminal stenting and directional atherectomy. Am J Cardiol 1992;70:161-167.

118. Hinohara T, Robertson GC, Selmon MR, et al: Restenosis after directional coronary atherectomy. J Am Coll Cardiol 1992;20:623-632.

119. Untereker WJ, Litvack F, Margolis JR, et al: Excimer laser coronary angioplasty of saphenous vein grafts. Circulation 1991;84(Suppl II):II-249.

120. Meany T, Kramer B, Knopf W, et al: Multicenter experience of atherectomy of saphenous vein grafts: Immediate results and follow-up. J Am Coll Cardiol 1992;19(Suppl A):262.

121. Miranda CP, Rutherford BD, McConahay DR, et al: Elective PTCA in post-bypass patients: Comparison between those undergoing native artery dilatations and those undergoing bypass graft dilatations. Circulation 1992;86(Suppl I):I-457.

122. de Feyter PJ, Serruys P, van den Brand M, et al: Percutaneous transluminal angioplasty of a totally occluded bypass graft: A challenge that should be resisted. Am J Cardiol 1989;64:88-90.

123. Levine DJ, Sharaf BL, Williams DO: Late follow-up of patients with totally occluded saphenous vein bypass grafts treated by prolonged selective urokinase infusion. J Am Coll Cardiol 1992;19(Suppl A):292A.

124. Hartmann J, McKeever L, Teran J, et al: Prolonged infusion of urokinase for recanalization of chronically occluded aortocoronary bypass grafts. Am J Cardiol 1988;61:189-191.

125. Marx M, Armstrong W, Brent B, et al: Transcatheter recanalization of a chronically occluded saphenous aortocoronary bypass graft. AJR Am J Roentgenol 1987;148:375-377.

126. Hartmann JR, McKeever LS, Stamato NJ, et al: Recanalization of chronically occluded aortocoronary saphenous vein bypass grafts by extended infusion of urokinase: Initial results and short-term clinical follow-up. J Am Coll Cardiol 1991;18:1517-1523.

127. Gurley JC, MacPhail BS: Acute myocardial infarction due to thrombolytic reperfusion of chronically occluded saphenous vein coronary bypass grafts. Am J Cardiol 1991;68:274-275.

128. McKeever LS, Hartmann JR, Bufalino VJ, et al: Acute myocardial infarction complicating recanalization of aortocoronary bypass grafts with urokinase therapy. Am J Cardiol 1989;64:683-685.

129. Margolis JR, Mogensen L, Mehta S, et al: Diffuse embolization following percutaneous transluminal coronary angioplasty of occluded vein grafts: The blush phenomenon. Clin Cardiol 1991;14:489-493.

130. Blankenship JC, Modesto TA, Madigan NP: Acute myocardial infarction complicating urokinase infusion for total saphenous vein graft occlusion. Cathet Cardiovasc Diagn 1993;28:39-43.

131. Taylor MA, Santoian EC, Ali J, et al: Intracerebral hemorrhage complicating urokinase infusion into an occluded aortocoronary bypass graft. Cathet Cardiovasc Diagn 1994;431:206-210.

132. Pitney MR, Cumpston N, Mews GC, et al: Use of twenty-four hour infusions of intracoronary tissue plasminogen activator to increase the application of coronary angioplasty. Cathet Cardiovasc Diagn 1992;26:255-259.

133. Kahn JK, Rutherford BD, McConahay DR, et al: PTCA of totally occluded saphenous vein grafts: Safety and success. J Am Coll Cardiol 1992;19(Suppl A):350A.

134. Bedotto JB, Rutherford BD, Hartzler GO: Intramyocardial hemorrhage due to prolonged intracoronary infusion of urokinase into a totally occluded saphenous vein bypass graft. Cathet Cardiovasc Diagn 1992;25:52-56.

135. Hartmann JR, McKeever LS, O'Neill WW, et al: Recanalization of Chronically Occluded Aortocoronary Saphenous Vein Bypass Grafts with Long-Term, Low-Dose Direct Infusion of Urokinase (ROBUST): A serial trial. J Am Coll Cardiol 1996;27:60-66.

136. Berger PB, Bell MR, Simari R, et al: Immediate and long-term clinical outcome in patients undergoing angioplasty of occluded vein grafts. J Am Coll Cardiol 1996;26(Suppl A):180A.

137. Glazier JJ, Bauer HH, Kiernan FJ, et al: Recanalization of totally occluded saphenous vein grafts using local urokinase delivery with the Dispatch catheter. Cathet Cardiovasc Diagn 1995;36:326-332.

138. Heuser RR: Recanalization or occluded SVGs: Is there light at the end of the graft? Cathet Cardiovasc Diagn 1995;36:333-334.

139. Sullebarger JT, Puleo J: Extraction atherectomy for the recanalization of totally occluded aortocoronary saphenous vein grafts. Cathet Cardiovasc Diagn 1995;36:339-343.

140. Margolis JR, Mehta S, Kramer B, et al: Extraction atherectomy for the treatment of recent totally occluded saphenous vein grafts. J Am Coll Cardiol 1994;23(Suppl A):405A.

141. Chapekis AT, George BS, Candela RJ: Rapid thrombus dissolution by continuous infusion of urokinase through an intracoronary perfusion wire prior to and following PTCA: Results in native coronaries and patent saphenous vein grafts. Cathet Cardiovasc Diagn 1991;23:89-92.

142. Coronary Artery Surgery Study (CASS) and Their Associates: A randomized trial of coronary artery bypass: Quality of life in patients randomly assigned to treatment groups. Circulation 1983;68:951-956.

143. Maynard C, Weaver WD, Litwin P, et al: Acute myocardial infarction and prior coronary artery surgery in the Myocardial Infarction Triage and Intervention Registry: Patient characteristics, treatment, and outcome. Coron Artery Dis 1991;2:443-448.

144. Peterson LR, Chandra NC, French WJ, et al: Reperfusion therapy in patients with acute myocardial infarction and prior coronary artery bypass graft surgery (National Registry of Myocardial Infarction-2). Am J Cardiol 1999;84:1287-1291.

145. Wiseman A, Waters DD, Walling A, et al: Long-term prognosis after myocardial infarction in patients with previous coronary artery bypass surgery. J Am Coll Cardiol 1988;12:873-880.

146. Little WC, Gwinn NS, Burrows MT, et al: Cause of acute myocardial infarction late after successful coronary artery bypass grafting. Am J Cardiol 1990;65:808-810.

147. Grines CL, Booth DC, Nissen SE, et al: Mechanism of acute myocardial infarction in patients with prior coronary artery bypass grafting and therapeutic implications. Am J Cardiol 1990;65:1292-1296.

148. Reiner JS, Lundergan CF, Kopecky SL, et al: Ineffectiveness of thrombolysis for acute MI following vein graft occlusion. Circulation 1996;94(Suppl I):I-570.

149. Stone GW, Brodie B, Griffin J, et al: Primary angioplasty in patients with prior bypass surgery. Circulation 1996;94(Suppl I):I-243.

150. Stone GW, Brodie BR, Griffin JJ, et al: Clinical and angiographic outcomes in patients with previous coronary artery bypass graft surgery treated with primary balloon angioplasty for acute myocardial infarction. J Am Coll Cardiol 2000;35:605-611.

151. Kavanaugh KM, Topol EJ: Acute intervention during myocardial infarction in patients with prior coronary bypass surgery. Am J Cardiol 1990;65:924-926.

152. Kleiman NS, Berman DA, Gaston WR, et al: Early intravenous thrombolytic therapy for acute myocardial infarction in patients with prior coronary artery bypass grafts. Am J Cardiol 1989;63:102-104.

153. Kahn JK, Rutherford BD, McConahay DR, et al: Usefulness of angioplasty during acute myocardial infarction in patients with prior coronary artery bypass grafting. Am J Cardiol 1990;65:698-702.

154. Brodie BR: Reperfusion therapy for acute myocardial infarction in patients with prior bypass surgery. Am Heart J 2001;142:381-383.

155. Suwaidi JA, Velianou JL, Berger PB, et al: Primary percutaneous coronary interventions in patients with acute myocardial infarction and prior coronary artery bypass grafting. Am Heart J 2001;142:452-459.

156. Watson PS, Hadjipetrou P, Cox SV, et al: Angiographic and clinical outcomes following acute infarct angioplasty on saphenous vein grafts. Am J Cardiol 1999;83:1018-1021.

157. Gunnar RM, Bourdillon PD, Dixon DW, et al: Guidelines for the early management of patients with acute myocardial infarction. J Am Coll Cardiol 1990;16:249-292.

158. Ryan TJ, Anderson JL, Antman EM, et al: ACC/AHA guidelines for the management of patients with acute myocardial infarction: A report of the American College of Cardiology/American Heart Association Task Force on Practice Guidelines (Committee on Management of Acute Myocardial Infarction). J Am Coll Cardiol 1996;28:1328-1428.

159. Iakovau I, Dangas G, Mintz GS, et al: Relation of final lumen dimensions in saphenous vein grafts after stent implantation to outcome. Am J Cardiol 2004;93:963.

160. Thomas WJ, Cowley MJ, Vetrovec GW, et al: Effectiveness of rotational atherectomy in aortocoronary saphenous vein grafts. Am J Cardiol 2000;86:88-91.

161. Ellis SG, Brener SJ, DeLuca S, et al: Late myocardial ischemia events after saphenous vein graft intervention—Importance of initially "nonsignificant vein graft lesions." Am J Cardiol 1997;79:1460-1464.

162. Stratienko AA, Ginsberg R, Schatz RA, et al: Technique for shortening angioplasty guide catheter length when therapeutic catheter fails to reach target stenosis. Cathet Cardiovasc Diagn 1993;30:331-333.

163. Satler LF: The advantage of anticipating the need for a short guiding catheter. Cathet Cardiovasc Diagn 1996;37:76.

164. Linnemeier TJ: Biliary stents for saphenous vein grafts: Reducing the risk of stent implantation [abstract]. Cathet Cardiovasc Diagn 1995;35:354.

165. Moscucci M, Punamiya K, Ricciardi MJ, et al: Guiding catheter thrombectomy during percutaneous coronary interventions for acute coronary syndromes. Catheter Cardiovasc Interv 2000;49:192-196.

166. Strauss BH, Natarajan MK, Batchelor WB, et al: Early and late quantitative angiographic results of vein graft lesions treated by excimer laser with adjunctive balloon angioplasty. Circulation 1995;92:348-356.

167. Hong MK, Wong SC, Popma JJ, et al: Favorable results of debulking followed by immediate adjunct stent therapy for high risk saphenous vein graft lesions. J Am Coll Cardiol 1996;27(Suppl A):A179.

168. Moses JW, Teirstein PS, Sketch MH Jr, et al: Angiographic determinants of risk and outcome of coronary embolus and myocardial infarction (MI) with the transluminal extraction catheter (TEC): A report from the New Approaches to Coronary Intervention (NACI) Registry. J Am Coll Cardiol 1994;24:220A.

169. Safian RD, Grines CL, May MA, et al: Clinical and angiographic results of transluminal extraction coronary atherectomy in saphenous vein bypass grafts. Circulation 1994;89:302-312.

170. Meany TB, Leon MB, Kramer BL, et al: Transluminal extraction catheter for the treatment of diseased saphenous vein grafts: A multicenter experience. Cathet Cardiovasc Diagn 1995;34:112-120.

171. Dooris M, Hoffmann M, Glazier S, et al: Comparative results of transluminal extraction coronary atherectomy in saphenous vein graft lesions with and without thrombus. J Am Coll Cardiol 1995;25:1700-1705.

172. Al-Shaibi KF, Goods CM, Jain SP, et al: Does transluminal extraction atherectomy reduce distal embolization in saphenous vein grafts? Circulation 1995;92(Suppl I):I-329.

173. Khan MA, Liu MW, Chio FL, et al: Effect of abciximab on cardiac enzyme elevation after transluminal extraction atherectomy (TEC) in high-risk saphenous vein graft lesions: Comparison with a historical control group. Catheter Cardiovasc Interv 2001;52:40-44.

174. Stone GW, Cox DA, Babb J, et al: Prospective, randomized evaluation of thrombectomy prior to percutaneous intervention in diseased saphenous vein grafts and thrombus-containing coronary arteries. J Am Coll Cardiol 2003;42:2007-2013.

175. Kramer B: Optimal therapy for degenerated saphenous vein graft disease. J Invasive Cardiol 1995;7(Suppl D):14D-20D.

176. George BS: TEC for old grafts, TEC for new clots: If you don't like it, you're not using it right. J Invasive Cardiol 1995;7(Suppl D):21D-24D.

177. Kaplan BM, Safian RD, Goldstein JA, et al: Efficacy of angioscopy in determining the effectiveness of intracoronary urokinase and TEC atherectomy thrombus removal from an occluded saphenous vein graft prior to stent implantation. Cathet Cardiovasc Diagn 1995;36:335-337.

178. Kaplan BM, Safian RD, Grines CL, et al: A prospective study of stent implantation in high risk lesions utilizing adjunctive extraction atherectomy and angioscopy guidance [abstract]. J Invasive Cardiol 1996;8:38.

179. Hong MK, Mintz GS, Popma JJ, et al: Angiographic results and late clinical outcomes utilizing a stent synergy (pre-stent atheroablation) approach in complex lesion subsets. J Invasive Cardiol 1996;8:15-22.

180. Cundey PE, Whitlock RR, Norman J, et al: Prolonged intragraft urokinase with a new infusion wire: Improved short-term results. Cathet Cardiovasc Diagn 1994;31:150-152.

181. Fischell TA, Haddad N, Baskerville S, et al: Ultrasound thrombolysis for the treatment of thrombotic occlusion of degenerated saphenous vein grafts. Catheter Cardiovasc Interv 2000;50:90-95.

182. Rosenschein U, Gaul G, Erbel R, et al: Percutaneous transluminal therapy of occluded saphenous vein grafts: Can the challenge be met with ultrasound thrombolysis? Circulation 1999;99:26-29.

183. Denardo SJ, Morris NB, Rocha-Singh KJ: Safety and efficacy of extended urokinase infusion plus stent deployment for treatment of obstructed, older saphenous vein grafts. Am J Cardiol 1995;76:776-780.

184. McKay RG: Site-specific, catheter-based thrombolysis: A new technique for treating intracoronary thrombus and thrombus-containing stenosis. J Invasive Cardiol 1995;7(Suppl E):36E-43E.

185. Mitchel JF, Fram DB, Palme DF, et al: Enhanced intracoronary thrombolysis with urokinase using a novel, local drug delivery system. Circulation 1995;91:785-793.

186. Barness GW, Buller C, Ohman EM, et al: Reduced thrombus burden with abciximab delivered locally before percutaneous intervention in saphenous vein grafts. Am Heart J 2000;139:824-829.
187. Huang RI, Patel P, Walinsky P, et al: Efficacy of intracoronary nicardipine in the treatment of no-reflow during percutaneous coronary intervention. Cathet Cardiovasc Interv 2006;68:671-676.
188. Piana RN, Paik GY, Moscucci M, et al: Incidence and treatment of "no-reflow" after percutaneous coronary intervention. Circulation 1994;89:2514-2518.
189. Waksman R, Scott NA, Douglas JS Jr, et al: Distal embolization is common after directional atherectomy in coronary arteries and vein grafts. Circulation 1993;88(Suppl I):I-299.
190. Michaels AD, Dauterman K, Malik F, et al: Pretreatment with intragraft verapamil prior to percutaneous coronary intervention of saphenous vein graft lesions: Results of the randomized, controlled Vasodilator Prevention of No Reflow (VAPOR) trial. J Am Coll Cardiol 2001;37(Suppl A):24A.
191. Marzilli M, Marraccini P, Gliozheni E, et al: Intracoronary adenosine as an adjunct to combined use of primary angioplasty in acute myocardial infarction: Beneficial effects on angiographically assessed no-reflow [abstract]. J Am Coll Cardiol 1996;27(Suppl A):81A.
192. Hillegass WB, Dean NA, Liao L, et al: Treatment of no-reflow and impaired flow with the nitric oxide donor nitroprusside following percutaneous coronary interventions: Initial human clinical experience. J Am Coll Cardiol 2001;37:1335-1343.
193. Kotani J, Nanto S, Ohara T, et al: Plaque gruel of atheromatous coronary lesions may contribute to the no-reflow phenomenon in patients with acute coronary syndrome. Circulation 2001;20;104(Suppl II):II-67.
194. Muhlestein JB, Gomez MA, Karagonuis LA, et al: "Rescue ReoPro": Acute utilization of abciximab for the dissolution of coronary thrombus developing as a complication of coronary angioplasty. Circulation 1995;92(Suppl I):I-607.
195. Kahn JK, Hartzler GO: Retrograde coronary angioplasty of isolated arterial segments through saphenous vein bypass grafts. Cathet Cardiovasc Diagn 1990;20:88-93.
196. Brown RIG, Galligan L, Penn IM, et al: Right internal mammary artery graft angioplasty through a right brachial artery approach using a new custom guide catheter: A case report. Cathet Cardiovasc Diagn 1992;25:42-45.
197. Almagor Y, Thomas J, Colombo A: Balloon expandable stent implantation of a stenosis at the origin of the left internal mammary artery graft. Cathet Cardiovasc Diagn 1991;24:256-258.
198. Bajaj RK, Roubin GS: Intravascular stenting of the right internal mammary artery. Cathet Cardiovasc Diagn 1991;24:252-255.
199. Ernst S, Bal E, Plokker T, et al: Percutaneous balloon angioplasty (PBA) of a left subclavian artery stenosis or occlusion to establish adequate flow through the left internal mammary artery for coronary bypass purposes. Circulation 1991;84(Suppl II):II-591.
200. Belz M, Marshall JJ, Cowley MJ, et al: Subclavian balloon angioplasty in the management of the coronary-subclavian steal syndrome. Cathet Cardiovasc Diagn 1992;25:161-163.
201. Shapira S, Braun S, Puram B, et al: Percutaneous transluminal angioplasty of proximal subclavian artery stenosis after left internal mammary to left anterior descending artery bypass surgery. J Am Coll Cardiol 1991;18:1120-1123.
202. Miller RM, Knox M: Patient tolerance of ioxaglate and iopamidol in internal mammary artery arteriography. Cathet Cardiovasc Diagn 1992;25:31-34.
203. Kent KM, Bentivoglio LG, Block PC, et al: Percutaneous transluminal coronary angioplasty: Report from the registry of the National Heart, Lung, and Blood Institute. Am J Cardiol 1982;49:2011-2020.
204. Detre K, Holubkov R, Kelsey S, et al: Percutaneous transluminal coronary angioplasty in 1985-1986 and 1977-1981: The National Heart, Lung, and Blood Institute Registry. N Engl J Med 1988;318:265-270.

205. Weintraub WS, Jones EL, Morris DC, et al: Outcome of reoperative coronary bypass surgery versus coronary angioplasty after bypass surgery. Circulation 1997;95:868-877.
206. Weintraub WS, Mauldin PD, Becker E, et al: Cost vs. outcome for redo coronary surgery vs. coronary angioplasty for clinical recurrence after coronary surgery. J Am Coll Cardiol 1996;27(Suppl A):318A.
207. Stephan WJ, O'Keefe JH Jr, Piehler JM, et al: Coronary angioplasty versus repeat coronary artery bypass grafting for patients with previous bypass surgery. J Am Coll Cardiol 1996;28:1140-1146.
208. Morrison DA, Sethi G, Sacks J, et al: Percutaneous coronary intervention versus repeat bypass surgery for patients with medically refractory myocardial ischemia: AWESOME randomized trial and registry experience with post-CABG patients. J Am Coll Cardiol 2002;40:1951-1954.
209. Cole JH, Jones EL, Craver JM, et al: Outcomes of repeat revascularization in diabetic patients with prior coronary surgery. J Am Coll Cardiol 2002;40:1968-1975,
210. Abhyankar A, Bernstein L, Harris PJ, et al: Reintervention and clinical events after saphenous vein graft angioplasty—a comparison of optimal PTCA versus stenting. Circulation 1996;94(Suppl I):I-686.
211. Holmes DR, Topol EJ, Califf RM, et al: A multicenter, randomized trial of coronary angioplasty versus directional atherectomy for patients with saphenous vein graft lesions. Circulation 1995;91:1966-1974.
212. Lefkovits J, Holmes DR, Califf RM, et al: Predictors and sequelae of distal embolization during saphenous vein graft intervention from the CAVEAT-II Trial. Circulation 1995;92:734-740.
213. Bittl JA, Sanborn TA, Yardley DE, et al: Predictors of outcome of percutaneous excimer laser coronary angioplasty of saphenous vein bypass graft lesions. Am J Cardiol 1994;74:144-148.
214. Wong SC, Popma JJ, Hong MK, et al: Procedural results and long term clinical outcome in aorto-ostial saphenous vein graft lesions after new device angioplasty. J Am Coll Cardiol 1995;25(Suppl A):394A.
215. Eigler NL, Weinstock B, Douglas JS Jr, et al: Excimer laser coronary angioplasty of aorto-ostial stenoses: Results of the Excimer Laser Coronary Angioplasty (ELCA) Registry in the first 200 patients. Circulation 1993;88:2049-2057.
216. Douglas JS Jr, Ghazzal ZMB, Bal Albaki HA, et al: Excimer laser coronary angioplasty of ostial lesions. Cathet Cardiovasc Diagn 1991;23:74-75.
217. Strauss BH, Natarajan MK, Batchelor WB, et al: Early and late quantitative angiographic results of vein graft lesions treated by excimer laser with adjunctive balloon angioplasty. Circulation 1995;92:348-356.
218. Hong MK, Wong SC, Popma JJ, et al: Favorable results of debulking followed by immediate adjunct stent therapy for high risk saphenous vein graft lesions. J Am Coll Cardiol 1996;27(Suppl A):A179.
219. Stone GW, Cox DA, Babb J, et al: Prospective, randomized evaluation of thrombectomy prior to percutaneous intervention in diseased saphenous vein grafts and thrombus-containing coronary arteries. J Am Coll Cardiol 2003;42:2007-2013.
220. Carrozza JP, Kuntz RE, Levine MJ, et al: Angiographic and clinical outcome of intracoronary stenting: Immediate and long-term results from a large single-center experience. J Am Coll Cardiol 1992;20:328-337.
221. Fenton SH, Fischman DL, Savage MP, et al: Long-term angiographic and clinical outcome after implantation of balloon-expandable stents in aortocoronary saphenous vein grafts. Am J Cardiol 1994;74:1187-1191.
222. Piana RN, Moscucci M, Cohen DJ, et al: Palmaz-Schatz stenting for treatment of focal vein graft stenosis: Immediate results and long-term outcome. J Am Coll Cardiol 1994;23:1296-1304.
223. Wong SC, Baim DS, Schatz RA, et al: Acute results and late outcomes after stent implantation in saphenous vein graft lesions: The multicenter USA Palmaz-Schatz stent experience. J Am Coll Cardiol 1995;26:704-712.

224. Savage MP, Douglas JS Jr, Fischman DL, et al: Stent placement compared with balloon angioplasty for obstructed bypass grafts. Saphenous Vein De novo Trial Investigators. N Engl J Med 1997;337:740-747.

225. Ahmed JM, Hong MK, Mehran R, et al: Influence of diabetes mellitus on early and late clinical outcomes in saphenous vein graft stenting. J Am Coll Cardiol 2000;36:1186-1193.

226. de Scheerder JK, Strauss BH, de Feyter PJ, et al: Stenting of venous bypass grafts: A new treatment modality of patients who are poor candidates for reintervention. Am Heart J 1992;23:1296-1304.

227. Strauss BH, Serruys PW, Bertrand ME, et al: Qualitative angiographic follow-up of the coronary Wallstent in native vessel bypass grafts. Am J Cardiol 1992;69:475-481.

228. de Jaegere PP, van Domburg RT, de Feyter PJ, et al: Long-term clinical outcome after stent implantation in saphenous vein grafts. J Am Coll Cardiol 1996;28:89-96.

229. Choussat R, Black AJR, Boss I, et al: Long-term clinical outcome after endoluminal reconstruction of diffusely degenerated saphenous vein grafts with less-shortening Wallstents. J Am Coll Cardiol 2000;36:387-394.

230. Fortuna R, Heuser RR, Garrat KN, et al: Wiktor intracoronary stent: Experience in the first 101 graft patients. Circulation 1993;88(Suppl I):I-308.

231. Hanekamp CEE, Koolen JJ, Den Heyer P, et al: A randomized comparison between balloon angioplasty and elective stent implantation in venous bypass grafts: The VENESTENT study. J Am Coll Cardiol 2000;35(Suppl A):9A.

232. Safian RD, Kaplan B, Schreiber T, et al: Interim results of the Wallstent endoprosthesis in saphenous vein graft trial. Circulation 1998;98(Suppl I):I-662.

233. Le May MR, Labinaz M, Marquis JF, et al: Predictors of long-term outcome after stent implantation in a saphenous vein graft. Am J Cardiol 1999;83:681-686.

234. Dharmadhikari A, Di Mario C, Tzifos V, et al: Comparison of procedural and one-year outcome with only balloon angioplasty, covered stents, and non-covered stents in saphenous vein grafts. J Am Coll Cardiol 2000;35(Suppl A):26A.

235. Baldus S, Koster R, Elsner M, et al: Treatment of aortocoronary vein graft lesions with membrane-covered stents: A multicenter surveillance trial. Circulation 2000;102:2024-2027.

236. Nishida T, Colombo A, Briguouri C, et al: Contemporary percutaneous treatment of saphenous vein graft stenosis: Immediate and late outcomes. J Invasive Cardiol 2000;12:505-512.

237. Bhargava B, Kornowski R, Mehran R, et al: Procedural results and intermediate clinical outcomes after multiple saphenous vein graft stenting. J Am Coll Cardiol 2000;35:389-397.

238. Urban P, Sigwart U, Golf S, et al: Intravascular stenting for stenosis of aortocoronary venous bypass grafts. J Am Coll Cardiol 1994;23:1296-1304.

239. Rechavia E, Litvack F, Macko G, Eigler NL: Stent implantation of saphenous vein graft aorto-ostial lesions in patients with unstable ischemic syndromes: Immediate angiographic results and long-term clinical outcome. J Am Coll Cardiol 1995;25:866-870.

240. Rocha-Singh K, Morris N, Wong SC, et al: Coronary stenting for treatment of ostial stenoses of native coronary arteries or aortocoronary saphenous venous grafts. Am J Cardiol 1995;75:26-29.

241. Ahmed JM, Hong MK, Mehran R, et al: Comparison of de-bulking followed by stenting versus stenting alone for aortic-ostial lesions: Immediate and one-year clinical outcomes. J Am Coll Cardiol 2000;35:1560-1568.

242. Brenner SJ, Ellis SG, Apperson-Hansen C: Compared with balloon angioplasty of saphenous vein grafts, stenting is associated with highly favorable results [abstract]. J Invasive Cardiol 1996;8:38.

243. Hong MK, Mehran R, Dangas G, et al: Are we making progress with percutaneous saphenous vein graft treatment? J Am Coll Cardiol 2001;38:150-154.

244. Keeley EC, Velez CA, O'Neill WW, et al: Long-term clinical outcome and predictors of major adverse cardiac events after percutaneous interventions on saphenous vein grafts. J Am Coll Cardiol 2001;38:659-665.

245. Roffi M, Mukherjee D, Bhatt DL, et al: Percutaneous interventions of coronary bypass grafts have doubled major adverse events. J Am Coll Cardiol 2001;37(Suppl A):6A.

246. Ahmed JM, Dangas GD, Mehran R, et al: Clinical, angiographic and intravascular ultrasound predictors of target vessel revascularization and late cardiac events after stent implantation in saphenous vein grafts. J Am Coll Cardiol 2001;37(Suppl A):20A.

247. Ashfaq S, Ghazzal Z, Douglas JS, et al: Impact of diabetes on five-year outcomes after vein graft intervention performed prior to the drug-eluting stent era. J Invasive Cardiol 2006;18:100-105.

248. Costa M, Angiolillo DJ, Teirstein P, et al: Sirolimus-eluting stents for treatment of complex bypass graft disease: Insights from the SECURE registry. J Invasive Cardiol 2005;17:396-398.

249. Hoye A, Lemos PA, Arampatzis CA, et al: Effectiveness of the sirolimus-eluting stent in the treatment of saphenous vein graft disease. J Invasive Cardiol 2004;16:230-233.

250. Ge L, Lakovou I, Sangiorgi GM, et al: Treatment of saphenous vein graft lesions with drug-eluting stents: Immediate and midterm outcome. J Am Coll Cardiol 2004;45:989-994.

251. Sousa JE, Abizaid A, Gershlick AH, et al: Real world use of sirolimus-eluting stents in saphenous vein graft disease: Data from the e-Cypher registry. Am Coll Cardiol 2005;45(Suppl A):26A.

252. Lasala J: ARRIVE II: Taxus registry. Paper presented at the meeting of the American College of Cardiology, March 2006, Atlanta, GA.

253. Lee MS, Shah AP, Aragon J, et al: Drug-eluting stenting is superior to bare metal stenting in saphenous vein grafts. Catheter Cardiovasc Interv 2005;66:507-511.

254. Vermeersh P, Pierfrancesco A, Verheye S, et al: Randomized double-blind comparison of sirolimus-eluting stent versus bare-metal stent implantation in diseased saphenous vein grafts: Six-month angiographic, intravascular ultrasound, and clinical follow-up of the RRISC trial. J Am Coll Cardiol 2006;48:2423-2431.

255. Selvanayagam JB, Channon K, Petersen SE, et al: Troponin elevation after percutaneous coronary intervention directly represents the extent of irreversible myocardial injury. Circulation 2005;111:1027-1032.

256. El-Jack S, Suwatchai P, Ruygrok PM, et al: Distal embolization during native vessel and vein graft coronary intervention with a vascular protection device: Predictor of high risk lesions. J Am Coll Cardiol 2006;47:(Suppl A):213A.

257. Prasad A, Singh M, Lerman A, et al: Isolated elevation in troponin T after percutaneous coronary intervention is associated with higher long-term mortality. J Am Coll Cardiol 2006;48:1765-1770, 2006.

258. Kalon KL, Carrozza JP, Popma JJ, et al: Creatine-kinase MB isoform (CK-MB) elevations following single vessel percutaneous revascularization of saphenous vein grafts. Circulation 1998;98(Suppl I):I-353.

259. Leon MB, Ellis SG, Moses J, et al: Interim report from the Reduced Anticoagulation Vein Graft Sent (RAVES) study. Circulation 1996;94(Suppl I):I-683.

260. Liu MW, Douglas JS Jr, King SB III, et al: Angiographic predictors of coronary embolization in the PTCA of vein graft lesions. Circulation 1989;80(Suppl I):II-172.

261. Giugliano GR, Kuntz RE, Popma JJ, et al: Determinants of 30-day adverse events following saphenous vein graft intervention and without a distal occlusion emboli protection device. Am J Coll Cardiol 2005;95:173-177.

262. Hong MK, Mehran R, Dangas G, et al: Creatine kinase-MB enzyme elevation following successful saphenous vein graft intervention is associated with late mortality. Circulation 1999;100:2400-2405.

263. Topol EJ, Yadav JS: Recognition of the importance of embolization in atherosclerotic vascular disease. Circulation 2000;101:570-580.

264. Webb JG, Carere RG, Virmani R, et al: Retrieval and analysis of particulate debris following saphenous vein graft intervention. J Am Coll Cardiol 1999;34:461-467.

265. Baim DS, Wahr D, George B, et al: Randomized trial of a distal embolic protection device during percutaneous intervention

of saphenous vein aorto-coronary bypass grafts. Circulation 2002;105:512-590.

266. Salloum J, Reddy B, Vaughn DE, et al: Elimination of soluble vasoactive factors by the PercuSurge GuardWire distal protection device during percutaneous coronary intervention of saphenous vein graft. J Am Coll Cardiol 2004;43:71A.

266a. Leineweber K, Bose D, Vogelsang M, et al: Intense vasoconstriction in response to aspirate from stented saphenous vein aortocoronary bypass grafts. J Am Coll Cardiol 2006;47: 981-986.

267. Gorog DA, Foale RA, Malik I, et al: Distal myocardial protection during percutaneous coronary intervention. When and where? J Am Coll Cardiol 2005;46:1434-1445.

268. Weisz G, Halkin A, Costantini CO, et al: Coronary blood flow velocity and myocardial perfusion with balloon occlusion and filter-based distal protection devices in saphenous vein graft stenting: Early experience of two centers. J Am Cardiol 2004;43:52A.

269. Giugliano GR, Prpic R, Cutlip D, et al: Does the beneficial effect of distal protection in saphenous vein graft interventions vary with lesion length? A SAFER (Saphenous Vein Graft Angioplasty Free of Emboli Randomized) substudy. J Am Coll Cardiol 2002;39:9A.

270. Giri S, Kuntz RE, Eisenhauer C, et al: Effect of baseline thrombus in the SAFER (Saphenous Vein Graft Angioplasty Free of Emboli Randomized) trial. J Am Coll Cardiol 2002; 39:52A.

271. Cohen DJ, Murphy SA, Baim DS, et al: Cost-effectiveness of distal embolic protection for patients undergoing percutaneous intervention of saphenous vein bypass grafts: Results from the SAFER trial. J Am Coll Cardiol 2004;44:1801-1808.

272. Senter SR, Nathan S, Grupta A, et al: Clinical and economic outcomes of embolic complications and strategies for distal embolic protection during percutaneous coronary intervention in saphenous vein grafts. J Invasive Cardiol 2006;18:49-53.

273. Klein LW, Brindis RG, Kutcher MA, et al: Intervention in saphenous vein grafts: A predictive model based on clinical presentation of 5,899 consecutive cases in the ACC-NCDR Registry. J Am Coll Cardiol 2002;39:8A.

274. Stone GW, Rogers C, Hermiller J, et al: Randomized comparison of the distal protection with a filter-based catheter and a balloon occlusion and aspiration system during percutaneous intervention of diseased saphenous vein arto-coronary bypass grafts. Circulation 2003;108:548-553.

275. Weizsz G, Rogers C, Hermiller, et al: Predilatation before distal protection device placement is associated with increased procedure-related myocardial infarction: Analysis from FIRE trial. J Am Coll Cardiol 2004;43:52A.

276. Rogers C, Huynh R, Siefert PA, et al: Embolic protection with filtering or occlusion balloons during saphenous vein graft stenting retrieves identical volumes and sizes of particulate debris. Circulation 2004;109:1735-1740.

277. Choudhury RP, Porto I, Banning AP: Debris trapped by a distal protection device may mimic no-reflow during percutaneous coronary intervention. Circulation 2004;109: 801-802.

278. Carrozza JP, Mumma M, Breall JA, et al: Randomized evaluation of the TriActiv Balloon-Protection flush and extraction system for the treatment of saphenous vein graft disease. J Am Coll Cardiol 2005;46:1677-1683.

279. Rogers C: Proximal protection during saphenous vein graft intervention using the Proxis embolic protective system: A randomized, prospective, multicenter clinical trial (PROXIMAL). Presented at TCT 2005, Washington, D.C. 2004. J Am Coll Cardiol 44:1801.

280. Dixon SR: Saphenous vein graft protection in a distal embolic protection randomized trial. Paper presented at the Transcatheter Cardiovascular Therapeutics meeting, 2005, Washington, DC.

281. O'Neill WW, for the TRAP Investigators: A randomized, controlled, multicenter trial of saphenous vein graft intervention with or without distal protection using the TRAP Vascular Filtration System. Paper presented at the Annual Scientific Session of the American College of Cardiology, March 2003, Chicago, IL.

282. Hillegass WB, Lyerly MJ, Patel NJ, et al: Frequency and predictors of post-procedural myonecrosis in saphenous vein graft intervention in the stent era: A meta-regression. Circulation 2006;114(Suppl II):II-733.

283. Ho PC, Leung CY: Rheolytic thrombectomy with distal filter embolic protection as adjunctive therapies to high-risk saphenous vein graft intervention. Catheter Cardiovasc Interv 2004;61:202-205.

284. Stankovic G, Colombo A, Presbito P, et al: Randomised evaluation of polytetrafluoroethylene-covered stents in saphenous vein grafts: The Randomised Evaluation of Polytetrafluoroethylene-Covered Stent in Saphenous Vein Grafts (RECOVERS) trial. Circulation 2003;108:37-42.

285. Schächinger V, Hamm CW, Muzel T, et al: A randomized trial of polytetrafluoroethylene-membrane covered stents compared with conventional stents in aortocoronary saphenous vein grafts. J Am Coll Cardiol 2003;42:1360-1369.

286. Stone GW: The Barricade trial. Randomized comparison of PTFE covered JoStent with bare metal stent in saphenous vein grafts. Paper presented at the American College of Cardiology Annual Scientific Sessions, 2005, Orlando, Florida.

287. Buchbinder M, Turco M, for the Symbiot III Investigators: Symbiot III randomized SVG trial. Paper presented at the Transcatheter Cardiovascular Therapeutics meeting, 2004, Washington, DC.

288. Turco MA, Buchbinder M, Popma JJ, et al: Pivotal, randomized U.S. study of the Symbiot covered stent system in patients with saphenous vein graft disease: Eight-month angiographic and clinical results of the Symbiot III trial. Catheter Cardiovasc Interv 2006;68:379-388.

289. Petrie MC, Peels JOJ, Jessurun G: The role of covered stents: More than an occasional cameo? Catheter Cardiovasc Interv 2006;68:21-26.

290. Colombo A: Covered stents: No class IA indication but "thank God they still exist!" Catheter Cardiovasc Interv 2006;68:27-28.

291. Kao J, Lincoff AM, Topol EJ, et al: Direct thrombin inhibition appears to be a safe and effective anticoagulant for percutaneous bypass graft interventions. Catheter Cardiovasc Interv 2006;68:352-356.

292. Ellis SG, Lincoff AM, Miller D, et al: Reduction in complications of angioplasty with abciximab occurs largely independently of baseline lesion morphology. J Am Coll Cardiol 1998;32:1619-1623.

293. Roffi M, Mukherjee D, Chew DP, et al: Lack of benefit from intravenous platelet glycoprotein IIb/IIIa receptor inhibition as adjunctive treatment for percutaneous interventions of aortocoronary bypass grafts: A pooled analysis of five randomized clinical trials. Circulation 2002;106: 3063-3067.

294. Jonas M, Stone GW, Mehran R, et al: Platelet glycoprotein IIb/IIIa receptor inhibition as adjunctive treatment during saphenous vein graft stenting: Differential effects after randomization to occlusion or filter-based embolic protection. Eur Heart J 2006;27:920-928.

295. Morrison DA, Thai H, Goldman S, et al: Percutaneous coronary intervention of or through saphenous vein grafts or internal mammary arteries: The impact of stents, adjunctive pharmacology, and multicomponent distal protection. Catheter Cardiovasc Interv 2006;67:571-579.

296. Assali A, Sdringlola S, Moustapha A, et al: Percutaneous intervention in saphenous vein grafts: In-stent restenosis lesions are safer than de novo lesions. J Invasive Cardiol 2001;13:446-450.

297. Dangas G, Mehran R, Lansky AJ, et al: Acute and long-term results of treatment of diffuse in-stent restenosis in aortocoronary saphenous vein grafts. Am J Cardiol 2000;86: 777-779.

298. Rha SW, Kuchulakanti P, Agani AE, et al: Three-year follow-up after intravascular gamma radiation for in-stent restenosis in saphenous vein grafts. Cathet Cardiovasc Interv 2005;65:257-262.

299. Weintraub WS, Cohen CL, Curling PE, et al: Results of coronary surgery after failed elective coronary angioplasty in patients with prior coronary surgery. J Am Coll Cardiol 1990;16:1341-1347.

300. Kahn JK, Rutherford BD, McConahay DR, et al: Outcome following emergency coronary artery bypass grafting for failed elective balloon coronary angioplasty in patients with prior coronary bypass. Am J Cardiol 1990;66:285-288.
301. Ellis SG, Roubin GS, King SB III, et al: Angiographic and clinical predictors of acute closure after native vessel coronary angioplasty. Circulation 1988;77:372-379.
302. Drummer E, Furey K, Hollman J: Rupture of a saphenous vein bypass graft during coronary angioplasty. Br Heart J 1987; 58:78-81.
303. Teirstein PS, Hartzler GO: Nonoperative management of aortocoronary saphenous vein graft rupture during percutaneous transluminal coronary angioplasty. Am J Cardiol 1987;60:377-378.
304. Namay DL, Roubin GS, Tommaso CL, et al: Saphenous vein graft rupture during percutaneous transluminal angioplasty. Cathet Cardiovasc Diagn 1988;14:258-262.
305. Subraya RG, Tannenbaum AK: Successful sealing of perforation of saphenous vein graft by coronary stent. Catheter Cardiovasc Interv 2000;50:460-462.
306. Lansky AJ, Stone GW, Grube E, et al: A multicenter registry of the JoStent® PTFE stent graft for the treatment of arterial perforations complicating percutaneous coronary interventions [abstract]. J Am Coll Cardiol 2000;35:26A.
307. Caputo RP, Amin N, Marvasti M, et al: Successful treatment of a saphenous vein graft perforation with an autologous vein-covered stent. Catheter Cardiovasc Interv 1999;48: 382-386.
308. Hernandez-Antolin RA, Banuelos C, Alfonso F, et al: Successful sealing of an angioplasty-related saphenous vein graft rupture with a PTFE-covered stent. J Invasive Cardiol 2000;12:589-593.

CHAPTER

26 Abrupt Vessel Closure

A. Michael Lincoff

KEY POINTS

- Abrupt closure of a target or adjacent segment of coronary vessel remains an important cause of mortality and morbidity associated with percutaneous coronary intervention.
- Although some characteristics are predictive of an increased risk of abrupt closure, the occurrence of most ischemic complications remains unforeseeable.
- Stents reduce obstructive mechanisms of abrupt closure due to coronary dissection or recoil, and routine use of stents is the most effective means of preventing abrupt closure.
- Although less prone to mechanical causes of abrupt closure, stents are susceptible to thrombotic occlusion.

- Stent thrombosis is associated with high rates of death and myocardial infarction.
- Contemporary periprocedural antiplatelet and anticoagulant regimens are critical for minimizing the risk of stent thrombosis or other ischemic complications.
- Routine use of stenting and advanced antithrombotic therapies has markedly diminished the need for emergency coronary bypass surgery after coronary intervention. Nevertheless, emergency bypass surgery in this setting, if required, is associated with high rates of mortality and morbidity.

Since the introduction of percutaneous coronary revascularization into clinical practice, improvements in equipment design and operator experience have led to primary success rates in excess of 90%, despite the increasing proportion of patients with unstable ischemic syndromes, complex coronary disease, poor ventricular function, and other clinical risk factors undergoing this procedure. Abrupt vessel closure, the sudden occlusion of a target or adjacent segment of a coronary vessel during or after the angioplasty procedure, has historically been an important limitation of this technique. This complication is a consequence of the arterial injury that is to an extent inseparable from the therapeutic mechanism of percutaneous revascularization techniques. With the emergence of elective coronary stenting as the predominant method of coronary intervention, there has been a shift in the profile of abrupt vessel closure. Although stents reduce or eliminate the obstructive mechanisms of closure, they appear to provide an intrinsically more thrombogenic stimulus than balloon angioplasty or atherectomy. The evolution of optimal stent deployment techniques and enhanced antiplatelet therapy has substantially diminished the risk of stent thrombosis and improved the overall safety of percutaneous coronary revascularization. Nevertheless, by virtue of its unpredictability and clinical sequelae of death, myocardial infarction (MI), and emergency coronary bypass surgery, abrupt vessel closure remains a feared clinical event. Effective strategies for the prevention and management of this complication continue to be important in the armamentarium of interventional cardiologists.

MECHANISMS

Insights into the extensive pathophysiologic changes resulting from coronary angioplasty are relevant to understanding the mechanisms underlying the development of acute coronary occlusion. Almost universally, coronary balloon dilation produces endothelial denudation and intimal fissuring; penetration into the media usually remains localized, but extensive disruption of this layer may lead to the formation of obstructive dissection flaps or intramural hematoma. Exposure of subendothelial components causes platelet deposition and activation with formation of thrombin; occlusive thrombosis may occur alone or in association with blood stasis produced by medial dissection flaps. In some patients, particularly those with unstable ischemic syndromes, propagation of preexistent mural thrombus at the treatment site may be the predominant mechanism of coronary obstruction. Some degree of local coronary vasoconstriction may occur from a combination of release of platelet- and endothelium-derived vasoactive factors and loss of endothelium-derived relaxant factors.

Direct assessment of the mechanism of abrupt closure in living patients is limited by the relative insensitivity and nonspecificity of coronary arteriography in the evaluation of arterial wall morphology.

Findings considered diagnostic for medial dissection include curvilinear or spiral-shaped filling defects or extraluminal protrusion of contrast material; thrombus may be visualized as a progressively enlarging or mobile intraluminal lucency surrounded by contrast. The most common specific angiographic feature is that of obstructive coronary dissection, with an incidence ranging from 35% to 80% of reported closures after balloon angioplasty or atherectomy.

In contrast to the setting of balloon angioplasty, dissections rarely become obstructive during stenting, except in some instances at the proximal or distal stent borders (Fig. 26-1) or within side branches. Thrombosis is the most common mechanism of abrupt closure after stent implantation (Fig. 26-2). The importance of platelet activity in the pathogenesis of stent thrombosis was highlighted by a study of hemostatic predictors by Neumann and colleagues.[1] These investigators demonstrated that elevated baseline expression of platelet surface glycoprotein (GP) IIb/IIIa predicted an increased risk of subacute stent thrombosis, whereas no correlation was found between thrombotic events and markers of plasma thrombin activity.

INCIDENCE

Depending on the definition employed, the reported incidences of abrupt closure after balloon angioplasty or atherectomy have ranged from 2.0% to 13.5% (Table 26-1). Two thirds or more of these closures take place while the patient is within the catheterization laboratory; out-of-laboratory closure occurs most commonly within the first 6 hours after coronary angioplasty. The various atherectomy devices have not been shown to favorably influence the incidence of abrupt closure and may even be associated with increased risk for mechanical complications.

Stents, by virtue of their ability to scaffold disruptions in the arterial wall, potently reduce the incidence of abrupt closure. This benefit of stenting was made possible only by an important evolution in deployment technique and adjunctive pharmacologic therapies. Early animal experiments demonstrated the feasibility and long-term patency of metal stents within the vasculature, although a substantial incidence of thrombosis suggested that these devices might be intrinsically thrombogenic. The outcome of initial clinical experience with stenting highlighted the risks associated with the use of stents in coronary

arteries,[2] with the observation of a prohibitively high subacute thrombotic occlusion rate of about 15%. These findings led to the adoption of intensive anticoagulation regimens consisting of aspirin, dipyridamole, dextran, and intravenous heparin for several days after stent placement, followed by aspirin, dipyridamole, and warfarin for 1 to 3 months after hospital discharge. Although reduced by aggressive anticoagulation, subacute thrombosis continued to occur in approximately 4% to 5% of patients after elective stent placement,[3] and this therapy resulted in frequent and often serious vascular and bleeding complications, prolonged hospitalizations, and substantially increased costs.

Evidence then emerged from intravascular ultrasound studies that most stents were inadequately deployed by traditional balloon inflation pressures (6 to 8 atm), with poor apposition of stent struts to the arterial wall. Based on these findings and the hypothesis that stent thrombosis may arise primarily at sites of poorly supported atherosclerotic plaque or stent struts protruding into the arterial lumen, feasibility of diminishing and ultimately eliminating postprocedural anticoagulant therapy after optimal stent implantation was demonstrated.[4,5] An enhanced antiplatelet regimen of aspirin combined with ticlopidine for several weeks was considered a key component of this reduced anticoagulation regimen. The pivotal Intracoronary Stenting and Anticoagulation Regimen (ISAR) trial showed that combined antiplatelet therapy with aspirin and ticlopidine was associated with remarkably lower rates of ischemic and hemorrhagic complications than traditional warfarin anticoagulation after optimal stent implantation,[6] findings that were confirmed in subsequent studies.[7] Rates of abrupt closure or stent thrombosis in contemporary series and trials of coronary stenting have typically been in the range of about 1%.[8,9] Most abrupt closures due to stent thrombosis occur after the patient leaves the cardiac catheterization laboratory, representing subacute thrombosis events. In a large series of 53 stent thromboses occurring among 6186 patients, most events had occurred within 2 days of the procedure, and only two occurred after day 8.[8]

There remains substantial controversy about whether the risk of stent thrombosis is increased with drug-eluting stents (DESs). DESs, by virtue of controlled local administration of antiproliferative agents such as sirolimus or paclitaxel into the arterial wall, have transformed the field of interventional cardiology with markedly reduced (by about 60%) rates of restenosis and repeat revascularization relative to those achieved with bare metal stents (BMSs). In the early experience with these devices, however, isolated reports of stent thromboses raised concerns that delayed endothelialization and enhanced platelet activation with DESs might lead to an increased risk of stent thrombosis.[10] Most single-center studies,[11] individual randomized trials, or pooled analyses of randomized trials of DESs versus BMSs[9,12] failed to show a difference in rates of stent thrombosis between

Table 26-1. Incidence of Abrupt Closure After Balloon Angioplasty or Atherectomy

Location	Years	Patients (N)	Closure Rate (%)
Beth Israel[71]	1981-1986	1160	4.7
Emory University[14]	1982-1986	4772	4.4
Thoraxcenter[15]	1986-1988	1423	7.3
University of Michigan[16]	1988-1990	1319	8.3
Beth Israel[17]	1989-1991	1919	4.2

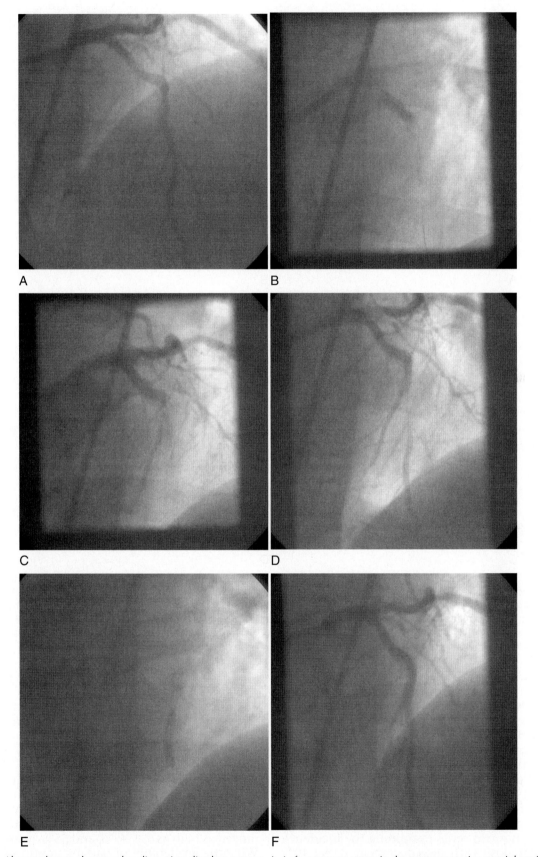

Figure 26-1. Abrupt closure due to edge dissection distal to a stent. **A,** Left coronary artery in the posteroanterior cranial projection with the left anterior descending (LAD) artery in the center. An eccentric 70% stenosis is present in the proximal vessel. **B,** Stent implantation in the proximal LAD at the stenosis. **C,** After stent placement, abrupt closure of the LAD occurs distally, with faint filling of only a septal branch. **D,** After balloon angioplasty distal to the stent, some improvement of flow is observed, with apparent residual obstructive spiral dissection. **E,** Stent placement distal to the first stent at the site of dissection. **F,** Final result, with resolution of abrupt closure and restoration of distal flow.

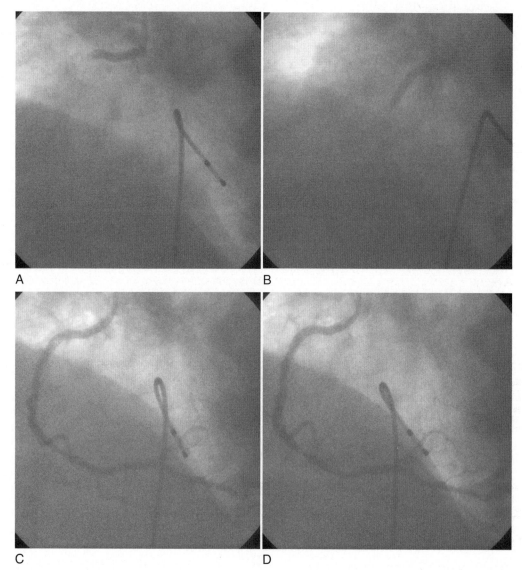

Figure 26-2. Subacute stent thrombosis. **A,** Right coronary artery in the left anterior oblique projection 7 days after stenting. The stent is visible in the proximal vessel. The patient discontinued aspirin and clopidogrel 2 days after stent placement and developed acute inferior myocardial infarction on day 7. Angiography shows stent occlusion. Notice the haziness and filling defect immediately proximal to the stent, consistent with thrombus. **B,** Balloon angioplasty within the stent with adjunctive glycoprotein IIb/IIIa receptor blockade. **C,** Recanalization of the right coronary artery, with a residual filling defect within the stent that suggests thrombus. **D,** After additional balloon inflations, the filling defect has resolved, and distal coronary flow is restored.

BMSs and DESs, although at least one large, prospective, observational study documented a cumulative 9-month incidence of stent thrombosis of 1.3% and suggested that thrombosis risk in "real world" patients was higher than that reported in randomized trials. Moreover, there is some evidence that the timing of stent thrombosis may differ between DESs and BMSs. The issue of late stent thrombosis is the topic of another chapter (see Chapter 31), but it is relevant to mention that two series examining the incidence of stent thrombosis with DESs documented that 40% to 50% of events occurred more than 30 days after implantation.[12,13] Although most analyses fail to show differences in rates of stent thrombosis between BMSs and DESs, it remains unknown whether DESs are more prone to develop late thrombotic occlusion after the typical follow-up period of clinical trials.

CLINICAL CONSEQUENCES

Abrupt vessel closure is an important cause of major ischemic complications associated with coronary intervention. Before the use of stents, rates of death, MI, and emergency bypass surgery after abrupt closure ranged as high as 5%, 45%, and 55%, respectively.[14-17] With the availability of bailout stenting for complicated balloon angioplasty, rates of referral for emergency bypass surgery after abrupt closure have declined dramatically. In a large series reported from the Cleveland Clinic, rates of referral for emergency bypass surgery declined from 1.5% of interventional procedures in 1992 to only 0.14% in 2000.[18] The incidences of death and MI have also been reduced by stenting for abrupt closure. However, if stent thrombosis does occur, the short-term consequences remain severe. In a pooled analysis of six trials of bare metal coronary stenting, 19% of patients who had experienced acute stent thrombosis died within 30 days, and 57% suffered an MI.[8] Similarly, two studies of outcomes after stent thrombosis with DESs have documented mortality rates ranging from 32% to 45%, with MI occurring in another 50% or more.[9,13]

PREDICTORS

A number of studies have identified clinical and angiographic parameters that are associated with abrupt vessel closure and consequent morbidity or mortality during percutaneous coronary intervention (Table 26-2). Recognition of these factors may improve patient selection or guide application of adjunctive pharmacologic or mechanical support techniques.

Correlates of Abrupt Closure during Balloon Angioplasty

A large body of data regarding predictors of ischemic complications relates to coronary balloon angioplasty. Variables associated with heightened risk for abrupt closure in this setting, however, may or may not have predictive value with other device modalities such as

Table 26-2. Predictors or Correlates of Abrupt Closure

Correlates of Abrupt Closure During Balloon Angioplasty
Unstable angina
Diabetes mellitus
Female gender
Advanced age
Intraluminal thrombus
American College of Cardiology/American Heart Association score
Lesion length two luminal diameters or >10 mm
Excessive proximal tortuosity
Bend point of 45 degrees
Branch point
Other stenoses 50% in same vessel
Multivessel disease
Ostial right coronary artery
Degenerated saphenous vein grafts
"Inoperable" surgical status
Collaterals originating from target vessel
Preangioplasty stenosis of 90% to 99%

Correlates of Stent Thrombosis
Unplanned (bailout) stenting
Unstable angina
Diabetes mellitus
Low ejection fraction
Renal failure
Small vessel diameter
Long lesions (long stents or multiple stents)
Bifurcation stenoses
Large plaque volume
Stented vessel perfusing poorly functioning myocardium
Residual uncovered dissection
Slow flow or poor distal runoff
Suboptimal final post-procedural lumen

atherectomy or stenting. Clinical characteristics that have been associated with abrupt closure include unstable angina, diabetes mellitus, female gender, and advanced age. Although such clinical parameters may be useful in delineating high-risk subgroups of patients, coronary angiographic assessment provides a more powerful means of preprocedural risk stratification.[14,19] Intracoronary thrombus has been shown to be a strong correlate of acute coronary occlusion, occurring in up to 73% of patients with this angiographic finding.[14,19,20] Among the 7917 patients in a pooled analysis of eight clinical trials, those with angiographically visible thrombus more frequently suffered abrupt closure (5.9% versus 3.9%, $P < .001$) and in-hospital death or MI (8.4% versus 5.5%, $P < .001$).[20] Several investigators have demonstrated that percutaneous coronary revascularization is associated with local activation of platelets and coagulation factors; the increased hazard of angioplasty in the setting of preexistent thrombus may be related to the liberation of clot-bound thrombin after mechanical disruption by a balloon catheter. Balloon dilation of diffusely diseased saphenous vein grafts carries an increased risk of abrupt closure or distal coronary embolization,[21] likely due in part to the frequent presence of thrombus within these degenerated vessels.

Several series have demonstrated that coronary dissection developing during balloon angioplasty is strongly correlated with the development of abrupt closure.[14,22] Ischemic risk after dissection is influenced by the length of tear (with closure of up to 57% of dissections 15 mm or longer), residual stenosis, vessel diameter, and the occurrence of transient in-laboratory closure.[22] Angiographic features predictive of subsequent progression to frank closure may be considered as constituting "threatened closure"; although distal coronary flow may be preserved and manifestations of ischemia absent, corrective mechanical interventions such as bailout stenting are strongly indicated.

Correlates of Stent Thrombosis and Abrupt Closure

Several predictors of stent thrombosis have been identified from clinical series or trials, although these findings must be considered in a historical perspective. With the development of optimal stent deployment techniques and enhanced antiplatelet therapy, the magnitude of risk imparted by any of these predictive factors has generally declined. Moreover, stent thrombosis occurs infrequently in the current era, rendering most contemporary analyses underpowered to fully assess the extent to which risk factors predispose to this event.

Before the use of high-pressure balloon inflations and dual-antiplatelet therapy, the indication for stenting was strongly associated with the risk of thrombotic closure. The relationship between indication for stenting and thrombosis risk has not been as consistent in more contemporary reports. In neither the Standard Treatment with Alteplase to Reverse Stroke (STARS) Registry[23] nor a large, single-center series[24] was abrupt closure or dissection before stenting associated with increased risk for stent thrombosis. However, large French[4] and Italian[25] registries documented a more than threefold increase in subacute thrombosis rates if stents were placed for coronary dissection; similarly, thrombosis occurred in 2.4% of patients stented for the indication of abrupt or threatened closure versus 0.7% of those stented for elective indications in a pooled analysis of more than 6000 patients enrolled in six modern multicenter stent trials.[8]

The influence of clinical setting on the risk of stent thrombosis has also been controversial. Even in early studies, rates of thrombosis were not consistently elevated among patients with unstable angina compared with those treated for stable symptoms, despite the intuitive expectation that the prothrombotic state during an unstable ischemic syndrome would confer additional risk. Similarly, findings in the current stent era have been mixed. Although the incidence of stent thrombosis was found to be higher among patients with unstable angina in the French (2.2% versus 1.1%) and Italian registries (threefold increase in risk),[4,25] unstable angina was not a significant risk factor in the large pooled analysis of randomized trials (OR = 1.1; 95% CI: 0.6 to 1.9).[8] Moreover, several trials have confirmed that thrombosis risk is not increased when stents are placed during primary intervention for acute MI, a setting that is generally considered to represent an intense thrombotic milieu. In the Controlled Abciximab and Device Investigation to Lower Late Angioplasty Complications (CADILLAC) trial, the largest stent versus angioplasty trial in acute MI, rates of thrombosis of uncoated stents were only 0.9% to 1.0% using aspirin and thienopyridine antiplatelet regimens.[26]

Coronary angiographic characteristics have been observed to predict increased risk for stent thrombosis. Prominent among these is vessel diameter.[8,9,27] Cutlip and colleagues,[8] for example, documented a twofold increase in thrombosis rates for stents placed with a final diameter of less than 3.0 mm compared with 3.0 mm or more in their pooled clinical trial analysis.[8] Several studies in the early and contemporary stent eras have correlated stent thrombosis with greater stented lesion length and variably with the use of multiple stents.[8,12,13] Among more than 2000 patients treated with DESs in one prospective study, each 1-mm increase in stent length was associated with a 1.03 greater risk of thrombosis.[13] Thrombosis risk with multiple or long stents may relate in part to increased surface area exposed to thrombus formation or difficulties in ensuring that stents are fully deployed in contact with the vessel wall over a long zone. Other angiographic features that have been linked to increased thrombosis risk include stents placed at bifurcation stenoses, an association that may be particularly strong with DESs.[9,13,27] The hazard of bifurcation stenoses may be accentuated in the setting of acute MI, for which one group documented an odds ratio of 12.9 for development of subacute stent thormbosis.[9]

Procedural factors probably influence the likelihood of subsequent closure. A prospective study using intravascular ultrasound among 7484 patients undergoing stenting identified an apparent procedural cause in 78% of those who subsequently suffered subacute stent thrombosis; luminal compromise was observed due to proximal or distal dissection, thrombus, tissue protrusion through stent struts, or inadequate stent expansion. Prior studies had also identified the hazard conferred by residual uncovered dissection, with a fourfold increase in risk in the French registry,[4] STARS trial,[7] and clinical trials pooled analysis.[8]

PREVENTION

Although clinical and angiographic correlates of abrupt closure may serve to stratify groups of patients according to anticipated risk, these criteria generally have a low positive and negative predictive value;[19] closure often remains unforeseeable. The high-risk characteristics are encountered commonly in clinical practice and may be present in patients for whom percutaneous intervention remains the preferred option for revascularization. Careful attention to a number of preventive measures may limit the incidence of abrupt closure and improve outcome in low- and high-risk patient subsets.

Pharmacologic Techniques

Pharmacologic approaches to prevent abrupt closure have focused on suppression of platelet aggregation and thrombus formation at the angioplasty site, as well as preprocedural resolution of intracoronary thrombi in patients with acute ischemic syndromes.

Aspirin

The efficacy of aspirin in reducing the ischemic complications of coronary angioplasty has been clearly established. Aspirin irreversibly acetylates and inactivates platelet cyclooxygenase, thereby inhibiting production of thromboxane A_2. In a retrospective analysis of 220 patients, the incidence of occlusive intracoronary thrombi after successful balloon angioplasty was significantly lower for the patients pretreated with aspirin (1.8% versus 10.7%).[28] Subsequently, a randomized trial compared therapy with aspirin and dipyridamole with placebo for the prevention of restenosis; although restenosis occurred with equal frequency in the two groups, the incidence of periprocedural Q wave MI was significantly lower (1.6% versus 6.9%) among patients receiving antiplatelet agents.[29]

Heparins

Heparins are indirect inhibitors of factor Xa and thrombin, exerting their anticoagulant effect by complexing with antithrombin and converting this circulating cofactor from a slow to a rapid inactivator. Unfractionated heparin has equal activity against factors Xa and IIa (thrombin). Systemic heparinization has been employed since the advent of coronary intervention, although few randomized trial data exist to guide the optimal level of anticoagulation. Individual responses to heparin vary considerably, and the adequacy of heparin anticoagulation may be affected by body size, previous heparin therapy, and concurrent nitroglycerin therapy. Retrospective analyses have associated the lowest rates of periprocedural ischemic complications with activated clotting times (ACTs) longer than 300 to 350 seconds,[30] although the risk of periprocedural hemorrhagic complications increases substantially at these levels of anticoagulation. Moreover, reductions in ischemic complications with increasing degrees of heparin anticoagulation during coronary intervention have not been consistently observed, and low rates of ischemic complications have been observed in some prospective series or small-scale clinical trials.[31]

Although early observational reports suggested that ischemic complications might be reduced among patients with acute coronary syndromes by 3 to 7 days of continuous heparin therapy *before* coronary intervention, efficacy of such an approach has never been demonstrated in a randomized trial, and the strategy of heparin pretreatment has been largely supplanted by administration of more potent periprocedural antithrombotics (discussed later). Similarly, there are no data to support a role for postprocedural heparin infusions. Prospective, randomized trials[32] failed to demonstrate a decrease in the incidence of ischemic complications among patients treated with intravenous heparin for 12 to 24 hours after uncomplicated angioplasty, and bleeding complications were more common among patients randomized to heparin infusion.

Low-molecular-weight heparins offer several theoretical advantages over unfractionated heparin. Their primary action is directed against factor Xa, with less activity against thrombin. Low-molecular-weight heparins generally have better bioavailability than unfractionated heparin when administered subcutaneously and are more suitable for long-term administration. Therapeutic monitoring of low-molecular-weight heparins cannot be performed with conventional partial thromboplastin time or prothrombin time measurements, but it may not be necessary in most settings. Randomized trials have demonstrated that one low-molecular-weight heparin, enoxaparin, is superior to unfractionated heparin in preventing ischemic complications among conservatively treated (i.e., without routine revascularization) patients with acute ischemic syndromes.[33,34] During invasive management and revascularization, an advantage of enoxaparin over unfractionated heparin has been more difficult to demonstrate. Among more than 10,000 patients with high-risk acute non-ST-segment elevation coronary syndromes in the Superior Yield of the New strategy of Enoxaparin,

Revascularization, and Glycoprotein IIb/IIIa inhibitors (SYNERGY) trial, 47% of whom underwent percutaneous intervention, no difference in ischemic outcomes (death or MI in 14.0% versus 14.5% of patients treated with enoxaparin and unfractionated heparin, respectively, $P = .40$), but higher rates of major bleeding (9.1% versus 7.6%, $P = .008$) with enoxaparin were observed.[35] Rates of abrupt closure (1.3% versus 1.7%) or "threatened closure" (1.1% versus 1.0%) were the same in the two treatment arms. The dose of enoxaparin used in that trial was 1 mg/kg given subcutaneously every 12 hours, with an additional 0.3-mg/kg intravenous dose before percutaneous intervention if 8 hours or more had elapsed since the previous dose. A lower dose of enoxaparin (0.75 mg/kg) was compared with unfractionated heparin among 3528 patients undergoing elective percutaneous intervention in the Safety and Efficacy of Enoxaparin in Percutaneous Coronary Intervention Patients (STEEPLE) trial. No differences were observed between ischemic end points in the two treatment arms, although enoxaparin in this trial was associated with lower rates of major bleeding (1.2% versus 2.8%, $P = .007$). The consistent finding is of no advantage or disadvantage of enoxaparin relative to unfractionated heparin with regard to suppression of ischemic complications during coronary intervention for elective or urgent indications. Reasons for the divergent outcomes with regard to hemorrhagic complications in the SYNERGY and STEEPLE trials are unclear, but they may relate to duration of therapy (i.e., acute coronary syndrome patients in SYNERGY were treated for a median of 23 hours before coronary intervention, whereas patients in STEEPLE received only a single dose of enoxaparin immediately before their procedure), dose reduction, or concomitant use of other antithrombotics such as platelet GP IIb/IIIa inhibitors (discussed later).

Fondaparinux is a synthetic molecule consisting of the essential pentasaccharide sequence of heparin that binds to and induces the conformational change in circulating antithrombin. Fondaparinux exclusively inhibits factor Xa and has no activity against thrombin. Large-scale trials have evaluated fondaparinux versus enoxaparin in patients with non-ST-segment elevation acute coronary syndromes (Organization to Assess Strategies for Ischemic Syndromes [OASIS]-5)[36] and fondaparinux versus heparin in the setting of ST-segment elevation MI (OASIS-6).[37] In both trials, evidence emerged that fondaparinux does not provide adequate protection against thrombotic complications during percutaneous coronary intervention. In OASIS-5, an excess incidence of new angiographically apparent thrombus (2.5% versus 1.1%) or catheter-related thrombus (1.1% versus 0.5%) during percutaneous coronary intervention led to a trial protocol amendment specifying that unfractionated heparin should be administered to patients in the fondaparinux arm during these procedures.[36] Similarly, although treatment with fondaparinux rather than unfractionated heparin among patients with acute MI in OASIS-6 was associated with a trend toward less frequent ischemic events during medical management, there was no benefit of fondaparinux over heparin among patients undergoing percutaneous coronary intervention.[37] As was observed in OASIS-5, fondaparinux therapy in OASIS-6 resulted in more frequent guide catheter thromboses (1.2% versus 0%, $P < .001$) and "coronary complications" (14.3% versus 11.9%, $P = .04$) than unfractionated heparin. The results of the OASIS-5 and -6 trials suggest that factor Xa inhibition alone is insufficient to prevent thrombus formation when coronary arteries are instrumented with catheters and guidewires and that at least some degree of thrombin inhibition is required during percutaneous coronary revascularization.

Thrombolytic Agents

Although administration of fibrinolytic agents is intuitively appealing as a means to reduce preexistent thrombus burden and prevent new thrombus formation within a treated coronary vessel, the potential of these agents for thrombin generation, platelet activation, and bleeding complications appears to limit their effectiveness. No large-scale, randomized trials have been performed to assess the efficacy of thrombolytic therapy during coronary intervention, but synthesis of the data from small prospective trials or retrospective series does not demonstrate a benefit of thrombolysis in reducing acute or chronic ischemic complications. The largest study of thrombolysis during coronary intervention was the Thrombolysis and Angioplasty in Unstable Angina (TAUSA) trial, in which 469 patients with rest angina were randomized to receive intracoronary urokinase or placebo before balloon angioplasty.[38] No difference in the incidence of intracoronary thrombus formation was observed between treatment groups, but patients receiving urokinase paradoxically had higher rates of abrupt vessel closure (10.2% versus 4.3%, $P < .02$) and ischemic clinical events (12.9% versus 6.3%, $P < .02$), particularly with the higher dose. Although speculative, the apparent unfavorable effects of thrombolytic therapy in this and other studies may have been caused by exacerbation of subintimal hemorrhage or inhibition of dissection adherence to the vessel wall.

Thienopyridines: Ticlopidine and Clopidogrel

Thienopyridines block platelet aggregation by selectively and irreversibly inhibiting the P2T subunit of the ADP receptor. The efficacy of combination therapy with a thienopyridine and aspirin in preventing subacute thrombosis after coronary stenting was demonstrated in two randomized trials. In the ISAR trial, a regimen of aspirin and ticlopidine was associated with significant reductions in the risk of stent occlusion, from 5.4% to 0.8% ($P = .002$), compared with the traditional regimen of aspirin, prolonged heparinization, and warfarin.[6] These findings were confirmed in the larger STARS trial, in which stent thrombosis rates were 3.6%, 2.7%, and 0.5% in the aspirin-only, aspirin plus warfarin, and aspirin plus ticlopidine groups, respectively ($P = .01$ for the comparison between ticlopidine and warfarin).[7] Clopidogrel is closely related structurally to ticlopidine, but it causes less gastrointestinal intolerance or bone marrow suppression and has a more rapid onset of peak action. Clopidogrel has virtually replaced ticlopidine in catheterization laboratories after stent implantation. Ticlopidine has been compared with two regimens of clopidogrel with aspirin after stenting; no differences in clinical outcome were observed, but tolerability was better with clopidogrel.[39] Several nonrandomized studies have also indicated comparable efficacy of clopidogrel and ticlopidine in this setting.

Large-scale clinical studies have shown that long-term therapy (9 to 12 months) with aspirin and clopidogrel reduces ischemic complications compared with aspirin alone among patients undergoing percutaneous coronary revascularization for elective indications[40] or in the setting of acute coronary syndromes.[41] Although 2 to 4 weeks of therapy may be sufficient to prevent subacute thrombosis of BMSs, trials of drug-eluting stents have used a minimum of 3 to 6 months of clopidogrel therapy to prevent late thrombosis due to delayed or incomplete neointimal coverage.[42] Strikingly, the most potent predictor of late stent thrombosis among 2229 patients after successful DES implantation, with a hazard ratio of 89.8 (95% CI: 30 to 270) was premature discontinuation (before 3 to 6 months) of antiplatelet therapy;[13] similar findings were reported in another series of 2974 patients undergoing DES placement.[27] On the basis of occasional reports of stent thrombosis after discontinuation of dual antiplatelet therapy even 6 or more months after DES placement (see Chapter 31), many interventionalists prolong administration of aspirin and clopidogrel for at least a year in this setting.

Several lines of evidence suggest that the greatest suppression of ischemic events in patients undergoing percutaneous coronary revascularization is achieved if a loading dose of clopidogrel is administered 2 to 6 hours before starting the interventional procedure.[41,43] This pretreatment period likely reflects the time required for clopidogrel to achieve a nearly maximal antiplatelet effect. Studies also suggest that the efficacy of clopidogrel may be improved by using a loading dose of 600 mg or more, rather than 300 mg. In a small-scale trial of 255 patients randomized to 300- or 600-mg clopidogrel bolus doses 4 to 8 hours before percutaneous coronary intervention, significantly fewer ischemic events and less frequent myocardial enzyme elevations were observed with the higher bolus dose.[44]

Glycoprotein IIb/IIIa Inhibitors

The integrin GP IIb/IIIa receptor on the platelet surface membrane binds circulating fibrinogen or von Willebrand factor and cross-links adjacent platelets as the final common pathway to platelet aggregation. Selective inhibition of the GP IIb/IIIa receptor potently inhibits platelet aggregation and thrombus formation. The administration of GP IIb/IIIa antagonists in addition to aspirin, heparin, and postprocedural thienopyridines was tested in a series of placebo-controlled, randomized trials, demonstrating unequivocal reductions in the 30-day risk of death, MI, or repeat urgent intervention by as much as 50% to 60% among patients undergoing balloon angioplasty or stenting for elective, urgent, or emergency indications.[45,46] Although improved outcome with GP IIb/IIIa blockade was observed in every patient subgroup, clinical benefit was enhanced among patients with high-risk characteristics such as unstable ischemic syndromes and diabetes mellitus. Excess hemorrhagic risk associated with this therapy in early trials has been markedly attenuated by weight adjustment and reduction of conjunctive heparin dosing.[45] At least one of the GP IIb/IIIa inhibitors, abciximab, has been associated with a reduction in mortality over long-term (>1 year) follow-up.[47]

Later investigations have suggested that improvements in interventional techniques and adjunctive antithrombotic therapies may diminish the clinical benefit to be derived from GP IIb/IIIa blockade during elective coronary intervention. In a trial of 2159 patients pretreated with 600 mg of clopidogrel at least 2 hours before stenting, no differences were observed in ischemic end points between patients randomized to abciximab with low-dose heparin (70 U/kg) or high-dose heparin (140 U/kg) alone.[48] However, patients with high-risk characteristics (i.e., recent MI, unstable angina, bypass graft interventions, angiographic thrombus, poor left ventricular function, hemodynamic instability, or diabetes mellitus) were excluded from that trial. In a subsequent trial testing the same treatment regimens among 2022 patients with acute coronary syndromes, abciximab was associated with a significant reduction in the incidence of death, MI, or urgent revascularization (8.9% versus 11.9% in the abciximab and heparin arms, respectively, $P = .03$).[49] Even after pretreatment with high-dose clopidogrel, abciximab provides important clinical benefit among high-risk patients undergoing contemporary percutaneous coronary revascularization.

Direct Thrombin Inhibitors

The anticoagulant potency of heparins is intrinsically limited by steric hindrance of the heparin-antithrombin complex, poorly predictable biophysical availability, and susceptibility to inhibitors released by activated platelets. Direct thrombin inhibitors specifically bind to and inactivate one or more of the active sites on the thrombin molecule.

The peptide inhibitor bivalirudin is approved for clinical use as an alternative to heparin in percutaneous coronary revascularization. In an early study of 4312 patients undergoing balloon angioplasty, ischemic events were decreased by 22% and hemorrhagic complications by 62% with bivalirudin compared with heparin.[50] In the Randomized Evaluation in PCI Linking Angiomax to reduced Clinical Events-2 (REPLACE-2) trial, more than 6000 patients undergoing contemporary coronary intervention were randomized to bivalirudin with provisional GP IIb/IIIa inhibitor (administered in 7.2% of patients for intraprocedural ischemic complication) or to heparin and a routine GP IIb/IIIa inhibitor. Statistical criteria for superiority to (imputed) heparin and noninferiority to heparin plus GP IIb/IIIa were satisfied for the ischemic composite end point (death, MI, or urgent revascularization), and major bleeding rates were significantly reduced from 4.1% to 2.4% with bivalirudin compared with heparin plus GP IIb/IIIa blockade.[51] Rates of angiographic complications were similar in the bivalirudin versus the heparin plus GP IIb/IIIa inhibitors arms: abrupt closure in 0.7% versus 0.5%, obstructive dissection in 2.8% versus 2.5%, and thrombus formation in 1.3% versus 1.1%. By 1 year, mortality rates trended to be lower among patients who had received bivalirudin (2.5% versus 1.9%, $P = .16$).[52] Bivalirudin with selective GP IIb/IIIa blockade is an effective alternative to heparin and routine GP IIb/IIIa inhibition as an anticoagulation strategy during percutaneous coronary revascularization, with advantages with regard to bleeding risk and potentially cost and ease of administration.

Mechanical Techniques

The planned use of stents is the most effective means of preventing abrupt closure during percutaneous coronary intervention, with rates of thrombosis or abrupt closure of about 1% in most contemporary series or trials. Srinivas and colleagues[53] compared the outcomes of 857 patients undergoing contemporary percutaneous coronary intervention within the National Heart, Lung, and Blood Institute Dynamic Registry (in which stents and GP IIb/IIIa inhibitors were used in 76% and 24% of patients, respectively) with those of 904 comparable patients treated with balloon angioplasty (and no GP IIb/IIIa inhibitors) in the Bypass Angioplasty Revascularization Investigation (BARI). Rates of abrupt closure were reduced from 9.5% in the BARI trial to 1.5% in the Dynamic Registry ($P < .001$). Ischemic complications of in-hospital coronary artery bypass graft surgery (0.8% versus 2.1%, $P < .001$) and MI (0.8% versus 2.1%, $P = .025$) were also less frequent in the more contemporary Registry. Similarly, in a retrospective study of two cohorts of patients treated during time periods before (1988-1992, $n = 3617$ patients) and during (1994-1997, $n = 4518$ patients) the unrestricted availability of stents at the Mayo Clinic, the risk of abrupt closure was observed to be reduced (4% versus 7%, P < .0001), as were rates of in-hospital mortality and major adverse cardiac events.[54] In a series of patients undergoing coronary intervention at the Cleveland Clinic, contemporary stent use was associated with a markedly diminished need for emergency bypass surgery (OR = 0.14; 95% CI: 0.09 to 0.20).[18]

MANAGEMENT

Coronary Artery Bypass Surgery for Abrupt Closure

Notwithstanding the expansion of percutaneous techniques for treatment of abrupt closure, emergency surgical revascularization after coronary angioplasty may infrequently be required for patients experiencing refractory myocardial ischemia in whom other methods have failed to reverse vessel closure or for those with certain high-risk anatomic features. Particularly relevant in this regard is the patient with abrupt closure involving the left main coronary artery. Although infrequent, left main closure has been reported to occur as a consequence of guide (or diagnostic) catheter manipulation, intervention within the left main trunk itself, or retrograde dissection or thrombosis during angioplasty of the proximal left anterior descending or circumflex arteries. Given the amount of myocardium typically served by this vessel, rates of mortality and morbidity after left main coronary artery closure are relatively high. Traditionally, these patients are referred for immediate emergency bypass surgery, with the transition to the operating room stabilized, if possible, by balloon angioplasty. Successful stenting may obviate the need for immediate coronary artery bypass grafting; nevertheless, it remains unknown whether long-term outcome is optimized by eventual definitive surgical revascularization, given the potential catastrophic consequences of subacute stent thrombosis or late restenosis.

Several series have documented the high rates of complications among patients treated with emergency bypass surgery for failed coronary angioplasty (Table 26-3). Mortality rates ranged as high as 19%, and perioperative Q-wave MI occurred in up to 57%

of patients. These data emphasize the inability of emergency surgical revascularization to prevent MI, even at the most experienced, high-volume centers.[18,55] In a review of 18,593 interventional procedures performed between 1992 and 2000, emergency bypass surgery was required in 113 (0.61%) cases.[18] Major indications for surgery were extensive dissection (54%), recurrent acute closure (20%), or perforation or tamponade (20%). Of patients undergoing emergency surgery, 15% died, 12% suffered perioperative Q-wave MIs, and 5% had strokes. The risk of complications of emergency surgery did not improve over the period under study; at least one complication occurred in 35% of patients requiring surgery from 1992 to 1996 and in 38% of patients undergoing surgery from 1997 to 2000.

Ongoing ischemia, as judged by the presence of refractory angina, electrocardiographic abnormalities, or hemodynamic instability, is the most important preoperative determinant of in-hospital outcome of patients treated with emergency bypass surgery for complicated angioplasty.[55,56] In the Emory University series,[55] for example, MI rates among patients with and without ischemia were 25% and 4%, respectively. Patients with preoperative cardiogenic shock or intractable cardiac arrest were at increased risk for death in other reports.

Pharmacologic Management of Abrupt Closure

Although pharmacologic agents are effective in preventing coronary closure during percutaneous intervention, the success of pharmacologic therapy as the sole means of managing established abrupt closure has been limited. For the rare instances of vessel occlusion due primarily to coronary spasm, vasodilator agents may be efficacious. Most pharmacologic therapies for treating coronary occlusion, however, focus on antithrombotic approaches.

Heparin

Although adequate anticoagulation with heparin or other thrombin antagonists appears to be a critical factor in the prevention of ischemic complications during coronary angioplasty, the value of additional

Table 26-3. In-Hospital Results of Emergency Coronary Bypass Surgery for Failed Coronary Angioplasty

Location	Years	Patients (N)	Ischemia (%)	Death (%)	Q-Wave MI (%)
NHLBI I[72]	1979-1982	202	NR	6	26
Texas Heart[73]	1979-1983	157	45	3.8	8
Mid-America Heart[74]	1979-1984	115	NR	11	43
Des-Moines, IA[75]	1979-1986	126	NR	2.4	15
Mayo Clinic[76]	1979-1986	146	62	2.7	39
Emory University[55]	1980-1986	430	80	1.4	21
Vandoeuvre-les-Nancy, France[56]	1980-1990	100	83	19	57
Cleveland Clinic[18]	1992-2000	113	NR	15	12

Ischemia, patients with ongoing ischemia on arrival to operating room as assessed by electrocardiographic criteria or persistence of angina or hemodynamic instability; MI, myocardial infarction; N, number of patients undergoing emergency (within 24 hours of angioplasty procedure) coronary bypass surgery; NHLBI, National Heart, Lung, and Blood Institute; NR, not reported.

heparin in the treatment of abrupt closure has not been investigated in a systematic manner. Scattered reports describe patients in whom additional boluses of heparin led to successful resolution of thrombotic closure, but adequacy of anticoagulation or other antithrombotic therapies are not well defined. It is likely that administration of additional heparin for abrupt closure is of little utility for patients in whom intraprocedural therapeutic heparin anticoagulation has been carefully maintained.

Thrombolytic Therapy

There are no prospective, randomized data evaluating the efficacy of thrombolytic therapy in the treatment of abrupt closure, and observational results are unconvincing. Some noncomparative reports have suggested a benefit of repeat balloon angioplasty with adjunctive thrombolytic therapy in this setting,[57] whereas other investigators have found thrombolytic therapy to be of limited or no value in the management of abrupt closure.[16,58] A key concern about the use of thrombolytic therapy in the treatment of complicated angioplasty is the potentiation of bleeding complications or the diminished use of the internal mammary artery in the event of emergency coronary bypass surgery.

Glycoprotein IIb/IIIa Receptor Antagonists

Animal data and limited clinical experience suggest that the platelet glycoprotein IIb/IIIa receptor antagonist abciximab may have a disaggregatory influence on the platelets within an immature thrombus, leading to thrombus dissolution.[59] In phase II studies of patients with acute MI, rates of Thrombolysis in Myocardial Infarction 3 (TIMI 3) reperfusion 60 to 90 minutes after treatment with abciximab alone (i.e., no thrombolytic) have ranged as high as 32%,[60] comparable to the patency rates achieved with streptokinase. These findings, as well as the extraordinary clinical efficacy of GP IIb/IIIa blockade in *preventing* ischemic complications of coronary intervention when administered prophylactically, have led to the clinical use of these agents in an unplanned fashion for complications of coronary angioplasty. Small observational series of patients treated with "rescue" or "bailout" abciximab for thrombosis during coronary intervention have been reported.[61-63] Garbarz and colleagues[61] described 138 patients who required rescue abciximab during coronary angioplasty or stenting, usually for persistent thrombosis (20 with stent thrombosis) or abrupt closure. The proportion of patients with TIMI 3 flow in the affected artery increased from 32% to 88% after abciximab, and clinical success was achieved in 83%. Similar rates of success with bailout abciximab have been reported in 29 patients with thrombotic complications during balloon angioplasty[62] and 10 patients with acute stent thrombosis.[63]

Although rescue administration of GP IIb/IIIa inhibitors may improve outcome among patients with thrombotic abrupt closure, the experience from the REPLACE-2 trial[51] suggests that "provisional" use of these agents does not completely ameliorate the adverse consequences of procedural complications. In that trial, which enrolled more than 6000 patients undergoing elective percutaneous coronary revascularization, antithrombotic treatment with bivalirudin (a direct thrombin inhibitor) and provisional GP IIb/IIIa blockade was found to be noninferior to the traditional regimen of heparin plus routine GP IIb/IIIa inhibition. Provisional GP IIb/IIIa use was required in 7.2% of patients in the bivalirudin treatment group, most commonly for complications of obstructive dissection, thrombosis, or diminished distal coronary flow. Compared with those who did not require the provisional drug, patients who received provisional GP IIb/IIIa inhibition had higher rates of MI (15.5% versus 5.9%), repeat revascularization (5.6% versus 2.5%), major bleeding (6.7% versus 3.0%), and blood product transfusions (4.5% versus 1.9%) during the first 30 days after their interventional procedures. These findings argue that use of GP IIb/IIIa inhibitors should be planned in patients considered to be at high risk for development of abrupt closure.

Mechanical Approaches to Management of Abrupt Closure

Device-based techniques are generally directed at stabilization of the disrupted angioplasty site and obstructive dissection flaps, although thrombotic vessel occlusion and excessive coronary spasm may also prove amenable to mechanical recanalization.

Repeat Balloon Angioplasty

Early experience with repeat balloon dilation for acute coronary occlusion met with modest and various degrees of success; moreover, rates of *clinical* stabilization (freedom from death, MI, or emergency bypass surgery) were usually 10% to 30% lower than the reported rates of *angiographic* resolution as a result of intraprocedural MI or later deterioration of the angioplasty site. Nevertheless, prolonged balloon inflations are commonly performed in the setting of abrupt coronary closure during balloon angioplasty,[15,16] and they may induce improved adhesion of dissection flaps to the vessel wall or substantial compression of intraluminal thrombi.

Stents

Stent placement for abrupt or threatened coronary closure during balloon or atherectomy interventions is a highly effective means of improving procedural outcome and reducing the risk of ischemic complications. By virtue of their ability to "tack down" obstructive dissection flaps, minimize contact between blood and thrombogenic subintimal arterial wall components, limit elastic recoil or spasm, and

Table 26-4. In-Hospital Results of Stent Implantation for Failed Coronary Angioplasty

Study	Patients (N)	Stent	Indication	Anticoagulation Regimen	Angiographic Success (%)	Death (%)	MI (%)	Emergency Surgery (%)	Subacute Thrombosis (%)
Roubin et al,[64] 1992	115	GR	AVC: 10% TVC: 73%	Asp, Dip, Dex, Hep, War	93	1.7	16	4.2	7.6
Reifart et al,[77] 1992	112	PS, ST	AVC: 28% TVC: 72%	Asp, Dip, Dex, Hep, War	96	7.7	2.6	5.4	12.6
George et al,[78] 1993	518	PS	AVC: 30% TVC: 65%	Asp, Dip, Dex, Hep, War	95	2.2	5.5	4.3	8.7
Hearn et al,[79] 1993	116	GR	AVC: 44% TVC: 56%	Asp, Dip, Dex, Uro, Hep, War	89	4.9	4.8	9.5	8.6
Schomig et al,[65] 1994	339	PS	AVC: 12% TVC: 88%	Asp, Hep, War	96	1.3	4.0	1.0	6.9
Lablanche et al,[68] 1996	133	PS, WI, GR, AV	NR	Asp, Hep, Dex, Tic	88	0.8	5.4	2.7	5.4
Dean et al,[80] 1997	118	GR	AVC: 17% TVC: 83%	NR	94	4.2	17.8	11	NR
Antoniucci et al,[67] 1997	120	PS, GR, AV, FR	AVC: 28% TVC: 72%	Asp, Hep, Tic	96	0.8	1.7	0.8	0.8

Asp, aspirin; AV, AVE stent; AVC, acute vessel closure (TIMI 0 or 1 flow); Dex, low-molecular-weight dextran; Dip, dipyridamole; FR, Freedom stent; GR, Gianturco-Roubin stent; Hep, heparin; MI, myocardial infarction; NR, not reported; PS, Palmaz-Schatz stent; ST, Strecker stent; Tic, ticlopidine; TVC, threatened vessel closure (significant dissection with diminished coronary flow or ischemia); Uro, urokinase; War, warfarin sodium; WI, Wiktor stent.

optimize blood flow dynamics, the various stent designs have been shown to produce excellent angiographic resolution of acute coronary occlusion or major dissection.

A number of studies have been reported in which different stent designs were applied in patients with abrupt or threatened coronary closure (Table 26-4). Angiographic success rates ranged from 88% to 96%. Clinical complications were not eliminated after stent placement, but they were commensurate with or lower than those reported in historical series using other techniques of management: death of 0.8% to 4.2% of patients, Q-wave MI in 1.7% to 18%, and emergency bypass surgery in 0.8% to 11%. Angiographic restenosis by 6 months' follow-up was documented in 28% to 41% of successfully treated patients.[64-68] A retrospective review of 2242 consecutive patients undergoing percutaneous coronary revascularization at one center demonstrated substantial reductions in ischemic complication rates coincident with the availability of bailout stents (death: 1.1% versus 0.7%; Q-wave MI: 0.5% versus 0.3%; and emergency bypass surgery: 2.9% versus 1.1%, during the time periods before and after stent availability, respectively).[69]

The principal limitation of intracoronary stenting in early series was the risk of subacute stent thrombosis, occurring in 7% to 13% of patients (see Table 26-4) and associated with substantial morbidity. Moreover, the aggressive anticoagulation regimen used during this period resulted in bleeding complications in up to 38% of patients. The efficacy of stenting for abrupt closure has been demonstrated to be markedly improved in the current era of optimal deployment and enhanced antiplatelet therapy.[67,68,70] A secondary analysis of the ISAR study showed that

the incidence of adverse cardiac events among high-risk patients (defined by acute ischemic syndromes, "difficult procedures," or suboptimal final results) was only 2% with antiplatelet therapy, compared with 12.6% with the traditional anticoagulant regimen.[70] Among 120 patients undergoing stenting with antiplatelet therapy for abrupt or threatened closure in a report from Italy,[67] rates of death, MI, and bypass surgery (0.8%, 1.7%, and 0.8%, respectively) were the lowest of any published series; only 1 patient suffered subacute thrombosis, and only 2 experienced major bleeding complications. With contemporary techniques of deployment and antithrombotic therapy, stenting can be expected to reverse abrupt vessel closure in a large proportion of cases with low rates of ischemic complications.

Atherectomy Devices

The application of directional coronary atherectomy to the treatment of abrupt vessel closure in a limited number of patients has been reported. Directional atherectomy may be particularly useful for treating abrupt closure at lesion sites poorly suited for stent implantation, such as at bifurcations. An important complication observed with bailout use of this device, however, has been coronary perforation, particularly in the presence of extensive dissections, likely resulting from resection of nondiseased vessel wall.

Newer devices designed to aspirate or pulverize intracoronary thrombus have also been applied to the management of stent thrombosis. Case reports describe favorable outcomes for patients treated with ultrasound thrombolysis, thrombus aspiration, or rheolytic thrombectomy.

SUMMARY

Although the incidence of abrupt vessel closure has declined, this complication continues to have important clinical consequences. Patients at elevated risk for coronary occlusion may be identified, but abrupt closure remains largely unpredictable.

The last several years have witnessed important advances in the field of interventional cardiology, many of which are directly relevant to the prevention and treatment of abrupt vessel closure. Newer methods for intracoronary imaging and critical analyses of long-term outcomes of patients enrolled in large-scale clinical trials have led to an improved understanding of the mechanisms of percutaneous coronary revascularization and a more sophisticated appreciation of the pathophysiology and consequences of periprocedural coronary closure and MI. The introduction into clinical practice of potent antithrombotic agents and optimal techniques for coronary stenting have proved to be effective strategies for the prevention of abrupt closure. Expectations for benefit from other pharmacotherapies and "new devices" for coronary intervention have become more realistic and enlightened, with refinements in the indications and applications of these techniques. The most reliable means of obtaining sustained patency in the event of abrupt closure is stent implantation, and GP IIb/IIIa inhibition likely confers additional benefit in this setting. Emergency bypass surgery remains the ultimate therapy for refractory coronary closure, but the frequency of this procedure among patients with abrupt closure appears to have been significantly diminished by the expansion of catheterization laboratory technologies. It is realistic to expect continued progress in the development of techniques to improve short- and long-term outcomes among patients with complicated percutaneous coronary revascularization.

REFERENCES

1. Neumann FJ, Gawaz M, Ott I, et al: Prospective evaluation of hemostatic predictors of subacute stent thrombosis after coronary Palmaz-Schatz stenting. J Am Coll Cardiol 1996;27:15-21.
2. Serruys PW, Strauss BH, Beatt KJ, et al: Angiographic follow-up after placement of a self-expanding coronary-artery stent. N Engl J Med 1991;324:13-17.
3. Savage MP, Fischman DL, Schatz RA, et al: Long-term angiographic and clinical outcome after implantation of a balloon-expandable stent in the native coronary circulation. J Am Coll Cardiol 1994;24:1207-1212.
4. Karrillon G, Morice M, Benveniste E, et al: Intracoronary stent implantation without ultrasound guidance and with replacement of conventional anticoagulation by antiplatelet therapy. 30-day clinical outcome of the French Multicenter Registry. Circulation 1996;74:1519-1527.
5. Colombo A, Hall P, Nakamura S, et al: Intracoronary stenting without anticoagulation accomplished with ultrasound guidance. Circulation 1995;91:1676-1688.
6. Schomig A, Neumann FJ, Kastrati A, et al: A randomized comparison of antiplatelet and anticoagulant therapy after the placement of coronary-artery stents. N Engl J Med 1996;334:1084-1089.
7. Leon MB, Baim DS, Popma JJ, et al: A clinical trial comparing three antithrombotic-drug regimens after coronary-artery stenting. N Engl J Med 1998;339:1665-1671.
8. Cutlip D, Baim DS, Ho KKL, et al: Stent thrombosis in the modern era. A pooled analysis of multicenter coronary stent clinical trials. Circulation 2001;103:1967-1971.
9. Ong AT, Hoye A, Aoki J, et al: Thirty-day incidence and six-month clinical outcome of thrombotic stent occlusion after bare-metal, sirolimus, or paclitaxel stent implantation. J Am Coll Cardiol 2005;45:947-953.
10. Virmani R, Farb A, Kolodgie FD. Histopathologic alterations after endovascular radiation and antiproliferative stents: Similarities and differences. Herz 2002;27:1-6.
11. Jeremias A, Sylvia B, Bridges J, et al: Stent thrombosis after successful sirolimus-eluting stent implantation. Circulation 2004;109:1930-1932.
12. Moreno R, Fernandez C, Hernandez C, et al: Drug-eluting stent thrombosis. J Am Coll Cardiol 2005;45:954-959.
13. Iakovou I, Schmidt T, Bonizzoni E, et al: Incidence, predictors, and outcome of thrombosis after successful implantation of drug-eluting stents. JAMA 2005;293:2126-2130.
14. Ellis SG, Roubin GS, King SB, et al: Angiographic and clinical predictors of acute closure after native vessel coronary angioplasty. Circulation 1988;77:372-379.
15. de Feyter PJ, van den Brand M, Jaarman GJ, et al: Acute coronary artery occlusion during and after percutaneous transluminal coronary angioplasty. Frequency, prediction, clinical course, management, and follow-up. Circulation 1991;83:927-936.
16. Lincoff AM, Popma JJ, Ellis SG, et al: Abrupt vessel closure complicating coronary angioplasty: Clinical, angiographic, and therapeutic profile. J Am Coll Cardiol 1992;19:926-935.
17. Kuntz RE, Piana R, Pomerantz RM, et al: Changing incidence and management of abrupt closure following coronary intervention in the new device era. Cathet Cardiovasc Diagn 1992;27:189-190.
18. Seshadri N, Whitlow PL, Acharya N, et al: Emergency coronary artery bypass surgery in the contemporary percutaneous coronary intervention era. Circulation 2002;106:2346-2350.
19. Tenaglia AN, Fortin DF, Califf RM, et al: Predicting the risk of abrupt vessel closure after angioplasty in an individual patient. J Am Coll Cardiol 1994;24:1004-1011.
20. Singh M, Reeder GS, Ohman EM, et al: Does the presence of thrombus seen on a coronary angiogram affect outcome after percutaneous coronary angioplasty? An angiographic trials pool data experience. J Am Coll Cardiol 2001;38:624-630.
21. Reeves F, Bonan R, Cote G, et al: Long-term angiographic follow-up after angioplasty of venous coronary bypass grafts. Am Heart J 1991;122:620-627.
22. Black AJR, Namay DL, Niederman AL, et al: Tear of dissection after coronary angioplasty—morphologic correlates of an ischemic complication. Circulation 1989;79:1035-1042.
23. Cutlip DE, Leon MB, Ho KK, et al: Acute and nine-month clinical outcomes after "suboptimal" coronary stenting: Results from the STent Anti-thrombotic Regimen Study (STARS) registry. J Am Coll Cardiol 1999;34:698-706.
24. Moussa I, DiMario C, Reimers B, et al: Subacute stent thrombosis in the era of intravascular ultrasound-guided coronary stenting without anticoagulation: Frequency, predictors, and clinical outcome. J Am Coll Cardiol 1997;29:6-12.
25. De Servi S, Repetto S, Klugmann S, et al: Stent thrombosis: Incidence and related factors in the R.I.S.E. Registry (Registro Impianto Stent Endocoronarico). Catheter Cardiovasc Interv 1999;46:13-18.
26. Stone GW, Grines CL, Cox DA, et al: Comparison of angioplasty with stenting, with or without abciximab, in acute myocardial infarction. N Engl J Med 2002;346:957-966.
27. Kuchulakanti PK, Chu WW, Torguson R, et al: Correlates and long-tem outcome of angiographically proven stent thrombosis with sirolimus- and paclitaxel-eluting stents. Circulation 2006;113:1108-1113.
28. Barnathan ES, Schwartz JS, Taylor L, et al: Aspirin and dipyridamole in the prevention of acute coronary thrombosis complicating coronary angioplasty. Circulation 1987;76:125-134.

29. Schwartz L, Bourassa MG, Lesperance J, et al: Aspirin and dipyridamole in the prevention of restenosis after percutaneous transluminal coronary angioplasty. N Engl J Med 1988;318:1714-1719.

30. Chew DP, Bhatt DL, Lincoff AM, et al: Defining the optimal activated clotting time during percutaneous coronary intervention. Circulation 2001;103:961-966.

31. Boccara A, Benamer H, Juliard J-M, et al: A randomized trial of a fixed high dose versus a weight-adjusted low dose of intravenous heparin during coronary angioplasty. Eur Heart J 1997;18:631-635.

32. Friedman HZ, Cragg DR, Glazier SM, et al: Randomized prospective evaluation of prolonged versus abbreviated intravenous heparin therapy after coronary angioplasty. J Am Coll Cardiol 1994;24:1214-1219.

33. Antman EM, Cohen M, Radley D, et al: Assessment of the treatment effect of enoxaparin for unstable angina/non-Q-wave myocardial infarction. TIMI 11B-ESSENCE meta analysis. Circulation 1999;100:1602-1608.

34. Antman EM, Morrow DA, McCabe CH, et al: Enoxaparin versus unfractionated heparin with fibrinolysis for ST-elevation myocardial infarction. N Engl J Med 2006;354:1477-1488.

35. SYNERGY Trial Investigators. Enoxaparin vs. unfractionated heparin in high-risk patients with non-ST-segment elevation acute coronary syndromes managed with an intended early invasive strategy. JAMA 2004;292:45-54.

36. OASIS-5 Investigators: Comparison of fondaparinux and enoxaparin in acute coronary syndromes. N Engl J Med 2006;354:1464-1476.

37. OASIS-6 Trial Group: Effects of fondaparinux on mortality and reinfarction in patients with acute ST-segment elevation myocardial infarction. JAMA 2006;295:1519-1530.

38. Ambrose JA, Almeida OD, Sharma SK, et al: Adjunctive thrombolytic therapy during angioplasty for ischemic rest angina: Results of the TAUSA trial. Circulation 1994;90:69-77.

39. Bertrand ME, Rupprecht HJ, Gershlick AH, et al: Double-blind study of the safety of clopidogrel with and without a loading dose in combination with aspirin compared with ticlopidine in combination with aspirin after coronary stenting: The Clopidogrel Aspirin Stent International Cooperative Study (CLASSICS). Circulation 2000;102:624-629.

40. Steinhubl SR, Berger PB, Mann JT, et al: Early and sustained dual oral antiplatelet therapy following percutaneous coronary intervention. A randomized controlled trial. JAMA 2002;288:2411-2420.

41. Mehta SR, Yusuf S, Peters GR, et al: Effects of pretreatment with clopidogrel and aspirin followed by long-term therapy in patients undergoing percutaneous coronary intervention: The PCI-CURE study. Lancet 2001;358:527-533.

42. Kotani J, Awata M, Nanto S, et al: Incomplete neointimal coverage of sirolimus-eluting stents. J Am Coll Cardiol 2006;47:2108-2111.

43. Steinhubl SR, Berger PB, Brennan DM, et al: Optimal timing for the initiation of pre-treatment with 300 mg clopidogrel before percutaneous coronary intervention. J Am Coll Cardiol 2006;47:939-943.

44. Patti G, Colonna G, Pasceri V, et al: Randomized trial of high loading dose of clopidogrel for reduction of periprocedural myocardial infarction in patients undergoing coronary intervention: Results from the ARMYDA-2 (Antiplatelet therapy for Reduction of MYocardial Damage during Angioplasty). Circulation 2005;111:2099-2106.

45. EPISTENT Investigators: Randomised placebo-controlled and balloon-angioplasty-controlled trial to assess safety of coronary stenting with use of platelet glycoprotein IIb/IIIa blockade. Lancet 1998;352:87-92.

46. ESPRIT Investigators: Novel dosing regimen of eptifibatide in planned coronary stent implantation (ESPRIT): A randomised, placebo-controlled trial. Lancet 2000;356:2037-2044.

47. Topol EJ, Mark DB, Lincoff AM, et al: Enhanced survival with platelet glycoprotein IIb/IIIa blockade in patients undergoing coronary stenting: one year outcomes and health care economic implications from a multicenter, randomized trial. Lancet 1999;354:2019-2024.

48. Kastrati A, Mehilli J, Schühlen H, et al: A clinical trial of abciximab in elective percutaneous coronary intervention after pretreatment with clopidogrel. N Engl J Med 2004;350:232-238.

49. Kastrati A, Mehilli J, Neumann F, et al: Abciximab in patients with acute coronary syndromes undergoing percutaneous coronary intervention after clopidogrel pretreatment. JAMA 2006;295:1531-1538.

50. Bittl JA, Chaitman BR, Feit F, et al: Bivalirudin versus heparin during coronary angioplasty for unstable or post-infarction angina: Final report reanalysis of the Bivalirudin Angioplasty Study. Am Heart J 2001;142:952-959.

51. Lincoff AM, Bittl JA, Harrington RA, et al: Bivalirudin and provisional glycoprotein IIb/IIIa blockade compared with heparin and planned glycoprotein IIb/IIIa blockade during percutaneous coronary intervention. The REPLACE-2 trial. JAMA 2003;289:853-863.

52. Lincoff AM, Kleiman NS, Kereiakes DJ, et al: Long-term efficacy of bivalirudin and provisional glycoprotein IIb/IIIa blockade vs heparin and planned glycoprotein IIb/IIIa blockade during percutaneous coronary revascularization. REPLACE-2 randomized trial. JAMA 2004;292:696-703.

53. Srinivas VS, Brooks MM, Detre KM, et al: Contemporary percutaneous coronary intervention versus balloon angioplasty for multivessel coronary artery disease. A comparison of the National Heart, Lung and Blood Institute Dynamic Registry and the Bypass Angioplasty Revascularization (BARI) study. Circulation 2002;106:1627-1633.

54. Suh WW, Grill DE, Rihal CS, et al: Unrestricted availability of intracoronary stents is associated with decreased abrupt vascular closure rates and improved early clinical outcomes. Catheter Cardiovasc Interv 2002;55:294-302.

55. Talley JD, Weintraub WS, Roubin GS, et al: Failed elective percutaneous transluminal coronary angioplasty requiring coronary artery bypass surgery. In-hospital and late clinical outcome at 5 years. Circulation 1990;82:1203-1213.

56. Buffet P, Danchin N, Villemot JP, et al: Early and long-term outcome after emergency coronary artery bypass surgery after failed coronary angioplasty. Circulation 1991;84(Suppl III):III-254-III-259.

57. Gulba DC, Caniel WG, Simon R, et al: Role of thrombolysis and thrombin in patients with acute coronary occlusion during percutaneous transluminal coronary angioplasty. J Am Coll Cardiol 1990;16:563-568.

58. Hasdai D, Garratt KN, Holmes DR, et al: Coronary angioplasty and intracoronary thrombolysis are of limited efficacy in resolving early intracoronary thrombosis. J Am Coll Cardiol 1996;28:361-367.

59. Gold HK, Garabedian HD, Dinsmore RE, et al: Restoration of coronary flow in myocardial infarction by intravenous chimeric 7E3 antibody without exogenous plasminogen activators. Observations in animals and humans. Circulation 1997;95:1755-1761.

60. SPEED Trial Investigators: Randomized trial of abciximab with and without low-dose reteplase for acute myocardial infarction. Circulation 2000;101:2788-2794.

61. Garbarz E, Farah B, Vuillemenot A, et al: "Rescue" abciximab for complicated percutaneous transluminal coronary angioplasty. Am J Cardiol 1998;82:800-803.

62. Muhlestein JB, Karagounis LA, Treehan S, et al: "Rescue" utilization of abciximab for the dissolution of coronary thrombus developing as a complication of coronary angioplasty. J Am Coll Cardiol 1997;30:1729-1734.

63. Casserly IP, Hasdai D, Berger PB, et al: Usefulness of abciximab for treatment of early coronary artery stent thrombosis. Am J Cardiol 1998;82:981-984.

64. Roubin GS, Cannon AD, Agrawal SK, et al: Intracoronary stenting for acute and threatened closure complicating percutaneous transluminal coronary angioplasty. Circulation 1992;85:916-927.

65. Schomig A, Kastrati A, Dietz R, et al: Emergency coronary stenting for dissection during percutaneous transluminal coronary angioplasty: Angiographic follow-up after stenting and after repeat angioplasty of the stented segment. J Am Coll Cardiol 1994;23:1053-1060.

66. Schomig A, Kastrati A, Mudra H, et al: Four-year experience with Palmaz-Schatz stenting in coronary angioplasty complicated by dissection with threatened or present vessel closure. Circulation 1994;90:2716-2724.

67. Antoniucci D, Valenti R, Santoro G, et al: Bailout coronary stenting without anticoagulation or intravascular ultrasound guidance: Acute and six-month angiographic results in a series of 120 consecutive patients. Cathet Cardiovasc Diagn 1997;41:14-19.

68. Lablanche J, McFadden E, Bonnet J, et al: Combined antiplatelet therapy with ticlopidine and aspirin. A simplified approach to intracoronary stent management. Eur Heart J 1996;17:1373-1380.

69. Altmann DB, Racz M, Battleman DS, et al: Reduction in angioplasty complications after the introduction of coronary stents: Results from a consecutive series of 2242 patients. American Heart J 1996;132:503-507.

70. Schühlen H, Hadamitzky M, Walter H, et al: Major benefit from antiplatelet therapy for patients at high risk for adverse cardiac events after coronary Palmaz-Schatz stent placement: Analysis of a prospective risk stratification protocol in the Intracoronary Stenting and Antithrombotic Regimen (ISAR) trial. Circulation 1997;95:2015-2021.

71. Sinclair IN, McCabe CH, Sipperly ME, et al: Predictors, therapeutic options, and long-term outcome of abrupt reclosure. Am J Cardiol 1988;61:61G-66G.

72. Cowley MJ, Dorros G, Kelsey SF, et al: Emergency coronary bypass surgery after coronary angioplasty: The National Heart, Lung, and Blood Institute's Percutaneous Transluminal Coronary Angioplasty Registry experience. Am J Cardiol 1984;53:22C-26C.

73. Reul GJ, Cooley DA, Hallman GL, et al: Coronary artery bypass for unsuccessful percutaneous transluminal coronary angioplasty. J Thorac Cardiovasc Surg 1984;88:685-694.

74. Killen DA, Hamaker WR, Reed WA: Coronary artery bypass following percutaneous transluminal coronary angioplasty. Ann Thorac Surg 1985;40:133-138.

75. Phillips SJ, Kongtahworn C, Zeff RH, et al: Disrupted coronary artery caused by angioplasty: Supportive and surgical considerations. Ann Thorac Surg 1989;47:880-883.

76. Connor AR, Vlietstra RE, Schaff HV, et al: Early and late results of coronary artery bypass after failed angioplasty. Actuarial analysis of late cardiac events and comparison with initially successful angioplasty. J Thorac Cardiovasc Surg 1988;96:191-197.

77. Reifart N, Langer A, Storger H, et al: Strecker stent as a bailout device following percutaneous transluminal coronary angioplasty. J Interv Cardiol 1992;5:79-83.

78. George BS, Voorhees WD, Roubin GS, et al: Multicenter investigation of coronary stenting to treat acute or threatened closure after percutaneous transluminal coronary angioplasty: Clinical and angiographic outcomes. J Am Coll Cardiol 1993;22:135-143.

79. Hearn J, King S, Douglas J, et al: Clinical and angiographic outcomes after coronary artery stenting for acute or threatened closure after percutaneous transluminal coronary angioplasty. Initial results with a balloon-expandable stainless steel design. Circulation 1993;88:2086-2096.

80. Dean LS, George CJ, Roubin GS, et al: Bailout and corrective use of Gianturco-Roubin flex stents after percutaneous transluminal coronary angioplasty. J Am Coll Cardiol 1997;29:934-940.

27 Periprocedural Myocardial Infarction and Embolism-Protection Devices

Khaled M. Ziada and Debabrata Mukherjee

Periprocedural Myocardial Infarction

KEY POINTS

◼ The contemporary definition of periprocedural myocardial infarction (PMI) is based on the rise and fall of biomarkers (e.g., total creatine kinase, creatine kinase–myocardial band isoenzyme [CK-MB], troponin) after percutaneous coronary intervention (PCI).

◼ The incidence of PMI is about 25%; this rate varies according to the biomarker and the preset threshold used for diagnosis.

◼ The primary underlying mechanism of PMI is embolization into the microcirculation distal to the PCI target segment, with platelet aggregation or activation playing a significant role in subsequent myonecrosis.

◼ Risk factors for development of PMI include acute presentation, heightened systemic inflammation, and advanced coronary or noncoronary atherosclerotic disease. Atheroablation devices (directional or rotational) are associated with higher rates of PMI, followed by stent implantation and balloon angioplasty.

◼ Side branch closure and abrupt vessel closure are associated with PMI, although most PMIs are diagnosed after apparently uncomplicated procedures.

◼ PMI is associated with increased late mortality, and the association is more robust when the CK-MB or troponin levels exceed five times the upper limit of normal.

◼ Potent antiplatelet therapies (e.g., intravenous glycoprotein IIb/IIIa inhibitors, oral thienopyridine inhibitors) decrease the incidence of PMI, especially in high-risk procedures.

◼ Pretreatment with statins reduces the incidence of PMI because of their anti-inflammatory effects.

◼ Embolism protection devices are the only nonpharmacologic intervention known to reduce PMI in saphenous vein graft PCI.

Over the last decade, major acute ischemic complications of percutaneous coronary intervention (PCI) have been significantly reduced by advances in pharmacologic therapies and interventional devices. The rates of Q-wave myocardial infarction (MI), emergent bypass grafting, and in-hospital mortality have been reduced to 1% to 2% of PCI procedures.[1,2] The reduced incidence of these complications can be attributed in large part to the invaluable role of coronary stents in the treatment of abrupt closure and the aggressive use of antiplatelet therapies during the past decade. This improvement in outcomes is remarkable considering ever-increasing number and complexity of patients and lesions undergoing PCI compared with 10 to 20 years ago. However, periprocedural release of cardiac biomarkers is still observed in a considerable proportion of patients undergoing otherwise successful PCI procedures.[2,3] Although the cause and clinical significance of the periprocedural release of cardiac markers are topics for debate, the rise and fall of serum levels of cardiac biomarkers can only indicate as a procedure-related acute MI.[3]

DEFINITION

The definition of periprocedural myocardial infarction (PMI) has been a subject of debate and has evolved over the past decade. Traditionally, PMI was defined along the same lines as acute MI not related to revascularization, using at least two of three criteria: prolonged chest pain, electrocardiographic q waves, and rise in the levels of serum markers. Subsequently, numerous publications demonstrated that creatine kinase (CK) and creatine kinase–myocardial band isoenzyme (CK-MB) elevations had prognostic implications, even in absence of pathologic q waves. The cutoff values of CK and CK-MB used to define PMI in these studies varied widely. Numerous investigators used the cutoff value of three times the upper limit of normal (ULN) of CK or CK-MB as the defining threshold of PMI, although it has been traditional to report more than one times the ULN, more than five times the ULN, and occasionally, more than eight times the ULN values.[4,5] Later studies used troponin and myoglobin levels, considered to be more sensitive markers for myonecrosis, to define PMI. With the consensus redefinition of acute MI,[3] it has become accepted that *any* rise and fall in cardiac biomarkers above the ULN on serial sampling should be considered a PMI.

The definition of PMI is further complicated by the current practice of earlier referral of acute MI patients and those with acute coronary syndromes to the catheterization laboratory. In those situations, detection of abnormal levels of cardiac markers after PCI may not necessarily be related to the procedure, but instead reflect the ongoing myonecrosis caused by thrombosis or distal embolization leading to the procedure. In acute coronary syndrome patients, biomarker levels may rise after an initially negative sample, which commonly coincides with the time when angiography and PCI are performed.[6]

Such a rise and fall in biomarker levels at the time of PCI is not a mere laboratory finding; there is solid qualitative and quantitative evidence of irreversible myocardial injury that correlates with the rise in the serum level of the biomarker. In a small study using contrast-enhanced magnetic resonance imaging (MRI) to directly visualize areas of myonecrosis, Ricciardi and colleagues[7] reported that there was MR evidence of hyperenhancement (equivalent to approximately 2 g of myocardium) in nine of nine patients in whom there was a minor procedure-related CK-MB level elevation (approximately two times the ULN). In the five control patients who did not have any elevation of the CK-MB level, there was no MR evidence of hyperenhancement in the target vessel perfusion territory. None of the patients in whom hyperenhancement was detected as evidence of myonecrosis developed electrocardiographic q waves.[7]

In a more contemporary and rigorous study, 48 patients underwent cardiac MRI before and after PCI to detect newly developed hyperenhancement as evidence of procedure-related myonecrosis.[8] One half of the patients underwent a third MR scan at a median of 8 months. Findings were correlated with serum troponin levels recorded 24 hours after the index PCI. All patients were preloaded with clopidogrel and received abciximab at the time of PCI, but the incidence of troponin elevation above the ULN was 37% (14 patients). There was evidence of new MR hyperenhancement in the target vessel territory in all 14 patients. In patients with no troponin elevation after PCI, there was no evidence of hyperenhancement on MR scans. There was also a linear correlation between the troponin level at 24 hours after PCI and the mass of newly hyperenhanced myocardium (measured in grams) on the early post-PCI scan and on the delayed 8-month scan, confirming the correlation between periprocedural biomarker release and irreversible myocardial damage (Fig. 27-1).[8]

In addition to confirming the irreversible nature of the myocardial injury, the location of MR hyperenhancement in relation to the PCI target segment may give insight into the pathophysiologic mechanism underlying PMI. When hyperenhancement is visualized in proximity of the treated segment, side branch occlusion (SBO) is the more likely explanation, but when the myocardial injury or damage is downstream from the treated segment, PMI can be best explained by distal microembolization and adverse platelet and inflammatory reactions in the microcirculation.[7,9]

INCIDENCE

As with its definition, the reported incidence of PMI has varied widely from one published report to another (Table 27-1). This variation can be attributed to several factors: the choice of biomarker assayed, the threshold value used to define PMI, and routine versus clinically driven biomarker assays. When the incidence of PMI is reported for a consecutive series of patients undergoing PCI (irrespective of their clinical condition after the procedure), it is invariably higher than in other series in which biomarkers were assayed only in patients who developed certain symptoms or signs of ischemia. This is the result of detection of a fairly larger proportion of clinically silent events, with small-magnitude biomarker release.[10] The PCI guidelines update published by the American College of Cardiology (ACC), American Heart Association (AHA), and European Society of Cardiology (ESC) experts in 2005 recommends the routine assay of CK-MB and troponin in every patient undergoing PCI 8 to 12 hours after the procedure, irrespective of presence or absence of symptoms of MI.[2] In nonselected patient series excluding patients with initially positive markers, the average incidence of PMI using CK-MB, troponin T, and troponin I

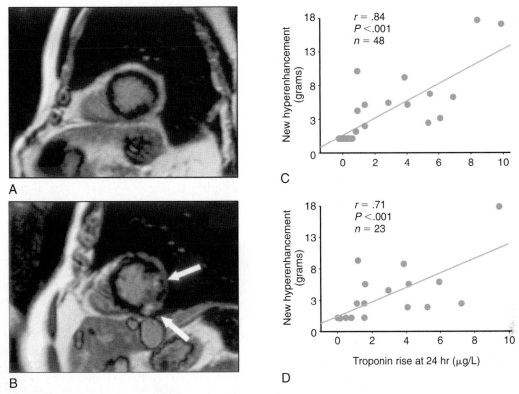

Figure 27-1. Apical ventricular short-axis image **(A)**, which was obtained in a patient before left circumflex/obtuse marginal bifurcation percutaneous coronary intervention (PCI), showed no hyperenhancement. Another image **(B)** demonstrated two regions of new hyperenhancement in the distribution of the obtuse marginal branch artery after PCI *(arrows)*. Correlations are demonstrated between the 24-hour post-PCI troponin I value and the mass of new myocardial hyperenhancement early **(C)** and late **(D)** after PCI. (From Selvanayagam JB, Porto I, Channon K, et al: Troponin elevation after percutaneous coronary intervention directly represents the extent of irreversible myocardial injury: Insights from cardiovascular magnetic resonance imaging. Circulation 2005;111:1027-1032.)

Table 27-1. Incidence of Periprocedural Myocardial Infarction in Selected Large Series of Patients

Study	Patients *(N)*	Type of PCI	Biomarker Definition of PMI	Incidence of PMI(%)
Abdelmeguid et al[10]	4664	PTCA, DCA	CK 2-5 × ULN	2.6
Ghazzal et al[14]	15637	PCI	CK 1-2 × ULN	4.6
			CK >3 × ULN	1.6
Harrington et al[15]	1012	PTCA	CK-MB × 2 ULN	3.8
		DCA		10.3
Simoons et al[16]	5025	PTCA	CK-MB 1-3 × ULN	13.2
Roe et al[11]	2384	PCI	CK-MB 1-3 × ULN	21.3
			CK-MB 3-5 × ULN	6.0
			CK-MB 5-10 × ULN	7.1
			CK-MB >10 × ULN	9.5
Stone et al[17]	7147	PTCA	CK-MB >4	25.1
		Stent		34.4
		Ablation		37.8
		Ablation + stent		48.8
Ellis et al[18]	8409	PCI	CK-MB >8.8	17.2
Ntarajan et al[19]	1128	PCI	Tn I >0.5	16.8
Nallamothu et al[12]	1157	PCI	Tn I 1-3 × ULN	16.0
			Tn I 3-5 × ULN	4.6
			Tn I 5-8 × ULN	2.0
			Tn I ≥8 × ULN	6.5
Cavallini et al[13]	3494	PCI	Tn I >0.15	44.2
			CK-MB >5	16.0

CK-MB, creatine kinase–myocardial band isoenzyme; PCI, percutaneous coronary intervention; PMI, periprocedural myocardial infarction; PTCA, percutaneous transluminal coronary angioplasty; Tn, troponin; ULN, upper limit of normal; DCA, directional coronary atherectomy.

values more than the ULN was 23% ± 12 %, 23% ± 12%, and 27% ± 12%, respectively.[9]

Using a lower biomarker cutoff value to define PMI increases the proportion of patients labeled as having PMI.[11,12] Similarly, using troponin assays reported a higher incidence of PMI (up to 44%) than other studies defining PMI using the more traditional CK or CK-MB.[13] Other important factors that contribute to the heterogeneity of the conclusions of the various published series include the widely disparate baseline and procedural characteristics in the studied populations, inclusion or exclusion of patients with antecedent MI, and the timing of blood sampling.[6,9]

There may be discrepancies in the reported incidences of PMI according to the time frame in which various reports were published, the anticoagulation or antiplatelet therapy, and the devices used for PCI. Large Q-wave PMI were reduced from 2.1% in the Bypass Angioplasty Revascularization Investigation (BARI) trial population to 0.8% in BARI-like patients selected from the more contemporary National Heart, Lung, and Blood Institute (NHLBI) dynamic registry. The reduction was primarily driven by contemporary liberal use of stents in the NHLBI Registry, which effectively treated abrupt closure and flow-limiting dissections.[20] In the Evaluation of Platelet IIb/IIIa Inhibitor for Stenting (EPISTENT) randomized, controlled trial, use of abciximab reduced Q-wave PMI during stenting by more than 40% (1.4% versus 0.8%).[21]

UNDERLYING PATHOPHYSIOLOGIC MECHANISMS

Magnetic resonance myocardial imaging in patients who develop biomarker release after PCI reveals two types of PMI, according to the distribution of hyperenhancement indicative of acute injury. In the more commonly seen *distal type* of PMI, hyperenhancement is in the distal distribution downstream from the treated segment. In the *proximal type* of PMI, the injury is primarily detected adjacent to the treated segment.[7,22] Proximal PMI is usually linked to flow impairment in a side branch arising from the treated segment, whereas the more commonly seen distal PMI results from microvascular obstruction in the distribution of the artery subjected to PCI.

Distal Embolization and Periprocedural Myocardial Infarction

Although distal embolization associated with endothelial injury has been recognized for years, the importance of this phenomenon in relation to PCI has not been fully appreciated until the last decade.[23] Platelet aggregates have been identified in the distal microcirculation and atherosclerotic debris retrieved from arteries downstream from the site of angioplasty using filter devices (Fig. 27-2).

Clinically, intravascular ultrasound (IVUS) studies provided further insight into the relationship between embolization of plaque material and PMI. Prati and

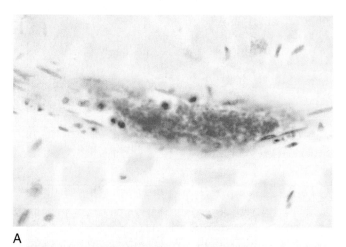

A

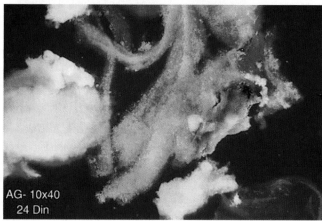

AG- 10x40
24 Din

B

Figure 27-2. A, The histologic specimen of an intramyocardial microvessel filled with platelets, stained positive for platelet GP IIb/IIIa, was from patient who had sudden cardiac death. **B,** Atherosclerotic particulate embolic material was retrieved from percutaneous coronary revascularization with an Angioguard guidewire filter. (From Topol EJ, Yadav JS: Recognition of the importance of embolization in atherosclerotic vascular disease. Circulation 2000;101:570-580.)

coworkers[24] examined the relationship between change in plaque volume before and after stenting and the degree of CK-MB release in 54 patients. In patients with unstable angina, there was a more significant reduction in plaque volume, but more importantly, such reduction significantly correlated with CK-MB release, even after adjusting for other variables influencing PMI.[24] A later and more sophisticated analysis of 62 patients undergoing complex PCI by Porto and associates[22] demonstrated a significant association between the change in target lesion plaque area by IVUS and the mass of myonecrosis assessed by hyperenhancement on MRI after PCI. The investigators also correlated impaired microvascular flow (Thrombolysis in Myocardial Infarction [TIMI] perfusion grade 0 or 1) with MR evidence of hyperenhancement downstream from the treated segment, suggesting that particulate matter from the atherosclerotic plaque disrupted by angioplasty drift downstream, leading to microvascular obstruction and myonecrosis.

The development and clinical use of embolism protection devices provided additional evidence of distal embolization, because particulate matter from the atherosclerotic plaque subjected to angioplasty could be collected, measured, and analyzed. The embolized material primarily consists of debris (i.e., atherosclerotic plaque and thrombotic elements), with particles ranging in size from about 50 to more than 600 µm. Neutrophils and macrophages are also identified. Although these devices are more frequently used in the setting of PCI in saphenous vein grafts, distal embolization in routine native vessel PCI is probably just as common, producing debris that is similar in quantity and composition.[25,26]

Role of the Platelet

Platelet activation plays a critical role in the development and perpetuation of coronary microvascular obstruction after PCI. By definition, the interventional devices used to treat an epicardial stenosis result in a break in the endothelial surface and release of debris into the coronary bloodstream. The exposed intraplaque contents stimulate platelet activation and aggregation at the site of PCI and probably in the downstream microvasculature. The platelet aggregates plugging the microcirculation cause mechanical obstruction and lead to biochemical responses due to their interaction with the injured endothelium, the neutrophils, and with more platelets. The release of vasoactive substances such as serotonin and endothelin-1 from the activated platelets and the injured endothelium lead to intense microvascular vasoconstriction, which accentuates the ischemic injury and resultant myonecrosis.[9,23]

One study of aspirin resistance emphasized the role of platelet aggregation in the pathophysiology of PMI. Patients deemed to be resistant to aspirin therapy were found to have a significantly higher incidence of PMI, defined as any increase in the degree of CK-MB (51.7% versus 24.6%, $P = .006$).[27] The odds of developing PMI in this cohort of 151 patients presenting for nonurgent PCI increase threefold if they are found to be aspirin-resistant before the procedure.[27]

Other Pathophysiologic Mechanisms

Distal embolization of plaque debris and platelet activation, with all its local metabolic consequences, probably are the primary mechanisms leading to distal PMI in absence of PCI complications such as side branch closure or flow-limiting dissections. However, other intriguing mechanisms may interact with embolism and platelet activation. These mechanisms have been suggested by analysis of coronary sinus blood samples obtained before and after PCI, reflecting the local metabolic derangements that result from the intervention. For instance, there is evidence of neutrophil activation in the coronary

sinus samples after PCI and an increase in serum levels of C-reactive protein (CRP) and interleukin-6 (IL-6). The increase in inflammatory marker levels was associated with post-PCI troponin release.[28] This demonstrates a local inflammatory response at the level of the myocardium in response to PCI and suggests a potential contribution to the process of myocyte damage.[9,28] Concentration of isoprostanes (i.e. stable end products of oxygen free radical mediated-lipid peroxidation) also increased in coronary sinus blood after PCI, which demonstrates an increase in oxygen free radical production during PCI.[29] The extent to which this inflammatory response and increased oxidative stress contribute to myonecrosis remains unclear.

RISK FACTORS PREDISPOSING TO PERIPROCEDURAL MYOCARDIAL INFARCTION

Clinical trials examining the role of newer interventional devices and GP IIb/IIIa inhibitors, as well as patient series investigating the incidence and significance of PMI, have identified certain subsets of patients who are at higher risk for PMI. These subsets can be identified based on clinical, lesion-related, procedural, or device-related variables.

Clinical Characteristics

The risk of PMI is significantly increased in patients with evidence of more severe atherosclerotic disease. Multivessel disease or more diffuse coronary artery disease is associated with an approximately 50% increase in the relative risk for developing PMI.[11,14,30] IVUS evidence of increased plaque burden is also a risk factor for development of PMI.[22,24] This may explain why diabetics are at a higher risk for PMI.[31] Evidence of advanced noncardiac atherosclerotic disease has been associated with an even higher relative risk for PMI.[30]

The clinical presentation at the time of PCI may also play a role in determining the risk of PMI and other adverse events during and after the procedure. Patients with acute coronary syndromes are more likely to develop PMI.[9] However, studies examining the incidence of PMI in this patient population have been limited by certain methodologic difficulties. First, it is difficult and more controversial to define PMI when patients present with elevated markers before PCI. Most of the studies on this topic excluded these patients from the analysis. Second, even if patients with elevated markers are excluded, it is conceivable that those with negative markers who were referred to PCI within a few hours of presentation might have been having a spontaneous infarction that was appreciated only after the PCI.[9,11]

A heightened systemic inflammatory state before PCI is also a major predictor of adverse outcomes, including PMI. Most of the evidence supporting this hypothesis is based on correlations between pre-PCI CRP levels and evidence of PMI. A small study of 85 patients with stable angina undergoing PCI

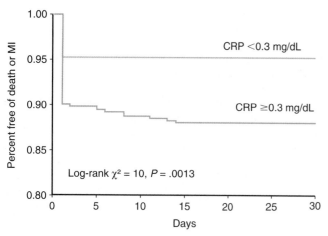

Figure 27-3. Kaplan-Meier survival curves for 30-day death or myocardial infarction stratified by the baseline C-reactive protein (CRP) level. Most events and the separation of the curves occur within the first 1 to 2 days (i.e., the difference is primarily driven by the incidence of periprocedural myocardial infarction. (From Chew DP, Bhatt DL, Robbins MA, et al: Incremental prognostic value of elevated baseline C-reactive protein among established markers of risk in percutaneous coronary intervention. Circulation 2001;104:992-997.)

demonstrated that PMI (defined by an elevated troponin level) was significantly more common in patients with elevated CRP levels; 46% of those with elevated CRP but only 18% of those with a normal CRP developed the complication.[32] Chew and colleagues[33] examined the relationship between the preprocedural CRP level and the adverse events (i.e., death and MI) in the first 30 days after PCI in a larger series of 727 consecutive patients. The highest quartile of CRP was predictive of worse outcome (OR = 3.68; 95% CI: 1.5 to 9.0), and that association persisted even after adjusting for other variables influencing outcome. The event-free survival curves separated within 24 hours and were primarily driven by a reduction in MI, suggesting that patients with elevated CRP levels are more susceptible to development of PMI (Fig. 27-3).[33]

Lesion-Related Risk Factors

Saphenous vein graft lesions are notorious for the risk of development of PMI, probably because of the increased incidence of macroembolization and microembolization, with subsequent slow flow and no reflow. In absence of embolism protection devices, the risk of PMI (defined as a CK-MB level more than three times the ULN) in the contemporary era can be as high as 13.7%. This rate almost doubles if the threshold cutoff value to define PMI is any increase in the CK-MB level.[34] The introduction of embolism protection devices in the past few years has significantly reduced the risk of PMI in those patients.[34,35]

Several lesion characteristics are traditionally associated with a higher risk of PMI, primarily features suggesting lesion instability (e.g., eccentricity, irregular contour, visible thrombosis). Complex lesions (ACC/AHA type C) usually contain one or more of those features and are associated with a significantly increased risk of PMI.[4,10] Lesions involving the ostium of a major side branch are usually among the more complex lesion types and more prone to result in PMI due to the higher risk of side branch closure. Other lesion characteristics that confer a higher risk of PMI include features that suggest a higher plaque burden, such as multiplicity of lesions, long lesions, and diffusely diseased arteries.

Procedural Complications and Risk of Periprocedural Myocardial Infarction

SBO, flow-limiting dissections, and transient abrupt closure have been the most recognizable procedural complications that result in relatively large PMIs.[4,10,14,36] However, these complications are rare, and most detected PMIs follow routine procedures with no obvious angiographic complications.[9,23] With routine use and universal availability of stents, abrupt closure has become rare (<1% of cases in contemporary PCI).[23] The effectiveness of stenting and the availability of potent antiplatelet therapies are probably the primary mechanisms by which large (q-wave) PMIs and need for emergent coronary surgery have been reduced by almost 50%.[20,37] Abrupt closure or no reflow have not been found to affect outcome when treated promptly with no subsequent PMIs.[36]

SBO has been and remains the most common angiographically recognizable procedural complication resulting in PMI.[10,14] Unlike abrupt closure, the incidence of SBO has not decreased with routine use of coronary stenting. With increasing stent use, SBO has become the most likely cause of acute occlusion during PCI.[38] Major SBO can be associated with large (possibly q-wave) infarctions, but even smaller branch occlusions have been associated with evidence of small areas of MR hyperenhancement, diagnostic of small areas of PMI. The distribution of hyperenhancement in these cases is different from that seen with distal embolization downstream of the target lesion for PCI. With SBO, hyperenhancement is adjacent rather than distal to the location of the PCI. The likelihood of development of new hyperenhancement increases 16-fold when SBO can be angiographically recognized.[22]

There have been some intriguing observations regarding SBO and PMI in the era of PCI of complex lesions using drug-eluting stents. In the TAXUS V trial that randomized 1172 patients to receive a paclitaxel-eluting (Taxus) or a bare metal stent, complex lesion subsets (more than 35% type C) were treated in both groups, and more than 30% of patients received more than one stent. In the subgroup of patients receiving multiple stents, the incidence of 30-day MI was significantly higher with paclitaxel-eluting stents (8.3% versus 3.3%, P = .047). Core laboratory angiographic analysis of this patient subset revealed a significantly higher incidence of side branch compromise or SBO with paclitaxel-eluting stents than with bare metal stents (42.6% versus 30.6%, $P = .03$), resulting in a higher incidence of greater than TIMI 3 flow in the paclitaxel-eluting stent group. Why paclitaxel-eluting stents are associated with more side branch compromise and subsequent PMI remains unclear. Possible explanations include the increasing thickness of the stent struts caused by the drug-eluting polymer, increased platelet deposition, and paclitaxel-induced spasm.[39]

Risk of Periprocedural Myocardial Infarction by Interventional Device

Some of the earliest investigations sparking interest in PMI and its significance were in the context of comparing newer interventional devices with standard balloon angioplasty. Data from the CAVEAT-I trial demonstrated that directional coronary atherectomy (DCA) was associated with more abrupt closure, evidence of PMI, and a subsequently higher rate of clinical adverse events compared with balloon angioplasty.[15,40] These findings were confirmed in the Balloon Angioplasty Versus Optimal Atherectomy (BOAT) trial, in which a more refined technique of DCA was supposed to demonstrate its superiority to percutaneous transluminal coronary angioplasty (PTCA). However, the incidence of PMI was still significantly higher with DCA than with balloon angioplasty (16% versus 6%).[41] DCA is associated with more distal embolization, particularly in saphenous vein graft interventions.[42] There is also evidence of a higher degree of platelet activation with DCA,[43] with its subsequent mechanical obstruction and thrombotic and inflammatory responses in the downstream microcirculation. Similarly, rotational atherectomy is associated with more platelet activation and distal embolization of plaque debris than balloon angioplasty owing to its mechanism of action.[44]

Although the routine use of coronary stents has dramatically reduced the incidence of most PCI complications (i.e., abrupt closure, flow-limiting dissections, need for emergent bypass surgery, and restenosis), stenting increases the incidence of PMI compared with balloon angioplasty, with a relative risk increase of about 20%.[9,23,45] In patients undergoing PCI of the left anterior descending coronary artery who were randomly assigned to balloon angioplasty or stenting, there was evidence of a higher degree of platelet and neutrophil surface activation after stenting.[46] High-pressure inflations aiming to overexpand stents and reduce restenosis can instead lead to higher CK-MB levels. In a study of approximately 1000 patients undergoing IVUS-guided stenting, the incidence of PMI (defined as a CK-MB level that was three times the ULN) was 16%, 18%, and 25% in three groups of patients in whom the final stent to reference lumen area was less than 70%, 70% to 100%, and more than 100%, respectively.[47]

Prognostic Implications of Periprocedural Myocardial Infarction

Although there is much controversy about the definition and prevalence of PMI with everyday PCI, there is no dispute that significant PMI is associated with an increased mortality risk. The controversy still exists about the pathophysiologic mechanisms underlying this association, the definition, and the size of PMI that would confer such increased risk. However, there is convincing evidence that any PMI is associated with some degree of increased risk of death, particularly with longer follow-up durations.

The pioneering work of Abdelmeguid and coworkers[10] had demonstrated that CK and CK-MB level elevation after PCI (primarily balloon angioplasty and DCA in this report) were associated with an approximately 30% relative increase in 3-year mortality. Three-year follow-up of the Evaluation of 7E3 for the Prevention of Ischemic Complications (EPIC) trial patients (also undergoing angioplasty and DCA) revealed an incremental long-term risk of death with increasing degrees of PMI. Among the 2001 patients enrolled in the trial, the mortality risk increased from 7.3% for those with no CK elevation to 13.1% when the CK level was more than three times the ULN and to 16.5% with a CK level of more than 10 times the ULN.[48] In the EPISTENT trial, in which stenting was routinely employed in two thirds of the patients, the 1-year mortality rate doubled between patients with no or minimal PMI (CK-MB level more than 1 times the ULN) and those with a CK-MB level more than 3 to 10 times the ULN (1.5% versus 3.4%).[21] Subsequently, similar conclusions were made by examining outcomes of patients enrolled in PCI clinical trials and large-scale, single-center patient registries (see Table 27-1).[11,14,15,18,21,49]

Although the association between PMI and mortality has not been disputed, the mechanisms that can explain this association are not clear. The magnitude of myonecrosis is limited, but it may provide a nidus for arrhythmogenesis. It has been suggested that the association between PMI and late mortality merely represents a reflection of increased risk in a group of patients with more advanced disease.[6] The latter hypothesis can be criticized by the fact that aggressive preprocedural platelet inhibition (by thienopyridine pretreatment or intravenous GP IIb/IIIa inhibitors) reduces PMI and subsequent risk of death and adverse events, suggesting that this is a modifiable risk.

The threshold above which a PMI is considered prognostically significant has been a subject of some debate. It has been traditional to define a PMI when the CK-MB level exceeds three times the ULN, although the recent PCI guidelines suggest that a CK-MB level more than five times the ULN should be the threshold for defining a PMI.[2] In the large series of Ghazzal and colleagues,[14] minor elevation of total CK (more than three times the ULN) did not confer a statistically significant increase in risk of late mortality.[14] Brener and coworkers[50] suggested that only massive CK-MB release (more than 10 times the ULN) predicts an increased risk of death over a 3-year period. However, there has been strong evidence that smaller CK-MB elevations are associated with increasing risk of death. Abdelmeguid and colleagues[10] examined that question specifically and concluded that any increase in CK-MB above normal limits confers some degree of risk. In a later meta-analysis, any increase in CK-MB, even less than three times the ULN, was associated with a statistically significant increase in the risk of death (OR = 1.5). Patients with a CK-MB level between three and five times the ULN and those with levels more than five times the ULN had even higher relative risks of dying over the 3-year follow-up.[51] Similarly, in the large meta-analysis by Roe and colleagues,[11] the increased mortality risk was associated with increasing CK-MB levels expressed as a continuous variable (i.e., with no specific thresholds above or below which the risk changes) (Fig. 27-4).

Frequently, very large PMIs (i.e., CK-MB levels more than 8 to 10 times the ULN) are associated with significant complications or an unsuccessful procedural result. The association between PMI and mortality has been attributed to the impact of an unsuccessful procedure on mortality and not considered to be an independent effect. In a study of approximately 6000 patients, the incidence of PMI was three times more frequent when the procedure was unsuccessful and the size of the infarction was also significantly larger. After adjusting for the success of the procedure (defined as residual stenosis less than 50%, achievement of TIMI 3 flow, and absence of significant residual dissection and need for urgent revascularization or stent thrombosis within 24 hours), the presence or absence of PMI was not statistically related to 1-year mortality.[52] However, the study examined only 1-year mortality, and in many investigations examining PMI, the effect on mortality was observed only with longer-term follow-up. The initial studies by Abdelmeguid and colleagues[4,10] that established a relationship between PMI and death have excluded unsuccessful procedural results from their analyses. In the CK-MB and PCI study examining the significance of post-PCI troponin elevation, unsuccessful procedures doubled the odds of 2-year mortality, but the effect of post-PCI CK-MB levels remained a strong and significant predictor of mortality.[13]

The association between mortality and PMI defined by elevated serum troponin levels is less robust. The updated PCI guidelines propose that a PMI becomes clinically significant if the troponin level exceeds five times the ULN.[2] In a study of 1157 patients (>77% receiving stents), 1-year mortality risk increased only in the group of patients with troponin I levels greater than eight times the ULN (≥16 ng/mL).[12] However, in the largest multicenter, prospective study (almost 3500 patients) addressing the significance of post-PCI

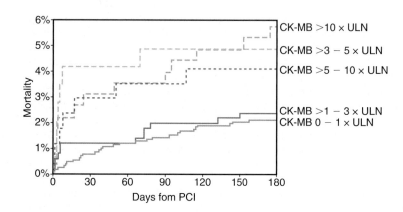

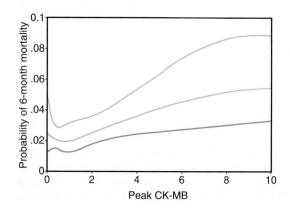

Figure 27-4. *Top,* The Kaplan-Meier curves for 6 months' unadjusted mortality after percutaneous coronary intervention (PCI) for increments of post-PCI creatine kinase–myocardial band isoenzyme (CK-MB). *Bottom,* Continuous unadjusted relationship between peak CK-MB (as times the upper limit of normal [ULN]) and 6 months' mortality. The *thin lines* represent the 95% confidence intervals. (From Roe MT, Mahaffey KW, Kilaru R, et al: Creatine kinase-MB elevation after percutaneous coronary intervention predicts adverse outcomes in patients with acute coronary syndromes. Eur Heart J 2004;25:313-321.)

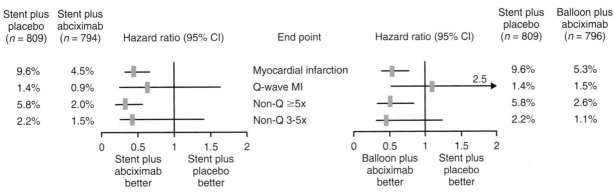

Figure 27-5. Kaplan-Meier estimates and hazard ratios (95% confidence intervals) for myocardial infarction in the EPISTENT trial. (From the EPISTENT investigators: Randomised placebo-controlled and balloon-angioplasty-controlled trial to assess safety of coronary stenting with use of platelet glycoprotein-IIb/IIIa blockade. Evaluation of Platelet IIb/IIIa Inhibitor for Stenting [EPISTENT]. Lancet 1998;352: 87-92.)

troponin levels, there was no statistically significant association between troponin I elevation and the 2-year mortality rate. As expected, the incidence of troponin I elevation after PCI was significantly higher than that of CK-MB, indicating the higher sensitivity of that marker in detecting myonecrosis. However, this high sensitivity appears to reduce the ability of troponin elevation to predict prognosis.[13]

PREVENTION AND MANAGEMENT OF PERIPROCEDURAL MYOCARDIAL INFARCTION

In most cases of PMI, the event is clinically silent, and the diagnosis is made on the basis of routine collection of cardiac biomarkers after PCI. Little can be done to treat the event by any specific measures different from those that should be employed with any patient undergoing PCI (i.e., effective β-blockade, antiplatelet therapy, lipid lowering, and aggressive risk factor control). In the event of a relatively large PMI (e.g., CK-MB level more than five times the ULN), an additional day of telemetry monitoring and more adequate β-blockade (with a target heart rate of about 60 beats/min) may be indicated.

Given the adverse prognostic implications, it is significantly more important to develop strategies to prevent rather than treat PMI. In the past decade, there have been significant successes in this field. Successful strategies to prevent PMI include pharmacologic and nonpharmacologic approaches. The primary pharmacologic interventions that achieved significant success include aggressive antiplatelet therapy (primarily intravenous GP IIb/IIIa inhibitors and oral thienopyridine inhibitors) and statin therapy. Nonpharmacologic approaches include the use of embolism protection devices in the setting of saphenous vein graft intervention.

Intravenous Glycoprotein IIb/IIIa Platelet Inhibitors

Periprocedural use of GP IIb/IIIa inhibitors provides immediate and near-complete inhibition of platelet aggregation. The intravenous administration of the appropriate doses and the targeting of the final common receptor for the aggregation process (the GP IIb/IIIa receptor) ensure an extremely high bioavailability and a very predictable and complete response. Abciximab, the prototype of this class of antiplatelet agents, has been shown in many clinical trials to reduce the incidence of post-PCI myonecrosis. In the seminal trials (EPIC, EPISTENT, and Evaluation in Percutaneous Transluminal Coronary Angioplasty to Improve Long-Term Outcome with Abciximab GP IIb/IIIa Blockade [EPILOG]), the cutoff threshold for defining PMI was a CK-MB level of three times the ULN. The relative risk reduction in MI at 30 days ranged between 40% and 60%, with differences appearing as early as the first day, indicating a significant reduction in PMI (Fig. 27-5).[21,40] In the Chimeric c7E3 Fab Antiplatelet Therapy in Unstable Refractory Angina (CAPTURE) trial, refractory unstable angina patients were randomized to receive abciximab or placebo many hours before and during PCI. In this trial, pre-PCI incidence of MI was reduced significantly in the abciximab arm, and the incidence of PMI was reduced by more than 50% in the abciximab arm (2.6% versus 5.5%, P = .009).[53] With rotational atherectomy, which consistently results in distal microembolization, abciximab bolus and infusion demonstrated a significant advantage over anticoagulation alone in reducing postprocedural elevations of CK and CK-MB levels.[44]

Similar effects have been demonstrated with the synthetic small-molecule GP IIb/IIIa inhibitors eptifibatide and tirofiban. The impact of eptifibatide on PMI was significantly better when the dosing regimen was adjusted from one bolus in the Platelet IIb/IIIa in Unstable Angina: Receptor Suppression Using Integrilin Therapy (PURSUIT-PCI) trial to the double-bolus regimen followed in the ESPRIT trial, emphasizing the importance of the near-complete inhibition that is required if an impact on distal embolization is to be expected. In the PURSUIT trial, the incidence of PMI was reduced by 25%, whereas the reduction with the double-bolus regimen was 40%. In both trials, PMI was defined as a CK-MB level three times the ULN, and the incidence of PMI in the placebo group was similar in both trials (≈9%).[54,55] In the Randomized Efficacy Study of Tirofiban for Outcomes and Restenosis (RESTORE) trial examining the role of tirofiban in patients with acute coronary syndromes, there was a small but significant reduction in PMI at the 48-hour mark. However, there was no statistically significant difference in the incidence of the primary end point (i.e., 30-day death, MI, or revascularization for recurrent ischemia and use of stents for threatened or abrupt closure) between tirofiban and placebo.[56] With a higher-dose tirofiban bolus, a small study of 202 high-risk patients undergoing PCI demonstrated that PMI defined by troponin level rise decreased by about 34% and that the average CK-MB level (expressed in absolute units) was reduced by more than 50%.[57]

Thienopyridine Platelet Inhibitors

The undisputed effect of GP IIb/IIIa platelet inhibitors in reducing PMI supports the central role of platelet aggregation and activation in the pathophysiology of PMI. This is further emphasized by the very high incidence of PMI and other adverse cardiac events in patients with aspirin resistance. Dual-antiplatelet therapy using thienopyridine platelet inhibitors (i.e., ticlopidine and clopidogrel) has been advocated. As with other antiplatelet agents, the timing and dosing of these agents seem to have a dramatic impact on their value in reducing PMI and other post-PCI adverse events. Steinhubl and coworkers[58] reported a significant reduction in the incidence of PMI with pre-PCI administration of ticlopidine. The longer the duration of therapy, the lower the incidence was, and among patients pretreated with ticlopidine, the odds ratio for development of PMI was 0.18 when the duration of pretreatment was 3 days or longer. Subsequently, the questions of dosing and duration of pretreatment with another thienopyridine inhibitor, clopidogrel, were addressed in the Clopidogrel for the Reduction of Events During Observation (CREDO) trial. The study randomized patients undergoing elective PCI to receive a 300-mg clopidogrel loading dose or placebo 3 to 24 hours before PCI. All patients were on aspirin, and most of them did undergo PCI. A second randomization to 28 days versus 9 months of dual-antiplatelet therapy was performed for those in the clopidogrel arm. The results demonstrated a reduction in 30-day major adverse events (primarily early MIs) only in patients who received the loading dose 6 hours or more before PCI (Fig. 27-6).[59] The timing of the loading dose significantly affected the beneficial effect of thienopyridine on PCI outcomes. In PCI-CURE trial, 30% of patients underwent PCI at the discretion of the treating cardiologists. The subgroup of the larger trial included 2658 patients with non-ST-segment elevation MI from non-U.S. centers, where the time between admission for acute coronary syndrome and PCI averaged 10 days. In this setting, the 30-day incidence of MI was reduced by more than 50% for

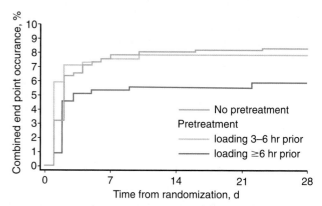

Figure 27-6. The 28-day combined end point of death, myocardial infarction, or urgent revascularization in the Clopidogrel for the Reduction of Events During Observation (CREDO) trial is stratified by use and timing of a clopidogrel loading dose. The curves separate within 48 hours, primarily because of differences in incidence of periprocedural myocardial infarction. (From Steinhubl SR, Berger PB, Mann JT 3rd, et al: Early and sustained dual oral antiplatelet therapy following percutaneous coronary intervention: A randomized controlled trial. JAMA 2002;288:2411-2420.)

patients receiving clopidogrel (2.9% versus 6.2%), suggesting that longer duration of pretreatment, particularly in high-risk patients, is associated with better protection against procedure-related MI.[60]

In the past few years, several groups have demonstrated that a higher loading dose (600 mg) of clopidogrel can achieve two important goals: reach higher levels of platelet inhibition and achieve that target within 2 hours of oral administration.[61] The improved efficacy of the higher loading dose is at least partly attributed to the fact that about one third of patients do not adequately respond to the inhibitory effect of the 300-mg dose.[61] The second Antiplatelet Therapy for Reduction of Myocardial Damage during Angioplasty (ARMYDA-2) trial established the superiority of the 600-mg loading dose of clopidogrel in reducing PMI and improving 30-day outcomes. This study enrolled 255 patients undergoing PCI and randomized them to 300-mg or to 600-mg loading doses of clopidogrel 4 to 8 hours before PCI. The primary end point of death, MI, or urgent revascularization at 30 days was reduced by 66% in the high-loading-dose arm (4% versus 12%, P = .04). The benefit almost entirely resulted from the marked reduction in PMI, a reduction of approximately 50% in a multivariable model adjusting for all variables influencing the incidence of PMI (OR = 0.48; 95% CI: 0.15 to 0.97; P = .044).[62] It remains controversial whether a higher loading dose of clopidogrel (i.e., 900 mg) can lead to further improvement in PMI and other ischemic complications.[63,64]

Clopidogrel, Glycoprotein IIb/IIIa inhibitors, and Periprocedural Myocardial Infarction

As the evidence for the role of clopidogrel in reducing procedural complications mounted, it became clear that there was some degree of overlap between the roles of clopidogrel and intravenous GP IIb/IIIa inhibitors in aggressive platelet inhibition before and during PCI procedures. Whether such high degrees of platelet inhibition are needed to achieve satisfactory PCI results remained unclear for some time. In sequential investigations, the Intracoronary Stenting and Antithrombotic Regimen: Rapid Early Action for Coronary Treatment (ISAR-REACT) trials, the interaction between clopidogrel loading and abciximab infusion for peri-PCI platelet inhibition was examined in low-risk and then in higher-risk patient populations. In ISAR-REACT-1, more than 1000 stable patients with no evidence of instability or infarction were included. They were randomized to receive clopidogrel loading plus placebo versus clopidogrel loading plus abciximab bolus and infusion. At 30 days, there was no statistically significant difference between the two groups in the incidence of MI or death.[65] However, the very low incidence of adverse events in the placebo group (compared with the investigators' estimates for sample size calculation) diminished the statistical power of the study to detect differences between the groups.

In the following study, ISAR-REACT-2, more than 2000 patients with non-ST-segment elevation acute coronary syndromes were enrolled. All patients received clopidogrel pretreatment, and then one half of them were randomized to abciximab bolus plus infusion. Unlike ISAR-REACT-1, there was a significant reduction in the 30-day composite end point (i.e., death, MI, or urgent revascularization) in favor of abciximab. This included a more than 20% reduction in infarctions, most of which were PMIs (8.1% versus 10.5%). Based on the results of those two investigations, it seems that a more complete degree of platelet inhibition is needed in patients at higher risk for PMI and procedural complications. In addition to the more complete platelet inhibition ensured by the use of abciximab, its cross-reactivity with $\alpha_v\beta_3$ (vitronectin) and $\alpha_M\beta_2$ (Mac-1) receptors may provide potent anti-inflammatory effects. This appears to be associated with a significant reduction in the degree of rise of inflammatory markers such as CRP, IL-6, and tumor necrosis factor-α (TNF-α) in the 1 to 2 days after PCI, an effect that may contribute to the reduction in PMI seen with abciximab use during PCI.[66]

Impact of Statin Therapy

The inflammatory response of distal embolization and platelet aggregate interaction with leucocytes contributes to the degree of myonecrosis that is frequently seen after PCI. The observations made in PCI registries demonstrated a reduction in PMI in patients who have been receiving statins at the time of their PCI.[67] Proposed mechanisms that can explain this finding include an anti-inflammatory effect and the ability of statins to enhance nitric oxide production.[68] In an analysis of 803 patients undergoing rota-

tional atherectomy, the incidence of any myonecrosis was reduced by statin therapy from 52% to 24%, and the incidence of PMI (CK-MB level of three times the ULN) was reduced from 22% to 7.5%.[69] These observations were eventually confirmed in two prospective, randomized trials. In both trials, statin therapy was started several days before scheduled PCI in the active therapy arm. In one report of the results for 451 patients, statin therapy was not restricted to any specific agents. The median post-PCI troponin level was 0.13 ng/mL in the statin group and 0.21 ng/mL in the control group ($P = .03$). Similarly, the incidence of troponin I levels more than five times the ULN was significantly reduced with statin therapy (23.5% versus 32% in the control group, $P = .04$).[70] In the similarly designed ARMYDA trial, a smaller number of stable angina patients were randomized to receive atorvastatin versus placebo. There was a more than 50% reduction in incidence of PMI, as measured by CK-MB, troponin I, or myoglobin in the atorvastatin group.[71] In ARMYDA-2, there was an incremental benefit of statin and high-dose loading clopidogrel, leading to an impressive 80% reduction in PMI.[62]

A subgroup analysis of the ARMYDA trial confirms the anti-inflammatory role of statins in reducing myonecrosis post-PCI. In 138 patients, serum levels of adhesion molecules (e.g., ICAM, VCAM, E-selectin) were similar in patients in the atorvastatin group and the placebo group before PCI. However, after PCI, the rise in the levels of ICAM and E-selectin was significantly attenuated with atorvastatin therapy. This attenuated rise in adhesion molecules paralleled the protective effect against myonecrosis, providing some evidence that the anti-inflammatory effect of statins contributes to its observed protective effect against myonecrosis and early mortality, which cannot be attributed to its 3-hydroxy-3-methylglutaryl coenzyme A (HMG-CoA) reductase inhibitory effect.[72]

Other Pharmacologic Interventions

Controversy still exists about the role of preprocedural β-blocker therapy and PMI. There is evidence that β-blockade has a favorable impact on survival after PCI. Ellis and associates[73] supported this finding in a study of 6200 patients undergoing PCI, concluding that β-blocker therapy improved survival in the post-PCI patients. However, after adjustment for multiple variables and using propensity analysis, there was no evidence that patients with β-blocker therapy had reduced risk of or reduced size of PMI.[73]

The use of bivalirudin as a primary anticoagulant for PCI procedures is gaining popularity for various reasons, but there is no evidence that this agent reduces the risk of PMI. In the Randomized Evaluation in PCI Linking Angiomax to Reduced Clinical Events-2 (REPLACE-2) trial examining the role of bivalirudin in low-risk PCI patients, the incidence of MI was slightly higher in the bivalirudin arm: 7.0%

compared with 6.2% to the control arm of heparin and GP IIb/IIIa inhibitors. That difference was not statistically significant.[74] In the Randomized Trial to Evaluate Relative Protection against Post-PCI Microvascular Dysfunction and Post-PCI Ischemia among Anti-Platelet and Anti-Thrombotic Agents (PROTECT-TIMI-30), bivalirudin alone was associated with improved coronary reserve, but eptifibatide therapy (with heparin or enoxaparin) was associated with improved perfusion grades and shorter duration of ischemia after PCI as measured by Holter monitoring. CK-MB levels were not significantly different between the two arms.[75]

Nonpharmacologic Approaches

Very few mechanical options to prevent PMI are available. Direct stenting (without balloon predilation) was proposed to reduce plaque trauma and distal embolization. A small study compared direct stenting with conventional predilation followed by stent deployment and demonstrated a significant reduction in PMI.[76] Subsequent larger trials did not confirm any concrete advantages of this approach in reducing myonecrosis or any other adverse events.[77]

Another concept that has been subjected to clinical testing is trapping plaque debris by using stents covered with microporous polymer. Several of these stents are commercially available and are approved by the U.S. Food and Drug Administration (FDA) as an emergency treatment of life-threatening coronary perforation. However, when used to reduce distal embolization and PMI in vein graft PCI, these devices failed to demonstrate any benefit over bare metal stents—the restenosis rates were slightly higher.[78]

Emboli protection devices have been the only significant nonpharmacologic interventions with a proven advantage in reduction of periprocedural myonecrosis, particularly in saphenous vein graft intervention. These devices are discussed in the following section.

PMI is not uncommon after an apparently uncomplicated PCI. The reported incidence varies according to the biomarker used, the threshold for diagnosis, and the timing of sample collection. Distal embolization of atherosclerotic debris and platelet aggregates is the most plausible mechanism underlying PMI. There is no dispute that PMI is associated with late mortality, and the larger the PMI, the more robust is the association. Potent platelet inhibitor therapy (intravenous or oral), statins (as anti-inflammatory agents), and embolism protection devices (in saphenous vein graft PCI) had the most success in reducing the incidence of PMI.

Embolism Protection Devices

KEY POINTS

- Embolism protection devices (EPDs) include distal occlusive balloons, filter devices, and proximal flow-reversal systems; all aim to trap embolized debris from the site of angioplasty before reaching the distal microvascular bed.
- Clinical trials have demonstrated that EPD protection during vein graft PCI leads to a significant reduction in PMI and is cost effective; it has become the standard of care for those patients.
- Several randomized trials failed to show any benefit of EPD protection in the setting of acute MI PCI, highlighting the complexity of the mechanisms of myonecrosis and injury in those settings.

- There is good evidence that EPD protection reduces cerebral embolism during carotid stenting, but there has not been a conclusive randomized trial based on clinical end points to confirm the benefit.
- Comparison of carotid stenting using EPD protection with carotid endarterectomy has been difficult, and results of the randomized trials have been inconclusive. Ongoing clinical trials may provide more definitive answers to the lingering questions in this field.
- Clinical trials testing the potential advantages of EPD use during interventions in other vascular beds (e.g., renal, peripheral) are ongoing.

With the wider acceptance of the significance of distal embolization during PCI, efforts to reduce the incidence and impact of this phenomenon have been underway. Effective antiplatelet therapy with GP IIb/IIIa inhibitors and thienopyridine inhibitors has resulted in significant progress in reducing procedure-related myonecrosis. Despite routine use of these pharmacologic agents, a small PMI is not uncommon, even after uncomplicated procedures. This is of particular concern in the setting of saphenous vein graft interventions, which have a high propensity for distal embolization, no-reflow phenomenon, and PMI. Lesions with a high thrombus burden are another subgroup of procedures with a higher risk of distal embolization with any interventional device. The prototype of such procedures is PCI in the setting of acute MI. Over the past few years, several innovative designs for embolism protection devices (EPDs) have been developed to improve outcomes for these subsets of patients and in other clinical settings.

DESIGNS OF EMBOLISM PROTECTION DEVICES

There are three basic designs of EPDs: distal occlusion balloons, distal filters, and proximal occlusion devices (Fig. 27-7). Table 27-2 summarizes the differences between the various features of EPDs.

Distal Occlusion Devices

The PercuSurge GuardWire system (Medtronic, Santa Rosa, CA), the prototype of the balloon occlusion devices, consists of a 0.014-inch, hollow guidewire with an occlusion balloon toward the distal end and a 2.5-cm steerable tip beyond the balloon (see Fig. 27-7). The PercuSurge GuardWire is used to cross the lesion, and the balloon is positioned distal to the lesion in a relatively disease-free segment. The balloon then is inflated at a low pressure of about 1 atm to create a seal; the occlusion diameter ranges from 3 to 6 mm. Angioplasty, stenting, and postdilation are performed as necessary. The aspiration catheter is then advanced over the wire, and any dislodged debris is removed with a slow distal-to-proximal pull-back. The balloon is deflated, and the GuardWire is withdrawn. Angiography is performed to confirm distal flow.

Distal Filter Devices

All nonocclusive devices consist of a guidewire and filter. The Angioguard filter wire (Cordis, Inc.), the prototype of the filter devices, consists of a 0.014-inch wire that has a filter basket near its distal end (see Fig. 27-7). Beyond the filter protrudes a short portion of guidewire that can be shaped. The currently used version has pores that are 100 μm in diameter. The smallest nominal filter basket size is 4 mm, which can be used for vessels that are more than 3.0 mm but less than 3.5 mm, and the largest basket size is 8 mm. In principle, the filter should be oversized by about 0.5 to 1.0 mm compared with the vessel reference diameter. Before introducing the wire into the guiding catheter, it is pulled into a sheath under water to collapse the filter basket and get rid of the air bubbles. After the wire crosses the lesion and the filter basket is in a relatively disease-free portion of the artery, the sheath is retracted, and the basket is released to deploy in the artery. The sheath is removed over the wire, which then serves as a standard angioplasty wire. During the intervention, blood flow through the pores of the filter is preserved, and injecting contrast for visualization is

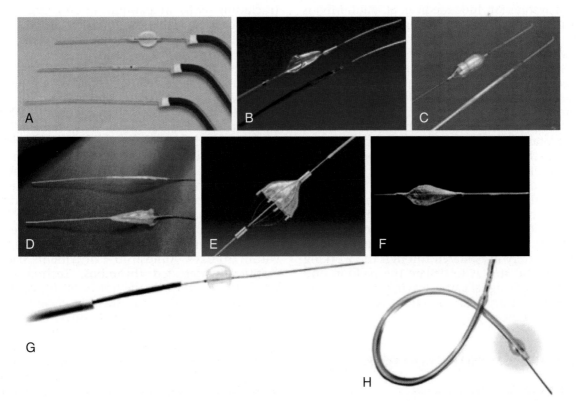

Figure 27-7. Embolism protection devices. **A,** The Medtronic PercuSurge GuardWire. **B,** The Boston Scientific FilterWire. **C,** The Abbott MedNova Emboshield. **D,** The eV3 Spider. **E,** The Cordis Angioguard. **F,** The Abbott Accunet. **G,** The Kensey-Nash Triactiv ShieldWire and FlushCatheter. **H,** The St. Jude Proxis catheter. (Modified from Mauri L, Rogers C, Baim DS: Devices for distal protection during percutaneous coronary revascularization. Circulation 2006;113:2651-2656.)

Table 27-2. Characteristics of Different Concepts in Embolism Protection Devices

Characteristic	Distal Filter	Distal Balloon Occlusion	Proximal Occlusion
Antegrade perfusion	Uninterrupted	Temporarily interrupted*	Temporarily interrupted*
Visualization of the distal vessel	Unhindered	Not possible during inflation	Possible by means of the inner sheath
Efficacy of emboli protection	May allow passage of emboli smaller than pore size (100 μm)†	Once inflated, traps all emboli	All particles can be aspirated
Vasoactive substances	Pass unimpeded	Can be aspirated completely	Can be aspirated completely
Crossing profile	0.040-0.050 inch	0.026-0.033 inch	No crossing, deployed proximal to the lesion
Embolization during device positioning	Likely to occur	Less likely to occur	None, because device does not cross the lesion
Retrieval profile	Occasionally difficult if filter full of debris	Not a problem after balloon deflation	Not a problem, device is proximal to the lesion
Flexibility of guidewire use	None, because filter is attached to wire	None, because balloon is attached to wire	Excellent, device can be used with any wire
Effect of distal disease on device	May not be feasible if no disease-free segment	May not be feasible if no disease-free segment	Device is proximal, distal disease irrelevant

*Transient ischemia while the embolism protection system is being used, unless there are adequate retrograde collaterals.
†The filter can trap particles smaller than its pore size because of clumping of the particles. Numerous trials have demonstrated no clinically significant differences between distal balloon occlusion and distal filter concepts.

not affected by the deployed filter. When the interventional procedure is complete, a retrieval sheath is advanced over the wire and used to collapse the filter basket securely. The retrieval sheath and the collapsed filter trapping the embolic debris inside it are then removed as one unit.

Proximal Occlusion Devices

The Proxis system (St. Jude Medical, St. Paul, MN) is the only device of this group that is approved by the FDA. The system contains an inner working sheath that is about 7 Fr in diameter and that is advanced through the guiding catheter. An inflatable balloon is attached to the end and the external surface of the inner sheath. Inflation of this balloon in the target artery proximal to the lesion provides a seal that prevents antegrade flow through the target artery. A second inflatable balloon is more proximal and is used to seal the inner sheath to the inside of the guiding catheter. After the system is in place, the intervention can be performed through the inner working sheath using the wire, balloon, and stent of choice. Small contrast injections for visualization are feasible. At the end of the procedure, the interventional devices are removed, and the stagnant blood in the target artery is aspirated through the working sheath. The final step is to deflate the balloon and remove the working sheath, leaving the guiding catheter in the artery after aspiration of debris and vasoactive substances.

USES OF EMBOLISM PROTECTION DEVICES

Saphenous Vein Graft Percutaneous Coronary Intervention

Traditionally, vein graft PCI is considered a high-risk procedure due to the increased risk of distal macro-

embolization and microembolization, with subsequent slow flow or no reflow and PMI. One of the most potent interventions to reduce risk of PMI in native coronary PCI, GP IIb/IIIa inhibitors, appears to be ineffective in the setting of vein graft PCI. A pooled analysis of several of GP IIb/IIIa inhibitor trials demonstrated that, compared with placebo, the use of a GP IIb/IIIa inhibitor was not associated with any significant reduction in ischemic complications (including PMI) in patients undergoing vein graft PCI.[79] A retrospective examination of the Cleveland Clinic Registry confirms these findings in a larger cohort vein graft PCI patients.[80]

Several small studies testing the efficacy of EPDs (particularly the PercuSurge GuardWire system) demonstrated that particulate matter could be aspirated in most cases. The observed incidence of PMI in these cases was significantly lower than what was expected historically with vein graft PCI.[81] Based on these findings, 801 patients from 47 centers were randomized to undergo vein graft PCI with the GuardWire protection or to no EPD in the SVG Angioplasty Free of Emboli Randomized (SAFER) trial.[34] The primary end point was death, Q-wave MI, non-Q-wave MI (CK-MB level more than three times ULN), emergent bypass surgery, or target vessel revascularization within 30 days. Almost 40% of patients had angiographically detected thrombus. Technical success was achieved with the device in 90.1% of the cases. The primary end point was significantly reduced with use of the PercuSurge GuardWire (from 16.5% to 9.6%, $P = .004$), a benefit primarily driven by the approximately 50% reduction in non-Q-wave MI (from 13.7% to 7.4%) (Fig. 27-8). Several important secondary end points were also favorably influenced; most importantly, no-reflow was reduced dramatically (9.0% versus 3.0%, $P = .02$).[34] Moreover, a cost-effectiveness analysis of the SAFER trial demonstrated that the reduction in ischemic complications led to shorter hospital stays and reduced early costs, com-

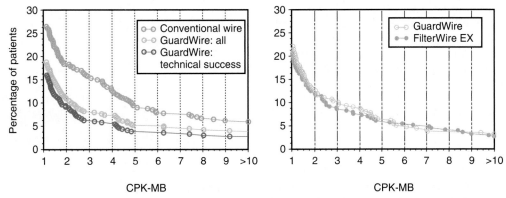

Figure 27-8. Impact of embolic protection device use on periprocedural myocardial infarction (PMI) in vein graft PCI. *Left,* The Saphenous Vein Graft Angioplasty Free of Emboli Randomized (SAFER) trial: cumulative distribution function curve of peak cardiac enzyme values after assignment to placebo (395 patients), GuardWire (406 patients), and the per-protocol subgroup with technically successful GuardWire use (366 patients). The creatine phosphokinase–myocardial band isoenzyme (CPK-MB) level is represented as multiples of the upper limit of normal. There is a significantly lower incidence of PMI of any size with GuardWire use. *Right,* The FilterWire EX Randomized Evaluation (FIRE) trial: a similar plot for patients randomized to distal protection with the FilterWire EX or to the GuardWire, showing noninferiority of the FilterWire. (Data from Baim DS, Wahr D, George B, et al: Randomized trial of a distal embolic protection device during percutaneous intervention of saphenous vein aorto-coronary bypass grafts. Circulation 2002;105:1285-1290; Stone GW, Rogers C, Hermiller J, et al: Randomized comparison of distal protection with a filter-based catheter and a balloon occlusion and aspiration system during percutaneous intervention of diseased saphenous vein aorto-coronary bypass grafts. Circulation 2003;108:548-553.)

pensating for most of the added expense of the EPD. The projected improved survival on the basis of reduced early complications (i.e., reduced PMI) was calculated to cost less than $4000 per year of life saved, which makes the use of EPD in vein graft PCI a very cost-effective strategy.[82]

The significant improvement in outcome with the use of the GuardWire occlusion device ushered a new era in which EPD use has become the standard of care with vein graft PCI. Because of ethical considerations, it was not feasible for developers of other EPD designs to test their devices against the conventional angioplasty wire, as was the case in the SAFER trial. The randomized, controlled trials leading to FDA approval of other EPDs for use in vein graft PCI were designed as noninferiority trials, with the GuardWire used in the active control arm. In a controlled trial, 651 patients undergoing vein graft PCI were randomized to receive the FilterWire EX or the GuardWire. Use of GP IIb/IIIa inhibitors was left to the discretion of the operators. The primary end point was a composite similar to that used in the SAFER trial. At 30 days, the incidence of any MI was 9% with the FilterWire versus 10% in the GuardWire arm (P = .49). There was a statistically insignificant reduction in the 1-year end point in the FilterWire arm (9.9% versus 11.6%, P = .53 for superiority; P = .0008 for noninferiority) (see Fig. 27-8).[35] An examination of these results demonstrated a favorable interaction between the use of GP IIb/IIIa inhibitors and FilterWire use, but not with GuardWire use. This may be related to the improved flow seen with GP IIb/IIIa inhibitor administration in patients receiving FilterWire protection, probably due to reducing the degree of platelet aggregation and deposition on the surface of the filter.[83]

Similarly designed trials were conducted to test the efficacy of the Triactiv device (Kensey Nash), the Proxis system (St. Jude Medical), MedNova Emboshield (Abbott), and the Spider device (eV3, Inc.). In those trials, the 30-day primary end point was reached in 8% to 11% of patients, achieving the preset standard for noninferiority compared with the GuardWire or FilterWire in all studies.[84]

Percutaneous Coronary Intervention for Acute Myocardial Infarction

The concept of EPD use in primary PCI is attractive and intuitive. These are the prototypical thrombotic lesions with a very high likelihood for distal embolization. The success of EPDs in vein graft PCI led to clinical trials examining the feasibility of the concept. In a small study of 72 patients with acute MI, the PercuSurge GuardWire was used during primary stenting of the infarct-related artery in 42 patients, with 30 patients undergoing primary stenting after thrombectomy with no EPD. The GuardWire group of patients had a significantly better corrected TIMI frame counts and TIMI myocardial perfusion grades. At 3 weeks, the GuardWire group also demonstrated a significantly better ejection fraction, improvement in ejection fraction, and improvement in wall motion abnormality.[85]

However, the larger randomized trials did not confirm the initial favorable impression regarding EPD use in primary PCI. The Enhanced Myocardial Efficacy and Removal by Aspiration of Liberated Debris (EMERALD) trial was an international multicenter, prospective, randomized trial enrolling 501 patients with ST-segment elevation MI undergoing primary or rescue PCI. Patients were randomized to

PCI with the PercuSurge GuardWire distal protection or to PCI without EPD. Two co-primary end points were prespecified: ST-segment resolution after PCI assessed by continuous Holter monitoring and infarct size measured by nuclear imaging between days 5 and 14. Secondary end points included major adverse cardiac events. Among 252 patients assigned to the GuardWire protection, debris was retrieved in 73% of cases. Disappointingly, there was no difference between the two groups in any of the primary or secondary end points (ST resolution: 63% versus 62%; infarct size: 12% versus 9.5%; *P* = NS for both). At 6 months, the frequency of major adverse cardiac events in the distal protection and control groups was similar (10.0% versus 11.0%, *P* = .66).[86]

Another trial tested the efficacy of the FilterWire distal protection in the setting of PCI for acute MI (i.e., Protection Devices in PCI treatment of Myocardial Infarction for Salvage of Endangered Myocardium [PROMISE]). However, the methodology of PROMISE was distinct from that of the EMERALD trial. Only 200 patients were randomized: 68% with ST-segment elevation MI, with the remainder diagnosed with non-ST-segment elevation MI. The primary end points were the coronary flow velocity measured by an intravascular Doppler wire and the size of the infarction measured by hyperenhancement on MRI scans 3 days after the procedure. Similar to the EMERALD trial, there was no difference between the patients randomized to the PCI with FilterWire protection and those who did not receive any EPD.[87]

There are several potential explanations for the disappointing results of the EMERALD and PROMISE trials. Using EPD may delay restoration of epicardial flow, and the devices may cause further embolization while crossing the lesion, negating any favorable effects of subsequent protection. The incomplete aspiration of liberated debris or leaking of vasoactive substances released from the ruptured plaques may lead to further downstream damage at the time of EPD removal. Embolization into side branches may play a role, particularly in cases with acute thrombotic occlusion, leading to initial TIMI flow grade 0 and absence of visualization of the distal artery at the time of EPD positioning. These results also indicate a relative underestimation of the degree of existing damage and the role of reperfusion injury in determining the final infarct size after primary PCI.[88]

Carotid Stenting

Although the clinical implications of embolization were first elucidated for coronary interventions, the paradigm is applicable in angioplasty procedures in other arterial beds. Interventional procedures in the carotid and renal arteries are two areas where embolization may be particularly significant. Embolization appears to occur much more frequently after carotid stenting than carotid endarterectomy (CEA). Using transcranial Doppler (TCD) monitoring, microscopic embolization occurs at least eight times more fre-

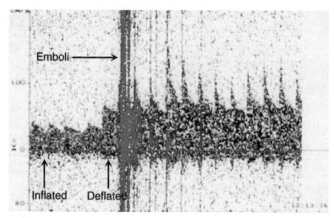

Figure 27-9. Transcranial Doppler monitoring of middle cerebral artery flow during elective carotid artery stenting. The high-intensity transients observed at the time of balloon deflation represent a surge of microemboli from the extracranial site of angioplasty to the intracranial circulation. (From Topol EJ, Yadav JS: Recognition of the importance of embolization in atherosclerotic vascular disease. Circulation 2000;101:570-580.)

quently with carotid angioplasty and stenting than with CEA.[89] Most patients undergoing carotid stenting have TCD evidence of microembolization (Fig. 27-9). Similar to embolization related to coronary interventions, it appears that evidence of systemic inflammatory response can lead to more embolization. In a small study of 43 patients undergoing carotid stenting with TCD monitoring of the ipsilateral middle cerebral artery, there was a positive correlation between TCD-identified microembolism and the preprocedural leukocyte count, a marker of systemic inflammation. This correlation remained significant even after adjusting for age, gender, comorbidities, medical therapy, and use of EPDs.[90]

Potentially, even small embolic particles are poorly tolerated by the cerebral microcirculation.[91] In an ex vivo model of carotid angioplasty, particles generated from human carotid plaques were injected into the cerebral circulation of rats. Stenting produced almost twice as much embolization as balloon angioplasty in this model; passage of the guidewire also produced embolization, although only about one fourth as many emboli as balloon angioplasty. Particles less than 200 μm in diameter did not cause cerebral ischemia during the first 3 days after the procedure, whereas particles 200 to 500 μm in diameter did cause neuronal death. However, at 7 days, injury was detected by fragments of both sizes. If smaller sizes of emboli are relevant in humans, an occlusion device may be better than a filter device. Although filters can be designed with smaller pore sizes, the disadvantage is that this can increase the risk of thrombosis by the filter itself and decrease distal flow.

Several EPDs were designed for use in conjunction with carotid angioplasty and stenting in the hope of reducing the incidence of procedure-related strokes. By designing a safe and effective EPD, the high-risk percutaneous procedure can be converted into a low-risk procedure comparable to, or even safer than, the current standard of care, carotid endarterectomy. Reimers and colleagues[92] reported their initial experience with three filter designs (i.e., Angioguard, Neurosheild, and FilterWire) in 84 patients undergoing carotid stenting. Macroscopic debris was collected in 53% of filters, and histologic analysis of the debris revealed lipid-rich macrophages, fibrin, and cholesterol clefts. The early experience with the balloon occlusion–variety of EPDs (e.g., PercuSurge Guard-Wire) was reported for a series of 75 patients. In this series, macroscopic debris was collected from all cases (100%), and histologic analysis was very similar to particles obtained from filter devices.[93]

In addition to retrieval of macroscopic and microscopic debris, there is evidence that the use of EPDs during carotid stenting effectively reduces embolism to the cerebral microcirculation. These data have been gleaned from studies using magnetic resonance diffusion-weighted imaging (DWI), which is the most sensitive imaging modality for detection of early cerebral ischemia.[94,95] Comparison of DWI scans before and after carotid stenting reveals that use of EPDs significantly reduces the incidence and number of new lesions identified on the postprocedural scan. Most new lesions were small (<10 mm) and asymptomatic (Fig. 27-10). In a study of 206 patients, there was no difference in incidence of stroke between patients who did or did not receive EPD protection, but the number of DWI-detected new lesions was significantly higher among patients who did develop a stroke.[95]

There has been no completed randomized trial comparing outcomes of carotid stenting with or without EPD protection. Based on large, multicenter registries, there is convincing evidence that EPD use has resulted in a significant reduction in neurologic adverse events. In a systematic review of published reports, Kastrup and coworkers[95] compared outcomes of 2357 patients undergoing carotid stenting without EPD protection to 839 patients in whom stenting was performed with an EPD in place. There was a significant reduction in 30-day death and stroke rate with EPD use (1.8% versus 5.5%, P < .001). Minor and major strokes were significantly reduced in patients receiving EPD protection (minor stroke: 0.5% versus 3.7%, P < .001; major stroke: 0.3% versus 1.1%, P < .05). The larger carotid stent global registry surveys the major interventional centers worldwide and collects self-reported data on technical details and outcomes. In the latest update, 6753 patients had undergone stenting without EPD protection, whereas 4221 patients had received EPD protection. The 30-day incidence of stroke and procedure-related death was reduced by more than 50% (from 5.3% to 2.2%). Despite EPD protection, symptomatic patients remained at higher risk for developing stroke or procedure-related death compared with the asymptomatic subgroup (2.7% versus 1.75%).[96]

Few randomized trials have compared contemporary carotid artery stenting with CEA. The Stenting and Angioplasty with Protection in Patients at High Risk for Endarterectomy (SAPPHIRE) trial randomized patients to endarterectomy or to carotid stenting with the Angioguard filter device. Symptomatic and asymptomatic patients were included if they had a coexisting condition that placed them at a higher risk for complications during a carotid endarterectomy. The primary composite end point was death, stroke, or MI at 30 days plus death due to neurologic causes or ipsilateral stroke between day 31 and 1 year. The trial was terminated after randomizing 334 patients because of slowing recruitment. In this high-risk population, the primary composite end point (i.e., death, stroke, or MI at 30 days plus ipsilateral

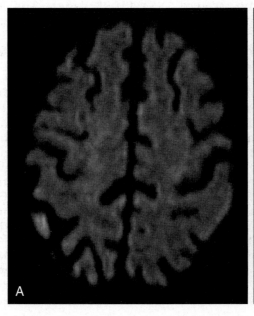
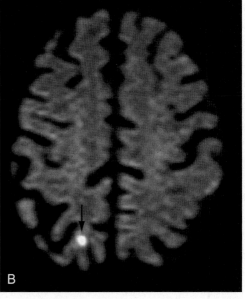

Figure 27-10. Preprocedural (a) and postprocedural (b) axial diffusion-weighted imaging of the brain. Despite carotid stenting with an embolic protection device, an ipsilateral hyperintense lesion *(arrow)* related to silent cerebral embolism is appreciable at the cortical-subcortical junction of the right parietal lobe. (From Cosottini M, Michelassi MC, Puglioli M, et al: Silent cerebral ischemia detected with diffusion-weighted imaging in patients treated with protected and unprotected carotid artery stenting. Stroke 2005;36:2389-2393.)

stroke or neurologic death between 31 days and 1 year) was reduced in the stent group compared with the surgical group (12.2% versus 20.1%, $P = .004$ for noninferiority, $P = .053$ for superiority). At 30 days, the incidence of stroke was 3.6% and 3.1% in the stent and CEA arms, respectively. This reduction in the primary end point was driven primarily by a reduction in MI in the stent arm, rather than by differences in cerebral events.[97]

The Stent-Supported Percutaneous Angioplasty of the Carotid Artery versus Endarterectomy (SPACE) was a larger, randomized, noninferiority trial that enrolled patients requiring carotid revascularization to stenting or CEA.[98] Unlike SAPPHIRE, all patients were symptomatic and the risk status of the patient was not a factor in determining eligibility. The primary end point was death or ipsilateral stroke at 30 days. Of the 599 patients who underwent carotid stenting, EPD was used in only 151 (25%). In the intention-to-treat analysis of the randomized 1183 patients, the primary end point was reached in 6.84% and 6.34% of patients in the stenting and CEA arms, respectively (absolute difference of 0.51%; 95% CI: −1.9% to 2.9%, $P = .09$ for noninferiority). The investigators concluded that carotid stenting cannot be considered noninferior and that in this population of symptomatic (but not necessarily high-risk) patients, endarterectomy remains the gold standard.

The Endarterectomy versus Angioplasty in Patients with Symptomatic Severe Carotid Stenosis (EVA-3S) trial was a multicenter, French study that randomized patients with symptomatic severe carotid stenosis to receive endarterectomy or stenting (with or without EPD protection). The primary end point was the incidence of death or any stroke within 30 days of revascularization. After enrolling 80 patients in the stenting arm, the safety committee discontinued carotid stenting without EPD protection because of an excess of adverse events. At that point, there were 4 strokes in the 15 patients treated without EPDs, compared with 5 in the 58 patients who received EPDs.[99] The EVA-3S was eventually prematurely stopped after enrolling 527 patients after it failed to demonstrate noninferiority of carotid stenting compared with endarterectomy. The 30-day incidence of any stroke or death was significantly higher in the stenting group (9.6% versus 3.9%, $P = .01$).[100]

There were significant differences among the conclusions reached by the SAPPHIRE, SPACE, and EVA-3S trials regarding the role of EPDs and carotid stenting in general. The differences are in part due to the difference in the patient populations enrolled in each study. In SAPPHIRE, although patients were at high risk for complications, most of the enrolled patients were asymptomatic from a neurologic perspective. SPACE and EVA-3S enrolled patients with symptomatic carotid disease (i.e., patients at higher risk for neurologic events without specific inclusion or exclusion based on anticipated risk of complications during surgery). Most adverse events in the stent arm of SPACE and a significant portion of the

strokes in EVA-S3 trial carotid stent group occurred in patients in whom there was no EPD protection. In SAPPHIRE, all patients received Angioguard filter protection. The definition of MI in the SAPPHIRE trial was based on periprocedural biomarker elevation, whereas the EVA-3S trial used the World Health Organization (WHO) definition requiring two of three criteria (i.e., pain, biomarker elevation, and electrocardiographic changes); the reported incidence of MI was significantly higher in SAPPHIRE than that reported in the EVA-3S trial. The SPACE investigators did not systematically record biomarker or electrocardiographic changes and were unable to report the incidence of MI in that study. MI was included in the primary composite end point in SAPPHIRE, and the incidence of MI was much higher in the endarterectomy arm, which contributed to the favorable impression of carotid stenting. There was significant heterogeneity in the level of expertise of the operators, the types of stents, and the types of protection devices in the EVA-3S, whereas SPACE and SAPPHIRE were performed in selected centers with experienced operators. In SAPPHIRE, only one stent and one EPD design were used. Unfortunately, all three trials were stopped prematurely (i.e., before reaching the number of patients that was proposed to achieve adequate statistical power), and no definitive conclusions regarding the role of carotid stenting with EPD protection can be reached at this time. Two major randomized trials are ongoing in this field: The Carotid Revascularization Endarterectomy versus Stent Trial (CREST) and International Carotid Stenting Study (ICSS or CAVATAS-2). Both studies are large, have broad inclusion criteria, and avoid many of the issues raised by the available data sets.

To gain FDA approval, several manufacturers of EPD and stent designs initiated a group of large patient registries to demonstrate safety and efficacy of their novel devices. Most of the registries enrolled patients at high risk for complications, similar to the SAPPHIRE design. The low incidence of death or stroke compared with historic adverse event rates for carotid endarterectomy resulted in the eventual FDA approval of many of these devices.[101,102]

Renal and Peripheral Interventions

Although there are fewer data demonstrating the importance of atheroembolism in the renal vasculature, emboli are also detrimental in this arterial bed. A study by Krishnamurthi and colleagues[103] examined the impact of embolization after surgical revascularization for renal artery stenosis. In this series, evidence of atheroembolism was detected in 16 of 44 patients. For those patients, 5-year survival was significantly worse than for patients with no evidence of distal embolism (54% versus 85%, $P = .001$), suggesting that this phenomenon is clinically relevant to the outcome of renal revascularization.[103] Although difficult to prove, there is little doubt that embolization also occurs in the setting of percutaneous renal revascularization and is likely associated with worse patient outcomes. It is estimated that 25% of patients have worse renal function after renal intervention. Although the reason for this decrease in renal function is probably multifactorial, embolization is likely part of the problem.

The PercuSurge GuardWire and the FilterWire systems have been used successfully during renal intervention. In one series, 65 renal arteries in 56 hypertensive patients were successfully stented with EPD protection (i.e., GuardWire, FilterWire, and Angioguard devices). Visible debris was aspirated with the 100% of cases with GuardWire protection and 80% of those in whom filter devices were used. The mean particle number was 98.1 ± 60.0 per procedure (range, 13 to 208). At 3 years, only two patients developed worsening renal function.[104]

Despite the growing number of renal artery procedures in the past few years, there is no conclusive evidence that the indiscriminate use of this procedure is better than medical therapy in all patients. Patients are being enrolled in the Cardiovascular Outcomes in Renal Artery Lesions (CORAL) trial, which aims to randomize 1080 patients with significant renal artery stenosis to stenting with the Angioguard device protection or medical therapy. The end points will include left ventricular hypertrophy and function measures, renal function measures, and mortality.

Early experiences with EPDs in lower extremity percutaneous revascularization procedures have been reported.[105,106] In most cases, filter devices were deployed and retrieved successfully. There was macroscopic and microscopic debris in all cases, suggesting a potential benefit of these devices in lower extremity procedures, particularly in cases of acute or subacute ischemia with large thrombus burden and high risk of distal showering.

CONCLUSIONS

Embolism protection devices have gained widespread acceptance in the interventional cardiology and vascular surgery community over the past decade. There is solid evidence that they are safe to use and effective in reducing distal embolism during interventional procedures. Clinical outcomes have been excellent in vein graft PCI, and EPD protection has become the standard of care. For various reasons, results of EPD use in the setting of primary and rescue PCI have been disappointing, and there does not seem to be a future for those devices in acute MI intervention. Controversy remains regarding the role of carotid stenting and the use of EPDs during such procedures, although there is reasonable evidence that carotid stenting with EPD protection represents an advance in this field. With more innovation in EPD design and as the ongoing clinical trials are completed, there is the potential for future application of EPDs in other settings of coronary and peripheral interventions.

REFERENCES

1. Togni M, Balmer F, Pfiffner D, et al: Percutaneous coronary interventions in Europe 1992-2001. Eur Heart J 2004;25:1208-1213.
2. Smith SC Jr, Feldman TE, Hirshfeld JW Jr, et al: ACC/AHA/SCAI 2005 guideline update for percutaneous coronary intervention: A report of the American College of Cardiology/American Heart Association Task Force on Practice Guidelines (ACC/AHA/SCAI Writing Committee to Update 2001 Guidelines for Percutaneous Coronary Intervention). Circulation 2006;113:e166-e286.
3. Alpert JS, Thygesen K, Antman E, et al: Myocardial infarction redefined—A consensus document of The Joint European Society of Cardiology/American College of Cardiology Committee for the redefinition of myocardial infarction. J Am Coll Cardiol 2000;36:959-969.
4. Abdelmeguid AE, Ellis SG, Sapp SK, et al: Defining the appropriate threshold of creatine kinase elevation after percutaneous coronary interventions. Am Heart J 1996;131:1097-1105.
5. Califf RM, Abdelmeguid AE, Kuntz RE, et al: Myonecrosis after revascularization procedures. J Am Coll Cardiol 1998;31:241-251.
6. Cutlip DE, Kuntz RE: Does creatine kinase-MB elevation after percutaneous coronary intervention predict outcomes in 2005? Cardiac enzyme elevation after successful percutaneous coronary intervention is not an independent predictor of adverse outcomes. Circulation 2005;112:916-922; discussion 922.
7. Ricciardi MJ, Wu E, Davidson CJ, et al: Visualization of discrete microinfarction after percutaneous coronary intervention associated with mild creatine kinase-MB elevation. Circulation 2001;103:2780-2783.
8. Selvanayagam JB, Porto I, Channon K, et al: Troponin elevation after percutaneous coronary intervention directly represents the extent of irreversible myocardial injury: Insights from cardiovascular magnetic resonance imaging. Circulation 2005;111:1027-1032.
9. Herrmann J Peri-procedural myocardial injury: 2005 update. Eur Heart J 2005;26:2493-2519.
10. Abdelmeguid AE, Topol EJ, Whitlow PL, et al: Significance of mild transient release of creatine kinase-MB fraction after percutaneous coronary interventions. Circulation 1996;94:1528-1536.
11. Roe MT, Mahaffey KW, Kilaru R, et al: Creatine kinase-MB elevation after percutaneous coronary intervention predicts adverse outcomes in patients with acute coronary syndromes. Eur Heart J 2004;25:313-321.
12. Nallamothu BK, Chetcuti S, Mukherjee D, et al: Prognostic implication of troponin I elevation after percutaneous coronary intervention. Am J Cardiol 2003;91:1272-1274.
13. Cavallini C, Savonitto S, Violini R, et al: Impact of the elevation of biochemical markers of myocardial damage on long-term mortality after percutaneous coronary intervention: Results of the CK-MB and PCI study. Eur Heart J 2005;26:1494-1498.
14. Ghazzal Z, Ashfaq S, Morris DC, et al: Prognostic implication of creatine kinase release after elective percutaneous coronary intervention in the pre-IIb/IIIa antagonist era. Am Heart J 2003;145:1006-1012.
15. Harrington RA, Lincoff AM, Califf RM, et al: Characteristics and consequences of myocardial infarction after percutaneous coronary intervention: Insights from the Coronary Angioplasty Versus Excisional Atherectomy Trial (CAVEAT). J Am Coll Cardiol 1995;25:1693-1699.
16. Simoons ML, van den Brand M, Lincoff M, et al: Minimal myocardial damage during coronary intervention is associated with impaired outcome. Eur Heart J 1999;20:1112-1119.
17. Stone GW, Mehran R, Dangas G, et al: Differential impact on survival of electrocardiographic Q-wave versus enzymatic myocardial infarction after percutaneous intervention: A device-specific analysis of 7147 patients. Circulation 2001;104:642-647.

18. Ellis SG, Chew D, Chan A, et al: Death following creatine kinase-MB elevation after coronary intervention: Identification of an early risk period: Importance of creatine kinase-MB level, completeness of revascularization, ventricular function, and probable benefit of statin therapy. Circulation 2002;106:1205-1210.

19. Natarajan MK, Kreatsoulas C, Velianou JL, et al: Incidence, predictors, and clinical significance of troponin-I elevation without creatine kinase elevation following percutaneous coronary interventions. Am J Cardiol 2004;93:750-753.

20. Srinivas VS, Brooks MM, Detre KM, et al: Contemporary percutaneous coronary intervention versus balloon angioplasty for multivessel coronary artery disease: A comparison of the National Heart, Lung and Blood Institute Dynamic Registry and the Bypass Angioplasty Revascularization Investigation (BARI) study. Circulation 2002;106:1627-1633.

21. Randomised placebo-controlled and balloon-angioplasty-controlled trial to assess safety of coronary stenting with use of platelet glycoprotein-IIb/IIIa blockade. The EPISTENT Investigators. Evaluation of Platelet IIb/IIIa Inhibitor for Stenting. Lancet 1998;352:87-92.

22. Porto I, Selvanayagam JB, Van Gaal WJ, et al: Plaque volume and occurrence and location of periprocedural myocardial necrosis after percutaneous coronary intervention: Insights from delayed-enhancement magnetic resonance imaging, thrombolysis in myocardial infarction myocardial perfusion grade analysis, and intravascular ultrasound. Circulation 2006;114:662-669.

23. Topol EJ, Yadav JS: Recognition of the importance of embolization in atherosclerotic vascular disease. Circulation 2000;101:570-580.

24. Prati F, Pawlowski T, Gil R, et al: Stenting of culprit lesions in unstable angina leads to a marked reduction in plaque burden: A major role of plaque embolization? A serial intravascular ultrasound study. Circulation 2003;107:2320-2325.

25. Rogers C, Huynh R, Seifert PA, et al: Embolic protection with filtering or occlusion balloons during saphenous vein graft stenting retrieves identical volumes and sizes of particulate debris. Circulation 2004;109:1735-1740.

26. Angelini A, Rubartelli P, Mistrorigo F, et al: Distal protection with a filter device during coronary stenting in patients with stable and unstable angina. Circulation 2004;110:515-521.

27. Chen WH, Lee PY, Ng W, et al: Aspirin resistance is associated with a high incidence of myonecrosis after non-urgent percutaneous coronary intervention despite clopidogrel pretreatment. J Am Coll Cardiol 2004;43:1122-1126.

28. Bonz AW, Lengenfelder B, Jacobs M, et al: Cytokine response after percutaneous coronary intervention in stable angina: Effect of selective glycoprotein IIb/IIIa receptor antagonism. Am Heart J 2003;145:693-699.

29. Iuliano L, Pratico D, Greco C, et al: Angioplasty increases coronary sinus F2-isoprostane formation: Evidence for in vivo oxidative stress during PTCA. J Am Coll Cardiol 2001;37:76-80.

30. Kini A, Marmur JD, Kini S, et al: Creatine kinase-MB elevation after coronary intervention correlates with diffuse atherosclerosis, and low-to-medium level elevation has a benign clinical course: Implications for early discharge after coronary intervention. J Am Coll Cardiol 1999;34:663-671.

31. Zairis MN, Ambrose JA, Ampartzidou O, et al: Preprocedural plasma C-reactive protein levels, postprocedural creatine kinase-MB release, and long-term prognosis after successful coronary stenting (four-year results from the GENERATION study). Am J Cardiol 2005;95:386-390.

32. Saadeddin SM, Habbab MA, Sobki SH, et al: Association of systemic inflammatory state with troponin I elevation after elective uncomplicated percutaneous coronary intervention. Am J Cardiol 2002;89:981-983.

33. Chew DP, Bhatt DL, Robbins MA, et al: Incremental prognostic value of elevated baseline C-reactive protein among established markers of risk in percutaneous coronary intervention. Circulation 2001;104:992-997.

34. Baim DS, Wahr D, George B, et al: Randomized trial of a distal embolic protection device during percutaneous intervention of saphenous vein aorto-coronary bypass grafts. Circulation 2002;105:1285-1290.

35. Stone GW, Rogers C, Hermiller J, et al: Randomized comparison of distal protection with a filter-based catheter and a balloon occlusion and aspiration system during percutaneous intervention of diseased saphenous vein aorto-coronary bypass grafts. Circulation 2003;108:548-553.

36. Abdelmeguid AE, Whitlow PL, Sapp SK, et al: Long-term outcome of transient, uncomplicated in-laboratory coronary artery closure. Circulation 1995;91:2733-2741.

37. Yang EH, Gumina RJ, Lennon RJ, et al: Emergency coronary artery bypass surgery for percutaneous coronary interventions: Changes in the incidence, clinical characteristics, and indications from 1979 to 2003. J Am Coll Cardiol 2005;46:2004-2009.

38. Almeda FQ, Nathan S, Calvin JE, et al: Frequency of abrupt vessel closure and side branch occlusion after percutaneous coronary intervention in a 6.5-year period (1994 to 2000) at a single medical center. Am J Cardiol 2002;89:1151-1155.

39. Stone GW, Ellis SG, Cannon L, et al: Comparison of a polymer-based paclitaxel-eluting stent with a bare metal stent in patients with complex coronary artery disease: A randomized controlled trial. JAMA 2005;294:1215-1223.

40. Topol EJ, Leya F, Pinkerton CA, et al: A comparison of directional atherectomy with coronary angioplasty in patients with coronary artery disease. The CAVEAT Study Group. N Engl J Med 1993;329:221-227.

41. Baim DS, Cutlip DE, Sharma SK, et al: Final results of the Balloon vs Optimal Atherectomy Trial (BOAT). Circulation 1998;97:322-331.

42. Lefkovits J, Holmes DR, Califf RM, et al: Predictors and sequelae of distal embolization during saphenous vein graft intervention from the CAVEAT-II trial. Coronary Angioplasty Versus Excisional Atherectomy Trial. Circulation 1995;92:734-740.

43. Dehmer GJ, Nichols TC, Bode AP, et al: Assessment of platelet activation by coronary sinus blood sampling during balloon angioplasty and directional coronary atherectomy. Am J Cardiol 1997;80:871-877.

44. Kini A, Reich D, Marmur JD, et al: Reduction in periprocedural enzyme elevation by abciximab after rotational atherectomy of type B2 lesions: Results of the Rota ReoPro randomized trial. Am Heart J 2001;142:965-969.

45. Bhatt DL, Topol EJ: Does creatine kinase-MB elevation after percutaneous coronary intervention predict outcomes in 2005? Periprocedural cardiac enzyme elevation predicts adverse outcomes. Circulation 2005;112:906-915; discussion 923.

46. Inoue T, Sohma R, Miyazaki T, et al: Comparison of activation process of platelets and neutrophils after coronary stent implantation versus balloon angioplasty for stable angina pectoris. Am J Cardiol 2000;86:1057-1062.

47. Iakovou I, Mintz GS, Dangas G, et al: Increased CK-MB release is a "trade-off" for optimal stent implantation: An intravascular ultrasound study. J Am Coll Cardiol 2003;42:1900-1905.

48. Topol EJ, Ferguson JJ, Weisman HF, et al: Long-term protection from myocardial ischemic events in a randomized trial of brief integrin beta3 blockade with percutaneous coronary intervention. EPIC Investigator Group. Evaluation of Platelet IIb/IIIa Inhibition for Prevention of Ischemic Complication. JAMA 1997;278:479-484.

49. Tardiff BE, Califf RM, Tcheng JE, et al: Clinical outcomes after detection of elevated cardiac enzymes in patients undergoing percutaneous intervention. IMPACT-II Investigators. Integrilin (eptifibatide) to Minimize Platelet Aggregation and Coronary Thrombosis-II. J Am Coll Cardiol 1999;33:88-96.

50. Brener SJ, Lytle BW, Schneider JP, et al: Association between CK-MB elevation after percutaneous or surgical revascularization and three-year mortality. J Am Coll Cardiol 2002;40:1961-1967.

51. Ioannidis JP, Karvouni E, Katritsis DG: Mortality risk conferred by small elevations of creatine kinase-MB isoenzyme after percutaneous coronary intervention. J Am Coll Cardiol 2003;42:1406-1411.

52. Jeremias A, Baim DS, Ho KK, et al: Differential mortality risk of postprocedural creatine kinase-MB elevation following

successful versus unsuccessful stent procedures. J Am Coll Cardiol 2004;44:1210-1214.

53. Randomised placebo-controlled trial of abciximab before and during coronary intervention in refractory unstable angina: The CAPTURE Study. Lancet 1997;349:1429-1435.

54. Inhibition of platelet glycoprotein IIb/IIIa with eptifibatide in patients with acute coronary syndromes. The PURSUIT Trial Investigators. Platelet Glycoprotein IIb/IIIa in Unstable Angina: Receptor Suppression Using Integrilin Therapy. N Engl J Med 1998;339:436-443.

55. Novel dosing regimen of eptifibatide in planned coronary stent implantation (ESPRIT): A randomised, placebo-controlled trial. Lancet 2000;356:2037-2044.

56. Effects of platelet glycoprotein IIb/IIIa blockade with tirofiban on adverse cardiac events in patients with unstable angina or acute myocardial infarction undergoing coronary angioplasty. The RESTORE Investigators. Randomized Efficacy Study of Tirofiban for Outcomes and REstenosis. Circulation 1997;96:1445-1453.

57. Valgimigli M, Percoco G, Barbieri D, et al: The additive value of tirofiban administered with the high-dose bolus in the prevention of ischemic complications during high-risk coronary angioplasty: The ADVANCE Trial. J Am Coll Cardiol 2004;44:14-19.

58. Steinhubl SR, Lauer MS, Mukherjee DP, et al: The duration of pretreatment with ticlopidine prior to stenting is associated with the risk of procedure-related non-Q-wave myocardial infarctions. J Am Coll Cardiol 1998;32:1366-1370.

59. Steinhubl SR, Berger PB, Mann JT 3rd, et al: Early and sustained dual oral antiplatelet therapy following percutaneous coronary intervention: A randomized controlled trial. JAMA 2002;288:2411-2420.

60. Mehta SR, Yusuf S, Peters RJ, et al: Effects of pretreatment with clopidogrel and aspirin followed by long-term therapy in patients undergoing percutaneous coronary intervention: The PCI-CURE study. Lancet 2001;358:527-533.

61. Muller I, Besta F, Schulz C, et al: Prevalence of clopidogrel non-responders among patients with stable angina pectoris scheduled for elective coronary stent placement. Thromb Haemost 2003;89:783-787.

62. Patti G, Colonna G, Pasceri V, et al: Randomized trial of high loading dose of clopidogrel for reduction of periprocedural myocardial infarction in patients undergoing coronary intervention: Results from the ARMYDA-2 (Antiplatelet therapy for Reduction of MYocardial Damage during Angioplasty) study. Circulation 2005;111:2099-2106.

63. von Beckerath N, Taubert D, Pogatsa-Murray G, et al: Absorption, metabolization, and antiplatelet effects of 300-, 600-, and 900-mg loading doses of clopidogrel: Results of the ISAR-CHOICE (Intracoronary Stenting and Antithrombotic Regimen: Choose Between 3 High Oral Doses for Immediate Clopidogrel Effect) Trial. Circulation 2005;112:2946-2950.

64. Montalescot G, Sideris G, Meuleman C, et al: A randomized comparison of high clopidogrel loading doses in patients with non-ST-segment elevation acute coronary syndromes: The ALBION (Assessment of the Best Loading Dose of Clopidogrel to Blunt Platelet Activation, Inflammation and Ongoing Necrosis) trial. J Am Coll Cardiol 2006;48:931-938.

65. Kastrati A, Mehilli J, Schuhlen H, et al: A clinical trial of abciximab in elective percutaneous coronary intervention after pretreatment with clopidogrel. N Engl J Med 2004;350:232-238.

66. Lincoff AM, Kereiakes DJ, Mascelli MA, et al: Abciximab suppresses the rise in levels of circulating inflammatory markers after percutaneous coronary revascularization. Circulation 2001;104:163-167.

67. Chang SM, Yazbek N, Lakkis NM: Use of statins prior to percutaneous coronary intervention reduces myonecrosis and improves clinical outcome. Catheter Cardiovasc Interv 2004;62:193-197.

68. Jones SP, Gibson MF, Rimmer DM 3rd, et al: Direct vascular and cardioprotective effects of rosuvastatin, a new HMG-CoA reductase inhibitor. J Am Coll Cardiol 2002;40:1172-1178.

69. Gurm HS, Breitbart Y, Vivekanathan D, et al: Preprocedural statin use is associated with a reduced hazard of postproce-dural myonecrosis in patients undergoing rotational atherectomy—A propensity-adjusted analysis. Am Heart J 2006;151: e1031-e1036.

70. Briguori C, Colombo A, Airoldi F, et al: Statin administration before percutaneous coronary intervention: Impact on periprocedural myocardial infarction. Eur Heart J 2004;25:1822-1828.

71. Pasceri V, Patti G, Nusca A, et al: Randomized trial of atorvastatin for reduction of myocardial damage during coronary intervention: Results from the ARMYDA (Atorvastatin for Reduction of MYocardial Damage during Angioplasty) study. Circulation 2004;110:674-678.

72. Patti G, Chello M, Pasceri V, et al: Protection from procedural myocardial injury by atorvastatin is associated with lower levels of adhesion molecules after percutaneous coronary interventions: Results from the ARMYDA-CAMs (Atorvastatin for Reduction of MYocardial Damage during Angioplasty-Cell Adhesion Molecules) substudy. J Am Coll Cardiol 2006;48:1560-1566.

73. Ellis SG, Brener SJ, Lincoff AM, et al: beta-blockers before percutaneous coronary intervention do not attenuate postprocedural creatine kinase isoenzyme rise. Circulation 2001;104:2685-2688.

74. Lincoff AM, Bittl JA, Harrington RA, et al: Bivalirudin and provisional glycoprotein IIb/IIIa blockade compared with heparin and planned glycoprotein IIb/IIIa blockade during percutaneous coronary intervention: REPLACE-2 randomized trial. JAMA 2003;289:853-863.

75. Gibson CM, Morrow DA, Murphy SA, et al: A randomized trial to evaluate the relative protection against post-percutaneous coronary intervention microvascular dysfunction, ischemia, and inflammation among antiplatelet and antithrombotic agents: The PROTECT-TIMI-30 trial. J Am Coll Cardiol 2006;47:2364-2373.

76. Ballarino MA, Moreyra E Jr, Damonte A, et al: Multicenter randomized comparison of direct vs. conventional stenting: The DIRECTO trial. Catheter Cardiovasc Interv 2003;58:434-440.

77. Ijsselmuiden AJ, Serruys PW, Scholte A, et al: Direct coronary stent implantation does not reduce the incidence of in-stent restenosis or major adverse cardiac events: Six month results of a randomized trial. Eur Heart J 2003;24:421-429.

78. Turco MA, Buchbinder M, Popma JJ, et al: Pivotal, randomized U.S. study of the Symbiot covered stent system in patients with saphenous vein graft disease: Eight-month angiographic and clinical results from the Symbiot III trial. Catheter Cardiovasc Interv 2006;68:379-388.

79. Roffi M, Mukherjee D, Chew DP, et al: Lack of benefit from intravenous platelet glycoprotein IIb/IIIa receptor inhibition as adjunctive treatment for percutaneous interventions of aortocoronary bypass grafts: A pooled analysis of five randomized clinical trials. Circulation 2002;106:3063-3067.

80. Karha J, Gurm HS, Rajagopal V, et al: Use of platelet glycoprotein IIb/IIIa inhibitors in saphenous vein graft percutaneous coronary intervention and clinical outcomes. Am J Cardiol 2006;98:906-910.

81. Webb JG, Carere RG, Virmani R, et al: Retrieval and analysis of particulate debris after saphenous vein graft intervention. J Am Coll Cardiol 1999;34:468-475.

82. Cohen DJ, Murphy SA, Baim DS, et al: Cost-effectiveness of distal embolic protection for patients undergoing percutaneous intervention of saphenous vein bypass grafts: Results from the SAFER trial. J Am Coll Cardiol 2004;44:1801-1808.

83. Jonas M, Stone GW, Mehran R, et al: Platelet glycoprotein IIb/IIIa receptor inhibition as adjunctive treatment during saphenous vein graft stenting: Differential effects after randomization to occlusion or filter-based embolic protection. Eur Heart J 2006;27:920-928.

84. Mauri L, Rogers C, Baim DS: Devices for distal protection during percutaneous coronary revascularization. Circulation 2006;113:2651-2656.

85. Nakamura T, Kubo N, Seki Y, et al: Effects of a distal protection device during primary stenting in patients with acute anterior myocardial infarction. Circ J 2004;68:763-768.

86. Stone GW, Webb J, Cox DA, et al: Distal microcirculatory protection during percutaneous coronary intervention in

acute ST-segment elevation myocardial infarction: A randomized controlled trial. JAMA 2005;293:1063-1072.

87. Gick M, Jander N, Bestehorn HP, et al: Randomized evaluation of the effects of filter-based distal protection on myocardial perfusion and infarct size after primary percutaneous catheter intervention in myocardial infarction with and without ST-segment elevation. Circulation 2005;112:1462-1469.

88. Ali OA, Bhindi R, McMahon AC, et al: Distal protection in cardiovascular medicine: Current status. Am Heart J 2006;152:207-216.

89. Jordan WD Jr, Voellinger DC, Doblar DD, et al: Microemboli detected by transcranial Doppler monitoring in patients during carotid angioplasty versus carotid endarterectomy. Cardiovasc Surg 1999;7:33-38.

90. Aronow HD, Shishehbor M, Davis DA, et al: Leukocyte count predicts microembolic Doppler signals during carotid stenting: A link between inflammation and embolization. Stroke 2005;36:1910-1914.

91. Rapp JH, Pan XM, Sharp FR, et al: Atheroemboli to the brain: Size threshold for causing acute neuronal cell death. J Vasc Surg 2000;32:68-76.

92. Reimers B, Corvaja N, Moshiri S, et al: Cerebral protection with filter devices during carotid artery stenting. Circulation 2001;104:12-15.

93. Whitlow PL, Lylyk P, Londero H, et al: Carotid artery stenting protected with an emboli containment system. Stroke 2002;33:1308-1314.

94. Cosottini M, Michelassi MC, Puglioli M, et al: Silent cerebral ischemia detected with diffusion-weighted imaging in patients treated with protected and unprotected carotid artery stenting. Stroke 2005;36:2389-2393.

95. Kastrup A, Nagele T, Groschel K, et al: Incidence of new brain lesions after carotid stenting with and without cerebral protection. Stroke 2006;37:2312-2316.

96. Wholey MH, Al-Mubarek N, Wholey MH: Updated review of the global carotid artery stent registry. Catheter Cardiovasc Interv 2003;60:259-266.

97. Yadav JS, Wholey MH, Kuntz RE, et al: Protected carotid-artery stenting versus endarterectomy in high-risk patients. N Engl J Med 2004;351:1493-1501.

98. Ringleb PA, Allenberg J, Bruckmann H, et al: 30-Day results from the SPACE trial of stent-protected angioplasty versus carotid endarterectomy in symptomatic patients: A randomised non-inferiority trial. Lancet 2006;368:1239-1247.

99. Mas JL, Chatellier G, Beyssen B: Carotid angioplasty and stenting with and without cerebral protection: Clinical alert from the Endarterectomy Versus Angioplasty in Patients With Symptomatic Severe Carotid Stenosis (EVA-3S) trial. Stroke 2004;35:e18-e20.

100. Mas JL, Chatellier G, Beyssen B, et al: Endarterectomy verus stenting in patients with symptomatic severe carotid stenosis. N Engl J Med 2006;355:1660-1671.

101. Gray WA, Hopkins LN, Yadav S, et al: Protected carotid stenting in high-surgical-risk patients: The ARCHeR results. J Vasc Surg 2006;44:258-268.

102. White CJ, Iyer SS, Hopkins LN, et al: Carotid stenting with distal protection in high surgical risk patients: The BEACH trial 30 day results. Catheter Cardiovasc Interv 2006;67:503-512.

103. Krishnamurthi V, Novick AC, Myles JL: Atheroembolic renal disease: Effect on morbidity and survival after revascularization for atherosclerotic renal artery stenosis. J Urol 1999;161:1093-1096.

104. Henry M, Henry I, Klonaris C, et al: Renal angioplasty and stenting under protection: The way for the future? Catheter Cardiovasc Interv 2003;60:299-312.

105. Wholey MH, Toursarkissian B, Postoak D, et al: Early experience in the application of distal protection devices in treatment of peripheral vascular disease of the lower extremities. Catheter Cardiovasc Interv 2005;64:227-235.

106. Siablis D, Karnabatidis D, Katsanos K, et al: Outflow protection filters during percutaneous recanalization of lower extremities' arterial occlusions: A pilot study. Eur J Radiol 2005;55:243-249.

CHAPTER
28 Access Management and Closure Devices

Fernando Cura

KEY POINTS

- The most common catheterization problems are access-site complications, which can also increase hospital stays and medical costs.
- Selection of the appropriate access site is frequently a key issue for the successful completion of coronary or peripheral vascular procedures. Selection depends on the target vessel, the patient's preferences, and the operator's skills.
- The operator should be careful in choosing the site of cannulation of the femoral artery. Ideally, the femoral artery is to be entered about 1 to 2 cm below the inguinal ligament.

- The most commonly used femoral closure devices provide two types of mechanisms for percutaneously controlling bleeding: deploying sutures or staples to close the femoral puncture site or using resorbable collagen plugs to temporarily seal the arteriotomy.
- Hemostasis accelerators, which are based on the electrical attractive forces between the patch and the erythrocytes, produce more rapid clot formation.
- Vascular closure devices have improved patient comfort by enabling early ambulation, and their use has decreased the burden on the medical staff, but they have not demonstrated a reduction in groin complication rates.

The steady increase in percutaneous interventional procedures for the treatment of cardiovascular diseases in a variety of vascular territories is associated with closer attention to access-site management. The more aggressive level of anticoagulation used during therapeutic procedures requires the achievement of safe and reliable hemostasis of the access site. Coronary interventions are usually performed by the femoral approach; however, to reduce complications and increase patient comfort, radial access is increasingly used and is becoming the preferred access site by many interventionalists.[1,2] Patients undergoing the femoral approach are usually immobilized overnight, which may result in significant discomfort because of increased back pain and the need for analgesics. Noncompliance of patients regarding strict bedrest after the procedure has been reported to be a substantial factor for femoral complications.[3]

The most common catheterization problem involves the access site. Major access-site complications also increase the length of hospital stay and medical costs. The use of manual or mechanical compression was until recently the only way to control bleeding by allowing clot formation at the arteriotomy site. The clinical use of vascular closure devices for rapid hemostasis after femoral access was first reported in

1991. Since then, these devices have improved patient comfort by enabling early ambulation, and their use has decreased the burden of the medical staff. However, they have not produced a reduction in groin complication rates. This chapter summarizes the concepts of arterial access puncture, the use of arterial closure devices, and the postprocedural management.

PLANNING ACCESS

The selection of an appropriate access site is frequently a key issue for the successful completion of coronary or peripheral vascular procedures. Proficiency with all available vascular puncture techniques is therefore a basic requirement for the interventionalist.

It is important to review clinical reports and perform preprocedural vascular assessment of the quality of all peripheral pulses, presence of bruits, blood pressure difference between arms, and other pertinent findings, such as skin color, trophic changes, ulcerations, or the presence of intermittent claudication. Body habitus, such as extreme obesity, may dictate the use of the radial artery instead of the femoral approach. This important decision deserves full analysis of the target vessel for treatment, consideration of the patient's preference, and assessment of the interventionalist's skills. Some aspects of the vascular access are crucial to the safety and success of the procedure.

The retrograde femoral access and radial access, with the choice based on the patient's limitations or the operator's preferences, are the two preferred approaches for coronary interventions. There are several techniques for endovascular peripheral therapies according to the target treatment vessel: crossover femoral approach for contralateral iliofemoral treatment; anterograde femoral puncture for ipsilateral treatment of below-the-knee arteries; femoral retrograde access for aortic, carotid, iliac, and renal vessels; and local puncture for dialysis access treatment.

Retrograde Puncture Technique for the Femoral Artery

The common femoral artery is preferred for percutaneous arterial cannulation because it is large, accessible, and easily compressible. However, strict adherence to meticulous vascular access technique is necessary to avoid vascular complications while using manual compression or femoral closure devices.

The mean luminal diameter of the common femoral artery is between 6 and 7 mm. This is theoretically large enough to comfortably accommodate the typical range of femoral sheath sizes for most diagnostic and interventional procedures. Diabetics and women have disproportionately smaller common femoral arteries. The vascular access is generally the only painful part of the procedure. Patient sedation and generous local anesthesia are needed, as well as adequate pressure and rhythm monitoring. The operator should be careful in choosing the site of cannulation of the femoral artery. When drawing an imaginary line between the anterior superior iliac supine and the pubis, the arterial pulsation is near or at the midpoint of the line. It is important not to rely on the inguinal crease for selection of the puncture site because the distance from the inguinal ligament to the inguinal crease varies, particularly in overweight patients. Fluoroscopy should be used to ascertain the relative location of the femoral head and pelvic brim in this subgroup of patients. Puncture at or just above the center of the femoral head is particularly important.

Ideally, the femoral artery is entered about 1 or 2 cm below the inguinal ligament (Fig. 28-1). Cannulation of the artery too low increases the chance of entering the superficial femoral artery rather than the common femoral artery. This entry site may predispose to dissection, arterial occlusion, pseudoaneurysm, bleeding, and arteriovenous fistula formation. Entering the artery above the inguinal ligament may lead to problems in compressing the artery against the inguinal ligament, increasing the risk of hematoma formation and favoring retroperitoneal hemorrhage. The use of femoral closure devices is

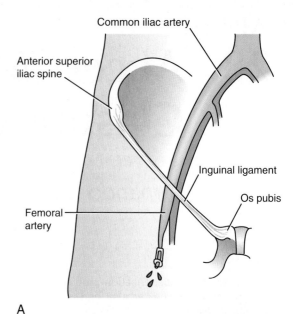

A

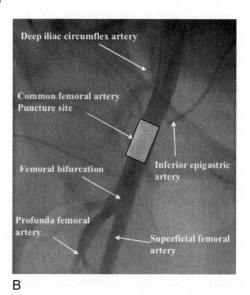

B

Figure 28-1. Accessing the femoral artery. **A,** An imaginary line between the superior anterior crest and the pubis is constructed. This imaginary line usually corresponds to the location of the inguinal ligament. The needle should enter approximately 1 cm below the imaginary line while advancing at a 30- to 45-degree angle. **B,** An excellent method for localizing the puncture site is to use fluoroscopy of the femoral head. The needle point should be over the lower inner quadrant.

contraindicated in higher or lower femoral punctures. The other important aspect is careful puncture of only the anterior wall of the femoral artery with open-bore needles, which have the advantage of demonstrating blood return immediately. Appropriate vascular hemostasis can be achieved with the use of manual compression or femoral closure devices (Fig. 28-2).

The reduction in the sheath size was presumed to result in fewer access complications, but there was not a clear association with a reduction in the bleed-

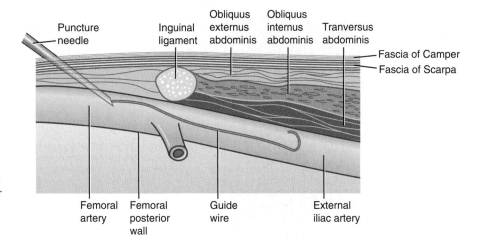

Figure 28-2. The femoral artery must be entered using a large-bore needle with backflow of blood. As soon as the needle passes into the vessel through the anterior wall, brisk, pulsatile flow occurs. The guidewire is advanced. It prevents occult bleeding through the posterior wall.

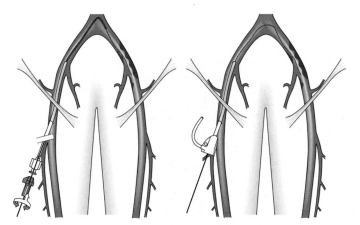

Figure 28-3. Retrograde femoral access for a contralateral approach.

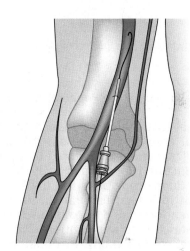

Figure 28-4. Puncture technique for the brachial artery.

ing rate. Retrograde femoral access can be considered the standard technique for coronary, renal, iliac, and crossover for contralateral femoral interventions (Fig. 28-3).

Puncture Technique for the Radial Artery

Miniaturization of the procedural equipment led to a revival of the transradial approach. Despite the considerable training needed, this approach remarkably improves patient comfort and decreases bleeding complications, particularly among patients with aggressive anticoagulation regimens.[1,4] This approach provides an alternative for coronary angiography and angioplasty and for vertebral and internal mammary interventions. This technique is addressed in Chapter 29.

Puncture Technique for the Brachial Artery

Brachial access is an alternative technique that can be used for coronary interventions. However, the radial access is usually preferred because of a higher rate of the brachial access-site complications, such as artery occlusion or hematoma. Puncture of the bra-

chial artery should be performed in its distal part above the antecubital fossa, where the artery is relatively superficial. At this level, after sheath removal, the artery can be compressed against the humerus to obtain hemostasis (Fig. 28-4). Direct puncture of the axillary artery, which has been performed in the past, has largely been abandoned.

Anterograde Puncture Technique for the Femoral Artery

The anterograde puncture technique provides more direct access to many lesions in the femoropopliteal segment and the infraglenoidale arteries. It allows reduction of the volume of contrast and provides stronger support for superficial femoral artery chronic occlusions. However, anterograde puncture is technically far more challenging. Although a high puncture of the common femoral artery is required to have enough space for navigation of the guidewire into the superficial femoral artery, suprainguinal puncture should be avoided because of the higher risk for retroperitoneal bleeding (Fig. 28-5). Injection of contrast through the needle usually helps to identify the femoral bifurcation anatomy.

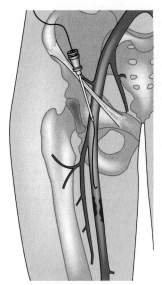

Figure 28-5. Anterograde puncture technique for the femoral artery.

Puncture Technique for the Popliteal Artery

Transpopliteal access becomes useful when the superficial femoral artery cannot be crossed using other techniques. The patients are placed in a prone position. The puncture is performed with the assistance of roadmap fluoroscopy after the injection of contrast from an ipsilateral femoral sheath (Fig. 28-6). Particular attention should be paid to achieving complete hemostasis after intervention. The incidence of access-site complications is potentially higher with transpopliteal access than with conventional techniques.

HEMOSTATIC METHODS AFTER PERCUTANEOUS CARDIOVASCULAR PROCEDURES

Proper technique is essential for achieving successful femoral artery hemostasis without complications. Methods used to achieve hemostasis after a percutaneous procedure include manual compression, mechanical compression, vascular plugs, percutaneous vascular suturing or staples, and topical hemostasis accelerators.

Manual Compression

Digital compression should be considered the gold standard for compressive methods. Performed properly, it can prevent bleeding and maintain distal perfusion. This procedure may be performed by a physician, nurse, or technician who has received formal training.

Before sheath removal, the distal pulses and the access site are assessed for signs of an existing hematoma. The duration of manual compression and the time of immobilization are proportional to the size of the introducer sheath and the level of anticoagulation. Although manual compression technique is

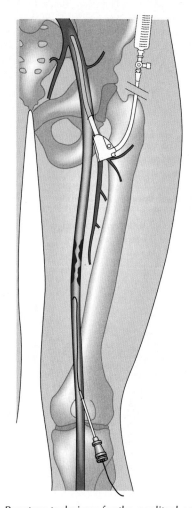

Figure 28-6. Puncture technique for the popliteal artery.

effective with smaller sheath sizes, it becomes more challenging and hazardous with increasing sheath sizes. The recommended compression time should be 10 minutes of "firm" pressure, 2 to 5 minutes of "less firm" pressure, and 2 minutes of light pressure while doing the pressure dressing. If bleeding continues, another 15 minutes of pressure should be applied.

Risk factors for prolonged bleeding include severe atherosclerosis at the puncture site and a loss of elasticity without adequate approximation of the vessel edges after removing the sheath. Other risk factors for bleeding include the sheath size, anticoagulation level at the time of sheath removal, aortic regurgitation, elevated blood pressure, obesity, and older age. The use of manual compression has the advantage of continuous observation and modulation of vascular compression. However, it has the disadvantage of requiring a staff member to be available, prolonged immobilization, and bedrest increasing patient discomfort and length of hospital stay. The Compass System (Advanced Vascular Dynamics, Vancouver, WA) is a manual compression-assist device developed to enhance comfort for patients and practitioners. It includes a handle and the detachable sterile and

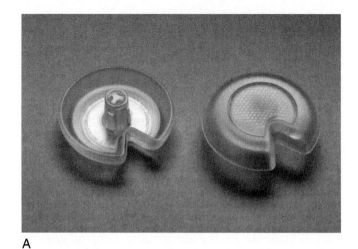

A

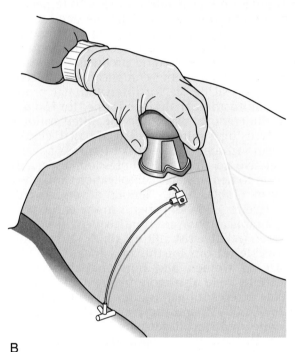

B

Figure 28-7. A, Compass compression assist device. **B,** The Compass is placed over the femoral sheath before pulling it. Then, more comfortable manual pressure is applied. (Photo courtesy of Advanced Vascular Dynamics, Vancouver, WA, 2006.)

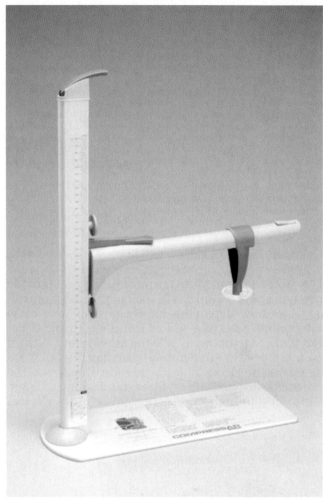

Figure 28-8. The C-clamp is a mechanical compressor system for femoral puncture sites. The disk that applies pressure rests on the vessel entry point. (Photo courtesy of Advanced Vascular Dynamics, Vancouver, WA, 2006.)

disposable disk. Practitioners apply external pressure using the Compass in much the same way that they would apply manual pressure (Fig. 28-7).

A vascular C-clamp (Advanced Vascular Dynamics) may be substituted for manual compression (Fig. 28-8). It consists of a flat, metal base; a pivoting metal shaft attached to the base; and an adjustable arm lever to hold the desired level of pressure. Disposable plastic compression disks, which are attached to the arm, apply pressure over the desired area. This approach has the advantage of freeing up personnel for other functions. It provides pressure over a relatively small area. Its limitations include the inability to modulate pressure easily and some discomfort from the device.

The Femo-Stop (RADI Medical Systems, Reading, MA) is a pneumatic pressure device that uses a clear plastic compression bag that molds to skin contours (Fig. 28-9). The Femo-Stop is composed of a plastic arch, inflatable transparent dome, connection tubing, a stopcock, an elastic or adjustable belt, and a hand-held manometer. It is held in place by straps passing around the hip. The amount of applied pressure may be modulated and observed with sphygmomanometer gauge. It allows visualization of the puncture site. The Femo-Stop is frequently indicated for compression to repair pseudoaneurysms.

The Safeguard (Datascope Interventional, Mahwah, NJ) is a product for post-hemostasis puncture-site management that combines a built-in inflatable bulb and a sterile dressing providing adjustable pressure to the site. The device has a clear window that allows staff to easily assess the site without removing the device. Safeguard is ideal for noncompliant patients or overweight patients (Fig. 28-10).

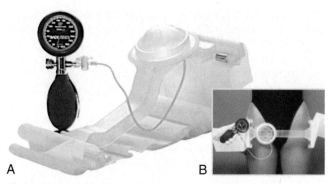

Figure 28-9. A, The Femo-Stop pressure system with the sphygmomanometer. **B,** The belt should be aligned with the puncture site equally across both hips.

Femoral Closure Devices

The most commonly used hemostasis devices provide two types of mechanisms for percutaneously controlling bleeding: deploying sutures or staples to close the femoral puncture site or using resorbable collagen plugs to temporarily seal the arteriotomy. A third group of devices are hemostasis accelerators that are based on the electrical attractive forces between the closure device and the erythrocytes, leading to more rapid clot formation. Arteriotomy closure devices

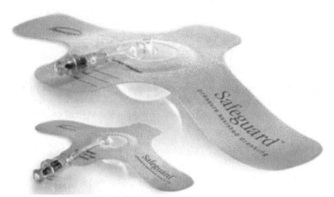

Figure 28-10. The Safeguard dressing is applied with the access site visible under the plastic window. The center bulb is inflated with air to the desired amount of pressure, and the syringe is removed.

have emerged as an alternative to traditional mechanical compression after percutaneous cardiovascular intervention. These devices have the potential to reduce the time to hemostasis, facilitate patient mobilization, decrease hospital length of stay, and improve patient satisfaction.

Although older, single-center studies and randomized trials have shown mixed results regarding the safety of arterial closure devices compared with manual compression, later data show decreased complications with closure devices. This difference may result from increased operator experience with arterial closure devices and improved device technology. A meta-analysis including 30 selected studies that have included a total of 37,066 patients (12,596 and 24,470 patients in the device and control groups, respectively) found no significant risk with respect to vascular complications between closure devices and mechanical compression in the setting of diagnostic or interventional procedures. The complication rate appears similar for the leading products, Angioseal and Perclose, with a higher complication rate seen with the VasoSeal device for interventional procedures.[5,6] A multivariate analysis performed for 156,853 patients undergoing diagnostic or interventional procedures using suture or collagen-based closure devices demonstrated a lower risk of serious adverse events relative to manual compression, especially with respect to hemorrhagic complications and pseudoaneurysm (Table 28-1).[7] Serious adverse events were reported in 1.56% of patients in the entire population. Complications were more frequent in women than in men (relative risk [RR]=2.13; $P<.001$) (Table 28-2). Possible reasons for this may include smaller vessel size in women and hormonal differences. Complications were also more frequent in patients who had interventional cardiac catheterization (RR=2.26; $P<.0001$), and they were less frequent in patients who used the collagen plug devices (RR=0.62; $P<.001$) or the suture device (RR=0.87; $P=.02$) compared with manual compression (Table 28-3).[7]

A study comparing the benefits and cost-effectiveness of suture-mediated closure devices and manual compression found that the use of closure devices of the femoral arterial access site was safe and cost saving.[8] All closure devices have been reported to be

Table 28-1. Risk of Adverse Events after Cardiac Catheterizations by Hemostasis Device in 2001: The American College of Cardiology–National Cardiovascular Disease Registry

Complications	Incidence in the Whole Population*	Collagen Plug	Suture Device	Manual Compression	P Value
Bleeding (%)	1.13	0.78	1.15	1.20	<.001
Vessel occlusion (%)	0.07	0.07	0.07	0.07	NS
Dissection (%)	0.02	0.01	0.02	0.03	NS
Pseudoaneurysm (%)	0.37	0.17	0.24	0.45	<.001
Arteriovenous fistula (%)	0.05	0.04	0.05	0.06	NS
Associated death (%)	0.09	0.03	0.10	0.10	<.001
Any vascular complication (%)	1.56	1.05	1.48	1.70	<.001

*N=166,680.
NS, not significant.

Table 28-2. Risk of Adverse Events after Cardiac Catheterizations by Gender in 2001: The American College of Cardiology–National Cardiovascular Disease Registry

Complications	Male Gender	Female Gender	*P* Value
Bleeding (%)	0.78	1.70	<.001
Vessel occlusion (%)	0.05	0.10	<.001
Dissection (%)	0.02	0.03	.03
Pseudoaneurysm (%)	0.25	0.56	<.001
Arteriovenous fistula (%)	0.05	0.06	NS
Associated death (%)	0.05	0.14	<.001
Any vascular complication (%)	1.09	2.32	<.001

*$N=166,680$.
NS, not significant.

safe in patients receiving glycoprotein IIb/IIIa inhibitors.[9-11] However, some reports have raised concerns about an increased risk of bleeding complications with the use of vascular closure devices among patients treated with a combination of anticoagulation drugs such as enoxaparin, clopidogrel, aspirin, and GP IIb/IIIa inhibitors compared with manual compression.[12-14]

Despite the advances in techniques and the introduction of new products, vessel closure technologies have failed to penetrate most diagnostic and interventional cases. However, the use of these devices is increasing in the diagnostic and interventional fields from 23% in 2003 up to an estimated 40% in 2009 (Fig. 28-11). Although the overall use of femoral closure devices has increased, the rates at which they are employed throughout the world are very different (Fig. 28-12).

Suture-Based Closure Devices

The percutaneous suture-mediated closure device represents one of several attempts to develop a method to achieve arteriotomy hemostasis in a safe and timely manner. Several studies have shown the efficacy of percutaneous suture-mediated closure devices in decreasing time to hemostasis and time to ambulation without increasing the rate of access-site complications.[5] However, experience suggests that

the devices may result in infrequent but challenging vascular complications of the groin, such as retroperitoneal hemorrhage, arterial thromboses, infections, dissections, and large pseudoaneurysms.[15,16] Proper training and operator skills are necessary for the successful use of these suture-based closure devices. The use of standard aseptic techniques in all cases, along with a single dose of prophylactic intravenous antibiotics during placement of the percutaneous suture-mediated closure device in high-risk patients, appears to prevent infectious complications.

The Perclose (Abbott Vascular Devices, Redwood City, CA) was the first suture-based closure device in the market, and it is based solely on sutures (Fig. 28-13). The main advantage of Perclose compared with other closure devices is that no material is left at the puncture site, except for the nonabsorbable sutures. Needles are used to guide the sutures through the vessel wall. The previous Prostar device used four needles and two sutures; the newer Techstar and later devices use two needles and one suture. They can be used with 6- to 10-Fr sheaths. Perclose consists of several components, including a 0.035-inch guidewire, an automatic knot-pushing tool, and the suture-containing device itself. This tool consists of a sheath connected to a handle by a guide that is introduced into the vessel by means of the 0.035-inch guidewire after the angioplasty sheath has been removed. When the intravascular position has been achieved, the device is secured by pulling the lever and releasing the anchor. Using the needle plunger, needles are inserted through the vessel wall and grip the sutures. The needles are then retracted until they are outside of the skin with the sutures. Each of the two suture ends can be retrieved, tied together, and pulled down to the surface of the artery with the help of a knot pusher. This improved device has shortened the time of deployment and improved handling. After it is apparent that hemostasis will be achieved, the guidewire is removed with further sequential tightening of the suture pairs.

The SuperStitch (Sutura, Inc., Fountain Valley, CA) is a suture-mediated device that is able to close 6- to 12-Fr sheaths (Fig. 28-14). It applies polypropylene sutures with a system of needles and ends in a flexible nylon shaft. This shaft can be inserted into the

Table 28-3. Risk of Adverse Events after Cardiac Catheterizations by Procedure in 2001: The American College of Cardiology–National Cardiovascular Disease Registry

Complications*	Diagnostic	Interventional	P Value
Bleeding (%)	0.59	1.55	<.001
Vessel occlusion (%)	0.07	0.07	NS
Dissection (%)	0.02	0.03	NS
Pseudoaneurysm (%)	0.21	0.49	<.001
Arteriovenous fistula (%)	0.07	0.10	.03
Associated death (%)	0.07	0.10	.03
Any vascular complication (%)	0.91	2.07	<.001

*Among the total population ($N=166,680$).
NS, not significant.

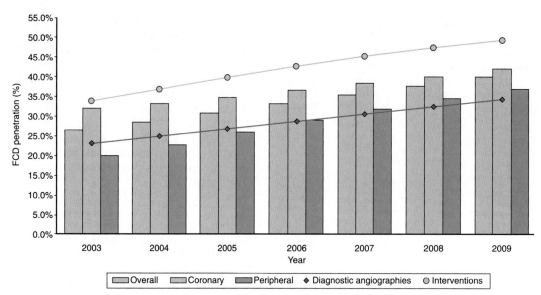

Figure 28-11. Estimated trends from 2003 to 2009 for the penetration of femoral closure devices (FCDs) in diagnostic and interventional procedures. (Graphic courtesy of Millennium Research Group, Toronto, Ontario, Canada, 2006.)

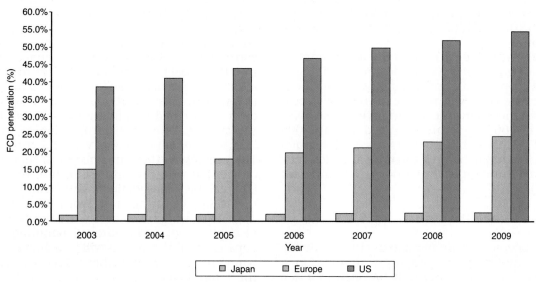

Figure 28-12. Estimated trends from 2003 to 2009 for the penetration of femoral closure devices (FCDs) in different market regions. (Graphic courtesy of Millennium Research Group, Toronto, Ontario, Canada, 2006.)

vascular access sheath to preserve the arteriotomy, reducing the risk of infection. Application is simplified by an applicator with a thumb plunger and finger rings. The sutures are positioned with rotating movements; after withdrawing the sheath and the device, the needles are deployed, and the sutures are retrieved. The knot is tied outside and delivered to the vessel with a knot pusher. Experimental comparison of the Sutura SuperStitch and the Perclose Closer showed that contrary to the normal angiographic findings, both devices incited periadventitial fibrosis, which creates a fibrous hood around the suture and vessel.[17] Studies showed a highly successful deployment rate with immediate hemostasis in most patients.[18]

The Angiolink (Medtronic, Santa Rosa, CA) and the Starclose (Abbott Vascular Devices, Redwood City, CA) represent a new concept of extravascular, clip-based femoral closure devices (Fig. 28-15). The clips are made of titanium or nitinol alloy; both are highly biocompatible materials that are deployed through the existing procedural sheath. The extravascular approach closes by apposing the tissue at and above the arteriotomy site, leaving nothing in the arterial lumen. The artery may be accessed again shortly after hemostasis has been achieved.

Collagen-Based Sealing Devices

Collagen is considered one of the most thrombogenic components of vascular wall. It attracts and binds platelets. Collagen also plays an important role in healing wounds by carrying growth factors and by

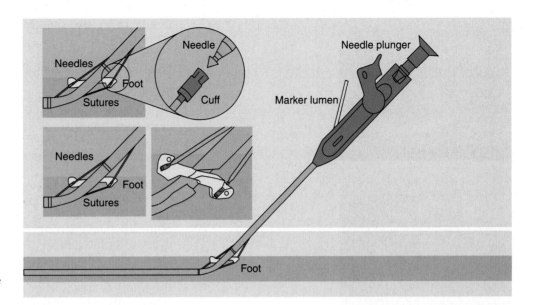

Figure 28-13. Perclose closure device.

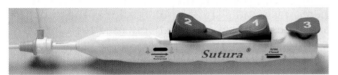

Figure 28-14. SuperStitch device (Sutura, Inc., Fountain Valley, CA).

providing a matrix for cellular proliferation. Because it is highly compatible and easily manufactured in many different forms, collagen is an ideal component for hemostasis products. Collagen can be used alone to plug the vessel wall or tissue tract, or it can be combined with thrombin or gel-foam. Thrombin converts fibrinogen to fibrin, accelerating and strengthening clot formation.

The Angioseal (St. Jude Medical, St. Paul, MN)[19] mechanically closes the site by sandwiching the arteriotomy site between a bioabsorbable polymer anchor inside the vessel and an extravascular collagen sponge covering the arterial surface within the skin tract (Fig. 28-16). It consists of four components within a delivery device: anchor, collagen plug, connecting suture, and a tamper. All three components deployed into the patient are completely resorbable. The small plug contains only about 15 mg of collagen, and the anchor is made from polyglycolic and polylactic acids. Before Angioseal deployment, the access site should be assessed by injecting contrast through the sheath under fluoroscopy. If the introducer enters the femoral artery above the inguinal ligament, at the bifurcation, at a branch vessel, or at an atherosclerotic vessel, there is an increased risk of device failure or embolization, and an alternative method for hemostasis should be used. Proper technique must be followed to avoid bleeding complications, anchor embolization, thrombosis, and infection.[20]

The VasoSeal (Datascope Corporation, Mahwah, NJ) was the first femoral closure device introduced in the market (Fig. 28-17). The VasoSeal ES device contains a temporary arteriotomy locator, a sheath and tissue dilator assembly, an introducer, and two cartridges, each containing a plug of purified bovine collagen. The device permits delivery of the collagen into the tissue tract created by removal of a sheath device and onto the exterior surface of the artery. The collagen interacts with the platelets to create a hemostatic seal directly over the puncture wound in the artery. The sterile and nonpyogenic collagen remains totally extravascular. No foreign material is left inside the artery, and the remaining collagen is absorbed within a few weeks.[21] The VasoSeal is indicated for use in procedures using 5- to 8-Fr sheaths. As with any foreign substance, use of collagen in contaminated sites may lead to infection, and special attention should be paid to the use of sterile and antiseptic applications. In the setting of diagnostic cardiac catheterization, the risk of vascular complications related to arterial access site was similar with the VasoSeal device compared with mechanical compression and other femoral closure devices. However, the rate of complications after interventional procedures was higher with VasoSeal compared with mechanical compression.[5] The On-Site (Datascope Corporation, Mahwah, NJ) precision closure device is a newer-generation, single-operator, over-the-wire technology that delivers an extravascular collagen sponge plug at the femoral arterial puncture site to achieve hemostasis. A temporary intra-arterial disk is used to locate the arteriotomy and to ensure precise collagen placement.

The Duett device (Vascular Solutions, Minneapolis, MN) met the challenge of simultaneously sealing the puncture hole in the artery and in the tissue track by generating a thrombus (Fig. 28-18). It incorporates a unique, low-profile, balloon-positioning catheter in combination with a biologic, procoagulant-containing bovine collagen and thrombin. The suspension incorporating both of these hemostatic agents is designed to have a viscosity suitable for

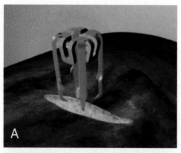

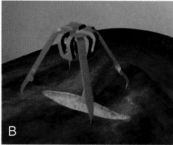

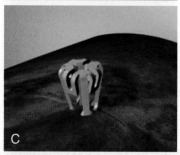

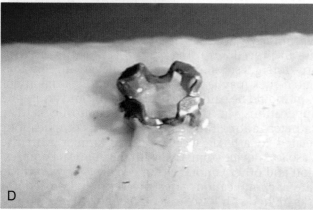

Figure 28-15. Expanding Angiolink staple-based closure device. **A,** Staple tracks small through a sterile delivery system, reducing the chance of touch contamination. **B,** It expands wide above the arteriotomy to close a 6- to 8-Fr arteriotomy. **C,** It purses the arteriotomy closed to promote healing. It does not remodel the vessel and has no intraluminal components to impede flow. **D,** The staple gathers the full thickness of the vessel media and adventitia for a secure mechanical closure. (Photograph courtesy of Medtronic, Minneapolis, MN, 2006.)

injecting through the side arm of vascular sheaths but has a consistency that would be likely to maintain the procoagulant at the desired location in the periarterial space at the puncture site. When the device is inflated, the balloon assumes an elliptical shape with a significantly larger diameter and a relatively shorter length. With this balloon size, a single

device can close sheath diameters in the range of 5 to 9 Fr.

Electrical-Based Sealing Pads

The patch technologies are a new form of biologically active, superficially applied therapies that accelerate local hemostasis at the puncture site.[22] The use of noninvasive closure devices for interventional procedures has rapidly increased in the past few years (Fig. 28-19). One of the substances used in these pads is chitosan, derived from the deacetylation of chitin. Chitin is obtained from the shells of lobsters, crab, and shrimp. Chitin has a slightly positive charge, and chitosan has a strong positive charge, but erythrocytes and platelets are negatively charged. Because of their positive charges, chitin and chitosan attract negatively charged platelets and red blood cells to the applied area. Other hemostatic pads are impregnated with chemicals such as bovine thrombin or potato starch. These agents, combined with effective manual compression, may result in a shorter time to hemostasis and a stronger blood clot at the puncture site. These devices are effectively used for adjunctive closure devices or as hemostatic accelerators for manual compression of the access site. The simple application and the low cost make this system attractive. The reliability of these devices, however, still needs to be evaluated in larger number of patients.

Chito-Seal Topical Hemostasis Pad (Abbott Vascular Devices, Redwood City, CA) is intended for use in the management of bleeding wounds such as vascular access sites. The pad is coated with chitosan gel, which is a powerful hemostatic agent twice as chemically active as chitin. The Clo-sur P.A.D. (Scion Cardio-Vascular, Miami, FL) is a pad consisting of hydrophilic, naturally occurring biopolymer polyprolate acetate. It also activates electrical interference between erythrocytes and the pad, leading to red blood cell agglutination and clot formation. The SyvekPatch (Marine Polymer Technologies, Danvers, MA), an external device used to control bleeding from vascular access sites, consists of a poly-N-acetyl glucosamine polymer, which is isolated from a microalga. The mechanism of action involves clot formation and local vasoconstriction as part of its hemostatic effect.

ACCESS-SITE COMPLICATIONS

Local vascular complications at the site of catheter insertion constitute the most common adverse events after cardiovascular interventions. Vascular complications can extend the patient's length of hospitalization and increase the associated procedural costs. Vascular access complications include external bleeding, hematoma, pseudoaneurysm, arteriovenous fistula, vessel dissection, acute vessel closure, retroperitoneal hemorrhage, neural damage, infection, and venous thrombosis.

One way to prevent femoral access complications is to carefully select patients and access sites. The

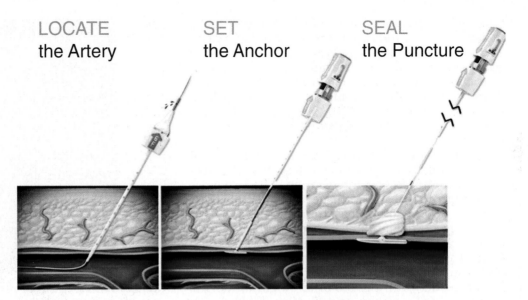

LOCATE
the Artery

SET
the Anchor

SEAL
the Puncture

Figure 28-16. Angioseal hemostasis system. The anchor is deployed, and retraction of the system secures the anchor against the anterior vessel wall. The collagen plug is deployed outside of the artery. The suture is cut at the skin line, leaving the subcutaneous vascular closure components hidden. (Image courtesy of St. Jude Medical, St. Paul, MN, 2006.)

American College of Cardiology-National Cardiovascular Data Registry (ACC-NCDR) reported an overall in-hospital serious adverse event rate related to vascular access of 1.56% among 166,680 patients after manual compression or the use of hemostasis devices (see Table 28-1).

Before vascular closure device placement, a femoral artery angiogram through the sheath should be obtained to assess the puncture site, vessel diameter, and presence and severity of atherosclerosis. It can help to identify patients at higher risk for groin complications. Femoral closure devices should be avoided when the artery diameter is less than 5 mm and in cases of higher or lower femoral punctures.

Bleeding complications occur more frequently while obtaining access and positioning sheaths or early after removal when local pressure is not properly achieved. Several comorbid conditions have been associated with groin complications. The presence of peripheral vascular disease, renal failure, myocardial

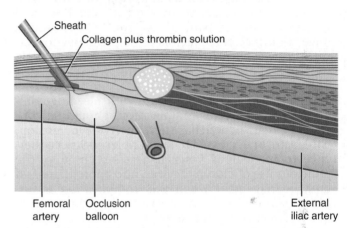

Figure 28-18. Duett hemostatic device uses a low-profile, balloon-positioning catheter in combination with a biologic, procoagulant-containing bovine collagen and thrombin solution.

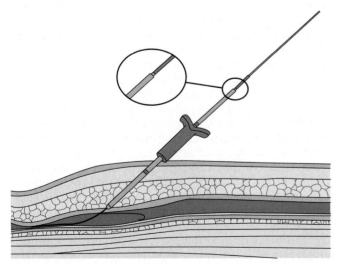

Figure 28-17. Vasoseal closure device. (Courtesy of Datascope Corp., Montvale, NJ.)

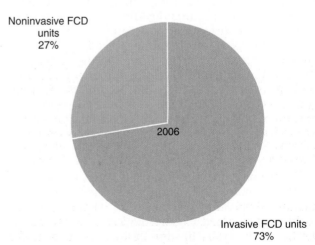

Noninvasive FCD units 27%

2006

Invasive FCD units 73%

Figure 28-19. Use of invasive and noninvasive femoral closure devices (FCDs) in interventional procedures in 2006. (Graphic courtesy of Millennium Research Group, Toronto, Ontario, Canada, 2006.)

infarction, emergency indication for the procedure, and shock as an indication for the procedure demonstrated statistically significant associations with access-site bleeding complications. Hematoma is considered a significant complication when it has a diameter of more than 6 cm. The incidence of local hematoma varies from 1% to 5%, and most hematomas require only observation and no further intervention.

Retroperitoneal hemorrhage remains an infrequent but occasionally devastating consequence of percutaneous cardiovascular intervention. The incidence of retroperitoneal hemorrhage is 0.6%; of these patients, 73% require blood transfusions, and 10% die during hospitalization.[23] Retroperitoneal hemorrhage was independently associated with "high femoral artery stick" when femoral artery sheaths are placed superior to the inferior epigastric artery, with female gender, with the use of an Angioseal device, with the use of a glycoprotein IIb/IIIa inhibitor, with a presentation of acute myocardial infarction, and inversely with the patient's weight.[23] Other studies have confirmed three factors to be predictive for retroperitoneal hemorrhage (female gender, low body weight, and high femoral puncture), whereas the use of glycoprotein IIb/IIIa, sheath size, and the use of a closure device did not correlate with bleeding complications.[24] Bleeding complications should be considered when a patient has a new onset of hypotension, flank pain, or decreased hematocrit level. Strict adherence to meticulous vascular access technique, the judicious use of closure devices, and appropriate and rapid management when this complication is suspected should lessen the occasionally serious consequences related to this problem.

A major cause of retroperitoneal bleeding is a puncture above the inguinal ligament. When the posterior arterial wall is punctured, blood can spread into the retroperitoneal space. The location of the inferior epigastric artery may be helpful in judging the location of the puncture with regard the inguinal ligament. The inferior border of this vessel defines the border of the inguinal ligament and represents a marker by which femoral punctures can be assessed for possible risk of retroperitoneal bleeding. The inferior epigastric artery arises from the distal external iliac artery just before it crosses under the inguinal ligament to enter the thigh and become the femoral artery. It typically originates opposite the deep iliac circumflex branch and bears a direct relation to the inferior extent of the peritoneal transversalis fascia (Fig. 28-20). When the entry site of the sheath is superior to the origin of the inferior epigastric artery, the sheath passes through various layers of the anterior abdominal wall, including superficial fascia and muscles, before entering the artery (Fig. 28-21). The collagen plug–based closure devices may not reach the wall of the artery in some cases, and the operator should be careful in choosing the site of cannulation of the femoral artery. Fluoroscopy can be used to ascertain the relative location of the femoral head and pelvic brim in that endeavor (see Fig. 28-1). The

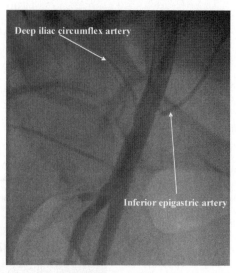

Figure 28-20. Angiogram through the sheath to assess the femoral artery and puncture location. The right anterior oblique, 30-degree projection of a typical femoral artery access site shows the inferior epigastric entry in relation to its surrounding anatomy. The inferior epigastric artery arises from the distal external iliac artery just before it crosses under the inguinal ligament. The inferior border of this vessel defines the border of the inguinal ligament.

retroperitoneal space appears to be able to sequester large amounts of blood.

Volume and blood product support and correction of thrombin and platelet inhibition are central to management when this complication is suspected. Although computed tomography (CT) or other forms of imaging are occasionally useful in diagnosing retroperitoneal hemorrhage, this modality is usually not required, and it may delay treatment. Peripheral vascular surgery or endovascular treatment is appropriate if blood product transfusion does not result in hemodynamic stabilization or if there is clinically significant organ or nerve compression.

The incidence of iatrogenic femoral pseudoaneurysms after percutaneous procedures ranges from 0.5% for diagnostic procedures to 1% to 2% for therapeutic interventions. A pseudoaneurysm is a hematoma that remains in continuity with the artery, allowing flow in and out of the hematoma. It can be differentiated from a simple hematoma by the presence of a bruit and a palpable pulsatile mass. Pseudoaneurysms are normally detected by ultrasound (Fig. 28-22). Older age, obesity, female gender, larger sheath size, peripheral vascular disease, a low arterial puncture site below the common femoral bifurcation, and the level of anticoagulation are associated with this complication. A pseudoaneurysm larger than 3 cm in diameter usually is treated by mechanical compression, thrombin injection, or surgery. Smaller pseudoaneurysms can be followed by serial ultrasound. Ultrasound-guided manual or mechanical compression is often used to convert the pseudoaneurysm to a thrombosed hematoma by compressing the neck connecting it to the artery. Ultrasound-guided, low-dose thrombin injection appears to be

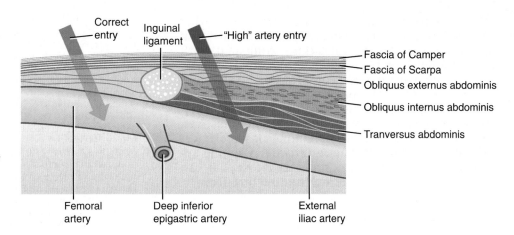

Figure 28-21. The diagram depicts the relation between the high entry and the correct puncture site related to the inguinal ligament and inferior epigastric artery. The placement of sheath in a high puncture site crosses over the fascia of Camper, fascia of Scarpa, obliquus externus abdominis muscle, obliquus internus abdominis muscle, and the transverses abdominis muscle.

more effective in reducing the need for surgical repair, is better tolerated by the patients, and requires a shorter hospital stay.[25]

Arteriovenous fistula is defined as an abnormal connection between an artery and vein. This may be caused by trauma, improper removal of adjacent arterial and venous sheaths, or inadvertent puncture of a vein while accessing an artery. It is an uncommon and low-risk groin complication that is suspected by the detection of a continuous bruit at the access site, and it is diagnosed by ultrasound. In cases of arterial insufficiency, the fistula can be treated with ultrasound-guided compression, endovascular stenting, or surgical repair.

Occasionally, hematoma-mediated femoral nerve compression accompanying limb weakness may occur. It resolves spontaneously within 2 to 3 weeks.

Vessel occlusion associated with manual compression may occur because of excessive occlusive pressure during the compression process. Patients with diabetes, female patients, or those with peripheral vascular disease have arteries with reduced lumen diameters and may be more susceptible to this complication. Vessel occlusion is characterized by a sudden onset of pain and possible paresthesia. The affected limb is cyanotic, is cool, and has diminished or absent pulses. Treatment methods for vessel occlusion include administration of heparin or lytic agents or an endovascular or surgical thrombectomy procedure.

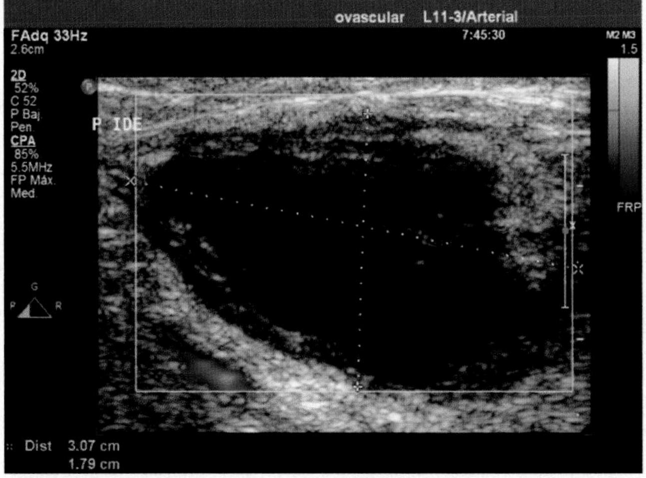

Although relatively uncommon, vascular closure device–related infection is an emerging and serious phenomenon with a high morbidity rate. It requires aggressive medical and surgical intervention to achieve cure.[16,26] Access-site infections manifest with high fever, femoral abscess, septic thrombosis, and mycotic aneurysm. The predominant source of pathogens is the endogenous flora of the patient's skin. Attention to skin preparation is part of the infection prevention strategy. Diabetes mellitus and obesity are the most common associated comorbidities. Infectious groin complications are significantly increased with suture-based closure devices.[27] Surgical removal of the percutaneous closure device and débridement to normal arterial wall are recommended for all patients with suspected femoral endarteritis. Before inserting a closure device, it is recommended to again prepare the skin insertion site and remove any pooled blood before beginning the arterial closure, especially in the case of a prolonged procedure. If compromise of sterile technique is suspected, the operator should consider a change of gloves before beginning the arterial closure and a change of towels around the skin insertion site, especially if the drape has become saturated with blood. Although some differences may exist regarding local complications with the use of femoral closure systems, neither device has been shown to reduce major local complications.

CONCLUSIONS AND FUTURE TRENDS

Several femoral access closure technologies are on the market, and more on the horizon offer at least equivalent patient outcomes compared with manual compression. The ease of use is continuing to improve. Sealing and suturing closure devices have been shown to shorten hemostasis time, reduce the discomfort of

Figure 28-22. Pseudoaneurysm arising from the common femoral artery is assessed by duplex ultrasound.

manual or mechanical compression, and allow earlier ambulation after cardiovascular procedures without increasing vascular complications compared with conventional compression techniques. Improved devices that assist manual compression are also continuing to evolve. The patch technologies are a new form of biologically active, superficially applied therapies that have found acceptance in many practices. Ultimately, the acceptance of femoral closure devices will depend on which device provides a simple approach with reliable hemostasis at a cost that can justify their incorporation into routine practice.

REFERENCES

1. Cantor WJ, Puley G, Natarajan MK, et al: Radial versus femoral access for emergent percutaneous coronary intervention with adjunct glycoprotein IIb/IIIa inhibition in acute myocardial infarction—The RADIAL-AMI pilot randomized trial. Am Heart J 2005;150:543-549.
2. Krone RJ, Johnson L, Noto T: Five year trends in cardiac catheterization: A report from the Registry of the Society for Cardiac Angiography and Interventions. Cathet Cardiovasc Diagn 1996;39:31-35.
3. Bogart MA, Bogart DB, Rigden LB, et al: A prospective randomized trial of early ambulation following 8 French diagnostic cardiac catheterization. Catheter Cardiovasc Interv 1999;47:175-178.
4. Agostoni P, Biondi-Zoccai GG, de Benedictis ML, et al: Radial versus femoral approach for percutaneous coronary diagnostic and interventional procedures: Systematic overview and meta-analysis of randomized trials. J Am Coll Cardiol 2004;44:349-356.
5. Nikolsky E, Mehran R, Halkin A, et al: Vascular complications associated with arteriotomy closure devices in patients undergoing percutaneous coronary procedures: A meta-analysis. J Am Coll Cardiol 2004;44:1200-1209.
6. Park Y, Roh HG, Choo SW, et al: Prospective comparison of collagen plug (Angio-Seal) and suture-mediated (the Closer S) closure devices at femoral access sites. Korean J Radiol 2005;6:248-255.
7. Tavris DR, Dey S, Albrecht-Gallauresi B, et al: Risk of local adverse events following cardiac catheterization by hemostasis device use—phase II. J Invasive Cardiol 2005;17:644-650.
8. Rickli H, Unterweger M, Sutsch G, et al: Comparison of costs and safety of a suture-mediated closure device with conventional manual compression after coronary artery interventions. Catheter Cardiovasc Interv 2002;57:297-302.
9. Boccalandro F, Assali A, Fujise K, et al: Vascular access site complications with the use of closure devices in patients treated with platelet glycoprotein IIb/IIIa inhibitors during rescue angioplasty. Catheter Cardiovasc Interv 2004;63:284-289.
10. Exaire JE, Dauerman HL, Topol EJ, et al: Triple antiplatelet therapy does not increase femoral access bleeding with vascular closure devices. Am Heart J 2004;147:31-34.
11. Applegate RJ, Grabarczyk MA, Little WC, et al: Vascular closure devices in patients treated with anticoagulation and IIb/IIIa receptor inhibitors during percutaneous revascularization. J Am Coll Cardiol 2002;40:78-83.
12. Exaire JE, Tcheng JE, Kereiakes DJ, et al: Closure devices and vascular complications among percutaneous coronary intervention patients receiving enoxaparin, glycoprotein IIb/IIIa inhibitors, and clopidogrel. Catheter Cardiovasc Interv 2005;64:369-372.
13. Assali AR, Sdringola S, Moustapha A, et al: Outcome of access site in patients treated with platelet glycoprotein IIb/IIIa inhibitors in the era of closure devices. Catheter Cardiovasc Interv 2003;58:1-5.
14. Michalis LK, Rees MR, Patsouras D, et al: A prospective randomized trial comparing the safety and efficacy of three commercially available closure devices (Angioseal, Vasoseal and Duett). Cardiovasc Intervent Radiol 2002;25:423-429.
15. Wagner SC, Gonsalves CF, Eschelman DJ, et al: Complications of a percutaneous suture-mediated closure device versus manual compression for arteriotomy closure: A case-controlled study. J Vasc Interv Radiol 2003;14:735-741.
16. Sohail MR, Khan AH, Holmes DR Jr, et al: Infectious complications of percutaneous vascular closure devices. Mayo Clin Proc 2005;80:1011-1015.
17. Hofmann LV, Sood S, Liddell RP, et al: Arteriographic and pathologic evaluation of two suture-mediated arterial closure devices in a porcine model. J Vasc Interv Radiol 2003;14:755-761.
18. Eggebrecht H, Naber C, Woertgen U, et al: Percutaneous suture-mediated closure of femoral access sites deployed through the procedure sheath: Initial clinical experience with a novel vascular closure device. Catheter Cardiovasc Interv 2003;58:313-321.
19. Abando A, Hood D, Weaver F, Katz S: The use of the Angioseal device for femoral artery closure. J Vasc Surg 2004;40:287-290.
20. Applegate RJ, Sacrinty M, Kutcher MA, et al: Vascular complications with newer generations of angioseal vascular closure devices. J Interv Cardiol 2006;19:67-74.
21. Shammas NW, Rajendran VR, Alldredge SG, et al: Randomized comparison of Vasoseal and Angioseal closure devices in patients undergoing coronary angiography and angioplasty. Catheter Cardiovasc Interv 2002;55:421-425.
22. Hirsch JA, Reddy SA, Capasso WE, Linfante I: Non-invasive hemostatic closure devices: "Patches and pads." Tech Vasc Interv Radiol 2003;6:92-95.
23. Ellis SG, Bhatt D, Kapadia S, Lee D, et al: Correlates and outcomes of retroperitoneal hemorrhage complicating percutaneous coronary intervention. Catheter Cardiovasc Interv 2006;67:541-545.
24. Farouque HM, Tremmel JA, Raissi Shabari F, et al: Risk factors for the development of retroperitoneal hematoma after percutaneous coronary intervention in the era of glycoprotein IIb/IIIa inhibitors and vascular closure devices. J Am Coll Cardiol 2005;45:363-368.
25. Olsen DM, Rodriguez JA, Vranic M, et al: A prospective study of ultrasound scan-guided thrombin injection of femoral pseudoaneurysm: A trend toward minimal medication. J Vasc Surg 2002;36:779-782.
26. Geary K, Landers JT, Fiore W, Riggs P: Management of infected femoral closure devices. Cardiovasc Surg 2002;10:161-163.
27. Heck DV, Muldowney S, McPherson SH: Infectious complications of Perclose for closure of femoral artery punctures. J Vasc Interv Radiol 2002;13:430-431.

29 Transradial Percutaneous Coronary Intervention for a Major Reduction of Bleeding Complications

Farzin Beygui and Gilles Montalescot

KEY POINTS

- Bleeding complications after percutaneous coronary intervention (PCI) are associated with poor outcomes, including death.
- The transradial approach to PCI is associated with a dramatic reduction of the risk of access-site complications and virtually no access-site bleeding.

- After an initial short learning period, the procedural success rates of the transradial approach become similar to those of the transfemoral approach.
- The transradial approach can be used in any clinical condition for all procedures and devices compatible with 5-, 6-, 7-, and even 8-Fr guiding catheters.

Diagnostic coronary angiography and percutaneous coronary interventions (PCIs) are most commonly performed through transfemoral access in most catheterization laboratories. Initial reports in the late 1980s demonstrated the feasibility and safety of diagnostic coronary angiography by means of a transradial approach.[1] The use of highly active antithrombotic regimens, which were associated with a major reduction in the thrombotic complications of PCI, and a significant increase in femoral access-site–related bleeding complications led to the development of the transradial approach to PCI during the past decade. The use of 6- and 5-Fr guide catheters with 6- or 5-Fr–compatible balloons, coronary stents, and other devices such as rotational atherectomy, thrombectomy, or distal protection devices, has allowed treatment of complex lesions by means of the transradial approach, which can be learned in a relatively short period.

RATIONALE FOR THE TRANSRADIAL APPROACH TO PERCUTANEOUS CORONARY INTERVENTION

Anatomic Considerations

The radial and ulnar arteries are usually terminal branches of the brachial artery and originate below the elbow. In some cases, the radial artery originates from the upper brachial artery or even directly from the axillary artery. It follows the external margin of the forearm to reach the wrist, where it divides into two branches that join branches of the ulnar artery through the superficial and deep palmar arches. The palmar arches may also be irrigated by branches of the common interosseous artery, a higher branch of the ulnar artery. Coursing superficially all along this path, the radial artery is covered by the brachioradialis muscle proximally. It becomes very superficial and accessible in its 3- to 5-cm distal portion before the wrist, which is considered to be the puncture site. The satellite radial nerve changes direction at this point, making puncture-related nerve injury unlikely. The absence of major veins around the radial artery reduces the risk of arteriovenous fistula. Because of this anatomy, the transradial approach to PCI appears to be safe.

Feasibility

The feasibility and safety of the transradial approach to coronary diagnostic or interventional procedures have been widely demonstrated. The data from these studies are summarized in Table 29-1. Because the transradial approach requires some training,

Table 29-1.   Transradial Percutaneous Coronary Intervention Feasibility Studies

Study	Type of Procedure	N	Catheter Size (Fr)	Success Rate (%)	Access-Site Complication Rate (%)
Molinari et al[17]	Diagnostic±PCI in patients >70 years old	250	6	Unknown	1
Kiemeneij and Laarman[44]	Stenting	20	6	100	0
Kiemeneij et al[21]	POBA (?)	100	6	94	2
Kiemeneij and Laarman[45]	Stenting	100	6	96	3
Lotan et al[46]	Diagnostic±PCI	100	6	93	2
Saito et al[4]	Unselected patient PCI	1360	6/7/8	92	0.2
Kim et al[18]	Primary PCI	30	6	90	0
Louvard et al[47]	Primary PCI	277	6	95	0
Mulukutla and Cohen[48]	Primary PCI (GP IIb/IIIa inhibitors in 75%)	41	6	100	0
Valsecchi et al[19]	Primary PCI	163	6	97	0
Valsecchi et al[20]	Unselected				
	≥70 years old	323	6	98.8	0.4
	<70 years old	80	6	99	0

PCI, percutaneous coronary intervention; POBA, plain old balloon angioplasty.

experienced operators have higher rates of procedural success and lower operative durations and x-ray exposure times.[2]

Overall, the feasibility of the transradial approach for diagnostic or interventional coronary procedures is high (>90%), especially in experienced centers (>95%). In a series of 1119 consecutive South Korean patients, the mean radial artery diameter measured by ultrasound was 2.6±0.41 mm in men and 2.43±0.38 mm in women.[3] In another series of 250 Japanese patients, the radial artery diameter was larger than 7- and 8-Fr catheters in 71.5% and 44.9% of male patients and in 40.3% and 24% of female patients, respectively.[4] Although these data may not be extrapolated to all other populations, they underline the fact that the transradial approach can be used in most patients with 5-, 6-, or 7-Fr catheters. In some patients, 8-Fr catheters may be used if needed.

The transradial approach has been used for different types of procedures and with various devices, such as intravascular ultrasound (IVUS)–guided stenting, coronary brachytherapy, distal protection, embolectomy, rotational atherectomy, myocardial biopsy, and bifurcated stents. The approach is incompatible with the intra-aortic balloon pump and all other devices or procedures needing access that is larger than an 8-Fr catheter.

Transradial versus Transfemoral Approaches for Percutaneous Coronary Intervention

The transfemoral approach represents an easily accessible, superficial arterial access point, through which large catheters delivering all types of devices can be introduced. Compared with the transfemoral approach, transradial access is associated with fewer vascular complications, more comfort for patients, and the possibilities of rapid ambulation, lower procedure costs, and reduced length of hospitalization.

Several randomized trials comparing advantages and disadvantages of each method are summarized in Table 29-2.

A meta-analysis of 11 published and unpublished randomized, controlled trials, which included 3224 patients, showed that the overall rates of postprocedural major ischemic coronary events were comparable with both methods; the procedural success rate was higher with the transfemoral approach (98% versus 93%, P=.0009); and all studies and the pooled analysis demonstrated a significant advantage for the transradial approach in terms of bleeding complications, mainly an 89% risk reduction for entry-site complications (0.3% versus 3%, P<.0001).[5] The meta-analysis also shows a clear ongoing trend toward equalization of procedural success rates for the two approaches. This finding is probably explained by improvements in the materials and in operators' skills with experience. However, the average length of exposure to x-rays was longer for the transradial approach (8.9 versus 7.8 minutes, P<.001).

Many advantages make the transradial approach the method of choice for outpatient PCI, which has been reported to be highly feasible and safe.[6,7] The transradial approach is also of particular interest for patients at high risk for bleeding, such as elderly patients, women, those with renal failure, obese patients, or those on multiple antithrombotic agents, especially glycoprotein (GP) IIb/IIIa inhibitors. For example, the transradial approach has been associated with fewer vascular complications in obese patients (multivariate OR=0.12; 95% CI: 0.02 to 0.94; P=.043) in a retrospective series of 5234 diagnostic or interventional (56.6%) procedures,[8] as well as in the elderly (1.6% versus 6.5%, P=.03).[9] Other patients may be better served by the radial rather than femoral approach, including those with severe or proximal peripheral arterial disease, patients with bilateral aortofemoral bypass grafts, those with aortic aneurysms, and patients with a history of femoral complications

Table 29-2.   Randomized Trials Comparing Transradial and Transfemoral Approaches for PCI

Study	Type of Procedure	N	Successful Procedure		Access-Site Complication		Other End Points
			TR	TF	TR	TF	
Mann et al[49]	POBA	152	91%	96%	0%	5%	TR reduced length of stay and total cost
Kiemeneij et al[10]	POBA	600	92%	91%	0%	2%	Similar procedure, hospital stay, and x-ray exposure length
Benit et al[11]	Elective stenting	112	89%	98%	0%	10%	Similar procedure, hospital stay, and x-ray exposure length
Mann et al[50]	Stenting in ACS	152	96%	96%	0%	4%	TR reduced length of stay and total cost
Mann et al[51]	stenting TR vs. TF with Perclose	218			0%	3.4%	TR reduced length of procedure, hospital stay, and total cost Perclose: inadequate in 18%, failure of hemostasis in 10% of patients
Louvard et al[52]	Diagnostic± ad hoc PCI in 43%	210	100%	100%	2%	6%	TR reduced length of stay, total cost, and was patient preferred but increased x-ray exposure length
Saito et al[53]	Primary stenting	149	96%	97%	0%	3%	Comparable in-hospital MACE rates
Louvard et al[9]	PCI in patients >80 years old	371	89%	91%	1.6%	6.6%	Trend to longer TR procedure duration
Agostoni et al[5]	Diagnostic or PCI	2845	93%	98%	0.3%	2.8%	Shorter hospital stay, lower hospital costs, longer fluoroscopy times with TR

ACS, acute coronary syndrome; MACE, major acute coronary event; PCI, percutaneous coronary intervention; POBA, plain old balloon angioplasty; TF, transfemoral; TR, transradial.

after catheterization. The transradial approach is also of particular interest in the setting of primary PCI (see Tables 29-1 and 29-2) performed by experienced operators in patients treated by aggressive antithrombotic regimens, because life-threatening, access-site bleeding complications can be avoided by such an approach.

The RIVIERA PCI registry (unpublished data presented at the European Society of Cardiology, in Barcelona, Spain, in 2006) prospectively included 7962 unselected patients. Results showed that the transradial approach appeared to be an independent predictor of better in-hospital outcomes (OR for death or myocardial infarction=0.16; 95% CI: 0.05 to 0.50).

Transradial versus Transbrachial Approaches

Two randomized trials included a group of patients treated by means of a transbrachial approach. A randomized comparison of percutaneous transluminal coronary angioplasty by means of the radial, brachial, and femoral approaches (ACCESS study)[10] reported comparable procedural success rates, equipment use, and procedural and fluoroscopy time for the three approaches to PCI. The transbrachial approach was associated with higher rates of vascular complications compared with the transradial approach (2% versus 0%, P=.035). The Brachial, Radial, or Femoral Approach for Elective Palmaz-Schatz Stent Implantation (BRAFE) study compared transradial and transfemoral approaches with a transbrachial cut-down approach and reported no local vascular complications with the latter approach.[11] The brachial approach is not commonly used, and the percutaneous transbrachial approach appears to be a hazardous method. In a series of 55 patients

undergoing such an approach, the global and major complication rates of 36% and 6%, respectively, appear to be unacceptably high.[12]

Transradial versus Transulnar Approaches

The transulnar approach to coronary procedures has been feasible in 91% of patients after confirmation of adequate collateral radial artery circulation by the reverse Allen test.[13] The Transulnar versus Transradial Artery Approach for Coronary Angioplasty (PCVI-CUBA) study randomized 413 patients with a normal direct or reverse Allen test result to undergo coronary angiography, followed or not by PCI by means of the transradial or transulnar approach. The two methods were associated with similar access success (96% versus 93%), PCI success (96% versus 95%), and asymptomatic access-site artery occlusion (5% versus 6%) rates.[14] Vascular complications occurred only in two patients in the transulnar group. If confirmed by additional data, the transulnar approach appears to be an alternative to the transradial approach for PCI.

PRACTICAL CONSIDERATIONS FOR THE TRANSRADIAL APPROACH

Contraindications to the Transradial Approach

Contraindications to a transradial approach include the presence of a forearm arteriovenous fistula or proven absence of collateral ulnar circulation, which can be evaluated as described later. The transradial approach should be considered with caution and after assessing the possibilities of other access-site complications and the risk of radial access in end-stage renal disease patients with potential forearm arteriovenous fistulas and in patients with small or heavily calcified radial arteries.

Assessment of Ulnopalmar Arterial Arches

Assessment of collateral ulnar circulation is usually recommended before undertaking the transradial approach to PCI. Early postprocedural occlusion of the radial artery can occur in 0% to 19% of patients, depending on the clinical or ultrasound assessment of radial artery patency, the diagnostic or interventional type of procedure, the use of anticoagulation regimens, and the sizes of the catheters.[4,15-20] In 40% to 60% of cases, the pulse could be detected within hours to weeks after the occlusion, which remains asymptomatic in most patients.[21,22] Nevertheless, incomplete palmar arches[23] and rare cases of transient or definitive hand or finger ischemia leading to amputation have been reported, justifying systematic evaluation of the ulnopalmar arch before the radial puncture.[24] Although assessment of the collateral ulnar circulation is recommended, the low specificity of the Allen test and the absence of serious ischemic complications in many very large series of patients means that this recommendation is not followed in many centers regularly using the radial approach.

The Allen Test

The adequacy of the collateral ulnar circulation can be determined by using the modified Allen test (Fig. 29-1A and B). The test consists of the simultaneous compression of radial and ulnar arteries, followed by several flexion-extension movements of the fingers leading to blanching of the palm. The ulnar compression is then ceased. The time for restoration of color of the palm after the end of the ulnar artery compression defines the Allen test results: normal is less than 5 seconds, intermediate is 5 to less than 10 seconds, and abnormal is 10 seconds or more. The reverse Allen test, comprising the same steps with the exception of a transient radial instead of ulnar compression, can be used in the case of a transulnar approach. In clinical practice the transradial approach can be attempted in patients with normal or intermediate results. Although the prognostic relevance of the Allen test is still controversial, one study demonstrated reduced blood flow and increased capillary lactate levels in the thumb after 30 minutes of occlusive compression of the radial artery in patients with an abnormal Allen test result compared with those with a normal test result.[25] Although such findings suggest potential ischemic complications in patients with abnormal test results, the relationship of the findings to the safety of the procedure remains to be shown. An abnormal Allen test result should be considered a contraindication to the transradial approach and cause the operator to seek another access point. However, abnormal Allen test results have been

reported for about 6%[26] of patients referred for transradial coronary procedures.

Plethysmo-oximetric Test

A potentially more accurate method for the evaluation of the ulnopalmar arch may be the plethysmo-oximetric test (see Fig. 29-1C and D). The radial artery is compressed after the detector is positioned on the thumb. Persistent damping of the plethysmographic curve and a decrease in blood oxygen saturation signal inadequate ulnar collateral circulation. Barbeau and colleagues[26] compared this method with the Allen test in 1010 consecutive patients. The study showed that 6.3% of patients would be excluded based on the Allen test results, whereas only 1.5% had abnormal plethysmo-oximetric test results.

Direct assessment of the palmar circulation by color Doppler ultrasonography is another method for selecting candidates based on collateral circulation. It has been reported to be more accurate than the Allen test.[27]

Considering the exceptionally low rates of symptomatic radial artery occlusion-related complications among thousands of patients undergoing transradial procedures or radial harvest for coronary artery bypass grafting, the specificity of these tests remains doubtful. Because of the rare occurrence of radial artery occlusion and the exceptionally symptomatic character of such a complication, the prognostic value of the previously described tests has not been demonstrated, and many operators use the transradial approach without prior evaluation of the ulnopalmar arch. Nevertheless, the Allen test is recommended before all procedures.

Right versus Left Transradial Approach

Left radial access may have some advantages over the right transradial approach:

- More comfort and less risk in the case of hand ischemia for the right-handed majority of patients
- Easier coronary cannulation using standard Judkins catheters
- Less guidewire use
- Lower rates of unusual artery branching or vessel tortuosity, requiring less catheter manipulation
- Shorter procedure and fluoroscopy times
- Selective opacification of left internal thoracic artery bypass grafts

In a randomized trial comparing 232 left and 205 right transradial diagnostic procedures, the left approach was associated with shorter durations of catheter manipulation, procedure, and fluoroscopy and with lower rates of guidewire use, suggesting increased procedural efficacy.[28] Nevertheless, the right transradial approach is more ergonomic for the majority of operators, and the choice between the two approaches may not rely on clinical evi-

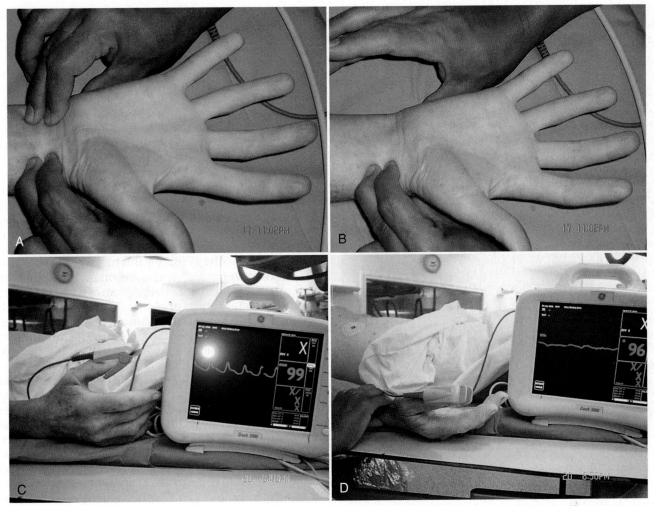

Figure 29-1. Ulnopalmar arch assessment. **A,** The Allen test: compression of the radial and ulnar arteries. **B,** The Allen test: homogenous recoloration of the palm after ulnar artery decompression in a patient with a normal palmar arch. **C,** Plethysmo-oximetric test: before radial artery compression. **D,** Plethysmo-oximetric test: dumping of the plethysmographic curve and decrease of oxygen saturation of the thumb after radial compression in a patient with an incomplete palmar arch.

dence. The choice of the side remains mainly a matter of operator preference.

Patient Preparation, Arterial Puncture, and Sheath Insertion

Explanations and premedication should be given to patients based on local practice. Because excessive anxiety may favor radial artery spasm, premedication may be used before radial artery puncture.

When possible, local anesthesia of the puncture site with an anesthetic cream administered 30 to 60 minutes before the puncture may improve the patient's comfort and reduce the risk of radial artery spasm and cannulation failure. Some operators recommend local vasodilation by apposition of a nitrate patch or paste on the puncture site.

The forearm should be shaved if necessary and aseptically prepared. Usually, the groins are also prepared in case of an eventual failure of the radial access or in case material larger than 7 Fr is needed.

The arm and wrist rest are supported by an armrest. A roll of gauze can be inserted under the wrist to make the puncture easier.

Before puncture, a dose of 0.5 to 2 mL of a 1% or 2% lidocaine solution is injected at the puncture site. The artery is punctured with a short, 18- to 19-gauge entry needle or a 20-gauge venous-type catheter entry needle, usually one with a 30-degree angle to the horizontal plane (Fig. 29-2). The needle is advanced until blood appears, and it is then stopped. The inner needle is then retrieved in case a venous-type needle is used. The needle or the catheter is then retrieved until pulsatile blood flow appears. A 0.025-inch, straight, preferably hydrophilic-coated guidewire is introduced through the needle or the catheter, which is then removed. A 70-mm-long arterial sheath is introduced on the wire eventually after making a very small, superficial skin incision. The use of hydrophilic-coated sheaths and the smallest sheath size— 4 Fr for diagnostic and 5 Fr for PCI, with further upsizing if needed to 6, 7, or 8 Fr—is recommended

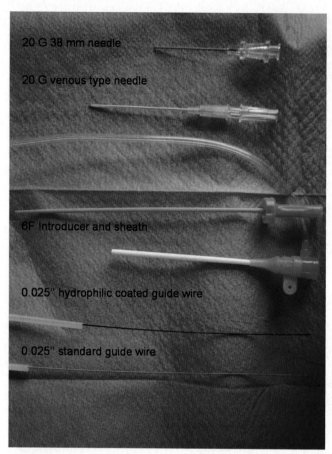

Figure 29-2. Transradial approach kit (Terumo Medical Corporation, Tokyo, Japan).

because these parameters are associated with less radial artery occlusion, spasm, and extraction force at removal.[29-31]

Prevention of Radial Artery Spasm

An intra-arterial spasmolytic drug or cocktail is injected through the sheath after its introduction. Different drug cocktails have been evaluated for various treatments, and they may include nitroglycerin, nitroprusside, molsidomine, phentolamine, diltiazem, or verapamil, used alone or in combination.

In a randomized trial including 406 patients, the rates of clinically or angiographically determined radial artery spasm were significantly reduced by the intra-arterial injection of 100 μg of nitroglycerin with or without combination therapy with 1.25 mg of verapamil (3.8% and 4.4%, respectively) compared with placebo (20.4%).[32]

In a randomized trial that included 1219 patients, the combination of 2.5 mg of verapamil and 1 mg of molsidomine was associated with less radial spasm (4.9%) compared with 2.5 or 5 mg of verapamil (8.3% and 7.9%) or 1 mg of molsidomine (13.3%) alone and compared with placebo (22.2%).[33] In another randomized trial, 2.5 mg of verapamil alone was more effective in the prevention of radial artery

spasm than 2.5 mg of the α-blocker phentolamine (spasm rates of 13.8% and 23.2%, respectively).[34]

The combination of the direct NO donor nitroprusside and nitroglycerin compared with either medication alone appears to be of no benefit in patients receiving intra-arterial heparin, lidocaine, and diltiazem.[35] The intra-arterial injection of verapamil, nitroglycerin, or a combination of the two seems to be associated with the lowest spasm rates and can be recommended for all patients after the introduction of the sheath in the radial artery.

Anticoagulation

Because of the potential risk of radial artery occlusion and the need for control of local bleeding complications, full-dose anticoagulation is administered after the arterial sheath is placed in the radial artery and before diagnostic and interventional procedures in patients who are not already on anticoagulation therapy. In a series of 415 consecutive patients, Spaulding and coworkers[15] showed a high correlation between heparin therapy and the prevention of postprocedural radial artery occlusion, occurring in 71% of untreated patients, 24% of patients receiving 2000 to 3000 IU, and only 4.3% of those receiving 5000 IU of unfractionated heparin.[15] No specific data concerning other regimens of anticoagulation in the specific setting of the transradial PCI are available. A small pilot study has reported the efficacy and safety of an ad hoc PCI strategy with bivalirudin after initial angiography with low-dose unfractionated heparin (1000 or 2500 IU).[36] This strategy requires validation by further studies. Full anticoagulation is recommended for all patients undergoing transradial procedures, and different regimens should be considered based on validated guidelines and local practice, such as fixed dose, weight-adjusted, or ACT-adjusted unfractionated heparin; weight-adjusted low-molecular-weight heparin; or bivalirudin. Anticoagulants may be injected through the arterial sheath or by means of venous access.

Glycoprotein IIb/IIIa Inhibitors and Fibrinolytics

Because of its extremely low rate of vascular-site complications, the transradial approach to PCI is the method of choice in the setting of highly active antithrombotic regimens and early or rescue PCI after thrombolysis.

In a series of mostly acute coronary syndrome patients undergoing PCI with abciximab through transradial (n=83) or transfemoral access (n=67), the 1-month major acute coronary events rate was similar for the two approaches. However, bleeding complications occurred in 0% of the transradial access procedures, compared with 7.4% of the transfemoral access procedures (P=.04).[37]

In another consecutive series of 119 patients undergoing primary PCI with systematic GP IIb/IIIa inhibition by abciximab, compared with the transfemoral approach (n=55), the transradial approach (n=67) was associated with fewer major access-site complications (5.5% versus 0%, P=.03), shorter hospital stays, and comparable procedural times but with higher x-ray exposure times and dose products.[38]

A retrospective analysis of post-thrombolysis rescue PCI with adjuvant GP IIb/IIIa inhibitor therapy in 111 patients, 47 of whom had a transradial approach, showed lower rates of access-site bleeding (0% versus 9%, P=.04) and lower rates of transfusion (4% versus 19%, P=.02) compared with procedures using transfemoral access. The fluoroscopy time, the contrast volume, and the time to first balloon inflation were comparable for the two approaches.[39]

A small, randomized pilot trial comparing transradial and transfemoral approaches for urgent PCI in 50 patients after thrombolysis (66% of patients) or GP IIb/IIIa inhibitors (94%), or both, reported comparable results in procedural success rates (only one failure in the transradial group) and vascular complication rates (one pseudoaneurysm in each group) but slightly longer average local anesthesia to first balloon time in the transradial group (32 versus 26 minutes, P=.04).[40] Despite the absence of adequately sized randomized trials in the specific setting of transradial PCI with GP IIb/IIIa inhibitors or after thrombolysis, the extremely low rate of access-site–related bleeding complications associated with such an approach firmly suggests its use in patients with these highly active antithrombotic therapies.

Guide Catheters

The guidewire used for the transradial approach is usually a standard 0.032- to 0.035-inch wire. In case of anatomic difficulties, such as radial or subclavian loops (Video 29-1), a hydrophilic-coated guidewire can be used. Progression of guidewires, especially with hydrophilic-coated guidewires, should be done under fluoroscopic control. The catheter exchange can be done using a long, 260- to 300-cm exchange guidewire or with a standard wire placed in the aortic root using a flush syringe to inject through the catheter, retrieved down to the tip of the wire. The syringe and the catheter are retrieved during the flush injection under fluoroscopic control. These exchange methods are extremely useful when difficult anatomic access is encountered.

Cannulation of the coronary arteries by the left or right transradial approach can be done using standard Judkins right and left catheters in most patients (Table 29-3). Cannulation of both right and left coronary ostia is similar for the left radial and the transfemoral approaches, and all standard catheters can be used through these approaches. In a series of 412 consecutive left transradial diagnostic procedures, only 5.5% of the left main and 3% of the right coronary ostia needed to be cannulated by catheters other than standard left or right Judkins coronary catheters.[15]

Using the right transradial approach, both left and right Judkins catheters usually end up in the right coronary or the noncoronary sinuses. The Judkins right catheters can be manipulated similar to the approach used for gaining transfemoral access, intubating the right coronary ostia after a slight clockwise rotation. For cannulation of the left main coronary ostium, clockwise rotation is needed initially, eventually followed by a gentle pull or push and then by a slight counterclockwise rotation.

In most high-volume centers, the guide catheters used are the long-tip Extra-backup 4 or 3.5 for left and Judkins right 4 for right coronary PCI. Several other guide catheters have been used for transradial PCI, such as the Amplatz left 2, the Champ, or the Multipurpose catheter, which is used for left and right transradial approaches. Specific transradial guide catheters have been developed, although most operators use standard catheters. The guide catheters

Table 29-3.   Guiding Catheters Used for Transradial Percutaneous Coronary Intervention

Guiding Catheter (Curves)	Left Coronary	Right Coronary	Bypass Grafts
Standard Catheters			
Judkins left (3.5 or 4)	+	– (+3.5 curve)	–
Judkins right (4)	–	++++	Left or right IMA
Amplatz left (2)	++	+	Left SVG
Amplatz right	–	+	–
Extra-backup (3.0 or 3.5)	++++	–	–
Multipurpose	+	+	Right SVG
Internal mammary	–	–	Left or right IMA
LCB/RCB	–	–/+	Left or right SVG
Specific Catheters			
Kimny (Boston Scientific)	+	+	–
MUTA L/R (Boston Scientific)	+	+	–
Radial curve (Boston Scientific)	+	+	–
Fajadet's L/R (Cordis)	+	+	–
Mann IM (Boston Scientific)	–	–	Left or right IMA
Barbeau L/R (Cordis)	+	+	–
Brachial type K (Terumo)	+	+	–
Tiger II (Terumo)	+	+	–

IMA, internal mammary artery; LCB, left coronary bypass; RCB, right coronary bypass; SVG, saphenous vein graft; –, unsuitable; +, suitable; ++, very suitable; ++++, recommended; –/+, suitable in some cases.

Table 29-4. Anatomic Abnormalities

Anatomic Difficulties	Solution
Forearm	
Lateral position of the radial artery on the wrist	Change puncture site or access site
Hypoplasic radial artery	Change access site
Radial artery remnants	Guidewire progression under angiographic control
Radial artery loops (see Fig. 29-4)	Hydrophilic-coated guidewires under angiographic control
Arm	
Brachial artery remnants	Guidewire progression under angiographic control
High origin of the radial artery	Guidewire progression under angiographic control
Brachial artery loops	Hydrophilic-coated guidewires under angiographic control or use of percutaneous coronary intervention 0.014-inch wire
Shoulder and Thorax	
Axillary or subclavian artery loops	Hydrophilic-coated guidewires under angiographic control, deep inspiration
Arteria lusoria (retroesophageal right subclavian artery)	Hydrophilic-coated guidewires under angiographic control, deep inspiration
Brachiocephalic arterial trunk abnormalities	Guidewire progression under angiographic control, deep inspiration
Posterior origin	
Bicarotidian trunks	
Thoracic aortic rotations	Guidewire progression under angiographic control, deep inspiration

used for the transradial approach are provided in Table 29-4.

The diameter of the guide catheter must be considered. In a randomized trial comparing 6- and 5-Fr guide catheters for PCI, 171 patients showed comparable procedural success rates (95.4% versus 92.9%) and almost statistically significant trends toward lower rates of radial artery occlusion (1.1% versus 5.9%, $P=.05$), spasm (1.1% versus 4.8%, $P=.08$), and minor nonsurgical access-site hematoma (1.1% versus 4.8%, $P=.07$) in favor of 5-Fr catheters.[41] The limitations of the 5-Fr catheters compared with the 6-Fr catheters are weaker backup due to higher flexibility of the catheters and incompatibility with some devices (e.g., rotational atherectomy, thrombectomy, and distal protection devices; larger than 4-mm coronary stents) or procedures (e.g., kissing stents, balloons for bifurcation lesions). Special attention should be paid to the possibility of bubble formation due to the Venturi effect when balloons or devices are rapidly removed from the catheter. Deep arterial intubation can be performed with 5-Fr catheters when needed, such as for crossing calcified coronary curves.

Difficult Anatomy

Variations in the arterial circulation of the upper limb are common among patients. During the initial phase of training in the procedure, failure of the transradial approach usually is caused by unsuccessful puncture, whereas for experienced operators, failure usually is related to difficult radial artery anatomy.

In a series of 1191 consecutive cases, the following anatomic situations were reported[3]:
- Anomalous upper branching of the radial artery: 3.2%
- High origin of the radial artery: 2.4%
- Radial or brachial artery tortuosity: 4.2% (S and Ω shapes, 31% each)

The most common anatomic variations and difficulties are listed in Table 29-5, and some examples are shown in Figures 29-3 to 29-6.

Repetition of Transradial Procedures

Because of the risk of postprocedural radial artery occlusion, although such complications are rare and usually asymptomatic, the repetition of transradial procedures may be questioned. In a series of 812 Japanese patients with a first successful transradial approach, the rates of access failure through the same radial artery in men and women were 3.5% and 7.9%, respectively, for the second attempt; 10% and 20% for the third attempt; and 30% and 50% for a fifth attempt.[42] These data should be considered with caution because the number of patients with multiple procedures was very low in the study. In another series of 117 repeated ipsilateral transradial procedures, the success rate for the second procedure was similar to the first, although the rates of postprocedural radial artery occlusion assessed by ultrasound were higher after the second procedure (2.6%, versus 0%, $P=.01$).[43]

These findings suggest that the transfemoral approach may be considered in patients with a low risk for femoral access-site complications and high risk for repeated procedures, such as those with complex, multivessel lesions with a high risk of restenosis or heart transplant recipients undergoing systematic annual angiography.

Complications

Transradial access is associated with a very low rate of major access-site–related complications. The most common complications are radial artery spasms (Fig. 29-7), which are often related to painful procedures or excessive catheter manipulations and asymptomatic, often reversible radial artery occlusion that may occur in 3.8% to 22% and 0% to 19% of patients,

Table 29-5. Transradial Approach-Related Complications

Complications	Frequency	Prevention	Solution
Asymptomatic loss of radial pulse (reversible in 50% of cases)	0-9%	Spasmolytic cocktail 5-Fr catheters	—
Radial artery spasm	4-23%	Avoid excessive catheter manipulation and change Preventive spasmolytic cocktail Hydrophilic-coated sheath and catheters	Spasmolytic cocktail, general sedation
Radial artery extraction (refractory spasm)	Exceptional	Avoid excessive force to remove catheter or sheath	Spasmolytic cocktail, general sedation
Radial artery false aneurysm	Exceptional	—	Local compression, surgery
Arteriovenous fistula	Exceptional	Avoid perforation	Local compression, surgery
Symptomatic finger or hand ischemia	Exceptional	Avoid radial puncture if inadequate Allen test result 5-Fr catheters Adequate antithrombotic cocktails Spasmolytic cocktails	Anticoagulation, surgery
Bleeding at the puncture site	0-2%	—	Local compression
Forearm hematoma	Exceptional	Control progression of guidewire, long arterial sheath to stop the bleeding in case of perforation, covered stent in case of uncontrollable perforation	Surgery, leeches
Vascular injury or dissection (radial, brachial, subclavian, carotid arteries)	Exceptional	Control progression of guidewire, especially hydrophilic-coated wires	Anticoagulation, stent, surgery

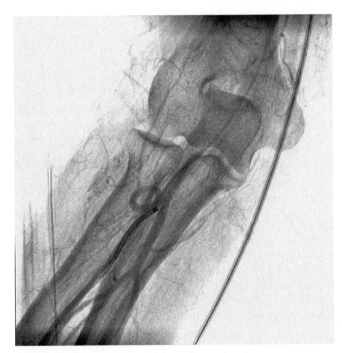

Figure 29-3. Radial artery: Ω-shaped complete loop.

respectively.[4,20-22,32-35] Female gender, diabetes, small body surface area, smoking history, diameter of the radial artery, and 6-Fr versus 5-Fr catheters have been related to radial artery spasm,[24,31,35,41] whereas the reported predictors of radial artery occlusion are small radial artery diameter, low difference between the radial artery and sheath diameters, diabetes, no or low-dose anticoagulation, and repeated procedures using the same access site.[15,22,24,41,43] A list of reported transradial access–related complications is provided in Table 29-5.

CONCLUSIONS

Bleeding complications after PCI have been associated with higher rates of serious clinical events, including death. The transradial approach, which is associated with a 89% risk reduction for entry-site complications compared with the transfemoral approach,[5] appears to be the easiest, safest, and most cost-effective way to control bleeding complications and to improve clinical outcomes after PCI. Transradial access is associated with easy entry-point hemostasis, more comfort for patients, quick postprocedural ambulation, and the possibility of outpatient procedures.

The only contraindication to using the transradial approach is inadequate ulnar collateral circulation detected by the Allen test, which continues to be recommended before the procedure even though many operators proceed without the test because of its unverified value in predicting postprocedural complications. Although the radial artery may appear to be a more difficult access site compared with the femoral artery, after initial training in the procedure and becoming aware of potential anatomic difficulties and ways to overcome such difficulties, the procedural success rates for the transradial approach

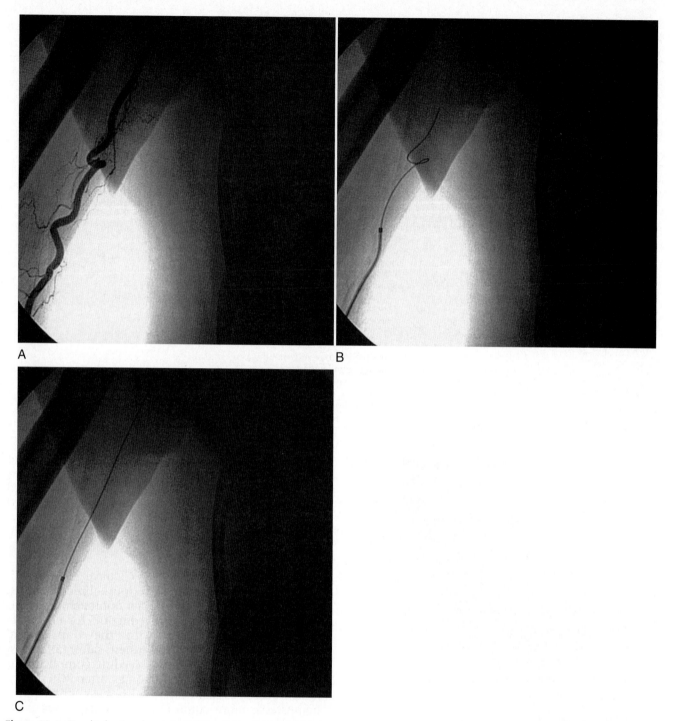

Figure 29-4. Brachial artery loop. **A,** Before wiring. **B,** During wiring. **C,** Artery unlooped by a hydrophilic-coated guidewire. (See Videos 29-2 and 29-3.)

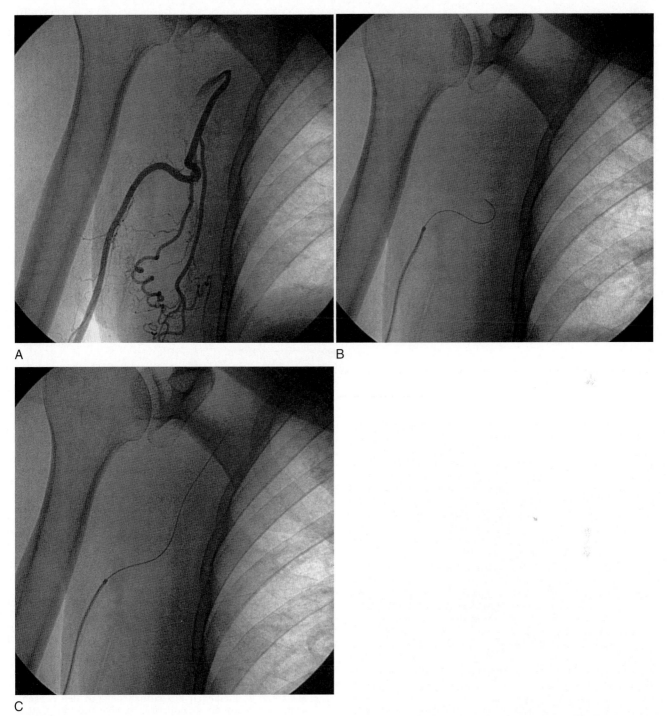

Figure 29-5. High brachial artery loop. **A,** Before wiring. **B,** During wiring. **C,** Artery unlooped by a hydrophilic-coated guidewire. (See Video 29-4.)

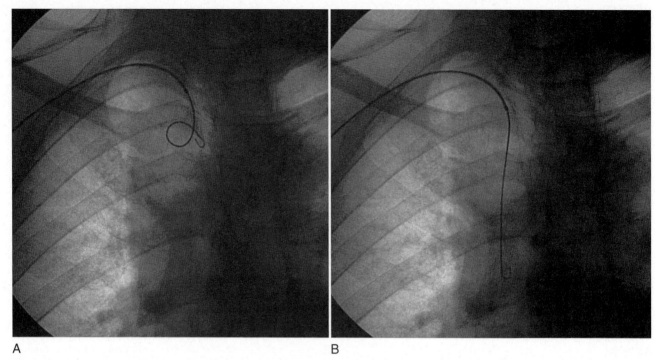

A   B

Figure 29-6. Subclavian loop. **A,** During wiring. **B,** Artery unlooped by the guidewire.

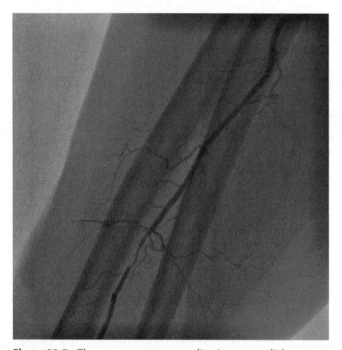

Figure 29-7. The most common complications are radial artery spasms. (See Video 29-5.)

become virtually identical to those for the transfemoral approach, without the access-site complications.

The transradial approach, which was initially considered to be an alternative to transfemoral access, has become the preferred method for PCI in many centers. Its choice as the first-line method is likely to be only a matter of time.

REFERENCES

1. Campeau L: Percutaneous radial artery approach for coronary angiography. Cathet Cardiovasc Diagn 1989;16:3-7.
2. Hildick-Smith DJ, Lowe MD, Walsh JT, et al: Coronary angiography from the radial artery—Experience, complications and limitations. Int J Cardiol 1998;64:231-239.
3. Yoo BS, Yoon J, Ko JY, et al: Anatomical consideration of the radial artery for transradial coronary procedures: Arterial diameter, branching anomaly and vessel tortuosity. Int J Cardiol 2005;101:421-427.
4. Saito S, Miyake S, Hosokawa G, et al: Transradial coronary intervention in Japanese patients. Catheter Cardiovasc Interv 1999;46:37-41; discussion 42.
5. Agostoni P, Biondi-Zoccai GG, de Benedictis ML, et al: Radial versus femoral approach for percutaneous coronary diagnostic and interventional procedures: Systematic overview and meta-analysis of randomized trials. J Am Coll Cardiol 2004;44:349-356.
6. Kiemeneij F, Laarman GJ, Slagboom T, van der Wieken R: Outpatient coronary stent implantation. J Am Coll Cardiol 1997;29:323-327.
7. Slagboom T, Kiemeneij F, Laarman GJ, van der Wieken R: Outpatient coronary angioplasty: Feasible and safe. Catheter Cardiovasc Interv 2005;64:421-427.
8. Cox N, Resnic FS, Popma JJ, et al: Comparison of the risk of vascular complications associated with femoral and radial access coronary catheterization procedures in obese versus nonobese patients. Am J Cardiol 2004;94:1174-1177.
9. Louvard Y, Benamer H, Garot P, et al: Comparison of transradial and transfemoral approaches for coronary angiography and angioplasty in octogenarians (the OCTOPLUS study). Am J Cardiol 2004;94:1177-1180.
10. Kiemeneij F, Laarman GJ, Odekerken D, et al: A randomized comparison of percutaneous transluminal coronary angioplasty by the radial, brachial, and femoral approaches: The ACCESS study. J Am Coll Cardiol 1997;29:1269-1275.
11. Benit E, Missault L, Eeman T, et al: Brachial, radial, or femoral approach for elective Palmaz-Schatz stent implantation: A randomized comparison. Cathet Cardiovasc Diagn 1997;41:124-130.

12. Hildick-Smith DJ, Khan ZI, Shapiro LM, Petch MC: Occasional-operator percutaneous brachial coronary angiography: First, do no arm. Catheter Cardiovasc Interv 2002;57:161-165; discussion 166.

13. Aptecar E, Dupouy P, Chabane-Chaouch M, et al: Percutaneous transulnar artery approach for diagnostic and therapeutic coronary intervention. J Invasive Cardiol 2005;17:312-317.

14. Aptecar E, Pernes JM, Chabane-Chaouch M, et al: Transulnar versus transradial artery approach for coronary angioplasty: The PCVI-CUBA study. Catheter Cardiovasc Interv 2006;67:711-720.

15. Spaulding C, Lefevre T, Funck F, et al: Left radial approach for coronary angiography: Results of a prospective study. Cathet Cardiovasc Diagn 1996;39:365-370.

16. Bagger H, Kristensen JH, Christensen PD, Klausen IC: Routine transradial coronary angiography in unselected patients. J Invasive Cardiol 2005;17:139-141.

17. Molinari G, Nicoletti I, De Benedictis M, et al: Safety and efficacy of the percutaneous radial artery approach for coronary angiography and angioplasty in the elderly. J Invasive Cardiol 2005;17:651-654.

18. Kim MH, Cha KS, Kim HJ, et al: Primary stenting for acute myocardial infarction via the transradial approach: A safe and useful alternative to the transfemoral approach. J Invasive Cardiol 2000;12:292-296.

19. Valsecchi O, Musumeci G, Vassileva A, et al: Safety, feasibility and efficacy of transradial primary angioplasty in patients with acute myocardial infarction. Ital Heart J 2003;4:329-334.

20. Valsecchi O, Musumeci G, Vassileva A, et al: Safety and feasibility of transradial coronary angioplasty in elderly patients. Ital Heart J 2004;5:926-931.

21. Kiemeneij F, Laarman GJ, de Melker E: Transradial artery coronary angioplasty. Am Heart J 1995;129:1-7.

22. Nagai S, Abe S, Sato T, et al: Ultrasonic assessment of vascular complications in coronary angiography and angioplasty after transradial approach. Am J Cardiol 1999;83:180-186.

23. Cambron BA, Ferrada P, Walcott R, et al: Images in cardiovascular medicine. Demonstration of unilateral absence of the palmar arch without collateral circulation. Circulation 2006;113:e6-e7.

24. Hildick-Smith DJ, Walsh JT, Lowe MD, et al: Transradial coronary angiography in patients with contraindications to the femoral approach: An analysis of 500 cases. Catheter Cardiovasc Interv 2004;61:60-66.

25. Greenwood MJ, Della-Siega AJ, Fretz EB, et al: Vascular communications of the hand in patients being considered for transradial coronary angiography: Is the Allen's test accurate? J Am Coll Cardiol 2005;46:2013-2017.

26. Barbeau GR, Arsenault F, Dugas L, et al: Evaluation of the ulnopalmar arterial arches with pulse oximetry and plethysmography: Comparison with the Allen's test in 1010 patients. Am Heart J 2004;147:489-493.

27. Yokoyama N, Takeshita S, Ochiai M, et al: Direct assessment of palmar circulation before transradial coronary intervention by color Doppler ultrasonography. Am J Cardiol 2000;86:218-221.

28. Kawashima O, Endoh N, Terashima M, et al: Effectiveness of right or left radial approach for coronary angiography. Catheter Cardiovasc Interv 2004;61:333-337.

29. Koga S, Ikeda S, Futagawa K, et al: The use of a hydrophilic-coated catheter during transradial cardiac catheterization is associated with a low incidence of radial artery spasm. Int J Cardiol 2004;96:255-258.

30. Dery JP, Simard S, Barbeau GR: Reduction of discomfort at sheath removal during transradial coronary procedures with the use of a hydrophilic-coated sheath. Catheter Cardiovasc Interv 2001;54:289-294.

31. Fukuda N, Iwahara S, Harada A, et al: Vasospasms of the radial artery after the transradial approach for coronary angiography and angioplasty. Jpn Heart J 2004;45:723-731.

32. Chen CW, Lin CL, Lin TK, Lin CD: A simple and effective regimen for prevention of radial artery spasm during coronary catheterization. Cardiology 2006;105:43-47.

33. Varenne O, Jegou A, Cohen R, et al: Prevention of arterial spasm during percutaneous coronary interventions through radial artery: The SPASM study. Catheter Cardiovasc Interv 2006;68:231-235.

34. Ruiz-Salmeron RJ, Mora R, Masotti M, Betriu A: Assessment of the efficacy of phentolamine to prevent radial artery spasm during cardiac catheterization procedures: A randomized study comparing phentolamine vs. verapamil. Catheter Cardiovasc Interv 2005;66:192-198.

35. Coppola J, Patel T, Kwan T, et al: Nitroglycerin, nitroprusside, or both, in preventing radial artery spasm during transradial artery catheterization. J Invasive Cardiol 2006;18:155-158.

36. Venkatesh K, Mann T: Transitioning from heparin to bivalirudin in patients undergoing ad hoc transradial interventional procedures: A pilot study. J Invasive Cardiol 2006;18:120-124.

37. Choussat R, Black A, Bossi I, et al: Vascular complications and clinical outcome after coronary angioplasty with platelet IIb/IIIa receptor blockade. Comparison of transradial vs transfemoral arterial access. Eur Heart J 2000;21:662-667.

38. Philippe F, Larrazet F, Meziane T, Dibie A: Comparison of transradial vs. transfemoral approach in the treatment of acute myocardial infarction with primary angioplasty and abciximab. Catheter Cardiovasc Interv 2004;61:67-73.

39. Kassam S, Cantor WJ, Patel D, et al: Radial versus femoral access for rescue percutaneous coronary intervention with adjuvant glycoprotein IIb/IIIa inhibitor use. Can J Cardiol 2004;20:1439-1442.

40. Cantor WJ, Puley G, Natarajan MK, et al: Radial versus femoral access for emergent percutaneous coronary intervention with adjunct glycoprotein IIb/IIIa inhibition in acute myocardial infarction—The RADIAL-AMI pilot randomized trial. Am Heart J 2005;150:543-549.

41. Dahm JB, Vogelgesang D, Hummel A, et al: A randomized trial of 5 vs. 6 French transradial percutaneous coronary interventions. Catheter Cardiovasc Interv 2002;57:172-176.

42. Sakai H, Ikeda S, Harada T, et al: Limitations of successive transradial approach in the same arm: The Japanese experience. Catheter Cardiovasc Interv 2001;54:204-208.

43. Yoo BS, Lee SH, Ko JY, et al: Procedural outcomes of repeated transradial coronary procedure. Catheter Cardiovasc Interv 2003;58:301-304.

44. Kiemeneij F, Laarman GJ: Percutaneous transradial artery approach for coronary Palmaz-Schatz stent implantation. Am Heart J 1994;128:167-174.

45. Kiemeneij F, Laarman GJ: Transradial artery Palmaz-Schatz coronary stent implantation: Results of a single-center feasibility study. Am Heart J 1995;130:14-21.

46. Lotan C, Hasin Y, Salmoirago E, et al: The radial artery: An applicable approach to complex coronary angioplasty. J Invasive Cardiol 1997;9:518-522.

47. Louvard Y, Ludwig J, Lefevre T, et al: Transradial approach for coronary angioplasty in the setting of acute myocardial infarction: A dual-center registry. Catheter Cardiovasc Interv 2002;55:206-211.

48. Mulukutla SR, Cohen HA: Feasibility and efficacy of transradial access for coronary interventions in patients with acute myocardial infarction. Catheter Cardiovasc Interv 2002;57:167-171.

49. Mann JT 3rd, Cubeddu MG, Schneider JE, Arrowood M: Right RADIAL ACCESS for PTCA: A prospective study demonstrates reduced complications and hospital charges. J Invasive Cardiol 1996;8(Suppl D):40D-44D.

50. Mann T, Cubeddu G, Bowen J et al: Stenting in acute coronary syndromes: A comparison of radial versus femoral access sites. J Am Coll Cardiol 1998;32:572-576.

51. Mann T, Cowper PA, Peterson ED, et al: Transradial coronary stenting: Comparison with femoral access closed with an arterial suture device. Catheter Cardiovasc Interv 2000;49:150-156.

52. Louvard Y, Lefevre T, Allain A, Morice M: Coronary angiography through the radial or the femoral approach: The CARAFE study. Catheter Cardiovasc Interv 2001;52:181-187.

53. Saito S, Tanaka S, Hiroe Y, et al: Comparative study on transradial approach vs. transfemoral approach in primary stent implantation for patients with acute myocardial infarction: Results of the test for myocardial infarction by prospective unicenter randomization for access sites (TEMPURA) trial. Catheter Cardiovasc Interv 2003;59:26-33.

CHAPTER

30 Surgical Standby: State of the Art

Paolo Angelini

KEY POINTS

- Surgical standby was originally instituted as a routine prerequisite for coronary angioplasty in the late 1970s.
- With the introduction of newer techniques and devices over the past 10 years, surgical standby has become almost obsolete. It is currently used in 0.1% to 0.3% of percutaneous coronary interventions (PCIs).
- Initial evidence suggests that low-risk PCIs can be safely performed in the absence of on-site surgical standby, but the discussion is ongoing.
- Complex anatomic or clinical conditions continue to indicate the need for selective on-site surgical standby and for improved methods of subclassifying PCI risk.

Catheter-based angioplasty of the coronary arteries was developed in the late 1970s, under the most unlikely conditions, by Dr. Andreas Grüntzig, who was initially an epidemiologist and a radiologist at the University Hospital in Zurich. In 1977, Grüntzig used a large-profile balloon catheter with a fixed-tip wire to treat coronary stenosis in an alert patient.[1] This crude device, designed to be used on the beating heart, was largely untested, and great institutional pressure soon came to bear on Grüntzig's work. His pioneering efforts would not have been possible without the generous support of Ake Senning and Marko Turina, who headed the cardiovascular surgical department.[2]

During Grüntzig's early experience with percutaneous coronary intervention (PCI), 17% of his patients needed emergency coronary bypass surgery because the procedure could not be completed successfully.[2] Consequently, surgical standby became a generally accepted prerequisite. During PCI, a cardiovascular surgical service had to be present on the premises (i.e., the on-site team); a surgical suite was kept staffed and a surgical team activated, ready for emergent use if angioplasty failed.[3] In the next decade, with improvements in technology and techniques, there was a substantial reduction in the need for emergency surgery, and the practice of surgical standby was gradually relaxed. For economical and practical reasons, it was considered sufficient to require only the presence of a cardiovascular department on the premises. The first available surgical suite and team would be activated on demand from the catheterization laboratory.[2-7] An important step in the evolution of this practice was that in 1993, the Federal Health Care Finance Administration, which administers Medicare and Medicaid services in the United States, ended reimbursement for standby services.[8]

Undoubtedly, the most innovative technology designed to substantially reduce complications during PCI was the Gianturco-Roubin stent, which was initially approved for "bailout" of sudden vessel reclosure during PCI.[9] Soon after this stent's introduction, stent placement became the standard practice for most PCIs (Fig. 30-1).[2,10-13] As a result of stenting, the in-hospital success rate for uncomplicated PCI in our experience rose from 91% in 1993 (before the introduction of stenting) to 96% in 1997 (when stents were used in 72% of PCIs) (Fig. 30-2).[8] The inability to deliver and deploy a drug-eluting stent is commonly considered a hallmark of an unsuccessful PCI. The incidence of emergency surgery for failed PCI decreased from about 10% in the early 1980s to 2.9% in the early 1990s and to 0.3% in the early 2000s (Fig. 30-3).[12]

Although the incidence of PCI-related Q-wave myocardial infarction and death have substantially decreased, complications requiring emergency surgical intervention continue to be reported, although rarely. In 2005, the American Heart Association (AHA) and American College of Cardiology (ACC),[11] the main de facto international authorities for establishing professional guidelines in cardiology, continued to recommend that all elective PCIs be done at

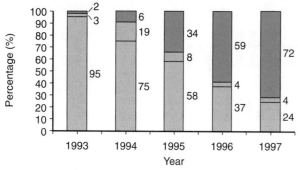

Figure 30-1. Yearly percutaneous interventions at St. Luke's/Texas Heart Institute, broken down by the type of intervention, as a percentage of each annual total. PCI, percutaneous catheter intervention.

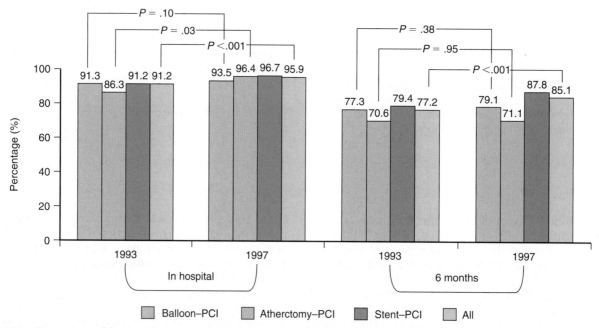

Figure 30-2. Comparison of freedom from major adverse events (i.e., death, myocardial infarction, redo balloon-PCI, or aortocoronary bypass), excluding angiographic failure, in hospital and at 6 months, after percutaneous catheter intervention (PCI) performed in 1993 and in 1997. Figures are provided for each type of PCI and for all PCIs.

institutions with well-developed cardiovascular services, although active standby is no longer required.

RISKS OF PERCUTANEOUS CORONARY INTERVENTION

Performance of a revascularization procedure in the catheterization laboratory on an awake, unsupported patient involves multiple risks, as listed in Table 30-1. Not all of these complications require urgent or emergent surgical intervention or can even be treated surgically. The indications for emergency surgery have been evaluated in detail by Yang and coworkers (Table 30-2).[12] The advisability of bailout surgical intervention requires careful evaluation in the specific context of a given case. The mortality rate for emergency coronary revascularization after failed PCI continues to average about 9% to 15% (Fig. 30-4).[11-14]

PCI sometimes inevitably necessitates emergency surgery because of myocardial compromise (e.g., acute myocardial infarction) or hemodynamic complications (e.g., shock, heart failure).

The management of anticoagulants during and after such emergency surgery is an especially critical issue because of contrasting simultaneous requirements. Typically, a newly deployed stent requires prompt antiplatelet treatment (i.e., a loading dose of clopidogrel and perhaps GP IIb/IIIa platelet receptor inhibitors), whereas postoperative bleeding necessitates protamine administration and aggressive platelet transfusion.

In view of the persistently high morbidity and mortality rates for emergency surgery for failed PCI and the gradually more aggressive indications for PCI in coronary artery disease, operators have taken advantage of an array of measures that have become available in the catheterization laboratory as adjuncts

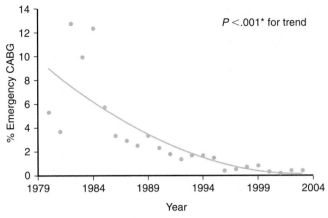

Figure 30-3. Percentage of patients requiring emergency coronary artery bypass grafting after percutaneous coronary intervention from 1979 to 2003 ($N = 23,087$). The Armitage test for trend is indicated by an *asterisk*. (From Yang EH, Gumina RJ, Lennon RJ, et al: Emergency coronary artery bypass surgery for percutaneous coronary interventions: Changes in the incidence, clinical characteristics, and indications from 1979 to 2003. J Am Coll Cardiol 2005;46:2004-2009.)

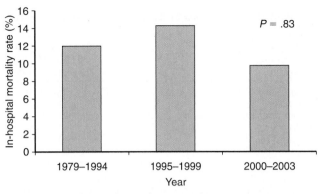

Figure 30-4. In-hospital mortality rates of patients requiring emergency coronary artery bypass grafting after percutaneous coronary intervention from 1979 to 2003 ($N = 335$). (From Yang EH, Gumina RJ, Lennon RJ, et al: Emergency coronary artery bypass surgery for percutaneous coronary interventions: Changes in the incidence, clinical characteristics, and indications from 1979 to 2003. J Am Coll Cardiol 2005;46:2004-2009.)

or alternatives to surgical options (Table 30-3).[2,15,16] An example of a case involving a major complication in which aggressive catheterization laboratory management obviated the need for bailout surgery is provided on the accompanying DVD (Video 30-1). Patients who have a high preoperative risk profile and those whose status may become compromised

Table 30-1. Risks of Percutaneous Coronary Intervention

1. Pain (ischemic or nonischemic)
2. Cardiovascular instability (e.g., onset of arrhythmias, hypotension, shock, cardiac failure) resulting from different mechanisms (mainly ischemia)
3. Myocardial ischemia, caused by multiple mechanisms, especially in
   a. Large arteries that become severely obstructed or occluded
   b. Small side or terminal branches that develop clots, plaque shifting, dissection, a clot/plaque embolism, or stent coverage or jailing
4. Guiding catheter-related dissection of a proximal vessel with possible extension to the ascending aorta
5. Guidewire-related perforation of a coronary branch, resulting in a subepicardial or intramural hematoma or hemopericardium
6. Balloon or other device-related trauma leading to perforation of a target coronary segment and causing a subadventitial hematoma, intramural hemorrhage, or pericardial bleeding
7. Intracoronary clot–related complications, with sudden (re)closure or stenosis
8. Coronary spasm; the no-reflow phenomenon
9. Retained intracoronary foreign bodies or devices
10. Entry-site or approach-vessel complications, mainly hematoma, arteriovenous fistula, pseudoaneurysm; dissection of an extracardiac vessel; clot- or spasm-related obstruction of a peripheral artery; extracardiac arterial perforation (e.g., retroperitoneal hematoma)
11. Systemic embolization (especially resulting in a stroke)
12. Hemorrhagic diathesis
13. Acute renal failure
14. Postoperative venous thrombosis at the entry site, with or without a pulmonary embolism

during PCI may need a higher level of protection than can be afforded by intra-aortic balloon counterpulsation.[17]

As a successor to the Hemopump (Nimbus Medical, Inc., Rancho Cordova, CA),[18] the portable cardiopulmonary support oxygenator/pump (C. R. Bard, Inc., Covington, GA),[19] and other early circulatory support systems, the TandemHeart Percutaneous Transseptal Ventricular Assist system (Cardiac Assist, Inc., Pittsburgh, PA)[20,21] (Fig. 30-5) appears to be the most important addition to the interventional cardiologist's armamentarium, offering more safety and control in the catheterization laboratory and thereby further eroding the need for surgical standby. The TandemHeart uses a venous access cannula that is advanced transseptally into the left atrium to sump arterial blood and a return cannula that is inserted into an iliac artery. Because blood is sampled from the left atrium, no oxygenator is required. A centrifugal, continuous-flow pump provides an output of up to 4 L/min, enabling critical support of the cardiac output, unloading of the left ventricle, and providing relief of pulmonary congestion, while effectively preventing the consequences of severe arrhythmias. Encouraging early results have been obtained in "nonoperable patients" with acute myocardial infarction complicated by shock or pulmonary edema, a low ejection fraction (<30%), or complicated left main coronary artery lesions.[22] The accompanying DVD provides a demonstrative case in which the TandemHeart enabled a salvage intervention in the catheterization laboratory (Video 30-2).

From a medicolegal viewpoint, before a PCI is carried out, it is important that the patient receive adequate, detailed information about the involved risks and the availability of corrective actions, including surgical standby. Alternative treatment options should be explained. Patients who are to undergo diagnostic coronary angiography and "possible PCI" should not be fully sedated until the specific intervention indicated by the angiography is clearly

Table 30-2. Indications for Emergency Coronary Bypass Surgery after Failed Percutaneous Coronary Intervention

	Periods		
Indication	**1979-1994** (*n* = 258 of 8905)	**1995-1999** (*n* = 56 of 7605)	**2000-2003** (*n* = 21 of 6577)
Abrupt vessel closure	55 (21%)	2 (4%)	3 (14%)
Dissection	88 (34%)	12 (22%)	3 (14%)
Incomplete revascularization	26 (10%)	7 (13%)	4 (19%)
Perforation	1 (0.5%)	1 (2%)	2 (9%)
Unsuccessful dilation	67 (26%)	28 (50%)	7 (33%)
Other	21 (8%)	6 (10%)	2 (9%)

Modified from Yang EH, Gumina RJ, Lennon RJ, et al: Emergency coronary artery bypass surgery for percutaneous coronary interventions: Changes in the incidence, clinical characteristics, and indications from 1979 to 2003. J Am Coll Cardiol 2005;46:2004-2009.

Table 30-3. Protective or Supportive Measures during Percutaneous Coronary Interventions

Preoperative Planning
1. Appropriate informed consent and communication with the family and patient
2. A clear plan of action before, during, and after percutaneous coronary intervention (PCI); considerations include
   a. Clopidogrel antiplatelet loading (dosing and time); IIb/IIIa platelet receptor inhibitors, and antithrombin medication
   b. The operative approach
   c. Target vessel and lesions and their diameters and lengths
   d. Types of required devices and the sequence for their use
3. Supportive or protective systems and techniques (if needed or possibly needed)
   a. Intra-aortic balloon counterpulsation
   b. Per-catheter hemoperfusion systems
   c. General anesthesia
   d. Percutaneous left ventricular support devices
   e. Surgical standby consultation

Perioperative Technical Considerations
1. Careful guiding-catheter management (i.e., avoiding proximal artery damage or obstruction)
2. Careful guidewire manipulation (e.g., avoiding perforation of small branches, induction of spasms, embolization)
3. Optimal anticoagulation and monitoring
4. Careful handling of side branches
   a. Double wiring, double stenting; recognition of essential versus expendable side branches; left main (and equivalent) stenting
   b. Use of filter wires
5. Predilation and postdilation, especially in stent PCI; use of intravascular ultrasound imaging
6. Follow-up postoperative observation in the catheter laboratory; evaluation of any new symptoms, the final angiographic or ultrasonographic anatomy, the electrocardiogram
7. Care of the vascular entry site; assessment of the anticoagulation status; intra-aortic balloon counterpulsation frequently used to treat hemodynamically unstable patients before, during, and after direct PCI

Table 30-4. ST-Elevation Myocardial Infarction: Prerequisites for Percutaneous Coronary Intervention in a Facility without an On-Site Cardiovascular Service

1. An experienced catheterization team is required.
2. An experienced operator should be specifically credentialed for percutaneous coronary intervention (PCI) and should follow a prudent protocol. The operator should regularly perform more than 75 elective PCIs per year at a remote surgical center.
3. A 7-day/week on-call schedule is needed for emergency, direct PCI.
4. A state-of-the-art catheterization laboratory should have digital imaging capability, a full array of interventional equipment, and intra-aortic balloon pump availability. This laboratory should perform more than 36 primary PCIs per year in patients with acute myocardial infarctions.
5. A proven plan is needed for transporting a patient to a cardiac operating room at a nearby hospital within 60 minutes, with appropriate hemodynamic support during transfer. The medical center should have a proven ability to perform balloon inflation within 90 minutes after the patient arrives.
6. The nonsurgical center should be committed to offering primary PCI for ST-elevation myocardial infarction patients as a treatment of choice, according to established protocols.
7. The program should be subjected to regular, periodic outcome and case-review analysis by a peer-review committee.

Data from Smith SC Jr, Feldman TE, Hirshfeld JW Jr, et al: ACC/AHA/SCAI 2005 guidelines update for percutaneous coronary intervention. J Am Coll Cardiol 2006;47:216-235.

myocardial infarction (not elective PCI) and only under the conditions listed in Table 30-4.

CONSIDERATIONS REGARDING THE SURGICAL STANDBY REQUIREMENT

The decision of the AHA/ACC[11] to continue recommending on-site surgical standby for elective PCIs was based on limited studies. In the future, this policy may change[23] after the publication of new, adequate data that reflect the improved results achieved by well-trained operators using contemporary equipment and techniques and that are currently available only for pilot studies.[14,24-26]

The Mayo Clinic reported a unique prospective investigation,[14] undertaken to evaluate 1000 PCIs carried out in a 150-bed community hospital coordinated with a tertiary care center 85 miles away (the Mayo Clinic's main campus). Unique conditions and protocols were realized by a team of operators trained and credentialed at the Mayo Clinic. The patients

explained. If that intervention involves an increased risk, a two-stage procedure should be considered. These interventions may necessitate an adequate discussion, perhaps including a preliminary surgical consultation, outside the catheterization laboratory. In particular, the patient should be aware of the availability of on-site surgical standby (or the lack of it), especially in cases of elective PCI. The 2005 ACC/AHA guidelines[11] allow the occasional use of facilities that lack an on-site cardiovascular service, but only in the context of PCI for an ST-segment elevation

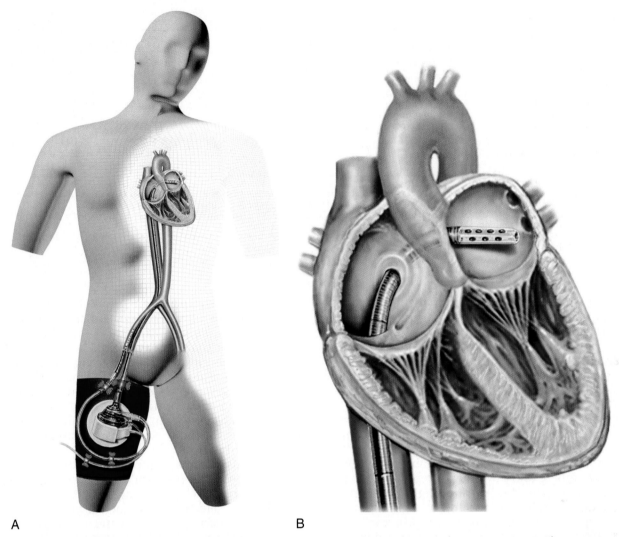

A   **B**

Figure 30-5. A, Schematic representation of the TandemHeart Percutaneous Transseptal Ventricular Assist system. **B,** The venous cannula is introduced percutaneously through a femoral vein and is advanced by means of a transseptal approach into the left atrium. The arterial sheath usually is introduced into the opposite femoral artery. The centrifugal pump (without an oxygenator) can handle outputs of 0 to 5 L/min. (Courtesy of Cardiac Assist, Inc., Pittsburgh, PA.)

included only persons with mild- to moderate-risk lesions undergoing elective or primary PCI, who were matched for preoperative risk with a similar population at the tertiary care center. All the patients received at least one stent (mean, 1.4 stents). Table 30-5 shows the comparative clinical outcomes. For the purpose of this discussion, the most important finding was that the mortality and morbidity rates in the two populations or environments were essentially identical. No patient from the community center needed to be transferred to the tertiary center for surgery, and "most of the deaths" were reported as "unrelated to procedural complications or the absence of on-site cardiac surgery."[14]

To appreciate how the lack of on-site surgical standby can affect a "real-world" PCI, we briefly review the experience at our hospital, a tertiary referral center with strong surgical and interventional cardiology services (data on file at St. Luke's Episcopal Hospital, Houston, TX) (Table 30-6).

Approximately 65 operators perform PCI under a wide range of clinical circumstances, and their surgical colleagues generally provide surgical standby under a "first available room" policy. This review involves a continuous series of 3653 PCIs performed during 2004 and 2005. In 12.5% of these cases, a surgical consultation was requested preoperatively, and surgical standby was arranged; in the other cases, no specific notice was provided to the surgical department before PCI was undertaken. The incidence of emergency surgery was 0.4% (11 of 1528 and 5 of 2125 in 2004 and 2005, respectively). For the patients with prearranged standby, the incidence of actual emergency surgery during those 2 years was similarly low (0.15% for patients with surgical standby and 0.3% for those without it). The mortality rate in the catheterization laboratory was 0.4% (13 of 3653) and was essentially for patients with acute myocardial infarction (about 8.5% of the patients underwent primary PCI for acute myocardial infarction). Even

Table 30-5. In-Hospital Clinical Outcomes

	Elective PCI			Primary PCI		
Variable	**SMH (n = 722)**	**ISJ (n = 722)**	**P Value**	**SMH (n = 285)**	**ISJ (n = 285)**	**P Value**
Angiographic success, n (%)*	707 (98%)	717 (99%)	.035	279 (98%)	280 (98%)	.76
Procedural success, n (%)†	686 (95%)	701 (97%)	.046	274 (96%)	266 (93%)	.085
In-hospital death, n (%)	1 (0.1%)	2 (0.3%)	.56	4 (1%)	10 (4%)	.050
Any in-hospital MI, n (%)	21 (3%)	15 (2%)	.27			
In-hospital Q-wave MI, n (%)	4 (1%)	0 (0%)	.019			
Recurrent in-hospital Q-wave MI, n (%)				1 (0.4%)	2 (1%)	.56
Any recurrent in-hospital MI, n (%)				1 (0.4%)	4 (1%)	.17
In-hospital emergency CABG, n (%)	1 (0.1%)	0 (0%)	.24	0 (0%)	0 (0%)	—

*Angiographic success defined as less than 20% residual stenosis (stent-treated lesion) or less than 50% residual stenosis (non–stent-treated lesion).
†Procedural success defined as angiographic success and without in-hospital death, any myocardial infarction, or emergency CABG.
CABG, coronary artery bypass grafting; ISJ, Immanuel St. Joseph's Hospital–Mayo Health System, Mankato, Minnesota; MI, myocardial infarction; PCI, percutaneous coronary intervention; SMH, St. Mary's Hospital, Rochester, Minnesota.
From Ting HH, Raveendran G, Lennon RJ, et al: A total of 1,007 percutaneous coronary interventions without onsite cardiac surgery: Acute and long-term outcomes. J Am Coll Cardiol 2006;47:1713-1721.

allowing for a wide spectrum of preoperative risk profiles, these numbers suggest that the current risk of major complications in the catheterization laboratory during PCI is quite low. The preoperative estimation of the risk of requiring emergency surgery is apparently still low, as evidenced by the equally low incidence of surgery in the patients with prearranged surgical standby compared with those without.

Reviews of mortality rates in surgical versus remote PCI centers continue to show that surgical centers have a definite, although small, advantage.[27,28] In analyzing the national Medicare database for 1999 to 2001, Wennberg and coworkers[28] reported that 943 hospitals were providing on-site surgical backup services and that 178 were not. In both environments, the mortality rate was similar for primary PCI in acute myocardial infarction, but it increased by 38% for elective PCIs performed at nonsurgical centers. In the opinion of the AHA/ACC's Writing Committee,[11] this difference is "small" in absolute terms, but it implies that elective procedures done without surgical standby involve a "medically unnecessary" increased risk.

In confirming the traditional requirement for surgical standby in elective PCI, the Writing Committee's leading concern was patient safety. The decision also appears reasonable, however, for discouraging the proliferation of sophisticated, expensive centers merely for convenience or profit, in a health care system such as ours, which essentially lacks a planning and prioritizing capacity.[29] In other settings (i.e., countries that have a national health care plan), discussions about the need for surgical standby may be less important in professional arenas, because the regulatory agency deals with these matters according to a comprehensive scheme.[30-35] In Canada, France, England, Italy, and Spain, the proportion of interventional centers without on-site cardiovascular services is approaching 50%.[29-35]

Prospective studies aimed at concluding the discussion about the need for surgical standby should avoid the reservations that are usually implied with respect to a selection bias. Such a bias tends to be seen in comparisons that involve centers in which well-trained interventionalists perform PCIs without on-site surgical services, but the selection criteria for intervention are prudent and restrictive (i.e., high-risk patients are routinely referred to a surgical center). This practice only confirms the need for the presence of surgical standby in the interventional cardiology arena. A possible option is to create a two-tiered interventional cardiology system in a given community; one center would have on-site cardiovascular services, and the other center would lack such services but would be coordinated with the first center. The nonsurgical center would be enabled to perform

Table 30-6. Percutaneous Coronary Intervention: The 2004-2005 Experience at the Texas Heart Institute

	Year		
Procedure	**2004 Apr-Dec**	**2005 Jan-Dec**	**Total**
Number of PCIs	1528	2125	3653
With surgical standby	241 (15.8%)	215 (10.1%)	456 (12.5%)
Without surgical standby	1287 (84.2%)	1910 (89.9%)	3197 (87.5%)
Emergency operations	11 (0.72%)	5 (0.24%)	16 (0.44%)
With surgical standby	6 (0.39%)	1 (0.05%)	7 (0.19%)
Without surgical standby	5 (0.33%)	4 (0.19%)	9 (0.25%)

PCIs, percutaneous coronary interventions.

low-risk PCIs in a continuous collaboration with the surgical center. The Mayo Clinic experience[14] could serve as a reasonable model in this respect.

CONCLUSIONS

Coronary angioplasty has reached a sufficiently mature stage of technologic and professional development, at least in centers of excellence, that operators can soon safely declare independence from surgical standby. Nevertheless, surgery continues to provide viable options for several types of patients with coronary artery disease. In particular, optimal treatment for multivessel coronary artery disease must be discussed in professional seminars and with patients in light of ongoing prospective and randomized studies that include the routine use of drug-eluting stents and arterial multivessel grafting.[36]

The relationship between interventional cardiologists and cardiovascular surgeons is likely to remain essential and privileged. The availability of on-site cardiovascular surgical standby will probably evolve to become more a sign of excellence (i.e., offering optimal coordination and continuity of service) than a condition for safe PCI. Safety in the PCI environment will increasingly depend on improved catheterization laboratory instrumentation, updated training, and ongoing education, as well as continual monitoring of quality and efficacy.

REFERENCES

1. Grüntzig AR, Senning A, Siegenthaler WE: Nonoperative dilatation of coronary artery stenosis: Percutaneous transluminal coronary angioplasty. N Engl J Med 1979;301:61-68.
2. Meier B: Surgical standby for percutaneous transluminal coronary angioplasty. In Topol EJ (ed): Textbook of Interventional Cardiology, 4th ed. Philadelphia, Elsevier Science, 2003, pp 475-479.
3. Angelini P: Complications during angioplasty. In Angelini P (ed): Balloon Catheter Coronary Angioplasty. Mount Kisco, NY, Futura, 1987, pp 135-154.
4. Ullyot DJ: Surgical standby for percutaneous coronary angioplasty. Circulation 1987;76:III-149-III-152.
5. Angelini P: Guidelines for surgical standby for coronary angioplasty: Should they be changed? J Am Coll Cardiol 1999;33:1266-1268.
6. Shannon FL, Sakwa MC: Emergency bypass surgery for failed PTCA. In Safian RD, Freed MS (eds): Manual of Interventional Cardiology, 3rd ed. Royal Oak, MI, Physicians' Press, 2001, pp 431-437.
7. Wilson JM, Dunn EJ, Wright CB, et al: The cost of simultaneous surgical standby for percutaneous transluminal coronary angioplasty. J Thorac Cardiovasc Surg 1986;91:362-370.
8. Angelini P, Vaughn WK, Zaqqa M, et al: Impact of the "stent-when-feasible" policy on in-hospital and 6-month success and complication rates after coronary angioplasty: Single-center experience with 17,956 revascularization procedures (1993-1997). Tex Heart Inst J 2000;27:337-345.
9. Macander PJ, Agrawal SK, Roubin GS: The Gianturco-Roubin balloon-expandable intracoronary flexible coil stent. J Invasive Cardiol 1991;3:85-94.
10. Shubrooks SJ Jr, Nesto RW, Leeman D: Urgent coronary bypass surgery for failed percutaneous coronary intervention in the stent era: Is backup still necessary? Am Heart J 2001;142:190-196.
11. Smith SC Jr, Feldman TE, Hirshfeld JW Jr, et al: ACC/AHA/SCAI 2005 guidelines update for percutaneous coronary intervention. J Am Coll Cardiol 2006;47:216-235.
12. Yang EH, Gumina RJ, Lennon RJ, et al: Emergency coronary artery bypass surgery for percutaneous coronary interventions: Changes in the incidence, clinical characteristics, and indications from 1979 to 2003. J Am Coll Cardiol 2005;46:2004-2009.
13. Seshadri N, Whitlow PL, Acharya N, et al: Emergency coronary artery bypass surgery in the contemporary percutaneous coronary intervention era. Circulation 2002;106:2346-2350.
14. Ting HH, Raveendran G, Lennon RJ, et al: A total of 1,007 percutaneous coronary interventions without onsite cardiac surgery: Acute and long-term outcomes. J Am Coll Cardiol 2006;47:1713-1721.
15. Zavala-Alarcon E, Cecena F, Ashar R, et al: Safety of elective—including "high risk"—percutaneous coronary interventions without on-site cardiac surgery. Am Heart J 2004;148:676-683.
16. Shannon FL, Sakula MP: Emergency bypass surgery for failed PTCA. In Safian RD, Freed MS (eds): Manual of Interventional Cardiology, 3rd ed. Royal Oak, MI, Physicians' Press, 2001, pp 431-437.
17. Trost JC, Hillis LD: Intra-aortic balloon counterpulsation. Am J Cardiol 2006;97:1391-1398.
18. Dubois-Rande JL, Teiger E, Garot J, et al: Effects of the 14F Hemopump on coronary hemodynamics in patients undergoing high-risk coronary angioplasty. Am Heart J 1998;135:844-849.
19. Teirstein PS, Vogel RA, Dorros G, et al: Prophylactic versus standby cardiopulmonary support for high risk percutaneous transluminal coronary angioplasty. J Am Coll Cardiol 1993;32:590-596.
20. Babic UU, Grujicic SN, Djurisic Z, et al: Non-surgical left-atrial aortic bypass. Lancet 1988;2:1430-1431.
21. Vranckx P, Foley DP, de Feijter PJ, et al: Clinical introduction of the TandemHeart, a percutaneous left ventricular assist device, for circulatory support during high-risk percutaneous coronary interventions. Int J Cardiovasc Intervent 2003;5:35-39.
22. Kar B, Adkins LE, Civitello AB, et al: Clinical experience with the TandemHeart percutaneous ventricular assist device. Tex Heart Inst J 2006;33:111-115.
23. Ryan TJ: Percutaneous coronary interventions without on-site cardiac surgery: A stretch for much-needed evidence. Am Heart J 2003;145:214-216.
24. Wharton TP Jr, McNamara NS, Fedele FA, et al: Primary angioplasty for the treatment of acute myocardial infarction: Experience at two community hospitals without cardiac surgery. J Am Coll Cardiol 1999;33:1257-1265.
25. Aversano T, Aversano LT, Passamani E, et al: Thrombolytic therapy vs. primary percutaneous coronary intervention for myocardial infarction in patients presenting to hospitals without on-site cardiac surgery: A randomized controlled trial. JAMA 2002;287:1943-1951.
26. Wharton TP Jr, Grines LL, Turco MA, et al: Primary angioplasty in acute myocardial infarction at hospitals with no surgery on-site (the PAMI-No SOS study) versus transfer to surgical centers for primary angioplasty. J Am Coll Cardiol 2004;43:1943-1950.
27. Lofti M, Mackie K, Dzavik V, et al: Impact of delays to cardiac surgery after failed angioplasty and stenting. J Am Coll Cardiol 2004;43:337-342.
28. Wennberg DE, Lucas FL, Siewers AE, et al: Outcomes of percutaneous coronary interventions performed at centers without and with onsite coronary artery bypass graft surgery. JAMA 2004;292:1961-1968.
29. Dehmer GJ, Gantt DS: Coronary intervention at hospitals without on-site cardiac surgery: Are we pushing the envelope too far? J Am Coll Cardiol 2004;43:343-345.
30. Baduini G, Belli R, de Benedictis M, et al: Coronary angioplasty in an Italian hospital without on-site cardiac surgery: The results and outlook. G Ital Cardiol 1994;24:1537-1539.
31. Meier B, Urban P, Dorsaz PA, et al: Surgical standby for coronary balloon angioplasty. JAMA 1992;268:780-781.
32. Iniguez A, Macaya C, Hernandez R, et al: Comparison of results of percutaneous transluminal coronary angioplasty with and without selective requirement of surgical standby. Am J Cardiol 69:1161-1165.

33. Coronary angioplasty: Guidelines for good practice and training. Joint Working Group on Coronary Angioplasty of the British Cardiac Society and British Cardiovascular Intervention Society. Heart 2000;83:224-235.

34. Turgeman Y, Atar S, Suleiman K, et al: Diagnostic and therapeutic percutaneous cardiac interventions without on-site surgical backup-review of 11 years experience. Isr Med Ass J 2003;5:89-93.

35. Loubeyre C, Morice MC, Berzin B, et al: Emergency coronary artery bypass surgery following coronary angioplasty and stenting: Results of a French multicenter registry. Catheter Cardiovasc Interv 1999;47:441-448.

36. Mercado N, Wijns W, Serruys PW, et al: One-year outcomes of coronary artery bypass graft surgery versus percutaneous coronary intervention with multiple stenting for multisystem disease: A meta-analysis of individual patient data from randomized clinical trials. J Thorac Cardiovasc Surg 2005; 130:512-519.

31 Late Stent Thrombosis

Anthony A. Bavry

KEY POINTS

- Although late stent thrombosis is relatively uncommon, it is a significant problem because of its associated high morbidity and mortality rates.
- Drug-eluting stents are at increased risk for late thrombosis compared with bare metal stents.
- Drug-eluting stents have largely been studied in stable patients with simple or focal lesions, but their unrestricted use in the setting of complex revascularization procedures may further potentiate late thrombosis.

- Additional risk factors that further increase the risk for late thrombosis include bifurcation lesions, in-stent restenosis, renal insufficiency, radiation therapy, adjacent vulnerable plaques, long total stent length, and penetration of a necrotic core.
- The optimal duration of dual-antiplatelet therapy is unclear, although the recommendation for 12 to 24 months of therapy or even longer appears reasonable.

Coronary stents were designed to reduce abrupt vessel closure and restenosis, but their initial introduction was associated with an unacceptably high rate of stent thrombosis.[1] Attempts to reduce stent thrombosis with aggressive anticoagulation were modestly successful, but this approach resulted in longer hospitalizations and more bleeding complications. The use of high-pressure balloon inflation coupled with dual-antiplatelet therapy reduced the incidence of stent thrombosis to less than 1%.[2,3] Despite these pharmacologic and technical advances, stent thrombosis remains a concern of coronary revascularization procedures, and increased attention has been given to this problem due to reports of very late stent thrombosis.

Although the greatest risk for stent thrombosis is in the first several weeks after percutaneous coronary intervention, late events also occur (Fig. 31-1).[4] Late thrombosis first gained attention with the use of intracoronary irradiation,[5,6] although most attention has focused on the use of drug-eluting stents. Despite the concern about late thrombosis, more than 1 million drug-eluting stents have been deployed worldwide, and they are used in more than 80% of current stent-based procedures.[7]

Stent thrombosis is a significant problem because of the associated high morbidity and mortality rates.[4] Late events are particularly troublesome because of their protracted course and unpredictable nature. Current percutaneous coronary interventions are more complex and are performed in sicker patients than earlier revascularization procedures. These factors may also be contributing to the incidence of late stent thrombosis. Given the vast number of revascularization procedures performed worldwide,

the impact of this uncommon but potentially deadly event is considerable.

Because stent thrombosis is often a catastrophic event, it is important to understand its epidemiology, predictors, and pathologic mechanisms for its occurrence. This chapter briefly reviews early stent thrombosis, but the primary focus is on late events. An understanding of late thrombosis may help to limit the occurrence of this problem while retaining the efficacy of percutaneous coronary interventions.

DEFINITIONS

Stent thrombosis is defined as an abrupt onset of cardiac symptoms (i.e., an acute coronary syndrome) along with an elevation in levels of biomarkers or electrocardiographic evidence of myocardial injury after stent deployment. A definite or angiographic stent thrombosis is accompanied by angiographic evidence of a flow-limiting thrombus near a previously placed stent. When an acute coronary syndrome exists, although an angiogram cannot be performed, the event is called a *possible* or *clinical stent thrombosis* if another cause for the acute coronary syndrome is unlikely. The former definition may lack sensitivity by underestimating the true stent thrombosis rate, whereas the latter definition may overestimate the true incidence of stent thrombosis.

There are limited data that clinical stent thrombosis is a reasonable surrogate for angiographically proven events. An analysis of more than 6000 patients in the bare metal stent era documented that 85% of clinical stent thromboses were able to be confirmed angiographically.[4] In contrast to events that do not occur in the context of an acute coronary syndrome,

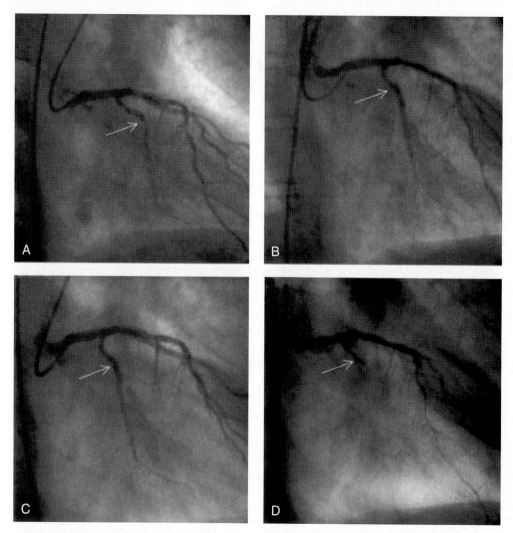

Figure 31-1. A, Baseline angiogram shows 95% narrowing of middle left circumflex coronary artery (LCx, *arrow*). **B,** Two overlapping Cypher stents (3 × 18 and 2.5 × 18 mm) *(arrow)* were placed. **C,** Stents *(arrow)* were widely patent 8 months after deployment and were similar to those in the angiogram in **B. D,** At 18 months, there was total occlusion at the site of the proximal Cypher stent *(arrow)*. (From Virmani R, Guagliumi G, Farb A, et al: Localized hypersensitivity and late coronary thrombosis secondary to a sirolimus-eluting stent: Should we be cautious? Circulation 2004;109:701-705.)

clinically silent vessel closures documented during follow-up angiography are usually not referred to as stent thromboses.

For drug-eluting stents, *premature interruption of antiplatelet therapy* is defined as cessation of one or both antiplatelet agents less than 6 months after implantation. Some investigators further specify premature interruption as less than 3 months for sirolimus and less than 6 months for paclitaxel, although for uniformity, the former definition is preferable. *Complete termination of antiplatelet therapy* is defined as interruption of antiplatelet therapy more than 6 months after implantation. In general, an *early stent thrombosis* is an event that occurs within 30 days of implantation (events within 24 hours of implant are called *acute thromboses,* and events occurring in 1 to 30 days are called *subacute thromboses*). Events that occur more than 30 days after stent implantation are *late thromboses,* and those occurring beyond 12 months are *very late thromboses.*

EARLY THROMBOSIS

A pooled analysis of 6186 patients performed in the bare metal stent era documented a 30-day incidence of stent thrombosis of 0.9%. Most events occurred within 1 week at a median of 1 day.[4] Using multivariate analysis, the investigators identified several predictors for early stent thrombosis. The strongest risk factor was residual dissection at the end of the procedure. The presence of dissection increased the hazard of stent thrombosis almost fourfold (OR = 3.8; 95% CI: 1.9 to 7.7). Smaller final lumen dimension and long stent length increased the risk for subsequent thrombosis. For every additional 10 mm in total stent length, there was a 30% increase in the hazard for early stent thrombosis (OR = 1.3; 95% CI: 1.2 to 1.5).

An intravascular ultrasound (IVUS) study in 7484 patients documented an incidence of subacute thrombosis within 1 week of revascularization of 0.4%.[8] This study similarly revealed residual dissection after stent deployment as the most frequent cause of early stent thrombosis. No cause for stent thrombosis could be identified in 22% of cases. Other important causes for early stent thrombosis included stent underexpansion, stent malapposition (i.e., positive remodeling), the presence of thrombus after stent deployment, tissue protrusion through stent struts, persistent slow flow, and reduced left ven-

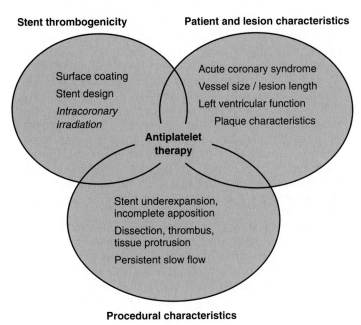

Figure 31-2. Multifactorial causes for early thrombosis. (From Honda Y, Fitzgerald PJ: Stent thrombosis: An issue revisited in a changing world. Circulation 2003;108:2-5.)

tricular function.[9] Relative resistance to antiplatelet therapy has also been described.[10] The hazard for early thrombosis appears to be similar for drug-eluting stents compared with bare metal stents as long as dual-antiplatelet therapy is continued.[11,12] Bare metal and drug-eluting stents are at increased risk for early thrombosis if dual-antiplatelet therapy is prematurely discontinued.[13,14]

Based on earlier studies from the bare metal stent era, Honda and Fitzgerald[15] proposed a multifactorial model for predicting early stent thrombosis (Fig. 31-2). During this period, most incidents of early stent thrombosis are caused by technical aspects of stent implantation. Late thrombosis is largely a separate phenomenon due to a different set of mechanisms from those of early thrombosis. The remainder of this chapter reviews the epidemiology, predictors, outcomes, and pathologic mechanisms of late thrombosis.

LATE THROMBOSIS

Late Thrombosis and Intracoronary Irradiation

The phenomenon of late thrombosis was initially recognized with the use of intracoronary radiation therapy. Although intracoronary irradiation decreased restenosis, this technology was limited by a high incidence of late thrombosis. One of the first descriptions of this association was an observational study on 108 patients with stable angina due to de novo coronary lesions who were revascularized with balloon angioplasty or stents followed by intracoronary beta radiation therapy.[5] In this study, ticlopidine was administered for 2 to 4 weeks along with indefinite aspirin therapy. The investigators docu-

mented a 6.6% incidence of late coronary occlusion and an 8.8% incidence of late stent thrombosis 2 to 15 months after the revascularization procedure. No placebo group was reported in this study, although the late thrombosis rate was much higher than expected in the era of high-pressure balloon inflation and dual-antiplatelet therapy.

The association between intracoronary irradiation and late thrombosis was strengthened by results of the GAMMA 1 clinical trial, which studied the efficacy and safety of gamma radiation for treating restenosis of stents in coronary arteries.[16] This trial randomized 252 patients with in-stent restenosis to receive intracoronary gamma radiation or to receive placebo. Both groups received conventional revascularization techniques, including balloon angioplasty, atheroablation (i.e., rotational atherectomy), or additional stents (i.e., bare metal). Study protocol required that patients receive aspirin indefinitely and a thienopyridine drug for 8 weeks. At a mean follow-up of 9 months, late thrombosis occurred in 5.3% of the radiation therapy group, compared with 0.8% of the placebo group ($P = .07$). Most stent thromboses occurred 3 to 4 months after radiation therapy, although one patient suffered an event 9 months after percutaneous coronary intervention. Late thrombosis frequently resulted in adverse cardiac events. The incidence of myocardial infarction was 9.9% in the radiation therapy group, compared with 4.1% in the placebo group ($P = .09$), and the incidence of death was 3.1%, compared with 0.8%, respectively ($P = .17$). All late events occurred in patients who had received an additional stent for the treatment of in-stent restenosis, and almost one half of all events were in patients who had prematurely discontinued their thienopyridine before 8 weeks. No late thromboses occurred while an individual was on dual-antiplatelet therapy.

The Washington Hospital Center performed a pooled analysis on six randomized, placebo-controlled trials enrolling 473 patients with in-stent restenosis who received intracoronary beta or gamma radiation therapy.[17] Aspirin and a thienopyridine were used for 1 month. The mean time of late thrombosis was 5.4 ± 3.2 months, and the incidence of late thrombosis was 9.1% among patients who received radiation therapy, compared with 1.2% among placebo patients ($P < .0001$).

The Washington Radiation for In-Stent Restenosis Trial plus 6 Months of Clopidogrel (WRIST PLUS) trial was designed to test whether prolonged dual-antiplatelet therapy could reduce the incidence of late thrombosis from radiation therapy to a more acceptable level.[18] These studies each examined 120 patients with diffuse in-stent restenosis treated by intracoronary gamma radiation. Patients were additionally revascularized by balloon angioplasty, atheroablation (i.e., rotational atherectomy), or additional stents (placed in approximately one third of each study cohort). In the WRIST PLUS study, patients were treated with dual-antiplatelet therapy for 6 months and compared with patients who received only 1 month of aspirin and a thienopyridine. At 6 months of follow-up, prolonged antiplatelet therapy was successful in reducing late thrombosis compared with a shorter duration of therapy. Late thrombosis after intracoronary irradiation was reduced from 9.6% with 1 month of dual-antiplatelet therapy to 2.5% with 6 months of dual-antiplatelet therapy (P = .02). The incidence of late thrombosis among placebo-treated patients was only 0.8%. Only one patient developed late thrombosis while on dual-antiplatelet therapy.

The Washington Radiation for In-Stent Restenosis Trial-12 (WRIST 12) trial tested an even longer duration (i.e., 12 months) of dual-antiplatelet therapy on reducing late thrombotic events after intracoronary irradiation.[19] At 15 months of follow-up, patients who received 12 months of dual-antiplatelet therapy had a 3.3% incidence of late thrombosis, compared with 4.2% for patients who received 6 months of therapy (P = .72). Although the incidence of late thrombosis was similar between the two groups, prolonged dual-antiplatelet therapy reduced major adverse cardiac events and target lesion revascularization compared with a shorter duration of therapy. Although these analyses showed that late thrombosis could be modulated with the use of prolonged antiplatelet therapy, an unacceptably high rate of late events continued to accrue from the use of radiation therapy despite 6 or even 12 months of dual-antiplatelet therapy. Despite efficacy with intracoronary irradiation, the safety issues pertaining to late thrombosis have contributed to this treatment modality falling out of favor.

Late Thrombosis and Bare Metal Stents

Patients with bare metal stents are often treated with a shorter duration of dual-antiplatelet therapy than those with drug-eluting stents because of the low risk for late stent thrombosis.[20] Accordingly, there are relatively few data on late thrombosis with the use of bare metal stents. One report on late thrombosis in nonirradiated patients with bare metal stents was issued from the Fuqua Heart Center.[21] Heller and colleagues[21] examined almost 1900 patients who had at least one coronary stent implanted. Patients were treated with aspirin indefinitely and with at least 3 weeks of a thienopyridine. Similar to previous reports, the investigators found that one half of all thromboses occurred within the first week after intervention, and two thirds occurred within 2 weeks. Late thrombosis continued to occur during 12 months of follow-up, producing an incidence of 0.65%. The mean time of late events was 2.4 months, with the latest occurrence at 9 months. The investigators were unable to identify any specific predictors for late thrombosis, although they documented a high incidence of mortality (16.7%), shock (16.7%), Q-wave myocardial infarction (58.3%), and stroke (8.3%) caused by late stent thrombosis.

Another study examined more than 1000 patients who received bare metal stents for complex coronary lesions and reported an incidence of late thrombosis of 0.76% over 13.6 months of follow-up.[22] Most revascularizations were performed for de novo lesions, and none of the patients had received brachytherapy. The mean time of late thrombosis was 3.6 months. Dual-antiplatelet therapy was used for only 2 to 4 weeks, although all patients were on aspirin monotherapy at the time of their events. Patients with early thrombosis received longer stents (i.e., 36 mm) and had a smaller final minimal lumen diameter (i.e., 2.8 mm) compared with those with late thrombosis (i.e., length of 21 mm and diameter of 3.2 mm). No specific predictors were identified for late thrombosis.

These two studies indicated that late bare metal stent thrombosis is uncommon (i.e., <1%) and found that the mean time of events is 2.4 to 3.6 months. Late thrombosis after bare metal stent implantation without prior radiation therapy that occurs beyond 6 months is rare, in contrast to the pattern of late thrombosis with drug-eluting stents.

Late Thrombosis and Drug-Eluting Stents

McFadden and colleagues[23] initially cautioned others about late thrombosis occurring after drug-eluting stent implantation in a 2004 publication. Their series reported two cases of late paclitaxel thrombosis (days 343 and 442) and two cases of late sirolimus thrombosis (days 335 and 375) that occurred after interruption of antiplatelet therapy. Although the incidence of late thrombosis was not reported because there was no control group, this article signaled a potential problem with drug-eluting stents that had not been previously seen with nonirradiated bare metal stents (Table 31-1).

The Thoraxcenter complemented this series by reporting their experience with more than 2000 patients who had received paclitaxel- or sirolimus-eluting stents.[24] Patients with paclitaxel-eluting stents were treated with dual-antiplatelet therapy for 6 months, and those with sirolimus-eluting stents were treated for 3 to 6 months (6 months of therapy was used for more complex procedures). Over a mean follow-up of 1.5 years, the incidence of late thrombosis was 0.35%. All stent thromboses manifested as ST-segment elevation myocardial infarctions. The mean time of stent thrombosis was 12.4 months, and two events occurred more than 2 years after implantation. The later two events also resulted in deaths of the patients. A common theme with all events was interruption of antiplatelet therapy. This study reinforced the idea that very late thrombosis can occur (i.e., around 1 year) and that events are frequently related to complete termination of dual-antiplatelet therapy.

Investigators at the Washington Center Hospital reported their experience with the use of drug-eluting stents in a cohort of 2974 patients who were treated with dual-antiplatelet therapy for at least 6 months.[25] During 12 months of follow-up, the incidence of late drug-eluting stent thrombosis was 0.27%, with a

Table 31-1. Incidence and Time of Late Drug-Eluting Stent Thrombosis

Study	Patients (N)	Type of Study	Clinical Follow-up (months)	Late DES Incidence (%)	Late BMS Incidence (%)	Mean Time of Thrombosis (months)
McFadden et al[23]	4	Case series	Approx. 12	NA	NA	12.5
Ong et al[24]	2006	Observational study	Mean, 18	0.35	NA	12.4
Kuchulakanti et al[25]	2974	Observational study	Mean, 12	0.27	NA	5.1
Park et al[26]	1911	Observational study	Median, 19.4	0.6	NA	6.1*
Rodriguez et al[27]	225	Observational study	Mean, 18.3	1.8	NA	11.7
Bavry et al[28]	6675	Meta-analysis of randomized clinical trials	Range, 9 to 48	0.5	0.28	18*
Iakovou et al[32]	2229	Observational study	Mean, 9	0.7	NA	1.9*
Moreno et al[43]	5030	Meta-analysis of randomized clinical trials	Range, 9 to 12	0.27	0.27	NA

*Median time of late stent thrombosis.
BMS, bare metal stent; DES, drug-eluting stent; NS, not available.

mean time of late thrombosis of 5.1 months. This contrasts with a report from the Asan Medical Center in Korea, where the investigators documented an incidence of late stent thrombosis of 0.6%, with a median time to thrombosis of 6.1 months.[26] Similarly, the third Argentine Randomized Trial of Percutaneous Transluminal Coronary Angioplasty Versus Coronary Artery Bypass Surgery in Multivessel Disease (Estudio Randomizado Argentino de Angioplastia vs. Cirugía [ERACI III]) registry reported a cumulative incidence of drug-eluting stent thrombosis of 3.1%, and late stent thrombosis of 1.8%. In 86% of these cases, stent thrombosis was related to interruption of antiplatelet therapy.[27]

Although all these studies are compelling, they are limited by uncontrolled or residual confounding factors that could influence the true incidence of late stent thrombosis. For example, current revascularization procedures frequently involve longer total stent length, are used in more complex lesions, and are performed in patients with greater comorbidities. The only way to correct for these confounding factors would be to perform an appropriately powered, randomized clinical trial with late thrombosis as the primary outcome. With such a low incidence for events, tens of thousands of patients would need to be enrolled to detect a clinically meaningful difference in the rate of stent thrombosis between drug-eluting and bare metal stents.

A meta-analysis was performed to examine the risk of late thrombosis in a clinical trial population.[28] This study examined 14 randomized clinical trials enrolling a total of 6675 patients. Each trial randomized patients to drug-eluting stents (paclitaxel or sirolimus) or to bare metal stents. Aspirin and clopidogrel were mandated for 2 to 3 months in the sirolimus trials and for 6 months in paclitaxel trials. Eight of the 14 trials reported more than 12 months of follow-up, and the longest duration of follow-up extended to 48 months. The overall incidence of late thrombosis among patients who received drug-eluting stents was 0.5%, compared with 0.28% among those who received bare metal stents (RR = 1.56; 95% CI:

0.77 to 3.16; $P = .22$). Although this association did not achieve statistical significance, there was a marked difference in the time of late stent thrombosis. The median time of late thrombosis was 18 months for drug-eluting stents and 3.5 months for bare metal stents ($P = .0003$) (Fig. 31-3). The latest documented thrombosis occurred 18.3 months after paclitaxel-eluting stent implantation, 25.8 months after sirolimus-eluting stent implantation, and 6 months after bare metal stent implantation. When the analysis was restricted to events after 6 months of follow-up, there was an almost fourfold increased risk for late drug-eluting stent thrombosis (Fig. 31-4). During this period, the incidence of late thrombosis among patients with drug-eluting stents was 0.44%, compared with 0.06% among those with bare metal stents (RR = 3.67; 95% CI: 1.30 to 10.38; $P = .014$). There

Median time of late stent thrombosis

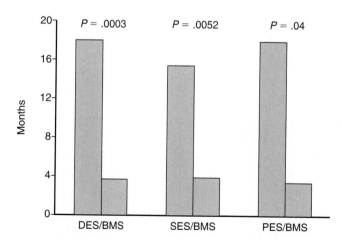

Figure 31-3. The course for drug-eluting stent (DES) thrombosis is markedly protracted compared with that for a bare metal stent (BMS). PES, paclitaxel-eluting stent; SES, sirolimus-eluting stent. (From Bavry AA, Kumbhani DJ, Helton TJ, et al: Late thrombosis of drug eluting stents: A meta-analysis of randomized clinical trials. Am J Med 2006;119:1056-1061.)

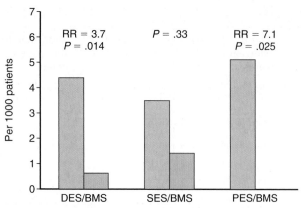

Figure 31-4. There is a 3.7-fold increased risk for late thrombosis (>6 months) for drug-eluting stents (DESs) compared with bare metal stents (BMSs). PES, paclitaxel-eluting stent; SES, sirolimus-eluting stent. (From Bavry AA, Kumbhani DJ, Helton TJ, et al: Late thrombosis of drug eluting stents: A meta-analysis of randomized clinical trials. Am J Med 2006;119:1056-1061.)

was a markedly increased hazard for very late thrombosis when the analysis was restricted to 12 months or more of follow-up (Fig. 31-5). During this period, there were no thromboses for the late bare metal stent group, but the incidence of late thrombosis for the drug-eluting group was 0.5% (RR = 5.02; 95% CI: 1.29 to 19.52; P = .02). This analysis showed that the incidence of late thrombosis for drug-eluting stents in a relatively low-risk clinical trial population is approximately 0.5%, even 1 year or more after stent implantation. This corresponds to a fourfold to five-fold increased risk for late thrombosis compared with the risk after bare metal stent implantation. Based on available data, the risk for thrombosis appears to be similar between paclitaxel- and sirolimus-eluting stents, although to definitively address this question, a large-scale, head-to-head trial with long-term follow-up would be required.[29]

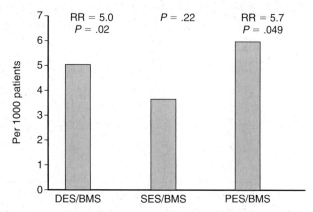

Figure 31-5. There is a fivefold increased risk for very late (>1 year) drug-eluting stent (DES) thrombosis compared with that for bare metal stents (BMSs). PES, paclitaxel-eluting stent; SES, sirolimus-eluting stent. (From Bavry AA, Kumbhani DJ, Helton TJ, et al: Late thrombosis of drug eluting stents: A meta-analysis of randomized clinical trials. Am J Med 2006;119:1056-1061.)

ANTIPLATELET THERAPY AND DRUG-ELUTING STENTS

Unfortunately, the meta-analysis previously described was unable to provide information on whether patients were on dual-antiplatelet therapy, aspirin monotherapy, or no antiplatelet therapy at the time of the stent thrombosis. Premature interruption of dual-antiplatelet therapy may carry the greatest hazard for late stent thrombosis, because several studies have reported this to increase the odds for thrombosis by as much as 25- to 90-fold (Table 31-2).

Complete termination of dual-antiplatelet therapy is often requested before surgical procedures or occurs because of patient noncompliance, but this also increases the hazard for stent thrombosis. In the Korean registry experience, 6.3% of patients had completely terminated antiplatelet therapy at a median of 7.4 months, and 3.3% of them experienced a stent thrombosis (HR = 5.4; 95% CI: 1.71 to 16.83).[26] In the e-Cypher registry, 4.4% of patients had completely terminated antiplatelet therapy by 1 year (43% remained on dual-antiplatelet therapy, and 52.6% were only on aspirin).[30] Using available data from published case reports, stent thrombosis may occur at a mean of 9.1 days after complete termination of dual-antiplatelet therapy (Table 31-3). Complete termination of dual-antiplatelet therapy may account for approximately one third of late events, which highlights the importance of proper patient selection for long-term use of antiplatelet therapy and effective communication with our surgical colleagues.[24,26]

Limited data are available on late stent thrombosis that occurs on aspirin monotherapy. These events appear to be more idiosyncratic in nature, because they have been described 1 to 92 weeks after termination of clopidogrel (Table 31-4). In the Thoraxcenter report, this accounted for most of the events. In this study, two thirds of stent thromboses occurred on aspirin monotherapy,[24] but in the Korean registry, only one third of events occurred on aspirin monotherapy.[26]

Although the exact frequency is unknown, late events have also been described on dual-antiplatelet therapy. In the Korean registry, an alarming one third of late stent thromboses occurred on dual-antiplatelet therapy.[26] This has previously been underappreciated and needs to be carefully monitored in the future.

OUTCOMES OF LATE THROMBOSIS

Late thrombosis is frequently a catastrophic event. The Washington Center Hospital identified late stent thrombosis as a significant predictor for both morbidity and mortality.[25] At 6 months of follow-up, stent thrombosis resulted in a 72% incidence of myocardial infarction, compared with 12% among those who did not have a thrombotic event (P < .001). Mortality was also significantly increased by stent thrombosis compared with no stent thrombosis (29%

Table 31-2. Predictors of Late Stent Thrombosis from Multivariate Logistic Regression

Study	Predictors	Hazard Ratio (95% CI)	Type of Stent
Waksman et al[17]	Intracoronary irradiation	7.5 (1.8 to 31.1)	Bare metal stents
	Treatment of in-stent restenosis with additional stent	2.55 (1.0 to 5.1)	
	Long coronary lesions	1.15 (1.0 to 1.2)	
Kuchulakanti et al[25]	Premature termination of antiplatelet therapy*,‡	4.7 (2 to 11)	Drug-eluting stents
	Bifurcation lesion*	4.4 (2.0 to 10.0)	
	Renal failure*	3.8 (1.2 to 11.3)	
	In-stent restenosis*	4.5 (1.8 to 11.4)	
Park et al[26]	Premature termination of antiplatelet therapy‡	24.8 (7.5 to 81.8)	Drug-eluting stents
	Renal failure	8.4 (1.8 to 39.1)	
	Primary stenting in acute myocardial infarction*	12.2 (1.7 to 89.7)	
	Total stent length (mm)*	1.02 (1.0 to 1.04)	
Ong et al[31]	Bifurcation stenting during acute myocardial infarction§	12.9 (4.7 to 35.8)	Drug-eluting stents
Iakovou et al[32]	Premature termination of antiplatelet therapy†	57.1 (14.8 to 220.0)	Drug-eluting stents
	Bifurcation lesion	8.1 (2.5 to 26.3)	
	Left ventricular dysfunction	1.06 (1.0 to 1.1)	
	Premature termination of antiplatelet therapy*,†	89.78 (29.9 to 269.6)	
	Renal failure*	6.49 (2.6 to 16.2)	
	Diabetes*	3.71 (1.7 to 7.9)	
Moreno et al[43]	Long stent length	Curve fit regression analysis	Drug-eluting stents

*Cumulative stent thrombosis that includes early and late thrombotic events.
†Premature termination defined as less than 3 months of dual-antiplatelet therapy for sirolimus stents and less than 6 months for paclitaxel stents.
‡Premature termination defined as less than 6 months of dual-antiplatelet therapy for sirolimus and paclitaxel stents.
§Early stent thrombosis.

Table 31-3. Late Events after Complete Termination of Dual-Antiplatelet Therapy

Case Report	Events (N)	Time of Stent Thrombosis (months)	Time from Antiplatelet Therapy Termination until Thrombosis (days)	Reason for Discontinuation	Stent Type
McFadden et al[23]	4	11.4	5	Urologic surgery	3.0 × 16 PES
		14.7	7	Gastrointestinal surgery	3.5 × 16 PES
		12.5	14	Patient noncompliance	3.0 × 33 SES
		11.2	4	Colonoscopy	3.0 × 18 SES
Ong et al[24]	3	2	5	Patient noncompliance	2.5 × 23 SES
		11	5	Surgical procedure	3.0 × 16 PES
		14.5	7	Surgical procedure	3.5 × 20 PES
Rodriguez et al[27]	4	6.8	7	Surgery	3.0 × 24 PES
		1.6	4	Urologic surgery	2.5 × 16 PES
		30.9	45	Gastrointestinal surgery	2.5 × 33 SES
		7.6	7	NA	2.5 × 23 SES
Waters et al[44]	2	8.1	7	Urologic surgery	3.5 × 13 SES
		17.8	13	Colonoscopy	3.3 × 23 SES
Stabile et al[45]	2	12	14	Patient noncompliance	3.0 × 33 SES
		11	4	Colonoscopy	3.0 × 18 SES
Nasser et al[46]	2	4	10	General surgery	3.0 × 18 & 3.0 × 33 SES
		21	10	Orthopedic surgery	3.0 × 13 SES
Lee et al[47]	3	8	3	Patient noncompliance	2.5 × 24 PES
		16	3	Gastrointestinal endoscopy	2.25 × 32 PES
		5	7	Patient noncompliance	4.0 × 12 & 3.5 × 32 PES

NA, not available; PES, paclitaxel-eluting stent; SES, sirolimus-eluting stent.

versus 5%, $P < .001$), as well as target lesion revascularization (32% versus 2%, $P < .001$). A registry study has reported late thrombotic events over 9 months of follow-up.[32] During this follow-up, stent thrombosis was associated with a 45% incidence of mortality. The e-Cypher registry has also reported high morbidity and mortality rates for thrombosis of sirolimus-eluting stents.[30] At 1 year of follow-up, stent thrombosis resulted in a 42% incidence of mortality and a 44% incidence of myocardial infarction.

The Prospective Registry Evaluating Myocardial Infarction: Events and Recovery (PREMIER registry)

collected data on 500 patients who received drug-eluting stents during an acute myocardial infarction and compared outcomes during the next year of those who discontinued thienopyridine therapy by 30 days and those who remained on dual-antiplatelet therapy.[33] The investigators found that 13.6% of individuals discontinued clopidogrel by 30 days, despite the recommendation for 3 to 6 months of therapy. Those who discontinued thienopyridine therapy were more likely to be elderly (64 versus 60 years, $P = .03$), less likely to have completed high school (73% versus 89%, $P < .001$), less often married (56% versus

Table 31-4. Late Events on Aspirin Monotherapy after Discontinuation of Clopidogrel

Case Report	Time of Stent Thrombosis (months)	Time from Termination of Clopidogrel until Thrombosis (weeks)	Stent Type
Ong et al[24]	7	4	3.0 × 68 PES
	6	3	3.0 × 32 PES
	8	8	3.0 × 20 PES
	25	76	3.0 × 46 SES
	26	92	3.0 × 36 SES
Waters et al[44]	6.4	1.7	2.5 × 13 SES
Lee[47]	13	28	3.0 × 24 PES
Karvouni[48]	17	32	3.0 × 8 SES & 2.75 × 8 SES
Kang[49]	14	6	3.0 × 32 PES

PES, paclitaxel-eluting stent; SES, sirolimus-eluting stent.

71%, $P = .01$), more likely to avoid heath care because of cost issues (24% versus 13%, $P = .02$), more likely to have preexisting cardiovascular disease (49% versus 30%, $P = .003$), and more likely to have anemia at presentation (19% versus 7%, $P = .001$). Not completing high school was the only factor independently associated with discontinuing thienopyridine therapy (OR = 1.79; 95% CI: 1.01 to 3.1). Discharge instructions and referral to cardiac rehabilitation reduced the likelihood of discontinuing thienopyridine. Premature discontinuation of thienopyridine therapy was associated with a ninefold increased hazard for death over the ensuing year. The 12-month mortality rate, adjusted for the propensity to discontinue thienopyridine therapy at 30 days, was 7.5% among those who discontinued medication and 0.7% for those who continued this medication (adjusted HR = 9.02; 95% CI: 1.3 to 60.6; $P = .02$). Premature discontinuation of thienopyridine also increased rehospitalizations (23% versus 14%; adjusted HR = 1.5; 95% CI: 0.78 to 3.0).

PREDICTORS AND MECHANISMS OF LATE THROMBOSIS

Angioscopic evaluation has revealed incomplete neointimal coverage and mural thrombi (not detected on angiography) 3 to 6 months after implantation of sirolimus stents.[34,35] Only 13% of sirolimus eluting stents had complete neointimal coverage, in contrast to bare metal stents, which all showed complete neointimal coverage with no angioscopic thrombi.[34] The Armed Forces Institute of Pathology has reported two valuable autopsy series on late stent thrombosis (Table 31-5).[36,37] One report is specific to bare metal stents[36] and the other to drug-eluting stents.[37] In the bare metal stent series, 13 cases of late thrombosis were described. No information on dual-antiplatelet therapy was given. The cause of death was mostly sudden cardiac death, with the remainder of deaths attributable to acute myocardial infarction and heart failure. Pathologic analysis revealed that delayed neointimal healing was present in every case of late stent thrombosis, except for one case that was characterized by diffuse in-stent restenosis. In the cases of delayed neointimal healing, associated risk factors for thrombosis included stenting near a bifurcation lesion, prior radiation therapy, disruption of a vulnerable plaque near the stent, and penetration of a stent strut deep into a necrotic core (Fig. 31-6). The mean stent length was 19.3 ± 9.3 mm, and the overall mean time from stent implantation to thrombosis was 3.6 ± 3.5 months, which is consistent with the time range reported in the earlier bare metal stent observational studies. Late thrombosis occurred relatively sooner when there was penetration into a

Table 31-5. Predictors of Late Stent Thrombosis from Case Series and Autopsy Studies

Study	Predictors	Type of Study	Stent Type
Farb et al[36]	Bifurcation lesion Radiation therapy Disruption of vulnerable plaque near stent Stent strut penetration of necrotic core Diffuse in-stent restenosis	Autopsy series	Bare metal
Jeremias et al[14]*	Premature termination of antiplatelet therapy	Case series	Sirolimus eluting
McFadden et al[23]	Interruption of long-term antiplatelet therapy	Case series	Drug eluting
Ong et al[24]	Interruption of long-term antiplatelet therapy	Case series	Drug eluting
Joner et al[37]	Long stent length Bifurcation lesion Localized hypersensitivity vasculitis Vessel malapposition or incomplete expansion Stent strut penetration of necrotic core Diffuse in-stent restenosis	Autopsy series	Drug eluting

*Early stent thrombosis.

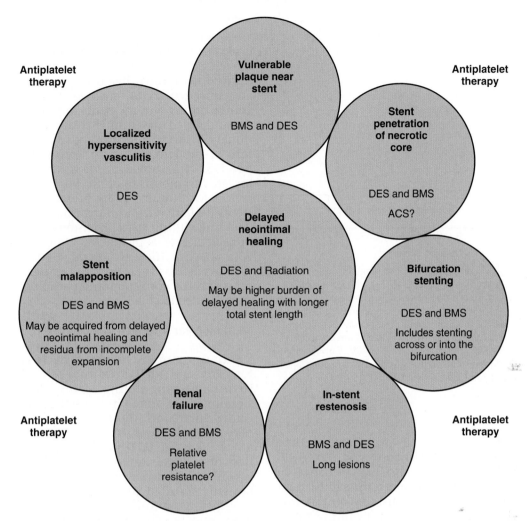

Figure 31-6. Multifactorial causes for late thrombosis. ACS, acute coronary syndrome; BMS, bare metal stent; DES, drug-eluting stent.

necrotic core (mean, 1.2 ± 0.007 months) or the stent was implanted near a bifurcation lesion (2.3 ± 1.3 months) and relatively later with prior radiation therapy (3.5 ± 1.1 months) or stent implantation near a vulnerable plaque (1.1-12.8 months). The one case of stent thrombosis that was caused by diffuse in-stent restenosis occurred at 10 months.

In the drug-eluting stent series, 14 cases of late thrombosis in paclitaxel- and sirolimus-eluting stents were described. One half of these events apparently occurred while patients remained on dual-antiplatelet therapy, 2 of the 14 events occurred on aspirin or clopidogrel monotherapy, and the remaining events occurred with no antiplatelet therapy. The cause of death was divided between sudden cardiac death and acute myocardial infarction. Mean stent length was significantly longer for drug-eluting stents than for bare metal stents (32.1 ± 17.3 versus 20.2 ± 11.9 mm, $P = .01$), and delayed neointimal healing was significantly greater among drug-eluting stents compared with bare metal stents. This was characterized by higher fibrin scores (2.3 ± 1.1 versus 0.9 ± 0.8, $P = .0001$) and percentage of struts surrounded by fibrin ($49.3\% \pm 30.8\%$ versus $22.3\% \pm 17.8\%$, $P =$

.0005). Eosinophilic infiltration was more common with drug-eluting stents than with bare metal stents. This was characterized by the number of eosinophils that surrounded struts (5.6 ± 11.1 versus 0.6 ± 2.3 per strut, $P = .01$). There was a lower percentage of endothelialized stent struts for drug-eluting stents compared with bare metal stents ($55.8\% \pm 26.5\%$ versus $89.8\% \pm 20.9\%$, $P = .0001$). Regardless of the duration of stent implantation, drug-eluting stents showed less endothelialization than bare metal stents, which were completely endothelialized by 6 to 7 months (Figs. 31-7 and 31-8). Even 40 months after stent implantation, drug-eluting stents were not completely re-endothelialized.

Neointimal healing was delayed in each case, along with an additional associated cause for late stent thrombosis: stent implant near a bifurcation lesion, localized hypersensitivity vasculitis, stent penetration into a necrotic core, stent malapposition (i.e., positive remodeling) or stent underexpansion, and diffuse in-stent restenosis (see Fig. 31-6). In 21% of patients, no additional cause for thrombosis was identified. There were two late bare metal stent thromboses in this series that were both caused by

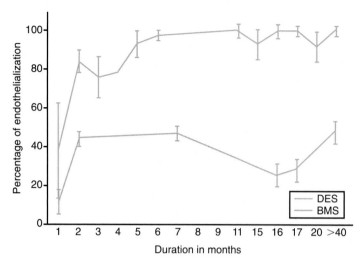

Figure 31-7. Line chart comparing the percentage of endothelialization in drug-eluting stents (DESs) with bare-metal stents (BMSs) as a function of time. The DESs *(purple line)* consistently show less endothelialization compared with BMSs *(blue line)*, regardless of the time point. Even beyond 40 months, DESs are not fully endothelialized, whereas BMSs are completely covered by 6 to 7 months. (From Joner M, Finn AV, Farb A, et al: Pathology of drug-eluting stents in humans: Delayed healing and late thrombotic risk. J Am Coll Cardiol 2006;48:193-202.)

diffuse in-stent restenosis. The overall mean time until drug-eluting stent thrombosis was 6.6 ± 4.6 months. Among those who also had evidence of hypersensitivity vasculitis, the mean time until stent thrombosis was 9.1 ± 6.9 months, and in patients with a bifurcation stent, the mean time until thrombosis was 10 ± 4.7 months.

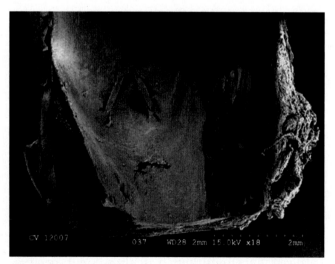

Figure 31-8. Scanning electron micrograph of a portion of a stent surface that has not become endothelialized 4 years after implantation. In this example, there is endothelial disruption over a stent strut. (From Sousa JE, Costa MA, Farb A, et al: Images in cardiovascular medicine. Vascular healing 4 years after the implantation of sirolimus-eluting stent in humans: A histopathological examination. Circulation 2004;110:e5-e6.)

In summary, the common pathologic finding of late stent thrombosis is usually delayed neointimal healing. Diffuse in-stent restenosis is seen in a minority of cases (see Table 31-5). For bare metal stents, delayed neointimal healing appears to be caused by an associated factor, such as radiation therapy. In contrast, drug-eluting stents appear to more directly cause delayed neointimal healing because no additional risk factors for thrombosis are identified in one fifth of the late events. In the multifactorial model (see Fig. 31-6), one or more risk factors are required for late thrombosis to occur, but when additional risk factors for thrombosis are present (e.g., drug-eluting stent implanted in a bifurcation lesion), the risk for late drug-eluting stent thrombosis may be markedly increased over a protracted time course compared with that for the bare metal stents. The following sections discuss the associated causes for late thrombosis and the corresponding pathologic mechanisms in more detail.

Stenting Near a Branch Vessel

Stenting near or in a branch vessel is a common cause for early and for late thrombosis with bare metal stents and drug-eluting stents. When bifurcation stenting is performed in the setting of an acute myocardial infarction, there is a further increase in the odds for early stent thrombosis (OR = 12.9; 95% CI: 4.7 to 35.8; $P < .001$)[31] compared with revascularization of a nonacute coronary syndrome bifurcation lesion, which increases the odds for late stent thrombosis by fourfold to eightfold (see Table 31-4).[25,32] Bifurcation stenting that employs the crush technique may be especially problematic (Fig. 31-9). This technique is associated with a high incidence (1.3%) of intraprocedural stent thrombosis and an even higher incidence (3.0%) of late stent thrombosis.[38,39] The mean time of late stent thrombosis was 4.6 ± 2.1 months, and most of the patients (4 of 7) were still on dual-antiplatelet therapy at the time of their events. Left main stem coronary artery bifurcation stenting was independently associated with increased odds for major adverse cardiac events (OR = 3.79; 95% CI: 1.76 to 8.14; $P = .001$).

The TAXUS V trial randomized 1172 patients with relatively complex coronary disease to paclitaxel-eluting stents versus bare metal stents.[40] One third of the overall cohort received multiple overlapping stents (mean stent length, 43.9 ± 10 mm). At 30 days of follow-up, overlapping paclitaxel stents were associated with a significant increase in myocardial infarction compared with bare metal stents (8.3% versus 3.3%, $P = .047$). Blinded angiographic evaluation revealed that paclitaxel stents compromised side branch vessels due to slow flow, a severe side branch stenosis, or side branch occlusion. Although the result raised concerns, it did not translate into an increased risk of late drug-eluting stent thrombosis. A registry study similarly revealed that overlapping left anterior descending artery drug-eluting stents (mean paclitaxel stent length, 74 ± 14 mm; mean sirolimus stent

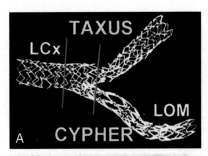
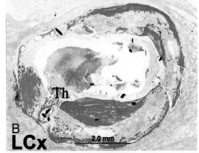
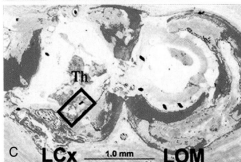
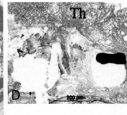

Figure 31-9. A 68-year-old woman had stents implanted in the left circumflex (LCx) and left obtuse marginal (LOM) arteries using the crush technique (Taxus in the LCx and Cypher in the LOM) 172 days before death. She presented 2 days before her death with acute myocardial infarction and was taken to the catheterization laboratory, where a 90% occlusion of the LCx near the LOM takeoff was found. The LCx artery was opened with balloon angioplasty, but the patient died of complications shortly thereafter. Cypher struts within LOM and fracture of the Taxus stent **(A)** after the LOM takeoff. Histologic sections taken proximal to the bifurcation **(B)** and at the LCx/LOM bifurcation **(C)** show thrombus (Th) in the LCx (i.e., Taxus stent), whereas the Cypher stent is covered by neointimal growth. Two struts with overlying thrombus are shown at high power **(D).** Notice the absence of neointimal coverage of the Taxus struts with overlying thrombus. (From Joner M, Finn AV, Farb A, et al: Pathology of drug-eluting stents in humans: Delayed healing and late thrombotic risk. J Am Coll Cardiol 2006;48:193-202.)

length, 84 ± 22 mm) were associated with a 17% incidence of in-hospital myocardial infarction.[41]

Although the crush technique is problematic, bifurcation lesions may be at risk for late stent thrombosis regardless of the revascularization technique employed. In the Armed Forces Institute of Pathology's report, several cases were described in which no stent was placed in the branch vessel or the branch vessel was stented without using the crush technique. In one case, a bare metal stent was implanted in the left anterior descending artery and a second stent was implanted in a major diagonal branch so that only a small portion of the diagonal stent protruded into the left anterior descending artery (Fig. 31-10). Numerous cases were also described in which a stent was not placed in the major branch vessel, but implanted only in the parent vessel. In this technique, the ostium of the side branch was partially or completely crossed (i.e., jailed) by the parent stent. Some cases in these reports include a jailed obtuse marginal artery (Fig. 31-11), a jailed diagonal artery (Fig. 31-12), and a jailed ostial circumflex artery (Fig. 31-13). All interventions were described as successful with Thrombolysis in Myocardial Infarction (TIMI) 3 flow in the jailed side branches at the completion of the procedure. Unfortunately, postprocedural information such as percent stenosis of the side branch was not given.

Pathologically, all thrombi that occurred in association with bifurcation lesions were occlusive and platelet rich. There was also evidence for ongoing thrombosis and delayed neointimal formation overlying the stent struts. This was characterized by fibrin deposition interspersed with smooth muscle cells and extracellular matrix. Bare stent struts were frequently observed across the ostia of the branch vessels.

Radiation Therapy

Observational studies and randomized clinical trials have documented an unacceptably high incidence of late stent thrombosis after intracoronary irradiation (see Table 31-4). In the Armed Forces Institute of Pathology's report, radiation therapy was a frequent cause for late thrombosis. Two cases in this report were caused by prior intracoronary irradiation, but one case was caused by external beam radiation therapy that was used to treat Hodgkin's disease. All cases were associated with fibrin-rich thrombi with infrequent platelet-rich thrombi (Fig. 31-14). One case was additionally characterized by diffuse in-stent restenosis. Most stent struts were uncovered, which provided evidence for delayed re-endothelialization and neointimal healing.

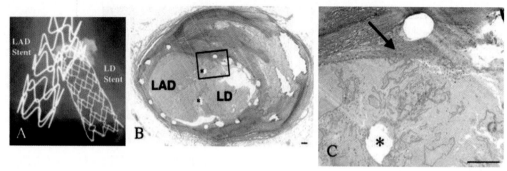

Figure 31-10. A 64-year-old man underwent bifurcation stenting of the left anterior descending artery (LAD) with an AVE stent and of the diagonal branch (LD) with an NIR stent after an acute myocardial infarction. Sudden death occurred 31 days after stenting. **A,** Postmortem radiography shows protrusion of the proximal portion of the LD stent into the LAD. **B,** Thrombosis of the bifurcation is demonstrated (low power, struts indicated by asterisks); the *boxed area* shows an organizing neointima with smooth muscle cells. **C,** High-power view of the boxed area shows proteoglycan-rich matrix *(arrow)* and platelet-rich thrombus around an uncovered strut *(asterisks).* (From Farb A, Burke AP, Kolodgie FD, Virmani R: Pathological mechanisms of fatal late coronary stent thrombosis in humans. Circulation 2003;108:1701-1706.)

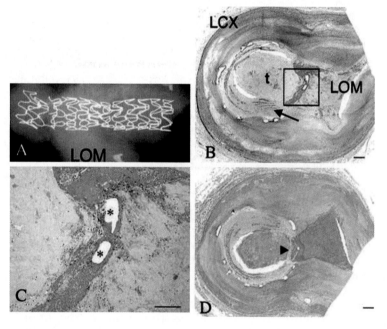

Figure 31-11. A 31-year-old man died suddenly 3 months after left circumflex coronary (LCX) stenting. Postmortem radiography **(A)** shows a Multi-Link stent crossing the ostium of the left obtuse marginal (LOM) branch. B and C are Low-power **(B)** and high-power **(C,** *boxed area* in **B)** views of an occlusive, platelet-rich thrombus (t) at the ostium of the LOM. Stent struts across the ostium **(C,** *asterisks)* are not covered by neointima. Struts in contact with the LCX plaque are covered with alternating layers of neointima and fibrin **(B,** *arrow).* A deeper section **(D)** demonstrates in-stent restenosis, a neointima with layered fibrin overlying the LOM ostium *(arrowhead),* and an occlusive luminal thrombus. (From Farb A, Burke AP, Kolodgie FD, Virmani R: Pathological mechanisms of fatal late coronary stent thrombosis in humans. Circulation 2003;108:1701-1706.)

Vulnerable Plaque Disruption Proximal or Distal to the Stent

An infrequent cause of late thrombosis is disruption of vulnerable plaque proximal or distal to the stented segment. Rupture of a vulnerable plaque near a stent can result in primary coronary occlusion and a subsequent acute coronary syndrome that is not directly attributable to the stent itself (Fig. 31-15). If a vulnerable plaque ruptures and tracks under a stent, it can destabilize an infrastent lipid-rich core and result in stent thrombosis.

Stenting a Necrotic Plaque with Lipid Core Prolapse

The Institute of Pathology identified deployment of a stent in a highly necrotic core as a risk factor for late thrombosis. In two cases, the lipid-rich core

occupied 38% and 47% of the total plaque area and caused prolapse of necrotic core between stent struts. This resulted in delayed healing of neointima overlying the stent and was characterized by an inconsistent smooth muscle cell–rich proteoglycan and collagen matrix (Fig. 31-16).

In-Stent Restenosis

In-stent restenosis is a predictor of late stent thrombosis. Analysis of patients who received drug-eluting stents identified the treatment of in-stent restenosis to be associated with more than fourfold increased odds for late thrombosis (OR = 4.5; 95% CI: 1.8 to 11.4; *P* = .0003) (see Table 31-4).[25] This was also shown in earlier intracoronary irradiation studies.[17] The pooled analysis from the Washington Center Hospital revealed a late thrombosis rate of 14.6%

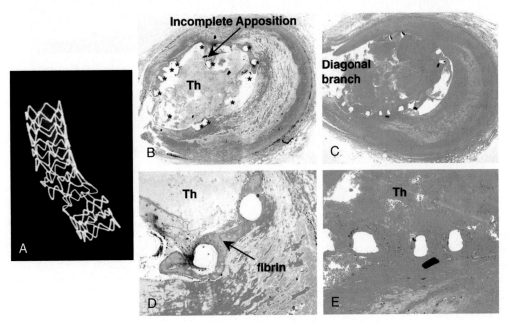

Figure 31-12. A 38-year-old woman had intervention in the proximal left anterior descending artery (LAD) with a 3.0 × 12 mm Taxus stent 6 months before death. The patient had been taking clopidogrel and aspirin, but she presented to a local emergency room with severe chest pain and shortly thereafter went into ventricular fibrillation and died. **A,** Radiograph of the stented LAD. **B** and **C,** Proximal and middle sections of the stented LAD stained with Movat pentachrome and hematoxylin and eosin, respectively. There is total occlusion of the lumen by platelet-rich thrombus (Th) and absence of healing of the stent strut regions, which are surrounded by fibrin. The stent is placed across the orifice of the diagonal branch. High-power views of the stent struts stained with Movat pentachrome **(D)** and with hematoxylin and eosin **(E)** show peristrut fibrin with an absence of smooth muscle, endothelial cells, and inflammatory cells. (From Joner M, Finn AV, Farb A, et al: Pathology of drug-eluting stents in humans: Delayed healing and late thrombotic risk. J Am Coll Cardiol 2006;48:193-202.)

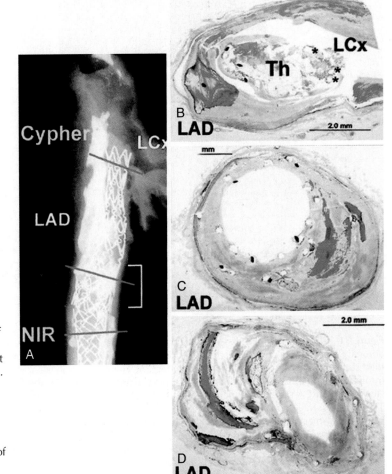

Figure 31-13. A 77-year-old man had two stents placed in the native left anterior descending coronary artery (LAD) for stable angina 450 days before sudden cardiac death. **A,** Radiograph of the LAD with two stents in place, a proximal Cypher and a distal bare metal stent (NIR). The Cypher stent struts protrude into the ostium of the left circumflex artery (LCx). **B,** Movat pentachromic–stained section taken from the proximal Cypher stent that is totally occluded by a platelet-rich thrombus *(asterisks)*. **C,** Distally, the stent is patent, with minimal neointimal tissue growth. **D,** The NIR stent in the distal LAD demonstrates 50% in-stent area stenosis consisting of neointimal tissue composed of smooth muscle cells in a proteoglycan and collagen matrix with an absence of fibrin. (From Joner M, Finn AV, Farb A, et al: Pathology of drug-eluting stents in humans: Delayed healing and late thrombotic risk. J Am Coll Cardiol 2006;48:193-202.)

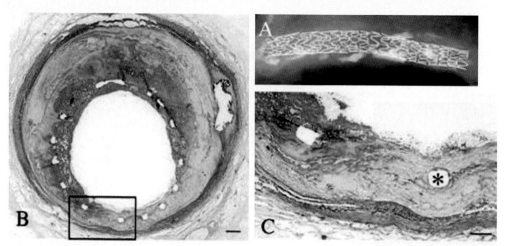

Figure 31-14. A 53-year-old woman presented with an acute myocardial infarction and underwent left anterior descending artery (LAD) stenting 18 weeks antemortem. Mediastinal adenopathy was observed at the time of stenting, and she was diagnosed with stage IIIB Hodgkin's disease (treated with chemotherapy and 20 Gy of mediastinal radiation therapy). Fourteen days antemortem, she presented with an acute myocardial infarction and cardiogenic shock. Angiography showed LAD stent occlusion, which was treated with balloon angioplasty. The patient died of multiorgan failure. **A,** At autopsy, a Multi-Link stent was identified in the proximal LAD. **B,** A fibrin-rich, nonocclusive mural thrombus was focally present between the stent and the underlying vessel. **C,** Most stent struts were uncovered by neointima except for those indicated (*asterisk* in **C,** *boxed area* in B). (From Farb A, Burke AP, Kolodgie FD, Virmani R: Pathological mechanisms of fatal late coronary stent thrombosis in humans. Circulation 2003;108:1701-1706.)

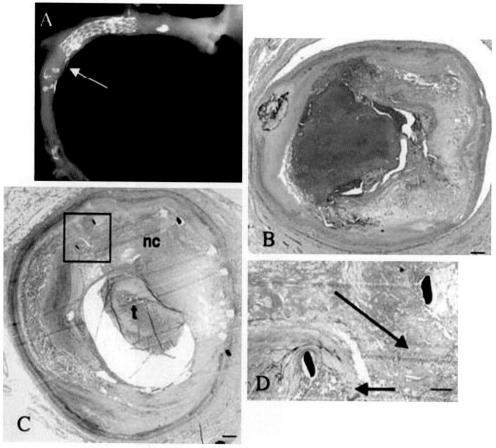

Figure 31-15. A 61-year-old man with angina after myocardial infarction underwent stenting of 90% stenotic lesions in middle right coronary artery (RCA) and middle left anterior descending artery (LAD). He presented with asymptomatic ventricular tachycardia and died suddenly 1 day later (32 days after stenting). **A,** The BX Velocity stent is shown in the middle RCA. **B,** Plaque rupture and acute thrombosis of the RCA were present in a lipid-rich plaque just distal to the RCA stent (*arrow* in **A**). **C,** A subocclusive thrombus (t) is shown in the RCA stent; the underlying plaque is markedly necrotic, with stent struts deeply embedded into the necrotic core (nc). The intimal surface remained unhealed. Stent struts were covered by a fibrin-rich thrombus, and a confluent smooth muscle cell–rich extracellular matrix had not formed. **D,** High-power view (of *boxed area* in **C**) shows fibrous cap rupture *(short arrow)* and plaque prolapse *(long arrow)* covered by fibrin thrombus. The LAD stent (not shown) was widely patent, with a healing neointima overlying the stent struts. (From Farb A, Burke AP, Kolodgie FD, Virmani R: Pathological mechanisms of fatal late coronary stent thrombosis in humans. Circulation 2003;108:1701-1706.)

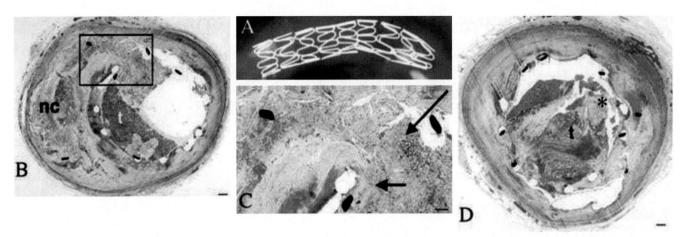

Figure 31-16. A 59-year-old man with angina and a positive stress test result underwent left anterior descending artery stenting with an AVE stent **(A)** and died suddenly 33 days later. The proximal portion of the stent **(B)** demonstrates a large necrotic core (nc), extensive plaque prolapse, and a subocclusive thrombus (t). The *boxed area* in **B** (magnified in **C**) shows the ruptured fibrous cap *(short arrow)* and plaque prolapse between struts *(long arrow)*; neointima is absent. An occlusive thrombus (t) is present in an adjacent section **(D)**, and plaque prolapse is indicated *(asterisk)*. (From Farb A, Burke AP, Kolodgie FD, Virmani R: Pathological mechanisms of fatal late coronary stent thrombosis in humans. Circulation 2003;108:1701-1706.)

among irradiated patients who received new stents compared with 3.8% among irradiated patients who did not receive new stents. This translated into more than twofold increased odds for late thrombosis from the treatment of in-stent restenosis with the use of additional stents (OR = 2.55; 95%CI: 1.0 to 5.1; P = .04). The development of diffuse in-stent restenosis can also lead to late thrombosis. Histopathologic analysis has revealed that diffuse and extensive in-stent restenosis is characterized by fibrin-rich thrombi with focal hemorrhage into infrastent plaques. Delayed neointimal healing does not appear to be a characteristic of this cause of late thrombosis.

Localized Hypersensitivity Vasculitis

A localized hypersensitivity reaction characterized by extensive eosinophilic infiltration has been described after implantation of drug-eluting stents (Fig. 31-17). Virmani and colleagues[42] first brought attention to this problem by reporting the histopathologic findings 18 months after an individual received a sirolimus-eluting stent for unstable angina. The patient was enrolled in the Sirolimus-Eluting Bx-Velocity Balloon Expandable Stent in the Treatment of Patients with De Novo Native Coronary Artery Lesions (E-SIRIUS) trial, which afforded baseline and follow-up angiograms and IVUS analysis (see Fig. 31-1). At the 8-month follow-up, there was minimal restenosis, but IVUS demonstrated positive arterial wall remodeling that resulted in malapposition of the stented segment. At 18 months, the patient suffered stent thrombosis and died during attempted revascularization. An autopsy revealed the stented arterial segment to be aneurysmally dilated. Severe inflammatory infiltrate was characterized by lymphocytes, plasma cells, macrophages, giant cells, and eosinophils within the intima, media, and adventitia. A thick

layer of fibrin-rich thrombus was found between the stent and the underlying arterial wall and was occlusive proximally. Incomplete stent expansion may also be related to late malapposition, highlighting the importance of a properly sized and expanded stent to the reference vessel diameter.[50]

Renal Failure

The presence of renal failure is associated with 3.8-fold increased odds for late stent thrombosis (OR = 3.8; 95% CI: 1.2 to 11.3; P = .018) (see Table 31-4). No pathologic correlation for stent thrombosis due to renal failure has been described. Although it is unknown how renal failure contributes to late thrombosis, it may be related to increased thrombogenicity or relative resistance to antiplatelet therapy.

Long Total Stent Length

In a meta-analysis of randomized clinical trials, curve-fit regression analysis revealed that increased stent length was associated with subsequent stent thrombosis (see Table 31-4). In the report of the Armed Forces Institute of Pathology, thrombosed drug-eluting stents were compared with patent drug-eluting stents implanted at a similar duration (mean, 6.6 ± 4.6 versus 6.0 ± 4.5 months, P = NS). The mean stent length was longer in drug-eluting stents that thrombosed than in the patent, drug-eluting stents (38.8 ± 18.1 versus 23.6 ± 12.2 mm, P = .0009). Thrombosed stents compared with patent stents were also characterized by more inflammation (fibrin score, 3.0 ± 0.9 versus 1.9 ± 1.1, P = .03) and less endothelialization (27.1% ± 25.9% versus 66.1% ± 25.4%, P = .001). Longer total stent length with multiple overlapping drug-eluting stents is also more likely to compromise side branch vessels and

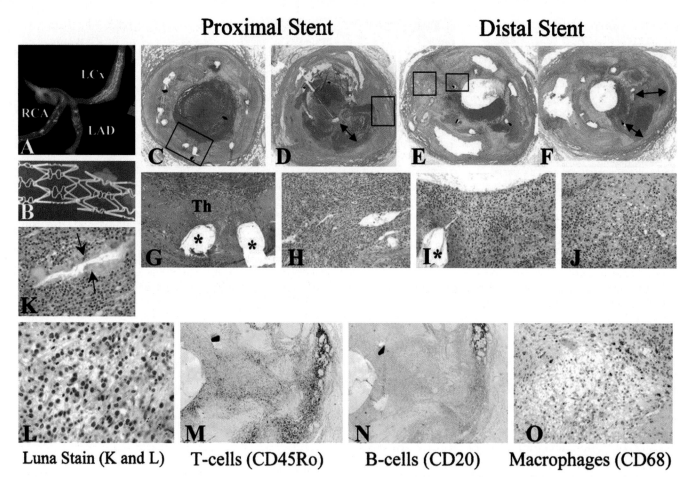

Proximal Stent   Distal Stent

Luna Stain (K and L)   T-cells (CD45Ro)   B-cells (CD20)   Macrophages (CD68)

Figure 31-17. Postmortem radiographs (**A** and **B**) show two left circumflex coronary artery (LCx) Cypher stents; notice the absence of stent overlap (**B**). Photomicrographs of representative cross sections of proximal (**C** and **D**) and distal (**E** and **F**) Cypher stents. Focal strut malapposition with aneurysmal dilation (*double arrows* in **D** and **F**) and occlusive luminal thrombosis (Th, **C** and **G**) are present. High-power views (**G** through **J**) of stented arteries from the *boxed areas* of the proximal (**C** and **D**) and distal (**E**) views. Luminal thrombus (Th) above stent struts (**G**) with absence of smooth muscle cells. There is diffuse inflammation within the intima and media (**H**, *boxed area* in **D**). Extensive inflammation (**I**, right boxed area in **E**) consists primarily of eosinophils and lymphocytes with a focal giant cell reaction around the stent strut *(asterisk)* and surrounding polymer. Marked inflammation is similarly present in the intima, media, and adventitia (**J**, left *boxed area* in **E**). Luna staining (**K** and **L**) shows giant cells *(arrowheads)* around a polymer remnant that has separated from stent strut and numerous eosinophils within the arterial wall. Immunohistochemical identification (**M** through **O**) of T cells (CD45Ro), B cells (CD20), and macrophages (CD68), respectively; T lymphocytes are the predominant inflammatory cell type. (From Joner M, Finn AV, Farb A, et al: Pathology of drug-eluting stents in humans: Delayed healing and late thrombotic risk. J Am Coll Cardiol 2006;48:193-202.)

result in myocardial infarction, which was discussed earlier.

CONCLUSIONS

Late stent thrombosis is a rare but potentially life-threatening complication of an otherwise successful coronary revascularization procedure. Late stent thrombosis first gained attention with the use of intracoronary irradiation, but the introduction and widespread acceptance of drug-eluting stents has created a resurgence of concern about this problem. Drug-eluting stents have been shown to increase the risk for late stent thrombosis compared with bare metal stents in a largely stable clinical trial population with relatively simple lesions. The unrestricted use of drug-eluting stents in unstable patients with complex lesions, including the use of longer total stent lengths, may further magnify the incidence of late thrombosis. Assuming a conservative incidence for late thrombosis of 0.5% and a case fatality rate of 45%, this translates into a few thousand deaths for every million drug-eluting stents implanted.

The premature termination of dual-antiplatelet therapy markedly increases the risk for drug-eluting stent thrombosis. Premature termination is usually defined as less than 3 months of dual-antiplatelet therapy for sirolimus-eluting stents and 6 months for paclitaxel-eluting stents. Assessing patient compliance with dual-antiplatelet therapy before stent implantation can help reduce stent thrombosis from this cause. Very late thrombotic events, occurring more than 1 year after stent implantation, have been described soon after complete termination of dual-antiplatelet therapy. Instructions should be provided to patients before they are discharged from the hospital that warn against complete termination of dual-antiplatelet therapy (e.g., preoperatively) without the direction of a cardiologist. Long-term dual-antiplatelet therapy is required because late idiosyncratic events may still occur on aspirin monotherapy or even on dual-antiplatelet therapy. The optimal duration of dual-antiplatelet therapy is unclear, but the recommendation for 12 to 24 months of therapy or even longer appears reasonable.

Certain high-risk patient and lesion characteristics have been identified that can help to gauge the risk for late thrombosis and the need for ongoing dual-antiplatelet therapy. Upfront, the presence of several high-risk thrombotic characteristics should temper the enthusiasm for the use of drug-eluting stents, especially if the patient is at low risk for restenosis (i.e., nondiabetic, vessel diameter more than 3.0 mm, and a focal lesion).[51]

If a patient is at increased risk for late stent thrombosis, although the use of a drug-eluting stent is still preferred, IVUS guidance to optimize stent deployment should be strongly considered.[50] IVUS should also be considered during stent deployment in critical coronary lesions such as the ostium of the left anterior descending artery, in which a stent thrombosis can be fatal.

Bifurcation lesions have been identified in many studies to increase the risk for late thrombosis. The crush technique may be especially problematic, but the use of noncrush techniques or jailing the side branch also increases the risk for late thrombosis. Histopathologically, most cases of late thrombosis are characterized by delayed neointimal healing with incomplete re-endothelialization. Less commonly, the development of diffuse in-stent restenosis may result in late thrombosis. The treatment of in-stent restenosis with the use of additional stents is also a risk factor for late events. It remains to be seen whether drug-eluting stent implantation during an acute coronary syndrome increases the risk for late events. Vulnerable plaque rupture close to a stent implanted earlier can lead to thrombosis and highlights the need for aggressive risk factor modification. Long total stent length has been implicated in late thrombosis, potentially by magnifying the effects of localized hypersensitivity vasculitis or because they would be more likely to cross side branches, which can become stenosed or occluded by drug-eluting stents.

Overall, late thrombosis remains a significant and potentially catastrophic problem for the interventional community. The unrestricted use of drug-eluting stents may further potentiate late thrombosis. Before coronary revascularization, patients' risk for late thrombosis should be assessed along with their ability to take long-term dual-antiplatelet therapy. The presence of multiple risk factors for late thrombosis in a patient at low risk for restenosis should influence the decision to implant a drug-eluting stent. All patients who receive drug-eluting stents should receive discharge instructions emphasizing the importance of long-term and uninterrupted dual-antiplatelet therapy. Further research is needed to determine the optimal duration of aspirin and clopidogrel.

REFERENCES

1. Serruys PW, Kutryk MJ, Ong AT: Coronary-artery stents. N Engl J Med 2006;354:483-495.
2. Colombo A, Hall P, Nakamura S, et al: Intracoronary stenting without anticoagulation accomplished with intravascular ultrasound guidance. Circulation 1995;91:1676-1688.
3. Leon MB, Baim DS, Popma JJ, et al: A clinical trial comparing three antithrombotic-drug regimens after coronary-artery stenting. Stent Anticoagulation Restenosis Study Investigators. N Engl J Med 1998;339:1665-1671.
4. Cutlip DE, Baim DS, Ho KK, et al: Stent thrombosis in the modern era: A pooled analysis of multicenter coronary stent clinical trials. Circulation 2001;103:1967-1971.
5. Costa MA, Sabate M, van der Giessen WJ, et al: Late coronary occlusion after intracoronary brachytherapy. Circulation 1999;100:789-792.
6. Waksman R: Late thrombosis after radiation. Sitting on a time bomb. Circulation 1999;100:780-782.
7. Colombo A, Corbett SJ: Drug-eluting stent thrombosis: Increasingly recognized but too frequently overemphasized. J Am Coll Cardiol 2006;48:203-205.
8. Cheneau E, Leborgne L, Mintz GS, et al: Predictors of subacute stent thrombosis: Results of a systematic intravascular ultrasound study. Circulation 2003;108:43-47.
9. Moussa I, Di Mario C, Reimers B, et al: Subacute stent thrombosis in the era of intravascular ultrasound-guided coronary stenting without anticoagulation: Frequency, predictors and clinical outcome. J Am Coll Cardiol 1997;29:6-12.
10. Wenaweser P, Dorffler-Melly J, Imboden K, et al: Stent thrombosis is associated with an impaired response to antiplatelet therapy. J Am Coll Cardiol 2005;45:1748-1752.
11. Bavry AA, Kumbhani DJ, Helton TJ, Bhatt DL: What is the risk of stent thrombosis associated with the use of paclitaxel-eluting stents for percutaneous coronary intervention? A meta-analysis. J Am Coll Cardiol 2005;45:941-946.
12. Bavry AA, Kumbhani DJ, Helton TJ, Bhatt DL: Risk of thrombosis with the use of sirolimus-eluting stents for percutaneous coronary intervention (from registry and clinical trial data). Am J Cardiol 2005;95:1469-1472.
13. Kaluza GL, Joseph J, Lee JR, et al: Catastrophic outcomes of noncardiac surgery soon after coronary stenting. J Am Coll Cardiol 2000;35:1288-1294.
14. Jeremias A, Sylvia B, Bridges J, et al: Stent thrombosis after successful sirolimus-eluting stent implantation. Circulation 2004;109:1930-1932.
15. Honda Y, Fitzgerald PJ: Stent thrombosis: An issue revisited in a changing world. Circulation 2003;108:2-5.
16. Leon MB, Teirstein PS, Moses JW, et al: Localized intracoronary gamma-radiation therapy to inhibit the recurrence of restenosis after stenting. N Engl J Med 2001;344:250-256.
17. Waksman R, Bhargava B, Mintz GS, et al: Late total occlusion after intracoronary brachytherapy for patients with in-stent restenosis. J Am Coll Cardiol 2000;36:65-68.
18. Waksman R, Ajani AE, White RL, et al: Prolonged antiplatelet therapy to prevent late thrombosis after intracoronary gamma-radiation in patients with in-stent restenosis: Washington Radiation for In-Stent Restenosis Trial plus 6 months of clopidogrel (WRIST PLUS). Circulation 2001;103:2332-2335.
19. Waksman R, Ajani AE, Pinnow E, et al: Twelve versus six months of clopidogrel to reduce major cardiac events in patients undergoing gamma-radiation therapy for in-stent restenosis: Washington Radiation for In-Stent restenosis Trial (WRIST) 12 versus WRIST PLUS. Circulation 2002;106:776-778.
20. Berger PB, Bell MR, Hasdai D, et al: Safety and efficacy of ticlopidine for only 2 weeks after successful intracoronary stent placement. Circulation 1999;99:248-253.
21. Heller LI, Shemwell KC, Hug K: Late stent thrombosis in the absence of prior intracoronary brachytherapy. Catheter Cardiovasc Interv 2001;53:23-28.

22. Wang F, Stouffer GA, Waxman S, Uretsky BF: Late coronary stent thrombosis: Early vs. late stent thrombosis in the stent era. Catheter Cardiovasc Interv 2002;55:142-147.

23. McFadden EP, Stabile E, Regar E, et al: Late thrombosis in drug-eluting coronary stents after discontinuation of antiplatelet therapy. Lancet 2004;364:1519-1521.

24. Ong AT, McFadden EP, Regar E, et al: Late angiographic stent thrombosis (LAST) events with drug-eluting stents. J Am Coll Cardiol 2005;45:2088-2092.

25. Kuchulakanti PK, Chu WW, Torguson R, et al: Correlates and long-term outcomes of angiographically proven stent thrombosis with sirolimus- and paclitaxel-eluting stents. Circulation 2006;113:1108-1113.

26. Park DW, Park SW, Park KH, et al: Frequency of and risk factors for stent thrombosis after drug-eluting stent implantation during long-term follow-up. Am J Cardiol 2006;98:352-356.

27. Rodriguez AE, Mieres J, Fernandez-Pereira C, et al: Coronary stent thrombosis in the current drug-eluting stent era: Insights from the ERACI III trial. J Am Coll Cardiol 2006;47:205-207.

28. Bavry AA, Kumbhani DJ, Helton TJ, et al: Late thrombosis of drug eluting stents: A meta-analysis of randomized clinical trials. Am J Med 2006;119:1056-1061.

29. Kastrati A, Dibra A, Eberle S, et al: Sirolimus-eluting stents vs paclitaxel-eluting stents in patients with coronary artery disease: Meta-analysis of randomized trials. JAMA 2005;294:819-825.

30. Urban P, Gershlick AH, Guagliumi G, et al: Safety of coronary sirolimus-eluting stents in daily clinical practice: one-year follow-up of the e-Cypher registry. Circulation 2006;113:1434-1441.

31. Ong AT, Hoye A, Aoki J, et al: Thirty-day incidence and six-month clinical outcome of thrombotic stent occlusion after bare-metal, sirolimus, or paclitaxel stent implantation. J Am Coll Cardiol 2005;45:947-953.

32. Iakovou I, Schmidt T, Bonizzoni E, et al: Incidence, predictors, and outcome of thrombosis after successful implantation of drug-eluting stents. JAMA 2005;293:2126-2130.

33. Spertus JA, Kettelkamp R, Vance C, et al: Prevalence, predictors, and outcomes of premature discontinuation of thienopyridine therapy after drug-eluting stent placement: Results from the PREMIER registry. Circulation 2006;113:2803-2809.

34. Kotani J, Awata M, Nanto S, et al: Incomplete neointimal coverage of sirolimus-eluting stents: Angioscopic findings. J Am Coll Cardiol 2006;47:2108-2111.

35. Tsimikas S: Drug-eluting stents and late adverse clinical outcomes: Lessons learned, lessons awaited. J Am Coll Cardiol 2006;47:2112-2115.

36. Farb A, Burke AP, Kolodgie FD, Virmani R: Pathological mechanisms of fatal late coronary stent thrombosis in humans. Circulation 2003;108:1701-1706.

37. Joner M, Finn AV, Farb A, et al: Pathology of drug-eluting stents in humans: Delayed healing and late thrombotic risk. J Am Coll Cardiol 2006;48:193-202.

38. Hoye A, Iakovou I, Ge L, et al: Long-term outcomes after stenting of bifurcation lesions with the "crush" technique: Predictors of an adverse outcome. J Am Coll Cardiol 2006;47:1949-1958.

39. Ge L, Airoldi F, Iakovou I, et al: Clinical and angiographic outcome after implantation of drug-eluting stents in bifurcation lesions with the crush stent technique: Importance of final kissing balloon post-dilation. J Am Coll Cardiol 2005;46:613-620.

40. Stone GW, Ellis SG, Cannon L, et al: Comparison of a polymer-based paclitaxel-eluting stent with a bare metal stent in patients with complex coronary artery disease: A randomized controlled trial. JAMA 2005;294:1215-1223.

41. Tsagalou E, Chieffo A, Iakovou I, et al: Multiple overlapping drug-eluting stents to treat diffuse disease of the left anterior descending coronary artery. J Am Coll Cardiol 2005;45:1570-1573.

42. Virmani R, Guagliumi G, Farb A, et al: Localized hypersensitivity and late coronary thrombosis secondary to a sirolimus-eluting stent: Should we be cautious? Circulation 2004;109:701-705.

43. Moreno R, Fernandez C, Hernandez R, et al: Drug-eluting stent thrombosis: Results from a pooled analysis including 10 randomized studies. J Am Coll Cardiol 2005;45:954-959.

44. Waters RE, Kandzari DE, Phillips HR, et al: Late thrombosis following treatment of in-stent restenosis with drug-eluting stents after discontinuation of antiplatelet therapy. Catheter Cardiovasc Interv 2005;65:520-524.

45. Stabile E, Cheneau E, Kinnaird T, et al: Late thrombosis in Cypher stents after the discontinuation of antiplatelet therapy. Cardiovasc Radiat Med 2004;5:173-176.

46. Nasser M, Kapeliovich M, Markiewicz W: Late thrombosis of sirolimus-eluting stents following noncardiac surgery. Catheter Cardiovasc Interv 2005;65:516-519.

47. Lee CH, Lim J, Low A, et al: Late angiographic stent thrombosis of polymer based paclitaxel eluting stent. Heart 2006;92:551-553.

48. Karvouni E, Korovesis S, Katritsis DG: Very late thrombosis after implantation of sirolimus eluting stent. Heart 2005;91:e45.

49. Kang WC, Han SH, Choi KR, et al: Acute myocardial infarction caused by late stent thrombosis after deployment of a paclitaxel-eluting stent. J Invasive Cardiol 2005;17:378-380.

50. Mintz GS, Weissman NJ: Intravascular ultrasound in the drug-eluting stent era. J Am Coll Cardiol 2006;48:421-429.

51. Bavry AA, Bhatt DL: Bare metal stents: No longer passé? J Invasive Cardiol 2006;18:403-404.

CHAPTER
32 Restenosis

Marco A. Costa and Daniel I. Simon

Nature does nothing without purpose or uselessly.

—Aristotle, 384-322 BC

KEY POINTS

■ Mechanisms of restenosis are different for balloon angioplasty, bare metal stents, and drug-eluting stents.

■ Intimal hyperplasia with smooth muscle cell proliferation is the key mechanism of restenosis after implantation of bare metal stents.

■ The biology of restenosis after drug-eluting stents varies, and tissue may have different cellular compositions (e.g., T lymphocytes) and fibrin deposition.

■ The relative contribution of procedural and mechanical factors in the development of clinical restenosis is amplified after implantation of drug-eluting stents.

■ Intimal hyperplasia after implantation of drug-eluting stents may appear as a homogeneous echolucent image

on intravascular ultrasound and may be unnoticed during routine examination.

■ The rates of restenosis and in-stent late lumen loss are lower with drug-eluting stents than with bare metal stents.

■ The rates and patterns of restenosis are different for the various drug-eluting stent platforms.

■ The best treatment for restenosis of drug-eluting stents remains to be determined, but emerging anti-restenosis strategies include catheter-based drug delivery systems and the use of biodegradable stents with or without combination drug therapy.

Restenosis is the arterial wall healing response to mechanical injury, which has plagued cardiologists since the introduction of balloon angioplasty by Grüntzig and collaborators.[1] This chapter describes the clinical features, mechanisms, and new facets of restenosis in contemporary percutaneous coronary intervention (PCI).

DEFINITIONS

Angiographic Restenosis

Angiographically detected obstruction of 50% diameter stenosis (DS) or more at the site of a previously treated coronary segment has been historically considered as representing restenosis.[2] This arbitrary cutoff point was founded on good scientific evidence; physiologic experimental studies demonstrated that when the arterial lumen diameter was reduced to 50% or less, coronary flow reserve became impeded.[3] For purposes of scientific studies, many definitions of angiographic restenosis have been used, although the classic binary definition based on the percentage of DS is the most widely accepted. Unfortunately, this measurement does not depict the degree of deterioration in lumen diameter and does not convey a

measure of the vessel response to injury.[4,5] The use of the term percentage DS itself carries with it the assumption of normal-appearing reference segments, which is known to be an erroneous assumption given the diffuse aspect of coronary disease and neointimal proliferation. Binary restenosis assumes that a patient with 51% DS and another one with 49% DS have different intimal hyperplasia responses and outcomes.

In view of these considerations, clinical restenosis studies have been adopting a more comprehensive approach in reporting findings from both perspectives (categorical and continuous) to determine whether the agent under investigation had restraining or inhibitory effect and whether the ultimate clinical or angiographic outcome has been improved by the use of any new therapy. However, the more subtle facets of potent antiproliferative devices such as drug-eluting stents (DESs) challenge the validity of conventional angiographic parameters.[6-8]

Late loss is a continuous angiographic measure of lumen deterioration. Late loss is conventionally calculated by subtracting the minimal lumen diameter (MLD) value at follow-up from the postprocedural MLD. These computations are made irrespective of the locations of MLD measurements. Late loss has

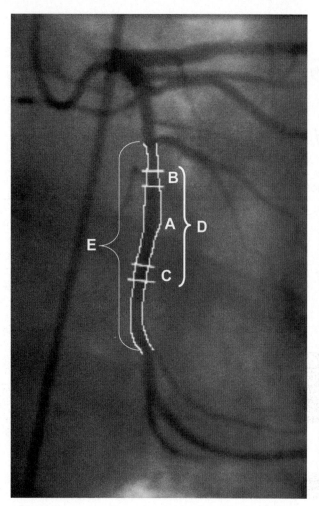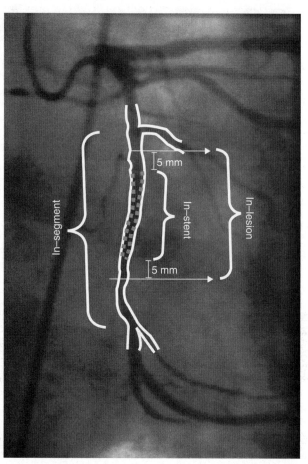

Figure 32-1. Coronary angiography and a schematic model illustrate a segmental approach to analyzing and reporting the effects of drug-eluting stents on coronary arteries. A, in-stent, which better describes the antiproliferative effect of the biologic agent; B, proximal edge (5 mm); C, distal edge (5 mm); and D, in-lesion sites determine potential paradoxical effects of low drug concentrations at traumatized stent edges (i.e. the edge effect); E, in-segment analysis is the ultimate determinant of angiographic success from a patient's perspective. (From Sousa JE, Serruys PW, Costa MA: New frontiers in cardiology: Drug-eluting stents. Part II. Circulation 2003;107:2383-2389.)

traditionally served as a major outcome measure in bare metal stent (BMS) trials and continues to play a similar role in the era of DESs.[9,10] It represents a surrogate marker of neointimal hyperplasia when measurements are performed within stented segments, because stents abolish the remodeling component of the restenotic process (discussed later).[4,11]

However, conventional late loss measurements may be methodologically flawed because of changes in the location of MLD between postprocedural and follow-up measurements.[8,12] As a result, late loss frequently is derived from measurements performed in different (unmatched) locations in the target segment. Sites with higher degrees of lumen deterioration and neointimal proliferation may be overlooked, potentially leading to inaccurate conclusions regarding the antiproliferative efficacy of a given device.

Angiographic restenosis parameters have been reported by means of in-lesion and in-stent analyses (Fig. 32-1). It is important to notice that in-lesion late loss will not necessarily be higher than in-stent late loss. These somewhat conflicting data, given that in-

lesion analysis encompassed the stented segment and 5 mm distally and proximally in an attempt to depict edge restenosis, happen because of the MLD relocation phenomenon. In-lesion late loss also is affected by vascular remodeling or vessel spasm, and it cannot be used as a surrogate for intimal hyperplasia or to determine antiproliferative device efficacy.

Quantitative coronary angiography (QCA) has been used largely to determine restenosis parameters in the clinical context,[13] because visual assessment may lead to overestimation of the degree of narrowing in severe lesions and underestimation of the severity in mild or moderate lesions.[14] Digital systems permit online QCA in the catheterization laboratory, providing fast, easy, objective, and clinically relevant information for patient care.

Clinical Restenosis

Although angiography has been widely used as the guiding tool for coronary disease management, the clinician should also consider functional, invasive or noninvasive assessment of the restenotic lesion before referring the patient to additional coronary revascularization. Grüntzig and coworkers observed that most clinical ischemic events related to vessel renarrowing occurred between 3 and 9 months after balloon angioplasty. This seminal observation illustrates the delay between the biologic process and symptomatic presentation of restenosis, which results in a 70% increase in the incidence of repeat revascularization between 6 and 12 months after the procedure.[15,16] Potent antiproliferative strategies may delay the biologic response to injury and extend the timeframe for developing clinical signs of restenosis. Intimal proliferation after brachytherapy seems to have a different time course.[17] Likewise, restenosis after DES implantation may be delayed, although a late catch-up restenotic phenomenon has not been observed in the initial studies.[18,19]

Restenosis may cause no symptoms in up to 50% of patients, although silent ischemia may be present and should be treated.[20] Exercise electrocardiographic testing has limited value for detecting silent restenotic lesions. Other noninvasive tests such as thallium scintigraphy and cardiac and stress echocardiography have been used to improve the sensitivity and specificity of noninvasive assessment of restenosis.[21] On the other end of the clinical spectrum, restenosis may manifest in the form of acute coronary syndrome in up to one third of patients, which challenges the notion that restenosis is benign.[22] This is of particular concern after left main PCI because of the risk of sudden cardiac death associated with early silent restenosis. As a result, routine 3- to 6-month angiographic follow-up should be considered for patients undergoing unprotected left main coronary artery PCI.

Target lesion revascularization (TLR), defined as any repeat percutaneous intervention of the treated coronary segment or bypass surgery of the target vessel, has been proposed as the most specific clinical restenosis end point among other clinical markers (i.e., death, myocardial infarction, symptom recurrence, or combined major adverse cardiac events).[4] Target vessel revascularization (TVR) expands the definition of TLR to include repeat percutaneous intervention of the target vessel, irrespective of the location of the stenosis within the treated segment.

In routine clinical practice, noninvasive assessment of recurrence of restenosis (i.e., symptomatic status and ischemia tests) appears to be an appropriate approach. This recommendation is based on a series of previous observations. Routine angiographic follow-up may have increased, albeit small, morbidity and mortality rates; asymptomatic patients with nonfunctional angiographic restenosis experience a benign course[23]; and the so-called occulostenotic reflex leads to a higher rate of repeat revascularization with no clear clinical benefit at 12 months after the initial intervention.[24] If repeat angiography is carried out without clear clinical evidence of ischemia, sensor-tipped guidewires for measurements of distal flow velocity or pressure may be useful for

assessing the functional status of restenotic lesions in the catheterization laboratory and can assist physiologically based decision-making regarding the need for reintervention.[25]

MECHANISMS OF RESTENOSIS

The pathophysiology of restenosis is characterized by neointimal proliferation and negative vascular remodeling. The later contributes only to restenosis after PCI without stent implantation because the scaffold properties of stents abolish the remodeling process. It is nevertheless important to understand that the proliferative vascular response is enhanced by the persistent stimuli of rigid metallic struts in the vessel wall.

Neointimal hyperplasia was originally proposed to be a general wound-healing response.[26] Platelet aggregation, inflammatory cell infiltration, release of growth factors, medial smooth muscle cell (SMC) modulation and proliferation, proteoglycan deposition, and extracellular matrix remodeling were identified as the major milestones in the temporal sequence of this response. Initially, thrombosis was considered the main trigger of SMC proliferation after angioplasty. Platelet-derived growth factor (PDGF), which may also be secreted by endothelial cells and macrophages, is a potent promoter of SMC migration.[27] However, a more prominent effect of inflammation on SMC proliferation has been proposed.

Smooth Muscle Cell Proliferation and Restenosis

The SMC has long been implicated in the healing process after arterial injury[28] because of its ability to migrate, proliferate, and synthesize extracellular matrix (ECM) on stimulation.[29] After shifting from the contractile to the synthetic phenotype, SMCs may proliferate 24 hours to 2 to 3 months after vascular injury, returning to the contractile phenotype after this period. Adventitial myofibroblasts (α-actin–staining cells) also proliferate and migrate into the neointimal layer[30] and appear to play an important role in supplying the intima layer with proliferative cellular elements for new lesion formation. Through fracture of the internal elastic membrane, these cells migrate into the intima, where they may continue to proliferate and synthesize ECM, which will ultimately constitute the bulk of the restenotic lesion. ECM is composed of various collagen subtypes and proteoglycans[31] and constitutes the major component of the restenotic lesion; neointimal hyperplasia has been shown to be predominantly a low-cellular tissue.[32]

Cellular proliferative status in atherectomy specimens of restenotic lesions has been demonstrated by use of antibodies to proliferating cell nuclear antigen (PCNA), cyclin E, and cyclin-dependent kinase 2 (CDK2).[33] There is also evidence that cells of a monocyte-macrophage lineage (HAM-56+) proliferate within human in-stent restenotic tissue.[34] The central

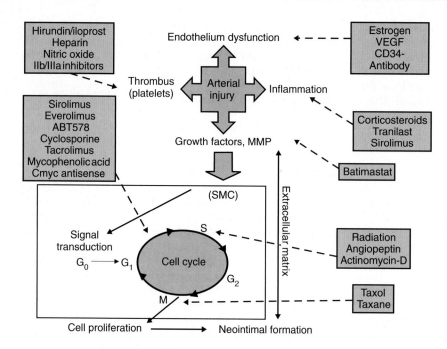

Figure 32-2. The leading processes of restenosis *(solid lines)* and corresponding inhibitory *(dashed lines)* effects of different anti-restenosis agents. MMP, matrix metalloproteinase; SMC, smooth muscle cell; VEGF, vascular endothelial growth factor. (From Sousa JE, Serruys PW, Costa MA: New frontiers in cardiology: Drug-eluting stents. Part I. Circulation 2003;107:2274-2279).

role of vascular cells in the restenotic process provided the basis for anti-restenosis pharmacologic strategies targeting cell cycle division early after stent implantation (Fig. 32-2).

Cell Cycle and Restenosis

The cell cycle is a common hub of the different phases of the restenosis process. The unprecedented clinical successes of recent anti-restenosis approaches targeting cellular division pathways illustrate its central role in the formation of neointimal hyperplasia. DES technologies deliver high concentrations of immunosuppressive or antitumor agents locally into the vessel wall. The specific molecular and cellular effects of these agents have been discussed in detail elsewhere.[6]

SMCs are quiescent and exhibit very low levels of proliferative activity. However, mechanical injury triggers the SMC progress through the G_1/S transition of the cell cycle.[35] The different phases of the cell cycle of eukaryotic cells are regulated by a series of protein complexes composed of cyclins (D, E, A, B), cyclin-dependent kinases (CDKs: CDK4, CDK2, CDC2 [p34]), and their cyclin-dependent inhibitors (CKIs: CDKN1B [p27 or KIP1], RPS6KB2 [p 70 or S6Kb], CDKN2A [INK4 or p16]). The function of CKIs is regulated by changes in their concentration and by their localization in the cell.[36] CDKN1B (i.e., p27 or KIP1) is downregulated after arterial injury when cell proliferation increases. CDKN1A (i.e., p21 or CIP1) is not observed in normal arteries, but it is upregulated along with CDKN1B in later phases of arterial healing response and is associated with a significant decline in cell proliferation and an increase in procollagen and transforming growth factor-beta (TGF-β) synthesis.[36] These findings suggest that CDKN1B and CDKN1A are endogenous regulators of G_1 transit in

vascular SMC and inhibit cell proliferation after arterial injury. CDKN1B and CDKN1A bind and alter the activities of cyclin D–, cyclin E–, and cyclin A–dependent kinases (CDK2) in quiescent cells, leading to failure of G_1/S transition and cell cycle arrest.[37,38] Overexpression of CDKN1B results in cell cycle arrest in the G_1 phase. Conversely, inhibition of CDKN1B increases the number of cells in S phase.[39]

The level of CDKN1B is also regulated by constituents of the ECM. Mature collagen (i.e., polymerized type 1 collagen) suppresses RPS6KB2 and has been shown to increase the levels of CDKN1B, whereas monomeric collagen, which is present during degradation of ECM in the synthesis phase of restenosis, downregulates CDKN1B. The cell cycle also regulates SMC migration. These cells migrate during G_1 but not in later phases of the cell cycle.

Inflammation and Restenosis

The central role of autocrine or paracrine inflammatory mediators on SMC proliferation has been proposed.[41] Leukocyte recruitment and infiltration occur early at sites of vascular injury, where the lining endothelial cells have been denuded and platelets and fibrin have been deposited. The initial tethering and rolling of leukocytes on platelet P-selectin[42] are followed by their firm adhesion and transplatelet migration, processes that depend on leukocyte Mac-1[43] and platelet glycoprotein (GP) Ibα.[44] The precise cellular and molecular mechanisms of inflammation after arterial injury depend on the specific type of injury (i.e., stent versus balloon and mechanical versus atherogenesis). Experimental stent deployment in animal arteries causes a sustained elevation of MCP-1 after injury (≈14 days) compared with balloon-injured arteries (<24 hours).[45] Antibody-mediated blockade of CCR2, a primary leukocyte

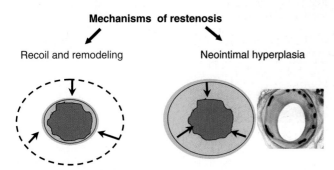

Mechanisms of restenosis

Recoil and remodeling   Neointimal hyperplasia

Figure 32-3. The two main mechanisms of restenosis, negative vessel remodeling and elastic recoil, are mainly observed after balloon angioplasty, whereas in-stent restenosis is mainly associated with intimal hyperplasia. In-stent restenosis histology is shown on the *right.*

receptor for MCP-1, markedly diminished neointimal thickening after stent-induced injury but not after balloon-induced injury in nonhuman primates.[46]

Investigators have pursued anti-restenosis strategies using systemic anti-inflammatory therapies, including liposome-encapsulated bisphosphonates,[47] prednisone,[48] anti-CD18 or anti-CCR2 blockade,[46] and the PPARG (PPAR-γ) activator rosiglitazone. Experimental observations support a causal relationship between inflammation and experimental restenosis. Antibody-mediated blockade[49] or selective absence of Mac-1[50] diminished leukocyte accumulation and limited neointimal thickening after experimental angioplasty or stent implantation. Corticosteroids reduce the influx of mononuclear cells, inhibit monocyte and macrophage function, and influence SMC proliferation.[51] However, clinical trials with systemic steroid therapy to prevent restenosis have shown disappointing results.[52]

Remodeling and Restenosis

The term *remodeling* has been applied largely to describe vascular shrinkage or enlargement. The definition proposed by Schwartz and colleagues,[53] in which remodeling is characterized in a continuous spectrum by any change in vascular dimension, may better describe this compensatory phenomenon. Studies using intravascular ultrasound provided the first evidence of the key role of negative remodeling (i.e., vessel shrinkage) on lumen deterioration after nonstented PCI.[54,55] Adventitial myofibroblasts, which are capable of collagen synthesis and tissue contraction as seen in wound healing,[56,57] may play an important role in negative vessel remodeling observed in restenosis after balloon angioplasty.

Remodeling is virtually absent after stenting as observed by volumetric intravascular ultrasound (IVUS) (Fig. 32-3).[58,59] The superior outcomes of bare metal stents compared with angioplasty result mainly from the scaffold property of these metallic prostheses, which prevents vessel shrinkage (i.e., elastic recoil and negative remodeling) despite inducing an enhanced neointimal hyperplasia response.

Specific Mechanisms of Bare Metal Stent Restenosis

The initial consequences immediately after stent placement are de-endothelialization, crush of the plaque (often with dissection into the tunica media and occasionally adventitia), and stretch of the entire artery.[60] A layer of platelets and fibrin are then deposited at the injured site. Activated platelets on the surface expressing adhesion molecules such as P-selectin attach to circulating leukocytes by means of platelet receptors, such as selectin P ligand (SELPLG, also called PSGL-1), and begin a process of rolling along the injured surface. Leukocytes then bind tightly to the surface through the leukocyte integrin class of adhesion molecules by direct attachment to platelet receptors such as GP Ibα and through cross-linking with fibrinogen to the GP IIb/IIIa receptor. Migration of leukocytes across the platelet-fibrin layer and diapedesis into the tissue is driven by chemical gradients of chemokines released from SMCs and resident macrophages.

The granulation or cellular proliferation phase occurs next. Growth factors are released from platelets, leukocytes, and SMCs that stimulate migration of SMCs from the media and adventitia into the intima layer. The resultant neointima consists of SMCs, extracellular matrix, and macrophages recruited over a several-week period. Cellular division takes place in this phase, which appears to be essential for the subsequent development of restenosis. Over a longer period, the artery enters a phase of remodeling involving ECM protein degradation and resynthesis (Fig. 32-4). Accompanying this phase is a shift to fewer cellular elements and greater production of ECM. In stented arteries, re-endothelialization of at least part of the injured vessel surface may occur.

Specific Mechanisms of Drug-Eluting Stent Restenosis

Our understanding on the mechanisms of restenosis after DES implantation is limited. However, the biology of restenosis is probably altered by the potent antiproliferative agents released from these devices. The variations in drug distribution, degree of injury, and tissue composition along the target vessel wall provide substrates for heterogeneous local vessel wall responses, which has been observed after balloon angioplasty.[61] We have found that the cellular composition of human DES restenotic tissue may vary from a T-lymphocyte infiltrate to tissues containing predominantly SMCs, similar to the pattern in bare metal stent restenosis. It remains largely unknown which clinical, anatomic, and local vascular factors govern the distinct vascular responses after DES, and it has yet to be elucidated whether these biologic features lead to different clinical consequences.

An echolucent intimal hyperplasia, called the *black hole,* has been identified in patients treated with DESs (Fig. 32-5).[62,63] The molecular mechanisms involved in the development of the black hole are not understood but likely represent an altered cellular response

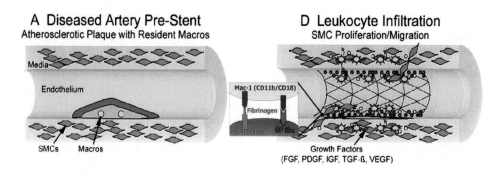

A Diseased Artery Pre-Stent
Atherosclerotic Plaque with Resident Macros

D Leukocyte Infiltration
SMC Proliferation/Migration

B Immediate Post-Stent
Endothelial Denudation, Platelet/Fibrinogen Deposition

E Neointimal Growth
Continued SMC Proliferation and Macro Recruitment

C Leukocyte Recruitment
Cytokine Release

F Restenotic Lesion
More ECM Rich Over Time

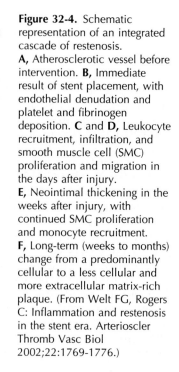

Figure 32-4. Schematic representation of an integrated cascade of restenosis. **A,** Atherosclerotic vessel before intervention. **B,** Immediate result of stent placement, with endothelial denudation and platelet and fibrinogen deposition. **C** and **D,** Leukocyte recruitment, infiltration, and smooth muscle cell (SMC) proliferation and migration in the days after injury. **E,** Neointimal thickening in the weeks after injury, with continued SMC proliferation and monocyte recruitment. **F,** Long-term (weeks to months) change from a predominantly cellular to a less cellular and more extracellular matrix-rich plaque. (From Welt FG, Rogers C: Inflammation and restenosis in the stent era. Arterioscler Thromb Vasc Biol 2002;22:1769-1776.)

to vascular injury. One possible explanation is the preservation of secretion properties of a few resident SMCs and inflammatory cells despite impairment of the cell cycle division. Regions of acellular, plasma-like collections were observed at 30 and 90 days after sirolimus-eluting stent implantation in porcine coronary arteries.[64] Experimental models have also shown increased fibrin deposition after DES implantation, which is considered a characteristic of delayed healing.[65] Fibrin accumulation was found at the site of a black hole in a patient who developed restenosis after DES treatment and was treated with atherectomy (Y. Oikawa, personal communication, 2006). Fibrin deposition was found in two cases of drug-eluting stent restenosis in our laboratory. Hypocellularity and the homogeneous characteristics of proteoglycans, fibrin, and plasma are likely responsible for the lack of ultrasound signal (i.e., echolucent). The black hole is a rare event and not always identified in DES restenosis tissue. This further supports the notion that the cellular mechanisms of restenosis after DES vary considerably.

Procedural Factors Associated with Restenosis

The "bigger is better" philosophy,[66] in which the lumen size obtained after PCI ultimately determines the occurrence of restenosis, has been largely accepted in the BMS era. The use of IVUS to guide optimal stent expansion, however, has not been shown to impact restenosis after BMS. Nevertheless, the Multicenter Ultrasound Stenting in Coronaries (MUSIC) IVUS study reported a 8.3% incidence of restenosis, which is likely the lowest rates ever reported in patients treated with BMS.[67] This study enrolled a much selected population and applied strict IVUS criteria of optimal stent deployment, which is difficult to achieve in routine practice.

Somewhat paradoxically, the potent antiproliferative effects of DESs exposed the mechanical- and procedural-related factors as major causes of restenosis. Neointimal hyperplasia is mostly abolished within the DES. As a result, the clinical signs of neointimal proliferation or negative remodeling in response to vessel trauma or untreated disease at the segments

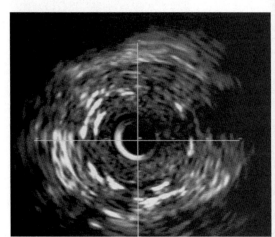

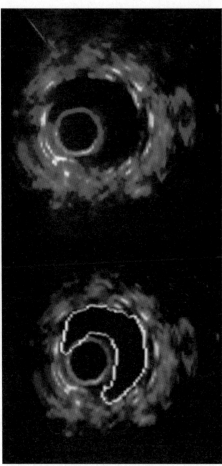

Figure 32-5. Example of a black hole *(left)* after implantation of a sirolimus-eluting stent, as detected by intravascular ultrasound (IVUS). The black hole has a homogeneous black appearance, but its differentiation from the lumen requires careful evaluation of the IVUS image. The typical IVUS appearance of intimal hyperplasia is shown after implantation of a bare metal stent *(right)*.

adjacent to the DES become amplified (Fig. 32-6). The deleterious clinical impact of suboptimal PCI techniques when applying antiproliferative devices was initially realized after the introduction of intracoronary radiation therapy.[68,69] At the time, the term *geographic miss* (GM) was used to describe a failure to fully cover the injured or diseased arterial segment with the radiation treatment source. There was a fourfold increase in the incidence of coronary-edge restenosis in patients with GM compared with those without GM undergoing intracoronary radiation therapy.[68,69] The STLLR study (i.e., prospective evaluation of the impact of stent deployment techniques on clinical outcomes of patients treated with the Cypher stent) was a large-scale ($N = 1567$, 43 participating institutions) study prospectively investigating sirolimus-eluting stent deployment technique and its relationship to clinical outcomes in the modern PCI era. This study reported a high incidence of GM as defined by the mismatching of lesion and injury vascular targets with subsequent sirolimus-eluting stent treatment deployment sites and provided the first scientific evidence of the negative impact of procedural related factors on clinical restenosis. Other mechanical-related failures that may trigger restenosis include stent underexpansion[70] and strut fracture.

Clinical Factors Linked to Restenosis

Identification of factors associated with a higher risk for restenosis may be useful in counseling patients about selecting PCI or other therapeutic strategies (i.e., clinical treatment or bypass surgery). Unfortunately, there have been inconsistencies in linking restenosis to baseline demographic and clinical characteristics. Diabetes mellitus has consistently been demonstrated to be an important clinical risk factor for restenosis after angioplasty and BMS implantation.[71] Some anatomic features have also been implicated with an increased likelihood of restenosis; saphenous vein graft disease, small vessel diameter, long lesions, and chronic total occlusion have been associated with a higher incidence of angiographic restenosis after BMS.[72-76] Although prior knowledge of the subset of patients at higher risk for restenosis may be useful for clinical decision-making, angiographic and IVUS studies have extensively demonstrated that the principal determinant of restenosis is the lumen size achieved at the end of the procedure.[77,78]

Although DES has drastically reduced angiographic and clinical restenosis across broad lesion and patient subsets, certain anatomic and clinical scenarios, such as patients with diabetes mellitus, restenotic lesions

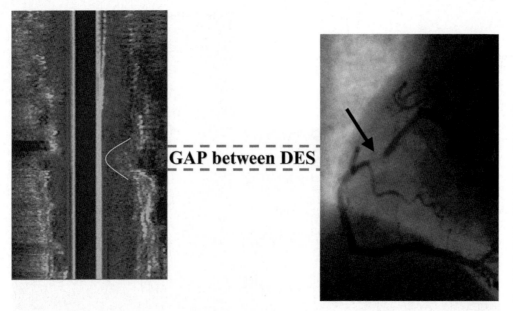

Figure 32-6. Longitudinal intravascular ultrasound (IVUS) image shows a focal intimal hyperplasia formation *(delineated)* in a gap between two sirolimus-eluting stents. Notice the lack of intimal hyperplasia within the stents. The corresponding angiographic illustration *(right)* shows restenosis *(arrow)*. Mechanical and procedural factors are key determinants of restenosis after implantation of drug-eluting stents (DESs).

after brachytherapy or DES implantation,[79] bypass graft disease,[80] and bifurcations, continue to be problematic.[81,82] Studies have reported a higher propensity for restenosis after implantation of paclitaxel-eluting stents than with sirolimus-eluting stents.[82-84]

INCIDENCE AND PATTERNS OF RESTENOSIS

The incidences of binary restenosis rate and late loss in key stent clinical trials are described in Table 32-1.[10,67,82,84-92] The differences in time of follow-up assessment, the percentage of patients with angiographic follow-up data, and the patient population should be considered when interpreting clinical trial restenosis data.

In-stent restenosis has been characterized angiographically as focal (≤10 mm long), diffuse (>10 mm), proliferative (>10 mm extending outside the stent), or total occlusion in patients treated with Palmaz-Schatz BMSs. This classification correlated with outcomes after reintervention and was largely adopted in the era of BMSs.[93] Focal restenosis occurred in 42% of patients, diffuse restenosis in 21%, proliferative restenosis in 30%, and total occlusion in 7% after Palmaz-Schatz stent implantation.[93,94] The mid-stent articulation, which provides less scaffolding support, was likely associated with the somewhat high frequency of focal restenosis in Palmaz-Schatz stents. The same classification has been used to evaluate restenosis after DES implantation, although modern stents do not have articulations and longer stents are used. Nevertheless, the pattern of in-stent restenosis has changed with DESs, and it appears to be specific for each type of device. Restenosis after implantation of sirolimus-eluting stents is mostly (>90%) focal and usually located at the stent edges,[95,96] whereas diffuse intimal proliferation or total occlusion accounts for approximately one half of the restenosis cases after using polymer-coated, paclitaxel-eluting stents.[97]

Assuming that intimal hyperplasia is almost completely blocked in nondiabetic patients with de novo, short (<20 mm) stenosis located in nonbifurcated native coronary arteries, restenosis is likely caused by technique-related failures. Restenosis would be mostly focal and observed at the stent edges or gaps between stents in these noncomplex cases (see Fig. 32-6). Biologic and mechanical failures likely contribute to more diffuse patterns of in-stent restenosis, seen mostly in more challenging clinical scenarios such as patients with in-stent BMSs, bypass graft disease, or diabetes mellitus. An exception to this rule is restenosis after bifurcation PCI, which should be classified separately because it is usually associated with focal stenosis at the ostium of the side branch.[98]

TREATMENT

Restenosis after balloon angioplasty has a relatively benign outcome after PCI. The 18% rate of repeat restenosis for patients treated with BMSs compares favorably with the data after treatment of de novo lesions (see Table 32-1).[99] Conversely, treatment of in-stent restenosis has been associated with high (>35%) rates of repeat TLR.[100] At 4 years of follow-up, the event-free survival rate was 69% after repeat BMS implantation and 64% after balloon angioplasty.[101]

Intracoronary radiation therapy was the sole therapeutic approach that proved clinically its efficacy for the treatment of BMS restenosis.[102] However, the treatment paradigm for in-stent restenosis changed recently, and DES implantation became the treatment of choice for restenosis of BMSs. Sirolimus-eluting stents and paclitaxel-eluting stents have been shown to be superior to brachytherapy for the treatment of BMS restenosis.[103-105] No data are available on the use of DESs for the treatment of postangioplasty restenosis.

Table 32-1. Summary of Clinical Data for Drug-Eluting Stents

Study	Randomized	Drug or Agent	Device Type	In-Stent Late Loss* (Follow-up Time)	In-Lesion Restenosis (Follow-up Time)
Pivotal Stent Trials					
STRESS (N = 410)	Yes	None	Palmaz-Schatz	0.74 mm (6 mo)[†]	31.6% (6 mo)
			Balloon angioplasty	0.38 mm (6 mo)[†]	42.1% (6 mo)
BENESTENT (N = 520)	Yes	None	Palmaz-Schatz	0.65 mm (6 mo)[†]	22% (6 mo)
			Balloon angioplasty	0.32 mm (6 mo)[†]	42% (6 mo)
MUSIC (N = 161)	No	None	IVUS-guided, Palmaz-Schatz	0.77 mm (6 mo)	8.3% (6 mo)
Pivotal DES Trials					
RAVEL (N = 238)	Yes	Sirolimus	BX Velocity	−0.01 mm (6 mo)	0% (6 mo)
			BX Velocity	0.8 mm (6 mo)	26.6% (6 mo)
SIRIUS (N = 1058)	Yes	Sirolimus	BX Velocity	0.17 mm (8 mo)	8.9% (9 mo)
	Yes	None	BX Velocity		
TAXUS II (N = 536)	Yes	Paclitaxel	NIR	0.31 mm (SR, 6 mo)	5.5% (6 mo)
				0.3 mm (MR, 6 mo)	8.6% (6 mo)
	Yes	None	NIR		
TAXUS IV (N = 1314)	Yes	Paclitaxel	Express 2	0.39 mm (SR, 9 mo)	7.9% (9 mo)
		None	Express 2	0.92 mm(9 mo)	26.6% (9 mo)
ENDEAVOR II (N = 1197)	Yes	Zotarolimus	Driver	0.61 mm (9 mo)	13.2% (9 mo)
		None	Driver	1.03 mm (9 mo)	35% (9 mo)
Head-to-Head Trials					
REALITY (N = 1386)	Yes	Sirolimus	BX Velocity	0.09 mm (8 mo)	9.6% (8 mo)
		Paclitaxel	Express 2	0.31 mm (8 mo)	11.1% (8 mo)
SIRTAX (N = 1012)	Yes	Sirolimus	BX Velocity	0.13 mm (9 mo)	6.7% (9 mo)
		Paclitaxel	Express 2	0.25 mm (9 mo)	11.9% (9 mo)
Diabetes Trials					
DIABETES-I (N = 160)	Yes	Sirolimus	BX Velocity	0.08 (9 mo)	7.7% (9 mo)
		None	BX Velocity	0.66 mm (9 mo)	33% (9 mo)
DIABETES-II (N = 80)	No	Paclitaxel	Express 2	0.42 mm (9 mo)	7.6% (9 mo)
ISAR-DIABETES (N = 250)	Yes	Sirolimus	BX Velocity	0.19 mm (6 mo)	6.9% (6 mo)
	Yes	Paclitaxel	Express 2	0.49 mm (6 mo)	16.5% (6 mo)

* Pivotal trials data provided for the active treatment groups only.
[†]In-lesion late loss is provided for bare metal stent studies because in-stent angiographic measurements were not applied. Drug-eluting stent figures reflect in-stent late loss.
BENESTENT, Belgian Netherlands Stent Study; DES, drug-eluting stent; DIABETES, Diabetes and Sirolimus-Eluting Stent Trial; ENDEAVOR II, Comparison of the Endeavor ABT-578 Drug Eluting Stent with a Bare Metal Stent for Coronary Revascularization; FR, fast release; ISAR, Intracoronary Stenting and Antithrombotic Regimen; IVUS, intravenous ultrasound; MUSIC, Multicenter Ultrasound Stenting in Coronaries Study; RAVEL, Randomized Study with the Sirolimus-Eluting Velocity Balloon Expandable Stent; REALITY, Prospective, Randomized Multicenter Head-to-Head Comparison of the Sirolimus-Eluting Stent (Cypher) and the Paclitaxel-Eluting Stent (Taxus); SIRIUS, Sirolimus-Eluting Bx-Velocity Balloon Expandable Stent in the Treatment of Patients with De Novo Native Coronary Artery Lesions; SIRTAX, Sirolimus-Eluting Stent Compared with Paclitaxel-Eluting Stent for Coronary Revascularization; SR, slow release; STRESS, Stent Restenosis Study; TAXUS, Taxus stent studies.

Newer approaches using balloon systems coated with hydrophobic agents such as paclitaxel have been tested in humans with promising results. A pilot study including a limited number of patients (N = 52) with BMS in-stent restenosis showed that recurrent restenosis rates were lower in patients treated with paclitaxel-coated balloon catheters compared with conventional balloon angioplasty (Fig. 32-7).[106] Larger studies comparing catheter-based versus stent-based delivery systems for the treatment of BMS restenosis are needed. Catheter-based strategies may also become an alternative treatment for DES restenosis in the future.

Modern interventional cardiologists must deal with a much less frequent, but still vexing, problem of restenosis after DES implantation, and the most appropriate treatment strategy has not been defined. Repeat restenosis rates up to 51% have been reported for repeat PCI of DES restenotic lesions. Outcomes appear to be associated with the pattern of the stenosis, with the highest repeat restenosis rates observed in patients with diffuse patterns.[107,108] Although the strategy of repeat DES implantation has been largely used, the safety of exposing the vessel wall to another potent antiproliferative therapy such as irradiation or a DES remains to be determined. The use of IVUS may be helpful in defining the mechanism associated with DES restenosis and should be considered by the physician. If mechanical failures are encountered, and the stenosis is discrete, properly sized balloon angioplasty may suffice. If the disease is mostly outside the stent (i.e., edge restenosis), another DES may be effective. A safe and effective strategy for the rare cases of diffuse or proliferative DES restenosis remains to be established.

FUTURE DIRECTIONS

There is room for improvement in the current DES delivery systems. Better flexibility and conformability are likely high on the wish list of most modern interventional cardiologists, who no longer fear

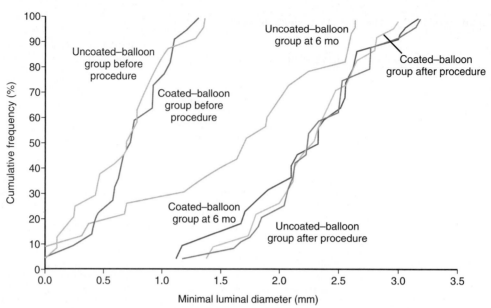

Figure 32-7. Cumulative frequency distribution of in-segment minimal luminal diameter on quantitative coronary angiography. Data are shown for the uncoated-balloon group and the coated-balloon group before the procedure, after the procedure, and at 6 months. (From Scheller B, Hehrlein C, Bocksch W, et al: Treatment of coronary in-stent restenosis with a paclitaxel-coated balloon catheter. N Engl J Med 2006;355:2113-2124. Copyright 2006 Massachusetts Medical Society. All rights reserved.)

restenosis but lack the appropriate tools to treat more complex disease.

Future anti-restenosis strategies will need to reconcile antiproliferative strategies with positive healing effects. Delayed endothelial dysfunction may persist for months after vascular injury and is likely more pronounced after DES implantation than with BMSs or balloon angioplasty.[109,110] Investigators have pursued diverse strategies, including pharmacologic combinations, tissue engineering, gene and stem cell therapies, and even procedural modifications (i.e., direct stenting) to limit endothelial injury and accelerate endothelial cell regeneration.[111-113]

Combination chemotherapy (i.e., use of multiple agents to optimize efficacy and limit toxicity) is the principal treatment strategy in oncology. Single-drug approaches have dominated DES programs, but there is emerging experimental evidence that combination anti-restenosis strategies may be effective in reducing neointimal thickening after stenting.[114] The use of antithrombotic agents associated with cell cycle inhibitors also may improve the safety of DES implantation.[115]

The catheter-based drug delivery approach has been resurrected. Local drug-delivery systems may provide high concentrations of antiproliferative drugs at the site of vascular injury without the undesirable persistence of a metallic prosthesis, which may remain prone to thrombosis if re-endothelialization does not occur. However, initial catheter-based local drug-delivery therapies have been unsuccessful in humans because of the rapid washout of the drug downstream into the coronary circulation and the potential flow- or pressure-mediated vessel wall injury.[116] The use of balloon-coating technology and hydrophobic drugs, which may minimize jet-induced injury and increase drug retention, produced satisfactory results in patients with in-stent restenosis (discussed earlier).[106] However, balloon-based PCI does not provide scaffold support, and vessels may be prone to dissection and abrupt closure. The predictability of the acute results of stent-based PCI is likely the main reason for the widespread acceptance of BMSs in the early days. A combination of balloon-based strategies and stents may play an important role in the future. Antithrombotic or prohealing agents may be used in conjunction with BMSs or DESs. Alternatively, the balloon may be coated with potent antiproliferative agents for early release, and the stents may carry healing drugs to trigger re-endothelialization.

Biodegradable DESs, which dissolve slowly after implantation, represents the ultimate stent technology. Theoretically, biodegradable or erodable stents provide initial scaffolding support to prevent vessel recoil and negative remodeling without the undesirable continuous vessel injury caused by a permanent, rigid foreign body. However, polymeric stents have yet to achieve the mechanical strength or surface properties of current stent technologies, and vessel toxicity remains a major limitation for polymeric biodegradable stents.[117] Biocorrosion of magnesium AE21 alloy containing 2% aluminum atoms and 1% rare earth elements (e.g., Ce, Pr, Nd) was well tolerated in pig coronary arteries,[118] although the vessel toxicity and hydrogen formation that may be associated with the corrosion of magnesium remains a concern.

SUMMARY

DESs represent a major breakthrough in the treatment of coronary disease and prevention of restenosis. However, restenosis has not been completely eradicated as initially thought, and the best treatment strategy for diffuse DES restenosis remains controversial. From better deliverability to biodegradable devices, DES platforms can improve considerably in the future. The current challenge of anti-restenosis strategies is to establish their long-term safety.

REFERENCES

1. Gruntzig AR, Senning A, Siegenthaler WE: Nonoperative dilatation of coronary-artery stenosis: Percutaneous transluminal coronary angioplasty. N Engl J Med 1979;301:61-68.

2. Roubin GS, King SB 3rd, Douglas JS Jr: Restenosis after percutaneous transluminal coronary angioplasty: The Emory University Hospital experience. Am J Cardiol 1987;60:39B-43B.

3. Gould KL, Lipscomb K, Hamilton GW: Physiologic basis for assessing critical coronary stenosis. Instantaneous flow response and regional distribution during coronary hyperemia as measures of coronary flow reserve. Am J Cardiol 1974;33:87-94.

4. Kuntz RE, Baim DS: Defining coronary restenosis. Newer clinical and angiographic paradigms. Circulation 1993;88:1310-1323.

5. Rensing BJ, Hermans WR, Deckers JW, et al: Which angiographic variable best describes functional status 6 months after successful single-vessel coronary balloon angioplasty? J Am Coll Cardiol 1993;21:317-324.

6. Costa MA, Simon DI: Molecular basis of restenosis and drug-eluting stents. Circulation 2005;111:2257-2273.

7. Sousa JE, Costa MA, Tuzcu EM, et al: New frontiers in interventional cardiology. Circulation 2005;111:671-681.

8. Costa MA, Sabate M, Angiolillo DJ, et al: Relocation of minimal luminal diameter after bare metal and drug-eluting stent implantation: Incidence and impact on angiographic late loss. Catheter Cardiovasc Interv 2006;69:181-188.

9. Mehilli J, Kastrati A, Wessely R, et al: Randomized trial of a nonpolymer-based rapamycin-eluting stent versus a polymer-based paclitaxel-eluting stent for the reduction of late lumen loss. Circulation 2006;113:273-279.

10. Morice MC, Serruys PW, Sousa JE, et al: A randomized comparison of a sirolimus-eluting stent with a standard stent for coronary revascularization. N Engl J Med 2002;346:1773-1780.

11. Strauss BH, Serruys PW, de Scheerder IK, et al: Relative risk analysis of angiographic predictors of restenosis within the coronary Wallstent. Circulation 1991;84:1636-1643.

12. Sabate M, Costa MA, Kozuma K, et al: Methodological and clinical implications of the relocation of the minimal luminal diameter after intracoronary radiation therapy. Dose Finding Study Group. J Am Coll Cardiol 2000;36:1536-1541.

13. Brown BG, Bolson E, Frimer M, Dodge HT: Quantitative coronary arteriography: Estimation of dimensions, hemodynamic resistance, and atheroma mass of coronary artery lesions using the arteriogram and digital computation. Circulation 1977;55:329-337.

14. Fleming RM, Kirkeeide RL, Smalling RW, Gould KL: Patterns in visual interpretation of coronary arteriograms as detected by quantitative coronary arteriography. J Am Coll Cardiol 1991;18:945-951.

15. Serruys PW, Luijten HE, Beatt KJ, et al: Incidence of restenosis after successful coronary angioplasty: A time-related phenomenon. A quantitative angiographic study in 342 consecutive patients at 1, 2, 3, and 4 months. Circulation 1988;77:361-371.

16. Cutlip DE, Chauhan MS, Baim DS, et al: Clinical restenosis after coronary stenting: Perspectives from multicenter clinical trials. J Am Coll Cardiol 2002;40:2082-2089.

17. Teirstein PS, Massullo V, Jani S, et al: Three-year clinical and angiographic follow-up after intracoronary radiation: Results of a randomized clinical trial. Circulation 2000;101:360-365.

18. Sousa JE, Costa MA, Abizaid A, et al: Four-year angiographic and intravascular ultrasound follow-up of patients treated with sirolimus-eluting stents. Circulation 2005;111:2326-2329.

19. Fajadet J, Morice MC, Bode C, et al: Maintenance of long-term clinical benefit with sirolimus-eluting coronary stents: Three-year results of the RAVEL trial. Circulation 2005;111:1040-1044.

20. Ruygrok PN, Webster MW, de Valk V, et al: Clinical and angiographic factors associated with asymptomatic restenosis after percutaneous coronary intervention. Circulation 2001;104:2289-2294.

21. Wijns W, Serruys PW, Simoons ML, et al: Predictive value of early maximal exercise test and thallium scintigraphy after successful percutaneous transluminal coronary angioplasty. Br Heart J 1985;53:194-200.

22. Chen MS, John JM, Chew DP, et al: Bare metal stent restenosis is not a benign clinical entity. Am Heart J 2006;151:1260-1264.

23. Popma JJ, van den Berg EK, Dehmer GJ: Long-term outcome of patients with asymptomatic restenosis after percutaneous transluminal coronary angioplasty. Am J Cardiol 1988;62:1298-1299.

24. Ruygrok PN, Melkert R, Morel MA, et al: Does angiography six months after coronary intervention influence management and outcome? BENESTENT II Investigators. J Am Coll Cardiol 1999;34:1507-1511.

25. Kruger S, Koch KC, Kaumanns I, et al: Clinical significance of fractional flow reserve for evaluation of functional lesion severity in stent restenosis and native coronary arteries. Chest 2005;128:1645-1649.

26. Forrester JS, Fishbein M, Helfant R, Fagin J: A paradigm for restenosis based on cell biology: Clues for the development of new preventive therapies. J Am Coll Cardiol 1991;17:758-769.

27. Libby P, Warner SJ, Salomon RN, Birinyi LK: Production of platelet-derived growth factor-like mitogen by smooth-muscle cells from human atheroma. N Engl J Med 1988;318:1493-1498.

28. Murray M, Schrodt GR, Berg HG: Role of smooth muscle cells in healing of injured arteries. Arch Pathol 1966;82:138-146.

29. Thyberg J, Hedin U, Sjolund M, et al: Regulation of differentiated properties and proliferation of arterial smooth muscle cells. Arteriosclerosis 1990;10:966-990.

30. Scott NA, Cipolla GD, Ross CE, et al: Identification of a potential role for the adventitia in vascular lesion formation after balloon overstretch injury of porcine coronary arteries. Circulation 1996;93:2178-2187.

31. Riessen R, Isner JM, Blessing E, et al: Regional differences in the distribution of the proteoglycans biglycan and decorin in the extracellular matrix of atherosclerotic and restenotic human coronary arteries. Am J Pathol 1994;144:962-974.

32. Schwartz RS, Huber KC, Murphy JG, et al: Restenosis and the proportional neointimal response to coronary artery injury: Results in a porcine model. J Am Coll Cardiol 1992;19:267-274.

33. Kearney M, Pieczek A, Haley L, et al: Histopathology of in-stent restenosis in patients with peripheral artery disease. Circulation 1997;95:1998-2002.

34. Rogers C, Seifert P, Edelman ER: The neointima provoked by human coronary stenting: Contributions of smooth muscle and inflammatory cells and extracellular matrix in autopsy specimens over time. Circulation 1998;98:I-182.

35. Nabel EG, Boehm M, Akyurek LM, et al: Cell cycle signaling and cardiovascular disease. Cold Spring Harb Symp Quant Biol 2002;67:163-170.

36. Tanner FC, Yang ZY, Duckers E, et al: Expression of cyclin-dependent kinase inhibitors in vascular disease. Circ Res 1998;82:396-403.

37. Polyak K, Kato JY, Solomon MJ, et al: p27Kip1, a cyclin-Cdk inhibitor, links transforming growth factor-beta and contact inhibition to cell cycle arrest. Genes Dev 1994;8:9-22.

38. Sherr CJ, Roberts JM: CDK inhibitors: Positive and negative regulators of G1-phase progression. Genes Dev 1999;13:1501-1512.

39. Coats S, Flanagan WM, Nourse J, Roberts JM: Requirement of p27Kip1 for restriction point control of the fibroblast cell cycle. Science 1996;272:877-880.

40. Koyama H, Raines EW, Bornfeldt KE, et al: Fibrillar collagen inhibits arterial smooth muscle proliferation through regulation of Cdk2 inhibitors. Cell 1996;87:1069-1078.

41. Libby P, Schwartz D, Brogi E, et al: A cascade model for restenosis. A special case of atherosclerosis progression. Circulation 1992;86:III-47-III-52.

42. McEver RP, Cummings RD: Role of PSGL-1 binding to selectins in leukocyte recruitment. J Clin Invest 1997;100:S97-S103.

43. Diacovo TG, Roth SJ, Buccola JM, et al: Neutrophil rolling, arrest, and transmigration across activated, surface-adherent platelets via sequential action of P-selectin and the beta 2-integrin CD11b/CD18. Blood 1996;88:146-157.

44. Simon DI, Chen Z, Xu H, et al: Platelet glycoprotein Ibalpha is a counterreceptor for the leukocyte integrin Mac-1 (CD11b/CD18). J Exp Med 2000;192:193-204.

45. Welt FG, Tso C, Edelman ER, et al: Leukocyte recruitment and expression of chemokines following different forms of vascular injury. Vasc Med 2003;8:1-7.

46. Horvath C, Welt FG, Nedelman M, et al: Targeting CCR2 or CD18 inhibits experimental in-stent restenosis in primates: Inhibitory potential depends on type of injury and leukocytes targeted. Circ Res 2002;90:488-494.

47. Danenberg HD, Golomb G, Groothuis A, et al: Liposomal alendronate inhibits systemic innate immunity and reduces in-stent neointimal hyperplasia in rabbits. Circulation 2003;108:2798-2804.

48. Versaci F, Gaspardone A, Tomai F, et al: Immunosuppressive Therapy for the Prevention of Restenosis after Coronary Artery Stent Implantation (IMPRESS Study). J Am Coll Cardiol 2002;40:1935-1942.

49. Rogers C, Edelman ER, Simon DI: A mAb to the beta2-leukocyte integrin Mac-1 (CD11b/CD18) reduces intimal thickening after angioplasty or stent implantation in rabbits. Proc Natl Acad Sci U S A 1998;95:10134-10139.

50. Simon DI, Chen Z, Seifert P, et al: Decreased neointimal formation in Mac-1(–/–) mice reveals a role for inflammation in vascular repair after angioplasty. J Clin Invest 2000;105:293-300.

51. Berk BC, Gordon JB, Alexander RW: Pharmacologic roles of heparin and glucocorticoids to prevent restenosis after coronary angioplasty. J Am Coll Cardiol 1991;17:111B-117B.

52. Holmes DR Jr, Savage M, LaBlanche JM, et al: Results of Prevention of Restenosis with Tranilast and its Outcomes (PRESTO) trial. Circulation 2002;106:1243-1250.

53. Schwartz RS, Topol EJ, Serruys PW, et al: Artery size, neointima, and remodeling: Time for some standards. J Am Coll Cardiol 1998;32:2087-2094.

54. Di Mario C, Gil R, Camenzind E, et al: Quantitative assessment with intracoronary ultrasound of the mechanisms of restenosis after percutaneous transluminal coronary angioplasty and directional coronary atherectomy. Am J Cardiol 1995;75:772-777.

55. Mintz G, Popma J, Pichard A, et al: Arterial remodeling after coronary angioplasty: A serial intravascular ultrasound study. Circulation 1996;94:35-43.

56. Staab ME, Srivatsa SS, Lerman A, et al: Arterial remodeling after experimental percutaneous injury is highly dependent on adventitial injury and histopathology. Int J Cardiol 1997;58:31-40.

57. Labinaz M, Pels K, Hoffert C, et al: Time course and importance of neoadventitial formation in arterial remodeling following balloon angioplasty of porcine coronary arteries. Cardiovasc Res 1999;41:255-266.

58. Dussaillant GR, Mintz GS, Pichard AD, et al: Small stent size and intimal hyperplasia contribute to restenosis: A volumetric intravascular ultrasound analysis. J Am Coll Cardiol 1995;26:720-724.

59. Costa MA, Sabaté M, Kay IP, et al: Three-dimensional intravascular ultrasonic volumetric quantification of stent recoil and neointimal formation of two new generation tubular stents. Am J Cardiol 2000;85:135-139.

60. Welt FG, Rogers C: Inflammation and restenosis in the stent era. Arterioscler Thromb Vasc Biol 2002;22:1769-1776.

61. Costa MA, Kozuma K, Gaster AL, et al: Three dimensional intravascular ultrasonic assessment of the local mechanism of restenosis after balloon angioplasty. Heart 2001;85:73-79.

62. Costa MA, Sabate M, Angiolillo DJ, et al: Intravascular ultrasound characterization of the "black hole" phenomenon after drug-eluting stent implantation. Am J Cardiol 2006;97:203-206.

63. Costa J de R Jr, Mintz GS, Carlier SG, et al: Frequency and determinants of black holes in sirolimus-eluting stent restenosis. J Invasive Cardiol 2006;18:348-352.

64. Carter AJ, Aggarwal M, Kopia GA, et al: Long-term effects of polymer-based, slow-release, sirolimus-eluting stents in a porcine coronary model. Cardiovasc Res 2004;63:617-624.

65. Joner M, Finn AV, Farb A, et al: Pathology of drug-eluting stents in humans: Delayed healing and late thrombotic risk. J Am Coll Cardiol 2006;48:193-202.

66. Kuntz RE, Safian RD, Carrozza JP, et al: The importance of acute luminal diameter in determining restenosis after coronary atherectomy or stenting. Circulation 1992;86:1827-1835.

67. de Jaegere P, Mudra H, Figulla H, et al: Intravascular ultrasound-guided optimized stent deployment. Immediate and 6 months clinical and angiographic results from the Multicenter Ultrasound Stenting in Coronaries Study (MUSIC study). Eur Heart J 1998;19:1214-1223.

68. Sabate M, Costa MA, Kozuma K, et al: Geographic miss: A cause of treatment failure in radio-oncology applied to intracoronary radiation therapy. Circulation 2000;101:2467-2471.

69. Sianos G, Kay IP, Costa MA, et al: Geographical miss during catheter-based intracoronary beta-radiation: Incidence and implications in the BRIE study. Beta-Radiation In Europe. J Am Coll Cardiol 2001;38:415-420.

70. Castagna MT, Mintz GS, Leiboff BO, et al: The contribution of "mechanical" problems to in-stent restenosis: An intravascular ultrasonographic analysis of 1090 consecutive in-stent restenosis lesions. Am Heart J 2001;142:970-974.

71. Abizaid A, Kornowski R, Mintz GS, et al: The influence of diabetes mellitus on acute and late clinical outcomes following coronary stent implantation. J Am Coll Cardiol 1998;32:584-589.

72. Hirshfeld JW Jr, Schwartz JS, Jugo R, et al: Restenosis after coronary angioplasty: A multivariate statistical model to relate lesion and procedure variables to restenosis. The M-HEART Investigators. J Am Coll Cardiol 1991;18:647-656.

73. Foley DP, Melkert R, Serruys PW: Influence of coronary vessel size on renarrowing process and late angiographic outcome after successful balloon angioplasty. Circulation 1994;90:1239-1251.

74. Violaris AG, Melkert R, Serruys PW: Long-term luminal renarrowing after successful elective coronary angioplasty of total occlusions. A quantitative angiographic analysis. Circulation 1995;91:2140-2150.

75. Kastrati A, Schomig A, Elezi S, et al: Predictive factors of restenosis after coronary stent placement. J Am Coll Cardiol 1997;30:1428-1436.

76. Kastrati A, Elezi S, Dirschinger J, et al: Influence of lesion length on restenosis after coronary stent placement. Am J Cardiol 1999;83:1617-1622.

77. de Feyter PJ, Kay P, Disco C, Serruys PW: Reference chart derived from post-stent-implantation intravascular ultra-

sound predictors of 6-month expected restenosis on quantitative coronary angiography. Circulation 1999;100: 1777-1783.

78. Serruys PW, Kay IP, Disco C, et al: Periprocedural quantitative coronary angiography after Palmaz-Schatz stent implantation predicts the restenosis rate at six months: Results of a meta-analysis of the BElgian NEtherlands Stent study (BENESTENT) I, BENESTENT II Pilot, BENESTENT II and MUSIC trials. Multicenter Ultrasound Stent In Coronaries. J Am Coll Cardiol 1999;34:1067-1074.

79. Lemos PA, Hoye A, Serruys PW: Recurrent angina after revascularization: An emerging problem for the clinician. Coron Artery Dis 2004;15(Suppl 1):S11-S15.

80. Costa M, Angiolillo DJ, Teirstein P, et al: Sirolimus-eluting stents for treatment of complex bypass graft disease: Insights from the SECURE registry. J Invasive Cardiol 2005;17: 396-398.

81. Lemos PA, Hoye A, Goedhart D, et al: Clinical, angiographic, and procedural predictors of angiographic restenosis after sirolimus-eluting stent implantation in complex patients: An evaluation from the Rapamycin-Eluting Stent Evaluated At Rotterdam Cardiology Hospital (RESEARCH) study. Circulation 2004;109:1366-1370.

82. Kastrati A, Dibra A, Eberle S, et al: Sirolimus-eluting stents vs paclitaxel-eluting stents in patients with coronary artery disease: Meta-analysis of randomized trials. JAMA 2005; 294:819-825.

83. Kastrati A, Dibra A, Mehilli J, et al: Predictive factors of restenosis after coronary implantation of sirolimus- or paclitaxel-eluting stents. Circulation 2006;113:2293-2300.

84. Windecker S, Remondino A, Eberli FR, et al: Sirolimus-eluting and paclitaxel-eluting stents for coronary revascularization. N Engl J Med 2005;353:653-662.

85. Serruys PW, de Jaegere P, Kiemeneij F, et al: A comparison of balloon-expandable-stent implantation with balloon angioplasty in patients with coronary artery disease. BENESTENT study group. N Engl J Med 1994;331:489-495.

86. Fischman DL, Leon MB, Baim DS, et al: A randomized comparison of coronary-stent placement and balloon angioplasty in the treatment of coronary artery disease. Stent Restenosis Study Investigators. N Engl J Med 1994;331: 496-501.

87. Moses JW, Leon MB, Popma JJ, et al: Sirolimus-eluting stents versus standard stents in patients with stenosis in a native coronary artery. N Engl J Med 2003;349:1315-1323.

88. Stone GW, Ellis SG, Cox DA, et al: A polymer-based, paclitaxel-eluting stent in patients with coronary artery disease. N Engl J Med 2004;350:221-231.

89. Fajadet J, Wijns W, Laarman GJ, et al: Randomized, double-blind, multicenter study of the Endeavor zotarolimus-eluting phosphorylcholine-encapsulated stent for treatment of native coronary artery lesions: Clinical and angiographic results of the ENDEAVOR II trial. Circulation 2006;114: 798-806.

90. Sabate M, Jimenez-Quevedo P, Angiolillo DJ, et al: Randomized comparison of sirolimus-eluting stent versus standard stent for percutaneous coronary revascularization in diabetic patients: The diabetes and Sirolimus-Eluting Stent (DIABETES) trial. Circulation 2005;112:2175-2183.

91. Colombo A, Drzewiecki J, Banning A, et al: Randomized study to assess the effectiveness of slow- and moderate-release polymer-based paclitaxel-eluting stents for coronary artery lesions. Circulation 2003;108:788-794.

92. Morice MC, Colombo A, Meier B, et al: Sirolimus- vs paclitaxel-eluting stents in de novo coronary artery lesions: The REALITY trial: A randomized controlled trial. JAMA 2006; 295:895-904.

93. Mehran R, Dangas G, Abizaid AS, et al: Angiographic patterns of in-stent restenosis: Classification and implications for long-term outcome. Circulation 1999;100:1872-1878.

94. Alfonso F, Cequier A, Angel J, et al: Value of the American College of Cardiology/American Heart Association angiographic classification of coronary lesion morphology in patients with in-stent restenosis. Insights from the Restenosis Intra-stent Balloon angioplasty versus elective Stenting

95. Lemos PA, Saia F, Ligthart JM, Arampatzis CA, et al: Coronary restenosis after sirolimus-eluting stent implantation: Morphological description and mechanistic analysis from a consecutive series of cases. Circulation 2003;108:257-260.

96. Colombo A, Orlic D, Stankovic G, et al: Preliminary observations regarding angiographic pattern of restenosis after rapamycin-eluting stent implantation. Circulation 2003;107: 2178-2180.

97. Corbett SJ, Cosgrave J, Melzi G, et al: Patterns of restenosis after drug-eluting stent implantation: Insights from a contemporary and comparative analysis of sirolimus- and paclitaxel-eluting stents. Eur Heart J 2006;27:2330-2337.

98. Steigen TK, Maeng M, Wiseth R, et al: Randomized study on simple versus complex stenting of coronary artery bifurcation lesions: The Nordic bifurcation study. Circulation 2006;114:1955-1961.

99. Erbel R, Haude M, Hopp HW, et al: Coronary-artery stenting compared with balloon angioplasty for restenosis after initial balloon angioplasty. Restenosis Stent Study Group. N Engl J Med 1998;339:1672-1678.

100. Alfonso F, Zueco J, Cequier A, et al: A randomized comparison of repeat stenting with balloon angioplasty in patients with in-stent restenosis. J Am Coll Cardiol 2003;42:796-805.

101. Alfonso F, Auge JM, Zueco J, et al: Long-term results (three to five years) of the Restenosis Intrastent: Balloon angioplasty versus elective Stenting (RIBS) randomized study. J Am Coll Cardiol 2005;46:756-760.

102. Waksman R, Ajani AE, White RL, et al: Five-year follow-up after intracoronary gamma radiation therapy for in-stent restenosis. Circulation 2004;109:340-344.

103. Sousa JE, Costa MA, Abizaid A, et al: Sirolimus-eluting stent for the treatment of in-stent restenosis: A quantitative coronary angiography and three-dimensional intravascular ultrasound study. Circulation 2003;107:24-27.

104. Holmes DR Jr, Teirstein P, Satler L, et al: Sirolimus-eluting stents vs vascular brachytherapy for in-stent restenosis within bare-metal stents: The SISR randomized trial. JAMA 2006; 295:1264-1273.

105. Stone GW, Ellis SG, O'Shaughnessy CD, et al: Paclitaxel-eluting stents vs vascular brachytherapy for in-stent restenosis within bare-metal stents: The TAXUS V ISR randomized trial. JAMA 2006;295:1253-1263.

106. Scheller B, Hehrlein C, Bocksch W, et al: Treatment of coronary in-stent restenosis with a paclitaxel-coated balloon catheter. N Engl J Med 2006;355:2113-2124.

107. Lemos PA, van Mieghem CA, Arampatzis CA, et al: Post-sirolimus-eluting stent restenosis treated with repeat percutaneous intervention: Late angiographic and clinical outcomes. Circulation 2004;109:2500-2502.

108. Cosgrave J, Melzi G, Biondi-Zoccai GG, et al: Drug-eluting stent restenosis: The pattern predicts the outcome. J Am Coll Cardiol 2006;47:2399-2404.

109. van Beusekom HM, Whelan DM, Hofma SH, et al: Long-term endothelial dysfunction is more pronounced after stenting than after balloon angioplasty in porcine coronary arteries. J Am Coll Cardiol 1998;32:1109-1117.

110. Drachman DE, Edelman ER, Seifert P, et al: Neointimal thickening after stent delivery of paclitaxel: Change in composition and arrest of growth over six months. J Am Coll Cardiol 2000;36:2325-2332.

111. Rogers C, Parikh S, Seifert P, Edelman ER: Endogenous cell seeding: Remnant endothelium after stenting enhances vascular repair. Circulation 1996;94:2909-2914.

112. Kawamoto A, Gwon HC, Iwaguro H, et al: Therapeutic potential of ex vivo expanded endothelial progenitor cells for myocardial ischemia. Circulation 2001;103:634-637.

113. Kutryk MJ, Foley DP, van den Brand M, et al: Local intracoronary administration of antisense oligonucleotide against c-myc for the prevention of in-stent restenosis: Results of the randomized Investigation by the Thoraxcenter of Antisense DNA using Local Delivery and IVUS after Coronary

Stenting (ITALICS) trial. J Am Coll Cardiol 2002;39: 281-287.

114. Alt E, Haehnel I, Beilharz C, et al: Inhibition of neointima formation after experimental coronary artery stenting: A new biodegradable stent coating releasing hirudin and the prostacyclin analogue iloprost. Circulation 2000;101:1453-1458.

115. Lin CE, Garvey DS, Janero DR, et al: Combination of paclitaxel and nitric oxide as a novel treatment for the reduction of restenosis. J Med Chem 2004;47:2276-2282.

116. Lincoff AM, Topol EJ, Ellis SG: Local drug delivery for the prevention of restenosis. Fact, fancy, and future. Circulation 1994;90:2070-2084.

117. Vogt F, Stein A, Rettemeier G, et al: Long-term assessment of a novel biodegradable paclitaxel-eluting coronary polylactide stent. Eur Heart J 2004;25:1330-1340.

118. Heublein B, Rohde R, Kaese V, et al: Biocorrosion of magnesium alloys: A new principle in cardiovascular implant technology? Heart 2003;89:651-656.

CHAPTER
33 Vascular Brachytherapy for Restenosis

Ron Waksman

KEY POINTS

- Vascular brachytherapy uses local radiation administration as an adjunct intervention for the prevention of restenosis.
- Isotopes that have been tested and used clinically were ^{192}I (gamma source) and ^{32}P, ^{90}Sr/^{90}Y, and ^{188}Re (beta sources).
- Extensive preclinical testing detected efficacy in the reduction of neointima formation after vascular brachytherapy in peripheral and coronary arteries.
- Vascular brachytherapy was proved to be safe and effective for the treatment of in-stent restenosis using beta and gamma emitters and was approved for marketing by the U.S. Food and Drug Administration (FDA) for this indication only.
- Studies using vascular brachytherapy for de novo lesions had mixed results; it was effective as an adjunct to balloon angioplasty and deleterious with stent implantation.

- The use of vascular brachytherapy in the superficial femoral artery as an adjunct to balloon angioplasty showed positive but not conclusive results.
- The main complications of vascular brachytherapy are stent thrombosis, edge-effect stenosis, and late restenosis. These complications can be corrected by administering prolonged antiplatelet therapy, covering the entire injured segment, and increasing dosage.
- Drug-eluting stents obviate the need for vascular brachytherapy because of lower restenosis rates and competitiveness in efficacy and logistics for the treatment of bare metal stent restenosis.
- The use of vascular brachytherapy is limited to patients with drug-eluting stent restenosis or patients with restenosis who are not candidates for drug-eluting stent implantation.

Vascular brachytherapy (VBT) after angioplasty for the prevention of restenosis was introduced in 1992 by several investigators who performed a series of preclinical studies and demonstrated consistently profound reduction of neointima formation after balloon injury (Fig. 33-1).[1-22] In these experiments, radiation was delivered into the vessel wall by high-dose rate catheter-based systems or by low-dose rate radioactive implants, such as radioactive stents. The results of these preclinical trials were encouraging and facilitated the initiation of feasibility clinical trials first in the peripheral arteries, later in coronary arteries through pivotal trials, and then in commercialization of the technology for clinical use in Europe in 1999. In November 2000, the U.S. Food and Drug Administration (FDA) approved VBT for in-stent restenosis.

Restenosis after angioplasty has been the major limitation confronting interventional cardiology. The three major components of restenosis after balloon angioplasty are an exuberant cellular proliferation and matrix synthesis (i.e., intimal hyperplasia) triggered by injury to the vessel wall,[23-26]

acute elastic recoil immediately after balloon deflation, and late vascular contraction (i.e., remodeling) resulting in a decrease in total vessel diameter.[27-30] Coronary stenting eliminates elastic recoil and vessel contraction by acting as a mechanical scaffold within the vessel, reducing the restenosis rate.[31,32] However, stents are associated with a higher degree of proliferative response and increased lumen late loss.[33]

With the use of stents in almost 90% of coronary intervention, in-stent restenosis, after it occurs, is the major challenge in prevention and treatment. Conventional treatments such as repeat balloon angioplasty, ablative treatment with atherectomy devices, laser angioplasty, or cutting balloon have been disappointing, with recurrence rates averaging 25% to 50% for focal restenosis and up to 65% for diffuse restenosis. Drug-eluting stents (DESs) reduced significantly the rate of restenosis and the need for repeat revascularization when compared with bare metal stents, but they are also associated with a modest degree of restenosis (up to 18%), especially for complex lesions and subset populations and recently

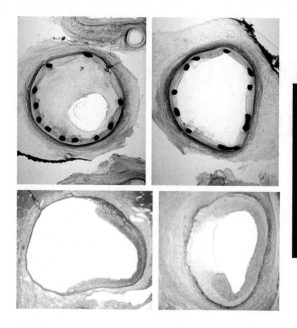

- Reduce intimal hyperplasia (overgrowth of tissue)
- Positively impact vessel remodeling
- Delayed vessel healing

Figure 33-1. Results from preclinical trials, including reduced intimal hyperplasia, positive impact on vessel remodeling, and delayed vessel healing. (From Waksman R, Robinson KA, Crocker IR, et al: Endovascular low-dose irradiation inhibits neointima formation after coronary artery balloon injury in swine. A possible role for radiation therapy in restenosis prevention. Circulation 1995;91:1533-1539.)

reported to be associated with a new phenomenon of very late stent thrombosis.

Ionizing radiation occurs in many forms, ranging from lightly ionizing x-rays, electrons, and beta or gamma rays to more densely ionizing neutrons, alpha particles, and other heavy particles. VBT has emerged as a promising means for reducing the restenosis recurrence rate. For years, the growth-inhibiting properties of ionizing radiation have been used successfully to control benign proliferative disorders such as keloid formation, ophthalmic pterygium, macular malformations, arteriovenous (AV) malformations, and heterotopic ossification.[34,35] Based on this experience, the intravascular delivery of radiation was viewed as a viable solution to inhibit neointimal hyperplasia and reduce the restenosis rate.

RADIATION BIOLOGY AND MECHANISM

For the prevention of restenosis, radiation biology intervenes in the cell cycle to cause cell death to radiosensitive cells, especially those undergoing mitosis after vascular injury. The cell death results from chromosomal damage, which depends on the cumulative dose, the dose rate, and the cell cycle. Cells in the M and G_2 phases are the most sensitive to radiation, those in G_1 are sensitive only in the early G_1 phase, and cells in G_0 are radioresistant (Fig. 33-2).

Ionizing radiation can cause tissue damage directly and indirectly. Direct injury occurs when an ionizing particle interacts with and is absorbed by a target biologic macromolecule such as DNA, RNA, or protein enzymes. In the process of indirect injury, the ionizing radiation interacts with cellular water to form a highly reactive hydroxyl free radical. The free radicals interact and damage the biologic macromolecules. Radiation causes different types of DNA damage: change or loss of a base and breakage of the

hydrogen bond between the two chains of the DNA molecule. For some cells, radiation-induced apoptosis (i.e., programmed cell death) occurs, although this may not be the main mechanism for the effect of radiation on myofibroblasts.[36] Hall and colleagues[37] have shown that human endothelial and smooth muscle cells (SMCs) have similar survival curves and suggested that inhibition of SMCs would result in inhibition of endothelial cells. Because cells can repair radiation damage, subtherapeutic doses may only delay restenosis, and the surviving cells will continue to divide and eventually occupy the lumen wall. Lower dose rates are less effective and require higher cumulative doses to reach the therapeutic window. The half-time for repair is probably about one-half hour, and a minimum dose rate is necessary to intervene in the cell cycle to stop cell division.[37]

Modeling studies suggest that comparatively few cell doublings of SMCs are needed to result in restenosis. This is consistent with the fact that a radiation dose of about 18 Gy (corresponding to a surviving fraction of about 10^5 cells) successfully inhibits reste-

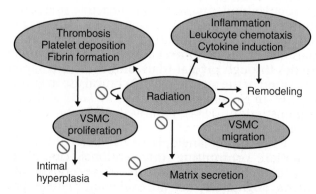

Figure 33-2. Biology of ionizing radiation. VSMC, vascular smooth muscle cell.

nosis. There appears to be a relatively narrow therapeutic window between the minimum dose needed to slow down the proliferation of SMCs and the maximum dose that can be tolerated before late sequelae occur in the vessel wall. The latter dose is not known with any certainty; the best estimates come from external radiation subtherapeutic doses that may have a potential to cause a stimulatory effect in vessels that were exposed to injury. Some of the features of endovascular radiation include delayed healing with accumulation of fibrin deposition, the potential of thrombosis and accelerated atherosclerosis, and the recurrence of late restenosis. Other late effects of VBT may be seen 5 to 10 years after treatment. Among the potential late effects are late thrombosis, fibrosis, thinning of the media, and aneurysm formation.[38]

Some of the potential mechanisms by which radiation may reduce restenosis were examined in a series of studies performed on pig coronary arteries by Waksman and coworkers.[36] After balloon overstretch injury, the arteries were treated with $^{90}Sr/^{90}Y$ (14 or 28 Gy prescribed to a depth of 2 mm). The animals were sacrificed 3, 7, and 14 days later. 5-Bromo-2-deoxyuridine (BrdU) was administered 24 hours before sacrifice to label proliferating cells. By 3 days after injury, cell proliferation, assessed by BrdU immunostaining, was significantly reduced in the media and the adventitia of irradiated vessels compared with the control arteries. However, there were no significant differences in the adventitia or the media of the irradiated arteries by 7 days compared with controls. The degree of α-actin staining for SMCs and myofibroblasts, which was used as an index for remodeling, was lower in the adventitia of the irradiated vessels by 2 weeks after the injury. A larger vessel perimeter was found in irradiated vessels in a dose-dependent fashion, suggesting favorable remodeling. Terminal deoxynucleotidyl transferase-mediated dUTP nick end labeling (TUNEL) detected apoptosis at 3 and 7 days in injured arteries and irradiated injured segments, with no significant difference in the degree of apoptosis between these two groups.[36] The degree of apoptosis at earlier or later time points has not been analyzed. However, it is possible that earlier on day 1 or later on day 14, there would be a significant difference between irradiated and nonirradiated vessels. It is not expected that substantial apoptosis will be detected with long-term (>6 months) follow-up. These studies suggest that endovascular radiation reduces restenosis by inhibiting the first wave of cell proliferation in the adventitia and the media and by inducing favorable remodeling.

Wang and associates[39] have suggested that macrophages are an important target for VBT. They argue that macrophages are very sensitive to radiation and may make up more than 30% of the cells in an advanced atherosclerotic lesion subjected to angioplasty. They have cited Ross's response to injury hypothesis, which holds that macrophage growth factors contribute significantly to vascular lesion for-

mation. Wilcox[39a] states that the adventitial myofibroblast is the critical cell affected by radiation therapy and suggests that doses of radiation that fail to block myofibroblast proliferation and recruitment also fail to inhibit constrictive vascular remodeling and restenosis. Most likely, radiation blocks restenosis and vascular remodeling after angioplasty through an induction of cell cycle arrest, possibly by increasing p21 expression in adventitial cells.[39] Radiation may be effective because it works as a central mechanism that blocks cell proliferation induced by a variety of stimuli, including macrophages, platelets, and other growth factors. Christen and colleagues[40] claim that SMCs derived from the media are the main component of the neointima formation after balloon angioplasty and stent implantation. They investigated the expression of smooth muscle myosin heavy-chain isoform 1 and 2, desmin and smoothelin, and found expression of smoothelin at the media and neointima of stented and balloon-injured arteries. Long-term studies will be necessary to determine whether this effect is long lasting or merely delays intimal proliferation and negative remodeling. Additional studies will also be necessary to determine whether proinflammatory cytokines such as interferon-γ (IFN-γ), tumor necrosis factor-α (TNF-α), and interleukin-1 (IL-1), as well as anti-inflammatory cytokines such as transforming growth factor-β1 (TGF-β1), known to be induced by radiation, are involved in the anti-restenotic effect of endovascular radiation.

RADIATION PHYSICS AND SYSTEMS

Different isotopes on various platforms and systems have been developed for the use of endovascular brachytherapy. The main platforms that deliver radiation are catheter-based systems such as line source wires, radioactive seeds, radioactive gas- and liquid-filled balloons, or stents using beta or gamma emitters. Isotope selection and dosimetry for intracoronary brachytherapy are derived from the anatomy of the vessel and the treated lesion, and by knowing the target tissue for this therapy. Other important parameters are the diameter and the curvature of the vessel, the eccentricity of the plaque, lesion length, composition of the plaque, amount of calcium, and the presence or absence of a stent in the treated segment. Gamma- and beta-emitting radionuclides being investigated and used in the clinical trials for VBT are presented in Table 33-1.

Requirements for an ideal radioisotope in VBT include dose distribution of a few millimeters from the source with minimal dose gradient, low-dose levels to the surrounding tissues, treatment time of less than 10 minutes, and a sufficient half-life for multiple applications when used in a catheter-based system. Among the considerations of source selection are the source energy half-life, available activity, penetration and dose distribution, radiation exposure to the patient and the operator, shielding requirement, availability, and cost.

Table 33-1.   Radionuclides for Vascular Brachytherapy*

Isotope	Emission	Half-Life	Beta Energy (MeV)		Photon Energy (MeV)	
			Average	Maximum	Average	Maximum
192Ir	Beta, photon	74 days	0.18	0.67	0.37	1.06
125I	Photon	60 days	—	—	0.028	0.035
103Pd	Photon	17 days	—	—	0.020	0.021
90Sr/Y	Beta	29 years	0.93	2.28	—	—
90Y	Beta	64 hours	0.93	2.28	—	—
32P	Beta	14 days	0.69	1.71	—	—
188W/Re	Beta, photon	69 days	0.77	2.12	0.16	0.93
133Xe	Beta, photon	5 days	0.10	0.35	0.056	0.081
186Re	Beta	91 hours	0.35	1.08	—	—
188Re	Beta, photon	17 hours	0.77	2.12	0.16	0.93
106Rh	Beta, photon	130 days	1.42	3.54	0.57	3.2

*The term ionizing photon radiation is preferred to x-rays or gamma rays as this implies photon radiation of sufficient energy to produce medically significant ionization, independent of the origin within the atom.

Understanding Gamma Radiation

Gamma rays are photons that originate from the center of the nucleus, as opposed to x-rays, which originate from the orbital outside of the nucleus. Gamma rays have deeply penetrating energies between 20 keV and 20 MeV, which require an excess of shielding, compared with beta and x-ray emitters. The only gamma ray isotope in use is ^{192}Ir. Other isotopes that emit both gamma rays and x-rays are ^{125}I and ^{103}P, which have lower energies and require higher activities to deliver the prescribed dose in an acceptable dwell time (<20 minutes). The latter isotopes are not available in such activities or are too expensive for this application. The dosimetry of ^{192}Ir is well understood, and because of less falloff in dose compared with beta emitters, the dose gradient at the area of interest is acceptable. ^{192}Ir is available in activities of up to 10 Ci, but because of the high penetration, the average shielding of a catheterization laboratory cannot handle more than the activity of a 500-mCi source. This limitation is associated with dwell times of more than 12 minutes for doses of more than 15 Gy when prescribed at a 2-mm radial distance from the source.

Understanding Beta Radiation

Beta rays are high-energy electrons emitted by nuclei that contain too many or too few neutrons. These negatively charged particles have a wide variety of energies, including transition energy, particularly between parent-daughter cells, and have a wide variety of half-lives, from several minutes (^{62}Cu) to 30 years (^{90}Sr/^{90}Y). Beta emitters rapidly lose their energy to the surrounding tissue, and their range is within 1 cm of tissue. They are associated with a higher gradient to the near wall. The use of beta sources for vascular application is attractive in terms of radiation exposure and safety.

Several dosimetry issues remain controversial: the choice of isotope, beta- versus gamma-emitting radioisotopes, centering versus noncentering devices, and administration of high- versus low-dose rates of radiation. To determine an accurate dosimetry, it is essential to first determine the treatment dose and the potential target: the plaque, the media, or the adventitia.

Despite the notion that the adventitia is the target,[36] it is hard to ignore that the wall and the residual plaque receive much higher doses, which may be essential to obtain efficacy. The doses prescribed today in clinical studies are empirical and are based on animal studies and the limited experience gained from treating other benign diseases. Because a wide variety of doses demonstrated effectiveness in preclinical studies, there must be a therapeutic window that allows for some flexibility in selecting the isotope for this application.

Dosimetric Considerations

Measurement standardization of ionizing radiation is essential. The dosimetry measurements determine the absorbed dose at a point in a medium. Radiation detection devices used in VBT include radiochromic film, thermoluminescence dosimeters, plastic scintillators, and extrapolation chambers. Isotope selection should take into account variables such as the effective energy, penetration properties, different dose gradients to the potential target areas, and the differences in the half-life across the beta and gamma isotopes. Ignoring these dosimetric considerations may result in treatment failure. A clinical example of underdosing the adventitia due to a fall in dose gradient with ^{90}Y, which resulted in the lack of effectiveness in reduction of the restenosis rate despite the use of a centering delivery system, has been reported.[41] A modification in the dose prescription, from 18 Gy to the surface of the balloon to a distance of 1.2 mm from the balloon, resulted in complete inhibition of neointima formation in stented and balloon injured coronary arteries in the porcine model. Intravascular ultrasound (IVUS) can assist in treatment planning and dosing, because it determines the actual lumen size and distances from the source to the lumen and the adventitia. Nevertheless, fixed radial prescription point seems to be easier and more practical without compromising the outcome. Most dose prescriptions have assumed a linear source centered in the vessel and a homogeneous, water-equivalent absorbing media. Some situations differ from these assumptions, which may potentially alter the dose delivered to the vessel wall. Significant dose perturbations in the dose distributions can occur from the presence of stent wires. The dose perturbation is more significant for beta emitters than for gamma emitters. Amols[41a] reported that the average dose rate could be reduced up to 14% for some stents, with the most severe homogeneity occurring near the stent surface. Beyond 0.5 mm from the stent surface, the dose distribution was similar to the unstented dose. Other considerations should be the presence of calcification in the vessel wall, vessel curvature, centering versus noncentering of the source in the vessel wall, the length of the treated segment, and the need for stepping.

Brachytherapy in Animal Models

External Radiation Therapy

The data from studies using external radiation therapy for the prevention of restenosis in animal models are not conclusive. Schwartz and coworkers[41] administered radiation (400 to 800 cGy) with an orthovoltage x-ray unit to the coronary vessels after stent placement in the porcine stent model of restenosis. In their study, external radiation treatment administered after coronary stent placement accentuated the development of neointimal hyperplasia. The degree of injury and lack of precise delivery to moving epicardial arteries are potential explanations for these findings. In later studies, higher doses of 21 Gy to the entire heart, which completed inhibition of the neointima formation, was demonstrated in the same model. Because this approach is associated with higher volumes of radiation, which may result in late fibrosis to the whole heart, the approach of external radiation is less attractive compared with the endovascular approach.

Catheter-Based Systems

Several groups using catheter-based systems have obtained consistent evidence for the efficacy of radiation in preventing restenosis using both gamma and beta emitters. Waksman and colleagues,[1,2] Wiedermann and coworkers,[3,4] and Mazur and associates[5] conducted separate studies using the gamma emitter [192]Ir. These studies showed marked reduction in neointimal hyperplasia after balloon injury in the short term (2 to 4 weeks) as assessed by histomorphometric studies in the porcine restenosis model. Waksman and colleagues[1,2] and Wiedermann and coworkers[3,4] delivered radiation through a hand-loading ^{192}Ir ribbon, whereas Mazur and associates[5] used a high-dose-rate afterloader to deliver similar doses using the same isotope. In two of the studies, the reduction

in the neointimal hyperplasia in the irradiated arteries was shown at 6 months.[1,4]

Several safety-related aspects of endovascular brachytherapy have been examined. In the previously cited studies, there was no evidence of malignant or premalignant transformation in the treated animals. There was no evidence of excess fibrosis or aneurysm formation in any of the arteries. Wiedermann and coworkers[6] studied endothelial function with intracoronary infusion of acetylcholine immediately after irradiation and at 4 weeks' follow-up. Vasoconstriction was demonstrated in response to acetylcholine in the noninjured, irradiated arteries, implying immediate stunning or impairment of endothelial function. However, the normal vasodilatory response to acetylcholine was restored in these arteries at 4 weeks. Moreover, Waksman and colleagues[1] demonstrated complete re-endothelialization by electron microscopy at 2 weeks in balloon-injured and irradiated arteries (dose of 14 Gy). However, incomplete re-endothelialization was seen after stent implantation with similar doses.

Lower doses can cause stimulatory effects in injured arteries. Wiedermann[3] demonstrated that low doses of 10 Gy could stimulate hyperplasia in porcine injured arteries. Several preclinical studies have been conducted with beta emitters in different animal models. Verin and coworkers[8] delivered intra-arterial radiation by means of ^{90}Y and a centering balloon catheter in atherosclerotic rabbit iliac and carotid arteries. They used doses of 6, 12, and 18 Gy and demonstrated a reduction in neointimal cells in all treated groups. At 6 weeks, however, the reduction in neointima was maintained only in the rabbits that received 18 Gy. Waksman and colleagues.[9] demonstrated reduction in neointima in a dose-dependent manner (7 to 56 Gy) with ^{90}Sr/^{90}Y, a pure beta emitter, in porcine coronary arteries. A consistent effect of reduction of neointima was seen with doses above 21 Gy, without an increase in adverse effects. Raizner[11] showed a similar effect of reduction of neointima formation, post balloon and stent injury with another pure beta emitter, ^{32}P, using doses of 32 Gy. The beta and gamma emitters appear to be equally effective in stented arteries, particularly when radiation is delivered before stent implantation.

Long-Term Animal Studies

Results of long-term animal studies using beta and gamma emitter sources were disappointing. Wiedermann[4] reported that at 6 months, arteries subjected to gamma radiation using ^{192}Ir had less neointima formation compared with control. Similar observations were reported by Waksman and associates[2] using the same source, ^{192}Ir, with 14 Gy. Six-month studies using ^{32}P in balloon injury model had similar findings, but studies with beta emitters (^{32}P and ^{90}Sr/^{90}Y) in a stented porcine coronary artery model were associated with increased mortality, thrombosis, and neointima formation compared with control. Similarly, 6-month studies with radioactive stents demonstrated an excess of neointima formation in the radioactive stents compared with control. Few of the observations in long-term animal studies are reproduced in humans. Among them are the late thrombosis phenomenon, delayed restenosis, and inferior results using stent and radiation versus balloon and radiation. The discrepancy between the long-term animal results and the human results at 3 to 5 years' follow-up can be explained by the differences in the species—normal porcine coronary arteries versus atherosclerotic human coronary arteries and the age of the animals (younger animals subjected late radiation effects).

RADIATION SYSTEMS FOR THE PERIPHERAL VASCULAR SYSTEM

The vessel size of the peripheral arterial system favored the use of gamma radiation because of the penetration characteristics of the emitter. Most investigational work performed in the peripheral arterial system used ^{192}Ir in doses of 14 to 18 Gy prescribed at 2 mm from the source center. Several radiation systems for peripheral endovascular brachytherapy have been suggested and are under development and testing.

External Radiation Therapy

External beam radiation is a viable option for the treatment of peripheral vessels. It allows a homogeneous dose distribution with the possibility of fractionation.

External radiation therapy is currently used in a few centers for the treatment of in-stent restenosis of the superficial femoral artery (SFA). Preliminary reports are encouraging, although caution should be applied to this strategy because of the potential for radiation injury to the nerve, vein, and the skin. Preliminary attempts with external radiation for the treatment of AV dialysis grafts failed to reduce the restenosis rate. This unsuccessful attempt was attributed to the conservative use of low doses and thrombosis of these grafts. Using stereotactic techniques to localize the radiation to the target area may improve the results of this approach.

In their study, Therasse and associates[42] tested the theory that external beam radiation would be more practical to administer than VBT after percutaneous transluminal angioplasty (PTA) in reducing restenosis. After femoropopliteal PTA without stent placement, 99 patients were randomly assigned to 0 Gy (placebo, $n = 24$), 7 Gy ($n = 24$), 10.5 Gy ($n = 6$), or 14 Gy ($n = 25$) of external beam radiation of the PTA site (with a 3-cm margin at both extremities) in one session 24 hours after PTA. Restenosis of more than 50% was present in 50%, 65%, 48%, and 25% of patients, respectively, for the 0-, 7-, 10.5-, and 14-Gy groups ($P = .072$). At 18 months, repeated revascularizations were required in 25% of patients in the 0-Gy group versus 12% of patients in the 14-Gy group ($P = .24$). It was found that a single session of external beam radiation of 14 Gy to the femoropopliteal

angioplasty site significantly reduced restenosis at 1 year.[42]

Catheter-Based Gamma Systems

The most common catheter-based system used for SFA application is the MicroSelectron HDR system (Nucletron-Odelft, Delft, The Netherlands), which uses a computerized, high-dose-rate afterloader system that delivers a 3-mm stepping, 10-Ci dose of ^{192}Ir into a closed-lumen radiation catheter (Fig. 33-3). The peripheral brachytherapy centering catheter (Paris catheter, Guidant Corporation, Indianapolis, IN) is a 7-Fr, double-lumen catheter with multiple centering balloons near its distal tip that enable the catheter to be in the center of the lumen of large peripheral vessels during inflation. The Paris catheter is no longer available. The only closed-end lumen catheter available is that used for oncology applications.

Catheter-Based Beta Systems

The only catheter-based beta system available is the BetaCath system (Novoste, Norcross, GA), with a source train of up to 60 mm, which can be pulled back to allow coverage of long lesions (Fig. 33-4). The main limitation of the system is the penetration of the beta emitter, which is weakened significantly beyond 5 mm. This system can be used for below-the-knee applications or for other small vessels, including in-stent renal stenosis. It is recommended to perform the radiation before the intervention to ensure better centering and a higher dose to the treated proliferating tissue.

Other innovative catheter-based radiation system developments have been halted because of the declining interest in the VBT field or slow recruitment into clinical trials. Included among these halted developments was the Radiance balloon system (Radiance Medical Systems, Irvine, CA), which was particularly attractive for peripheral applications because it is associated with apposition of a solid beta ^{32}P source attached to the inner balloon surface into the surface of the vessel wall. Another approach was the use of low x-ray energy delivered intraluminally through a catheter. The emitter was 5 mm long and 1.25 to 2.0 mm in diameter and could be administered distally to the lesion and pulled back to cover the entire lesion length. The Corona system, a modification of the BetaCath system, was used to accommodate beta systems with the ^{90}Sr/^{90}Y emitter in the peripheral system. In this system, the balloon was filled with carbon dioxide, allowing centering and preventing dose attenuation. A clinical study in SFA for in-stent restenosis lesions (More Patency with Beta In the Lower Extremity [MOBILE]) was terminated because of poor enrollment. The Corona system was also used in the Beta Radiation after Balloon Angioplasty for Improving Life Span of Recurrent Failed Arteriovenous Fistulas (BRAVO) study for patients with AV dialysis grafts.

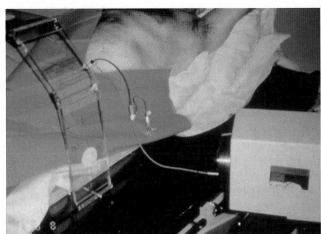

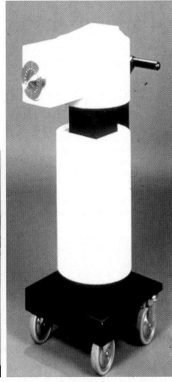

Figure 33-3. MicroSelectron high-dose-rate automatic afterloader.

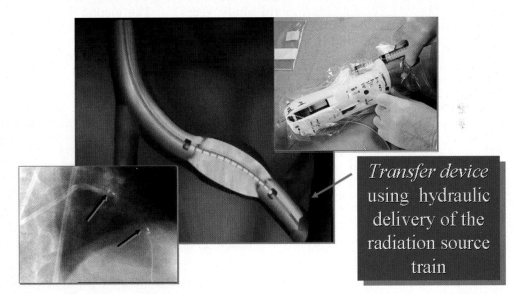

Transfer device using hydraulic delivery of the radiation source train

Figure 33-4. The Novoste Beta-Cath system. (Courtesy of the Novoste Corporation, Norcross, GA.)

CLINICAL TRIALS

Superficial Femoral Artery

Liermann and Schopohl were the first to perform VBT for the treatment of in-stent restenosis in the peripheral arteries. Known as the Frankfurt Experience, this pilot study was conducted in 30 patients with in-stent restenosis in their SFAs.[43-46] Patients underwent atherectomy and PTA, followed by endovascular radiation using the MicroSelectron HDR afterloader and a noncentering catheter with [192]Ir. No adverse effects from the radiation treatment were reported at up to 7 years' follow-up. The 5-year patency rate of the target vessel was 82%, with only 11% stenosis within the treated segment reported. Late total occlusion developed in 7% of the treated vessels after 37 months.

The Vienna Experience

A series of studies was conducted at the University of Vienna. Most were randomized studies targeting the SFA with or without stents using the MicroSelectron HDR afterloader with or without a centering catheter

Table 33-2. Superficial Femoral Artery Irradiation Trials

Study	N	Random.	Center Cath.	Dose (Gy)	Dose Depth (mm)	Patency Control (%)	Patency VBT (%)
Frankfurt[43]	40	—	—	12	3	—	82
Vienna 1[47]	10	—	No	12	3	—	60
Vienna 2[48]	113	Yes	No	12	r + 0	—	72
Vienna 3[49]	134	Yes	Yes	18	r + 2	46	77
Vienna 4[50]	33	No	Yes	14	r + 2	—	79
Vienna 5[50]	98	Yes	Yes	14	r + 2	45	88*
Bern II for restenotic lesions[53]	100	Yes	—	12	r + 2	58	77
PARIS pilot[51]	40	No	Yes	14	r + 2	—	88
PARIS randomized[51]	300	Yes	Yes	14	r + 2	80	76
Swiss 4-arm study[54]	346	Yes	Yes	12	r + 2	58	83

*Excluding the thrombosis cases.
Cath., catheterization; r, radius; Random., randomized; VBT, vascular brachytherapy.

using different doses. The results of these studies are displayed in Table 33-2.

Vienna I was a pilot study with an indication of radiation safety after PTA that showed only 60% patency at 1 year.[47] The Vienna II trial had 113 patients with de novo or recurrent femoropopliteal lesions who were randomized to PTA plus brachytherapy (n = 57) or PTA alone (n = 56). The rate of the primary end point of cumulative patency rates at 12-month follow-up was higher in the PTA plus brachytherapy group (63.6%) compared with the PTA group (35.3%). The patients from this study were followed-up to 36 months and demonstrated durability of the results (Fig. 33-5).[48] In Vienna III, a centering catheter that was used for the same patient population with a dose of 18 Gy showed a restenosis rate of 23.4% in the irradiated group compared with 53.3% in the placebo arm.[49] Vienna IV was a pilot study examining radiation with stenting of the SFA; and Vienna V was a randomized study for similar indications. Both Vienna IV and V demonstrated an increase rate of subacute and late thrombosis when stents were combined with radiation, with up to 16.7% in the radiation group versus 4.3% in the control stenting without radiation group. After thrombosis was controlled, the radiation group had less restenosis.[50]

The Vienna trials demonstrated efficacy of gamma radiation in reduction of restenosis after PTA to the SFA. However, these studies also demonstrated late catch-up of restenosis and late thrombosis in arteries that underwent stenting and radiation therapy.

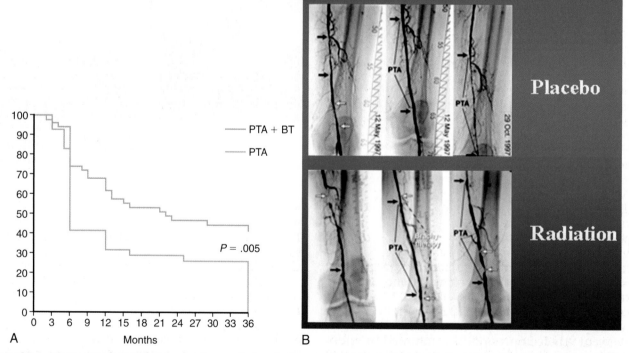

Figure 33-5. Vienna II radiation therapy for de novo lesions in the superficial femoral artery. **A,** Restenosis-free survival curves. **B,** Patterns of restenosis. BT, brachytherapy; PTA, percutaneous transluminal angioplasty. (**B** from Minar E, Pokrajac B, Maca T, et al: Endovascular brachytherapy for prophylaxis of restenosis after femoropopliteal angioplasty: Results of a prospective randomized study. Circulation 2000;102:2694-2699.)

The PARIS Trials

The Paris Radiation Investigational Study (PARIS) is the first FDA-approved, multicenter, randomized, double-blind, controlled study involving 300 patients after PTA to SFA stenosis using a gamma radiation ^{192}Ir source. Using the MicroSelectron high-dose-rate afterloader, a treatment dose of 14 Gy was delivered through a centered segmented end-lumen balloon catheter. The primary objectives of this study were to determine angiographic evidence of patency and a reduction of more than 30% of the restenosis rate of the treated lesion at 6 months. A secondary end point was to determine the clinical patency at 6 and 12 months by treadmill exercise and by the ankle-brachial index (ABI). In the feasibility phase of PARIS, 40 patients with claudication were enrolled. The mean lesion length was 9.9 ± 3.0 cm, with a mean reference vessel diameter of 5.4 ± 0.5 mm. The 6-month angiographic follow-up was completed for 30 patients; 13.3% of them had evidence of clinical restenosis.[51]

Because of poor enrollment, only 203 patients with claudication and femoropopliteal disease were enrolled in the study. After successful PTA, a segmented centering balloon catheter was positioned to cover the PTA site. The patients were transported to the radiation oncology suite and randomized to receive radiation therapy using the MicroSelectron HDR afterloader with ^{192}Ir at a dose of 14 Gy at 2 mm into the vessel wall (105 patients) or treatment with a sham control in 98 patients. Patients were followed for 12 months, with clinic visits at 1, 6, and 12 months and follow-up angiography at 12 months. The restenosis rate at follow-up was similar in both groups (28.6% for brachytherapy versus 27.5% for placebo). There was no significant difference in minimal lumen diameter (MLD), late lumen loss, or the number of total occlusions. Exercise ABI, resting ABI, and maximum walking time were not different between treatment groups. For patients older than 65 years, maximum walking times at 6 and 12 months were better in the brachytherapy group. In the subgroups of patients with diabetes, male patients, or patients receiving clopidogrel or who have a proximal or medial lesion, maximum walking time in the brachytherapy group was better than in the placebo at 6 months but not different at 12 months.

More studies to support the effectiveness of gamma radiation for in-stent restenosis were published by Krueger and coworkers.[52] In this study, 30 patients who underwent PTA for de novo femoropopliteal stenoses were randomly assigned to undergo 14 Gy centered endovascular irradiation (irradiation group, $n = 15$) or no irradiation (control group, $n = 15$). Intra-arterial angiography was performed 6, 12, and 24 months after treatment, and duplex ultrasonography was performed the day before and after PTA and at 1, 3, 6, 9, 12, 18, and 24 months later. Baseline characteristics did not differ significantly between the two groups. Mean absolute individual changes in degree of stenosis compared with the degrees of stenosis shortly after PTA in the irradiation group versus in the control group were $-10.6\% \pm 22.3\%$ versus $39.6\% \pm 24.6\%$ ($P < .001$) at 6 months, $-2.0\% \pm 34.2\%$ versus $40.6\% \pm 32.6\%$ ($P = .002$) at 12 months, and $7.4\% \pm 43.2\%$ versus $37.7\% \pm 34.5\%$ ($P = .043$) at 24 months. The rates of target lesion restenosis at 6 months ($P = .006$) and 12 months ($P = .042$) were significantly lower in the irradiation group. The investigators concluded that endovascular radiation was effective for patients who were treated with angioplasty for de novo femoropopliteal lesions.

Restenotic Lesions and Vascular Brachytherapy

The effectiveness of VBT for restenotic SFA lesions was examined in another randomized study reported by Zehnder and associates.[53] In this study, gamma radiation was used at a dose of 12 Gy. The primary end point was more than 50% restenosis at 12 months assessed by duplex Doppler. The recurrence rate in the radiation arm was 23% versus 42% in the PTA alone group.[53] This study demonstrated that VBT can be effective in restenotic lesions.

Brachytherapy and Probucol

In another randomized, four-arm study for patients with PTA lesions, patients were randomized to VBT, VBT and probucol, probucol alone, or placebo. The recurrence rate was 17% in the radiation-only arm, 20% for VBT and probucol, 27% for probucol alone, and 42% for the placebo group. This study confirms prior observations regarding the effectiveness of VBT for the treatment of SFA lesions without additional benefit of probucol when compared with PTA alone.[54]

Studies with Beta Radiation for Superficial Femoral Artery Stenosis

Two studies that used the Corona system were the MOBILE study that targeted in-stent restenosis lesions and the Limb Ischemia Treatment and Monitoring after Vascular Brachytherapy to Prevent Restenosis (LIMBER) study. These two studies were both terminated prematurely, therefore no data are available. Like the Corona system, a strategy to use the Beta Cath System for the treatment of chronic limb ischemia is in the planning stages.

Arteriovenous Dialysis Studies

An initial study at Emory University in 1994 to treat patients who had failed PTA of arteriovenous dialysis grafts using the MicroSelectron HDR afterloader reported 40% patency rate at 44 weeks,[55] but the long-term results of this study were similar to stand-alone PTA without irradiation. Similar disappointing results were reported by Parikh and colleagues[56] from a pilot study using external radiation doses of 12 and 18 Gy for AV dialysis shunts in 10 patients. At 6 months, target lesion revascularization (TLR) was 40%, but at 18 months, all grafts failed and required intervention. Cohen and associates[57] randomized 31 patients to PTA or stent placement alone followed by external radiation of 14 Gy in two 7-Gy fractions and reported restenosis rates of 45% versus 67% in the irradiated and control groups, respectively, at 6 months. New studies are currently underway using low-dose external radiation therapy to reduce restenosis of vascular access for AV grafts in hemodialysis patients, as are other studies using a centering device to deliver an accurate homogenous dose of radiation after PTA. BRAVO was a pilot study using the Corona system with a $^{90}Sr/^{90}Y$ beta emitter. In the study of 10 patients with an average of 3.9 previous angioplasties to their AV graft, there was 60% primary patency and cumulative patency of 80% at 12-month mean follow-up.[58]

Radiation for Renal In-Stent Restenosis

Several investigators reported on the efficacy of gamma radiation for the treatment of in-stent renal stenosis.[59,60] In their study, Kuchulakanti and colleagues[61] aimed to assess the safety and efficacy of gamma brachytherapy for the treatment of in-stent restenosis in renal arteries. Eleven patients who presented with renal in-stent restenosis from January 2003 to March 2004, documented by selective renal angiography, were assigned to treatment with gamma brachytherapy using ^{192}Ir, followed by balloon angioplasty, laser, or restenting. The patients were followed clinically at 1, 3, 6, and 9 months, and duplex ultrasound was conducted at 9 months. Procedural success was 100% and free of complications. Clinical follow-up was available in all patients and duplex ultrasound in 10 patients. No significant changes in blood urea nitrogen, serum creatinine, creatinine clearance, or the number of antihypertensive medications was observed at follow-up. One patient (9.1%) required TLR at 9 months. It was found that gamma brachytherapy as adjunct therapy for the treatment of renal artery in-stent restenosis appears safe and feasible. However, the clinical benefit of this therapy has to be proven in a large, randomized clinical trial.[61]

Other reports for the use of VBT in the peripheral arterial system include the Scripps Coronary Radiation to Inhibit Proliferation Post-Stenting (SCRIPPS) experience in which endovascular radiation therapy was used for the prevention of restenosis after TIPS for patients with portal hypertension. Overall, the restenosis rate due to intimal hyperplasia of TIPS at 6 months has been reported to be as high as 70%. Complete thrombosis as early as 2 weeks after the procedure has been reported.[62]

Trials of Gamma Radiation

The Venezuelan Experience

The first study of intracoronary radiation in human coronary arteries was conducted in 1994 by Condado and associates,[63] in which 21 patients (22 lesions—77.3% were de novo lesions) were treated with ^{192}Ir

after routine balloon angioplasty. On angiographic follow-up at 6 months, a binary restenosis rate of 28.6% was reported, which remained the same at 5 years. Angiographic complications included four aneurysms (two were procedure related and two occurred within 3 months). At 3 and 5 years, all aneurysms except one remained unchanged, and no other angiographic complications were observed.[64]

Gamma Radiation for In-Stent Restenosis

The only gamma emitter used for the prevention of restenosis in clinical trials is ^{192}Ir. The efficacy of ^{192}Ir in reducing clinical and angiographic restenosis in patients with in-stent restenosis has been confirmed by a number of studies, including two single-center trials, SCRIPPS and Washington Radiation for In-Stent restenosis Trial (WRIST); two multicenter trials, GAMMA 1 and GAMMA 2; and the Angiorad Radiation Therapy for In-Stent Restenosis Trial In Coronaries (ARTISTIC). All of these trials were performed using a manual delivery system with a noncentering catheter with IVUS-based or fixed-depth dosimetry.

SCRIPPS Trials

The SCRIPPS trial was the first randomized trial to evaluate the safety and efficacy of intracoronary gamma radiation as adjunctive therapy to stents. Follow-up at 6 months and 3 years showed significantly lower restenosis rates in the ^{192}Ir group (17% and 33%, respectively) compared with placebo (54% and 63%). A subgroup analysis of the 35 patients enrolled because of in-stent restenosis showed a 70% reduction in the recurrence rate in the irradiated group compared with the placebo.[65,66] There were no evident clinical complications resulting from the radiation treatment, and clinical benefits were maintained at 5 years, with a significant reduction in the need for TLR.[67]

SCRIPPS II for in-stent restenosis in diffuse lesions (30 to 80 mm), SCRIPPS III with prolonged antiplatelet therapy (6 to 12 months of Plavix), and SCRIPPS IV to evaluate higher doses (17 versus 14 Gy) followed the original SCRIPPS study and have shown, respectively, that irradiation is effective for diffuse lesions, that prolonged platelet therapy reduces late thrombosis and additional stenting is to be avoided, and that optimization of radiation dose improves the outcomes further in diffuse lesions.

Gamma Dose-Finding Study

After coronary intervention, 336 patients with in-stent restenosis were randomly assigned to receive intracoronary radiation therapy (IRT) with 14 or 17 Gy at 2 mm from an ^{192}Ir source. At the 8-month follow-up, fewer patients in the 17-Gy group underwent TLR (15.2% versus 27.2%), had target vessel revascularization (TVR) (21.3% versus 33.1%), or reached the composite end point of death, myocardial infarction (MI), thrombosis, or TLR (17.1% versus 28.4%). There were no differences in late thrombosis or mortality between treatment groups. There was a strong trend toward reduced in-lesion late loss (0.36 ± 0.63 mm versus 0.51 ± 0.64 mm) and a significantly lower rate of binary restenosis (23.9% versus 38.1%) in the high-dose group.[68]

Washington Radiation for In-Stent restenosis Trial Series

WRIST was the first study to evaluate the effectiveness of radiation therapy in patients with in-stent restenosis. In this study, 130 patients (100 with native coronaries and 30 with saphenous vein grafts [SVGs]) with in-stent restenosis lesions (up to 47 mm long) were randomized to receive ^{192}Ir or placebo. At 6 months, the radiation therapy group showed a reduction in restenosis (19% versus 58% in placebo) and a 79% and 63% reduction in the need for revascularization and major adverse cardiac events (MACEs), respectively, compared with placebo.[69] Extended follow-up of these patients showed durable beneficial effect of radiation at 1 year, 3 years,[70] and 5 years[71] in MACE rates compared with placebo. Between 6 and 60 months, patients treated with IRT compared with placebo had more TLR (IRT, 21.6% versus placebo, 4.7%) and TVR (21.5% for IRT versus 6.1% for placebo) At 5 years, the MACE rate was significantly reduced with IRT (46.2% versus 69.2%).

Other landmark trials in this series were SVG-WRIST, which evaluated the effect of radiation therapy in patients with diffuse in-stent restenosis lesions in SVGs[72]; Long WRIST in patients with diffuse in-stent restenosis in native coronary arteries (lesion lengths of 36 to 80 mm)[73]; Long WRIST High Dose, which tested the efficacy of an 18-Gy dose of radiation; WRIST Plus and WRIST 12, which tested the efficacy of prolonged clopidogrel therapy (up to 6 and 12 months, respectively) to reduce the incidence of late thrombosis; and WRIST 21, which tested whether the escalation of radiation dose to 21 Gy would improve the clinical outcomes beyond Long WRIST High Dose. These studies have demonstrated superiority of radiation therapy in the treatment of in-stent restenosis in vein graft disease (SVG-WRIST) and diffuse lesions (Long WRIST). The Long WRIST High Dose registry showed that a 3-Gy increase in the dose, from 15 to 18 Gy, provided additional reduction in MACE rates.[74] The strategy of prolonged antiplatelet therapy for 6 months in WRIST Plus reduced thrombosis rates from 9.6% to 2.5%—levels comparable to nonirradiated controls.[75] WRIST 12 has demonstrated further reduction in MACEs and TLRs with 12 months of clopidogrel therapy.[76] Based on these observations, it has become standard practice to provide at least 12 months of clopidogrel therapy for patients undergoing radiation therapy for in-stent restenosis. The WRIST 21 trial aimed to examine whether an escalation in dose of intracoronary gamma radiation to 21 Gy is safe and confers additional benefit in reducing repeat revasculariza-

tion and MACEs in patients with diffuse in-stent restenosis. Forty-seven patients with diffuse in-stent restenosis (lesion length of 20 to 80 mm) in native coronary arteries (n = 25) and SVG (n = 22) underwent PTA or additional stents, or both, followed by gamma radiation using the Checkmate system (Cordis) with a dose of 21 Gy. Follow-up at 6 months revealed nonsignificant but lower late loss (in-stent: 0.33 ± 0.7 mm; in-lesion: 0.41 ± 0.6 mm) in the 21-Gy group compared with the 18-Gy group; and at 12 months revealed a trend toward less overall MI, although repeat revascularization and MACE rates were similar.[77]

GAMMA 1

GAMMA 1 was a multicenter, randomized trial of 252 patients with in-stent restenosis treated with 8 to 30 Gy, that was hand delivered using IVUS-guided dosimetry. This trial showed significant reductions in the in-stent (21.6%) and in-lesion (32.4%) restenosis rates compared with 50.5% and 55.3% in the control group at 6-month angiographic follow-up. The greatest benefit was obtained in patients with long lesions or diabetes, or both. Although TLR rates were lower in GAMMA 1, the rates of death and acute MI were higher in the irradiated group compared with control. These complications were related in part to the late thrombosis phenomenon, which was more frequent in patients treated with radiation therapy than with placebo (5.3% versus 0.8%). All patients in the ^{192}Ir group who presented with late thrombosis had new stents placed within the in-stent target lesion at the time of the procedure.[78] This trial demonstrated the efficacy of intracoronary gamma radiation for the prevention of in-stent restenosis recurrence, and increased awareness regarding the correlation between late thrombosis and an increased risk of MI.

GAMMA 2

GAMMA 2, a registry of 125 patients including complex lesions such as calcific lesions requiring rotablation, used a fixed dose of 14 Gy at 2 mm from the center of the source and showed a reduction of 52% and 40% in in-stent and in-lesion restenosis, respectively, and a reduction of 48% and 36% in TLR and MACE rates, respectively.[79]

Prpic and coworkers[80] analyzed all patients enrolled in the GAMMA 1 and GAMMA 2 brachytherapy trials who underwent repeat percutaneous TLR because of restenosis. Subjects were divided into two cohorts: those who had received ^{192}Ir brachytherapy and those who had been randomized to placebo. Forty-five (17.6%) of a total of 256 patients whose index treatment was IRT and 36 (29.8%) of 121 patients whose index treatment was placebo required repeat percutaneous TLR. Acute procedural success occurred in 100% of irradiated patients and 94% of placebo controls (P = .19). After the first TLR, a subsequent TLR was required in 15 (33.3%) of 45 brachytherapy patients versus 17 (47.2%) of 36 placebo failure

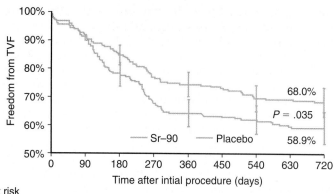

Figure 33-6. The Stents and Radiation Therapy (START) trial: 720-day event-free survival (i.e., major adverse cardiac events). TVF, target vessel failure.

patients (P = .26). Investigators concluded that in those patients who "failed" [192]Ir brachytherapy for in-stent restenosis, treatment with ^{192}Ir delayed the time to first TLR. They also found that repeat percutaneous intervention in these patients is safe and efficacious in the short term, with acceptable long-term results.[80]

Clinical Trials of Beta Radiation

Large-scale clinical studies testing the effectiveness of beta radiation for de novo, restenotic and in-stent restenosis lesions, and vein grafts have paralleled the encouraging results of gamma radiation.

Beta Radiation for In-Stent Restenosis

Beta WRIST
Beta WRIST showed that beta radiation was effective in the treatment of in-stent restenosis in 50 patients. These patients had a 58% reduction in the rate of TLR and a 53% reduction in TVR at 6 months compared with the historical control group of WRIST.[81] The clinical benefit was maintained at 2 years' follow-up with a reduction in TLR (42 % versus 66%), TVR (46% versus 72%), and MACE (46 % versus 72%) compared with placebo. This study showed that the efficacy of beta and gamma emitters for the treatment of in-stent restenosis appeared similar at longer-term follow-up.

START and START 40/20
In the Stents and Radiation Therapy (START) trial, 476 patients were randomized to placebo or to an active radiation train 30 mm long using the BetaCath system.[82] Late thrombosis as a complication of brachytherapy was first recognized during this trial and antiplatelet therapy was prolonged to at least 90 days. Angiographic restenosis rates at 8 months were 24% in the irradiated segments versus 46% in the placebo group. The rates of TLR, TVR, and MACE were 13%, 16%, and 18% in the irradiated group and 22%, 24%, and 26% in the control

group, respectively. START demonstrated continued significance in favor of the ^{90}Sr group for MACE and TVR through 3 and almost 4 years, and by 5 years, although statistical significance was not reached, the results numerically were in favor of [90]Sr (Fig. 33-6).[83]

During multiple studies of radiation, including START, the medical community became aware of the mismatch between the interventional injury length and radiation length—the so-called geographic miss phenomenon—with the potential to compromise clinical outcome.[84] START 40/20 was a 207-patient registry that mirrored START and ensured an adequate irradiation margin with 10 mm of radiation therapy applied proximal and distal to the injury zone (i.e., additional 5 mm each end). Compared with the control arm of START, patients in START 40/20 had a reduction of 44% in restenosis in the analysis segment, 50% reduction in TLR, 34% reduction in TVR, and 26% reduction in MACEs. This registry demonstrated no deleterious effects of adding 10 mm of length to the source train, but there was a lack of a relationship between geographic miss and clinical or angiographic outcomes for in-stent restenosis.

INHIBIT and Galileo INHIBIT
The Intimal Hyperplasia Inhibition with Beta In-stent Trial (INHIBIT) examined the efficacy of the Galileo system for the treatment of in-stent restenosis in 332 patients.[85] At 9 months, treatment with ^{32}P reduced binary restenosis by 67% and 50% in the stented and analysis segments, respectively. There were no differences in the edge-effect rates between the active and control-treated groups. At 9 months, ^{32}P significantly reduced rates of TLR and MACE. Tandem positioning to cover diffuse lesions larger than 22 mm with ^{32}P was safe and effective.

Galileo INHIBIT was an international, multicenter registry of 120 patients with in-stent restenosis in which ^{32}P was delivered at 20 Gy at 1 mm into the vessel wall. There was a reduction in the primary clinical end point defined as MACE-TLR by 49% and a reduction in the angiographic end point of binary restenosis by 74% in the stented segment and by 27% in the analysis segment.[86] The thrombosis rate was low (1.5%) and similar to that of the control group (1.2%).

Balloon Catheter–Based Beta Radiation Trials for In-Stent Restenosis

BRITE, BRITE-II, SVG BRITE, and 4R

Beta radiation using the Radiance system was administered in 32 patients in the feasibility study Beta Radiation to Prevent In-Stent Restenosis (BRITE). Seventy percent of the dose was administered when the balloon was inflated. At 6 months, TVR (3%), MACE (3%), and in-stent binary restenosis rates (0%) were the lowest reported in any VBT series. Investigators concluded that beta radiation delivered with a balloon ^{32}P source design for patients with in-stent restenosis resulted in lower-than-expected rates of angiographic and clinical restenosis and the absence of late complications.[87]

The BRITE II study evaluated the efficacy of beta radiation using the RDX system in 429 patients randomized to irradiation ($n = 321$) or placebo ($n = 108$). The RDX system demonstrated safety characterized by high technical success rates (>95%), low periprocedural complications (<1%), and a low 30-day MACE rate (<1%). The most prevalent location of restenosis was within the radiated vessel outside the injured zone despite lower rates of geographic miss (8.5%).[88] The RDX system demonstrated a very low in-stent restenosis rate (10.9% versus 46.1%) and proved to optimize the results when compared with historical studies.

SVG BRITE

The SVG BRITE study examined the RDX system using ^{32}P emitter at a dose of 20 Gy at 1 mm from the balloon surface in SVG of 49 patients, 24 of whom were treated for de novo lesions. New stents were implanted in most patients with de novo lesions. The outcome of the patients with de novo lesions was encouraging, with only 8% requiring TVR at 12 months' follow-up and a 13% angiographic restenosis rate for the entire analysis segment (allowing for edge effect). These data warrant further investigation of this promising application, especially as the efficacy of potential alternatives, such as DESs, has not yet been investigated in SVG lesions.[89]

4R

4R, a South Korean registry, evaluated beta radiation therapy with ^{188}Re-MAG$_3$-filled balloons after rotational atherectomy for diffuse in-stent restenosis in 50 patients. The mean dose was 15 Gy, and the mean irradiation time was 201.8 ± 61.7 seconds. No adverse events occurred during the follow-up period. The 6-month binary angiographic restenosis rate was 10.4%. The investigators concluded that beta irradiation using a ^{188}Re-MAG$_3$-filled balloon after rotational atherectomy is safe and feasible in patients with diffuse in-stent restenosis, and it may improve their clinical and angiographic outcomes.[90]

Tungsten WRIST

The Tungsten WRIST study aimed to determine the safety and feasibility of IRT using tungsten (^{188}W), a beta emitter. A total of 30 patients with angiographic evidence of in-stent restenosis in a previously treated native coronary artery underwent percutaneous coronary intervention (PCI) (i.e., balloon angioplasty, ablation by atherectomy, or laser angioplasty). After the intervention, a noncentered delivery catheter with a side, 0.014-inch guidewire carrying a tungsten (^{188}W) coil, with an active length of 33 mm, was inserted. Patients were randomized to a radiation dose of 18, 22, or 25 Gy at 2 mm from the center of the source. At 6 months' follow-up, the overall binary angiographic restenosis rate was 18.8%. The TVR rate was 23%, and the TLR-MACE rate was 13.3%, without any intergroup differences. The investigators concluded that VBT with ^{188}W was feasible and safe; the 6-month clinical outcomes are similar to those for the original WRIST radiation group.[91]

Beta Radiation for De Novo Lesions

Several clinical studies were undertaken to test the effectiveness of beta radiation for de novo lesions concurrent to the trials of in-stent restenosis. Important early studies included the Geneva trial,[92] the dose-finding Beta Energy Restenosis Trial (BERT) that used ^{90}Y,[93] and the Proliferation Reduction with Vascular Energy Trial (PREVENT)[94] that used ^{32}P.

BERT was a feasibility study of 23 patients using the Novoste system with prescribed doses of 12, 14, or 16 Gy and treatment times of less than 3.5 minutes. Investigators concluded that the administration of endovascular beta radiation after angioplasty was safe and feasible and substantially altered the postangioplasty late lumen loss, resulting in a lower-than-expected rate of restenosis.[93] The Canadian arm of this study included 30 patients, and at 6 months' follow-up, the angiographic restenosis rate was 10% with negative late loss and late loss index.[95] The European arm of BERT (BERT 1.5)[96] was conducted at the Thoraxcenter in Rotterdam, The Netherlands, and involved an additional 30 patients who were treated successfully with balloon angioplasty. Angiographic restenosis in this cohort was higher than reported in the U.S. and Canadian trials. Overall, the restenosis rate based on 64 of the 80 patients in the BERT series was 17%, and the late loss and late loss indexes were below 5%. More than 50% of the patients had larger MLD at follow-up compared with control, and a substudy involving IVUS demonstrated vessel remodeling at the irradiated site.

PREVENT was a randomized study of 105 patients with de novo (70%) or restenotic (30%) lesions. Angiographic restenosis at 6 months was 8.2% (target site) and 22.4% (target site plus adjacent segments) compared with 39.1% and 50.0% in the control group, respectively. The 1-year MACE rate (death, MI, and TLR) was less in the radiation group, although the difference was not statistically significant. The occurrence of MI due to thrombotic events after discharge occurred in seven patients who received radiotherapy and in none in the control group. Investigators determined that beta radiotherapy with a centered ^{32}P source is safe and highly effective in inhibiting restenosis at the target site after stent or balloon angioplasty. However, minimizing edge narrowing and late thrombotic events must be accomplished to maximize the clinical benefit of this modality.[94]

Dose-Finding Study Group

In this study, 183 patients were randomized; 181 received beta radiation (9 to 18 Gy) with ^{90}Y at a tissue depth of 1 mm. Stenting after radiation was required in 47% of the patients because of residual stenosis or major dissection. At 6 months' angiographic follow-up, a significant dose-dependent benefit was evident. Thrombosis or late occlusion of the target vessel occurred in 3.3% of patients who were treated with only balloon angioplasty and in 14.3% of patients who received new stents. This study demonstrated a marked reduction in restenosis in nonstented arteries after administration of 18 Gy of beta radiation, especially in patients who underwent plain balloon angioplasty, suggesting that beta radiation therapy should be evaluated as an adjunct to PTA.[97]

BetaCath

In the large, randomized BetaCath study, 1455 patients with suboptimal results after balloon angioplasty were treated with a stent and then assigned to $^{90}Sr/^{90}Y$ or placebo treatment.[98] In patients treated with balloon angioplasty alone, those receiving radiation treatment ($n = 264$) tended to have lower target vessel failure (TVF) (14.2%) compared with placebo (20.4%, $n = 240$). In the 452 patients treated with extended antiplatelet therapy who received a new stent, there were no differences in the 240-day TVF rate. Comparison of placebo and radiation treatment from pooled PTA and stent groups (antiplatelet therapy for 60 days or more) showed similar 8-month TLR and TVF-MACE rates. An interesting point in this study was the low TVF in the irradiated balloon-only group. This was attributed to a reduction in angiographic restenosis within the initial lesion site in these patients (21.4% versus 34.3% in the placebo group), although the restenosis rates were similar in the analysis segment (i.e., treated segment plus the radiation margins). The loss of benefit at the treatment margins is attributable to geographic miss because of the relatively short treatment length in the study. This was the first study to identify the higher-than-expected rate of late stent thrombosis when radiation was used with new stent implantation.

ECRIS

The Endocoronary Rhenium Irradiation Study (ECRIS) was a randomized trial in which 225 patients (71% de novo lesions) were randomly assigned to receive 22.5 Gy of beta irradiation to a depth of 0.5 mm using a ^{188}Re-filled balloon catheter ($n = 113$) or no additional intervention ($n = 112$). Clinical and procedural data were not different between the groups except that there was a higher rate of stenting in the control group (63%) compared with the ^{188}Re group (45%). At 6 months' follow-up, late loss was significantly lower in the irradiated group compared with the control group, both of the target lesion (0.11 ± 0.54 versus 0.69 ± 0.81 mm) and of the total segment (0.22 ± 0.67 versus 0.70 ± 0.82 mm). This was also evident in the subgroup of patients with de novo lesions and was independent of stenting. Binary restenosis rates and TVR were significantly lower after ^{188}Re brachytherapy compared with the control group. Investigators found that intracoronary beta brachytherapy with the ^{188}Re-liquid-filled balloon was safe and efficiently reduced restenosis and revascularization rates after coronary angioplasty.[99]

BRIDGE

The Beta-Radiation Investigation with Direct Stenting and Galileo (BRIDGE) study was a multicenter, randomized, controlled trial of 112 patients that evaluated the acute and long-term efficacy of VBT with ^{32}P (20 Gy to a depth of 1 mm in the coronary wall) immediately after direct stenting in de novo lesions. TVR and MACE rates at 1 year in the irradiated group (20.4% and 25.9%, respectively) were higher than rates in the control group (12.1% and 17.2%, respectively). Investigators found that despite the optimization of preprocedural, periprocedural, and postprocedural factors, and despite the relative efficacy of the brachytherapy for the prevention of the intrastent neointimal hyperplasia, the clinical outcome of the irradiated group was less favorable than that of the control group.[100]

Vascular Brachytherapy versus Drug-Eluting Stents

Vascular Brachytherapy for Failed Drug-Eluting Stents

RESCUE

Radiation for Eluting Stents in Coronary Failure (RESCUE) is an international, Internet-based registry of 61 patients who presented with in-stent restenosis of a DES and were assigned to intravascular radiation therapy with commercially available systems after PCI. The outcomes of these patients were compared with a consecutive series of 50 patients who presented with in-stent restenosis of a DES and were assigned to repeat DES (r-DES) treatment. At 8 months, there were fewer MACEs overall in the IRT group compared with the r-DES group (9.8% versus 24%, $P = .044$). The need for TVR and TLR was similar in both groups at 8 months. There has been no report of subacute thrombosis in either group. IRT as adjunct therapy to PCI for patients presenting with in-stent restenosis of a DES was found to be safe, and it should be considered an alternative therapeutic option for this difficult subset of patients.[101]

In this in vitro study, the study authors investigated the effect of gamma and beta radiation doses typically used in VBT on the performance of the TAXUS Express(2) paclitaxel-eluting stent (PES), including polymer and drug degradation and the release of the paclitaxel from the polymer carrier. The brachytherapy catheters used were the BetaCath System using beta radiation (^{90}Sr/^{90}Y) and the Checkmate System (Cordis, Miami, FL) using gamma radiation (^{192}Ir). It was determined that there were no statistically significant changes to in vitro paclitaxel release from the stent exposed to radiation compared with controls subjected to the same conditions except for the radiation exposure. The molecular weight of the Translute polymer carrier matrix and the level of paclitaxel degradants were not changed after exposure to radiation doses up to twice what is typically used in intravascular VBT. Beta and gamma radiation doses typically used in intravascular VBT had no significant effect on the Translute polymer carrier, paclitaxel degradation, or paclitaxel release in this in vitro model.[102]

Vascular Brachytherapy versus Drug-Eluting Stents for In-Stent Restenosis of Bare Metal Stents

TAXUS V
Patients were randomly assigned to undergo angioplasty followed by VBT with a beta source ($n = 201$) or PES implantation ($n = 195$). Follow-up at 9 months was completed for 194 patients in the VBT group and 191 patients in the PES group (96.5% and 97.9%, respectively). For VBT and PES, respectively, the number of events and 9-month rates for ischemic TLR were 27 (13.9%) and 12 (6.3%); for ischemic TVR, 34 (17.5%) and 20 (10.5%); and for overall MACE, 39 (20.1%) and 22 (11.5%), with similar rates of cardiac death or MI of 10 (5.2%) and 7 (3.7%) and target vessel thrombosis of 5 (2.6%) and 3 (1.6%). Angiographic restenosis at 9 months was 31.2% (53 of 170 patients) with VBT and 14.5% (25 of 172 patients) with PES. Investigators found that treatment of bare metal in-stent restenotic lesions with PES rather than angioplasty followed by VBT reduced clinical and angiographic restenosis at 9 months and improved event-free survival.[103]

SISR
SISR was a prospective, multicenter, randomized trial of 384 patients with in-stent restenosis who were enrolled between February 2003 and July 2004 at 26 academic and community medical centers. Intervention included VBT ($n = 125$) or the sirolimus-eluting stent (SES, $n = 259$). Procedural success was 99.2% (124 of 125) in the VBT group and 97.3% (250 of 257) in the SES group ($P = .28$). The rate of TVF was 21.6% (27 of 125) with VBT and 12.4% (32 of 259) with the SES. TLR was required in 19.2% (24 of 125) of the VBT group and 8.5% (22 of 259) of the SES group. At follow-up angiography, the rate of binary angiographic restenosis for the analysis segment was 29.5% (31 of 105) for the VBT group and 19.8% (45 of 227) for the SES group. It was found that the SES results in superior clinical and angiographic outcomes compared with VBT for the treatment of restenosis within a bare metal stent.[104]

Drug-Eluting Stents versus Vascular Brachytherapy for Failed Vascular Brachytherapy

A cohort of 88 patients who were previously treated with brachytherapy for in-stent restenosis and presented with angina and recurrence of angiographic restenosis were evaluated for treatment with DES implantation (SES or PES, $n = 34$) or PCI and repeat irradiation (gamma or beta radiation, $n = 54$). The two groups had similar baseline clinical and angiographic characteristics. The in-hospital outcomes were similar between both groups. At long-term follow-up of 9.7 ± 4.1 months for the DES group and 10.3 ± 3.5 months for the repeat IRT group, there were no deaths or MIs. There was a trend toward more TVR-MACEs in the DES group ($P = .09$). The patients in the DES group had a significantly lower survival rate compared with those in the repeat IRT group ($P = .018$). For patients who had recurrent in-stent restenosis after IRT, DES implantation or repeat irradiation was safe and was associated with excellent immediate outcomes. However, at long-term follow-up, repeat IRT was associated with fewer recurrences and a reduced need for repeat revascularization compared with DES implantation (Fig. 33-7).[105] A summary

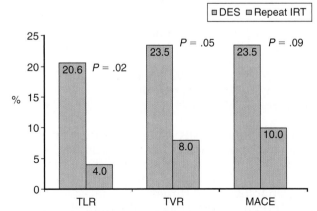

Figure 33-7. Drug-eluting stent (DES) implantation versus vascular brachytherapy for failed intracoronary radiation therapy (IRT) long-term outcomes. MACE, major adverse cardiac events; TLR, target lesion revascularization; TVR, target vessel revascularization. (From Chu WW, Torguson R, Pichard AD, et al: Drug-eluting stents versus repeat vascular brachytherapy for patients with recurrent in-stent restenosis after failed intracoronary radiation. J Invasive Cardiol 2005;17:659-662.)

Table 33-3.   Results of Major Clinical Trials with Gamma and Beta Radiation

Study	No. of Patients (No. Irradiated)	Year	Isotope	Dose (Gy)	In-Stent Late Loss (mm)	In-Stent Restenosis (%)	TLR (%)	TVR (%)	MACE (%)
Gamma Radiation Studies									
SCRIPPS[67]	55 (26)	1997	[192]Ir	≥8-<30	0.38 ± 1.06	8.3	12	NA	15
WRIST[70]	130 (65)	2000	[192]Ir	15-18	0.22 ± 0.84	19	13.8	26	29
GAMMA 1[78]	252 (131)	2001	[192]Ir	≥8-<30	0.73 ± 0.79	21.6	24.4	31.3	28.2
ARTISTIC[106]	26 (26)	2001	[192]Ir	12-18	NA	19	7.6	NA	15
WRIST PLUS[75]	120 (120)	2001	[192]Ir	14	0.58 ± 0.57	26	20.8	23.3	23.3
SVG WRIST[72]	120 (60)	2002	[192]Ir	15-18	0.23 ± 0.75	15	17	28	32
WRIST 12[76]	120 (120)	2002	[192]Ir	14	NA	NA	12.6	14.3	13.4
LONG WRIST[73]	120 (120)	2003	[192]Ir	15	0.67 ± 0.88	34	39	NA	42
LONG WRIST[73]	120 (120)	2003	[192]Ir	18 (*)	0.48 ± 0.88	25	19.6	NA	21.7
High Dose[74]					0.27 ± 0.74	23	19.6	NA	19.6
WRIST 21[77]	47 (47)	2005	[192]Ir	21	0.33 ± 0.7	17.4	15.2	28.3	28.3
Beta Radiation Studies									
BERT[93]	23(23)	1998		12-16	0.005	10	8.6	13	13
Beta WRIST[81]	50 (50)	2000	[90]Y	20.6	0.37 ± 0.8	22	28	34	34
PREVENT[94]	105 (80)	2000	[32]P	16-24	0.2 ± 0.6	8	6	21	26
4R[90]	50 (50)	2001	[188]Rh	15	0.37 ± 0.65	10.4	—	—	2
Dose Finding	183 (181)	2001	[90]Y	9	0.37 ± 0.7	28.6	—	13.3	13.3
Study Group[97]				12	0.25 ± 0.1	21.4	—	8.8	11.1
				15	0.21 ± 0.09	15.9	—	10.8	10.8
				18	0.18 ± 0.12	15	—	11.1	15.5
START[82]	476 (244)	2002	[90]Sr/[90]Y	18-23	0.21 ± 0.61	14.2	13.9	17	19.1
INHIBIT[85]	332 (166)	2002	[32]P	20	0.41 ± 69	34	8	19	21
BRITE I[87]	32 (32)	2002	[32]P	20	-0.05 ± 0.41	0	3	3	3
BRIE[107]	149 (149)	2002	[32]P	14-18	0.26	9.9	NA	15.4	28.2
SVG BRITE[89]	49 (49)	2003	[32]P	20 (†)	NA	11.8	4.2	8.3	12.5
					NA	25	36	36	48
ECRIS[99]	225 (113)	2003	[188]Rh	22.5	0.11 ± 0.54	6.3	1.8	8	14.2
RENO[108]	1098 (1098)	2003	[90]Sr/[90]Y	16-25	NA	24.5	—	7.6	18.7
BRIDGE[100]	112 (54)	2004	[32]P	20	0.43 ± 0.75	12.7	3.7	11.1	25.9
Tungsten WRIST[91]	30 (30)	2004	[188]W	18-25	0.14 ± 0.88	11	13	23	23

*Upper row: patients with 1-month dual-antiplatelet therapy; lower row: patients with 6 months of therapy.
†Upper row: de novo lesions; lower row: in-stent restenosis lesions.
ARTISTIC, Angiorad Radiation Therapy for In-Stent Restenosis Trial In Coronaries; BERT, Beta Energy Restenosis Trial; BRIDGE, Beta-Radiation Investigation with Direct Stenting and Galileo study; BRIE, Beta Radiation in Europe; BRITE, Beta Radiation to Prevent In-Stent Restenosis; ECRIS, Endocoronary Rhenium Irradiation Study; GAMMA, studies of efficacy and safety of gamma radiation for treating reclogged stents in coronary arteries; INHIBIT, Intimal Hyperplasia Inhibition with Beta In-stent Trial; MACE, major adverse cardiac event; NA, not available; PREVENT, Proliferation Reduction with Vascular Energy Trial; RENO, Registry Novoste; SCRIPPS, Scripps Coronary Radiation to Inhibit Proliferation Post-Stenting; START, Stents and Radiation Therapy; SVG, saphenous vein graft; TLR, target lesion revascularization; TVR, target vessel revascularization; WRIST PLUS, Washington Radiation for In-Stent Restenosis Trial plus 6 Months of Clopidogrel; WRIST, Washington Radiation for In-Stent Restenosis; 4R, South Korean registry evaluating beta radiation therapy.

of the landmark clinical trials conducted with gamma and beta emitters is presented in Table 33-3.

LESSONS FROM THE VASCULAR BRACHYTHERAPY EXPERIENCE AND FUTURE PERSPECTIVES

Although clinical trials using VBT for coronary and peripheral applications have demonstrated positive results in reducing restenosis rates, these trials have also identified two major complications related to the technology: late thrombosis and edge stenosis. Late thrombosis probably results from the delay in healing associated with radiation. It has been estimated that late thrombosis can be remedied through the prolonged administration of antiplatelet therapy after intervention. Over the years we have learned how to optimize the VBT treatment by applying the right dose, covering the edges of the injured segment, minimizing the use of stenting, and prolonging the

antiplatelet administration for the prevention of late thrombosis. It is interesting that some of the lessons from VBT, such as late catch-up and late thrombosis, are seen now with DES and perhaps some of the solutions to solve these complications will be similar to those used in the VBT field.

Evidence is favorable for the efficacy of DES to reduce restenosis in de novo lesions and in-stent restenosis of bare metal stents. With expanding indications of use for DES, there will more DES failures. The data on how to treat DES failure are limited, but they are favorable for VBT, and it may have a niche in the era of DES. VBT will remain an alternative for difficult cases that continue to restenose with conventional therapy. The future of VBT depends on the degree of restenosis seen with DES. It is anticipated that over time, up to 5% of the population undergoing DES implantation will require additional therapy to handle the restenosis. Tertiary centers should hold onto their VBT systems to be able to offer this therapy for patients who present with restenosis.

REFERENCES

1. Waksman R, Robinson KA, Crocker IR, et al: Endovascular low-dose irradiation inhibits neointima formation after coronary artery balloon injury in swine. A possible role for radiation therapy in restenosis prevention. Circulation 1995; 91:1533-1539.
2. Waksman R, Robinson KA, Crocker IR, et al: Intracoronary radiation before stent implantation inhibits neointima formation in stented porcine coronary arteries. Circulation 1995;92:1383-1386.
3. Wiedermann JG, Marboe C, Amols H, et al: Intracoronary irradiation markedly reduces restenosis after balloon angioplasty in a porcine model. J Am Coll Cardiol 1994;23: 1491-1498.
4. Wiedermann JG, Marboe C. Amols H, et al: Intracoronary irradiation markedly reduces neointimal proliferation after balloon angioplasty in swine: Persistent benefit at 6-month follow-up. J Am Coll Cardiol 1995;25:1451-1456.
5. Mazur W, Ali MN, Khan MM, et al: High dose rate intracoronary radiation for inhibition of neointimal formation in the stented and balloon injured porcine models of restenosis: Angiographic, morphometric and histopathological analyses. Int J Radiat Oncol Biol Phys 1996;36:777-788.
6. Wiedermann JG, Leavy JA, Amols H, et al: Effects of high dose intracoronary irradiation on vasomotor function and smooth muscle histopathology. Am J Physiol 1994;267 (Heart Circ Physiol 36):H125-132.
7. Waksman R, Robinson KA, Crocker IR, et al: Intracoronary radiation decreases new additional intimal hyperplasia in a repeat balloon angioplasty swine model of restenosis. Int J Radiat Oncol Biol Phys 1997;376:767-777.
8. Verin V, Popowski Y, Urban P, et al: Intra-arterial beta irradiation prevents neointimal hyperplasia in a hypercholesterolemic rabbit restenosis model. Circulation 1995;92: 2284-2290.
9. Waksman R, Robinson KA, Crocker IR, et al: Intracoronary low-dose beta-irradiation inhibits neointima formation after coronary artery balloon injury in the swine restenosis model. Circulation 1995;92:3025-3031.
10. Wienberger J, Amols H, Ennis RD, et al: Intracoronary irradiation: Dose response for the prevention of restenosis in swine. Int J Radiat Oncol Biol Phys 1996;36:767-775.
11. Raizner A: Endovascular radiation: The Baylor experience. Highlights in intracoronary radiation therapy. Presented at the Thoraxcenter, December 10-11, 1996, Rotterdam, The Netherlands.
12. Fischell TA, Kharma BK, Fischell DR, et al: Low dose beta particle emission from stent wire results in complete localized inhibition of smooth muscle cell proliferation. Circulation 1994;90:2956-2963.
13. Hehrlein C, Kniser S, Kollum M, et al: Effects of very low dose endovascular irradiation via an activated guidewire on neointima formation after stent implantation. Circulation 1995;92:I-69.
14. Hehrlein C, Gollan C, Donges K, et al: Low dose radioactive endovascular stents prevent smooth muscle cell proliferation and neointimal hyperplasia in rabbits. Circulation 1995; 92:1570-1575.
15. Laird JR, Carter AJ, Kufs WM, et al: Inhibition of neointimal proliferation with low-dose irradiation from a beta-particle-emitting stent. Circulation 1996;93:529-536.
16. Carter AJ, Laird JR, Bailey LR, et al: Effects of endovascular radiation from a beta-particle-emitting stent in a porcine coronary restenosis model. A dose-response study. Circulation 1996;94:2364-2368.
17. Waksman R, Chan RC, Vodovotz Y, et al: Radioactive 133-xenon gas-filled angioplasty balloon: A novel intracoronary radiation system to prevent restenosis. J Am Coll Cardiol 1998;31:356A.
18. Weinberger J: Solution-applied beta emitting radioisotope (SABER) system. In Waksman R, Serruys P (eds): Handbook of Vascular Brachytherapy. London, Martin Dunitz, 1998.
19. Robinson KA, Pipes DW, Bibber RV, et al: Dose response evaluation in balloon injured pig coronary arteries of a beta emitting ^{186}Re liquid filled balloon catheter system for endovascular brachytherapy. Advances in Cardiovascular Radiation Therapy II, March 8-10, 1998, Washington, DC.
20. Makkar R, Whiting J, Li A, et al: A beta-emitting liquid isotope filled balloon markedly inhibits restenosis in stented porcine coronary arteries. J Am Coll Cardiol 1998;31:350A.
21. Kim HS, Cho YS, Kim JS, et al: Effect of transcatheter endovascular holmium-166 irradiation on neointimal formation after balloon injury in porcine coronary artery. J Am Coll Cardiol 1998;31:277A.
22. Waksman R, Saucedo JF, Chan RC, et al: Yttrium-90 delivered via a centering catheter and remote afterloader, uniformly inhibits neointima formation after balloon injury or stenting in swine coronary arteries. J Am Coll Cardiol 1998;31:278A.
23. Pickering JG, Weir L, Janowski J, et al: Proliferative activity in peripheral and coronary atherosclerotic plaque among patients undergoing percutaneous revascularization. J Clin Invest 1993;91:1469-1480.
24. Karas SP, Gravanis MB, Santoian EC, et al: Coronary intimal proliferation after balloon injury and stenting in swine: An animal model of restenosis. J Am Coll Cardiol 1992;20: 467-474.
25. Schwartz R, Huber K, Murphy J, et al: Restenosis and the proportional neointima response to coronary artery injury results in the porcine model. J Am Coll Cardiol 1992; 19:267-274.
26. Anderson HR, Maeng M, Thorwest M, et al: Remodeling rather than neointimal formation explains luminal narrowing after deep vessel wall injury. Circulation 1996;93:1716-1724.
27. Scott, NA, Cipolla GD, Ross CE, et al: Identification of potential role for the adventitia in vascular lesion formation after balloon overstretch injury of porcine coronary arteries. Circulation 1996;93:2178-2187.
28. Lafont A, Guzman LA, Whitlow PL, et al: Restenosis after experimental angioplasty: Intimal, medial, and adventitial changes associated with constrictive remodeling. Circ Res 1995;76:996-1002.
29. Mintz GS, Popma JJ, Pichard AD, et al: Arterial remodeling after coronary angioplasty: A serial intravascular ultrasound study. Circulation 1996;94:35-43.
30. Mintz GS, Pichard AD, Kent K, et al: Endovascular stents reduce restenosis by eliminating geometric arterial remodeling: A serial intravascular ultrasound study. J Am Coll Cardiol 1995;35A:701-705.
31. Serruys PW, de Jaegere P, Kiemeneij F, et al, for the BENESTENT Study Group: A comparison of balloon-expandable stent implantation with balloon angioplasty in patients with coronary artery disease. N Engl J Med 1994;331:489-495.
32. Fischman DL, Leon MB, Baim D, et al, for the STRESS Trial Investigators: A randomized comparison of coronary-stent placement and balloon angioplasty in the treatment of coronary artery disease. N Engl J Med 1994;331:496-501.
33. Mintz GS, Hoffmann R, Mehran R, et al: In-stent restenosis: The Washington Hospital Center experience. Am J Cardiol 1998;81(Suppl 7A):7E-13E.
34. Inalsingh CHA: An experience in treating 501 patients with keloids. Johns Hopkins Med J 1974;134:284-290.
35. Van den Brenk HAS: Results of prophylactic postoperative irradiation in 1300 cases of pterygium. Am J Radiol 1968;103:723-733.
36. Waksman R, Rodriquez JC, Robinson KA, et al: Effect of intravascular irradiation on cell proliferation, apoptosis and vascular remodeling after balloon overstretch injury of porcine coronary arteries. Circulation 1997;96:1944-1952.
37. Hall EJ, Miller RC, Brenner DJ: The basic radiobiology of intravascular irradiation. In Waksman R Vascular Brachytherapy, 2nd ed. Armonk, NY, Futura Publishing, 1999, pp 63-72.

38. Gillette EL, Powers BE, McChensey SM, et al: Response of aorta and branch arteries to experimental intraoperative irradiation. Int J Radiat Oncol Biol Phys 1989;17:1247-1255.

39. Wang H, Griendling KK, Scott NA, et al: Intravascular radiation inhibits cell proliferation and vascular remodeling after angioplasty by increasing the expression of p21 in adventitial myofibroblasts. Circulation 1999;100:I-700.

39a. Wilcox JN: Mechanisms by which vascular brachytherapy prevents postangioplasty restenosis. Front Radiat Ther Oncol 2001;35:172-191.

40. Christen T, Verin V, Bochaton-Piallat M, et al: Mechanisms of neointima formation and remodeling in the porcine coronary artery. Circulation 2001;103:882-888.

41. Schwartz RS, Koval TM, Edwards WD, et al: Effect of external beam irradiation on neointimal hyperplasia after experimental coronary artery injury. J Am Coll Cardiol 1992;19:1106-1113.

41a. Amols HI, Trichter F, Weinberger J: Intracoronary radiation for prevention of restenosis: Dose perturbations caused by stents. Circulation 1998;98:2024-2029.

42. Therasse E, Donath D, Lesperance J, et al: External beam radiation to prevent restenosis after superficial femoral artery balloon angioplasty. Circulation 2005;111:3310-3315.

43. Liermann DD, Bottcher HD, Kollath J, et al: Prophylactic endovascular radiotherapy to prevent intimal hyperplasia after stent implantation in femoropopliteal arteries. Cardiovasc Interv Radiol 1994;17:12-16.

44. Bottcher HD, Schopohl B, Liermann D, et al: Endovascular irradiation—a new method to avoid recurrent stenosis after stent implantation in peripheral arteries: Technique and preliminary results. Int J Radiat Oncol Biol Phys 1994;29:183-186.

45. Liermann D, Kirchner J, Schopohl B, et al: Brachytherapy with iridium-192 HDR to prevent restenosis in peripheral arteries: An update. Herz 1998;23:394-400.

46. Sidawy AN, Weiswasse JM, Waksman R: Peripheral vascular brachytherapy. J Vasc Surg 2002;35:1041-1047.

47. Minar E, Pokrajac B, Ahmadi R, et al: Brachytherapy for prophylaxis of restenosis after long-segment femoropopliteal angioplasty: Pilot study. Radiology 1998;208:173-179.

48. Minar E, Pokrajac B, Maca T, et al: Endovascular brachytherapy for prophylaxis of restenosis after femoropopliteal angioplasty: Results of a prospective randomized study. Circulation 2000;102:2694-2699.

49. Pokrajac B, Schmid R, Poetter R, et al: Endovascular brachytherapy prevents restenosis after femoropopliteal angioplasty: Results of the Vienna-3 multicenter study. Int J Radiat Oncol Biol Phys 2003;57(Suppl):S250.

50. Wolfram RM, Pokrajac B, Ahmadi R, et al: Endovascular brachytherapy for prophylaxis against restenosis after long-segment femoropopliteal placement of stents: Initial results. Radiology 2001;220:724-729.

51. Waksman R, Laird JR, Jurkovitz CT, et al: Intravascular radiation therapy after balloon angioplasty of narrowed femoropopliteal arteries to prevent restenosis: Results of the PARIS feasibility clinical trial. J Vasc Interv Radiol 2001;12:915-921.

52. Krueger K, Zaehringer M, Bendel M, et al: De novo femoropopliteal stenoses: Endovascular gamma irradiation following angioplasty—angiographic and clinical follow-up in a prospective randomized controlled trial. Radiology 2004;231:546-554.

53. Zehnder T, von Briel C, Baumgartner I, et al: Endovascular brachytherapy after percutaneous transluminal angioplasty of recurrent femoropopliteal obstructions. J Endovasc Ther 2003;2:304-311.

54. Gallino A, Do DD, Alerci M, et al: Effects of probucol versus aspirin and versus brachytherapy on restenosis after femoropopliteal angioplasty: The PAB randomized multicenter trial. J Endovasc Ther 2004;11:595-604.

55. Waksman R, Crocker IR, Lumsden AB: Long term results of endovascular radiation therapy for prevention of restenosis in the peripheral vascular system [abstract]. Circulation 1996;94:I-300.

56. Parikh S, Nori D, Rogers D, et al: External beam radiation therapy to prevent postangioplasty dialysis access restenosis: A feasibility study. Cardiovasc Radiat Med 1999;1:36-41.

57. Cohen GS, Freeman H, Ringold MA: External beam irradiation as an adjunctive treatment in failing dialysis shunts. J Vasc Interv Radiol 2000;11:321-326.

58. Bonan R: BRAVO. Paper presented at the Cardiovascular Revascularization Therapies meeting, 2004, Washington, DC.

59. Jahraus CD, Meigooni AS: Vascular brachytherapy: A new approach to renal artery in-stent restenosis. J Invasive Cardiol 2004;4:224-227.

60. Stoeteknuel-Friedli S, Do DD, von Briel C, et al: Endovascular brachytherapy for prevention of recurrent renal in-stent restenosis. J Endovasc Ther 2002;9:350-353.

61. Kuchulakanti PK, Laird JR, Dieter R, et al: Gamma brachytherapy for the treatment of in-stent restenosis of renal arteries. Vasc Dis Manage 2006;3:178-183.

62. Raat H, Stockx L, Ranschaert E, et al: Percutaneous hydrodynamic thrombectomy of acute thrombosis in transjugular intrahepatic portosystemic shunt (TIPS): A feasibility study in five patients. Cardiovasc Interv Radiol 1997;20:180-183.

63. Condado JA, Waksman R, Gurdiel O, et al: Long-term angiographic and clinical outcome after percutaneous transluminal coronary angioplasty and intracoronary radiation therapy in humans. Circulation 1997;96:727-732.

64. Condado JA, Waksman R, Saucedo JF, et al: Five-year clinical and angiographic follow-up after intracoronary iridium-192 radiation therapy. Cardiovasc Radiat Med 2002;3:74-81.

65. Teirstein PS, Massullo V, Jani S, et al: Catheter-based radiotherapy to inhibit restenosis after coronary stenting. N Engl J Med 1997;336:1697-1703.

66. Teirstein PS, Massullo V, Jani S, et al: Two-year follow-up after catheter-based radiotherapy to inhibit coronary restenosis. Circulation 1999;99:243-247.

67. Grise MA, Massullo V, Jani S, et al: Five-Year Clinical Follow-Up After Intracoronary Radiation, Results of a Randomized Clinical Trial. Circulation 2002;105:2737-2740.

68. Price MJ, Moses JW, Leon MB, et al: A multicenter, randomized, dose-finding study of gamma intracoronary radiation therapy to inhibit recurrent restenosis after stenting. J Invasive Cardiol 2006;18:169-173.

69. Waksman R, White RL, Chan RC: Intracoronary radiation therapy for patients with in-stent restenosis: 6-month follow-up of a randomized clinical study [abstract]. Circulation 1998;98:I-651.

70. Ajani AE, Waksman R, Sharma AK, et al: Three-year follow-up after intracoronary gamma radiation therapy for in-stent restenosis. Original WRIST. Washington Radiation for In-Stent Restenosis Trial. Cardiovasc Radiat Med 2001;2:200-204.

71. Waksman R, Ajani AE, White RL, et al: Five-year follow-up after intracoronary gamma radiation therapy for in-stent restenosis. Circulation 2004;109:340-344.

72. Waksman R, Ajani AE, White RL, et al: Intravascular gamma radiation for in-stent restenosis in saphenous-vein bypass grafts. N Engl J Med 2002;346:1194-1199.

73. Waksman R, Cheneau E, Ajani AE, et al: Intracoronary radiation therapy improves the clinical and angiographic outcomes of diffuse in-stent restenotic lesions: Results of the Washington Radiation for In-Stent Restenosis Trial for Long Lesions (Long WRIST) studies. Circulation 2003;107:1744-1749.

74. Javed MH, Mintz GS, Waksman R, et al: Serial intravascular ultrasound assessment of the efficacy of intracoronary γ radiation therapy for preventing recurrence of very long, diffuse, in-stent restenosis lesions. Circulation 2000;104:856-859.

75. Waksman R, Ajani AE, White RL, et al: Prolonged antiplatelet therapy to prevent late thrombosis after intracoronary gamma-radiation in patients with in-stent restenosis: Washington Radiation for In-Stent Restenosis Trial plus 6 months of clopidogrel (WRIST PLUS). Circulation 2001;103:2332-2335.

76. Waksman R, Ajani AE, Pinnow E, et al: Twelve Versus Six Months of Clopidogrel to Reduce Major Cardiac Events in Patients Undergoing γ-Radiation Therapy for In-Stent Restenosis. Washington Radiation for In-Stent restenosis Trial (WRIST) 12 versus WRIST PLUS. Circulation. 2002;106: 776-778.

77. Kuchulakanti P, Torguson R, Canos D, et al: Optimizing dosimetry with high-dose intracoronary gamma radiation (21 Gy) for patients with diffuse in-stent restenosis. Cardiovasc Revasc Med 2005;6:108-112.

78. Leon MB, Teirstein PS, Moses JW, et al: Localized intracoronary gamma-radiation therapy to inhibit the recurrence of restenosis after stenting. N Engl J Med 2001;344:250-256.

79. Kim HS, Ajani AE, Waksman R. Vascular brachytherapy for in-stent restenosis. J Interv Cardiol 2000;13:417-423.

80. Prpic R, Teirstein PS, Reilly JP, et al: Long-term outcome of patients treated with repeat percutaneous coronary intervention after failure of gamma-brachytherapy for the treatment of in-stent restenosis. Circulation 2002;106:2340-2345.

81. Waksman R, Bhargava B, White L, et al: Intracoronary beta radiation therapy inhibits recurrence of in-stent restenosis. Circulation 2000;101:1895-1898.

82. Popma J: Late clinical and angiographic outcomes after use of ^{90}Sr/^{90}Y beta radiation for the treatment of in-stent restenosis: Results from the ^{90}Sr treatment of angiographic restenosis (START) trial. J Am Coll Cardiol 2000;36:311.

83. Bonan R; for the START Investigators: Efficacy of ^{90}Sr/^{90}Y beta radiation for the treatment of in-stent restenosis: 5 years' clinical outcomes from the Stents and Radiation Therapy (START) trial. Presented at the Cardiovascular Revascularization Therapies meeting, 2006, Crystal City, VA.

84. Kim HS, Waksman R, Cottin Y, et al: Edge stenosis and geographical miss following intracoronary gamma radiation therapy for in-stent restenosis. J Am Coll Cardiol 2001;15: 1026-1030.

85. Waksman R, Raizner AE, Yeung AC, et al: Use of localized intracoronary beta radiation in treatment of in-stent restenosis: The INHIBIT randomized controlled trial. Lancet 2002; 359:551-557.

86. Waksman R, on behalf of the Galileo INHIBIT and INHIBIT Investigators: Manual stepping of 32P-emitter for diffuse in-stent restenosis lesions, tandem versus single position. Clinical and angiographic outcome from a multicenter randomized study. Paper presented at the annual meeting of the American Heart Association, 2001, Anaheim, CA.

87. Waksman R, Buchbinder M, Reisman M, et al: Balloon-based radiation therapy for treatment of in-stent restenosis in human coronary arteries: Results from the BRITE I study. Cathet Cardiovasc Interv 2002;57:286-294.

88. Waksman R, for the BRITE II Investigators: Balloon based radiation for coronary in-stent restenosis: 9 months results from the BRITE II study. Paper presented at the annual meeting of the American College of Cardiology, 2003, Chicago.

89. Stone GW, Mehran R, Midei M, et al: Usefulness of beta radiation for de novo and in-stent restenotic lesions in saphenous vein grafts. J Am Coll Cardiol 2003;92:312-314.

90. Park S-W, Hong M-K, Moon DH, et al: Treatment of diffuse in-stent restenosis with rotational atherectomy followed by radiation therapy with a rhenium-188-mercaptoacetyltriglycine-filled balloon. J Am Coll Cardiol 2001;38:631-637.

91. Dilcher C, Satler LF, Pichard AD, et al: Intracoronary radiation therapy using a novel beta emitter for in-stent restenosis: Tungsten WRIST. Cardiovasc Revasc Med 2005;6:52-57.

92. Verin V, Urban P, Popowski Y, et al: Feasibility of intracoronary beta-irradiation to reduce restenosis after balloon angioplasty: A clinical pilot study. Circulation 1997;95: 1138-1144.

93. King SB III, Williams DO, Chougule P, et al: Endovascular beta-radiation to reduce restenosis after coronary balloon angioplasty: Results of the beta energy restenosis trial (BERT). Circulation 1998;97:2025-2030.

94. Raizner AE, Oesterle SN, Waksman R, et al: Inhibition of restenosis with beta-emitting radiotherapy report of the Proliferation Reduction with Vascular Energy Trial (PREVENT). Circulation 2000;102:951-958.

95. Bonan R, Arsenault A, Tardif JC, et al: Beta energy restenosis trials, Canadian arm. Circulation 1997;96:I-219.

96. Gijzel AL, Wardeh AJ, van der Giessen WJ, et al: Beta-energy to prevent restenosis: The Rotterdam contribution to the BERT 1.5 trial—1 yr. follow up [abstract]. Eur Heart J 1999;370: 1945.

97. Verin V, Popowski Y, de Bruyne B, et al: Endoluminal beta-radiation therapy for the prevention of coronary restenosis after balloon angioplasty. N Engl J Med 2001;344:243-249.

98. Results from late-breaking clinical trials sessions at ACC 2001. J Am Coll Cardiol 2001;38:595.

99. Höher M, Wöhrle J, Wohlfrom M, et al: Intracoronary beta-irradiation with a rhenium-188-filled balloon catheter: A randomized trial in patients with de novo and restenotic lesions. Circulation 2003;7:3022-3027.

100. Serruys PW, Wijns W, Sianos G, et al: Direct stenting versus direct stenting followed by centered beta-radiation with IVUS-guided dosimetry and long-term antiplatelet treatment; results of a randomized trial: Beta-Radiation Investigation with Direct Stenting and Galileo in Europe (BRIDGE). J Am Coll Cardiol 2004;44:528-537.

101. Torguson R, Sabate M, Deible R, et al: Intravascular brachytherapy versus drug-eluting stents for the treatment of patients with drug-eluting stent restenosis. Am J Cardiol 2006;98:1340-1344.

102. Dilcher C, Chan R, Hellinga D, et al: Effect of ionizing radiation on the stability and performance of the TAXUS Express(2) paclitaxel-eluting stent. Cardiovasc Radiat Med 2004;5: 136-141.

103. Stone GW, Ellis SG, O'Shaughnessy CD, et al, for the TAXUS V ISR Investigators: Paclitaxel-eluting stents vs vascular brachytherapy for in-stent restenosis within bare-metal stents: The TAXUS V ISR randomized trial. JAMA 2006;295: 1253-1263.

104. Holmes DR Jr, Teirstein P, Satler L, et al, for the SISR Investigators: Sirolimus-eluting stents vs vascular brachytherapy for in-stent restenosis within bare-metal stents: The SISR randomized trial. JAMA 2006;295:1264-1273.

105. Chu WW, Torguson R, Pichard AD, et al: Drug-eluting stents versus repeat vascular brachytherapy for patients with recurrent in-stent restenosis after failed intracoronary radiation. J Invasive Cardiol 2005;17:659-662.

106. Waksman R, Porrazzo MS, Chan RC, et al: Results from the ARTISTIC feasibility study of 192-Iridium gamma radiation to prevent recurrence of in-stent restenosis. Circulation 1998;98:17,I-442:2327.

107. Sianos G, Kay P, Costa MA, et al: Geographical miss during catheter-based intracoronary beta-radiation: Incidence and implications in the BRIE study. J Am Coll Cardiol 2000;38:415-420.

108. Coen V, Serruys P, Sauerwein W, et al for the RENO Investigators: RENO, a European postmarker surveillance registry, confirms effectiveness of coronary brachytherapy in routine clinical practice. Int J Radiat Oncol Biol Phys 2003;55:1019-1026.

CHAPTER
34 Bioabsorbable Stents

Pranab Das and Debabrata Mukherjee

KEY POINTS

- Bioabsorbable stents herald another significant step forward in the advancement of stent technology.
- Several agents are being evaluated as bioabsorbable stents. The polymer of poly-L-lactic acid (PLLA) is the most promising.
- Because bioabsorbable stents leave no permanent implant, repeat percutaneous or surgical revascularization may be accomplished easily if needed at a later time.
- The best-in-class bioabsorbable stent appears to have solved the tissue response issues seen with early bioabsorbable stent designs.
- Bioabsorbable stents are compatible with magnetic resonance imaging and with computed tomography angiography.
- Bioabsorbable stents are likely to be useful in younger patient populations, for whom repeat percutaneous or surgical revascularization of the stented segment of the vessel is often needed, and therefore appear promising in the field of pediatric cardiology.
- Bioabsorbable stents may provide temporary scaffolding of vulnerable plaques and prevent their rupture.
- Bioabsorbable stents appear particularly attractive for lesions of the superficial femoral artery, in which traditional metallic stents have had a high incidence of strut fracture.

One of the major advances in the field of interventional cardiology has been the development of coronary stents. A conventional metallic stent, by providing mechanical scaffolding to the vessel, prevents abrupt closure of the vessel, a major safety concern with balloon angioplasty. Disruption of the endothelium invariably ensues after angioplasty or stenting, requiring in most cases about 12 weeks for complete re-endothelialization and intimal healing.[1] Although stents have significantly reduced acute vessel closure compared with angioplasty, there are several drawbacks. Besides leaving a permanent implant, stenting in the long term may also prevent favorable arterial remodeling.[2] Stenting of long lesions, which is commonly performed, may preclude future surgical or percutaneous revascularization if needed and may interfere with image interpretations of magnetic resonance angiography (MRA) and computed tomography angiography (CTA) because of metallic artifacts. Because conventional metallic stents provide stimuli for smooth muscle cell proliferation, neointimal hyperplasia leading to in-stent restenosis occurs in up to 30% of patients at 6 months.[3-5] Drug-eluting stents, based on the platform of metallic stents, markedly reduce the rate of in-stent restenosis by eluting antiproliferative drugs such as rapamycin, rapamycin analogues, or paclitaxel.[6,7] Although drug-eluting stents have significantly overcome the hurdles of in-stent restenosis

and reduced the rate of revascularization, they may result in increased early and late stent thrombosis because of long-term, ongoing inflammation or other factors.[8-10] Combinations of antiplatelet therapy with aspirin and clopidogrel are therefore recommended for at least 3 to 6 months after drug-eluting stent implantation to minimize the risks of stent thrombosis.[9,10]

Another significant step forward in stent technology is the development of biodegradable or bioabsorbable stents. Bioabsorbable stents are made of materials capable of gradual degradation in the body, leaving no residual implant within the arteries. A bioabsorbable stent should provide adequate scaffolding for a clinically relevant period and then disappear. This avoids the potential disadvantages of a permanent metallic implant. An effective bioabsorbable stent must perform acutely like a current-generation drug-eluting metallic stent and provide the same long-term safety profile. Only after these criteria have been met will the advantages of bioabsorption encourage the widespread adoption of the bioabsorbable stents. A successful design is a combination of numerous factors, including material selection, absorption profile, drug efficacy, deliverability of the stent system, and acute mechanical performance of the stent. Table 34-1 lists the advantages and disadvantages of bioabsorbable stents compared with traditional metallic stents.

Table 34-1. Advantages and Disadvantages of Bioabsorbable Stents

Advantages	Disadvantages
Long lengths of vessel can be treated without worries of forming a permanent "full metal jacket," resulting in more physiologic repair.	Loss of scaffolding too early may lead to restenosis from vessel remodeling
Provide scaffolding only when needed during vessel healing	May cause local tissue reaction with inflammation and neointimal proliferation, leading to restenosis
Avoid long-term complications of permanent stent implant, such as late remodeling	Not visible on radiographs without markers or contrast embedding
Restore local vascular compliance	Sensitivity to heat and solvents may limit choices of the drug or the coating
Do not interfere with cardiac magnetic resonance angiography or computed tomography angiography imaging	Thick struts needed to improve mechanical strength may impede the deliverability of the stents in smaller vessels
May reduce the risk of late stent thrombosis	
Do not preclude future surgical or percutaneous revascularization and allow reintervention	
May afford new treatment options for diffuse disease and unstable or vulnerable plaque	
May be used repetitively in a single vessel because there will be no permanent implant	
Suitable for pediatric use and for use in a younger population	
May be suitable for vessels with complex anatomy and vessels of lower extremities	

BIOABSORBABLE MATERIALS

Beginning in the 1960s with absorbable sutures, bioabsorbable polymers have been employed in a wide variety of medical devices. Polymers manufactured from lactide- and glycolide-based polymers are the most commonly used materials for clinically approved devices. The safety of these polymers as vascular and nonvascular device ingredients has been well demonstrated, with hundreds of devices being approved for human use over the past 4 decades.

Mechanical properties of a polymer include tensile strength, modulus and strain-to-failure effect recoil, expansibility, flexibility, and deliverability of a stent. A suitable polymer should have high tensile strength, high modulus effect, and optimal elongation to allow creation of a low-profile, balloon-expandable stent design. Degradation rate and degradation products of the polymer affect the duration of vessel support and degree of tissue reaction. Chemical and thermal properties affect the type of degradation products and the type of processing and sterilization methods that can be used. The characteristics of a suitable polymer for intravascular stenting are listed in Table 34-2.[11]

Physical properties of a polymer are determined by its hydrophilicity, crystallinity, molecular-weight distribution, end groups, and presence of residual monomers or additives.[12-14] Table 34-3 describes the physical properties of commonly used biodegradable polymers. Polyglycolic acid (PGA), the polymer of glycolic acid, is the simplest linear aliphatic polyester. PGA is highly crystalline, with a high melting point and a degradation period of 6 to 12 months. Polylactide (PLA) is the polymer of lactic acid. Lactic acid has two optical isomers, L-lactic acid the naturally occurring isomer, D-lactic acid. Poly-D,L-lactide (PDLLA) contains D-lactide and L-lactic acid. Poly-L-lactic acid (PLLA) is the homopolymer of L-lactide. The degradation time of PLLA is much longer than that of PDLLA. Because PDLLA is amorphous with a low tensile strength, higher elongation time, and rapid degradation rate, it is very suitable for a drug-delivery system. Table 34-4 illustrates the ideal properties of a polymer suitable for drug elution. PLLA is a semicrystalline substance with a slower degradation rate and higher tensile strength that appears ideal for use as a stent.

The tissue response to the degradation products depends on the rate of degradation, size and site of the implant, and local tissue microenvironment (e.g., pH, acidity). Lactide- and glycolide-based polymers undergo degradation by hydrolysis, which leads to

Table 34-2. Characteristics of an Ideal Bioabsorbable Stent Material

1. The stent material should have a moderate degradation rate in a predictable fashion over a finite period (6 to 12 months), leaving no residual matrices.
2. The degradation products should be biocompatible, nontoxic, and devoid of significant inflammatory reaction.
3. The stent material should have high tensile strength and strain-to-failure ability before degradation to allow creation of a low-profile, balloon-expandable design for easy deliverability and flexibility.
4. The stent material should possess adequate radial strength and mechanical properties for vessel support during local healing.
5. The stent material should not be thrombogenic and should release no emboli.
6. The stent material should perform acutely and over the long term like metal stents and should be equal to or better than drug-eluting metal stents with respect to restenosis and clinical outcomes.
7. The stent material should be easily processed and sterilizable.
8. The stent material should have an acceptable shelf life.

Modified from Zidar J, Lincoff A, Stack R. Biodegradable stents. In Topol EJ (ed): Textbook of Interventional Cardiology, 2nd ed. Philadelphia, WB Saunders, 1994, pp 787-802.

Table 34-3. Physical Properties of Bioabsorbable Polymers Used for Bioabsorbable Stents

Polymer	Crystallinity	Tensile Strength (MPa)	Tensile Modulus (GPa)	Melting Point (°C)	Elongation (%)	Degradation Rate (mo)	Degradation Products
PGA	Semi-crystalline	60-80	7	225-230	15-20	6 to 12	Glycolic acid
PLLA	Semi-crystalline	60-70	2.7	173-178	5-10	>24	Lactic acid
PDLLA	Amorphous	40-50	1.9	—	3-10	12 to 16	Lactic acid

PGA, polyglycolic acid; PLLA, poly-L-lactic acid; PDLLA, poly-D,L-lactic acid.
Modified from Middleton JC, Tipton J: Synthetic biodegradable polymers as orthopedic devices. Biomaterials 2000:21:2335-2346.

Table 34-4. Ideal Characteristics of a Drug-Eluting Bioabsorbable Polymer

- Linear degradation profile
- Fast degradation rate (<6 months)
- Compatible with hydrophilic and hydrophobic drugs
- Stable under different pH conditions
- Good film-forming properties
- Soluble in common solvents
- No toxic metabolic end products

the formation of water-soluble, low-molecular-weight components that are metabolized into carbon dioxide and water. Bulk erosion occurs when the rate at which water penetrates the device exceeds that at which the polymer is converted into water-soluble materials, resulting in erosion throughout the device. Strongly hydrophobic polymers undergo mostly surface erosion, a process that occurs when the rate at which water penetrates the device is slower than the rate of conversion of the polymer into water-soluble materials, leading to device thinning over time while maintaining its bulk integrity.[15-17] Figures 34-1 and 34-2 portray the degradation process of bioabsorbable polymers.

The search for potential alternatives to bioabsorbable polymers as stent materials has led the scientists to investigate the scope of absorbable metals. An ideal absorbable metal stent candidate should have mechanical properties similar to conventional metal stents and should have sustained mechanical integrity, have steerable kinetics, induce normal endothelial function with minimal or zero inflammatory or thrombogenic response, and degrade into nontoxic by-products. Magnesium and iron satisfy most of these properties and have been further evaluated. These two metals, even at an overdose by several-fold, have no cytotoxic or genotoxic effects, are devoid of acute systemic toxicity, and are hemocompatible with no signs of chronic toxicity. In general, metallic stents are found to have a higher collapse pressure and smaller degree of recoil, providing efficient scaffolding.[18]

POLYMER-BASED BIOABSORBABLE STENTS

The first biodegradable stent, made of a polymer of PLLA, was developed in the early 1980s by Stack and colleagues[19] and implanted in animal models at Duke University in the 1990s. Although this stent could withstand up to 1000 mm Hg of crush pressure,

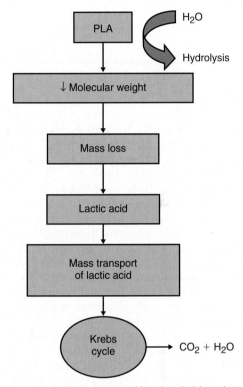

Figure 34-1. Metabolic pathways of bioabsorbable polymers. Bioabsorbable polymers are degraded in the body with hydrolysis into carbon dioxide and water. PLA, polylactide.

almost twice as much a Palmaz-Schatz stent, it maintained its radial strength for 1 month and degraded completely by 9 months; further progress in the research with this polymeric stent was somewhat slow. The Duke bioabsorbable stent was the prototype of the PLA stent used in canine femoral arteries and was self-expanding. The long-term degradation of this stent caused little thrombotic response, minimal neointimal hyperplasia, and minimal inflammatory reaction.[19] The Kyoto University biodegradable stent, made of polyglycolic acid, was more thrombogenic when implanted in a canine model.[20] The Cleveland Clinic/Mayo/Thoraxcenter biodegradable stent, consisting of five biodegradable polymers (i.e., poly D,L-lactic acid, polyorthoester, poly-hydroxybutyrate/hydroxyvalerate, polycaprolactone, and polyethylene oxide) exhibited marked inflammatory reactions (Fig. 34-3) with neointimal proliferation in porcine coronary arteries.[21] This intense local reaction, demonstrated by a marked inflammatory reaction, neointimal proliferation, medial necro-

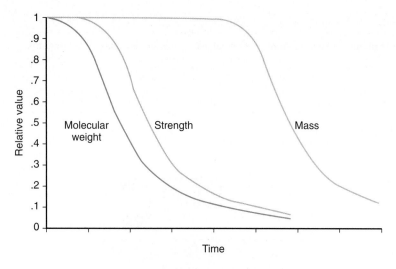

Figure 34-2. During the degradation process, bioabsorbable polymers undergo reduction in molecular weight, loss of strength, and loss of mass.

sis, and pseudoaneurysm formation, was observed for bioabsorbable and biodurable polymers. The observed response (at 28 days) therefore is not caused by the formation of degradation products. The inflammatory response most likely resulted from the use of nonsterile implants combined with a less than ideal geometry. When the results obtained in this study are compared with the low thrombotic and low inflammatory response obtained with the Duke PLLA stent, it becomes apparent that the vessel response is driven by a combination of parameters. An effective bioabsorbable stent must therefore combine an ideal material, adequate sterilization techniques, and an optimal design to achieve desirable results.

In a further evaluation of bioabsorbable stents, Lincoff and colleagues[22] demonstrated that the differential degree of local reaction in a porcine coronary injury model depends on the size of the polymers, with lighter PLLA polymers (molecular mass ≈80 kd) being more inflammatory and heavier polymers (molecular mass ≈321 kd) being less so. Yamawaki and coworkers[23] coated the biodegradable stent with an antiproliferative drug, a tyrosine kinase inhibitor (i.e., tranilast) to suppress this local reaction and found there was a reduced risk of stenosis with the drug-polymer combination.

Poly-L-Lactic Acid Bioabsorbable Stents

Poly-L-Lactic Acid Coronary Stents

The collapse pressure of the PLLA stents are almost equal to that of stainless steel metal stents, making these polymers suitable for bioabsorbable stents.[15] The Igaki-Tamai stent (Fig. 34-4), another monofilamentous, PLLA-based biodegradable stent of 183 kd, has been improved from its earlier versions with a zigzag, helical-coiled design that may minimize tissue injury and thereby reduce local tissue reaction and thrombus formation.[23-26] A combination of the heat-expandable and balloon-expandable properties of the stent allowed its initial self-expansion in response to heat (transmitted by a delivery balloon inflated with a 70°C contrast-water mixture [50°C at the balloon site]) and subsequent re-expansion with a moderate degree of balloon inflation (6 to 14 atm). Continued expansion of the stent to its normal size over 20 to 30 minutes at 37°C generated a radial strength similar to that of the Palmaz-Schatz stent. After initial success with implantation in animal models characterized by minimal inflammatory response,[25] Tamai and colleagues[27] extended their experience to humans and implanted 25 of these stents in 19 lesions in 15 patients electively, with angiographic follow-up by intravascular ultrasound at day 1, 3 months, and 6 months. Angiographic restenosis rates of 5.3% and 10.5% with rates of target vessel revascularization per lesion of 6.3% and 10.5% were associated with a loss index of 0.44 and 0.48 mm at 3 and 6 months, respectively (Table 34-5). No deaths, myocardial infarctions, or coronary artery bypass grafting (CABG) were reported. Although self-expansion of the stent continued up to the third month after implantation, the stent maintained its scaffolding even at 6 months. Vessel wall injury from the initial heat delivered for rapid stent expansion, with resultant stent thrombosis or neointimal proliferation, remained the major concern but was not observed in this study at 6 months of follow-up.

In further follow-up, Tamai and coworkers[27] reported long-term outcomes of 63 lesions in 50 patients undergoing elective stenting with PLLA Igaki-Tamai stent between September 1998 and April 2003 (Table 34-6). This pilot study showed that even at long-term follow-up to 48 months, Igaki-Tamai biodegradable stents appear safe and effective, and they may be a feasible alternative to conventional metal stents for clinical use.

Drug-Eluting Poly-L-Lactic Acid Stents

Poly-L-Lactic Acid–Tranilast Stents

In an attempt to reduce the local inflammatory reaction at the site of stent implantation, Yamawaki and associates[23] incorporated ST 638 (tranilast, a specific

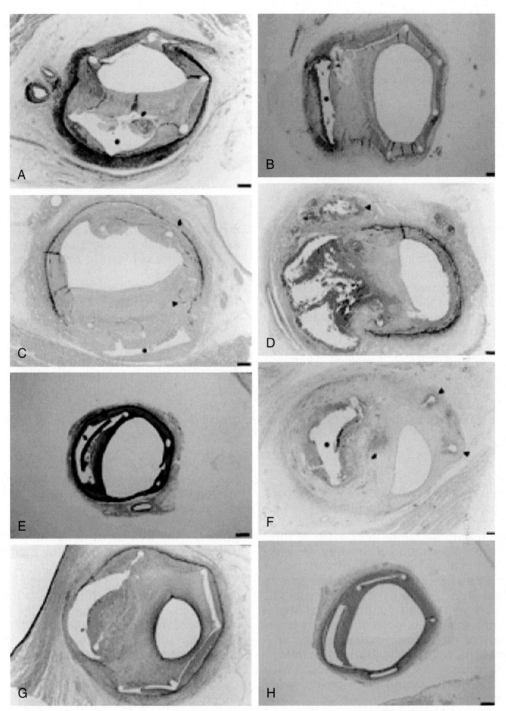

Figure 34-3. Various tissue responses to the individual biodegradable (**A** to **E**) and nonbiodegradable (**F** to **H**) polymer test samples. In each panel, the *bar* indicates 375 µm. **A,** With PGLA, the large open area was occupied by the polymer and proteinaceous debris and was covered by a distinct fibrocellular layer (elastic stain). **B,** PCL showed a smaller polymer artifact but a more pronounced eccentric fibrocellular response (hematoxylin and eosin stain). **C,** With PHBV, at the site of the polymer implant, the media ruptured, but at the opposite side, lysis of the elastic membranes occurred as a result of the inflammatory response (elastic stain). **D,** POE induced an immense inflammatory response with a granulomatous appearance that extended into the adventitia and resulted in destruction of the architecture of the vessel (elastic stain). **E,** With PEO/PBTP, the vascular response to the polymer was limited in nature and had a more benign character (elastic stain). F, PUR demonstrated a circumferential inflammatory reaction to the polymer and damaging bare wire that extended into the neointima (hematoxylin and eosin stain). **G,** With SIL, in contrast to the reaction to PUR, the intense inflammatory response was restricted to the polymer but with a circumferential fibrocellular response (elastic stain). **H,** PETP produced a benign tissue response and limited neointimal growth (hematoxylin and eosin stain).

Table 34-5. Results of Quantitative Intravascular Ultrasound Analysis of Patients at 3 and 6 Months after Igaki-Tamai Stent Placement

Characteristics	Immediate Post Stenting $n = 19$	1-day Post Stenting $n = 19$	3-Month Follow-up $n = 18$	6 Month Follow-up $n = 18$
Stent CSA (mm²)	7.42 ± 1.51	7.37 ± 1.44	8.18 ± 2.42*	8.13 ± 2.52*
Neointimal area (mm²)	—	—	2.51 ± 0.94	2.50 ± 0.65
Lumen CSA (mm²)	7.42 ± 1.51	7.37 ± 1.44	5.67 ± 2.42†	5.63 ± 2.70‡

*$P < .1$ versus after stenting.
†$P < .005$ versus after stenting.
‡$P < .001$ versus after stenting.
CSA, cross-sectional area.
Modified from Colombo A, Karvouni E: Biodegradable stents "fulfilling the mission and stepping away." Circulation 2000;102:371-373.

tyrosine kinase inhibitor) or ST 494 (an inactive metabolite of ST 638) into Igaki-Tamai PLLA stents and evaluated the stents in a porcine coronary artery model for 21 days. Three weeks after the implantation of the stents, coronary stenosis was assessed by coronary angiography followed by histologic examination. Coronary stenosis was significantly less with the ST638 stent than the ST 494 stent. Histological examination of the vessels also showed less neointimal proliferation and a lesser degree of geometric remodeling at the ST 638 sites compared with ST 494 stent sites.[23] Antiproliferative agents incorporated into the bioabsorbable stents may be an effective way of minimizing tissue inflammatory reactions and thereby reducing the degree of subsequent restenosis.

Poly-L-Lactic Acid–Paclitaxel Stents
Vogt and colleagues[28] developed a novel balloon-expandable, biodegradable, double-helical PDLLA stent (Fig. 34-5) using controlled expansion of saturated polymers (CESP) for better integration of thermally sensitive polymers and longer drug delivery. Twelve paclitaxel-loaded (170 μg of paclitaxel, with a release rate of 5 to 8 μg initially and tapering to 1 μg at 4 weeks and 0 at 3 months) PDLLA stents, 12 unloaded PDLLA stents, and 12 bare metal stents (316L) were implanted in 36 porcine coronary arteries. Six animals of each group were sacrificed at 3 weeks and 3 months, respectively. During this follow-up, coronary stenosis was significantly reduced with paclitaxel-eluting stents compared with unloaded and bare metal stents (Fig. 34-6). Although early endothelialization of the stents were evident and

mechanical integrity was maintained at 3 months, a local inflammatory response to the polymer stent was the major concern in this animal study.

Poly-L-Lactic Acid–Sirolimus Stents
Tamai and associates[27] have studied drug-eluting, PLLA-based stents in a porcine coronary artery model. A total of 26 stents were implanted in porcine coronaries, 8 of which were loaded with a sirolimus analogue, 12 with tranilast, and 6 with no drug. After a follow-up of 4 weeks, the neointimal thickness and neointimal area were significantly less with the drug-eluting stents compared with controls, and between the two drugs, the sirolimus analogue performed better than tranilast.[24]

Poly-L-Lactic Acid–Everolimus Stents
The Bioabsorbable Vascular Solutions (BVS) everolimus-eluting stent (Fig. 34-7) is a major advancement in the field of bioabsorbable stents and is the first drug-eluting bioabsorbable stent to undergo clinical studies. The BVS stent is a fully bioabsorbable, balloon-expandable, drug-eluting stent that performs acutely like a metallic drug-eluting stent (Fig. 34-8). No special techniques are required to deliver and deploy the stent. With thin struts, a low profile, and a plastic-like polymeric material, the BVS stent is a highly deliverable and conformable stent. It is a high-molecular-weight, PLLA-based stent, with a PDLLA coating serving as a bioabsorbable matrix for an everolimus-eluting layer. Mounted on the ML Vision SDS Balloon, the stent includes two platinum radiopaque markers on end rings of the stent for

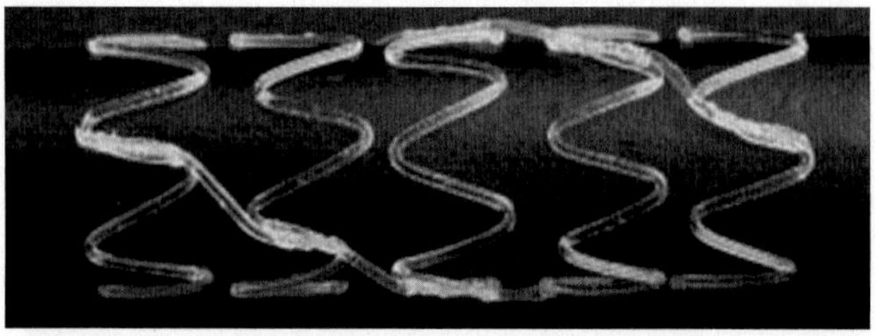

Figure 34-4. The Igaki-Tamai stent is a premounted, balloon-expandable poly-L-lactic acid stent with the ability for self-expansion. It has a helical, zigzag design.

Table 34-6. Clinical Follow-up Data at 4 Years after Igaki-Tamai Stent Placement

Results	Incidence (%)
Death	1/50 (2%)
Q-wave myocardial infarction	1/50 (2%)
Coronary artery bypass graft surgery	0
Stent thrombosis	1/50* (2%)
Repeat percutaneous coronary intervention	
6 months	6/50 (12%)
12 months	7/50 (14%)
48 months	9/50 (18%)

*In-hospital, same patient.

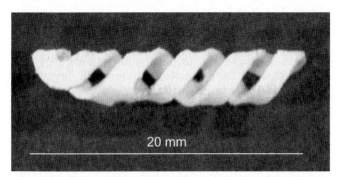

Figure 34-5. Double-helical geometry of the poly-D,L-lactic acid (PDLLA) stent.

enhanced visibility. Because of its semicrystalline nature, PLLA has a much higher mechanical strength and is well suited for use as a stent material. PDLLA is an amorphous polymer and is well suited for drug-delivery applications. The polymeric material of the BVS stent allows it to be visible with MR and CT imaging, offering the potential for noninvasive patient follow-up in the future.

The BVS everolimus-eluting coronary stent system contains 100 µg of everolimus per 1 cm² of surface area. Everolimus is a sirolimus analogue that inhibits mammalian target of rapamycin (mTOR). Everolimus has been shown in porcine and rabbit models and in clinical trials to be effective in reducing neointimal

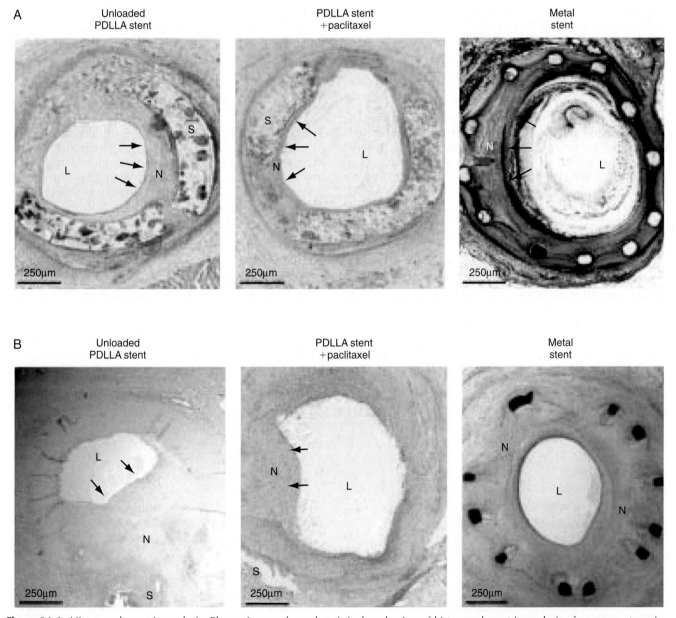

Figure 34-6. Histomorphometric analysis. Photomicrographs and statistical evaluation of histomorphometric analysis of coronary stenosis after implantation of unloaded poly-D,L-lactic acid (PDLLA) stents *(left)*, paclitaxel-loaded PDLLA stents *(middle)*, or metal stents *(right)* (magnification ×40) after 3 weeks (a) and after 3 months (b). L, lumen; N, neointima; S, stent; *arrows*, neointimal areas.

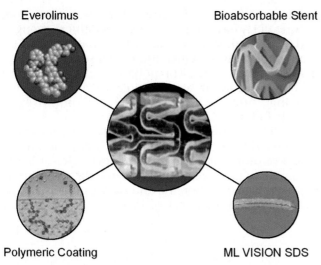

Figure 34-7. Bioabsorbable Vascular Solutions' everolimus-eluting stent is a balloon-expandable, drug-eluting (i.e., everolimus) bioabsorbable stent composed of polylactide polymers and copolymers mounted on a standard delivery system. (Courtesy of Abbott Vascular.)

effect that was resolved by 90 days and indicated drug elution off of the stent. This observation was similar to that seen with metallic drug-eluting systems. Complete luminal endothelialization was observed at all time points evaluated (28 days to 12 months), with minimal inflammation and no medial necrosis (data obtained from Abbott Vascular, Santa Clara, CA) (Figs. 34-9 to 34-12).

The BVS everolimus-eluting coronary stent system's first-in-humans clinical trial, the ABSORB trial,[31] is a prospective, open-labeled trial enrolling patients with visually estimated nominal vessel diameters of 3.0 mm. The investigators have enrolled 30 patients to date. The primary outcomes are ischemia-driven MACEs at 30, 180, and 270 days and at 1, 2, 3, 4, and 5 years; ischemia-driven target vessel failure (TVF) at 30, 180, and 270 days and at 1, 2, 3, 4, and 5 years; and acute success (i.e., clinical device and clinical procedure). Twenty-six patients have already been enrolled in the trial. The trial is ongoing, and final results will be announced at major conferences.

thickness and neointimal area in response to angioplasty or stenting.[29,30] The clinical trials investigated the use of an everolimus-eluting metallic stent containing an ultrathin coating of a poly-(lactic acid) bioabsorbable polymer used for drug delivery. Everolimus appears to be a potential therapeutic agent for the reduction of restenosis after angioplasty and stenting. The vascular response of the BVS everolimus-eluting stent in porcine and rabbit arterial models was characterized by a thin, well-healed neointima composed of compact smooth muscle cells in a proteoglycan-collagen matrix. Peristrut fibrin deposition was observed at 28 days, consistent with a drug

Poly-ʟ-Lactic Acid Peripheral Stents

The peripheral Igaki-Tamai stent is undergoing testing in humans.[27] This stent has a zigzag helical coil, strut thickness of 0.24 mm, and two radiopaque gold markers, and it is available only with a 36-mm length and with 5-, 6-, 7-, and 8-mm diameters. Hietala and colleagues[32] reported the long-term follow-up results for a copolymeric polylactide stent (PLA 96, L/D ratio 96/4) implanted in the rabbit aorta model for 34 months. Complete endothelialization of the stents occurred at 3 months with no inflammatory reaction, and hydrolyzation was evident at 12 months, with complete degradation occurring by 24 months.

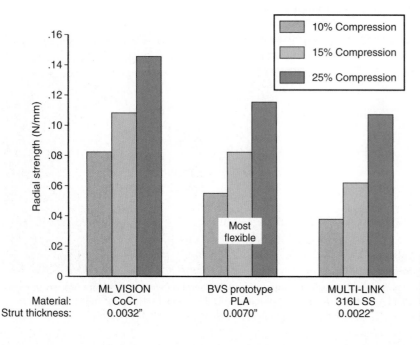

Figure 34-8. Radial strength testing of bioabsorbable stents is compared with that of bare metal stents, and results show that bioabsorbable stents are more flexible, even in graded compression testing.

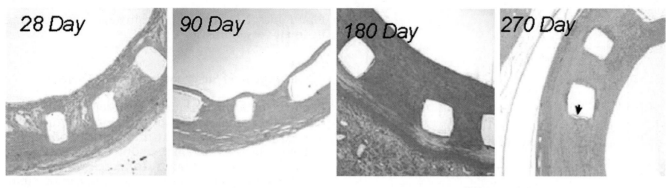

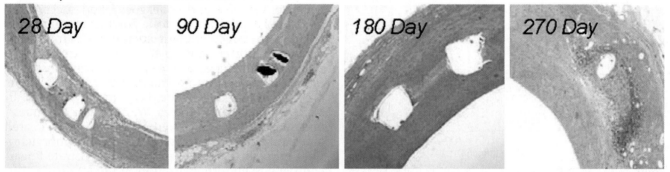

Figure 34-9. Neointimal responses to the Bioabsorbable Vascular Solutions everolimus-eluting stents *(top)* at 3 months, 6 months, and 9 months in a porcine coronary model show minimal neointimal thickness and minimal inflammation compared with sirolimus-eluting stents *(bottom)*. (Courtesy of Abbott Vascular.)

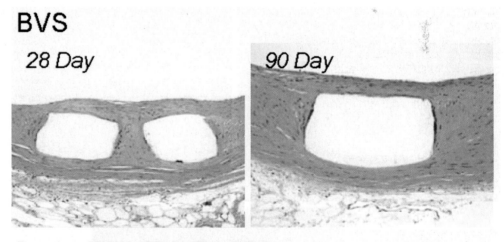

Figure 34-10. Neointimal responses to the Bioabsorbable Vascular Solutions (BVS) everolimus-eluting stents and sirolimus-eluting stents (Cypher) in a rabbit iliac artery model show benign neointimal response to the BVS stent with a minimal giant cell reaction. The response to the Cypher stent was marked with a giant-cell reaction. (Courtesy of Abbott Vascular.)

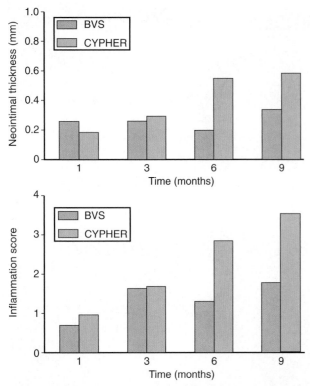

Figure 34-11. Neointimal responses to the Bioabsorbable Vascular Solutions (BVS) everolimus-eluting stents and Cypher stents at 6 months and 9 months in a porcine coronary model show minimal inflammatory response to BVS stents compared with the Cypher stents at all time points.

PLA96 may be another promising agent for stenting in small-vessel disease.

Poly-L-Lactic Acid Stents for Local Gene Delivery

Rapid re-endothelialization in response to tissue injury after angioplasty or stenting may prevent restenosis and inhibit stent thrombosis. Endothelial mitogens such as vascular endothelial growth factor (VEGF) have been found to accelerate this re-endothelialization process.[33,34] Stent technology may provide an excellent scaffold for the catheter-based approach of gene transfer. Bioabsorbable stents with genetic manipulation appear to be appealing for local gene delivery. Ye and colleagues[35] had successfully used a PLLA/polycaprolactone polymer stent impregnated with a recombinant adenovirus carrying the beta-Gal reporter gene to transfer and express this nuclear-localizing gene in cells of the arterial walls of rabbits. DNA-eluting polymer-based coronary stents provide localized gene delivery and expression in porcine coronary arteries.[36] Walter and colleagues[37] had successfully transferred VEGF-2 plasmid-coated bioabsorbable polymer stents (i.e., phosphorylcholine) into rabbit iliac arteries and demonstrated near-complete re-endothelialization of the arteries within 10 days compared with the control groups (i.e., polymer stents with no VEGF coating) and transgene

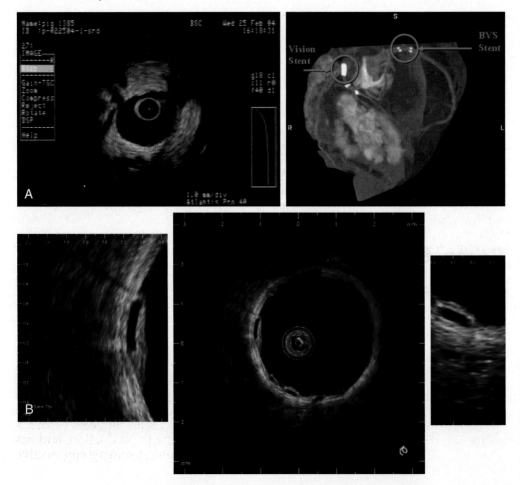

Figure 34-12. Visualization of a Bioabsorbable Vascular Solutions (BVS) everolimus-eluting stent with intravascular ultrasound **(A)**, computed tomography (CT) angiography **(B)**, and optical coherence tomography **(C).** (Courtesy of Abbott Vascular.)

expression was also detectable in the vessel wall within 10 days with improvement of endothelial cell function. Despite these promising animal data, efficacy of human gene therapy for the prevention of restenosis has not been demonstrated. Moreover, gene therapy may have the hazards of potential malignant transformation from oncogene activation and several other risks.

Poly-L-Lactic Acid Stents for Vulnerable Plaque Treatment

Vulnerable plaques are advanced atherosclerotic lesions with a lipid-rich core and abundant inflammatory cells and proteins.[38] Because these lesions are responsible for most life-threatening acute vascular syndromes, prompt identification by a suitable imaging modality is crucial for containment of the process. Intravascular ultrasound and optical coherence tomography (OCT) are useful for diagnosing vulnerable plaques.[39,40] Bioabsorbable stents may explore a future innovation in treatment of vulnerable plaques by covering them and preventing plaque rupture and acute coronary syndromes.

Non–Poly-L-Lactic Acid Bioabsorbable Coronary Stents

A tyrosine-derived polycarbonate is the bioabsorbable polymer of the stent developed by REVA Medical.[41] This polymer, developed at Rutgers University, delivers good stent performance and doubles as a drug-delivery matrix, with complete drug release from the polymer. The stent contains iodine to allow x-ray visibility, polyethylene glycol to make the material less adhesive to components and less thrombogenic, and an acidic co-monomer to control biodegradation. The nondeforming nature of its slide-and-lock design (Fig. 34-13) results in a stent with exceptional strength and flexibility but with reduced stent strut thickness and conformability to the vessel wall. It also allows for standard balloon deployment. As the stent is resorbed, the degradation products are safely excreted from the body. In the preclinical study, the polymer was found to have a molecular weight loss of 80% at 1 year, thereby providing adequate vessel support while sparing natural vessel mechanics. The stent is visible by x-ray radiography or fluoroscopy, and it does not interfere with MRA and CTA imaging, allowing less invasive diagnostic and clinical imaging in the future. The REVA stent is being developed in a non–drug-eluting and a paclitaxel-eluting version. The paclitaxel-eluting version has the paclitaxel contained in the same polycarbonate polymer coating. The randomized endovascular study of REVA bioabsorbable stent (RESORB), a first-in-humans clinical trial, will evaluate the safety of the new stent platform (i.e., slide-and-lock technology) in native coronary arteries and may be a promising alternative in biodegradable stent technology.

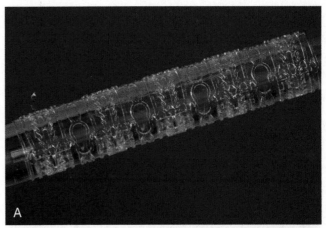

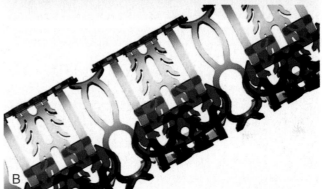

Figure 34-13. Photograph of the REVA bioabsorbable stent **(A)** and its unique slide-and-lock design **(B)**. (Courtesy of REVA Medical.)

NON–POLYMER-BASED BIOABSORBABLE STENTS

Because bioabsorbable polymer stents need to be bulkier with thicker struts compared with bare metal stents to generate adequate mechanical properties for its sustenance in the vessels, biodegradable metallic stents appear to be quite promising. Only two bioabsorbable metal alloys have been considered for this application: magnesium and iron. Both metals are essential elements in the human body, and the degradation products are likely to be less toxic and more biocompatible than metallic drug-eluting stents.

Bioabsorbable Magnesium Stents

Magnesium is one of the most important micronutrients in our body. The physiologic plasma magnesium concentration is 1.4 to 2.1 mEq/L (0.70 to 1.05 mmol/L), and metabolic conversion of magnesium to its chloride, oxide, sulfate, or phosphate salts is well tolerated. Biodegradation products of magnesium in the body are unlikely to cause any serious side effects. Magnesium can also act as a systemic and coronary vasodilator. It is a physiologic calcium antagonist, and it prevents an intracellular calcium load during ischemia and platelet aggregation. Magnesium may prevent endothelin-induced vasoconstriction, can inhibit endothelin production, and has been found to be safe in patients undergoing elective

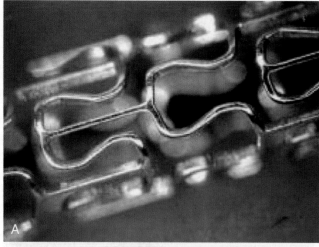

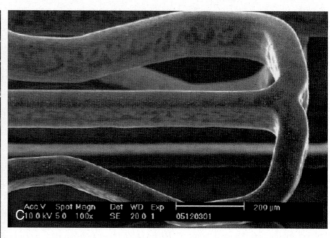

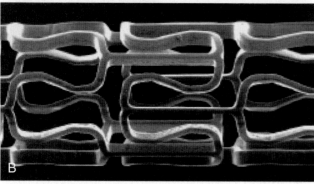

Figure 34-14. A, Photograph of the tubular-slot, balloon-expandable, magnesium alloy stent after electropolishing. The stent is characterized by circumferential noose-shaped structures connected by unbowed cross-links along the longitudinal axis. **B,** Electron microscope picture of a magnesium alloy stent at low magnification. **C,** Electron microscope picture of the magnesium stent at high magnification. Diameters: 3 mm, 3.5 mm; lengths: 10 mm, 15 mm; elastic recoil: ≤8%; collapse pressure: ≥0.5 bar, foreshortening: ≤5%.

percutaneous coronary intervention (PCI).[42-43] Magnesium alloys contain magnesium of 3 to 6 mg per stent, depending on the stent length, and various amounts of other metals. Magnesium alloy AE21 contains 2% aluminum and 1% rare earth elements (Ce, Pr, Nd) and has an anticipated mass loss of only 50% during the first 6 months. In the first animal model with this magnesium alloy stent, 20 stents were implanted in coronaries of 16 pigs through 8-Fr guiding catheters and followed for up to 56 days with angiograms, intravascular ultrasound, and histopathologic evaluation. The initial procedural success rate was 100%, and there was no evidence of any thromboembolic events during follow-up; however, there was a significant 40% loss of perfused lumen diameter between days 10 and 35 due to neointima formation and a significant 25% luminal re-enlargement between days 35 and 56 due to vascular remodeling from loss of stent integrity. Moreover, uneven and asymmetric expansion of the stent with protrusion of the stent struts within the adventitia caused inflammation and exaggerated intimal hyperplasia in areas with the greatest concentration of degradation products.[44] Further improvements of the stent by prolonging the rate of metal degradation and enhancing its mechanical integrity were therefore necessary.

The Lekton Magic coronary stent (Biotronik, Bulach, Switzerland) was an upgrade from the earlier magnesium alloy stent, made of the WE43 magnesium alloy with zirconium (<5%), yttrium (<5%), and rare earths (<5%). The stent has circumferential, noose-shaped elements connected by unbowed cross-links along its longitudinal axis.[45] Mounted on a dedicated balloon, it can be delivered with a 6-Fr system. It has a diameter of 1.2 mm, and for a 3-mm stent, the elastic recoil is approximately 5% with a collapse pressure of 0.8 atm. In a preclinical study, two Lekton Magic stents (Fig. 34-14) and one control stent (Lekton Motion, Biotronik) were implanted in each of 33 minipigs. The angiographic mean luminal diameter of the magnesium stent at 4 weeks was 1.49 mm, compared with 1.33 mm for the control, and at 3 months, the mean luminal diameter of the magnesium stent was 1.68 mm, compared with 1.33 mm for the control ($P < .001$). The anticipated rate of complete degradation of the stent was less than 3 months.

Absorbable Magnesium Coronary Stents

The first absorbable magnesium stent (Fig. 34-15) implanted in humans was evaluated in the Clinical Performance and Angiographic Results of the Coronary Stenting with Absorbable Magnesium Stents (PROGRESS-AMS) trial of 63 patients from seven European centers with stable or unstable angina pectoris without myocardial infarction. The result of this feasibility study was reported at the American College

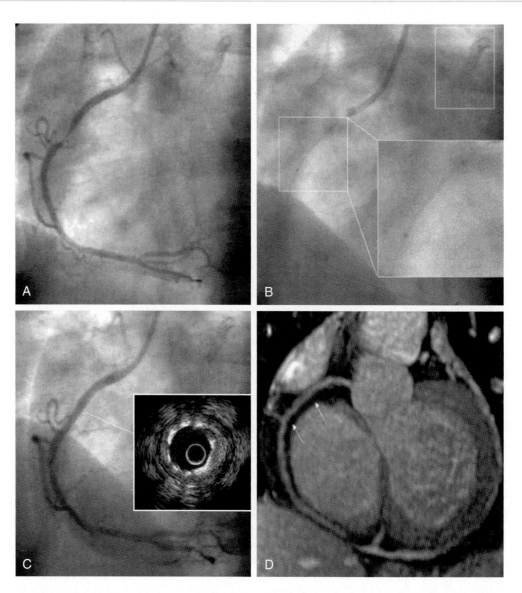

Figure 34-15. A, Preinterventional coronary angiogram shows a high-grade stenosis in the proximal segment of the right coronary artery. **B,** Fluoroscopy immediately after implantation of the absorbable magnesium alloy stent. The implantation balloon is still in place, indicating the position of the implanted stent. Notice that the magnesium alloy stent is completely radiolucent and cannot be visualized on radiographs, in contrast to the stainless steel stent in the left anterior descending coronary artery. **C,** Postinterventional angiographic result without residual stenosis. Intravascular ultrasound showed complete expansion of the magnesium alloy stent. **D,** Contrast-enhanced magnetic resonance angiography of the right coronary artery 1 week after stent placement. The stented segment *(arrows)* can be well visualized by magnetic resonance imaging because of the absence of metallic artifacts.

of Cardiology 2006 annual convention in Atlanta, Georgia.[46] The primary end point of the study was a composite of death, nonfatal myocardial infarction, and ischemia-driven target lesion revascularization. Lesions that were 3.0 to 3.5 mm in diameter and less than 15 mm long with 50% or more stenosis were included in this trial. The right coronary artery was treated in 36% and the left anterior descending artery in 34% of the patients. Clopidogrel was given for 6 months, and aspirin was recommended indefinitely. The expected degradation of the stent was 2 to 3 months, and follow-up with intravascular ultrasound had demonstrated complete endothelialization at 2 to 3 months. The designated noninferiority criterion was less than 30% of the primary end point, and the study reported 23% of patients meeting the primary end point. The angiographic success rate was 100%, and no patients experienced myocardial infarction or cardiac death during this short follow-up. Although the stent was shown to be safe with no acute or sub-acute stent thrombosis, the rates of ischemia-driven target lesion revascularization and all target lesion

revascularizations of about 24% and 38%, respectively, were rather disappointing considering that the lesions treated were mostly of type A lesions, with an expected low risk for restenosis (Table 34-7). The late lumen loss of 1.09 mm at 4 months and mean diameter stenosis of 48% at 4 months also suggests that absorbable magnesium stents may not prevent restenosis.

Absorbable Magnesium Peripheral Stents

Absorbable magnesium stents were studied in the PROGRESS-AMS trial for critical limb ischemia from high grade infrapopliteal stenoses (80% to 100%) in 20 patients.[47] Angiographic procedural success was achieved in 100% of the patients. Primary clinical patency was maintained in 90% and 78% of patients at 3 and 6 months, respectively. No major or minor amputation was needed in any of the patients at 3 months, whereas at 6 months, one patient had undergone amputation of the

Table 34-7. Angiographic and Clinical Outcome Data at 4 Months for Patients after Absorbable Magnesium Coronary Stent Implantation

Characteristic	Baseline: Preprocedural (*n* = 63)	At 4-Month Follow-up (*n* = 63)
Reference vessel diameter (mm)	2.76 ± 0.47	2.66 ± 0.46
Minimal lumen diameter (mm)	1.05 ± 0.38	1.37 ± 0.52
Late loss (mm)	—	1.09 ± 0.51
Target lesion revascularization		
Total	—	38%
Ischemia-driven	—	24%
Stent thrombosis, death, or myocardial infarction	0	0
MACE (primary end point)*		24%

Major adverse cardiovascular events (MACE) constituted the prespecified primary end point (i.e., composite of death, nonfatal myocardial infarction, and ischemia-driven target lesion revascularization). At 4 months, the incidence of MACE needed to be less than 30% to meet the inferiority criteria compared with bare metal stents.

index limb. Duplex ultrasound and MRI demonstrated complete absorption of the stents at 3 months. The average improvement in Rutherford class was 2.3 at 3 months. These results were very encouraging, and they may open up avenues for treatment of critical limb ischemia with bioabsorbable metal stents.

Drug-Eluting Absorbable Metal Stent System

Although absorbable metal stents were found to have adequate mechanical strength, the lack of superior efficacy in reducing restenosis has been disappointing. A strategy of impregnating an antiproliferative agent into the magnesium stents to prevent the rate of stenosis is warranted. Drug-eluting absorbable metal stent concept resulted in bioabsorbable magnesium alloy impregnated with bioabsorbable polymer matrix carrying discrete drug-delivery reservoirs with pimecrolimus. Pimecrolimus, an antiinflammatory agent (not an mTOR inhibitor), binds with high affinity to FKBP-12 and inhibits calcineurin, which inhibits T-cell activation by blocking the transcription of early cytokines.[48] Because it does not inactivate mTOR, it does not affect cell cycle regulation. In the porcine coronary model, pimecrolimus has been shown to be effective in inhibiting restenosis at 28 days (Table 34-8) compared with bare metal controls.[49] Further evaluation of the efficacy of pimecrolimus in the reduction of restenosis is

ongoing in a multicenter, randomized study of patients with stable or unstable angina eligible for PCIs. Pimecrolimus promises to be an effective antistenotic, and the magnesium alloy can provide the scaffolding and radial strength in the stent.[50] The unique reservoir-based drug-delivery system (Conorized reservoir system) within the bioabsorbable polymer matrix may allow the polymer release and drug release to continue independent of magnesium bioabsorption.

Magnesium Stents for Noncoronary Applications

Conventional stents leave a permanent implant at the vessel site, and if used in the pediatric population, they may be outgrown as the vessel size grows appropriately with age. This may lead to a fixed mechanical obstruction of the vessel with the implanted metal stents and may necessitate surgical intervention to relieve this obstruction. Bioabsorbable stents, because of a lack of any permanent implantation and of any casting of the index vessel, may offer an attractive choice for percutaneous interventions of congenital heart diseases, which are treated mostly by surgical procedures. Case reports of successful and uneventful deployment of absorbable magnesium stents in the treatment of ligated pulmonary artery in a preterm baby and in relief of critical recoarctation of the aorta in a newborn (Fig. 34-16) reaffirm these promises.[51,52]

Table 34-8. Differential Effects of Pimecrolimus-Eluting Stents and Bare Metal Stents on Inflammation and Restenosis in a Porcine Coronary Model

Characteristic	Bare Metal	Slow-Release Pimecrolimus	Intermediate-Release Pimecrolimus	*P* Value
Intimal thickness (mm)	0.40 ± 0.17	0.26 ± 0.14	0.22 ± 0.13	<.0002 DES vs. BMS
Area stenosis (%)	42 ± 17	31 ± 15	26 ± 13	< .05, DES vs. BMS
Injury score	0.77 ± 0.63	0.62 ± 0.29	0.47 ± 0.46	NS
Inflammation score	1.46 ± 1.53	0.33 ± 0.73	0.27 ± 0.52	<.0004, DES vs. BMS
Intimal fibrin	0.57 ± 0.74	0.70 ± 0.67	0.70 ± 0.99	NS
Endothelialization (%)	89 ± 15	85 ± 17	84 ± 22	NS

BMS, bare metal stent; DES, drug-eluting stent; NS, not significant.
From Waksman R: Drug-eluting pimecrolimus eluting absorbable meta-stents (DREAMS) concept. Presented at the European Paris Course on Revascularization (EuroPCR), May 2006, Paris.

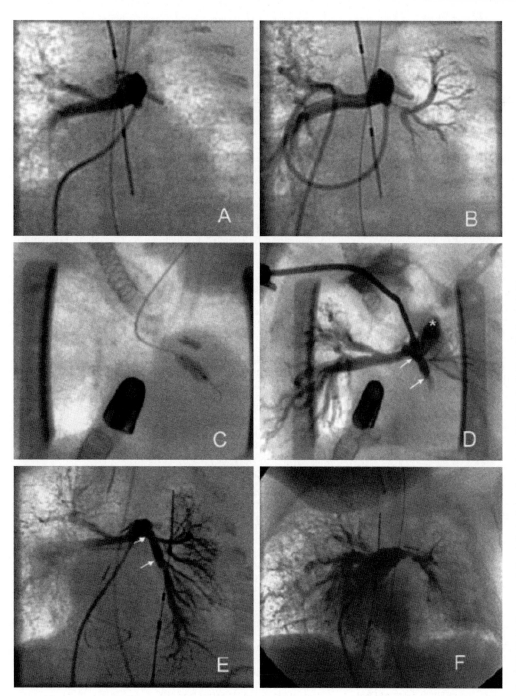

Figure 34-16. A, Complete occlusion of the left pulmonary artery after debanding and closure of the arterial duct with a clip (the device with three markers is for calibration purposes). **B,** After crossing the stenosis with a guidewire, angiography revealed reperfusion. **C,** Implantation procedure with a contrast-filled balloon catheter. **D,** Immediately after implantation, only minimal perfusion of the left upper lobe artery was detectable by angiography. The left lower lobe artery was still completely occluded at 4 mm distal to the stent. Both ends of the stent are marked by *arrows*. The *asterisk* marks some extravascular contrast agent. **E,** At 1-week follow-up, the left lung was reperfused. **F,** At the latest follow-up (33rd day after stent implantation), after the circumferential integrity of the stent had resolved, left lung perfusion persisted with a curved course within the stented area.

Absorbable Iron Stents

Iron is an essential nutrient and acts as an essential cofactor for a multitude of enzymes involved in oxygen binding, DNA synthesis, and redox enzyme activity. The process of iron degradation involves ferrous ion to be oxidized to ferric ion or an interaction with nearby cells. Iron released from biodegradable iron stents have been shown to reduce the vascular smooth muscle cell proliferation rate by influencing growth-related gene expression and may play a potential role in reducing restenosis in vivo.[53] The degradation rate of iron is slow. This slow degradation and the small amount of iron in a stent (40 mg) in relation to the iron load of the whole body (400 to 500 mg/L) make any systemic toxicity unlikely. Corrodible iron appears to offer an attractive concept for formulation of bioabsorbable stents. Peuster and colleagues[54] used corrodible iron (>99.8% iron) to produce iron stents (NOR-I) and implanted these stents in the native descending aorta of 16 New Zealand white rabbits (mean luminal diameter of 3.4 mm; balloon diameter to vessel diameter ratio of 1.13). During the 6 to 18 months' follow-up, no adverse events and no thromboembolic complications were reported and all the stents were patent in follow-up angiographic evaluation at 6, 12, and 18 months. Moreover, these stents had produced no systemic iron toxicity, no local inflammation, and no neointimal proliferation. Iron stents appear to be promising and feasible based on preliminary animal data.

CONCLUSION AND FUTURE DIRECTIONS

Bioabsorbable stents have the potential to herald the next revolution in percutaneous coronary and endovascular interventions. Although further refinements of the drug-delivery system and stent mechanics are needed, available data appear encouraging. With further progress in polymer technology, bioabsorbable stents may replace traditional metallic stents in the future. The scope of PCI in the pediatric population with these temporary stents offers promise in treating congenital heart disease. Impregnation of bioabsorbable stents with antiproliferative and anti-inflammatory drugs to reduce inflammation and restenosis by synergistic effects appears very promising to further reduce tissue reaction after bioabsorbable stent implantation. These stents may also have a role in treating vulnerable plaques, and they appear to be particularly attractive for lesions of the superficial femoral arteries, for which traditional metallic stents have a very high strut fracture rate.

ACKNOWLEDGEMENTS

We wish to acknowledge Ms. Donna Gilbreath for her editorial support, Ms. Christine Fernandez and Connie Stellar from Abbott Vascular for providing us with Figures 34-7 to 34-12, and Ms. Cheryl Liberatore of REVA Medical for providing Figure 34-13.

REFERENCES

1. Grewe PH, Deneke T, Machraoui A, et al: Acute and chronic tissue response to coronary stent implantation: Pathologic findings in human specimen. J Am Coll Cardiol 2000;35:157-163.
2. Hoffmann R, Mintz G, Popma J, et al: Chronic arterial responses to stent implantation: A serial intravascular ultrasound analysis of Palmaz-Schatz stents in native coronary arteries. Circulation. 1996;1134-1139.
3. Fischman D, Leon M, Baim D, et al: A randomized comparison of coronary stent placement and balloon angioplasty in the treatment of coronary artery disease. The STRESS trial. N Engl J Med 1994;331:496-501.
4. Serruys PW, de Jaegere P, Kiemeneij F, et al, for the BENESTENT Study Group. A comparison of balloon expandable stent implantation with balloon angioplasty in patients with coronary artery disease. N Engl J Med 1994;331:489-495.
5. Ellis SG, Savage M, Fischman D, et al: Restenosis after placement of Palmaz-Schatz stents in native coronary arteries. Initial results of a multicenter experience. Circulation 1992;86:1836-1844.
5. Stone GW, Ellis SG, Cox DA, et al: A polymer-based paclitaxel-eluting stent in patients with coronary artery disease. N Engl J Med. 2004;350:221-231.
7. Moses JW, Leon MB, Popma JJ, et al: Sirolimus-eluting stents versus standard stents in patients with stenosis in a native coronary artery. N Engl J Med 2003;349:1315-1323.
8. Farb A, Burke AP, Kolodgie ED, Virmani R: Pathological mechanisms of fatal late coronary stent thrombosis in humans. Circulation 2003;108:1701-1706.
9. Ong AT, McFadden EP, Regar E, et al: Late angiographic stent thrombosis (LAST) events with drug-eluting stents. J Am Coll Cardiol. 2005;45:2088-2092.
10. Pfisterer ME: Masel stent cost-effectiveness trial—Late thrombotic events (BASKET-LATE). Presented at the American College of Cardiology summit, 2006, Atlanta, GA.
11. Zidar J, Lincoff A, Stack R. Biodegradable stents. *In* Topol EJ (ed): Textbook of Interventional Cardiology, 2nd ed. Philadelphia, WB Saunders, 1994, pp 787-802.
12. Middleton JC, Tipton J: Synthetic biodegradable polymers as orthopedic devices. Biomaterials 2000;21:2335-2346.
13. Eberhart RC, Su SH, Nguyen KT, et al: Bioresorbable polymeric stents: Current status and future promise. J Biomater Sci Polym Ed 2003;14:299-312.
14. Pietrzak WS, Sarver D, Verstynen M: Bioabsorbable implants: Practical considerations. Bone 1996;19(Suppl 1)109S-119S.
15. Venkatraman S, Poh TL, Vinalia T, et al: Collapse pressure of biodegradable stents. Biomaterials 2003;24:2105-2111.
16. Nuutinen JP, Clerc C, Reinikainen R, Törmälä P: Mechanical properties and in vitro degradation of bioabsorbable self-expanding braided stents. J Biomater Sci Polym Ed 2003;14:255-266.
17. Grizzi L, Garreau H, Li S, Vert M: Hydrolytic degradation of devices based on poly(DL-lactic acid) size-dependence. Biomaterials 1995:16:305-311.
18. Koolen J, Bonnier H, Waksman R, Heublein B: Absorbable magnesium stents. Paper presented at the Transcatheter Cardiovascular Therapeutics meeting, 2004, Washington, DC.
19. Stack RE, Califf RM, Phillips HR, et al: Interventional cardiac catheterization at Duke Medical Center. Am J Cardiol 1988;62(Suppl F):3F-24F.
20. Susawa T, Shiraki K, Shimizu Y: Biodegradable intracoronary stents in adult dogs [abstract]. J Am Coll Cardiol 1993;21:483A.
21. Van der Giessen W, Lincoff M, Schwartz R, et al: Marked inflammation sequelae to implantation of biodegradable and nonbiodegradable polymers in porcine coronary arteries. Circulation 1996;94:1690-1697.
22. Lincoff AM, Furst JG, Ellis SG, et al: Sustained local delivery of dexamethasone by a novel intravascular eluting stent to prevent restenosis in the porcine coronary injury model. J Am Coll Cardiol 1997;29:808-816.
23. Yamawaki T, Shimokawa H, Kozai T: Intramural delivery of a specific tyrosine kinase inhibitor with biodegradable stent suppresses the restenotic changes of the coronary artery in pigs in vivo. J Am Coll Cardiol. 1998;32:780-786.
24. Tamai H, Igaki K, Tsuji T, et al: A biodegradable poly-L-lactic acid coronary stent in porcine coronary artery. J Interv Cardiol 1999;12:443-449.
25. Tamai H, Igaki K, Kyo E, et al: Initial and 6-month results of biodegradable poly-L-lactic acid coronary stents in humans. Circulation 2000;102:399-404.
26. Colombo A, Karvouni E: Biodegradable stents "fulfilling the mission and stepping away." Circulation 2000;102:371-373.
27. Tamai H: Biodegradable stents: Four-year follow up. Paper presented at the Transcatheter Cardiovascular Therapeutics meeting, 2004, Washington, DC.
28. Vogt F, Stein A, Rettemeier G, et al: Long-term assessment of a novel biodegradable paclitaxel-eluting coronary polylactide stent. Eur Heart J 2004;25:1330-1340.
29. Costa RA, Lansky AJ, Mintz GS, et al: Angiographic results of the first human experience with everolimus-eluting stents for the treatment of coronary lesions (the FUTURE I trial). Am J Cardiol 2005;95:113-116.
30. Storger H, Grube E, Hofmann M, et al: Clinical experiences using everolimus-eluting stents in patients with coronary artery disease. J Interv Cardiol 2004;17:387-390.
31. ABSORB FIM trial information. Available at www.clinicaltrials.gov
32. Hietala EM, Salminen US, Stahls A, et al: Biodegradation of the copolymeric polylactide stent: Long-term follow-up in a rabbit aorta model. J Vasc Res 2001;38:361-369.
33. Asahara T, Chen D, Tsurumi Y, et al: Accelerated restitution of endothelial integrity and endothelium dependant function after phVGEF165 gene transfer. Circulation 1996;94:3291-3302.

34. Van Belle E, Tio FO, Chen D, et al: Passivation of metallic stents following arterial gene transfer of phVGEF165 inhibits thrombus formation and intimal thickening. J Am Coll Cardiol 1997;29:1371-1379.
35. Ye YW, Landau C, Willard JE, et al: Bioresorbable microporous stents deliver recombinant adenovirus gene transfer vectors to the arterial wall. Ann Biomed Eng 1998;26:398-408.
36. Klugherz BD, Jones PL, Cui X, et al: Gene delivery from a DNA controlled-release stent in porcine coronary arteries. Nat Biotechnol 2000;18:1181-1185.
37. Walter DH, Cejna M, Diaz-Sandoval L, et al: Local gene transfer of phVGEF2 plasmid by gene-eluting stents: An alternative strategy for inhibition of restenosis. Circulation 2004;110: 36-45.
38. Virmani R, Burke AP, Farb A, Kolodgie FD: Pathology of the vulnerable plaque. J Am Coll Cardiol 2006;47:C13-C18.
39. Tearney GJ, Jang IK, Bouma BE: Optical coherence tomography for imaging the vulnerable plaque. J Biomed Opt 2006; 11:21002.
40. Badiman JJ, Fuster V: Can we image the active thrombus? Arterioscler Thromb Vasc Biol 2002;22:1753-1754.
41. REVA bioabsorbable stent. Available at www.teamreva.com
42. Ruksin V, Azarbal B, Shah PK, et al: Intravenous magnesium in experimental stent thrombosis in swine. Arterioscler Thromb Vasc Biol 2001;12:1544-1549.
43. Rukshin V, Santos R, Gheorghiu M, et al: A prospective, non-randomized, open-labelled pilot study investigating the use of magnesium in patients undergoing non acute percutaneous coronary intervention with stent implantation. J Cardiovasc Pharmacol Ther 2003;8:193-200.
44. Heublein B, Rohde R, Kaese V, et al: Biocorrosion of magnesium alloys: A new principle in cardiovascular implant technology? Heart 2003;89:651-656.
45. Di Mario C, Griffiths H, Goktekin O, et al: Drug-eluting bioabsorbable magnesium stent. J Interv Cardiol 2004;17: 391-395.
46. Erbel R, Bonnier JJ, Koolen C, et al, on behalf of the PROGRESS-1 investigators group. Late breaking clinical trial: Bioabsorbable magnesium-alloy stent in human coronary arteries [abstract 2405-9]. Paper presented at the American College of Cardiology Summit, 2006, Atlanta, GA.
47. Peeters P, Bosiers M, Verbist J, et al: Preliminary short term results after application of absorbable metal stents in patients with critical limb ischemia. J Endovasc Ther 2005;12:1-5.
48. Donners M, Daemen M, Cleutjens K, Heeneman S: Inflammation and restenosis: Implications for therapy. Ann Med 2003;35:523-531.
49. Aragon J, Berg R, Kar S, et al: Pimecrolimus eluting cobalt stent decreases inflammation and restenosis in porcine model. Am J Cardiol 2005;96(Suppl 7A):23H.
50. Waksman R: Drug-eluting pimecrolimus eluting absorbable meta-stents (DREAMS) concept. Presented at the European Paris Course on Revascularization (EuroPCR), May 2006, Paris.
51. Zartner P, Cesnjevar R, Singer H, et al: First successful implantation of a biodegradable metal stent into the left pulmonary artery of a preterm baby. Catheter Cardiovasc Interv 2005;66: 590-594.
52. Schranz D, Zartner P, Michel-Behnke I, Akinturk HL: Bioabsorbable metal stents for percutaneous treatment of critical recoarctation of the aorta in a newborn. Catheter Cardiovasc Interv 2006;67:671-673.
53. Mueller PP, May T, Perz A et al: Control of smooth muscle cell proliferation by ferrous iron. Biomaterials 2006;27:2193-2200.
54. Peuster M, Wohlsein P, Brugmann M, et al: A novel approach to temporary stenting: Degradable cardiovascular stents produced from corrodible metal-results 6-18 months after implantation into New Zealand white rabbits. Heart 2001;86: 563-569.

35 Role of Adjunct Devices: Cutting Balloon, Thrombectomy, Laser, Ultrasound, and Atherectomy

John A. Bittl

KEY POINTS

- Pivotal mechanistic studies have claimed that atheroablative techniques and thrombectomy devices achieve better angiographic results than percutaneous transluminal coronary angioplasty.
- Randomized trials have failed to show that atheroablative techniques and thrombectomy devices achieve better clinical outcomes than percutaneous transluminal coronary angioplasty.
- Certain advantages of atheroablative and thrombectomy procedures have not been amenable to study in large, multicenter studies and may yet have a role in selected patients.
- The technical advantage of cutting balloon angioplasty over conventional balloon angioplasty is reduced slippage within target lesions.
- Rheolytic thrombectomy is superior to urokinase in treating thrombus-containing lesions, but the routine use of

thrombectomy during acute myocardial infarction has failed to achieve improved clinical outcomes.
- Laser angioplasty ablates tissue predominantly through a photoacoustic effect, which may facilitate stenting of resistant or undilatable lesions.
- Optimal use of directional coronary atherectomy achieves low restenosis rates, but this has not translated into improved clinical outcomes.
- Rotational atherectomy continues to play a useful role in the contemporary treatment of undilatable lesions.
- The use of atheroablative devices is associated with a slightly increased risk of coronary perforation compared with the use of conventional balloon angioplasty.
- The hypothesis that atheroablative procedures improve clinical outcomes is either untrue or untestable in the setting of multicenter, randomized trials.

Atheroablative approaches emerged before the modern era of coronary stenting to overcome the limitations of percutaneous transluminal coronary angioplasty (PTCA). Experimental studies[1] showed that the healing response of treated coronary arteries was directly proportional to the degree of underlying injury. Angiographic analyses[2] suggested that the restenosis response was uniform for any amount of gain achieved for a broad range of interventional devices.

The 20-year search for mechanical approaches to excise or section atheromatous plaque tested the hypothesis that tissue ablation would improve clini-

cal outcomes and lower restenosis rates. In 1987, directional coronary atherectomy (DCA) entered coronary trials, and several other mechanical approaches rapidly followed. In 1988, excimer laser coronary angioplasty (ELCA), percutaneous transluminal rotational atherectomy (PTRA), and transluminal extraction coronary atherectomy (TEC) appeared. Holmium laser angioplasty (HLA) premiered in 1990, cutting balloon angioplasty (CBA) debuted in 1991, rheolytic thrombectomy appeared in 1992, and ultrasound angioplasty emerged in 1994. Although each device used a different mechanism for modifying thrombus or atheromatous plaque, the common goal was to obtain better acute results and lower restenosis rates than could be achieved with PTCA.

The process of device development and evaluation constituted a great experiment in medicine. Hundreds of reports of case series, registries, and mechanistic studies demonstrated the efficacy and safety of adjunct atheroablative devices during percutaneous coronary intervention (PCI). Dozens of randomized clinical trials attempted to generalize the results of the pivotal mechanistic studies by evaluating the premise that routine use of atheroablative devices would improve clinical outcomes after PCI.

Despite initial enthusiasm, several events resulted in a reduction in the use of atheroablative approaches. The totality of evidence from dozens of randomized trials comparing atheroablative approaches with PTCA (Table 35-1), most of which have been published,[3-32] raised serious concerns about the ability of atheroablative procedures to trump PTCA in the contemporary practice of interventional cardiology.[33] Coronary stenting, particularly the use of drug-eluting stents (see Chapter 15), rapidly became the default treatment for most coronary interventions. Although lesion preparation before stenting has remained important to facilitate stent delivery and to enhance stent expansion,[34,35] the development of lower-profile, trackable, high-pressure balloon catheters (see Chapter 16) has made PTCA the default method for lesion preparation before and after coronary stenting, and in many cases, no lesion preparation is required before stent deployment.

In the previous edition of this textbook,[36] separate chapters were devoted to the individual topics of directional coronary atherectomy, percutaneous transluminal rotational atherectomy, ultrasound angioplasty, and laser angioplasty. This edition departs from the earlier format and combines within a single chapter discussions of each device with evidence from randomized trials or updated references from 2002 onward to provide a perspective on the use of atheroablative devices in the contemporary practice of PCI.

CUTTING BALLOON ATHEROTOMY

CBA, or atherotomy, is a variation of conventional PTCA in which three or four sharp metal microtome blades mounted on a noncompliant balloon incise and score coronary atheroma during the process of balloon dilation. The purpose of using cutting balloon atherotomy is to reduce the risk of uncontrolled longitudinal tears in the vessel wall induced by conventional balloon dilation.

Mechanism of Action

Compared with conventional PTCA, CBA makes controlled microincisions in the atheromatous plaque at lower pressures and may cause less barotrauma. Hoop stress is the force required to expand a tube or artery. Overcoming hoop stress by PTCA causes stretching and dissections of the vessel wall. After the balloon is deflated, the artery undergoes elastic recoil. After the artery is torn and stretched in certain places, the lumen remains larger.

Small mechanistic studies suggest that lesions can be dilated at lower pressures with cutting balloon catheters than conventional PTCA.[30,37] The mechanism of lumen enlargement after CBA was determined by intravascular ultrasound (IVUS) in 180 lesions from the Restenosis Reduction by Cutting Balloon Evaluation (REDUCE I) trial.[38] Lower balloon pressure was used during CBA than after PTCA, but the increase in the cross-sectional area of plaque plus media was larger after CBA. In noncalcified lesions, CBA achieved similar luminal dimensions with larger plaque reduction and less vessel expansion than PTCA. In calcified lesions, CBA achieved larger lumen gain than PTCA.[38]

Equipment

The Cutting Balloon Ultra-2 is a monorail device, and the Flextome Cutting Balloon (both from Boston Scientific, Natick, MA) is an over-the-wire device (Fig. 35-1). The Flextome device contains a flex point every 5 mm along the length of the atherotomes for greater flexibility and deliverability.

The balloons are available in balloon lengths of 6, 10, and 15 mm. The cutting blades, or atherotomes, are mounted longitudinally along the balloon surface. The atherotomes are not directly affixed to the balloon but bonded to a pad mounted on the balloon. The double bond ensures that atherotomes remain firmly fixed in place but allows flexibility. The number of atherotomes depends on balloon diameter. Three atherotomes are in place on balloons 2.0 to 3.25 mm in diameter, and four atherotomes are in place on balloons 3.5 or 4.0 mm in diameter.

Technique

The guidewires, catheters, and techniques used for cutting balloon angioplasty are similar to those for conventional PTCA (see Chapter 16). The cutting balloon catheters are less compliant than and may not track as well as conventional balloon catheters. Cutting balloons are not recommended in very tortuous proximal anatomy or when balloon-sizing flexibility is required. Slow inflation and deflation of the cutting balloon and avoiding balloon pressures at or above the rated burst pressure should reduce the risk of blade fracture and retention.[39]

Clinical Results

Small Trials

Several small, but positive, single-center trials of CBA have been reported or published. Ergene and colleagues[30] randomized patients with stenoses in vessels less than 3.0 mm to CBA (n = 36) or to PTCA (n = 35) and observed a 54% reduction in angiographic restenosis at 6 months (Fig. 35-2). Molstad and colleagues[31]

Table 35-1. Acronyms of Randomized Trials Evaluating Adjunct Atheroablative and Thrombectomy Devices

Eponym	Definition	Primary End Point*	Patients (N)	Year†	Indications	Comparison
AIMI[3]	AngioJet in Myocardial Infarction	Sestamibi-measured infarct size	480	2004	Infarct artery	RT/PCI
AMIGO[4]	Atherectomy before Multi-Link Improves Luminal Gain and Clinical Outcomes	Binary restenosis	753	2002	Native vessel	DCA/PTCA
AMRO[5]	Amsterdam Rotterdam Randomised Trial	6-month MACE	308	1993	Native vessel	ELA/PTCA
ARTIST[6]	Angioplasty/Rotational Atherectomy for Treatment of Diffuse In-Stent Restenosis Trial	6-month MACE	298	2002	In stent	PTRA/PTCA
ATLAS[7]	Acolysis During Treatment of Lesions Affecting Saphenous Vein Bypass Grafts	Successful procedure	189	2000	Infarct artery	UT/PTCA
BOAT[8]	Balloon/Optimal Atherectomy Trial	Binary restenosis	989	1995	Native vessel	DCA/PTCA
CAPAS[9]	Cutting Balloon Atherotomy vs. Plain Old Balloon Angioplasty Study	Binary restenosis	232	1997	Native vessel	CBA/PTCA
CARAT[10]	Coronary Angioplasty and Rotablator Atherectomy Trial	Postprocedural diameter stenosis	222	2000	Native vessel	PTRA/PTRA
CAVEAT-I[11]	Coronary Angioplasty versus Excisional Atherectomy Trial I	Binary restenosis	1012	1992	Native vessel	DCA/PTCA
CAVEAT-II[12]	Coronary Angioplasty versus Excisional Atherectomy Trial II	Binary restenosis	305	1993	SVG	DCA/PTCA
CBASS[13‡]	Cutting Balloon for Small Size Vessels	Binary restenosis	99	1999	Native vessels <2.6 mm	CBA/PTCA
CCAT[14]	Canadian Coronary Atherectomy Trial	Binary restenosis	274	1992	LAD	DCA/PTCA
COBRA[15]	Comparison of Balloon Angioplasty/Rotational Atherectomy	Binary restenosis	502	1996	Native vessel	PTRA/PTCA
CUBA[13‡]	Cutting Balloon versus Conventional Balloon Angioplasty Trial	Binary restenosis	306	1997	Native vessel	CBA/PTCA
DART[16]	Dilation/Ablation Revascularization Trial	Binary restenosis	446	1998	Small vessel	PTRA/PTCA
DESIRE[17‡]	Debulking and Stenting in Restenosis Elimination	Binary restenosis				
ERBAC[18]	Excimer Rotablator Balloon Angioplasty Comparison	Procedural success	454†	1996	Native vessel	ELA/PTCA
ERBAC[18]	Excimer Rotablator Balloon Angioplasty	Procedural success	453†	1996	Native vessel	PTRA/PTCA
GRT[19]	Global Randomized Trial	Binary restenosis	1238	1997	Native vessel	CBA/PTCA
LAVA[20]	Laser Angioplasty/Coronary Angioplasty	6-month MACE	215	1997	Native vessel	HLA/PTCA
REDUCE 1[21‡]	Restenosis Reduction by Cutting Balloon Evaluation 1	Binary restenosis	802	2001	Native vessel	CBA/PTCA
REDUCE 2[13‡]	Restenosis Reduction by Cutting Balloon Evaluation 2	Binary restenosis	492	2002	In stent	CBA/PTCA
REDUCE 3[22‡]	Restenosis Reduction by Cutting Balloon Evaluation 3	Binary restenosis	521	2003	Stenting	CBA/PTCA
RESCUT[23]	Restenosis Cutting Balloon Evaluation	Binary restenosis	428	2002	In stent	CBA/PTCA
ROSTER[24]	Rotational Atherectomy versus Balloon Angioplasty for Diffuse In-Stent Restenosis	Target lesion revascularization	200	2001	Diffuse in stent	PTRA/PTCA
SPORT[25‡]	Stenting Post Rotational Atherectomy Trial	30-day MACE	735	1999	Stenting in calcified vessels	PTRA/PTCA
STRATAS[26]	Study to Determine Rotablator System and Transluminal Angioplasty Strategy	Acute success	497	2000	Native vessel	PTRA/PTRA
VeGAS 2[27]	Vein Graft AngioJet Study	30-day modified MACE	349		Thrombus-containing lesions	RT/PTCA
X-AMINE-ST[28]	X-Sizer in AMI for Negligible Embolization and Optimal ST Resolution	ST-segment resolution	201		ST-segment elevation MI	MT/PTCA
X-TRACT[29‡]	X-Sizer for Treatment of Thrombus and Atherosclerosis in Coronary Applications Trial	30-day death, MI, TVR, or salvage IIb/IIIa or X-Sizer use	797	2002	Thrombus-containing lesions	MT/PTCA

*If the primary end point was not explicitly stated, or if multiple primary end points were listed, the end point used in power calculations for sample size estimation was used.
†Year patient recruitment was completed; otherwise, the year the study was reported or published.
‡Unpublished.
CBA, cutting balloon atherotomy; DCA, directional coronary atherectomy, ELCA, excimer laser coronary angioplasty, HLA, holmium laser angioplasty, PTCA, percutaneous transluminal coronary angioplasty; LAD, proximal segment of the left anterior descending artery; MACE, major adverse cardiac event (death, myocardial infarction, or revascularization); modified MACE, death, Q-wave myocardial infarction, revascularization, stroke, or stent thrombosis; MI, myocardial infarction; MT, mechanical thrombectomy, PTRA, percutaneous transluminal rotational atherectomy; RT, rheolytic thrombectomy; STEMI, ST-segment elevation myocardial infarction; successful procedure (ATLAS), final diameter stenosis of 30% or less by quantitative coronary angiography, achievement of Thrombolysis in Myocardial Infarction (TIMI) 3 flow (by quantitative coronary angiography), and freedom from major adverse cardiac events (MACE) (a composite of cardiac death, Q-wave and non-Q-wave myocardial infarction, emergency bypass, repeat target lesion revascularization, and disabling stroke) within 30 days of treatment; SVG, saphenous vein graft; TVR, target vessel revascularization; UT, ultrasound thrombolysis.

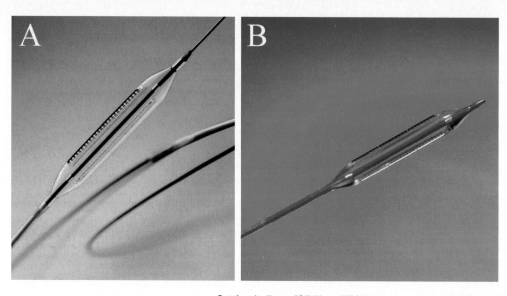

Figure 35-1. The Cutting Balloon Ultra-2 **(A)** is a monorail device, and the Flextome Cutting Balloon **(B)** is an over-the-wire catheter. (Courtesy of Boston Scientific, Natick, MA.)

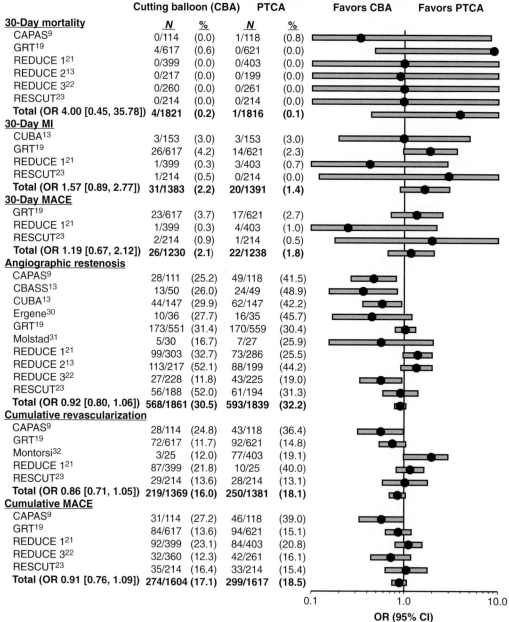

	Cutting balloon (CBA)		PTCA		Favors CBA / Favors PTCA
30-Day mortality	**N**	**%**	**N**	**%**	
CAPAS[9]	0/114	(0.0)	1/118	(0.8)	
GRT[19]	4/617	(0.6)	0/621	(0.0)	
REDUCE 1[21]	0/399	(0.0)	0/403	(0.0)	
REDUCE 2[13]	0/217	(0.0)	0/199	(0.0)	
REDUCE 3[22]	0/260	(0.0)	0/261	(0.0)	
RESCUT[23]	0/214	(0.0)	0/214	(0.0)	
Total (OR 4.00 [0.45, 35.78])	4/1821	(0.2)	1/1816	(0.1)	
30-Day MI					
CUBA[13]	3/153	(3.0)	3/153	(3.0)	
GRT[19]	26/617	(4.2)	14/621	(2.3)	
REDUCE 1[21]	1/399	(0.3)	3/403	(0.7)	
RESCUT[23]	1/214	(0.5)	0/214	(0.0)	
Total (OR 1.57 [0.89, 2.77])	31/1383	(2.2)	20/1391	(1.4)	
30-Day MACE					
GRT[19]	23/617	(3.7)	17/621	(2.7)	
REDUCE 1[21]	1/399	(0.3)	4/403	(1.0)	
RESCUT[23]	2/214	(0.9)	1/214	(0.5)	
Total (OR 1.19 [0.67, 2.12])	26/1230	(2.1)	22/1238	(1.8)	
Angiographic restenosis					
CAPAS[9]	28/111	(25.2)	49/118	(41.5)	
CBASS[13]	13/50	(26.0)	24/49	(48.9)	
CUBA[13]	44/147	(29.9)	62/147	(42.2)	
Ergene[30]	10/36	(27.7)	16/35	(45.7)	
GRT[19]	173/551	(31.4)	170/559	(30.4)	
Molstad[31]	5/30	(16.7)	7/27	(25.9)	
REDUCE 1[21]	99/303	(32.7)	73/286	(25.5)	
REDUCE 2[13]	113/217	(52.1)	88/199	(44.2)	
REDUCE 3[22]	27/228	(11.8)	43/225	(19.0)	
RESCUT[23]	56/188	(52.0)	61/194	(31.3)	
Total (OR 0.92 [0.80, 1.06])	568/1861	(30.5)	593/1839	(32.2)	
Cumulative revascularization					
CAPAS[9]	28/114	(24.8)	43/118	(36.4)	
GRT[19]	72/617	(11.7)	92/621	(14.8)	
Montorsi[32]	3/25	(12.0)	77/403	(19.1)	
REDUCE 1[21]	87/399	(21.8)	10/25	(40.0)	
RESCUT[23]	29/214	(13.6)	28/214	(13.1)	
Total (OR 0.86 [0.71, 1.05])	219/1369	(16.0)	250/1381	(18.1)	
Cumulative MACE					
CAPAS[9]	31/114	(27.2)	46/118	(39.0)	
GRT[19]	84/617	(13.6)	94/621	(15.1)	
REDUCE 1[21]	92/399	(23.1)	84/403	(20.8)	
REDUCE 3[22]	32/360	(12.3)	42/261	(16.1)	
RESCUT[23]	35/214	(16.4)	33/214	(15.4)	
Total (OR 0.91 [0.76, 1.09])	274/1604	(17.1)	299/1617	(18.5)	

OR (95% CI) 0.1 — 1.0 — 10.0

Figure 35-2. Systematic overview of randomized trials of cutting balloon angioplasty (CBA) versus percutaneous transluminal coronary angioplasty (PTCA). Pooled odds ratios (OR) and 95% confidence intervals (CI) were calculated to estimate the overall effect of CBA versus that of PTCA using an empirical Bayes model. The empirical Bayes model is a random-effects model that coincides with a fixed-effects model when all studies are homogeneous. Trial abbreviations are given in Table 35-1. (Data from Bittl JA, Chew DP, Topol EJ, et al: Meta-analysis of randomized trials of percutaneous transluminal coronary angioplasty versus atherectomy, cutting balloon atherotomy, or laser angioplasty. J Am Coll Cardiol 2004;43:936-942.)

randomized patients with type A or B lesions to CBA ($n = 32$) or to PTCA ($n = 32$) and reported a 43% reduction in restenosis at 6 months. The Cutting Balloon Angioplasty for Small-Size Vessels (CBASS) study[13] claimed a 63% reduction in restenosis (99 patients), the Cutting Balloon vs. Conventional Angioplasty (CUBA) study[13] reported a 41% reduction in restenosis ($n = 194$), and the Cutting Balloon Angioplasty versus Plain Old Balloon Angioplasty Randomized Study in Small Coronary Arteries (CAPAS) study[9] claimed a 53% reduction in angiographic restenosis ($n = 229$).

Large, Multicenter Trials

Several large, but negative, multicenter trials of CBA have been carried out, and in contrast to the small-trial experience, only a few have been published (see Fig. 35-2). The Cutting Balloon Global Randomized Trial (GRT)[19] randomized 1238 patients and reported no difference in angiographic restenosis between CBA (31.4%) and PTCA (30.4%). The Restenosis Cutting Balloon Evaluation Trial (RESCUT) study[23] enrolled 428 patients with in-stent restenosis and reported no difference in restenosis between CBA (29.8%) and PTCA (31.2%). The REDUCE I study enrolled 802 patients and reported slightly higher restenosis rates with CBA than with PTCA (32.7% versus 25.5%). The REDUCE 2 study enrolled 416 patients and also observed a trend toward higher restenosis rates (52.1% versus 44.2%). The REDUCE III study randomized 453 patients undergoing coronary stenting and reported lower restenosis rates after the use of CBA than after PTCA (11.8% versus 19.0%).

Lesion Selection

Several comparative and a few small, randomized trials have suggested that cutting balloon angioplasty may be appropriate in small vessels.[30,37] Ostial lesions have been a customary challenge to conventional PTCA because of the elastic nature of these lesions and high likelihood of recoil. They may be responsive to CBA, but firm evidence for this recommendation is lacking.[40]

The optimal approach to bifurcation lesions has not been defined. Plaque shift and high restenosis rates remain current limitations. Cutting balloon angioplasty may be superior to conventional PTCA for bifurcation lesions, as shown in a small nonrandomized series of 87 patients with restenosis of 40% after CBA versus 67% after PTCA,[41] but a general recommendation for using CBA in this setting has not been supported by evidence.[40]

The treatment of in-stent restenosis often entails the use of a drug-eluting stent (Chapter 15). When balloon dilation is required, however, cutting balloons are much less likely to slip inside narrowed stents and offer a clear technical advantage over conventional balloons. Although CBA has only a slightly increased risk of coronary perforation over that for PTCA (0.8% versus 0.0%), as reported in the Global Randomized Trial,[19] the complication can occur in the setting of in-stent restenosis as well (Fig. 35-3).

THROMBECTOMY

The pathogenesis of acute coronary syndromes such as unstable angina and myocardial infarction involves plaque rupture and intracoronary thrombus formation. Conventional approaches using PTCA or stents for thrombus-containing lesions in saphenous vein grafts (SVGs) or native coronary arteries carries a high risk for complications such as abrupt closure, late re-occlusion, periprocedural myocardial infarction, emergent coronary bypass surgery, and death. Various approaches designed to remove thrombus have emerged, including mechanical compression by balloon angioplasty, mechanical removal using extraction and atherectomy devices, and ultrasound thrombolysis.

Equipment

Several innovative approaches have been designed to remove thrombus from coronary arteries during PCI based on aspiration, rheolytic, or cut-and-aspirate mechanisms (Table 35-2). Several aspiration catheters are available and share many common design features (Fig. 35-4). The catheters usually contain two lumens. The primary lumen, which is used to apply suction and aspirate thrombus, is open at the distal end and attached on the proximal end by means of an extension tube to a large syringe with a locking stopcock. The second lumen accommodates a guidewire, which is used to position the catheter within the target artery. The catheter shaft tends to become flexible near the tip for negotiating tortuous catheter segments. Most aspiration catheters are compatible with 6-Fr guiding catheters and have a radiopaque tip marker.

The AngioJet (Possis, Minneapolis, MN) uses the mechanism of rheolytic thrombectomy to break up and extract thrombus (Fig. 35-5). The mechanism of action of the AngioJet catheter is based on Bernoulli's principle of a high-pressure jet producing a zone of low pressure. The catheter is attached to a drive unit with a piston pump that generates pulses of saline at a high pressure of 10,000 psi at a rate of 60 mL/min through a hypotube (see Fig. 35-5). The hypotube ejects the saline pulses against a loop in the catheter tip, which deflects the jets into an exhaust lumen and creates a vortex by means of the Bernoulli effect to capture and extract thrombus fragments through the catheter.

The cut-and-aspirate approach is exemplified by the X-Sizer catheter (eV3, Plymouth, MN), which has undergone coronary investigation but has been approved by the U.S. Food and Drug Administration (FDA) only for dialysis graft intervention. The system consists of a dual-lumen catheter shaft connected to

Table 35-2.   Thrombectomy Devices

Use	Device	Company	FDA Indication
Aspiration thrombectomy			
	Diver CE Clot Extraction	eV3 (Plymouth, MN)	Thrombi in arterial systems
	Export catheter	Medtronic AVE (Santa Rosa, CA)	Thrombi in saphenous vein grafts
	Pronto V3	Vascular Solutions (Minneapolis, MN)	Thrombus in arterial systems
	Rescue thrombus management system	Boston Scientific International (La Garenne Colombes Cedex, France)	Investigational
	Rio	Boston Scientific (Natick, MA)	Thrombi in arterial systems
	Rinspirator	Kerberos Proximal Solutions (Cupertino, CA)	Dialysis grafts
Cut and aspirate			
	Transluminal Extraction Catheter (TEC)	Boston Scientific (Natick, MA)	No longer marketed
	X-Sizer	eV3 (Plymouth, MN)	Dialysis graft intervention
Venturi-Bernoulli effects			
	Hydrolyzer	Cordis/Johnson & Johnson (Miami Lakes, FL)	Dialysis access
	AngioJet	Possis Medical (Minneapolis, MN)	Thrombi in coronary arteries and saphenous vein grafts
Ultrasonic			
	Acolysis	Vascular Solutions (Minneapolis, MN)	Investigational

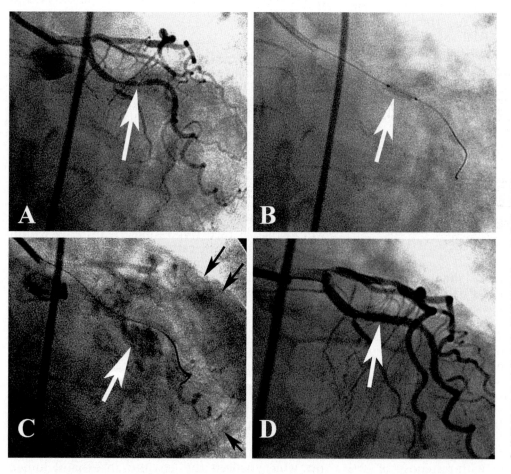

Figure 35-3. Perforation after cutting balloon angioplasty. The first marginal branch had been stented with a 3.0-mm bare stent, showing moderate restenosis 7 months later *(A, arrow)* associated with angina. A 3.0-mm cutting balloon was positioned within the stented segment *(B, arrow)*, but inflation was complicated by free perforation *(C, white arrow)*, circumferential hemopericardium *(C, black arrows)*, and cardiac tamponade. The patient was rapidly stabilized with pericardiocentesis and placement of a polytetrafluoroethylene-covered stent *(D, arrow)* to seal the coronary perforation.

a hand-held control module. The catheter is available in two sizes of 1.5 mm (7 Fr compatible) and 2-mm (8 Fr compatible). The X-Sizer catheter can be inserted over a 0.014-inch guidewire. The inner lumen contains a helical cutter rotated at 2100 rpm. Activation of the system leads to fragmentation of thrombus, which is removed by vacuum through the outer lumen.

Clinical Results with Thrombectomy Devices

The second Vein Graft AngioJet Study (VeGAS 2 trial)[27] compared AngioJet treatment with urokinase for patients undergoing PCI of lesions in native coronary arteries or SVGs with angiographically visible thrombus. The use of the AngioJet produced higher procedural success (86% versus 72%, $P = .002$) than

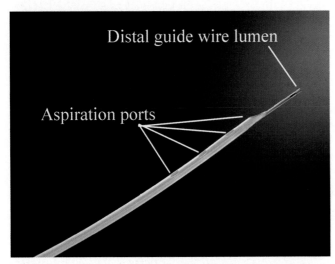

Figure 35-4. Aspiration thrombectomy catheter. The Diver Clot Extraction (CE) catheter is a rapid-exchange, thrombus-aspirating catheter that has a distal guidewire lumen and a primary lumen with multiple distal ports to extract thrombus when the proximal port is connected to a large locking syringe under negative pressure. (Courtesy of eV3, Plymouth, MN.)

did urokinase treatment. Bradycardia occurred in 24% of those treated with AngioJet and 2% of those treated with urokinase, and it was successfully managed with intravenous atropine and temporary pacing. Although no difference was seen in the incidence of the primary composite end point of death, Q-wave myocardial infarction, revascularization, stroke, or stent thrombosis (29% versus 30%), the occurrence of major adverse events, bleeding, and vascular complications was lower in the AngioJet group.[27]

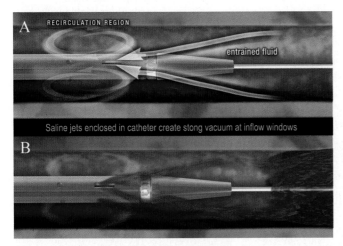

Figure 35-5. Rheolytic thrombectomy. The AngioJet operates on the principle of a high-pressure jet producing a zone of low pressure. The catheter is attached to a drive unit with a piston pump that generates pulses of saline at a high pressure. A hypotube ejects the saline pulses against a loop at the catheter tip, which deflects the jets into an exhaust lumen and creates a vortex by means of the Bernoulli effect to capture and remove thrombus fragments through the catheter. (Courtesy of Possis Medical, Minneapolis, MN.)

The AngioJet Rheolytic Thrombectomy in Patients Undergoing Primary Angioplasty for Acute Myocardial Infarction (AIMI) trial[3] tested the benefit of AngioJet as an adjunct to direct PCI in patients with ST-segment elevation myocardial infarction. Patients presenting within 12 hours of symptom onset were randomized to AngioJet treatment (*n* = 240) or to usual care during PCI (*n* = 240). The group assigned to the AngioJet had larger infarct sizes (12.5% ± 12.1% versus 9.8% ± 10.9%, *P* = .03), worse angiographic measures, and a higher incidence of adverse clinical events than patients assigned to usual care.[3]

The X-Sizer for Treatment of Thrombus and Atherosclerosis in Coronary Applications Trial (X-TRACT study) evaluated mechanical thrombectomy with the X-Sizer catheter. A total of 797 consecutive patients undergoing stent implantation in SVGs (72%) or native coronary arteries containing thrombus (28%) were prospectively randomized to thromboatherectomy with the X-Sizer catheter or to usual care followed by PCI. The rates of no reflow (2.2% versus 3.2%), distal emboli (3.2% versus 3.4%), myocardial infarction (15.8% versus 16.9%), and the 30-day rate of major adverse cardiac events (17.4% versus 17.0%) were similar between the treatment groups.[29]

Lefevre and colleagues[28] evaluated the adjunctive use of the X-Sizer in the X-Amine trial before PCI in 201 patients with myocardial infarction of less than 12 hours' duration. The primary end point of the study was the magnitude of ST-segment resolution at 1 hour, which was improved in the X-Sizer group compared with conventional therapy (7.5 versus 4.9 mm, *P* = .033). Although the occurrence of distal embolization was reduced with the use of the X-Sizer (2% versus 10%, *P* = .033), equivalent rates were seen for Thrombolysis in Myocardial Infarction (TIMI) flow grade 3 (96% versus 89%), myocardial blush grade 3 (30% versus 31%), and 6-month major adverse cardiac and cerebral events (13% versus 13%).

Antoniucci and colleagues[42] reported a randomized trial evaluating the X-Sizer catheter before direct PCI in 100 patients with a first acute myocardial infarction. The primary end point of early ST-segment elevation resolution was seen in 90% of the patients in the X-Sizer group and in 72% in the placebo group (*P* = .022). Infarct size was smaller in the thrombectomy group (13.0% ± 11.6% versus 21.2% ± 18.0%, *P* = .010).

Several other single-center studies have evaluated thrombectomy devices during coronary intervention. The Rescue thrombus management system produced a normal myocardial blush grade in 4 (13%) of 30 patients with myocardial infarction and angiographic evidence of thrombus.[43] The Diver Clot Extraction reduced thrombus burden in 50 patients with myocardial infarction and angiographic evidence of thrombus.[44] The Pronto aspiration device has been used successfully for thrombus extraction in three patients with stent thrombosis.[45]

Recommendations

Most randomized trials evaluating adjunctive thrombectomy have enrolled small numbers of patients and used surrogate end points. Four randomized trials using aspiration thrombectomy have produced conflicting results. Three studies showed improved myocardial perfusion with thrombectomy, but one showed larger infarct size. There is no compelling evidence to recommend thrombectomy procedures routinely in patients undergoing PCI for acute myocardial infarction, but certain indications may exist.

The failure of thrombectomy to improve clinical outcomes seems counterintuitive but has been attributed to several factors. The conventional metrics used in randomized trials, such as infarct size, are probably too insensitive to measure small amounts of myocardial salvage against a preexisting background of a large amount of myocardial necrosis. The commonly recommended technique of a distal-to-proximal thrombectomy motion for rheolytic thrombectomy used in many clinical trials[3,27] may cause distal embolization. The increased rate of serious clinical events with rheolytic thrombectomy seen in some trials[3] may be attributed to adjunctive therapies required. In AIMI, pacemakers were used more commonly with rheolytic thrombectomy than after conventional PCI (58% versus 14%). It is not certain whether hemopericardium, cardiac tamponade, or other complications from pacemaker insertion affected the outcomes. Other drawbacks of the devices are failure to reach target lesions, reduced coronary flow from microembolization, and perforation.

Some randomized trials[3] started the randomization process after diagnostic angiography. Many investigators concluded that patients with a large thrombus burden should not be enrolled and should be treated with a thrombectomy device. This approach is clinically sound, especially when large filling defects are seen and strong contraindications exist against the use of high-dose anticoagulants or platelet glycoprotein IIb/IIIa inhibitors (Fig. 35-6).

ULTRASOUND

The concept of delivering high-intensity, low-frequency ultrasound through catheters for atheroablation has been investigated for more than 20 years.

Principles

The frequency of catheter-based therapeutic ultrasound (19 to 50 kHz) is several orders of magnitude lower than the frequency of IVUS used for diagnostic purposes (20 to 30 MHz). Higher power intensities and lower frequencies result in higher amplitudes of probe motion (20 to 110 μm), causing mechanical ablation characteristics not seen with the higher-frequency diagnostic application. The potential effects of catheter-delivered therapeutic ultrasound with a vibrating metal probe on tissue are thought to be caused by mechanical disruption, cavitation, and heating of tissue.

Clinical Results

The Acolysis during Treatment of Lesions Affecting Saphenous Vein Bypass Grafts (ATLAS) trial[7] compared coronary ultrasound thrombolysis with abciximab in 181 patients with acute coronary syndromes undergoing saphenous vein graft intervention. The primary end point of a successful procedure and freedom from major adverse cardiac events was

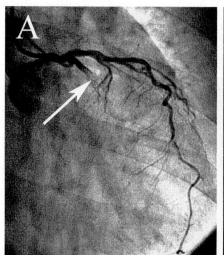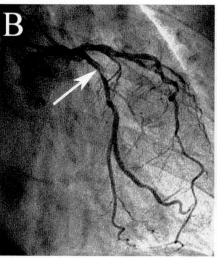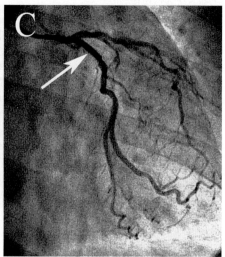

Figure 35-6. Aspiration thrombectomy for acute ST-segment elevation myocardial infarction after a subdural hematoma. Three weeks after experiencing a subdural hematoma, this 84-year-old woman developed an inferoposterolateral myocardial infarction from thrombotic occlusion of the left circumflex coronary artery (**A,** *arrow*), complicated by mitral regurgitation and congestive heart failure. The emergency use of the Export aspiration catheter (Medtronic AVE, Santa Rosa, CA) and adjunctive emergency use of aspirin, clopidogrel, and bivalirudin resulted in recovery of moderate thrombus and reperfusion (**B,** *arrow*). The placement of a bare metal stent produced a good angiographic result (**C,** *arrow*), with immediate resolution of chest pain and congestive heart failure.

achieved in 63% of patients treated with ultrasound thrombolysis and in 82% of patients treated with abciximab ($P = .008$). The incidence of major adverse cardiac events at 30 days was 25% with ultrasound thrombolysis and 12% with abciximab ($P = .036$). The use of therapeutic ultrasound in vein graft lesions in patients with acute coronary syndrome had poor angiographic outcomes and increased the incidence of acute ischemic complications.

LASER

The use of laser during coronary interventions and in other areas of medicine and surgery carries a cachet based on the lay perception of precise effects and predictable results. The systematic study of laser-tissue interaction, however, has revealed minimal photochemical but predominant photoacoustic effects.

Principles

Absorption of the laser energy by the atherosclerotic plaque, thrombus, or water in the target tissue is necessary for a laser effect.[46] The holmium:yttrium aluminum garnet laser (Ho:YAG) used in coronary angioplasty operated at a wavelength of 2.1 μm in the infrared range of the electromagnetic spectrum. The holmium system delivered pulses of 250-μsec duration at a repetition rate of 3.5 Hz and generated energies of 300 to 500 mJ per pulse. The resulting fluence, or energy density, was 1.0 to 1.7 J/mm^2. Because radiation at a wavelength of 2.1 μm was avidly absorbed by water but had insufficient energy per photon to break macromolecular covalent bonds, the predominant tissue effect of holmium laser angioplasty was to vaporize water and generate prominent thermal and acoustic effects.[46]

The XeCl excimer laser used in coronary angioplasty operates at a wavelength of 308 nm in the ultraviolet portion of the electromagnetic spectrum. The excimer system delivers pulses of 125-nsec duration at a repetition rate up to 40 Hz and generates fluences up to 60 mJ/mm^2. Radiation at 308 nm is absorbed by water and by the nonaqueous components of atherosclerotic plaque containing protein and nucleic acids. Although excimer laser light carries

enough energy to break individual molecular bonds, most of the energy is converted into heat. Microscopically, intracellular water is vaporized, causing cells to explode.

Although tissue absorption patterns vary between the near-infrared and the excimer lasers, several similar phenomena occur when either is used in biologic tissue.[46] Powerful, high-frequency acoustic compressions occur up to several thousand bars of pressure at a frequency of 107 Hz, propagating shock waves in the tissue. These acoustic waves may cause dissections and perforations. A rapidly expanding and collapsing vapor bubble with a 2.5-mm diameter appears within 100 μsec in the tissue as a by-product of debulking. A single pulse of an excimer laser on the rabbit femoral artery produces a necrotic zone 200 to 750 μm deep, which is more than an order of magnitude greater than the penetration depth of up to 30 to 100 μm of laser light and therefore reflects the collateral effect of excimer laser radiation.[46] The relatively high incidence of dissection accompanying pulsed-wave laser angioplasty has been attributed to the rapid expansion and implosion of vapor bubbles (Fig. 35-7). The detrimental consequences of pulsed-laser ablation have been ascribed to a combination of acoustic shock-wave creation, microplasma formation, and volume expansion and implosion of gas bubbles.

Technique

Catheters are selected (Table 35-3) to be less than two thirds of or 1.0 mm less than the reference diameter of the target vessel. For severe stenoses, the smaller laser catheters are recommended to increase the likelihood of successful crossing.

The elimination of blood and contrast from the coronary artery during laser angioplasty has reduced the extent of collateral damage during angioplasty.[47] This is achieved by flushing all lines with saline and injecting saline at a rate of 2 to 3 mL/sec during laser activation. Slow catheter advancement rate of 0.2 mm/sec yields maximal ablation of plaque (Fig. 35-8). If advancement through the lesion cannot be maintained at a steady pace, the maximum fluence should be tried. If no advancement is apparent after

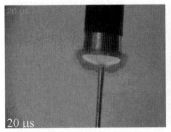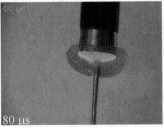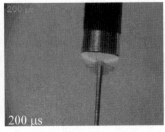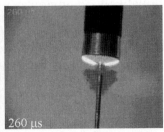

Figure 35-7. Bubble formation during excimer laser angioplasty. Excimer laser light is absorbed by tissue in a disk-shaped layer about 100 μm deep and with an area equal to that of the beam, typically the diameter of the catheter. Although some energy is converted into the process of photochemical dissociation, most is converted into heat. The steam forms a rapidly expanding vapor bubble that is typically two times the diameter of the catheter tip. After reaching a maximum diameter within approximately 100 microseconds after the laser pulse, the bubble implodes. (Courtesy of Spectranetics, Colorado Springs, CO.)

Table 35-3. Excimer Laser Catheters for Cardiovascular Applications

Coronary Catheter	No. of Fibers	Fiber Core (µm)	Fluence Range (mJ/mm²)	Repetition Rate (Hz)	Guidewire (inch)	Guide Catheter (inch)
0.9-mm Extreme (OTW)	65	50	30-60	25-40	0.014	0.060
0.9-mm Vitesse (RX)	65	50	30-60	25-40	0.014	0.060
1.4-mm Vitesse Cos (RX + OTW)	108	61	30-60	25-40	0.014	0.072
1.7-mm Vitesse Cos (RX + OTW)	136	61	30-60	25-40	0.014	0.080
2.0-mm Vitesse Cos (RX + OTW)	250	61	30-60	25-40	0.014	0.088
1.7-mm Vitesse E (RX + OTW)	185	50	30-60	25-40	0.014	0.080
2.0-mm Vitessee E (RX + OTW)	290	50	30-60	25-40	0.014	0.088
Prima Laserwire	12	45	30-80	25-80	NA	0.060

NA, not available; OTW, over the wire; RX, rapid exchange.

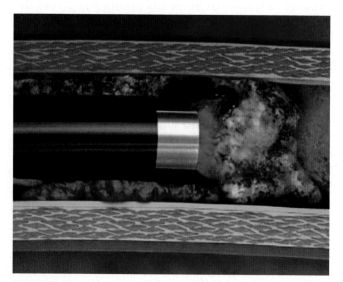

Figure 35-8. Schematic rendition of an excimer laser angioplasty procedure. (Courtesy of Spectranetics, Colorado Springs, CO.)

several seconds, forceful pushing may increase the risk of vessel perforation.

Clinical Results

Several randomized studies have compared pulsed-wave lasers with other treatment modalities. In the Excimer Laser-Rotational Atherectomy-Balloon Angioplasty Comparison (ERBAC trial),[18] 685 patients with moderately complex lesions in native vessels were randomized to undergo treatment with conventional balloon angioplasty (222 patients), rotational atherectomy (231 patients), or excimer laser angioplasty (232 patients). The primary end point of procedural success was 80% for balloon angioplasty, 89% for rotational atherectomy, and 78% for excimer laser angioplasty. The incidence of major adverse coronary events and restenosis was slightly higher for ELCA than for PTCA (Fig. 35-9).

In the Laser Angioplasty Versus Angioplasty trial (LAVA) trial,[20] patients with unstable or stable angina were randomized to treatment with holmium:YAG laser angioplasty or PTCA. The planned 500-patient study was stopped after slow enrollment of 208 patients. Holmium laser angioplasty was associated

with more in-hospital complications than PTCA (17.5% versus 2.1%, $P < .0001$), but the primary end point of major adverse cardiac events at 6 months was only slightly higher for holmium laser angioplasty than for PTCA (see Fig. 35-9).

In the Amsterdam-Rotterdam (AMRO) study,[5] 308 patients with stable angina and lesions longer than 10 mm were randomly assigned to treatment with ELCA or balloon angioplasty. The rate of the primary end point of major adverse cardiac adverse events at 6 months was similar for the two treatment groups (see Fig. 35-9).

Lesion Selection

Although ELCA has been approved for seven lesion types—long lesions, moderately calcified lesions, in-stent restenosis before brachytherapy, undilatable lesions (Fig. 35-10), saphenous vein graft lesions, ostial lesions, and total occlusions—the prominent use is for SVG lesions, for which the rate of embolization appears to be very low. Ablative technologies such as excimer laser coronary angioplasty may also facilitate angioplasty and stent deployment in patients with aorto-ostial vein graft stenoses.[40]

DIRECTIONAL CORONARY ATHERECTOMY

Atherectomy refers to the excision and removal of obstructive, fibrotic, noncalcified atheromatous tissue by a transcatheter technique. The DCA device was approved by the FDA in 1990 as the first nonballoon percutaneous coronary interventional device based on uncontrolled multicenter registry data defining safety and efficacy of the approach.

Mechanism of Action

Although directional atherectomy was designed to remove obstructive atheroma, early studies suggested that two thirds of the angiographic improvement was attributed to an angioplasty mechanism caused by vessel wall stretching from advancing the relatively large device and by inflating the low-pressure balloon. The amount of tissue removed (<20 mg on average[48]) could not explain the entire angiographic lumen gain. A small IVUS study suggested that more

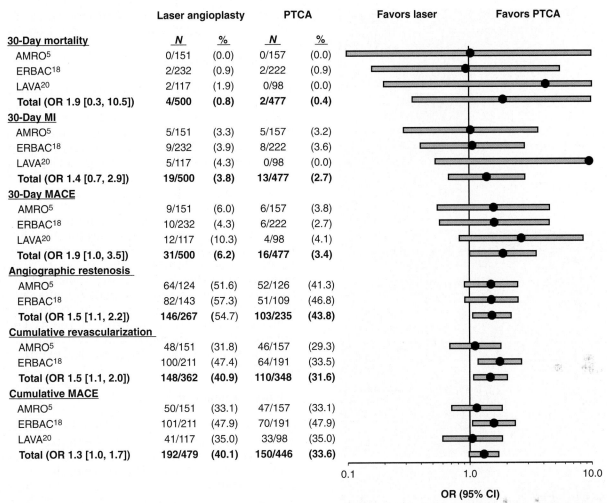

	Laser angioplasty		PTCA		Favors laser		Favors PTCA
30-Day mortality	**_N_**	**%**	**_N_**	**%**			
AMRO[5]	0/151	(0.0)	0/157	(0.0)			
ERBAC[18]	2/232	(0.9)	2/222	(0.9)			
LAVA[20]	2/117	(1.9)	0/98	(0.0)			
Total (OR 1.9 [0.3, 10.5])	**4/500**	**(0.8)**	**2/477**	**(0.4)**			
30-Day MI							
AMRO[5]	5/151	(3.3)	5/157	(3.2)			
ERBAC[18]	9/232	(3.9)	8/222	(3.6)			
LAVA[20]	5/117	(4.3)	0/98	(0.0)			
Total (OR 1.4 [0.7, 2.9])	**19/500**	**(3.8)**	**13/477**	**(2.7)**			
30-Day MACE							
AMRO[5]	9/151	(6.0)	6/157	(3.8)			
ERBAC[18]	10/232	(4.3)	6/222	(2.7)			
LAVA[20]	12/117	(10.3)	4/98	(4.1)			
Total (OR 1.9 [1.0, 3.5])	**31/500**	**(6.2)**	**16/477**	**(3.4)**			
Angiographic restenosis							
AMRO[5]	64/124	(51.6)	52/126	(41.3)			
ERBAC[18]	82/143	(57.3)	51/109	(46.8)			
Total (OR 1.5 [1.1, 2.2])	**146/267**	**(54.7)**	**103/235**	**(43.8)**			
Cumulative revascularization							
AMRO[5]	48/151	(31.8)	46/157	(29.3)			
ERBAC[18]	100/211	(47.4)	64/191	(33.5)			
Total (OR 1.5 [1.1, 2.0])	**148/362**	**(40.9)**	**110/348**	**(31.6)**			
Cumulative MACE							
AMRO[5]	50/151	(33.1)	47/157	(33.1)			
ERBAC[18]	101/211	(47.9)	70/191	(47.9)			
LAVA[20]	41/117	(35.0)	33/98	(35.0)			
Total (OR 1.3 [1.0, 1.7])	**192/479**	**(40.1)**	**150/446**	**(33.6)**			

0.1   1.0   10.0

OR (95% CI)

Figure 35-9. Systematic overview of randomized trials of laser angioplasty (LA) versus percutaneous transluminal coronary angioplasty (PTCA). Pooled odds ratios (OR) and 95% confidence intervals (CI) were calculated to estimate the overall effect of laser angioplasty versus that of PTCA using an empirical Bayes model. Trial abbreviations are given in Table 35-1. (Data from Bittl JA, Chew DP, Topol EJ, et al: Meta-analysis of randomized trials of percutaneous transluminal coronary angioplasty versus atherectomy, cutting balloon atherotomy, or laser angioplasty. J Am Coll Cardiol 2004;43:936-942.)

aggressive tissue removal in some cases accounts for up to 90% of the luminal enlargement after DCA and leads to positive remodeling.[49]

Equipment

Since initial FDA approval, five generations of improvements have been made in the design of the catheter and ancillary hardware for DCA. The prototype atherectomy catheter was the Simpson Coronary AtheroCath, which consisted of a metal housing with a low-pressure balloon, a nose-cone collection chamber, and a central lumen accommodating a 0.014-inch guidewire. A cup-shaped cutter inside the housing was connected to a flexible drive shaft and rotated at 2500 rpm, powered by a hand-held, battery-operated motor drive unit. The AtheroCath was initially marketed by Devices for Vascular Intervention (DVI, Redwood City, CA). The current iteration is the Flexi-Cut Directional Debulking System, and it can be acquired with Viking Optima 8-Fr guiding cathe-

ters from Guidant Corporation (St. Paul, MN), which has recently become a part of Abbott Vascular (Chicago, IL). The various iterations of atherectomy catheters share several key components (Fig. 35-11).

The 6-Fr Flexi-Cut catheter has a larger cutting window than the previous GTO AtheroCath device and a titanium nitride–coated cutter to remove more tissue and treat mildly calcified lesions. In a series of 143 lesions in 117 patients,[50] luminal diameters were larger (2.92 ± 0.79 versus 2.52 ± 0.64 mm, $P < .0001$) after treatment with the Flexi-Cut catheter than after using the GTO device in 277 lesions in 212 previously treated consecutive patients.

A novel plaque excision system called the Silver-Hawk (FoxHollow Technologies, Redwood City, CA), based on the concept of atherectomy, has had extensive uncontrolled experience in the treatment of peripheral artery disease (see Chapter 39) and preliminary experience in human coronary cases.[51] The theoretical advantages of the SilverHawk include the use of a hinge mechanism and avoidance of balloon

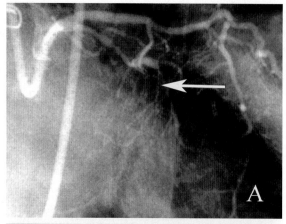

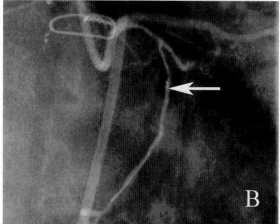

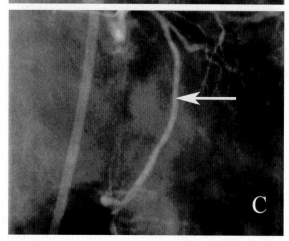

Figure 35-10. Long, undilatable lesion treated with excimer laser angioplasty. The occluded left circumflex coronary artery (**A,** *arrow*) was crossed with a guidewire and treated with a 1.4-mm excimer laser catheter (**B,** *arrow*), followed by percutaneous transluminal coronary angioplasty (**C,** *arrow*).

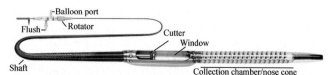

Figure 35-11. Flexi-Cut Directional Debulking System for atherectomy. (Courtesy of Abbott Vascular, Chicago, IL.)

barotrauma, variable cut length, and more efficient cutting with a carbide blade spinning at 8000 rpm.

Guiding Catheters

The original line of 11-Fr guiding catheters has been replaced by 8-Fr guiding catheters with enhanced torque response. In contrast to the conventional Judkins catheters, DCA guiding catheters for the left coronary artery have gentle C curves, which permit easy cornering of the more rigid device. Standard sizes for the left coronary artery include JCL 3.5, JCL 4.0, JCL 4.5, and JCL 5.0, depending on the diameter of the aortic root. For the right coronary artery, the JCR4 is available in standard-length and short-tip (JCR4S) designs. Additional guides for the right coronary artery include the JCR4IF (for inferior takeoff), the hockey stick (for horizontal, anterior, or superior takeoffs), and the JCRGRF (for a superior takeoff or shepherd crook origin). For bypass grafts, available guiding catheters include the JCRGRF (for anterior grafts with gentle upward takeoffs), the JCLGRF (for anterior grafts with marked superior takeoffs), and the multipurpose guide (for grafts with vertical inferior takeoffs).

Ancillary Equipment

Other ancillary equipment for DCA includes a large-bore rotating hemostatic valve, the motor drive unit, and 0.014-inch High-Torque Flexi-Wires with distal polytetrafluoroethylene (PTFE) coating to prevent device binding.

Technique

Because of the caliber and rigidity of the directional atherectomy catheter, proper guiding catheter position is critical. The most important feature is coaxial alignment of the tip of the guide with the vessel ostium, and guiding catheter maneuvers such as overrotation and deep seating increase the risk of vessel injury.

A gentle screwing motion helps to advance the atherectomy device into the target lesion. If the atherectomy catheter does not cross the target lesion, predilating with a 2.0-mm balloon or 1.5-mm rotational atherectomy burr may improve crossing.

Contrast injections under fluoroscopy ensure optimal positioning of the atherectomy catheter before initial cuts are made. For initial cuts, the window should be oriented toward the plaque, and the balloon should be inflated at low pressure (10 to 15 psi, or 0.5 to 1 atm). Balloon expansion pushes the window against the plaque, allowing part of the plaque to protrude into the housing. Slow advancement of the cutter at a rate of approximately 1 mm/sec avoids tearing the tissue and provides a smooth cut. The balloon is deflated and the window reoriented by turning the proximal part of the atherectomy catheter. After reorientation of the window, the balloon is reinflated with low pressure (10 psi) before retraction of the cutter to avoid distal embolization of excised tissue. With subsequent cuts, the operator may increase balloon inflation pressures to 20 to 30 psi, based on vessel size and angiographic findings. Usually, 8 to 12 cuts are made if the patient tolerates ischemia during device insertion. When the plaque has extremely eccentric morphology, the window must be oriented toward the eccentric plaque to achieve an arc of 180 degrees by repositioning the window. When the plaque is concentric, cuts should be made in a 360-degree arc.

Free mobility of the distal guidewire should be maintained at all times. Loss of wire mobility after several cuts suggests that the nose-cone collection chamber is full. Forceful removal of the device at this point increases the risk of guidewire fracture. If free mobility cannot be achieved, the guidewire and directional atherectomy catheter should be removed together as a single unit. It is important to withdraw the guide catheter slightly when the device is retracted to avoid the risk of deeply seating the guide catheter.

Adjunctive Medical Therapy

Adjunctive medical therapy for DCA is similar to that for PTCA, including preprocedural aspirin (325 mg/day, starting at least 1 day before DCA) and intraprocedural heparin monitored by the activated clotting time (ACT). Long-acting nitrates or calcium antagonists are administered at the discretion of the operator to minimize vasospasm. If a satisfactory angiographic result is obtained, heparin is discontinued at the end of the case, and the vascular sheaths are removed 4 to 6 hours later.

Clinical Results

Early Pivotal Studies and Randomized Trials

Several randomized trials have evaluated DCA versus PTCA with and without coronary stenting (Fig. 35-12). The first Coronary Angioplasty vs. Excisional Atherectomy Trial (CAVEAT I) study[11] compared DCA with PTCA for de novo lesions in native coronary arteries. Although the use of DCA was associated with higher procedural success than PTCA and larger

gains in lumen diameter (Table 35-4), the primary end point of angiographic restenosis was not convincingly lower in the DCA group (50% versus 57%, $P = .06$).

The Canadian Coronary Atherectomy Trial (CCAT) study[14] was a randomized trial comparing DCA with PTCA in primary lesions in the proximal segment of the left anterior descending artery. Although DCA resulted in better immediate lumen enlargement and higher procedural success (see Table 35-4), the primary end point of angiographic restenosis was identical in the two treatment groups (see Fig. 35-12).

The CAVEAT II study[12] compared DCA with PTCA for stenoses in saphenous vein bypass grafts. Although DCA resulted in better immediate lumen enlargement and higher procedural success, the incidence of non-ST-segment-elevation myocardial infarction was higher than after PTCA, and no differences in angiographic restenosis or clinical outcomes were seen at 6 months (see Fig. 35-12).

Optimal Atherectomy Trials

The failure of DCA to improve the prospectively defined primary end points in CAVEAT I,[11] CCAT,[14] and CAVEAT II[12] was attributed to several factors. In several registry reports and small comparative trials in a variety of settings with or without stents (Table 35-5), DCA resulted in better immediate lumen enlargement and lower restenosis rates than PTCA (see Tables 35-4 and 35-5). Adjunctive PTCA, initially discouraged after DCA, actually improved the acute outcome of DCA.[48] In the Optimal Atherectomy Restenosis Study (OARS), 199 patients prospectively treated with DCA using ultrasound guidance and adjunctive PTCA if necessary achieved a post-treatment diameter stenosis of 7%, major complication rate of 2.5%, and perforations in 0.9%.[52]

The Balloon Angioplasty versus Optimal Atherectomy Trial (BOAT study)[8] tested the strategy of optimal atherectomy, and similar to CAVEAT and CCAT, BOAT demonstrated better immediate lumen enlargement and higher procedural success after DCA (see Table 35-4). Despite a lower rate of angiographic restenosis, no differences were seen in late outcomes or the rates of target lesion revascularization (see Fig. 35-12).

Table 35-4. Angiography Results from Randomized Trials of Directional Atherectomy

Characteristic	CAVEAT-I[11]		CAVEAT-II[12]		CCAT[14]		BOAT[8]		AMIGO[4]	
	DCA	PTCA	DCA	PTCA	DCA	PTCA	DCA	PTCA	DCA/Stent	Stent Alone
No. of patients	512	500	149	156	138	136	497	492	381	372
Acute gain (mm)*	1.05	0.86	1.45	1.12	1.45	1.16	1.75	1.30	1.77	1.74
MLD (mm)	2.02	1.80	2.43	2.22	2.34	2.10	2.82	2.33	2.67	2.61
Perforation (%)	0.4	0.2	0.7	0.7	—	—	1.4	0.0	—	—

*Acute gain equals the postprocedural minimum lumen diameter (MLD) minus the preprocedural MLD.
DCA, directional coronary atherectomy; PTCA, percutaneous transluminal coronary angioplasty.

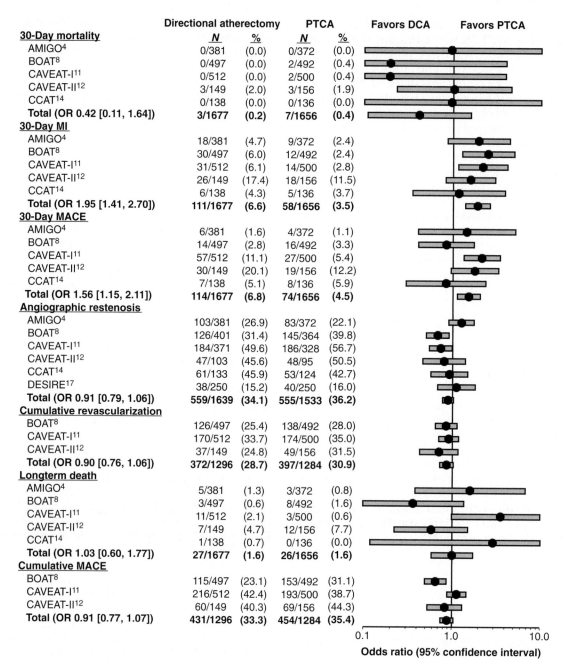

Figure 35-12. Systematic overview of randomized trials of directional coronary atherectomy (DCA) versus percutaneous transluminal coronary angioplasty (PTCA). Pooled odds ratios (OR) and 95% confidence intervals (CI) were calculated to estimate the overall effect of directional coronary atherectomy versus that of PTCA using an empirical Bayes model. Trial abbreviations are given in Table 35-1. (Data from Bittl JA, Chew DP, Topol EJ, et al: Meta-analysis of randomized trials of percutaneous transluminal coronary angioplasty versus atherectomy, cutting balloon atherotomy, or laser angioplasty. J Am Coll Cardiol 2004;43:936-942.)

Table 35-5. Pivotal Mechanistic Trials of Directional Coronary Atherectomy

Characteristic	ABACAS[57]		START[58]		OARS[52]	AtheroLink[59]	Bramucci et al[60]		SOLD[61]	
	DCA Alone	DCA/PTCA	DCA	DCA/Stent	DCA	DCA	DCA/Stent	PTCA/Stent	DCA/Stent	PTCA/Stent
N	106	108	57	61	216	167	94	94	75	75
Acute gain (mm)*	—	—	1.88	1.80	1.85	2.6	2.43	2.20	2.63	2.30
MLD (mm)	2.60	2.88	2.89	2.80	1.96	3.60	2.26	2.00	2.57	2.14
Perforation (%)	0.0	0.9	1.4	0.0	1.0	1.2	—	—	—	—
Restenosis (%)	19.6	23.6	15.8	32.8	28.9	10.8	6.8	30.5	11	21

*Acute gain equals the postprocedural minimum lumen diameter (MLD) minus the preprocedural MLD.
DCA, directional coronary atherectomy; PTCA, percutaneous transluminal coronary angioplasty.

In the Atherectomy before Multi-link Improves Lumen Gain and Clinical Outcomes (AMIGO) trial,[4] a total of 753 patients with de novo lesions in native vessels were randomized to DCA followed by coronary stenting or to coronary stenting alone. The use of DCA appeared to have no effect on angiographic (see Table 35-4) or clinical outcomes (see Fig. 35-12).

The failure of optimal atherectomy to achieve better clinical outcomes than PTCA was attributed to several factors. In BOAT,[8] more aggressive debulking was associated with reduced rates of angiographic restenosis, but this was not associated with reduced target-vessel revascularization or improved clinical outcome. In the AMIGO trial,[4] in which the primary end point of angiographic restenosis was numerically higher in the group treated with directional atherectomy plus stenting (27%) than in the group treated with stents alone (22%), protocol-prescribed aggressive debulking as defined by less than 20% stenosis, was achieved in only 27% of lesions after atherectomy. A retrospective analysis of two centers in the AMIGO trial where more optimal atherectomy was performed showed binary restenosis rates were significantly lower (14%) in the group treated with stents plus aggressive atherectomy than in the stent-alone group (32%).

Complications

The incidence of perforation after DCA has been approximately 1% (see Tables 35-4 and 35-5), which is higher than the 0.2% incidence after PTCA. The incidence of non-ST-segment myocardial infarction has been 4.7% to 17.4%, caused by embolization of atheromatous material during atherectomy. The risk of myocardial infarction has been approximately twice as high after DCA than after PTCA (see Fig. 35-12).

A contentious issue has been the relation between procedural myocardial infarction and late mortality. The body of evidence from randomized trials suggests that long-term mortality rates after DCA are similar to those after PTCA (see Fig. 35-12).

Lesion Selection

The strategy of aggressive debulking with DCA before coronary stenting was evaluated by IVUS in a series of 187 patients.[53] Although the postprocedural lumen cross-sectional area was largest after DCA plus stenting (11.2 ± 2.7 mm²) and DCA (10.8 ± 2.5 mm²) than stenting alone (9.0 ± 2.9 mm²) (P < .0005), rates of binary restenosis were not different among the three groups (DCA plus stent: 12.5%; DCA: 18.3%; stent: 18.8%; P = .57). Debulking with directional atherectomy before stenting has been theoretically attractive to achieve full stent expansion and reduce restenosis,[34,35] but no evidence exists to recommend the approach routinely.[40] One drawback of aggressive debulking before stenting is that the beat-to-beat movement in the stent-delivery device within the

treated target lesion may increase the risk of a geographic miss.

The use of DCA for bifurcation lesions remains unsettled. Although uncontrolled experiences supported the use of the device for bifurcation lesions,[54] other studies reported a higher incidence of side branch closure and clinical complications after DCA than after PTCA.[55] The routine use of DCA for treating bifurcation lesions may appear theoretically sound, but no consistent evidence exists to support DCA for this indication.[40]

A unique feature of DCA compared with other interventional techniques is that it provides a directional approach for lesion excision. Extremely eccentric or ulcerated lesions can be excised selectively by directional positioning of the window, which may reduce elastic recoil in patients who cannot undergo stenting or tolerate thienopyridine therapy (Fig. 35-13). Nevertheless, most operators prefer stents for lesions with abnormal contours because of the simplicity of stenting compared with DCA.

Although DCA has been used to treat in-stent restenosis,[56] no data suggest its superiority over conventional PTCA.[40] There have been several instances

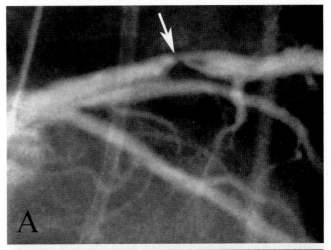

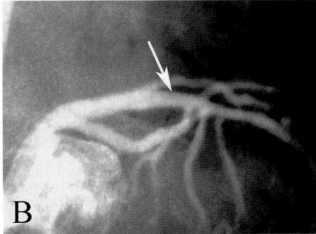

Figure 35-13. Directional coronary atherectomy for complex eccentric lesion (**A,** *arrow*) followed by balloon angioplasty (**B,** *arrow*).

of partial excision of stent struts and complete extraction of stent coils. Histologic studies of DCA for in-stent restenosis confirm a high incidence of intimal hyperplasia, virtually identical to that observed after restenosis following other interventions.

PERCUTANEOUS TRANSLUMINAL ROTATIONAL ATHERECTOMY

Rotational atherectomy involves the excavation of inelastic, calcified atherosclerotic tissue in much the same way as a dental drill is able to bore into enamel and leave pulp unharmed. The rotational atherectomy system cuts inelastic plaque inside coronary arteries and retains the integrity of the elastic artery wall. The plaque is abraded into small particles ranging in size to less than 5 µm in diameter, which are taken up by the reticuloendothelial system.

Mechanism

Rotational atherectomy preferably ablates atherosclerotic plaque according to the theory of differential cutting. This is the ability of a device to cut one material selectively while maintaining the integrity of the adjacent tissues. Rotary ablation preferentially attacks hard, calcified atherosclerotic plaque because of its selective differential cutting effect. Elastic tissue is more difficult to cut because it deflects underneath the spinning burr without cutting. Hard tissue is not able to deflect, and microfissures appear at the zone of contact with the burr.

Equipment

The Rotablator (Scimed, Boston Scientific, Natick, MA) system includes an advancer that houses the air turbine, drive shaft, and burr and a console to monitor and control the rotation by regulating the air supply to the advancer and the DynaGlide foot pedal. The abrasive tip is welded to a long, flexible drive shaft covered by a plastic sheath, and it tracks along a central, flexible guidewire. The Rotalink burr catheter is 135 cm long and contains a 0.058-inch outer sheath. The nickel-coated brass burr is elliptical and has 2000 to 3000 microscopic diamond crystals on the leading face (Fig. 35-14). The diamond crystals are 20 µm in diameter, with only 5 µm protruding from the nickel coating. The trailing edge of the burr is smooth. The burrs are available for coronary use in 0.25-mm increments from 1.25 to 2.50 mm in diameter. Rotational energy is transmitted by a compressed air motor that drives the flexible, helical shaft at speeds up to 200,000 rpm.

The number of revolutions per minute is measured by a fiberoptic light probe and displayed on a control panel. The speed of rotation and the speed of advancement of the burr are controlled by the operator. During rotation, saline solution irrigates the catheter sheath to lubricate and cool the rotating parts. The burr and the drive shaft move freely over a central coaxial guidewire (0.009 inch in diameter and 3 m

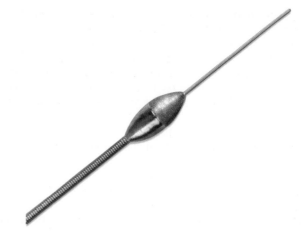

Figure 35-14. Rotablator burr. (Courtesy of Boston Scientific, Natick, MA.)

long) with a flexible radiopaque platinum distal part (20 mm long) that does not rotate with the burr during abrasion. The wire and the abrasive tip can be advanced independently, which allows the wire to be placed in a safe distal location before the burr is advanced into the diseased artery. With the Rotalink system and a single advancer, an operator can use multiple burrs. The exchange of burrs is easier, saves time, and promotes use of a multiburr approach.

A console displays the rotational speed in revolutions per minute. The DynaGlide foot pedal is important for withdrawal. Tanks, regulators, and attachments drive the system. The Advancer has preset delimiters for retraction and advancement. The WireClip torquer and guidewires are critical components of the system. RotaGlide lubricant is useful for crossing resistant lesions.

Procedure

All patients are pretreated with aspirin and a calcium antagonist. A sheath is inserted into the femoral artery under local anesthesia, and 6-, 7-, or 8-Fr guide catheters are used, depending on the size of the burr. The 1.25-mm burr advances freely through the 0.070-inch inner lumen of the 6-Fr Runway Guide (Boston Scientific, Natick, MA), allowing easy conversion to salvage atherectomy for any coronary intervention that becomes stymied by an undilatable or uncrossable lesion. When treating large coronary arteries, particularly the right coronary artery, prophylactic insertion of a temporary pacemaker is recommended because of the frequency of bradyarrhythmias.

Rotary ablation begins by placing the Rotawire across the lesion to a safe distal vessel location not in a side branch. The burr and the drive shaft are then manually advanced over the guidewire to the site of the lesion, and rotation is begun. When an adequate speed of rotation (140,000 rpm) has been achieved, the abrasive tip is advanced gently over the guidewire. If resistance is encountered, the tip is moved backward and forward to maintain a high speed of rotation. The lower rotational speed of

140,000 rpm may be associated with less platelet activation and aggregation. Excessive decelerations of greater than 5000 rpm below the platform speed must be avoided, because they increase the risk of vessel trauma, formation of large particles, and creation of ischemic complications related to frictional heat. Several slow passes are usually required to achieve maximum plaque removal.

Clinical Results

The Study to Determine Rotablator and Transluminal Angioplasty Strategy (STRATAS)[26] compared an aggressive PTRA strategy using a burr-to-artery ratio of 0.7 to 0.9 followed by balloon inflation of less than 1 atm (or none at all) versus a moderate debulking strategy using a burr-to-artery ratio of less than 0.7 followed by conventional balloon angioplasty. The clinical success was similar, but the aggressive strategy caused more myocardial infarctions (11% versus 7%) and a higher rate of restenosis (58% versus 52%).

The Coronary Angioplasty and Rotablator Atherectomy Trial (CARAT)[10] compared a large-burr strategy using a burr-to-artery ratio of greater than 0.7 with a small-burr strategy using a burr-to-artery ratio of less than 0.7. The large-burr strategy achieved similar immediate lumen enlargement and rate of target vessel revascularization as the small-burr strategy but caused more angiographic complications (12.7% versus 5.2%, $P < .05$).

The Dilatation vs Ablation Revascularization Trial Targeting Restenosis (DART)[16] was a multicenter, randomized trial comparing PTRA with PTCA in noncomplex lesions (types A and B1) in vessels 2.0 to 2.9 mm in diameter. Although the rate of procedural success was high (99%), the primary end point of angiographic restenosis was identical in the PTRA and PTCA groups (Fig. 35-15).

The Angioplasty versus Rotational Atherectomy for Treatment of Diffuse In-stent Restenosis Trial (ARTIST)[6] was a randomized trial comparing PTRA with PTCA in 298 patients with in-stent restenosis. In-hospital complications were more frequent (14.5% versus 6.8%, $P = .04$), and the restenosis rate was significantly higher (65% versus 51%) after PTRA than PTCA (see Fig. 35-15). At the 6-month follow-up, the event-free survival rate was lower for the PTRA group than the PTCA group (79.6% versus 91.1%).

Rotational Atherectomy versus Balloon Angioplasty for Diffuse In-Stent Restenosis (ROSTER)[24] was a randomized trial comparing PTRA with PTCA in 200 patients with diffuse in-stent restenosis (see Fig. 35-15). At follow-up, the primary end point of target lesion revascularization was lower after PTRA than after PTCA (32% versus 45%, $P = .04$).

Lesion Selection

About 1% to 3% of lesions that can be crossed with guidewires are uncrossable with balloon catheters or undilatable at balloon pressures higher than 20 atm.

Rotational atherectomy successfully improves the compliance of most of these resistant lesions, allowing balloon dilation and stent implantation to be completed successfully (Fig. 35-16). For long calcified lesions, small burrs are recommended to modify the compliance of the vessel, completing the procedure with balloon inflations and performing spot stenting on the segments with dissection. Although rotational atherectomy has been recommended as a strategy before stenting of bifurcation lesions,[34,35] no evidence exists to support this approach.[40]

Certain precautions about rotational atherectomy need emphasis. Angulated lesions located in a bend of more than 60 degrees are a contraindication to the use of PTRA because of the risk of dissection or perforation. When rotational atherectomy is performed in nonangulated lesions, the rotating burr should never be advanced to the point of contact with the spring tip of the Rotawire. The rotating burr should not be allowed to remain in one location within the artery; gentle retraction and advancement motion is needed to avoid dissection formation and welding. The rotating burr should not be advanced within the guide catheter. Rotational atherectomy should be avoided in dissected segments after balloon angioplasty, in lesions with visible thrombus, and in degenerated saphenous vein grafts.

DECONSTRUCTING DEBULKING

The published and unpublished randomized trials reported during the past 20 years were evaluated to define the clinical and angiographic advantages of ablative techniques over the common comparator of PTCA. The pooled results of dozens of studies, which are generalizable across several centers and directly compared with the benchmark therapy of PTCA, suggest that ablative techniques have not been able to achieve prospectively defined end points.

Several explanations exist to reconcile the negative results of dozens of randomized trials with the generally favorable results of scores of pivotal mechanistic studies. Randomized trials produce only general principles about treatment effects, not the fine details of how the treatment should be used. Randomized trials can generate firm conclusions about whether the use of an ablative device can produce a lower rate of restenosis than PTCA, but retrospective secondary analyses focusing on how devices were used in individual centers in multicenter trials must be viewed as tentative, exploratory, or hyperbole.

Randomized trials have been the benchmark of evidence for device development in the subspecialty of interventional cardiology, but no field of medicine has seen such a surfeit of negative results (except perhaps medical oncology). The evidence for using atheroablative devices in interventional cardiology has been generated in registries and small trials. It is possible that too much reliance on luminology in mechanistic trials has missed the importance of counting clinical events. Although multicenter, ran-

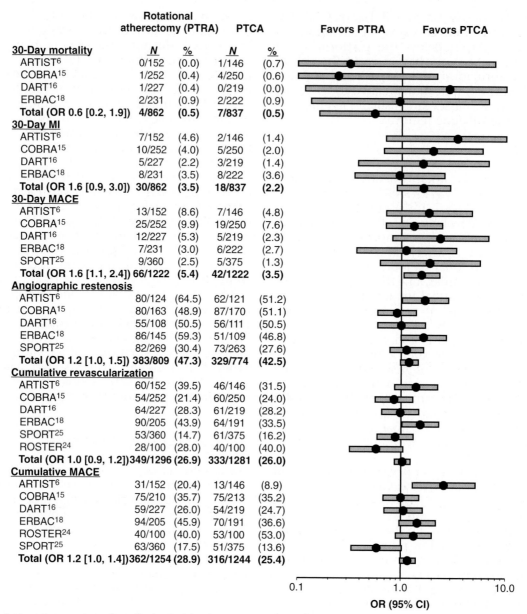

Figure 35-15. Systematic overview of randomized trials of percutaneous transluminal rotational atherectomy (PTRA) versus percutaneous transluminal coronary angioplasty (PTCA). Pooled odds ratios (OR) and 95% confidence intervals (CI) were calculated to estimate the overall effect of percutaneous transluminal rotational atherectomy versus that of PTCA using an empirical Bayes model. Trial abbreviations are given in Table 35-1. (Data from Bittl JA, Chew DP, Topol EJ, et al: Meta-analysis of randomized trials of percutaneous transluminal coronary angioplasty versus atherectomy, cutting balloon atherotomy, or laser angioplasty. J Am Coll Cardiol 2004;43:936-942.)

domized trials remain the best mechanism to control for confounding factors during the evaluation of new therapies, they may not be the optimal venue for studying relatively complex ablative techniques that depend on operator expertise and selection of appropriate lesions for ablation, such as bifurcation lesions, ostial stenoses, certain calcified stenoses, or undilatable lesions. The techniques used in various centers in randomized trials may not have uniformly achieved desired degrees of debulking.

The main goal of any randomized study is to measure the primary end point. The most commonly

studied end point in the randomized trials of atheroablative techniques was binary restenosis (see Table 35-1). A systematic overview of binary restenosis versus trial size (Fig. 35-17) reveals several insights into the tentative evidence for atheroablative procedures. First, smaller studies claimed the larger relative reductions in restenosis than larger studies. Selective reliance on results of mechanistic studies, small randomized trials, and opinions of thought leaders could lead to the conclusion that atheroablative treatments are clinically beneficial. Secondly, directional coronary atherectomy was associated with

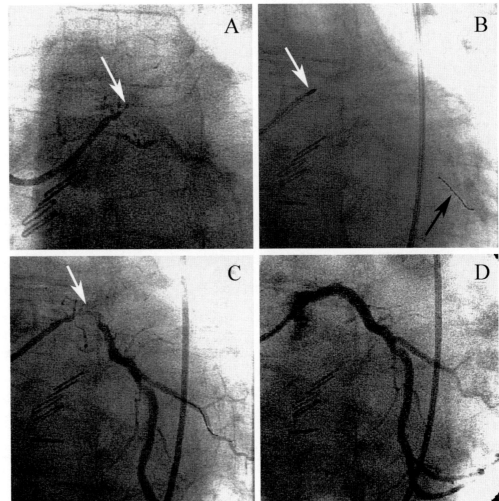

Figure 35-16. Rotational atherectomy for an uncrossable left main stenosis. The left main occlusion jeopardized a large, unbypassed left circumflex coronary artery, which could be crossed with a guidewire but could not be crossed with a balloon catheter *(A, arrow)*. After placement of a Rotawire with the tip positioned distally *(B, black arrow)*, a 1.25-mm burr was advanced to the left main occlusion *(B, white arrow)*. The residual stenosis *(C, arrow)* was successfully treated with a sirolimus-eluting stent and then dilated to 4.0 mm, achieving the final result *(D)*.

reduced restenosis in large trials, but its use was not associated with improved clinical outcomes (see Fig. 35-12). Commonly repeated theories such as "bigger is better" or "debulking reduces restenosis" acquire the raiment of accepted truth if they are cited often enough. The totality of scientific evidence, however, proves the contrary position—that the routine use of mechanical approaches for plaque modification has not been able to improve clinical outcomes.

The results and analyses presented in this chapter raise the larger biologic issue of why atheroablative procedures have failed to achieve better clinical outcomes than PTCA. It is possible that these techniques are more injurious than initially thought. For example, laser angioplasty was originally proposed to ablate atheromatous plaque by the benign process of photochemical dissociation, but this was disproved when both excimer and holmium laser angioplasty were shown to cause significant collateral injury with minimal plaque removal in experimental studies.[46] Likewise, rotational atherectomy was observed to injure vascular tissue from excessive heat generation, and more aggressive application of rotational ather-

ectomy was more injurious than a light approach.[10,26] Aggressive DCA performed in BOAT[53] produced a larger relative increase in the rate of periprocedural myocardial infarctions than that seen in CAVEAT I.[11] DCA doubled the rates of embolization in SVGs compared with PTCA in CAVEAT II (13.4% versus 5.1%).[12] Coronary perforation probably occurs more often after the use of atheroablative devices than after PTCA. The incidence of perforation has been reported to be 0.10% to 0.20% with balloon angioplasty, 0.25% to 0.70% with DCA, 0.0% to 1.3% with rotational atherectomy, and 1.9% to 2.0% after excimer laser coronary angioplasty.[40]

Because mechanical approaches involving plaque ablation or sectioning have not been associated with improved clinical outcomes or lower restenosis in randomized trials, innovations in tissue ablation should be identified before any new large clinical trials are launched. The solution to the problem of restenosis in native coronary arteries has come not from mechanical removal of atheromatous plaque, but from molecular interventions such as drug-eluting stents that alter vascular biology (Chapter 15).

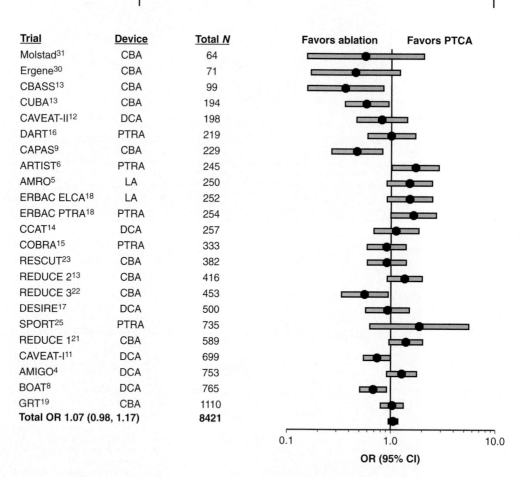

Figure 35-17. Systematic overview of binary restenosis comparing the treatment effect with trial size for randomized trials of atheroablative therapies versus percutaneous transluminal coronary angioplasty (PTCA). Pooled odds ratios (OR) and 95% confidence intervals (CI) were calculated to estimate the overall effect of atheroablative therapies versus that of PTCA using an empirical Bayes model. The empirical Bayes model is a random-effects model that coincides with a fixed-effects model when all studies are homogeneous. Trial acronyms are given in Table 35-1. CBA, cutting balloon angioplasty; DCA, directional coronary atherectomy; LA, laser angioplasty; PTRA, percutaneous transluminal rotational atherectomy. (Data from Bittl JA, Chew DP, Topol EJ, et al: Meta-analysis of randomized trials of percutaneous transluminal coronary angioplasty versus atherectomy, cutting balloon atherotomy, or laser angioplasty. J Am Coll Cardiol 2004;43:936-942.)

REFERENCES

1. Schwartz RS, Huber KC, Murphy JC, et al: Restenosis and the proportional neointimal response to coronary artery injury: Results in a porcine model. J Am Coll Cardiol 1992;18: 267-274.
2. Kuntz RE, Gibson CM, Nobuyoshi M, et al: A generalized model of restenosis following conventional balloon angioplasty, stenting, and directional atherectomy. J Am Coll Cardiol 1993;21:15-25.
3. Ali A, Cox D, Dib N, et al: Rheolytic thrombectomy with percutaneous coronary intervention for infarct size reduction in acute myocardial infarction: 30-day results from a multicenter randomized study. J Am Coll Cardiol 2006;48:244-252.
4. Stankovic G, Colombo A, Bersin R, et al: Comparison of directional coronary atherectomy and stenting versus stenting alone for the treatment of de novo and restenotic coronary artery narrowing. Am J Cardiol 2004;93:953-958.

5. Appelman YEA, Piek JJ, Strikwerda S, et al: Randomised trial of excimer laser versus balloon angioplasty for treatment of obstructive coronary artery disease. Lancet 1996;347: 79-84.
6. vom Dahl J, Dietz U, Haager PK, et al: Rotational atherectomy does not reduce recurrent in-stent restenosis: Results of the Angioplasty Versus Rotational Atherectomy for Treatment of Diffuse In-stent Restenosis Trial (ARTIST). Circulation 2002; 105:583-588.
7. Singh M, Rosenschein U, Ho KK, et al: Treatment of saphenous vein bypass grafts with ultrasound thrombolysis: A randomized study (ATLAS). Circulation 2003;107:2331-2336.
8. Baim DS, Cutlip DE, Sharma SK, et al: Final results of the Balloon vs Optimal Atherectomy Trial. Circulation 1998;97: 322-331.
9. Izumi M, Tsuchikane E, Funamoto M, et al: Final results of the CAPAS trial. Am Heart J 2001;142:782-789.
10. Safian RD, Feldman T, Muller DW, et al: Coronary Angioplasty and Rotablator Atherectomy Trial (CARAT): Immediate and

late results of a prospective multicenter randomized trial. Catheter Cardiovasc Interv 2001;53:213-220.

11. Topol EJ, Leya F, Pinkerton CA, et al: A comparison of balloon angioplasty with directional atherectomy in patients with coronary artery disease. N Engl J Med 1993;329:221-227.

12. Holmes DR Jr, Topol EJ, Califf RM, et al: A multicenter, randomized trial of coronary angioplasty versus directional atherectomy for patients with saphenous vein bypass graft lesions. CAVEAT-II Investigators. Circulation 1995;91:1966-1974.

13. Chin K: Cutting balloons. *In* Ellis SG, Holmes DR Jr (eds): Strategic Approaches in Coronary Intervention, 3rd ed. Philadelphia, Lippincott Williams & Wilkins, 2006, pp 125-142.

14. Adelman AG, Cohen EA, Kimball BP, et al: A comparison of coronary atherectomy with coronary angioplasty for lesions of the proximal left anterior descending coronary artery. N Engl J Med 1993;329:228-233.

15. Dill T, Dietz U, Hamm CW, et al: A randomized comparison of balloon angioplasty versus rotational atherectomy in complex coronary lesion (COBRA study). Eur Heart J 2000;21:1759-1766.

16. Mauri L, Reisman M, Buchbinder M, et al: Comparison of rotational atherectomy with conventional balloon angioplasty in the prevention of restenosis of small coronary arteries: Results of the Dilatation vs Ablation Revascularization Trial Targeting Restenosis (DART). Am Heart J 2003;145:847-854.

17. Aizawa T: The Debulking and Stenting in Restenosis Elimination trial (DESIRE). Circulation 2001;104:2954A.

18. Reifart N, Vandormael M, Krajcar M, et al: Randomized comparison of angioplasty of complex lesions at a single center. Excimer Laser, Rotational Atherectomy, and Balloon Angioplasty Comparison (ERBAC) study. Circulation 1997;19:91-98.

19. Mauri L, Bonan R, Weiner BH, et al: Cutting balloon angioplasty for the prevention of restenosis: Results of the Cutting Balloon Global Randomized Trial. Am J Cardiol 2002;90:1079-1083.

20. Stone GW, de Marchena E, Dageforde D, et al: Prospective, randomized, multicenter comparison of laser-facilitated balloon angioplasty versus stand-alone balloon angioplasty in patients with obstructive coronary artery disease. The Laser Angioplasty Versus Angioplasty (LAVA) Trial Investigators. J Am Coll Cardiol 1997;30:1714-1721.

21. Yamaguchi T: REDUCE 1 trial: Final results. Presented at the Transcatheter Therapeutics meeting, 2001; Washington, DC.

22. Ozaki Y, Suzuki T, Yamaguchi T, et al: Can intravascular ultrasound guided cutting balloon angioplasty before stenting be a substitute for a drug eluting stent? Final results of the prospective randomized multicenter trial comparing cutting balloon with balloon angioplasty before stenting (REDUCE III). J Am Coll Cardiol 2004;43:82A.

23. Albiero R, Silber S, Di Mario C, et al: Cutting balloon versus conventional balloon angioplasty for the treatment of in-stent restenosis: Results of the restenosis cutting balloon evaluation trial (RESCUT). J Am Coll Cardiol 2004;43:943-949.

24. Sharma SK, Kini A, Mehran R, et al: Randomized trial of Rotational Atherectomy Versus Balloon Angioplasty for Diffuse In-stent Restenosis (ROSTER). Am Heart J 2004;147:16-22.

25. Buchbinder M, Fortuna R, Sharma SK, et al: Debulking prior to stenting: Long-term clinical and angiographic results from the SPORT Trial [abstract]. Circulation 2000;102:II-663.

26. Whitlow PL, Bass TA, Kipperman RM, et al: Results of the Study to Determine Rotablator and Transluminal Angioplasty Strategy (STRATAS). Am J Cardiol 2001;87:699-705.

27. Kuntz RE, Baim DS, Cohen DJ, et al: A trial comparing rheolytic thrombectomy with intracoronary urokinase for coronary and vein graft thrombus (the Vein Graft AngioJet Study [VeGAS 2]). Am J Cardiol 2002;89:326-330.

28. Lefevre T, Garcia E, Reimers B, et al: X-Sizer for thrombectomy in acute myocardial infarction improves ST-segment resolution: Results of the X-Sizer in AMI for negligible embolization and optimal ST resolution (X AMINE ST) trial. J Am Coll Cardiol 2005;46:246-252.

29. Stone GW, Cox DA, Babb J, et al: Late-breaking clinical trial abstracts: The X-TRACT trial: A prospective, randomized comparison of stent implantation in thrombotic native coronary arteries and saphenous vein grafts with versus without thromb-atherectomy. Circulation 2002;106:2986A.

30. Ergene O, Seyithanoglu BY, Tastan A, et al: Comparison of angiographic and clinical outcome after cutting balloon and conventional balloon angioplasty in vessels smaller than 3 mm in diameter: A randomized trial. J Invasive Cardiol 1998;10:70-75.

31. Molstad P, Myreng Y, Golf S, et al: The Barath cutting balloon versus conventional angioplasty. A randomized study comparing acute success rate and frequency of late restenosis. Scand Cardiovasc J 1998;32:79-85.

32. Montorsi P, Galli S, Fabbiocchi F, et al: Randomized trial of conventional balloon angioplasty versus cutting balloon for in-stent restenosis. Acute and 24-hour angiographic and intravascular ultrasound changes and long-term follow-up. Ital Heart J 2004;5:271-279.

33. Bittl JA, Chew DP, Topol EJ, et al: Meta-analysis of randomized trials of percutaneous transluminal coronary angioplasty versus atherectomy, cutting balloon atherotomy, or laser angioplasty. J Am Coll Cardiol 2004;43:936-942.

34. Moses JW, Carlier SG, Moussa I: Lesion preparation prior to stenting. Rev Cardiovasc Med 2004;5(Suppl 2):S16-S21.

35. Sharma S, Bagga RS, Kini AS: Debulking approaches prior to stenting in interventional cardiology. *In* Ellis S, Holmes, DR Jr (eds): Philadelphia, Lippincott Williams & Wilkins, 2006, pp 116-124.

36. Topol EJ (ed): Textbook of Interventional Cardiology, 4th ed. Philadelphia, WB Saunders, 2003.

37. Iijima R, Ikari Y, Wada M, et al: Cutting balloon angioplasty is superior to balloon angioplasty or stent implantation for small coronary artery disease. Coron Artery Dis 2004;15:435-440.

38. Okura H, Hayase M, Shimodozono S, et al: Mechanisms of acute lumen gain following cutting balloon angioplasty in calcified and noncalcified lesions: An intravascular ultrasound study. Catheter Cardiovasc Interv 2002;57:429-436.

39. Haridas KK, Vijayakumar M, Viveka K, et al: Fracture of cutting balloon microsurgical blade inside coronary artery during angioplasty of tough restenotic lesion: A case report. Catheter Cardiovasc Interv 2003;58:199-201.

40. ACC/AHA/SCAI guideline update for percutaneous coronary intervention: A report of the American College of Cardiology/American Heart Association Task Force on Practice Guidelines (ACC/AHA/SCAI Writing Committee to Update the 2001 Guidelines for Percutaneous Coronary Intervention). J Am Coll Cardiol 2006;47:el-121.

41. Takebayashi H, Haruta S, Kohno H, et al: Immediate and 3-month follow-up outcome after cutting balloon angioplasty for bifurcation lesions. J Interv Cardiol 2004;17:1-7.

42. Antoniucci D, Valenti R, Migliorini A, et al: Comparison of rheolytic thrombectomy before direct infarct artery stenting versus direct stenting alone in patients undergoing percutaneous coronary intervention for acute myocardial infarction. Am J Cardiol 2004;93:1033-1035.

43. Vijayalakshmi K, Kunadian B, Wright RA, et al: Successful thrombus extraction with the Rescue thrombus management system during acute percutaneous coronary intervention improves flow but does not necessarily restore optimal myocardial tissue perfusion. Catheter Cardiovasc Interv 2006;67:879-886.

44. Burzotta F, Trani C, Romagnoli E, et al: A pilot study with a new, rapid-exchange, thrombus-aspirating device in patients with thrombus-containing lesions: The Diver C.E. study. Catheter Cardiovasc Interv 2006;67:887-893.

45. Siddiqui DS, Choi CJ, Tsimikas S, et al: Successful utilization of a novel aspiration thrombectomy catheter (Pronto) for the treatment of patients with stent thrombosis. Catheter Cardiovasc Interv 2006;67:894-899.

46. van Leeuwen TG, van Erven L, Meertens JH, et al: Origin of arterial wall dissections induced by pulsed excimer and mid-infrared laser ablation in the pig. J Am Coll Cardiol 1992;19:1610-1618.

47. Deckelbaum LI, Natarajan MK, Bittl JA, et al: Effect of intracoronary saline on dissection during excimer laser coronary

angioplasty: A randomized trial. J Am Coll Cardiol 1995;26:1264-1269.

48. Suzuki T, Hosokawa H, Katoh O, et al: Effects of adjunctive balloon angioplasty after intravascular ultrasound-guided optimal directional coronary atherectomy: The result of Adjunctive Balloon Angioplasty After Coronary Atherectomy Study (ABACAS). J Am Coll Cardiol 1999;34:1028-1035.

49. Oikawa Y, Kirigaya H, Aizawa T, et al: Mechanisms of acute gain and late lumen loss after atherectomy in different preintervention arterial remodeling patterns. Am J Cardiol 2002;89:505-510.

50. Takagi T, Di Mario C, Stankovic G, et al: Effective plaque removal with a new 8 French-compatible atherectomy catheter. Catheter Cardiovasc Interv 2002;56:452-459.

51. Ikeno F, Hinohara T, Robertson GC, et al: Early experience with a novel plaque excision system for the treatment of complex coronary lesions. Catheter Cardiovasc Interv 2004;61:35-43.

52. Simonton CA, Leon MB, Baim DS, et al: "Optimal" directional coronary atherectomy: Final results of the Optimal Atherectomy Restenosis Study (OARS). Circulation 1998;97:332-339.

53. Kawamura A, Asakura Y, Ishikawa S, et al: Stenting after directional coronary atherectomy compared with directional coronary atherectomy alone and stenting alone: A serial intravascular ultrasound study. Circ J 2004;68:455-461.

54. Dauerman HL, Higgins PJ, Sparano AM, et al: Mechanical debulking versus balloon angioplasty for the treatment of true bifurcation lesions. J Am Coll Cardiol 1998;32:1853-1854.

55. Brener SJ, Leya FS, Apperson-Hansen C, et al: A comparison of debulking versus dilatation of bifurcation coronary arterial narrowings (from the CAVEAT I trial). Coronary Angioplasty Versus Excisional Atherectomy Trial-I. Am J Cardiol 1996;78:1039-1041.

56. Airoldi F, Di Mario C, Stankovic G, et al: Effectiveness of treatment of in-stent restenosis with an 8-French compatible atherectomy catheter. Am J Cardiol 2003;92:725-728.

57. Suzuki S, Matsuo T, Kobayashi H, et al: Antithrombotic treatment (argatroban vs. heparin) in coronary angioplasty in angina pectoris: Effects on inflammatory, hemostatic, and endothelium-derived parameters. Thromb Res 2000;98:269-279.

58. Tsuchikane E, Sumitsuji S, Awata N, et al: Final results of the Stent Versus Directional Coronary Atherectomy Randomized Trial (START). J Am Coll Cardiol 1999;34:1058-1060.

59. Hopp HW, Baer FM, Ozbek C, et al: A synergistic approach to optimal stenting: Directional coronary atherectomy prior to coronary artery stent implantation—The AtheroLink Registry. AtheroLink Study Group. J Am Coll Cardiol 2000;36:1853-1859.

60. Bramucci E, Angoli L, Merlini PA, et al: Adjunctive stent implantation following directional coronary atherectomy in patients with coronary artery disease. J Am Coll Cardiol 1998;32:1855-1860.

61. Moussa I, Moses J, Di Mario C, et al: Stenting after optimal lesion debulking (SOLD) registry. Angiographic and clinical outcome. Circulation 1998;98:1604-1609.

CHAPTER

36 Support Devices for High-Risk Percutaneous Coronary Interventions

Victor M. Mejia, Srihari S. Naidu, and Howard C. Herrmann

KEY POINTS

- Clinical characteristics of the high-risk patient include older age, history of myocardial infarction, low ejection fraction, congestive heart failure, and renal insufficiency.
- High-risk angiographic characteristics include left main or multivessel coronary artery disease, complex lesions, decreased Thrombolysis in Myocardial Infarction (TIMI) flow, and thrombotic lesions.
- The decision to use a circulatory support device should be made within the context of the risk profile of the specific patient and in concert with the appropriate surgical consultation.
- Intra-aortic balloon pump support provides up to 0.5 L/min of cardiac output and is optimal for use in patients with stable cardiac rhythm.

- Cardiopulmonary support can completely support the circulation, provides support irrespective of the cardiac rhythm, and can be instituted quickly by experienced practitioners, but it leads to high rates of vascular and access-site complications.
- The TandemHeart device provides an intermediate level of support, reaching flows of up to 3.5 L/min, and it can be used for extended periods.
- The percutaneous Impella device can provide up to 2.5 L/min of circulatory support, but remains investigational under restricted use.

BACKGROUND AND RATIONALE

Complications of balloon angioplasty that threaten coronary blood flow, called *acute and threatened occlusion,* usually require urgent surgical intervention and are the main causes of procedure-related morbidity and mortality. Before the advent of stents as a bailout treatment for impending vessel closure, this complication occurred in about 6% of balloon angioplasty procedures. Patients who required emergent surgery in this setting had a 50% likelihood of suffering myocardial infarction (MI), with mortality rates as high as 10%.[1]

In these early studies, patient characteristics, including compromised ventricular function, left main and multivessel disease, and older age, were identified as risk factors for balloon angioplasty–related mortality.[2,3] With the development of coronary stents to seal dissections and improve blood flow in thrombotic lesions, the need for urgent surgery was reduced with a concomitant reduction in percutaneous coronary intervention (PCI)–related morbidity and mortality.[4]

Later studies have demonstrated that the need for urgent surgery after PCI has been reduced to less than 1%, with a marked reduction in procedure-related mortality.[5] In one comparison of patients treated between 1997 and 1998 with those treated between 1985 and 1986, the rate of in-hospital deaths, MI, and coronary artery bypass grafting (CABG) fell from 7.9% to 4.9%, despite the treatment of more complex lesions and stent use in only 71% of patients.[6] Most of the difference between treatment periods was accounted for by the reduction in the need for emergent CABG from 3.7% to 0.4%.[6] Nonetheless, morbidity and mortality rates for patients who required emergent CABG remained high.[5]

The increased confidence afforded interventionalists by stents has prompted interventions in more complex lesions and patients with more severe cardiac and noncardiac disease. It has therefore become essential to identify the predictors of risk and to consider the use of hemodynamic support for patients at high risk for procedural complications.

Although several investigators have used common sense definitions to classify patients at high risk,[7,8] two studies systematically developed risk models that are discussed in more detail here.[9,10] In the Mayo Clinic model, eight clinical and angiographic variables were used to predict in-hospital complications after PCI. The variables were age, shock, renal insufficiency, urgent procedures, heart failure, thrombus, and left main coronary artery (LMCA) and multivessel disease. A score based on these factors predicted the risk of complications and identified a highest-risk group with an event rate that exceeded 25%.[10]

In a similar study of 46,000 procedures in the New York State–required PCI reporting system, investigators included nine factors in a risk score: ejection fraction, previous MI, gender, age, hemodynamic state, peripheral arterial disease, congestive heart failure, renal failure, and LMCA disease. Using this risk score, a graded risk for in-hospital mortality was derived and validated. About 2% of all patients had a risk for in-hospital death of more than 5%, and about 4% of patients had a risk of more than 3%.[9]

Other studies have confirmed these risk factors for PCI-related complications.[3,11,12] Angiographic factors of lesion complexity (e.g., thrombus, calcification, bifurcations) have been associated with more dissections, distal embolization, and side branch occlusions, resulting in a threefold increase in the risk for in-hospital death.[13] Two patient characteristics deserve separate discussion. Although female gender was initially associated with complications in early studies of balloon angioplasty,[14,15] later studies failed to demonstrate this very important effect on outcome.[9,10] Similarly, diabetics have more complex lesion characteristics and risk factors, but there was no increase in in-hospital mortality after multivariable adjustment.[16]

Despite major advances in the technical and procedural performance of modern PCI, clinical and angiographic predictors of significant morbidity and mortality can be identified (Table 36-1). These data provide the rationale for hemodynamic support during complex or high-risk PCI. The remainder of this chapter discusses the approach to such patients, the devices that are available to provide support, and the results that are achieved using them.

APPROACH TO THE PATIENT

Mechanical circulatory support at the time of PCI has historically been instituted in one of two settings: electively for presumed high-risk intervention and emergently for periprocedural hemodynamic instability. Specific indications, however, remain controversial owing to limitations in performing large-scale, randomized trials and evaluating specific devices in individual patient subsets. Nevertheless, a review of the existing literature provides guidelines for patient and device selection when evaluating patients for elective or emergent support.

Electively placed mechanical support is aimed at improving procedural success and thereby reducing mortality rates for high-risk, preselected patient subsets. In this setting, prophylactic insertion of the

Table 36-1. Predictors of Risk during Percutaneous Coronary Intervention

Factor	References
Clinical and Patient Related Factors	
Older age	3, 9, 10, 41
Cardiogenic shock	6, 9, 10, 41
Recent myocardial infarction	6, 9, 10, 41
Congestive heart failure	9-11, 41
Prior coronary artery bypass grafting or revascularization	66
Peripheral vascular disease	9, 41
Chronic renal insufficiency	9, 10, 41
Angiographic Factors	
Left main coronary artery or multivessel disease	9, 10, 41, 67, 68
Complex lesions (bifurcation, calcification, total occlusion)	13
Decreased Thrombolysis in Myocardial Infarction (TIMI)–defined flow	69
Left ventricular dysfunction	6, 9, 11, 12, 41
Thrombus	10, 13

intra-aortic counterpulsation balloon pump (IABP) appeared to improve procedural success with a minimal increase in complications.[17-21]

More familiar to interventional cardiologists is the use of mechanical circulatory support in the emergent setting for patients with documented hemodynamic instability or cardiogenic shock. Instability may be present before PCI or develop as a consequence of procedural complications, such as coronary dissection, poor coronary reflow, or thromboembolism.

Determining which device to use in specific settings remains controversial. Device selection is based on several factors, including ease and rapidity of institution, level of invasiveness and complications, physician familiarity, requisite technical expertise, and level of anticipated circulatory support. Although IABP is the least invasive and may be instituted rapidly, it provides the least support, averaging a 0.5-L/min augmentation in cardiac output.[22] It may be left in place for several days, with an associated vascular complication rate of 15%.[23] Conversely, full cardiopulmonary support (CPS) is significantly more invasive, requiring timely surgical and perfusionist collaboration for institution and removal, but it can produce greater improvement in cardiac output, approximating normal physiology. CPS cannot be maintained indefinitely, and hematologic and pulmonary complications increase as bypass time approaches 6 hours.[23]

Percutaneous ventricular assist devices (pVADs), such as the TandemHeart or Impella, provide an intermediate level of support (approaching 2.5 to 4 L/min) and can be placed emergently in the catheterization laboratory without surgical backup. Unlike the Impella, the TandemHeart (Cardiac Assist Inc., Pittsburgh, PA) requires transseptal puncture to deliver the inflow cannula into the left atrium. Only those skilled in this technique are able to use the device. The cannulas are large and may result in significant vascular morbidity. However, unlike full CPS, use of pVADs has been successful for intermediate periods (up to 14 days). Smaller cannulas, as with the Impella device, are likely to reduce femoral complications.

In most patients, elective, high-risk PCI can be performed safely with IABP support. In selected patients who appear to require additional circulatory support, CPS or pVAD may be considered, with the caveat that the inherent increase in delay and invasiveness may partially offset the benefit. For patients who develop severe hemodynamic instability, cardiogenic shock, or frank arrest during PCI, bailout use of the IABP appears beneficial and is the most familiar and rapid strategy. Full CPS may be considered in catheterization laboratories equipped and staffed for timely initiation. In the emergent setting, pVADs appear promising, but they require specialized technical expertise.

DEVICES

Intra-Aortic Counterpulsation Balloon Pump

The IABP was first used clinically in cardiogenic shock by Kantrowitz in 1968.[24] As its application expanded to include refractory angina,[24] severe hemodynamic compromise, and postcardiotomy pump failure[25] and with the advent of percutaneous insertion,[26] the IABP was one of the first hemodynamic devices used to support high-risk coronary interventions.

Rapid filling of the balloon in early diastole augments diastolic pressure and leads to increased coronary perfusion pressure, whereas deflation of the balloon at end-diastole reduces effective aortic volume and decreases aortic systolic pressure, leading to lower left ventricular afterload. The net effect is a decrease in myocardial oxygen requirements from lower systolic wall tension and an increase in coronary perfusion pressure, improving the myocardial supply and demand balance. Cardiac output increases because of improved myocardial contractility as a result of the increased coronary blood flow and the reduced afterload.[27,28]

Insertion Technique

Evaluation of the iliac and femoral arteries is recommended to exclude significant arterial disease. Access in the common femoral artery is obtained by means of the Seldinger technique. The balloon can be inserted through an 8- or 9-Fr sheath or, alternatively, directly in a sheathless fashion. Before insertion, all air in the balloon should be evacuated with a large syringe attached to the one-way valve to maintain the lowest possible profile during insertion. The balloon catheter is advanced under angiographic guidance over a stiff, 0.021-inch guidewire until the radiopaque tip marker reaches a level just distal to

the left subclavian artery. After removal of the guidewire, the central lumen is flushed and connected to a pressure transducer. The balloon is then connected to the console, the system is purged with helium, and counterpulsation is started. Proper placement and inflation of the balloon should be done fluoroscopically, and the timing of inflation and deflation should be optimized to achieve peak hemodynamic support.

Clinical Trials

Much of the data on the use of IABP during high-risk PCI, as well as the other support circulatory support devices, comes from the prestent era of coronary interventions. Voudris and colleagues[19] showed that support with IABP during elective high-risk angioplasty was safe and feasible. During a 13-month period from 1987 to 1988, 27 patients, who were considered to be high risk because of decreased left ventricular function or multivessel disease, underwent angioplasty with IABP support. Primary success according to contemporary American College of Cardiology (ACC) guidelines was achieved in all 27 patients. There were no major cardiac events during the hospitalization, and only one IABP-related vascular complication occurred. After a mean follow-up period of 13 months, there were two deaths, one cardiac transplantation, and six cases of symptom-driven target vessel revascularization (22% rate of recurrent angina), which was also successfully performed with IABP support.[19]

Similar outcomes were reported by Kahn and coworkers[18] for a group of 28 high-risk patients during the same period. The most common high-risk feature in this cohort of patients was severe left ventricular dysfunction, but some patients had critical stenoses in the LMCA or a single remaining coronary artery. The procedural success rate was 96% (90 of 94 lesions were successfully dilated). There were 11 cases of intraprocedural hypotension, although the augmented diastolic pressure was maintained over 90 mm Hg in all cases, and the angioplasty was completed in all patients. There were vascular complications associated with the IABP in 11% of the patients. In another series of 21 patients with similar high-risk features,[20] 90% of lesions attempted were successfully dilated without hemodynamic compromise. Device-related complications (e.g., hematoma) occurred in 10% of cases, and procedure-related complications occurred in 14% of cases.[20]

The beneficial effects of IABP support were also shown in high-risk coronary rotational atherectomy.[29] In a retrospective analysis, 28 patients scheduled to undergo rotational atherectomy were placed on IABP support before the coronary intervention. This group was compared with 131 patients with high-risk coronary lesions who did not have an IABP placed a priori. Patients in the group that received a planned IABP were older, had more left ventricular dysfunction, and had a higher incidence of multivessel disease. Although systolic hypotension occurred in 11% of the patients in the study group, diastolic pressure augmentation provided by the IABP allowed successful completion of the procedure in all patients. Hypotension necessitating IABP placement occurred in 7% of the patients in the comparison group. Slow flow occurred at a similar rate in both groups, but 27% of the patients in the comparison group who experienced slow flow developed a non-Q-wave MI, compared with none in the study group. There were no differences in the rate of transfusion requirements or vascular complications.[29]

In a study by Brodie and colleagues,[2] IABP was shown to reduce periprocedural events. The group studied consisted of 213 patients presenting with an acute MI who received an IABP. In contrast to the earlier studies discussed, most patients in this study were treated with stents, and about one third were treated with abciximab, reflecting the use of more contemporary treatments. Although the indication for the IABP in most cases was cardiogenic shock, there were 80 patients who were hemodynamically stable but were considered high risk because of left ventricular dysfunction. In this group, the use of IABP support led to a decreased incidence of prolonged hypotension, cardiac arrest, and ventricular fibrillation, but the difference was not statistically significant because of the low number of patients in this group. IABP use was associated with an increased risk of major bleeding and with higher transfusion rates.

Although IABP use during high-risk coronary interventions has been shown to be effective in supporting the circulation,[19,29] the increased rates of vascular and hemorrhagic complications associated with its use demand careful patient selection.[2,18,21] For this reason, a strategy of provisional IABP support was compared with prophylactic placement of IABP in high-risk interventions in a retrospective, nonrandomized study.[30] Sixty-one patients who received elective IABP were compared with 72 patients in whom support was initiated only if clinically necessary. The patients in the elective IABP group were slightly older, but other high-risk features were similar, including severity of left ventricular dysfunction (ejection fraction [EF] <30%) and rates of multivessel disease and of unstable angina. Rates of stent and glycoprotein inhibitor use were similar for the two groups. Although rates of slow flow were similar in both groups, hemodynamic deterioration occurred only in patients (15%) in the provisional IABP group, and all received urgent IABP support. Rates of vascular complications were low in this study, with only two patients in the provisional IABP group developing groin hematomas. There were no cases of major bleeding. Although not statistically significant, three patients in the provisional IABP group who required urgent placement of an IABP died, compared with one death in the elective group.[30] A summary of the trials using IABP during high-risk PCI is provided in Table 36-2.

Percutaneous Cardiopulmonary Support

Introduction of the portable Bard CardioPulmonary Bypass Support (CR Bard, Inc., Murray Hill, NJ) system in 1985 expanded the application of percutaneous CPS.[31] Although the most common application for temporary circulatory support is for patients who cannot be weaned from cardiopulmonary bypass after cardiac surgery, CPS has also been implemented in the catheterization laboratory emergently as a bridge to cardiac surgery or prophylactically to support high-risk coronary interventions.

CPS circulates and oxygenates blood and can temporarily substitute for the entire circulation, irrespective of cardiac rhythm. CPS unloads the right ventricle but does not unload the left ventricle.[31] The pulmonary and systolic aortic pressures have been shown to decrease, whereas the diastolic and mean systemic arterial pressures remain unchanged.[31,32] In normal-functioning hearts, the reduction in preload and small increase in afterload produced by the arterial inflow reduces wall stress and produces smaller end-diastolic left ventricular volumes because the left ventricle is able to eject the blood it receives. However, in dilated and poorly contracting hearts, especially

Table 36-2. Intra-Aortic Counterpulsation Balloon Pump Clinical Trials

Study	Year	Coronary Intervention	Patients (N)	Revascularization Success Rate (%)	Device-Related Complication Rate (%)	In-Hospital Mortality Rate (%)
Anwar et al[17]	1990	PTCA	97	85.6	2	1
Kahn et al[18]	1990	PTCA	28	96	11	7.1
Voudris et al[19]	1990	PTCA	27	100	3.7	0
Kreidieh et al[20]	1992	PTCA	21	90	9.5	0
Kaul et al[46]	1995	PTCA	20	95	0	5
O'Murchu et al[29]	1995	ROTO/PTCA	28	100	7.1	0
Schreiber et al[47]	1998	PTCA	91	87	27	8.7
Brodie et al[2]	1999	PTCA/stent*	108[†]	89.8	8[‡]	37[§]
Briguori et al[30]	2003	PTCA/stent	61	94	0	8

*Stents used in the last 3 years of the study.
[†]Includes patients with shock or congestive heart failure; the number of patients undergoing high-risk coronary intervention was not defined.
[‡]Includes patients who received intra-aortic balloon pump therapy after percutaneous transluminal coronary angioplasty.
[§]Thirty-day mortality that includes patients with cardiogenic shock.
PTCA, percutaneous transluminal coronary angioplasty; ROTO, rotational atherectomy.

after cardiac arrest, the increase in afterload may impair left ventricular emptying, and another means of assisting emptying of the left ventricle (e.g., IABP) may be necessary. Studies have also shown that CPS does not increase coronary perfusion in the setting of an occlusion, and bypass surgery should be considered if circulation is unable to be restored percutaneously.

Insertion Technique

Before arterial cannulation, angiography of the ilio-femoral arteries is performed to exclude significant arterial disease. Care should be taken to access the artery below the inguinal ligament in the common femoral artery. Invasive monitoring with a pulmonary artery catheter is recommended during support. After venous and arterial access is obtained with a flexible, 0.038-inch guidewire and an 8-Fr dilator, anticoagulation is started with heparin. The flexible wire is replaced with a stiff, 0.038-inch guidewire, and the vein and artery are progressively dilated with a 12- and 14-Fr dilator. Finally, the 18-Fr cannulas are placed, the inflow cannula at the level of the right atrium and the outflow cannula at the level of the aortic bifurcation. The cannulas are then clamped before connecting to the primed perfusion circuit. Priming of the circuit should be performed by a perfusionist while access is being obtained. After carefully de-airing the system, the cannulas are connected to the perfusion circuit, and support is started at 2.0 L/min and progressively advanced by 0.5-L/min increments as needed.[32] After successful coronary intervention, CPS is weaned quickly, usually over 15 minutes, by gradually reducing the flow rate. Volume is infused to increase the left ventricular filling pressure to at least 8 to 10 mmHg or to prebypass levels (whichever is less). If necessary, inotropic agents may be used to allow weaning of support. An intra-aortic balloon can also be used if weaning proves difficult to tolerate.

The Bard percutaneous cardiopulmonary support system (CPS, CR Bard, Murray Hill, NJ) is a portable, battery-operated system that consists of a centrifugal pump (Biomedicus pump), heat exchanger, and membrane oxygenator. Venous inflow is achieved by active suction, not gravity like the classic cardiopulmonary bypass system, making it essential that patients be well hydrated. Central venous access should be avoided while the pump is operating. Percutaneous CPS can be performed only for 6 hours. After 6 hours, platelet aggregation, hemolysis, and increased capillary permeability with plasma loss become major complications.

Clinical Trials

Early reports on a small number of patients showed that using CPS for high-risk angioplasty was feasible, albeit with high rates of femoral access-site complications.[33-35] The national registry of elective supported angioplasty reported data on 801 patients who underwent elective angioplasty with CPS in 25 centers from 1988 to 1992. The suggested inclusion clinical criteria were the presence of severe or unstable angina, at least one likely dilatable coronary artery stenosis, and a left ventricular ejection fraction [LVEF] less than 25% or a target vessel supplying more than one half of the viable myocardium, or both.[36]

Although the initial angioplasty success rate was high in this registry, so were the rates of device-related complications. The strategy was changed to one of standby support for these high-risk interventions. Prophylactic support was implemented in 73% of the patients, and the last 27% of the patients registered had standby support. The overall primary success rate was 93%, and the success rate in the group who had standby support was 91%.[37] The rates of vascular complications (15% versus 6.1%) and transfusions (31% versus 14%) decreased with the change in strategy from prophylactic to standby support. The rates of death (6.3% versus 6%) and emergent bypass surgery (2.5% versus 3.2%) did not change, however, reflecting the high-risk profile of the patients in the registry. Only 16 (7.4%) of 217 patients in the standby strategy required emergency initiation of bypass support. Of these 16 patients, 75% had successful angioplasty without the need for bypass surgery, suggesting that standby support reduced the need for emergency bypass surgery. The only group of patients for whom there was a clear benefit in using prophylactic support was the group with an LVEF of 20% or less. Among these patients, those treated with prophylactic placement of CPS before coronary intervention had a lower mortality rate than those who had CPS on standby (7% versus 18%, $P < .05$).

A separate analysis of the 42 patients in the registry with 60% or more LMCA stenosis who underwent angioplasty of the LMCA were compared with high-risk patients who had another vessel dilated.[38] The hospital mortality rate was 14.3% for patients who had angioplasty of the LMCA, significantly higher than the 4.6% hospital mortality rate for patients who did not have significant LMCA disease and had angioplasty of another vessel ($P < .001$).[38] In the prestent era, adding support with CPS did not improve the outcome of PCI in LMCA disease.

As the insertion technique evolved from requiring surgical cut-down to a percutaneous approach as described by Shawl and associates,[39] the experience with CPS continued to grow in the catheterization laboratory. His group reported one of the largest series of supported angioplasty from 1988 to 1991.[39-41] In the first 51 patients, 94% had three-vessel disease, 70% had an LVEF of 35% or less, and most had been turned down for bypass surgery.[39] All the patients tolerated the coronary intervention, with the mean coronary stenosis improving from 89% to 21%. The hospital mortality rate was 6%, which compared well with the 6.9% mortality rate for patients undergoing coronary bypass surgery with an EF of 35% or less at that time.[42] The most frequent complication was bleeding requiring transfusion, which occurred in 40% of the patients. Other complications included pseudoaneurysm (8%), hematoma (2%), and femoral nerve weakness (8%). With improvement in the cannula removal technique, the requirement for transfusion decreased in later patients to 4% and eliminated the occurrence of femoral nerve injury.[40] In patients with particularly high-risk disease (mean LVEF ≤19.5% ± 3.5%; 54% had dilation of the single remaining patent artery; 17% had dilation of an unprotected LMCA), CPS showed promising short-term and long-term results.[41] Angiographic success was achieved in 98.7% of the arteries attempted in 105 patients (98%). Despite the occurrence of asystole in 5 (4.6%) patients and of electromechanical dissociation in 40 (37%) with balloon inflation, there were no procedural deaths, and all patients were weaned off CPS after the angioplasty. The hospital mortality rate was 4.7%. After a mean follow-up of 24 ± 13 months, 97% of patients were in Canadian Cardiovascular Society (CCS) functional class I or II, compared with only 3% before the intervention (P < .001).[41]

Because of the high rate of complications, attention was turned to using CPS on a standby basis. Two retrospective analyses showed that the incidence of hemodynamic collapse requiring support during angioplasty was less than 1%.[35,43] Subsequently, the National Registry of Elective Cardiopulmonary Support compared the utility of prophylactic with standby PCPS in patients undergoing high-risk angioplasty.[44] The mortality rates were similar: 6.4% in the prophylactic group and 6.1% in the standby group. The rates of procedural success were also similar in the two groups. However, morbidity was significantly higher in the prophylactic CPS group, with 42% of patients sustaining femoral access-site complications or requiring blood transfusions, compared with only 11.7% of patients in the standby group. Of 180 patients in the standby group, only 13 (7.2%) suffered irreversible hemodynamic collapse, and emergency CPS was initiated in less than 5 minutes in 12 of the 13 patients. The patients who did benefit from prophylactic CPS were those with an ejection fraction of 20% or less; a lower mortality rate was associated with support initiated before angioplasty (4.8% versus 18.8%, P < .05).[44]

A later European study evaluated the utility of CPS during the stent era.[45] The report included two groups of patients. Group I comprised 68 patients undergoing elective high-risk coronary intervention. Group II consisted of 24 patients presenting with acute MI and cardiogenic shock. In the elective group, primary success was achieved in 66 (97%) patients, with complete revascularization obtained in 44% of the group. Four patients (6%) developed femoral artery complications, and one patient (1.4%) died before discharge. After 28 ± 19 months of follow-up, major adverse cardiac events occurred in 30% of patients, including seven deaths (10%). Compared with the previous literature on supported angioplasty with CPS, this study showed that CPS can be used effectively during coronary stenting and demonstrated an improvement in the rate of complications.

Two studies compared CPS and IABP for high-risk coronary interventions. One prospective trial randomized patients to CPS or IABP support during PCI, which was considered high risk because of the presence of unstable angina with poor left ventricular function in a target vessel supplying more than one half of the remaining viable myocardium.[46] Between June 1991 and November 1993, 40 patients were randomized. All patients had a history of a prior MI, most had three-vessel disease, and the mean ejection fraction in both groups was lower than 25%. All patients were treated with angioplasty using balloon inflations longer than 2 minutes. Patients in both groups tolerated balloon inflations lasting 2 to 3 minutes without hemodynamic decompensation. Primary success was achieved in 19 of 20 patients in both groups, with similar angiographic results. There were no vascular or hemorrhagic complications in the IABP group, whereas two patients assigned to CPS developed vascular complications requiring surgical repair, and five other patients required blood transfusions.[46] There was one death in each group, thought to be caused by acute vessel closure after discontinuation of support. The study authors concluded that IABP and CPS were effective in supporting high-risk coronary interventions, with IABP having lower rates of complications.

Schreiber and colleagues[47] reported retrospective, observational data comparing outcomes in a larger group of patients who had undergone high-risk PCI with hemodynamic support.[47] Over a 4-year period, 149 patients who had a high-risk PCI underwent prophylactic placement of an IABP (91) or CPS (58). Patients presenting with acute MI, unstable angina, and stable angina were included if they were hemodynamically stable before the procedure. Patients were considered high risk if they had poor ventricular function, had a culprit vessel supplying most of myocardium, or required multivessel PCI. Patients who received CPS were more likely to be male (91% versus 73%, P < .01), have a history of chronic angina (91% versus 69%, P = .003), have congestive heart failure (59% versus 35%, P = .008), and have a lower mean ejection fraction (26% ± 13% versus 32% ± 14%, P < .01). Multivessel PCI was performed more often in the CPS group (40% versus 20%, P < .01). Despite the greater severity of disease in the CPS group, successful angioplasty was achieved more often in the CPS group compared with the IABP group (99% versus 87% of lesions, P = .005). Major cardiac events (i.e., MI, CABG, stroke, and death) occurred at similar rates in both groups, although the rate of CABG trended higher in the IABP group without reaching statistical significance (1.7% versus 6.5%, P = .33). The rate of death was high in both groups (12% in the CPS group versus 8.7% in the IABP group, P = .71).[47] As in the study of Kaul and associates,[46] access-site complications and transfusions occurred more frequently in the CPS group. The

Table 36-3. Cardiopulmonary Support (CPS) Clinical Trials

Study	Year	Coronary Intervention	Patients (N)	Revascularization Success Rate (%)	Device-Related Complication Rate (%)	Transfusion Rate (%)	In-Hospital Mortality Rate (%)	Bypass Time (min)
Vogel et al[70]	1988	PTCA	9	100	11	100	11	NR
Shawl et al[39]	1989	PTCA	51*	100	14	38	5.8	37
Shawl et al[40]	1990	PTCA	121[†]	NR	9.9	29.7	NR	37[‡]
Teirstein et al[44]	1993	PTCA	389[§]	88.7	12.6	39	6.4	NR
Sivananthan et al[34]	1994	PTCA	13	83	83	100	7.7	92.8 ± 46
Kaul et al[46]	1995	PTCA	20	95	10	25	5	NR
Vogel et al[37]	1995	PTCA	801[¶]	93	15[¶]	31[¶]	6.9	NR
Shawl et al[41]	1996	PTCA	107	98	4.7	1.9	4.7	46 ± 30
Schreiber et al[47]	1998	PTCA	58	99	50	60	12	60 ± 45
de Lezo et al[71]	2002	PTCA	68**	97	6	NR	1.5	NR

*Includes 20 patients with a left ventricular ejection fraction ≤25% who were included in the 1996 report.
[†]A total of 121 patients reported, 101 of whom underwent elective coronary interventions.
[‡]Time reported for the elective interventions.
[§]Number of patients with prophylactic percutaneous CPS placement.
[¶]Twenty-seven percent of patients were treated with a standby strategy.
[¶]Complication and transfusion rate reported for the group with percutaneous CPS placed prophylactically.
**A total of 92 patients were reported, 68 of whom had elective procedures.
NR, not reported; PTCA, percutaneous transluminal coronary angioplasty.

higher angioplasty success rate in the CPS group is likely explained by the longer duration of balloon inflation tolerated by this group. This difference would likely be overcome with the use of stents. The studies describing CPS in high-risk PCI are summarized in Table 36-3.

Percutaneous Left Ventricular Assist Devices

Left Atrial to Femoral Artery Bypass

The most recent innovation in circulatory support that is available to interventionalists is the pVAD. The left atrial to femoral artery bypass strategy was first described in 1962 by Dennis and was initially used in patients who could not be weaned from cardiopulmonary bypass after surgery.[48-50] A dedicated system with a compact centrifugal pump (i.e., TandemHeart pVAD) was developed to allow rapid percutaneous institution of left atrial to femoral artery bypass (Fig. 36-1). The pump cycles oxygenated blood from the left atrium to the femoral artery without the need for an external oxygenator or heat exchanger.

The left atrial to femoral artery bypass system directly unloads the left ventricle and decreases cardiac filling pressures, cardiac workload, and myocardial oxygen demand.[51,52] Previous studies have shown a decrease in infarct size in acutely ischemic myocardium with the use of a transseptal left ventricular assist device. Right ventricular failure is a contraindication to use of a transseptal left ventricular assist device.

Insertion Technique

After angiography of the distal aorta and iliac vessels to exclude significant arterial occlusive disease, access in the femoral vein is obtained. After a transseptal puncture is performed, the interatrial septum is dilated with a two-stage 14- and 21-Fr dilator, and the 22-Fr inflow cannula is advanced to the left atrium under angiographic and echocardiographic guidance.[51,53] The outflow 15- to 17-Fr cannula is then inserted by the Seldinger technique over a stiff guidewire and advanced to the common iliac artery. The cannulas are de-aired and connected to the pump.

The TandemHeart pVAD is a continuous-flow centrifugal pump that operates at 7500 rpm and provides up to 3.5 L/min of blood flow. The pump contains a single moving part (i.e., impeller) suspended by a magnetic force on a thin, lubricating film of fluid.[54] A continuous infusion of heparinized saline solution provides the hydrodynamic bearing for the pump and local anticoagulation and cooling of the motor.

Clinical Trials

A small, prospective feasibility study evaluated the hemodynamic effects of the TandemHeart pVAD in short-term stabilization of patients with cardiogenic shock.[52] The device was safely implanted in 18 patients, with a mean duration of support of 4 ± 3 days. Hemodynamic indices, including pulmonary capillary wedge pressure (PCWP), peak airway pressure, cardiac output, and systemic blood pressure, showed a significant improvement on pVAD support. During support, there was negligible hemolysis; bleeding requiring transfusion occurred in five patients, and two with peripheral arterial disease required surgical placement of an antegrade perfusion cannula to relieve limb ischemia.

There are only a few case reports and small series on the experience with the left atrial to femoral artery bypass system to support high-risk coronary interventions[51,53-57] (see "Case Study"). In these series, the

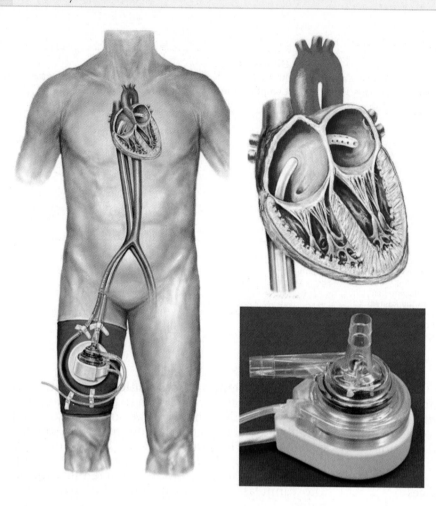

Figure 36-1. TandemHeart percutaneous left ventricular assist device. The inflow cannula to the centrifugal pump is inserted transseptally to the left atrium, and the outflow is inserted in the femoral artery.

pVAD has been shown to be easily implanted by experienced interventionalists and to provide the circulatory support to allow high-risk coronary interventions to be done successfully in a controlled fashion (Table 36-4). Because of the transseptal puncture required, the TandemHeart pVAD will likely be best suited for elective initiation of hemodynamic support because insertion times tend to be longer than for IABP or CPS.

CASE STUDY

An 80-year-old man with severe chronic obstructive pulmonary disease, chronic renal insufficiency, and carotid artery disease presented with unstable angina. Echocardiography revealed severe left ventricular dysfunction (ejection fraction of 10%), anterior wall akinesis, and moderate mitral regurgitation. Positron emission tomography showed lateral wall ischemia and high anterolateral viability. Cardiac catheterization revealed 95% distal LMCA disease involving the ostia of the left anterior descending (LAD) and left circumflex arteries (LCx) (Fig. 36-2) and a 50% stenosis in the middle right coronary artery. The patient was thought to be at high risk for surgical revascularization, and we proceeded with hemodynamically supported LMCA intervention with the TandemHeart pVAD. After transseptal placement of a 21-Fr inflow cannula in the left atrium and placement of a 15-Fr

outflow cannula in the right common iliac artery, left atrial to distal aorta bypass was achieved with a nonpulsatile flow rate of 3.0 L/min. Bifurcation stenting of the LAD and LCx arteries was performed with two sirolimus-eluting stents deployed simultaneously using the kissing technique (Figs. 36-3 and 36-4). There was a significant decrease in aortic pulse pressure due to diminished stroke volume, but the mean perfusion pressure was maintained, and the patient remained hemodynamically stable without angina or arrhythmia (Fig. 36-5). The patient was discharged 2 days after the procedure and remained angina free at 1 month of follow-up.*

Transvalvular Left Ventricular Assist Devices

In 1988, Wampler and colleagues[58] described a catheter-mounted transvalvular left ventricular assist device, which was initially placed surgically through the femoral artery. Development of a smaller (13- or 14-Fr) system allowed percutaneous insertion of the device. Two investigational devices, the Impella and

---

*The case study is adapted from Naidu SS, Rohatgi S, Herrmann HC, Glaser R: Unprotected left main "kissing" stent implantation with a percutaneous ventricular assist device. J Invasive Cardiol 2004;16:683-684.

Table 36-4. Left Atrial to Femoral Artery Bypass Clinical Trials

Study	Year	Patients (N)	Insertion Time (min)	Revascularization Success Rate (%)	Mean Support Duration	In-Hospital Mortality Rate (%)	Other Complications
Glassman et al[57]*	1993	13	†	100	43 ± 17 min	0	Transfusion in 1 of 13 patients Small left to right shunts in 2 of 13 patients
Lemos et al[53]	2003	7‡	31 to 69	92.3	55 ± 96 hr	1	Bleeding in 4 of 7 patients Hypothermia in 2 of 7 patients
Aragon et al[51]	2005	8	†	100	§	1	Acute renal failure requiring hemodialysis in 1 of 8 patients
Kar et al[56]	2006	5	†	100	107 min +¶	1	Blood transfusions in all patients Groin hematomas in 2 of 5 patients

*The device used in this series was not the TandemHeart percutaneous ventricular assist device (pVAD).
†Not reported.
‡Five patients were hemodynamically stable before insertion of the pVAD.
§Not reported, but all patients had the pVAD removed in the catheterization laboratory at the end of the coronary intervention. The mean procedure time was 169 ± 21 minutes.
¶Excludes duration of support for one patient who required support for an additional 48 hours because of persistent poor left ventricular function.

Hemopump, have been tested clinically, but only the Impella remains available for restricted use as part of research protocols.

The Impella Recover LP 2.5 (Impella Cardiotechnik, Aachen, Germany) is a micro-axial rotary blood pump that unloads the left ventricle by directly expelling blood from the left ventricle to the aorta (Fig. 36-6). The device can deliver an output of up to 2.5 L/min. The Impella device has been shown to unload the left ventricle by decreasing the end-diastolic pressure, decreasing end-diastolic and end-systolic volume, and increasing cardiac output.[59,60]

Insertion Techniques
Before the procedure, an echocardiogram should be performed to exclude left ventricular thrombus, especially because the patient that would be considered for this type of support is at higher risk for having a thrombus because of decreased ventricular function. Angiography of the distal aorta and iliac vessels should also be performed before insertion of the femoral sheath. The percutaneous device is available in 12- and 13-Fr sizes. After inserting an appropriate-sized sheath in the femoral artery, an exchange-length (300-cm), 0.014-inch guidewire is delivered to the left ventricle with an angiographic catheter (e.g.,

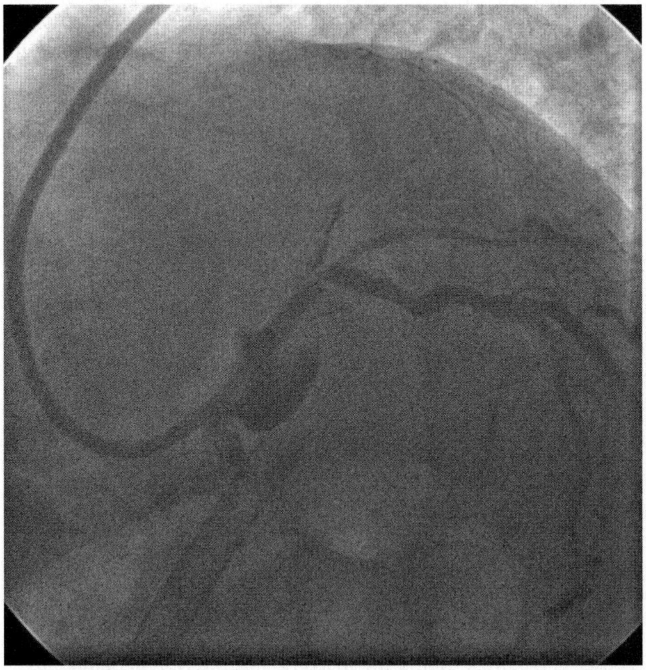

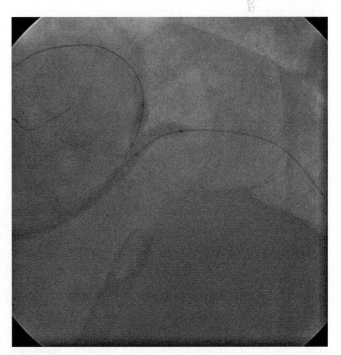

Figure 36-2. Baseline angiography showing distal left main coronary artery stenosis and subtotal occlusion of the proximal left anterior descending coronary artery.

Figure 36-3. Percutaneous coronary intervention using two sirolimus-eluting stents in a kissing technique

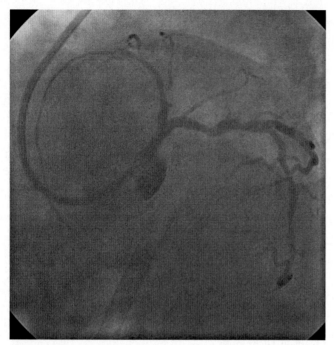

Figure 36-4. Final angiography showing reconstruction of the distal left main, proximal left anterior descending coronary, and left circumflex coronary arteries.

JR4, MPA). The device is then advanced over the wire and positioned across the aortic valve under angiographic guidance. Proper placement is critical to prevent damage to the aortic valve leaflets. The proximal part of the catheter connects to a portable mobile console that provides power and allows control of the pump.[60]

The Impella Recover LP 2.5 device is mounted on a 9-Fr pigtail catheter (see Fig. 36-6), which sits in the left ventricular cavity. The device provides flows up to 2.5 L/min at its maximal rotational speed of 50,000 rpm, and it can be safely left in place for up to 5 days.[59] A heparinized 20% dextrose solution continuously lubricates the pump.

Clinical Trials

A recent study evaluated the hemodynamic effects of the Impella Recover LP 2.5 left ventricular assist device. In 10 high-risk patients who had successful placement of the device, a 7-Fr pressure-conductance catheter was also placed in the left ventricle for hemodynamic assessment. At maximum support, the Impella device did not significantly affect end-systolic pressure, end-systolic or end-diastolic volume, or cardiac output. There was no significant effect on brain natriuretic peptide levels during or after device support, which lasted a mean of 144 ± 88 minutes.[61] The investigators argued that perhaps having the additional 7-Fr catheter across the aortic valve decreased the effect of the device on the measured hemodynamic indices.

A multicenter, nonrandomized, prospective trial assessed the safety and efficacy of the Impella device in patients presenting with cardiogenic shock and in patients undergoing elective high-risk coronary revascularization (PCI or off-pump coronary artery bypass).[62] Of a total of 36 patients who were studied, 23 patients were hemodynamically stable before a scheduled revascularization. The high-risk features in the patients who underwent PCI included LMCA or single-remaining-vessel disease with poor left ven-

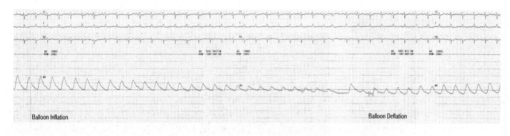

Balloon Inflation

Balloon Deflation

Figure 36-5. Aortic pressure tracing during balloon inflation shows a significant decrease in pulse pressure due to diminished stroke volume, with preserved mean perfusion pressure by means of the TandemHeart bypass circuit.

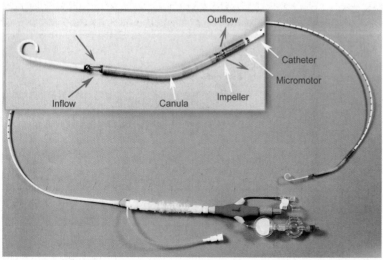

Outflow

Catheter

Micromotor

Inflow

Canula

Impeller

Figure 36-6. Impella Recover LP 2.5 device. (Modified from Valgimigli M, Steendijk P, Sianos G, et al: Left ventricular unloading and concomitant total cardiac output increase by the use of percutaneous Impella Recover LP 2.5 assist device during high-risk coronary intervention. Catheter Cardiovasc Interv 2005;65:263-267.)

Table 36-5. Transvalvular Left Ventricular Assist Device Clinical Trials

Study	Year	Patients (N)	Revascularization Success Rate	Device-Related Complication	Hemolysis	Support Duration (hr)
Dens et al[62]*	2006	23	100%	17%	22%	2.1 ± 1.6
Valgimigli[61]	2006	10	100%	30%†	60%	2.4 ± 1.5
Henriques[22]	2006	19	100%	5%	NR	2‡

*Revascularization strategy included percutaneous coronary intervention and off-pump coronary artery bypass grafting.
†Four of 10 patients also received a transfusion.
‡Maximum support time reported.

Table 36-6. Comparison of Circulatory Support Modalities

Support Type	Insertion Technique	Major Complications	Effect on Circulation	Length of Support	Advantages	Limitations	Contraindications
IABP	Percutaneous or surgical	Limb ischemia, aortic dissection	Augment CO by up to 1 L/min	Up to 14 days	More prolonged support duration, unloads the LV	Requires stable rhythm, lowest level of hemodynamic support	Moderate to severe AI, aortic disease, uncontrolled sepsis, coagulopathy, PAD
CPS	Percutaneous or surgical	Bleeding, hemolysis, stroke, embolus	Provide complete circulatory support	Up to 6 hours	Independent of rhythm, allows controlled transfer to the OR, full support	Limited duration of support, requires perfusionist, does not unload the LV	Moderate to severe AI, PAD, coagulopathy
pVAD	Percutaneous	Pericardial hemorrhage, aortic puncture, limb ischemia	Augment CO by up to 3.5 L/min	Up to 14 days	Prolonged support duration, full LV support, does not require external oxygenation or heater	Large arterial cannulas, requires transseptal puncture	VSD, PAD, RV failure
Transvalvular LVAD	Percutaneous or surgical	Aortic valve damage	Augment CO by up to 2.5 L/min	Up to 5 days	Unloads the LV	Aortic stenosis	LV thrombus, VSD, aortic valve disease, hypertrophic obstructive CM

AI, aortic insufficiency; CM, cardiomyopathy; CO, cardiac output; CPS, cardiopulmonary support; IABP, intra-aortic balloon pump; LV, left ventricle or left ventricular; LVAD, left ventricular assist device; OR, operating room; PAD, peripheral artery disease; pVAD, percutaneous ventricular assist device; RV, right ventricular; VSD, ventricular septal defect.

tricular function. The overall rate of bleeding was 8%, and hemolysis was seen in 25% of patients. Technical pump failure occurred in 5 of the 36 patients, including a cannula fracture. In the elective revascularization group, a small but significant decrease in filling pressures occurred with device support (PCWP decreased from 14.3 ± 5.8 to 10 ± 2.9 mm Hg, P = .327), but the mean arterial pressure did not change significantly.[62]

Another safety and feasibility trial in Amsterdam[22] showed that the device could be used to provide circulatory support during high-risk coronary interventions. The device was used in 19 patients, 17 of whom were scheduled to have an elective coronary intervention. The guiding catheter was successfully engaged and remained stable during the procedure in all patients. Maximum support time was 120 minutes, excluding one patient who could not be weaned from bypass after cardiac surgery and had the Impella placed for 30 hours. There was only one case of access-site hematoma requiring a transfusion. No significant increase in or development of aortic insuf-

ficiency occurred in 12 patients who had evaluation of the aortic valve during the procedure, but there was no follow-up evaluation. Table 36-5 provides a summary of these trials.

The Hemopump system (Medtronic, Minneapolis, MN) also expels blood from the left ventricle to the aorta by use of a rotating turbine that imparts a rotational and longitudinal velocity to the blood. This device has been shown to increase the cardiac output and reduce mean pulmonary artery pressure in clinical trials.[63-65] However, the Hemopump was not shown to significantly affect coronary blood flow velocities before or after angioplasty.[64] Small feasibility trials have shown the Hemopump to be safe in supporting high-risk interventions.[63,64]

CONCLUSIONS

With the development of stents and technical improvements in coronary wires, guide catheters, and balloons, the rates of abrupt closure and of hemodynamic collapse during PCI have decreased. However, the improved technology has also allowed cardiologists to undertake higher-risk procedures that in the early days of coronary angioplasty would have been referred for bypass surgery. No formal guidelines exist to direct the use of circulatory support devices during high-risk coronary interventions, and the decision to implement them remains that of the individual interventionalist. The first step in using the devices described is a thorough understanding of the clinical characteristics and angiographic factors that portend a high-risk procedure. The choice of support device requires an understanding the level of support provided by each device and the specific risks associated with its use (Table 36-6).

REFERENCES

1. Herrmann H, Hirshfeld J: Emergent stenting for failed percutaneous transluminal coronary angioplasty. *In* Herrmann H, Hirshfeld J (eds): Clinical Use of the Palmaz-Schatz Intracoronary Stent. Mount Kisco, NY, Futura Publishing, 1993, pp 93-109.
2. Brodie BR, Stuckey TD, Hansen C, et al: Intra-aortic balloon counterpulsation before primary percutaneous transluminal coronary angioplasty reduces catheterization laboratory events in high-risk patients with acute myocardial infarction. Am J Cardiol 1999;84:18-23.
3. Cohen HA, Williams DO, Holmes DR Jr, et al: Impact of age on procedural and 1-year outcome in percutaneous transluminal coronary angioplasty: A report from the NHLBI Dynamic Registry. Am Heart J 2003;146:513-519.
4. Herrmann HC, Buchbinder M, Clemen MW, et al: Emergent use of balloon-expandable coronary artery stenting for failed percutaneous transluminal coronary angioplasty. Circulation 1992;86:812-819.
5. Seshadri N, Whitlow PL, Acharya N, et al: Emergency coronary artery bypass surgery in the contemporary percutaneous coronary intervention era. Circulation 2002;106:2346-2350.
6. Williams DO, Holubkov R, Yeh W, et al: Percutaneous coronary intervention in the current era compared with 1985-1986: The National Heart, Lung, and Blood Institute Registries. Circulation 2000;102:2945-2951.
7. Hartzler GO, Rutherford BD, McConahay DR, et al: "High-risk" percutaneous transluminal coronary angioplasty. Am J Cardiol 1988;61:33G-37G.
8. Block PC, Peterson ED, Krone R, et al: Identification of variables needed to risk adjust outcomes of coronary interventions: Evidence-based guidelines for efficient data collection. J Am Coll Cardiol 1998;32:275-282.
9. Wu C, Hannan EL, Walford G, et al: A risk score to predict in-hospital mortality for percutaneous coronary interventions. J Am Coll Cardiol 2006;47:654-660.
10. Singh M, Rihal CS, Selzer F, et al: Validation of Mayo Clinic risk adjustment model for in-hospital complications after percutaneous coronary interventions, using the National Heart, Lung, and Blood Institute dynamic registry. J Am Coll Cardiol 2003;42:1722-1728.
11. Holper EM, Blair J, Selzer F, et al: The impact of ejection fraction on outcomes after percutaneous coronary intervention in patients with congestive heart failure: An analysis of the National Heart, Lung, and Blood Institute Percutaneous Transluminal Coronary Angioplasty Registry and Dynamic Registry. Am Heart J 2006;151:69-75.
12. Keelan PC, Johnston JM, Koru-Sengul T, et al: Comparison of in-hospital and one-year outcomes in patients with left ventricular ejection fractions < or = 40%, 41% to 49%, and > or = 50% having percutaneous coronary revascularization. Am J Cardiol 2003;91:1168-1172.
13. Wilensky RL, Selzer F, Johnston J, et al: Relation of percutaneous coronary intervention of complex lesions to clinical outcomes (from the NHLBI Dynamic Registry). Am J Cardiol 2002;90:216-221.
14. Bergelson BA, Jacobs AK, Cupples LA, et al: Prediction of risk for hemodynamic compromise during percutaneous transluminal coronary angioplasty. Am J Cardiol 1992;70:1540-1545.
15. Myler RK, Shaw RE, Stertzer SH, et al: Lesion morphology and coronary angioplasty: Current experience and analysis. J Am Coll Cardiol 1992;19:1641-1652.
16. Laskey WK, Selzer F, Vlachos HA, et al: Comparison of in-hospital and one-year outcomes in patients with and without diabetes mellitus undergoing percutaneous catheter intervention (from the National Heart, Lung, and Blood Institute Dynamic Registry). Am J Cardiol 2002;90:1062-1067.
17. Anwar A, Mooney MR, Stertzer SH, et al: Intra-aortic balloon counterpulsation support for elective coronary angioplasty in the setting of poor left ventricular function: A two center experience. J Invasive Cardiol 1990;2:175-180.
18. Kahn JK, Rutherford BD, McConahay DR, et al: Supported "high risk" coronary angioplasty using intraaortic balloon pump counterpulsation. J Am Coll Cardiol 1990;15:1151-1155.
19. Voudris V, Marco J, Morice MC, et al: "High-risk" percutaneous transluminal coronary angioplasty with preventive intra-aortic balloon counterpulsation. Cathet Cardiovasc Diagn 1990;19:160-164.
20. Kreidieh I, Davies DW, Lim R, et al: High-risk coronary angioplasty with elective intra-aortic balloon pump support. Int J Cardiol 1992;35:147-152.
21. Osterne EC, Alexim GA, da Motta VP, et al: Intraaortic balloon pump support during coronary angioplasty. Initial experience. Arq Bras Cardiol 1999;73:191-200.
22. Henriques JP, Remmelink M, Baan J Jr, et al: Safety and feasibility of elective high-risk percutaneous coronary intervention procedures with left ventricular support of the Impella Recover LP 2.5. Am J Cardiol 2006;97:990-992.
23. Mulukutla SR, Pacella JJ, Cohen HA: Percutaneous mechanical assist devices for severe left ventricular dysfunction. *In* Hasdai E, Berger PB, Battler A, Holmes DR Jr (eds): Contemporary Cardiology: Cardiogenic Shock: Diagnosis and Treatment. Totowa, NJ, Humana Press, 2002.
24. Kantrowitz A, Tjonneland S, Freed PS, et al: Initial clinical experience with intraaortic balloon pumping in cardiogenic shock. JAMA 1968;203:113-8.
25. Bolooki H: Current status of circulatory support with an intra-aortic balloon pump. Cardiol Clin 1985;3:123-133.
26. Bregman D, Casarella WJ: Percutaneous intraaortic balloon pumping: Initial clinical experience. Ann Thorac Surg 1980;29:153-155.
27. Weber KT, Janicki JS: Intraaortic balloon counterpulsation. A review of physiological principles, clinical results, and device safety. Ann Thorac Surg 1974;17:602-636.
28. Buckley MJ, Leinbach RC, Kastor JA, et al: Hemodynamic evaluation of intra-aortic balloon pumping in man. Circulation 1970;41(Suppl):II-130-II-136.
29. O'Murchu B, Foreman RD, Shaw RE, et al: Role of intra-aortic balloon pump counterpulsation in high risk coronary rotational atherectomy. J Am Coll Cardiol 1995;26:1270-1275.
30. Briguori C, Sarais C, Pagnotta P, et al: Elective versus provisional intra-aortic balloon pumping in high-risk percutaneous transluminal coronary angioplasty. Am Heart J 2003;145:700-707.
31. Litzie A: Extracorporeal cardiopulmonary bypass support: A historical and current perspective. *In* Shawl F (ed): Supported Complex and High Risk Coronary Angioplasty. Dordrecht, The Netherlands, Kluwer Academic Publishers, 1991, pp 35-46.
32. Shawl F: Percutaneous cardiopulmonary bypass support: Technique, indications and complications. *In* Shawl F (ed): Supported Complex and High Risk Coronary Angioplasty. Dordrecht, The Netherlands, Kluwer Academic Publishers, 1991, pp 65-100.
33. Vogel RA: The Maryland experience: Angioplasty and valvuloplasty using percutaneous cardiopulmonary support. Am J Cardiol 1988;62:11K-14K.

34. Sivananthan MU, Rees MR, Browne TF, et al: Coronary angioplasty in high risk patients with percutaneous cardiopulmonary support. Eur Heart J 1994;15:1057-1062.

35. Ferrari M, Scholz KH, Figulla HR: PTCA with the use of cardiac assist devices: Risk stratification, short- and long-term results. Cathet Cardiovasc Diagn 1996;38:242-248.

36. Vogel RA, Shawl F, Tommaso C, et al: Initial report of the National Registry of Elective Cardiopulmonary Bypass Supported Coronary Angioplasty. J Am Coll Cardiol 1990;15:23-29.

37. Vogel RA: Cardiopulmonary bypass support of high risk coronary angioplasty patients: Registry results. J Interv Cardiol 1995;8:193-197.

38. Tommaso CL, Vogel JH, Vogel RA: Coronary angioplasty in high-risk patients with left main coronary stenosis: Results from the National Registry of Elective Supported Angioplasty. Cathet Cardiovasc Diagn 1992;25:169-173.

39. Shawl FA, Domanski MJ, Punja S, et al: Percutaneous cardiopulmonary bypass support in high-risk patients undergoing percutaneous transluminal coronary angioplasty. Am J Cardiol 1989;64:1258-1263.

40. Shawl FA, Domanski MJ, Wish MH, et al: Percutaneous cardiopulmonary bypass support in the catheterization laboratory: Technique and complications. Am Heart J 1990;120:195-203.

41. Shawl FA, Quyyumi AA, Bajaj S, et al: Percutaneous cardiopulmonary bypass-supported coronary angioplasty in patients with unstable angina pectoris or myocardial infarction and a left ventricular ejection fraction < or = 25%. Am J Cardiol 1996;77:14-19.

42. Alderman EL, Fisher LD, Litwin P, et al: Results of coronary artery surgery in patients with poor left ventricular function (CASS). Circulation 1983;68:785-795.

43. Guarneri EM, Califano JR, Schatz RA, et al: Utility of standby cardiopulmonary support for elective coronary interventions. Catheter Cardiovasc Interv 1999;46:32-35.

44. Teirstein PS, Vogel RA, Dorros G, et al: Prophylactic versus standby cardiopulmonary support for high risk percutaneous transluminal coronary angioplasty. J Am Coll Cardiol 1993;21:590-596.

45. Suarez de Lezo J, Pan M, Medina A, et al: Percutaneous cardiopulmonary support in critical patients needing coronary interventions with stents. Catheter Cardiovasc Interv 2002;57:467-475.

46. Kaul U, Sahay S, Bahl VK, et al: Coronary angioplasty in high risk patients: Comparison of elective intraaortic balloon pump and percutaneous cardiopulmonary bypass support—A randomized study. J Interv Cardiol 1995;8:199-205.

47. Schreiber TL, Kodali UR, O'Neill WW, et al: Comparison of acute results of prophylactic intraaortic balloon pumping with cardiopulmonary support for percutaneous transluminal coronary angioplasty (PCTA). Cathet Cardiovasc Diagn 1998;45:115-119.

48. Killen DA, Piehler JM, Borkon AM, et al: Bio-Medicus ventricular assist device for salvage of cardiac surgical patients. Ann Thorac Surg 1991;52:230-235.

49. Pavie A, Leger P, Nzomvuama A, et al: Left centrifugal pump cardiac assist with transseptal percutaneous left atrial cannula. Artif Organs 1998;22:502-507.

50. Edmunds LH Jr, Herrmann HC, DiSesa VJ, et al: Left ventricular assist without thoracotomy: Clinical experience with the Dennis method. Ann Thorac Surg 1994;57:880-885.

51. Aragon J, Lee MS, Kar S, et al: Percutaneous left ventricular assist device: "TandemHeart" for high-risk coronary intervention. Catheter Cardiovasc Interv 2005;65:346-352.

52. Thiele H, Lauer B, Hambrecht R, et al: Reversal of cardiogenic shock by percutaneous left atrial-to-femoral arterial bypass assistance. Circulation 2001;104:2917-2922.

53. Lemos PA, Cummins P, Lee CH, et al: Usefulness of percutaneous left ventricular assistance to support high-risk percutaneous coronary interventions. Am J Cardiol 2003;91:479-481.

54. Vranckx P, Foley DP, de Feijter PJ, et al: Clinical introduction of the TandemHeart, a percutaneous left ventricular assist device, for circulatory support during high-risk percutaneous coronary intervention. Int J Cardiovasc Interv 2003;5:35-39.

55. Kar B, Butkevich A, Civitello AB, et al: Hemodynamic support with a percutaneous left ventricular assist device during stenting of an unprotected left main coronary artery. Tex Heart Inst J 2004;31:84-86.

56. Kar B, Forrester M, Gemmato C, et al: Use of the TandemHeart percutaneous ventricular assist device to support patients undergoing high-risk percutaneous coronary intervention. J Invasive Cardiol 2006;18:93-96.

57. Glassman E, Chinitz LA, Levite HA, et al: Percutaneous left atrial to femoral arterial bypass pumping for circulatory support in high-risk coronary angioplasty. Cathet Cardiovasc Diagn 1993;29:210-216.

58. Wampler RK, Moise JC, Frazier OH, et al: In vivo evaluation of a peripheral vascular access axial flow blood pump. ASAIO Trans 1988;34:450-454.

59. Valgimigli M, Steendijk P, Sianos G, et al: Left ventricular unloading and concomitant total cardiac output increase by the use of percutaneous Impella Recover LP 2.5 assist device during high-risk coronary intervention. Catheter Cardiovasc Interv 2005;65:263-267.

60. Reesink KD, Dekker AL, Van Ommen V, et al: Miniature intracardiac assist device provides more effective cardiac unloading and circulatory support during severe left heart failure than intraaortic balloon pumping. Chest 2004;126:896-902.

61. Valgimigli M, Steendijk P, Serruys PW, et al: Use of Impella Recover LP 2.5 left ventricular assist device during high-risk percutaneous coronary interventions; clinical, haemodynamic and biochemical findings. EuroIntervention 2006;2:91-100.

62. Dens J, Meyns B, Hilgers RD, et al: First experience with the Impella Recover LP 2.5 micro axial pump in patients with cardiogenic shock or undergoing high-risk revascularization. EuroIntervention 2006;2:84-90.

63. Scholz KH, Dubois-Rande JL, Urban P, et al: Clinical experience with the percutaneous Hemopump during high-risk coronary angioplasty. Am J Cardiol 1998;82:1107-1110, A6.

64. Dubois-Rande JL, Teiger E, Garot J, et al: Effects of the 14F hemopump on coronary hemodynamics in patients undergoing high-risk coronary angioplasty. Am Heart J 1998;135(Pt 1):844-849.

65. Smalling RW, Sweeney M, Lachterman B, et al: Transvalvular left ventricular assistance in cardiogenic shock secondary to acute myocardial infarction: Evidence for recovery from near fatal myocardial stunning. J Am Coll Cardiol 1994;23:637-644.

66. Bourassa MG, Detre KM, Johnston JM, et al: Effect of prior revascularization on outcome following percutaneous coronary intervention; NHLBI Dynamic Registry. Eur Heart J 2002;23:1546-1555.

67. Lee RJ, Lee SH, Shyu KG, et al: Immediate and long-term outcomes of stent implantation for unprotected left main coronary artery disease. Int J Cardiol 2001;80:173-177.

68. Silvestri M, Barragan P, Sainsous J, et al: Unprotected left main coronary artery stenting: Immediate and medium-term outcomes of 140 elective procedures. J Am Coll Cardiol 2000;35:1543-1550.

69. Mehta RH, Harjai KJ, Cox D, et al: Clinical and angiographic correlates and outcomes of suboptimal coronary flow in patients with acute myocardial infarction undergoing primary percutaneous coronary intervention. J Am Coll Cardiol 2003;42:1739-1746.

70. Vogel RA, Tommaso CL, Gundry SR: Initial experience with coronary angioplasty and aortic valvuloplasty using elective semipercutaneous cardiopulmonary support. Am J Cardiol 1988;62(Pt 1):811-813.

71. de Lezo JS, Medina A, Romero M, et al: Effectiveness of percutaneous device occlusion for atrial septal defect in adult patients with pulmonary hypertension. Am Heart J 2002;144:877-880.

37 Regional Centers of Excellence for the Care of Patients with Acute Ischemic Heart Disease

Dean J. Kereiakes and Alice K. Jacobs

KEY POINTS

- Coronary heart disease is the leading cause of death and disability in the United States. Specialized centers of care have been implemented for patients with trauma or stroke, but the lack of specialized centers of care for patients with acute ischemic heart disease is not commensurate with the magnitude of this public health problem.

- Regional care for patients with acute coronary syndromes implies "meaningful networking" associations between community and rural hospitals that do not provide tertiary cardiovascular services and a tertiary cardiovascular service provider. The definition of *networking* ranges from being a merged affiliate (i.e., same hospital system) to sharing common patient care protocols, as well as tracking, reporting, and auditing clinical practice guideline compliance, core measures, and clinical outcomes.

- A direct relationship exists between annual volumes of cardiovascular procedures (e.g., coronary bypass surgery, coronary angioplasty, stenting) achieved by either physician operators or hospital facilities and optimal clinical outcomes, including survival. Physicians and hospitals that perform the highest annual volumes of procedures have the best outcomes.

- Medical resources are limited. There exists a critical shortage of subspecialized nurses for intensive cardiovascular care and cardiovascular physician providers. The trend toward proliferation of smaller "heart centers" under the guise of patient convenience is counter to the well-established link between higher procedural volumes and better clinical outcomes, and it further taxes the already limited resource pools of subspecialty nurses and cardiologists.

- The prehospital phase of acute ST-segment elevation myocardial infarction (STEMI) is critically important. The performance and transmission of a 12-lead electrocardiogram by emergency medical service providers in the field at the point of first medical contact can significantly reduce the time delays to initiation of STEMI treatment with fibrinolytic or primary percutaneous coronary interventions and thereby reduce mortality.

- The American College of Cardiology/American Heart Association recommended door-to-needle (<30 minutes) or door-to-balloon (<90 minutes) times to starting treatment do not represent the optimal delays before beginning treatment, but instead should be considered the longest acceptable delays before initiating therapy.

- Most concerns regarding strategies to regionalize care for patients with acute coronary syndromes have focused on the lack of a clear consensus regarding the specific nature of regionalization and on the economic and market impacts of such a strategy. The most likely initial focus of a regionalized strategy for acute coronary syndrome care would be STEMI, which has more definitive electrocardiographic and clinical diagnostic criteria and represents a more widely acknowledged medical emergency for which efficacy of treatment is time dependent. The process for development of and for credentialing systems of care for STEMI patients has been initiated by the American Heart Association, and recommendations should be forthcoming.

The past decade has witnessed a remarkable evolution in our understanding of the pathogenesis of acute coronary syndromes (ACS) and in therapeutic innovation for catheter-based technologies and adjunctive pharmacotherapies. Concomitantly, great strides have been made in our ability to risk-stratify patients who present with ACS.

Spontaneous plaque rupture is followed by platelet adherence, activation, and aggregation with fibrin incorporation, leading to thrombus propagation.[1] The severity of the resultant clinical syndrome manifests in direct proportion to the degree of restriction in coronary blood flow and ranges from asymptomatic (i.e., insignificant restriction) to non-ST-segment elevation ACS (NSTEACS), including unstable angina and non-ST-segment elevation myocardial infarction (NSTEMI), which are associated with severe coronary flow restriction, and with ST-segment elevation myocardial infarction (STEMI), which usually results from complete coronary occlusion.[2]

Because the pathogenesis of coronary flow restriction is multifactorial (i.e., platelets, thrombus, vasomotion, and mechanical obstruction), it is best addressed by a multimodal approach to therapy (i.e., antiplatelet, anticoagulant, fibrinolytic, and percutaneous catheter-based interventions) implemented in a timely manner. The rapid restoration of normal coronary blood flow by means of pharmacologic or mechanical recanalization of an occluded coronary artery limits the extent of myocardial necrosis and reduces mortality. However, a concerted, integrated approach to therapy for patients with ACS is complicated by the diversity and extent of resources required for the comprehensive treatment of this disease spectrum and by the various settings (i.e., urban, suburban, and rural) in which care is delivered. Potential therapeutic strategies and systems of care for ACS must consider resource availability (i.e., technical facilities and manpower) and logistic and economic concerns.

The concept of regional centers of excellence is a primary concern for physicians and hospitals caring for patients with ACS, and the wisdom of this approach is actively debated. In this chapter, we address the issues and evidence that fuel this controversy.

Regional implies meaningful networking associations between community and rural hospitals that do not provide tertiary cardiovascular services, including percutaneous coronary intervention (PCI), and a tertiary cardiovascular service provider. The definition of *meaningful networking* ranges from being a merged affiliate (i.e., same hospital system) to sharing common protocols for patient care, as well as tracking, auditing, and reporting clinical practice guideline compliance, core measures, and clinical outcomes.. These "networks" should have well-defined and rehearsed systems for patient transport that will differ depending on whether care is delivered in an urban/suburban or rural setting.

SCOPE OF THE PROBLEM

Creating specialized centers of care for treating victims of trauma has been shown to improve clinical outcomes.[3] Trauma victims treated in a trauma center had significantly lower mortality rates compared with patients treated in a nontrauma center. Specialized centers for care of stroke patients have been implemented with the standard of care established by the American Heart Association and with a formal process provided through the Joint Commission on Accreditation of Healthcare Organizations (JCAHO) for the certification of primary stroke centers.[4] The number of deaths from coronary heart disease in the United States alone exceeds (sevenfold) that for all-cause trauma and (fourfold) for stroke in the general population and is 20-fold and fivefold higher for trauma and stroke, respectively, for persons 65 years old or older (Fig. 37-1).[5] In 2003, there were 865,000 new and recurrent heart attacks in the United States, with 35% to 40% attributed to STEMI.[6] In this context, the lack of specialized regional centers of care for patients with acute ischemic heart disease is not commensurate with the magnitude of this public health problem.

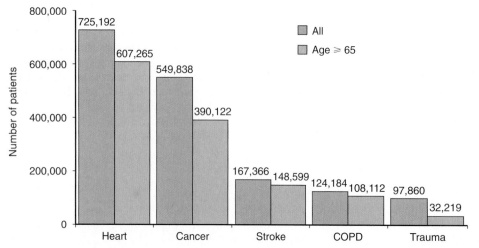

Figure 37-1. Deaths in the United States stratified by cause for all individuals and for individuals older than 65 years. COPD, chronic obstructive pulmonary disease. (Modified from Anderson RN: Anderson RN: Deaths: Leading causes for 1999. National Vital Statistics Report, vol 49, no. 11. Hyattsville, MD, National Center for Health Statistics, October 12, 2001.)

THE CASE FOR AND AGAINST REGIONALIZED CARE FOR ACUTE CORONARY SYNDROMES

Where and how patients with acute ischemic heart disease are treated have been the subjects of debate. Some believe that "the real issue is not whether the creation of specialized centers for care of those [ACS] patients would provide an important advance, but how to create them,"[7-9] Others contend that "clear, compelling evidence of the benefits of ACS regionalization within the United States and a better understanding of its potential consequences are needed before implementing a national policy of regionalized ACS care."[10,11] Proponents assert that the treatment of patients with ACS at regional centers with dedicated facilities will save lives by providing higher-quality care and by improving access to new technologies and to specialist physicians.[7-9] These beliefs are in large part based on the precedent U.S. experience with trauma and stroke, as well as on the experiences gleaned from many European countries, where regionalized systems for ACS care have been developed.[12-14] Although efficiency of process and quality outcomes have been demonstrated in several European systems, the generalizability of these data to current practice in the United States has been questioned.[10,11] Because European health care systems are characterized by centralized financing and control of hospital and emergency transportation organizations, they avoid the financial reimbursement issues and other control barriers present in the U.S. health care system. The logistics of providing regionalized care in the United States, where the population is more geographically dispersed, may present additional challenges. Nevertheless, the state of Maryland has begun planning for regionalized care of patients with ACS.[15] The American Heart Association has convened an acute myocardial infarction advisory working group to examine the feasibility of developing strategies to increase the number of patients with STEMI who receive timely primary PCI and to explore systems and centers of care in conjunction with its goal of reducing deaths from coronary heart disease and stroke by 25% by the year 2010.[16]

These initiatives are in part prompted by studies that demonstrate shortfalls in the current use of quality-assured, guideline-driven care for ACS patients and by the wide variability in the treatments administered based on age, gender, race, geographic locale, and time of presentation.[17-19] A treatment-risk paradox has been demonstrated for the use of an early angiography and coronary revascularization treatment strategy in patients who present with NSTEACS.[20,21] Although clinical trials have demonstrated that the benefit of an early invasive treatment strategy in this patient population is directly proportional to the patient's risk profile, the likelihood of receiving such treatment is greatest for patients at lower risk. This pattern may be attributed to physicians' misconceptions regarding benefit-harm tradeoffs or concerns about treatment complications. An analysis suggests that at least 25% of opportunities to initiate guide-line-based care are missed in contemporary community practice.[22]

The process of care for patients with ACS has been further complicated by the fact that coronary heart disease is the major determinant of financial well-being for many U.S. hospitals. Profitability from a cardiovascular service is often used to offset deficits incurred by the provision of other important but less profitable services (e.g., mental health, obstetrics, emergency medicine).[16]

Potential Advantages of Regional Centers

Practice Makes Perfect: Relationship between Volume and Outcomes

In general, patients have better clinical outcomes when treated in centers that commonly encounter the clinical problem with which the patient is afflicted.[23,24] A direct relationship has been demonstrated between physician-operator and facility procedural volumes and optimal clinical outcomes for elective and primary PCI procedures and for coronary bypass surgery.[25-29] A similar relationship has been demonstrated between the volume of ACS patients treated at a hospital and clinical outcomes and adherence to the American College of Cardiology/American Heart Association (ACC/AHA) guidelines for recommended care.[30,31] The doctors and hospitals performing the highest volumes of procedures demonstrate the best clinical outcomes, including survival rates. Higher-volume PCI centers demonstrate lower risk-adjusted, in-hospital mortality rates and less frequent need for emergency coronary bypass surgery, even in the current era of coronary stenting.[28,29,32] The relative benefit of primary PCI compared with fibrinolysis for the treatment of STEMI may be completely lost when primary PCI is performed in a low-volume institution.[25,33] Data from the New York statewide database demonstrate that the physician-operator volume significantly influences the success rate for primary PCI procedures and that hospital volume influences (by 50%) in-hospital mortality rates after the procedure.[34] These observations have led to the belief that PCI "generally should not be conducted in low-volume hospitals unless there are substantial overriding concerns about geographic or socioeconomic access"[27] and to recommendations for hospitals performing primary PCI for STEMI to satisfy specific minimum requirements for the volume of procedures.[35] A pooled analysis of multiple studies involving more than 1 million PCI procedures confirms the relationship between lower procedural volumes (<200 cases) and an increase in in-hospital mortality rates and the requirement for emergency coronary bypass surgery after PCI (Fig. 37-2).[29]

Others have suggested that institutional volume credentialing at a level of 200 or more cases yearly may be too low. For example, an analysis of 37,848 PCI procedures performed at 44 centers in 2001 and 2002 as part of the Greater Paris area PTCA registry

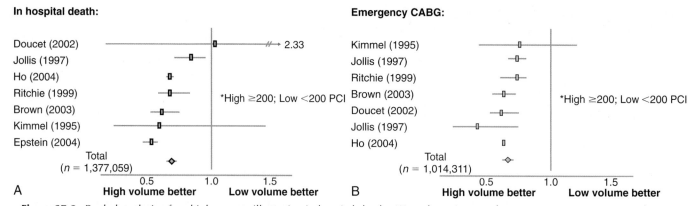

In hospital death:

Emergency CABG:

A High volume better — Low volume better

B High volume better — Low volume better

Figure 37-2. Pooled analysis of multiple reports illustrating in-hospital deaths (**A**) and requirement for emergency coronary artery bypass grafting (CABG) stratified by institutional volume of percutaneous coronary intervention (PCI) (**B**). All programs were stratified as high volume (>200 PCIs/year) or low volume (<200 PCIs/year). (Modified from Keeley EC, Grines CL: Should patients with acute myocardial infarction be transferred to a tertiary center for primary angioplasty or receive it at qualified hospitals in the community? The case for emergency transfer for primary percutaneous coronary intervention. Circulation 2005;112:3520-3532.)

demonstrated an increased incidence of major adverse cardiovascular events after elective and primary PCI procedures performed in centers doing fewer than 400 procedures yearly.[32] In-hospital mortality after primary PCI was increased at the lower volume (<400 PCI/year). The investigators concluded, "Tolerance of low-volume thresholds for angioplasty centers with the purpose of providing primary PCI in acute myocardial infarction should not be recommended, even in underserved areas."[32] The established link between procedural volumes and quality outcomes remains despite the advent of coronary stenting and improvements in adjunctive pharmacotherapies. The volume of institutional intra-aortic balloon pump procedures has been inversely correlated with the in-hospital mortality rate for patients who present with STEMI complicated by cardiogenic shock.[38]

Adherence to Practice Guidelines

The process of care as measured by ACC/AHA guideline adherence has been linked to in-hospital and late (6 to 12 months) survival after presentation with ACS.[38,39] An analysis of hospital composite guide-line adherence quartiles demonstrates an inverse relationship between the adherence to guideline-compliant care and the risk-adjusted, in-hospital mortality rate.[22] For every 10% increase in guideline adherence, a 10% relative reduction in in-hospital mortality was observed (Fig. 37-3).[22] This observation supports the central hypothesis of hospital quality improvement: better adherence to evidence-based care practices results in better outcomes for patients who are treated.[40]

The current system of nonregionalized care has been suboptimal in promoting and achieving guideline adherence, even for ACS patients who present with high-risk indicators.[41] For example, only 33.8% and 44.2% of patients with elevated serum troponin levels in the Can Rapid Risk Stratification of Unstable Angina Patients Suppress Adverse Outcomes with Early Implementation of the ACC/AHA guidelines (CRUSADE) registry received early (<24 hours) glycoprotein IIb/IIIa inhibitor therapy or early (<48 hours) cardiac catheterization, respectively.[42] Similarly, although a direct correlation exists between the presence and magnitude of serum troponin elevation with in-hospital mortality, no correlation was observed between troponin levels and the

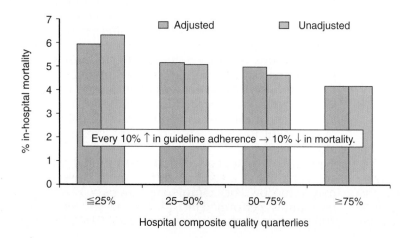

Figure 37-3. Hospital composite quarterly quartiles for American College of Cardiology/American Heart Association guideline adherence correlated with in-hospital mortality that is adjusted (for age; gender; body mass index; race; insurance status; family history of coronary disease; hypertension; diabetes; smoking; hypercholesterolemia; prior myocardial infarction, angioplasty, coronary bypass surgery, congestive heart failure, or stroke; renal insufficiency; blood pressure; heart rate; ST-segment shift; and positive cardiac biomarkers) and unadjusted. Increments in clinical practice guideline adherence are associated with a reduction in mortality. (Modified from Peterson ED, Roe MT, Mulgund J, et al: Association between hospital process performance and outcomes among patients with acute coronary syndromes. JAMA 2006:295:1912-1920.)

Figure 37-4. Relationship between in-hospital mortality **(A)** and the frequency of in-hospital cardiac catheterization within 48 hours of hospital admission **(B),** stratified by the presence and degree of troponin level elevation. A graded relationship exists between the presence and magnitude of troponin elevation and in-hospital mortality. No significant relationship is defined between the presence or magnitude of troponin elevation and the performance of early (<48 hours) cardiac catheterization. Data are derived from the Can Rapid Risk Stratification of Unstable Angina Patients Suppress Adverse Outcomes with Early implementation of the ACC/AHA Guidelines (CRUSADE) registry for non-ST-segment elevation acute coronary syndromes. (Modified from Roe MT, Newby LK, Peterson ED, et al: Suboptimal treatment of patients with non-ST elevation acute coronary syndromes presenting with positive baseline troponin values. [abstract]. J Am Coll Cardiol 2004;43:300A.)

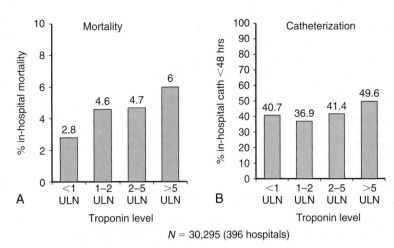

$N = 30,295$ (396 hospitals)

performance of early (<48 hours) coronary angiography (Fig. 37-4), which has a class I ACC/AHA guideline recommendation for NSTEACS patients with high-risk indicators (including elevated troponin).[43]

Compliance with clinical practice guidelines and the ability to monitor or audit guideline adherence appear to be enhanced in higher-volume, regional programs.[30] Lower-volume, small community hospitals are unlikely to allocate the capital resources and personnel required to adequately track, collate, and report clinical outcomes or process measures (i.e., guideline compliance). From the perspective of national or regional payers and that of the Centers for Medicare and Medicaid Services, the prospect of monitoring and auditing data derived from multiple small hospitals versus fewer, larger, networked systems has different orders of magnitude in complexity. In a survey commissioned by the American Heart Association, only slightly more than one half of the hospitals queried were systematically tracking times to STEMI treatment (i.e., door-to-needle or door-to-balloon times), infection rates, readmission or stroke rates (to 30 days after the procedure), and recurrent myocardial infarction or mortality rates after PCI or coronary bypass surgery.[16] This observation is made more meaningful by the fact that multiple national initiatives such as Get with the Guidelines, the Cardiac Hospitalization Atherosclerosis Management (CHAMPS), the Guidelines Applied to Practice (GAP) project, the National Registry of Myocardial Infarction (NRMI), and the CRUSADE project have emphasized system quality through systematic measurement of care processes and clinical outcomes.[9]

Percutaneous Coronary Intervention Centers without On-site Cardiac Surgery

The current trend toward proliferation of PCI centers that lack on-site cardiac surgical facilities for the performance of primary PCI in STEMI may be associated with suboptimal clinical outcomes. In an analysis of 625,854 Medicare patients undergoing PCI, in-hospital and 30-day mortality rates were significantly increased in centers without on-site cardiac surgery (Fig. 37-5),[44] and the increase was primarily confined to hospitals performing a low number (≤50) of PCI procedures in Medicare patients. Even in the context of a completely integrated community hospital and tertiary hospital system, the performance of primary PCI without on-site cardiac surgery was associated with a trend toward increased hospital mortality compared with primary PCI performed at the tertiary center (Table 37-1).[45] This observation is made more meaningful by the fact that patients with STEMI complicated by refractory cardiogenic shock or ventricular arrhythmias were excluded from having primary PCI at the hospital without on-site cardiac surgery. Although single-center studies have reported excellent outcomes for patients undergoing primary PCI at hospitals without on-site cardiac surgery, the one randomized trial that compared fibrinolysis to primary PCI at hospitals without on-site surgery was flawed by an inadequate sample size and by a majority of patients being enrolled at a single site.[47] Based on these and other data, the ACC/AHA guidelines for the performance of PCI designate a class III (i.e., practice may be harmful and is not recommended) indication for elective PCI and a class IIb (i.e., usefulness or efficacy is less well established by evidence/opinion) for primary PCI in hospitals without on-site cardiac surgical facilities and mention the need for additional trials and registries to increase the evidence base.[35]

Of particular concern has been the proliferation of new, low-volume cardiac surgical programs to support PCI programs despite the general decline in cardiac surgical volumes observed nationwide. This proliferation of surgical programs has exaggerated the average per capita (center) decline in procedural volumes, with a consequent adverse effect on clinical outcomes. Data have shown that for bypass surgery and PCI, the removal of a certificate of need requirement has led to the proliferation of low-volume centers with a corresponding increase in risk-adjusted mortality rates compared with states that maintained a certificate of need program.[48] Certificate of need laws

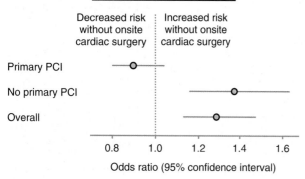

In-hospital and 30-day mortality

Decreased risk without onsite cardiac surgery | Increased risk without onsite cardiac surgery

Primary PCI

No primary PCI

Overall

0.8   1.0   1.2   1.4   1.6

Odds ratio (95% confidence interval)

Jan 1999–Dec 2001 625,854 medicare patients
178 hospitals (no CABG) vs. 943 (CABG)

Figure 37-5. Analysis of 625,854 Medicare recipients undergoing percutaneous coronary intervention in 178 hospitals without on-site coronary artery bypass grafting (CABG) facilities and 943 hospitals with on-site CABG facilities. In-hospital and 30-day mortality is stratified by procedural acuity (i.e., primary percutaneous coronary intervention [PCI] for ST-segment elevation myocardial infarction versus elective no primary PCI) and by the presence or absence of on-site cardiac surgical facilities. A significant increase in mortality is observed after PCI performed in hospitals without on-site coronary bypass surgical facilities. (Modified from Wennberg DE, Lucas FL, Siewers AE, et al: Outcomes of percutaneous coronary interventions performed at centers without and with onsite coronary artery bypass graft surgery. JAMA 2004;292:1961-1968).

provide a platform for state health planning agencies to review access, quality, and costs of health care services before the development of additional services. Certificates of need represent a form of regionalization by which specialized procedures (e.g., coronary bypass surgery, PCI) are deliberately distributed in a presumably rational and efficient geographic context.

In the current free-market approach to health care in the United States, only one half of the states have such requirements. Certificate of need regulations have been entirely repealed by 19 states and repealed specifically for cardiac surgery in 25 states.[16] An analysis of 1,139,792 Medicare beneficiaries 68 years old or older who were hospitalized for the diagnosis of acute myocardial infarction by the certificate of need status of their respective states provides insight into the influence of such certificates on the process and quality of care.[49] In states with certificates of need, Medicare patients who presented with acute myocardial infarction were less likely to be admitted to hospitals with coronary revascularization services and were less likely to undergo revascularization at the admitting hospital. These individuals were more likely to have revascularization at a transfer hospital, with the net effect that they were less likely to undergo revascularization within 2 days of hospital admission. Despite lower rates of early revascularization in states with certificates of need, the risk-adjusted 30-day mortality rate was no different from that observed in states without certificate of need regulations. This observation appears counter to the results of randomized clinical trials that have clearly demonstrated the benefits of early revascularization in patients with acute myocardial infarction. The potential explanations offered by the study authors were that hospitals in states with certificates of need had higher volumes of revascularization procedures, that higher volumes are associated with better outcomes, and that at least some of the revascularization procedures that were performed in states without certificates of need involved patient subsets who derived marginal benefit.[49] The higher facility or institutional procedural volumes in states with certificates of need (accompanied by better clinical outcomes) may counteract any adverse effects of limiting access to revascularization services.[50] Alternatively, certificates of need may decrease the use of revascularization in patients least likely to derive benefit.

Table 37-1. Primary Percutaneous Coronary Intervention for Patients Presenting with ST-Segment Elevation Myocardial Infarction

Characteristic	Primary Percutaneous Coronary Intervention*		
	SMH (*n* = 285)	SJH (*n* = 285)	*P* Value
Angiographic success	279 (98%)	280 (98%)	0.76
Procedural success	274 (96%)	266 (93%)	0.08
In-hospital death	4 (1%)	10 (4%)	0.05
Any recurrent in-hospital MI	1 (0.4%)	4 (1%)	0.17
Recurrent in-hospital Q-wave MI	1 (0.4%)	2 (1%)	0.56
In-hospital emergency CABG	0 (0%)	0 (0%)	—

*Primary percutaneous coronary intervention for patients presenting with ST-segment elevation myocardial infarction to Saint Mary's Hospital of the Mayo Clinic, a tertiary cardiovascular service provider, or to Saint Joseph's Hospital, a community hospital 80 miles away with no on-site cardiovascular surgery support. Both hospitals are completely integrated with respect to imaging and information technology and share protocol-driven algorithms for patient care and physician and ancillary personnel. Figures for both hospitals are presented as the number of patients (*n*) and the percentage (%) of the total.
CABG, coronary artery bypass grafting; SJH, Saint Joseph's Hospital; MI, myocardial infarction; SMH, Saint Mary's Hospital.
From Ting HH, Raveendran G, Lennon RJ, et al: A total of 1,007 percutaneous coronary interventions without onsite cardiac surgery: acute and long-term outcomes. J Am Coll Cardiol 2006;47:1713-1721.

Limited Medical Resources

The trend for proliferation of small "heart centers" under the guise of patient convenience runs counter to the well-established link between higher procedural volumes and better clinical outcomes, and it further taxes critically limited resource pools, including specialized nurses and subspecialty-trained physician providers.[51] Patients with more complex cardiovascular illness (e.g., congestive heart failure, acute myocardial infarction) fare better with subspecialty (cardiologist) care compared with care by generalists.[8,9,52] One strategy for dealing with the mismatch between the emerging evidence in favor of an interventional (catheter-based) approach to the treatment of ACS and the ability to deliver such care is to construct regionalized centers for ACS care.[8,9,23,53] These centers would provide state-of-the-art radiographic equipment, a broad array of PCI supplies and intra-aortic balloon pumps, and experienced ancillary staff well versed in their use and maintenance. Subspecialized nurses and trained cardiologists are in limited supply.[51,54,55]

During the past 5 years, the numbers of ambulances diverted away from major hospitals has reached an all time high because of a lack of "available" beds. The absence of vacant beds or limited bed capacity is not the problem; it is instead the lack of available trained nursing staff to cover beds that remain unfilled.[56] The proliferation of small PCI or "heart" programs with duplication of services further taxes already limited resource pools and may diminish the ability of established tertiary care centers to provide quality care. The development of more PCI programs, particularly those without on-site cardiac surgical facilities, may be unnecessary in light of recent information that more than 80% of the adult U.S. population lives within a 60-minute commute of an existing PCI center.[57]

Potential Disadvantages of Regional Centers

Most concerns regarding strategies to regionalize care for patients with ACS have focused on the lack of clear consensus on the specific nature of regionalization and on the economic and market impacts of such a strategy. Will this policy focus on STEMI (as planned in Maryland) or encompass all patients with suspected ACS?[10,11] Cardiac services supplement low profit margins in other services for many U.S. hospitals. The operating margins for PCI procedures performed at community hospitals and system-affiliated hospitals were 3.6% and 9.5%, respectively, in 2002.[16] Similarly, cardiac surgical procedures yielded operating margins of 8.7% and 14.1%, respectively, which compares favorably to the overall operating margin for all U.S. hospitals of 4.3% in 2002.[16] The loss of PCI or cardiac surgical volumes could lower a hospital's case-mix index, which would lower the overall rate of Medicare reimbursement. A reduced case-mix index could also affect commercial insurance reimbursement. At the extreme, a local hospital that does not provide PCI could be forced to close and thereby limit access to other needed services in the community. Financial incentives for the local hospital to transfer patients to regional centers and assurance of the return of the patient to the local practice would need to be part of any system of care.

The potential financial losses to individual hospitals must be weighed against the potential societal benefits in terms of reduced morbidity and mortality with a regionalized care strategy. For example, if even one half of the approximately 30% of patients who present with STEMI who do not receive reperfusion therapy would be able to undergo primary PCI in an integrated, regionalized system and an absolute risk reduction of 4% (compared with no reperfusion) could be achieved, approximately 2600 lives per year could be saved.[16] When primary PCI is performed in a timely fashion at experienced, high-volume centers, approximately 20 lives are saved per 1000 patients treated (compared with fibrinolytic therapy). If even one half of the 31% of STEMI patients who currently receive fibrinolytic therapy would undergo primary PCI, an additional 1240 lives could be saved. The implementation of strategies that increase the number of patients with timely access to PCI could save approximately 4000 lives each year.[16] In evaluating the cost-effectiveness of primary PCI, it has been suggested that this strategy is cost-effective at hospitals with existing catheterization laboratories and is not cost-effective at low-volume or redundant catheterization laboratories.[16]

It is not clear how hospital capacity will need to be reallocated to make regionalized ACS care feasible. It has been suggested that restricting the treatment of ACS patients to hospitals with PCI facilities and on-site cardiac surgery would require transfer of almost 65% of Medicare beneficiaries hospitalized for myocardial infarction nationwide in 1994 through 1996.[10] Extrapolation of these data to the 768,495 patients hospitalized for the diagnosis of acute myocardial infarction in 2000 suggests that almost 500,000 patients would need to undergo treatment at different hospitals.[10] Even such crude estimates raise serious questions about the feasibility of transferring such a large number of patients and the available capacity of existing tertiary centers to care for them. ACS regionalization will require a national redistribution of cardiovascular resources.

Although concentrating ACS care at fewer hospitals may reduce the cost to the global health care system through economies of scale, such a strategy may have an offsetting effect by "increasing hospital market power" and by enabling designated ACS centers to charge private payers more for ACS care.[10,11] However, a regionalized approach to care has been endorsed and validated for improving clinical outcomes of trauma patients. A similar approach for developing specialized centers for care of stroke and a credentialing process has been proposed by the American Heart Association. The collaborative spirit encountered among community hospitals participating in integrated regional systems for trauma or stroke may be facilitated by the stark reality that trauma and stroke patients are frequently not profitable.[58] Stroke patients generate few high-profit-margin procedures, and they often have protracted, complicated hospital stays. The current scheme for relatively disproportionate reimbursement for cardiovascular procedures constrains the evolution of an optimal care process for ACS, similar to the processes that have evolved for trauma or stroke.

The regionalization of care for the global burden of ACS may be an unrealistic objective to begin with for several reasons. First, ACS is distinct from trauma in that ACS may not be an obvious diagnosis. Second, less than 5% of patients transported by emergency medical services (EMS) for "chest pain" are having a myocardial infarction.[16] Extrapolation from these observations suggests that regional ACS centers would likely be overwhelmed with patients, most of whom would not have coronary heart disease. The burden of non-ACS patients in this scenario could easily exhaust the ACS center's capacity and resources, with consequent impairment in care for true ACS patients. The diagnosis of unstable angina is frequently obscure at the time of hospital presentation, and the diagnosis of non-STEMI often requires serial measurements of blood enzyme levels over time. The most likely (and manageable) initial focus of a regionalized strategy for ACS care appears to be STEMI.[23,59] STEMI has more definitive electrocardiogram (ECG) and clinical diagnostic criteria, and it represents a more widely acknowledged medical emergency. The treatment of STEMI has more time-dependent efficacy, and STEMI patients have higher short-term mortality rates.

REGIONAL CENTERS OF CARE FOR PATIENTS WITH ST-SEGMENT ELEVATION MYOCARDIAL INFARCTION

The technology available to EMS providers that enables transmission of a prehospital 12-lead ECG makes the diagnosis of STEMI evident at the time and place of first medical contact. The integration of EMS and incorporation of the prehospital phase for ACS evaluation and diagnosis are integral components of a regionalized system for STEMI care. STEMI is the logical initial objective for a regionalized ACS treatment strategy because 5 of Medicare's 10 quality indicators focus on STEMI care.[16] Several system process or quality measures are already in place to provide a performance incentive to define regional networks for STEMI care. The development of such regional networks for STEMI care should facilitate adherence to clinical practice guidelines and the ability to monitor, audit, and adjudicate data. Combinations of evidence-based therapies (e.g., antiplatelet agents, β-blockers, lipid-lowering agents, angiotensin-converting enzyme inhibitors) provide an incremental survival advantage to 1 year after presentation with an ACS, especially STEMI.[38,39] The comparison of adherence to clinical practice guidelines and clinical outcomes among regional facilities or networks can contribute to the continuous cycle for quality improvement and therapeutic development (Fig. 37-6).[22,40] Greater adherence to clinical practice guidelines has been observed in hospitals with higher STEMI volumes.[30] Smaller centers are unlikely to allocate the resources necessary to track, audit, and report these measures.

Model Systems of Care

A regionalized approach to the provision of primary PCI therapy for STEMI has been successfully implemented in major metropolitan areas of the United States, such as Minneapolis.[23,60] Through partnership with community hospitals in protocol-driven algorithms for care, designated transport systems, and enhanced multidisciplinary communication (e.g., EMS staff, emergency physicians, interventional cardiologists), the Minneapolis Heart Institute at Abbott

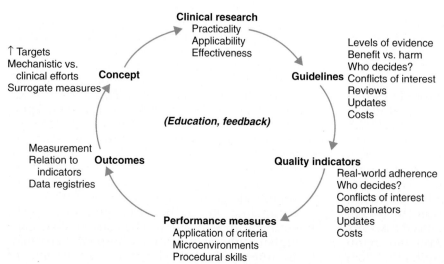

Figure 37-6. The cycle of continuous quality improvement and therapeutic development involves the determination of quality indicators, assessment of performance measures and outcomes, and integration of clinical research and leading-edge technologies. These factors contribute to the construct of clinical practice guidelines, which set boundaries for the process of care. (Modified from Califf RM, Peterson ED, Gibbons RM, et al: Integrating quality into the cycle of therapeutic development. J Am Coll Cardiol 2002;40: 1895-1901.)

Northwestern Hospital has demonstrated the ability to promptly access and treat STEMI patients who originate from a broad area (90- to 120-minute transit). By focusing on collaboration and integration of resources, community hospitals initiate adjunctive pharmacotherapies in patients who present with STEMI and emergently transport these patients to the interventional team waiting at Abbott Northwestern Hospital. Using this approach, remarkably short total door-to-balloon times (i.e., door at community hospital to balloon therapy at Abbott Northwestern Hospital) and good clinical outcomes have been achieved (Fig. 37-7 and Table 37-2).[60]

Other cities such as Chicago and Ann Arbor are planning similar initiatives. A statewide approach is being used in North Carolina with the Reperfusion of Acute Myocardial Infarction in North Carolina Emergency Department (RACE) program that is similar to the Minnesota model. The Initiative uses standardized protocols and integrated systems for the treatment and timely transfer of patients with STEMI in five regions in North Carolina. Regional centers play a key role in the systems, but the goal is to effectively apply the ACC/AHA STEMI guidelines.

This experience stands in stark contrast to the NRMI-3 and NRMI-4 data for STEMI patients who first present to a community hospital and are subsequently transported to a tertiary facility for PCI.[61] In the absence of a well-defined, integrated system with protocol-driven algorithms for care and dedicated

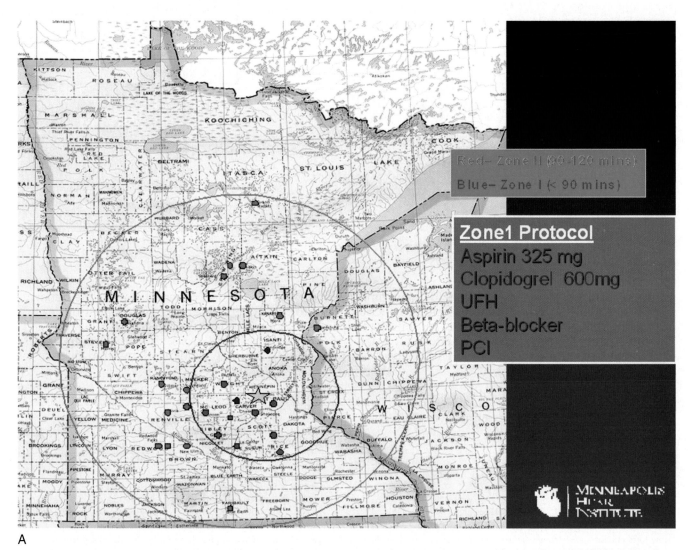

A

Figure 37-7. Demographic distribution of multiple community hospitals participating in a network for providing primary percutaneous coronary intervention for ST-segment elevation myocardial infarction with the Minneapolis Heart Institute in Minneapolis, Minnesota. The protocol-driven algorithm for adjunctive pharmacotherapies is illustrated for patients originating within a 90-minute radius for ground transport (zone 1) **(A)** and for patients originating within a 90- to 120-minute radius (zone 2) **(B).** Participating centers have an established, rehearsed mechanism for patient transport. Angiographic and clinical outcomes after transport are comparable to those observed for patients admitted directly to Abbott Northwestern Hospital in Minneapolis (see Table 37-2).

Continued

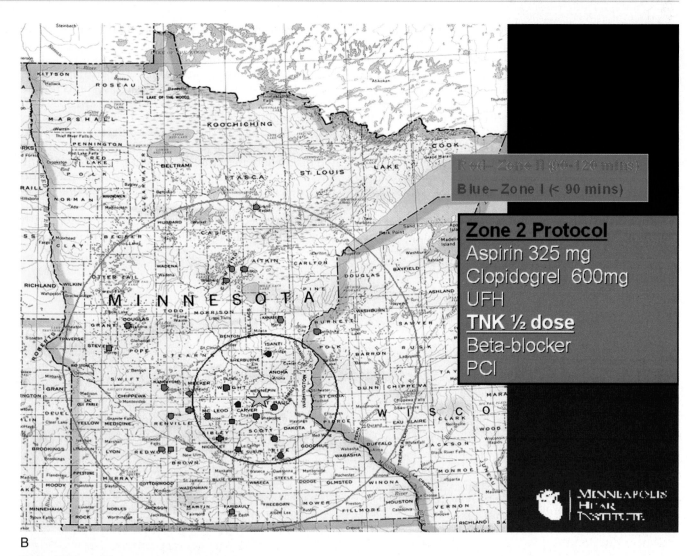

B

Figure 37-7, cont'd

transport facilities, the median door-to-balloon time from NRMI-3 and -4 is 180 minutes, and only 15% of patients receive PCI therapy within 120 minutes. The discrepancy between current practice and what can be achieved through collaboration in the absence of marked duplication of services offers the opportunity for improvement and begs the question regarding the optimal process for ACS care.

The striking limitations of the current process for STEMI care are evidenced by the absence of

Table 37-2. Time to Treatment and Outcomes for Patients Presenting with ST-Segment Elevation Myocardial Infarction

Treatment*	Preintervention TIMI 3/2 (%)	Postintervention TIMI 3 (%)	Stroke at 30 Days	Reinfarction or Ischemia at 30 Days	Mortality at 30 Days	Major Bleeding
Facilitated PCI (zone II) n = 176	43/29	96	0%	0%	3.8%	0%
ANW (direct admission) n = 158	15/16	93	2.5%	3.8%	6.3%	0%
P value	<.0001	NS	NS	NS	NS	NS

*Time to treatment and outcomes for patients presenting with ST-segment elevation myocardial infarction directly to Abbott-Northwestern Hospital (ANW) who underwent primary percutaneous coronary intervention (PCI) and those admitted to peripheral community hospitals in zone 11 (i.e., 90- to 120-minute ground transport time) who were emergently transferred to ANW for primary PCI. Patients admitted to community hospitals were administered aspirin (325 mg PO) and clopidogrel (600 mg PO) and were given half-dose tenecteplase, unfractionated heparin, and β-blockade therapy intravenously before transfer. Rates (%) of TIMI flow grades 2 or 3 before and after PCI, as well as stroke, reinfarction, death, and major bleeding to 30 days of follow-up are shown for both patient cohorts.

NS, not significant; TIMI, Thrombolysis in Myocardial Infarction.

From Larson DM, Menssen KM, Newell MC, et al: Long distance transfer for direct percutaneous coronary intervention: a facilitated approach [abstract]. J Am Coll Cardiol 2006;47:174A.

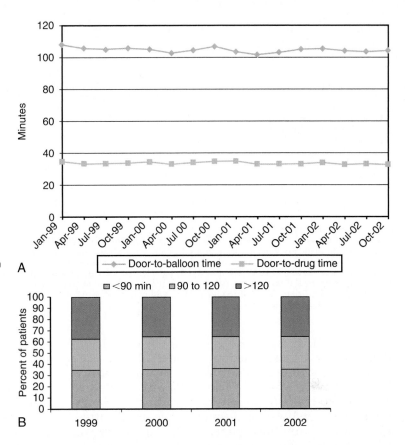

Figure 37-8. Pooled analysis of data derived from the National Registry of Myocardial Infarction (NRMI) between January 1999 and October 2002, summarizing mean door-to-balloon times and the mean door-to-thrombolytic drug infusion treatment times **(A)**. Throughout a 4-year period of observation, no differences in the percentage of patients observed to have American College of Cardiology/American Heart Association guideline compliant treatment time (door-to-balloon time <90 minutes) was observed despite the publication of Clinical Practice Guidelines **(B)**. (Modified from McNamara RL, Herrin J, Bradley EH, et al, for the NRML Investigators: Hospital improvement in time to reperfusion in patients with acute myocardial infarction, 1999 to 2002. J Am Coll Cardiol 2006;47:45-51.)

improvement in prolonged times to treatment despite widespread dissemination of benchmark goals for therapy (door-to-fibrinolytic infusion or door-to-balloon times) in the form of clinical practice guidelines.[62] These recommended times to treatment (30 minutes for door-to-fibrinolytic infusion and 90 minutes for door-to-balloon treatment) are not ideal times, but rather the longest times that should be considered acceptable by the medical system.[63] No improvement in overall times to treatment or the percentage of patients who received clinical practice guidelines–compliant care has been observed with our current process for ACS care (Fig. 37-8). Considering the direct relationship between treatment delays and short- and long-term mortality rates after infarction[64,65] (Fig. 37-9 and Table 37-3), the need for improvement in the current process for ACS care is clear.

The realization that "all hospitals are not equal" for the care of STEMI[36] and the demonstration of improved patient outcomes in specialized centers for care of trauma and stroke have shattered the antiquated concept that patients with suspected myocardial infarction should be transported to the nearest hospital. Several U.S. cities such as Boston have begun directing public EMS to transport such patients to a limited few "centers of excellence" for heart attack care.[66]

In addition to concentrating high-volume expertise and technology, these centers are integrated with the EMS so that the diagnosis of infarction can be made more rapidly and the system for providing PCI is more responsive. The prehospital care for ACS,

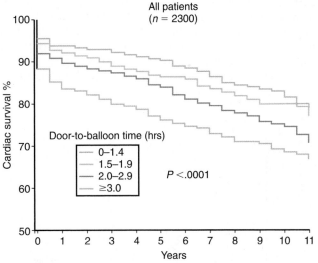

Figure 37-9. Cardiac survival to 11 years after primary percutaneous coronary intervention for ST-segment elevation myocardial infarction, stratified by door-to-balloon time treatment delay. Prolonged door-to-balloon time significantly influences late survival. (Modified from Brodie BR, Hansen C, Stuckey TD, et al: Door-to-balloon time with primary percutaneous coronary intervention for acute myocardial infarction impacts late cardiac mortality in high-risk patients and patients presenting early after the onset of symptoms. J Am Coll Cardiol 2006;47:289-295.)

Table 37-3. Cumulative Analysis of Four Trials of Primary Percutaneous Coronary Intervention for ST-Segment Elevation Myocardial Infarction

Characteristic	Door-to-Balloon Times (min)*				P Value
	<60	60-90	90-120	>120	
Patients (n)	183	296	304	403	
Prior myocardial infarction	9%	12%	9%	8%	NS
Anterior myocardial infarction	43%	40%	45%	41%	NS
Onset-to-door (min)	197 ± 182	140 ± 140	141 ± 151	113 ± 124	<.0001
Door-to-balloon (min)	44 ± 12	75 ± 9	103 ± 8	156 ± 30	
Onset-to-balloon (min)	235 ± 180	216 ± 140	244 ± 150	269 ± 126	<.0001
Death 30 days	0.6%	0.7%	4.7%	2.5%	.0037
MACE at 30 days	1.6%	2.4%	7.6%	5.5%	.0034
Infarct size (% of left ventricle)	14.2 ± 15.8	13.2 ± 14.6	18.0 ± 18.0	17.4 ± 18.0	.0023

*Analysis was performed for four trials of primary percutaneous coronary intervention for ST-segment elevation myocardial infarction: Enhanced Myocardial Efficacy and Recovery by Aspiration of Liberated Debris (EMERALD); Cooling as an Adjunctive Therapy to Percutaneous Intervention in Patients with Acute Myocardial Infarction (COOL-MI); Acute Myocardial Infarction with Hyperoxemic Therapy (AMI-HOT); Intravascular Cooling Adjunctive to Percutaneous Coronary Intervention (ICE-IT). The trials showed patient demographics and outcomes stratified by door-to-balloon times. The major adverse cardiovascular events (MACE) include death, recurrent myocardial infarction, urgent revascularization, or stroke, and infarct size was determined by nuclear scintigraphy (single photon emission computed tomography).
From O'Neill WW, Grines CL, Dixon SR, et al: Does a 90-minute door-to-balloon time matter? Observations from four current reperfusion trials [abstract]. J Am Coll Cardiol 2005;45:225A.

especially STEMI, is critically important. Earlier STEMI diagnosis by a transmitted prehospital 12-lead ECG facilitates in-hospital STEMI treatment with fibrinolysis or PCI (Fig. 37-10).[67-69] Hospitals with the shortest door-to-balloon times in the United States incorporate prehospital diagnosis (i.e., transmitted ECG) with a multidisciplinary team approach, in which the emergency physician activates the cardiac catheterization laboratory before cardiology consultation.[70] Facilitation of in-hospital PCI treatment for patients with a transmitted prehospital ECG has resulted in a significant reduction in door-to-balloon times and in improvement of survival rates.[71] The consistent and significant relationships demonstrated

for earlier STEMI diagnosis, more rapid treatment, and improved outcomes has prompted a National Heart, Lung, and Blood Institute consensus recommendation for the implementation of prehospital 12-lead ECG systems by all EMS providers.[72]

However, the rapid transport of patients with STEMI to the nearest appropriate facility for their care may be hampered by several factors. First, only 4% to 5% of EMS-transported patients with chest pain have STEMI.[16] Second, only about 10% of EMS systems have 12-lead ECG capabilities.[16] Third, a precedent mandate exists for transport of the patient to the nearest facility, even when fibrinolysis may be contraindicated and the facility does not provide

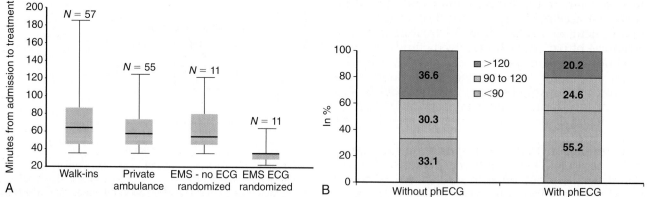

Figure 37-10. Prehospital diagnosis of ST-segment elevation myocardial infarction expedites the initiation of in-hospital thrombolytic therapy (i.e., reduced door-to-needle time), as demonstrated in a randomized, controlled trial (**A**). Emergency medical system (EMS) transport without the performance of a prehospital transmitted electrocardiogram (ECG) alone did not significantly reduce time to treatment (**B**). Analysis of data derived from the National Registry of Myocardial Infarction-4 (NRMI-4) registry demonstrates that among patients who have a prehospital 12-lead ECG transmitted (with phECG), there is a significant increase in the percentage of patients receiving primary percutaneous coronary intervention (PCI) with a door-to-balloon time of less than 90 minutes compared with patients without a transmitted prehospital ECG (without phECG). (**A,** modified from Kereiakes DJ, Gibler WB, Martin LH, et al: Relative importance of emergency medical system transport and the pre-hospital electrocardiogram on reducing hospital time delay to therapy for acute myocardial infarction: A preliminary report from the Cincinnati Heart Project. Am Heart J 1992;123:835-840; **B,** modified from Curtis JP, Portnay EL, Wang Y, et al, for the National Registry of Myocardial Infarction-4: The pre-hospital electrocardiogram and time to reperfusion in patients with acute myocardial infarction, 2000-2002: Findings from the National Registry of Myocardial Infarction-4. J Am Coll Cardiol 2006;47:1544-1552.)

primary PCI. Rapid evolution in the current process of prehospital care is further complicated by the fact that there are 329 different EMS regions in the United States with at least 993 hospital-based EMS systems.[16] Hospital-based EMS systems represent only 6.5% of all EMS providers; the remainder are private, third-party systems (48.6%) and fire station–based systems (44.9%).[16] Although the transport time to a specialized center of excellence may appear long, it can be more than counterbalanced by an integrated EMS system and prenotification. A doubling of the recommended transport time has been proposed for suspected STEMI patients who are transported to a center of excellence, for which the target door-to-balloon time is 60 minutes or less.[53] Such a level of efficiency can be achieved only through an integrated system for STEMI care that incorporates a prehospital ECG for earlier diagnosis.

Future Care of Patients with ST-Segment Elevation Myocardial Infarction

The lack of a coordinated system of care denies many patients the benefit of primary PCI. A coordinated system for the provision of PCI could prevent an estimated six to eight major adverse cardiovascular or cerebrovascular events per 100 STEMI patients treated and therefore could affect 35,000 patients yearly.[23] However, the current scheme for cardiovascular reimbursement could penalize community hospitals without cardiac catheterization laboratories when patients are transferred or admitted directly to a regional center.[16] An adjustment to the reimbursement strategy, possibly to include regional networks of partnering community and tertiary care centers, must be addressed. Hospitals without PCI capabilities could be incentivized to risk-stratify and transfer STEMI patients based on risk, transport time, and distance. Such contractually defined networks could provide similar quality-assured and monitored, protocol-driven algorithms for care with predefined systems for prompt patient transport. Issues of case-mix index could be defined by systems rather than individual hospitals.

Credentialing and criteria for the development of a level I heart attack center should include the established ability to provide prehospital diagnosis of STEMI with a transmitted 12-lead ECG by means of integration with local or regional EMS.[16,23] Suggested criteria for level 1 heart attack centers are listed in Table 37-4. To be successful, a system for care of STEMI patients should have many integral components (Table 37-5), including a patient care focus, enhanced operational efficiency, appropriate system incentives i.e., ("pay for performance" or "pay for value"), specific outcome and process measures, and mechanisms for quality review with continuous quality improvement. Professional societies and organizations can and should develop the credentialing criteria for these centers. State and local government agencies could be charged with the oversight of legitimacy for regional STEMI networks. Clinical practice

Table 37-4. Criteria for a Level 1 Heart Attack Center

- 24-Hour cardiac catheterization laboratory availability
- 24-Hour cardiovascular surgery availability
- Comprehensive interventional cardiology and cardiovascular surgery services
- More than 200 PCI patients/year (>36 STEMI) per hospital
- More than 75 PCI patients/year per interventional cardiologist
- EMS integration with prehospital 12-lead electrocardiographic transmission
- Standardized protocols at referral and receiving hospitals
- Transfer agreements in place
- Education and training programs for transport, referral, and receiving hospital personnel
- Quality-assurance program

EMS, emergency medical services; PCI, percutaneous coronary intervention; STEMI, ST-segment elevation myocardial infarction.
Modified from Henry TD, Atkins JM, Cunningham MS, et al: ST-segment elevation myocardial infarction: Recommendations on triage of patients to heart attack centers—Is it time for a national policy for the treatment of ST-segment elevation myocardial infarction? J Am Coll Cardiol 2006;47:1339-1345.

guidelines adherence and monitoring could be performed by established systems rather than individual hospitals or centers.

The process for development of systems of care for STEMI patients has already been initiated by the AHA and is the subject of ongoing stakeholder meetings. The AHA has issued a call to action to improve the implementation and timeliness of infarct reperfusion with primary PCI that carefully considers the ideal system from the perspective of each constituent, including the patient, physician, EMS staff, non–PCI-capable hospitals, PCI-capable centers, and payers. Given the importance of time to treatment for STEMI patients, the ideal system of care will likely be different for various geographic locales (e.g., urban, suburban, rural) and will consider the risk of the myocardial infarction in an individual patient. Recommendations for additional research and

Table 37-5. Integral Components of a System for Care of Patients with ST-Segment Elevation Myocardial Infarction

- Patient-centered care as the number 1 priority
- High-quality care that is safe, effective, and timely
- Stakeholder consensus on systems' infrastructure
- Increased operational efficiencies
- Appropriate incentives for quality, such as pay for performance, pay for value, or pay for quality
- Measurable patient outcomes
- An evaluation mechanism to ensure quality-of-care measures reflect changes in evidence-based research, including consensus-based treatment guidelines
- A role for local community hospitals to avoid a negative impact that could eliminate critical access to local health care
- A reduction in disparities of health care delivery, such as those across economic, educational, racial or ethnic, and geographic lines

From Jacobs AK, Antman EM, Ellrodt G, et al: Recommendation to develop strategies to increase the number of ST-segment elevation myocardial infarction patients with timely access to primary percutaneous coronary intervention—The American Heart Association's acute myocardial infarction (AMI) Advisory Working Group. Circulation 2006;113:2152-2163.

requisite changes in policy to support the construct and implementation of systems that will improve quality of care and outcomes for STEMI patients should be forthcoming.

REFERENCES

1. Fuster V, Badimon L, Badimon JJ, et al: The pathogenesis of coronary artery disease and the acute coronary syndromes. N Engl J Med 1992;326:242-250.
2. Braunwald E, Antman EM, Beasley JW, et al: American College of Cardiology/American Heart Association Task Force on Practice Guidelines (Committee on the Management of Patients With Unstable Angina). ACC/AHA guideline update for the management of patients with unstable angina and non-ST-segment elevation myocardial infarction—2002: Summary article: A report of the American College of Cardiology/American Heart Association Task Force on Practice Guidelines (Committee on the Management of Patients With Unstable Angina). Circulation 2002;106:1893-1900.
3. MacKenzie EJ, Rivara FP, Jurkovich GJ, et al: A national evaluation of the effect of trauma-center care on mortality. N Engl J Med 2006;354:366-378.
4. Schwamm LH, Pancioli A, Acker JE III, et al: American Stroke Association's task force on the development of stroke systems. Recommendations for the establishment of stroke systems of care: Recommendations from the American Stroke Association's task force on the development of stroke systems. Circulation 2005;111:1078-1091.
5. Anderson RN: Deaths: Leading causes for 1999. National Vital Statistics Report, vol 49, no. 11. Hyattsville, MD, National Center for Health Statistics, October 12, 2001.
6. American Heart Association: Heart disease and stroke statistics—2006 update. Circulation 2006;113:e85-e151.
7. Willerson JT: Centers of excellence. Circulation 2003;107:1471-1472.
8. Topol EJ, Kereiakes DJ: Regionalization of care for acute ischemic heart disease—A call for specialized centers. Circulation 2003;107:1463-1466.
9. Califf RM, Faxon DP: Need for centers to care for patients with acute coronary syndromes. Circulation 2003;107:1467-1470.
10. Rathore SS, Epstein RJ, Volpp KGM, et al: Regionalization of care for acute coronary syndromes—More evidence is needed. JAMA 2005;293:1383-1387.
11. Rathore SS, Epstein AJ, Nallamouthu BK, et al: Regionalization of ST-segment elevation acute coronary syndromes care—Putting a national policy in proper perspective. J Am Coll Cardiol 2006;47:1346-1349.
12. Widimsky P, Groch L, Zelizko M, et al: Multicenter randomized trial comparing transport to primary angioplasty vs. immediate thrombolysis vs. combined strategy for patients with acute myocardial infarction presenting to a community hospital without a catheterization laboratory. The PRAGUE study. Eur Heart J 2000;21:823-831.
13. Widimsky P, Budesinsky T, Vorac D, et al: Long distance transport for primary angioplasty vs. immediate thrombolysis in acute myocardial infarction—PRAGUE-2. Eur Heart J 2003;24:94-104.
14. Andersen HR, Nielsen TT, Rasmussen K, et al: A comparison of coronary angioplasty with fibrinolytic therapy in acute myocardial infarction. N Engl J Med 2003;349:733-742.
15. Williams DO: Treatment delayed is treatment denied. Circulation 2004;109:1806-1808.
16. Jacobs AK, Antman EM, Ellrodt G, et al: Recommendation to develop strategies to increase the number of ST-segment elevation myocardial infarction patients with timely access to primary percutaneous coronary intervention—The American Heart Association's acute myocardial infarction (AMI) Advisory Working Group. Circulation 2006;113:2152-2163.
17. Vaccarino V, Rathor SS, Wenger NK, et al: Sex and racial differences in the management of acute myocardial infarction, 1994 through 2002. N Engl J Med 2005;353:671-682.
18. Magid DJ, Wang Y, Herrin J, et al: Relationship between time of day, day of week, timeliness of reperfusion, and in-hospital mortality for patients with acute ST-segment elevation myocardial infarction. JAMA 2005;294:803-812.
19. Rathore SS, Masoudi FA, Havranek EP, et al: Regional variations in racial differences in the treatment of elderly patients hospitalized with acute myocardial infarction. Am J Med 2004;117:811-812.
20. Yan AT, Yan RT, Tan M, et al: Despite the temporal increases, coronary angiography and revascularization remain paradoxically directed towards low risk non-ST elevation acute coronary syndrome patients [abstract]. J Am Coll Cardiol 2005;45:190A.
21. Roe MT, Peterson ED, Newby LK, et al: The influence of risk status on guideline adherence for patients with non-ST-segment elevation acute coronary syndromes. Am Heart J 2006;151:1205-1213.
22. Peterson ED, Roe MT, Mulgund J, et al: Association between hospital process performance and outcomes among patients with acute coronary syndromes. JAMA 2006:295:1912-1920.
23. Henry TD, Atkins JM, Cunningham MS, et al: ST-segment elevation myocardial infarction: Recommendations on triage of patients to heart attack centers—Is it time for a national policy for the treatment of ST-segment elevation myocardial infarction? J Am Coll Cardiol 2006;47:1339-1345.
24. Nallamothu BK, Wang Y, Magid DJ, et al: Relation between hospital specialization with primary percutaneous coronary intervention and clinical outcomes in ST-segment elevation myocardial infarction: National Registry of Myocardial Infarction-4 analysis. Circulation 2006;113:222-229.
25. Magid DJ, Calonge GN, Rumsfeld JS, et al: Relation between hospital primary angioplasty volume and mortality for patients with acute MI treated with primary angioplasty vs. thrombolytic therapy. JAMA 2000;284:3131-3138.
26. Moscucci M, Share D, Smith D, et al: Relationship between operator volume and adverse outcome in contemporary percutaneous coronary intervention practice: An analysis of a quality-controlled multicenter percutaneous coronary intervention clinical database. J Am Coll Cardiol 2005;456:625-632.
27. Jollis JG, Romano PS: Volume-outcome relationship in acute myocardial infarction: The balloon and the needle. JAMA 2000;284:3169-3171.
28. Hannan EL, Wu C, Walford G, et al: Volume-outcome relationships for percutaneous coronary interventions in the stent era. Circulation 2005;112:1171-1179.
29. Keeley EC, Grines CL: Should patients with acute myocardial infraction be transferred to a tertiary center for primary angioplasty or receive it at qualified hospitals in the community? The case for emergency transfer for primary percutaneous coronary intervention. Circulation 2005;112:3520-3532.
30. Lewis WR, Sorof SA, Super DM: Practice makes perfect: ACC/AHA guideline adherence is higher in hospitals with high acute myocardial infarction volume [abstract]. J Am Coll Cardiol 2006;47:255A.
31. Kugelmass A, Brown P, Becker E, et al: How do acute percutaneous coronary intervention complication rates vary in hospitals ranked in the top versus the bottom quartiles of hospitals [abstract]? J Am Coll Cardiol 2005;45:339A.
32. Morice MC, Spalding C, Lancelin B, et al: Does hospital PTCA volume influence mortality and complication rates in the era of PTCA with systematic stenting? Results of the Greater Paris Area PTCA registry [abstract]. J Am Coll Cardiol 2006:47:192A.
33. Cannon CP, Gibson CM, Lambrew CT, et al: Relationship of symptom-onset-to-balloon time and door-to-balloon time with mortality in patients undergoing angioplasty for acute myocardial infarction. JAMA 2000;283:2941-2947.
34. Vakili BA, Brown DL: 1995 Coronary angioplasty reporting system of the New York State Department of Health. Relation between hospital primary angioplasty volume and mortality for patients with acute MI treated with primary angioplasty vs thrombolytic therapy. Am J Cardiol 2003;91:726-728.
35. Smith S, Feldman TD, Hirshfeld JW, et al: ACC/AHA/SCAI 2005 Guideline update for percutaneous coronary intervention—Summary article. A report of the American College of Cardiology/American Heart Association Task Force on Practice

Guidelines (ACC/AHA/SCAI Writing Committee to update the 2001 Guidelines for Percutaneous Coronary Intervention). Circulation 2005;113:156-175.

36. Weaver WD: All hospitals are not equal for treatment of patients with acute myocardial infarction. Circulation 2003; 108:1768-1771.

37. Chen EW, Canto JG, Parsons LS, et al: Relation between hospital intra-aortic balloon counterpulsation volume and mortality in acute myocardial infarction complicated by cardiogenic shock. Circulation 2003;108:951-957.

38. Mukherjee D, Fang J, Chetcuti S, et al: Impact of combination evidence-based medical therapy on mortality in patients with acute coronary syndromes. Circulation 2004;109:745-749.

39. Tay E, Chan MY, Tan WD, et al: Impact of combination evidence-based medical therapy on mortality following myocardial infarction in patients with and without renal dysfunction [abstract]. J Am Coll Cardiol 2006;47:161A.

40. Califf RM, Peterson ED, Gibbons RM, et al: Integrating quality into the cycle of therapeutic development. J Am Coll Cardiol 2002;40:1895-1901.

41. Roe MT, Peterson ED, Newby LK, et al: The influence of risk status on guideline adherence for patients with non-ST-segment elevation acute coronary syndromes. Am Heart J 2006;151:1205-1213.

42. Roe MT, Peterson ED, Li Y, et al: Suboptimal adherence to the ACC/AHA non-ST-elevation acute coronary syndrome practice guidelines for patients with positive troponin levels [abstract]. J Am Coll Cardiol 2003;41:390A.

43. Roe MT, Peterson ED, Yui L, et al: Relationship between risk stratification by cardiac troponin level and adherence to guidelines for non-ST-segment elevation acute coronary syndrome. Arch Intern Med 2005;165:1870-1876.

44. Peterson ED, Roe MT, Mulgund J, et al: Association between hospital process performance and outcomes among patients with acute coronary syndromes. JAMA 2006:295:1912-1920.

45. Ting HH, Raveendran G, Lennon RJ, et al: A total of 1,007 percutaneous coronary interventions without onsite cardiac surgery: Acute and long-term outcomes. J Am Coll Cardiol 2006;47:1713-1721.

46. Wharton TP Jr: Should patients with acute myocardial infarction be transferred to a tertiary center for primary angioplasty or receive it at qualified hospitals in community? The case for community hospital angioplasty. Circulation 2005;12:3509-3520.

47. Aversano T, Aversano LT, Passamani E, et al: Thrombolytic therapy vs primary percutaneous coronary intervention for myocardial infarction in patients presenting to hospitals without on-site cardiac surgery: A randomized controlled trial. JAMA 2002;287:1943-1951.

48. Vaughan-Sarrazin MS, Hannan EL, Gormley CJ, Rosenthal GE: Mortality in Medicare beneficiaries following coronary artery bypass graft surgery in states with and without certificate of need regulation. JAMA 2002;288:1859-1866.

49. Popescu I, Vaughan-Sarrazin MS, Rosenthal GE: Certificate of need regulations and use of coronary revascularization after acute myocardial infarction. JAMA 2006;295:2141-2147.

50. Hannan EL: Evaluating and improving the quality of care for acute myocardial infarction—Can regionalization help? JAMA 2006;295:2177-2179.

51. Kereiakes DJ, Willerson JT: The United States cardiovascular care deficit. Circulation 2004;109:821-823.

52. Greenfield S, Kaplan SH, Kahn R, et al: Profiling care provided by different groups of physicians: Effects of patient case-mix (bias) and physician-level clustering on quality assessment results. Ann Intern Med 2002;136:111-121.

53. Jacobs AK: Primary angioplasty for acute myocardial infarction: Is it worth the wait? N Engl J Med 2003;349:798-800.

54. Bonow RO, Smith SC: Cardiovascular manpower—The looming crisis. Circulation 2004;109:817-820.

55. Fye WB: Cardiology's workforce shortage—Implications for patient care and research. Circulation 2004;109:813-816.

56. The Lewin Group Analysis of AHA, ED and Hospital Capacity Survey: 2002. Available at http://www.ahrq.gov/news/ulp/hospital/weinick.ppt/ Accessed 2006.

57. Nallamothu BK, Bates ER, Wang Y, et al : Driving times and distances to hospitals with percutaneous coronary intervention in the United States—Implications for pre-hospital triage of patients with ST-elevation myocardial infarction. Circulation 2006;113:1189-1195.

58. Kereiakes DJ, Antman EM: Clinical guidelines and practice: In search of the truth. J Am Coll Cardiol 2006;48:1129-1135.

59. Jacobs AK: Regionalized care for patients with ST-elevation myocardial infarction—It's closer than you think. Circulation 2006;113:1159-1169.

60. Larson DM, Menssen KM, Newell MC, et al: Long distance transfer for direct percutaneous coronary intervention: A facilitated approach [abstract]. J Am Coll Cardiol 2006;47: 174A.

61. Nallamothu BK, Bates ER, Herrin J, et al: Times to treatment in transfer patients undergoing primary percutaneous coronary intervention in the United States: National Registry of Myocardial Infarction (NRMI)-3/4 analysis. Circulation 2005; 111;761-767.

62. McNamara RL, Herrin J, Bradley EH, et al, for the NRML Investigators: Hospital improvement in time to reperfusion in patients with acute myocardial infarction, 1999 to 2002. J Am Coll Cardiol 2006;47:45-51.

63. Antman EM, Anbe DJ, Armstrong PW, et al: ACC/AHA guidelines for the management of patients with ST-elevation myocardial infarction: A report of the American College of Cardiology/American Heart Association Task Force on Practice Guidelines (Committee to Revise the 1999 Guidelines for the Management of Patients with Acute Myocardial Infarction). Circulation 2004;110:e82-e292.

64. O'Neill WW, Grines CL, Dixon SR, et al: Does a 90-minute door-to-balloon time matter? Observations from four current reperfusion trials [abstract]. J Am Coll Cardiol 2005;45: 225A.

65. Brodie BR, Hansen C, Stuckey TD, et al: Door-to-balloon time with primary percutaneous coronary intervention for acute myocardial infarction impacts late cardiac mortality in high-risk patients and patients presenting early after the onset of symptoms. J Am Coll Cardiol 2006;47:289-295.

66. Moyer P, Feldman J, Levine J, et al: Implications of the mechanical (PCI) vs thrombolytic controversy for ST segment elevation myocardial infarction on the organization of emergency medical services. Crit Pathways Cardiol 2004;3: 53-61.

67. Kereiakes DJ, Gibler WB, Martin LH, et al: Relative importance of emergency medical system transport and the pre-hospital electrocardiogram on reducing hospital time delay to therapy for acute myocardial infarction: A preliminary report from the Cincinnati Heart Project. Am Heart J 1992;123: 835-840.

68. Bush HS, Brown A, Fromkin K, et al: "Cath alert" and transmission of a pre-hospital 12-lead electrocardiogram can shorten door-to-balloon times in patients with ST-segment elevation acute myocardial infarction [abstract]. J Am Coll Cardiol 2005;45:222A.

69. Curtis JP, Portnay EL, Wang Y, et al, for the National Registry of Myocardial Infarction-4: The pre-hospital electrocardiogram and time to reperfusion in patients with acute myocardial infarction, 2000-2002: Findings from the National Registry of Myocardial Infarction-4. J Am Coll Cardiol 2006;47:1544-1552.

70. Bradley EH, Roumanis SA, Radford, MJ, et al: Achieving door-to-balloon times that meet quality guidelines: How do successful hospitals do it? J Am Coll Cardiol 2005;46: 1236-1241.

71. Bjorklund E, Stenestrand U, Landback J, et al: A pre-hospital diagnostic strategy reduced time to treatment and mortality in real life patients with ST-elevation myocardial infarction treated with primary percutaneous coronary intervention [abstract]. J Am Coll Cardiol 2006;47:192A.

72. Garvey JL, MacLead BA, Dopko G, et al: Pre-hospital 12-lead electrocardiography programs: A call for implementation by emergency medical services systems providing advanced life support—National Heart Attack Alert Program (NHAAP) Coordinating Committee; National Heart, Lung, and Blood Institute (NHLBI); National Institutes of Health. J Am Coll Cardiol 2006;47:485-491.

38 Percutaneous Revascularization Procedures

Motoya Hayase

KEY POINTS

- Despite advances in percutaneous interventions and coronary bypass surgery for coronary artery disease, many patients are unable to be optimally revascularized because of clinical or anatomic characteristics that limit procedural success and durability. These so-called refractory patients pose an increasing challenge to cardiologists worldwide.
- Investigators have attempted to address this need by exploring options for achieving myocardial revascularization through novel techniques, such as diverting blood to the ischemic myocardium from alternative routes.
- The coronary venous system has been investigated as a source of in situ conduits for diverting blood to the ischemic myocardium. Two of these approaches, percutane-

ous coronary venous arterialization (PICVA) and percutaneous in situ coronary artery bypass (PICAB), source blood from the native coronary circulation and use the coronary veins as an in situ bypass graft. A third method, catheter-based ventricle-to-coronary vein bypass (VPASS), directs blood from the ventricular chambers to the coronary vein in an attempt to retroperfuse the ischemic territory.
- Despite promising results from preclinical studies, all of the techniques have been dropped from further development. This chapter describes the anatomy, rationale, and history of the coronary veins as bypass conduits and provides a critical and historical perspective on these procedures.

BACKGROUND

Coronary artery disease affects millions of patients worldwide each year. More than one million percutaneous interventions and an additional half-million surgical coronary bypass procedures are performed in the United States annually for treatment of disease not adequately managed by medical therapies.[1] However, many patients are unable to be optimally revascularized as a result of clinical or anatomic characteristics that limit procedural success and durability. These patients are often subjected to surgical bypass, even with expectations of suboptimal results, or they may be categorized as "nonrevascularizable" because of poor target vessels and diffuse disease. Investigators have attempted to address this need by exploring options for achieving myocardial revascularization through alternate means, such as diverting blood to the ischemic myocardium from alternate routes. Such novel, mainly percutaneous procedures have the potential to be alternatives to costly, invasive surgical approaches, especially for patients who

have been determined to have no conventional treatment options.

Several strategies have been investigated to address this patient population. Two of these approaches, percutaneous coronary venous arterialization (PICVA) and percutaneous in situ coronary artery bypass (PICAB), source blood from the native coronary circulation and use the coronary veins as an in situ bypass graft. A third method, catheter-based ventricle-to-coronary vein bypass (VPASS), directs blood from the ventricular chambers to the coronary vein.

Despite recognition of the need for such devices to meet the needs of an underserved patient population and almost a decade of effort to develop these techniques, none has yet passed the stage of small feasibility studies in humans. All of the techniques discussed in this chapter have recently been dropped from further development. Inclusion of a discussion of these topics in this book is therefore intended to provide historical perspective, describing the effort that went into their development and the state of the art at the time when they were dropped. Because these techniques took advantage of segments of coronary veins as a source of in situ conduits for diverting blood from one place to another, it is germane to first discuss the anatomy, rationale, and history of the coronary veins as bypass conduits.

CORONARY VENOUS BYPASS

Anatomy

The epicardial coronary venous system comprises three major networks: the coronary sinus (CS) and its tributaries (draining the anterolateral surface of the heart), the middle cardiac vein (MCV) and its tributaries (draining the posterior portion of the heart), and the auricular veins (draining the atria).[2,3] The epicardial veins are extensively collateralized and tolerate segmental ligation well.[4-9] The epicardial coronary arteries, with a few exceptions, closely parallel the epicardial veins. The left anterior descending coronary artery (LAD) parallels the anterior interventricular vein (AIV), the left circumflex coronary artery (LCx) runs with the great cardiac vein (GCV), and the posterior descending coronary artery runs with the MCV (Fig. 38-1). The AIV often branches in the region of the mid-LAD and receives blood from several branching diagonal veins. The AIV enlarges and crosses the LCx to become the oblique vein of Marshall near a venous valve known as Vieussens' valve (named after the early 18th century anatomist Raymond de Veiussens). This marks the beginning of the true CS, which receives blood from the posterior surface of the heart through the MCV and ultimately drains into the right atrium. The site of CS drainage into the right atrium is usually guarded by another venous valve, the valve of Thebesius (named after Adam Thebesius, another early eighteenth century

anatomist). Because of the "milking" action of myocardial contraction (endocardium to epicardium, apex to base) to facilitate coronary venous flow,[10,11] the valves of Vieussens and Thebesius are minimally functional and believed to represent remnant tissue. They remain noteworthy, however, as minor obstacles to percutaneous access to the coronary venous system during interventional procedures. In approximately 25% of patients, the MCV drains directly into the right atrium, not into the CS. Aside from rich collateralizations within the epicardial venous networks, an additional redundancy exists in the coronary venous system: the Thebesian venous system (Fig. 38-2). These veins, described by Vieussens in 1706 and by Thebesius in 1708, have direct connections to arteries, veins, and capillary networks and drain blood from the myocardium directly into the heart chambers. This system can drain up to 90% of the myocardial blood supply, if necessary, to offload selectively ligated epicardial veins.[12] The proximate and parallel nature of the epicardial coronary veins to arteries and the multiple redundancies for coronary venous drainage make the epicardial coronary veins appealing targets for in situ bypass procedures.

History of Coronary Venous Bypass

Pratt, in 1893, first suggested that the heart could receive adequate nutrition by retroperfusion from the coronary veins and thebesian network.[13] In 1935, Robertson and colleagues[14] pursued this concept by evaluating the effects of CS and sequential epicardial coronary venous ligation on the coronary microcirculation. These investigators suggested several possible mechanisms of benefit, the most noteworthy being that segmental ligation of coronary veins forces arterial blood to underperfused myocardium rather

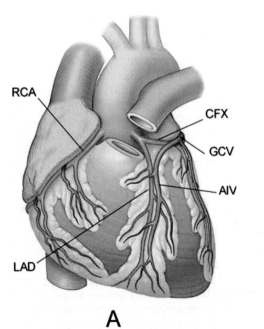

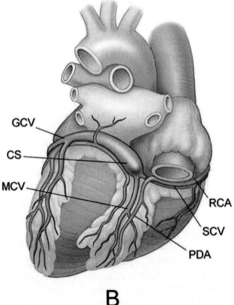

A   **B**

Figure 38-1. Anterior (**A**) and posterior (**B**) views of the epicardial coronary circulation, demonstrating the relationship between arterial and venous systems. AIV, anterior interventricular vein; CFX, left circumflex coronary artery; CS, coronary sinus; GCV, great cardiac vein; LAD, left anterior descending coronary artery; MCV, middle cardiac vein; PDA, posterior descending coronary artery; RCA, right coronary artery; SCV, small cardiac vein. (From Oesterle SN, Reifart N, Hauptmann E, et al: Percutaneous in situ coronary venous arterialization: Report of the first human catheter-based coronary artery bypass. Circulation 2001;103: 2539-2543.)

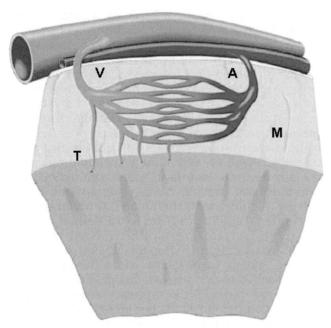

Figure 38-2. Thebesian venous system. Thebesian veins (T) provide an alternate venous drainage route through the myocardium (M) into the cardiac chambers. A arterioles; V, venules. (Courtesy of TransVascular, Inc., Menlo Park, CA.)

than through the lower resistance venous routes. Subsequently, several reports suggested that although complete ligation may be deleterious, myocardial infarct size could be attenuated by partial ligation of the CS.[15,16]

Roberts and coworkers[17] performed the first animal investigations of surgical venous retroperfusion ("venous arterialization") in 1943. They demonstrated that the anterior myocardial wall could be retroperfused by a surgical arterial conduit to the CS, despite experimental occlusion of the LAD. Glass microspheres and labeled erythrocytes proved that perfusion occurred from the capillaries and that blood was not preferentially shunted into sinusoids or thebesian networks.

Beck and colleagues[18-20] performed the first human clinical investigations of this approach. Their procedure was refined to a staged procedure, known as the Beck II operation, in which an aortocoronary vein bypass was followed by partial CS ligation.

Observational clinical follow-up (3 months to 5 years) of more than 200 patients in whom the Beck II procedure was performed suggested that approximately 90% of patients thought that their symptoms were improved by the procedure. Bakst and associates[21-24] evaluated the Beck II procedure in a dog model. They demonstrated a mortality reduction from 90% in control to 20% in Beck II–treated animals, respectively, who had subsequent LAD ligation.

Although other surgeons described excessive surgical mortality associated with the Beck II procedure, the feasibility of coronary venous bypass was established. Subsequently, several investigators evaluated

the prospect of selective, rather than global, venous arterialization. Several animal studies[9,25-29] of selective venous arterialization produced mixed results. However, reductions in infarct size and regions of ischemia along with improved myocardial perfusion were consistently demonstrated. One study reported by Marco and colleagues[29] demonstrated a proclivity for intimal fibrosis, thrombosis, and anastomotic failure of the arterialized vein.

Hochberg and colleagues[4-7] performed an extensive series of animal studies that demonstrated that retrograde perfusion could restore almost 30% of normal myocardial blood flow to all myocardial layers and could reduce ischemia present on electrocardiography. In contrast to the results of Marco and colleagues,[29] Hochberg's group[7] did not encounter problems with anastomotic failure and hypothesized that it was a complication of beating heart bypass (rather than his experiments of arrested hearts on cardiopulmonary bypass) and not an intrinsic problem with venous arterialization.

Park and associates[8] performed the first selective surgical venous bypass in six patients with diffuse disease. These patients were reported to be doing well at the 1-year follow-up. Another small series and a retrospective clinical survey of 55 American heart surgeons who had performed venous bypass procedures supported these findings.[30-33]

Despite these apparent successes, selective surgical bypass of coronary veins was ultimately overshadowed by widespread enthusiasm for direct coronary arterial bypass surgery and was never widely adopted. It is only with recent recognition of the fact that a significant number of patients have diffuse coronary disease not amenable to arterial bypass or percutaneous intervention that interest in coronary venous retroperfusion and related concepts became renewed.

INTERVENTION METHODS

Percutaneous Coronary Venous Arterialization

One novel approach that targets patients with no options (i.e., poor distal target vessels, diffuse disease, or excessive comorbidity) is to produce selective venous arterialization and myocardial retroperfusion by means of a catheter-based procedure. The concept of percutaneous coronary venous arterialization (PICVA) (Fig. 38-3) has been proposed based on innovative technologies developed by TransVascular (Menlo Park, CA).[34-36] This method requires the following:

1. CS and selective guiding catheters, developed to access the coronary sinus and maintain a stable platform for introduction of interventional devices into the coronary venous system
2. A TransAccess catheter, which is a unique catheter designed to obtain access of a guidewire from one vessel (e.g., an artery) to a neighboring vessel (e.g., a vein) with a

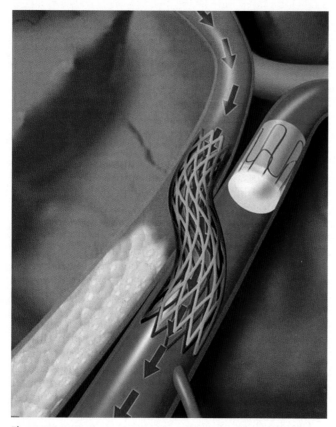

Figure 38-3. Percutaneous in situ coronary venous arterialization (PICVA). With the connection of the left anterior descending artery to the anterior interventricular vein, oxygenated blood that normally perfuses the ventricular apex by an arterial route is instead rerouted (retrograde) through the venous segment. An occlusion device is implanted to direct blood flow toward the apex instead of the coronary sinus. (Courtesy of TransVascular, Inc., Menlo Park, CA.)

high-precision, vessel-to-vessel needle puncture and transvascular guidewire exchange system that uses phased-array intravascular ultrasound (IVUS) guidance
3. A venous blocking device to prevent shunting of arterial blood entering the epicardial venous network back to the CS, directing it through the targeted in situ venous conduit
4. Channel creation and maintenance devices, designed to be delivered over a 0.014-inch arteriovenous guidewire to create permanent conduits between the vessels
5. Standard coronary guiding catheters and angioplasty balloons, used to deliver devices into the coronary arteries and intermittently to predilate and postdilate the channel during the procedure

After proper anticoagulation, coronary arteriography is performed at the onset of each procedure, with emphasis on acquiring images throughout the venous follow-through phase. This gives important information on the coronary anatomy, the relationships of the coronary arteries and their companion veins, anomalous venous drainage patterns, and the loca-

tion of the CS. The CS is accessed from a femoral approach, with a diagnostic catheter being placed within the right ventricle and slowly withdrawn with clockwise rotation. The tip is thus directed posteriorly as the catheter is prolapsed across the tricuspid valve, typically falling into the CS. A 0.035-inch, hydrophilic-coated guidewire with a J-shaped tip is securely placed through the CS, and the diagnostic catheter is exchanged with standard over-the-wire technique with specialized CS and subselective guide catheters. These CS and subselective guiding catheters are used to maintain access throughout the procedure and provide backup support for device delivery. A guidewire is then placed through the coronary arterial guiding catheter to the desired location and the 6-Fr TransAccess catheter is advanced to the desired location. Using the phased-array IVUS imaging system incorporated near the tip of the TransAccess catheter, an extendable nitinol needle is advanced through the coronary artery into the adjacent companion vein. Because the puncture is subadventitial, blood does not escape into the pericardium. A 0.014-inch arteriovenous guidewire secures this initial connection, and the needle is withdrawn into its protective sheath. The TransAccess catheter is withdrawn over the exchange-length guidewire, and a small angioplasty balloon is used to predilate the arteriovenous channel. A connector device is then used to create a permanent connection between the artery and vein. This connector is sized differently on its two ends to accommodate the larger vein relative to the artery. This connector is postdilated as necessary. A blocker device is delivered through the CS and subselective catheters to a position near the connector to prevent shunting of the arterial blood back through the CS. The goal is that oxygenated blood retroperfuses the myocardium through the arterialized venous system. Final arteriography is performed to confirm procedural success.

The PICVA procedure has allowed pigs to survive acute proximal occlusion of the LAD, which is generally fatal in this model.[34] In 2001, Oesterle and colleagues[35,36] reported a 1-year follow-up of the first patient to have this PICVA procedure. The patient was a 53-year-old diabetic man with Canadian Cardiovascular Society class IV angina despite medical therapy. At baseline, he was able to perform at 50 to 80 W on an exercise bicycle, and sestamibi imaging demonstrated a previous apical infarct with apical ischemia. This patient had a proximal total occlusion of the LAD (Fig. 38-4A) that was unable to be crossed with a guidewire despite multiple attempts for standard percutaneous revascularization. This patient was seen by the cardiac surgical team and determined not to be a candidate for this approach because of diffuse disease in the LAD and poor distal targets. After informed consent was obtained, the patient was enrolled in the phase I PICVA trial, which was performed at the Krankenhause der Barmherzingen Bruder in Trier, Germany. The PICVA procedure was successfully completed (see Fig. 38-4B), and the in

Figure 38-4. First successful human percutaneous in situ coronary venous arterialization (PICVA). **A,** An angiogram taken before intervention shows the left coronary system in the left anterior oblique, cranial projection. The left anterior descending coronary artery *(arrow A)* is occluded after the second large diagonal. **B,** In the angiogram taken immediately after PICVA, *arrow B* indicates an arterialized anterior interventricular vein, and *arrow C* indicates the site of arteriovenous connection. **C,** In the angiogram taken at the 3-month follow-up, *arrow D* indicates persistent arterialization of the coronary vein. (From Oesterle SN, Reifart N, Hauptmann E et al: Percutaneous in situ coronary venous arterialization: Report of the first human catheter-based coronary artery bypass. Circulation 2001;103:2539-2543.)

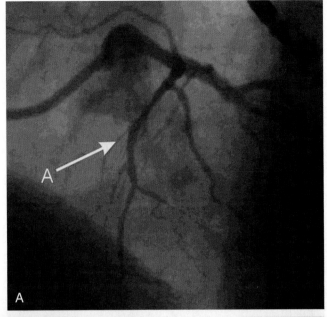

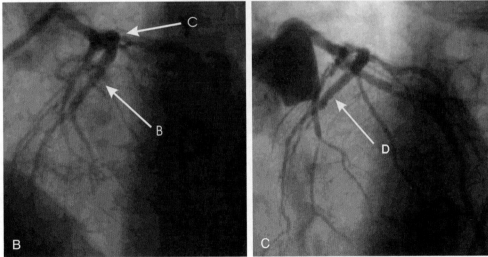

situ bypass conduit remained widely patent at 3-month follow-up angiography (see Fig. 38-4C). The patient remained completely free of angina at the 12-month follow-up and was able to exercise to 120 W on exercise bicycle testing without chest pain.

Small-scale feasibility clinical studies were initiated.[35,36] Eleven patients were enrolled, and PICVA was successfully completed in five patients, but several issues emerged. Two of the five treated patients died within 48 hours after the procedure, reportedly due in part to venous congestion (i.e., venous hyperperfusion or hemorrhagic infarction), raising important safety questions regarding this procedure. An additional issue related to anatomic variation of the relationship between the AIV and LAD. The procedure could not be completed in six of the enrolled patients because of vessel crossovers and unexpected distances (>6 to 8 mm). Other complications included tamponade and migration of the venous blocker

toward the coronary sinus requiring deployment of an additional blocker, which may have contributed to the trauma. These factors, in addition to the fact that the procedure was difficult to perform, lead the investigators and sponsors to abandon further evaluation of this approach.

Percutaneous In Situ Coronary Artery Bypass

Percutaneous in situ coronary artery bypass (PICAB) (Fig. 38-5) is another method based on technologies developed by TransVascular that uses the companion coronary vein as an in situ bypass graft for the diseased artery.[34] PICAB is intended to address patients requiring revascularization in whom the technical success or durability by standard percutaneous interventional techniques is suboptimal. This typically includes a population of patients believed to be best treated by surgical coronary artery bypass. It was intended that PICAB patients would have

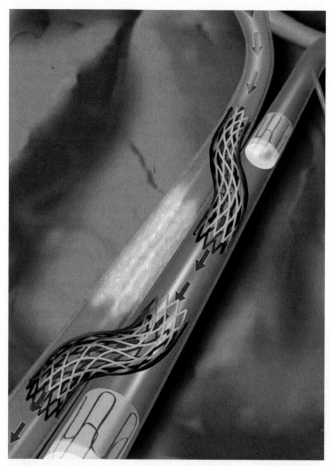

Figure 38-5. Percutaneous in situ coronary artery bypass (PICAB) is shown. The native cardiac vein has been used as the bypass conduit. (Courtesy of TransVascular, Inc., Menlo Park, CA.)

appropriate distal vessels and outflow for the distal venoarterial connection. PICAB shares many of the same devices and techniques previously described for the PICVA procedure. In PICAB, most procedural work is performed within the coronary veins.

Preparation, sedation, anticoagulation, and femoral artery and venous access are similar to those in the PICVA procedure. The CS is likewise cannulated, and the CS catheter is positioned over a 0.035-inch exchange-length hydrophilic guidewire. A subselective guiding catheter is placed farther within the coronary venous system to facilitate device exchange and positioning. The TransAccess catheter is advanced over a 0.014-inch guidewire to the appropriate position, and transvenous needle puncture is performed under phased-array IVUS guidance into the companion artery distal to the target arterial stenosis. A venoarterial guidewire is placed to secure position, and the needle is withdrawn. A distal blocker is deployed within the coronary veins beyond this distal puncture to prevent shunting of arterial blood to the distal venous system. The TransAccess catheter is withdrawn into the vein to an area proximal to the arterial stenosis, and an IVUS-guided needle puncture and guidewire passage from vein to artery are performed in a similar manner. At this point, venoarterial access is maintained by guidewires proximal and distal to the arterial stenosis. The distal and proximal venoarterial anastomoses are dilated with standard angioplasty balloons, and connectors are placed and postdilated appropriately to ensure full expansion and size matching for the newly formed, permanent, dual arteriovenous conduits. A blocker is deployed proximal to the most proximal connector. In effect, this allows blood to bypass the culprit arterial stenosis using the segment of the companion coronary vein as an in situ bypass conduit.

When feasible, the PICAB procedure theoretically has a potential advantage over PICVA because of the maintenance of normal arterial perfusion patterns and decreased likelihood of shunting. Peripheral experience with veins as in situ bypass conduits suggest that durability is good, likely because the vein is not harvested from its natural bed and blood supply.[37,38] The PICAB procedure has been performed successfully in pig models. It is particularly appealing as an approach to a vessel with a chronic total occlusion when antegrade guidewire passage in the native artery has failed. PICAB also looms as a potential alternative to redo bypass surgery. However, this procedure was never performed for coronary bypass in human subjects.

Ventricular Sourcing Bypass

The concept of treating heart disease by redirecting blood to the myocardium independent of the coronary arteries was first conceived more than 50 years ago.[18,39] Vineberg and, later, Beck recognized that there were large sources of oxygenated blood directly adjacent to the ischemic heart wall (i.e., within the left ventricular cavity or in arteries near the heart). Vineberg's approach involved implanting an internal mammary artery directly into the ischemic myocardium. Later, Sen and coworkers[40] proposed a technique in which blood was directed to the myocardium from the left ventricle through an acupuncture-like technique, for which holes were created in the ischemic tissue. Horvath and colleagues,[41] among others,[42] attempted to perfuse the myocardium by drilling channels in the heart wall using a laser. These channels occluded almost immediately,[43] and the mechanism responsible for potential clinical benefit was unclear. No increased survival was observed with this technique when the procedure was compared with medical management.[44]

Ventricular sourcing of blood to perfuse coronary arteries is an alternative approach for improving myocardial perfusion that is aimed at relieving ischemia by delivering oxygenated blood directly from the left ventricle of the heart to a coronary vessel through a communication in the heart wall. Ventricular sourcing was first proposed by Goldman[45] and Massimo[46] in the 1950s and then further studied by Munro and Allen in 1969.[47] Munro's experimental model consisted of inserting a long polymeric tube into the left ventricle and then looping the tube, external to the heart, to a coronary artery. They reported an average flow rate into the coronary artery of only 30% of the baseline flow and concluded "any attempts to revascularize the wall of the left ventricle direct from the cavity of the ventricle are likely to be functional failures, even if technically feasible."

Unlike conventional techniques, ventricular sourcing delivers blood to the coronary vessels during systole (i.e., the high-pressure ejection phase of the heart's pumping action). During systole, blood is forced through the conduit and into the coronary vessel. During diastole (i.e., the low-pressure filling phase) some blood within the coronary vessel returns to the ventricle because there is no valve to maintain perfusion pressure during diastole.

There has been renewed interest in the development of ventricular sourcing as an alternative myocardial revascularization technique. New device designs have emerged that overcome the limitations observed in Munro's studies resulting in improved flow[48,49] and function.[50] Studies by Tweden and colleagues[48] and Emery and coworkers[49] used an L-shaped hollow tube with one end implanted directly into the left ventricle and the other connected to a coronary artery. They observed flow to the coronary vessel approximately 70% of baseline with their improved device design and concluded, contrary to Munro, that ventricular sourcing is feasible. In similar studies of ventricular sourcing using a ventricle-to-coronary artery conduit, Suehiro and colleagues[50] observed a direct relationship between flow and function. Net flow between 50% and 70% was achieved in their studies. Myocardial perfusion and regional contractility were measured to evaluate function. Their studies showed that 70% of regional function could be maintained with 70% flow from the ventricular source, further demonstrating that ventricular sourcing is feasible.

Yi and colleagues[51] examined the retroperfusion through a direct left ventricle–to–great cardiac vein (GCV) conduit in dogs. The left ventricular GCV flow was established using an extracorporeal circuit. Left ventricular pressure, aortic pressure, regional myocardial segment length, and circuit blood flow were measured before LAD ligation, after LAD ligation, and after left ventricular GCV circuit placement. To eliminate backward flow during diastole, an in-line flow regulator was placed. The study results showed that a left ventricular GCV circuit could significantly restore regional function to the acutely ischemic myocardium. An in-line valve that eliminated backward diastolic flow improved regional function even further.[51]

Percardia (Merrimack, NH) developed a surgically deliverable implant (VSTENT myocardial implant) for ventricular sourcing. The company's VSTENT implant is a balloon-expandable device inserted in the myocardium, creating a connection between the left ventricle and a coronary artery. In a study published in *Circulation*, Boekstegers and colleagues[52] examined the flow and function of the VSTENT implant in juvenile pigs. They found that approximately 70% of baseline flow and function could be

provided by the VSTENT implant when the coronary vessel was totally occluded. They also observed preservation of flow and function under increased oxygen demand, especially in the presence of a high-degree stenosis, similar to that typically encountered in patients with clinically significant coronary artery disease. Boekstegers and associates[52] concluded that the VSTENT implant for ventricular sourcing is feasible. Later clinical results[53,54] with this surgically based technique confirmed that ventricular sourcing is feasible, but the overall efficacy of the device was limited by an unacceptably high rate of stenosis within the expanded polytetrafluoroethylene (ePTFE)–covered device. In this initial clinical study, the restenosis rate approached 50% at 6 months' follow-up. Although the stenotic processes appeared to be predominantly an intimal hyperplastic response, it could not be determined whether this response was caused by flow disturbances, material issues, injury response, or a combination of all these factors. Additional clinical studies of this technique are not being pursued.

Many patients with advanced coronary artery disease cannot be effectively treated using conventional revascularization methods. This group of patients is often described as "no option" or "medically refractory." There are patients who, although they have been revascularized, have one or more vessels that could not be repaired, resulting in an "incomplete revascularization." The reasons that these patients are not candidates for standard revascularization therapy include chronic total occlusions (CTOs), diffuse disease, comorbidities that make them poor candidates for surgery, poor target vessels, lack of conduits, and lack of an acceptable site in the target vessel for treatment. For example, these patients would not be treatable by PICAB, but they would be potential candidates for PICVA. Percardia also developed a treatment for these patients suffering from refractory angina using an implant (VPASS myocardial implant) to connect the left ventricle to a coronary vein. Delivered percutaneously (VPASS Percutaneous Delivery System), this novel bypass technique provides blood flow from the ventricle through the coronary venous system and retroperfuses the myocardium (Fig. 38-6).

Important differences exist between PICVA and Percardia's VPASS approach, suggesting potential safety improvements for VPASS. By sourcing from the ventricle rather than an artery, the VPASS myocardial implant exposes the venous system to a lower mean pressure. When connected to an artery, the venous system is exposed to arterial pressure (e.g., mean pressure of about 100 mm Hg). Alternatively with the VPASS implant, the venous system is exposed to mean ventricular pressure (e.g., mean pressure of about 50 mm Hg). The low pressure within the left ventricle during diastole represents a natural pressure-relief mechanism for the VPASS implant perfused venous system. Preclinical studies have demonstrated that Percardia's VPASS implant approach is safe and does not result in venous

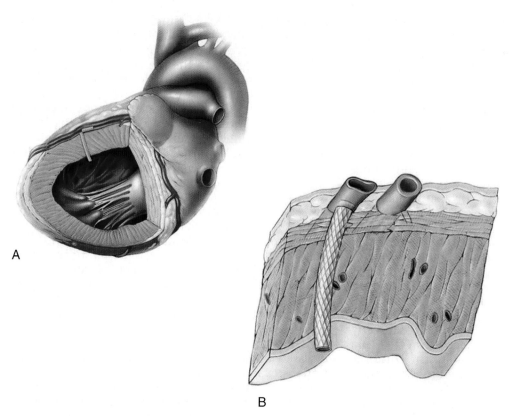

A

B

Figure 38-6. The ventricle-to-coronary venous bypass is achieved with a VPASS myocardial implant. **A,** The VPASS myocardial implant sources blood from the left ventricle to the target vessel (i.e., the anterior interventricular vein[58]). **B,** Close-up view of the VPASS implant– anterior interventricular vein (AIV) anastomosis. (Courtesy of Percardia, Inc., Merrimack, NH.)

congestion, as determined by gross observation and histopathologic analyses. Several groups have evaluated the potential of using ventricular sourced blood for perfusing the ischemic heart through the coronary sinus. Martin[55,56] evaluated a prosthetic left ventricle–to–coronary sinus shunt designed to provide retrograde perfusion of the venous system. The shunt was shown to reduce infarct size by up to 73% in pigs made ischemic by acute occlusion of the left anterior diagonal vessels. Patel[57] demonstrated the technical feasibility of creating a left ventricle–to–coronary artery shunt in dogs using percutaneous endovascular techniques. Preclinical studies have demonstrated that Percardia's VPASS implant-based perfusion may be effective at enhancing nutritive blood flow to the myocardium as evidenced by magnetic resonance imaging (MRI) perfusion studies[58,59] and maintenance of myocardial function.[60]

Catheter-Based Ventricle-to-Coronary Vein Bypass

In catheter-based ventricle-to-coronary vein bypass (VPASS), preparation, sedation, anticoagulation, and femoral artery and venous access are similar to those for the PICVA procedure. Through the right femoral vein, the CS is selectively cannulated with a CS catheter and a 0.035-inch exchange-length hydrophilic-coated guidewire. The wire is then advanced from the CS to the AIV. Over the exchange wire, a CS guide catheter with dilator is delivered to the ostium of the CS. The exchange wire is then replaced with a 300-cm, 0.014-inch guidewire. A 6.2-Fr TransAccess CrossPoint-CX catheter (Medtronic, Minneapolis,

MN) is advanced to the middle of the AIV over the 0.014-inch guidewire through the CS guiding catheter. Using solid-state, 64-element, phased-array IVUS imaging element (20 MHz), the CrossPoint-CX catheter is oriented in the direction toward the left ventricular chamber.[58] The catheter is rotated until the LAD is located between 8- and 9-o'clock positions and the pericardium between the 4- and 5-o'clock positions. The puncture needle is then oriented toward the left ventricular chamber at the 12-o'clock position (Fig. 38-7A). A 24-gauge nitinol needle is then extended 9 mm into the myocardium and extended incrementally up to 17 mm based on the myocardial thickness. After the needle exits the myocardium into the left ventricle, the 300-cm, 0.014-inch guidewire is advanced through the needle lumen into the left ventricle and then further advanced through the left ventricular chamber into the ascending aorta for support during the VPASS implant. The CrossPoint-CX catheter is removed, and a 3.0-mm balloon catheter is advanced within a subselective catheter and inflated to 10 atm to dilate the myocardial channel. After balloon deflation, a VPASS delivery system (see Fig. 38-7B and C) is tracked to the target location. The VPASS delivery system design allows tactile feedback in combination with fluoroscopic guidance to place a section of the VPASS implant in the AIV and the remaining length in the myocardium. The delivery system is a double-balloon system consisting of a balloon to inflate the AIV VPASS implant section and a balloon to inflate the myocardial VPASS implant section. The total length of the VPASS implant in the myocardium is approximately 28 mm.

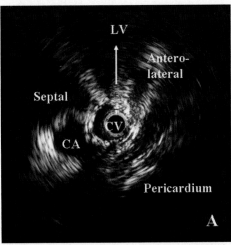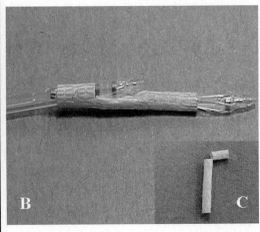

Figure 38-7. A, Intravascular imaging shows that the CrossPoint-CX catheter is placed in the coronary vein. The *white arrow* indicates the needle direction. The best puncture direction is achieved when the coronary artery is located between the 8- and 9-o'clock positions on the image. **B,** The ventricle-to-coronary vein bypass (VPASS) system. The VPASS delivery catheter has two semicompliant balloons, each mounted on a separate shaft: a 4.0-mm-diameter balloon for the myocardial segment and a 3.0-mm-diameter balloon for the vein segment. The VPASS delivery system is supplied with a premounted VSTENT myocardial implant. This is accomplished by the balloons bifurcating as the myocardial balloon enters the myocardium and the venous balloon is positioned in the vein. This allows for precise positioning of the VPASS delivery system. **C,** The VSTENT implant consists of three important components: a metal stent scaffold, a covering, and a hemocompatible coating. The expandable stent scaffold provides the mechanical strength necessary to resist the cyclical compressive forces generated within the myocardium while providing for ease of deployment. The biocompatible covering minimizes tissue invasion into the channel, resists leakage of blood into interstitial spaces, and facilitates healing. The hemocompatible coating prevents thrombotic closure of the channel and enhances long-term patency and function. The metal scaffold is laser-cut from a 316 L stainless steel tube, creating an expandable device with high resistance to compression. The vein segment of the VSTENT has a balloon-expandable stent connected to the myocardial segment by a 316 L-covered flexible hinge. The hinge connection enables seating the myocardial segment of the VSTENT implant at the vessel floor and minimizes the risk that the device will migrate after implantation. The VSTENT metal scaffold is encapsulated between two thin layers of expanded polytetrafluoroethylene (ePTFE). The ePTFE layers are laminated to each other between the openings between the struts of the metal scaffold, completely encapsulating the metal stent, and the connecting hinge is also covered with ePTFE. CA, coronary artery; CV, coronary vein.

After final positioning, the VPASS implant is deployed. Fluoroscopic orthogonal views are used to confirm that the VPASS implant is deployed satisfactorily. A venogram is used to confirm that a connection has been made from the AIV to the left ventricle with flow distal to the VPASS implant.[58]

Hayase and colleagues[58] demonstrated that the VPASS procedure could be safely and effectively performed in a large-animal model. Contrast injection after VPASS placement demonstrates implant patency and capillary blush and contrast in the left ventricle (Fig. 38-8A and B). This animal underwent VPASS and LAD occlusion. Figure 38-8 demonstrates the systolic left ventriculogram (see Fig. 38-8C) and diastolic left ventriculogram (see Fig. 38-8D) 10 minutes after completing the VPASS procedure. The left ventricular ejection fraction was 32% by quantitative analysis, and anterior wall motion was preserved by the VPASS procedure, even in the setting of mid-LAD occlusion. There were no ischemic changes on electrocardiography or clinical signs of heart failure. The black arrows show the patent flow in the distal AIV 10 minutes after completing the VPASS procedure (see Fig. 38-8C). The blocker position within the vein is identified by the place where the contrast flow stops on the left ventriculogram (see Fig. 38-8C). In this case, placement was approximately 10 mm beyond the VSTENT implant in the proximal AIV.

Angiography at 1 month demonstrated a patent and functioning VSTENT with AIV flow in systole (see Fig. 38-8E) and preserved left ventricular function (LVEF = 59%). VPASS implant deployment achieved equalization of the AIV and left ventricular systolic pressures and creation of retrograde flow in the distal AIV. These investigators have also reported that the VPASS implant provided oxygenated blood into the ischemic myocardium during concomitant LAD and AIV occlusions.[58,59]

Hayase and coworkers[58] assessed the ability of venous perfusion to preserve myocardial viability in a porcine model of acute myocardial infarction. VPASS myocardial implants were deployed percutaneously in the AIV of juvenile swine connecting the left ventricle with the AIV. The AIV was occluded toward the coronary sinus by implanting a vessel blocker proximal to the VPASS implant. An embolic coil was placed in the LAD to create an acute infarction model. On deploying an embolic coil in the LAD, animals typically exhibit ST-segment elevation indicative of an evolving infarct. Importantly, the animals in which a VPASS implant had been placed before occlusion of the LAD appeared to have a stable electrocardiogram (Fig. 38-9). This indicates that the VPASS implant was providing sufficient flow acutely to support myocardial viability during the acute arterial occlusion.

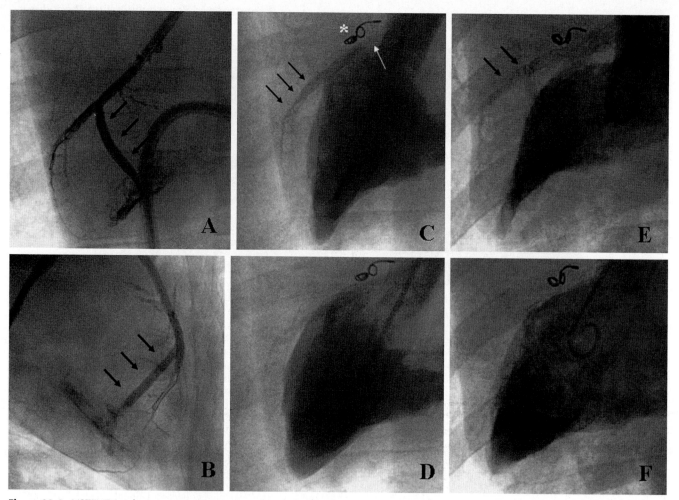

Figure 38-8. VSTENT implant venography. Venography after VSTENT implantation with a 9-Fr subselective guiding catheter. **A,** Left anterior oblique (LAO), 30-degree view. **B,** In the right anterior oblique (RAO), 90-degree view, the *black arrows* indicate the patent VSTENT. The left ventriculogram (LVG) was obtained after the VPASS procedure. The systolic LVG (LAO, 30-degree view) **(C)** and diastolic LVG **(D)** were obtained 10 minutes after VPASS procedure with left anterior descending coronary artery occlusion. The *black arrows* show the contrast flow in the anterior interventricular vein (AIV) in systole. The blocker position was identified by where the contrast flow stops from the LVG **(C).** The *white arrow* shows the position of the blocker, and an *asterisk* shows the emboli coil. Systolic LVG (LAO, 30-degree view) **(E)** and diastolic LVG **(F)** were obtained 1 month after the VPASS procedure. The *black arrow* shows the contrast flow in the AIV in systole.

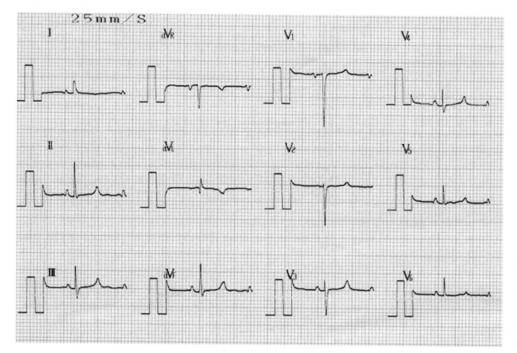

Figure 38-9. Electrocardiogram 30 minutes after occluding the left anterior descending coronary artery in a pig previously implanted with a ventricle-to-coronary vein bypass (VPASS) implant. Notice the absence of any significant abnormalities in the electrocardiographic waveform.

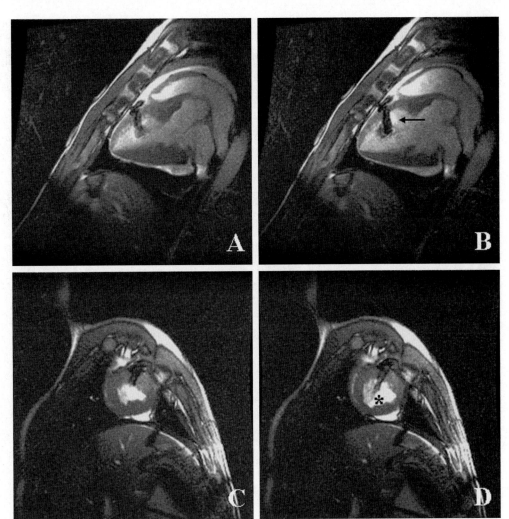

Figure 38-10. FIESTA magnetic resonance images 1 month after ventricle-to-coronary vein bypass (VPASS) and left anterior descending coronary artery occlusion. Upper images show the long-axis view in systole (**A**) and in diastole (**B**). Lower images show the short-axis view in systole (**C**) and in diastole (**D**). The *black arrow* indicates the VSTENT artifact (**B**). The flow *(asterisk)* is coming back through the VSTENT into the left ventricle in diastole (**D**).

After VPASS and occlusion of the LAD, animals were allowed to recover, and they survived for 30 days. Figure 38-10 shows examples of MR images obtained 30 days after the VPASS device had been implanted in addition to a proximal AIV blocker, and the embolic coil had been deployed within the LAD. In these animals at this time, MRI showed hypokinetic anterior wall motion and normal wall thickness. The first-pass perfusion imaging showed myocardial blood flow distal to the VPASS implant. Delayed contrast enhancement showed almost no infarcted area. Good flow was apparent in the VPASS implant. These studies indicate that the VPASS myocardial implant was able to preserve myocardial function in a porcine infarct model. Figure 38-11 shows the fast imaging employing steady-state acquisition (FIESTA) (see Fig. 38-11A to C), the perfusion (see Fig. 38-11D to F), and the delayed, enhanced images (see Fig. 38-11G to J) from one animal of this study. Myocardial thickness was preserved, and the epicardial and mid-myocardial areas were viable. A small focal perfusion defect was observed in the subendomyocardium, and a delayed, enhanced area was observed in the anterior subendomyocardium. Figure 38-12. shows the FIESTA, delayed enhanced images, and gross images from another animal. Myocardial thickness was preserved and

there was no obvious infarction area with the delayed enhanced images.

Figure 38-13 shows Masson's trichrome staining of the left ventricular slice distal to the VPASS implant. The myocardial thickness was preserved and Masson's trichrome staining demonstrated fibrous infarction in the subendomyocardium.

The first pilot study in humans was initiated in late 2005 to investigate the safety and performance of the VPASS myocardial implant as a potential therapy for no-option patients with chronic refractory angina. The procedure was attempted in five patients at five sites around the globe (one patient per site). The procedure could not be completed in the first two patients because of insufficient AIV diameter and thick myocardium. The procedure was completed in the other three patients. Clinical follow-up is being performed, but the study was terminated because of slow enrollment, making it unlikely that a sufficient number of patients would be studied in a reasonable time to fully assess the clinical impact of this approach.

CONCLUSIONS

Millions of surgical and percutaneous revascularization procedures are performed each year for the treat-

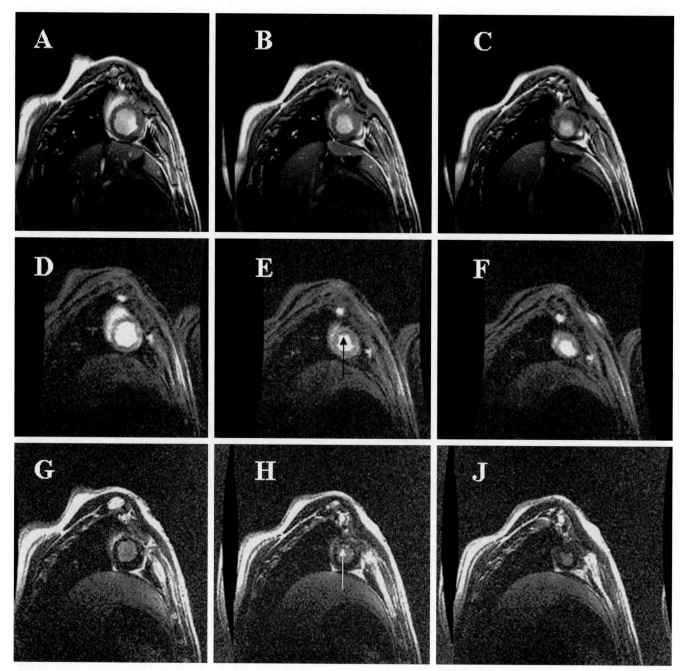

Figure 38-11. FIESTA magnetic resonance images in the upper row (**A** to **C**) were obtained 1 month after ventricle-to-coronary vein bypass (VPASS) and left anterior descending coronary artery occlusion. Perfusion is shown in the middle three images (**D** to **F**). Delayed enhancement is demonstrated in the lower three images (**G** to **J**). *Left to right:* Base to apex, a small focal perfusion defect was observed in the subendomyocardium (**E,** *black arrow*), and a delayed enhanced area was observed in the anterior subendomyocardium (**H,** *white arrow*).

ment of coronary artery disease. These techniques are often constrained by clinical and anatomic characteristics that limit procedural success and durability to restore perfusion in areas supplied by arteries with complex coronary stenoses. Development of innovative concepts of alternate strategies to restore perfusion to such regions of the myocardium attempted to launch a new era in the treatment of no-option patients with coronary disease and medically refractory angina. Although it is recognized that such technologies are needed to address this underserved

patient population and much effort has been expended to develop these technologies, none has yet emerged as a viable option. Techniques such as PICVA, PICAB, and VPASS (applied to coronary arteries or veins) have been evaluated only in the context of small clinical trials. Technical challenges and safety concerns faced in those early studies led to termination of further clinical evaluation. However, it is possible that these concepts can be revisited in future efforts, especially if new technical approaches are conceived. Based on studies performed in animal

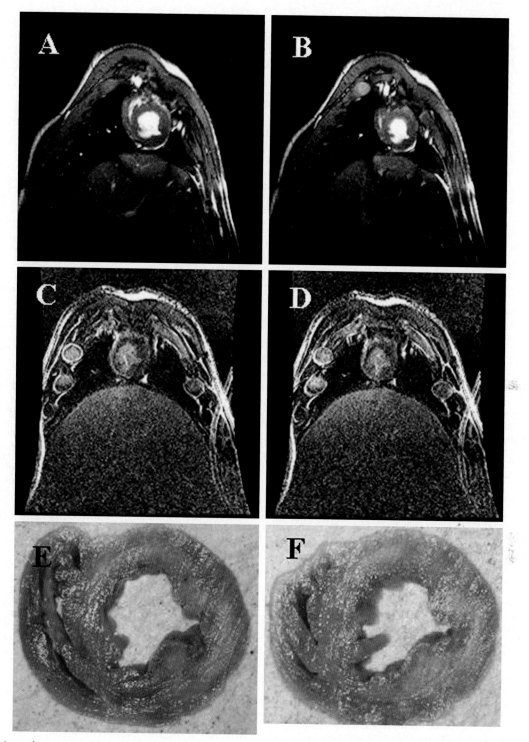

Figure 38-12. Magnetic resonance imaging and gross anatomy. FIESTA (**A** and **B**) and delayed, enhanced images (**C** and **D**). Myocardial thickness was preserved (**A, B, E,** and **F**), and there was no obvious infarction area with the delayed, enhanced images (**C** and **D**).

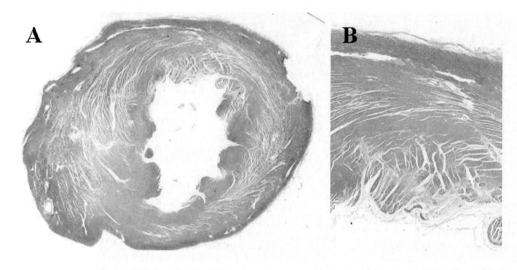

Figure 38-13. Masson's trichrome staining demonstrated the focal fatty fibrosis in the subendomyocardium. **A,** Low magnification (×7). **B,** high magnification (×1.25).

models of chronic ischemia, there is every reason to think that one or more of the techniques discussed in this chapter may ultimately provide clinical benefit to patients with no other treatment option.

REFERENCES

1. American Heart Association: 2001 Heart and Stroke Statistical Update. Dallas, TX, American Heart Association, 2001.
2. von Ludinghausen M: Clinical anatomy of cardiac veins, Vv. cardiacae. Surg Radiol Anat 1987;9:159-168.
3. von Ludinghausen M, Schott C: Microanatomy of the human coronary sinus and its major tributaries. *In* Meerbaums (ed): Myocardial Perfusion, Rertoperfusion, Coronary Venous Retroperfusion. Darmstadt, Germany, Steinkopff, 1990, pp 93-122.
4. Hochberg MS: Hemodynamic evaluation of selective arterialization of the coronary venous system. An experimental study of myocardial perfusion utilizing radioactive microspheres. J Thorac Cardiovasc Surg 1977;74:774-783.
5. Hochberg MS, Austen WG: Selective retrograde coronary venous perfusion: An encouraging approach documented by microsphere flow studies. Surg Forum 1978;29:261-262.
6. Hochberg MS, Roberts WC, Morrow AG, Austen WG: Selective arterialization of the coronary venous system. Encouraging long-term flow evaluation utilizing radioactive microspheres. J Thorac Cardiovasc Surg 1979;77:1-12.
7. Hochberg MS, Austen WG: Selective retrograde coronary venous perfusion. Ann Thorac Surg 1980;29:578.
8. Park SB, Magovern GJ, Liebler GA, et al: Direct selective myocardial revascularization by internal mammary artery-coronary vein anastomosis. J Thorac Cardiovasc Surg 1975;69:63-72.
9. Rhodes GR, Syracuse DC, McIntosh CL: Evaluation of regional myocardial nutrient perfusion following selective retrograde arterialization of the coronary vein. Ann Thorac Surg 1978;25:329-335.
10. Tiedt N, Litwin J, Skolasinska K: The dynamics of the coronary venous pressure in the dog. Pflugers Arch Gesamte Physiol Menschen Tiere 1966;288:27-42.
11. Klassen GA, Armour JA: Canine coronary venous pressures: Responses to positive inotropism and vasodilation. Can J Physiol Pharmacol 1983;61:213-221.
12. Wearn J: The role of the thebesian vessels in the circulation of the heart. J Exp Med 1927;47:293-318.
13. Pratt F. The nutrition of the heart through the vessels of Thebesius and the coronary veins. Am J Physiol 1893;1:86-103.
14. Robertson H: The re-establishment of cardiac circulation during progressive coronary occlusion. Am Heart J 1935;10:533-541.
15. Gross L, Blum L, Silverman G: Experimental attempts to increase the blood supply to the dog's heart by means of coronary sinus occlusion. J Exp Med 1936;65:91-108.
16. Beck C, Mako A: Venous stasis in the coronary circulation: Experimental study. Am Heart J 1941;21:767-779.
17. Roberts J, Browne R, Roberts G: Nourishment of the heart by way of coronary veins. Fed Proc 1943;2:90.
18. Beck C, Stanton E: Revascularization of the heart by graft or systemic artery to the coronary sinus. JAMA 1948;65:477-495.
19. Beck C, Stanton E: Nourishment of the myocardium by way of the coronary veins. Fed Proc 1948;2:90.
20. Beck C, Leighninger D: Operations for coronary artery disease. JAMA 1954;13:1226-1233.
21. Bakst AA, Adam A, Goldberg H, Bailey CP: Arterialization of the coronary sinus in occlusive coronary artery disease. III. Coronary flow in dogs with aorticocoronary sinus anastomosis of six months' duration. J Thorac Surg 1955;29:188-196.
22. Bakst AA, Bailey CP: Arterialization of the coronary sinus in occlusive coronary artery disease. IV. Coronary flow in dogs with aorticocoronary sinus anastomosis of twelve months' duration. J Thorac Surg 1956;31:559-568.
23. Bakst AA, Costas-Durieux J, Goldberg H, Bailey CP: Protection of the heart by arterialization of the coronary sinus. II. Coronary flow in dogs with aorticocoronary sinus anastomosis. J Thorac Surg 1954;27:442-454.
24. Bakst AA, Costas-Durieux J, Goldberg H, Bailey CP: Protection of the heart by arterialization of the coronary sinus. I. Coronary collateral flow in normal dogs and in dogs having had previous nondescript cardiac surgery. J Thorac Surg 1954;27:433-441.
25. Arealis EG, Volder JG, Kolff WJ: Arterialization of the coronary vein coming from an ischemic area. Chest 1973;63:462-463.
26. Bhayana JN, Olsen DB, Byrne JP, Kolff WJ: Reversal of myocardial ischemia by arterialization of the coronary vein. J Thorac Cardiovasc Surg 1974;67:125-132.
27. Chiu CJ, Mulder DS: Selective arterialization of coronary veins for diffuse coronary occlusion: An experimental evaluation. J Thorac Cardiovasc Surg 1975;70:177-182.
28. Kay EB, Suzuki A: Coronary venous retroperfusion for myocardial revascularization. Ann Thorac Surg 1975;19:327-330.
29. Marco JD, Hahn JW, Barner HB, et al: Coronary venous arterialization: Acute hemodynamic, metabolic, and chronic anatomical observations. Ann Thorac Surg 1977;23:449-454.
30. Moll JW, Dziatkowiak AJ, Edelman M, et al: Arterialization of the coronary veins in diffuse coronary arteriosclerosis. J Cardiovasc Surg (Torino) 1975;16:520-525.
31. Moll JW, Iljin W, Ratajczyk-Pakalska E, et al: Experimental and clinical experiences in the arterialisation of the heart veins. Surgical modification of the left ventricle in coronary sclerosis. Zentralbl Chir 1976;101:112-117.

32. Hochberg M, Roberts A, Parsonnet V, Fisch D: Selective arterialization of the coronary veins: Clinical experience of 55 American heart surgeons. Clin CSI 1986;1:195-201.
33. Benedict JS, Buhl TL, Henney RP: Cardiac vein myocardial revascularization. An experimental study and report of 3 clinical cases. Ann Thorac Surg 1975;20:550-557.
34. Fitzgerald PJ, Hayase M, Yeung AC, et al: New approaches and conduits: In situ venous arterialization and coronary artery bypass. Curr Interv Cardiol Rep 1999;1:127-137.
35. Oesterle SN, Reifart N, Hauptmann E, et al: Percutaneous in situ coronary venous arterialization: Report of the first human catheter-based coronary artery bypass. Circulation 2001;103:2539-2543.
36. Oesterle SN, Reifart N, Hayase M, et al: Catheter-based coronary bypass: A development update. Catheter Cardiovasc Interv 2003;58:212-218.
37. Rosenthal D, Dickson C, Rodriguez FJ, et al: Infrainguinal endovascular in situ saphenous vein bypass: Ongoing results. J Vasc Surg 1994;20:389-394; discussion 394-395.
38. Rosenthal D, Herring MB, O'Donovan TG, et al: Endovascular infrainguinal in situ saphenous vein bypass: A multicenter preliminary report. J Vasc Surg 1992;16:453-458.
39. Vineberg AM: The development of an anastomosis between the coronary vessels and a transplanted internal mammary artery. Can Med Assoc J 1946;55:117-119.
40. Sen PK, Udwadia TE, Kinare SG, Parulkar GB: Transmyocardial acupuncture: A new approach to myocardial revascularization. J Thorac Cardiovasc Surg 1965;50:181-189.
41. Horvath KA, Cohn LH, Cooley DA, et al: Transmyocardial laser revascularization: Results of a multicenter trial with transmyocardial laser revascularization used as sole therapy for end-stage coronary artery disease. J Thorac Cardiovasc Surg 1997;113:645-653; discussion 653-654.
42. Allen KB, Dowling RD, DelRossi AJ, et al: Transmyocardial laser revascularization combined with coronary artery bypass grafting: A multicenter, blinded, prospective, randomized, controlled trial. J Thorac Cardiovasc Surg 2000;119:540-549.
43. Fisher PE, Khomoto T, DeRosa CM, et al: Histologic analysis of transmyocardial channels: Comparison of CO_2 and holmium:YAG lasers. Ann Thorac Surg 1997;64:466-472.
44. Schofield PM, Sharples LD, Caine N, et al: Transmyocardial laser revascularisation in patients with refractory angina: A randomised controlled trial. Lancet 1999;353:519-524.
45. Goldman A, Greenstone SM, Preuss FS, et al: Experimental methods for producing a collateral circulation to the heart directly from the left ventricular. J Thorac Surg 1956;31:364-374.
46. Massimo C, Boffi L: Myocardial revascularization by a new method of carrying blood directly from the left ventricular cavity into the coronary circulation. J Thorac Surg 1957;34:257-264.
47. Munro I, Allen P: The possibility of myocardial revascularization by creation of a left ventriculocoronary artery fistula. J Thorac Cardiovasc Surg 1969;58:25-32.
48. Tweden KS, Eales F, Cameron JD, et al: Ventriculocoronary artery bypass (VCAB), a novel approach to myocardial revascularization. Heart Surg Forum 2000;3:47-54; discussion 54-55.
49. Emery RW, Eales F, Van Meter CH Jr, et al: Ventriculocoronary artery bypass results using a mesh-tipped device in a porcine model. Ann Thorac Surg 2001;72:S1004-S1008.
50. Suehiro K, Shimizu J, Yi GH, et al: Direct coronary artery perfusion from the left ventricle. J Thorac Cardiovasc Surg 2001;121:307-315.
51. Yi GH, He KL, Dang NC, et al: Direct left ventricle to great cardiac vein retroperfusion: A novel alternative to myocardial revascularization. Heart Surg Forum 2006;9:E579-E586.
52. Boekstegers P, Raake P, Al Ghobainy R, et al: Stent-based approach for ventricle-to-coronary artery bypass. Circulation 2002;106:1000-1006.
53. Boekstegers P, Steinbeck G, Bengel FM, et al: First human experience with stent-based ventricle-to-coronary artery bypass. Catheter Cardiovasc Interv 2004;62:198-200.
54. Vicol C, Reichart B, Eifert S, et al: First clinical experience with the VSTENT: A device for direct left ventricle-to-coronary artery bypass. Ann Thorac Surg 2005;79:573-579; discussion 579.
55. Martin JS: A new treatment for acute experimental coronary artery occlusion: LV powered coronary sinus retroperfusion. Surg Forum 1998;49:260-263.
56. Martin JS: LV-powered coronary sinus retroperfusion reduces infarct size in acutely ischemic pigs. Ann Thorac Surg 2000;69:84-89.
57. Patel NH: Percutaneous transmyocardial intracardiac retroperfusion shunts: Technical feasibility in a canine model. J Vasc Interv Radiol 2000;11:382-390.
58. Hayase M, Kawase Y, Yoneyama R, et al: Catheter-based ventricle-coronary vein bypass. Catheter Cardiovasc Interv 2005;65:394-404.
59. Yoneyama R, Kawase Y, Hoshino K, et al: Magnetic resonance assessment of myocardial perfusion via catheter-based ventricle-coronary vein bypass in porcine myocardial infarction model. Catheter Cardiovasc Interv 2006;67:58-67.
60. Raake P, Hinkel R, Kupatt C, et al: Percutaneous approach to a stent-based ventricle to coronary vein bypass (venous VPASS): Comparison to catheter-based selective pressure-regulated retro-infusion of the coronary vein. Eur Heart J 2005;26:1228-1234.

"Big Artery" Vascular Interventions

CHAPTER
39 Lower Extremity Interventions

Nezar Falluji and Debabrata Mukherjee

KEY POINTS

- Despite recent advances in noninvasive evaluation of peripheral artery disease (PAD) of the lower extremities, contrast angiography remains the gold standard for definitive evaluation.
- Occlusive disease confined to the iliac arteries appears to occur in relatively young patients and may have a greater impact on productivity and lifestyle.
- The excellent intermediate- to long-term patency rates after percutaneous intervention of the lower extremity arteries has led to its emergence as an attractive alternative to surgery in patients with suitable lesions.
- A strategy of primary as opposed to provisional stenting is generally recommended for aorto-ostial lesions.
- Technical and clinical success rates of endovascular interventions for iliac artery stenosis exceed 90%, and intermediate- and long-term patency are fairly comparable to

those of surgical revascularization, making them the initial therapy of choice for most iliac stenoses.
- Surgery remains the preferred strategy for patients with common femoral and proximal profunda femoris obstructive PAD.
- The lower durability of percutaneous intervention may be offset by the less invasive nature of endovascular interventions and the resultant decreased morbidity and mortality compared with vascular surgery.
- Interventions can be repeatedly performed if they fail, but repeat surgery is technically more challenging and may be limited by availability of conduit.
- In patients with anatomically appropriate lesions, most practitioners use endovascular interventions preferentially as the initial therapy of choice.

EPIDEMIOLOGY AND NATURAL HISTORY

Peripheral arterial disease (PAD) of the lower extremities is a common health problem. Epidemiologic studies have mostly used intermittent claudication (IC) as a symptomatic marker of the disease and an abnormal ankle-brachial index (ABI) to define the burden of asymptomatic PAD. The prevalence of the disease is dependent on the age of the population studied and the underlying atherosclerotic risk profile of the cohort. It is estimated that the overall disease prevalence is in the range of 3% to 10%, increasing to about 15% to 20% in persons older than 70 years of age. More than half of all patients with lower extremity PAD are asymptomatic.[1-7]

History (including standardized questionnaires such as the Rose Claudication Questionnaire used in the Framingham Heart Study) and physical examination may grossly underestimate the true burden of lower extremity PAD.[1] Criqui and colleagues evaluated the prevalence of lower extremity PAD in a population of 613 men and women in southern California, using four different modalities (the Rose questionnaire, pulse examination, ABI, and pulse-wave

velocity). The detection rate of PAD with ABI and pulse-wave velocity was two to seven times higher than the detection rate of the Rose questionnaire. However, clinical examination of the pulse overestimated the prevalence of PAD by twofold.[8]

To optimally manage patients with lower extremity PAD, whether symptomatic or asymptomatic, it is important to understand the global vascular disease burden, the natural history of the disease process, its impact on the patient's lifestyle, and the risk factors for an individual patient. Such knowledge is key in reducing the mortality and morbidity of the individual patient.

VASCULAR ANATOMY OF THE LOWER EXTREMITY

The abdominal aorta bifurcates at the level of the fourth lumbar vertebra into two branches, the right and the left common iliac arteries. The common iliac arteries divide into the external iliac artery, which normally follows the same axis as the common iliac artery, and the internal iliac arteries, which take a posteromedial track in relation to the common iliac

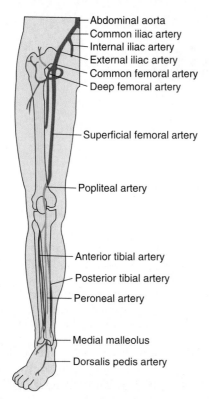

- Abdominal aorta
- Common iliac artery
- Internal iliac artery
- External iliac artery
- Common femoral artery
- Deep femoral artery
- Superficial femoral artery
- Popliteal artery
- Anterior tibial artery
- Posterior tibial artery
- Peroneal artery
- Medial malleolus
- Dorsalis pedis artery

Figure 39-1. Arterial tree of the lower extremity. (Redrawn from http://www.gehealthcare.com/usen/ultrasound/images/cmeadi_fig1_500.jpg. Accessed April 9, 2007.)

artery. In addition to its terminal branches, the common iliac artery gives branches to the surrounding tissues, peritoneum, psoas muscle, ureter, and nerves. Occasionally, the common iliac artery provides accessory renal arteries to a normal or ectopic kidney. Figure 39-1 depicts the arterial circulation of the lower extremity.

The external iliac arteries are larger than the internal iliac arteries. They descend along the medial border of the psoas major muscle, entering the thigh posterior to the inguinal ligament and becoming the common femoral arteries (CFAs). The inferior epigastric artery arises medially from the distal external iliac artery and ascends behind the rectus abdominis muscle. This vessel is a useful landmark for predicting higher bleeding risk in arterial punctures that are proximal to its origin.[9] The external iliac artery gives off other branches, namely the deep circumflex, cremasteric, and several muscular and cutaneous branches, before it continues as the CFA. Together, the common iliac and external iliac arteries contribute to the inflow of the lower extremity.

The CFA starts as a continuation of the external iliac artery, giving multiple branches to surrounding tissues, such as the pudendal arteries and the superficial circumflex artery, then it becomes the superficial femoral artery (SFA) after giving rise to the profunda femoris artery (PFA), roughly 3.5 cm distal to the inguinal ligament. The PFA arises laterally and posteriorly from the CFA, whereas the SFA continues its pathway, to end as the popliteal artery when it passes through the abductor canal. The PFA gives off perforating branches (usually three, with the end of the PFA as the fourth perforating branch), the circumflex (lateral and medial) arteries, and muscular branches. The popliteal artery continues through the abductor's canal, and, after giving off muscular, cutaneous, genicular, and sural branches, it terminates into the anterior tibial artery and the tibioperoneal trunk. The CFA, the SFA, the PFA, and the popliteal artery make up the outflow of the lower extremity.

The anterior tibial artery runs between the two heads of the tibialis posterior muscle and then through the upper part of the interosseous membrane to the front of the leg, medial to the head of the fibula. It descends down to the ankle and then continues to the dorsum of the foot, where it becomes the dorsalis pedis artery. The posterior tibial artery arises from the popliteal artery, distal to the origin of the anterior tibial artery, as the tibioperoneal trunk. After giving rise to the peroneal artery, the tibioperoneal trunk continues as the posterior tibial artery behind the leg. It passes behind the medial malleolus to end by giving rise to the arteries of the foot—namely the calcaneal artery, which anastomoses with the calcaneal and malleolar branches of the peroneal, and the medial and lateral planter arteries. The anterior tibial artery, the posterior tibial artery, and the peroneal artery are considered the runoff vessels.

DIAGNOSIS OF LOWER EXTREMITY PERIPHERAL ARTERIAL DISEASE

History and Physical Examination

Patients with lower extremity PAD may be asymptomatic (with PAD detected during physical examination or screening tests), or they may present with IC, rest pain, nonhealing ulcers, or intractable foot infections. In light of the limitations of clinical assessment, additional assessment of patients with risk factors for atherosclerosis may be required to identify patients with asymptomatic advanced PAD. Symptomatic patients can be classified based on the severity of ischemia by either the Fontaine stages or the Rutherford categories (Table 39-1).

Ankle-Brachial Index

ABI is a ratio of the blood pressure in either the dorsalis pedis or the posterior tibial artery (whichever is higher) to the blood pressure in the brachial artery. ABI measurement is one of the most cost-effective methods in assessing PAD of the lower extremity and typically is done with a handheld Doppler ultrasound device. This is a noninvasive, fairly reproducible, and inexpensive test. The most widely accepted definition of lower extremity PAD is a resting ABI of less than 0.9. A resting ABI of less than 0.9 is usually associated with 50% or greater angiographic arterial stenosis, with a reported sensitivity of 95% and

Table 39-1. Fontaine and Rutherford Classification of Lower extremity PAD

Stage	Fontaine Clinical	Rutherford Grade	Rutherford Category	Clinical
I	Asymptomatic	0	0	Asymptomatic
IIa	Mild claudication	I	1	Mild claudication
IIb	Moderate-severe claudication	I	2	Moderate claudication
		I	3	Severe claudication
III	Ischemic rest pain	II	4	Ischemic rest pain
IV	Ulceration or gangrene	III	5	Minor tissue loss
		IV	6	Ulceration or gangrene

From Dormandy JA, Rutherford RB: Management of peripheral arterial disease (PAD). TASC Working Group. Trans-Atlantic Inter-Society Consensus (TASC). J Vasc Surg 2000;31(1 Pt 2):S1-S296.

Table 39-2. Grading Lower Extremity PAD by Ankle-Brachial Index*

	Supine Resting ABI	Post-exercise ABI
Normal	>1.0	>1.0
Mild	0.8-0.9	>0.4
Moderate	0.4-0.8	>0.2
Severe	<0.4	<0.2

*Postexercise ankle-brachial index (ABI) is measured after treadmill exercise, at 1 to 2 mph with 10% to 12% grade, for 5 minutes or until symptom limited.
From Mukherjee D, Yadav JS: Update on peripheral vascular diseases: From smoking cessation to stenting. Cleve Clin J Med 2001;68:723-733, Table 2.

almost 100% specificity.[7] A resting ABI of 0.4 to 0.9 is suggestive of mild to moderate PAD, and an ABI of less than 0.4 is suggestive of severe PAD (Table 39-2). Resting ABI measurement can be artifactually high in the setting of tibial artery calcification, usually seen in diabetics. In that setting, the toe-brachial index (TBI) may be used. A TBI of less than 0.7 is considered abnormal.

The use of exercise ABI may be helpful in equivocal cases. For this, the patient walks on the treadmill at a constant speed of 1 to 2 mph and with a 10% to 12% incline for 5 minutes. Alternatively, the exercise can be done with active pedal plantar flexion. A decrease of at least 15 mm Hg in the ankle systolic pressure after the exercise challenge is considered an abnormal test. Patients with no significant PAD are expected to have an increase or no change in their ankle systolic pressure.

Pulse Volume Recording

Plethysmography is used to detect volumetric changes in lower extremity blood flow. It is performed with pressure cuffs inflated to 60 to 65 mm Hg at various segments of the lower extremity. Normal tracings show a rapid systolic upstroke and downstroke, with a prominent dicrotic notch. This pattern changes as PAD develops and progresses, with a noted attenuation and widening of the arterial waveform. Ultimately, the waveform becomes flat (nonpulsatile) in patients with advanced PAD (Fig. 39-2).

Segmental Blood Pressure

For the segmental blood pressure test, a series of blood pressure cuffs are placed at the level of the thigh (one or two cuffs), calf, ankle, foot, and big toe. These cuffs are inflated sequentially to about 20 mm Hg above the systolic pressure in that segment. The cuff pressure is then released slowly, and a continuous-wave Doppler probe is used to obtain the pressure at each segment. A decrease between two consecutive levels of 30 mm Hg or more indicates the presence of a stenosis in the segment proximal to the blood pressure cuff. Also, the presence of a 20 to 30 mm Hg difference in the pressure at one limb, compared with the contralateral limb at the same level, is suggestive of significant PAD proximal to the cuff in that limb.

Duplex Ultrasonography

Duplex ultrasound uses a 5 to 7.5 MHz transducer to assess and characterize suprainguinal and infrainguinal PAD with a high sensitivity and specificity (>90%). Doppler velocities are obtained (60-degree Doppler angle) to complement two-dimensional ultrasonography. Traditionally, arteries are classified into five categories: normal, 1% to 19% stenosis, 20% to 49% stenosis, 50% to 99% stenosis, and total occlusion. Duplex ultrasonography may be useful to operators in planning access to a lesion that is amenable to endovascular therapy. It is also very helpful in identifying iatrogenic traumatic lesions and pseudoaneurysms. Direct ultrasound-guided compression or thrombin injection to repair femoral artery pseudoaneurysms is widely used in treating such lesions without the need for surgical procedures. One important limitation of Duplex ultrasonography is that it may overestimate residual stenosis after interventions, limiting its usefulness as a follow-up tool in this setting.

Computed Tomography Angiography

The use of spiral computed tomographic angiography (CTA) in assessing lower extremity PAD has 93%

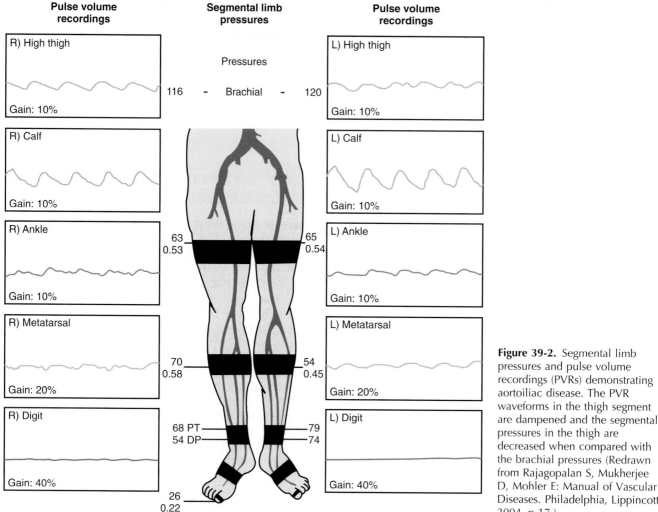

Pulse volume recordings

Segmental limb pressures

Pulse volume recordings

R) High thigh — Gain: 10%

L) High thigh — Gain: 10%

Pressures

116 — Brachial — 120

R) Calf — Gain: 10%

L) Calf — Gain: 10%

R) Ankle — Gain: 10%

L) Ankle — Gain: 10%

63 0.53   65 0.54

R) Metatarsal — Gain: 20%

L) Metatarsal — Gain: 20%

70 0.58   54 0.45

R) Digit — Gain: 40%

L) Digit — Gain: 40%

68 PT   79
54 DP   74

26 0.22

Figure 39-2. Segmental limb pressures and pulse volume recordings (PVRs) demonstrating aortoiliac disease. The PVR waveforms in the thigh segment are dampened and the segmental pressures in the thigh are decreased when compared with the brachial pressures (Redrawn from Rajagopalan S, Mukherjee D, Mohler E: Manual of Vascular Diseases. Philadelphia, Lippincott, 2004, p 17.)

sensitivity and 96% specificity for detection of stenoses greater than 50%, with high accuracy when compared to digital subtraction angiography (DSA). This technology and its role in the management of lower extremity PAD is at an early development stage, and its use in routine clinical practice is not yet well established.[7] Although the role of magnetic resonance angiography (MRA) is better defined, CTA has advantages over MRA in the setting of patients with pacemakers and defibrillators and in those with metal clips, stents, or prostheses (no significant artifact is seen in CTA), and it is significantly faster to perform. However, CTA requires the use of a fairly large dose of iodinated contrast material, and it entails exposure to ionizing radiation (although the dose may be lower than in contrast angiography).[10]

Magnetic Resonance Angiography

Gadolinium-enhanced magnetic resonance angiography (GEMRA) (Fig. 39-3) in the assessment of lower extremity PAD has been compared with standard catheter angiography and has a reported sensitivity of about 90% and a specificity of 100% for detection

of stenoses greater than 50%. Most contemporary studies report an agreement of 91% to 97% between MRA and catheter angiography. GEMRA is superior to duplex ultrasound in detecting stenotic lesions of greater than 50% (sensitivity, 98% vs. 88%; specificity, 96% vs. 95%).[7]

Limitations of this technology include the tendency to overestimate the severity of stenosis; metal clips may give the impression of total occlusion, and metal stents can also obscure vascular flow. In addition, a certain subset of patients cannot be studied with MRA, including those with pacemakers or defibrillators and those with certain types of cerebral aneurysm clips.[7] The principal role of MRA is in the initial evaluation for PAD, especially for patients with inflow disease, using "bolus chase" three-dimensional imaging in which a single bolus of contrast material is followed to the foot.

Contrast Angiography

Despite recent advances in the noninvasive evaluation of lower extremity PAD, contrast angiography remains the gold standard. Traditionally, a pelvic/

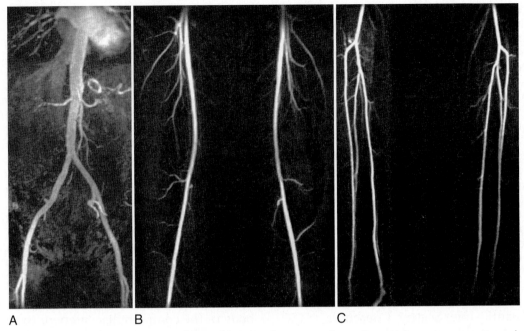

Figure 39-3. Maximal-intensity projection images of three-dimensional contrast-enhanced magnetic resonance angiography in a patient with normal lower extremities runoff. (From Rajagopalan S, Mukherjee D, Mohler E: Manual of Vascular Diseases. Philadelphia, Lippincott, 2004, p 65.)

abdominal aortogram in the anteroposterior projection is done using a straight pigtail catheter (5 or 6 Fr) placed at the level of the L1-L2 vertebrae. Between 10 and 15 mL of an iso-osmolar contrast agent is injected at a rate of 15 mL/sec with DSA technology. This allows an excellent view of the distal aorta and the origin of the common iliac arteries and the external iliac and CFA. Angulated views (30 degrees left anterior oblique) can then be used to visualize the iliac and femoral bifurcations without overlap. Next, the pigtail catheter is placed above the aortic bifurcation (L3-L4), and digital subtraction with bolus chase, 8 mL/sec for 10 seconds (total ~80 mL contrast), is used to assess the outflow and distal runoff. Selective injections and sheath injections can then be used to further define the territory of interest as needed. "Roadmap" technology may be employed subsequently to help operators in their intervention and in the placement of balloons and stents.

Contrast angiography remains the most readily used and most widely available imaging technique for patients with PAD of the lower extremity in whom revascularization is contemplated. Noninvasive technologies such as MRA or CTA may be used before contrast angiography to help identify the potential culprit lesion and plan a best approach (e.g., access point, catheter selection) to study it invasively.[7] Contrast angiography may be associated with vascular access complications (bleeding, infections, pseudoaneurysms, and vascular disruption), and atheroembolism, as well as contrast nephropathy and contrast-induced anaphylactoid reactions. These complications, although rare, should be considered in the decision-making process with regard to the assessment of PAD.

INTERVENTIONS

Percutaneous or surgical interventions are indicated for severe lifestyle-limiting symptoms, to reduce tissue breakdown in the context of critical limb ischemia (CLI), or for salvage in the context of acute limb ischemia.

Iliac Artery Intervention (Inflow Disease)

Indications

The indication for iliac artery (or aortoiliac) percutaneous intervention include symptom relief in patients with IC for whom medical therapy has failed, management of CLI (rest pain, ulceration, or gangrene), as part of the preparation for a planned distal lower extremity bypass surgery to restore or preserve the inflow to the lower extremity or for other invasive procedures such as the placement of an intra-aortic balloon pump, and for the treatment of flow-limiting dissection after invasive catheterization-based procedures.

Revascularization Options

Occlusive disease confined to the iliac arteries appears to occur in relatively young patients and may therefore have a greater impact on productivity and lifestyle. For instance, the mean age of the cohort in the Dutch Iliac Stent Trial was approximately 59 years.[11] These patients (>90% of whom were smokers) were otherwise healthy compared to those with infrainguinal disease or more diffuse PAD. In general, any type of revascularization for this subset of patients can offer satisfactory long-term results. Historically, aortobifemoral bypass surgery has been the gold standard for PAD involving the iliac arteries, because it is associated with excellent long-term patency rates (85%-90% at 5 years, 75%-80% at 10 years, and 60% at 20 years); however, it may be associated with an intraoperative mortality rate of approximately 1% to 3% and a major complication rate of 5% to 10%. These disadvantages, combined with the excellent intermediate- to long-term patency rates after percutaneous intervention, have led to the emergence of percutaneous revascularization as an attractive alternative to surgery in patients with suitable lesions for such intervention. In the Swedish randomized controlled trial (RCT), in which 37% of randomized patients had iliac artery stenosis, there was equivalence in outcomes between PTA and surgery.[12] In the iliac disease subgroup, the patency rate at 1 year was 90% in the PTA arm and 94% in the surgical arm. Table 39-3 summarizes the recommendation of the Trans-Atlantic Inter-Society Consensus (TASC) working group for the revascularization strategy of iliac lesions.

Techniques

Access and Recanalization Techniques
In patients with a unilateral stenotic iliac lesion that does not involve the CFA, ipsilateral access through the CFA with retrograde percutaneous transluminal angioplasty (PTA) is usually preferred, because it provides direct access to the diseased segment and allows a coaxial alignment of the equipment (Fig. 39-4). Contralateral accesses with the use of a crossover sheath is reserved for instances in which the disease involves the ipsilateral CFA (Fig. 39-5), there are plans to intervene on more distal lesions in the same limb, or there is concern about jeopardizing the flow to the affected limb by placement the sheath in the ipsilateral CFA. Various crossover sheaths are available. The ArrowFlex (Arrow International) sheath is more flexible, a feature that can be helpful in crossing over acute aortic bifurcation angles, but it provides less support than the RAABE (Cook) or the Balkin (Cook) sheath, which provide more support but are less compliant.

If the iliac artery is occluded, then either or both approaches may be needed. For aortic bifurcation lesions, a bilateral retrograde approach is used; the placement of kissing balloons, and subsequently kissing stents, is the optimal approach in this setting.

For lesions distal to the aortic bifurcation (in the body of the common iliac artery or the external iliac artery) PTA is attempted. If satisfactory results are achieved (<5 mm Hg residual gradient and <30% residual stenosis with no flow-limiting dissection), stenting may not be indicated. However, ostial lesions of the common iliac arteries (i.e.. aortoiliac bifurcation lesions) are preferably stented with kissing stents. Usually, 0.035-mm guidewires are used for PTA and stenting of the iliac arteries, but 0.018 or 0.014 guidewires may be used. For nonocclusive lesions, a regular nonhydrophilic guidewire may be used, but, if crossing such lesions is difficult, then the use of hydrophilic wires is indicated.

Table 39-3. Recommendations* of the Trans-Atlantic Inter-Society Consensus (TASC) Working Group for the Revascularization Strategy of Aortoiliac and Femoropopliteal Lesions

Type	Iliac Disease	Femoral Lesions
TASC A	Single lesion, <3 cm of CIA or EIA (unilateral/bilateral)	Single lesion, ≤3 cm in length, not involving SFA or popliteal
TASC B	1. Single lesion, 3-10 cm, not extending into the CFA 2. Two stenoses <5 cm long in CIA and/or EIA not extending to CFA 3. Unilateral CIA occlusion	1. Single stenosis or occlusion 3-5 cm long, not involving the distal popliteal artery 2. Heavily calcified lesion ≤3 cm or multiple stenoses or occlusions, each <3 cm 3. Single or multiple lesions in the absence of continuous tibial runoff
TASC C	1. Bilateral 5-10 cm stenosis of CIA and/or EIA, not extending to CFA 2. Unilateral EIA occlusion or stenosis not extending into the CFA 3. Bilateral CIA occlusion	1. Single stenosis/occlusion >5 cm 2. Multiple stenoses or occlusions 3-5 cm, with or without heavy calcification
TASC D	1. Lesions >10 cm or diffuse, multiple unilateral stenoses involving the CIA, EIA, and CFA 2. Unilateral occlusion involving both the CIA and the EIA 3. Bilateral EIA occlusions 4. Diffuse disease involving the aorta and both iliac arteries or lesions in a patient requiring aortic or iliac surgery (AAA)	Complete CFA or SFA occlusions

*Endovascular procedure is the treatment of choice for type A, and surgery is the procedure of choice for type D. At present, endovascular treatment is more commonly used in type B lesions, and surgical treatment is more commonly used in type C lesions. There is insufficient evidence to make firm recommendations, particularly in the case of types B and C.
AAA, abdominal aortic aneurysm; CFA, common femoral artery; CIA, common iliac artery; EIA, external iliac artery; SFA, superficial femoral artery.
From Dormandy JA, Rutherford RB: Management of peripheral arterial disease (PAD). TASC Working Group. Trans-Atlantic Inter-Society Consensus (TASC). J Vasc Surg 2000;31(1 Pt 2):S1-S296.

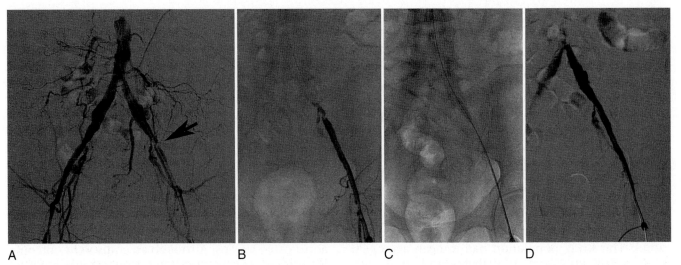

Figure 39-4. Left external iliac artery intervention. **A,** Abdominal aortogram with runoffs where the lesion is noted (*arrow*). **B,** By means of an ipsilateral approach, the lesion is crossed with a guidewire. **C,** Angioplasty is done. **D,** Successful final result with resolution of the obstructive lesion and no flow-limiting dissection or significant elastic recoil. (See Video 39-1.)

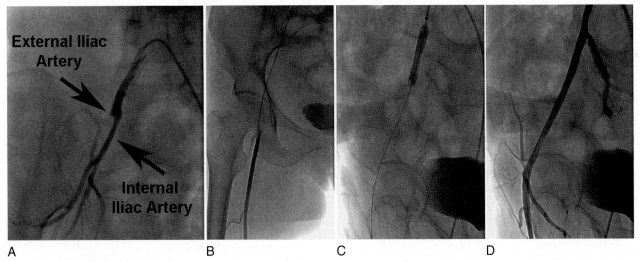

Figure 39-5. Ostial external iliac artery occlusion. **A,** The lesion is approached from a contralateral access point with the use of a crossover sheath. **B,** The lesion is crossed with a hydrophilic guidewire; a balloon is placed at the level of the noted distal external iliac artery lesion; and angioplasty is done. **C,** The first stent deployed, and a second, more proximal, stent is placed. **D,** Final result after stent placement. (See Video 39-2.)

Stent Choice

Both balloon-expandable and self-expandable stents may be used in aortoiliac disease. The balloon-expandable stent is advantageous in the context of an aortic bifurcation lesion, where kissing stents are usually placed. It is also superior to self-expandable stents if precision in stent placement is needed. The self-expanding stent provides flexibility in flexion points, reducing the risk of stent deformity and fracture, and is ideal in the setting of common iliac lesions not involving the ostium, as well as lesions in the external iliac artery.

Clinical Data

Percutaneous revascularization in the management of IC secondary to iliofemoral disease (specifically PTA without stenting) has been compared with conservative management (specifically with exercise training, smoking cessation counseling, and antiplatelet therapy with aspirin). The results revealed two important findings. First, PTA can effectively alleviate patients' symptoms, improve treadmill distance, and improve ABI during a short-term follow-up period, but these benefits are mostly lost within

2 years. The second observation was that, although PTA improves perfusion to the feet, which may confer protection particularly for populations at higher risk for limb loss (e.g., diabetics), supervised exercise improves functional outcome and at the same time enhances global conditioning. These two strategies should therefore be considered complementary to each other, because they address different but inter-related issues.[13-15]

Overall, for iliofemoral lesions, the clinical results of percutaneous revascularization are generally comparable to those of surgical bypass or reconstruction. The Swedish trial randomized patients with threatened limb loss (40% with rest pain or gangrene) or claudication that did not improve with exercise training (60%) to either PTA or surgical revascularization.[16] The study population had a mean age of 70 years, a 26% prevalence of diabetes, and an average symptom duration of 18 months. There were no differences between the PTA or surgery treatment groups with regard to 1-year primary and secondary patency rates, which were 61% and approximately 72%, respectively. The complications rates were not statistically different between treatment groups, although most of the adverse events involved patients who presented with rest pain or gangrene, highlighting the impact of baseline limb status on subsequent outcomes. Adverse events included a 1-year death rate of approximately 10% and a reocclusion rate of 5% (in both treatment groups), a major amputation rate of 5.7% for PTA versus 16% for surgery, and a hematoma rate of 7.5% for PTA versus 4.1% for surgery. The infection and embolization rates were 8.2% each; these complications were seen only in the surgical group and not with PTA.

The Swedish trial findings were corroborated by the Veterans Administration (VA) Cooperative study, which randomized 255 male patients with iliac or femoropopliteal disease and claudication or rest pain. To be eligible, patients needed to be suitable for either PTA or surgery, which may have resulted in a case mix with less diffuse disease compared to the typical vascular surgery population.[17] The average age was 61.5 years; 29% of the subjects had diabetes, 20% had a history of myocardial infarction, more than a quarter had previous surgery or PTA for PAD, and 99% were current or previous smokers (approximately 48 pack-years each). There were three study-related deaths, all in the surgery group (n=126). Among the 129 patients randomized to PTA, no deaths occurred, but there were 20 (15.4%) procedural failures: inability to cross the lesion with wire in 7.8%, inability to dilate the lesion in 2.3%, thrombosis within 24 hours in 3.9%, and no hemodynamic improvement after PTA in 1.6%. No stents were available for this trial. Seventeen of the failed PTA patients subsequently underwent successful surgical revascularization. At a median follow-up of 2 years, there was no statistically significant difference between PTA and surgery groups with regard to death or major amputations. This pattern of equivalent outcome also held true at 4 years follow-up. However, the rate of repeat revascularization in the target limb at 2 years was higher after PTA compared with surgery.[13]

In a review of the available literature from 1989 to 1997, Bosch and Hunink reported a higher technical success with stenting and found no difference in complication rates or 30-day mortality rates in their meta-analysis of six studies that included 2116 patients with IC secondary to aortoiliac disease.[18] The severity-adjusted primary patency rates were 65% with PTA versus 77% with stenting for treatment of stenotic lesions; for occlusions, the rates were 54% with PTA versus 61% with stenting.

A strategy of primary stenting, as opposed to provisional stenting, is generally recommended for aorto-ostial lesions. Although an equivalent outcome for primary versus provisional stenting was reported in the Dutch Iliac Stent Trial, only 57% of patients randomized to PTA did not require stenting.[19] In comparison, a strategy of routine implantation of the same stent (Palmaz balloon-expandable) gave results that were superior to PTA in an RCT of 185 patients by Richter and colleagues.[20] The authors reported a 4-year patency rate of 94% in the stent arm, compared with 69% in the PTA arm. Cumulative clinical success, defined as improvement in clinical stage of one level or more, was 89% for stenting and 67% PTA. Major periprocedural complications were noted in four patients in the stent group and three patients in the PTA group (3.7% overall). These findings were confirmed in the meta-analysis by Bosch and Hunink, in which stenting offered superior technical success rate and long-term patency compared with PTA in occluded arteries.[18] The outcomes of two different self-expanding stents, the stainless steel Wallstent (Schneider) and the nitinol SMART stent (Cordis Endovascular) for the treatment of iliac artery lesions were compared in a multicenter prospective randomized trial.[21] The acute procedural success rate was higher with SMART stent (98.2% vs. 87.5%; P=.002). The patency rate at 1 year was similar for both stents (Wallstent, 91.1%, and SMART stent, 94.7%), with similar complication rates (5.9% vs. 5.9%, respectively; P=not significant).

Overall, it is fair to say that the technical and clinical success rates of endovascular interventions for iliac artery stenosis exceed 90% (approaching almost 100% in focal iliac lesions) and that the intermediate- and long-term patency rates are comparable to those of surgical revascularization. Factors that negatively affect long-term patency for either modality are the quality of the distal runoff vessels, the severity of ischemia, and the length of the diseased segment.[22,23] Female gender has been associated with decreased patency after placement of external iliac stents.[24] Technical success is commonly defined as less than 30% residual stenosis (anatomic success), a postintervention mean translesional gradient of <5 mm Hg, and an increase in the ABI of at least 0.1 and/or a decrease in symptoms by one category (hemodynamic success). Another criterion that has been suggested (clinical success) is an improvement of at least one category of symptoms.[25]

Complications and Their Management

Complication rates are generally low in aortoiliac interventions. These include access site complications (e.g., groin hematoma, retroperitoneal bleed, pseudoaneurysm, arteriovenous fistula formation), thrombosis at the site of PTA, arterial rupture, and distal embolization. These complications happen at a rate of less than 5% to 6% in most series.[26] Death, contrast-induced nephropathy, myocardial infarction, and cerebrovascular accident occur at a rate of less than 0.5%. The need for urgent vascular repair is reported to be about 2%. With regard to serious complications, rupture seems to be reported more frequently with the iliac arteries than with percutaneous interventions in other lower extremity arteries.[26,27]

When to Refer to Surgery

Surgery is usually reserved for patients with diffuse disease and those with long total occlusions. It is also the appropriate approach for those with associated infrarenal aortic aneurysms. Table 39-3 summarizes the recommendations of the TASC working group for the appropriate revascularization strategy of iliac lesions.

Femoropopliteal Intervention (Outflow Disease)

In general, CFA revascularization should preferably be done surgically. Concerns about elastic recoil and dissection after PTA and concerns about mechanical compression of stents and acute stent thrombosis have limited endovascular intervention in this territory. PTA has been used in case of severe fibrotic lesions after previous surgery.

The SFA and the proximal popliteal artery are the most common anatomic sites of stenosis and occlusion in patients with IC. It is estimated that slightly more than a quarter of diseased SFAs progress over a 3-year period, and 17% may go on to occlusion. Predictors of progression are continued smoking, worsening symptoms, and the presence of an already occluded contralateral SFA.[24] For patients who have disease confined to the SFA, a supervised exercise program might offer a functional outcome that is equivalent or even superior to that of percutaneous revascularization. This could be due to preserved iliac inflow in the PFA, which is a common and important source of collaterals for patients with SFA stenoses or occlusion. Surgery remains the gold standard when therapy is indicated, because primary femoropopliteal graft patency rates of about 80% at 5 years have been documented.[24] Continued improvements in technology, including metal alloys with shape memory and superelastic properties and stents coated with antiproliferative agents, are helping surmount

the problem of poor long-term durability, which is currently the main limitation of endovascular techniques. Femoropopliteal angioplasty may be considered for discrete single lesions smaller than 10 cm, or 5 cm for calcified stenosis, or 3 cm for multiple lesions, so long as the SFA origin or distal popliteal artery is not involved. Factors that have been found to adversely impact long-term patency are CLI (gangrene or rest pain) presentation, multiple stenoses or diffuse disease, and poor distal runoff.[28,29]

Indications

The low morbidity and mortality of endovascular intervention makes this strategy the preferred choice in patients with suitable lesions (see Table 39-3). It is an appropriate option in the management of symptomatic femoropopliteal lesions in the following situations: (1) single lesions less than 10 cm in length (unilateral or bilateral), (2) multiple stenosis or occlusion of less than 5 cm (not involving the trifurcation), (3) single stenosis of less than 15 cm (not involving the trifurcation), and (4) before surgery in patients with no continuous tibial runoffs in order to improve inflow for surgical bypass.

Techniques

Common Femoral Artery
Access is usually obtained via the contralateral femoral artery (with a crossover sheath) or via the brachial artery. Lesions involving the bifurcation of the CFA represent a challenging problem, and sometimes kissing balloons are needed to achieve desirable angiographic outcome.

Stents are not recommended but may be used in salvage situations, with the flexible self-expanding stent being the appropriate choice in this vessel. Stenting should be avoided, if possible, because stent compression or fracture can occur and may render future surgical repair more complicated. It is important to point out that, although restenosis rates are high in the CFA (>50%), restenosis may be associated with less limiting symptoms in patients who needed the PTA for persistent or critical symptoms.

Profunda Femoris Artery
Revascularization of the PFA may be needed in the setting of total occlusion of the SFA or of a femoropopliteal bypass graft, because this vessel plays an important role as a source of collaterals to the lower extremity. Surgery is the preferred strategy in this vessel, but PTA may be tried in the setting of severe limb-threatening ischemia if surgery is contraindicated or if the disease involves the distal portion of the descending branch of the PFA, which is less accessible to the surgeons.

Access via the contralateral femoral artery (with a crossover sheath) or via the brachial artery may be used. The interventions are usually done in the context of limb-threatening ischemia, so it is important to emphasize that a rather conservative approach with regard to balloon sizing is used in this setting, especially with no available data regarding the placement of stents in the PFA. Stents are used provisionally in the context of flow-limiting dissections or severe residual lesions.

Superficial Femoral Artery

There are four possible approaches to accessing the SFA. The lesion may be approached through a contralateral femoral artery (with a crossover sheath) approach, an ipsilateral antegrade CFA approach, a retrograde popliteal approach, or a brachial artery approach. By accessing the contralateral CFA and then using a curved catheter (such as the internal mammary, Judkins right, Cobra, or Simmons catheter) to engage the ostium of the common iliac artery of the diseased limb, a kink-resistant long sheath (Balkin, RAABE, or ArrowFlex) may be placed. The contralateral approach is more popular, because it provides excellent support and helps access other segment (iliac or infrainguinal vessels) on the same limb. The antegrade CFA access, which is relatively more challenging than the retrograde approach, also remains widely used. The antegrade brachial approach might be the only viable option in patients with bilateral iliofemoral disease. The popliteal approach is the least used, because it is associated with a higher risk of complications owing to the smaller size of the popliteal artery and the nearby vital structures that may be injured; it is also uncomfortable for the patient. In general, familiarity with all of the various approaches is necessary, because the underlying anatomy of each patient determines the feasible vascular access points. Figure 39-6 is an example of SFA intervention.

Stent Choice

Stenting as a primary approach for femoropopliteal lesions is not indicated. Stenting is indicated as a salvage procedure after complicated PTA (i.e., for flow-limiting dissection or thrombosis), because primary stenting has not been shown to be superior to PTA-only with bailout stenting.[30] If stenting is indicated, then self-expanding stents are generally used in SFA lesions, in light of the high risk of stent compression and fracture. Stainless steel stents, nitinol stents, and sirolimus stents have been used in the management of femoropopliteal lesions.[30,31] The use of sirolimus-eluting SMART stents for SFA occlusion was evaluated in the Sirolimus-Eluting versus Bare Nitinol Stent for Obstructive Superficial Femoral Artery Disease (SIROCCO II) study and did not show any significant differences in clinical outcome compared with bare metal stents.[31] Stent/strut fractures were reported in about 8% of patients in both arms of the study. The coated stent proved to be safe and was not associated with any serious adverse events when compared with noncoated stents.[31]

Specific Techniques

Although anecdotal experiences and reported case series have suggested some benefits with laser atherectomy, Silver Hawk atherectomy, and so on, the use of directional atherectomy and laser angioplasty has not been shown to offer clear advantage over PTA in femoropopliteal PAD.[32-34]

Clinical Data

RCTs in patients with IC and femoropopliteal disease that compared medical therapy with PTA consistently revealed that PTA offers early symptomatic

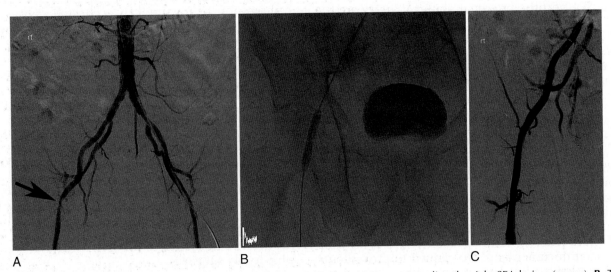

Figure 39-6. Right superficial femoral artery (SFA) intervention. **A,** Abdominal aortogram revealing the right SFA lesion *(arrow).* **B,** The lesion is crossed, and angioplasty is done using a contralateral access point. **C,** Successful percutaneous transluminal angioplasty result with no significant residual lesion or flow-limiting dissection. (See Video 39-3.)

Table 39-4. Estimated Pooled Primary Patency Rates after Balloon Dilatation and Stent Implantation in Patients with Intermittent Claudication or Critical Limb Ischemia Secondary to Femoropopliteal Stenosis

		Balloon Dilation		Stent Implantation	
Lesion Type	Years after Treatment	Patency (%)*	Range (%)†	Patency (%)*	Range (%)†
Intermittent Claudication					
Stenosis	0	100 (1.0)	98-100	100 (1.2)	99-100
	1	77 (1.7)	78-80	75 (2.2)	73-79
	2	66 (2.0)	63-71	67 (2.4)	65-71
	3	61 (2.2)	55-68	66 (2.7)	64-70
	4	57 (2.5)	54-63	NA	NA
	5	55 (2.8)	52-62	NA	NA
Occlusion	0	88 (2.9)	81-94	99 (2.3)	92-100
	1	65 (3.0)	55-71	73 (2.8)	69-75
	2	54 (3.1)	45-61	66 (3.0)	61-68
	3	48 (3.3)	40-55	64 (3.2)	59-67
	4	44 (3.5)	36-53	NA	NA
	5	42 (3.7)	33-51	NA	NA
Critical Limb Ischemia					
Stenosis	0	83 (3.7)	69-88	100 (3.3)	94-100
	1	60 (4.0)	46-63	74 (3.8)	68-80
	2	49 (4.0)	35-54	66 (3.9)	59-72
	3	43 (4.1)	30-51	65 (4.1)	58-71
	4	40 (4.3)	26-46	NA	NA
	5	38 (4.5)	24-44	NA	NA
Occlusion	0	70 (3.5)	62-75	98 (3.2)	94-100
	1	47 (3.5)	41-51	73 (3.6)	68-75
	2	36 (3.6)	28-41	65 (3.7)	60-68
	3	30 (3.7)	20-37	63 (3.9)	58-68
	4	27 (3.9)	16-34	NA	NA
	5	25 (4.1)	13-32	NA	NA

*The number in parentheses is the standard error.
†Ranges are derived from sensitivity analyses.
NA, not available.
From Muradin GS, et al: Balloon dilation and stent implantation for treatment of femoropopliteal arterial disease: Meta-analysis. Radiology 2001;221:137-145.

relief at 3 to 6 months compared with medical therapy, and outcomes were similar at 2 years.[35,36] Clinical acute success rates of PTA for femoropopliteal disease in the contemporary era exceed 95%.[30] Contemporary endovascular approaches that include stenting offer acute technical success rates of up to 99%, and short- to medium-term patency rates are superior to those achieved with PTA alone.[31] The mid-term to long-term data of endovascular interventions in patients with IC or CLI and femoropopliteal disease are summarized in Table 39-4.

The advantage of placing a stent in the SFA is that it limits elastic recoil, scaffolds flow-limiting dissection, and provides a higher acute technical support. However, these advantages are counterbalanced by the stent-induced enhanced endothelial hyperplasic response, which may result in in-stent restenosis and negate the noted advantages of stenting on long-term follow-up. Restenosis after endovascular interventions depends on the severity of the disease (total occlusion versus patent vessel with a high-grade lesion), the status of the distal runoffs, and the length of the lesion. Whether a different stent material and/or drug elution with antiproliferative agents would result in improved outcomes remains to be seen in future investigations. Restenosis remains a limiting factor in achieving optimal intermediate- to long-term patency. The use of brachytherapy in treating

in-stent restenosis resulted in a 50% reduction in the restenosis rate with no noted increased risk in late thrombosis. The use of sirolimus-eluting stents was not associated with superior results when compared with bare-metal stents.[31] Nitinol (an alloy of nickel and titanium) is flexible and more likely to recover from being crushed than stainless steel. A small single-center clinical trial compared the use of the self-expanding nitinol stent versus PTA with optional stenting (with 32% receiving stents in this arm) in patients with symptomatic SFA disease (i.e., severe IC or chronic limb ischemia). The use of stents was associated with a lower rate of angiographic restenosis at 6 months (24% vs. 43%, P=.05) and improved treadmill time at 6 to 12 months. This study was limited by its small size and short-term follow-up.[37] Figure 39-7 lists the overall success and patency rates of PTA (with and without stenting) versus surgery in all claudicants.

There are limited RCTs comparing PTA versus surgery in the management of infrainguinal PAD. This is partly because the choice of revascularization modality depends on how extensive the disease is in the individual patient, with surgery being the most likely route of action in the setting of extensive or long lesions and in those with CLI. In a multicenter RCT of 263 men, Wolf and colleagues reported three operative deaths in the surgical arm (n=126) and

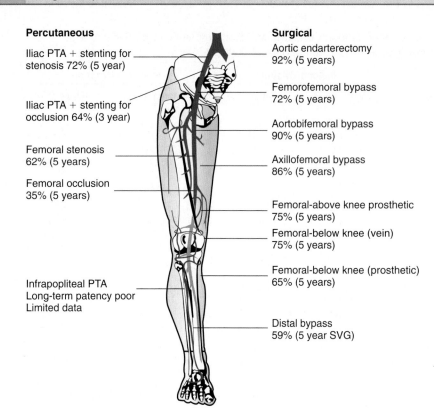

Percutaneous

Iliac PTA + stenting for stenosis 72% (5 year)

Iliac PTA + stenting for occlusion 64% (3 year)

Femoral stenosis 62% (5 years)

Femoral occlusion 35% (5 years)

Infrapopliteal PTA Long-term patency poor Limited data

Surgical

Aortic endarterectomy 92% (5 years)

Femorofemoral bypass 72% (5 years)

Aortobifemoral bypass 90% (5 years)

Axillofemoral bypass 86% (5 years)

Femoral-above knee prosthetic 75% (5 years)

Femoral-below knee (vein) 75% (5 years)

Femoral-below knee (prosthetic) 65% (5 years)

Distal bypass 59% (5 year SVG)

Figure 39-7. Patency rates for percutaneous and bypass procedures in intermittent claudication. Data adapted from TASC recommendation. (Redrawn from Dormandy JA, Rutherford RB: Management of peripheral arterial disease (PAD). TASC Working Group. Trans-Atlantic Inter-Society Consensus (TASC). J Vasc Surg 2000;31(1 Pt 2): S1-S296.)

none in the PTA arm (*n*=129). No difference in survival was noted, although there was a trend in favor of the PTA arm. Whereas patients in both arms had sustained improvement in their hemodynamics and in their quality of life, there was higher reported success rate in the surgical arm and more limb salvage than in the PTA arm. No differences were reported in clinical outcome on median follow-up of 4 years.[13] In a small randomized trial, a 1-year patency rate of 43% in the PTA arm (*n*=30) versus 82% in the surgical arm (*n*=24) was reported.[38]

Complications and Their Management

Dissection, perforation, and distal embolization are the complications encountered in femoropopliteal interventions. Although the use of stenting is discouraged as a primary strategy, its use as a bailout strategy in the context of flow-limiting dissections and perforations is well established. The appropriate use of anticoagulation and antiplatelet therapy safeguards against acute and subacute thrombosis and may limit the incidence and consequences of distal embolization.

When to Refer to Surgery

Surgery remains the preferred strategy for patients with CFA and proximal PFA obstructive PAD. It is also the preferred strategy for patients with heavily calcified or completely occluded CFA, femoropop-

liteal calcified stenosis, or occlusions that are longer than 15 cm, total occlusions of SFA that are longer than 20 cm, and total occlusion of the popliteal artery or of the proximal trifurcation.[1,7] It is important to point out that a strategy of initial PTA in lieu of surgery in selected patients is reasonable.[16]

Infrapopliteal Intervention (Runoff Disease)

Indications

Despite the fact that the first reported case of endovascular intervention in the management of infrapopliteal PAD was in 1964 by Dotter and Judkins, endovascular therapy has had a limited role in the management of infrapopliteal PAD. In patients with IC secondary to infrapopliteal PAD, medical therapy is the most appropriate initial strategy.[7] Tibioperoneal angioplasty is limited by recurrence and also by the need for highly skilled operators, because the possibility for emergency surgical bailout is associated with considerable risk that cannot be justified in patients with stable IC, especially when medical management is known to produce similar outcomes with limited risk.[1] However, in carefully selected patients and in the hands of experienced operators, an acute success rate of 95% (98% for stenoses, 86% for total occlusion) with less than 1% of patients experiencing significant complications can be achieved.[23,39-41] The role of angioplasty in patients with CLI is more promising and justified, because its results are comparable, if not superior, to those of infrapopliteal/tibial bypass surgery.[41] Endovascular techniques can therefore be used as a primary therapy or as an adjunctive therapy with bypass surgery to improve segments with inflow disease or to improve the outflow. Up to a quarter of patients with CLI have lesions isolated to arteries below the knee, and these occur mostly in patients with diabetes and other comorbid conditions. Historically, the main concerns with regard to endovascular interventions of the infrapopliteal vessels were the long-term patency of such interventions, complications, and technical failure. With improved equipment, appropriate patient selection, and meticulous technical approach, acute success rates greater than 90% and 5-year limb salvage rates of almost 90% are now possible on a more consistent basis, particularly in the context of a comprehensive strategy that includes medical, endovascular, and surgical modalities as well as long-term lesion surveillance.[39]

Techniques

Access and Recanalization Techniques and Devices

Antegrade ipsilateral femoral access is usually used for infrapopliteal interventions. The advantages of such access include a straight-line approach to the lesion, a shorter length of catheter or balloon shaft, more torque control, and a better mechanical advantage and "pushability" for occlusions or lesions that are difficult to cross. This approach requires experience to minimize complications at the access site. If combined below-knee and above-knee PTA is necessary, angioplasty of the tibioperoneal arteries initially might lower the risk of peripheral embolization. In the Uppsala series,[41a] 6 of the initial 40 procedures had embolization that required either transcatheter embolectomy or local streptokinase infusion. After altering their practice to performing distal angioplasty before more proximal lower limb angioplasty, the authors saw no embolization in their subsequent 54 procedures.

Because occlusion of these end-arteries jeopardizes the foot and leaves no surgical bailout options, the characteristics of reported successful series must be carefully considered. In the series of Dorros and colleagues,[41] tibioperoneal lesions had to be less than 10 cm in length, and distal vessels were visualized. Occlusions were less successfully opened than stenoses (73% vs. 98%). A residual stenosis of up to 50% was acceptable for these relatively small vessels. Complete multivessel revascularization may not be necessary, especially if a significant improvement in ABI is already documented. If angioplasty results in straight-line flow to the foot, clinical success rates of up to 80% at 24 months have been reported. Conversely, the lack of straight-line flow portends failure within 11 months. Vasospasm usually abates with intra-arterial nitroglycerin or verapamil.

Stent Choice

Stents are not recommended in the management of infrapopliteal disease. However, stent placement may be used as a bailout in the context of flow-limiting dissections.

Specific Techniques

Case series of the use of atherectomy in treatment of tibial lesions have shown dismal results.[42] Therefore, atherectomy is not recommended. The use of Silver Hawk atherectomy has shown promise but needs to be evaluated prospectively.

Clinical Data

Despite advances in the modern aggressive revascularization techniques, the mortality and morbidity rates for this cohort of patients have remained substantial, with 30-day mortality rates of approximately 4% to 10%, a 6% to 14% amputation rate, and a 90-day graft failure rate of almost 5%[43] The 5-year patency rate for femoral below-knee bypass is about 75% (vein graft) to 60% (prosthetic grafts), whereas for distal bypass it is about 50%.[1] An important contributor to these poor outcomes is the substantial disease burden in this cohort of patients, who have a preponderance of coronary artery disease, diabetes mellitus, and baseline tissue loss (foot ulcer, gangrene, or nonhealing wound).[1,43,44]

There are no RCTs comparing strategies for the treatment of below-knee arterial occlusive disease. Dorros and colleagues reported the largest prospective series of infrapopliteal angioplasty on 284 limbs with CLI (Fontaine stages III and IV) in 235 patients between 1983 and 1996.[44] The mean age was 67 years; 69% of the patients were men, half had diabetes, more than a quarter had previous myocardial infarction, a third had prior coronary artery bypass surgery, and 39% had prior peripheral vascular surgery. The overall acute technical success rate was 100% for inflow lesions and 92% for infrapopliteal lesions. The success rate was 98% for stenoses, but only 73% for occlusions. Complications were infrequent: the authors reported 0.7% in-hospital all-cause mortality, 0.7% emergency vascular surgery, 9% in-hospital major amputation, and 0.4% (one case) each of compartment syndrome, major infection, and transfusion. In a more contemporary series (n=60) reported by Soder and colleagues, the patients were older (mean age, 72 years) and sicker: more than three fourths had diabetes, almost a quarter had baseline renal insufficiency, 90% presented with minor (81%) or major (9.7%) tissue loss, and the majority were not eligible for distal bypass surgery (no runoff in 70 limbs, single-vessel runoff in 2 limbs.[39] The authors reported a primary angiographic success rate of 84% (102/121) for stenosis and 61% (41/67) for occlusions, with corresponding restenosis rates of 32% and 52% at follow-up angiography performed at a mean of 10 months after primary PTA. The rate of major complications was 2.8% (access site pseudoaneurysms in two patients). The primary clinical success was 63% (45/72). A 48% cumulative primary patency rate, a 56% secondary patency rate, and an

80% cumulative limb salvage rate were reported at 18 months. Factors that independently correlated with continued lesion patency up to 12 months were angiographic improvement to the site of most severe ischemia (6-month primary patency of 68% vs. 16%; *P*=.001) and absence of renal insufficiency (patency of 63% vs. 24%; *P*=.06). Clinical success, defined as relief of claudication or avoidance of major amputation, was achieved in only 45 (63%) of 72 limbs acutely, but this is comparable to results from surgical series. No patient in this series had a subsequent surgical bypass operation for the limbs, largely because of poor distal targets or pedal arteries.[39]

When to Refer to Surgery

In the management of infrapopliteal disease, bypass surgery has been associated with disappointing results. Just as with PTA, the patency rate of bypass grafting remains inferior to that of bypass grafting in more proximal PAD, as shown in Figure 39-7.[1] Success in achieving limb salvage with minimal periprocedural complications is dependent on the status of the distal circulation and the overall risk profile of the patient. Amputation (primary if no antecedent attempt at revascularization is made, or secondary after failure of revascularization) may be necessary in patients with CLI complicated by intractable infections or uncontrollable rest pain.

ACUTE LIMB ISCHEMIA

Acute limb ischemia (ALI) is defined as a sudden or rapidly developing loss of limb perfusion resulting in the development or worsening symptoms and signs of limb ischemia with an imminent threat to the limb viability. ALI may be the first manifestation of PAD in previously asymptomatic patients.[7] More commonly, patients with IC experience progression in their disease, with development of rest pain, ischemic ulcers, and eventually gangrene. This progression, although it may be gradual, is usually the result of recurrent acute ischemic events. Two mechanisms are implicated in ALI: embolism and in situ thrombosis. Differentiation based on history and clinical examination alone may be clinically impossible in 10% to 15% of cases. Although there is little information on the incidence of ALI in the general population, it is estimated to be 14 per 100,000, and ALI is

the indication for 10% to 16% of all vascular procedures performed. Patients with embolic ALI are more likely to die than those with thrombosis, usually secondary to underlying cardiac disease, whereas patients with thrombotic ALI are more likely to lose their limbs.

The natural history of ALI has remained largely unchanged despite the advances in surgical, endovascular, and pharmacologic therapies. Patients presenting with ALI continue to have a particularly poor short-term outlook both in terms of loss of the leg and mortality, with 30-day amputation rates of between 10% and 30% and a mortality rate of 15%. The fact that overall mortality rates after intervention for acute ischemia have not improved dramatically over the past 20 years reflects the severity of the underlying atherosclerotic burden in these high-risk patients.[1,7,45]

Embolic events complicate atrial fibrillation, myocardial infarction with left ventricular thrombus, or peripheral pseudoaneurysm. Thrombosis in situ is usually encountered in patients with PAD and tenuous collateral circulation, or it may be seen in patients with prior bypass surgery who have an acute thrombosis of the graft. Also of importance are other mechanisms of ALI, such as septic or cardiac tumor emboli, trauma (e.g., popliteal artery disruption), and dissection of large vessels with distal progression (e.g., aortic dissection with iliac artery occlusion).

Table 39-5 shows a recommended classification of ALI that is useful in estimating the impact of ALI for the individual patient and determining the prognosis of the limb at the time of presentation.[46]

Management Strategies

In approaching patients with suspected ALI, the history and physical examination should be focused on establishing the underlying mechanism of the ALI and on categorizing the patient based on the underlying leg symptoms and signs in addition to the Doppler assessment of the peripheral pulses. Once the diagnosis of ALI is made, the objective should be to prevent thrombus propagation and worsening ischemia. Therefore, anticoagulation (if not contraindicated) with heparin is the first step in the management. The next step (for viable limbs in class I or II) is restoration of the flow as soon as possible, either pharmacologic or endovascular versus open catheter thromboembolectomy. If the patient has a true late

Table 39-5. Classification of Acute Limb Ischemia

Category	Description	Neuromuscular Findings	Doppler Findings
I	Viable	No sensory or muscle weakness	Audible arterial and venous
IIa	Threatened (marginally)	Minimal	Often inaudible arterial, audible venous
IIb	Threatened (immediately)	Mild to moderate, associated with pain	Usually inaudible arterial, audible venous
III	Irreversible	Profound deficit	No signals

From Thrombolysis in the management of lower limb peripheral arterial occlusion: A consensus document. J Vasc Interv Radiol 2003;14(9 Pt 2): S337-S349.

Table 39-6. Recommended Doses of Antiplatelet, Antithrombotic Medications and Thrombolytics for Management of Limb Ischemia

Medication	Route	Dosage	Laboratory Studies
Aspirin	PO/PR	325 mg	None
Heparin	IV	60 U/kg bolus, then 12 U/kg/hr	aPTT, platelets, Hct
Mannitol	IV	12.5-25 g	Creatinine
Plasminogen activator	IA	Depends on agent*	Hct, fibrinogen, FSP
Urokinase	IA	80,000-200,000 U/hr tapered infusion	Hct, fibrinogen, FSP

*Depends on thrombolytic agent: retaplase, 0.25-1.0 U/hr; alteplase 0.2-1.0 mg/hr; tenecteplase 0.25-0.5 mg/hr.
aPTT, activated partial thromboplastin time; FSP, fibrin split products; Hct, hematocrit; IA, intra-arterial; IV, intravenous; PO, oral; PR, rectal.
From Rajagopalan S, Mukherjee D, Mohler E: Manual of Vascular Diseases. Philadelphia, Lippincott, 2004, p 92.

nonviable limb (class III), then amputation is the only option, because revascularization of such limbs in of no benefit and is associated with a high risk of mortality. Table 39-6 lists the recommended medications and doses of thrombolytic therapy. In general, patients with a clear embolic etiology and a discernible location of obstruction by physical examination are taken to surgery for open embolectomy. If there is no clear embolic etiology, an arteriogram should be performed, and the decision should be made, based on the findings, regarding endovascular versus surgical intervention.

Interventional Treatment

Pharmacologic Thrombolysis

Although systemic thrombolysis has no role in the management of ALI, catheter-directed thrombolytic therapy is effective in the management of class I and class IIa ischemia. This approach is clearly less invasive, has less morbidity and mortality than open surgery, and may reduce the risk of reperfusion injury. The choice of lytic therapy depends on the location, anatomy, and patient comorbidities. Contraindication to thrombolysis should be observed.

Percutaneous Aspiration Thrombectomy

Percutaneous aspiration thrombectomy (PAT) is an alternative nonsurgical modality to treat ALI. It uses large-lumen catheters and suction with a 50-mL syringe to remove embolus or thrombus from native vessels, bypass grafts, and runoff vessels. PAT devices such as the Amplatz "clot buster" (BARD-Microvena), and the Straub Rotarex System (Straub Medical) have been used with fibrinolysis to reduce the time and dose of the fibrinolytic agent or as a stand-alone procedure.

Percutaneous Mechanical Thrombectomy

The concept of creating a "hydrodynamic recirculation vortex" that would dissolute a thrombus and remove its fragment is the underlying thought behind most PMT devices, such as the AngioJet (Possis

Medical), Hydrolyser (Cordis) and Oasis (Boston Scientific/Medi-tech) thrombectomy systems. The efficacy of PMT depends on the age of the thrombus: fresh thrombi can be efficiently removed, as opposed to old, organized thrombi.

Surgery

The indications for surgery include patients with a clear embolic etiology in whom an open embolectomy can be performed and patients with CLI (class IIb and III). Surgery is associated with the risks of infection, hemorrhage, and periprocedural cardiovascular adverse events.

CRITICAL LEG ISCHEMIA

Critical leg (or limb) ischemia is characterized by persistent rest pain with or without ongoing tissue loss, ischemic ulceration, or gangrene. The term CLI is traditionally used to describe patients with ischemic symptoms lasting longer than 2 weeks. Patients with CLI usually have an ankle systolic pressure of less than 40 mm Hg, a toe systolic pressure of less than 30 mm Hg, and/or a reduced transcutaneous oxygen concentration ($TCPo_2$) of less than 50 mm Hg.

In general, the underlying etiology is almost exclusively atherosclerosis; frequently, multivessel and multisegment disease is present. Smoking and diabetes are the most potent risk factors and are associated with higher rates of amputation. The prognosis in patients with CLI is poor secondary to comorbid conditions, with mortality rates approaching 10% per year and amputation rates of 25% to 45% at 1 year.[1,7]

Interventional Treatment and Surgery

The decision regarding management of CLI depends on the risk profile of the patient (e.g., expected operative mortality, underlying renal function and the risk of contrast nephropathy) and the anatomic profile of the patient (e.g., multisegment and/or multivessel disease, number of runoffs, suitability of the disease to PTA versus surgery). Figure 39-8 outlines a general approach to the management of CLI.

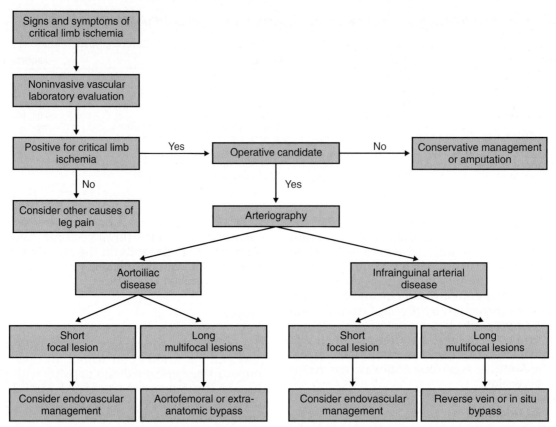

Figure 39-8. Treatment algorithm for patients with critical limb ischemia. (Redrawn from Rajagopalan S, Mukherjee D, Mohler E: Manual of Vascular Diseases. Philadelphia, Lippincott, 2004, p 92.)

Periprocedural Antithrombotic Therapy

PTA and stenting are usually conducted with weight-based heparinization to achieve an activated clotting time (ACT) of 200 to 250 seconds. A front load of aspirin and clopidogrel (300 mg) at least 12 hours before intervention is widely used. Glycoprotein IIb/IIIa may be useful in the context of diabetes, evidence of angiographic thrombus, or ulceration and in patients with poor runoff (one vessel or none), to prevent distal embolization. After PTA and stenting, lifelong aspirin therapy is recommended because of the high rate of cardiovascular events in patients with advanced PAD. Most clinicians prescribe adjunctive clopidogrel for 1 to 12 months after a lower extremity percutaneous intervention.

Complications after Peripheral Bypass Surgery

Various types of vascular bypass grafts are used in the management of lower extremity PAD. A detailed discussion of this subject is beyond the scope of this chapter; however, interventionalists are likely to encounter graft-related complications, the most serious of which is ALI secondary to graft thrombosis.

In general, acute thrombosis of bypass grafts occurs secondary to technical problems, usually manifests in the early postoperative period, and requires an urgent intervention. In this setting, patients should be anticoagulated and then evaluated for balloon catheter thrombectomy. Mature graft thrombosis occurs at a rate of 10% at 5 years and rarely causes ALI. Such patients are managed with thrombolytic therapy to clear the thrombus burden, after which the underlying etiology should be addressed through an endovascular intervention or open surgery.[47]

MISCELLANEOUS CONDITIONS

Buerger's Disease (Thromboangiitis)

Buerger's disease is a nonatherosclerotic inflammatory vasculitis of the small and medium size arteries, veins, and nerves. It can affect upper and lower extremities and occurs most commonly in young male smokers. The etiology is uncertain, although there is a clear and strong association with smoking and tobacco use. The mainstay of therapy is smoking cessation, and in fact, without complete cessation of smoking and tobacco use, the prognosis for limb salvage is dismal.[48] Medical therapy with antiplatelets, immunosuppressant (cyclophosphamide), and analgesics has been used.

Surgical revascularization of the lower extremity in the context of Buerger's disease has a limited role in the light of the diffuse nature of the disease and its tendency to involve distal small vessels before progressing proximally. Bypass surgery, if feasible, should be done with an autogenous vein and veins not affected by the disease process. Percutaneous intervention has no clear role in the management of patients with Buerger's disease.

Peripheral Aneurysm

The most common cause of peripheral aneurysm formation is atherosclerosis. Other predisposing factors include hypertension, inflammatory and infectious processes, trauma, connective tissue diseases, and familial tendencies. Although most aneurysms are asymptomatic, they may become the source of distal embolization, may become infected, may compress surrounding tissues, and may rupture. Aneurysms of the lower extremity have particular complications depending on their location.

Iliac artery aneurysms are associated with atheroembolism, obstructive uropathies, iliac vein obstruction, and perineal or groin pain. MRA or multidetector contrast computed tomography is the preferred strategy for diagnosis. Traditionally, surgical resection is indicated if the aneurysm is symptomatic or is more than 3 cm in diameter. Endovascular treatment (using a variety of options that are available today, such as coil embolization and stent-graft placement) may now be an alternative to surgery. Early experience indicates that endovascular treatment is safe and effective in the hands of skilled operators; however, large, long-term follow-up studies are needed to determine whether this approach is a practical alternative to open surgery.[49]

Femoral artery aneurysm is associated with atheroembolism and venous obstruction. It can be diagnosed with ultrasound and is managed surgically if symptomatic. Case series of endovascular interventions have been reported, but the data are limited, and larger studies with long-term follow-up are needed to help identify the role of this approach in the setting of femoral artery aneurysm.[50]

Popliteal artery aneurysm is associated with thrombosis, atheroembolism, venous obstruction, popliteal neuropathy, and infection. These aneurysms are bilateral in 50% of patients. Ultrasound may be used to make the diagnosis, although contrast angiography is usually needed before surgery to assess the proximal and distal circulation. Once diagnosed, popliteal aneurysm should be resected to prevent its potentially devastating thromboembolic complications. Endovascular repair of popliteal artery aneurysms is a new technique that has emerged as an alternative to open surgical bypass. The evidence to support its use is limited, and long-term follow up data are lacking, but early results have been promising, with high rates of initial treatment success.[50,51]

Atheroembolism

Atheroembolism refers to the occlusion of arteries secondary to the detachment and embolization of atheromatous debris, including cholesterol crystals, platelets, fibrin, and calcium. Atheroemboli can originate from any atherosclerotic segment, although typically they originate from aortic atheromas and from aneurysms of large and medium size arteries. They tend to occlude small end-arteries and arterioles, such as those of the kidneys, retina, brain, and extremities.

Clinical features of this disorder are usually reflective of acute ischemic complications and depend on the affected organ. Atheroembolic events in the lower extremity result in painful cyanotic toes (blue toe syndrome) and are associated with digital and foot ulcerations in addition to multiorgan dysfunction depending on the extent of the embolic burden. Livedo reticularis is commonly (up to 50%) encountered in patients with atheroembolism as well. It is important to point out that, because atheroemboli occlude smaller, more distal vessels, distal pulses remain intact, in contrast to CLI and ALI secondary to thromboembolism, in which pulses are usually abnormal. The differential diagnosis includes many conditions such as vasculitis and prothrombotic conditions such as anti-phospholipid syndrome and heparin-induced thrombocytopenia.

Affected patients may have an elevated erythrocyte sedimentation rate, thrombocytopenia, eosinophilia, eosinophiluria, and hypocomplementemia. The finding of cholesterol crystals in small arteries is a pathognomonic sign when found in skin or muscle biopsies. Transesophageal echocardiography, computed tomography, and MRA can be used to image the aorta (searching for shaggy mobile atheromas) and to assess for aneurysms as part of the workup to identify the source of the emboli if possible.

If the source cannot be identified, then no definitive therapy exists, but antiplatelet therapy with aspirin has been advocated. If the source is identified, then surgical removal or endovascular isolation of the source is the only definitive therapy.[52]

CONCLUSIONS AND FUTURE DIRECTIONS

PAD of the lower extremity is a serious health problem associated with significant morbidity and is a reflection of advanced atherosclerosis that often affects other vascular trees. Whereas the management of IC is based an integrated exercise program and pharmacologic modification of the associated risk factors, percutaneous interventions have emerged as an alternative modality to surgical revascularization in patients who remain symptomatic or progress to CLI. Advances in technology will likely continue to optimize the role of percutaneous interventions in the management of PAD. Although such interventions are already very effective in the management of IC caused by iliofemoral disease, there remains room for improvement in the use of such interventions in the management of infrapopliteal disease and of acute and chronic limb ischemia.

REFERENCES

1. Dormandy JA, Rutherford RB: Management of peripheral arterial disease (PAD). TASC Working Group. TransAtlantic Inter-Society Consensus (TASC). J Vasc Surg 2000;31(1 Pt 2): S1-S296.
2. Management of peripheral arterial disease (PAD). TransAtlantic Inter-Society Consensus (TASC). Section D: Chronic critical limb ischaemia. Eur J Vasc Endovasc Surg 2000;12(Suppl A): S144-S243.
3. Hirsch AT, Hiatt WR: PAD awareness, risk, and treatment: New resources for survival—The USA PARTNERS program. Vasc Med 2001;6(3 Suppl):9-12.
4. Selvin E, Erlinger TP: Prevalence of and risk factors for peripheral arterial disease in the United States: Results from the National Health and Nutrition Examination Survey, 1999-2000. Circulation 2004;110:738-743.
5. Fowkes FG, et al: Edinburgh Artery Study: Prevalence of asymptomatic and symptomatic peripheral arterial disease in the general population. Int J Epidemiol 1991;20:384-392.
6. Willigendael EM, et al: Peripheral arterial disease: Public and patient awareness in The Netherlands. Eur J Vasc Endovasc Surg 2004;27:622-628.
7. Hirsch AT, et al: ACC/AHA 2005 Practice Guidelines for the management of patients with peripheral arterial disease (lower extremity, renal, mesenteric, and abdominal aortic): A collaborative report from the American Association for Vascular Surgery/Society for Vascular Surgery, Society for Cardiovascular Angiography and Interventions, Society for Vascular Medicine and Biology, Society of Interventional Radiology, and the ACC/AHA Task Force on Practice Guidelines. Circulation 2006;113:e463-e654.
8. Criqui MH, et al: The prevalence of peripheral arterial disease in a defined population. Circulation 1985;71:510-515.
9. Sherev DA, Shaw RE, Brent BN: Angiographic predictors of femoral access site complications: Implication for planned percutaneous coronary intervention. Catheter Cardiovasc Interv 2005;65:196-202.
10. Rubin GD, et al: Multi-detector row CT angiography of lower extremity arterial inflow and runoff: Initial experience. Radiology 2001;221:146-158.
11. Whyman MR, et al: Randomised controlled trial of percutaneous transluminal angioplasty for intermittent claudication. Eur J Vasc Endovasc Surg 1996;12:167-172.
12. Whyman MR, et al: Is intermittent claudication improved by percutaneous transluminal angioplasty? A randomized controlled trial. J Vasc Surg 1997;26:551-557.
13. Wolf GL, et al: Surgery or balloon angioplasty for peripheral vascular disease: A randomized clinical trial. Principal Investigators and their Associates of Veterans Administration Cooperative Study Number 199. J Vasc Interv Radiol 1993;4: 639-648.
14. Lundgren F, et al: Intermittent claudication—Surgical reconstruction or physical training? A prospective randomized trial of treatment efficiency. Ann Surg 1989;209:346-355.
15. Perkins JM, et al: Exercise training versus angioplasty for stable claudication: Long and medium term results of a prospective, randomised trial. Eur J Vasc Endovasc Surg 1996;11:409-413.
16. Holm J, et al: Chronic lower limb ischaemia: A prospective randomised controlled study comparing the 1-year results of vascular surgery and percutaneous transluminal angioplasty (PTA). Eur J Vasc Surg 1991;5:517-522.
17. Wilson SE, Wolf GL, Cross AP: Percutaneous transluminal angioplasty versus operation for peripheral arteriosclerosis: Report of a prospective randomized trial in a selected group of patients. J Vasc Surg 1989;9:1-9.
18. Bosch JL, Hunink MG: Meta-analysis of the results of percutaneous transluminal angioplasty and stent placement for aortoiliac occlusive disease. Radiology 1997;204:87-96.
19. Tetteroo E, et al: Randomised comparison of primary stent placement versus primary angioplasty followed by selective stent placement in patients with iliac-artery occlusive disease. Dutch Iliac Stent Trial Study Group. Lancet 1998;351: 1153-1159.

20. Richter GM, et al: (Initial long-term results of a randomized 5-year study: Iliac stent implantation versus PTA). Vasa Suppl 1992;35:192-193.
21. Ponec D, et al: The Nitinol SMART stent vs Wallstent for suboptimal iliac artery angioplasty: CRISP-US trial results. J Vasc Interv Radiol 2004;15:911-918.
22. Sacks D, et al: Reporting standards for clinical evaluation of new peripheral arterial revascularization devices. Technology Assessment Committee. J Vasc Interv Radiol 1997;8(1 Pt 1):137-149.
23. Management of peripheral arterial disease (PAD). TransAtlantic Inter-Society Consensus (TASC). Int Angiol 2000;19(1 Suppl 1):I-XXIV, 1-304.
24. Taylor LM Jr, Porter JM: Clinical and anatomic considerations for surgery in femoropopliteal disease and the results of surgery. Circulation 1991;83(2 Suppl):I63-I69.
25. Walsh DB, et al: The natural history of superficial femoral artery stenoses. J Vasc Surg 1991;14:299-304.
26. Ballard JL, et al: Complications of iliac artery stent deployment. J Vasc Surg 1996;24:545-553; discussion 553-555.
27. Creasy TS, et al: Is percutaneous transluminal angioplasty better than exercise for claudication? Preliminary results from a prospective randomised trial. Eur J Vasc Surg 1990;4: 135-140.
28. Matsi PJ, et al: Percutaneous transluminal angioplasty in femoral artery occlusions: Primary and long-term results in 107 claudicant patients using femoral and popliteal catheterization techniques. Clin Radiol 1995;50:237-244.
29. Ljungman C, et al: A multivariate analysis of factors affecting patency of femoropopliteal and femorodistal bypass grafting. Vasa 2000;29:215-220.
30. Muradin GS, et al: Balloon dilation and stent implantation for treatment of femoropopliteal arterial disease: Meta-analysis. Radiology 2001;221:137-145.
31. Duda SH, et al: Sirolimus-eluting versus bare nitinol stent for obstructive superficial femoral artery disease: The SIROCCO II trial. J Vasc Interv Radiol 2005;16:331-338.
32. Vroegindeweij D, et al: Directional atherectomy versus balloon angioplasty in segmental femoropopliteal artery disease: Two-year follow-up with color-flow duplex scanning. J Vasc Surg 1995;21:255-268; discussion 268-269.
33. Nakamura S, et al: A randomized trial of transcutaneous extraction atherectomy in femoral arteries: Intravascular ultrasound observations. J Clin Ultrasound 1995;23:461-471.
34. Fisher CM, et al: No additional benefit from laser in balloon angioplasty of the superficial femoral artery. Eur J Vasc Endovasc Surg 1996;11:349-352.
35. Vroegindeweij D, et al: Recanalization of femoropopliteal occlusive lesions: A comparison of long-term clinical, color duplex US, and arteriographic follow-up. J Vasc Interv Radiol 1995;6:331-337.
36. Vroegindeweij D, et al: Patterns of recurrent disease after recanalization of femoropopliteal artery occlusions. Cardiovasc Intervent Radiol 1997;20:257-262.
37. Schillinger M, et al: Balloon angioplasty versus implantation of nitinol stents in the superficial femoral artery. N Engl J Med 2006;354:1879-1888.
38. van der Zaag ES, et al: Angioplasty or bypass for superficial femoral artery disease? A randomised controlled trial. Eur J Vasc Endovasc Surg 2004;28:132-137.
39. Soder HK, et al: Prospective trial of infrapopliteal artery balloon angioplasty for critical limb ischemia: Angiographic and clinical results. J Vasc Interv Radiol 2000;11:1021-1031.
40. Matsi PJ, et al: Chronic critical lower-limb ischemia: Prospective trial of angioplasty with 1-36 months follow-up. Radiology 1993;188:381-387.
41. Dorros G, et al: The acute outcome of tibioperoneal vessel angioplasty in 417 cases with claudication and critical limb ischemia. Cathet Cardiovasc Diagn 1998;45:251-256.
41a. Löfberg AM, et al: The use of below-knee percutaneous transluminal angioplasty in arterial occlusive disease causing chronic critical limb ischemia. Cardiovasc Intervent Radiol 1996;19:317-322.
42. Jahnke T, et al: Treatment of infrapopliteal occlusive disease by high-speed rotational atherectomy: Initial and mid-term results. J Vasc Interv Radiol 2001;12:221-226.

43. Holdsworth RJ, McCollum PT: Results and resource implications of treating end-stage limb ischaemia. Eur J Vasc Endovasc Surg 1997;13:164-173.

44. Dorros G, et al: Tibioperoneal (outflow lesion) angioplasty can be used as primary treatment in 235 patients with critical limb ischemia: Five-year follow-up. Circulation 2001;104:2057-2062.

45. Dormandy J, Heeck L, Vig S: Acute limb ischemia. Semin Vasc Surg 1999;12:148-153.

46. Thrombolysis in the management of lower limb peripheral arterial occlusion: A consensus document. J Vasc Interv Radiol 2003;14(9 Pt 2):S337-S349.

47. Weaver FA, et al: Surgical revascularization versus thrombolysis for nonembolic lower extremity native artery occlusions: Results of a prospective randomized trial. The STILE Investigators. Surgery versus Thrombolysis for Ischemia of the Lower Extremity. J Vasc Surg 1996;24:513-521; discussion 521-523.

48. Olin JW, Shih A: Thromboangiitis obliterans (Buerger's disease). Curr Opin Rheumatol 2006;18:18-24.

49. Sakamoto I, et al: Endovascular treatment of iliac artery aneurysms. Radiographics 2005;25(Suppl 1);S213-S227.

50. Saxon RR, et al: Endograft use in the femoral and popliteal arteries. Tech Vasc Interv Radiol 2004;7:6-15.

51. Siauw R, Koh EH, Walker SR: Endovascular repair of popliteal artery aneurysms: Techniques, current evidence and recent experience. A N Z J Surg 2006;76:505-511.

52. Smyth JS, Scoble JE: Atheroembolism. Curr Treat Options Cardiovasc Med 2002;4:255-265.

40 Upper Extremities and Aortic Arch

Samuel L. Johnston and Robert S. Dieter

KEY POINTS

- Significant anatomic variation in the proximal arch and upper extremity arteries occurs in 30% of the population.
- Subclavian steal syndrome (SSS) occurs when there is retrograde vertebral artery blood flow away from the cerebral posterior circulation to accommodate demand for blood in the ipsilateral subclavian artery beyond a tight proximal stenosis.
- Coronary SSS and other forms of iatrogenic steal phenomena are increasing in prevalence.
- Indications for intervention in patients with SSS are predicated on the presence of symptoms.
- Percutaneous intervention for occlusive diseases of the aortic arch vessels and upper extremities has become a successful, safe, and durable alternative to surgical intervention and is reasonable as first-line therapy.

- Thoracic outlet syndrome (TOC) occurs when there is a symptomatic compression of the neurovascular bundle as it exits the thorax. Most cases are primarily neurogenic, rather than vascular.
- Thoracic outlet diagnostic maneuvers have a high false-positive rate.
- Most patients with TOC are adequately treated with conservative measures.
- The most common cause of axillary aneurysm is crutch syndrome.
- The most common source of emboli to the upper extremities is arterial aneurysm of the proximal arch or proximal upper extremity vessels.

In the past decade, the scope of interventional cardiology has widened to encompass almost the whole realm of vascular medicine, including arterial diseases of the proximal arch and upper extremity. The extension of cardiology to peripheral artery disease (PAD) has been a natural outgrowth for several reasons. First, the major risk factors for PAD are identical to those for coronary artery disease (CAD), and, hence, there is considerable overlap in the affected patient populations. There is a high degree of correlation in the extent of atherosclerosis in the brachial, carotid, and coronary arteries.[1] The cardiologist invariably will have initial exposure to these patients when they present for health care. Second, patients with PAD are at extremely high risk for morbidity and mortality from myocardial infarction and stroke and should arguably be regularly monitored by a cardiologist for medical care.[2-5] Indeed, most patients with PAD do not require surgical or catheter-based intervention and will derive their greatest benefits in terms of decreased morbidity and mortality simply from risk factor reduction and best medical therapy. Third, the tools and techniques that work for intervention in atherosclerosis of the coronary arteries are

translatable to the large arteries of the peripheral vasculature. In most cases, the same standard catheter skills that are used for coronary cases can be applied to noncoronary arch and upper extremity cases.[6] There is high primary success in treating proximal arch and upper extremity occlusive disease and reasonable long-term patency (Fig. 40-1). In some cases, catheter-based therapies have become superior to traditional surgical techniques.[7]

It has been estimated that atherosclerosis of the *upper* limbs accounts for 5% of PAD affecting the extremities.[8,9] Even so, if one considers that 25% to 40% of patients seen in a typical cardiology clinic have significant PAD,[2,3,5] it becomes apparent that proximal arch and upper extremity arterial diseases constitute a significant disease burden. The Peripheral Artery Disease Detection, Awareness, and Treatment in Primary Care (PARTNERS) trial revealed that PAD is underdiagnosed and undertreated[2]; this is especially true for arterial diseases of the proximal arch and upper extremities.

Unlike PAD of the lower extremities, which is almost exclusively caused by atherosclerosis, the differential diagnosis for arterial disease of the proximal

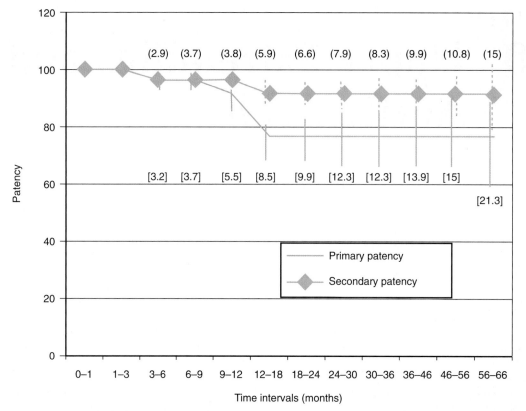

Figure 40-1. Long-term patency of subclavian artery stenting. (From Brountzos EN, Petersen B, Binkert C, et al: Primary stenting of subclavian and innominate artery occlusive disease: A single center's experience. Cardiovasc Intervent Radiol 2004;27:616-623.)

arch and upper extremities is extensive. Whereas the relative infrequency of significant atherosclerosis in the proximal arch vessels and upper extremities (compared with the lower extremities) probably represents underlying differences in pathophysiology (e.g., turbulence, inflammation, oxidative stress, density of receptors), its low prevalence is probably also a result of our collective failure to diagnose it. The relatively low prevalence of symptomatic arterial disease affecting the proximal arch and upper extremities, combined with the complex differential diagnosis underlying these diseases, makes timely and accurate diagnosis problematic. Many of these patients, such as those with subclavian steal (coronary or vertebral artery) or thoracic outlet syndrome (TOS), are misdiagnosed and/or inappropriately treated. With correct diagnosis, these patients are highly treatable, and, in the cases of atherosclerotic PAD, stand to benefit greatly in terms of decreased rates of cardiovascular events by receiving the appropriate medical therapy.

OBJECTIVES

The objectives of this chapter are as follows:
- Review the normal anatomy of the aortic arch, upper extremities, and the anatomic variants.
- Discuss the wide differential diagnosis that must be considered when evaluating a patient with suspected aortic arch or upper extremity arterial disease and see how tackling these problems frequently requires a multidisciplinary approach.

- Review the pertinent aspects of the patients' history, physical examination findings with special maneuvers, and initial laboratory workup.
- Introduce diagnostic modalities that are used in the peripheral vascular laboratory, and review the application of several common imaging modalities as they are applied to PAD.
- Discuss the application of catheter-based techniques for the diagnosis and treatment of arterial diseases of the proximal arch and upper extremities.
- Focus individually on the most common diseases: subclavian steal syndrome (SSS), coronary SSS, arm claudication, TOS, axillary artery stenosis/ crutch syndrome, and embolic diseases.

Other vascular conditions, such as trauma, small-vessel vasculitis, hemodialysis access interventions, and venous and lymphatic disorders will not be emphasized.

NORMAL ANATOMY

The arterial system of the upper extremities (Fig. 40-2) is analogous to that of the lower extremities. In 70% of the population,[10] the proximal arch arteries are the brachiocephalic (innominate) artery on the right (which quickly divides into the right subclavian artery and the right common carotid artery) and the left common carotid artery and left subclavian artery, which come off the arch separately, on the left. The subclavian artery becomes the axillary artery at the lateral border of the 1st rib. The

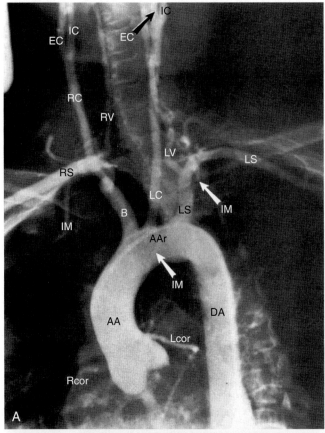

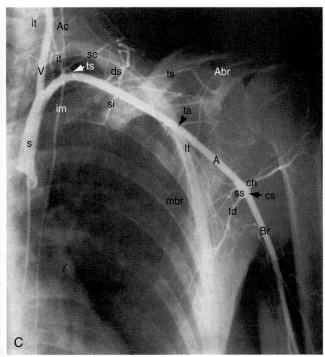

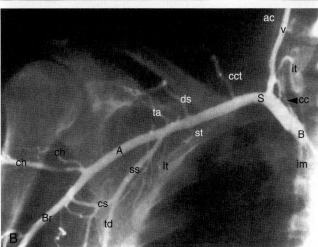

Figure 40-2. Normal anatomy. **A,** Left anterior oblique aortogram of the aortic arch. **B,** Right subclavian arteriogram. **C,** Left subclavian arteriogram. A, axillary; AA, ascending aorta; AAr, aortic arch; Abr, acromial branch; Ac, ascending cervical; B, brachiocephalic artery; Br, brachial artery; CC, common carotid; cct, costocervical trunk; ch, circumflex humeral; cs, circumflex scapular; DA, descending aorta; ds, dorsal (descending) scapular; EC, external carotid artery; IC, internal carotid artery; IM or iM, internal mammary artery; IT, inferior thyroid; It, thoracic; LC, left common carotid artery; Lcor, left coronary artery; LS, left subclavian artery; LV, left vertebral artery; mbr, mammary branch of lateral thoracic; RC, right common carotid artery; Rcor, right coronary artery; RS right subclavian artery; RV, right vertebral artery; S, subclavian; sc, superficial cervical; ss, subscapular; st/si, superior (highest) thoracic; ta, thoracoacromial; td, thoracodorsal; ts, scapular (suprascapular); V, vertebral. (From Kadir S: Atlas of Normal and Variant Angiographic Anatomy. Philadelphia, Saunders, 1991.)

axillary artery becomes the brachial artery, the first intrinsic artery of the upper extremity, in the shoulder girdle at the border of the teres major muscle. The brachial artery is superficial and should be palpable throughout its course. It first lies medial to the humerus and then courses anterior to it. Just below the antecubital fossa, the brachial artery divides into the ulnar artery, which courses medially, and the radial artery, which courses laterally. The ulnar and radial arteries are also superficial and normally palpable. In the wrist, the distal ulnar artery forms the superficial palmar arch, and the distal radial artery forms the deep palmar arch. The palmar arches form

extensive anastomoses before giving off the true digital arteries (medial and lateral).[11]

There are extensive collaterals formed by lesser arteries around the shoulders, around the elbows, and in the palms. These collaterals form a parallel arterial circuit that allows normal perfusion in the upper extremities even if there is a significant occlusion—with one major exception. In contrast to most other large vascular beds, each upper extremity is supplied by only one artery coming off the aorta. Therefore, all anastomoses in the extremities are distal to the aortic branch point, resulting in the potential for ischemic vulnerability and various steal phenomena.

Anatomic Variants

The presence of anomalous circulation in the proximal arch and upper extremity arteries (cumulatively, about 30% of the population)[10,12] can lead to confusion in the catheterization laboratory and misdiagnosis. Anatomic variants associated with TOS are described later in the chapter. Other common anatomic variants are described here.

Bovine arch: The bovine arch is the most common anatomic variant of the aortic arch, occurring in 22% of the population and accounting for 73% of all arch vessel anomalies.[10,12] It consists of a common origin of the right brachiocephalic and left common carotid arteries (Fig. 40-3). It is not associated with any pathologic significance.

Double aortic arch: The double aortic arch is a rare anomaly that is caused by persistence of the fetal double aortic arch system. It is rarely associated with congenital heart disease.

Right aortic arch: The right aortic arch is a rare anomaly that results from the persistence of the right fourth brachial arch, most commonly in association with an aberrant left subclavian artery (described later).

Left vertebral artery originating from aorta: Normally, the left vertebral artery comes off the left subclavian artery. In 4% to 6% of the population, it originates directly from the aortic arch, accounting for 14% of arch vessel anomalies.[10,12] It is not associated with other anomalies and does not confer any pathologic predilection. However, it may predispose to more upper extremity symptoms in the presence of proximal left subclavian artery stenosis owing to the absence of a significant collateral pathway.

Aberrant right subclavian artery (ARSA): ARSA (or *arteria lusoria*) is an example of a vascular ring with pathologic significance (Fig. 40-4).[13-15] It is caused by the persistence of the posterior segment of the fourth

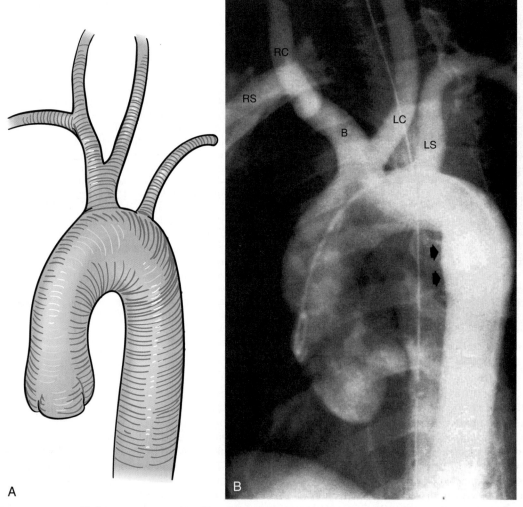

Figure 40-3. Common origin of left common carotid and brachiocephalic arteries (bovine arch). **A,** Schematic diagram. **B,** Left anterior oblique arch aortogram of a bovine arch. B, brachiocephalic artery; LC, left common carotid artery; LS, left subclavian artery; RC, right common carotid artery; RS, right subclavian artery. (From Kadir S: Atlas of Normal and Variant Angiographic Anatomy. Philadelphia, Saunders, 1991.)

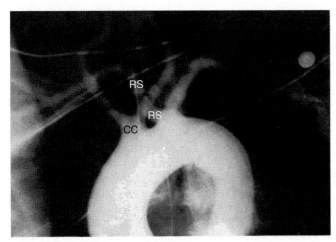

Figure 40-4. Aberrant right subclavian artery and a common carotid trunk. CC, common carotid trunk; RS, right subclavian artery. (From Kadir S: Atlas of Normal and Variant Angiographic Anatomy. Philadelphia, Saunders, 1991.)

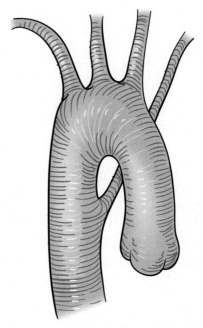

Figure 40-5. Right aortic arch with aberrant left subclavian artery (schematic). (From Kadir S: Atlas of Normal and Variant Angiographic Anatomy. Philadelphia, Saunders, 1991.)

aortic arch. It manifests as a right subclavian artery that arises from the left aortic arch *distal* to the origin of the left subclavian artery and follows a retroesophageal course. It occurs in fewer than 2% of the population and is associated with other anomalies of the arch vessels. The proximal section of an ARSA has a propensity for aneurysm (termed Kommerell's diverticulum) and may cause symptoms related to compression of nearby structures. The most common symptom is intermittent dysphagia *(dysphagia lusoria)*, caused by compression of the esophagus.[16] However, regardless of the presence of symptoms, the presence of Kommerell's diverticulum is an indication for surgical repair because of its significant risk of rupture.[17,18] Interestingly, surgical repair of ARSA by way of ligation of the anomalous origin has been described as an iatrogenic cause of the SSS.[18]

Aberrant left subclavian artery: An isolated left subclavian artery arises from a right aortic arch when there is interruption of the left fourth arch proximal to the seventh cervical intersegmental artery. This anomaly is a rare cause of upper extremity ischemia and has been associated with SSS (Fig. 40-5).[10,19] As for ARSA, repair of aberrant left subclavian artery has also been associated with development of the SSS.[18]

Brachial, radial, and ulnar arteries: In 20% of the population, the brachial artery is doubled during all or part of its course. Owing to extensive collateralization around the elbow, occlusion of one of these branches is generally well tolerated. In 15% to 20% of the population, the radial artery originates early on from the brachial artery, or even as high as the axillary artery (Fig. 40-6).[10] It is relatively uncommon, however, for the ulnar artery to branch off prematurely (prevalence, 1% to 3%). The ulnar artery is congenitally absent in 2% to 3% of the population. These variants confer no intrinsic pathologic significance.

CLASSIFICATIONS

Given the broad differential diagnosis that must be considered when approaching suspected proximal arch vessel or upper extremity arterial disease, it is useful to classify these diseases based on symptom acuity (time of onset) and size of the involved artery.

The diseases involving large or medium-sized arteries, such as those proximal to the wrist, are most relevant to the cardiologist, and they are caused by one of five mechanisms (Table 40-1). The small vessel diseases (i.e., those distal to the wrist) are frequently rheumatologic or hematologic disorders and include blood dyscrasias, Buerger's disease, Henoch-Schönlein purpura, the various hypercoagulable states, and multiple small-vessel vasculitides. It can be clinically difficult to distinguish between large vessel and small vessel disease. For example, although most think of Raynaud's phenomenon as a disease of the small arteries only, it is a common feature of both.

INITIAL EVALUATION

The history and physical examination rarely suffice in establishing a definitive diagnosis. Nonetheless, the broad differential diagnosis of proximal arch and upper extremity diseases can be significantly narrowed with good history-taking skills and a thorough examination. These fundamental skills remain essential to expediting a correct diagnosis, minimizing unnecessary testing, and making the necessary referrals.

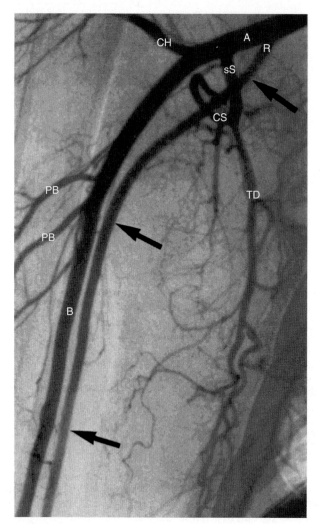

Figure 40-6. Radial artery *(arrows)* originating from axillary artery. A, axillary; B, brachial; CH, circumflex humeral; CS, circumflex scapular; PB, profunda brachial; R, radial; sS, subscapular; TD, thoracodorsal. (From Kadir S: Atlas of Normal and Variant Angiographic Anatomy. Philadelphia, Saunders, 1991.)

Table 40-1. Large and Medium Artery Disease

Mechanism	Site or Disease State
Atherosclerosis	Brachiocephalic artery
	Subclavian artery
	Axillary artery
Aneurysm	Thoracic outlet syndrome
	Trauma, "crutch" syndrome
	Vasculitis
	Fibromuscular dysplasia
Thromboembolism	Cardiac
	Aortic arch
	Proximal great vessels
Entrapment	Thoracic outlet syndrome
	Trauma
	Neoplasm
Vasculitis	Giant cell (temporal) arteritis
	Kawasaki's arteritis
	Takayasu's arteritis
	Radiation-induced arteritis

Adapted from Rajagopalan S, Mukherjee D, Mohler E: Manual of Vascular Diseases. Philadelphia, Lippincott, 2004, p 464.

History

Establishing the correct diagnosis in proximal arch and upper extremity disease is often facilitated by noting "the company it keeps." Indeed, an awareness of the patient's comorbid illnesses usually provides important clues. For instance, complaints of chronic or recurrent headache in a patient with tetralogy of Fallot and history of the Blalock-Taussig procedure is highly suggestive of the SSS.

Most commonly, a patient simply has a history of atherosclerosis or risk factors for it. Atherosclerosis is frequently a systemic process, so if a patient is already known to have CAD or PAD, one's suspicion for proximal arch vessel or upper extremity ischemia should be raised. Likewise, a prior diagnosis of atrial fibrillation, severe left ventricular dysfunction, aortic plaquing, or arterial aneurysm raises the probability that thromboembolic disease is the culprit. Previously diagnosed hematologic diseases, rheumatologic diseases, or malignancies all suggest vasospasm, vasculitis, or hypercoagulability.

Vasculitides, in general, tend to be systemic diseases and patients usually present with constitutional symptoms such as fever, weight loss, and fatigue in the early phase of disease. The presence of arthralgias and myalgias is also suggestive of vasculitis. The vasculitides, particularly Takayasu's, are uncommon and affect women more often than men. Takayasu's arteritis is more common in, but not exclusive to, the Asian races. Fibromuscular dysplasia may mimic Takayasu's arteritis but lacks the constitutional symptoms.

In terms of distinguishing the vasculitides, age is often the best initial discriminator. Kawasaki's disease is strictly a pediatric disease in onset; however, its sequelae, such as coronary and peripheral artery aneurysmal disease, can be significant in the adult population. Takayasu's arteritis usually occurs in patients younger than 40 years of age, whereas giant cell (temporal) arteritis is unlikely to affect patients younger than 65 years of age.

TOS is, perhaps, the most difficult entity to tease out from history alone. Its presence is suggested by an exacerbation of symptoms (e.g., pain or paresthesia) in the context of upper extremity movement, particularly abduction. Unfortunately, this feature hardly distinguishes it from the upper extremity claudication that is characteristic of subclavian or axillary artery stenosis. Except in cases of trauma, symptom onset is usually vague and slowly progressive.

During the initial evaluation, the clinician should inquire about timing of symptoms, symmetry, use of potentially vasospastic medications (Table 40-2), use of recreational drugs (including tobacco), prior external beam irradiation (as in the treatment of Hodgkin's disease, breast cancer or lung cancer), and occupational exposures (Table 40-3). It is essential to know these details before prescribing further testing.

Table 40-2. Medication-Induced Vasospasm

Class	Examples	Common Uses
5-HT agonists	Sumatriptan	Migraine headache
Ergot alkaloids	Methysergide	Migraine headache
	Ergonovine	Postpartum bleeding
Dopamine agonists	Bromocriptine	Parkinson's disease
		Acromegaly
		Hyperprolactinemia
Immunomodulators	α-Interferon (α-IFN)	Hepatitis C virus
		Hepatitis B virus
		Hematologic malignancies
Antiseizure agents	Phenytoin	Seizure treatment and prevention
	Carbamazepine	
Antibiotics	Trimethoprim/sulfamethoxazole	Antimicrobial
	Tetracycline, doxycycline	
Xanthine oxidase inhibitors	Allopurinol	Gout prophylaxis
		Tumor lysis syndrome
		Nephrolithiasis prophylaxis (calcium oxalate)
Diuretics (thiazides)	Hydrochlorothiazide	Congestive heart failure
	Chlorothiazide	Edema
	Chlorthalidone	Hypertension
	Metolazone	
Aldosterone receptor antagonists	Spironolactone	Congestive heart failure
		Edema
		Hypertension (systemic)
		Portal hypertension
		Hyperaldosteronism
Recreational	Nicotine	Recreational
	Cocaine	

5-HT, 5-hydroxytryptamine (serotonin).

The utility of gathering a comprehensive history from the patient with suspected proximal arch or upper extremity disease cannot be overstated. It is easy to be led astray by the large differential diagnosis that must be considered. Common sense dictates that common diseases occur commonly, and this line of thinking should be applied when approaching these patients. Nevertheless, one should be prepared to hunt for the occasional zebra. For instance, in the context of upper extremity symptoms, dysphagia may suggest a rheumatologic disorder, such as CREST syndrome, or an anatomic variant, such as ARSA with *dysphagia lusoria*.

Table 40-3. Occupational Exposures Associated with Proximal Arch and Upper Extremity Disease

Exposure	Disease State
Vinyl chloride	Raynaud's phenomenon
Vibratory tools	Raynaud's phenomenon
	Hypothenar hammer syndrome
Repetitive palmar pressure/trauma	Raynaud's phenomenon
	Hypothenar hammer syndrome
Sporting activities	Thoracic outlet syndrome
	Hypothenar hammer syndrome
Irradiation	Atherosclerosis
	Vasculitis

Physical Examination

As with a thorough history, careful attention to the physical examination usually narrows the differential diagnosis and reveals the best next step in the patient's workup. For example, noted absence of the brachial and radial pulses in a young Asian woman would be immediately be suggestive of Takayasu's arteritis.

For patients in whom proximal arch and upper extremity disease is already suspected, it is prudent to conduct a thorough (rather than focused) physical examination, because the underlying pathology is so frequently a systemic process. But given the high prevalence of PAD, it is reasonable to at least perform office-based screening for upper extremity disease on all patients who present to the cardiology clinic by measuring the pulses and blood pressures in both arms.

The physician should manually measure the blood pressure in both arms. A systolic gradient of more than 15 to 20 mm Hg is suspicious for significant proximal arch or upper extremity stenosis (although in patients with bilateral disease there may be no differential). The specificity of a 10 mm Hg differential in cuff pressure between arms is 85%, and the specificity of a 20 mm Hg differential is 94%.[20] The brachial, radial, and ulnar pulses should be palpable and symmetric throughout their course. Multiple pulse deficits in a young patient (as in the example just mentioned) are suggestive of Takayasu's arteritis.

TOS maneuvers, which typically involve palpation of the radial artery before and after a maneuver (usually involving arm abduction), are specifically discussed in the later section on TOS. Allen's test and capillary refill (<5 seconds) should be compared in each hand. Bilateral findings indicate a systemic disease process. The carotid arteries and supraclavicular fossae should be palpated and auscultated. A supraclavicular pulsatile mass raises the possibility of a subclavian artery aneurysm or associated cervical rib.

Fortunately, the signs of acute and chronic arterial insufficiency are usually distinct. Signs of acute arterial insufficiency are neatly summarized by the 5 Ps: pulselessness, pallor, poikilothermia, pain, and paresthesia. Signs of chronic arterial insufficiency include muscle atrophy, skin "bronzing," focal hair loss, and digital gangrene. Nonhealing skin ulcers are an exception to this rule, because they can result from either acute or chronic arterial insufficiency. The presence of skin ulceration should prompt one's consideration of atherosclerotic disease, embolic disease, Buerger's disease, or vasculitis.

Patients with vasculitis or malignancy often look chronically ill and may present with fever, unintentional weight loss, or frank cachexia. The presence of synovitis, nail pitting, prominent nailbed capillary loops, and skin lesions such as erythema nodosum, pyoderma gangrenosum, petechial rash or palpable purpura are highly suggestive of a vasculitis or other rheumatologic disease. However, the constellation of fever, rash, petechiae, and nail findings also warrants the consideration of infective endocarditis with embolization to the upper extremities. Splinter hemorrhages under the nail beds on the involved side indicate an atheroembolic process, such as originating from the heart or the ipsilateral subclavian/axillary arteries, or from infective endocarditis.

Laboratory

A few initial laboratory tests, such as a complete metabolic profile (CMP), a complete blood count (CBC), coagulation parameters, an erythrocyte sedimentation rate (ESR), and a lipid profile are useful in narrowing the differential diagnosis. Table 40-4 gives a comprehensive list of laboratory tests organized according to a system-based differential diagnosis.

Vascular Laboratory

Measuring Segmental Limb Pressures (with Continuous-Wave Doppler)

Segmental arm pressure measurements using a two-cuff system with continuous-wave Doppler (CWD) are available in most vascular laboratories. It is the most useful initial test to determine the level of obstruction, especially when symptoms are asymmetric. Proximal blood pressure cuffs are placed on each arm to occlude the brachial arteries, and distal cuffs are placed on each forearm to occlude the radial and ulnar arteries. CWD is applied to detect arterial

Table 40-4. Laboratory Tests

Cardiovascular	Rheumatologic
Atherosclerotic	CBC with differential
Basic metabolic profile	Rheumatoid factor
Lipid profile	Antinuclear antibody
Lipoprotein (a)	Anti-dsDNA antibodies
hsCRP	Extractable nuclear antigens
HbA$_{1c}$	ESR
	C-reactive protein
Cardiac emboli	Hepatitis virus screening
aPTT	Cryoglobulins
PT/INR	
	Hematologic
Cholesterol emboli	
CBC with differential	*Malignancy*
Urine eosinophils	Complete metabolic profile
	CBC with differential
Infectious	SPEP with immunofixation
CBC with differential	Serum free light chains
ESR	
C-reactive protein	*Hypercoagulability*
Blood cultures	CBC
	aPTT, PT/INR
Neurologic	Factor V Leiden
Vitamin B$_{12}$	Prothrombin 20210 gene mutation
RPR	Antithrombin III
TSH	Antiphospholipid antibodies
HgbA$_{1c}$	Protein C
hsCRP	Protein S
	Lupus anticoagulant

aPTT, activated partial thromboplastin time; CBC, complete blood count; dsDNA, double-stranded deoxyribonucleic acid; ESR, erythrocyte sedimentation rate; HbA$_{1c}$, glycosylated hemoglobin; hsCRP, high-sensitivity C-reactive protein; PT/INR, prothrombin time/International Normalized Ratio; RPR, rapid plasma reagin; SPEP, serum protein electrophoresis; TSH, thyroid-stimulating hormone.

flow, measure pressures, and visualize the arterial waveforms. One can see waveforms and pressures in each upper extremity at the level of the subclavian, axillary, brachial, radial, and ulnar arteries. Arterial occlusion is indicated by flattened waveforms and decreased amplitudes on CWD. The blood pressure differential between sides using this technique should be less than 10 mm Hg. The wrist-brachial index (WBI, analogous to the ankle-brachial index [ABI]) and the finger-brachial index (FBI) can also be calculated. A WBI of less than 0.85 or an FBI of less than 0.70 is abnormal and suggests arterial insufficiency. Like the ABI, the WBI and FBI can be falsely elevated in the presence of arterial calcinosis and other forms of arterial incompressibility.

Finger Pressure Pulse Contours/Photoplethysmography Waveforms

Measuring finger pressure pulse contours with photoplethysmography is an excellent technique for distinguishing normal arterial flow from obstructive disease or from vasospastic disease (Fig. 40-7). The normal arterial waveform is characterized by a rapid systolic upstroke, a sharp systolic peak, and a dicrotic notch on the downstroke. Arterial obstruction is typified by a reduced waveform amplitude, increased time to peak systole (decreased slope), and loss of the dicrotic notch. Vasospasm, as in Raynaud's phenom-

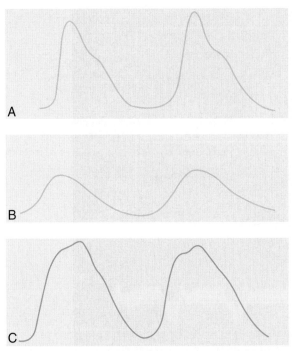

Figure 40-7. Arterial waveforms from finger pressure pulse contours. **A,** Normal waveform: rapid systole upstroke, sharp systolic peak, dicrotic notch on downstroke. **B,** Obstructive waveform: reduced waveform amplitude, time to peak systole increased, loss of dicrotic notch. **C,** Vasospastic Raynaud's syndome: peaked pulse ("nipple sign"), secondary ascending peak.

enon, is characterized by a secondary ascending peak that results in a marked widening of the whole waveform (the "nipple sign").

Imaging

Establishing the patient's diagnosis is almost always facilitated by obtaining an imaging study. Choice of optimum therapy depends on precisely defining the patient's anatomy to guide interventions and for follow-up. The gold standard remains digital subtraction angiography (DSA). But duplex ultrasonography remains the most popular initial imaging technique, and there is increasing application of computed tomographic angiography (CTA) and magnetic resonance imaging/angiography (MRI/MRA).

Duplex Ultrasonography

Duplex ultrasonography (combined two-dimensional B-mode ultrasound and pulsed-wave Doppler) is a noninvasive imaging technique that provides functional as well as anatomic detail based on the Doppler waveform and increases in peak systolic velocities (Fig. 40-8A). It is a relatively inexpensive test, is feasible for use in most patients, and can be performed in the clinic or at the bedside. Its primary disadvantage is that its results are highly operator dependent.

The standard probe uses a 10-MHz transducer (as opposed to the 3- to 5-MHz transducers used for adult echocardiography). With the exception of a blind spot behind the clavicle, one can use duplex to visualize the course of the upper extremity vasculature from the origin of the subclavian artery all the way to the palm (>10 MHz is needed to resolve the digital arteries). The sensitivity and specificity of duplex for detecting arterial stenosis is greater than 90%.

However, its utility is not limited to detecting arterial stenoses. Duplex can detect the flow reversal that is characteristic of steal phenomena, iatrogenic trauma (e.g., pseudoaneurysm, arterial dissection), and deep venous thrombosis. It is often used to assess whether a lesion is amenable to angioplasty and then for surveillance after therapy.

Tomographic Imaging Techniques

Tomographic imaging techniques such as CTA and MRA are excellent noninvasive, high-resolution imaging techniques that are useful tools for establishing the diagnosis of proximal arch and upper extremity vascular disease. They are capable of defining complex anatomy (as in the case of a congenital abnormality or prior intervention), allow visualization of the vasculature in multiple planes without the problem of overlap, and also show extravascular structures.

MRA has the advantage over CTA (and catheter-based angiography) in that it does not use ionizing radiation or nephrotoxic contrast dye. Gadolinium-enhanced magnetic resonance angiography (GEMRA) is the most useful MRI technique for assessing PAD. Its sensitivity and specificity for detecting occlusive arterial disease is greater than 95% (compared with catheter-based DSA). It is also highly sensitive and specific for assessing vascular wall inflammation. Phase-contrast MRA is a separate technique that provides simultaneous anatomic and functional data, similar to duplex ultrasonography. Phase-contrast MRA can quantify flow across a stenosis or a shunt and can measure turbulence. It is not typically included in MRI protocols at most institutions, so it must be specifically ordered.

There are a number of disadvantages to MRI. It is time-consuming, and imaging of the vasculature within the thorax requires prolonged breath-holding. Patients who are susceptible to claustrophobia cannot tolerate MRI or require prior treatment with anxiolytics. It is highly operator dependent and susceptible to artifact. The presence of permanent pacemakers, implantable cardiac defibrillators, Swan-Ganz catheters, and shrapnel are contraindications to MRI. However, contrary to the conventional wisdom, endovascular stents and most prosthetic cardiac valves are not contraindicated in magnetic resonance scanners.

CTA provides high-resolution multiplanar images that include perivascular structures, similar to MRI,

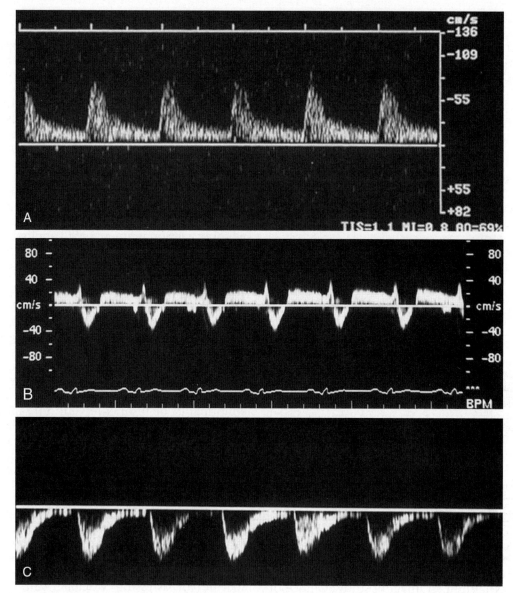

Figure 40-8. A, Normal vertebral artery duplex waveform. **B,** Intermittent vertebral artery flow reversal, as seen with subclavian steal. **C,** Permanent vertebral artery flow reversal, as seen with subclavian steal.

but is more widely available, less operator dependent, and less susceptible to artifact. Less patient cooperation is necessary compared with MRI, and claustrophobia and prolonged breath-holding are less problematic. Ferric metal is not a contraindication to CTA, but its presence may impair image gathering and cause artifacts. Unfortunately, multidetector CTA requires relatively high doses of ionizing radiation compared to catheter-based angiography, and, like catheter-based angiography, CTA requires the use of iodinated contrast dye that has the potential to cause nephrotoxicity and/or an allergic reaction.

Angiography/Digital Subtraction Angiography

Catheter-based angiography, in particular DSA, remains the gold standard for imaging the peripheral

vasculature, including the aortic arch, the great vessels, and the arteries of the upper extremities. It is the most definitive method of delineating the vasculature, and it allows one to measure intra-arterial blood pressures, gradients, and waveforms. It can facilitate the use of intravascular ultrasound (IVUS, discussed later) or a pressure-sensing wire.[21] If a lesion is significant and amenable to intervention, it is accessible at the time of the diagnostic catheterization. The disadvantages of catheter-based angiography include its invasiveness, exposure to ionizing radiation, and potential for complications (vascular trauma, bleeding, infection, contrast-induced nephropathy, and contrast-induced allergic reaction).

It is usually feasible and preferable to obtain vascular access through the femoral artery for percutaneous catheter-based angiography and angioplasty of the aortic arch and upper extremity vessels. In the case of a tight subclavian or axillary artery lesion, it may be necessary to obtain brachial artery access on the ipsilateral side.

An array of diagnostic catheters is available for accessing and imaging the great arch vessels and upper extremities. The pigtail catheter in conjunction with an AutoInjector is necessary to obtain good images of the aortic arch. Common projections are left anterior oblique (LAO) 30 degrees for origin of great vessels and right anterior oblique (RAO) 20 degrees for the brachiocephalic bifurcation. It is usually necessary to modify these angles to open up the arch. The arch vessels may be imaged with a variety of catheters, such as the Judkins right no. 4 (JR4), internal mammary (IMA), Vitek (VTK), Simmons, or multipurpose catheter. Injection rates for the arch are usually 30 to 40 mL over 2 seconds. The upper extremities may be selectively taken with hand injections.

SUBCLAVIAN STEAL SYNDROME

Definition, Historical Background, and Controversy

Subclavian steal is a result of the reversal of blood flow in vascular territories normally supplied by the subclavian artery. It is characterized by retrograde vertebral blood flow away from the cerebral posterior circulation to accommodate demand for blood in the ipsilateral subclavian artery beyond a tight proximal stenosis. The phenomenon was first described in 1960,[22] and it was quickly appreciated that it could cause symptoms consequent to a paucity of arterial blood flow to the cerebral posterior circulation, extremity, or heart.[23-25] In the classic description, blood may flow up the right brachiocephalic artery to the right carotid artery or right vertebral artery, through the circle of Willis, then down the left vertebral artery to the distal subclavian artery, where there is decreased arterial pressure (because of a proximal subclavian artery stenosis) and, hence, a gradient that results in the "stealing" of blood from the

posterior cerebral vascular territory.[26] In the context of *symptoms,* the phenomenon is called the subclavian steal *syndrome* (SSS). More commonly, however, it is a phenomenon found incidentally (by way of vascular studies) in an asymptomatic patient. When this occurs, it is sometimes referred to as "radiologic" subclavian steal to distinguish it from clinically significant steal. Recently, transient obstruction of the proximal segment of the subclavian artery with respiratory variation ("Dieter sign") has been described in some individuals (Fig. 40-9).[27]

The concept of SSS has not been without controversy, and some early papers suggested that the syndrome did not exist.[28,29] These authors pointed to evidence showing that even when there is reversal of blood flow in the vertebral artery, there is not an appreciable difference in total cerebral arterial flow.[28,29] That, indeed, may be the case for patients with an isolated severe proximal subclavian artery stenosis. Subsequent studies have shown that most patients affected by SSS have concurrent cerebrovascular lesions.[30] Up to 80% of patients who have SSS (i.e., symptomatic patients) also have concurrent stenosis in the contralateral carotid or vertebral artery. These patients presumably have inadequate cerebral arterial reserve in the context of increased demand from the affected extremity. The controversy has not ended with this discovery, however. There are many who speculate that these patients with symptoms of cerebral vascular ischemia in the context of both cerebrovascular lesions and a subclavian artery lesion are most likely to have symptoms intrinsic to the cerebrovascular lesions, and the subclavian lesion is merely incidental.

It is also important to note that some of the controversy surrounding the diagnosis of subclavian steal is a result of the disparity in reports on its prevalence. Early literature reported a low prevalence of vertebral artery flow reversal in patients with severe subclavian artery stenosis (as assessed by contrast angiography),[30,31] whereas more recent literature has reported a very high (although not necessarily clini-

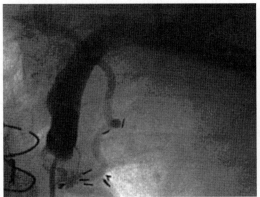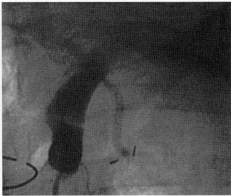

Figure 40-9. Dynamic left subclavian artery obstruction ("Dieter sign"). Exacerbation of proximal subclavian artery kink with expiration. Left subclavian arteriogram during inspiration *(left)* and expiration *(right)*. (From Dieter RS, et al: Description of a new angiographic sign: Dynamic left artery obstruction. Vasc Dis Manage 2006;3:298-299.)

cally significant) incidence of vertebral artery flow reversal in the same patient population.[32] These differences are hard to reconcile, but they most likely reflect an underdiagnosis of the phenomenon (but not necessarily the syndrome) before the widespread use of duplex ultrasonography.

Presentation

Most patients with SSS come to the physician's attention because of symptoms or abnormal physical findings. Symptoms are caused by vertebrobasilar insufficiency or ischemia of the upper extremity and may include syncope, dizziness, vertigo, ataxia, headache, visual disturbances, arm claudication, or paresthesia. These symptoms are generally worsened or precipitated by use of the extremity (as with exercise) or by compression of the vertebral artery (as with head rotation). Because symptoms are usually related to a *transient* paucity of arterial blood flow to either the cerebral posterior circulation or the upper extremity, stroke and severe limb ischemia are uncommon presentations for SSS. A thorough physical examination (as described earlier), with particular attention to the upper extremities and neurologic examination, is also often revealing.

Etiology

Subclavian steal is most commonly caused by an atherosclerotic narrowing of the proximal subclavian artery. The prevalence of significant subclavian artery atherosclerosis in patients with CAD is 17% to 23%.[6,31] Of these patients, only 2.5% are estimated to be symptomatic (and many more have radiologic steal). The left subclavian artery is affected three times more often than the brachiocephalic artery, possibly because of accelerated atherosclerosis caused by the more acute origin of the left subclavian artery and, hence, greater turbulence. The presence of subclavian steal is two times more common in men and reportedly has a peak incidence at 40 to 60 years of age.[33]

Subclavian steal can also be caused by a vasculitis, such as Takayasu's arteritis. This is less common, however, because the vasculitides typically involve a diffuse area of the artery. For example, if Takayasu's arteritis affects the subclavian artery, it is likely to involve a region both proximal *and* distal to the origin of the vertebral artery, rather than the focal proximal stenosis that is the substrate for the subclavian steal phenomenon.

TOS (discussed later) can also cause the SSS by causing compression or kinking of the proximal subclavian artery. This phenomenon is most common in athletes such as baseball pitchers, swimmers, golfers, and others who vigorously and repetitively abduct the upper extremity.

Congenital heart and vascular abnormalities (described earlier) can predispose an individual to SSS. A right aortic arch with isolation of the left subclavian artery and anomalies of the brachiocephalic arteries are the most common associations.

Iatrogenic causes of subclavian steal have been increasingly recognized. Prior vascular surgery is a significant risk factor for the development of SSS and should alert the physician to this and various other steal phenomena.[34] Classic examples include coronary artery bypass grafting (CABG) with a left internal mammary artery (IMA) conduit (see later discussion), arteriovenous fistula creation for hemodialysis access,[35] repair of tetralogy of Fallot with a Blalock-Taussig anastomosis,[34,36] and surgical repair of coarctation of the aorta.[37] There are numerous other inadvertent steal phenomena created by various surgical techniques that have been described previously.[18,26,34] External beam irradiation, as for the treatment of Hodgkin's disease, breast cancer, or lung cancer, is another potential iatrogenic cause of subclavian steal.[38] Intervention is usually warranted to correct iatrogenically created steal syndromes.[26,34]

Establishing the Diagnosis

The hallmark of the SSS is the presence of *symptoms*. If SSS is suspected, an initial evaluation with a noninvasive study of the carotid and vertebral arteries (with particular attention to the direction of blood flow) is warranted.

Flow reversal in the vertebral artery is most readily seen by duplex ultrasonography.[39] There are three classifications of vertebral artery flow abnormalities. Stage I describes reduced antegrade flow; stage II describes intermittent flow reversal, as with exercise (see Fig. 40-8B); and stage III describes permanent retrograde flow through the vertebral artery (see Fig. 40-8C).

Depending on the results of noninvasive studies, one may decide to proceed with catheter-based angiography of the aortic arch, brachiocephalic, subclavian, carotid, vertebral, and subclavian arteries. In patients who have had prior CABG using the left IMA as a conduit, the coronary arteries should also be evaluated (see later discussion of coronary SSS).

If the relative functional significance of a subclavian artery stenosis is unclear, as in the case of a concurrent ipsilateral vertebral artery stenosis, the use of a pressure-sensing wire can be helpful.[21] Noninvasive thallium-201 radionucleotide imaging of the upper extremities to determine the functional significance of subclavian artery stenosis after arm exercise (i.e., stress testing) has also been reported.[40] Finally, if there is a history of congenital heart disease or other complex anatomic variation, it may be helpful to obtain CTA or GEMRA before, or in lieu of, catheter-based angiography.

Prognosis

The long-term prognosis of the SSS is generally favorable with regard to progression of neurologic deficits and other associated symptoms.[32,41] However, if the cause is atherosclerosis, the prognosis of SSS (as with all cases of PAD) is surprisingly dismal over the 5-year interval after its diagnosis.[2-5] For these patients (i.e., the majority of patients with SSS), the greatest benefit in terms of decreasing morbidity and mortality will be derived from instituting best medical therapy and cardiovascular risk factor modification.

The prognosis for patients with SSS caused by Takayasu's arteritis is considerably better than for those who have SSS caused by atherosclerosis. The 5-year survival rate for patients with Takayasu's arteritis is 80% to 90%.[42-44] The long-term prognosis is excellent, even for patients who require surgical revascularization (mean survival, 19.8 years).[45] The favorable prognosis in these patients is contingent on lifelong surveillance and appropriate medical and surgical therapy.

Therapy

Intervention for subclavian steal should be reserved for symptomatic patients only. In the absence of symptoms (i.e., radiologic subclavian steal), the condition is generally benign. A relatively recent study reported the most common indications for subclavian artery revascularization, in order of decreasing prevalence, as SSS; arm claudication; coronary SSS (discussed later); and nonhealing wounds.[46]

In the four decades that have passed since SSS was first described, traditional surgical revascularization of the supra-aortic vessels has been largely supplanted by endovascular interventions. This shift has been catalyzed by fewer complications and shorter recovery times with catheter-based therapy. The first report on percutaneous transluminal angioplasty (PTA) for SSS was published in 1980.[47] The past quarter-century has brought forth significant progress in this area, and recent studies demonstrate high primary success and reasonable long-term patency for PTA and stenting of the subclavian artery in patients with SSS (see Fig. 40-1).[46,48] Primary success for subclavian artery stenting of *subtotal* occlusions is achieved in more than 98% of cases, with an incidence of major complications of less than 1%.[46,48]

With the use of conscious sedation and local anesthesia, subclavian stenoses can usually be approached via femoral access. In cases where there is complete or near-complete occlusion, access via a brachial or combined femoral-brachial approach may be necessary to cross the lesion. Crossing a totally occluded subclavian artery proves insurmountable in almost 50% of cases.[49] If the subclavian artery is selectively cannulated, a reference angiogram is performed to visualize the lesion and size the balloon. Many interventionalists advocate predilatation, although primary stenting is gaining popularity. Balloon-expandable stents are used for lesions in the proximal subclavian artery. Self-expanding stents are used for subclavian artery lesions distal to the origin of the vertebral artery.[50] Positioning of the stent can be guided by angiography, calcification, and road-mapping (Fig. 40-10).

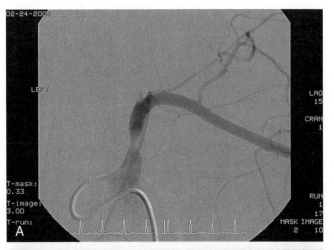

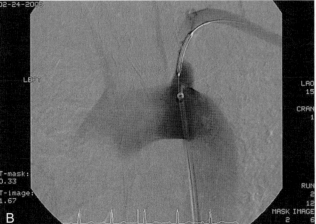

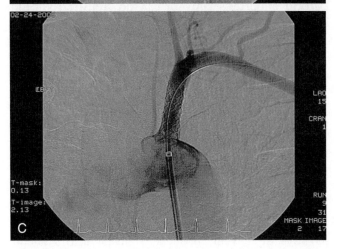

Figure 40-10. Proximal left subclavian artery stenosis **(A)**, stent deployment **(B)**, and view after stenting **(C)**.

Potential major complications of percutaneous intervention, albeit uncommon, include upper extremity embolization, transient ischemic attack and stroke, avulsion, perforation, dissection of the subclavian artery and aorta, and mycotic aneurysm.[46,48,49,51,52] Embolization to the vertebral artery or left IMA–left anterior descending (LAD) coronary artery graft can be catastrophic. However, given the rarity of major embolic complications, it has been suggested that there is persistent vertebral flow reversal for several seconds to minutes after PTA, which would provide some hemodynamic protection.[53] Nevertheless, some interventionalists prefer to use a distal protection device, such as a filter wire, in the vertebral artery via a radial/brachial approach.[54] The simplest method is balloon occlusion of the vertebral artery with a small, compliant balloon, which is deflated after the intervention and after the subclavian balloon is deflated (i.e., so that any debris embolizes the arm rather than the brain).[55] Likewise, some have advocated that a double-balloon technique be used during subclavian artery interventions to protect a left IMA graft.[56]

In most cases, the initial success of PTA with stent placement is equivalent to that of surgical revascularization, but with significantly lower morbidity and mortality. Furthermore, the long-term patency after PTA with stent placement (but not PTA alone) appears to be equivalent to the long-term patency with surgical revascularization.[7,46] However, there has not been a randomized trial comparing the two techniques at the time of this writing.

In complicated cases, such as the presence of a totally occluded subclavian artery, complex anatomy, or multiple lesions, a surgical or combined procedure may still be necessary. However, before a complex revascularization of the supra-aortic vessels is undertaken, correction of a significant carotid stenosis (by carotid endarterectomy or carotid stenting) should first be performed, because it will often be sufficient to resolve the patient's symptoms.[57]

The risks of surgical revascularization of the supra-aortic vessels are significant and have been published extensively. The traditional transthoracic approach with median sternotomy is associated with a 10% to 20% risk of stroke and/or death.[58,59] Nevertheless, this approach may be reasonable if the patient also requires CABG or in cases of complex brachiocephalic lesions. The potential for complications resulting from the transthoracic approach has spurred the development of safer extrathoracic approaches. Extrathoracic revascularization is now the most popular form of surgical correction. Overall patency for extrathoracic revascularization has been reported as 95% at 1 year, 86% at 3 years, and 73% at 5 years.[60] Although it carries less perioperative mortality than the transthoracic approach, extrathoracic revascularization is technically challenging owing to the intrinsic friability of the subclavian arteries and their tendency to tear.[26,61] The risk of major complication with extrathoracic bypass is 13% overall, with a 3% risk of stroke and a 2% risk of death.[7]

Medical therapy for SSS due to atherosclerosis is directed at cardiovascular event risk reduction, rather than symptomatic relief. Unlike PAD of the lower extremities, there is no established role for phosphodiesterase-III inhibitors (e.g., cilostazol). At least some data, by way of case reports, suggest that it is ineffective for SSS and upper extremity claudication.[40] Extrapolation from data for lower extremity PAD also suggests that there is no role for prostaglandin E_1 in the management of upper extremity ischemia.[62] Warfarin therapy should be reserved for the most severe and refractory cases, and it has never been studied in a prospective or randomized manner.

If a large vessel vasculitis, such as Takayasu's or giant cell (temporal) arteritis, is suspected, it is reasonable to initially treat with high-dose corticosteroids (prednisone 60 mg PO daily or equivalent). Early stages of vasculitis respond well to high-dose corticosteroids. Long-term therapy with a slow taper (e.g., a decrease in dose by 10% per week in responders) is necessary to prevent arterial stenosis. In the chronic stages of large vessel vasculitis, the artery becomes irreversibly stenosed and may require PTA or surgical bypass. Intervention tends to be more difficult, because the artery may be friable, fibrotic, or inflamed. Because establishing a definitive diagnosis of vasculitis can be challenging and a large percentage of cases of Takayasu's arteritis do not respond to corticosteroid treatment, consultation with a rheumatologist is recommended.

CORONARY SUBCLAVIAN STEAL SYNDROME

A similar steal phenomenon can occur in patients who have undergone CABG with an IMA conduit and also have proximal subclavian artery stenosis (or occlusion) (Fig. 40-11). In this variation, blood is shunted away from the coronary circulation retrograde through the IMA graft to supply the subclavian artery watershed. Classically, the patient experiences angina pectoris with exercise of the arm.[63,64] However, acute myocardial infarction in a patient with an IMA graft after occlusion of the subclavian artery has also been reported.[65]

Coronary SSS has become increasingly relevant over the past 2 decades as the use of the IMA has increased to 75% to 90% of all CABGs.[66] Given the prevalence of significant subclavian artery atherosclerosis (17%-23%) in patients with CAD,[6,31] one must consider coronary SSS in the differential diagnosis of patients who present with chest pain after CABG. Citing the low risk and potential benefits, some cardiologists have presented a strong argument for performing angiography of the left subclavian artery (with nonselective angiography of the left IMA) at the time of coronary angiography for all patients who are referred for CAGB.[6,67] In affected patients, it may be reasonable to perform subclavian artery stenting preoperatively to allow use of the left IMA or to use alternative conduits.

As with SSS and other cases of symptomatic subclavian artery stenosis, it is preferable to approach coronary SSS with a catheter-based intervention as a first approach. The surgical approaches for coronary SSS are similar to those for SSS.[68,69]

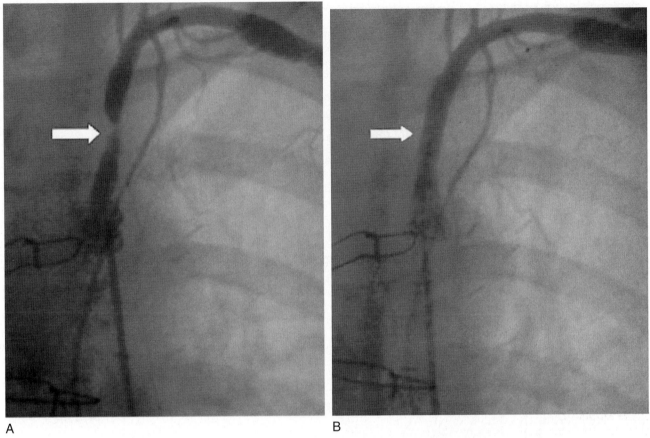

A   B

Figure 40-11. Coronary subclavian steal syndrome before intervention **(A)** and after intervention **(B)**. (From Bilku RS, Khogali SS, Been M: Subclavian artery stenosis as a cause for recurrent angina after LIMA graft stenting. Heart 2003;89:1429.)

THORACIC OUTLET SYNDROME

Definition

The TOS encompasses a heterogeneous group of disorders that result in symptomatic compression of the neurovascular bundle at any of several points as it traverses the cervicoaxillary canal through the scalene triangle and costoclavicular space to enter the upper extremity (Fig. 40-12).[70] The neurovascular bundle principally comprises the five roots of the brachial plexus, the subclavian artery, and the subclavian vein (some anatomists would also include the phrenic nerve, long thoracic nerve, and sympathetic chain). The roots of the brachial plexus, along with the subclavian artery, pass through the scalene triangle, which is bounded by the anterior and middle scalene muscles on each side and by the 1st rib at the base. The subclavian vein passes outside the scalene triangle, in front of the anterior scalene muscle and behind the pectoralis major muscle. The components of the neurovascular bundle then pass through the costoclavicular space, which is bounded by the clavicle, 1st rib, costoclavicular ligament, and middle scalene muscle. In practice, one finds the anatomy of the thoracic outlet highly variable among individuals.[71] Nine separate types of congenital bands and ligaments have been described within the scalene trian-gle.[72] Cervical ribs, which have a tendency to impinge on the structures exiting the thoracic outlet, occur in 0.5% to 1.5% of the general population.

Etiology and Prevalence

TOS is commonly classified as either neurogenic or vascular (Table 40-5). Neurogenic TOS, which refers to the symptomatic compression of the brachial plexus, is thought to account for 95% of cases. The site of compression is usually in the scalene triangle. Seventy percent of neurogenic TOS cases occur in female patients. Vascular TOS accounts for the remaining 5% of cases, with the majority of those affecting the subclavian artery and the minority affecting the subclavian vein. The site of compression in arterial TOS is most often an osseous narrowing in the costoclavicular space, as from a cervical rib. Compression of the subclavian artery at this point commonly results in aneurysm formation and embolization (Fig. 40-13). Unlike neurogenic TOS, arterial TOS occurs equally among men and women. For unknown reasons, venous TOS occurs twice as often in men as it does in women. The overall prevalence of TOS is unknown, because it represents an assortment of various rare disorders that are collectively difficult to definitively diagnose.

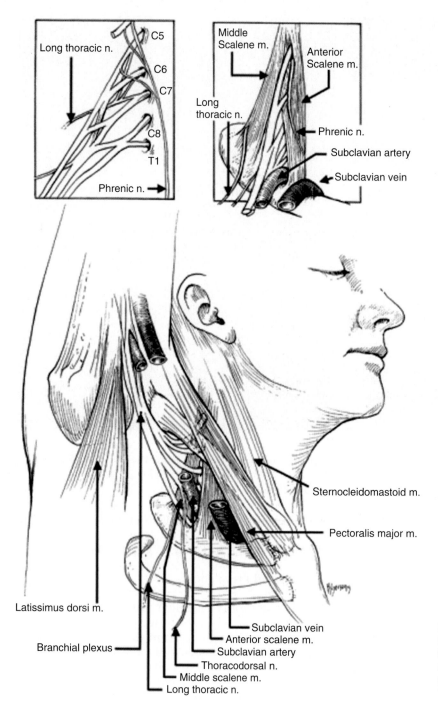

Figure 40-12. Anatomy of the thoracic outlet. (From Thompson RW, Petrinec D: Surgical treatment of thoracic outlet compression syndromes: Diagnostic considerations and transaxillary first rib resection. Ann Vasc Surg 1997;11:315-323.)

Table 40-5. Causes of Thoracic Outlet Syndrome

Bony	Cervical rib
	First thoracic rib
	Enlarged C7 transverse process
	Dislocation of the head of the humerus
	Clavicle (fracture, exostosis, bifid)
	Cervical spondylosis
	Crushing injury to upper thorax
Soft tissue	Fibrous bands
	Scalene muscles
	Omohyoid muscle
	Large, pendulous breasts

Adapted from Dieter RA Jr, O'Brien T, and Dieter RA III: Thoracic outlet syndrome. In Chang JB, et al (eds): Textbook of Angiology. New York, Springer, 2000, pp 635-643.

Age is a poor discriminator, but TOS tends to be most common in men and women between 20 and 40 years of age. Most of these patients have both an underlying anatomic predisposition for the disorder, such as a cervical rib or fibrous band, and an underlying mechanical feature, such as overuse or trauma. The chance of developing TOS is highest for those who have the susceptible anatomic substrate and engage in occupational or recreational activities that involve repetitive arm movements (e.g., painters, throwing athletes, rowers, weight lifters).

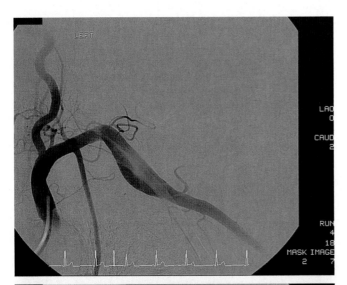

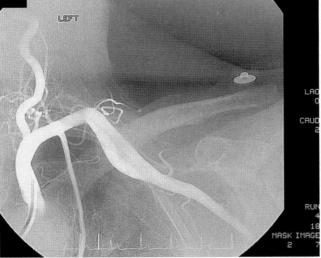

Figure 40-13. Arteriogram of the left subclavian artery shows a large subclavian aneurysm in a patient with a cervical rib and thoracic outlet syndrome.

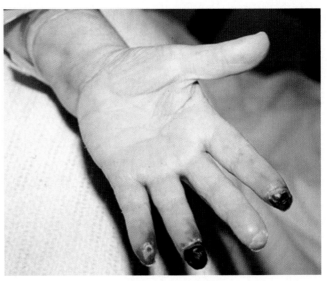

Figure 40-14. Atheroembolism as a complication of thoracic outlet syndrome. (From www.emedicine.com/cgi-bin/foxweb.exe/makezoom@/em/makezoom?picture=\websites\emedicine\med\images\Large\64775HAND.JPG&template=izoom2 Accessed June 2006.)

Presentation

The symptoms of TOS usually have an insidious onset and become progressively worse. Patients are likely to describe bouts of pain or paresthesias of the upper limb or limbs that occur in dermatomal patterns. The patient's dominant hand is most likely to be affected, although TOS occasionally occurs bilaterally or in the nondominant hand. Various arm movements, especially those involving abduction, may precipitate or exacerbate the patient's symptoms. In time, weakness and muscle atrophy may occur. Raynaud's phenomenon and other discoloration or coldness in one or both hands can occur. Extreme hypersensitivity or causalgia may be present. Headache is a common symptom and may represent referred pain to the occiput.[73] All of these symptoms may take hours to days to resolve after the precipitating arm movements. Because the symptoms of TOS are hardly unique and the disorder is relatively uncommon, patients are usually initially misdiagnosed as having a pure musculoskeletal disorder, or even PAD of the proximal arch or upper extremity.

Establishing the diagnosis of TOS may be further delayed because patients are late in seeking medical attention. Late presentations can be attributed to the insidious and subtle onset of symptoms, adaptive modifications (conscious or subconscious) in daily activities, and, in cases of arterial TOS, the presence of compensating arterial collaterals. The late presentation of vascular TOS occasionally manifests with catastrophic results (Fig. 40-14).

Diagnosis

The diagnosis of TOS is often challenging because of its lack of specific findings and its overall rarity. Indeed, there is no single test or pathognomonic finding to prove TOS. Most testing will either be negative or equivocal. Therefore, the diagnosis must be based on clinical pattern recognition and the exclusion of other diagnoses (Table 40-6). Commonly, the patient is seen by multiple specialists before the diagnosis is established.

In addition to the components of the physical examination that were emphasized earlier, there are numerous diagnostic maneuvers that have been described especially for TOS (Table 40-7). The common denominator among most of these maneuvers is some form of abducting the arm while palpating the radial pulse and noting its disappearance (Fig. 40-15). The external rotation-abduction stress test (EAST maneuver) is widely regarded as the most useful in diagnosing neurogenic TOS, whereas Adson's maneuver is most useful in identifying positional compression of the subclavian artery. All of the TOS maneuvers suffer from low specificity (15% false-positive rate overall).

Table 40-6. Differential Diagnosis for Thoracic Outlet Syndrome

Arterial	Embolic disease
	Aneurysms
	Atherosclerosis
	Arterial dissection
	Aberrant anatomy
	Reflex, vasomotor
	Raynaud's syndrome
	Vasculitis
	Radiation injury
Venous	Deep venous thrombosis
	Superior vena cava syndrome
	Other neoplastic compression
Cervical spine	Spinal cord tumor
	Ruptured intervertebral disk
	Degenerative joint disease/osteoarthritis
	Other neurologic diseases
Compressive syndromes	Carpal tunnel syndrome
	Ulnar nerve entrapment
	Trauma (brachial plexus injury, compartment syndrome, hyperextension)
	Rotator cuff injury
	Pancoast's tumor
Referred pain, Other	Coronary artery disease
	Esophageal spasm
Secondary gain	

Adapted from Dieter RA Jr, O'Brien T, Dieter RA III: Thoracic outlet syndrome. In Chang JB, et al (eds): Textbook of Angiology. New York, Springer, 2000, pp 635-643.

Table 40-7. Diagnostic Maneuvers for Thoracic Outlet Syndrome

Adson's maneuver	Sitting upright, patient takes a deep breath, looks upward, and turns face *toward* the affected side
External rotation-abduction stress test (EAST maneuver)	Arms extended, externally rotated and behind the head, patient repeatedly makes fists for 3 min while the radial pulses are palpated
Hyperabduction maneuver	Patient hyperabducts the affected extremity (evaluate for compression)
Costoclavicular maneuver	Patient thrusts both shoulders maximally backward and downward

In terms of diagnostic testing, it is reasonable to begin with chest radiographs and, possibly, a cervical spine radiographic series (Fig. 40-16). if vascular TOS is suspected, the patient should be referred to the vascular laboratory for photoplethysmography and duplex ultrasound to measure arterial patterns during provocative TOS maneuvers. Tomographic imaging may be useful, especially MRI, because it can identify soft tissue abnormalities such as congenital bands and ligaments, in addition to bony abnormalities. If there is a high suspicion of vascular TOS, the patient should proceed to bilateral arteriography (and possibly venography), sometimes with provocative maneuvers during angiography.

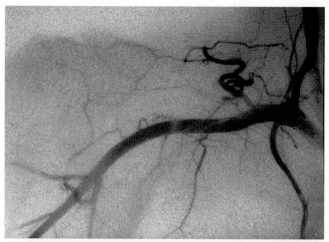

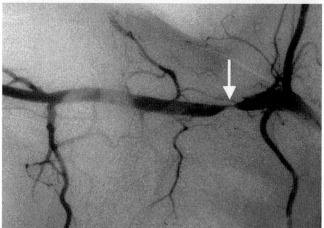

Figure 40-15. Right subclavian artery occlusion with arm abduction *(lower frame)* and absence of occlusion with arm relaxed *(upper frame)*. (From www.emedicine.com/cgi-bin/foxweb.exe/makezoom@/em/makezoom?picture=\websites\emedicine\med\images\Large\28642864ANGIO-UP.JPG&template=izoom2 Accessed June 2006.)

Therapy and Prognosis

In cases where TOS causes an acute vascular syndrome, therapy is directed at emergency surgical decompression of the subclavian artery and restoration of peripheral perfusion. Acute thromboembolism from a subclavian artery aneurysm can be treated by catheter-directed thrombolytic therapy (see later discussion) or embolectomy. However, it should be emphasized that there is no role for initial endovascular repair in cases of TOS (aside from thromboembolic complications).

Barring an acute vascular syndrome, the best initial approach to the treatment of patients with TOS is a conservative one. Most patients derive considerable benefit from noninvasive therapies and have a favorable long-term outcome (Table 40-8).[74] Surgical intervention is reserved for severe or refractory cases of TOS and is directed at releasing the scalene muscles and/or removing any bony obstruction.

The relevance of TOS to the interventional cardiologist lies primarily in recognizing how this heterogeneous group of disorders can masquerade as PAD of the proximal arch and upper extremity. Because

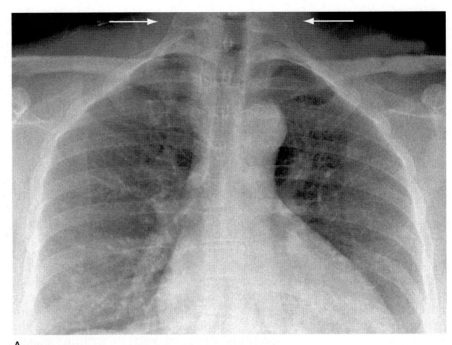

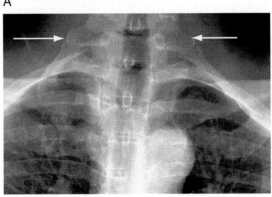

Figure 40-16. A and **B,** Chest radiographs demonstrating cervical ribs *(arrows).* (Courtesy of Terrence Demos, MD, Loyola University Medical Center.)

Table 40-8.   Therapies for Thoracic Outlet Syndrome

Physiotherapy	
Lifestyle changes	
Psychiatric therapy	
Medication	Acetaminophen
	Nonsteroidal anti-inflammatory drugs
	Muscle relaxants
	Opioids
	Anticoagulants
	Thrombolytics
Surgery	Rib resection
	Clavicle resection
	Scalenus transaction
	Breast reduction
	Thrombectomy/embolectomy
	Bypass graft
	Dorsal sympathectomy
	Neurolysis

Adapted from Dieter RA Jr, O'Brien T, Dieter RA III: Thoracic outlet syndrome. In Chang JB, et al (eds): Textbook of Angiology. New York, Springer, 2000, pp 635-643.

most cases of TOS are the result of nerve compression or related to musculoskeletal entrapment of the neurovascular bundle, most cardiologists prefer to delegate the management of these patients to their respective medical and surgical colleagues.

AXILLARY ARTERY DISEASE

The incidence of atherosclerosis is much lower in the axillary artery than it is in the subclavian artery. The most common pathologies of the axillary arteries are aneurysm and vasculitis.

The most common cause of axillary aneurysm in the United States is "crutch syndrome." As the name implies, long-term crutch use and compression of the axillary artery can lead to stenosis or aneurysm formation. Iatrogenic trauma to the axillary artery (as from catheter-based angiography, misdirected central line insertion, or pacemaker placement) can also result in vascular aneurysm formation.

Large vessel vasculitides commonly affect the axillary arteries and can result acutely in severe vasospasm and chronically in stenosis or aneurysm. Kawasaki's disease, a pediatric cause of vasculitis, frequently causes arterial aneurysms (including axillary artery aneurysms) that become symptomatic during adulthood. Aggressive treatment of Kawasaki's disease with immunosuppressive therapy, including gamma globulin, minimizes the formation of aneurysm. Takayasu's arteritis, a rare autoimmune-mediated vasculitis of young adults, commonly affects the subclavian and axillary arteries. Giant cell (temporal) arteritis is a disease of older adults that can involve the axillary arteries and occasionally affects arteries as distal as the radial. Axillary artery vasculitis may also be caused by external beam irradiation used to treat cancer (especially lung and breast cancer and Hodgkin's disease).

Axillary artery aneurysm commonly results in thrombus formation and embolization to the distal arteries of the upper extremity. Large or symptomatic axillary artery aneurysms should be treated, either percutaneously with self-expanding stents or with surgical correction. Embolic complications are discussed in the next section.

EMBOLIC DISEASE

Thromboembolism to the upper extremities is a vascular emergency. Clinical manifestations depend on the arterial segment affected by thromboembolism but often manifest as acute unilateral digital ischemia (see "Initial Evaluation").[75]

Raynaud's phenomenon is also a common finding. If the source of emboli is the heart or thoracic aorta, it is common for the patient to present with multiple arterial beds simultaneously involved.

Unlike atheroembolic disease in general, which is most often attributable to a cardiac source, embolism to the upper extremities is most often caused by aneurysmal disease of the proximal arch vessels. As previously discussed, the most common causes of proximal arch vessel aneurysm are "crutch syndrome," TOS, and the large vessel vasculitides. It should be noted that vasculitis-induced thromboembolic phenomena can occur in the absence of aneurysm.

The distal arteries of the upper extremity can also be affected by aneurysmal disease. The most common mechanism for this pathology is the hypothenar hand syndrome, an occupationally related repeated compression of the ulnar artery against the hamate bone. Affected patients usually have a history of using the heel of their hand as a hammer or of extensive use of vibratory tools. Involvement in certain sporting activities, such as martial arts and mountain biking, has also been implicated. As with aneurysmal disease in the proximal arteries, thromboembolism is a common complication.

Cardiac emboli are a slightly less common source of embolism to the upper extremities. However, approximately 30% of cardiac emboli travel to the upper extremities. Other potential sources of upper extremity emboli include atherosclerosis of the proximal arch vessels in the absence of aneurysm and atherosclerosis of the aortic arch.

The occurrence of thromboembolism must be diagnosed and treated swiftly. Treatment can be dependent on the source of embolism, so it is important to try to establish the source before initiating an intervention. Often, a focused history and physical examination along with an electrocardiogram can distinguish a proximal arch vessel source of embolization from a cardiogenic one. Duplex ultrasonography and/or transesophageal echocardiography may be useful adjuncts. Otherwise, procession to the catheterization laboratory to identify the occluded arterial segment should not be delayed.

Endovascular treatment options for atheroembolism to the upper extremities include catheter-directed thrombolytic therapy, Fogarty catheter-facilitated removal of emboli, and PTA with or without placement of a self-expanding stent. It is wise to alert one's surgical colleagues early in the management of complex cases, if the patient has a large embolic burden or is late in seeking medical attention. Surgical options for these patients include use of the Fogarty catheter, bypass grafting, and limb/digit amputation. After revascularization, a prolonged course of anticoagulation is often needed.

CONCLUSION

Cardiologists continue to enlarge their scope of knowledge and apply their skills to a wider field of practice. The management of arterial diseases of the proximal arch and upper extremity is one of the latest examples of this phenomenon. It represents a logical extension to our field of practice. However, diseases of the aortic arch and upper extremity are uniquely challenging. For the interventional cardiologist who pursues this realm of vascular medicine, it is vital to have an awareness of the differences from CAD and lower extremity PAD. The differential diagnosis for arterial diseases of the proximal arch and upper extremity is vast, and the potential for various (and often iatrogenic) steal phenomena exists. Nevertheless, when one understands these differences, the standard techniques for angiography and angioplasty that have been applied to the lower extremity can be applied with great success to the upper extremity. Percutaneous intervention for occlusive diseases of the aortic arch vessels and upper extremities has become a successful, safe, and durable alternative to surgical intervention and is reasonable as first-line therapy. The optimal techniques regarding stent deployment, type of stent, use of distal protection devices, and when to refer for surgery remain unknown and await randomized clinical trials.

REFERENCES

1. Sorensen KE, Kristensen IB, Celermajer DS: Atherosclerosis in the human brachial artery. J Am Coll Cardiol 1997;29:318-322.
2. Hirsch AT, Criqui MH, Treat-Jacobson D, et al: Peripheral arterial disease detection, awareness, and treatment in primary care. JAMA 2001;286:1317-1324.
3. Hirsch AT, Lenfant C, Creager M, Gloviczki P: NHLBI Workshop on Peripheral Arterial Disease (PAD): Developing a Public Awareness Campaign. Bethesda, MD, National Heart, Lung and Blood Institute, 2003.
4. Weitz JI, Byrne J, Clagett GP, et al: Diagnosis and treatment of chronic arterial insufficiency of the lower extremities: A critical review. Circulation 1996;94:3026-3049.
5. Dieter RS, Tomasson J, Gudjonsson T, et al: Lower extremity peripheral arterial disease in hospitalized patients with coronary artery disease. Vasc Med 2003;8:233-236.
6. Rigatelli G, Rigatelli G: Screening angiography of supraaortic vessels performed by invasive cardiologists at the time of cardiac catheterization: Indications and results. Int J Cardiovasc Imaging 2005;21:179-183.
7. Hadjipetrou P, Cox S, Piemonte T, Eigenhaver A: Percutaneous revascularization of atherosclerotic obstruction of aortic arch vessels. J Am Coll Cardiol 1999;33:1238-1245.
8. Rajagopalan S, Mukherjee D, Mohler E: Manual of Vascular Diseases. Philadelphia, Lippincott Williams & Wilkins, 2004, p 464.
9. Bogey WM, Demasi RJ, Tripp MD, et al: Percutaneous transluminal angioplasty for subclavian artery stenosis. Am Surg 1994;60:103-106.
10. Kadir S: Atlas of Normal and Variant Angiographic Anatomy. Philadelphia, Saunders, 1991, pp xi, 529.
11. Moore KL, Dalley AF, Agur AMR: Clinically Oriented Anatomy, 5th ed. Philadelphia, Lippincott Williams & Wilkins, 2006, pp xxxiii, 1209.
12. Blake HA, Manion WC: Thoracic arterial arch anomalies. Circulation 1962;26:251-265.
13. Grollman JH Jr, Harris CH, Hamilton LC: Congenital diverticula of the aortic arch. N Engl J Med 1967;276:1178-1182.
14. Klinkhamer AC: Aberrant right subclavian artery: Clinical and roentgenologic aspects. Am J Roentgenol Radium Ther Nucl Med 1966;97:438-446.
15. Kommerell B: Verlagernung des Ösophagus durch eine abnorm verlaufende arteria subclavia Dextra (arteria lusoria). Fortschr Geb Rontgenstr Nuklearmed Erganzungsband 1936;54:5905.
16. Brown DL, Chapman WC, Edwards WH, et al: Dysphagia lusoria: Aberrant right subclavian artery with a Kommerell's diverticulum. Am Surg 1993;59:582-586.
17. Verkroost MW, Hamerlijnck RP, Vermeulen FE: Surgical management of aneurysms at the origin of an aberrant right subclavian artery. J Thorac Cardiovasc Surg 1994;107:1469-1471.
18. Pifarre R, Dieter RA Jr, Niedballa RG: Definitive surgical treatment of the aberrant retroesophageal right subclavian artery in the adult. J Thorac Cardiovasc Surg 1971;61:154-159.
19. Tschirch E, Chaovi R, Waver RR, et al: Perinatal management of right aortic arch with aberrant left subclavian artery associated with critical stenosis of the subclavian artery in a newborn. Ultrasound Obstet Gynecol 2005;25:296-298.
20. English JA, Carell ES, Guidera SA, Tripp HF: Angiographic prevalence and clinical predictors of left subclavian stenosis in patients undergoing diagnostic cardiac catheterization. Catheter Cardiovasc Interv 2001;54:8-11.
21. Liu CP, Ling YH, Kao HL: Use of a pressure-sensing wire to detect sequential pressure gradients for ipsilateral vertebral and subclavian artery stenoses. AJNR Am J Neuroradiol 2005;26:1810-1812.
22. Contorni L: (The vertebro-vertebral collateral circulation in obliteration of the subclavian artery at its origin.). Minerva Chir 1960;15:268-271.
23. Reivich M, Holling HE, Roberts B, Toole JF: Reversal of blood flow through the vertebral artery and its effect on cerebral circulation. N Engl J Med 1961;265:878-885.
24. Fischer C: A new vascular syndrome: "The subclavian steal." N Engl J Med 1961;265:912-913.
25. Mannick JA, Suter CG, Hume DM: The "subclavian steal" syndrome: Further documentation. JAMA 1962;182:134-139.
26. Dieter RA Jr, Maganini RO, Dieter RA III: Subclavian steal syndrome. In Chang JB, et al (eds): Textbook of Angiology. New York, Springer, 2000, pp 629-634.
27. Dieter RS, Morshedi-Meibodi A, Ahmed MH, et al: Description of a new angiographic sign: Dynamic left artery obstruction. Vasc Dis Manage 2006;3:298-299.
28. Eklof B, Schwartz SI: Effects of subclavian steal and compromised cephalic blood flow on cerebral circulation. Surgery 1970;68:431-441.
29. Bornstein NM, Norris JW: Subclavian steal: A harmless haemodynamic phenomenon? Lancet 1986;2:303-305.
30. Lord RS, Adar R, Stein RL: Contribution of the circle of Willis to the subclavian steal syndrome. Circulation 1969;40:871-878.
31. Fields WS, Lemak NA: Joint study of extracranial arterial occlusion: VII. Subclavian steal: A review of 168 cases. JAMA 1972;222:1139-1143.
32. Hennerici M, Klemm C, Rautenberg W: The subclavian steal phenomenon: A common vascular disorder with rare neurologic deficits. Neurology 1988;38:669-673.
33. Ackermann H, Diener HC, Dichgans J: Stenosis and occlusion of the subclavian artery: Ultrasonographic and clinical findings. J Neurol 1987;234:396-400.
34. Dieter RA Jr, Kuzycz GB: Iatrogenic steal syndromes. Int Surg 1998;83:355-357.
35. Lee PY, Ng W, Chen WH: Concomitant coronary and subclavian steal caused by ipsilateral subclavian artery stenosis and arteriovenous fistula in a hemodialysis patient. Catheter Cardiovasc Interv 2004;62:244-248.
36. Kurlan R, Krall RL, Deweese JA: Vertebrobasilar ischemia after total repair of tetralogy of Fallot: Significance of subclavian steal created by Blalock-Taussig anastomosis. Vertebrobasilar ischemia after correction of tetralogy of Fallot. Stroke 1984;15:359-362.
37. Saalouke MG, Perry LW, Breckbill BL, et al: Cerebrovascular abnormalities in postoperative coarctation of aorta: Four cases demonstrating left subclavian steal on aortography. Am J Cardiol 1978;42:97-101.
38. Cavendish JJ, Berman BJ, Schnyder G, et al: Concomitant coronary and multiple arch vessel stenoses in patients treated with external beam radiation: Pathophysiological basis and endovascular treatment. Catheter Cardiovasc Interv 2004;62:385-390.
39. Kliewer MA, Hertzberg BS, Kim DH, et al: Vertebral artery Doppler waveform changes indicating subclavian steal physiology. AJR Am J Roentgenol 2000;174:815-819.
40. Wasson S, Bedi A, Singh A: Determining functional significance of subclavian artery stenosis using exercise thallium-201 stress imaging. South Med J 2005;98:559-560.
41. Ackermann H, Diener HC, Seboldt H, Huth C: Ultrasonographic follow-up of subclavian stenosis and occlusion: Natural history and surgical treatment. Stroke 1988;19:431-435.
42. Hall S, Barr W, Lie JT, Stanson AW, et al: Takayasu arteritis: A study of 32 North American patients. Medicine (Baltimore) 1985;64:89-99.
43. Ishikawa K: Natural history and classification of occlusive thromboaortopathy (Takayasu's disease). Circulation 1978;57:27-35.
44. Eichhorn J, Sima D, Thiele B, et al: Anti-endothelial cell antibodies in Takayasu arteritis. Circulation 1996;94:2396-2401.
45. Miyata T, Sato O, Koyama H, et al: Long-term survival after surgical treatment of patients with Takayasu's arteritis. Circulation 2003;108:1474-1480.
46. Bates MC, Broce M, Lavigne PS, Stone P: Subclavian artery stenting: Factors influencing long-term outcome. Catheter Cardiovasc Interv 2004;61:5-11.
47. Bachman DM, Kim RM: Transluminal dilatation for subclavian steal syndrome. AJR Am J Roentgenol 1980;135:995-996.
48. De Vries JP, Jager LC, Van den Berg JC, et al: Durability of percutaneous transluminal angioplasty for obstructive lesions of proximal subclavian artery: Long-term results. J Vasc Surg 2005;41:19-23.

49. Amor M, Eid-Lidt G, Chati Z, Wilentz JR: Endovascular treatment of the subclavian artery: Stent implantation with or without predilatation. Catheter Cardiovasc Interv 2004;63:364-370.

50. Brountzos EN, Petersen B, Binkert C, et al: Primary stenting of subclavian and innominate artery occlusive disease: A single center's experience. Cardiovasc Intervent Radiol 2004;27:616-623.

51. Bates MC, Almehmi A: Fatal subclavian stent infection remote from implantation. Catheter Cardiovasc Interv 2005;65:535-539.

52. Salerno JL, Vitek J: Fatal cerebral hemorrhage early after subclavian artery endovascular therapy. AJNR Am J Neuroradiol 2005;26:183-185.

53. Ringelstein EB, Zeumer H: Delayed reversal of vertebral artery blood flow following percutaneous transluminal angioplasty for subclavian steal syndrome. Neuroradiology 1984;26:189-198.

54. Gimelli G, Tefera G, Turnipseed WD: Vertebral artery embolic protection via ipsilateral brachial approach during left subclavian artery angioplasty and stenting: A case report. Vasc Endovascular Surg 2006;40:235-238.

55. Turi ZG: The way to a man's heart (or head) is through his shoulder. Catheter Cardiovasc Interv 2004;63:371-372.

56. Jones RD, Uberoi R: Subclavian artery angioplasty for the treatment of angina using a double balloon technique to protect a left internal mammary artery graft. Eur Radiol 2002;12:908-910.

57. Smith JM, Koury HI, Hafner CD, Welling RE: Subclavian steal syndrome: A review of 59 consecutive cases. J Cardiovasc Surg (Torino) 1994;35:11-14.

58. Berguer R, Morasch MD, Kline RA: Transthoracic repair of innominate and common carotid artery disease: Immediate and long-term outcome for 100 consecutive surgical reconstructions. J Vasc Surg 1998;27:34-41; discussion 42.

59. Vogt DP, Hertzer NR, O'Hara PJ, Beven EG: Brachiocephalic arterial reconstruction. Ann Surg 1982;196:541-552.

60. Salam TA, Lumsden AB, Smith RB 3rd: Subclavian artery revascularization: A decade of experience with extrathoracic bypass procedures. J Surg Res 1994;56:387-392.

61. Wittwer T, Wahlers T, Dresler C, Haverich A: Carotid-subclavian bypass for subclavian artery revascularization: Long-term follow-up and effect of antiplatelet therapy. Angiology 1998;49:279-287.

62. The ICAI Study Group: Prostanoids for chronic critical leg ischemia: A randomized, controlled, open-label trial with prostaglandin E1. Ischemia Cronica degli Arti Inferiori. Ann Intern Med 1999;130:412-421.

63. Bilku RS, Khogali SS, Been M: Subclavian artery stenosis as a cause for recurrent angina after LIMA graft stenting. Heart 2003;89:1429.

64. Fergus T, Pacanowski JP Jr, Fasseas P, Dieter RS: Coronary-Subclavian Steal: Presentation and Management. New Orleans, Loyola University Medical Center, 2006, p 6.

65. Barlis P, Brooks M, Hare DL, Chan RK: Subclavian artery occlusion causing acute myocardial infarction in a patient with a left internal mammary graft. Catheter Cardiovasc Interv 2006;68:326-331.

66. Ferguson TB Jr, Coombs LP, Peterson ED: Internal thoracic artery grafting in the elderly patient undergoing coronary artery bypass grafting: Room for process improvement? J Thorac Cardiovasc Surg 2002;123:869-880.

67. Speciale G, Pristipino C, Pasceri V, et al: A uncommon cause of angina during upper limb exercise. Ital Heart J 2004;5:548-550.

68. Norsa A, Gamba G, Ivic N, et al: The coronary subclavian steal syndrome: An uncommon sequel to internal mammary-coronary artery bypass surgery. Thorac Cardiovasc Surg 1994;42:351-354.

69. Saydjari R, Upp JR, Wolma FJ: Coronary-subclavian steal syndrome following coronary artery bypass grafting. Cardiology 1991;78:53-57.

70. Thompson RW, Petrinec D: Surgical treatment of thoracic outlet compression syndromes: Diagnostic considerations and transaxillary first rib resection. Ann Vasc Surg 1997;11:315-323.

71. Juvonen T, Satta J, Laitala P, et al: Anomalies at the thoracic outlet are frequent in the general population. Am J Surg 1995;170:33-37.

72. Roos DB: Congenital anomalies associated with thoracic outlet syndrome: Anatomy, symptoms, diagnosis, and treatment. Am J Surg 1976;132:771-778.

73. Raskin NH, Howard MW, Ehrenfeld WK: Headache as the leading symptom of the thoracic outlet syndrome. Headache 1985;25:208-210.

74. Dieter RA Jr, O'Brien T, Dieter RA III: Thoracic outlet syndrome. In Chang JB, et al (eds): Textbook of Angiology. New York, Springer, 2000, p 635-643.

75. Bryan AJ, Hicks E, Lewis MH: Unilateral digital ischaemia secondary to embolisation from subclavian atheroma. Ann R Coll Surg Engl 1989;71:140-142.

41 Carotid and Cerebrovascular Interventions

Ivan P. Casserly

KEY POINTS

- Cerebrovascular intervention has largely evolved for the treatment of atherosclerotic disease. The potential for serious neurologic complications during such procedures places a premium on careful studies documenting the overall clinical efficacy of intervention compared with medical therapy.
- Carotid bifurcation disease and intracranial atherosclerosis account for 15% to 20% of all ischemic strokes and represent an important target for stroke prevention.
- Contemporary carotid bifurcation intervention involves the use of self-expanding stents with embolic protection systems, to reduce the risk of distal embolization. The technique has been proven equivalent to carotid endarterectomy in high-risk patients, and data from

- randomized controlled trials in low-risk populations are emerging.
- Proximal vertebral artery disease may account for up to 10% of posterior circulation ischemic events. Intervention at this site is straightforward and safe but has not been proven superior to medical therapy alone.
- Intracranial intervention, when practiced by skilled and experienced operators, is technically feasible and reasonably safe. Randomized studies documenting superiority over medical therapy are needed.
- Further refinements in technique, technology, and patient selection, together with dedicated randomized controlled trials, will allow cerebrovascular intervention to realize its true potential in stroke prevention.

Stroke is the leading cause of adult disability and the third leading cause of death in North America, Europe, South America, and Asia. The vast majority of strokes (80%-85%) are ischemic in etiology. In the United States, atherosclerotic disease affecting the extracranial and intracranial arterial circulation is believed to account for approximately 20% of all ischemic strokes[1] (Fig. 41-1) and therefore is an important target in the fight to prevent stroke. Cerebrovascular intervention has evolved largely for the treatment of atherosclerotic disease with the goal of stroke prevention. Based on dramatic technological advances and increased operator expertise, these procedures can now be performed with a high rate of technical success. However, because of the potential for serious neurologic complications from endovascular intervention in the cerebrovascular circulation, clear documentation of the safety of these procedures and their overall clinical efficacy is of paramount importance. These considerations have obviously raised the bar for cerebrovascular intervention compared with other peripheral vascular procedures.

In the field of cerebrovascular intervention, carotid bifurcation intervention is unique in that the natural history of carotid artery bifurcation disease has been well defined, and large randomized trials have documented the clinical effectiveness of surgical revascularization for this disease. There is already a large evidence base supporting carotid intervention in specific patient subgroups, and several randomized trials are ongoing in the remaining patient populations. With more than 140,000 carotid endarterectomy (CEA) procedures performed each year in the United States, and 280,000 worldwide, the potential impact of percutaneous revascularization has captured the interest of endovascular specialists who are keen to offer an alternative to surgery.

In contrast, endovascular intervention in the cerebrovascular circulation outside of the carotid bifurcation has been hampered by two important considerations: the natural history of noncarotid cerebrovascular disease is less well defined, and there is a notable absence of randomized data documenting the benefit of revascularization compared with

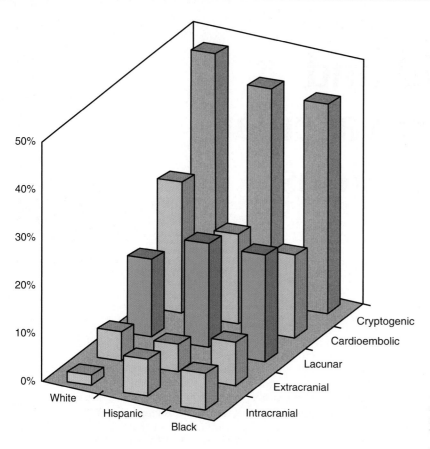

Figure 41-1. Proportion of ischemic stroke subtypes according to race in Northern Manhattan Study. (Redrawn from White H, Boden-Albala B, Wang C, et al: Ischemic stroke subtype incidence among whites, blacks, and Hispanics: The Northern Manhattan Study. Circulation 2005;111:1327-1331.)

Ischemic stroke subtype

medical therapy alone. Despite these obstacles, dramatic advances in the technical aspects of these interventions have been made, and there is an increased recognition of the need for well-designed clinical studies that address these deficiencies. What is often underappreciated is that non–carotid bifurcation cerebrovascular disease is responsible for at least the same number of ischemic strokes as carotid bifurcation disease and represents an equally important target for stroke prevention.

This chapter summarizes the current status of carotid bifurcation intervention and the most frequently performed non–carotid bifurcation cerebrovascular interventions, notably proximal vertebral artery and intracranial interventions.

CAROTID BIFURCATION INTERVENTION

Carotid Bifurcation Atherosclerosis and Stroke

The carotid bifurcation has a remarkable predilection for the development of atherosclerosis, which is typically located at the origin of the internal carotid artery (ICA) (Fig. 41-2). This plaque is similar to that found at other sites throughout the arterial system, in that it contains a dense cap of connective tissue with embedded smooth muscle cells and an underlying core of lipid and necrotic debris.[2] Histologic studies of plaque from the carotid bifurcation of symptomatic and asymptomatic individuals have revealed features associated with the development of symptoms that are similar to those associated with plaque vulnerability in the coronary circulation: reduced amounts of collagen, increased inflammation, thinning of the fibrous cap, and increased cholesterol in the necrotic core.[2,3] Based on current understanding, these processes result in plaque fissuring or rupture at the carotid bifurcation, causing either occlusive or nonocclusive thrombus formation. The dominant mechanism of stroke is believed be distal thromboembolism to the anterior cerebral circulation. However, a number of considerations, such as the size and composition of the embolus, the presence of contralateral disease, the anatomy of the circle of Willis, and the activity of fibrinolytic pathways, may attenuate or accentuate the clinical consequence of the pathologic event, such that a given event could result in a reversible neurologic deficit (i.e., transient ischemic attack [TIA]), an irreversible neurologic deficit (i.e., stroke), or no symptoms at all.

Natural History of Carotid Artery Bifurcation Disease

In clinical practice, two dominant factors are used to determine the risk of ischemic complications from a

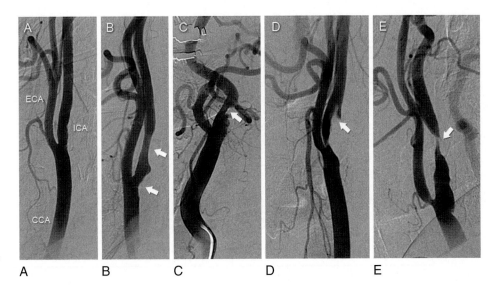

Figure 41-2. Angiographic images from the carotid bifurcation showing the spectrum of atherosclerotic disease at this site. **A,** Minimal disease at origin of internal carotid artery (ICA). **B,** Mild stenosis extending from distal common carotid artery (CCA) into proximal ICA. **C,** Moderate eccentric stenosis in proximal portion of ICA. **D,** Thrombotic lesion in proximal portion of ICA in patient with recent stroke. **E,** High-grade stenosis in proximal portion of ICA. Arrows indicate locations of plaque. Note that atherosclerotic plaque tends to accumulate in the posterior aspect of the ICA. ECA, external carotid artery.

carotid artery bifurcation lesion: the symptomatic status of the lesion and the severity of stenosis. Although most of these data are derived from the medical arm of the large randomized CEA trials performed between the late 1980s and early 2000s, these considerations continue to be used as the major criteria for choosing patients for endovascular procedures and enrollment in carotid endovascular trials.

Symptomatic carotid bifurcation lesions are associated with a high risk of recurrent ischemic stroke. Based on data from the NASCET (North American Symptomatic Carotid Endarterectomy Trial), the risk of any ipsilateral stroke at 2-year follow-up in medically treated patients with a symptomatic stenosis of 70% to 99% was 26%.[4] Among patients with a symptomatic stenosis of 50% to 69%, the 5-year risk of any ipsilateral stroke was 22.2%.[5] There is a close temporal relationship between these recurrent strokes and the index event, with a steep exponential decline in risk within the first months, followed by a more gradual decline and ultimate normalization of risk at 2 to 3 years (Fig. 41-3). By contrast, asymptomatic carotid bifurcation lesions are associated with a much lower risk of ischemic stroke. Over a 5-year period after the diagnosis of an asymptomatic carotid stenosis of greater than 60% by carotid ultrasound, the risk of any stroke among medically treated patients in the ACST (Asymptomatic Carotid Surgery Trial) was 11%.[6] Not surprisingly, the risk of stroke was constant over the duration of the study.

Among symptomatic patients, a close relationship between the severity of stenosis as assessed by careful angiographic methods and subsequent risk of ipsilateral stroke has been demonstrated.[7] The relationship is nonlinear, with a steep increase in risk associated with the tightest degree of stenosis (Fig. 41-4). However, for symptomatic patients with so-called near-occlusion of the ICA, defined as a stenosis causing sufficient obstruction to result in a decrease in ICA diameter beyond the lesion (Fig. 41-5), there are data to suggest that the risk of recurrent stroke is reduced compared with the risk in patients with severe stenosis without features of near-occlusion.[8] One potential explanation for this finding is the reduced likelihood of distal cerebral embolization caused by diminished flow velocities distal to the critical stenosis. Among asymptomatic patients, the association between stenosis severity and risk of subsequent stroke has been inconsistent.[6,9] This likely underscores the heterogenous nature of carotid plaque histology in asymptomatic patients, and it suggests that assessments of plaque vulnerability may be a more potent predictor of recurrent events than severity of stenosis in this patient group.

Recently, more sophisticated prediction models have been developed to predict the risk of stroke in patients with carotid disease, particularly for symptomatic patients.[10,11] In addition to stenosis severity, these models incorporate variables such as age, sex, nature of the presenting symptomatic event, time from index event, and plaque surface morphology to provide a more individualized estimate of risk.

Benefit of Carotid Revascularization

The benefit of carotid revascularization in patients with carotid artery disease has been documented in several randomized controlled trials (RCT) comparing medical therapy versus surgical revascularization (i.e., CEA). These data are extremely important in any discussion of endovascular therapy for carotid bifurcation disease, because they form the cornerstone justifying revascularization in certain subsets of patients with carotid artery disease.

In a pooled analysis of data from the three major RCTs in symptomatic patients,[12] CEA was associated with a significant reduction in the end point of stroke or operative death at 5-year follow-up in patients with a carotid stenosis of 50% or greater, as assessed by carotid angiography using the NASCET criteria (Fig. 41-6). This benefit was more pronounced in patients with 70% to 99% stenosis (absolute risk reduction [ARR]=15.3%; 95% confidence interval

50–69% Stenosis

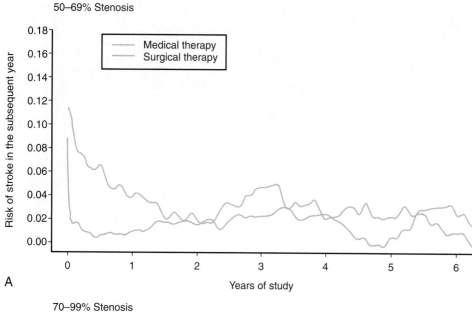

A

70–99% Stenosis

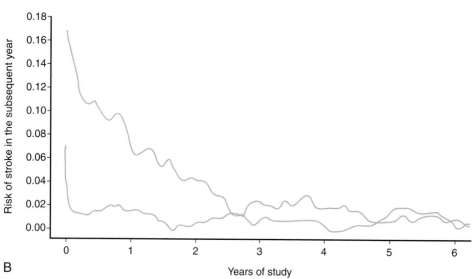

B

Figure 41-3. Change in risk of ipsilateral stroke over time in medically treated and surgically treated patients with symptomatic 50% to 69% stenosis (**A**) or 70% to 79% stenosis (**B**) in the NASCET trial. (Redrawn from Barnett HJ, Taylor DW, Eliasziw M, et al: Benefit of carotid endarterectomy in patients with symptomatic moderate or severe stenosis. North American Symptomatic Carotid Endarterectomy Trial Collaborators. N Engl J Med 1998;339: 1415-1425.)

[CI]: 9.8 to 20.7) compared with 50% to 69% stenosis (ARR=7.8%; 95% CI: 3.1 to 12.5). In addition, the crossover of the event-free curves occurs very early in the patient cohort with 70% to 99% stenosis (1-2 months) compared with 50% to 69% stenosis (1 year). The incidence of perioperative stroke and/or death in these studies was uniformly less than 6%, and the benefits derived from CEA are predicated on maintenance of similar procedural outcomes. No significant benefit was observed in patients with near-occlusion of the carotid artery (ARR=0.1%; 95% CI: 10.3 to 10.2), most likely related to the lower risk of recurrent stroke with medical therapy in this group. These studies were performed in the late 1980s and early to middle 1990s, and, as a result, the only stipulated medical therapy in the nonsurgical arm was aspirin. Contemporary medical therapy would likely attenuate the observed benefit associated with CEA. However, given the magnitude of the observed benefit associated with CEA in symptomatic patients, inves-

tigators have been reluctant to repeat randomized studies using contemporary medical therapy alone as a treatment arm.

Compared with medical therapy, CEA has also been demonstrated to significantly reduce the incidence of stroke or operative death at 5-year follow-up in asymptomatic patients with carotid stenosis of 60% or more as assessed by carotid ultrasound (11.8% vs. 6.4%; ARR=5.4%; 95% CI: 3 to 7.8).[6] It is important to emphasize that, in this asymptomatic population, the early hazard associated with revascularization persists up to 2 years from the time of CEA. If the life expectancy of a patient is less than 5 years, then significant benefit should not be anticipated. In addition, participation in these asymptomatic carotid trials required documentation of a perioperative stroke and death rate of less than 3% at the investigation site, and generalization of these findings is predicated on reproducing similar procedural outcomes.

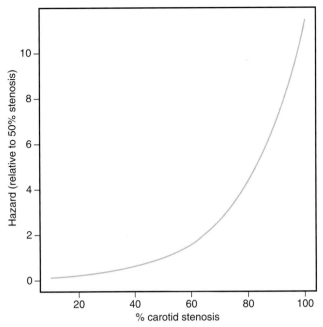

Figure 41-4. Hazard of ipsilateral ischemic stroke within 3 years after index transient ischemic attack or stroke as a function of percentage of carotid stenosis, as determined from biplane angiographic views. (Redrawn from Cuffe RL, Rothwell PM: Effect of nonoptimal imaging on the relationship between the measured degree of symptomatic carotid stenosis and risk of ischemic stroke. Stroke 2006;37:1785-1791.)

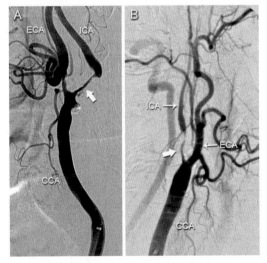

Figure 41-5. Angiographic appearance of "near-occlusion" of internal carotid artery. **A,** Reduction in diameter of internal carotid artery (ICA) compared with external carotid artery (ECA) reflects mild form of near-occlusion of ICA (arrow). **B,** Major collapse of ICA beyond critical stenosis (arrow) reflects severe form of near-occlusion of ICA and is often referred to as a "string sign".

Percutaneous Carotid Revascularization

Initial animal experimentation with percutaneous carotid revascularization began in the late 1970s, followed by the first clinical reports of carotid angioplasty in the early 1980s. The first rigorous clinical testing of percutaneous carotid revascularization began in the mid-1990s. Whereas the latter studies demonstrated the feasibility of the technique, two subsequent pivotal developments allowed percutaneous carotid revascularization to emerge as a viable alternative to CEA in the treatment of carotid disease: the ability to provide protection from distal embolization at the time of intervention using a variety of embolic protection devices, and the use of self-expanding stents. Carotid artery stenting (CAS) using self-expanding stents in combination with distal embolic protection represents the contemporary approach to carotid revascularization.[13]

Preprocedural Assessment

Before any CAS procedure, clinical assessment of the patient and anatomic assessment of the aortic arch and carotid/cerebral vasculature are essential. Advanced age (>80 years) has been associated with significantly worse outcomes with CAS and should be carefully considered in making decisions regarding the appropriateness of intervention.[14,15] Decreased cerebral reserve, manifested by the presence of dementia or cognitive impairment, or a history of prior strokes or lacunar infarcts increases the likelihood that distal embolization will be clinically manifested and is a relative contraindication for the procedure.[16]

Anatomic assessments can generally be made using noninvasive studies, notably computed tomographic angiography (CTA) and magnetic resonance angiography (MRA). CTA offers higher spatial resolution and superior visualization of the aortic arch compared with MRA, and it allows an assessment of the degree of calcification of the aortic arch and carotid bifurcation lesion that is not possible with MRA. The major advantage of MRA is the ability to use nonnephrotoxic contrast agents. Table 41-1 lists the anatomic features that should be reviewed when using these studies and highlights the importance of each. Overall, these anatomic features allow the operator to more accurately determine the procedural risk associated with the procedure and facilitate the planning of appropriate techniques for procedural success.

Baseline Angiography

Except in rare circumstances, CAS procedures are performed using femoral artery access. Although the extent of baseline angiography varies depending on the preprocedural noninvasive assessment, high-quality angiography of the carotid bifurcation, ipsilateral ICA, and intracranial anterior circulation is essential. I administer a heparin bolus of 25 units/kg before all diagnostic cerebrovascular procedures, in an effort to minimize the risk of thrombotic complications. A variety of catheter types are used to perform angiography, depending on the personal preference

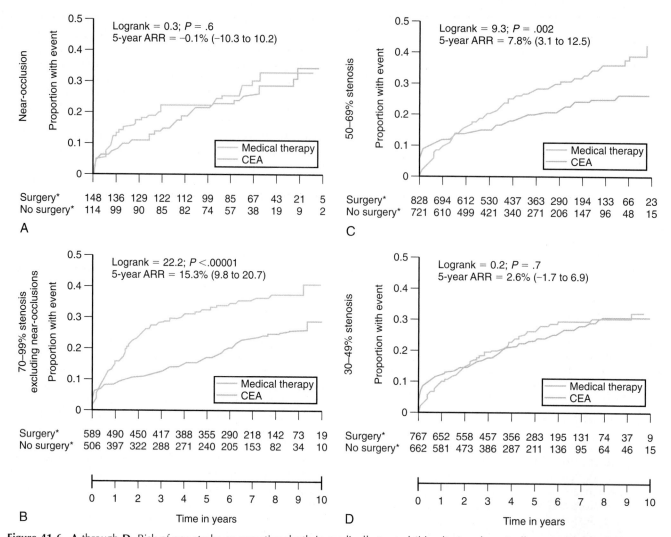

Figure 41-6. A through **D,** Risk of any stroke or operative death in medically treated (*blue line*) and surgically treated (*violet line*) symptomatic patients with varying degrees of carotid artery stenosis. CEA, carotid endarterectomy. (Redrawn from Rothwell PM, Eliasziw M, Gutnikov SA, et al: Analysis of pooled data from the randomised controlled trials of endarterectomy for symptomatic carotid stenosis. Lancet 2003;361:107-116.)

Table 41-1. Anatomic Assessments Recommended before Carotid Artery Stenting and Their Impact on Interventional Planning

Angiographic Assessment	Impact on Interventional Procedure
Arch Anatomy Type I, II, or III arch Anomalies of origin of great vessels Tortuosity of proximal portion of great vessels	Predict difficulty of percutaneous approach and influence strategy for delivery of guide or sheath to CCA
Lesion Characteristics Precise location of the lesion, with definition of the proximal and distal extent of lesion Lesion length Complex lesion ulceration Severity of stenosis Severity of lesion calcification Diameter of vessels proximal and distal to lesion	Influences planned location for stent placement and stent length Influences strategy for delivery of guide/sheath to distal CCA Influences choice of stent length Predicts difficulty of crossing lesion with filter device or wire Predicts need for predilation of lesion before filter delivery Predicts ability to achieve adequate stent expansion Influences choice of stent diameter
ICA Distal to Lesion Assess cervical portion of the ICA for presence of disease and tortuosity Diameter of cervical ICA	Influences the choice of landing zone for the filter or proximal occlusion EPD Increased tortuosity favors use of guide to provide support for delivery of filter Influences choice of diameter of filter-type or proximal occlusion EPD
ECA Patency of ECA	Influences strategy for delivery of guide/sheath to distal CCA

CCA, common carotid artery; ECA, external carotid artery; EPD, embolic protection device; ICA, internal carotid artery.

of the operator and the anatomy of the aortic arch and great vessels. For patients with uncomplicated anatomy (i.e., type I aortic arch, no tortuosity of great vessels), a Bernstein catheter functions well. For more complicated anatomies (i.e., type II or III arch, tortuosity of great vessels, bovine origin of left common carotid artery [CCA]), Vitek or Simmons catheters are generally required.

Interventional Technique

The technique for CAS placement follows a number of well-defined steps. All patients should receive aspirin and clopidogrel for at least 3 days before CAS placement. During the procedure, anticoagulation using unfractionated heparin to achieve an activated clotting time (ACT) of 275 to 300 seconds is standard.[17] For patients with a contraindication to heparin, a direct thrombin inhibitor such as bivalirudin is administered.[18] Currently, there are limited data documenting the safety of bivalirudin for *routine* use during CAS. Most operators perform the procedure without the administration of sedatives, which enhances the ability to screen for any neurologic change during the procedure.

Delivery of Sheath or Guide to Common Carotid Artery

In order to employ the range of contemporary equipment required for CAS, a 6-Fr sheath or 8-Fr guide must be delivered to the distal CCA. In patients with difficult aortic arch anatomy, bovine origin of the left CCA, occlusion of the external carotid artery (ECA), distal CCA lesions, or significant tortuosity of the great vessels, this can be one of the most technically challenging parts of the procedure. This portion of the procedure is "unprotected," in that there is no distal embolic protection device (EPD) and the safety of this step is therefore heavily operator dependent.

The standard procedure for delivery of a 6-Fr sheath in the CCA is as follows. A diagnostic catheter is used to engage the CCA of interest. A stiff angled Glidewire is advanced into the ECA, over which the diagnostic catheter is advanced. The Glidewire is exchanged for a superstiff Amplatz wire, followed by removal of the diagnostic catheter. Over this stiff

wire, the 6-Fr sheath and its dilator are delivered to the distal CCA, followed by removal of the dilator. This standard approach is sufficient for approximately 70% of cases, but a number of variations to the technique may be necessary, depending on the specific anatomic features of the individual patient. Much of the learning curve in CAS involves achieving experience with these variations and learning how to predict which variation is appropriate for an individual patient's anatomy. One of the pivotal dogmas in CAS is that guide wires and catheters should never be placed across the carotid lesion in order to deliver the sheath or guide to the CCA. It is preferable to refer the patient for CEA than to persist in risky attempts to deliver the guide or sheath.

Delivery of Embolic Protection Device

The use of EPDs is now considered the standard of care during CAS. Although there are no randomized trials comparing CAS with and without the use of EPDs, there are compelling data supporting this recommendation. Several studies demonstrate that distal embolization is a ubiquitous finding during CAS,[19,20] and observational series have reported significant decreases in periprocedural stroke and death rates with use of EPDs.[15,21]

Over the last decade, three different device systems that provide protection from distal embolization at the time of carotid intervention have been developed.[22,23] In clinical practice, the most popular and user-friendly of these systems is the filter-type EPD (Table 41-2; Fig. 41-7). This is largely based on the fact that these systems allow continued antegrade flow during carotid intervention, an important consideration for patients with compromised collateral flow to the ipsilateral carotid territory (e.g., patients with contralateral carotid artery disease or occlusion). Because most contemporary CAS registries and RCTs have used filter-type EPDs, they have the largest body of data to support their use in carotid intervention. Based on submission of these data to the U.S. Food and Drug Administration (FDA), five filter-type EPDs have been approved for use (Accunet, EmboShield, and Spider, Angioguard, and FilterWire), with several others awaiting approval.

Although there is some variation in the individual design of these devices, they typically contain a polyurethane membrane, with pores of fixed size ranging

Table 41-2. Filter-Type Embolic Protection Devices Used during Carotid Intervention

Filter	Manufacturer	Diameter (mm)	Pore size (μm)
Interceptor	Medtronic	4.5, 5.5, 6.5	100
Rubicon	Rubicon Medical Corporation	4, 5, 6	100
FilterWire EX FilterWire EZ	Boston Scientific	3.5-5.5	80
Angioguard XP Angioguard RX	Cordis	4, 5, 6, 7, 8	100
NeuroShield/EmboShield	Abbott Laboratories	3,4,5,6	140
Spider	ev3	3, 4, 5, 6, 7	50-200
Accunet OTW Accunet RX	Guidant Corporation	4.5, 5.5, 6.5, 7.5	120

OTW, over the wire; RX, monorail.

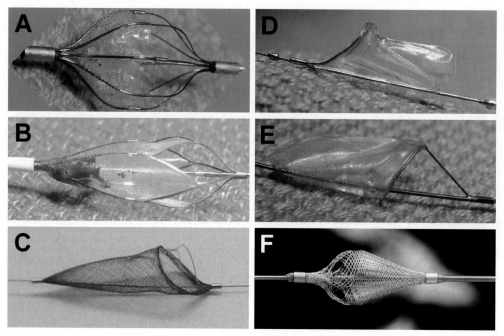

Figure 41-7. Examples of filter-type embolic protection devices used during carotid intervention. **A,** Angioguard XP (Cordis). **B,** Accunet (Guidant Corporation). **C,** Spider (ev3). **D,** FilterWire EX (Boston Scientific). **E,** FilterWire EZ (Boston Scientific). **F,** Interceptor (Medtronic). (From Casserly IP, Yadav JS: Carotid intervention. In Casserly IP, Sachar R, Yadav JS [eds]: Manual of Peripheral Vascular Intervention, 1st ed. Philadelphia, Lippincott Williams & Wilkins, 2005, pp 83-109.)

from 80 to 140 μm between devices, which is supported by a nitinol frame. The Spider and Interceptor EPDs are unique in that the filter pores are formed by a nitinol mesh. Each filter is designed such that it is integrated with a 0.014-inch guide wire and a 3- to 4-cm shapeable floppy tip. With the exception of the EmboShield and Spider devices, the filter is fixed to the wire.

The technique for delivery of the filter-type EPD varies according to the design of the system. In systems such as the Accunet, FilterWire EZ, and Angioguard, the filter is delivered in a collapsed form across the carotid lesion on the attached guide wire. With the EmboShield system, a unique 0.014-inch wire (BareWire) is used to cross the lesion first, and the filter is delivered in a collapsed form over this wire, then deployed over the distal portion of the wire. The Spider system allows the lesion to be crossed using any 0.014-inch wire, followed by a 2.9-Fr delivery catheter, which allows delivery of the Spider filter; the filter is integrated with a dedicated 0.014-inch wire that allows a small range of independent motion of the wire and filter. Predilatation of the carotid lesion before delivery of the filter-type EPD is required in fewer than 1% to 2% of cases. If required, a small-caliber coronary balloon (i.e., 2.0-mm diameter) that minimizes the risk of distal embolization should be used. Regardless of the filter-type EPD used, the filter should ideally be deployed in a straight and nondiseased portion of the cervical ICA, which is typically just proximal to the petrous portion of the vessel. The presence of tortuosity or disease in the cervical portion of the ICA may require an alternative placement, but there must be at least 3 to 4 cm of

distance between the proximal margin of the filter and the distal margin of the ICA lesion to allow subsequent delivery of interventional equipment.

The distal occlusion balloon EPD was the first type of EPD used during a carotid intervention (circa 1998). The only remaining example of this type of system is the Percusurge GuardWire device (Medtronic Vascular), which consists of a 0.014-inch angioplasty wire with a hollow nitinol hypotube and a distal compliant balloon that is inflated and deflated through the hypotube. The GuardWire is advanced across the carotid lesion with the balloon deflated. Complete interruption of antegrade flow is then achieved by inflating the balloon. After treatment of the carotid lesion, a monorail Export catheter is used to aspirate the column of blood proximal to the balloon, thus removing any debris that may have embolized from the treatment site. The balloon is then deflated and the GuardWire removed. There are no randomized comparisons of carotid intervention using distal occlusion versus filter-type EPDs. A retrospective comparison of outcomes from a large CAS registry showed no difference in in-hospital death or stroke between these systems (2.3% vs. 1.8%, respectively).[24]

The most recent group of EPDs developed for carotid intervention is the proximal occlusion devices, including the Parodi Anti-embolism System (ArteriA Medical Science) and the MO.MA system (Invatec). These systems attempt to protect the brain from distal embolization by generating retrograde flow in the ICA during the procedure, essentially generating an endovascular clamp.[25] Compliant balloons are inflated in the distal CCA and ECA, inter-

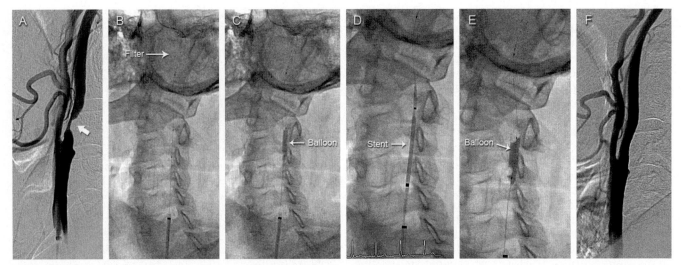

Figure 41-8. Angiographic images from carotid artery stent procedure. **A,** Baseline angiographic image showing severe internal carotid stenosis (*arrow*). **B,** Placement of filter-type embolic protection device (5.5-mm diameter Accunet filter, Guidant Corporation). **C,** Predilatation (4.0×20 mm Maverick balloon, Boston Scientific). **D,** Placement of 6- to 8-mm diameter, tapered, 30 mm long self-expanding nitinol stent (Acculink, Guidant Corporation). **E,** Postdilatation with 5.0×20 mm Aviator balloon (Cordis). **F,** Final angiographic appearance after removal of filter.

rupting antegrade carotid flow and allowing retrograde flow along the ICA from the circle of Willis. By connecting the lumen of the catheter whose tip is in the CCA and distal to the occlusive balloon to the femoral vein through a blood return system, a gradient for flow between the ICA and the femoral vein is generated, ensuring continued retrograde ICA flow. The success of such a system is predicated on adequate collateral circulation from the circle of Willis to ensure retrograde flow along the ICA. These systems appear particularly useful for cases in which tortuosity or disease distal to the carotid bifurcation lesion precludes the use of filter-type or distal balloon occlusion EPDs. Data with these systems are more limited, but the largest registry using a proximal balloon occlusion system (PRIAMUS, which enrolled 416 "real world" patients with carotid disease) reported a high rate of technical success (~99%) and acceptable clinical outcomes (4.5% incidence of in-hospital stroke, death, and myocardial infarction [MI]).[25a]

Angioplasty and Stenting

Predilatation. After placement of the EPD system, the lesion is usually predilated, to facilitate stent delivery (Fig. 41-8). Low-profile coronary balloons with diameters of 3.0 to 4.0 mm are typically used. Attempts to

deliver the stent without predilatation have been associated with a greater amount of athereombolism,[16] probably related to increased trauma to the lesion with forcible passage of the stent across a tight stenosis.

Stent Selection and Placement. As in other vascular territories, the ability to stent carotid lesions allowed operators to achieve a predictable angiographic result, to deal with procedural complications such as dissection and abrupt vessel closure, and to improve long-term patency by eliminating vessel recoil. Initial attempts at carotid stenting using relatively inflexible stainless steel balloon-expandable stents (e.g., Palmaz [Cordis]) were associated with acute technical success. However, their use was abandoned owing to the subsequent development of stent crushing, most likely related to compression of the superficially located carotid stent as a result of neck movements.[26] This led to the development and use of flexible self-expanding stents that could conform to the tortuous anatomy of the carotid bifurcation and vessel shape changes associated with neck movements (Table 41-3). The functional properties of these stents are defined by their metal composition and stent design.[27] Nitinol, a nickel-titanium alloy, is the most widely used material for carotid self-expanding stents;

Table 41-3. Self-Expanding Carotid Artery Stents

Stent	Manufacturer	Metal Composition	Design	Tapered Version Available
Carotid Wallstent	Boston Scientific	Cobalt chromium	Closed-cell	No
Exponent	Medtronic	Nitinol	Open-cell	No
NexStent	Endotex	Nitinol	Closed-cell	Yes
Precise	Cordis	Nitinol	Open-cell	No
Protégé	ev3	Nitinol	Open-cell	No
Acculink	Guidant	Nitinol	Open-cell	Yes
X-Act	Abbott Vascular	Nitinol	Closed-cell	Yes
Zilver	Cook	Nitinol	Open-cell	No

because of its large elastic range, it confers an ability to withstand significant elastic deformations. A variety of nitinol stents with either a closed- or an open-cell design are available. The closed-cell design offers superior scaffolding at a cost of reduced flexibility. A single cobalt-based alloy stent with a closed-cell design is currently available (e.g., Wallstent [Boston Scientific]). Both the metal composition and the design of this stent result in a more rigid stent with excellent scaffolding properties.

Carotid stents come in a variety of sizes that match the typical diameter of the ICA and CCA (5-10 mm), and they are usually 20 to 40 mm in length. The nominal diameter of the stent used should be 1 to 2 mm larger than the diameter of the largest treated vessel (usually the CCA). Stent lengths are chosen to provide complete lesion coverage. Initially, all carotid stents were cylindrical. However, tapered stents that conform to the size mismatch between the ICA and the CCA and facilitate treatment across the carotid bifurcation are now most commonly used. In most cases, tapered stents that are 6 to 8 mm or 7 to 9 mm in diameter and either 30 or 40 mm in length are used.

Usually, any of the available carotid stents will achieve similar technical success and clinical outcomes. In the remaining cases (~25%), assuming that all stents are available to the operator, the choice of stent should be individualized and is largely influenced by arterial anatomy and lesion morphology.[28] For example, stents with the greatest degree of flexibility (i.e., open-cell design nitinol stents with large open-cell areas and highly flexible interconnecting bridges, such as the Precise and Zilver stents) may be optimal for treating lesions in tortuous locations. Calcified lesions should be treated with stents that have a high radial force and a moderate outward expansive force, as provided by nitinol stents with a closed-cell design (e.g., Xact). And finally, lesions with the greatest risk for distal embolism should be treated with stents that provide greater vessel scaffolding, which are closed-cell nitinol or cobalt alloy stents (e.g., Wallstent, NexStent, X-Act).

Postdilatation. Postdilatation of the self-expanding stent is usually performed with the use of a 4.5- to 5.5-mm diameter, noncompliant balloon (e.g., Viatrec [Guidant Corporation], Aviator [Cordis], Sterling [Boston Scientific]). There is general agreement that postdilatation is associated with the greatest propensity for plaque embolization, and, as a result, experienced operators advocate a conservative approach to postdilatation balloon sizing. Residual stenosis of less than 20% is usually accepted.

After predilation, stent deployment, and postdilatation, contrast angiography is performed to assess the angiographic result and detect any potential complications. For filter-type EPDs, this practice allows the detection of "slow flow," which is an important finding that requires special management.[29] Slow flow is manifested by delayed antegrade flow in the ICA, and it may vary from complete cessation of antegrade flow to mild delay of ICA flow

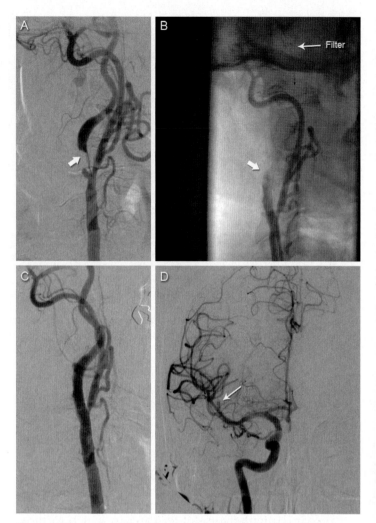

Figure 41-9. Angiographic appearance and complication of "slow flow" during carotid intervention. **A,** Baseline angiogram showing critical bulky stenosis at the origin of the right internal carotid artery (ICA) in a symptomatic patient. **B,** Angiographic appearance after post-stent dilatation showing cessation of flow in the ICA (*arrow*). Note complete filling of the external carotid artery. **C,** Angiographic appearance after aspiration of column of blood proximal to the filter and subsequent retrieval of the filter. **D,** Angiogram of middle cerebral artery after retrieval of the filter showing occlusion of a branch of middle cerebral artery (*arrow*).

compared with that in the ECA (Fig. 41-9). Most likely, this phenomenon is caused by excessive distal embolization of plaque elements that occlude the filter pores, compromising antegrade flow through the filter (Fig. 41-10). The phenomenon is frequent, occurring in 8% to 10% of cases,[29,30] and it is most commonly observed after postdilatation of the stent (~75% of cases) and stent deployment (~25% of cases). Predictors of this event include treatment of symptomatic lesions, increased patient age, and increased stent diameter.[29]

In patients with slow flow, the column of blood proximal to the filter has not been appropriately cleared by the filter EPD of debris that has embolized from the treatment site. In an effort to prevent distal embolization of this debris at the time of filter

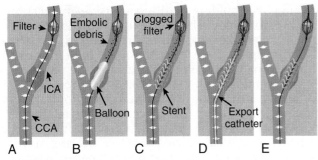

Figure 41-10. Schematic of proposed mechanism of slow flow and rationale for aspiration. **A,** Carotid bifurcation lesion with filter placed distally. **B** and **C,** Balloon angioplasty and stenting results in embolization of debris from the atherosclerotic plaque toward the filter, causing occlusion of filter pores and accumulation of debris in the column of blood proximal to the filter. **D** and **E,** Aspiration proximal to filter removes debris from the column of blood without affecting the debris causing occlusion of filter. (From Casserly IP, Abou-Chebl A, Fathi RB, et al: Slow-flow phenomenon during carotid artery intervention with embolic protection devices: Predictors and clinical outcome. J Am Coll Cardiol 2005;46:1466-1472.)

retrieval, it is recommended that 40 to 60 mL of blood be aspirated from the column of blood proximal to the filter, using an Export catheter, before retrieval of the filter EPD. If slow flow is observed after stent deployment, post-stent dilatation is discouraged because it will likely exacerbate the degree of embolization from the treatment site.

Removal of the Embolic Protection Device and Final Angiography

Removal of filter-type EPD devices is achieved by advancing a retrieval sheath over the interventional wire and collapsing the filter. The collapsed filter is then withdrawn carefully across the stent and removed. Most retrieval sheaths are available in a straight or angled shape to allow the retrieval sheath to advance past the stent. Rarely, the patient may have to turn his or her head, or external compression may have to applied to the carotid, to facilitate this maneuver.

Final angiography at the treatment site, the EPD landing zone, and the ipsilateral anterior cerebral circulation is performed to assess the procedural outcome and detect any procedural complication (e.g., distal embolization, spasm at filter site).

Postprocedural Care and Follow-up

At most centers, patients are admitted overnight to a step-down telemetry floor and typically discharged the following day. Neurologic and hemodynamic monitoring are the most important components of care. All patients should receive lifelong aspirin therapy unless contraindicated, and clopidogrel is recommended for a minimum of 4 weeks after the procedure. Patients are seen at 1 month and 12 months after the procedure for clinical assessment and carotid ultrasound to screen for in-stent stenosis.

Complications

Stroke

Stroke represents the dominant complication of CAS. The 30-day incidence of stroke after CAS in several studies of high-risk patients has been consistently reported to be in the range of 3.5% to 4.5%.[31-33] In this cohort, roughly 80% of strokes are ipsilateral to the treatment site, and, of these, 25% to 33% are major (persistence of neurologic deficit beyond 30 days or National Institutes of Health [NIH] Stroke Scale >3). The risk of stroke in low-risk patients is less certain, but data from the roll-in phase of the CREST trial (Carotid Revascularization Endarterectomy versus Stent Trial) reported an overall risk of stroke of 4% (30.7% of patients were symptomatic).[14] Although the time of occurrence is poorly documented in most studies, the majority of strokes occur at the time of the CAS procedure, based on my experience. This impression is corroborated by data from the CAVATAS trial (CArotid and Vertebral Artery Transluminal Angioplasty Study), in which 16 of the 22 ischemic strokes in the 30-day period after carotid intervention occurred within the first 24 hours of the procedure.[34] Beyond 30 days, the risk of ipsilateral stroke with CAS is extremely low. In the SAPPHIRE trial (Stenting and Angioplasty with Protection in Patients at High Risk for Endarterectomy), there were only two additional strokes (both minor) in the period between 30 days and 1 year after CAS among 167 patients,[33] emphasizing the long-term durability of the procedure.

The majority of procedure-related strokes (>80%) are ischemic in nature, with the dominant mechanism being distal embolization of plaque from manipulation of catheters and wires in the aortic arch and CCA and extrusion of plaque elements associated with angioplasty and stent placement at the treatment site. Hemorrhagic strokes accounted for 15% to 20% of all strokes in large high-risk stent registries.[31,32] The timing of these strokes is slightly later compared to ischemic strokes, and the dominant mechanism is probably cerebral hyperperfusion after CAS.

Neurologic deficits during the CAS procedure should be assumed to be ischemic in nature, and immediate cerebral angiography should be performed. A normal angiogram is associated with an excellent clinical outcome, and no further treatment should be instituted. In contrast, occlusion of a large artery (≥2-2.5 mm in diameter) is associated with poor neurologic outcome, and attempted recanalization using a combination of mechanical (i.e., angioplasty) and pharmacologic (i.e., thrombolytic, glycoprotein IIb/IIIa) therapies by suitably qualified interventionalists with experience in intracranial intervention is reasonable.[35] Even in qualified hands, the outcome of such rescue maneuvers is unpredictable, because conventional therapies have largely been designed to treat thrombus, and the occlusive emboli in the setting of CAS are composed of atheromatous debris.

Hemodynamic Depression

Baroreceptors located in the adventitia of the carotid sinus form part of the rapidly acting pressure-control mechanism of the body and are activated by increases in blood pressure. Signals from these receptors are transmitted through the glossopharyngeal nerve (cranial nerve IX) toward the vasomotor center in the medulla, which in turn activates the vagus nerve (cranial nerve X) and reticulospinal tract, resulting in peripheral vasodilatation, bradycardia, and decreased cardiac contractility (Fig. 41-11). Transient pressure from angioplasty and more prolonged pressure from self-expanding stents activate these baroreceptors and are responsible for the hypotension and bradycardia that is frequently associated with CAS. In general, these hemodynamic effects are seen immediately at the time of intervention, and in some patients they persist into the postprocedural period for 24 to 48 hours.[36-38] It is uncommon for significant effects to be seen beyond 48 to 72 hours, because the baroreceptors gradually adapt to the pressure from the self-expanding stent.

In a retrospective analysis of 500 consecutive CAS cases from a single center, the frequency of procedural hemodynamic depression, defined as a systolic blood pressure of less than 90 mm Hg or bradycardia of less than 60 beats/min, was 42%, with persistent hemodynamic depression after the procedure in 17% of cases.[36] Not surprisingly, the location of the lesion at the carotid bulb was a predictor of the event. Prior endarterectomy, which is associated with denervation of the carotid sinus, was associated with a reduced incidence of hemodynamic depression.

The management of hemodynamic depression is usually straightforward. Prophylactic measures include withholding antihypertensive medications on the morning of the procedure (provided that the baseline systolic blood pressure [SBP] is less than 160 mm Hg) and ensuring adequate hydration with intravenous fluids before and during the procedure. Some operators routinely administer atropine (0.25 to 0.5 mg intravenously) before the angioplasty and stenting portion of the procedure, whereas others restrict its use to patients that have critical aortic stenosis or critical coronary artery disease or who demonstrate an exaggerated hemodynamic response to angioplasty or stent deployment. In the presence of severe asymptomatic (i.e., SBP < 75 mm Hg) or any symptomatic hemodynamic depression, the use of intravenous pressors is indicated (e.g., Neo-Synephrine, dopamine, epinephrine). For less severe asymptomatic hemodynamic depression, oral pseudoephedrine (40-60 mg every 4-6 hours) may be used in an effort to avoid intravenous pressors.

For patients with persistent postprocedural hemodynamic depression, it is important to withhold routine antihypertensive medications and to carefully titrate these medications as the patient's blood pressure returns to baseline. Providing the patient with an automated blood pressure cuff and ensuring daily contact between the patient and the health care provider is advisable to optimize this management after hospital discharge.

Hyperperfusion Syndrome

Cerebral hyperperfusion syndrome is a rare but potentially life-threatening complication of carotid and vertebral revascularization procedures that provide improved flow to a chronically ischemic cerebral territory.[39] The syndrome is thought to be caused by significant increases in cerebral blood flow (>100%) after revascularization,[40] which, in combination with impaired cerebral autoregulation, results in transudation of fluid into the brain interstitium and cerebral edema (Fig. 41-12). Although hypertension is typically present in these patients, it is not a universal finding. Clinically, patients typically complain of a throbbing headache that is ipsilateral to the revascularization site, although the headache may be diffuse. Associated symptoms include nausea and vomiting, confusion, and visual disturbances. In the most severe cases, patients develop focal neurologic deficits and seizures. The feared complication of the hyperperfusion syndrome is intracerebral or subarachnoid hemorrhage, which is associated with a high mortality rate (40%-60%) and severe morbidity among survivors.

Several large retrospective case series have now reported the occurrence of cerebral hyperperfusion syndrome after CAS.[41,42] The incidence of the syndrome ranged from 1.1% to 5% in these series. There was some variation in the timing of the syndrome, but most cases manifested within 24 hours after the procedure, and cases occurring more than 2 to 4 days after the procedure were rare. Based on data from

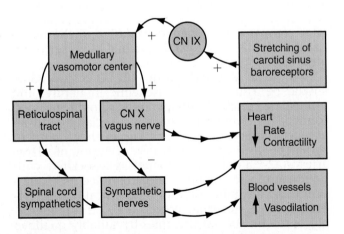

Figure 41-11. Diagrammatic representation of the effect of activation of mechanoreceptors in the carotid sinus during carotid intervention.

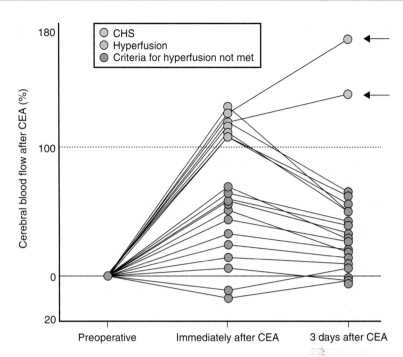

Figure 41-12. Graph showing increase in cerebral blood flow (CBF) after carotid endarterectomy. Increase in CBF>100% from baseline defines a patient group with cerebral hyperperfusion (*violet circles*). Within this group, two patients (*arrows*) developed clinical signs and symptoms consistent with cerebral hyperperfusion syndrome (CHS). (From van Mook WN, Rennenberg RJ, Schurink GW, et al: Cerebral hyperperfusion syndrome. Lancet Neurol 2005;4:877-888.)

carotid revascularization with CEA, an increased risk of the syndrome most likely persists for up to 28 days after CAS. Hemorrhagic complications of the syndrome after CAS appear to be high, with 25% to 60% of cases in the largest series being complicated by intraparenchymal or subarachnoid hemorrhage.[41,42] Because the absolute numbers of cases of hyperperfusion syndrome in these large series is small, multivariate analyses of predictors of the syndrome after CAS are problematic. Several risk factors have been reported in the CEA literature and probably also apply in patients undergoing CAS, including preexisting hypertension, postprocedural hypertension, contralateral carotid occlusion, critical ipsilateral carotid stenosis, and incomplete circle of Willis.[39]

The cornerstones of management of hyperperfusion syndrome are prompt diagnosis and emergent institution of therapy. The diagnosis is initially a clinical one, based on the patients' symptoms. Although confirmatory studies are helpful, the clinical diagnosis of hyperperfusion syndrome mandates immediate medical therapy. Because blood flow is pressure dependent in patients with cerebral hyperperfusion syndrome, the major focus of therapy is a reduction in systemic arterial pressure.[39] Several antihypertensive agents are associated with increased cerebral blood flow and are therefore contraindicated (e.g., glycerol trinitrate, nitroprusside, calcium channel antagonists, angiotensin-converting enzyme inhibitors). Recommended agents include β-blockers, labetalol (mixed α– and β–adrenergic antagonist), and clonidine (central α₂-adrenergic antagonist), which have favorable effects on cerebral blood flow and cerebral perfusion pressure in this clinical situation. Patients should be cared for in an intensive care setting that facilitates meticulous control of systemic arterial pressure. After institution of treatment, imaging studies (i.e., CT and MRI) are helpful to screen for hemorrhagic complications and assess for the presence of cerebral edema. In addition, transcranial Doppler documenting a significant increase in the ipsilateral middle cerebral artery (MCA) flow velocity (>150%-300%) is useful in confirming the diagnosis.

Adverse Cardiac Events

In earlier RCTs of CEA versus medical therapy, MI was not included in the outcomes analysis. However, the importance of MI as a component of the primary composite end point is underscored by the increased risk of death in patients who experience MI in the perioperative period after vascular surgery.[43,44] For this reason, the incidence of MI, as determined by preprocedural and postprocedural electrocardiograms and serial creatine kinase CK/CK-MB measurements, has been included in the end point of most high-risk CAS registries and trials. In this patient cohort, the 30-day incidence of MI is the range of 1% to 2.4%.[31-33,43,44] More than 80% of these are non–Q-wave in type. There appears to be significant and consistent reduction in MI with CAS versus CEA (2.4% vs. 6.1%; P=.04 in the SAPPHIRE trial[33]). The risk of MI in low-risk patients undergoing CAS is likely to be even lower, a contention that is supported by data from the CAVATAS trial, which reported no cases of MI in the endovascular arm.[34]

Restenosis

In-stent restenosis (ISR) is one of the most important late complications of CAS. Because of the sensitivity, safety, and accessibility of duplex ultrasound in screening for carotid ISR,[45] estimates of the frequency of ISR have largely been based on assessments using this imaging modality. With this method, the incidence of severe ISR (80% restenosis) is 3% to 4% at approximately 18 months of follow-up.[46,47] For less severe degrees of ISR, conventional ultrasound criteria for determining the degree of stenosis in non-stented carotid arteries may overestimate stenosis after CAS, because of alterations in the compliance of the stented artery.[48] In two large series, only 1 of 12 total patients with severe ISR (>80%) was symptomatic,[46,47] suggesting the low risk of clinical events associated with neointimal hyperplasia within the stent. A recent serial intravenous ultrasound (IVUS) study demonstrated that the immediate postprocedure minimum carotid stent area was negatively correlated with the percent restenotic area at follow-up.[49] Before that study, it was thought that such a relationship would not exist because of the large caliber of the carotid artery. This finding emphasizes the need to balance the short-term procedural risk of distal embolization and stroke from aggressive post-stent dilatation with the long-term risk of ISR.

Similar to the situation with restenosis after CEA, the clinical benefits of revascularization for ISR after CAS have not been demonstrated. Both of these pathologies appear to be associated with a relatively benign clinical outcome,[49] suggesting that a conservative approach is appropriate. Repeat revascularization is usually limited to patients with severe ISR and may be influenced by other considerations, such as the presence of contralateral disease or occlusion. A variety of interventional techniques have been reported for treating carotid ISR, including angioplasty, cutting balloon angioplasty, repeat stenting, and brachytherapy, with repeat recurrence rates of zero to 50%.[46,47,50,51]

Clinical Trial Data

Although the benefits of CEA over medical therapy have been clearly demonstrated in RCTs, these trials systematically excluded patients with certain baseline comorbidities or high-risk anatomic features (Table 41-4). Subsequent "real world" assessments of clinical outcomes with CEA suggested that the conclusions of these trials may not be broadly applicable in clinical practice. For example, Wennberg and colleagues analyzed outcomes in 113,000 Medicare patients undergoing CEA between 1992 and 1993 and reported mortality rates at least three times higher than those reported in RCTs.[52] A single-center CEA registry of more than 3000 patients demonstrated that the presence of comorbidities such as severe coronary artery disease, chronic obstructive pulmonary disease, and renal insufficiency were associated with an incidence of perioperative death, stroke, or MI of 7.4%, compared with 2.9% in a low-risk cohort of patients without these comorbidities.[53] Based on such data, initial attempts to demonstrate equipoise between contemporary percutaneous carotid revascularization and CEA focused on a "high-risk" patient cohort as the study population of inter-

Table 41-4. Criteria Used to Define "High-Risk" Populations in Carotid Artery Stent Studies

Clinical Criteria
Age >75-80 yr
Congestive heart failure (class III/IV)
Known severe left ventricular dysfunction, LVEF <30-35%
Planned CABG or heart valve surgery
Recent MI (>24 hr and <4-6 wk)
Unstable angina (CCS class III/IV)
Severe pulmonary disease*
Contralateral cranial nerve injury

Anatomic Criteria
Previous CEA with recurrent stenosis
Surgically inaccessible lesion
High cervical lesion (at or above C2)
Below the clavicle
Contralateral carotid occlusion
Radiation therapy to neck
Prior radical neck surgery
Severe tandem lesions
Spinal immobility of the neck

CABG, coronary artery bypass surgery; CCS, Canadian Cardiovascular Society; CEA, carotid endarterectomy; LVEF, left ventricular ejection fraction; MI, myocardial infarction.
*Defined as need for home oxygen, oxygen tension (pO_2) <60 mm Hg on room air, forced expiratory volume in 1 second (FEV_1) <30-50% of predicted.

est. Accepting that carotid revascularization has not been proven in RCTs to be more efficacious than medical therapy in this "high-risk" cohort, surgical CEA has been widely employed by vascular surgeons on the basis that a beneficial effect in this cohort could be extrapolated from trial data in "low-risk" patients.

Carotid Artery Stenting in High-Risk Patients

Among high-risk patients, outcomes of CAS using contemporary techniques have been reported in the form of case series, industry-sponsored registries, and a single RCT. In general, high-risk studies have grouped symptomatic and asymptomatic patients together, with the majority of patients being asymptomatic (~75%). The enrollment criteria used in these high-risk studies have relied heavily on data from prior RCTs in low-risk patients, with symptomatic patients who have greater than 50% carotid stenosis and asymptomatic with greater than 70% to 80% carotid stenosis being eligible for inclusion.

Case series were particularly helpful in the early stages of the development of CAS, but in general they suffer from a lack of stringent oversight. A large number of multicenter industry-sponsored registries with strict oversight have been performed (Table 41-5). Although the data have been presented at various national meetings and have formed the basis for submissions to U.S. and European regulatory bodies for device approval, only four studies have currently been published in peer-reviewed journals.[31,32,54,54a] The BEACH (Boston Scientific EPI: A Carotid Stenting Trial for High-Risk Surgical Patients), CREATE

Table 41-5. Registries of Carotid Artery Stenting with Embolic Protection in "High-Risk" Patients

Study	Sponsor	Sample Size	Stent	Embolic Protection Device	Status
SAPPHIRE (CAS registry)	Cordis	409	Precise	Angioguard	30-day and 1-yr outcomes presented
ARCHeR 2, 3	Guidant	ARCHeR 2: 278 ARCHeR 3: 145	Acculink (OTW & RX)	Accunet	1-yr outcomes published
SECuRITY	Abbott Vascular devices	320	MedNova Xact	MedNova NeuroShield/ EmboShield	1-yr outcomes presented
BEACH	Boston Scientific	480	Wallstent	FilterWire EX and EZ	30-day outcomes published
CABERNET	EndoTex	380	NexStent	FilterWire EX	1-yr outcomes presented
MAVErIC International	Medtronic	51	Exponent	Interceptor	1-yr outcomes published
MAVErIC II	Medtronic	Phase I: 99 Phase II: 399	Exponent	GuardWire	30-day outcomes presented
PASCAL	Medtronic	115	Exponent	Any CE Mark-approved device	30-day outcomes presented
CREATE	ev3	400	Protégé	Spider	30-day outcomes published
MO.MA*	Invatec	157	Any carotid stent	MO.MA	30-day outcomes presented

*75% of patients were "high-risk."
ARCHeR, Acculink for Revascularization of Carotids in High-Risk Patients; BEACH, Boston Scientific EPI: A Carotid Stenting Trial for High-Risk Surgical Patients; CABERNET, Carotid Artery Revascularization Using the Boston Scientific EPI FilteRwire EX/EZ and the EndoTex NexStent; CAS, carotid artery stenting; CREATE, Carotid Revascularization with ev3 Arterial Technology Evolution; MAVErIC, Evaluation of the Medtronic AVE Self-Expanding Carotid Stent System with Distal Protection in the Treatment of Carotid Stenosis; MO.MA, A Prospective Multicenter Clinical Registry for Carotid Stenting with a New Neuro-Protection Device based on Endovascular Clamping (MO.MA); OTW, over-the-wire; PASCAL, Performance And Safety of the Medtronic AVE Self Expandable Stent in Treatment of Carotid Artery Lesions; RX, monorail; SAPPHIRE, Stenting and Angioplasty with Protection in Patients at HIgh Risk for Endarterectomy; SECuRITY, Study to Evaluate the Neuroshield Bare Wire Cerebral Protection System and Xact Stent in Patients at High RIsk for Carotid EndarterecTomY.

(Carotid Revascularization with ev3 Arterial Technology Evolution), ARCHeR (Acculink for Resvascularization of Carotids in High-Risk Patients), and MAVErIC (Evaluation of the Medtronic AVE Self-Expanding Carotid Stent System with Distal Protection in the Treatment of Carotid Stenosis) trials reported 30-day outcomes using, respectively, the Boston Scientific Wallstent and FilterWire EZ/EX EPD, the ev3 Protégé stent and Spider embolic protection system, and the Exponent stent and Interceptor carotid filter system. Although the composite major adverse event end point and MI definition used in these four trials differed, the incidences of death and stroke were similar at approximately 1.8% and 4.5%, respectively, consistent with other unpublished registries (Fig. 41-13).

The SAPPHIRE trial is the sole randomized trial comparing CEA with CAS in high-risk patients.[33] Enrollment in this study differed from that of the multicenter industry-sponsored registries in one important respect: the carotid lesion had to be deemed amenable to revascularization by both surgical and percutaneous methods. As a result, the overall risk of the cohort in the randomized portion of this trial was probably somewhat less than in the registry-type studies. Given its randomized design, the SAPPHIRE trial provides the most robust data supporting the role of CAS with filter-type EPDs in high-risk patients. At 30-day and 1-year follow-up, there was a trend toward a reduction in the incidence of stroke or death and a significant reduction in the incidence of MI in the CAS arm (Table 41-6). Target lesion revascularization (0.7% vs. 4.6%; P=.04) and cranial nerve palsies (0% vs. 5.3%; P=.003) were also significantly reduced in the CAS arm. Overall, the data support the conclusion that CAS with embolic protection is at least equivalent to CEA in high-risk patients.

Based on the results of the BEACH, SAPPHIRE, CREATE, SECuRITY (A Registry Study to Evaluate the NeuroShield Bare Wire Cerebral Protection System

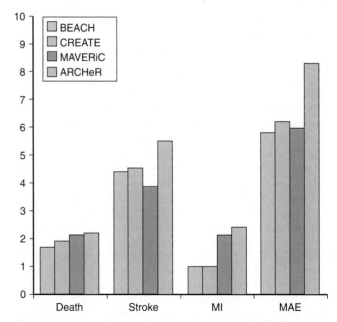

Figure 41-13. Incidence of death, stroke, myocardial infarction (MI), and all major adverse events (MAE) at 30 days in BEACH, CREATE, MAVErIC, and ARCHeR high-risk carotid artery stent registries. MAEs for the trials were defined differently: BEACH, non–Q-wave MI within 24 hours and 30-day incidence of death, stroke, or Q-wave MI; CREATE, procedure-related contralateral stroke and 30-day incidence of death, ipsilateral stroke, and MI; MAVErIC and ARCHeR, 30-day incidence of death, MI (Q-wave and non–Q-wave) or stroke.

Table 41-6. 30-Day and 1-Year Outcomes in the SAPPHIRE Trial (Based on Intention-to-Treat Analysis)

Outcome	CAS	CEA
30 Days		
Death	0.6	2.0
Stroke	3.1	3.3
MI	1.9	6.6
Death/Stroke/MI	4.4	9.9
1 Year		
Death	7.4	13.5
Stroke	6.2	7.9
MI	3.0	7.5
30-day Death/Stroke/MI + Death and ipsilateral stroke between 31 days and 1 yr	12.2	20.1

CAS, carotid artery stenting; CEA, carotid endarterectomy; MI, myocardial infarction; SAPPHIRE, Stenting and Angioplasty with Protection in Patients at HIgh Risk for Endarterectomy.

and Xact Stent in Patients at High RIsk for Carotid EndarterecTomY), and ARCHeR registries, the FDA Circulatory Systems Devices Panel voted for approval of CAS using the Wallstent, NexStent, Precise, Protégé, Xact, and Acculink stents in conjunction with the FilterWire, Angioguard, Spider, EmboShield, and Accunet EPD filter systems, respectively. These devices are currently available to qualified operators for clinical use. Several other carotid stent/EPD filter combinations will be seeking the same approval and are expected to become available in the next 1 to 2 years.

As part of the FDA approval process, rigorous post-marketing studies with each approved carotid stent/EPD filter system are being required to demonstrate the continued safety of the procedure in high-risk patients after the broad application of the technique with less experienced operators. The 30-day results have been reported from the CAPTURE (Carotid RX ACCULINK/RX ACCUNET Post-Approval Trial to Uncover Unanticipated or Rare Events) postapproval study, using the Acculink stent and the Accunet filter.[54b] At 30 days, the incidence of death and stroke was 5.7%, which compared favorably with 6.9% in the premarket pivotal registry. Also reassuring was the absence of any observed difference in the incidence of death and/or stroke in patients treated by physicians with differing predefined levels of experience. The EXACT (EmboShield and Xact Post Approval Carotid Stent Trial) postapproval study, using the Xact stent and EmboShield filter, is now completed, and several other postapproval studies are planned. These studies will add to the body of data supporting CAS in high-risk patients and hopefully will facilitate approval for reimbursement of the procedure in this entire patient cohort.

Carotid Artery Stenting in Low-Risk Patients

Carotid intervention remains investigational in low-risk patients. In contrast to high-risk CAS trials, studies in low-risk patients have usually studied symptomatic and asymptomatic patients in isolation, based on the clearly established difference in the natural history of patients based on symptomatic status. Additionally, all low-risk studies have had a randomized design and in general have compared CAS with CEA.

The CAVATAS trial was the first randomized trial in a low-risk, largely symptomatic, patient cohort with carotid disease.[55] However, because this study enrolled patients between 1992 and 1997, the endovascular arm largely employed a strategy of angioplasty alone, because EPDs were not yet available, and carotid stents became available only toward the end of the trial. Despite the lack of a contemporary technique, the 30-day incidence of death or disabling stroke was identical in each arm (6%). Not surprisingly, the low rate of stent usage was associated with a high rate of restenosis in the endovascular arm at 1 year (14% vs. 4%; $P<.001$). However, in long-term follow-up out to 3 years, the incidence of death or disabling stroke (including procedure-related events) was 14.3% in the endovascular arm and 14.2% in the CEA arm, indicating the absence of a significant clinical effect from this high rate of restenosis.

Several other RCTs in low-risk symptomatic patients using a more contemporary CAS technique have subsequently been performed or are in progress (Table 41-7). Two European trials were recently stopped prematurely, and the 30-day results were published.[56,57] The EVA-3S (Endarterectomy Versus Angioplasty in patients with Symptomatic Severe carotid Stenosis) trial reported a 30-day risk of stroke or death of 9.6% in the CAS arm versus 3.9% in the CEA arm (P=.01).[56] The SPACE (Stent-protected Percutaneous Angioplasty of the Carotid versus Endarterectomy) trial reported an incidence of ipsilateral stroke and death at 30 days in the CAS arm of 6.8%, compared with 6.3% in the CEA arm.[57] Based on predefined statistical rules to prove equivalency of CAS versus CEA, the SPACE investigators concluded that CAS failed to demonstrate equivalency; because enrollment would have had to be doubled to provide enough power to prove equivalence, they stopped further patient recruitment into the trial. Several issues relating to one or both of these studies have been raised, including study design (absence of a lead-in phase, inadequate credentialing of CAS operators, cessation of trial prior to completion of planned enrollment), the CAS technique employed (failure to mandate use of EPD, use of multiple stent and EPD systems, lack of balloon predilation), and periprocedural pharmacotherapy (failure to pre- and post-treat all patients with dual antiplatelet therapy, use of general anesthesia), that might explain the adverse outcomes in the CAS arms compared with the CEA arms of these trials. Despite these concerns, the results of SPACE and EVA-3S have heightened the importance of data from the ISIS (International Carotid Stenting Study) European trial[58] and the symptomatic arm of the North American CREST

Table 41-7. Carotid Artery Stent Trials in "Low-Risk" Patients

Trial	Planned Sample Size	Sites of Enrollment	Funding	Clinical Enrollment Criteria	Lesion Enrollment Criteria	Endovascular Strategy	Primary End Points	Status of Trial
ICSS (CAVATAS-2)	1500	Europe Australia Canada	Stroke Association, Sanofi Synthelabo, European Commission	TIA/stroke within 12 mo	>50% by NASCET method or equivalent noninvasive	CAS±EPD	30-Day death/stroke/MI 3 Yr death/disabling stroke	723 Patients enrolled by November 2005
EVA-3S	900	France	National Research Organization	TIA/stroke within 4 mo	>60% by NASCET or noninvasive equivalent	CAS+EPD	30-Day death/stroke 30-Day death/stroke+ipsilateral stroke at 2-4 yr	Enrollment stopped at 527 patients owing to safety concerns
SPACE	1900	Germany Austria Switzerland	Federal Ministry of Education and Research, German Research Foundation, industry funding	TIA/stroke within 6 mo	>50% by NASCET or 70% by Doppler	CAS±EPD	30-Day death/ipsilateral stroke	Enrollment halted at 1200
CREST	2500	No. America Europe	National Institute of Neurological Disorders and Stroke–NIH Guidant Corporation	Symptomatic Asymptomatic	>50% by NASCET >70% by ultrasound >60% by NASCET >70% by ultrasound	CAS+EPD	30-Day death/stroke/MI Ipsilateral stroke after 30 days	1250 Patients currently enrolled Completion anticipated in 2008
ACT 1	1540	No. America	Abbott Vascular	Asymptomatic	>70% by ultrasound	CAS+EPD	Stroke/death/MI within 30 days after procedure +ipsilateral stroke between 30 and 365 days after procedure	Enrollment began April 2005
TACIT	3700	No. America Europe	NIH, Pharma, device industry	Asymptomatic	>60% by ultrasound	CAS+EPD	Stroke/death at 3-5 yr follow-up	In planning stage

ACT I, Asymptomatic Carotid Stenosis, Stenting versus Endarterectomy Trial; CAS, carotid artery stenting; CREST, Carotid Revascularization Endarterectomy versus Stent Trial; EPD, embolic protection device; EVA-3S, Endarterectomy Versus Angioplasty in patients with Symptomatic Severe carotid Stenosis; ICSS, International Carotid Stenting Study; MI, myocardial infarction; NASCET, North American Symptomatic Carotid Endarterectomy Trial; NIH, National Institutes of Health; SPACE, Stent-Supported Percutaneous Angioplasty of the Carotid Artery versus Endarterectomy; TACIT, Transatlantic Asymptomatic Carotid Intervention Trial; TIA, transient ischemic attack.

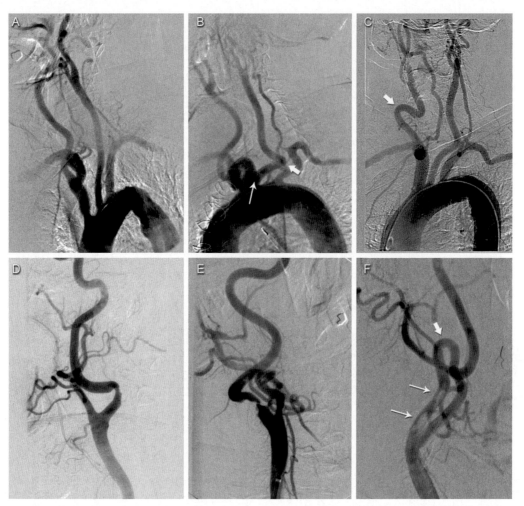

Figure 41-14. Examples of anatomic variations that increase procedural risk during carotid artery stenting. **A,** Type III aortic arch. **B,** Bovine origin of left common carotid artery (CCA) (*narrow arrow*) and severe tortuosity in left CCA (*thick arrow*). **C,** Severe tortuosity in right CCA (*arrow*). **D,** Marked angulation in internal carotid artery (ICA) at site of stenosis. **E,** Tandem areas of angulation distal to ICA stenosis. **F,** Dense circumferential calcification at lesion site (*narrow arrows*) and severe tortuosity distal to ICA stenosis (*thick arrow*).

trial[59] to help corroborate or refute the results of the EVA-3S and SPACE trials.

In low-risk patients with asymptomatic carotid artery disease, no trials of CAS versus CEA have been completed. Two trials are currently enrolling patients (the asymptomatic arm of CREST[59] and the ACT I.[60] A further RCT is in the planning stages (TACIT)[61] and, importantly, has incorporated medical therapy alone as one of the treatment arms.

Future Perspective

Realizing the potential of CAS will require further refinements in interventional tools and techniques. Perhaps more dramatic may be a re-evaluation of the current paradigm for choosing patients for carotid revascularization. We need to move beyond using symptomatic status and percent carotid stenosis as the sole determinants of the need for revascularization. Combining more sophisticated prediction models that incorporate multiple clinical variables

with advanced imaging studies of carotid plaque (e.g., tissue characterization with MRI or ultrasound) that allow a more accurate estimation of the individual's risk of recurrent neurologic events is necessary. Combining the latter with an estimate of the individual's procedural risk (for either CEA or CAS), based on clinical and anatomic assessments, will allow physicians make a more valid assessments of the risks and benefits for the individual patient (Fig. 41-14). Further, the current culture of viewing CAS and CEA as competitive strategies for carotid revascularization is counterproductive, and is reminiscent of the percutaneous coronary intervention versus coronary artery bypass surgery debate. Instead, these strategies should be viewed as complementary. The mode of revascularization that is most likely to achieve the safest procedural outcome for an individual patient should be chosen. Close examination of outcomes from trials of CAS versus CEA should help elucidate those variables that favor one mode of revascularization over the other.

PROXIMAL VERTEBRAL ARTERY INTERVENTION

Atherosclerotic disease of the vertebral artery (VA) is most commonly located at the origin and proximal V1 extracranial segment of the vessel. Typically, disease at this location represents extension of plaque from the subclavian artery into the proximal VA. In a large prospective registry of patients with symptomatic posterior circulation ischemia, proximal VA disease was deemed the primary mechanism of stroke in 9% of patients, underscoring the importance of atherosclerotic disease at this site.[62] The mechanism of stroke was attributed predominantly to either hemodynamic compromise or artery-to-artery embolism (i.e., VA to distal posterior circulation).

Contemporary surgical revascularization of proximal VA disease typically involves transposition of the VA to the ipsilateral CCA or ICA. Although some centers have reported excellent procedural and long-term results,[63] these surgical techniques have now been almost completely replaced by endovascular therapies. However, the lack of RCT data demonstrating a benefit of revascularization over medical therapy alone in patients with proximal VA disease makes clinical decision-making problematic. Moreover, there is almost a complete absence of data regarding the natural history of asymptomatic patients with proximal VA disease and a relative paucity of data regarding the natural history in symptomatic patients. Given these uncertainties, most operators restrict endovascular revascularization to symptomatic patients, especially those for whom medical therapy has failed. Intervention in asymptomatic patients should be strictly limited to patients who are deemed to be at high risk based on the appearance of the lesion, the presence of poor collateral flow from the carotid circulation, and the existence of contralateral VA disease.

Technique

Most proximal VA interventions are performed using femoral artery access,[64] but the ipsilateral brachial artery may also be used, particularly if the VA has a retroflexed origin off the subclavian artery (Fig. 41-15). A 6-Fr guide or 8-Fr sheath is delivered to the proximal subclavian artery, and the lesion is crossed using a soft-tipped 0.014-inch coronary wire. This wire is advanced to the distal V2 segment of the VA to provide support for device delivery. Predilatation with a coronary balloon is routinely performed to facilitate stent delivery. Stenting with a balloon-expandable stent is recommended to provide radial strength and reduce restenosis. For smaller-sized VAs (i.e., diameter <3.75 mm), I typically use a coronary stainless steel drug-eluting or bare metal stent. For larger sized VAs (>4 mm diameter), stainless steel or cobalt-chromium peripheral balloon-expandable stents may be used. There is a lack of consensus regarding the need for EPDs during proximal VA intervention. If the V2 segment of the vessel is sufficiently large to accommodate current-generation filter-type EPDs (i.e., ≥4 mm), and the ostial lesion has a high-risk appearance (e.g., ulceration), then the use of such devices is recommended.

Endovascular Outcomes

Data regarding the endovascular treatment of proximal VA disease is largely derived from a number of single-institution case series treating a symptomatic patient population.[64,65] Using contemporary stenting techniques, procedural success approaches 100%, and periprocedural neurologic complications are rare (Table 41-8). The high restenosis rates associated with angioplasty alone have been significantly improved with stenting, with most series reporting ISR in 3% to 10% of patients. Long-term follow-up shows a late stroke rate of less than 1%, reinforcing the overall safety of the procedure.

Coward and colleagues reported an analysis of a small subset of patients from the CAVATAS trial with proximal VA disease (mean stenosis, ~75%).[66] From a cohort of 16 patients, 8 received endovascular therapy (angioplasty in 6, stenting in 2), and 8 received medical therapy. There were two procedure-related

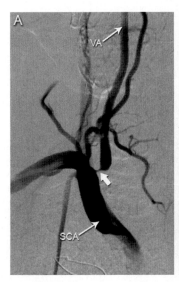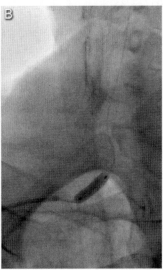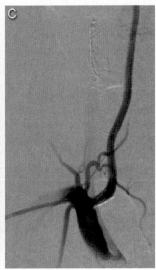

Figure 41-15. Vertebral artery intervention. **A,** Right subclavian artery (SCA) angiography showing severe stenosis at the origin of the right vertebral artery (VA). Because of the takeoff angle of the right VA, the decision was made to approach the lesion from the right brachial artery approach. **B,** Inflation of 5.0×12 mm Palmaz Blue (Cordis) balloon-expandable cobalt-chromium stent at ostium of right VA. **C,** Final angiographic appearance.

Table 41-8. Clinical Outcomes in Selected Series of Proximal Cerebral Artery Stenting

Author	N	Technical Success (%)	Procedural Complications	Improvement in Symptoms	Mean Follow-up (Mo)	Late Stroke	Restenosis
Mukherjee et al	12	100	None	12/12	6.4	0	1/12
Malek et al	13	100	1 TIA	11/13	20.7	0	N/A
Jenkins et al	32	100	1 TIA	31/32	10.6	0	1/32
Chastain et al	50	98	None	48/50	25	1	5/50
Qureshi et al	12	92*	None	N/R		1	0	N/R

*Technical success was defined as successful deployment of distal protection device and final residual stenosis of <30%.
N/A=not available; N/R, not reported; TIA, transient ischemic attack.
From Mukherjee D, Rosenfield K. Vertebral artery disease. In Casserly IP, Sachar R, Yadav JS: Manual of peripheral vascular intervention, 1st edition. Philadelphia: Lippincott Williams & Wilkins, 2005:110-119.

posterior circulation TIAs in the endovascular group and no neurologic events in the medically treated group. Although this trial involved a small number of patients and did not reflect contemporary endovascular techniques, it does reinforce the need for dedicated trials of endovascular revascularization versus medical therapy in patients with proximal VA disease to help define the benefit, if any, of endovascular revascularization in this patient cohort.

INTRACRANIAL INTERVENTION

Intracranial large vessel atherosclerosis is estimated to account for 5% to 10% of all ischemic strokes in the United States. In Asian, Hispanic, and Black populations, the incidence of intracranial atherosclerosis is significantly greater and accounts for a greater proportion of all ischemic strokes.[1,67] As in the extracranial circulation, atherosclerosis of the intracranial circulation has a predilection for specific anatomic sites. In the anterior cerebral circulation, these include the petrous, cavernous, and supraclinoid (Fig. 41-16) portions of the ICA and the main trunk of the MCA; in the posterior cerebral circulation, the distal VA (Fig. 41-17), the vertebrobasilar junction, and the midportion of the basilar artery are most commonly affected.

Intracranial atherosclerosis causes ischemic stroke by a variety of mechanisms, including hypoperfusion, thrombotic occlusion at the site of disease, distal embolization from the site of disease, and occlusion of small penetrating arteries due to plaque extension. Developing an understanding of the likely mechanism of stroke in each individual patient based on clinical evaluation, noninvasive imaging, and contrast angiography is important in identifying those patients most likely to benefit from revascularization therapy.

The natural history of asymptomatic intracranial atherosclerosis is largely unknown, but limited data

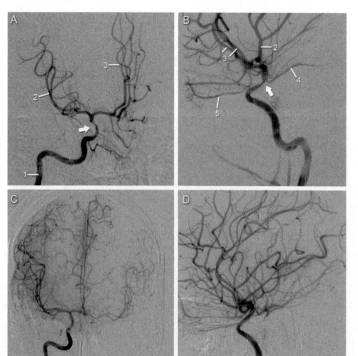

Figure 41-16. Intracranial intervention. Baseline cerebral angiography in posteroanterior cranial (**A**) and lateral (**B**) projections showing severe stenosis in supraclinoid portion of internal carotid artery (*arrows*). Cerebral angiography in posteroanterior cranial (**C**) and lateral (**D**) projections after placement of 3.0×8 mm balloon-expandable Multilink Vision stent (Guidant Corporation). 1, internal carotid artery; 2, middle cerebral artery; 3, anterior cerebral artery; 4, anterior choroidal branch; 5, ophthalmic branch.

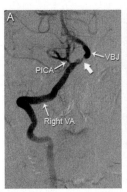
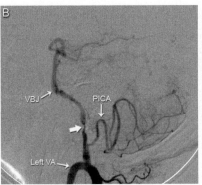
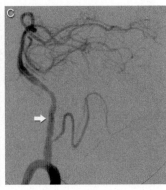

Figure 41-17. Intracranial intervention. **A** and **B,** Baseline right vertebral artery (VA) demonstrating severe stenosis in intracranial portion of vessel between origin of posterior inferior cerebellar artery (PICA) and vertebrobasilar junction (VBJ). **C,** VA angiography after placement of 3.0×12 mm Multilink stent (Guidant Corporation).

suggest a benign course.[68] By contrast, the WASID trial (Warfarin-Aspirin Symptomatic Intracranial Disease Trial) provides a reasonable estimate of the high risk of recurrent events in patients with a recent TIA or stroke caused by angiographically verified 50% to 99% stenoses of a major intracranial vessel.[69] In this cohort, the 1-year risk of an ischemic stroke in the distribution of the diseased intracranial artery in medically treated patients was approximately 12%. Additional retrospective studies have suggested a variety of clinical and angiographic variables to further risk-stratify patients with symptomatic intracranial atherosclerosis, including recurrent symptoms despite medical therapy,[70] lesion location (e.g., VA and ICA lesions proximal to major points of collateral supply have a lower risk than lesions involving the basilar artery or MCA), and severity of stenosis.[71]

Surgical revascularization of intracranial ICA and MCA disease was first performed in 1967 and subsequently tested in a large RCT of almost 1400 patients, which was reported in 1985.[72] Patients were randomized to surgical revascularization (by anastomosing branches of the ECA to the cortical branches of the MCA) versus medical therapy with aspirin (325 mg four times daily). Surgical therapy was associated with a 14% increase in the relative risk of nonfatal and fatal stroke and was subsequently abandoned as a therapy for the treatment of intracranial carotid disease. Despite this finding, initial attempts at percutaneous revascularization of intracranial disease were made in the 1980s. The initial experience was disappointing, with limited technical success and prohibitively high complication rates. However, by the mid-1990s, a variety of technological advances, borrowed from coronary intervention, and improved operator expertise resulted in a renewed enthusiasm for the technique. Technological advances included the availability of 0.014-inch wires that can negotiate the tortuous intracranial anatomy and low-profile flexible balloon dilation catheters. As in other vascular territories, stents were used to address some of the shortcomings associated with angioplasty of intracranial vessels (i.e., vessel recoil, abrupt vessel closure, and restenosis). However, the tortuosity of the intra-

cranial circulation presented a significantly greater challenge for stent delivery than that encountered in the coronary circulation, so it was not until the availability of third- and fourth-generation coronary stents with improved flexibility and lower crossing profiles that stenting of intracranial disease became more widespread. Today, a number of stents designed specifically for use in intracranial intervention, most notably the nitinol self-expanding WingSpan stent (Boston Scientific) and the stainless steel balloon-expandable Neurolink stent (Guidant Corporation), have been developed and tested in prospective studies.[72]

Although stenting offers an effective treatment for arterial dissection and vessel recoil and improves restenosis rates, the use of stents in intracranial vessels raises a number of unique concerns. Intracranial arteries are particularly fragile, owing to the sparse adventitia and elastic layers of the media, and hence are prone to perforation. Depending on the lesion location, such perforations result in either subarachnoid or intraparenchymal hemorrhage,[73] which is associated with high morbidity and mortality. Given this consideration, intracranial stents are generally undersized and inflated to lower pressures (4-8 atm). However, several studies of stenting in the coronary circulation have shown that the use of stents that are appropriately sized to the reference vessel diameter and inflated to high pressures (14-16 atm) is required for optimal stent deployment and apposition of stent struts to the vessel wall. The latter considerations are believed to minimize the risk of stent thrombosis and reduce the rate of restenosis. Hence, there are potentially serious consequences associated with the current practice of intracranial stenting. Moreover, stenting is associated with significantly more plaque shifting than angioplasty alone. Although the occlusion of small side-branches in the coronary circulation is generally a benign event, compromise of critical side branches from intracranial vessels (e.g., lenticulostriate branches of MCA, perforating branches of basilar artery) can have severe neurologic consequences.[74] Finally, significant complications may occur with attempts to deliver stents through the technically challenging vascular terrain

Table 41-9. Contemporary Clinical Series of Intracranial Angioplasty for Treatment of Atherosclerotic Disease

Study	Year	N	Lesions	Lesion Location		Mean Follow-up (mo)	Technical Success (%)	In-hospital Adverse Outcome (%)		
				Anterior	Posterior			Stroke	Hemorrhage	Death
Marks	2005	36	37	16	21	52.9	91	3	0	6
Connors	1999	50*	N/R	32	18	12	98	0	4	2
Clarke	1995	17	22	6	16	22	82	12	0	0
Mori	1998	42	42	29	13	‡	†	†	†	†
Alazzaz	2000	16	17	8	9	24	94	13	0	0

*Based on data from interventions performed since 1994.
†Outcome dependent on lesion type: type A lesions (concentric stenoses <5 mm in length, $n=12$)—procedural success 92%, complications 8%, restenosis 0%; type B lesions (stenoses 5-10 mm in length, occlusions <3 mo old, $n=21$)—procedural success 86%, complications 26%, restenosis 33%; type C lesions (lesion length >10 mm, occlusions >3 mo old, $n=9$)—procedural success 33%, complications 87%, restenosis 100%.
‡Mean follow-up not reported. Range of follow-up was 1 month to 6 years.
N/R, not reported.
From Casserly IP, Yadav JS. The approach to intracranial carotid artery intervention. In Saw J, Exaire JE, Lee DS et al (eds): Contemporary Cardiology: Handbook of Complex Percutaneous Carotid Intervention, 1st edition. Totowa, NJ: Humana Press Inc, 2006:189-209.

of the intracranial circulation (e.g., stent dislodgement, vessel dissection, and distal embolization of plaque).

Technique

Intracranial intervention is almost universally performed using femoral arterial access.[75] In contrast to other cerebrovascular interventions, most operators use general anesthesia, but the use of conscious sedation has been shown to be a viable alternative.[76] Preprocedural antiplatelet and procedural anticoagulation regimens mirror those practiced during carotid bifurcation intervention.

The first task during anterior or posterior circulation intracranial intervention is the delivery of a guide or sheath to the distal CCA or proximal subclavian artery, respectively. Sheaths are most commonly used (e.g., Shuttle sheath [Cook]), and the inner luminal diameter of a 6-Fr sheath is adequate for delivery of standard interventional equipment. For normal-sized individuals, a 70 cm length sheath is optimal, because longer sheath lengths may restrict the ability to treat distal intracranial lesions owing to limitations in the length of current balloon and stent delivery systems. Through this sheath, a 6-Fr Envoy guide is advanced over a 0.035-inch wire to the level of the distal cervical ICA for anterior circulation intracranial intervention, or to the distal V2 segment of the VA for posterior circulation intracranial intervention. Having achieved this platform, a variety of 0.010- to 0.014-inch wires (e.g., Synchro [Precision Therapeutics]) may be used to cross the intracranial lesion. To provide sufficient support for device delivery, the wire is usually advanced to the second- or third-order branches of the middle and posterior cerebral arteries, for anterior and posterior circulation interventions, respectively.

Angioplasty is performed using coronary balloons (e.g., Maverick [Boston Scientific]), and the angioplasty technique is modified to minimize the risk of vessel perforation. These modifications include using balloon diameters that are 70% to 80% of the vessel diameter and performing slow, prolonged inflation

of the balloon to less than nominal pressures (4-8 atm), followed by slow deflation. In addition, the minimal balloon length required to treat the lesion is chosen to minimize the risk of compromising flow in side or perforating branches. Whereas some operators adopt a practice of "provisional" stenting (i.e., stent only if the angioplasty result is suboptimal), an increasing number practice a strategy of primary stenting (stent placement regardless of the initial angioplasty result). Currently, the most popular stents being used for intracranial intervention include the recent generation of cobalt-chromium balloon-expandable coronary stents (e.g., Multilink Vision [Guidant], Driver [Medtronic]), which have superior deliverability compared with stainless steel coronary stents. Balloon-expandable stents are sized 0.5 mm smaller than the estimated vessel diameter and are inflated to moderate pressures (6-8 atm). The minimum stent length is used, to attenuate the risk of plaque shift into critical side or perforating branches. Final angiography of the lesion site and distal cerebral circulation is performed, and patients are sent for recovery in a neurointensive care setting.

Clinical Outcomes

The majority of data regarding intracranial intervention are derived from retrospective observational case series at a small number of institutions with highly experienced operators; as such, they have significant limitations. Case series from the late 1990s and early 2000s reported the experience with intracranial angioplasty. Rates of technical success varied from 80% to 95%, in-hospital death from 0% to 6%, and periprocedural stroke or intracranial hemorrhage from 3% to 13% (Table 41-9). The availability of balloon-expandable coronary stents appears to have improved the technical success rate to greater than 90%, without a significant increase in periprocedural complications (Table 41-10).[77,78] One small series (8 patients) using drug-eluting stents for the treatment of intracranial atherosclerosis has been published and reported acceptable medium-term outcomes.[79] It

Table 41-10. Contemporary Clinical Series of Intracranial Stenting for Treatment of Atherosclerotic Disease

| Study | Year | N | Lesions | Lesion Location | | Mean Follow-up (mo) | Technical Success (%) | In-hospital Adverse Outcome (%) | | | Restenosis (%) | Follow-up Stroke Rate (%) |
				Anterior	Posterior			Stroke	Hemorrhage	Death		
Mori	2000	10	12	4	8	12	80	0	0	0	0*	0
Levy	2001	11	11	—	11	4	63	1	0	36	14	0
Lylyk	2002	34	34	18	16	5	88	0	1	6	0[†]	0
De Rochemont	2004	18	20	9	11	6	90	0	6	0	—	0
Jiang	2004	40	42	42[‡]	—	10	98	0	7.5	2.5	12.5[§]	0
Straube	2005	12	12	6	6	N/R	92	0	0	3	0[¶]	0

*Based on angiography performed at mean of 4 months' follow-up.
[†]Based on a subset of seven patients who had clinical and angiographic follow-up.
[‡]All in MCA MI segment.
[§]Based on angiographic follow-up in eight patients with eight stented vessels.
[¶]Based on two patients with angiographic follow-up.
N/R, not reported.
From Casserly IP, Yadav JS. The approach to intracranial carotid artery intervention. In Saw J, Exaire JE, Lee DS et al (eds): Contemporary Cardiology: Handbook of Complex Percutaneous Carotid Intervention, 1st edition. Totowa, NJ: Humana Press Inc, 2006:189-209.

is unclear whether these stents are associated with a significant reduction in restenosis, and it remains to be seen whether the potential issues of vessel toxicity and delayed endothelialization will manifest clinically.

There have been two prospective studies of intracranial stenting with stringent neurologic assessment and angiographic follow-up.[80,81] In the SSYLVIA (Stenting of SYmptomatic Atherosclerotic Lesions in the Vertebral of Intracranial Arteries) trial, symptomatic patients with a greater than 50% culprit stenosis of an intracranial artery (n=43) or extracranial VA (n=18) underwent stenting of the culprit vessel, using the Neurolink balloon-expandable stent.[80] The stent was successfully deployed in 95% of all cases. In the outcome data reported for the whole group, the rates of stroke and death at 30 days were 6.6% and 0%, respectively. However, it would appear that all of the strokes (n=4) occurred in the intracranial intervention group, giving a 30-day incidence of stroke in the intracranial cohort of 9.3% (2.3% hemorrhagic, 7% ischemic). At 1 year, there were two additional strokes in the intracranial stent group (1-year incidence, 14%). Repeat angiography at 6 months documented a restenosis rate of 32% in the intracranial cohort. In the overall group, 39% of patients with restenosis were symptomatic (i.e., TIA or stroke).

More recently, the prospective multicenter Wing-Span study enrolled medically refractory patients with recurrent stroke due to a >50% intracranial stenosis (n=45).[81] Patients were stented using the self-expanding nitinol WingSpan stent (Smart Therapeutics/Boston Scientific). Procedural success was achieved in 97.7% of cases, with a 30-day incidence of ipsilateral stroke or death of 4.4%. At 6 months, the incidence of ipsilateral stroke or death was 7.0%. The restenosis rate (>50% by angiography) at 6 months was 7.5%. In contrast to the SSYLVIA study, all patients with restenosis were asymptomatic.

These prospective studies underscore the technical success of intracranial procedures that mirror the rates reported in observational series. However, the 6-month and 1-year rates of death and stroke in prospective series appear to be greater than in observational series, highlighting the potential bias in reporting in the latter studies. Indeed the 14% rate of stroke at 1 year in the SSYLVIA study is remarkably similar to the 1-year risk of stroke reported in the WASID trial in medically treated patients. Therefore, these prospective studies reinforce the urgent need for randomized studies of contemporary endovascular therapies versus optimal medical management for patients with stroke or TIA due to intracranial disease.

CONCLUSIONS

Cerebrovascular intervention has evolved dramatically over the last decade. It is clear that these procedures are feasible and are safe when performed by experienced endovascular specialists using contemporary interventional equipment and techniques. The challenge for the future is to advance understanding of the natural history of cerebrovascular atherosclerosis, and more accurately, to predict those patients who will develop recurrent events and refine the patient populations in whom endovascular revascularization provides meaningful clinical benefit.

REFERENCES

1. White H, Boden-Albala B, Wang C, et al: Ischemic stroke subtype incidence among whites, blacks, and Hispanics: The Northern Manhattan Study. Circulation 2005;111: 1327-1331.
2. Golledge J, Greenhalgh RM, Davies AH: The symptomatic carotid plaque. Stroke 2000;31:774-781.
3. Redgrave JN, Lovett JK, Gallagher PJ, Rothwell PM: Histological assessment of 526 symptomatic carotid plaques in relation to the nature and timing of ischemic symptoms: The Oxford Plaque Study. Circulation 2006;113:2320-2328.
4. Beneficial effect of carotid endarterectomy in symptomatic patients with high-grade carotid stenosis. North American Symptomatic Carotid Endarterectomy Trial Collaborators. N Engl J Med 1991;325:445-453.
5. Barnett HJ, Taylor DW, Eliasziw M, et al: Benefit of carotid endarterectomy in patients with symptomatic moderate or severe stenosis. North American Symptomatic Carotid Endarterectomy Trial Collaborators. N Engl J Med 1998;339: 1415-1425.
6. Halliday A, Mansfield A, Marro J, et al: Prevention of disabling and fatal strokes by successful carotid endarterectomy in patients without recent neurological symptoms: Randomised controlled trial. Lancet 2004;363:1491-1502.
7. Cuffe RL, Rothwell PM: Effect of nonoptimal imaging on the relationship between the measured degree of symptomatic carotid stenosis and risk of ischemic stroke. Stroke 2006;37: 1785-1791.
8. Fox AJ, Eliasziw M, Rothwell PM, et al: Identification, prognosis, and management of patients with carotid artery near occlusion. AJNR Am J Neuroradiol 2005;26:2086-2094.
9. Inzitari D, Eliasziw M, Gates P, et al: The causes and risk of stroke in patients with asymptomatic internal-carotid-artery stenosis. North American Symptomatic Carotid Endarterectomy Trial Collaborators. N Engl J Med 2000;342:1693-1700.
10. Rothwell PM: Risk modeling to identify patients with symptomatic carotid stenosis most at risk of stroke. Neurol Res 2005;27(Suppl 1):S18-S28.
11. Rothwell PM, Mehta Z, Howard SC, et al: Treating individuals 3: From subgroups to individuals. General principles and the example of carotid endarterectomy. Lancet 2005;365: 256-265.
12. Rothwell PM, Eliasziw M, Gutnikov SA, et al: Analysis of pooled data from the randomised controlled trials of endarterectomy for symptomatic carotid stenosis. Lancet 2003;361: 107-116.
13. Casserly IP, Yadav JS: Carotid intervention. In Casserly IP, Sachar R, Yadav JS (eds): Manual of Peripheral Vascular Intervention, 1st ed. Philadelphia, Lippincott Williams & Wilkins, 2005, pp 83-109.
14. Hobson RW 2nd, Howard VJ, Roubin GS, et al: Carotid artery stenting is associated with increased complications in octogenarians: 30-Day stroke and death rates in the CREST lead-in phase. J Vasc Surg 2004;40:1106-1111.
15. Roubin GS, New G, Iyer SS, et al: Immediate and late clinical outcomes of carotid artery stenting in patients with symptomatic and asymptomatic carotid artery stenosis: A 5-year prospective analysis. Circulation 2001;103:532-537.
16. Roubin GS, Iyer S, Halkin A, et al: Realizing the potential of carotid artery stenting: Proposed paradigms for patient selection and procedural technique. Circulation 2006;113: 2021-2030.

17. Saw J, Bajzer C, Casserly IP, et al: Evaluating the optimal activated clotting time during carotid artery stenting. Am J Cardiol 2006;97:1657-1660.

18. Katzen BT, Ardid MI, MacLean AA, et al: Bivalirudin as an anticoagulation agent: Safety and efficacy in peripheral interventions. J Vasc Interv Radiol 2005;16:1183-1187; quiz 1187.

19. Al-Mubarak N, Roubin GS, Vitek JJ, Iyer SS: Microembolization during carotid stenting with the distal-balloon antiemboli system. Int Angiol 2002;21:344-348.

20. Angelini A, Reimers B, Della Barbera M, et al: Cerebral protection during carotid artery stenting: Collection and histopathologic analysis of embolized debris. Stroke 2002;33:456-461.

21. Zahn R, Mark B, Niedermaier N, et al: Embolic protection devices for carotid artery stenting: Better results than stenting without protection? Eur Heart J 2004;25:1550-1558.

22. Gruberg L, Beyar R: Cerebral embolic protection devices and percutaneous carotid artery stenting. Int J Cardiovasc Intervent 2005;7:117-121.

23. Kasirajan K, Schneider PA, Kent KC: Filter devices for cerebral protection during carotid angioplasty and stenting. J Endovasc Ther 2003;10:1039-1045.

24. Zahn R, Ischinger T, Mark B, et al: Embolic protection devices for carotid artery stenting: Is there a difference between filter and distal occlusive devices? J Am Coll Cardiol 2005;45:1769-1774.

25. Bates MC, Dorros G, Parodi J, Ohki T: Reversal of the direction of internal carotid artery blood flow by occlusion of the common and external carotid arteries in a swine model. Catheter Cardiovasc Interv 2003;60:270-275.

25a. Coppi G, Moratou R, Silingardi R, et al: PRIAMUS—proximal flow blockage cerebral protection during carotid stenting. J Cardiovasc Surg 2005;46:219-227.

26. Mathur A, Dorros G, Iyer SS, et al: Palmaz stent compression in patients following carotid artery stenting. Cathet Cardiovasc Diagn 1997;41:137-140.

27. Stoeckel D, Bonsignore C, Duda S: A survey of stent designs. Min Invas Ther Allied Technol 2002;11:137-147.

28. Bosiers M, Deloose K, Verbist J, Peeters P: Carotid artery stenting: Which stent for which lesion? Vascular 2005;13:205-210.

29. Casserly IP, Abou-Chebl A, Fathi RB, et al: Slow-flow phenomenon during carotid artery intervention with embolic protection devices: Predictors and clinical outcome. J Am Coll Cardiol 2005;46:1466-1472.

30. Reimers B, Schluter M, Castriota F, et al: Routine use of cerebral protection during carotid artery stenting: Results of a multicenter registry of 753 patients. Am J Med 2004;116:217-222.

31. Safian RD, Bresnahan JF, Jaff MR, et al: Protected carotid stenting in high-risk patients with severe carotid artery stenosis. J Am Coll Cardiol 2006;47:2384-2389.

32. White CJ, Iyer SS, Hopkins LN, et al: Carotid stenting with distal protection in high surgical risk patients: The BEACH trial 30 day results. Catheter Cardiovasc Interv 2006;67:503-512.

33. Yadav JS, Wholey MH, Kuntz RE, et al: Protected carotid-artery stenting versus endarterectomy in high-risk patients. N Engl J Med 2004;351:1493-1501.

34. Endovascular versus surgical treatment in patients with carotid stenosis in the Carotid and Vertebral Artery Transluminal Angioplasty Study (CAVATAS): A randomised trial. Lancet 2001;357:1729-1737.

35. Wholey MH, Tan WA, Toursarkissian B, et al: Management of neurological complications of carotid artery stenting. J Endovasc Ther 2001;8:341-353.

36. Gupta R, Abou-Chebl A, Bajzer CT, et al: Rate, predictors, and consequences of hemodynamic depression after carotid artery stenting. J Am Coll Cardiol 2006;47:1538-1543.

37. Qureshi AI, Luft AR, Sharma M, et al: Frequency and determinants of postprocedural hemodynamic instability after carotid angioplasty and stenting. Stroke 1999;30:2086-2093.

38. Trocciola SM, Chaer RA, Lin SC, et al: Analysis of parameters associated with hypotension requiring vasopressor support after carotid angioplasty and stenting. J Vasc Surg 2006;43:714-720.

39. van Mook WN, Rennenberg RJ, Schurink GW, et al: Cerebral hyperperfusion syndrome. Lancet Neurol 2005;4:877-888.

40. Ogasawara K, Yukawa H, Kobayashi M, et al: Prediction and monitoring of cerebral hyperperfusion after carotid endarterectomy by using single-photon emission computerized tomography scanning. J Neurosurg 2003;99:504-510.

41. Abou-Chebl A, Yadav JS, Reginelli JP, et al: Intracranial hemorrhage and hyperperfusion syndrome following carotid artery stenting: risk factors, prevention, and treatment. J Am Coll Cardiol 2004;43:1596-1601.

42. Meyers PM, Higashida RT, Phatouros CC, et al: Cerebral hyperperfusion syndrome after percutaneous transluminal stenting of the craniocervical arteries. Neurosurgery 2000;47:335-343; discussion 343-345.

43. Kim LJ, Martinez EA, Faraday N, et al: Cardiac troponin I predicts short-term mortality in vascular surgery patients. Circulation 2002;106:2366-2371.

44. Lopez-Jimenez F, Goldman L, Sacks DB, et al: Prognostic value of cardiac troponin T after noncardiac surgery: 6-Month follow-up data. J Am Coll Cardiol 1997;29:1241-1245.

45. Goldman CK, Morshedi-Meibodi A, White CJ, Jaff MR: Surveillance imaging for carotid in-stent restenosis. Catheter Cardiovasc Interv 2006;67:302-308.

46. Lal BK, Hobson RW 2nd, Goldstein J, et al: In-stent recurrent stenosis after carotid artery stenting: Life table analysis and clinical relevance. J Vasc Surg 2003;38:1162-1168; discussion 1169.

47. Zhou W, Lin PH, Bush RL, et al: Management of in-sent restenosis after carotid artery stenting in high-risk patients. J Vasc Surg 2006;43:305-312.

48. Lal BK, Hobson RW 2nd, Goldstein J, et al: Carotid artery stenting: Is there a need to revise ultrasound velocity criteria? J Vasc Surg 2004;39:58-66.

49. Clark DJ, Lessio S, O'Donoghue M, et al: Mechanisms and predictors of carotid artery stent restenosis: A serial intravascular ultrasound study. J Am Coll Cardiol 2006;47:2390-2396.

50. Chan AW, Roffi M, Mukherjee D, et al: Carotid brachytherapy for in-stent restenosis. Catheter Cardiovasc Interv 2003;58:86-92.

51. Setacci C, de Donato G, Setacci F, et al: In-stent restenosis after carotid angioplasty and stenting: A challenge for the vascular surgeon. Eur J Vasc Endovasc Surg 2005;29:601-607.

52. Wennberg DE, Lucas FL, Birkmeyer JD, et al: Variation in carotid endarterectomy mortality in the Medicare population: Trial hospitals, volume, and patient characteristics. JAMA 1998;279:1278-1281.

53. Ouriel K, Hertzer NR, Beven EG, et al: Preprocedural risk stratification: Identifying an appropriate population for carotid stenting. J Vasc Surg 2001;33:728-732.

54. Hill MD, Morrish W, Soulez G, et al: Multicenter evaluation of a self-expanding carotid stent system with distal protection in the treatment of carotid stenosis. AJNR Am J Neuroradiol 2006;27:759-765.

54a. Gray WA, Hopkins LN, Yadav S, et al; ARCHeR Trial Collaborators: Protected carotid stenting in high-surgical-risk patients: The ARCHeR results. J Vasc Surg 2006;44:258-269.

54b. Gray WA, Yadav JS, Verta P, et al: The CAPTURE registry: Results of carotid stenting with enbolic protection in the post approval setting. Catheter Cardiovasc Interv 2007;69:341-348.

55. Randomised trial of endarterectomy for recently symptomatic carotid stenosis: Final results of the MRC European Carotid Surgery Trial (ECST). Lancet 1998;351:1379-1387.

56. Mas J, Chatellier G, Beyssen B, et al; EVA-3S Investigators: Endarterectomy versus stenting in patients with symptomatic severe carotid stenosis. N Engl J Med 2006;355:1660-1671.

57. SPACE Collaborative Group, Ringleb PA, Allenberg J, et al: 30 day results from the SPACE trial of stent-protected angioplasty versus carotid endarterectomy in symptomatic patients: A randomised non-inferiority trial. Lancet 2006;368:1239-1247.

58. Featherstone RL, Brown MM, Coward LJ: International carotid stenting study: Protocol for a randomised clinical trial comparing carotid stenting with endarterectomy in symptomatic carotid artery stenosis. Cerebrovasc Dis 2004;18:69-74.

59. Hobson RW 2nd: CREST (Carotid Revascularization Endarterectomy versus Stent Trial): Background, design, and current status. Semin Vasc Surg 2000;13:139-143.

60. Carotid Stenting vs. Surgery of Severe Carotid Artery Disease and Stroke Prevention in Asymptomatic Patients (ACT I). Available at: http://www.clinicaltrials.gov/ (accessed April 13, 2007.)

61. Katzen BT, for the TACIT Investigators: The Transatlantic Asymptomatic Carotid Intervention Trial. Endovascular Today 2005:49-50.

62. Wityk RJ, Chang HM, Rosengart A, et al: Proximal extracranial vertebral artery disease in the New England Medical Center Posterior Circulation Registry. Arch Neurol 1998;55:470-478.

63. Berguer R, Flynn LM, Kline RA, Caplan L: Surgical reconstruction of the extracranial vertebral artery: Management and outcome. J Vasc Surg 2000;31:9-18.

64. Mukherjee D, Rosenfield K: Vertebral artery disease. In Casserly IP, Sachar R, Yadav JS: Manual of Peripheral Vascular Intervention, 1st ed. Philadelphia, Lippincott Williams & Wilkins, 2005, pp 110-119.

65. Qureshi AI, Kirmani JF, Harris-Lane P, et al: Vertebral artery origin stent placement with distal protection: Technical and clinical results. AJNR Am J Neuroradiol 2006;27:1140-1145.

66. Coward LJ, Featherstone RL, Brown MM: Percutaneous transluminal angioplasty and stenting for vertebral artery stenosis. Cochrane Database Syst Rev 2005:CD000516.

67. Wong KS, Huang YN, Gao S, et al: Intracranial stenosis in Chinese patients with acute stroke. Neurology 1998;50:812-813.

68. Kremer C, Schaettin T, Georgiadis D, Baumgartner RW: Prognosis of asymptomatic stenosis of the middle cerebral artery. J Neurol Neurosurg Psychiatry 2004;75:1300-1303.

69. Chimowitz MI, Lynn MJ, Howlett-Smith H, et al: Comparison of warfarin and aspirin for symptomatic intracranial arterial stenosis. N Engl J Med 2005;352:1305-1316.

70. Thijs VN, Albers GW: Symptomatic intracranial atherosclerosis: Outcome of patients who fail antithrombotic therapy. Neurology 2000;55:490-497.

71. Prognosis of patients with symptomatic vertebral or basilar artery stenosis. The Warfarin-Aspirin Symptomatic Intracranial Disease (WASID) Study Group. Stroke 1998;29:1389-1392.

72. Failure of extracranial-intracranial arterial bypass to reduce the risk of ischemic stroke. Results of an international randomized trial. The EC/IC Bypass Study Group. N Engl J Med 1985;313:1191-1200.

73. Terada T, Tsuura M, Matsumoto H, et al: Hemorrhagic complications after endovascular therapy for atherosclerotic intracranial arterial stenoses. Neurosurgery 2006;59:310-318; discussion 310-318.

74. Levy EI, Chaturvedi S: Perforator stroke following intracranial stenting: A sacrifice for the greater good? Neurology 2006;66:1803-1804.

75. Casserly IP, Yadav JS: The approach to intracranial carotid artery intervention. In Saw J, Exaire JE, Lee DS, et al (eds): Contemporary Cardiology: Handbook of Complex Percutaneous Carotid Intervention, 1st ed. Totowa, NJ, Humana Press, 2006, pp 189-209.

76. Abou-Chebl A, Krieger DW, Bajzer CT, Yadav JS: Intracranial angioplasty and stenting in the awake patient. J Neuroimaging 2006;16:216-223.

77. Hartmann M, Jansen O: Angioplasty and stenting of intracranial stenosis. Curr Opin Neurol 2005;18:39-45.

78. Higashida RT, Meyers PM, Connors JJ, et al: Intracranial angioplasty and stenting for cerebral atherosclerosis: A position statement of the American Society of Interventional and Therapeutic Neuroradiology, Society of Interventional Radiology, and the American Society of Neuroradiology. J Vasc Interv Radiol 2005;16:1281-1285.

79. Abou-Chebl A, Bashir Q, Yadav JS: Drug-eluting stents for the treatment of intracranial atherosclerosis: Initial experience and midterm angiographic follow-up. Stroke 2005;36:e165-e168.

80. Stenting of Symptomatic Atherosclerotic Lesions in the Vertebral or Intracranial Arteries (SSYLVIA): Study results. Stroke 2004;35:1388-1392.

81. Henkes H, Miloslavski E, Lowens S, et al: Treatment of intracranial atherosclerotic stenoses with balloon dilatation and self-expanding stent deployment (WingSpan). Neuroradiology 2005;47:222-228.

42 Chronic Mesenteric Ischemia: Diagnosis and Intervention

Christopher J. White and Stephen R. Ramee

KEY POINTS

- Atherosclerotic stenoses commonly involve the major mesenteric arteries (celiac, superior mesenteric, and inferior mesenteric) but rarely cause symptomatic ischemia owing to an excellent collateral circulation between the visceral vascular beds.
- The classic presentation is postprandial abdominal pain with weight floss. Patients with functional bowel complaints rarely have significant weight loss.
- Patients with suspected chronic mesenteric ischemia commonly have atherosclerosis involving other vascular territories (i.e., coronary disease, stroke, renovascular disease, or lower extremity atherosclerotic disease).
- Single-vessel disease of the mesenteric circulation can cause symptomatic ischemia, particularly after abdominal surgery that interrupts the collateral circulation.

- Noninvasive testing with ultrasound, computed tomographic angiography, or magnetic resonance angiography is an appropriate screening test in patients with suspected chronic mesenteric ischemia.
- Invasive angiography requires a lateral view to visualize the origin of the mesenteric vessels.
- Recent studies suggest that percutaneous therapy with stents is the treatment of choice for this disease, with comparable efficacy to surgery and lower morbidity and mortality. The clinical recurrence rate appears to be about 1 in 5 patients, so careful follow-up is warranted in these patients.

Although the most common vascular disorder involving the intestines is ischemia, the clinical syndrome of chronic mesenteric ischemia (CMI) or chronic intestinal ischemia is very unusual. Other etiologies associated with this uncommon syndrome include fibromuscular dysplasia, Buerger's disease, and aortic dissection, but atherosclerosis is by the far the most common cause. Atherosclerotic disease of the aorta with associated aorto-ostial stenosis of the visceral vessels is a relatively common angiographic finding.

In a population-based prevalence study of mesenteric artery stenosis, 553 healthy Medicare beneficiaries were screened with abdominal ultrasound for evidence of mesenteric disease.[1] Significant (>50% diameter stenosis) narrowing of a mesenteric vessel, mostly (>97%) isolated celiac artery narrowing, was detected in 17.5% of the total cohort. There was no correlation between age, race, gender, or body mass index and the presence of mesenteric artery stenosis.

Only 1.3% of the patients had involvement of more than one mesenteric vessel.

Another natural history study reported on a group of 980 asymptomatic patients with mesenteric ischemia who were monitored clinically.[2] Only three patients eventually developed symptoms, and they all had three mesenteric vessels severely affected. The most likely explanation for the infrequent occurrence of CMI in clinical practice is the redundancy of the visceral circulation, which has multiple interconnections between the superior mesenteric artery (SMA) and the inferior mesenteric artery (IMA).

CLINICAL PRESENTATION

Women are much more commonly affected (70%) than men. The classic presentation of this disease is postprandial abdominal discomfort with significant weight loss (Fig. 42-1). The abdominal discomfort associated with eating leads these patients to avoid

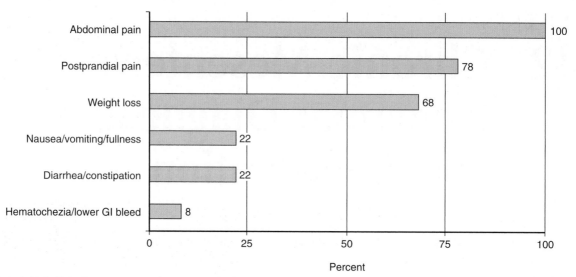

Figure 42-1. Initial clinical presentation of patients with chronic mesenteric ischemia. GI, gastrointestinal. (From Silva JA, White CJ, Collins TJ, et al: Endovascular therapy for chronic mesenteric ischemia. J Am Coll Cardiol 2006;47:944-950.)

food, and therefore they lose weight. Patients with CMI typically avoid food and demonstrate significant weight loss. However, patients with ischemic gastropathy may also present with atypical symptoms such as vomiting, diarrhea, constipation, ischemic colitis, and lower gastrointestinal bleeding. Most patients have evidence of atherosclerosis in other vascular beds and may have had prior myocardial infarction, stroke, or claudication.

Patients with atypical symptoms may be very difficult to diagnose, but a high degree of suspicion for CMI in patients with other manifestations of atherosclerosis and unexplained weight loss is appropriate. Often, the diagnosis is delayed in patients who are being evaluated for a possible malignancy as an explanation for their weight loss. Patients with functional bowel complaints rarely experience significant weight loss, which helps to differentiate them from patients with CMI. Evidence of significant obstruction of two or more of these vessels is often found when classic symptoms and endoscopy suggest bowel ischemia,[3] although single-vessel disease, usually of the SMA, has been described, particularly if collateral connections have been disrupted by prior abdominal surgery.

DIAGNOSIS

The diagnosis of CMI is a clinical one, based on symptoms and consistent anatomic findings. There is no laboratory test that can identify CMI. There are several ways to identify arterial stenoses or occlusions, including Doppler ultrasound (duplex) imaging and noninvasive angiography with computed tomographic angiography (CTA) and magnetic resonance angiography (MRA).

The ability to visualize the mesenteric vessels is technically challenging and requires a skilled and dedicated technologist. The reported accuracy with duplex imaging to identify significant stenoses of the celiac artery and the SMA approaches 90%.[4,5] With the relatively common application of CTA and MRA imaging for abdominal pathology, it is now possible to make the "anatomic" diagnosis without invasive angiography.[6]

Invasive angiography is useful for diagnosis, but a lateral aortogram is needed to visualize the ostia of the mesenteric vessels (Fig. 42-2). Occasionally, an enlarged collateral vessel connecting a branch of the IMA with the SMA (arc of Riolan) is seen on an anteroposterior aortogram and is an indication of proximal mesenteric artery disease. When critical stenoses (70%) are found in symptomatic patients, revascularization is appropriate. However, in patients with borderline lesions or questionable symptoms, there is no stress test to elicit an ischemic response.

TREATMENT

Revascularization has traditionally been done by open surgery with either endarterectomy or bypass grafting. As might be expected, however, this patient group has a high incidence of coronary artery disease, and the perioperative surgical mortality ranges from 3.5% to 15% (Table 42-1),[7-22] with the highest incidence of complications occurring in patients older than 70 years of age.[21]

Atherosclerotic aorto-ostial obstructions of the visceral vessels are similar to those of the renal arteries, and the technical considerations for percutaneous transluminal angioplasty (PTA) with stent placement are similar to those for renal artery intervention (Fig. 42-3). As with renal interventions, stent placement offers a superior late patency compared to PTA alone.[23] The endovascular approach circumvents the need for general anesthesia and the operative trauma

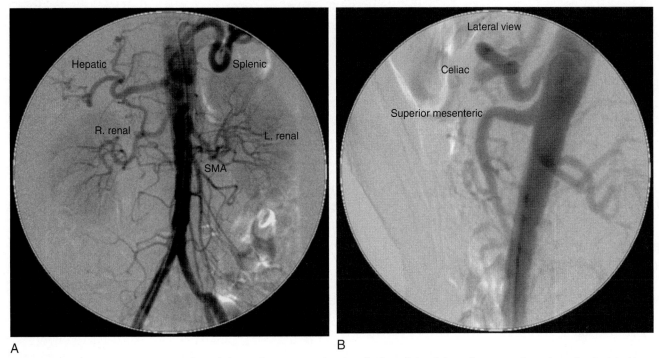

Figure 42-2. A, Anteroposterior view of an abdominal aortogram showing the branches of the celiac artery (hepatic and splenic), the renal arteries, and the superior mesenteric artery (SMA). **B,** Lateral view of an abdominal aortogram showing the origin of the celiac artery and the SMA.

associated with open surgery and, it is believed, will result in a lower acute mortality and morbidity (Table 42-2).[3,17,23-34]

Because of the relative infrequency of this disease, there are no randomized trials comparing surgery to endovascular treatment for CMI. The 20-year (1977-1997) Cleveland Clinic experience in 85 patients with CMI treated with surgery demonstrated an 8% perioperative mortality rate, and one third of the patients had a major complication of surgery.[16] Advanced age, hypertension, coronary disease, and disease in other vascular beds correlated with surgical complications. At late follow-up, 23% (*n*=18) had objective evidence of restenosis, 21% (*n*=16) had recurrent CMI symptoms, and 12% (*n*=9) underwent

target vessel revascularization. Interestingly, the use of vein conduit as graft material was associated with poorer patency and outcome than Dacron as a graft material. The 5-year survival rate was 64% (95% confidence interval [CI]: 53% to 75%), and the 3-year symptom-free survival rate was 81% (95% CI: 72% to 90%).

As a follow-up, a retrospective comparison of a 3-year percutaneous revascularization experience from the Cleveland Clinic with the surgical cohort reported by Mateo and colleagues[16] failed to show an advantage for the percutaneous treatment group.[29] Their 8% perioperative surgical mortality rate was not different from the 11% (3/28) mortality rate for the angioplasty and stent group. Two of the angioplasty

Table 42-1. Outcomes of Surgical Therapy for Chronic Mesenteric Ischemia

Author (Ref. No.)	Year	N	No. Vessels	Technical Success (%)	30-Day Mortality (%)	Symptom Relief (%)	Restenosis (%)
Kien (7)	1990	60	69	100	3.5	NA	25
Cormier (8)	1991	32	90	100	9	NA	9
Cunningham (9)	1991	74	194	100	12	86	NA
McAfee (10)	1992	58	119	100	10	90	10
Caideron (11)	1992	20	36	100	0	100	0
Christensen (12)	1994	90	109	100	13	NA	NA
Gentile (13)	1994	26	29	100	10	89	11
Johnson (14)	1995	21	43	100	0	NA	16
Moawad (15)	1997	24	38	100	4	78	23
Mateo (6)	1999	85	130	100	8	87	24
Sivamurthy (17)	2006	41	59	100	15	68	17

NA, not applicable.

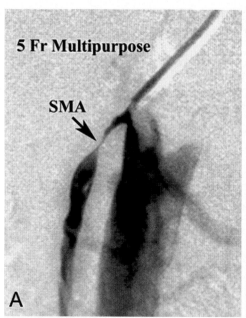
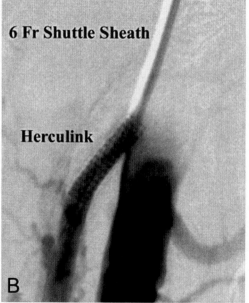

Figure 42-3. A, Baseline angiogram of tight proximal superior mesenteric artery (SMA) stenosis with brachial artery access. **B,** Final angiogram after deployment of balloon-expandable stent (Herculink, Guidant Corporation).

Table 42-2. Outcomes of Percutaneous Therapy for Chronic Mesenteric Ischemia

Author (Ref. No.)	Year	N	No. Vessels	Technical Success (%)	30-Day Mortality (%)	Symptom Relief (%)	Restenosis (%)
Matsumoto (3)	1995	19	20	79	0	52	NA
Hallisey (24)	1995	16	25	84	6	75	25
Allen (25)	1996	19	24	95	5	79	NA
Maspes (26)	1997	23	41	90	0	75	12
Nyman (27)	1998	5	6	100	0	80	60
Sheeran (28)	1999	12	13	92	8	75	16
Kasirajan (29)	2001	28	32	100	11	66	27
AbuRahma (30)	2003	22	24	95	0	67	30
Sharafuddin (31)	2003	25	26	96	4	85	8
Landis (23)	2005	29	33	97	6.9	90	16.3
Sivamurthy (17)	2006	21	29	95.3	16	27	32
Silva (32)	2006	59	79	96	1.7	83	29

NA, not applicable.

and stent patients who died developed bowel gangrene. There was no difference in length of hospital stay, suggesting that the angioplasty and stent group must have had severe comorbidities that perhaps made the cohorts not comparable. At follow-up, the restenosis rate for patients treated with a balloon alone was 33% but fell to 11.5% in the stent-treated patients. Late patency and survival were not different between the open surgery and the percutaneous therapy group.

A recently reported retrospective analysis of 14 patients undergoing percutaneous stent placement for CMI by vascular surgeons demonstrated an excellent procedural success rate, with no perioperative mortality or major morbidity, but 53% of patients required reintervention at 13 months. Despite the high recurrence rates, the surgeons concluded that patients with severe nutritional deficiency or high surgical risk should be offered percutaneous therapy as the initial choice of treatment, and then be re-considered for open surgery if re-treatment became necessary.

We reported the largest single series of patients with CMI treated percutaneously from the Ochsner Clinic in 59 patients and 79 vessels.[32] The technical success rate was 96%, and symptom relief was achieved in 88% of the patients. There was one perioperative death (1.7%) and two access site complications. At a mean follow-up of 38±15 months, 17% of the patients had recurrence of their symptoms, but none developed acute mesenteric ischemia. All patients with recurrent symptoms underwent successful retreatment without complication. The in-stent restenosis rate at 14±5 months, with 90% of the vessels imaged by either CTA, invasive angiography, or duplex ultrasound, was 29% (see Table 42-2). The rate of target vessel revascularization was 17%. The 5-year rates of cumulative freedom from death, symptom recurrence, or both were 72%, 79%, and 57%, respectively.

CONCLUSION

The infrequent occurrence of CMI has made randomized control trials comparing treatment outcomes very difficult to perform. Case series have shown that percutaneous therapy with stent placement offers the lowest morbidity and roughly equivalent long-term outcomes when compared with surgery. The current treatment recommendation is that patients who are candidates for either surgery or percutaneous therapy should receive percutaneous therapy with stent placement.

REFERENCES

1. Hansen KJ, Wilson DB, Craven TE, et al: Mesenteric artery disease in the elderly. J Vasc Surg 2004;40:45-52.
2. Thomas JH, Blake K, Pierce GE, et al: The clinical course of asymptomatic mesenteric arterial stenosis. J Vasc Surg 1998;27:840-844.
3. Matsumoto AH, Tegtmeyer CJ, Fitzcharles EK, et al: Percutaneous transluminal angioplasty of visceral arterial stenoses: Results and long-term clinical follow-up. J Vasc Interv Radiol 1995;6:165-174.
4. Bowersox JC, Zwolak RM, Walsh DB, et al: Duplex ultrasonography in the diagnosis of celiac and mesenteric artery occlusive disease. J Vasc Surg 1991;14:780-786; discussion 786-788.
5. Zwolak RM, Fillinger MF, Walsh DB, et al: Mesenteric and celiac duplex scanning: A validation study. J Vasc Surg 1998;27:1078-1087; discussion 1088.
6. Chow LC, Chan FP, Li KC: A comprehensive approach to MR imaging of mesenteric ischemia. Abdom Imaging 2002;27:507-516.
7. Kieny R, Batellier J, Kretz JG: Aortic reimplantation of the superior mesenteric artery for atherosclerotic lesions of the visceral arteries: sixty cases. Ann Vasc Surg 1990;4:122-125.
8. Cormier JM, Fichelle JM, Vennin J, et al: Atherosclerotic occlusive disease of the superior mesenteric artery: Late results of reconstructive surgery. Ann Vasc Surg 1991;5:510-518.
9. Cunningham CG, Reilly LM, Rapp JH, et al: Chronic visceral ischemia: Three decades of progress. Ann Surg 1991;214:276-287; discussion 287-288.
10. McAfee MK, Cherry KJ Jr, Naessens JM, et al: Influence of complete revascularization on chronic mesenteric ischemia. Am J Surg 1992;164:220-224.
11. Calderon M, Reul GJ, Gregoric ID, et al: Long-term results of the surgical management of symptomatic chronic intestinal ischemia. J Cardiovasc Surg (Torino) 1992;33:723-728.
12. Christensen MG, Lorentzen JE, Schroeder TV: Revascularisation of atherosclerotic mesenteric arteries: Experience in 90 consecutive patients. Eur J Vasc Surg 1994;8:297-302.
13. Gentile AT, Moneta GL, Taylor LM Jr, et al: Isolated bypass to the superior mesenteric artery for intestinal ischemia. Arch Surg 1994;129:926-931; discussion 931-932.
14. Johnston KW, Lindsay TF, Walker PM, Kalman PG: Mesenteric arterial bypass grafts: Early and late results and suggested surgical approach for chronic and acute mesenteric ischemia. Surgery 1995;118:1-7.
15. Moawad J, McKinsey JF, Wyble CW, et al: Current results of surgical therapy for chronic mesenteric ischemia. Arch Surg 1997;132:613-618; discussion 618-619.
16. Mateo RB, O'Hara PJ, Hertzer NR, et al: Elective surgical treatment of symptomatic chronic mesenteric occlusive disease: Early results and late outcomes. J Vasc Surg 1999;29:821-831; discussion 832.
17. Sivamurthy N, Rhodes JM, Lee D, et al: Endovascular versus open mesenteric revascularization: Immediate benefits do not equate with short-term functional outcomes. J Am Coll Surg 2006;202:859-867.
18. Foley MI, Moneta GL, Abou-Zamzam AM Jr, et al: Revascularization of the superior mesenteric artery alone for treatment of intestinal ischemia. J Vasc Surg 2000;32:37-47.
19. Jimenez JG, Huber TS, Ozaki CK, et al: Durability of antegrade synthetic aortomesenteric bypass for chronic mesenteric ischemia. J Vasc Surg 2002;35:1078-1084.
20. Kihara TK, Blebea J, Anderson KM, et al: Risk factors and outcomes following revascularization for chronic mesenteric ischemia. Ann Vasc Surg 1999;13:37-44.
21. Park WM, Cherry KJ Jr, Chua HK, et al: Current results of open revascularization for chronic mesenteric ischemia: A standard for comparison. J Vasc Surg 2002;35:853-859.
22. Leke MA, Hood DB, Rowe VL, et al: Technical consideration in the management of chronic mesenteric ischemia. Am Surg 2002;68:1088-1092.
23. Landis MS, Rajan DK, Simons ME, et al: Percutaneous management of chronic mesenteric ischemia: Outcomes after intervention. J Vasc Interv Radiol 2005;16:1319-1325.
24. Hallisey MJ, Deschaine J, Illescas FF, et al: Angioplasty for the treatment of visceral ischemia. J Vasc Interv Radiol 1995;6:785-791.
25. Allen RC, Martin GH, Rees CR, et al: Mesenteric angioplasty in the treatment of chronic intestinal ischemia. J Vasc Surg 1996;24:415-421; discussion 421-423.
26. Maspes F, Mazzetti di Pietralata G, Gandini R, et al: Percutaneous transluminal angioplasty in the treatment of chronic mesenteric ischemia: Results and 3 years of follow-up in 23 patients. Abdom Imaging 1998;23:358-363.
27. Nyman U, Ivancev K, Lindh M, Uher P: Endovascular treatment of chronic mesenteric ischemia: Report of five cases. Cardiovasc Intervent Radiol 1998;21:305-313.
28. Sheeran SR, Murphy TP, Khwaja A, et al: Stent placement for treatment of mesenteric artery stenoses or occlusions. J Vasc Interv Radiol 1999;10:861-867.
29. Kasirajan K, O'Hara PJ, Gray BH, et al: Chronic mesenteric ischemia: Open surgery versus percutaneous angioplasty and stenting. J Vasc Surg 2001;33:63-71.
30. AbuRahma AF, Stone PA, Bates MC, Welch CA: Angioplasty/stenting of the superior mesenteric artery and celiac trunk: Early and late outcomes. J Endovasc Ther 2003;10:1046-1053.
31. Sharafuddin MJ, Olson CH, Sun S, et al: Endovascular treatment of celiac and mesenteric arteries stenoses: Applications and results. J Vasc Surg 2003;38:692-698.
32. Silva JA, White CJ, Collins TJ, et al: Endovascular therapy for chronic mesenteric ischemia. J Am Coll Cardiol 2006;47:944-950.
33. Cognet F, Ben Salem D, Dranssart M, et al: Chronic mesenteric ischemia: Imaging and percutaneous treatment. Radiographics 2002;22:863-879; discussion 879-880.
34. Matsumoto AH, Angle JF, Spinosa DJ, et al: Percutaneous transluminal angioplasty and stenting in the treatment of chronic mesenteric ischemia: Results and longterm followup. J Am Coll Surg 2002;194(1 Suppl):S22-S31.

CHAPTER
43 Renal Artery Stenosis

Eduardo Infante de Oliveira and Christopher Bajzer

KEY POINTS

- Renal artery stenosis (RAS) is most commonly caused by atherosclerotic vascular disease involving the ostia of the renal artery and the abdominal aorta. Less frequently, RAS is caused by fibromuscular dysplasia (FMD).
- RAS usually manifests with the signs and/or symptoms of chronic ischemic renal disease. A normotensive presentation is possible, but moderate to severe hypertension is a usual clinical feature, and RAS is the most common curable cause for hypertension.
- FMD of the renal arteries has a pathognomonic angiographic appearance. Hypertension is the most common manifestation of this disease. Renal dysfunction and renal artery occlusion are uncommon consequences of FMD. Intervention for FMD is usually made on the basis of control of hypertension.
- Among the noninvasive means to screen for and conduct surveillance of RAS (duplex Doppler ultrasonography, computed tomographic angiography, and magnetic resonance angiography), duplex ultrasonography has competitive sensitivity and specificity with the lowest cost.

- Captopril nuclear renograms and renal vein renin sampling are no longer routinely used for screening and diagnosis of RAS.
- Renal arteriography is the gold standard method for diagnosis of RAS. Arteriography allows the option of percutaneous revascularization.
- Revascularization in the setting of unilateral RAS is not supported by conclusive scientific literature except in situations of renal salvage.
- Current accepted indications for renal artery revascularization include severe and refractory hypertension, recurrent flash pulmonary edema, and progressive renal insufficiency despite adequate medical therapy.
- Surgical revascularization is recommended in the setting of failed percutaneous revascularization, in the presence of multiple small renal arteries excluding the option of percutaneous revascularization, and in aneurysmal disease of the aorta.

Renal artery stenosis (RAS), in the context of either atherosclerosis or fibromuscular dysplasia (FMD), is associated with chronic renal ischemia and increased cardiovascular morbidity and mortality. Revascularization therapies aim to salvage renal function, treat hypertension, and reduce cardiovascular risk. The first percutaneous transluminal renal angioplasty was performed in 1977, the same year as the first coronary angioplasty.[1] Percutaneous intervention is presently the mainstream modality for revascularization, and it is one of the most common peripheral interventional procedures (Fig. 43-1). The equipment has changed dramatically in the last decade, and the procedure has become safer and reliably successful. However, many aspects of the technique remain controversial, such as adequate patient and lesion selection, benefits of stenting or embolic protection devices (EPDs), and impact on cardiovascular risk and renal function preservation. The inconsistency of scientific evidence surrounding some of these issues and the ongoing clinical trials that will bring new insights in the near future characterize this exciting field.

EPIDEMIOLOGY

RAS has mainly two causes, FMD, which accounts for fewer than 10% of cases, and atherosclerosis, which represents more than 90% of cases. Because no specific symptom or syndrome is associated with RAS, the problem is largely under-recognized and under-diagnosed. The true prevalence of RAS in the general population is unknown. Most studies include specific subsets of patients, and there is no efficient and economically viable way to screen large populations to determine the true prevalence of RAS.

In the United States, the prevalence and incidence of RAS based on administrative data in the general population older than 65 years of age (Medicare enrollees) are estimated to be 0.5% and 3.7% per 1000 patient-years, respectively.[2] There is a near-linear association between RAS and atherosclerosis in other territories. The prevalence of RAS increases in subsets of the population with high cardiovascular risk. The presence of RAS increases the likelihood of disease in other territories and is associated with increased cardiovascular morbidity and mortality. In

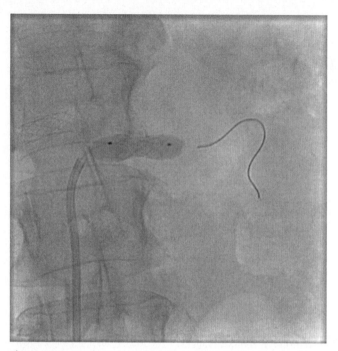

Figure 43-1. Implantation of a balloon-expandable stent in the left renal artery.

the Medicare population, patients with RAS presented with concurrent atherosclerotic coronary, cerebral vascular disease, and peripheral arterial disease in 67%, 37%, and 56% of the cases, respectively. The presence of atherosclerosis elsewhere in the body is 2 to 4 times higher in patients with RAS than in those without RAS, and the rates of cardiovascular events are 4 to 5 times higher in patients with RAS.[2]

A population-based study[3] evaluating individuals older than 65 years of age participating in the Cardiovascular Health Study used renal duplex ultrasonography and the criteria of renal artery peak systolic velocity greater than 1.8 m/sec to identify significant renal stenosis. A total of 870 individuals with a mean age of 77 years were studied. The overall prevalence rate of RAS was 6.8% (0.8% bilateral). RAS was independently associated with increasing age, low levels of high-density cholesterol, and increasing systolic blood pressure.

The first scientific data regarding the prevalence of RAS was provided by an anatomic/pathologic series.[4] In recent autopsy series, a prevalence of 4% has been reported for the general population (Western countries). Prevalence increases to 8.3% among patients with diabetes and to 10.1% among those with diabetes and hypertension.[5] Among patients with evidence of myocardial infarction, RAS is found in 12%, and its prevalence increases with the number of coronary vessels involved and with the presence of hypertension (39%).[6] Among patients with stroke older than 40 years of age, the prevalence of RAS is 10.4% and increases to 14.7%, 28.6%, and 23.9% in the presence of hypertension, renal failure, and aortic aneurysm, respectively.[7]

In series in which patients underwent abdominal aortography after coronary angiography, the prevalence of RAS with greater than or equal to 50% stenosis was 6.3% to 9.1%[8,9]; for RAS with 75% or greater stenosis, the prevalence was 4.8%,[8] and for bilateral stenosis it was 0.8% to 1.3%.[8,9] Increased stenosis severity and bilateral involvement were associated with increased mortality on 4-year follow-up.[8] Patients undergoing catheterization for peripheral arterial disease in other territories had a RAS prevalence of 33% to 39%.[10,11] Despite the angiographic evidence of RAS with its associated cardiovascular morbidity and mortality, 25% to 50% of these patients are not hypertensive and the clinical benefit of revascularization is unclear.[8,9]

Among patients presenting with hypertension, the prevalence of RAS varies according to the severity of the hypertension, the individual clinical setting, and the cardiovascular risk. Among patients with mild hypertension, RAS occurs in fewer than 1%,[12] but among patients with severe or malignant hypertension the prevalence of RAS increases to 10% to 45%.[13]

The burden associated with the loss of renal function provides a different perspective of the problem. It has been estimated that chronic ischemic renal vascular disease may be responsible for more than a quarter of the cases of end-stage renal failure; in some populations, it is the leading cause and is increasing faster than other causes.[14-18]

Rate of Progression of Stenotic Lesions

In a prospective study,[19] patients being screened for RAS were enrolled if at least one renal artery had Doppler velocities above the normal range as detected by duplex scanning. A total of 132 renal arteries were monitored. At baseline, 36 arteries were normal, 35 had less than 60% stenosis, and 61 had stenosis of 60% or greater. The cumulative incidence of progression from less than 60% to 60% or greater RAS was 30% at 1 year, 44% at 2 years, and 48% at 3 years. All renal arteries that progressed to occlusion had 60% or greater stenoses at the initial baseline visit, and for those arteries the cumulative incidence of progression to occlusion was 4% at 1 year, 4% at 2 years, and 7% at 3 years. Progression of RAS occurred at an average rate of 7% per year for all categories of baseline disease combined.

In another prospective study using duplex scanning,[20] 295 renal arteries were monitored. The cumulative incidence of RAS progression was 35% at 3 years and 51% at 5 years. The 3-year cumulative incidence of progression stratified by baseline disease classification was 18%, 28%, and 49% for renal arteries initially classified as normal, less than 60% stenosis, and 60% or greater stenosis, respectively. Only 3% of renal arteries occluded during the study. All of the renal artery occlusions occurred in renal arteries having 60% or greater stenosis at baseline. The risk of renal artery disease progression is highest in individuals with preexisting high-grade stenosis in either renal artery, elevated systolic blood pressure, and diabetes mellitus.[20] In both studies, approximately 7% of the arteries with 60% or greater stenosis at baseline occluded during the 3-year follow-up period.

These two prospective studies confirmed the conclusions of previous retrospective studies that renal artery disease progression is a frequent occurrence, especially in patients with high-grade stenosis.

Another prospective study addressed the risk of atrophy in kidneys with atherosclerotic RAS.[21] The 2-year cumulative incidence of renal atrophy was 5.5%, 11.7%, and 20.8% in kidneys with a baseline renal artery disease classification of normal, less than 60% stenosis, and 60% or greater stenosis, respectively. Other baseline factors associated with a high risk of renal atrophy were a systolic blood pressure higher than 180 mm Hg, a renal artery peak systolic velocity greater than 400 cm/second, and a renal cortical end-diastolic velocity less than or equal to 5 cm/second. The number of kidneys demonstrating atrophy per participant correlated with elevations in the serum creatinine concentration. Thus, persistent severe stenosis appears to carry the risk of long-term loss of renal mass.

Despite the frequent progression of atherosclerotic lesions by imaging criteria and the correlation with progressive loss of renal mass, there is no clear association with deterioration from the clinical point of view in most patients with RAS (i.e., on the basis of hypertensive medication requirements, renal function deterioration, or need for renal revascularization).[22] This is particularly true for patients with an incidental finding of RAS.[11] However, deterioration of renal function and mortality risk is greatest in patients with bilateral stenosis or stenosis to a solitary functioning kidney.[22,23]

Other studies[24,25] have reported a lack of association between renal artery anatomy and renal function in patients with RAS. However, patients in these studies usually had a diverse number of conditions that could induce renal parenchymal damage, and therefore RAS was not a solitary factor in declining renal function. This setting should be considered when revascularization procedures are contemplated, because irreversible parenchymal disease compromises the desired outcome of renal revascularization.

CLINICAL PRESENTATION

Some patients with RAS or chronic ischemic renal disease present with normal blood pressure without medical therapy, although moderate to severe hypertension treated with medical therapy usually dominates as the presenting clinical scenario. Certain features associated with hypertension are suggestive of the diagnosis of RAS:

- Onset of hypertension before 30 years of age (FMD)
- Onset of stage II or diastolic hypertension after 55 years of age

- Exacerbation of previously well-controlled hypertension
- Malignant hypertension (severe hypertension and signs of end-organ damage—acute renal failure, retinal hemorrhages or papilledema, heart failure, or neurologic disturbance)
- Refractory or resistant hypertension (inadequate blood pressure control despite compliance with adequate therapy with three or more antihypertensive agents)
- Azotemia shortly after the institution of therapy with angiotensin-converting enzyme (ACE) inhibitor or angiotensin receptor blocking agent (ARB) therapy—this phenomenon may occur also in the presence of nephrosclerosis
- Moderate to severe hypertension and an atrophic kidney or discrepancy in renal size (>1.5 cm)
- Moderate to severe hypertension and diffuse atherosclerosis
- Moderate to severe hypertension and recurrent episodes of acute (flash) pulmonary edema or unexplained heart failure
- Moderate to severe hypertension and a systolic-diastolic abdominal bruit that lateralizes to one side (sensitivity 40%, specificity 99%)[26]
- Moderate to severe hypertension and progressive unexplained azotemia (bland urine sediment with few cells or casts; mild to moderate proteinuria may be present)

Other associations with RAS that are not well understood include the following:

- Renal vascular hypertension and hyponatremia that seems to correlate inversely with plasma renin levels[27]
- Renal vascular hypertension and Caucasian race[28,29]

Ultimately, all the constellation of signs and symptoms associated with the cardiovascular consequences (e.g., angina pectoris, myocardial infarction, flash pulmonary edema, heart failure, stroke, aortic dissection) as well as the renal consequences (chronic renal insufficiency) of RAS may occur.

SCREENING AND DIAGNOSTIC TESTS

Despite being the most common curable cause of hypertension, RAS occurs in fewer than 1% of patients with mild hypertension.[12] However, the incidence of RAS varies dramatically according to the clinical setting. For instance, 10% to 45% of white patients with severe or malignant hypertension have RAS.[13] Ideally, all patients should be screened for curable causes of hypertension; however, this strategy would not be economically viable because of the high prevalence of idiopathic hypertension. Therefore, screening for RAS should be performed only in the appropriate clinical setting, where renal vascular hypertension is more likely to occur. The clinical clues previously noted should help to triage patients for RAS screening. A score system based on multiple weighted clinical factors has been proposed to identify high-risk patients.[30] The recent American College of Cardiology/American Heart Association (ACC/AHA)[31,32] guidelines recommended that patients be screened if a revascularization procedure is intended.

Renal arteriography is the gold standard for the diagnosis of RAS[31,32] and can be performed as a first-line examination for patients with a high probability of having RAS. However, most patients are initially evaluated with a noninvasive test that varies according to institutional and physician preferences and patient characteristics. A diverse number of noninvasive examinations have been used over the years, but at present only three alternatives should be considered for screening[31,32] for RAS: magnetic resonance angiography (MRA), computed tomographic angiography (CRA), and duplex Doppler ultrasonography.

MRA angiography is becoming more accessible and in many institutions is the preferred screening method for atherosclerotic RAS. Increasing evidence supports the use of MRA in patients who are likely to have atherosclerotic RAS. MRA should not be used as a screening tool in populations without clinical features suggestive of the disease, nor for FMD screening.[33,34] MRA is not adequate to visualize the middle and distal portions of the renal artery, which are typically affected in FMD.

Compared with intra-arterial digital subtraction arteriography (DSA) as the gold standard, MRA has a sensitivity of 100%[35-37] and a specificity between 71%[36] and 98%[37] for the detection of stenosis of the main renal arteries. The combination of three-dimensional gadolinium-enhanced MRA and cine phase-contrast flow measurement produces similar results to intra-arterial DSA for the ostium and proximal segment of the renal artery.[38] However, MRA misses most of the accessory renal arteries seen by intra-arterial DSA,[35,39] even when breath-hold MRA with paramagnetic contrast material is used.[37] Identification of accessory renal arteries is important for the interventional decision-making process.

Helical computed tomographic scanning with intravenous contrast injection (CTA) is another highly accurate noninvasive screening test for atherosclerotic RAS. Compared with the gold standard, CTA has a sensitivity between 90%[40] and 98%[41] and a specificity between 94%[41] and 97%[40] for the diagnosis of RAS (>50% stenosis). The test performance increases if only the main renal arteries are considered (sensitivity 100%, specificity 97%).[40] The test performance decreases in patients with compromised renal function,[41] in those with fibromuscular disease,[33,34] and in populations without clinical features suggestive of atherosclerotic RAS.[33,34] High-grade stenoses may appear as occlusions in both CTA and MRA. Other disadvantages include large-volume contrast requirements, prolonged breath-hold, and significant radiation exposure.

Duplex ultrasonography has a sensitivity of 93%[42] to 98%[43] and a specificity of 96%[42] to 98%,[3] compared with intra-arterial DSA in patients with a high likelihood of renal vascular disease.[42,43] Duplex ultrasound has several advantages: it provides anatomic and functional data, and it offers reasonably good visualization of the distal segment of the renal arteries and therefore is more adequate for FMD diagnosis and can be used to detect restenosis after angioplasty, stent implantation, or surgery. However, the accuracy is highly operator-dependent and a complete examination is time-consuming.

Several classic duplex ultrasound criteria are currently used to identify a significant RAS (60%-99%), such as renal-aortic ratio,[44] peak systolic velocity,[44,45] poststenotic turbulence, and abnormal renal artery hilar waveform. Several velocimetric indices have been tested as screening tools. In one study, the pulsatility index and resistive index failed to reach an adequate negative predictive value for a screening test.[46] However, the acceleration indices have higher negative predictive values and seem more appropriate to use for screening, especially the maximal acceleration index (ratio between maximal systolic acceleration and relative peak systolic velocity).[46]

Noninvasive tests that were used frequently in the past, including plasma renin activity, captopril renography, and intravenous pyelography, were abandoned for screening purposes because of inadequate sensitivity and specificity.[31,32]

SIGNIFICANCE OF RENAL ARTERY STENOSIS

Angiographically, a renal artery lesion is classified as significant if the stenosis is greater than or equal to 75%, or greater than or equal to 50% with poststenotic dilatation. However, such lesions may or may not be associated with renal vascular hypertension or chronic ischemic disease. An incidental finding of RAS is frequent in patients undergoing angiography to evaluate atherosclerosis in other territories. However, the clinical impact of these incidental lesions does not seem relevant in long-term follow-up.[11] The decision for renal revascularization is based in the assumption that the lesions are hemodynamically significant and that clinical benefit will ensue after revascularization. The appropriate clinical setting is usually the discriminator used to classify lesions as clinically significant. However, several other tests have been used to assess the hemodynamic significance of RAS lesions and to identify patients who will benefit from revascularization.

The ACE inhibitor scan or captopril renogram is a test used to assess the clinical significance of known renal artery lesions. The positive predictive value for a beneficial revascularization result may be as high as 80% to 93%.[47,48] Many institutions still include the ACE inhibitor scan after a positive imaging test in the algorithm to identify patients who are eligible for revascularization.

Renal vein renin measurement (captopril-stimulated renal vein renin ratio) is not sufficiently sensitive to enable prediction of which patients will respond to revascularization and is not specific enough to exclude patients who do not have renal vascular hypertension.[49] The exception is in the setting of bilateral RAS, where this test may be useful to determine which kidney contributes most to the presence of hypertension.

The resistive index determined by duplex ultrasound may determine the presence of irreversible parenchymal disease in the setting of RAS and predict the outcome with revascularization. One study[50] reported that patients treated successfully with percutaneous angioplasty had poor outcome if the resistive index values were greater than 0.8. Eighty percent of patients with a resistive index greater than 0.8 undergoing renal artery angioplasty had renal function decline, resulting in the need for chronic dialysis in half of the patients, and there was no decrease in blood pressure. Patients with a resistive index lower than 0.8 undergoing renal artery angioplasty had a significant decrease in blood pressure (94% of patients), and only 3% had renal function decline. Another study[51] revealed a relation between the resistive index by Doppler ultrasonography and arteriolosclerosis in damaged kidneys (biopsy). However, there is still controversy surrounding the use of this index, and contradictory evidence is found in the literature.[52]

Determination of a renal flow index and kidney volume by MRA has also been proposed as a useful tool to identify patients who respond to revascularization or, alternatively, do not respond to revascularization efforts and have irreversible renal disease.[53]

PERCUTANEOUS ANGIOPLASTY

The 2005 ACC/AHA guidelines[31,32] on peripheral arterial disease recommend stenting for atherosclerotic renal artery lesions in patients who meet the clinical indications for intervention (e.g., severe or refractory hypertension, recurrent episodes of flash pulmonary edema or cardiac disturbance syndrome, otherwise unexplained progressive renal insufficiency, progressive renal insufficiency despite lowering of blood pressure even with non-ACE inhibitor medical therapy). The guidelines state that renal artery revascularization should not be performed in the setting of an incidental finding of RAS during angiography to assess atherosclerosis in other territories. Surgical revascularization is recommended if angioplasty fails or in the presence of multiple small renal arteries or aortic disease (aneurysm, severe aortoiliac disease) that requires surgical reconstruction near the origin of the renal arteries. Correction of fibromuscular lesions is indicated only for hypertension control, because progression to total occlusion and severe bilateral involvement with renal failure is rare.

Despite the inconsistencies found in some of the medical literature, Medicare data indicate that between 1996 and 2000 the volume of percutaneous renal artery interventions increased rapidly (2.4-fold), whereas the volume of renal artery surgery declined (−45%). This phenomenon was mainly attributed to increased performance by cardiologists (increased annual volume, 3.9-fold).[54]

Percutaneous Transluminal Balloon Angioplasty Versus Medical Therapy

The Dutch Renal Artery Stenosis Intervention Cooperative (DRASTIC)[55] trial was a multicenter study that randomized 106 patients with RAS (≥50% stenosis) and difficult-to-treat hypertension to medical therapy or percutaneous transluminal balloon angioplasty. Based on intent-to-treat analysis, blood pressure, daily drug doses, and renal function were similar at 1 year. However, at 3 months, 22 (44%) of the 50 patients initially assigned to drug therapy required rescue angioplasty because of refractory hypertension.

The Essai Multicentrique Medicaments versus Angioplastie (EMMA) trial[56] randomized 49 patients with unilateral RAS to balloon angioplasty or medical therapy alone. At 6 months' follow-up, the ambulatory blood pressure was equivalent in the two groups. The main advantage of angioplasty was drug sparing: the number of patients requiring two or more antihypertensive medications was 8 of 23 in the angioplasty group (with 6 patients requiring no drug therapy), compared to 22 of 25 with medical therapy alone.

The Scottish and Newcastle Renal Artery Stenosis Collaborative Group[57] trial randomized 55 hypertensive patients with unilateral and bilateral atheromatous renal disease (≥50% stenosis) to percutaneous transluminal balloon angioplasty or medical therapy. Angioplasty resulted in a modest improvement in systolic blood pressure only in patients with bilateral disease, and renal function did not improve.

A meta-analysis[58] comparing balloon angioplasty versus medical therapy alone in the three mentioned trials, comprising a total of 210 patients with at least 50% stenosis in unilateral/bilateral RAS and poorly controlled hypertension, described a modest improvement of systolic and diastolic blood pressure and need for fewer antihypertensive medications in favor of angioplasty. There was no consistent difference in changes in renal function between the group treated with angioplasty and the group receiving medical therapy alone. Patency of the renal arteries after 12 months was more likely in the angioplasty group. A more recent study revealed that the modest decrease in antihypertensive medication did not have an impact in terms of quality of life improvement.[59]

Renal Artery Stent Placement after Unsuccessful Percutaneous Transluminal Balloon Angioplasty

The ASPIRE-2[60] study analyzed the safety and durability of renal stenting (balloon-expandable) after suboptimal/failed renal artery angioplasty in patients (n=208) with aorto-ostial atherosclerotic renal artery lesions. The stent procedure was immediately successful in 80.2% of lesions treated. The 9-month restenosis rate was 17.4%. Systolic/diastolic blood pressure decreased from 168±25/82±13 mm Hg to 149±24/77±12 mm Hg at 9 months (P<.001 vs. baseline), and to 149±25/77±12 mm Hg at 24 months ($P<.001$ vs. baseline). Mean serum creatinine concentration was unchanged from baseline values at 9 and 24 months. The 24-month cumulative rate of major adverse events was 19.7%.

Percutaneous Transluminal Balloon Angioplasty versus Renal Artery Stent Placement

A meta-analysis[61] of renal arterial stent placement and renal percutaneous transluminal balloon angioplasty studies performed until 1998, including a total of 1322 patients, revealed that stenting was technically superior and clinically comparable to balloon angioplasty alone. Stent placement had a higher technical success rate and a lower restenosis rate than did renal percutaneous angioplasty (98% vs. 77% and 17% vs. 26%, respectively; $P<.001$). The cure rate for hypertension was higher and the improvement rate for renal function was lower after stent placement than after renal percutaneous angioplasty (20% vs. 10% and 30% vs. 38%, respectively; $P<.001$).

A more recent multicenter randomized prospective trial compared balloon angioplasty alone versus balloon angioplasty with stent implantation in patients ($n=84$) with ostial RAS. The primary success rate of balloon angioplasty was 57%, compared with 88% for stenting. Complications were similar. At 6 months, the primary patency rate was 29% for balloon angioplasty and 75% for stenting. Restenosis after a successful primary procedure occurred in 48% of patients for balloon angioplasty and 14% for stenting. Patients who underwent secondary stenting for primary or late failure of balloon angioplasty within the follow-up period had a success rate similar to that of primary stenting. Primary stenting was better than balloon angioplasty to achieve vessel patency in ostial atherosclerotic RAS. Primary stenting and primary balloon angioplasty plus rescue stenting had similar clinical outcomes at 6 months (intention-to-treat analysis). However, the burden of repeat intervention after balloon angioplasty outweighed the potential savings of the cost of the stent in the original procedure.[62]

The renal function response seemed difficult to predict in these trials, and improvement, stabilization, or worsening each occurred in one third of patients. Certain subgroups seemed more prone to respond with improvement or stabilization, such as nondiabetic patients and patients with bilateral stenoses. A prospective trial that included 215 patients with ostial RAS of 70% or greater treated with stent-supported angioplasty identified the following independent predictors of improved renal function: baseline serum creatinine and left ventricular function.[63] Female gender, elevated baseline mean blood pressure, and normal renal parenchymal thickness were independent predictors for decreased mean blood pressure after stenting.[63] However, other prospective trials did not find any independent predictors of improved renal function.[64]

Despite the potential benefits, it is unclear whether angioplasty plus stent placement preserves renal function or slows the deterioration of renal function over time. The assumed correlation between angiographic improvement, lower restenosis rates, and enhanced long-term renal function has not been clearly proven.

Bare Metal Versus Drug-Eluting Renal Artery Stent Placement

Restenosis rates after bare metal stenting of the renal arteries vary between 6% and 20%,[65] depending significantly on the definition of restenosis. The renal artery diameter and the stent diameter are independent predictors of in-stent restenosis. Renal arteries with a diameter of 5 mm or less are particularly at risk, with a rate of restenosis of 20% or more.[65] Therefore, it is hypothesized that patients with small renal arteries might benefit with a lower restenosis rate from the use of drug-eluting stents.

The GREAT trial[66] (Palmaz Genesis peripheral stainless steel balloon-expandable stent: comparing a sirolimus coated vs. bare stent in REnal Artery Treatment) is the only completed study comparing the efficacy of drug-eluting versus bare metal stents in the setting of renal artery angioplasty and stenting. The results, partially published, show a 50% relative risk reduction of angiographic in-stent restenosis (7% with sirolimus-eluting stent vs. 14% with bare metal stent). The stents used were exclusively 5 mm and 6 mm in diameter.[66]

Drug-eluting stents may have a role in the treatment of small renal arteries, particularly in patients with impaired renal function in whom reintervention would lead to recurrent exposure to contrast agents or embolism. Another indication could be the treatment of in-stent restenosis, which until now has been treated with repeat balloon angioplasty or placement of a bare metal stent within the previously placed stent.

In renal arteries with a diameter of at least 6 mm, bare metal stenting should be the treatment of choice, because the rate of restenosis is considered to be low.[65]

Distal Protection Devices

The relatively frequent deterioration of renal function despite successful percutaneous renal artery revascularization is theorized to be a result of microembolization of atherothrombotic debris liberated during the percutaneous revascularization procedure. This theory forms the rationale for the use of a distal artery EPD during percutaneous renal revascularization procedures. No randomized controlled trials have yet been published regarding this theoretical improvement in percutaneous renal revascularization. Several small, noncontrolled studies using different EPDs (filter and occlusion devices) showed lower rates of postprocedure renal function deterioration (5%-10% at 1-3 months' follow-up)[67-69] than the rates published in the literature regarding renal artery intervention without distal protection. In most of the patients studied (60%-80%),[67-69] the devices successfully removed debris in the form of fresh thrombus, chronic thrombus, atheromatous fragments, and cholesterol clefts. Despite promising initial data, the use of these devices is not currently recommended, and additional investigation is needed before their use would become routine or mandatory.

Future Trials

Future trials should focus on demonstrating the impact of renal artery intervention on survival, major cardiovascular events, hypertension, and renal function. The role of EPDs and the benefit of drug-eluting stents should be clarified. Several ongoing trials should provide new insights into these matters.

The Cardiovascular Outcomes of Renal Artery Lesions (CORAL) trial[70] is a randomized clinical trial comparing medical therapy alone versus stenting with medical therapy on a composite cardiovascular and renal end point: cardiovascular or renal death, myocardial infarction, hospitalization for congestive heart failure, stroke, doubling of serum creatinine, and need for renal replacement therapy. Effectiveness of revascularization in important subgroups of patients, improvement in quality of life, cost-effectiveness, and correlation between stenosis severity and longitudinal renal function will also be analyzed. The study will include 1080 patients with significant RAS (at least 60% stenosis with 20 mm Hg systolic pressure gradient or at least 80% stenosis with no gradient necessary) and hypertension (systolic hypertension of at least 155 mm Hg with at least two antihypertensive medications).

The Nephropathy Ischemic Therapy (NITER) trial[71] is an ongoing prospective, multi-center, randomized trial that is comparing medical therapy alone (antihypertensive, lipid-lowering, antiplatelet medications) with medical therapy plus renal artery stent placement. The study includes patients with RAS (70% or greater stenosis), hypertension, and stable renal failure (glomerular filtration rate [GFR]=30 mL/min). The combined primary end point includes death, dialysis initiation, or reduction of 20% or more in the GFR.

ASTRAL[72] is another multicenter, prospective, randomized, controlled trial that will include about 1000 patients with atherosclerotic RAS treated with percutaneous revascularization (balloon angioplasty and/or stent placement) or best medical therapy. The follow-up will be between 1 and 5 years, and the primary comparison end point is the rate of progression of renal failure. Secondary analyses will include blood pressure changes and cardiovascular events. Prespecified subgroup analyses will try to clarify the influence of important baseline characteristics on renal function outcome (e.g., baseline renal function, severity of RAS, ultrasound renal length).

TECHNICAL ASPECTS

Contrast Agents

A low-osmolar or iso-osmolar, non-ionic contrast agent is sufficient for good visualization of the renal arteries. When DSA radiographic techniques are used, the contrast can be diluted (heparinized saline) to two-thirds strength and still produce a diagnostic-quality angiogram. Carbon dioxide or gadolinium may be used as a contrast agent to minimize iodinated contrast use in patients with compromised renal function (creatinine clearance <20 mL/min). However, the images produced with these agents are not of equal quality to those produced with the use of iodinated contrast material.

Another alternative is to use a 1:1 combination of gadolinium and an iodinated contrast agent. Carbon dioxide is a reasonable option for performing initial aortography to identify the number and location of renal arteries. Both of these alternatives, however, result in a compromise in image quality.

Access Site

The femoral approach is used in most cases (>90%), and some centers prefer to use contralateral access to the renal artery to be treated. Occasionally, upper extremity access (e.g., brachial approach) may be used in case of caudal takeoff of the renal artery, severe bilateral aortoiliac disease, or infrarenal abdominal aortic aneurysm.

Diagnostic Procedure

Usually a 4-, 5-, or 6-Fr sheath is used. Many authors prefer to use longer sheaths (23 cm) with radiopaque tips. For the aortogram, a 5-Fr Omniflush, straight flush, tennis racquet, or a pigtail catheter may by used. The catheter should be configured in the infrarenal abdominal aorta to minimize the likelihood of renal atheroembolism. The pigtail catheter and straight flush catheter sometimes result in more cephalic contrast injection, which could opacify the superior mesenteric artery and potentially obscure visualization of the renal arteries. The Omniflush catheter was designed to avoid this problem. The top of the flush catheter should be placed at the level of the superior margin of the first lumbar vertebra (L1) for optimal imaging. An alternative anatomic landmark is the superior apex of the left kidney, assuming that the right kidney is lower. DSA radiographic techniques should be used. The aortogram gives an idea about the configuration and the presence of pathology in the aorta. It identifies the number and location of renal arteries on either side and allows the operator to make an appropriate catheter selection for selective renal artery engagement. If a previous aortogram or renal angiogram is available for review, this first step should be skipped in the interest of reducing contrast volume and therefore minimizing the risk of contrast nephropathy. Previously deployed stents can also be used as reference to proceed directly to selective engagement of the renal arteries.

To selectively engage the renal arteries, a 4- to 5-Fr diagnostic catheter at least 80 cm long is usually used. The shape of the catheter selected depends on the anatomy of the aorta and geometry of the takeoff of the renal arteries. Catheter shapes available for renal use include the Judkins right catheters (e.g., JR4), internal mammary catheter, renal standard curve catheter, renal double curve catheter, Cobra catheter, and SOS Omni II catheter (for difficult angulation). Great care should be exercised in manipulating a catheter in the region of the renal artery ostium to minimize the likelihood of atheroemboli or dissection complications. Occasionally, a 0.014-inch steerable medium- to high-support guide wire is used to traverse the extraparenchymal length of the renal artery before performing selective angiography. This tends to hold the catheter in place and prevents the diagnostic catheter from backing out during injections. It also allows for convenient subsequent intervention. Once the selective diagnostic catheter is in the renal ostium, a gently ramped but brisk hand injection of a small volume of contrast material can be administered, and imaging should be continued until the nephrogram is seen in its entirety.

In terms of angiographic views, the preference varies among different institutions and physicians. Shallow ipsilateral oblique projections (10-20 degrees), straight posteroanterior (PA) projections, and shallow contralateral oblique projections have been used. However, an adequate perpendicular view to the plane of the renal artery and aorta is preferable to assess the severity of the lesion or lesions. A cross-sectional image obtained by CTA or MRA can sometimes provide a good estimate of the necessary angle.

Interventional Procedure

Several guiding catheter shapes may be used (e.g., hockey stick, internal mammary artery, JR4, renal standard curves, multipurpose, SOS Omni II), usually in a 6- or 7-Fr, 65-cm size. In the telescoping technique, the diagnostic catheter is introduced through the guiding catheter, which enables subsequent atraumatic engagement with the guiding catheter over the diagnostic catheter for proceeding with intervention. Alternatively, the "direct engagement technique" may be used. In this technique, the catheter is primarily advanced into the ostium, which may result in trauma and embolization. A variation of this technique is the "no touch" technique, in which the tip of the guide catheter is placed near the ostium of the renal artery using a 0.035-inch guide wire, avoiding direct contact between the tip of the catheter and the ostium of the renal artery. Once the guide catheter is in the vicinity of the renal artery ostium, a 0.014-inch guidewire is used to engage the artery. The guide catheter can be gently advanced using the 0.014-inch guidewire as a monorail.

Presently, there is a trend toward the use of 0.014-inch guide wires, balloons, and stents in percutaneous renal revascularization. This trend opens the wide range of coronary wires, balloons, and stents to the renal intervention arena, in addition to equipment specifically designed for renal artery intervention using the 0.014-inch platform. Alternatively, 0.035-inch or 0.018-inch guide wire platforms may be used with the appropriate balloon and stent system. Hydrophilic guide wires should be used only when difficulty crossing the renal ostium is encountered due to the risk of dissection or perforation. Once the hydrophilic wire has been used to accomplish access, it should be exchanged for a different wire with a nonhydrophilic tip.

Monorail (rapid exchange, RX) balloons are preferred when using a 0.014-inch system. Alternatively, over-the-wire (OTW) balloons with a short shaft may be used. Generally, balloons 3.5 mm to 4 mm in diameter and 8 to 15 mm in length are used for predilatation of a renal stenosis. Some centers use as reference 1 mm less than the apparent normal vessel diameter to choose the predilatation balloon diameter. Smaller-diameter balloons may be required for initial angioplasty for a high-grade stenosis, large volume plaque, or subtotal occlusion. Longer length balloons may create an unnatural force on the renal artery and ultimately cause spasm or even dissection. OTW balloons may be useful for exchanging wires, especially if the initial wire used was one with a hydrophilic tip (although these wires are generally to be avoided). Postdilation balloon size selection varies depending on the size of the artery and stent. However, it is a good idea to have balloons between 4 and 8 mm in diameter available (bearing in mind that many 8-mm balloons do not fit through a 6-Fr guiding catheter). Systematic postdilation is recommended after deployment of ostial stents in order to flare the proximal end of the stent at the ostium into the aorta.

Balloon-expandable stents are used and are generally available in lengths of 12 to 20 mm and in diameters of 5 and 7 mm. Self-expanding stents have been used in to treat midsegment lesions but are not recommended for ostial or proximal renal artery lesions. Although stents with an open-cell design have more flexibility, those with a closed-cell design are preferred because they provide, in general, the most radial strength at the renal ostium. In most cases, it is essential to ensure complete coverage of the renal ostium, and sometimes the proximal stent will have to extend back into the aorta by 1 to 2 mm in a segment (arc) to achieve full circumferential coverage of the renal ostium.

EPDs may be used, but they are not currently mandatory nor recommended. If the operator decides to use such a device in a patient considered to be at high risk for embolization, essential technical aspects must be kept in mind. An adequate landing zone for the EPD must be present downstream of the target lesion. The EPD must be of adequate diameter to appose the entire circumference of the renal artery (coronary distal protection devices may not be large enough to ensure complete vessel apposition). Early branching of the main renal trunk is highly unfavorable for the use of an EPD. It is useful to have a monorail version of the EPD available for use in the renal artery. On rare occasions, a "buddy" 0.014-inch wire is used if there is difficulty navigating through the lesion or the length of the artery. In the presence of a critical lesion, predilation may be necessary to safely advance the EPD.

In terms of the use of procedural anticoagulation and antiplatelet medication after the procedure, there is a paucity of scientific evidence. Many centers start antiplatelet aggregation monotherapy before the intervention. During the procedure, intravenous heparin is used as anticoagulation therapy and is titrated to maintain the activated clotting time (ACT) between 250 and 300 seconds. The use of glycoprotein IIb/IIIa inhibitors is not recommended, but they have been used in cases of acute thrombosis.[73] Bivalirudin was used in a prospective, single-arm study that showed it to be a safe alternative in terms of procedural anticoagulation.[74] Dual antiplatelet therapy (aspirin and clopidogrel) is currently used in many centers. The rationale for use of most of these therapeutic agents is extrapolated from coronary trials.

Complications and Follow-up

The equipment used to perform percutaneous renal artery revascularization has changed dramatically in the last decade, and the procedure has become safer and more reliably successful. However, deterioration in renal function is still the most important complication of the procedure and can be multifactorial (e.g., contrast toxicity, embolization, incorrect patient selection). Every effort should be made to avoid using an excessive volume of contrast material, and great care should be exercised in the manipulation of catheters and devices to reduce the risk of contrast nephropathy and embolic debris resulting in renal parenchymal damage. Both of these goals can be achieved by avoiding bilateral renal artery interventions in the same procedure. Other complications are less frequent but should also been kept in mind, because they can result in mortality and contribute to renal function deterioration.

Atheroembolism or thromboembolism to the distal renal artery branches: If embolization is documented during the procedure; treatment depends on the distal extent of the embolization. A more proximal, branch vessel embolus can be aspirated with commercially available aspiration catheters. A more distal or parenchymal-level embolus is more difficult to treat or manage. Infusion of a glycoprotein IIb/IIIa inhibitor may be used on a theoretical basis, but no direct clinical data exist to support its use in this setting.

Occlusion or thrombosis of renal artery: Either occurrence is another potential indication for the use of glycoprotein IIb/IIIa inhibitors and thrombectomy devices.

Renal artery dissection: If this occurs in the ostium or proximal artery segment, it should be treated by placing a stent. If a dissection occurs in a more distal (extraparenchymal) artery segment, then balloon angioplasty is the best option, because stent implantation compromises any possibility of a successful bailout surgery (though surgery usually is not an option if a distal bypass target is no longer present). If dissection occurs in a more distal (intraparenchymal) artery segment, only undersized balloon angioplasty is possible, because more aggressive angioplasty or stent implantation risks injury to the surrounding renal parenchyma.

Renal artery/aortic perforation: Extra caution and care is mandatory when stenting a renal artery adjacent to an aneurysm in the renal artery or aorta. Oversized stents or aggressive post-stent dilation should be avoided. Patient-reported flank pain during balloon inflation is usually a sign of reaching the maximum safe luminal diameter of the target artery, and further inflation is not recommended. The flank pain is the result of stretching the pain receptors located in the adventitia of the target artery segment. If a renal artery perforation does occur, a prolonged balloon inflation and/or reversal of procedural anticoagulation can safely treat a small perforation. In the setting of a larger perforation, a covered stent or a perfusion flow-balloon may be useful, and anticoagulation should be reversed. Surgery is a potential option for treatment of a larger perforation or a perforation that is not responsive to endovascular treatment. To maximize the benefit of the surgical option, early communication with a skilled surgeon is necessary.

Parenchymal perforations/perinephric hematoma/ retroperitoneal hematoma: Extra caution and care are mandatory when using hydrophilic coated or stiff guide wires. The distal tip of the guide wire should not be allowed to migrate out to the level of the renal cortex. Guide wire migration out to the level of the renal cortex increases the risk of distal artery perforation. Hemorrhage at this level can be intraparenchymal or extraparenchymal. Hemorrhage at either level results in local tissue injury and hydraulic tissue dissection, creating more sources of hemorrhage. If a distal artery perforation is noticed during the procedure, anticoagulation should be reversed and consideration made for temporary proximal flow occlusion with a balloon to control the hemorrhage. If proximal flow occlusion and reversal of procedural anticoagulation is unsuccessful in controlling the hemorrhage, prompt microparticle or microcoil embolization at the site of hemorrhage may be performed. If efforts at controlling hemorrhage are unsuccessful, the patient will require emergency surgery to control the hemorrhage and decompress the accumulated blood and clot. The risk of nephrectomy in such a circumstance is high.

Stent embolization: Dislodgement of the stent from the deployment balloon platform occurs less frequently with premounted or manufacturer-mounted stents compared with hand-crimping of a loose stent on an angioplasty balloon. In the event a stent becomes dislodged from the deployment balloon, subsequent actions are highly dependent on the circumstance and location of the dislodged stent. In some instances, successful positioning and stent deployment in the renal artery is possible. In other instances, the stent may be retrieved with or without the use of special retrieval efforts and devices such as snares. In other instances, the stent may not be retrievable and can be deployed in the iliac artery or, if not deployable, crushed behind a second stent. Surgery is required in very infrequent instances for removal of a dislodged stent.

Cholesterol embolization to the lower extremities and/ or mesenteric circulation: This type of embolization occurs with manipulation of guide wires and catheters in a juxtarenal aorta with significant atherosclerosis. The recognition that this type of embolization has occurred is usually delayed several days to weeks, because signs and symptoms (toe and foot ischemic changes and livedo reticularis in legs) do not occur immediately at the time of embolization. Clinically relevant signs or symptoms are treated with systemic anticoagulation. The most effective treatment is prevention. Here again, extra caution and care in minimizing excessive guide wire and catheter manipulation in a significantly diseased aorta will lower the risk of this complication.

Bleeding and access site complications: Prevention and management of these complications are similar to those encountered with coronary angiography and intervention and are discussed elsewhere in this text.

Infection: This is an exceedingly rare complication as long as strict adherence to sterile technique is followed and as long as preexisting infection is not present elsewhere in the body.

The follow-up strategy varies with the institution, and there is no clear evidence regarding this matter. Clinical (blood pressure) and renal function are universally monitored in follow-up. The need for anatomic assessment in follow-up is controversial. Some institutions perform anatomic assessment in follow-up only in the presence of uncontrolled high blood pressure or declining renal function. Others perform anatomic assessment by protocol (6-12 months after the procedure and yearly). Duplex ultrasonography is the preferred technique, but CTA may be used according with local expertise. MRA has limited use because of the stent artefact and a tendency to overestimate the degree of stenosis present.

FIBROMUSCULAR DYSPLASIA

FMD accounts for about 10% of all cases of RAS. FMD is most often diagnosed (60%-70% of cases) based on pathognomonic findings in the renal arteries (Fig. 43-2). Approximately 25% of patients have multiple arterial segments involved.[75] Among adults, there is a twofold to tenfold higher prevalence of FMD in women athan in men. There does not appear to be a female predominance in children.[76] Among patients

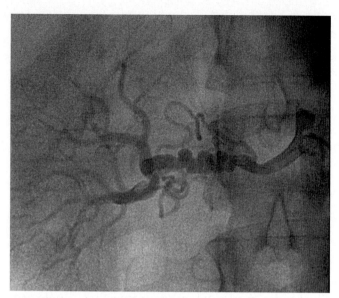

Figure 43-2. Pathognomonic angiographic appearance of fibromuscular dysplasia in the right renal artery.

with renal vascular hypertension, FMD accounts for 35% to 50% of cases in children and 10% to 15% of cases in adults before the age of 50 years.[30,77-80]

FMD of the renal arteries is bilateral in 35% to 50% of cases, and, among those with bilateral disease, almost half have extrarenal involvement.[75,76]

The precise cause of the disease remains unknown. However, a variety of factors have been implicated, including genetic predisposition, hormonal influence, mechanical factors, and ischemia. Fibrous lesions can be seen in different arterial layers and with different compositions. The most common dysplastic lesion is medial fibroplasia (75%-80% of cases), which angiographically is characterized by the classic "string of beads" appearance. This phenomenon is caused by alternating fibromuscular webs and aneurysmal dilation. In areas of aneurysmal dilation, there is absence of the internal elastic lamina, which is possibly the primary defect. The second most common dysplastic lesion is intimal fibroplasia (10%), which is caused by circumferential or eccentric deposition of collagen in the intima. Less frequent dysplastic lesions are perimedial fibroplasia and medial and periarterial hyperplasia.[81,82] Angiographic disease progression occurs in a significant number of patients (>30% of cases in some reports). Despite this, progressive worsening of kidney function and total occlusion of the renal arteries are rare (except for perimedial fibroplasia lesions).[83,84]

Renal FMD should be suspected in the appropriate clinical settings, particularly in women younger than 30 years of age. Hypertension is the most common manifestation of renal artery FMD, but the clinical presentation may include a myriad of symptoms related to other vascular territories. Azotemia symptoms are rarely associated with FMD, because renal artery occlusion and decline of kidney function are infrequent.

The gold standard for evaluating renal artery FMD, as for atherosclerotic RAS, is DSA. Different pathologic lesions have different angiographic patterns. Medial fibroplasia has the classic "string of beads" appearance, with the diameter of the beading larger than the diameter of the artery (aneurysmal). In perimedial fibroplasia, the beads are smaller than the diameter of the artery and less numerous than in medial fibroplasia. Medial hyperplasia and intimal fibroplasia manifest as concentric smooth stenosis, and periarterial fibroplasia shows as sharply localized tubular areas of stenosis.

Noninvasive imaging modalities that are used for the diagnosis of atherosclerotic RAS may be used with FMD of the renal arteries. However, some characteristics specific to FMD must be taken into account when assessing RAS caused by FMD. Renal artery duplex ultrasound can detect elevated blood flow velocities in the middle and distal portions of the artery, the most common locations for FMD.[43,85] Therefore, the value of duplex ultrasound is higher if FMD is suspected as the cause of RAS. CTA and MRA are not accurate techniques to detect stenosis in the distal portions of the renal arteries. Therefore, their use is limited if there is a high degree of suspicion for FMD.[33] Some technical improvements in these techniques may change this scenario in the future.

Patients with suspected renal artery FMD should first undergo renal artery duplex ultrasonography. However, the choice of the noninvasive test should be based on local expertise. If noninvasive tests are inconclusive and the pretest probability of FMD is high, the patient should undergo invasive angiography, using DSA techniques. Renal arteriography arguably could be the first diagnostic test in patients at high risk for renal vascular hypertension secondary to FMD, such as women between the ages of 15 and 50 years. The patient assessment should be limited to noninvasive tests if intervention would not be considered.

The two main rationales for renal artery revascularization, either by surgery or by percutaneous transluminal angioplasty, are control of hypertension and possibly delay or prevention of loss of renal mass, particularly in patients with intimal or perimedial FMD. The reported hypertension cure rate with renal artery revascularization in FMD (by either percutaneous angioplasty or surgery) ranges from 20% to 85%, and a large additional percentage of patients are clinically improved (better blood pressure control and use of fewer antihypertensive agents).[75,86,87] The rate of cure of hypertension may be lower if FMD affects multiple vascular beds or if the intraparenchymal renal vessels are involved. In one report, hypertension was cured after angioplasty in 62% of patients with unilateral, isolated renal FMD but in only 28% of those with systemic FMD.[75] Although revascularization does not reverse cortical thinning and loss of renal mass, limited data suggest that renal function remains stable.[88]

Based on these two rationales, it is generally recommended that the following patients have renal artery revascularization:

- Patients with recent-onset hypertension, in particular younger patients who are less likely to have underlying atherosclerotic disease, in whom the goal is to cure hypertension or significantly reduce the number of antihypertensive medications
- Patients whose blood pressure cannot be lowered to desired ranges despite compliance with a comprehensive medication regimen
- Patients who are unable to tolerate antihypertensive medications or are noncompliant with their medication regimen
- Patients with loss of parenchymal mass from ischemic nephropathy

In patients with relatively well-controlled hypertension, and in those with no loss of renal parenchymal mass, the risks of the procedure may outweigh the benefits. For eligible patients who do not undergo revascularization, it is probably useful to closely monitor blood pressure and renal filtration function and to periodically evaluate renal parenchymal mass.

Percutaneous transluminal angioplasty has largely supplanted surgery for management of significant RAS in FMD. The reported angiographic success rates for percutaneous angioplasty range from 89% to almost 100%.[79,88] Hypertension is usually cured (22%-52%) or improved (22%-74%) but fails to improve in a significant proportion of patients (12%-30%).[79,87,89-93] The rate of restenosis after percutaneous angioplasty ranges from 12% to 25% over follow-up intervals of 6 months to 2 years.[79,94] However, restenosis is not necessarily associated with recurrent hypertension, and recurrent hypertension may not be the result of restenosis. Renal artery stenting is indicated only in cases of suboptimal result with balloon angioplasty or flow-limiting dissection. Stent placement in the distal renal artery may limit the option for surgical revascularization should it become necessary.

Immediate technical success with percutaneous angioplasty is usually determined by visual inspection during the procedure. It may be difficult to determine whether balloon dilation has been adequate if multiple sequential stenoses are present. A number of additional methods are available to assist with the determination of technical success. Physiologic assessment may be performed using a pressure guide wire, with a mean gradient of less than 5 mm Hg across the treated segment suggesting a satisfactory result.[95] Intravascular ultrasound may be used to evaluate the elimination or reduction of various endoluminal defects.[96] Postprocedure renal duplex scanning has also been used to assess the adequacy of intervention. In successfully treated patients, the ratio of renal artery peak systolic velocity to aortic peak systolic velocity (i.e., the renal-aortic ratio, or RAR) decreases to less than 3.5, a value that classifies the diameter stenosis as less than 60%.[97]

The clinical response to percutaneous intervention is also an important indicator of success or failure. No improvement in blood pressure, or an initial improvement followed by recurrence of hypertension a few weeks after percutaneous angioplasty, may be the result of inadequate angioplasty.

Although both surgery and percutaneous angioplasty lead to similar technical success rates,[98,99] surgery is associated with markedly higher morbidity and mortality.[100] Therefore, surgical revascularization is usually reserved for patients who have failed percutaneous angioplasty or whose arterial anatomy is not amenable to percutaneous angioplasty. This includes patients who have disease in secondary branch vessels, a long stenotic segment, or aneurysm and therefore might need complex, sometimes ex vivo, reconstructions.

REFERENCES

1. Grüntzig A, Kuhlmann U, Vetter W, et al: Treatment of renovascular hypertension with percutaneous transluminal dilatation of a renal-artery stenosis. Lancet 1978;1:801-802.
2. Kalra PA, Guo H, Kausz AT, et al: Atherosclerotic renovascular disease in United States patients aged 67 years or older: Risk factors, revascularization, and prognosis. Kidney Int 2005; 68:293-301.
3. Hansen KJ, Edwards MS, Craven TE, et al: Prevalence of renovascular disease in the elderly: A population-based study. J Vasc Surg 2002;36:443-451.
4. Holley KE, Hunt JC, Brown AL Jr, et al: Renal artery stenosis. A clinical-pathologic study in normotensive and hypertensive patients. Am J Med 1964;37:14-22.
5. Sawicki PT, Kaiser S, Heinemann L, et al: Prevalence of renal artery stenosis in diabetes mellitus: An autopsy study. J Intern Med 1991;229:489-492.
6. Uzu T, Inoue T, Fujii T, et al: Prevalence and predictors of renal artery stenosis in patients with myocardial infarction. Am J Kidney Dis 1997;29:733-738.
7. Kuroda S, Nishida N, Uzu T, et al: Prevalence of renal artery stenosis in autopsy patients with stroke. Stroke 2000;31: 61-65.
8. Conlon PJ, Little MA, Pieper K, et al: Severity of renal vascular disease predicts mortality in patients undergoing coronary angiography. Kidney Int 2001;60:1490-1497.
9. Crowley JJ, Santos RM, Peter RH, et al: Progression of renal artery stenosis in patients undergoing cardiac catheterization. Am Heart J 1998;136:913-918.
10. Olin JW, Melia M, Young JR, et al: Prevalence of atherosclerotic renal artery stenosis in patients with atherosclerosis elsewhere. Am J Med 1990;88:46N-51N.
11. Leertouwer TC, Pattynama PM, van den Berg-Huysmans A: Incidental renal artery stenosis in peripheral vascular disease: A case for treatment? Kidney Int 2001;59:1480-1483.
12. Lewin A, Blaufox MD, Castle H, et al: Apparent prevalence of curable hypertension in the Hypertension Detection and Follow-up Program. Arch Intern Med 1985;145:424-427.
13. Mann SJ, Pickering TG: Detection of renovascular hypertension: State of the art—1992. Ann Intern Med 1992;117: 845-853.
14. Appel RG, Bleyer AJ, Reavis S, et al: Renovascular disease in older patients beginning renal replacement therapy. Kidney Int 1995;48:171-176.
15. Mailloux LU, Napolitano B, Bellucci AG, et al: Renal vascular disease causing end-stage renal disease—Incidence, clinical correlates, and outcomes: A 20-year clinical experience. Am J Kidney Dis 1994;24:622-629.
16. van Ampting JM, Penne EL, Beek FJ, et al: Prevalence of atherosclerotic renal artery stenosis in patients starting dialysis. Nephrol Dial Transplant 2003;18:1147-1151.
17. Valderrabano F, Berthoux FC, Jones EH, et al: Report on management of renal failure in Europe XXV: 1994 End stage renal disease and dialysis report. The EDTA-ERA Registry. European Dialysis and Transplant Association–European Renal Association. Nephrol Dial Transplant 1996;11(Suppl)1: 2-21.
18. Fatica RA, Port FK, Young EW: Incidence trends and mortality in end-stage renal disease attributed to renovascular disease in the United States. Am J Kidney Dis 2001;37: 1184-1190.
19. Zierler RE, Bergelin RO, Davidson RC, et al: A prospective study of disease progression in patients with atherosclerotic renal artery stenosis. Am J Hypertens 1996;9:1055-1061.
20. Caps MT, Perissinotto C, Zierler RE, et al: Prospective study of atherosclerotic disease progression in the renal artery. Circulation 1998;98:2866-2872.
21. Caps MT, Zierler RE, Polissar NL, et al: Risk of atrophy in kidneys with atherosclerotic renal artery stenosis. Kidney Int 1998;53:735-742.
22. Chabova V, Schirger A, Stanson AW, et al: Outcomes of atherosclerotic renal artery stenosis managed without revascularization. Mayo Clin Proc 2000;75:437-444.
23. Connolly JO, Higgins RM, Walters HL, et al: Presentation, clinical features and outcome in different patterns of atherosclerotic renovascular disease. Q J Med 1994;87:413-421.
24. Wright JR, Shurrab AE, Cheung C, et al: A prospective study of the determinants of renal functional outcome and mortality in atherosclerotic renovascular disease. Am J Kidney Dis 2002;39:1153-1161.
25. Suresh M, Laboi P, Mamtora H, et al: Relationship of renal dysfunction to proximal arterial disease severity in atherosclerotic renovascular disease. Nephrol Dial Transplant 2000;15:631-636.
26. Turnbull JM: The rational clinical examination: Is listening for abdominal bruits useful in the evaluation of hypertension? JAMA 1995;274:1299-1301.
27. Agarwal M, Lynn KL, Richards AM, et al: Hyponatremic-hypertensive syndrome with renal ischemia: An under-recognized disorder. Hypertension 1999;33:1020-1024.
28. Davis BA, Crook JE, Vestal RE, et al: Prevalence of renovascular hypertension in patients with grade III or IV hypertensive retinopathy. N Engl J Med 1979;301:1273-1276.
29. Svetkey LP, Kadir S, Dunnick NR, et al: Similar prevalence of renovascular hypertension in selected blacks and whites. Hypertension 1991;17:678-683.
30. Krijnen P, van Jaarsveld BC, Steyerberg EW, et al: A clinical prediction rule for renal artery stenosis. Ann Intern Med 1998;129:705-711.
31. Hirsch AT, Haskal ZJ, Hertzer NR, et al: ACC/AHA 2005 Practice Guidelines for the management of patients with peripheral arterial disease (lower extremity, renal, mesenteric, and abdominal aortic): A collaborative report from the American Association for Vascular Surgery/Society for Vascular Surgery, Society for Cardiovascular Angiography and Interventions, Society for Vascular Medicine and Biology, Society of Interventional Radiology, and the ACC/AHA Task Force on Practice Guidelines (Writing Committee to Develop Guidelines for the Management of Patients With Peripheral Arterial Disease). Endorsed by the American Association of Cardiovascular and Pulmonary Rehabilitation; National Heart, Lung, and Blood Institute; Society for Vascular Nursing; TransAtlantic Inter-Society Consensus; and Vascular Disease Foundation. Circulation 2006;113: e463-e654.
32. Hirsch AT, Haskal ZJ, Hertzer NR, et al: ACC/AHA 2005 Practice Guidelines for the management of patients with peripheral arterial disease (lower extremity, renal, mesenteric, and abdominal aortic): Executive summary. A collaborative report from the American Association for Vascular Surgery/Society for Vascular Surgery, Society for Cardiovascular Angiography and Interventions, Society for Vascular Medicine and Biology, Society of Interventional Radiology, and the ACC/AHA Task Force on Practice Guidelines (Writing Committee to Develop Guidelines for the Management of Patients With Peripheral Arterial Disease). Endorsed by the American Association of Cardiovascular and Pulmonary Rehabilitation; National Heart, Lung, and Blood Institute; Society for Vascular Nursing; TransAtlantic Inter-Society Consensus; and Vascular Disease Foundation. J Am Coll Cardiol 2006;47:1239-1312.

33. Vasbinder GB, Nelemans PJ, Kessels AG, et al: Accuracy of computed tomographic angiography and magnetic resonance angiography for diagnosing renal artery stenosis. Ann Intern Med 2004;141:674-682; discussion 682.

34. Textor SC: Pitfalls in imaging for renal artery stenosis. Ann Intern Med 2004;141:730-731.

35. Postma CT, Joosten FB, Rosenbusch G, et al: Magnetic resonance angiography has a high reliability in the detection of renal artery stenosis. Am J Hypertens 1997;10(9 Pt 1):957-963.

36. Rieumont MJ, Kaufman JA, Geller SC, et al: Evaluation of renal artery stenosis with dynamic gadolinium-enhanced MR angiography. AJR Am J Roentgenol 1997;169:39-44.

37. Thornton MJ, Thornton F, O'Callaghan J, et al: Evaluation of dynamic gadolinium-enhanced breath-hold MR angiography in the diagnosis of renal artery stenosis. AJR Am J Roentgenol. 1999;173:1279-1283.

38. Schoenberg SO, Knopp MV, Londy F, et al: Morphologic and functional magnetic resonance imaging of renal artery stenosis: A multireader tricenter study. J Am Soc Nephrol 2002;13:158-169.

39. Wasser MN, Westenberg J, van der Hulst VP, et al: Hemodynamic significance of renal artery stenosis: Digital subtraction angiography versus systolically gated three-dimensional phase-contrast MR angiography. Radiology 1997;202:333-338.

40. Kim TS, Chung JW, Park JH, et al: Renal artery evaluation: Comparison of spiral CT angiography to intra-arterial DSA. J Vasc Interv Radiol 1998;9:553-559.

41. Olbricht CJ, Paul K, Prokop M, et al: Minimally invasive diagnosis of renal artery stenosis by spiral computed tomography angiography. Kidney Int 1995;48:1332-1337.

42. Riehl J, Schmitt H, Bongartz D, et al: Renal artery stenosis: Evaluation with color duplex ultrasonography. Nephrol Dial Transplant 1997;12:1608-1614.

43. Olin JW, Piedmonte MR, Young JR, et al: The utility of duplex ultrasound scanning of the renal arteries for diagnosing significant renal artery stenosis. Ann Intern Med 1995;122:833-838.

44. Soares GM, Murphy TP, Singha MS, et al: Renal artery duplex ultrasonography as a screening and surveillance tool to detect renal artery stenosis: A comparison with current reference standard imaging. J Ultrasound Med 2006;25:293-298.

45. Kawarada O, Yokoi Y, Takemoto K, et al: The performance of renal duplex ultrasonography for the detection of hemodynamically significant renal artery stenosis. Catheter Cardiovasc Interv 2006;68:311-318.

46. Bardelli M, Veglio F, Arosio E, et al: New intrarenal echo-Doppler velocimetric indices for the diagnosis of renal artery stenosis. Kidney Int 2006;69:580-587.

47. Setaro JF, Saddler MC, Chen CC, et al: Simplified captopril renography in diagnosis and treatment of renal artery stenosis. Hypertension 1991;18:289-298.

48. Elliott WJ, Martin WB, Murphy MB: Comparison of two noninvasive screening tests for renovascular hypertension. Arch Intern Med 1993;153:755-764.

49. Roubidoux MA, Dunnick NR, Klotman PE, et al: Renal vein renins: Inability to predict response to revascularization in patients with hypertension. Radiology 1991;178:819-822.

50. Radermacher J, Chavan A, Bleck J, et al: Use of Doppler ultrasonography to predict the outcome of therapy for renal-artery stenosis. N Engl J Med 2001;344:410-417.

51. Ikee R, Kobayashi S, Hemmi N, et al: Correlation between the resistive index by Doppler ultrasound and kidney function and histology. Am J Kidney Dis 2005;46:603-609.

52. Voiculescu A, Schmitz M, Plum J, et al: Duplex ultrasound and renin ratio predict treatment failure after revascularization for renal artery stenosis. Am J Hypertens 2006;19:756-763.

53. Cheung CM, Shurrab AE, Buckley DL, et al: MR-derived renal morphology and renal function in patients with atherosclerotic renovascular disease. Kidney Int 2006;69:715-722.

54. Murphy TP, Soares G, Kim M: Increase in utilization of percutaneous renal artery interventions by Medicare beneficiaries, 1996-2000. AJR Am J Roentgenol 2004;183:561-568.

55. van Jaarsveld BC, Krijnen P, Pieterman H, et al: The effect of balloon angioplasty on hypertension in atherosclerotic renal-artery stenosis. Dutch Renal Artery Stenosis Intervention Cooperative Study Group. N Engl J Med 2000;342:1007-1014.

56. Plouin PF, Chatellier G, Darne B, et al: Blood pressure outcome of angioplasty in atherosclerotic renal artery stenosis: A randomized trial. Essai Multicentrique Medicaments vs. Angioplastie (EMMA) Study Group. Hypertension 1998;31:823-829.

57. Webster J, Marshall F, Abdalla M, et al: Randomized comparison of percutaneous angioplasty vs. continued medical therapy for hypertensive patients with atheromatous renal artery stenosis. Scottish and Newcastle Renal Artery Stenosis Collaborative Group. J Hum Hypertens 1998;12:329-335.

58. Nordmann AJ, Woo K, Parkes R, et al: Balloon angioplasty or medical therapy for hypertensive patients with atherosclerotic renal artery stenosis? A meta-analysis of randomized controlled trials. Am J Med 2003;114:44-50.

59. Krijnen P, van Jaarsveld BC, Hunink MG, et al: The effect of treatment on health-related quality of life in patients with hypertension and renal artery stenosis. J Hum Hypertens 2005;19:467-470.

60. Rocha-Singh K, Jaff MR, Rosenfield K: Evaluation of the safety and effectiveness of renal artery stenting after unsuccessful balloon angioplasty: The ASPIRE-2 study. J Am Coll Cardiol 2005;46:776-783.

61. Leertouwer TC, Gussenhoven EJ, Bosch JL, et al: Stent placement for renal arterial stenosis: Where do we stand? A meta-analysis. Radiology 2000;216:78-85.

62. van de Ven PJ, Kaatee R, Beutler JJ, et al: Arterial stenting and balloon angioplasty in ostial atherosclerotic renovascular disease: A randomized trial. Lancet 1999;353:282-286.

63. Zeller T, Frank U, Muller C, et al: Predictors of improved renal function after percutaneous stent-supported angioplasty of severe atherosclerotic ostial renal artery stenosis. Circulation 2003;108:2244-2249.

64. Burket MW, Cooper CJ, Kennedy DJ, et al: Renal artery angioplasty and stent placement: Predictors of a favorable outcome. Am Heart J 2000;139(1 Pt 1):64-71.

65. Zeller T, Rastan A, Rothenpieler U, et al: Restenosis after stenting of atherosclerotic renal artery stenosis: Is there a rationale for the use of drug-eluting stents? Catheter Cardiovasc Interv 2006;68:125-130.

66. Sapoval M, Zahringer M, Pattynama P, et al: Low-profile stent system for treatment of atherosclerotic renal artery stenosis: The GREAT trial. J Vasc Interv Radiol 2005;16:1195-1202.

67. Henry M, Henry I, Klonaris C, et al: Renal angioplasty and stenting under protection: The way for the future? Catheter Cardiovasc Interv 2003;60:299-312.

68. Holden A, Hill A: Renal angioplasty and stenting with distal protection of the main renal artery in ischemic nephropathy: Early experience. J Vasc Surg 2003;38:962-968.

69. Holden A, Hill A, Jaff MR, et al: Renal artery stent revascularization with embolic protection in patients with ischemic nephropathy. Kidney Int 2006;70:948-955.

70. Cooper CJ, Murphy TP, Matsumoto A, et al: Stent revascularization for the prevention of cardiovascular and renal events among patients with renal artery stenosis and systolic hypertension: Rationale and design of the CORAL trial. Am Heart J 2006;152:59-66.

71. Scarpioni R, Michieletti E, Cristinelli L, et al: Atherosclerotic renovascular disease—Medical therapy versus medical therapy plus renal artery stenting in preventing renal failure progression: The rationale and study design of a prospective, multicenter and randomized trial (NITER). J Nephrol 2005;18:423-428.

72. Angioplasty and Stent for Renal Arterial Lesions (ASTRAL) trial. Available at: http://www.astral.bham.ac.uk/trial/protocol/ (accessed April 12, 2007).

73. Berkompas DC: Abciximab combined with angioplasty in a patient with renal artery stent subacute thrombosis. Cathet Cardiovasc Diagn 1998;45:272-274.

74. Allie DE, Hall P, Shammas NW, et al: The Angiomax Peripheral Procedure Registry of Vascular Events Trial (APPROVE):

In-hospital and 30-day results. J Invasive Cardiol 2004;16: 651-656.

75. Luscher TF, Keller HM, Imhof HG, et al: Fibromuscular hyperplasia: Extension of the disease and therapeutic outcome. Results of the University Hospital Zurich Cooperative Study on Fibromuscular Hyperplasia. Nephron 1986;44(Suppl 1):109-114.

76. Estepa R, Gallego N, Orte L, et al: Renovascular hypertension in children. Scand J Urol Nephrol 2001;35:388-392.

77. Deal JE, Snell MF, Barratt TM, et al: Renovascular disease in childhood. J Pediatr 1992;121:378-384.

78. Piercy KT, Hundley JC, Stafford JM, et al: Renovascular disease in children and adolescents. J Vasc Surg 2005;41: 973-982.

79. Klow NE, Paulsen D, Vatne K, et al: Percutaneous transluminal renal artery angioplasty using the coaxial technique: Ten years of experience from 591 procedures in 419 patients. Acta Radiol 1998;39:594-603.

80. Pascual A, Bush HS, Copley JB: Renal fibromuscular dysplasia in elderly persons. Am J Kidney Dis 2005;45:e63-e66.

81. Stanley JC, Gewertz BL, Bove EL, et al: Arterial fibrodysplasia: Histopathologic character and current etiologic concepts. Arch Surg 1975;110:561-566.

82. Harrison EG Jr, McCormack LJ: Pathologic classification of renal arterial disease in renovascular hypertension. Mayo Clin Proc 1971;46:161-167.

83. Kincaid OW, Davis GD, Hallermann FJ, et al: Fibromuscular dysplasia of the renal arteries: Arteriographic features, classification, and observations on natural history of the disease. Am J Roentgenol Radium Ther Nucl Med 1968;104: 271-282.

84. Schreiber MJ, Pohl MA, Novick AC: The natural history of atherosclerotic and fibrous renal artery disease. Urol Clin North Am 1984;11:383-392.

85. Carman TL, Olin JW, Czum J: Noninvasive imaging of the renal arteries. Urol Clin North Am 2001;28:815-826.

86. Slovut DP, Olin JW: Fibromuscular dysplasia. N Engl J Med 2004;350:1862-1871.

87. Bonelli FS, McKusick MA, Textor SC, et al: Renal artery angioplasty: Technical results and clinical outcome in 320 patients. Mayo Clin Proc 1995;70:1041-1052.

88. Mounier-Vehier C, Haulon S, Devos P, et al: Renal atrophy outcome after revascularization in fibromuscular dysplasia disease. J Endovasc Ther 2002;9:605-613.

89. Birrer M, Do DD, Mahler F, et al: Treatment of renal artery fibromuscular dysplasia with balloon angioplasty: A prospective follow-up study. Eur J Vasc Endovasc Surg 2002;23: 146-152.

90. Surowiec SM, Sivamurthy N, Rhodes JM, et al: Percutaneous therapy for renal artery fibromuscular dysplasia. Ann Vasc Surg 2003;17:650-655.

91. Jensen G, Zachrisson BF, Delin K, et al: Treatment of renovascular hypertension: One year results of renal angioplasty. Kidney Int 1995;48:1936-1945.

92. Davidson RA, Barri Y, Wilcox CS: Predictors of cure of hypertension in fibromuscular renovascular disease. Am J Kidney Dis 1996;28:334-338.

93. de Fraissinette B, Garcier JM, Dieu V, et al: Percutaneous transluminal angioplasty of dysplastic stenoses of the renal artery: Results on 70 adults. Cardiovasc Intervent Radiol 2003;26:46-51.

94. Oertle M, Do DD, Baumgartner I, et al: Discrepancy of clinical and angiographic results in the follow-up of percutaneous transluminal renal angioplasty (PTRA). Vasa 1998;27: 154-157.

95. Gross CM, Kramer J, Weingartner O, et al: Determination of renal arterial stenosis severity: Comparison of pressure gradient and vessel diameter. Radiology 2001;220:751-756.

96. Gowda MS, Loeb AL, Crouse LJ, et al: Complementary roles of color-flow duplex imaging and intravascular ultrasound in the diagnosis of renal artery fibromuscular dysplasia: Should renal arteriography serve as the "gold standard"? J Am Coll Cardiol 2003;41:1305-1311.

97. Edwards JM, Zaccardi MJ, Strandness DE Jr: A preliminary study of the role of duplex scanning in defining the adequacy of treatment of patients with renal artery fibromuscular dysplasia. J Vasc Surg 1992;15:604-609; discussion 609-611.

98. Reiher L, Pfeiffer T, Sandmann W: Long-term results after surgical reconstruction for renal artery fibromuscular dysplasia. Eur J Vasc Endovasc Surg 2000;20:556-559.

99. Marekovic Z, Mokos I, Krhen I, et al: Long-term outcome after surgical kidney revascularization for fibromuscular dysplasia and atherosclerotic renal artery stenosis. J Urol 2004; 171:1043-1045.

100. Mackrell PJ, Langan EM 3rd, Sullivan TM, et al: Management of renal artery stenosis: Effects of a shift from surgical to percutaneous therapy on indications and outcomes. Ann Vasc Surg 2003;17:54-59.

44 Aortic Vascular Interventions (Thoracic and Abdominal)

Christoph A. Nienaber and Hüseyin Ince

KEY POINTS

- Acute aortic dissection is an uncommon but potentially catastrophic illness that occurs with an incidence of approximately 2.9/1000,000/year, with at least 7000 cases per year in the United States.
- The exact role of percutaneous stent-grafting in the treatment of aortic dissection is not fully established yet.
- Aortic stent-grafts are primarily used to reconstruct the compressed true lumen cranial to major aortic branches and to increase distal aortic flow. Therefore, proximal communications should be sealed to direct flow into the true lumen, depressurize the false lumen, and induce thrombosis in the false lumen with fibrotic transformation and subsequent remodeling of the aortic wall.
- Recent reports suggest that percutaneous stent-graft placement in the dissected aorta is safer and produces better results than surgery for type B dissection.
- The use of endovascular stent-grafts for repair of thoracic aortic aneurysms (TAAs) is emerging as a promising, less invasive therapeutic alternative to conventional surgical treatment.
- The evaluation of a patient for repair of a TAA considers the patient's overall risk profile, evidence of rapid enlargement of the aneurysm, diameter equal to or greater than 5.5 cm, and presence of symptoms. The suitability of the patient for endovascular repair is based on both clinical and anatomic considerations.
- Endoleaks are the most prevalent of TAA stent-graft treatment complications. Treatment options include transcatheter coil or glue embolization, balloon angioplasty, placement of endovascular graft extensions, and open repair.
- The key features of endovascular repair of abdominal aortic aneurysms (AAAs) that determines procedural success and long-term outcomes are proximal and distal fixation and sealing. Most of the devices use a metal skeleton throughout the graft that is made from stainless steel, nitinol, or Elgiloy.

AORTIC DISSECTION

INTERVENTIONAL TREATMENT OF AORTIC DISSECTION

Acute aortic dissection is an uncommon but potentially catastrophic illness that occurs with an incidence of approximately 2.9/100,000/year, with at least 7000 cases per year in the United States. Early mortality is as high as 1% per hour if untreated, but survival may be significantly improved by the timely institution of appropriate therapy. Prompt clinical recognition and definitive diagnostic testing are therefore essential in the management of aortic dissection. Conventional treatment of Stanford type A (De Bakey type I and II) dissection (Fig. 44-1) consists of surgical reconstruction of the ascending aorta with complete or partial resection of the dissected aortic segment. Therefore, in type A dissections, interventional endovascular strategies have no clinical application except to relieve critical malperfusion before surgery of the ascending aorta by distal endovascular interventions in cases of thoracoabdominal extension of a proximal dissection (De Bakey type I) with distal ischemic complications.

Conversely, stent-graft placement aims at remodeling of the thoracic descending aorta, typically in Stanford type B dissection, by sealing one (or multiple) proximal entry tears with a Dacron-covered stent, thus initiating thrombosis of the false lumen.[1-4] In addition, reconstruction of a collapsed true lumen might result in re-establishment of side branch flow (Fig. 44-2). Various scenarios of malperfusion syndrome are amenable to endovascular management. These include static or dynamic (by intima invagination) collapse of the aortic true lumen (so-called pseudocoarctation (Fig. 44-3); static or dynamic

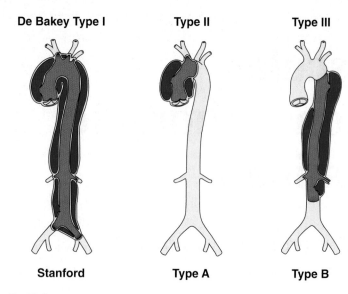

De Bakey Type I   Type II   Type III

Stanford   Type A   Type B

De Bakey

Type I   Originates in the ascending aorta, propagates at least to the aortic arch and often beyond it distally

Type II   Originates in and is confined to the ascending aorta

Type III   Originates in the descending aorta and extends distally down the aorta or, rarely, retrograde into the aortic arch and ascending aorta

Stanford

Type A   All dissections involving the ascending aorta, regardless of the site of origin

Type B   All dissections not involving the ascending aorta

Figure 44-1. The most common classifications of thoracic aortic dissection: Stanford and DeBakey.

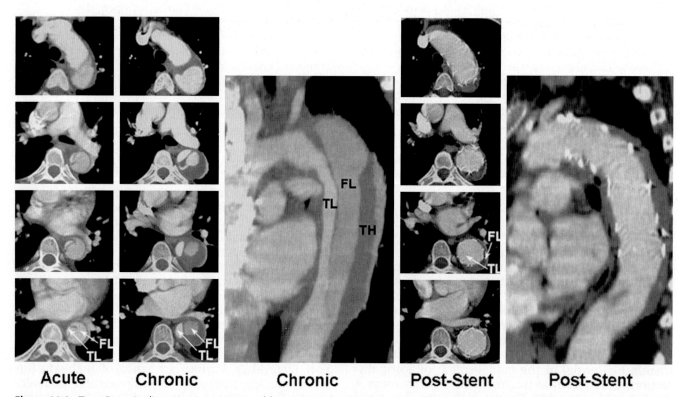

Acute   **Chronic**   **Chronic**   **Post-Stent**   **Post-Stent**

Figure 44-2. Type B aortic dissection in a 48-year-old man; note the dynamic obstruction of the true lumen (TL) in the acute phase. After stent-graft placement across the proximal thoracic entry, the entire true lumen of the thoracic aorta is reconstructed with time, with complete "healing" of the dissected aortic wall and shrinking of the completely thrombosed false lumen (FL). TH, thrombus.

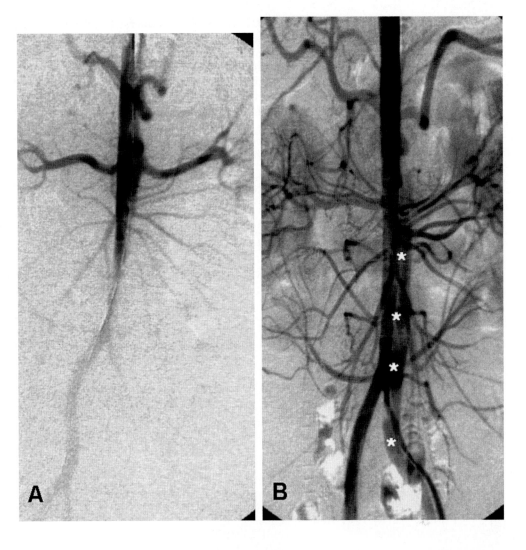

Figure 44-3. Digital subtraction angiography in thoracoabdominal type B dissection. **A,** Dynamic obstruction of the true lumen distally to the renal arteries causing malperfusion of the mesentery and both lower extremities. **B,** At follow-up (3 months after stent-graft placement in the proximal descending aorta), the true lumen has widened as a consequence of aortic remodeling and the patient is asymptomatic. However, the false lumen (white stars) in the abdominal aorta is not completely thrombosed.

occlusion of one or more vital side branches, and enlarging false aneurysm due to patent proximal entry tear.

Although peripheral pulse deficits can be acutely reversed with surgical repair of the dissected thoracic aorta in many cases, patients with signs of mesenteric or renal ischemia do not fare well. Mortality of patients with renal ischemia is 50% to 70%, and as high as 87% with mesenteric ischemia.[5-7] Surgical mortality rates in patients with acute peripheral vascular ischemic complications are similar to those of patients with mesenteric ischemia, reaching an 89% in-hospital mortality rate.[8-11] Operative mortality of surgical fenestration varies from 21% to 61%, which has encouraged percutaneous interventional management by endovascular balloon fenestration of a dissecting aortic membrane to treat mesenteric ischemia, a concept discussed as a niche indication in such complicated cases of malperfusion.[10-12]

Management of Stanford type B (De Bakey type III) dissection with the use of endovascular stent-grafts is evolving slowly in anticipation of an unknown risk of paraplegia from spinal artery occlusion, as seen in up to 18% of cases after open surgery.[11,12] With further technical improvement, a large series of patients has now been successfully treated in various specialized centers by endovascular stent-graft placement covering entry tears in the descending aorta and even in the aortic arch. Recent studies have demonstrated that closure of proximal entry tears is essential to reconstruct the aortic wall and reduce total aortic diameter. Entry tear closure promotes depressurization of the false lumen, thrombus formation in the false lumen (Fig. 44-4), and remodeling of the entire aorta.[2,3,12] In the near future, combined surgical and interventional procedures even for proximal dissection are likely to evolve.[13-15]

Current Indications for Endovascular Aortic Interventions

The exact role of percutaneous stent-grafting in the treatment of aortic dissection is not fully established yet. There appears to be a role for interventional management in the treatment of static or dynamic obstruction of aortic branch arteries. Static obstruction of a branch can be overcome by placing endovascular stents in the ostium of a compromised side branch, and dynamic obstruction may benefit from stents in the aortic true lumen, sometimes combined with side branch stenting and preferentially without any additional balloon fenestration, because fenestration does not improve stress and tension on the thin aortic wall.[16] Sometimes, bare stents deployed from the true lumen into side branches are useful to buttress the flap in a stable position.[17] In rare cases, fenestration may be helpful to create a reentry tear for the dead-end false lumen back into the true lumen, with the aim of preventing thrombosis of the false lumen and compromise of branches fed exclusively from the false lumen—however, this concept lacks clinical proof of benefit. Conversely, fenestration increases the long-term risk of aortic rupture, because a large reentry tear promotes flow in the false lumen and provides the basis for its aneurysmal expansion. There is also a risk of peripheral embolism from a patent but partly thrombosed false lumen.[17,18]

The most effective method to avoid an enlarging false lumen is the sealing of proximal entry tears with a customized stent-graft (Fig. 44-5); the absence of a distal reentry tear is desirable for optimal results but is not a prerequisite. Compression of the true aortic lumen cranial to the main abdominal branches with distal malperfusion (pseudocoarctation) is usually corrected by stent-grafts that expand the compressed true lumen and improve distal aortic blood flow.[2,3,10,12] Depressurization and shrinking of the false lumen is the most beneficial result to be gained, ideally followed by complete thrombosis of the false lumen and remodeling of the entire dissected aorta (see Fig. 44-2), in rare occasions even in retrograde type A dissection.[14]

Similar to previously accepted indications for open surgical repair in complicated type B dissection, scenarios such as intractable pain with descending dissection, rapidly expanding false lumen diameter, extra-aortic blood collection as a sign of imminent

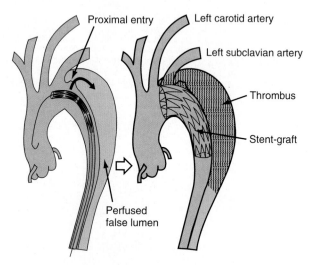

Figure 44-4. Concept of interventional reconstruction of the dissected aorta with sealing of the proximal entries, depressurization of the false lumen, and initiation of false lumen thrombosis.

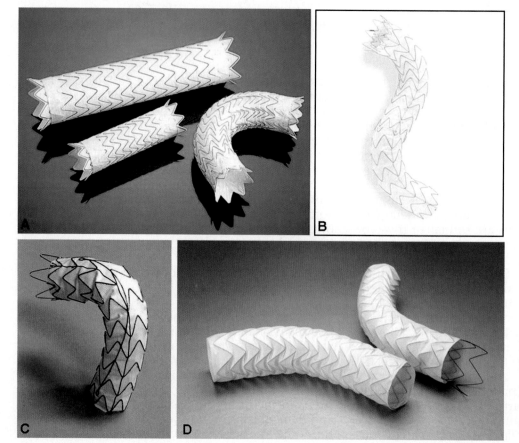

Figure 44-5. A selection of thoracic stent-grafts from American manufacturers currently available in Europe: **A,** TAG (Gore); **B,** Valiant (Medtronic AVE); **C,** Relay Thoracic Stent-Graft (Bolton Medical); **D,** EndoFit (LeMaitre Vascular).

Table 44-1. Considerations for Surgical, Medical, and Interventional Therapy in Aortic Pathologies

Surgery
Treatment of choice in acute type A dissection
Acute type B dissection complicated by the following:
  Retrograde extension into the ascending aorta
  Dissection in Marfan's syndrome
  Rupture or impending rupture (historically classic indication)
  Progression with compromise of vital organs

Medical therapy
Treatment of choice in uncomplicated type B dissection
Stable, isolated arch dissection
Stable type B dissection (chronic, ≥2 wk since onset)

Interventional therapy
Stent-grafts to seal entry to false lumen of aortic dissection and to
  enlarge compressed true lumen
  Complicated (unstable) type B dissection
  Malperfusion syndrome (proximal aortic stent-graft and/or distal
    fenestration/stenting of branch arteries)
  Stable type B dissection (under study)
Stent-grafts to exclude thoracic aortic aneurysm (≥5.5 cm)
Stent-grafts to cover perforating aortic ulcers (especially deep,
  progressive ulcers)
Stent-grafts to reconstruct the thoracic aorta after traumatic injury
Stent-grafts as an emergency treatment of evolving or imminent
  aortic rupture

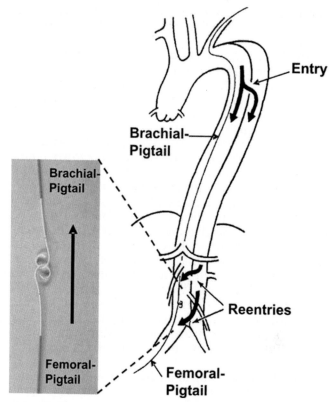

Figure 44-6. "Embracing pigtails" technique to ensure navigation of the guide wire in the true lumen before stent-graft placement. See text for details.

rupture, and distal malperfusion syndrome are at present accepted indications for emergent stent-graft placement.[15,17-19] Moreover, even late onset of complications such as malperfusion of vital aortic side branches is likely to justify endovascular stent-grafting of an occlusive lamella to improve distal true lumen flow as a first option, with surgery employed only after an unsuccessful attempt, considering that surgical repair failed to prove superior to interventional treatment even in uncomplicated cases; in complicated cases, the concept of endoluminal treatment is currently replacing open surgery in advanced aortic centers.[1-3,17-20] A summary of potential treatment options is listed in Table 44-1.

Technique of Aortic Stent-Graft Placement

Aortic stent-grafts are primarily used to reconstruct the compressed true lumen cranial to major aortic branches and to increase distal aortic flow. Therefore, proximal communications should be sealed to direct flow into the true lumen, depressurize the false lumen, and induce thrombosis in the false lumen with fibrotic transformation and subsequent remodeling of the aortic wall. Stent-graft placement across the origin of the celiac, superior mesenteric, and renal arteries may lead to fatal organ failure.

Based on the measurements obtained during angiography, transesophageal echography (mandatory for detection of small entries), contrast-enhanced spiral computed tomographic (CT) scanning (the best technique for unstable patients in an emergency situation), magnetic resonance (MR) angiography (contraindicated for patients with pacemakers or implantable defibrillators), or intravascular ultra-

sound, customized stent-grafts are available to both scaffold up to 20 cm of dissected aorta and cover major tears. The procedure is best performed in the catheterization and imaging laboratory using digital angiography and general anesthesia.

The femoral artery is the most popular access-site and can usually accommodate a 24-Fr stent-graft system. In the Seldinger technique, a 260-cm stiff wire is placed over a pigtail catheter that is navigated with a soft wire in the true lumen under both fluoroscopic and transesophageal ultrasound guidance. In complex cases with multiple reentries in the abdominal aorta, the "embracement technique," using two pigtail catheters, is useful (Fig. 44-6). A pigtail catheter that has been installed in the true aortic lumen via the left brachial artery picks up the femoral pigtail catheter in the true lumen of the abdominal aorta and pulls it up into the aortic arch. This procedure ensures definite positioning of the stiff guide wire in the true lumen, which is essential for correct deployment of the stent-graft. The stent is carefully advanced over the stiff wire, and the launching of the stent-graft is performed with systolic blood pressure lowered to 50 to 60 mm Hg by infusion of sodium nitroprusside or by rapid right ventricular pacing to prevent dislodgement.[21,22] After deployment, short inflation of a latex balloon can improve apposition of the stent struts to the aortic wall, but only if proximal sealing of thoracic communications is incomplete. Both Doppler ultrasound and contrast fluoroscopy are instrumental for documenting the immediate result or initiating adjunctive maneuvers.

For thoracic aortic aneurysm or ulcers the navigation of wires and instruments is easier, but dual imaging using ultrasound and fluoroscopy simultaneously is equally important. A frequent anatomic consideration is the short distance between the origin of the left subclavian artery (LSA) and the primary tear in type B dissections. Coverage of the ostium to the LSA has to be accepted at times to perform endovascular aortic repair in this aortic pathology adjacent to the LSA. According to observational evidence, prophylactic surgical maneuvers are not imperatively and always required for safety reasons but may be relegated to an elective measure after an endovascular aortic intervention if intolerable signs or symptoms of ischemia occur.[23] However, before intentional LSA occlusion, careful attention must be paid to potential supra-aortic variants (e.g., presence of a lusorian artery, a nonintact vertebral-basilar system, dominant left vertebral artery) that originate directly from the aortic arch and other pathologies recognized during preinterventional vascular staging.

Interventional Therapy in an Elective Setting

Recent reports suggest that percutaneous stent-graft placement in the dissected aorta is safer and produces better results than surgery for type B dissection.[24] Paraplegia may occur after use of multiple stent-grafts, but this still appears to be a rare phenomenon, especially when the stented segment does not exceed 16 cm. Results of short-term follow-up are excellent, with a 1-year survival rate of greater than 90%; tears can be readapted, and aortic diameters typically decrease with complete thrombosis of the false lumen. This suggests that stent placement may facilitate healing of the dissection, sometimes of the entire aorta, including abdominal segments (see Fig. 44-2). However, late reperfusion of the false lumen has been observed occasionally, underlining the need for stringent MR or CT follow-up imaging. Postinterventional imaging should be done 3 months and 12 months after the procedure, followed by further examinations at yearly intervals. In some patients, follow-up imaging has revealed tears that were initially overlooked but required additional stents.

Interventional Therapy in an Emergent Setting

Established criteria for endovascular treatment of acute type B aortic dissection. especially if emergent stent-graft placement is considered,[24-26] are as follows:

1. Identification of a least one patent primary entry tear in the descending thoracic aorta
2. Major tear located in the descending aorta proximal to the tenth thoracic vertebra
3. Absence of severe dilatation (>40 mm in diameter) and/or severe atherosclerotic alterations in the landing zone for stent-grafting

4. Exclusion of severe aortic regurgitation
5. Exclusion of coronary artery or aortic arch branch ischemia
6. Femoral and iliac arteries of sufficient size and quality (absence of kinking or significant stenosis) to permit passage of at least a 22-Fr catheter (vessel diameter ≥7.5 mm)

In recent reports, patients treated by emergent endovascular aortic repair of dissection were compared with controls subjected to conventional therapy. In all patients with acute type B aortic dissection complicated by loss of blood into the periaortic space, procedures were performed successfully with no evidence of periprocedural morbidity, leakage was aborted, and eventually successful reconstruction of the dissected aorta occurred; at a mean follow up of 15±6 months, no deaths had occurred in the stent-graft group, whereas four patients had died in the conventional treatment group.[18,27,28] Also, as previously seen in elective endovascular procedures, emergent aortic dissection stent-grafting was not associated with excessive peripheral or neurologic complications.[18]

Nevertheless, although patients with postsurgery aortic dissection who receive stent-grafts seem to show better outcome than those in whom a second surgical intervention is attempted,[29] endovascular repair in impending rupture or para-aortic leakage has not yet proved to be always effective. However, with endovascular aortic stenting and sometimes additional use of bare stents in aortic side branches, compromised flow can be restored in more than 90% (range, 92% to 100%) of vessels obstructed from aortic dissection. The average 30-day mortality rate is 10% (range, 0% to 25%), and additional surgical revascularization is rarely needed.[30] Most patients remain asymptomatic over a mean follow-up time of about 1 year. Fatalities related to the interventional procedure may occur as a result of nonreversible ischemic complications, progression of the dissection, or complications of additional reconstructive surgical procedures on the thoracic aorta.[1-3,17,20] Potential problems may arise from unpredictable hemodynamic alterations in the true and false lumina after fenestration and side branch stenting. These alterations can result in loss of previously well perfused arteries or loss of initially salvaged side branches.

Conclusion

The emergence of endovascular stent-grafting as an alternative therapy to the classic, formerly used open surgical repair of aortic dissection is an exciting new field. Although it is apparent that patients at high surgical risk will benefit from endovascular technology, the exact role of stent-grafting remains to be defined as long-term data and experience continue to accumulate and as devices and techniques evolve. Instead of replacing conventional surgical treatment completely, endovascular repair will likely play a complementary role and offer a less invasive option in the treatment armamentarium. It is clear that the limitations of both approaches are distinct. Although what is considered high risk for surgery is defined by clinical parameters in terms of comorbidities, contraindications for endovascular stent-graft treatment are defined by anatomic constraints. In this regard, both strategies will continue to coexist and may even merge to generate hybrid procedures.

DESCENDING THORACIC AORTIC ANEURYSM

Endovascular Repair by Stent-Grafts

Aortic aneurysms, both thoracic and abdominal, occur predominantly in the elderly and therefore have been increasing in incidence as the population ages and diagnostic capabilities advance.[31] With an incidence of 6 to 10 per 100,000 person-years, thoracic aortic aneurysms (TAAs) are less common than abdominal aortic aneurysms (AAAs) but remain life-threatening.[31,32] The natural history of TAAs is one of progressive expansion and weakening of the aortic wall, leading to eventual rupture.[33-35] With an associated mortality rate of 94%, TAA rupture is usually a fatal event.[32,36] The 5-year survival rate of unoperated TAA patients approximates 13%, whereas 70% to 79% of those who undergo elective

surgical intervention are alive at 5 years.[37-39] The risk of rupture mandates consideration for surgical treatment in all patients who are suitable candidates for operation. The use of endovascular stent-grafts for repair of TAAs is emerging as a promising, less invasive therapeutic alternative to conventional surgical treatment.

Endovascular treatment of aortic aneurysms is achieved by transluminal placement of one or more stent-graft devices across the longitudinal extent of the lesion (Fig 44-7). The prosthesis bridges the aneurysmal sac to exclude it from high-pressure aortic blood flow, thereby allowing for sac thrombosis around the endograft and possible remodeling of the aortic wall. Although the advent and ensuing rapid evolution of endovascular aortic repair techniques occurred initially in cases of AAA, efforts to adapt this technology for the thoracic aorta are ongoing. As is the case for AAA, a less invasive approach to TAA repair is highly desirable, because the patient population tends to be elderly and harbors multiple comorbidities.[35,39,40] Continued development of endovascular therapy for thoracic aneurysms is likely to provide greater benefits in patient outcomes than those observed with AAAs. Conventional surgical treatment of TAA is physiologically more demanding and

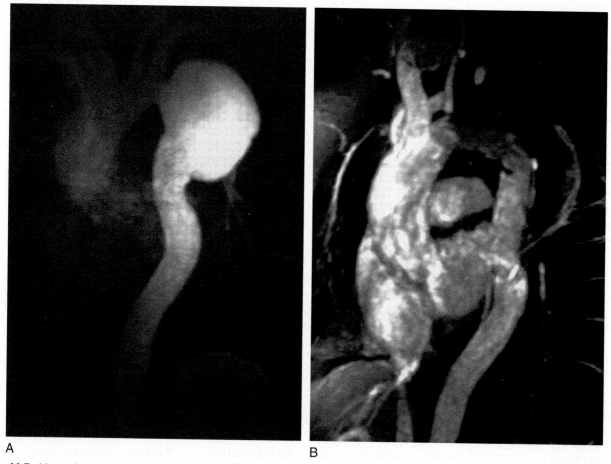

A   B

Figure 44-7. Magnetic resonance angiography before (**A**) and 16 months after (**B**) stent-graft exclusion of aneurysm late after surgical correction of aortic coarctation. Left subclavian artery is occluded without symptoms; aneurysm is completely thrombosed and shrunk.

carries a greater operative risk. It mandates open thoracotomy, aortic cross-clamping, resection of the aneurysm, and replacement with a prosthetic graft, and it often requires cardiopulmonary bypass.[41] Despite advances in operative technique, intraoperative monitoring, and postoperative care, the mortality and morbidity of surgery remain substantial and less favorable than outcomes for open AAA repair. Mortality for TAA surgical repair ranges from 5% to 20% in elective cases and up to 50% in emergent situations.[39,42-46] Major complications associated with surgical TAA treatment include renal and pulmonary failure, visceral and cardiac ischemia, stroke, and paraplegia. Paraplegia is a particularly devastating complication that is almost unique to the surgical treatment of thoracic aneurysms, occurring in 5% to 25% of cases, compared with less than 1% for AAAs.[37,39,45-48] For these reasons, a significant population of TAA patients are not candidates for open repair and have been without a treatment option until recently.

Endovascular aneurysm repair of the thoracic aorta is currently focused on the descending portion. Approximately half of TAAs are located in the descending thoracic aorta.[32,40] Anatomically, this aortic segment provides a substrate more amenable for endovascular stent-graft repair given its avoidance of the great vessels proximally and major visceral branches and aortic bifurcation distally. Despite these anatomic advantages and the ability to draw from early experiences with endovascular AAA repair, the development of stent-grafting in the thoracic aorta has progressed more slowly than that of its infrarenal counterpart. The thoracic aorta poses several unique challenges that have impeded simple adaptation of endovascular devices and techniques developed for the abdominal aorta.[49] First, the hemodynamic forces of the thoracic aorta are significantly more aggressive and place greater mechanical demands on thoracic endografts. The potential for device migration, kinking, and late structural failures are important concerns. Second, greater flexibility is required of thoracic devices to conform to the natural curvature of the proximal descending aorta and to lesions with tortuous morphology. Third, because larger devices are necessary to accommodate the diameter of the thoracic aorta, arterial access is more problematic. This is an important concern because a greater proportion of TAA patients, compared with AAA patients, are women, and in women access vessels tend to be smaller. Fourth, as with conventional open TAA repair, paraplegia remains a potential complication in the endovascular approach despite the absence of aortic cross-clamping.[50,51] Lastly, TAAs often extend beyond the boundaries of the descending thoracic aorta and involve more proximal or distal aorta than desired. Management of the LSA, in particular, has gained considerable attention.[52-54]

With these challenges in mind, significant progress has been achieved since the first stent-graft was deployed for TAA exclusion in 1992.[23,50,55]

Technical Aspects of Endovascular Repair

Early clinical experiences with stent-grafting of the thoracic aorta were based on the use of first-generation, homemade devices that were rigid and required large delivery systems (24 to 27 Fr).[55,56] Since then, several commercial manufacturers of abdominal endografts have created derivatives for the thoracic aorta with dramatic improvements over homemade devices. The endoprostheses are composed of a stent (nitinol or stainless steel) covered with fabric (polyester or polytetrafluoroethylene [PTFE]).

The evaluation of a patient for repair of a TAA considers the patient's overall risk profile, evidence of rapid enlargement of the aneurysm, diameter greater than or equal to 5.5 cm, and presence of symptoms. The suitability of the patient for endovascular repair is based on both clinical and anatomic considerations. Preprocedural imaging is essential to fully characterize the lesion and access route. Detailed imaging evaluation can be obtained with spiral CT or MR imaging. Measurements from imaging data are used to select the appropriate device diameter and length.

Determination of aneurysm location in relation to the LSA and celiac axis is of utmost importance. Successful TAA exclusion requires normal segments of native aorta at both ends of the lesion (the so-called landing zone or neck) of at least 15 to 25 mm to ensure adequate contact between the endoprosthesis and the aortic wall and formation of a tight circumferential seal. Landing zones that are markedly angled or conical or that contain thrombus can result in poor fixation. Devices are oversized by 10% in diameter to provide sufficient radial force for adequate fixation.

The vascular access route for device introduction and delivery to the pathologic target must be of sufficient size and of suitable morphology. Stent-grafts are most commonly introduced through the femoral artery. Small-diameter, tortuous, or excessively calcified iliac arteries may preclude such access, requiring more proximal retroperitoneal exposure and direct cannulation of or creation of a graft conduit to the common iliac or abdominal aorta. Additionally, severe stenosis and tortuosity of the abdominal and thoracic aorta distal to the target are contraindications for endovascular repair.

Despite these criteria, treatment failures can occur, but the specific contributing factors and frequencies are currently unknown, particularly over the long term. Therefore, follow-up surveillance with serial CT scans at 1, 6, and 12 months and annually thereafter is recommended to monitor changes in aneurysm morphology, identify device failures, and detect endoleaks.

Clinical Experience

The literature on thoracic stent-grafting consists mostly of small to medium-sized case series with short- to medium-term follow-up (Table 44-2). Nev-

Table 44-2. Summary Data on Studies of Endovascular Repair of TAA

Author, Year (Ref. No.)	N	Mean Follow-Up (mo)	Devices	Technical Success	30-Day Mortality (%)	Long-Term Survival (%)	Paraplegia (%)	Endoleak (%)
Dake, 1998 (56)	103	22	Homemade	83% complete thrombosis	9	73 (actuarial 2 yr)	3	24
Ehrlich, 1998 (57)	10	NA	Talent	80% complete thrombosis	10	NA	0	20
Cartes-Zumelzu, 2000 (58)	32	16	Excluder, Talent	90.6%	9.4	90.6 (32 mo)	3.1	15.4
Grabenwoger, 2000 (59)	21	NA	Talent, Prograft	100%	9.5	NA	0	14.3
Greenberg, 2000 (60)	25	15.4	Homemade	NA	20 (12.5 for elective, 33 for emergent)	NA	12	12
Temudom, 2000 (61)	14	5.5	Homemade, Vanguard, Excluder	78.6%	14.3	NA	7.1	14.3
Najibi, 2002 (62)	24	12	Excluder, Talent	94.7%	5.3	89.5 (1 yr)	0	0
Heijmen, 2002 (63)	28	21	Talent, AneuRx, Excluder	96.4%	0	96.4 (mean, 21 mo)	0	28.6
Schoder, 2003 (64)	28	22.7	Excluder	100%, 89.3% complete exclusion	0	96.1 (1 yr), 80.2 (3 yr)	0	25
Marin, 2003 (65)	94	15.4	Excluder, Talent	85.1%	NA	NA	NA	24
Lepore, 2003 (66)	21	12	Excluder, Talent	100%	9.5	76.2 (1 yr)	4.8	19
Sunder-Plassman, 2003 (67)	45	21	Corvita, Stenford, Vanguard, AneuRx, Talent, Excluder	NA	6.7	NA	2.2	22.2
Ouriel, 2003 (49)	31	6	Excluder, Talent, Other commercial	NA	12.9	81.6 (1 yr)	6.5	32.3
Bergeron, 2003 (68)	33	24	Excluder, Talent	NA	9.1	75.8 (mean 24 mo)	0	0
Czerny, 2004 (69)	54	38	Excluder, Talent	94.4%	9.3	63 (3 yr event free)	0	27.8
Makaroun, 2004 (70)	142	29.6	TAG	97.9%	1.5	75 (2-yr freedom from death)	3.5	8.8
Leurs, 2004 (71)	249	1-60	Excluder, Talent, Zenith, EndoFit	87%	10.4 (5.3 for elective, 27.9 for emergent)	80.3 (1 yr)	4	4.2

TAA, thoracic aortic aneurysm.

ertheless, these studies illustrate a consensual pattern of outcomes when viewed in aggregate. Overall, successful device deployment is achieved in 85% to 100% of cases, and periprocedural mortality ranges from 0% to 14%, falling within or below elective surgery mortality rates of 5% to 20%.[49,56-71] As expected, outcomes have improved over time with accumulated technical expertise, use of commercially manufactured devices, and improved patient selection criteria. The recently published collective experiences of the EUROSTAR and United Kingdom Thoracic Endograft registries, the largest series to date (N = 249), demonstrate successful deployment in 87% of cases, a 30-day mortality rate of 5% for elective cases, and paraplegia and endoleak rates of 4% each.[71] U.S. Food and Drug Administration (FDA) phase II trial data from exclusive deployment of the Gore TAG endograft in 142 patients with TAA revealed similar results: technical success in 98%, a 30-day mortality rate of 1.5%, paraplegia in 3.5%, and endoleak in 8.8%.[70]

These results cannot be directly compared with the outcomes of contemporary surgical studies. The majority of patients with TAA repaired by the endovascular approach in these studies were older and sicker, having been deemed either high-risk or not suitable for open surgical repair. For example, 52% of patients in the combined EUROSTAR and United Kingdom registries were preoperatively classified as ASA 3 or above by the American Society of Anesthesiologists' physical status classification that predicts procedural risk (1 to 2, low risk; 3, intermediate risk; 4 to 5, high risk; 6, organ donor).[71]

True comparisons between conventional therapy and the endovascular alternative can be made only after the completion of prospective, randomized, controlled trials. Although such trials are underway, a few studies have compared endovascular treatment with anatomically similar open-surgery historical controls. As part of the phase II Gore Excluder study, 19 TAA patients who were candidates for open repair received stent-graft therapy and were compared with a nonrandomized cohort of 10 patients who had undergone open repair before the availability of thoracic stent-grafts.[62] All aneurysms met the same inclusion/exclusion criteria for anatomic involvement. The 1-year survival rate was 89.5% in the endovascular group and 70% in the operative group. As expected, mean hospital stay (6.2 vs. 16.3 days) and length of intervention (155 vs. 256 minutes) were significantly less in those treated endovascularly. In a similar study, Ehrlich and colleagues found decreased 30-day mortality (10% vs. 31%), mean hospital stay (6 vs. 10 days), and mean intervention time (150 vs. 325 minutes) with endovascular repair; the paraplegia rate was also decreased (0% vs. 12%).[57]

Complications and Current Conclusions

With the avoidance of aortic cross-clamping and prolonged iatrogenic hypotension, endovascular TAA repair was expected to result in lower incidences of paraplegia relative to conventional treatment. Indeed, this has held true, with paraplegia rates generally ranging from 0% to 5% in endovascular studies,[49,56-71] compared with 5% to 25% in open repair cases.[37,39,45,46] Although low, these rates remain significant, especially because it is impossible to reimplant intercostal arteries in this setting. Some evidence suggests that the occurrence of paraplegia is associated with concomitant or prior surgical AAA repair and increased exclusion length due to the absence of lumbars and hypogastric collateral circulation.[60,72] Adjunctive measures to further reduce spinal cord ischemic complication rates in endovascular TAA repair are being investigated.[73]

Endoleaks are the most prevalent of TAA stent-graft treatment complications. However, their observed frequency is substantially less than that reported for AAA endograft repair.[74] Interestingly, the distribution of endoleak types also differs. TAA endoleaks occur more commonly at the proximal or distal attachment site (type I endoleak), whereas most AAA endoleaks are type II.[75] It is generally accepted that type I endoleaks are more serious and require expeditious intervention, because they represent direct communications between the aneurysm sac and aortic blood flow.[76] Treatment options include transcatheter coil or glue embolization, balloon angioplasty, placement of endovascular graft extensions, and open repair.[77,78]

Although current anatomic criteria limit thoracic stent-graft exclusion to lesions located at least 15 to 25 mm away from the origin of the LSA and celiac trunk, it is common for descending TAAs to be located within the proximal or distal neck length necessary for adequate fixation. At the proximal end, the landing zone can be extended by prophylactic transposition of the LSA to the left carotid artery or by bypass graft placement.[50] Alternatively, the uncovered proximal portion of the Talent endograft can be placed across the LSA origin to achieve fixation without blocking flow. However, case reports of inadvertent coverage of the LSA origin found no resulting complications,[79] and subsequent studies determined that such maneuvers may not be necessary as long as there is no obstruction of the right vertebral or carotid artery and the left internal mammary artery is not used as a coronary bypass conduit.[52-54] Complications such as left arm ischemia were found to be rare, possibly owing to collateral blood supply via retrograde left vertebral flow. Most centers now intentionally cover the LSA origin if necessary and reserve secondary revascularization procedures for treatment of related symptoms if they develop.[23,50]

For even more proximal TAAs involving the aortic arch, branched and fenestrated stent-grafts are being developed to accommodate perfusion through the great vessels.[80,81] Although feasibility has been demonstrated, it is already apparent that the required implantation techniques would be highly complex and would demand considerable technical expertise. Some centers have been investigating techniques to create fenestrations intraoperatively after device deployment and coverage of critical branches.[82]

In contrast, there are no easy management strategies to deal with a short distal neck. In this setting as well, fenestrated and branched grafts have been used in isolated cases, but the overall experience is very limited. Intentional coverage of the celiac artery is not recommended given the risk of hepatic and visceral ischemia. Although a normal superior mesenteric artery may provide collateral flow, no methods exist to predetermine whether such collateral supply would be sufficient. Furthermore, the celiac trunk may serve as a prominent source of retrograde endoleak if the artery is covered without adjunctive transcatheter occlusion. In distal aneurysms that involve both the descending thoracic and the abdominal aorta, combined open AAA repair and endovascular TAA exclusion is a novel treatment approach under investigation.

Stent-grafts are also being used to treat patients with diffuse aneurysmal disease involving the entire thoracic aorta. In such patients, the traditional surgical treatment is a two-stage procedure named the "elephant trunk technique."[83] In the first stage, the ascending aorta and aortic arch are repaired via a median sternotomy, and an extra-long graft is used for reconstruction, which leaves the excess portion of the graft, the elephant trunk, dangling within the lumen of the remaining diseased aorta. In the second stage, the lesion in the descending aorta is repaired via a left thoracotomy, and the graft replacement is connected to the elephant trunk proximally. To bypass the need for thoracotomy, a few centers have successfully deployed thoracic stent-grafts into the elephant trunk extension, altogether replacing the second stage of the traditional elephant trunk procedure.[84]

Following closely on the heels of early clinical experiences with stent-grafting for TAA repair, experimental application of this less invasive approach has been extended to a growing number of other pathologies of the thoracic aorta. Most noteworthy among these are aortic dissection,[3] traumatic aortic injury,[85] penetrating atherosclerotic ulcer,[86] and aortic rupture.[87] Some investigators believe that thoracic stent-graft technology may eventually yield the greatest impact on clinical care in the management of aortic dissections, because current treatment standards are far from optimal.

The emergence of endovascular stent-grafting as an alternative therapy to open surgical repair of thoracic aneurysms is an exciting advance. But the exact role of stent-grafting remains to be defined as long-term data and experience continue to accumulate and devices and techniques evolve.

ABDOMINAL AORTIC ANEURYSM

Therapeutic Strategies for Abdominal Aortic Aneurysm

Aneurysm of the abdominal aorta represent a potentially life-threatening scenario in an increasingly important segment of the aging patient population. With improved overall health care, many patients reach an advanced age despite severe cardiovascular, hypertensive, and/or pulmonary comorbidities, thus buying time for an AAA to enlarge to critical diameter and qualify for open surgical or endovascular treatment. Although surgical resection and interposition of an abdominal aortic prosthesis (Dacron or Gore-Tex) have long been considered standard treatment, despite a well known perioperative mortality risk, endovascular strategies have evolved over the last decade to be perceived as an accepted standard of care in patients considered too sick or too old for open surgery. Advanced technology, the ease of use, and the temptation of a fully percutaneous procedure have attracted a new breed of "endovascular surgeons," propelled by the prospect of both avoiding surgical risk and inducing reconstructive remodeling of the aneurysmatic aorta through depressurization and complete exclusion of the aneurysmal sac.

Once deployed, the stent-graft serves to bridge the region of the aneurysm, thereby excluding it from the circulation while allowing aortic blood flow to continue distally through the prosthetic stent-graft lumen. To begin with, only 30% to 60% of AAAs are anatomically suitable for endovascular repair. When such repair is undertaken, the rate of successful stent-graft implantation has ranged from 78% to 94%. One of the major technical difficulties associated with the stent-graft technique that has yet to be overcome is endoleaks, which occur in 10% to 20% of cases[88] and are seen angiographically as persistent contrast flow into the aneurysm sac due to failure to completely exclude the aneurysm from the aortic circulation. If left untreated, these endoleaks may potentially leave the patient at continued risk for aneurysm expansion or rupture. Indeed, in a follow-up study of outcomes at 12 months or longer among more than 1000 stent-graft recipients, the EUROSTAR investigators reported that almost 10% of patients per year required secondary interventions, suggesting that there should be caution in the broad application of endovascular aneurysm repair (EVAR).[89]

Patients and physicians have embraced EVAR as the method of choice to treat AAAs in patients at high risk. EVAR has great appeal for this older population, because it leads to faster recovery with fewer systemic complications than open repair.[90-95] Parodi and colleagues[96] reported the first endovascular repair of an AAA in a human in 1991; they used a graft fashioned from prosthetic vascular grafts and expandable stents. Current estimates are that more than 20,000 EVAR procedures take place each year in the United States, representing 36% of all AAA repairs. The estimate is that more than 12% of all procedures in Europe are with EVAR, and the expected annual growth is 15% at this time (Medtronic Marketing Department, personal communication, 2006). EVAR is the method of choice in high-risk older patients because of its minimal incisions, shorter operating time, and reduced blood loss.

Indications for Treatment

Most asymptomatic AAAs are discovered serendipitously, often on imaging examinations for other complaints. Increasing evidence indicates that there is value to screening patients for AAA, and it is likely that screening will be approved in the near future.[97] Once the diagnosis of AAA is made, two critical questions need to be answered: when to intervene and how to intervene. The availability of EVAR has made these decisions somewhat more complex while adding a significant treatment option.

Recent studies have questioned whether aneurysms smaller than 5 cm should be treated.[98] However, in general, the clinical recommendation remains to offer treatment for aneurysms between 5 and 5.5 cm, depending on the results of clinical trials.[99] An exception to this guideline is that intervention should be offered despite the size of the aneurysm if symptoms develop or if the aneurysm increases in size by 1 cm per year.[100] In addition, if the patient is a woman with smaller native vessels, the relative size that represents aneurysmal disease may be less than the conventional 5 to 5.5 cm range.

Patient selection has emerged as the most important factor related to successful EVAR. The assessment begins with consideration of the body habitus and gender of the patient; small body size and female gender have been associated with a higher risk of procedure abortion.[101,102] In addition, the comorbidities of the patient must be assessed, with careful attention to cardiac, pulmonary, and renal conditions. The use of risk stratification to analyze outcomes clearly indicates that survival for those at low to minimal risk is excellent over 10 years; those at highest risk succumb to cardiac disease or cancer, and survival is poorest for those patients.[103] EVAR has shown a reduction in 30-day mortality relative to that achieved with open repair (1.2% vs. 4.6%). Risk stratification determines survival in general and shows that both open surgery and EVAR decrease the risk of death from AAA rupture.[104]

The characteristics of the aneurysm must be matched to the most suitable device; this has a direct impact on outcomes and the complication profile of the procedure. The aneurysm is evaluated from a three-dimensional reconstruction CT scan or aortography with a calibrated catheter. There are at least four important features that must be assessed before a patient's eligibility for EVAR can be determined, and this analysis leads to a list of contraindications[105] (Table 44-3). Experienced interventionalists can deal with some of these challenges, but morphologic features of the aneurysm and access vessels may preclude EVAR.

The key features of endovascular repair of AAAs that determine procedural success and long-term outcomes are proximal and distal fixation and sealing. Most of the devices use a metal skeleton throughout the graft that is made from stainless steel, nitinol, or Elgiloy. Attachment is facilitated by the use of hooks or radial force.

Table 44-3. Evaluation for Endovascular Aneurysm Repair (EVAR)

Computed tomographic scan assessment for EVAR eligibility
Proximal neck: diameter, length, angle, presence or absence of thrombus
Distal landing zone: diameter and length
Iliac arteries: presence of aneurysms and occlusive disease
Access arteries: diameter, presence of occlusive disease

Contraindications for EVAR
Short proximal neck
Thrombus presence in proximal landing zone
Conical proximal neck
Greater than 120° angulation of the proximal neck
Critical inferior mesenteric artery
Significant iliac occlusive disease
Tortuosity of iliac vessels

Once the graft is inserted through the sheath, it can be deployed by a self-expanding mechanism or by balloon expansion. Some grafts attach superior to the renal arteries (suprarenal attachment), whereas most of the devices require at least 15 mm of proximal neck to achieve fixation and sealing in the infrarenal position. The grafts also differ in their "profile" or the size of the delivery system. Low-profile devices permit access through smaller arteries.

Most of the complications associated with EVAR are minor and can be watched carefully or treated easily with additional interventional procedures. Some complications occur during or soon after the procedure, whereas others may be noticed only during graft surveillance.[106] A study by Ohki and colleagues[107] analyzed complication and death rates within 30 days after EVAR and reported them to be 17.6% and 8.5%, respectively. This remains an active and important area of EVAR research, and standards have been developed to facilitate reporting of endovascular abdominal aortic repair complications.[108]

Endoleaks can have substantial clinical significance, because they carry an increased risk of symptoms or aneurysm rupture. Endoleak describes the continuation of blood flow into the extragraft portion of the aneurysm; this flow increases the size of the aneurysmal sac.[109] Endoleaks occur in either the acute setting during graft implantation or during the postoperative surveillance period. The majority of procedural endoleaks disappear without intervention.

Endoleaks are either graft related or non–graft related, and a classification system has been developed (Table 44-4).[110] Type I endoleaks occur when the attachment is not complete, either proximally or distally; blood is able to flow into the aneurysmal sac and is not completely occluded by endograft attachment to the arterial wall. Type II endoleaks result from continued backflow from aortic branches such as the inferior mesenteric artery and lumbar arteries. This flow occurs retrograde into the aneurysmal sac around the endograft. Type III endoleaks are caused by defects in the endograft structure that lead to leakage of blood flow from inside the endograft to

Table 44-4.   Classification of Endoleaks

Type I: Attachment site leaks
Proximal end of endograft
Distal end of endograft
Iliac occluder (plug)

Type II: Branch leaks (without attachment site connection)
Simple or to-and-fro (from only one patent branch)
Complex or flow-through (with two or more patent branches)

Type III: Graft defect
Junctional leak or modular disconnect
Fabric disruption (midgraft hole)
  Minor (<2 mm; e.g., suture holes)
  Major (≥2 mm)

Type IV: Graft wall (fabric) porosity (<30 days after graft placement)

the aneurysmal sac. Finally, type IV endoleaks are noted early after endograft placement and resolve when the fabric porosity is decreased by clotted blood. Because endovascular repair uses a relatively new technology, graft surveillance for complications such as endoleaks is essential. Endoleaks are diagnosed by a variety of techniques: arteriography, pressure monitoring during or after the procedure, CT scanning, and duplex scanning. The preferred method of detecting endoleaks is by CT scanning, An analysis of 2463 patients from the EUROSTAR registry revealed that 171 had an endoleak by the time of their 1-month postoperative evaluation, and 317 patients developed an endoleak at a later date.[111] Of these, 7.8% had a type II endoleak, and 12% had a type I, type III, or combination of endoleaks.

There are many different ways to treat endoleaks, including coil embolization, placement of stent-graft cuffs and extensions, laparoscopic ligation of inferior mesenteric and lumbar arteries, open surgical repair, and repeat EVAR procedures. Type I and III endoleaks require fairly urgent intervention, because blood flow and sac pressure will continue to increase and lead to rupture. Type IV endoleaks usually resolve on their own. The management of type II endoleaks is more controversial, because some of them will thrombose on their own, whereas others will lead to sac enlargement.

Endograft surveillance is important to document normal and abnormal morphologic changes in the repair and in the involved vessels. This process is vital for the detection of endoleaks, increased aneurysm diameter, and possible device migration.[112] The recommended surveillance routine includes a CT scan at 1, 6, and 12 months and annually thereafter. If an endoleak is detected, the frequency of the scans increases to every 6 months until resolution of the endoleak is detected.

The use of EVAR technology has led to a greater understanding of the basic science of aneurysmal disease. For example, Curci and Thompson[113] have been studying the relationship between the secretion of matrix metalloproteinases (MMPs) and AAAs. They have measured increased levels in the aneurysmal rather than the normal arterial wall.

Randomized Data and Current Conclusions

The EVAR study group has provided the community with important revelations from randomized studies on the treatment of a "moving target" called AAA, in the context of increasing age of patients, continuously refined technology, and improving operator skills. Whereas treatment of large AAAs with EVAR reduced the 30-day mortality rate to 1.7%, compared with 4.7% with open repair ($P<.009$) on an intention-to-treat basis, the authors were prudent to judge such early benefits only as a license to continue evaluation of EVAR by use of longer follow-up.[114] After 4 years, all-cause mortality was not improved with EVAR versus open repair of AAA despite an initial postinterventional benefit of EVAR; midterm aneurysm-related mortality was 4% with EVAR and 7% with open repair, a differential explained by the 3% higher mortality rate with open repair.[115] This marginal advantage (at the expense of a costly surveillance program) is consistent with results from the DREAM study,[116] but it led the authors to the sobering conclusion that EVAR may offer no advantage with respect to all-cause mortality and quality of life in patients with AAAs of 5.5 cm or larger who are fit for open surgery.[115]

Scores for measures of quality of life and sexual functioning favored EVAR only in the early postoperative period but equalized after 6 months in comparison to open repair, in parallel with a continued need for reinterventions with EVAR. A closer look, however, revealed that many late complications after successful EVAR were of low prognostic impact, such as endoleak type II requiring reintervention in only 17 of 79 cases. Severe complications such as graft rupture ($n=9$), graft migration ($n=12$), endoleak type I ($n=27$), and graft thrombosis ($n=12$), which required reintervention in 35 of 60 cases, were likely to be attributed to technical or procedural problems with the stent-graft or unsuitable anatomy, again reminding the medical community of the inherently immature nature of an emerging technology. Moreover, at least six different brands of endovascular devices were used by surgeons with different levels of experience.

The midterm results and outlook with EVAR may even be more sobering in the light of the outcome data of the EVAR-2 trial[117]: patients considered unfit for open repair of AAA did not benefit from EVAR in terms of improved survival, compared with no intervention, and the costs were higher. EVAR-2 patients were older and had more comorbidity than EVAR-1 patients; therefore, confounding variables of prognosis were strong and rendered the potential perioperative advantage of EVAR irrelevant, considering that only 9 aneurysm-related fatalities per 100 patient-years occurred among the patients randomized to observation in the control arm.

The data presented by the EVAR trialists (both 30-day and midterm outcomes in EVAR-1 and data from EVAR-2 in patients unfit for open surgery) are not just sobering, but provocative and revealing at the same time. In accordance with the DREAM studies,[115,118] EVAR-1 showed significant early survival benefit after 30 days with endovascular repair owing to reduced peri-interventional risk, corroborating previous observational evidence.[119-121] Although early euphoria has been severely dampened by midterm follow-up outcomes, on second sight careful analysis of randomized data provides highly valuable information:

1. Health status, comprising age, comorbidities, and prognostic confounders, was the most important denominator of individual prognosis, followed by, to a lesser degree, the nonsurgical nature of EVAR (which can be performed percutaneously in local anesthesia). Therefore, assessment of the general state of health of patients in the older and sicker population and serious attempts at improvement should precede EVAR; examples are cardiopulmonary workup, potentially including percutaneous coronary intervention, and respiratory improvement as an integral part of strategic planning. Under particular conditions, it appears justified to reject EVAR when conservative care is more appropriate.

2. The nature of complications requiring reinterventions after EVAR is often related to technical shortcomings with current-generation devices or to the use in nonsuitable anatomy. Physicians and industry must recognize those limitations and develop both better devices and improved selection algorithms for treatment with EVAR.

3. Eventually, although the endovascular community should always embrace the "Nihil nocere" principle (a classic in medicine and surgery) and avoid well-intended but harmful treatment, it should also realize the "moving target" nature of the problem. Some patients considered unfit for surgery can possibly improve and find themselves in a lower risk category and eventually fit for surgery or EVAR. EVAR technology and interventional skills constantly improve with training, and the short-term differential advantage over open surgery is likely to increase. More elderly patients may express a personal preference for a less traumatic procedure such as EVAR (if performed by an expert) despite lack of a clearcut midterm advantage and accept surveillance and interventions during follow-up. Finally, the higher costs for follow-up imaging with EVAR could be dramatically reduced with a smarter surveillance strategy based on clinical and ultrasound interrogation, instead of serial CT or MR imaging.

All things considered, even though at midterm EVAR may not improve AAA prognosis compared with classic surgery, resulting at present in a draw after an early advantage, EVAR is here to stay. Better staging and selection of patients, constantly improving technology,[120] and the expertise of centers of excellence for aortic diseases will enhance matching of a given patient with one of a variety of therapeutic options including EVAR or even conservative treatment. Thus, despite all the new technology, it is still wise to adhere to the old principles of responsible use of clinical judgment and offer especially the growing segment of older patients with multiple comorbidities an holistic approach with intelligent use of prognosticating tools and interdisciplinary cooperation. Whether the results of the EVAR trials and the cautious voice of Jonathan Michaels[122] will halt the trend of increasing use of EVAR instead of open surgery remains to be seen; it is certain, however, that the randomized data from EVAR-1 and EVAR-2 will refocus the debate on natural history and patient selection for a forward-moving technology.

REFERENCES

1. Ince H, Nienaber CA: The concept of interventional therapy in acute aortic syndrome. J Card Surg 2002;17:135-142.
2. Nienaber CA, Fattori R, Lund G, et al: Nonsurgical reconstruction of thoracic aortic dissection by stent-graft placement. N Engl J Med 1999;340:1539-1545.
3. Dake MD, Kato N, Mitchell RS, et al: Endovascular stent-graft placement for the treatment of acute aortic dissection. N Engl J Med 1999;340:1546-1552.
4. Walkers PJ, Miller DC: Aneurysmal and ischemic complications of type B (type III) aortic dissections. Semin Vasc Surg 1992;5:198-214.
5. Bossone E, Rampoldi V, Nienaber CA, et al: Usefulness of pulse deficit to predict in-hospital complications and mortality in patients with acute type A aortic dissection. Am J Cardiol 2002;89:851-855.
6. Cambria RP, Brewster DC, Gertler J, et al: Vascular complications associated with spontaneous aortic dissection. J Vasc Surg 1988;7:197-209.
7. Laas J, Heinemann M, Schaefers HJ, et al: Management of thoracoabdominal malperfusion in aortic dissection. Circulation 1991;84:20-24.
8. Miller DC: The continuing dilemma concerning medical versus surgical management of patients with acute type B dissections. Semin Thorac Cardiovasc Surg 1993;5:33-46.
9. Miller DC, Mitchell RS, Oyer PE, et al: Independent determinants of operative mortality for patients with aortic dissections. Circulation 1984;70:153-164.
10. Elefteriades JA, Hartleroad J, Gusberg RJ, et al: Long-term experience with descending aortic dissection: The complication-specific approach. Ann Thorac Surg 1992;53:11-20.
11. Walker PJ, Dake MD, Mitchell RS, et al: The use of endovascular techniques for the treatment of complications of aortic dissection. J Vasc Surg 1993;18:1042-1051.
12. Fann JI, Sarris GE, Mitchell RS, et al: Treatment of patients with aortic dissection presenting with peripheral vascular complications. Ann Surg 1990;212:705-713.
13. Yano H, Ishimaru S, Kawaguchi S, et al: Endovascular stent-grafting of the descending thoracic aorta after arch repair in acute type A dissection. Ann Thorac Surg 2002;73:288-291.
14. Kato N, Shimono T, Hirano T, et al: Transluminal placement of endovascular stent-grafts for the treatment of type A aortic dissection with an entry tear in the descending thoracic aorta. J Vasc Surg 2001;34:1023-1028.
15. Iannelli G, Piscione F, Di Tommaso L, et al: Thoracic aortic emergencies: Impact of endovascular surgery. Ann Thorac Surg 2004;77:591-596.
16. Saito S, Arai H, Kim K, et al: Percutaneous fenestration of dissecting intima with a transseptal needle: A new therapeutic technique for visceral ischemia complicating acute aortic dissection. Cathet Cardiovasc Diagn 1992;26:130-135.

17. Nienaber CA, Ince H, Petzsch M, et al: Endovascular treatment of thoracic aortic dissection and its variants. Acta Chir Belg 2002;102:292-298.

18. Nienaber CA, Ince H, Weber F, et al: Emergency stent-graft placement in thoracic aortic dissection and evolving rupture. J Card Surg 2003;18:464-470.

19. Beregi JP, Haulon S, Otal P, et al: Endovascular treatment of acute complications associated with aortic dissection: Midterm results from a multicenter study. J Endovasc Ther 2003;10:486-493.

20. Bortone AS, Schena S, D'Agostino D, et al: Immediate versus delayed endovascular treatment of post-traumatic aortic pseudoaneurysms and type B dissections: Retrospective analysis and premises to the upcoming European trial. Circulation 2002;106:234-240.

21. v Knobelsdorff G, Hoppner RM, Tonner PH, et al: Induced arterial hypotension for interventional thoracic aortic stent-graft placement: Impact on intracranial haemodynamics and cognitive function. Eur J Anaesthesiol 2003;20:134-140.

22. Koschyk DH, Nienaber CA, Knap M, et al: How to guide stent-graft implantation in type B aortic dissection? Comparison of angiography, transesophageal echocardiography, and intravascular ultrasound. Circulation 2005;112(Suppl I): I-260-I-264.

23. Rehders TC, Petzsch M, Ince H, et al: Intentional occlusion of the left subclavian artery during endovascular stent-graft implantation in the thoracic aorta: Risk and relevance. J Endovasc Ther 2004;11:659-666.

24. Eggebrecht H, Nienaber CA, Neuhauser M, et al: Endovascular stent-graft placement in aortic dissection: A meta-analysis. Eur Heart J 2006;27:489-498.

25. Shimono T, Kato N, Yasuda F, et al: Transluminal stent-graft placement for the treatments of acute onset and chronic aortic dissections. Circulation 2002;106:241-247.

26. Fattori R, Lovato L, Buttazzi K, et al: Evolving experience of percutaneous management of type B aortic dissection. Eur J Vasc Endovasc Surg 2006;31:115-122.

27. Dialetto G, Covino FE, Scognamiglio G, et al: Treatment of type B aortic dissection: Endoluminal repair or conventional medical therapy? Eur J Cardiothorac Surg 2005;27:826-830.

28. Duebener LF, Lorenzen P, Richardt G, et al: Emergency endovascular stent-grafting for life-threatening acute type B aortic dissections. Ann Thorac Surg 2004;78:1261-1266.

29. Pansini S, Gagliardotto PV, Pompei E, et al: Early and late risk factors in surgical treatment of acute type A aortic dissection. Ann Thorac Surg 1998;66:779-784.

30. Slonim SM, Nyman U, Semba CP, et al: Aortic dissection: percutaneous management of ischemic complications with endovascular stents and balloon fenestration. J Vasc Surg 1996;23:241-251.

31. Clouse WD, Hallett JW Jr, Schaff HV, et al: Improved prognosis of thoracic aortic aneurysms: A population-based study. JAMA 1998;280:1926-1929.

32. Bickerstaff LK, Pairolero PC, Hollier LH, et al: Thoracic aortic aneurysms: A population-based study. Surgery 1982;92: 1103-1108.

33. Coady MA, Rizzo JA, Goldstein LJ, Elefteriades JA: Natural history, pathogenesis, and etiology of thoracic aortic aneurysms and dissections. Cardiol Clin 1999;17:615-635.

34. Crawford ES, DeNatale RW: Thoracoabdominal aortic aneurysm: Observations regarding the natural course of the disease. J Vasc Surg 1986;3:578-582.

35. McNamara JJ, Pressler VM: Natural history of arteriosclerotic thoracic aortic aneurysms. Ann Thorac Surg 1998;26: 468-473.

36. Johansson G, Markstrom U, Swedenborg J: Ruptured thoracic aortic aneurysms: A study of incidence and mortality rates. J Vasc Surg 1995;21:985-988.

37. DeBakey ME, McCollum CH, Graham JM: Surgical treatment of aneurysms of the descending thoracic aorta: Long-term results in 500 patients. J Cardiovasc Surg (Torino) 1998; 19:571-576.

38. Hilgenberg AD, Rainer WG, Sadler TR Jr: Aneurysm of the descending thoracic aorta: Replacement with the use of a shunt or bypass. J Thorac Cardiovasc Surg 1981;81: 818-824.

39. Moreno-Cabral CE, Miller DC, Mitchell RS, et al: Degenerative and atherosclerotic aneurysms of the thoracic aorta: Determinants of early and late surgical outcome. J Thorac Cardiovasc Surg 1984;88:1020-1032.

40. Pressler V, McNamara JJ: Thoracic aortic aneurysm: Natural history and treatment. J Thorac Cardiovasc Surg 1980;79: 489-498.

41. Fann JI: Descending thoracic and thoracoabdominal aortic aneurysms. Coron Artery Dis 2002;13:93-102.

42. Svensson LG, Crawford ES, Hess KR, et al: Variables predictive of outcome in 832 patients undergoing repairs of the descending thoracic aorta. Chest 1993;104:1248-1253.

43. Borst HG, Jurmann M, Buhner B, Laas J: Risk of replacement of descending aorta with a standardized left heart bypass technique. J Thorac Cardiovasc Surg 1994;105:126-132.

44. Pressler V, McNamara JJ: Aneurysm of the thoracic aorta: Review of 260 cases. J Thorac Cardiovasc Surg 1985;89: 50-54.

45. Svensson LG, Crawford ES, Hess KR, et al: Experience with 1509 patients undergoing thoracoabdominal aortic operations. J Vasc Surg 1993;17:357-368.

46. Livesay JJ, Cooley DA, Ventemiglia RA, et al: Surgical experience in descending thoracic aneurysmectomy with and without adjuncts to avoid ischemia. Ann Thorac Surg 1985; 39:37-46.

47. Berg P, Kaufmann D, van Marrewijk CJ, Buth J: Spinal cord ischaemia after stent-graft treatment for infra-renal abdominal aortic aneurysms: Analysis of the EUROSTAR database. Eur J Vasc Endovasc Surg 2001;22:342-347.

48. Rosenthal D: Spinal cord ischemia after abdominal aortic operation: Is it preventable? J Vasc Surg 1999;30:391-397.

49. Ouriel K, Greenberg RK: Endovascular treatment of thoracic aortic aneurysms. J Card Surg 2003;18:455-463.

50. Dake MD: Endovascular stent-graft management of thoracic aortic diseases. Eur J Radiol 2001;39:42-49.

51. Gravereaux EC, Faries PL, Burks JA, et al: Risk of spinal cord ischemia after endograft repair of thoracic aortic aneurysms. J Vasc Surg 2001;34:977-1003.

52. Burks JA Jr, Faries PL, Gravereaux EC, et al: Endovascular repair of thoracic aortic aneurysms: Stent-graft fixation across the aortic arch vessels. Ann Vasc Surg 2002;16:24-28.

53. Gorich J, Asquan Y, Seifarth H, et al: Initial experience with intentional stent-graft coverage of the subclavian artery during endovascular thoracic aortic repairs. J Endovasc Ther 2002;9(Suppl 2):II39-II43.

54. Tiesenhausen K, Hausegger KA, Oberwalder P, et al: Left subclavian artery management in endovascular repair of thoracic aortic aneurysms and aortic dissections. J Card Surg 2003;18:429-435.

55. Dake MD, Miller DC, Semba CP, et al: Transluminal placement of endovascular stent-grafts for the treatment of descending thoracic aortic aneurysms. N Engl J Med 1994; 331:1729-1734.

56. Dake MD, Miller DC, Mitchell RS, et al: The "first generation" of endovascular stent-grafts for patients with aneurysms of the descending thoracic aorta. J Thorac Cardiovasc Surg 1998;116:689-703.

57. Ehrlich M, Grabenwoeger M, Cartes-Zumelu F, et al: Endovascular stent graft repair for aneurysms on the descending thoracic aorta. Ann Thorac Surg 1998;66:19-24.

58. Cartes-Zumelzu F, Lammer J, Kretschmer G, et al: Endovascular repair of thoracic aortic aneurysms. Semin Interv Cardiol 2000;5:53-57.

59. Grabenwoger M, Hutschala D, Ehrlich MP, et al: Thoracic aortic aneurysms: Treatment with endovascular self-expandable stent grafts. Ann Thorac Surg 2000;69:421-425.

60. Greenberg R, Resch T, Nyman U, et al: Endovascular repair of descending thoracic aortic aneurysms: An early experience with intermediate-term follow-up. J Vasc Surg 2000;31: 147-156.

61. Temudom T, D'Ayala M, Marin ML, et al: Endovascular grafts in the treatment of thoracic aortic aneurysms and pseudoaneurysms. Ann Vasc Surg 2000;14:230-238.

62. Najibi S, Terramani TT, Weiss VJ, et al: Endoluminal versus open treatment of descending thoracic aortic aneurysms. J Vasc Surg 2002;36:732-737.

63. Heijmen RH, Deblier IG, Moll FL, et al: Endovascular stent-grafting for descending thoracic aortic aneurysms. Eur J Cardiothorac Surg 2002;21:5-9.

64. Schoder M, Cartes-Zumelzu F, Grabenwoger M, et al: Elective endovascular stent-graft repair of atherosclerotic thoracic aortic aneurysms: Clinical results and midterm follow-up. AJR Am J Roentgenol 2003;180:709-715.

65. Marin ML, Hollier LH, Ellozy SH, et al: Endovascular stent graft repair of abdominal and thoracic aortic aneurysms: A ten-year experience with 817 patients. Ann Surg 2003;238:586-593.

66. Lepore V, Lonn L, Delle M, et al: Treatment of descending thoracic aneurysms by endovascular stent grafting. J Card Surg 2003;18:436-423.

67. Sunder-Plassmann L, Scharrer-Pamler R, Liewald F, et al: Endovascular exclusion of thoracic aortic aneurysms: Mid-term results of elective treatment and in contained rupture. J Card Surg 2003;18:367-374.

68. Bergeron P, De Chaumaray T, Gay J, Douillez V: Endovascular treatment of thoracic aortic aneurysms. J Cardiovasc Surg (Torino) 2003;42:349-361.

69. Czerny M, Cejna M, Hutschala D, et al: Stent-graft placement in atherosclerotic descending thoracic aortic aneurysms: Midterm results. J Endovasc Ther 2004;11:26-32.

70. Makaroun MS, Dillavou ED, Kee ST, et al: Endovascular treatment of thoracic aortic aneurysms: Results of the phase II multicenter trial of the GORE TAG thoracic endoprosthesis. J Vasc Surg 2005;41:1-9.

71. Leurs LJ, Bell R, Degrieck Y, et al: Endovascular treatment of thoracic aortic diseases: Combined experience from the EUROSTAR and United Kingdom Thoracic Endograft registries. J Vasc Surg 2004;40:670-679.

72. Mitchell RS, Miller DC, Dake MD: Stent-graft repair of thoracic aortic aneurysms. Semin Vasc Surg 1997;10:257-271.

73. Carroccio A, Marin ML, Ellozy S, Hollier LH: Pathophysiology of paraplegia following endovascular thoracic aortic aneurysm repair. J Card Surg 2003;18:359-366.

74. Thurnher SA, Grabenwoger M: Endovascular treatment of thoracic aortic aneurysms: A review. Eur Radiol 2002;12:1370-1387.

75. Resch T, Koul B, Dias NV, et al: Changes in aneurysm morphology and stent-graft configuration after endovascular repair of aneurysms of the descending thoracic aorta. J Thorac Cardiovasc Surg 2001;122:47-52.

76. Buth J, Harris PL, van Marrewijk C, Fransen G: The significance and management of different types of endoleaks. Semin Vasc Surg 2003;16:95-102.

77. Chuter TA, Faruqi RM, Sawhney R, et al: Endoleak after endovascular repair of abdominal aortic aneurysm. J Vasc Surg 2001;34:98-105.

78. Kato N, Semba CP, Dake MD: Embolization of perigraft leaks after endovascular stent-graft treatment of aortic aneurysms. J Vasc Interv Radiol 1996;7:805-811.

79. Hausegger KA, Oberwalder P, Tiesenhausen K, et al: Intentional left subclavian artery occlusion by thoracic aortic stent-grafts without surgical transposition. J Endovasc Ther 2001;8:472-476.

80. Stanley BM, Semmens JB, Lawrence-Brown MM, et al: Fenestration in endovascular grafts for aortic aneurysm repair: New horizons for preserving blood flow in branch vessels. J Endovasc Ther 2001;8:16-24.

81. Inoue K, Hosokawa H, Iwase T, et al: Aortic arch reconstruction by transluminally placed endovascular branched stent graft. Circulation 1999;100(Suppl II):II-316-II-321.

82. McWilliams RG, Murphy M, Hartley D, et al: In situ stent-graft fenestration to preserve the left subclavian artery. J Endovasc Ther 2004;11:170-174.

83. Heinemann MK, Buehner B, Jurmann MJ, Borst HG: Use of the "elephant trunk technique" in aortic surgery. Ann Thorac Surg 1995;60:2-6.

84. Fann JI, Dake MD, Semba CP, et al: Endovascular stent-grafting after arch aneurysm repair using the "elephant trunk." Ann Thorac Surg 1995;60:1102-1105.

85. Kato N, Dake MD, Miller DC, et al: Traumatic thoracic aortic aneurysm: Treatment with endovascular stent-grafts. Radiology 1997;205:657-662.

86. Eggebrecht H, Baumgart D, Schmermund A, et al: Penetrating atherosclerotic ulcer of the aorta: Treatment by endovascular stent-graft placement. Curr Opin Cardiol 2003;18:431-435.

87. Kato N, Hirano T, Ishida M, et al: Acute and contained rupture of the descending thoracic aorta: Treatment with endovascular stent grafts. J Vasc Surg 2003;37:100-105.

88. Brewster DC, Cronenwett JL, Hallett JW Jr, et al; Joint Council of the American Association for Vascular Surgery and Society for Vascular Surgery: Guidelines for the treatment of abdominal aortic aneurysms: Report of a subcommittee of the Joint Council of the American Association for Vascular Surgery and Society for Vascular Surgery. J Vasc Surg 2003;37:1106-1117.

89. Laheij RJ, Buth J, Harris PL, et al: Need for secondary interventions after endovascular repair of abdominal aortic aneurysms: Intermediate-term follow-up results of a European collaborative registry (EUROSTAR). Br J Surg. 2000;87:1666-1673.

90. Criado FJ, Fairman RM, Becker GJ: Talent LPS AAA stent graft: Results of a pivotal clinical trial. J Vasc Surg 2003;37:709-715.

91. Matsumura JS, Brewster DC, Makaroun MS, Naftel DC: A multicenter controlled clinical trial of open versus endovascular treatment of abdominal aortic aneurysm. J Vasc Surg 2003;37:262-271.

92. Ouriel K, Clair DG, Greenberg RK, et al: Endovascular repair of abdominal aortic aneurysms: Device-specific outcome. J Vasc Surg 2003;37:971-978.

93. Moore WS: The Guidant Ancure bifurcation endograft: Five-year follow-up. Semin Vasc Surg 2003;16:139-143.

94. Zarins CK, White RA, Moll FL, et al: The AneuRx stent graft: Four-year results and worldwide experience 2000. J Vasc Surg 2001;33:S135-S145.

95. Greenberg RK, Chuter TA, Sternbergh WC III, Fearnot NE: Zenith AAA endovascular graft: Intermediate-term results of the US multicenter trial. J Vasc Surg 2004;39:1209-1218.

96. Parodi JC, Palmaz JC, Barone HD: Transfemoral intraluminal graft implantation for abdominal aortic aneurysms. Ann Vasc Surg 1991;5:491-497.

97. Kent KC, Zwolak RM, Jaff MR, et al: Screening for abdominal aortic aneurysm: A consensus statement. J Vasc Surg 2004;39:267-269.

98. The UK Small Aneurysm Trial Participants: Mortality results for randomised controlled trial of early elective surgery or ultrasonographic surveillance for small abdominal aortic aneurysms. Lancet 1998;352:1649-1655.

99. Powell JT, Greenhalgh RM: Clinical practice: small abdominal aortic aneurysms. N Engl J Med 2003;348:1895-1901.

100. Scott RA, Tisi PV, Ashton HA, Allen DR: Abdominal aortic aneurysm rupture rates: A 7-year follow-up of the entire abdominal aortic aneurysm population detected by screening. J Vasc Surg 1998;28:124-128.

101. Mathison M, Becker GJ, Katzen BT, et al: The influence of female gender on the outcome of endovascular abdominal aortic aneurysm repair. J Vasc Interv Radiol 2001;12:1047-1051.

102. Mathison MN, Becker GJ, Katzen BT, et al: Implications of problematic access in transluminal endografting of abdominal aortic aneurysm. J Vasc Interv Radiol 2003;14:33-39.

103. Becker GJ, Kovacs M, Mathison MN, et al: Risk stratification and outcomes of transluminal endografting for abdominal aortic aneurysm: 7-Year experience and long-term follow-up. J Vasc Interv Radiol 2001;12:1033-1046.

104. Huber TS, Wang JG, Derrow AE, et al: Experience in the United States with intact abdominal aortic aneurysm repair. J Vasc Surg 2001;33:304-310.

105. Ohki T, Veith FJ: Patient selection for endovascular repair of abdominal aortic aneurysms: Changing the threshold for intervention. Semin Vasc Surg 1999;12:226-234.

106. Elkouri S, Gloviczki P, McKusick MA, et al: Perioperative complications and early outcome after endovascular and open surgical repair of abdominal aortic aneurysm. J Vasc Surg 2004;39:497-505.

107. Ohki T, Veith FJ, Shaw P, et al: Increasing incidence of midterm and long-term complications after endovascular

graft repair of abdominal aortic aneurysms: A note of caution based on a 9-year experience. Ann Surg 2001;234: 323-334.

108. Chaikof EL, Blankensteijn JD, Harris PL, et al: Reporting standards for endovascular aortic aneurysm repair. J Vasc Surg 2002;35:1048-1060.

109. White GH, Yu W, May J: Endoleak: A proposed new terminology to describe incomplete aneurysm exclusion by an endoluminal graft. J Endovasc Surg 1996;3:124-125.

110. Veith FJ, Baum RA, Ohki T, et al: Nature and significance of endoleaks and endotension: Summary of opinions expressed at an international conference. J Vasc Surg 2002;35: 1029-1035.

111. van Marrewijk C, Buth J, Harris PL, et al: Significance of endoleaks after endovascular repair of abdominal aortic aneurysms: The EUROSTAR experience. J Vasc Surg. 2002; 35:461-473.

112. Corriere MA, Feurer ID, Becker SY, et al: Endoleak following endovascular abdominal aortic aneurysm repair: Implications for duration of screening. Ann Surg 2004;239: 800-805.

113. Curci JA, Thompson RW: Adaptive cellular immunity in aortic aneurysms: Cause, consequence, or context? J Clin Invest 2004;114:168-171.

114. Greenhalgh RM, Brown LC, Kwong GP, et al: Comparison of endovascular aneurysm repair with open repair in patients with abdominal aortic aneurysm (EVAR trial 1), 30-day operative mortality results: Randomised controlled trial. Lancet 2004;364:843-848.

115. EVAR trial participants: Endovascular aneurysm repair versus open repair in patients with abdominal aortic aneurysm (EVAR trial 1): Randomised controlled trial. Lancet 2005; 365:2179-2186.

116. Prinssen M, Verhoeven ELG, Buth J, et al: A randomized trial comparing conventional and endovascular repair of abdominal aortic aneurysms. N Engl J Med 2004;351:1607-1618.

117. EVAR Trial Participants: Endovascular aneurysm repair and outcome in patients unfit for open repair of abdominal aortic aneurysm (EVAR trial 2): Randomised controlled trial. Lancet 2005;365:2187-2192.

118. Blankensteijn JD, de Jong SECA, Prinssen M, et al: Two-year outcomes after conventional or endovascular repair of abdominal aortic aneurysms. N Engl J Med 2005;352: 2398-2405.

119. Anderson PL, Arons RR, Moskowitz AJ, et al: A statewide experience with endovascular abdominal aortic aneurysm repair: Rapid diffusion with excellent early results. J Vasc Surg 2004;39:10-19.

120. Lee WA, Carter JW, Upchurch G, et al: Perioperative outcomes after open and endovascular repair of intact abdominal aortic aneurysms in the United States during 2001. J Vasc Surg 2004;39:491-496.

121. Hua HT, Campria RP, Chuang SK, et al: Early outcomes of endovascular versus open abdominal aortic aneurysm repair in the National Surgical Quality Improvement Program-Private Sector (NS-QIP-PS). J Vasc Surg 2005;41:382-389.

122. Michaels J: The future of endovascular aneurysm repair. Eur J Vasc Endovasc Surg 2005;30:115-118.

45 Venous Intervention

Mitchell J. Silver and Gary M. Ansel

KEY POINTS

- Typical symptoms of superior vena cava (SVC) syndrome include severe congestion and edema of the face, arms, and upper thorax and may progress to dyspnea, cognitive dysfunction, and headache.
- Thrombolytic therapy before SVC endovascular stenting has great utility. After the acute thrombus is resolved, one need stent only the remaining stenosis, which most of the time is shorter than the occluded segment that was occupied by thrombus.
- It is paramount, after successful treatment of an acute upper extremity deep venous thrombosis (UEDVT), that some form of imaging be undertaken to evaluate for the presence of vein compression.
- Patients with Paget-Schroetter syndrome develop spontaneous UEDVT, usually in their dominant arm, after strenuous physical activity. Heavy repetitive exertion causes microtrauma to the vessel intima and leads to activation of the coagulation cascade.
- Clinical pulmonary embolism occurs in 26% to 67% of patients with untreated proximal deep venous thrombosis

(DVT) and is associated with a mortality rate of 11% to 23% if not treated. Under treatment, the incidence of pulmonary embolism decreases to 5%, and the mortality rate to less than 1%.
- Catheter-directed thrombolysis (CDT), or the delivery of thrombolytic agents directly into the thrombus, offers significant advantages for lower extremity DVT over systemic therapy, which may fail to reach and penetrate an occluded venous segment.
- There is an expanding role for the prophylactic use of retrievable inferior vena cava filters during CDT for lower extremity DVT, particularly in patients with "free-floating" iliac vein thrombus and in those whose cardiopulmonary reserve is already compromised.
- Percutaneous mechanical thrombectomy is an important adjunct to CDT that may result in a shorter time to vein patency, shorter length of hospitalization, reduction in hemorrhagic risk, and overall cost savings.

As interventional cardiologists with training in peripheral vascular disease have expanded their "skill set" from coronary interventions to the endovascular management of peripheral vascular disease, venous intervention has gradually become a natural extension to the "global cardiovascular interventionalist." In fact, more and more interventional cardiologists have become interested in the management of venous disorders, which now include central venous stenosis, and in the endovascular treatment of upper and lower extremity deep venous thrombosis (DVT).

THE VENOUS SYSTEM: BASIC HISTOLOGY AND PHYSIOLOGY

Veins are larger in caliber and more numerous then arteries. The venous system has a much greater volume capacity than the arterial system. The walls of veins are thinner and less elastic than the walls of arteries. Most anatomists distinguish three layers in the walls of veins: tunica intima, tunica media, and tunica adventitia. The distinctions between the layers are subtle. The internal elastic membrane is poorly

defined, and the tunica media is not as developed as that of arteries.

There are three categories of veins: venules and small-size veins, medium-size veins, and large-size veins. Only medium- and large-size veins are discussed in this chapter; for a complete review of venous embryology and anatomy, please refer to an anatomy text book.

Medium-size veins range between 2 and 9 mm in diameter. These include veins from extremities distal to the axillary or inguinal crease and cutaneous veins. The intima consists of endothelium, basal lamina, and reticular fibers. The media consists of a very thin layer of circular smooth muscle and few collagen fibers. The adventitia is the thickest layer and consists of collagen and elastic fibers.

The large-size veins consist of veins central to the axillary or inguinal crease, the superior vena cava (SVC), the inferior vena cava (IVC), and the renal, hepatic, and azygos veins. The intima is similar to that in the medium-size veins. A tunica media is lacking in most of the large veins, with the exception of the veins of the gravid uterus and pulmonary veins. A thick adventitia makes up the greater part of the thickness of the wall. This layer is rich in elastic fibers and longitudinally oriented collagen. The IVC is exceptional in that its adventitia contains scattered longitudinal bundles of smooth muscle. Large-size veins get their nutrient blood supply from very small penetrating vessels called vasa vasorum.

Vein Valves

Valve leaflets are a thin fold of the intima, with a thin layer of collagen and a network of elastic fibers that extend toward the intima of the vessel wall. The space between the valve and the vessel wall is called the sinus of the valve. The wall of the vessel becomes thinner and slightly expanded just above the attachment of each valve cusp.

Only the medium-size veins have valves. Their main function is to ensure antegrade flow of blood, peripheral to central, and superficial to deep, and to prevent backflow of blood away from the heart. In general, small- and large-size veins have no valves. Valves have a bicuspid structure and are more numerous in the veins of the lower extremity, where the force of gravity is the greatest. Venous valves have cup-like endothelial flaps that fill when there is retrograde flow of blood. When filled, the valves completely block the lumen, preventing flow reversal.

Physiology

The venous system has a large capacity, accounting for approximately two thirds of the systemic blood. Veins, because of their unique vascular structure, can undergo a large change in volume with minimal change in transmural pressure. This characteristic is called venous capacitance.

Because of their low elastic tissue content and prominent collagen-containing adventitia, the veins are actually stiffer than arteries when compared at the same distending pressure. A person in a resting upright position has significantly elevated venous pressures at the level of the feet and calves, accumulating a large volume of blood in the lower extremities. In these cases, the calf muscles magnify the venous return by working as a pump system. During walking or exercise, calf muscle contraction pushes the accumulated blood toward the heart, decreasing the venous pressures to near-zero. The venous pressure remains low even during calf muscle relaxation. At this time, the venous valves come into play, preventing backflow of blood but allowing the inflow of blood to refill the system. It is imperative that the vein valves be competent for this pump system to work appropriately. This calf muscle pump works most efficiently when all venous valves are competent. A normal pump system reduces venous pressure and volume in the exercising muscle, increases venous return, and improves arterial perfusion.

Varicose Veins

Incompetent valves in the saphenous system permit reflux of blood from the central veins to the peripheral veins. As the vein dilates because of excessive volume of blood, each valve becomes incompetent. This valve incompetence occurs in the deep and superficial systems, creating a standing column of blood with a constant increase in pressure transmitted through the systems, resulting in varicose veins.

Chronic Venous Disease

Chronic venous insufficiency is a significant problem in the United States, affecting as much as a quarter of the population. Venous valve incompetence is central to the venous hypertension that appears to underlie most or all signs of chronic venous disease. Chronic venous disease afflicts a younger segment of the population, and the morbidity of edema, leg pain, and ulceration may result in lifestyle alterations, loss of work, and frequent hospitalizations. The prevalence of venous ulcerations is not restricted to the elderly but certainly increases with age.[1] It has been estimated that venous ulcers have a major negative economic impact, with the loss of approximately 2 million working days treatment costs of approximately 3 billion dollars per year in the United States.[2]

The chief clinical manifestations of chronic venous disease are aching, leg pain, heaviness, a sensation of swelling, itching, cramps, and restless legs. Chronic venous disease can be graded according to the descriptive clinical, etiologic, anatomic, and pathophysiologic (CEAP) classification, which provides an orderly framework for communication and decision-making (Table 45-1).[3,4]

The pathophysiology of chronic venous disease in regard to its clinical expression has been well described and involves venous valve incompetence, structural changes in the vein wall manifested as hypertrophy, and the effects of elevated venous pressure and shear stress.[5] Much newer work has been done on understanding the pathophysiology of the skin changes of chronic venous disease. These studies have validated that chronic inflammation has a key role in the skin changes of chronic venous disease.

Support for the role of chronic inflammation in chronic venous disease has come to be known as the microvascular leukocyte-trapping hypothesis. Elegant studies have shown elevated numbers of macrophages, T lymphocytes, and mast cells in skin biopsy specimens from lower limbs affected by chronic venous disease.[6,7] The chronic inflammatory state in patients with chronic venous disease is related to the skin changes that are typical of the condition.[5] Increased expression and activity of matrix metalloproteinases (MMPs), especially MMP2, has been reported in lipodermatosclerosis,[8] in venous leg ulcers,[9] and in wound fluid from nonhealing ulcers.[10]

Table 45-1. Revised Clinical Classification of Chronic Venous Disease of the Leg

Class	Definition	Comments
C_0	No visible or palpable signs of venous disease	
C_1	Telangiectases, reticular veins, malleolar flare	Telangiectases defined by dilated intradermal venules <1 mm diameter
		Reticular veins defined by dilated, nonpalpable, subdermal veins ≤3 mm diameter
C_2	Varicose veins	Dilated, palpable, subcutaneous veins generally >3 mm diameter
C_3	Edema without skin changes	
C_4	Skin changes ascribed to venous disease	
C_{4A}		Pigmentation, venous eczema, or both
C_{4B}		Lipodermatosclerosis, atrophic blanche, or both
C_5	Skin changes with healed ulceration	
C_6	Skin changes with active ulceration	

Adapted from Porter JM, Moneta GL: Reporting standards in venous disease: An update. J Vasc Surg 1995;21:635-645; and Eklof B, Rutherford RB, Bergan JJ, et al: Revision of the CEAP classification for chronic venous disorders: Consensus statement. J Vasc Surg 2004;40:1248-1252.

The treatment of chronic venous disease is beyond the scope of this chapter but would be aimed at preventing venous hypertension, venous reflux, and, now, chronic inflammation (Fig. 45-1). Compression stockings and devices are certainly the mainstay of controlling venous hypertension. New endovenous ablation procedures using laser or radiofrequency energy are available to treat venous reflux. Clinical research is being actively pursued to develop pharmacotherapeutic approaches to alleviate the chronic inflammatory state of chronic venous disease, particularly targeting the interaction of leukocytes and endothelial cells.

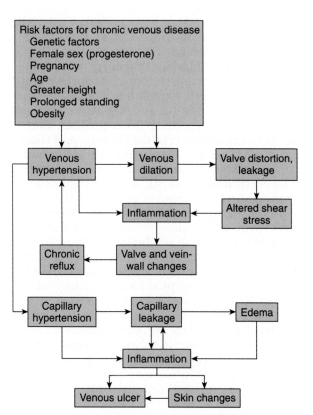

Figure 45-1. Venous hypertension as the hypothetical cause of the clinical manifestations of chronic venous disease, emphasizing the importance of inflammation.

CENTRAL VENOUS STENOSIS

SVC syndrome is a serious disorder resulting from impeded venous return from the upper body caused by obstruction of the SVC. The symptoms include severe congestion and edema of the face, arms, and upper thorax and may progress to dyspnea, cognitive dysfunction, and headache. A clinical classification system has been used by several clinicians and helps to classify symptom severity (Table 45-2). The SVC syndrome is usually caused by extrinsic or intrinsic obstruction of the SVC, although bilateral obstruction of both brachiocephalic venous segments can result in a similar syndrome.

Compression caused by mediastinal malignancy or lymphadenopathy is the most common cause of SVC syndrome.[11-13] The syndrome can also result from extension of central venous DVT to the SVC, usually in the presence of bilateral subclavian vein stenosis. Other benign causes include (1) thrombosis caused by underlying stenosis from long-term

Table 45-2. Clinical Scoring System for Central Venous Stenosis

Signs and Symptoms	Grade
Neurologic symptoms	
Stupor, coma, blackout	4
Blurry vision, headache, dizziness, amnesia	3
Changes in mentation	2
Uneasiness	1
Laryngotracheal or thoracic symptoms	
Orthopnea, laryngeal edema	3
Stridor, hoarseness, dysphagia, shortness of breath	2
Cough, pleural effusion	1
Nasal and facial signs or symptoms	
Lip edema, nasal stiffness, epistaxis, rhinorrhea	2
Facial swelling	1
Venous dilation	
Neck vein or arm vein distention, upper extremity swelling or upper body plethora	1

Modified from Kish K, Sonomura T, Mitsuzane K, et al: Self expandable metallic stent therapy for superior vein cava syndrome: Clinical observations. Radiology 1993;189:531-535.

indwelling central venous catheters or other transvenous instruments and (2) benign compressive or constrictive conditions of the mediastinum, such as adenopathy from earlier histoplasmosis, fibrosing mediastinitis, previous irradiation, tuberculosis, or histiocytosis.[14-19]

Diagnosis

The clinical presentation of SVC syndrome is relatively consistent. The diagnosis can be verified with multiple diagnostic modalities. Computed tomography (CT) is helpful for workup of SVC syndrome and often gives enough information to proceed directly to an endovascular procedure.[20] An upper extremity venogram reveals multiple collaterals if the obstruction has been long-standing, but with acute SVC obstruction there are often surprisingly few collaterals. With most causes, the venogram demonstrates the level of involvement, but it can still overestimate the length of involvement of the innominate veins, and even of the SVC, because of the high resistance to flow.

Magnetic resonance imaging (MRI) is helpful for the evaluation of SVC syndrome, and procedure planning can be based solely on MRI findings.[21,22] MRI gives good information regarding the extent of occlusion and collateral flow. Ultrasound, on the other hand, is not accurate in locating the central obstruction. The Doppler signal raises a suspicion of obstruction because of the flattened character of the waveform, but the level of obstruction is difficult or impossible to estimate with ultrasound, especially in the central portion of the SVC. Ultrasound with Doppler can, however, be a useful tool for follow-up after endovascular repair. In that setting, obstructive changes in the waveform raise suspicion of recurrent narrowing or occlusion of the recanalized vessel.

Technique

It is important to have a plan of approach before attempting SVC recanalization or stent placement. For a successful outcome, it is essential to take into account the patient's clinical presentation and preprocedure noninvasive imaging findings.

Many operators have used femoral vein access, but others have used jugular, subclavian,[23,24] arm vein, or even transhepatic venous approaches for stent delivery.[25] Any combination of these approaches may be used, but it is always paramount to have a guide wire "through and through," especially if the stenosis is severe and difficult to pass.[26,27] It certainly adds to the safety of the procedure to have a guide wire passing the right atrium into the IVC during stent delivery and dilation. This is particularly important in regard to preventing stent migration. This guide wire position prevents the stent from migrating into the right side of the heart or pulmonary artery. The stent is more likely to stay on the wire and can be more safely manipulated, removed, or moved to a different location.

Accessing the SVC from the right internal jugular vein or from upper extremity veins has several benefits. Manipulation is easier because of the limited space in the internal jugular vein compared with the right atrium, which one must work through when coming from a femoral vein access. The distance from the access site to the obstruction is also shorter, which can make it easier to cross a chronic total occlusion. An upper extremity access, such as via the brachial or basilic vein, is also a viable option. The entire venous intervention can be performed from this access, including thrombolysis, angioplasty, and stent placement in most cases.[28] This approach is also comfortable and well tolerated by most patients. Hemostasis is not usually problematic; placing a pressure dressing for 20 minutes or holding pressure for 5 to 10 minutes is usually successful. If double-barrel stenting is required to treat the SVC obstruction, bilateral upper extremity access is ideal, with the stents each traversing the brachiocephalic veins.

Several operators advocate using the common femoral vein for access, but it can be difficult to access an occluded or severely narrowed SVC from the femoral vein because of the anatomic relationship with the right atrium.[29-32] Some operators have, therefore, crossed the obstruction from the brachial veins, creating a through-and-through access from the femoral vein access by snaring the wire and pulling it through the femoral vein.[33] In addition, double-barrel stents into each of the brachiocephalic veins can easily be placed from bilateral common femoral vein access.

There is some experience performing thrombolytic therapy before and during SVC stent placement. Kee and colleagues[34] treated 27 patients with SVC syndrome with thrombolytic therapy. Six of the 27 patients did not have stents placed for the following reasons: one patient experienced failed treatment, one patient died secondary to massive pulmonary emboli presumably during thrombolysis, and four patients did not have residual stenosis and therefore did not require stent placement. The remaining 21 patients underwent stent placement subsequent to successful thrombolysis. All 27 patients were found to have acute thrombus on preprocedural venography. In the appropriate clinical setting, thrombolysis for SVC syndrome before endovascular therapy can have great utility. With resolution of the acute thrombus, one need stent only the underlying stenosis, which most of the time is shorter than the occluded segment that was occupied by thrombus. Therefore, a shorter segment of vessel must be stented, reducing the number of stents used and ultimately reducing the potential thrombogenic stent surface.

Gray and associates[35] reviewed the outcomes from thrombolysis of SVC thrombus in 16 patients and found no major complications and complete success in 56% of patients without stenting. Thrombolysis was effective in 73% of the cases. Stents were not used in any of the patients, which may explain many of the poor clinical outcomes. Many patients with SVC syndrome have central venous catheters in place on which they are dependent. Numerous reports describe pulling the catheters up from the SVC during the procedure, then placing the catheter down through the stent immediately after the procedure.[36-38]

Stent Selection

Early reports of SVC stenting described the use of Gianturco (Cook Incorporated) stents. This was the first stent in wide use, and it had diameters that were acceptable. Few complications were reported, but large sheath introducers are required for this stent, and it is used only in cases in which inflow vessels must be covered, because of the large spaces between the stent interstices.

Next, the Palmaz stent (Cordis Corporation) was released for use. This stent is balloon expandable and is now rarely used in the SVC. It has a higher radial force than self-expanding stents. On occasion, when extra radial force is needed, it can be used either primarily or secondarily within a deployed self-expanding stent that cannot sustain the radial force of SVC recoil.

In today's era of endovascular therapy, self-expanding stent delivery systems are now used for most SVC stenting (Fig. 45-2). The newer self-expanding stent delivery systems are easily deployed and come on a small, 6- to 7-Fr delivery system. The Wallstent (Boston Scientific Corporation) was one of the earlier versions of a self-expanding stent and is still widely used for SVC interventions. Its main shortcoming is that it foreshortens significantly on delivery, which makes precise placement difficult. Recent generations of self-expanding stents are made of nitinol and do not have this problem. Self-expanding nitinol stents include the Smart Stent (Cordis), the Luminex (Angiomed/Bard, Karlsruhe, Germany), and the Zilver (Cook). For the SVC, a 12- to 16-mm stent diameter is usually adequate.

Complications

In a group of 59 patients with malignant disease, Lanciego and coworkers reported six reocclusions, all of which were treated successfully with restenting in combination with thrombolysis.[23] One of the patients in this series had stent migration to the right atrium,

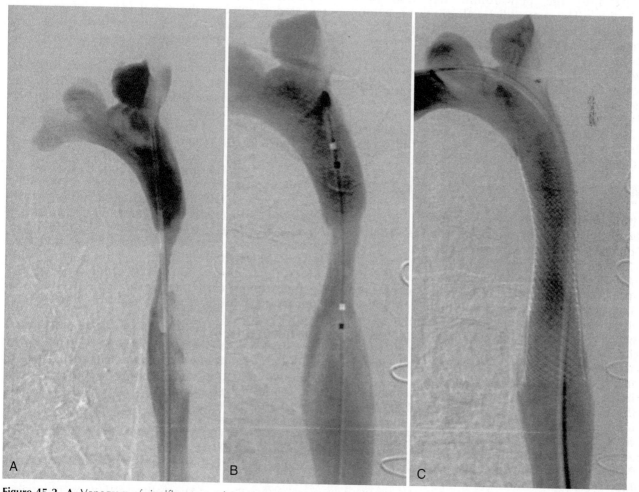

Figure 45-2. A, Venogram of significant superior vena cava (SVC) stenosis. **B,** Venogram of SVC after 12 mm percutaneous transluminal angioplasty. **C,** Venogram after placement of 14 mm Wallstent (Boston Scientific Corporation).

Table 45-3. Presenting Signs and Symptoms of UEDVT*

Condition	Symptoms	Signs
Axillary or subclavian vein thrombosis	Vague shoulder or neck discomfort Arm or hand edema	Supraclavicular fullness Palpable cord Arm or hand edema Extremity cyanosis Diluted cutaneous veins Jugular venous distention Unable to access central venous catheter
Thoracic outlet syndrome	Pain radiating to arm/forearm Hand weakness	Brachial plexus tenderness Arm or hand atrophy Positive Adson[†] or Wright[‡] maneuver

*The signs and symptoms of upper extremity deep venous thrombosis (UEDVT) are nonspecific and may be recognized with provocative maneuvers.
[†]Adson maneuver: The examiner extends the patient's arm on the affected side while the patient extends the neck and rotates the head toward the same side. The test is positive if there is weakening of the radial pulse with deep inspiration and suggests compression of the subclavian artery.
[‡]Wright maneuver: The patient's shoulder is abducted and the humerus is externally rotated. The test is positive if symptoms are reproduced and there is weakening of the radial pulse.

which was successfully treated. Nicholson and associates[30] reported on a patient who developed chronic shoulder pain after undergoing stenting of an SVC that extended into the subclavian vein.

Hemopericardium has been reported by several operators in the literature. This complication most commonly occurs during the procedure itself or immediately after stent placement,[39,40] but delayed bleeding into the pericardium has also been described.[41,42] The pericardial reflection can extend very high in the mediastinum, and the position is unpredictable.[43] In this regard, it is advisable to place stents high in the SVC, without compromising clinical results. If there is a high index of suspicion for hemopericardium, an echocardiogram or right heart catheterization should be done immediately.

In reviewing the literature, Martin and colleagues[40] found mention of 19 stent migrations, 6 fractured stents, 8 misplaced stents, and 3 cases of infection. There were also 3 cases of pulmonary emboli.

UPPER EXTREMITY DEEP VENOUS THROMBOSIS

Traditionally named after Paget and Von Shroetter, upper extremity deep venous thrombosis (UEDVT) was typically regarded as a rare and benign condition. As available case reports and literature grew in the 1990s, UEDVT became regarded as a more common and less benign disease, involved with serious complications such as pulmonary embolism, post-thrombotic syndrome, and death.[44-48] This change in viewpoint on UEDVT can be explained by a higher degree of clinical awareness and by increased effectiveness and availability of noninvasive diagnostic techniques.[49-52]

Primary UEDVT is a rare disorder (2 cases per 100,000 persons per year)[53] that comprises both effort thrombosis (Paget–Schroetter syndrome) and idiopathic UEDVT. Patients with Paget-Schroetter syndrome develop spontaneous UEDVT, usually in their dominant arm, after strenuous activity such as rowing, wrestling, weight lifting, or baseball pitching, but are otherwise young and healthy.[54] The heavy exertion causes microtrauma to the vessel

intima and leads to activation of the coagulation cascade. Significant thrombosis may occur with repeated insults to the vein wall, especially if mechanical compression of the vessel is also present.[55]

Thoracic outlet syndrome refers to compression of the neurovascular bundle (brachial plexus, subclavian artery, subclavian vein) as it exits the thoracic inlet.[54] Although this disorder may initially cause intermittent, positional extrinsic vein compression, repeated trauma to the vessel can result in dense, perivascular, fibrous scar tissue formation that compresses the vein persistently.[56] Compression of the subclavian vein typically develops in young athletes with hypertrophied muscles who do heavy lifting or completely abduct their arms. Cervical ribs, long transverse processes of the cervical spine, musculofascial bands, and clavicular or first rib anomalies are sometimes found in these patients. Therefore, cervical spine and chest plain films should be obtained in all patients undergoing evaluation for thoracic outlet syndrome.[57] Presenting signs and symptoms of UEDVT can be found in Table 45-3.

Secondary UEDVT is associated with both exogenous and endogenous risk factors and usually develops in older, ill patients, with a slightly higher incidence in women.[45,46,58] Among exogenous risk factors, the positioning of central venous lines, malignancy, previous or actual episodes of lower extremity DVT, treatment with oral contraceptives, and trauma appear to have the highest impact on the development of UEDVT.

Patients with indwelling central venous catheters constitute a particularly high-risk population, especially when undergoing chemotherapy, invasive hemodynamic monitoring, chronic parenteral nutrition, hemodialysis, or transvenous pacing, resulting in a more than 60% prevalence of either symptomatic or asymptomatic UEDVT.[59-62] In fact, ipsilateral catheter-related UEDVT accounts for up to 70% of all secondary UEDVT cases.[60-64]

Malignancy, either overt or undiagnosed, is also frequently associated with UEDVT (>40% of cases).[44-45,65] Recent data indicate that occult malignancy, especially lung cancer and lymphoma, may be discovered during follow-up in up to 24% of patients with UEDVT, mostly during the first week of hospital admission.[65]

A history of previous episodes or an ongoing DVT of the lower extremities is associated with UEDVT in up to 18% of cases.[60] In an ultrasound surveillance study, almost 30% of high-risk trauma patients developed UEDVT during the course of hospitalization, and up to 30% of them were asymptomatic.[66]

Treatment with oral contraceptives may represent a significant risk factor in women (up to 14%), although the data are conflicting.[45,67,68] Administration of recombinant gonadotropins during controlled ovarian hyperstimulation to induce ovulation was also suggested to increase the risk of UEDVT in subjects without known coagulation defects.[69,70]

Infrequently, UEDVT arises in carriers of peripheral venous catheters, usually from a superficial phlebitis spreading to the deep venous system,[71] or is associated with intravenous drug abuse, especially of cocaine.[72]

The prevalence of hypercoagulable states in patients with UEDVT is uncertain, because observational studies report varying results.[67,69,73,74] Furthermore, screening for coagulation disorders is controversial and has never been shown to be cost-effective.[54] The yield of these tests is highest for patients with idiopathic UEDVT; a family history of DVT; a history of recurrent, unexplained pregnancy loss; or a personal history of a prior DVT.

Diagnostic Testing

The gold standard for the diagnosis of UEDVT, which involves direct imaging of the whole deep venous system of the arm, is contrast venography. This is balanced by its invasive nature, inconvenience for patients, technical difficulty in performance and interpretation, and potential induction of contrast dye–related allergic reactions and thrombosis.

Several noninvasive methods are now available as alternatives to contrast venography and are highlighted in the following paragraphs.

Contrast Venography

Contrast venography is the standard reference for the diagnosis of UEDVT. Ideally, contrast injections should be made into the medial antecubital vein or more distally (e.g., in the back of the hand). This guarantees adequate opacification of the brachial, axillary, and subclavian veins. Hand injections should be used preferentially over power injectors to reduce the risk of serious contrast extravasation. A common pitfall of contrast venography is nonfilling of the cephalic segment, because isolated thrombosis of this venous segment could go unnoticed. It is essential to perform one series of the SVC during a single breath-hold.

Contrast venography may not be feasible in up to 20% of patients because of the inaccessibility of arm veins and contraindications for contrast agents (e.g., renal failure, hypersensitivity).

Despite some apparent disadvantages, venography may be required to confirm the diagnosis of UEDVT if suspicion for thrombosis remains high despite a negative noninvasive test. Venography is also required as a prelude to endovascular intervention, and is used to assess the response to these treatments, including thrombolytic therapy.

Duplex Ultrasonography

Duplex ultrasonography has largely replaced invasive venography for the diagnosis of DVT. It has many positive features: there is no requirement for nephrotoxic contrast agents, the test is noninvasive, and there is no need for ionizing radiation. In addition, it is widely available and can be performed at the bedside. Duplex ultrasonography has high sensitivity and specificity for peripheral (jugular, distal subclavian, axillary) UEDVT.[75] However, acoustic shadowing from the clavicle limit visualization of a segment of subclavian vein and may result in a false-negative study.[76]

Some technical recommendations regarding the use of duplex ultrasonography for the diagnosis of UEDVT include employing a combination of real-time compression gray-scale ultrasonography, color Doppler, and flow measurements using duplex technique with a 7.5 MHz linear-array probe.

When one is considering the diagnosis of UEDVT using duplex ultrasonography, the definition of thrombosis is critical. It is widely accepted that noncompressibility of a venous segment with or without visible thrombus constitutes thrombosis. There is a building body of evidence regarding isolated flow abnormalities; these are crucial because the entire venous system of the upper extremity cannot be followed beyond the clavicle.[77] Those flow abnormalities seen on duplex ultrasound are only suggestive of thrombosis, and contrast venography should be considered if there is a high clinical index of suspicion.

No studies have specifically addressed interobserver and intraobserver variability, but it is a widely known fact that ultrasonography is operator dependent in clinical practice and that imaging is more difficult in some patients, such as those with very extensive edema or obesity.

Magnetic Resonance Imaging

Magnetic resonance venography is an accurate, noninvasive method for detecting thrombus in the central chest veins, such as the SVC and brachiocephalic veins. Magnetic resonance venography provides a complete evaluation of central collaterals, central veins, and blood flow patterns. The correlation with traditional contrast venography is very good; therefore, magnetic resonance venography is a valuable imaging modality for the diagnosis of

UEDVT when contrast venography is contraindicated or impossible. The increased use of pacemakers and internal defibrillators does not make this imaging modality uniformly applicable.

Computed Tomographic Venography

As CT technology evolves with the use of multidetector CT equipment that can provide coronal and sagittal slice reformation and three-dimensional reconstruction, this imaging modality will likely play an important role in managing UEDVT. One major advantage of CT venography is the ability to assess for the presence of pulmonary emboli and other causes of upper extremity complaints during the same imaging session. Comparative studies evaluating the correlation of CT venography with digital subtraction venography for the diagnosis of UEDVT are underway.

Treatment Options

The optimal approach for the treatment of UEDVT remains unknown, but in general, there are two goals. The first goal is to prevent further propagation of thrombi, to reduce the risk of secondary events such as pulmonary embolus or disease recurrence. The second goal should be the preservation of normal venous anatomy by some form of recanalization of existing thrombus. It is quite likely that more patients with UEDVT will be approached with a multimodal effort. These treatment options will include, either individually or in combination, anticoagulant therapy, thrombolytic therapy, endovascular intervention, and vascular surgery.

Anticoagulation

Anticoagulation represents the mainstay of therapy for UEDVT. Anticoagulation helps maintain the patency of venous collaterals and reduces thrombus propagation even if the clot does not completely resolve.[78] However, anticoagulation rarely achieves recanalization and therefore leads to permanent obstruction of the upper extremity veins. Collateral veins often develop, but these are not accessible for placement of intravenous lines.

Standard anticoagulation typically includes the administration of unfractionated heparin or low-molecular-weight heparin (LMWH) for 5 to 7 days, as a "bridge" to oral warfarin. Warfarin is typically continued for a minimum of 3 months, with a goal being an international normalized ratio (INR) of 2.0 to 3.0. A longer duration of warfarin anticoagulation may be indicated if some form of coagulation abnormality is detected.

Thrombolytic Therapy

Because many patients with UEDVT are young, active, and healthy, consideration for thrombolytic therapy over conservative anticoagulation should be considered strongly on a case-to-case basis. Certainly, a young, healthy patient with UEDVT may have significant long-term morbidity if treated with only anticoagulation.[79] Thrombolysis restores venous patency early, minimizes damage to the vessel endothelium, and reduces the risk of long-term complications, especially the development of post-thrombotic syndrome, with its disabling chronic arm and hand aching and swelling. The obvious disadvantage of thrombolytic therapy is greater risk of a bleeding complication.

The ideal candidate for thrombolytic therapy for UEDVT is an otherwise healthy, young patient with a primary UEDVT. Those patients with an indwelling central venous catheter for whom it is essential to maintain patency for central venous access are also prime candidates.

Catheter-directed thrombolysis (CDT) achieves higher rates of complete clot resolution with lower doses of medication and reduces the risk for serious bleeding compared with systemic thrombolysis.[54] Thrombolysis has the best chance of success if it is used within 4 to 6 weeks after the onset of symptoms, because older organized thrombus is more resistant to thrombolysis. For CDT, the catheter should be directly placed within the entire length of thrombus; otherwise, the potential for collateral circulation to divert drug distribution away from the thrombus may lead to an unsuccessful procedure.

There are no randomized, prospective controlled clinical trials comparing different thrombolytic agents for the treatment of UEDVT. At our tertiary referral center, catheter-directed Retavase (reteplase, or r-PA) is usually administered at 0.25 to 0.5 U/h for 8 hours. Clinical examination and serial venography are used to assess the response to treatment. We often employ a percutaneous mechanical thrombectomy (PMT) device in combination with thrombolytic therapy. This adjunctive catheter-based thrombectomy has the benefit of extracting thrombus before thrombolytic therapy, which often initiates some blood flow, thereby improving drug distribution, reducing dose, and reducing the duration of thrombolytic therapy.[80] PMT devices are discussed thoroughly in a later section of this chapter.

The time required to achieve complete thrombolysis in subclavian vein thrombosis can be up to 72 hours. Oral anticoagulation (e.g., warfarin) should be used for 3 to 6 months after successful thrombolysis for UEDVT. The duration of warfarin therapy should be individualized on a case-to-case basis depending on the clinical situation.

Interventional Therapy

Catheter-based mechanical thrombectomy is an important adjunct to thrombolytic therapy, as stated earlier. It is theoretically advantageous in that instant debulking or removal of thrombus, and thereby restoration of flow, is very beneficial before CDT to

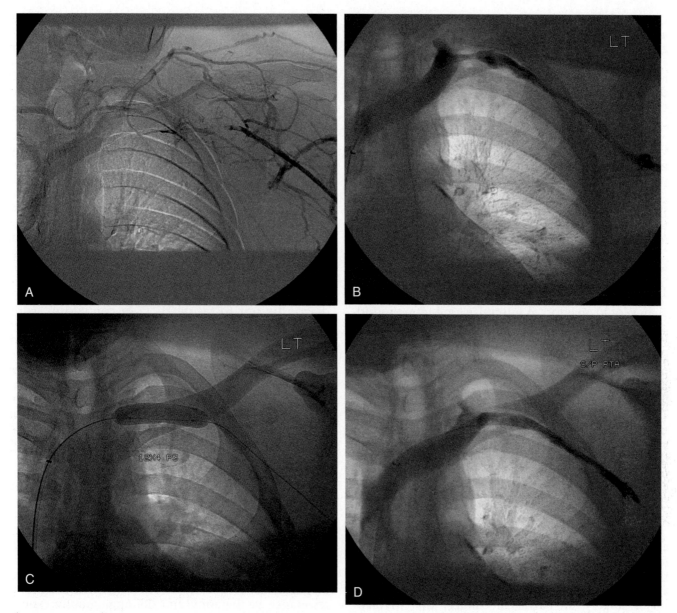

Figure 45-3. **A,** Left upper extremity venogram demonstrating acute left subclavian vein thrombosis. **B,** Placement of infusion catheter into left subclavian vein thrombus. **C,** Percutaneous transluminal angioplasty (PTA) of left subclavian vein with 12 mm balloon after thrombolysis. **D,** Completion venogram of left subclavian vein after successful catheter-directed thrombolysis with adjunctive PTA.

improve drug distribution and to decrease the dose and duration of thrombolytic therapy.

Adjunctive percutaneous transluminal angioplasty or stenting of the subclavian vein has utility especially for catheter-related stenosis when there is a hemodynamically significant pressure gradient after thrombolytic therapy. A flexible, self-expanding, oversized stent is best suited for this location. Intravascular ultrasound has proved to be very useful in determining stent sizing when treating subclavian vein stenosis. Figure 45-3 demonstrates CDT for a left subclavian DVT followed by adjunctive percutaneous transluminal angioplasty.

Surgical Therapy

Vein compression in patients with primary UEDVT is an important cause of recurrent thrombosis and long-term morbidity.[81] It is paramount, after successful treatment of an acute UEDVT, that some form of imaging be undertaken to evaluate for the presence of vein compression. After successful thrombolysis, venography in the neutral and shoulder-abducted positions can help demonstrate vein compression. Recent surgical series recommend surgical correction of extrinsic vein compression,[81,82] which typically requires resection of part of the first rib or clavicle.

Lysis of adhesions around the subclavian vein may also be required if anatomic anomalies have caused chronic, repeated trauma to the subclavian vein. Surgical thrombectomy is rarely required because of advancements in pharmacologic and catheter-based therapies. However, in symptomatic patients with UEDVT refractory to other therapies, surgical thrombectomy can restore venous patency.

Treatment of UEDVT is aimed at preservation of venous anatomy, prevention of potentially fatal pulmonary embolism, and decrease in the risk of post-phlebitic syndrome. Treatment is dependent on the cause, duration of thrombosis, and clinical circumstances. For most patients with UEDVT, anticoagulation with an antithrombin agent followed by 3 to 6 months of oral anticoagulation is usually sufficient.

However, there is a tendency to be more aggressive with thrombolytic therapy and catheter-based thrombectomy in individual cases, especially in younger patients who are at risk for chronic venous insufficiency, or in an effort to minimize long-term morbidity and optimize functionality. A structured physical therapy program to loosen muscles compressing the subclavian vein and weight loss, if appropriate, are other important adjuncts to complete therapy.

LOWER EXTREMITY DEEP VENOUS THROMBOSIS

DVT is a process that can affect each one of the deep veins of the body but is more frequently present in the deep veins of the lower extremity. Venous thrombus formation is initiated by intravascular clotting and is increased in the presence of risk factors. These risk factors were postulated more than 100 years ago by Virchow and are summarized by his classic triad of coagulation abnormalities, endothelial damage, and stasis. The main conditions contributing to the formation of venous thrombus in the deep veins of the legs are related to these three basic risk factors and include advanced age, prolonged bed rest, and major surgery. In particular, surgery that involves large abdominal operations, and especially orthopedic surgery; previous venous thrombosis; malignancy; trauma; varicose veins; chronic venous insufficiency; pregnancy and the postpartum period; use of contraceptive pills; and hypercoagulable states, either primary or secondary, are frequently implicated.

The main complications of lower extremity DVT are pulmonary embolism and post-thrombotic syndrome. Clinical pulmonary embolism occurs in 26% to 67% of cases of untreated proximal DVT and is associated with a mortality rate of 11% to 23% if not treated. Under treatment, the incidence of pulmonary embolism decreases to 5%, and the mortality rate to less than 1%. Post-thrombotic syndrome is a cause of increased morbidity and disability. Up to two thirds of patients with iliofemoral DVT develop edema and pain, with 5% developing ulcers despite adequate anticoagulation.[83] Early diagnosis and treatment of DVT is essential to prevent mortality and morbidity from pulmonary embolism and post-thrombotic syndrome.

Diagnosis of Acute Lower Extremity Deep Venous Thrombosis

Venous Duplex Ultrasound

The clinical diagnosis of lower extremity DVT is notoriously inaccurate, with the classic signs and symptoms of DVT being as common in patients without DVT as they are in those with confirmed DVT. Therefore, objective confirmation of clinically suspected DVT is required. Despite its many limitations, as noted earlier, ascending venography historically was the gold standard for the diagnosis of acute DVT. It is invasive, not easily repeatable, and impossible to perform or interpret in 9% to 14% of patients; fails to visualize all venous segments in 10% to 30% of studies; and is associated with interobserver disagreements in 4% to 10% of studies. Not surprisingly, therefore, venography has been replaced by venous duplex ultrasonography as the most widely used diagnostic test for acute DVT. In comparison with venography, duplex ultrasound has the advantages of being widely available, noninvasive, portable, and easily repeatable.

A complete ultrasound evaluation of the lower extremities includes an assessment of venous compressibility, intraluminal echoes, venous flow characteristics, and luminal color filling. Venous incompressibility, or failure to completely coapt the venous walls with gentle probe compression, is the most widely used diagnostic criterion for acute DVT. Adjunctive gray-scale findings include the appearance of echogenic thrombus within the vein lumen and dilation of an acutely thrombosed segment. Normal flow in the proximal veins should be spontaneous and should vary with respiration (increasing during expiration and decreasing during inspiration).

Other noninvasive imaging techniques for the diagnosis of lower extremity DVT include magnetic resonance venography and CT angiography. These modalities are comparable to conventional venography, but they cannot be done at the bedside, carry the risk of contrast allergy, and are more expensive than venous duplex ultrasonography.

Diagnostic Testing and Clinical Risk Stratification

D-Dimer, which is formed as a byproduct in the degradation of cross-linked fibrin by plasmin, reflects thrombus and has been proposed as an alternative or adjunct to initial diagnostic testing. Although D-dimer is sensitive for the diagnosis of DVT, measurements of D-dimer are nonspecific, and elevated levels may be associated with preeclampsia, malignancy, infection, trauma, or recent surgery. The high sensitivity of D-dimer measurements makes it theoretically possible to exclude a diagnosis of DVT; however, the low specificity and positive predictive value necessitate confirmatory noninvasive testing after a positive result.

A combined strategy using an assessment of clinical probability, D-dimer testing, and venous duplex ultrasonography may hold the greatest diagnostic promise. The negative predictive value of this approach is almost 100% in outpatients with a low pretest clinical probability for DVT.[84]

Goals of Therapy

There are four generally accepted goals for the treatment of lower extremity DVT. These treatment goals have expanded as understanding of the pathophysiology of venous thromboembolism has evolved, along with the constant refinement of endovascular devices and thrombotic therapy. Therapy for lower extremity DVT is undertaken to (1) diminish the severity and duration of lower extremity symptoms, (2) prevent pulmonary embolism, (3) minimize the risk of recurrent venous thrombosis, and/or (4) prevent the post-thrombotic syndrome.

Detailed monographs regarding the medical management of lower extremity DVT are numerous and readily available. There is uniform agreement that adequate initial anticoagulant therapy is required to prevent thrombus growth and pulmonary embolism. Intravenous unfractionated heparin is being replaced by LMWH as the anticoagulant of choice for the initial treatment of lower extremity venous thromboembolism. Both agents are relatively safe and effective when used to treat lower extremity DVT, with LMWH suitable for outpatient therapy because of improved bioavailability and more predictable anticoagulant response. Serious potential complications of heparin therapy, such as heparin-induced thrombocytopenia and osteoporosis, seem less common with LMWH.

Although medical therapy with anticoagulation is the mainstay of the initial management of lower extremity DVT, many patients, particularly those with large proximal iliofemoral DVT, have persistent leg edema, pain, and difficulty ambulating. These morbid symptoms arise from venous hypertension caused by outflow obstruction. Relief of outflow obstruction is one of the primary goals of therapy for lower extremity DVT, but this is not accomplished by anticoagulation alone, because thrombus regression occurs in only 50% of patients.[85] The newer endovascular techniques, including CDT, mechanical thrombectomy, and stenting, offer viable options in treating and restoring the pathway of thrombosed veins. The details of endovascular venous interventions that are targeted to restore venous patency, preserve valvular function, and possibly minimize the risk of late post-thrombotic complications are outlined in the following paragraphs.

Catheter-Directed Thrombolysis

In the early 1990s, Semba and Drake[86] first reported the feasibility of CDT for iliofemoral thrombosis as an alternative to systemic anticoagulation, systemic thrombolysis, or surgical venous thrombectomy.

CDT, or the delivery of thrombolytic agents directly into the thrombus, offers significant advantages over systemic therapy, which may fail to reach and penetrate an occluded venous segment. Because thrombolytic agents activate plasminogen within the thrombus, the delivery of the drug to that site enhances its effectiveness. CDT focuses the delivery of higher concentrations of the drug, resulting in improved lysis rates, reduced duration of treatment, and reduced complications associated with exposure of the patient to systemic thrombolytic therapy. After successful CDT, the implication is that preservation of valvular function and removal of the obstructing thrombus will facilitate a lower incidence of post-thrombotic syndrome. In addition, this endovascular approach allows for the detection and correction of any underlying venous obstructive lesions with balloon angioplasty and/or stents.

Currently, no thrombolytic agents have been approved for CDT by the U.S. Food and Drug Administration (FDA). The use of thrombolytic agents in CDT for venous thrombosis constitutes an "off label" use. There are five thrombolytic agents available in the United States that can be used during CDT for venous thrombosis. Although the various agents have unique properties that might theoretically imply superiority of one over another, there is no peer-reviewed consensus on a superior or "best choice" agent for CDT for venous thrombosis. The literature on CDT for venous thrombosis has a paucity of prospective randomized comparative trials. Therefore, the choice of thrombolytic agent is usually individualized based on the physician's discretion.

The largest published experience with CDT has come from the National Venous Thrombolysis Registry,[86] which included 287 patients treated with urokinase and monitored up for 1 year. Overall, 71% of the patients were treated for iliofemoral DVT. Complete dissolution of thrombus was achieved in 31% of cases, and partial thrombus dissolution was reported in an additional 52%. Primary patency at 1 year was 60%. Preservation of valvular competence was demonstrated in 72% of the patients with complete thrombolysis. Table 45-4 reviews the available clinical experience for CDT in the treatment of DVT.

The decision to perform CDT for lower extremity DVT must be individualized to each case based on a risk-benefit analysis. The technique for CDT for lower extremity DVT is not standardized; however, the primary goal is to deliver the lytic agent directly into venous clot.

The location of the lower extremity DVT and the patent's symptoms determine the access technique. For most cases of iliofemoral DVT, the ipsilateral popliteal vein is favored if the clinical situation allows. With the patient prone on the angiographic table, the venous access site should be accessed under ultrasound guidance with a small-gauge echogenic needle. Should the popliteal vein be thrombosed, the ipsilateral posterior tibial vein may be cannulated. After popliteal vein cannulation, a 5-Fr short sheath

Table 45-4. Catheter-Directed Thrombolysis for Deep Venous Thrombosis (Single-Center Case Studies)

Authors	N	Agent	Outcome (% Lysis)	Hemorrhage (%)
Molina et al.	12	UK	95	0
Comerota et al.	7	UK	71	0
Semba and Drake	27	UK	92	0
Bjarnason et al.	87	UK	86	6.9 major, 14 minor
Patel et al.	10	UK	100	0
Ouriel et al.	11	rPA	73	0
Castaneda et al.	25	rPA	92	4
Chang et al.	10	tPA	90	0
Horne et al.	10	tPA	90	30 minor
Razavi et al.	36	TNK	83	2.7 major, 8.3 minor

rPT, reteplase; TNK, tenecteplase; tPA, alteplase; UK, urokinase.

is introduced, through which all subsequent catheters are exchanged. Next, a baseline venogram is obtained using the venous sheath, and then a combination of 0.035-inch straight and curved glidewires are used to cross the occluded venous segment. After wire and then catheter traversal of the occluded venous segment, venography is repeated to confirm the intraluminal position of the catheter. The catheter is then exchanged for a 5-Fr infusing coaxial system, consisting of a proximal multiside-hole catheter and a distal infusion wire. It is essential to position the system directly into the thrombus to maximize plasminogen activation at the site of obstruction. Figure 45-4 illustrates the endovascular management of an acute right common iliac DVT.

The patient is monitored in the interventional recovery unit as the thrombolytic agent is infused. It is quite common, particularly with extensive thrombus burden, for the duration of therapy to exceed 24 hours. Follow-up venography should be performed every 12 hours to assess and/or reposition the infusion catheter directly into any remaining thrombus. Weighing the risk versus the benefit of lytic therapy, the infusion should be continued until complete lysis is achieved.

If venous patency is restored and there is no underlying stenotic/occlusive lesion, thrombolysis is discontinued and anticoagulation is initiated. Hemodynamically significant lesions that are uncovered in the iliac veins should be considered for endovascular stenting, although the long-term benefits of venous stenting are not known. However, if left untreated, a significant iliac vein stenosis appears to be a significant risk of early rethrombosis.

Indications for placement of an IVC filter during CDT for lower extremity DVT fall within the same spectrum as indications for routine prophylactic IVC filters. The use of IVC filters during lower extremity venous thrombolysis has always been controversial because of the low incidence of complications that occur when lysis is performed without filter protection. With the advent of retrievable IVC filters, we have been implementing them routinely when performing CDT for iliofemoral DVT. This seems particularly reasonable for patients in whom the venogram

defines a true "free-floating" iliac vein thrombus or for those with a documented pulmonary embolus and limited cardiopulmonary reserve for additional emboli.

If an underlying stenosis after successful CDT is believed to be secondary to iliac vein compression, stent deployment is required, because vein compression typically does not respond to stand-alone angioplasty. This iliac vein compression, or May-Thurner syndrome, involves extrinsic compression of the common iliac vein by the crossing iliac artery, usually on the left, at the iliocaval junction. Self-expanding stents are usually preferred because of their longitudinal flexibility and ability to conform to various venous configurations. Care should be exercised to avoid stenting across the common femoral vein, particularly at the saphenofemoral junction.

Percutaneous Mechanical Thrombectomy

Issues surrounding CDT for lower extremity DVT include the time to lysis, need for intensive care monitoring, hemorrhagic risks, cost, and lack of prospective, randomized clinical trials. With these issues in mind, PMT is conceptually attractive because such a technique may result in a shorter time to vein patency, shorter length of stay, reduction in hemorrhagic risk, and overall cost savings because of reduced hospitalization and elimination or reduction in thrombolytic drugs.

From a mechanistic standpoint, PMT devices can be categorized as rotational, hydrodynamic, or ultrasound-facilitated. Table 45-5 outlines current mechanical thrombectomy devices. In addition, with some of these PMT devices, simultaneous administration of thrombolytic therapy can be performed; this is known as pharmacomechanical thrombectomy.

Rotational thrombectomy devices employ a high-speed rotating basket or impeller to pulverize or fragment the thrombus. Preclinical evaluation of these devices focused on clot removal and assessment of potential valve injury. In one such study, the Arrow-Trerotola (Arrow) percutaneous thrombectomy device did not cause physiologically significant damage to valves 7 mm or larger in diameter.[87] In several cases, small particles have been documented to embolize to

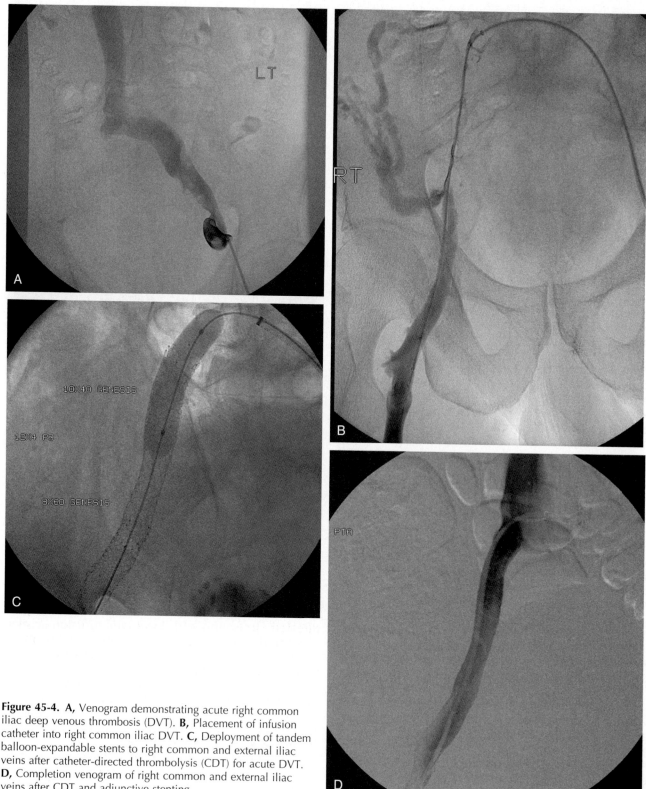

Figure 45-4. A, Venogram demonstrating acute right common iliac deep venous thrombosis (DVT). **B,** Placement of infusion catheter into right common iliac DVT. **C,** Deployment of tandem balloon-expandable stents to right common and external iliac veins after catheter-directed thrombolysis (CDT) for acute DVT. **D,** Completion venogram of right common and external iliac veins after CDT and adjunctive stenting.

the pulmonary circulation during rotational thrombectomy.[87-89] Because these rotational thrombectomy devices have the potential of damaging the endothelial lining of the vein, the Bacchus Fino device (Bacchus Vascular) was designed to use a rotating Archimedes screw that is protected from vessel wall

contact by a helically oriented nitinol framework. The screw fragments the thrombus, extracting much of it into a sheath through rotational motion.

Hydrodynamic or "rheolytic" recirculation devices have become a common treatment modality for lower extremity DVT. One of the PMT devices that

Table 45-5. Mechanical Thrombectomy Devices

Device	Manufacturer
Wall Contact Devices	
Arrow percutaneous thrombectomy device (PTD)	Arrow International, Reading, PA
Solera	Bacchus Vascular, Santa Clara, CA
Cleaner	Rex Medical, Fort Worth, TX
MTI-Castaneda Brush	Microtherapeutics, San Clemente, CA
Fino	Baccus Vascular, Santa Clara, CA
Cragg Brush	Microtherapeutics, San Clemente, CA
Prolumen	Datascope, Maheah, NJ
Hydrodynamic Thrombectomy Fragmentation Devices	
Amplatz thrombectomy device (ATD/Helix)	Microvena, White Bear Lake, MN
Rotarex catheter	Straub Medical, Wangs, Switzerland
Thrombex PMT	Edwards Lifesciences, Irvine, CA
Rheolytic (Flow-Based) Thrombectomy Devices	
AngioJet	Possis Medical, Minneapolis, MN
Oasis Thrombectomy System	Boston Scientific, Watertown, MA
Hydrolyzer	Cordis Corporation, Warren, NJ

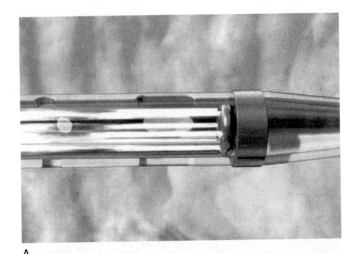

A

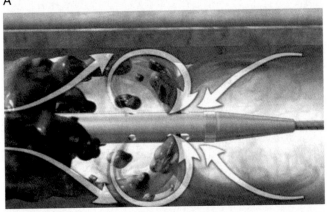

B

Figure 45-5. **A,** The AngioJet system (Possis Medical) emits high-velocity saline jets that are directed backward from the tip of the device to outflow channels in a coaxial fashion. **B,** A vacuum force is generated that draws the thrombus into the catheter.

have been shown to be effective in removal of acute thrombus is the AngioJet (Possis Medical) system. The principle of this device is based on the venturi effect, which creates rapidly flowing saline jets that are directed backward from the tip of the device to outflow channels in a coaxial fashion. This generates a vacuum force that draws the thrombus into the catheter (Fig. 45-5). One major advantage of this PMT device is that the thrombectomy catheter can be delivered through a 6-Fr introducer sheath, which reduces access-site complications. Devices based on "rheolytic" recirculation might possibly produce less valvular or endothelial damage than PMT devices that employ rotational thrombectomy, although these two mechanisms of thrombus removal have not been directly compared. Examples of other "rheolytic" recirculation devices include the Hydrolyser (Cordis Corporation) and the Oasis Thrombectomy System (Boston Scientific). The Hydrolyser system uses a conventional contrast power injector to inject saline solution through an injection lumen. The resultant pressure reduction at the nozzle tip creates a 360-degree vortex that fragments and aspirates thrombus into an exhaust lumen. The thrombotic material is then discharged through the exhaust lumen into a collection bag. The Oasis Thrombectomy System operates similarly to the AngioJet, using a venturi effect with thrombus fragmentation. However, the AngioJet system now has a "large-vessel" catheter that has the ability to extract a large amount of thrombus.

Despite great advances in PMT technologies, complete thrombus resolution rarely occurs, so adjunctive thrombolytic therapy is often required. In an effort to improve thrombus resolution, an ultrasound-based infusion system, the Lysus Infusion System (EKOS Corporation) was developed. The EKOS Lysus System combines high-frequency, low-power ultrasound with simultaneous catheter-directed thrombolytics to accelerate clot dissolution. The exposure of thrombus to nonfragmenting ultrasound has no lytic effect on its own. However, the combination of directed ultrasound with local lytic infusion accelerates the thrombolytic process.[90] The mechanism for accelerated thrombolysis is that the delivery of high-frequency, low-power ultrasound loosens the fibrin matrix to increase clot permeability and drive the thrombolytic agent deep into the thrombus for better drug distribution. In addition, the ultrasound energy penetrates venous valves and facilitates clearing of thrombus associated with them.

The EKOS System consists of a 5.2-Fr, multilumen drug delivery catheter with one central lumen and three separate infusion ports (Fig. 45-6). Each catheter has a matched ultrasound core wire that is placed in the central lumen and delivers the ultrasound energy evenly along the entire infusion pathway. After the catheter is positioned in the thrombus, an infusion of lytic agent is started, along with saline to serve as a coolant. Ultrasound is then started and delivered simultaneously with the lytic agent infusion.

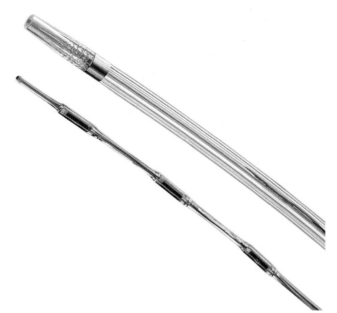

Figure 45-6. The Lysus multilumen drug delivery catheter and removable ultrasound core wire. Application of radial ultrasound energy along the axis of the infusion catheter enhances permeability and penetration of lytic agent into clot.

Another ultrasound-based technology, the Omni-Sonics Resolution Endovascular System (OmniSonics Medical Technologies) is based on ultrasound ablation of thrombus. Currently, ultrasound technology is routinely used for disintegration of renal and urethral calculi, aortic valve decalcification, and cataract phacoemulsion procedures. In regard to thrombus dissolution, there are many hypotheses regarding the mode of action of ultrasonic energy. In the case of intravascular ultrasound delivery catheters, cavitation, microstreaming, and mechanical effects are the primary mode of action of thrombolysis.[91]

The OmniSonics Resolution Endovascular System utilizes OmniWave Technology, which enables the creation of a standing transverse wave on the distal section of a small profile wire (Fig. 45-7).[92] The transverse wave creates ultrasonic energy circumferentially around the wire using very low power. The proprietary wire design converts the longitudinal motion to transverse motion in the treatment zone, producing

an extended region of ultrasonic activation. The system has a pump that irrigates fluid down the catheter to ensure that the system does not produce a temperature greater than 41°C. The Resolution Endovascular System is currently FDA-approved for declotting of hemodialysis grafts. It is being tested in large animal models in iliofemoral arteries and veins.

Pharmacomechanical thrombectomy, or the simultaneous administration of thrombolytics during PMT, represents true "combination therapy." This form of PMT has been reported with the AngioJet (Possis Medical) and the Trellis (Bacchus Vascular) devices.

In a small series, Uppot and colleagues[93] reported a technique of mixing the thrombolytic drug in the AngioJet saline infusion bag for direct administration during PMT. In 24 patients, complete or substantial thrombus removal was achieved. With more experience, this technique has been refined to develop the "Power Pulse technique." This technique involves placement of a stopcock on the AngioJet return port. The stopcock is closed for the Power Pulse technique to prevent thrombus and lytic drug aspiration. With the outflow port occluded, the AngioJet catheter effectively becomes a one-way infusion system, with dilute lytic agent pulsed into the clot. After delivery of the lytic agent throughout the thrombus, a period of up to 30 to 45 minutes is allowed to elapse, permitting maximal lytic time. After this period, the AngioJet is activated in a normal fashion, with the outflow port open to promote aspiration of thrombus.

The Bacchus Trellis (Bacchus Vascular) consists of a catheter with proximal and distal occlusion balloons (Fig. 45-8) and a sheath designed to aspirate contents between the balloons. A sinusoidal nitinol wire placed within the catheter is rotated to mix the blood between the balloons. The Trellis device, which combines a high concentration of thrombolytic medication with mechanical disruption of thrombus, has been used with success to treat patients with DVT.[94] The occlusive balloons limit leakage of thrombolytic agent into the systemic circulation, potentially reducing the risk of bleeding complications, whereas the central balloon is intended to reduce embolization of particulate matter to the pulmonary circulation. One limitation with this catheter system is that it cannot be used in large veins such as the common iliac or SVC.

Figure 45-7. The Lysus OmniSonics wire design converts the longitudinal motion to transverse motion in the treatment zone, producing an extended region of ultrasonic activation.

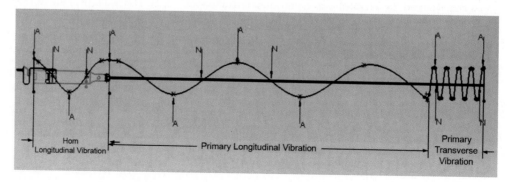

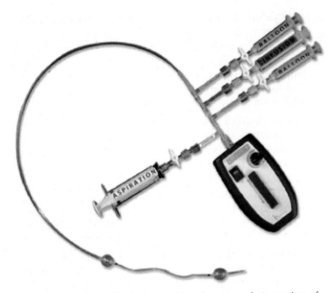

Figure 45-8. The Trellis 8 System (Bacchus Vascular) consists of proximal and distal balloons, balloon inflation syringes, a thrombolysis infusion port, the thrombus aspiration syringe, and a drive unit for mechanical dispersion of the thrombolytic agent.

These exciting combination strategies continue to be developed and investigated and with further follow-up will be better defined for their efficacy and role in PMT for DVT.

REFERENCES

1. Moffatt CJ, Franks PJ, Doherty DC, et al: Prevalence of leg ulceration in a London population. Q J Med 2004;97:431-437.
2. McGuckin M, Waterman R, Brooks J, et al: Validation of venous leg ulcer guidelines in the United States and United Kingdom. Am J Surg 2002;183:132-137.
3. Porter JM, Moneta GL: Reporting standards in venous disease: An update. J Vasc Surg 1995;21:635-645.
4. Eklof B, Rutherford RB, Bergan JJ, et al: Revision of the CEAP classification for chronic venous disorders: Consensus statement. J Vasc Surg 2004;40:1248-1252.
5. Bergan JJ, Schmid-Schonbein GW, Cooleridge Smith PD, et al: Chronic venous disease. N Engl J Med 2006;355:488-498.
6. Wilkinson LS, Bunker C, Edwards JC, et al: Leukocytes: Their role in the etiopathogenesis of skin damage in venous disease. J Vasc Surg 1993;17:669-675.
7. Pappas PJ, DeFouw DO, Venezio LM, et al: Morphometric assessment of the dermal microcirculation in patients with chronic venous insufficiency. J Vasc Surg 1997;26:784-795.
8. Herouy Y, May AE, Pornschlegel G, et al: Lipodermatosclerosis is characterized by elevated expression and activation of matrix metalloproteinases: Implications for venous ulcer formation. J Invest Dermatol 1998;111:822-827.
9. Norgauer J, Hildenbrand T, Idzko M, et al: Elevated expression of extracellular matrix metalloproteinase inducer (CD147) and membrane-type matrix metallaproteinases in venous leg ulcers. Br J Dermatol 2002;147:1180-1186.
10. Mwaura B, Mahendran B, Hynes N, et al: The impact of differential expression of extracellular matrix metalloproteinase inducer, matrix metalloproteinase-2, tissue inhibitor of matrix metalloproteinase-2 and PDGF-AA on the chronicity of venous leg ulcers. Eur J Vasc Endovasc Surg 2006;31:306-310.
11. Crowe MT, Davies CH, Gaines PA: Percutaneous management of superior vena cava occlusions. Cardiovasc Intervent Radiol 1995;18:367-372.
12. Kee ST, Kinoshita L, Razavi MK, et al: Superior vena cava syndrome: Treatment with catheter-directed thrombolysis and endovascular stent placement. Radiology 1998;206:187-193.
13. Lochridge SK, Knibbe WP, Doty DB: Obstruction of the superior vena cava. Surgery 1979;85:14-24.
14. Chamorro H, Rao G, Wholey M: Superior vena cava syndrome: A complication of transvenous pacemaker implantation. Radiology 1978;126:377-378.
15. Mocherla S, Wheat LJ: Treatment of histoplasmosis. Semin Respir Infect 2001;16:141-148.
16. Christenson ML, Franks TJ, Galvin JR: Fibrosing mediastinitis. Radiographics 2001;21:737-757.
17. Mahajan V, Strimlan V, Ordstrand HS, Loop FD: Benign superior vena cava syndrome. Chest 1975;68:32-35.
18. Qanadli SD, El Hajjam M, Mignon F, et al: Subacute and chronic benign superior vena cava obstructions: Endovascular treatment with self-expanding metallic stents. AJR Am J Roentgenol 1999;173:159-164.
19. Connell J, Muhm J: Radiographic manifestations of pulmonary histoplasmosis: A 10-year review. Radiology 1976;121:281-285.
20. Qanadli SD, El Hajjam M, Bruckert F, et al: Helical CT phlebography of the superior vena cava: Diagnosis and evaluation of venous obstruction. AJR Am J Roentgenol 1999;172:1327-1333.
21. Finn JP, Zisk JH, Edelman RR, et al: Central venous occlusion: MR angiography. Radiology 1993;187:245-251.
22. Hartnell GG, Hughes LA, Finn JP, Longmaid HE 3rd: Magnetic resonance angiography of the central chest veins: A new gold standard? Chest 1995;107:1053-1057.
23. Lanciego C, Chacon JL, Julian A, et al: Stenting as first option for endovascular treatment of malignant superior vena cava syndrome. AJR Am J Roentgenol 2001;177:585-593.
24. Miller JH, McBride K, Little F, Price A: Malignant superior vena cava obstruction: Stent placement via the subclavian route. Cardiovasc Intervent Radiol 2000;23:155-158.
25. Petersen BD, Uchida B: Long-term results of treatment of benign central venous obstructions unrelated to dialysis with expandable Z stents. J Vasc Interv Radiol 1999;10:757-766.
26. Link J, Brossmann J, Muller-Hulsbeck S, Heller M: Venous stent application with a simultaneous cubitofemoral approach. [German] Rofo 1995;163:81-83.
27. Dondelinger RF, Gofette P, Kurdziel JC, Roche A: Expandable metal stents for stenosis of the vena cava and large veins. Semin Interv Radiol 1991;8:252-263.
28. Smayra T, Otal P, Chabbert V, et al: Longer-term results of endovascular stent placement in the superior caval venous system. Cardiovasc Intervent Radiol 2001;24:388-394.
29. Kishi K, Sonomura T, Mitsuzane K, et al: Self-expandable metallic stent therapy for superior vena cava syndrome: Clinical observations. Radiology 1993;189:531-535.
30. Nicholson AA, Ettles D, Arnold A, et al: Treatment of malignant superior vena cava obstruction: Metal stents or radiation therapy. J Vasc Interv Radiol 1997;8:781-788.
31. Chatziioannou A, Alexopoulos TH, Mourikis D, et al: Stent therapy for malignant superior vena cava syndrome: Should be first line treatment or simple adjunct to radiotherapy. Eur J Radiol 2003;47:247-250.
32. Courtheoux P, Alkofer B, Al Refai M, et al: Stent placement in superior vena cava syndrome. Ann Thorac Surg 2003;75:158-161.
33. Hennequin L, Fade O, Fays JG, et al: Superior vena cava stent placement: Results with Wallstent endoprosthesis. Radiology 1995;196:353-361.
34. Kee ST, Kinoshita L, Razavi MK, et al: Superior vena cava syndrome: Treatment with catheter-directed thrombolysis and endovascular stent placement. Radiology 1998;206:187-193.
35. Gray BH, Olin JW, Graor RA, et al: Safety and efficiency of thrombolytic therapy for superior vena cava syndrome. Chest 1991;99:54-59.
36. Qanadli SD, Hajjam M, Mignon F, et al: Subacute and chronic benign superior vena cava obstructions: Endovascular treatment with self-expanding metallic stents. AJR Am J Roentgenol 1999;173:159-164.
37. Perno J, Putnam SG III, Cohen GS, Ball D: Endovascular treatment of superior vena cava syndrome without removing a

central venous catheter. J Vasc Interv Radiol 1999;10: 917-918.

38. Stocks L, Raat H, Donck J, et al: Repositioning and leaving in situ the central venous catheter during percutaneous treatment of associated superior vena cava syndrome: A report of eight cases. Cardiovasc Intervent Radiol 1999;22: 224-226.

39. Evans J, Saba Z, Rosenfeld H, et al: Aortic laceration secondary to Palmaz stent placement for treatment of superior vena cava syndrome. Catheter Cardiovasc Interv 2000;49:160-162.

40. Martin M, Baumgartner I, Kolb M, et al: Fatal pericardial tamponade after Wallstent implantation for malignant superior vena cava syndrome. J Endovasc Ther 2002;9;680-684.

41. Recto MR, Bousamra M, Yeh T Jr: Late superior vena cava perforation and aortic laceration after stenting to treat superior vena cava syndrome secondary to fibrosing mediastinitis. J Invasive Cardiol 2002;14:624-629.

42. Smith SL, Manhire AR, Clark DM: Delayed spontaneous superior vena cava perforation associated with a SVC Wallstent. Cardiovasc Intervent Radiol 2001;24:286-287.

43. Choe YH, Im JG, Park JH, et al: The anatomy of the pericardial space: A study in cadavers and patients. AJR Am Roentgenol 1987;149:693-697.

44. Hill SL, Berry RE: Subclavian vein thrombosis: A continuing challenge. Surgery 1990;108:1-9.

45. Prandoni P, Polistena P, Bernardi E, et al: Upper extremity deep-vein thrombosis risk factors, diagnosis, and complications. Arch Intern Med 1997;157:57-62.

46. Hingorani A, Ascher E, Lorenson E, et al: Upper extremity deep venous thrombosis and its impact on morbidity and mortality rates in a hospital-based population. J Vasc Surg 1997;26: 853-860.

47. Becker DM, Philbrick JT, Walker FB: Axillary and subclavian venous thrombosis: Prognosis and treatment. Arch Intern Med 1991;151:1934-1943.

48. Hingorani A, Ascher E, Hanson J, et al: Upper extremity versus lower extremity deep venous thrombosis. Am J Surg 1997; 174:214-217.

49. Sottiurai VS, Towner K, McDonnell AE, Zarins CK: Diagnosis of upper extremity deep vein thrombosis using noninvasive technique. Surgery 1982;91:582-585.

50. Knudson GJ, Wiedmeyer DA. Erickson SJ, et al: Color Doppler sonographic imaging in the assessment of upper extremity deep venous thrombosis. AJR Am J Roentgenol 1990;154: 399-403.

51. Fraser JD, Anderson DR: Deep venous thrombosis: Recent advances and optimal investigation with US. Radiology 1999;211:9-24.

52. Fielding JR, Nagel JS, Pomery O: Upper extremity DVT: Correlation of MR and nuclear medicine flow imaging. Clin Imag 1997;21:260-263.

53. Lindblad B, Tengborn L, Bergqvist D: Deep vein thrombosis of the axillary-subclavian veins: Epidemiologic data, effects of different types of treatment and late sequelae. Eur J Vasc Surg 1988;2:161-165.

54. Joffe HV, Goldhaber SZ: Upper-extremity deep vein thrombosis. Circulation 2002;106:1874-1880.

55. Zell L, Kindermann W, Marschall F, et al: Paget-Schroetter syndrome in sports activities: Case study and literature review. Angiology 2001;52:337-342.

56. Thompson RW, Schneider PA, Nelken NA, et al: Circumferential venolysis and paraclavicular thoracic outlet decompression for "effort thrombosis" of the subclavian vein. J Vasc Surg 1992;16:723-732.

57. Parziale JR, Akelman E, Weiss AP, et al: Thoracic outlet syndrome. Am J Orthop 2000;29:353-360.

58. Coon WW, Willis PW: Thrombosis of axillary and subclavian veins. Arch Surg 1966;94:657-663.

59. Lokich JJ, Becker B: Subclavian vein thrombosis in patients treated with infusion chemotherapy for advanced malignancy. Cancer 1983;52:1586-1589.

60. Marinella MA, Kathula SK, Markert RJ: Spectrum of upper-extremity deep venous thrombosis in a community teaching hospital. Heart Lung 2000;29:113-117.

61. Monreal M, Raventos A, Lerma R, et al: Pulmonary embolism in patients with upper extremity DVT associated to venous

central lines: A prospective study. Thromb Haemost 1994;72: 548-550.

62. Timsit JF, Farkas JC, Boyer JM, et al: Central vein catheter-related thrombosis in intensive care patients: Incidence, risk factors, and relationship with catheter-related sepsis. Chest 1998;114:207-213.

63. De Cicco M, Matovic M, Balestreri L, et al: Central venous thrombosis: An early and frequent complication in cancer patients bearing long-term Silastic catheter. A prospective study. Thromb Res 1997;86:101-113.

64. Martin C, Viviand X, Saux P, Gouin F: Upper-extremity deep vein thrombosis after central venous catheterization via the axillary vein. Crit Care Med 1999;27:2626-2629.

65. Girolami A, Prandoni P, Zanon E, et al: Venous thromboses of upper limbs are more frequently associated with occult cancer as compared with those of lower limbs. Blood Coagul Fibrinol 1999;10:455-457.

66. Hammers LW, Cohn SM, Brown JM, et al: Doppler color flow imaging surveillance of deep vein thrombosis in high-risk trauma patients. J Ultrasound Med 1996;15:19-24.

67. Martinelli I, Cattaneo M, Panzeri D, et al: Risk factors for deep vein thrombosis of the upper extremities. Ann Intern Med 1997;126:707-711.

68. Linblad B, Tengblom L, Bergqvist D: Deep vein thrombosis of the axillary-sublclavian veins, epidemiologic data, effects of different types of treatment and late sequelae. Eur J Vasc Surg 1988;2:161-165.

69. Heron E, Lozinguez O, Alhenc-Gelas M, et al: Hypercoagulable states in primary upper-extremity deep vein thrombosis. Arch Intern Med 2000;160:382-386.

70. de Mola JRL, Kiwi R, Austin C, Goldfarb JM: Subclavian deep vein thrombosis associated with the use of recombinant follicle-stimulating hormone (Gonal-F) complicating mild ovarian hyperstimulation syndrome. Fertil Steril 2000;73:1253-1255.

71. Ninet J, Demolombe-Rague S, Bureau du Colombier P, Coppere B: Les thromboses veineuses profondes des membres superieurs. Sang Thrombose Vaisseaux 1994;6:103-114.

72. Lisse JR, Davis CP, Thurmond-Anderle M: Cocaine abuse and deep venous thrombosis. Ann Intern Med 1989;110:571-572.

73. Leebeek FW, Stadhouders NA, van Stein D, et al: Hypercoagulability states in upper-extremity deep venous thrombosis. Am J Hematol 2001;67:15-19.

74. Ruggeri M, Castaman G, Tosetto A, et al: Low prevalence of thrombophilic coagulation defects in patients with deep vein thrombosis of the upper limbs. Blood Coagul Fibrinol 1997;8: 191-194.

75. Prandoni P, Polistena P, Bernardi E, et al: Upper-extremity deep vein thrombosis: Risk factors, diagnosis and complications. Arch Intern Med 1997;157:57-62.

76. Haire WD, Lynch TG, Lund GB, et al: Limitations of magnetic resonance imaging and ultrasound-directed (duplex) scanning in the diagnosis of subclavian vein thrombosis. J Vasc Surg 1991;13:391-397.

77. Baarslag HJ, van Beek EJR, Koopman MMW, Reekers JA: Prospective study of color duplex ultrasonography compared with contrast venography in patients suspected of having deep venous thrombosis of the upper extremities. Ann Int Med 2002;136:865-872.

78. Horattas MC, Wright DJ, Fenton AH, et al: Changing concepts of deep venous thrombosis of the upper extremity: Report of a series and review of the literature. Surgery 1988;104: 561-567.

79. Urschel HC, Razzuk MA: Paget-Schroetter syndrome: What is the best management? Ann Thorac Surg 2000;69:1663-1669.

80. Kasirajan K, Gray B, Ouriel K: Percutaneous AngioJet thrombectomy in the management of extensive deep venous thrombosis. J Vasc Interv Radiol 2001;12:179-185.

81. Hicken GJ, Ameli M: Management of subclavian-axillary vein thrombosis: A review. Can J Surg 1998;41:13-25.

82. Lee MC, Grassi CJ, Belkin M, et al: Early operative intervention after thrombolytic therapy for primary subclavian vein thrombosis, an effective treatment approach. J Vasc Surg 1998;27: 1101-1108.

83. Strandness DE, Langlois Y, Cromor M, et al: Long-term sequelae of acute venous thrombosis. JAMA 1983;250: 1289-1292.

84. Shields GP, Turnipseed S, Panacek EA, et al: Validation of the Canadian clinical probability model for acute venous thrombosis. Acad Emerg Med 2002;9:561-566.

85. Breddin HK, Hach-Wunderle V, Nakov R, et al: Effects of a low molecular-weight heparin on thrombus regression and recurrent thromboembolism in patients with deep-vein thrombosis. N Engl J Med 2001;344:626-631.

86. Semba CP, Drake M: Iliofemoral deep vein thrombosis: Aggressive therapy using catheter-directed thrombolysis. Radiology 1994;191:487-494.

87. McClennan G, Trerotola S. Davidson D, et al: The effects of a mechanical thrombolytic device on normal canine vein valves. J Vasc Interv Radiol 2001;12:89-94.

88. Trerotola SO, McLennan G, Davidson D, et al: Preclinical in vivo testing of the Arrow-Trerotola percutaneous thrombolytic device for venous thrombosis. J Vasc Interv Radiol 2001;12:95-103.

89. Delomez M, Beregi JP, Willoteaux S, et al: Mechanical thrombectomy in patients with deep venous thrombosis. Cardiovasc Intervent Radiol 2001;24:42-48.

90. Braaten JV, Goss RA, Francis CW: Ultrasound reversibly disaggregates fibrin fibers. Thromb Haemost 1997;78:1063-1068.

91. Altar S, Rosenschein U: Perspectives on the role of ultrasonic devices in thrombolysis. J Thrombosis Thrombolysis 2004;2:107-114.

92. Hallisey MJ: Ultrasonic energy treatment of deep vein thrombosis. J Endovasc Today 2006;4:80-82.

93. Uppot RN, Garcia MJ, Roe C, et al: Management of deep venous thrombosis using the AngioJet rheolytic thrombectomy system. J Vasc Interv Radiol 2002;13(S):S116.

94. Ramaiah V, Del Santo PB, Rodriguez-Lopez JA, et al: Trellis thrombectomy system for the treatment of iliofemoral deep venous thrombosis. J Endovasc Ther 2003;10:585-589.

46 Acute Stroke Intervention

Christopher J. White and Stephen R. Ramee

Stroke affects approximately 750,000 Americans each year and results in almost 150,000 deaths.[1] Stroke is the third leading cause of death in the United States, after heart disease and cancer; it is the number one cause of disability and the number one reason for rehabilitation. There are estimated to be more than 3 million stroke survivors in the United States, with a third of these being young adults with long-term disability.[2]

Stroke may be hemorrhagic, thrombotic, or embolic. In embolic strokes, the embolus may move from artery to artery or from a heart chamber (left atrium or ventricle) to an artery, particularly in patients with atrial fibrillation. One of the major tenets of treatment of ischemic stroke is that "time is brain." Variables that affect the extent of ischemic brain injury include the time from onset of symptoms to reperfusion; the presence of collateral circulation, including an intact circle of Willis; and the "penumbra of viability" surrounding the infarcted brain tissue. The penumbra is the region of brain surrounding the infarct area in which the blood supply is significantly reduced but energy metabolism is maintained owing to collateral flow. The viability of this area depends on both the severity and the duration of ischemia. If blood flow is rapidly restored, some ischemic brain tissue will be saved. For both ischemic and hemorrhagic

stroke, there are opportunities to minimize injury early after the onset of the stroke. This puts a premium on the rapid assessment of patients presenting with stroke (Table 46-1).[3,4]

Ischemic stroke therapy is designed to achieve reperfusion as quickly as possible and to minimize further damage. It consists of either intravenous (IV) thrombolysis or catheter-based reperfusion therapy, which can include intra-arterial thrombolysis, mechanical thrombectomy, or balloon angioplasty with or without stent placement (Table 46-2).

IV thrombolysis is indicated if less than 3 hours have passed since the onset of symptoms. It is widely available and does not require angiography, but it is restricted to patients who are without evidence of bleeding on computed tomographic (CT) imaging, who have blood pressure readings of 185/110 mm Hg or lower, and who are determined to be at low bleeding risk (Table 46-3). Catheter-based stroke therapies may be effective up to 6 hours from the time of onset of the stroke; these therapies are usually reserved for larger strokes and are particularly useful for patients in whom thrombolysis is contraindicated (Table 46-4).[5]

The National Institute of Neurological Disorders and Stroke (NINDS) conducted a landmark randomized trial for acute stroke comparing IV thrombolysis

Table 46-1. The Seven "D's" of Stroke Care

Detection
Dispatch
Delivery
Door (urgent triage in emergency department)
Data
Decision
Drug administration

Adams H, Adams R, Del Zoppo G, Goldstein LB: Guidelines for the early management of patients with ischemic stroke: 2005 Guidelines Update. A scientific statement from the Stroke Council of the American Heart Association/American Stroke Association. Stroke 2005;36:916-923.

and placebo. They randomized 524 patients within 3 hours after the onset of a stroke to receive either placebo or IV recombinant tissue plasminogen activator (rt-PA), 0.9 mg/kg (maximum, 90 mg), over a 1-hour period. At 24 hours, there was no benefit from the thrombolytic therapy. At 3 months, patients treated with rt-PA had less severe disability than the placebo group (odds ratio=1.7; 95% confidence interval [CI]: 1.2 to 2.6).[6] Patients treated with IV thrombolysis had a full recovery rate of 34%, compared with 21% in the placebo-treated group (34% relative improvement). There was no difference in mortality between the groups, but the rate of intracranial hemorrhage (ICH) was 6.4% for the rt-PA group versus 0.6% for the placebo group (P<.001).

It appears that the benefit for IV lytic treatment for stroke is restricted to early (≤3 hr) administration.[7] The benefit is balanced by the risk of a symptomatic ICH in 3.3% and asymptomatic ICH in 8.2% of those treated with IV lytic agents. The risk of ICH is increased in patients with larger strokes (i.e., middle cerebral artery sign on CT imaging), later treatment (>3 hr), older age (≥85 yr), and hypertension.

NEW IMAGING TECHNIQUES

The imaging choice for acute stroke patients is CT or magnetic resonance imaging (MRI). Imaging is the cornerstone for selecting candidates for stroke therapy. The purpose of the baseline CT is to detect conditions that make the patient ineligible for thrombolysis, such as subdural, subarachnoid, or parenchymal ICH. CT may also detect mass lesions or hemorrhagic infarctions.

A CT without contrast is an excellent tool to rule out hemorrhage, but its sensitivity for discriminating between ischemic and infarcted brain is not as good as MRI. MRI perfusion and diffusion techniques can distinguish ischemic brain at risk from the infarcted core, thereby identifying salvageable brain tissue. Diffusion imaging is of value in the rapid detection of infarction and in the differentiation of new versus old brain infarctions. Perfusion imaging with contrast CT is also available, although most experts believe that MRI is superior.

MANAGEMENT OF PHYSIOLOGIC VARIABLES

The management of acute stroke involves reducing the risk of recurrent events and minimizing the disability that occurs secondary to the established stroke. Acute therapy involves management of physiologic

Table 46-3. Eligibility for Thrombolysis in Stroke

Indication
Ischemic stroke, within 3 hr since onset of symptoms

Clinical Contraindications
Any history of intracranial hemorrhage
Blood pressure: systolic, >185 mm Hg; diastolic, >110 mm Hg
Rapid improvement in neurologic status
Mild neurologic impairment
Symptoms of subarachnoid bleeding
Stroke or head trauma within the last 3 mo
Gastrointestinal/genitourinary hemorrhage within last 3 wk
Major surgery within last 3 wk
Recent heart attack
Seizure with stroke
Taking oral anticoagulants
Received heparin within 48 hr

Radiologic Contraindications
Evidence of intracranial hemorrhage on computed tomography

Laboratory Contraindications
International normalized ratio (INR) >1.7
Platelet count <100,000/μL
Elevated activated partial thromboplastin time (aPTT)
Blood glucose <50 mg/dL

Table 46-2. Randomized Trials of Thrombolytic Therapy for Acute Ischemic Stroke

Name of Study	Treatment Window	Medications Tested	Delivery	Dose of Agent	No. of Patients
NINDS t-PA Stroke Trial (Parts 1 and 2)	3 h, 1/2 90 min	t-PA	IV	0.9 mg/kg over 1 h	624
ECASS I	6 h	t-PA	IV	1.1 mg/kg over 1 h	620
ECASS II	6 h	t-PA	IV	0.9 mg/kg over 1 h	800
Atlantis A62,63	6 h	t-PA	IV	0.9 mg/kg over 1 h	142
Atlantis B	0 to 5 h	t-PA	IV	0.9 mg/kg over 1 h	613 (313 h)
ASK	4 h	Streptokinase	IV	1.5 million units over 1 h	340
MAST I	6 h	Streptokinase	IV	1.5 million units over 1 h	622
MAST-E	6 h	Streptokinase	IV	1.5 million units over 1 h	310
PROACT II	6 h	Prourokinase plus IV heparin	IA	9 mg over 2 h	180

ASK, Australian Streptokinase Trial; ECASS, European Cooperative Acute Stroke Study; MAST, Multicenter Acute Stroke Trial—Europe; NINDS, National Institute of Neurological Diseases and Stroke; PROACT, PROlyse in Acute Cerebral Thromboembolism II; t-PA, tissue plasminogen activator.

Table 46-4. Comparison of "Real-World" Patients Undergoing Catheter-Based Therapy in the Ochsner Clinic Series with Patients Undergoing Intravenous and Intra-arterial Thrombolysis for Stroke in Treatment Trials

Study	N	Age (Yr), % Males	NIHSS Baseline	Symptomatic ICH (%)	Follow-up		
					No. Months	Mortality (%)	Good Outcome (%)
NINDS	168	69, 57%	14	6.4	3	17	39
STARS	389	69, 55%	13	3.3	1	13	35
PROACT II	121	64, 58%	17	10	3	25	26
Ochsner series	16	67, 44%	16	12.5	1	25	38

ICH, intracranial hemorrhage; NIHSS, National Institutes of Health Stroke Scale; NINDS, National Institute of Neurologic Disorders and Stroke; PROACT II, PROlyse in Acute Cerebral Thromboembolism II; STARS, Standard Treatment with Alteplase to Reverse Stroke Study.

variables, reperfusion of ischemic tissue, and reduction of ICH.

Hypertension

Arterial hypertension is present in most patients presenting with a stroke and is associated with a poorer outcome; however, lower blood pressure may result in decreased perfusion to the ischemic penumbra, thus extending the size of the infarction. There is a great deal of uncertainty regarding the treatment of hypertension during the acute stroke. Current recommendations include lowering blood pressure to at least 220 mm Hg systolic and 120 mm Hg diastolic.[8]

Hyperglycemia

Elevated blood sugar concentration is associated with worse outcome in acute stroke. This may be related to increased lactate production, which increases infarct size, reduces effectiveness of thrombolytic therapy, and may increase the risk of hemorrhagic transformation of infarcted brain tissue. Trials are in progress to determine optimal therapy, with current recommendations stating that glucose-containing fluids should not be used during the acute stroke period and that markedly elevated glucose concentrations should be lowered.

Fever

Fever is associated with poorer stroke outcome, possibly because of a detrimental effect on brain metabolism, increased free radical production, or deterioration of the blood-brain barrier function. Current recommendations are to use antipyretics to maintain normothermia.

REPERFUSION STRATEGIES

Intravenous Thrombolysis

IV administration of the thrombolytic agent, rt-PA, is the only therapy approved by the U.S. Food and Drug Administration (FDA) for acute ischemic stroke (see Table 46-2). IV rt-PA is an effective therapy for stroke. In a recent meta-analysis of 2775 patients treated with 6 hours after stroke onset, patients treated within 90 minutes after onset had an almost threefold increase in good outcome; this dropped to 1.6-fold for patients treated between 91 and 180 minutes after stroke onset. For those treated between 180 and 270 minutes, the odds ratio for benefit was 1.4 times greater than placebo. The risk of ICH was greater for the thrombolytic group (5.9%) compared with the placebo group (1.1%), but most of these hemorrhages were asymptomatic. The number of stroke patients needed to treat (NNT) with IV lysis in order to achieve an excellent outcome and avoid 1 stroke death or dependency was 7. For every 100 stroke patients treated with IV thrombolysis within 3 hours after stroke onset, 32 had a better outcome, although 3 experienced a significant ICH. At 1 year after treatment, those treated with IV lysis had a 30% increased likelihood of minimal or no disability compared with placebo; however, there was no difference in mortality, and the rate of recurrent stroke was not different.[9] The risk of hemorrhage was increased in elderly patients and in those with larger strokes, diabetes mellitus, a history of prior stroke, or thrombocytopenia.

The risk-to-benefit ratio for IV thrombolysis is narrow. About 11% more patients will benefit at 3 months from IV lysis, whereas 6.4% will experience ICH. In an attempt to improve the recanalization rate for IV thrombolysis, it has been combined with low-frequency ultrasound therapy. In animal studies, low-frequency ultrasound makes rt-PA–mediated clot degradation 50% more efficient when used transcranially. However, a recent human trial was stopped because of an excess of ICH events in the insonated group.[10]

The management of IV lysis in stroke includes admission to an intensive care unit with frequent monitoring of vital signs and neurologic status. Arterial, central venous, and bladder catheters should not be placed until at least 2 hours after completion of the IV lytic therapy. Elevated blood pressure may be lowered very cautiously. A head CT should be done if ICH is suspected. All antithrombotic and antiplatelet therapy should be withheld for at least 24 hours.

Intra-Arterial Thrombolysis

Intra-arterial thrombolysis involves direct catheterization of the intracerebral vessels and is analogous, in many ways, to the treatment of an acute myocardial infarction. However, there are also major differences between the catheter-based treatment of acute stroke and acute myocardial infarction. The benefit offered by catheter-based intra-cranial therapy is the ability to use smaller doses of lytic agents and to employ mechanical clot disruption techniques with guide wires, balloons, or thrombectomy devices.

The effectiveness of intra-arterial thrombolysis has been established in several trials. The PROACT II trial randomized patients presenting within 6 hours after stroke who had angiographically documented occlusion of the middle cerebral artery to 9 mg of intra-arterial pro-urokinase (pro-UK) plus unfractionated heparin (UFH) versus UFH alone. Successful reperfusion was achieved in 66% of the group treated with intracranial pro-UK, compared with only 18% of the control group ($P<.001$). The clinical benefit was that 40% of the pro-UK group had slight or no neurologic disability (modified Rankin scale [mRs] ≤2) at 90 days, compared with only 25% of the control group ($P=.04$). There were more symptomatic ICHs in the thrombolytic group (11% vs. 3%; $P=.03$). The NNT to make one patient independent was 7. This trial demonstrated efficacy of stroke treatment up to 6 hours, but only a small minority (2%) of all screened patients were enrolled. Contraindications to catheter-directed thrombolysis include recent brain surgery, unknown time of onset of the deficit, uncontrolled hypertension, and CT evidence of hemorrhage or tumor.

Mechanical Thrombectomy

An alternative strategy for reperfusion in stroke in patients who are not candidates for thrombolysis is mechanical clot removal or thrombectomy (Figs. 46-1 through 46-5). The MERCI device is a mechanical thrombectomy or embolectomy device that was tested for safety and efficacy in 151 acute stroke patients who were not candidates for thrombolysis.[11] Successful recanalization was achieved in 48% of treated patients, which is significantly higher than the historical control of 18% ($P<.001$). Significant procedural complications occurred in 7.1%, and symptomatic ICH was seen in 7.8%. Good (mRs=2) neurologic recovery at 90 days was seen in 46% of those with successful recanalization, compared with 10% of those with failed recanalization (relative risk [RR]=4.4; 95% CI: 2.1 to 9.3; $P<.0001$). There was also a mortality benefit for those with successful reperfusion (32% vs. 54%; RR=0.59; 95% CI: 0.39 to 0.89; $P=.01$).

Neuroprotection

Drugs and devices are under investigation to prolong the life of the penumbra, maintain the blood-brain barrier, and reduce hemorrhage and reperfusion injury. A promising free radical scavenger (NXY-059) was tested in a randomized trial of 1722 acute stroke patients and demonstrated a 20% reduction in disability at 90 days ($P=.038$) compared to placebo.[12]

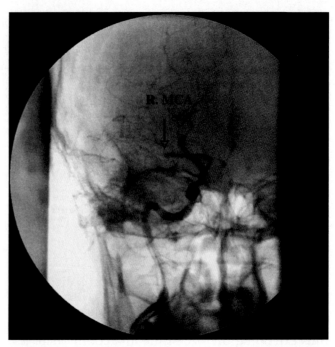

Figure 46-1. Atrial fibrillation with acute stroke and right middle cerebral artery (R MCA) occlusion.

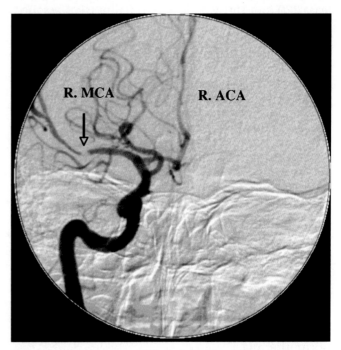

Figure 46-2. After intracranial administration of 2 mg rt-PA, there is partial recanalization (*arrow*) of the right middle cerebral artery (R MCA). R. ACA, right anterior cerebral artery.

Among patients who received IV thrombolysis, there was also reduction of hemorrhagic transformation and symptomatic ICH with NXY-059.

Hypothermia is an exciting and emerging therapy for stroke. Hypothermia functions as a neuroprotectant by decreasing cellular metabolism, limiting cytotoxicity, reducing free radical formation, and preventing breakdown of the blood-brain

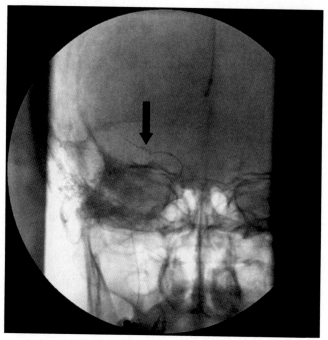

Figure 46-3. Placement of the MERCI thrombectomy catheter (*arrow*) in the right middle cerebral artery.

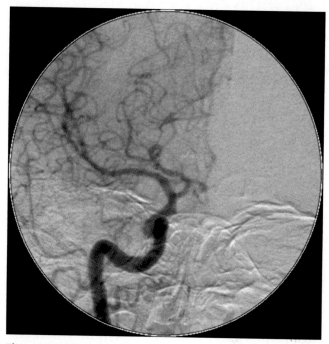

Figure 46-5. Final result with recanalization of right middle cerebral artery.

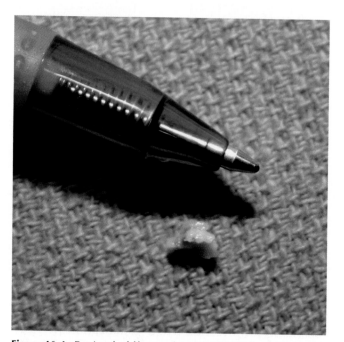

Figure 46-4. Retrieval of fibrous clot with MERCI thrombectomy device. The imprint of the left atrial appendage can be seen.

barrier. Mechanisms of cooling include invasive central venous catheters and surface methods. There is much evidence to support the neuroprotective effects of hypothermia in animal models but a lack of comparative data in humans. The benefits of hypothermia are facilitated by early initiation.[13]

THE ROLE OF CARDIOLOGY IN A STROKE PROGRAM

Fewer than 5% of patients with ischemic stroke receive IV thrombolysis, either because physicians are reluctant to commit them to this therapy with a narrow risk-to-benefit ratio or because patients present with contraindications to lytic therapy. Intra-arterial thrombolysis has been shown to be effective alone and after failed IV therapy in recanalizing culprit lesions and improving neurologic outcomes in acute stroke.[14]

Percutaneous angioplasty, including mechanical thrombectomy, as an adjunct to intra-arterial thrombolysis is feasible in acute stroke. We have reported our experience with emergent catheter-based treatment including local thrombolysis and/or mechanical therapy with balloon angioplasty/stenting for patients with acute ischemic stroke who are ineligible for IV thrombolysis.[5] Benefits related to catheter-based therapy in acute stroke include a higher rate of reperfusion than for IV thrombolysis, clinical benefit up to 6 hours from onset of symptoms, confirmation of the cerebral anatomy, treatment of the culprit lesion, and a low rate of ICH.

Differences between treatment of stroke and treatment of heart attack are that stroke thrombi are usually of embolic origin, making them older, more organized, and more resistant to lysis; the volume of clot is larger, and cerebral vessel tortuosity makes intervention more difficult than in the treatment of acute myocardial infarction.

The updated Ochsner Clinic series of "real-world" stroke patients with contraindications to thrombolysis includes the outcomes of 25 consecutive patients

Table 46-5. Ochsner Clinic Series of Consecutive Patients with Acute Stroke Intervention and Contraindications to Thrombolytic Therapy

Patients	
No.	25
Males (%)	52
Contraindications to IV lysis (%)	100
Time from onset to angiography (min)	219
Therapy employed (%)	
Intra-arterial lysis	28
Percutaneous transluminal angioplasty (PTA)	20
Both lysis and PTA	24
Neither lysis nor PTA (lacunar infarcts)	28
Outcomes (%)	
Acute intracranial hemorrhage	9
30-day survival	84
"Excellent" outcome	56

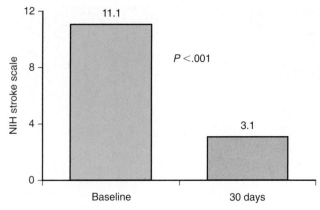

Figure 46-6. Improvement in National Institutes of Health Stroke Scale score after catheter-based therapy (*N*=25).

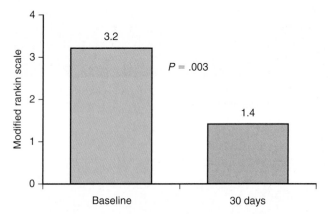

Figure 46-7. Improvement in functional status after catheter-based therapy (*N*=25).

with ischemic stroke (Table 46-5). A stroke neurologist in consultation with the interventional cardiologist/neuroradiologist determined the appropriateness of catheter-based treatment. Patients were considered eligible for catheter-based therapy if they were less than 7 hours from symptom onset, their National Institutes of Health Stroke Scale (NIHSS) was 4 or greater, and they had no evidence of ICH of the middle cerebral artery territory on CT.

Culprit lesion characteristics determined the recanalization strategy. After anticoagulation was achieved with intra-arterial heparin, balloon angioplasty and stenting was the primary strategy for stenotic lesions (90% diameter or greater stenosis and flow-limiting), with intra-arterial thrombolytic therapy being used in the presence of a thrombotic occlusion. The thrombolytic agent (urokinase or rt-PA) was administered via an infusion catheter placed in direct contact with the thrombus. After partial recanalization was achieved with thrombolysis, balloon angioplasty and stent placement were used at the discretion of the operator to manage any residual flow-limiting stenosis.

Intra-arterial lysis was administered to 7 patients (28%), angioplasty was the sole treatment for 5 patients (20%), 6 patients (24%) received both intra-arterial lysis and angioplasty, and 7 patients had no identifiable culprit lesion (lacunar strokes) (see Table 46-5). The most common reason for ineligibility for systemic thrombolysis was time from symptom onset greater than 180 minutes (48%), followed by recent surgery (24%), recent arteriotomy at a noncompressible site (16%), and recent gastrointestinal or genitourinary bleeding (12%). The culprit lesion was located in the anterior circulation in 13 patients (52%) and in the posterior circulation in 6 patients (24%). Culprit lesion recanalization was initiated at a median of 219 minutes from symptom onset. There was significant improvement in the NIHSS score (Fig. 46-6) and in the mRs score (Fig. 46-7) at 30 days.

We have demonstrated that skilled interventional cardiologists with carotid stent experience, working on a team with neurologists and neuroradiologists, can achieve reasonable safety and efficacy in the treatment of selected stroke patients. The neurologic severity at presentation of our patients was comparable to that of patients in the IV and intra-arterial thrombolytic trials (see Table 46-2). A favorable outcome was achieved in most of our patients, with 56% demonstrating a marked improvement in NIHSS score and 38% achieving independent survival at follow-up. The rate of symptomatic ICH was comparable to that seen in the IV thrombolysis studies, attesting to the safety of this strategy.

Our experience differs from that of prior intra-arterial thrombolysis studies in two regards. First, our patients had contraindications to systemic thrombolysis. Second, the recanalization strategy (local thrombolysis and/or mechanistic therapy with balloon angioplasty/stenting) was based on culprit lesion assessment. The implementation of a catheter-based treatment strategy requires a multidisciplinary, collaborative approach for patient selection, culprit lesion anatomy assessment, and postintervention management, as well as the availability of an interventional laboratory 24 hours a day, 7 days a week, 365 days a year (Fig. 46-8).

The most important problem facing stroke therapy today is a lack of on-demand interventional therapy for the majority of stroke patients who are not can-

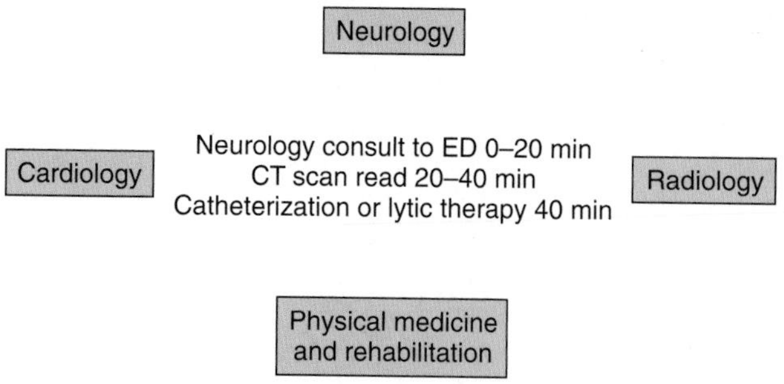

Neurology

Cardiology

Neurology consult to ED 0–20 min
CT scan read 20–40 min
Catheterization or lytic therapy 40 min

Radiology

Physical medicine
and rehabilitation

Figure 46-8. Ochsner Acute Stroke Intervention Service (OASIS). Structure and goals of the multidisciplinary service led and coordinated by Stroke Neurology personnel.

didates for lysis. This is, quite simply, due to the relatively few neuroradiologists who are available to provide 24/7 coverage in every hospital that treats stroke patients. One way to expand this service is to take advantage of the manpower available from interventional cardiology.

Interventional cardiologists are currently providing 24/7 interventional response for acute myocardial infarction (Table 46-6). Training and formation of a multidisciplinary stroke treatment group including neurology, radiology, and surgical specialties could significantly extend the treatment capability that is so badly needed in many communities. The other fortuitous factor is that many interventional cardiologists are currently performing carotid stent placement, including intracerebral angiography. It is a very achievable step to enable a person who is competent for carotid stent placement with cerebral angiography to perform acute stroke intervention. The cardiologist's role will be to provide on-demand stroke intervention service 24/7 as a skilled angiographer, a skilled interventionalist, and a member of a multidisciplinary team who can meet the challenge bringing reperfusion therapy to this devastating disease.

REFERENCES

1. 2005 American Heart Association Guidelines for Cardiopulmonary Resuscitation and Emergeny Cardiovascular Care. Circulation 2005;112:IV-1-203.
2. American Heart Association: Heart disease and stroke statistics—2004 Update. Dallas, TX, American Heart Association, 2003.
3. Adams HP Jr, Adams RJ, Brott T, et al: Guidelines for the early management of patients with ischemic stroke: A scientific statement from the Stroke Council of the American Stroke Association. Stroke 2003;34:1056-1083.
4. Adams H, Adams R, Del Zoppo G, Goldstein LB: Guidelines for the early management of patients with ischemic stroke: 2005 Guidelines Update. A scientific statement from the Stroke Council of the American Heart Association/American Stroke Association. Stroke. 2005;36:916-923.
5. Ramee SR, Subramanian R, Felberg RA, et al: Catheter-based treatment for patients with acute ischemic stroke ineligible for intravenous thrombolysis. Stroke 2004;35:e109-e111.
6. Tissue plasminogen activator for acute ischemic stroke. The National Institute of Neurological Disorders and Stroke rt-PA Stroke Study Group. N Engl J Med 1995;333:1581-1587.
7. Albers GW, Bates VE, Clark WM, et al: Intravenous tissue-type plasminogen activator for treatment of acute stroke: the Standard Treatment with Alteplase to Reverse Stroke (STARS) study. JAMA 2000;283:1145-1150.
8. Dawson J, Walters M: New and emerging treatments for stroke. Br Med Bull 2006;77-78:87-102.
9. Kwiatkowski TG, Libman RB, Frankel M, et al: Effects of tissue plasminogen activator for acute ischemic stroke at one year. National Institute of Neurological Disorders and Stroke Recombinant Tissue Plasminogen Activator Stroke Study Group. N Engl J Med 1999;340:1781-1787.
10. Daffertshofer M, Gass A, Ringleb P, et al: Transcranial low-frequency ultrasound-mediated thrombolysis in brain ischemia: Increased risk of hemorrhage with combined ultrasound and tissue plasminogen activator. Results of a phase II clinical trial. Stroke 2005;36:1441-1446.
11. Smith WS, Sung G, Starkman S, et al; for the MTI: Safety and efficacy of mechanical embolectomy in acute ischemic stroke: Results of the MERCI Trial. Stroke 2005;36:1432-1438.
12. Lees KR, Zivin JA, Ashwood T, et al; the Stroke-Acute Ischemic NXYTTI: NXY-059 for acute ischemic stroke. N Engl J Med 2006;354:588-600.
13. Berger C, Schramm P, Schwab S: Reduction of diffusion-weighted MRI lesion volume after early moderate hypothermia in ischemic stroke. Stroke 2005;36:e56-e58.
14. Shaltoni HM, Albright KC, Gonzales NR, et al: Is intra-arterial thrombolysis safe after full-dose intravenous recombinant tissue plasminogen activator for acute ischemic stroke? Stroke 2007;38:80-84.

Table 46-6. Strengths and Weaknesses of Cardiologists on the Stroke Intervention Team

Pro	Con
Excellent catheter skills	Limited knowledge of the following:
Manage risk factors for stroke	
Experience with carotid stent placement	Cerebral anatomy
Rapid response 24/7	CT and MRI interpretation
Manage coexistent cardiac disease	Localization of deficit
Stroke volume overwhelms neuroradiology	NIHSS and neurologic examination
	Management of intracranial hemorrhage

NIHSS, National Institutes of Health Stroke Scale.

Intracardiac Intervention

SECTION

5

Intracardiac Intervention

CHAPTER
47 Imaging for Intracardiac Interventions

Mehdi H. Shishehbor and Samir R. Kapadia

KEY POINTS

- Structural heart disease interventions require multimodality imaging in the cardiac catheterization laboratory, including fluoroscopy and echocardiography.
- Fluoroscopy allows the operator to monitor manipulation of radiopaque devices and visualize intracardiac structures with contrast injection as necessary. Echocardiography shows nonradiopaque cardiac structures in greater detail and helps with the safety and precision of the procedures.
- Fluoroscopy visualizes a large area of the heart with excellent temporal and spatial resolution and projects this three-dimensional (3D) information onto a two-dimensional (2D) screen. Therefore, multiple projections (commonly biplane imaging) may be needed to determine the precise locations of devices and structures in 3D space.
- Echocardiography shows cross-sectional information about soft tissues and devices in a 2D display. Precise

location in 3D space and trajectory of devices can be determined by viewing these structures in multiple views and mentally synthesizing this information (in future on-line 3D imaging may help).
- Echocardiography can be performed by an intracardiac (ICE) or a transesophageal (TEE) probe in the catheterization laboratory. ICE is currently used for septal interventions (transseptal puncture, patent foramen ovale, and atrial septal defect closures); however, its use for other interventions is increasing. Mitral valve interventions are primarily done under TEE guidance at the present time.
- Synthesis of fluoroscopic and echocardiographic images in the catheterization laboratory is becoming increasingly important with the growing number of percutaneous structural heart disease interventions.

Interventional cardiac procedures rely on various imaging modalities for their safety and efficacy. Traditionally, x-ray fluoroscopy and cineangiography have been used to guide coronary angioplasty procedures, and they remain an integral part of intracardiac interventions. Fluoroscopy creates a two-dimensional (2D) view of a three-dimensional (3D) object by creating superimposed images. Accurate position of an object in a 3D space can be determined by viewing multiple different projections or by observing motion of an object that is moving in a known direction (e.g., catheter). The major limitation of fluoroscopy is that only radiopaque objects are visible; to make the soft tissue structures such as myocardium, interatrial and interventricular septum, and cardiac valves visible, radiopaque dye must be injected.

Ultrasonography is the other imaging modality that is used to guide intracardiac interventions. Both transesophageal echocardiography (TEE) and intracardiac echocardiography (ICE) depict a 2D image from a 2D plane. Ultrasound-based imaging allows visualization of soft tissues without the injection of

contrast material; this allows for real-time imaging during device manipulation. Although the spatial resolution of ultrasound is not as good as that of cineangiography, it is adequate for visualization of most intracardiac structures. Precise location of an object in a 3D space can be obtained by viewing multiple planes or by manipulating the ultrasound probe in a known direction. A particular limitation of ICE and TEE imaging is the difficulty of recognizing the specific aspect of a device; for instance, the tip of a catheter may appear indistinguishable from the shaft just a few millimeters proximal to the tip. Other limitations include restricted areas where the probe can be placed (esophagus, cardiac chambers) and shadowing from metallic objects, calcium, and air. The most comprehensive approach to intracardiac imaging is the complementary use of fluoroscopy together with ultrasound imaging; this allows for combining the strengths of these imaging modalities while compensating for their weaknesses.

This chapter first highlights the structural anatomy using each of these imaging techniques and then

823

synthesizes imaging pearls for various intracardiac procedures.

FLUOROSCOPY

Left Ventriculogram

The left ventricle (LV) is typically divided into inflow and outflow segments.[1] The inflow consists of the mitral valve apparatus, and the outflow portion includes the apex, the left ventricular outflow tract (LVOT), and the aortic valve. The angle between the inflow and the outflow tract is about 30 degrees at a young age and increases with "unfolding of the aorta." Because the interventricular septum maintains its position while the aorta is transposed anteriorly and more horizontally, there can be "bulging" of the septum.

A left ventriculogram is frequently performed during cardiac catheterization to assess wall motion abnormality, degree of mitral valvular regurgitation, presence of ventricular septal defect, presence of hypertrophic cardiomyopathy, and LV thrombus. However, when performed for advanced intracardiac procedures, it requires detailed appreciation of each anatomic structure and its position relative to the neighboring structures. A good ventriculogram is performed by placing the catheter in the ventricle where it does not cause extrasystole. Most commonly, this location is in the inflow portion of the LV (mid-cavity), away from the septum, as appreciated in the left anterior oblique (LAO) projection (Fig. 47-1). A pigtail catheter is most commonly used for this procedure; however, it tends to unfold when contrast in injected, and this may cause extrasystole. Removing the slack in the catheter before injection (the last motion being withdrawal rather than advancement), selecting the appropriate rate of injection for the size of the ventricle, and confirming the position of the catheter with inspiration before injection (to avoid adjustment in catheter position during injection) are important for a good-quality ventriculogram. In addition, catheters with multiple side holes (pigtail catheter) are preferred, because the force of the contrast jet out of a single end-hole catheter (e.g., multipurpose catheter) can cause catheter recoil and ventricular ectopic beats. The injected volume of contrast depends on the size of the catheter, the ventricular size, and the pressure at which it is delivered. With small-size diagnostic catheters, adequate volume may not be delivered unless high pressure is used, and even then the rate of injection may be limited (e.g., for a typical 4-Fr catheter at 1200 psi, the maximum volume that can be delivered is about 15 mL/sec). In contrast to ventriculography performed for assessment of wall motion abnormalities or mitral regurgitation, the assessment of structural problems (e.g., ventricular septal defect) may require rapid injection of a large volume of contrast material (15-20 mL/sec for 1 sec), despite the fact that this may cause ventricular extrasystole.

Left ventriculography is typically performed in the 30-degree right anterior oblique (RAO) projection; however, different views should be considered, depending on the purpose of the procedure. The RAO projection separates the atriums from the ventricles. Various structures seen on the RAO projection are delineated in Figure 47-2. Anterior and inferior walls

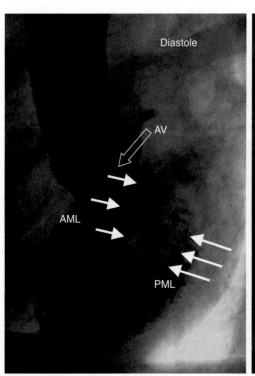 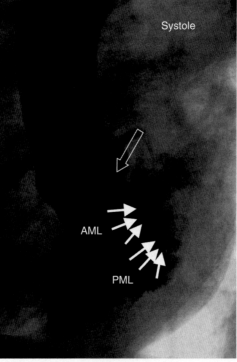

Figure 47-1. Sixty-degree left anterior oblique (LAO) view of left ventricle in diastole *(left panel)* and in systole *(right panel)*. The aortic valve *(open arrow)*, mitral valve *(solid white arrow)*, and papillary muscles are shown. In diastole, the mitral valve is open and there is clearance of contrast as the blood without contrast enters the left ventricle from the left atrium. Anterior and posterior leaflets are seen separated in diastole. In this view, lateral and septal walls can be assessed. AML, anterior mitral leaflet; AV, aortic valve; PML, posterior mitral leaflet.

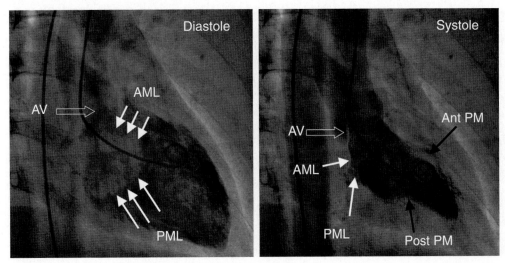

Figure 47-2. Thirty-degree right anterior oblique (RAO) view of left ventricle in diastole *(left panel)* and in systole *(right panel).* The aortic valve *(open arrow),* mitral valve *(solid white arrow),* and papillary muscles *(solid black arrows)* are shown. In diastole, the mitral valve is open and there is clearance of contrast as the blood enters the left ventricle from left atrium. Anterior and posterior leaflets are seen separated in diastole. In systole, the mitral valve is closed, and the aortic valve is open. In this view the anterior, apex, and inferior walls can be assessed. AML, anterior mitral leaflet; Ant PM, anterolateral papillary muscle; AV, aortic valve; PML, posterior mitral leaflet; Post PM, posterolateral papillary muscle.

as well as the apex are seen without overlap in this view. The lateral wall and septum are overlapped, and their motion is perpendicular to the x-ray beam, making it difficult to assess them. Anterior and posterior mitral valve leaflets are seen from the side in a longitudinal plane, along with the inflow portion of the ventricle. This relationship is critical to recognize for mitral valve intervention, because devices must be advanced coaxially in the inflow (e.g., Inoue balloon). Anterolateral and posteromedial commissures superimpose in this view, so there is significant overlap between various segments of the anterior and posterior leaflet of the mitral valve. The aortic valve and the coronary sinus can be appreciated in this view. Typically, the right coronary sinus is well separated from the posteriorly superimposed noncoronary and left sinuses. The noncoronary sinus is typically lower than the left sinus in this projection.

Various structures seen on the LAO view are outlined in Figure 47-1. In order to align mitral inflow to the apex of the ventricle, some caudal angulation can be added to the LAO projection, depending on patient habitus. This allows an end-on view of the LV in which papillary muscles as well as the anterior and posterior leaflets can be clearly identified. The left coronary sinus is seen clearly, but the right and noncoronary sinuses typically overlap in this projection.

Unconventional views allow better delineation of certain parts of the LV. The LAO cranial projection is typically better to assess the LVOT. The purpose of this projection is to see the anterior leaflet of the mitral valve in a longitudinal view when it does not overlap the interventricular septum. It is also the view of choice to see the interventricular septum in

the muscular portion for assessment of ventricular septal defect.

Right Ventriculogram

The right ventricle (RV) is trabeculated, with the inflow and outflow tracts at right angles to each other. Most typically, a right ventriculogram is performed in anteroposterior (AP) and lateral projections with the catheter positioned midcavity to prevent ventricular ectopy. A pigtail catheter or NIH catheter can be used to perform a right ventriculogram. The rate of injection must be higher to identify the details (>25 mL/sec). A right ventriculogram can be used to assess the pulmonary valve, the tricuspid valve, and right ventricular outflow tract (RVOT) obstruction (Fig. 47-3).

Right Atrial Angiogram

A right atrial angiogram is typically performed to look at the interatrial septum (IAS). A pigtail or NIH catheter with rapid injection rate is used. Various anatomic structures are shown in Figure 47-4. This procedure can be used for transseptal puncture and for patent foramen ovale (PFO) or atrial septal defect (ASD) closures. Right atrial angiography is used after ASD closure to determine the relation of the device to surrounding structures such as the aorta and left atrial wall.

Left Atrial Angiogram

A left atrial angiogram is rarely performed by direct injection, but the left atrium is frequently seen on the levo phase of the right-sided angiogram.

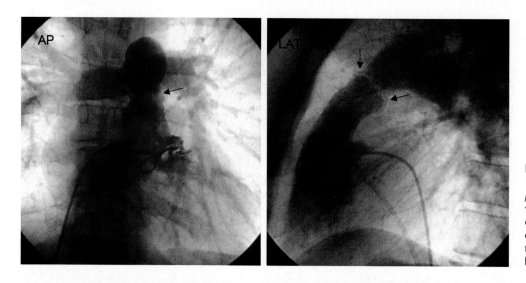

Figure 47-3. Anteroposterior *(left panel)* and lateral *(right panel)* views show the right ventricle with the pigtail catheter in the right ventricular outflow tract. Note doming of the pulmonary valve, as shown by the black arrows.

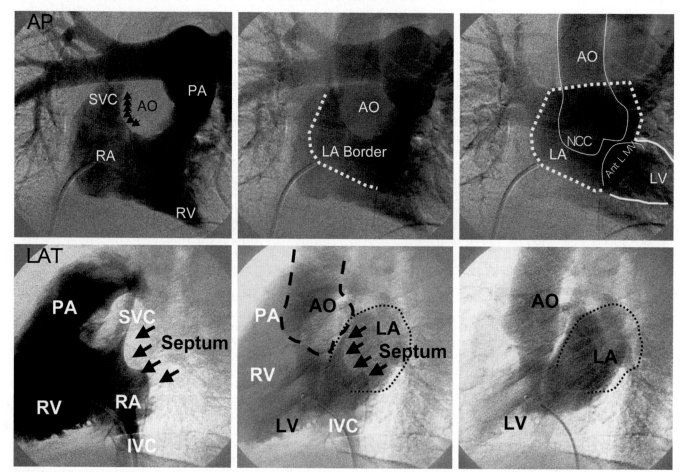

Figure 47-4. Anteroposterior *(top row)* and lateral *(bottom row)* views of a right atrial angiogram is shown in dextro phase *(left panels)*, in levo phase *(right panels)*, and with the two phases superimposed *(middle panels)*. Ant L MV, anterior leaflet of the mitral valve; AO, aorta; IVC, inferior vena cava; LA, left atrium; LV, left ventricle; NCC, noncoronary cusp; PA, pulmonary artery; RA, right atrium; RV, right ventricle; SVC, superior vena cava.

Frequently, a pulmonary artery angiogram is performed in the AP and lateral views to visualize the left atrium and assess pulmonary vein drainage before ASD closure (Fig. 47-5). Direct injection into the left atrial appendage (LAA) is performed to evaluate the anatomy before percutaneous closure (Fig. 47-6).

Typically, the RAO cranial view shows the LAA opening in the medial-lateral diameter, and the RAO caudal view delineates the superior-inferior opening diameter (see Fig. 47-6). These views are also important to study the shape of the LAA, which may determine the feasibility of percutaneous closure.

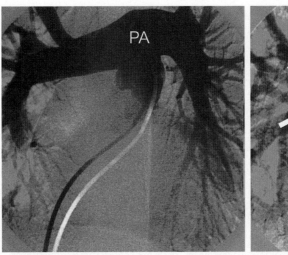

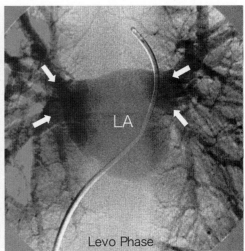

Figure 47-5. Normal pulmonary angiogram is shown in the anteroposterior view. A large volume of dye (40 mL/sec) is rapidly injected using an NIH catheter. The left panel shows the pulmonary artery trunk and the left and right pulmonary arteries and their branches. The right panel shows opacification of the left atrium in levo phase. Digital subtraction is used to visualize the pulmonary veins *(solid white arrows)*. LA, left atrium; PA, pulmonary artery.

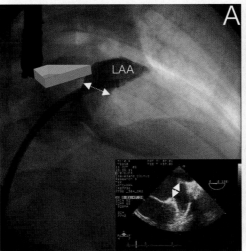

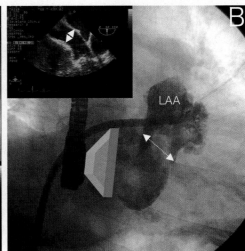

Figure 47-6. A, Right anterior oblique (RAO) cranial view of left atrial appendage (LAA) injection. The "width" of the LAA opening is shown by the dotted arrows and is also depicted in horizontal view by transesophageal echocardiography (TEE) in the inset. **B,** RAO caudal view of the LAA in the same subject, showing the "height" of the opening, which corresponds to the vertical view by TEE *(inset).*

Aortography

An ascending aortogram is performed to examine the aortic valve and root, aortic aneurysms, and, rarely, aortic dissections. An aortogram is performed in the RAO (30 degrees) and LAO (40 degrees) projections. A high rate of injection (20 mL/sec for 2-3 seconds) and proper catheter positioning allow assessment of the various aortic cusps. Aortography is usually performed with a multiside-hole pigtail catheter positioned 2 to 3 cm above the sinus of Valsalva (Fig. 47-7). Various anatomic relationships are important to recognize on fluoroscopy, including the relation of the noncoronary cusp to the IAS for transseptal puncture, the superior vena cava (SVC) for ICE imaging, and the anterior leaflet of the mitral valve for antegrade interventions. These relationships are well demonstrated in an AP view on a right atrial angiogram (see Fig. 47-4).

Pulmonary Angiogram

Pulmonary angiography is the gold standard technique for diagnosing pulmonary embolism.[2] In addition, it is used to assess a variety of other conditions, such as pulmonary valve stenosis, pulmonary artery stenosis, anomalous pulmonary venous return, and pulmonary arteriovenous malformation. Most commonly, a multiside-hole pigtail or NIH catheter is used with a high injection rate (40 mL/sec) to visualize the pulmonary veins. Dextro and levo phases of the injections are shown in Figure 47-5.

TRANSESOPHAGEAL ECHOCARDIOGRAPHY

TEE has become an integral part of invasive cardiac procedures including ASD and PFO closure, mitral valvuloplasty, aortic valvuloplasty, percutaneous aortic valve replacement, and mitral valve E-clip.[3] TEE is a relatively safe procedure; however, in rare cases, esophageal tear has been reported. Most patients in the catheterization laboratory tolerate this procedure in the supine position without endotracheal intubation. Judicious use of short-acting sedatives such as midazolam and good suction of the posterior pharynx are critical for patient comfort.

The TEE probe contains a 3- to 7.5-MHz ultrasound transducer at its tip and can be advanced to the

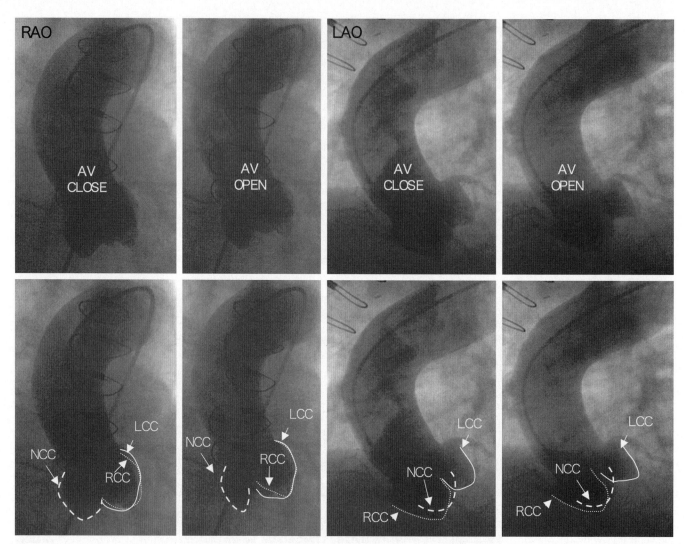

Figure 47-7. Shallow right (RAO) and left (LAO) anterior oblique aortograms in a subject with aortic stenosis and restricted leaflet motion are shown on the left and on the right, respectively. Various structures visualized in the top row are delineated by dashed lines and arrows in the bottom row of images. For each view, the aortic valve (AV) is shown in the closed and in the open position. Note the overlap of the left and right coronary cusps in the RAO projection and of the right and noncoronary cusps in the LAO projection. LCC, left coronary cusp; NCC, noncoronary cusp; RCC, right coronary cusp.

esophagus or stomach for proper visualization of cardiac structures.[4] The tip of the probe can be ante-flexed, retroflexed, or moved from side to side as needed. The currently available TEE transducers are multiplane and consist of a single array of crystals that can be rotated from 0 to 180 degrees. The common views include the 0, "40-60," 90, and 120 degree views. The common positions for the TEE transducer are the upper midesophagus, midesopha-gus, and transgastric positions.

Three important planes can be visualized at 0 degrees, starting from upper to lower esophagus (Fig. 47-8). From the upper midesophagus in a horizontal (0 degree) or basal short-axis view, the aortic arch, pulmonary artery, LAA, pulmonary veins, and aortic valve can be visualized by scanning from left to right. At 0 to 20 degrees mid-esophageal view or with the four-chamber view, the left atrium, LV, right atrium, RV, mitral valve, tricuspid valve, and IAS can be seen

(see Fig. 47-8). The 0-degree transgastric view shows a cross-section of the LV and the mitral valve (see Fig. 47-8).

At 40-60 degrees from upper to midesophageal view, two important planes can be seen (Fig. 47-9). From the 40-60 degree view, the aortic valve, RVOT, right atrium, IAS, and left atrium can be seen (see Fig. 47-9). From the 60-degree midesophageal level (the mitral commissural view), the mitral valve, LV, and left atrium can be seen (see Fig. 47-9). In this view, the posterior mitral leaflet is to the left of the image display, and the anterior leaflet is to the right (see Fig. 47-9). Typically, A2 is located in the middle of the LV inflow tract, with P1 and P3 on each side (see Fig. 47-9).

At 80-100 degrees from upper to lower esophagus, three important planes can be visualized (Fig. 47-10). From the 90-degree upper to midesophageal view (the bicaval view), the SVC, right atrium, inferior

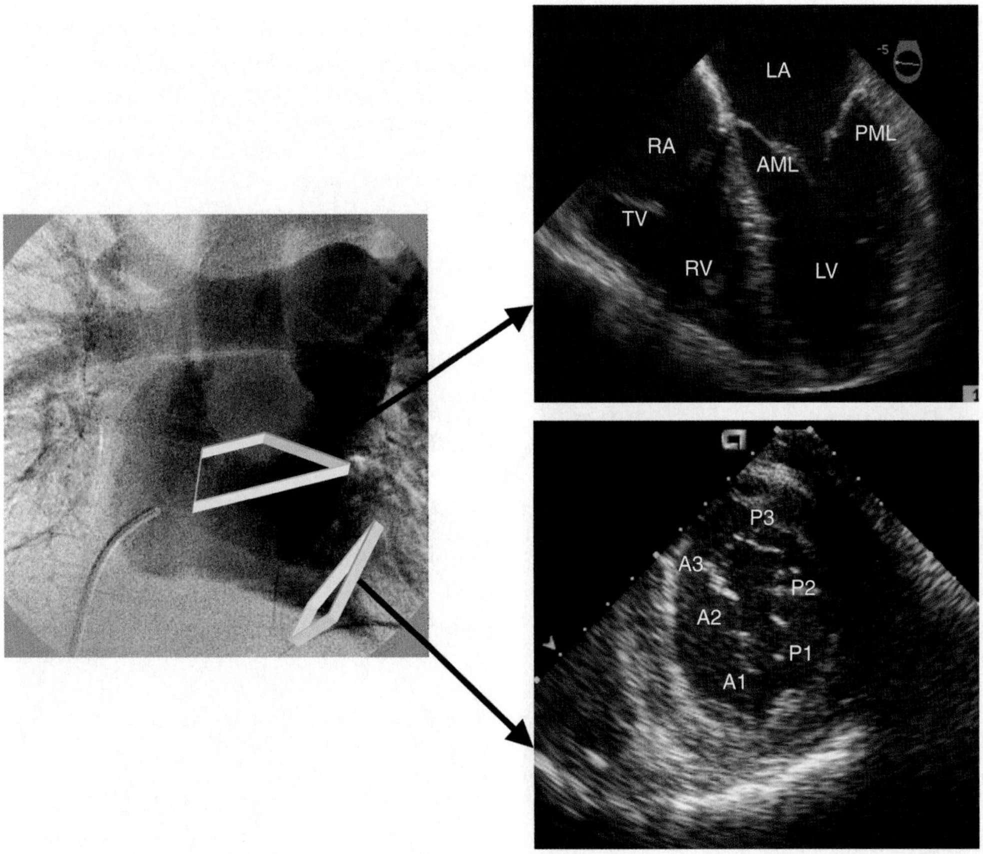

Figure 47-8. Transesophageal echocardiography shows "0 degree" (horizontal) midesophageal *(top right)* and transgastric *(bottom right)* views. On the left, the heart is shown in anteroposterior view (refer to Fig. 47-4 for orientation). Upper right panel provides the four-chamber view and the lower right panel a short-axis view of the mitral valve with the corresponding leaflet segments. The posterior leaflet is divided into P1 to P3 and the anterior leaflet into A1 to A3, from lateral to medial. AML, anterior mitral leaflet; LA, left atrium; LV, left ventricle; PML, posterior mitral leaflet; RA, right atrium; RV, right ventricle; TV, tricuspid valve.

vena cava (IVC), IAS, and left atrium can be seen (see Fig. 47-10). From the 80-100 degree midesophagus (two-chamber) view, the anterior and inferior LV walls, LAA, mitral valve, and coronary sinus can be visualized (see Fig. 47-10). In this view, the LAA can be examined for presence of thrombus. Similarly, in this view, P3 is to the left of the image display, and A1 is to the right (see Fig. 47-10).

In the 120-160 degree midesophagus (long-axis) view, the LV, left atrium, aortic valve, LVOT, mitral valve, and ascending aorta can be seen (Fig. 47-11). The most import TEE views are the four-chamber, long-axis, and two-chamber views.

INTRACARDIAC ECHOCARDIOGRAPHY ANATOMY

ICE provides excellent images of the intracardiac structures without the associated patient discomfort and airway issues that are present with other modalities such as TEE.[5] In addition, in certain situations ICE can produce a clearer, well-defined image compared to TEE. These include assessment of the posterior part of the IAS (where the TEE probe is too close to the area of interest), the pulmonary valve (due to its anterior position), the aortic arch for dissection (due to air shadowing from the bronchus), and some cases of mechanical aortic valve (because of shadowing). ICE is less optimal for evaluating mitral regurgitation, LAA, and LV wall motion (e.g., contrast distribution for alcohol ablation).

The two main ICE transducer systems are the mechanical/rotational and the phased-array systems. The mechanical transducers typically operate at 9 MHz or higher and produce a circular scan path perpendicular to the catheter. Mechanical catheters are imaging catheters without color or Doppler capabilities and are less useful than the phased-array systems, which allow complete evaluation comparable to TEE. In our catheterization laboratory, we exclusively use phased-array systems to guide structural heart disease interventions.

The phased-array system (Acuson) uses 64 piezoelectric elements with frequencies of 5.5, 7.5, 8.5, and 10 MHz to produce a single sector scan that is perpendicular to the long axis of the catheter. The probe is available as an 8 or 11 Fr catheter with "monoplane" imaging. Each device has two handles that allow the operator to move the probe tip anterior, posterior, or from side to side. Maximum tissue penetration with ICE is 10 to 12 cm.

ICE is currently being used for assessment of the IAS, pulmonary veins, crista terminalis, the eustachian valve, tricuspid annulus, coronary sinus ostium, aortic valve, ascending aorta, aortic arch, and mitral valve in some cases.

In general, there are three standard views; however, modification of these views by clockwise or counterclockwise rotation may be necessary. One can typically start from the SVC and pull the probe back caudally for visualization of various structures. The initial view is from the SVC when the transducer is

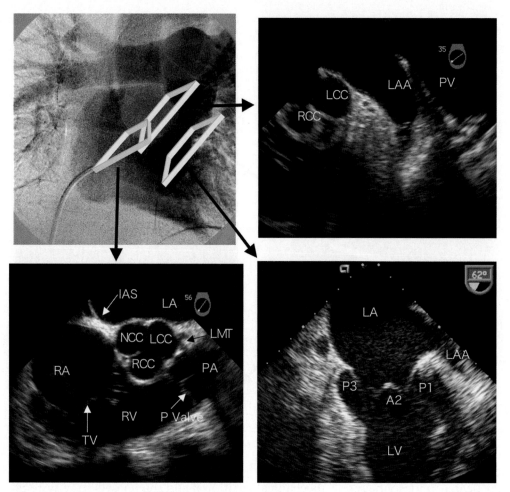

Figure 47-9. Transesophageal echocardiography "40-60 degree" views in the upper to midesophagus with the probe turned to the left *(top right),* at the upper to midesophageal junction with the probe directed anteriorly *(bottom left),* and in the midesophageal commisural view *(bottom right).* The top top left panel shows the heart in anteroposterior view (refer to Fig. 47-4 for orientation). IAS, interatrial septum; LA, left atrium; LAA, left atrial appendage; LCC, left coronary cusp; LMT, left main trunk; LV, left ventricle; NCC, noncoronary cusp; PV, pulmonary vein; RA, right atrium; RCC, right coronary cusp; RV, right ventricle; TV, tricuspid valve.

in the neutral position (Fig. 47-12). Subsequent counterclockwise rotation turns the transducer anteriorly, to where the ascending aorta, the aortic valve, part of the pulmonary trunk, and the tricuspid valve can be seen (see Fig. 47-12). Clockwise rotation from this neutral position rotates the transducer posteriorly, where the IAS, right pulmonary artery, and descending aorta may be seen (see Fig. 47-12). The next view is typically obtained from the right atrium at the level of the tricuspid valve (see Fig. 47-12), which shows the tricuspid valve and the ascending aorta. Further clockwise rotation delineates part of the IAS. To see the entire IAS, posterior flexion is applied to the probe. This allows enough depth so that the entire IAS can be visualized. The third standard view (anterior horizontal view) is obtained by flexing the probe in the middle right atrium with some clockwise rotation (Fig. 47-13). This generates a short-axis view of the aortic valve and produces a better visualization of the anteroposterior section of the septum. Further clockwise rotation demonstrates the mitral valve and its apparatus.

It is possible to see the aortic valve in cross-section by rotating the probe clockwise and posteriorly; however, this view is less reproducible than the anterior horizontal view (see Fig. 47-13). Occasionally, the mitral valve can be visualized from the coronary sinus, the RV, or the superior aspect of the right atrium.

SPECIFIC PROCEDURAL USES FOR INTRACARDIAC IMAGING

Transseptal Puncture

Transseptal puncture has become an integral part of many intracardiac procedures, including percutaneous mitral valvuloplasty, mitral valve repair, LAA closure, some cases of PFO closure, and ablation of atrial fibrillation.[6] The goal is to cross the IAS through the fossa ovalis, an area 2 cm in diameter that is bounded superiorly by the septum secundum, called the limbus. It is located posterior and inferior to the aortic root in the midportion of the IAS. The procedure is performed using the Brockenbrough needle (USCI), which is introduced through an 8-Fr Mullins sheath and dilator combination.

The procedure is performed primarily by fluoroscopic guidance, with ultrasound imaging as an important supplement. Fluoroscopically, the most important landmarks are the position of the aorta (determined by placing a catheter in the aortic root) and the margins of the right and left atria. These landmarks can be determined by right atrial angiog-

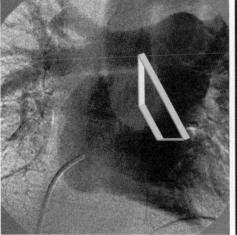

Figure 47-10. Transesophageal echocardiography shows the "90 degree" midesophageal view of the left atrial appendage *(upper right)*, the bicaval view *(lower left)*, and the two-chamber view *(lower right)* views as the probe is directed from left to right. The left panel shows the heart in anteroposterior view (refer to Fig. 47-4 for orientation). EV, eustachian valve; IAS, interatrial septum; IVC, inferior vena cava; LA, left atrium; LAA, left atrial appendage; LV, left ventricle; PV, pulmonary vein; RA, right atrium; RPA, right pulmonary artery; RV, right ventricle; SVC, superior vena cava.

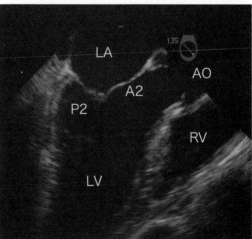

Figure 47-11. Transesophageal echocardiography shows "130 degree" midesophageal long-axis view of the ascending aorta *(right panel)*. Left panel shows the heart in anteroposterior view (refer to Fig. 47-4 for orientation). AO, aorta; LA, left atrium; LV, left ventricle; RV, right ventricle. P2 and A2 refer to the posterior and anterior middle scallops of mitral leaflets.

raphy in the AP and lateral projections (see Fig. 47-4). The needle is withdrawn caudally in the AP projection from the SVC; three medial drops are identified, corresponding, respectively, to the SVC-right atrial junction, the noncoronary sinus of the aorta, and the limbus of the fossa ovalis. The needle position is then checked in the lateral projection to ensure a posterior direction in relation to the aorta (Fig. 47-14). The needle is advanced to the left atrium, with close monitoring to ensure that there is no drop in pressure through the needle as it traverses the IAS. Staining of the septum can be very helpful if there is any

doubt regarding the location of the puncture site (see Fig. 47-14).

TEE can also help determine the appropriate location of the transseptal puncture site. The vertical distance from the mitral valve and from the aorta can be determined by the four-chamber and 45-60 degree views, respectively (Fig. 47-15). TEE is also helpful to rule out thrombus in the left atrium or the LAA and to monitor the pericardium for the presence of effusion. The puncture site must be identified through recognition of tenting, which indicates the correct needle tip position (see Fig. 47-15).

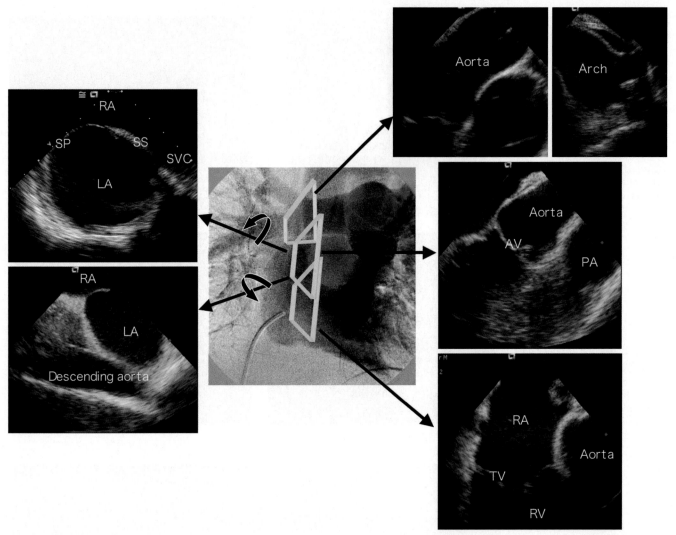

Figure 47-12. The basic views obtained by intracardiac echocardiography (ICE) in the neutral position *(right panel)* and with progressive clockwise rotation *(left panel)* are shown. The corresponding planes are shown on the fluoroscopic image *(center panel)*. Refer to Figure 47-4 for orientation of the fluoroscopic image. In the neutral position, the images were taken at the level of the superior vena cava *(top)*, the middle right atrium *(middle)*, and the tricuspid valve *(bottom)*. The images on the left were obtained by turning the probe clockwise from the middle right atrium to visualize the entire interatrial septum from anterior to posterior aspect. AV, aortic valve; PA, pulmonary artery; RA, right atrium; RV, right ventricle; SP, septum primum; SS, septum secundum; SVC, superior vena cava; TV, tricuspid valve.

ICE is now frequently used for this procedure, and it can clearly identify the IAS, pulmonary veins, and aorta. Typically, the ICE probe is kept in neutral view, with retroflexion as necessary to stay away from the septum, and it is rotated clockwise to identify the left pulmonary veins through the IAS. The presence of the left pulmonary veins opposite the ICE probe ensures posterior entry into the left atrium (see Fig. 47-14A). The appropriate site can also be confirmed in the anterior horizontal view (Fig. 47-16).[7]

Patent Foramen Ovale

The details of this procedure are covered in Chapter 48. Briefly, under normal embryologic processes, the septum primum and secundum (two independent, crescent-shaped membranes) make up the IAS. During fetal life, the mobile septum primum allows right-to-left shunting to maintain life. However, after birth, left atrial pressure increases and helps to fuse these two membranes. In about 15% to 20% of individuals, this fusion does not occur and allows occasional right-to-left shunting, which is called patent foramen ovale (PFO).

Fluoroscopy is used in conjunction with ICE for percutaneous PFO closure. The most common views are the shallow LAO (10-degree) cranial (10-degree) view and the lateral view (or the 60 degree LAO view), which allows better appreciation of the PFO orientation. Typically, a Gudel-Lubin catheter is used to cross the PFO; while the catheter is being pulled back, the injection is made to visualize the PFO on fluoroscopy (see Fig. 47-16). This allows visualization of the length of the tunnel (overlap between septum primum and secundum) and the thickness of the

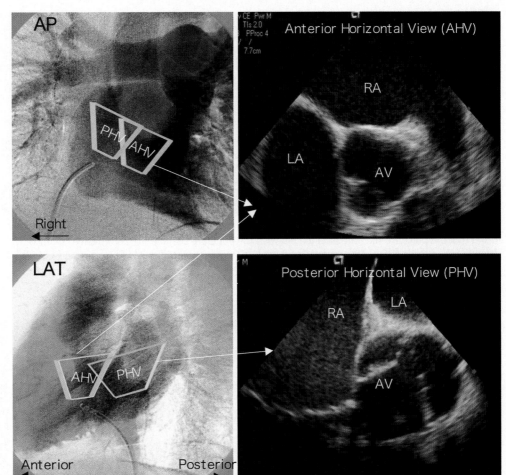

Figure 47-13. Intracardiac echocardiograms (ICE) in the anterior horizontal *(upper right)* and posterior horizontal *(lower right)* views are shown. The corresponding planes are shown in the anteroposterior *(upper left)* and lateral *(lower left)* fluoroscopic views (see text for details). AP, anteroposterior; AV, aortic valve; LA, left atrium; LAT, lateral; RA, right atrium.

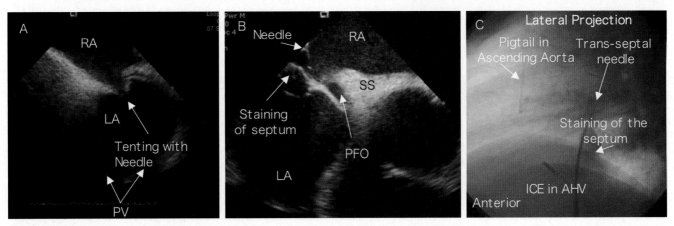

Figure 47-14. Intracardiac echocardiography (ICE) shows a good location for puncture, demonstrated by needle tenting opposite to the pulmonary veins **(A).** A transseptal puncture is made in a patent foreman ovale with a long tunnel. **B,** The needle with stained septum is shown. Note that the puncture site is close to the end of the septum secundum (SS). **C,** The position of the ICE probe and septal staining in the lateral projection are shown (same patient as in **B**). Note that the ascending aorta is anterior, whereas the Brockenbrough needle is pointing posteriorly. AHV, anterior horizontal view; LA, left atrium; PFO, patent foramen ovale; PV, pulmonary vein; RA, right atrium.

septum secundum. Additionally, balloon inflation in the PFO not only helps to determine the size of the PFO but also helps to delineate the shape and size of the tunnel and allows one to "feel" the quality of the tissue around the PFO (see Fig. 47-16). Deployment of the device is usually done in the shallow LAO cranial view (10-10 degrees), which allows perpen-

dicular visualization of the IAS. Lastly, injection of the contrast material under fluoroscopy from the guide catheter before release confirms good apposition (see Fig. 47-16).

ICE is commonly used to first assess the IAS in the longitudinal plane from top to bottom in the anterior and posterior directions. This is done by turning

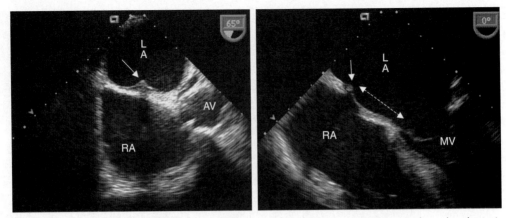

Figure 47-15. Transesophageal echocardiography in the "65 degree" (midesophagus) and "0 degree" (four-chamber) views shows the location of the puncture site. The distance between the puncture site and the aortic valve *(right)* or the mitral valve *(left)* can be determined on these views. The presence of tenting *(white arrow)* confirms the location and position of the needle. AV, aortic valve; LA, left atrium; MV, mitral valve; RA, right atrium.

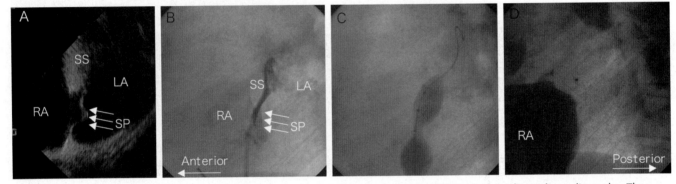

Figure 47-16. A, Patent foreman ovale with septum primum (SP) and septum secundum (SS) on intracardiac echocardiography. The image is rotated to match the fluoroscopic image **(B).** The SP is flimsy (atrial septal aneurysm). **B,** Lateral view on fluoroscopy shows a patent PFO. **C,** "Feeling" of the PFO with the sizing balloon. **D,** Proper positioning of the device with a right atrial angiogram before detachment. LA, left atrium; RA, right atrium.

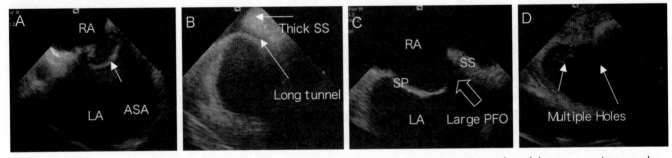

Figure 47-17. Intracardiac echocardiography shows the presence of an atrial septal aneurysm **(A);** overlap of the septum primum and septum secundum, showing the "tunnel" **(B);** the thickness of the septum secundum **(B);** the size of the patent foramen ovale (PFO) **(C);** and the presence of additional openings **(D).** ASA, atrial septal aneurysm; LA, left atrium; RA, right atrium; SP, septum primum; SS, septum secundum.

the probe in the clockwise and counterclockwise directions at various heights in the right atrium (see Fig. 47-12). Next, the probe is flexed anteriorly and the ultrasound beam is directed superiorly and posteriorly to visualize the anteroposterior length of the IAS (see Fig. 47-13). ICE should be carefully performed with following points in consideration:

1. The presence or absence of an atrial septal aneurysm (Fig. 47-17A)
2. The relationship of the septum primum to the septum secundum, to determine the length of the "tunnel" (see Fig. 47-17B)
3. The thickness of the septum secundum (see Fig. 47-17B)

4. The size of the PFO (see Fig. 47-17C)
5. The presence of additional openings (see Fig. 47-17D)
6. The degree of shunt
7. The presence of a prominent Chiari network
8. Assessment of other pathologies such as ascending aortic atheroma

ICE can also show whether the wire has crossed the PFO when other holes are present. Similarly, ICE can be very useful if transseptal puncture for a tunneled PFO is necessary (see Fig. 47-16). Typically, the puncture must be made fairly anterior, near the PFO, to adequately cover the PFO with the device.

Device deployment is typically performed under ICE and fluoroscopy guidance. Proper but not excessive tension during deployment of the device can make it sit well without the risk of deploying both disks in the left atrium. Once the device is deployed, proper interrogation of all margins provides reassurance that the device will not embolize. "Push and pull" is performed, and simultaneous imaging with ICE confirms that the atrial tissue is between the disks. Once the operator is satisfied, the device is released and bubbles are injected to document any residual shunt.

In our institution, almost all PFOs are closed using fluoroscopy and ICE guidance; however, TEE may also be used for this procedure. TEE is associated with greater patient discomfort and requires an additional operator. Two views are most helpful when using TEE: the (30-40 degree) midesophageal short-axis view of the aortic valve and IAS, and the (90-100 degree) midesophageal bicaval view, which shows the IVC, SVC, right atrium, and IAS (see Fig. 47-10). However, every patient is different, and subtle changes in these views and angles may be necessary for better visualization.

Secundum Atrial Septal Defect

Secundum ASD results from underdeveloped septum secundum, which can cause a true opening in the IAS. The key elements in the assessment of ASD with echocardiography for percutaneous closure are (1) location of the defect in the septum secundum (superior, inferior, anterior, or posterior), (2) adequacy of the rims (Fig. 47-18), (3) identification of multiple defects, and (4) size of the defect. Pulmonary angiography is the most helpful modality to identify anomalous venous drainage in the catheterization laboratory (see Fig. 47-5).

ICE is the preferred imaging method for this procedure.[8] In general, the two views described for PFO closure are also adequate for visualizing ASD and its structural detail. Individualization of views should be considered, because the ASD occurs in many different sizes and shapes. Obliteration of color flow with balloon inflation allows proper sizing without oversizing, as commonly happens when only the waist of the balloon is used with fluoroscopy (Fig. 47-19). Device deployment is guided by ICE, and proper gripping can be tested with "push and pull" maneuvers. Impingement of surrounding structures (e.g., mitral valve, SVC, roof of the LA, aorta, coronary sinus) should be carefully assessed before the device is released. Right atrial angiography with an end-on view of the device allows clear visualization of the device margins and their relationships to the left atrial walls and aorta (Fig. 47-20).

Mitral Valvuloplasty

Proper guidance with imaging can make percutaneous mitral valvuloplasty safer and more effective, especially in developed countries, where patients are older and valves are less optimal for balloon valvuloplasty.[9,10]

TEE is most helpful in guiding percutaneous mitral valvuloplasty (Fig. 47-21). It helps (1) guide transseptal puncture, (2) rule out clots in the LAA before the procedure, (3) monitor the degree and the mechanism of mitral regurgitation with balloon inflation, and (4) document the size of the hole at the site of interatrial puncture after removal of the balloon. We prefer to use TEE in the cardiac catheterization laboratory for this procedure.[11] This can be safely accomplished with the patient in the supine position without endotracheal intubation with proper sedation and suction of the posterior pharynx. Careful interrogation of the mitral valve with TEE in the esophageal as well as the transgastric view is helpful for determining the mechanism and severity of mitral

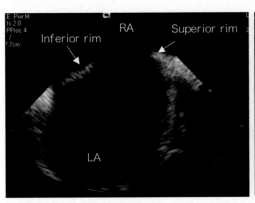
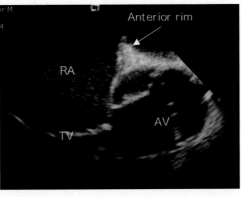

Figure 47-18. Intracardiac echocardiography shows the inferior and superior rims of secundum atrial septal defect *(left)*. Note the presence of a small anterior rim *(right)*. AV, aortic valve; LA, left atrium; RA, right atrium; TV, tricuspid valve.

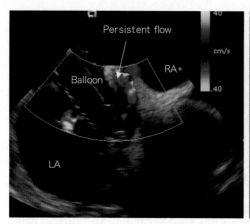

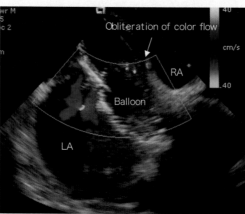

Figure 47-19. Intracardiac echocardiography shows the process of atrial septal defect (ASD) sizing. The balloon is inflated with color interrogation of the ASD. Initially, there is persistent flow around the ASD balloon *(left)*. The balloon is inflated further to barely obliterate the flow across the ASD, and the size is measured. This allows selection of the proper size of ASD closure device without oversizing. LA, left atrium; RA, right atrium.

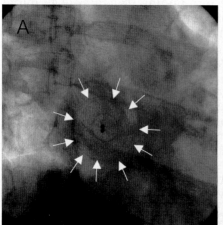

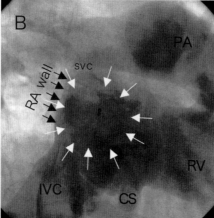

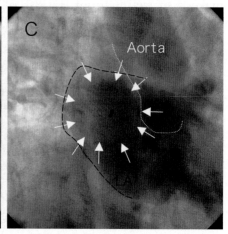

Figure 47-20. Right anterior oblique (RAO) caudal view of a right atrial angiogram shows the atrial septal defect (ASD) device "end-on" **(A)** with surrounding structures in the dextro **(B)** and levo **(C)** phases of contrast injection. Note the relation of the device with the right atrial walls, left atrial walls, and aorta. White arrows show the margin of the left atrial device disk. Black arrows point to the right atrial wall. The aortic silhouette is traced with a dashed white line. The left atrial border is shown by the dashed black line. CS, coronary sinus; IVC, inferior vena cava; LA, left atrium; PA, pulmonary artery; RA, right atrium; RV, right ventricle; SVC, superior vena cava.

regurgitation. Currently, ICE is not very helpful for mitral valve interrogation and assessment.

Fluoroscopy is also an important component of this procedure. LV angiography can assess the severity of mitral regurgitation; however, an adequate volume of dye must be injected, because patients with mitral stenosis have a large left atrium. Fluoroscopy is also used to ensure that the balloon is in proper position and that it is not entangled with the mitral subvalvular apparatus. The RAO projection on fluoroscopy is helpful to ensure coaxial entry of the balloon through the mitral valve without going through the chordae. Partial inflation of the Inoue balloon and advancement of the balloon to the cardiac apex in this view before engagement and inflation can ensure that the balloon is not entangled.

Aortic Valvuloplasty

Fluoroscopy plays a significant role in visualizing the aortic valve and its orifice. Using fluoroscopy in the LAO and RAO projections can help determine which

leaflet has the most motion (see Fig. 47-7). Typically the AL-1 catheter should be pointed under the moving leaflet to cross the valve with a straight wire. If the right coronary cusp is moving, this motion is best appreciated in RAO projection. If the left coronary cusp or the noncoronary cusp has the most motion, then the LAO projection is helpful. The LAO view is the safest view for crossing the aortic valve to prevent inadvertent entry into coronary ostia with a straight wire.

This procedure is done with fluoroscopy only.[12,13] Hemodynamic measurements are important to guide the aggressiveness of balloon valvuloplasty. In the event of complication, TEE or ICE can help determine the exact cause (e.g., severity and mechanism of aortic insufficiency).

Pulmonary Valvuloplasty

Pulmonary valve stenosis is a common congenital abnormality. Many of these patients undergo pulmonary valvuloplasty in adulthood. Cineangiography,

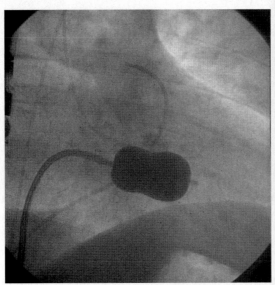

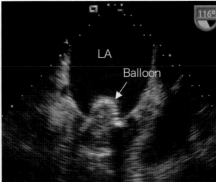

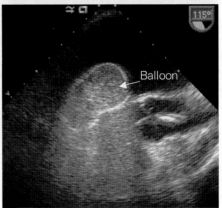

Figure 47-21. Mitral valvuloplasty using the Inoue balloon in the right anterior oblique (RAO) projection under fluoroscopy *(left panel)*. Upper and lower right panels show a stepwise balloon inflation in the 110-120 degree long-axis view under transesophageal echocardiography guidance. LA, left atrium.

transthoracic echocardiography, TEE, and ICE are helpful modalities used for this procedure.[14]

Pulmonary artery angiography in AP and lateral views is helpful to visualize the pulmonary annulus size and preexisting pulmonary insufficiency (Fig. 47-22). Occasionally, right ventriculography in the same views may be performed to assess the RVOT (Fig. 47-23). Severe subpulmonary hypertrophy may be associated with significant dynamic RVOT obstruction after pulmonary valvuloplasty.

Both transthoracic echocardiography and TEE can be helpful in assessing pulmonary valve annular size. ICE provides useful assessment of the pulmonary insufficiency and allows measurement of the annulus. However, for assessment of the pulmonary valve, the ICE probe should be placed in the RVOT (see Fig. 47-23).

Percutaneous Mitral Valve Repair

The mitral valve apparatus consists of the annulus, leaflets, chordae, and papillary muscles. The mitral annulus is saddle-shaped, with the trigonal part and lateral commissures as the highest points. There is some suggestion that the shape of the annulus changes when the left atrium and LV dilate. The anterior leaflet is larger in length but covers one third of the circumference of the annulus. The posterior leaflet is shorter in length but covers two thirds of the annulus.

For edge-to-edge percutaneous mitral valve repair,[15] TEE is used to guide transseptal puncture and to assess the proper medial-lateral, axial, and anterior-

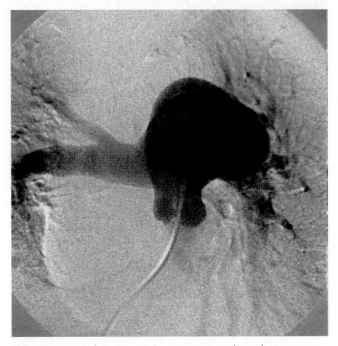

Figure 47-22. Pulmonary angiogram assesses the pulmonary valve using the NIH catheter. Note the presence of mild pulmonary insufficiency and poststenotic pulmonary artery dilation. Digital subtraction was used for better visualization.

posterior adjustment of the mitral system (Fig. 47-24). In addition, TEE can guide perpendicular alignment of the clip arms to the line of coaptation. It is also useful for assessment of mitral regurgitation with each attempt at treatment. The most common

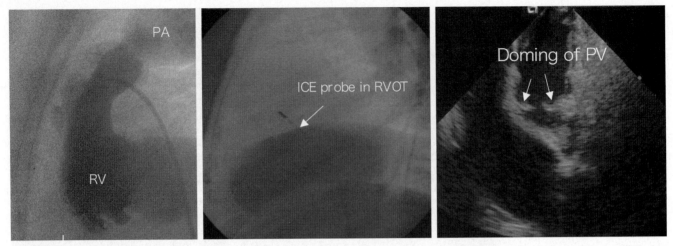

Figure 47-23. *Left,* Right ventriculogram showing pulmonary stenosis in the lateral view. *Middle,* Intracardiac echocardiogram (ICE) probe in the right ventricular outflow tract (RVOT) in the lateral view (same projection). *Right,* Pulmonary valve doming in the corresponding ICE view. PA, pulmonary artery; PV, pulmonary valve; RV, right ventricle.

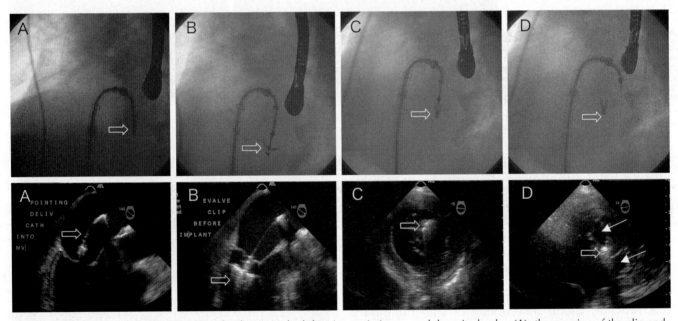

Figure 47-24. Images in the top row show the device in the left atrium pointing toward the mitral valve **(A)**, the opening of the clip and advancing across the mitral valve **(B)**, grabbing of the leaflet tips **(C)**, and releasing of the clip *(open arrow)* **(D)**. The corresponding images in the bottom row depict, respectively, the transesophageal echocardiography images of the device in the left atrium pointing toward the mitral valve, the opening of the clip and advancing across the mitral valve, the perpendicular orientation of the clip to the mitral valve coaptation line in transgastric view, and the final result with a double orifice *(two white arrows).*

views are the midesophageal short-axis view (typically for transseptal puncture and to guide catheter manipulation), the midesophageal commissural or two-chamber view, a midesophageal long-axis ("LVOT") view (multiplane angle of approximately 120-150 degrees), and a transgastric short-axis view (multiplane angle 0-30 degrees) at the mitral valve level.

For coronary sinus–related procedures, fluoroscopy and TEE are helpful for proper positioning of the device and evaluation of the effectiveness of any intervention. Angiography helps to determine left circumflex and coronary sinus relationships. Computed tomography (CT) can help patient selection by defining the relationship of the coronary sinus, mitral annulus, and left circumflex coronary artery.

The pericardial approach to mitral valve repair also is heavily dependent on proper use of various imaging modalities, including fluoroscopy, TEE, and ICE. Proper use of these techniques will only mature as human experience with these novel methods increases.

Percutaneous Aortic Valve Replacement

Percutaneous aortic valve replacement is becoming a reality in the 21st century.[16] Many different approaches are being investigated with balloon-

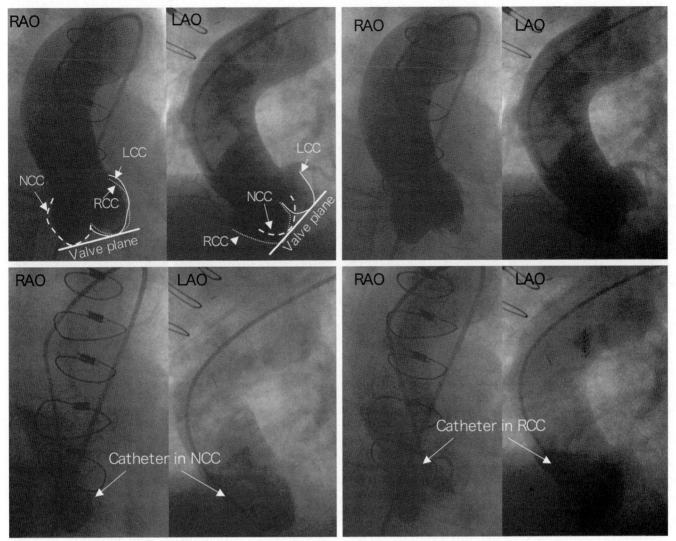

Figure 47-25. Left anterior oblique (LAO) cranial "40/20 degree" and right anterior oblique (RAO) caudal "20/20 degree" views of the aortic valve and its plane. The proper angulation of the camera must be customized in each patient so that the all cusps are superimposed. Note that the catheter is in different sinuses in different phases of injection. LCC, left coronary cusp; NCC, noncoronary cusp; RCC, right coronary cusp.

expandable or self-expanding stented or unstented valves. Accurate positioning of the valve is critical, especially for balloon-expandable valves; therefore, proper imaging in the catheterization laboratory is of paramount importance.

Several elements that are important to make this procedure accurate and reproducible. The aortic valve plane must be accurately defined (see Fig. 47-7). Fluoroscopy with minimal contrast injection at times can determine the appropriate angles so that the aortic valve plane is seen without any overlap of the sinuses (Fig. 47-25). Typically, LAO cranial and RAO caudal views are used. It is also important to note which leaflets and commissures are calcified and restricted.

Accurate definition of leaflet morphology may help to identify patients in whom compromise of coronary ostia is likely at the time of valve deployment. Injection of dye at the time of balloon valvuloplasty may also help to predict this relationship

(Fig. 47-26A). The ascending aortic slope (horizontal versus vertical in LAO projection) may determine the ease or difficulty in delivering the valve. Angiography is also important in determining size, calcification, and degree of tortuosity of the iliac and femoral vessels.

TEE is important for valve assessment (calcification, annulus size, and severity), accurate positioning of the valve, and assessment of the results of valve replacement (valvular or perivalvular leak and function). Again, complementary use of these imaging modalities is critical for the success of this procedure (see Fig. 47-26).

Four-dimensional cardiac CT may allow better visualization of the aortic valve, its relation to the coronary ostia, and its morphology and extent of leaflet calcification (Fig. 47-27). Additionally, CT scanning is critically helpful in assessing the iliac and femoral arteries for size, tortuosity, and extent of calcification.

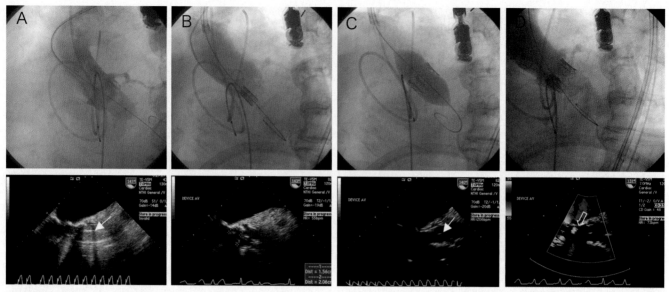

Figure 47-26. Percutaneous aortic valve replacement. The top row shows the left anterior oblique (LAO) cranial projection, and the bottom row shows the corresponding transesophageal echocardiography (TEE) images in aortic long-axis view (130 degrees). **A,** Valvuloplasty balloon in the aortic position with contrast injection depicting the distance from the aortic cusp tips to the coronary ostia. **B,** Positioning of the stent-valve. **C,** Once appropriately positioned, the valve is deployed with rapid pacing. **D,** Good final position of aortic valve with mild regurgitation *(open arrow)*.

Alcohol Septal Ablation

The details of this procedure are covered in a separate chapter. Preprocedural assessment with echocardiography, magnetic resonance imaging, and cardiac catheterization is paramount to proper patient selection. In the catheterization laboratory, selecting an appropriate septal perforator for injection is critical to success. Combining proper angiographic views with transthoracic echocardiography can help define the septal area that needs to be targeted. ICE has been used for this purpose and provides a visualization of the septum; however, its use for this procedure is tempered by cost, inability to reliably see all walls of the LV (i.e., whether the contrast agent is going in any unintended area), measurement of gradients, and at times difficulty in visualizing the mitral regurgitation. Importantly, there is no specific advantage of ICE if transthoracic images are of good quality.

Mechanical Prosthetic Valve Assessment

Occasionally, mechanical valves require a full assessment for the presence of dehiscence, vegetations, or obstruction secondary to thrombus or pannus formation. Although transthoracic echocardiography and TEE can provide valuable information, some limitations persist. These include shadowing, pressure recovery phenomena, and difficulty in visualizing the aortic valve secondary to its anterior location.

Fluoroscopy has been helpful in measuring opening and closing angles of the mechanical aortic valve. For this determination, fluoroscopy cameras should be positioned so that tangential views of the leaflets are obtained (Fig. 47-28). Because the rotational orientation can vary from patient to patient during the placement of the prosthetic aortic valve, there is no single view that can correctly visualize this valve. Therefore, we recommend a systematic approach,

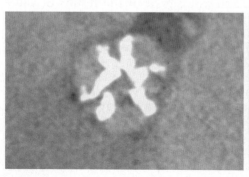
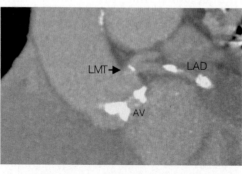

Figure 47-27. Four-dimensional computed tomography (CT) of the aortic valve (AV) in short axis *(left)* and in a longitudinal cut *(right)*. Note significant calcification on the AV and left anterior descending coronary artery (LAD). CT can also help to determine the distance between the aortic valve and the left main trunk (LMT).

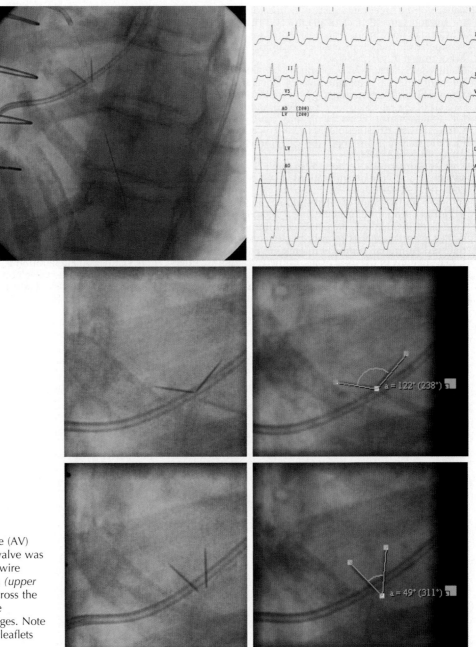

Figure 47-28. Prosthetic aortic valve (AV) assessment using fluoroscopy. The valve was crossed with a 0.014-inch pressure wire *(upper left).* Hemodynamic tracings *(upper right)* show a significant gradient across the AV. Opening and closing angles are measured in the lower block of images. Note that the valve is imaged so that the leaflets are seen end-on.

starting with the 20-30 degrees RAO caudal view and gradually increasing this angle toward a LAO cranial projection (see Fig. 47-28). Occasionally, ventriculography may be helpful to see the subvalvular pathology (e.g., pannus). In patients with a low-profile tilting disk (i.e., Bjork-Shiley, St. Jude, or Medtronic-Hall valve), transseptal puncture and pressure measurements with or without ventriculography may be necessary for better assessment of the prosthetic valve. Although the prosthetic aortic valve can be crossed with a 0.014-inch pressure wire, the safety of such a procedure is unclear. In situations where both the mitral and the aortic valves have mechanical prostheses, apical puncture or crossing of the aortic or mitral valve with pressure wire may be considered (see Fig. 47-28).

Cardiac CT scanning also allows assessment of the opening and closing angles of the mechanical prosthetic valves. ICE can be used to assess prosthetic aortic valve function. It is also possible to visualize the LVOT just below the mechanical aortic valve from right atrium using ICE.

REFERENCES

1. Hildner FJ, Furst A, Krieger R, et al: New principles for optimum left ventriculography. Cathet Cardiovasc Diagn 1986;12: 266-273.
2. Grollman JH Jr: Pulmonary arteriography. Cardiovasc Intervent Radiol 1992;15:166-170.
3. Shanewise JS, Cheung AT, Aronson S, et al: ASE/SCA guidelines for performing a comprehensive intraoperative multiplane transesophageal echocardiography examination: Recommen-

dations of the American Society of Echocardiography Council for Intraoperative Echocardiography and the Society of Cardiovascular Anesthesiologists Task Force for Certification in Perioperative Transesophageal Echocardiography. J Am Soc Echocardiogr 1999;12:884-900.

4. Shanewise JS, Cheung AT, Aronson S, et al: ASE/SCA guidelines for performing a comprehensive intraoperative multiplane transesophageal echocardiography examination: Recommendations of the American Society of Echocardiography Council for Intraoperative Echocardiography and the Society of Cardiovascular Anesthesiologists Task Force for Certification in Perioperative Transesophageal Echocardiography. Anesth Analg 1999;89:870-884.

5. Kort S: Intracardiac echocardiography: Evolution, recent advances, and current applications. J Am Soc Echocardiogr 2006;19:1192-1201.

6. Solomon SB: The future of interventional cardiology lies in the left atrium. Int J Cardiovasc Intervent 2004;6:101-106.

7. Cafri C, de la Guardia B, Barasch E, et al: Transseptal puncture guided by intracardiac echocardiography during percutaneous transvenous mitral commissurotomy in patients with distorted anatomy of the fossa ovalis. Catheter Cardiovasc Interv 2000;50:463-467.

8. Salome N, Braga P, Goncalves M, et al: Transcatheter device occlusion of atrial septal defects and patent foramen ovale under intracardiac echocardiographic guidance. Rev Port Cardiol 2004;23:709-717.

9. Guerios EE, Bueno R, Nercolini D, et al: Mitral stenosis and percutaneous mitral valvuloplasty (part 1). J Invasive Cardiol 2005;17:382-386.

10. Guerios EE, Bueno R, Nercolini D, et al: Mitral stenosis and percutaneous mitral valvuloplasty (part 2). J Invasive Cardiol 2005;17:440-444.

11. Roberts JW, Lima JA: Role of echocardiography in mitral commissurotomy with the Inoue balloon. Cathet Cardiovasc Diagn 1994;Suppl 2:69-75.

12. Feldman T: Transseptal antegrade access for aortic valvuloplasty. Catheter Cardiovasc Interv 2000;50:492-494.

13. Vahanian A: Balloon valvuloplasty. Heart 2001;85:223-228.

14. Shively BK: Transesophageal echocardiographic (TEE) evaluation of the aortic valve, left ventricular outflow tract, and pulmonary valve. Cardiol Clin 2000;18:711-729.

15. Feldman T, Wasserman HS, Herrmann HC, et al: Percutaneous mitral valve repair using the edge-to-edge technique: Six-month results of the EVEREST Phase I Clinical Trial. J Am Coll Cardiol 2005;46:2134-2140.

16. Cribier A, Eltchaninoff H, Tron C, et al: Percutaneous implantation of aortic valve prosthesis in patients with calcific aortic stenosis: Technical advances, clinical results and future strategies. J Interv Cardiol 2006;19:S87-S96.

48 Percutaneous Closure of Patent Foramen Ovale and Atrial Septal Defect

John M. Lasala, Alan Zajarias, and Srihari Thanigaraj

KEY POINTS

■ Although patent foramen ovale (PFO) and atrial septal defect (ASD) both involve an abnormal communication across the interatrial septum, their etiologic mechanisms are markedly different. PFO results from lack of fusion between the septum primum and the septum secundum, whereas a secundum ASD is caused by the absence of a segment of the atrial septum.

■ PFO has been associated with paradoxical embolization, cryptogenic stroke, migraine headache, decompression sickness, and platypnea orthodeoxia syndrome.

■ Until the results of ongoing clinical trials and registries are available, the routine closure of PFO can be recommended only for patients who participate in clinical trials or who have had a recurrent cerebrovascular event while being therapeutically anticoagulated.

■ Percutaneous closure of PFO or secundum ASD is a simple, safe, and effective treatment option for the appropriate candidates.

The advent of cardiopulmonary bypass support revolutionized the management of many structural cardiac abnormalities. Ever since the first surgical repair of an atrial septal defect (ASD) in 1952, surgical techniques have been refined steadily and now confer excellent short-term and long-term outcomes. Until recently, the management of ASD was considered to be primarily surgical. The last 2 decades have witnessed the growth of percutaneous techniques for management of coronary and other vascular pathology. The refinements in percutaneous interventional technology and recent advances in cardiac imaging techniques have permitted percutaneous treatment of selected structural cardiac defects. One of the most common congenital cardiac anomalies, ASD was the earliest to be approached percutaneously. The early attempts at percutaneous closure with devices such as the Rashkind and Das Angel Wings occluders date back to the 1980s, but they were limited by the large profile of the catheters and delivery sheath systems, which made the procedures less attractive.

Improvements in the technology over the ensuing 2 decades paved the way for newer generations of devices that made percutaneous closure of secundum ASD not only acceptable but preferable to the surgical approach. The closely related entity patent foramen ovale (PFO), which until now was rarely treated surgically despite its well known association with paradoxical embolism, also became accessible to percutaneous closure. In the 5 years since the U.S. Food and Drug Administration (FDA) approved selected devices for closure of ASD and PFO, a paradigm shift has occurred in the management of these two entities. ASD and PFO management shifted away from the surgical arena and into the catheterization laboratory when patient recovery time was found to be shortened, complications decreased, and treatment efficacy maintained. The associations of PFO with other disease processes (e.g., migraine) were also identified, opening the potential of new treatment options for a large portion of patients.

This chapter provides an introduction to the percutaneous closure of ASD and PFO. It includes an overview of their embryology, pathophysiology, and clinical associations, followed by a description of the available devices for closure. The procedure, its indications, and complications are also detailed.

EMBRYOLOGY

By the 18th day of gestation, the primordium of the heart becomes evident. At the end of the fourth week, the endocardial cushions fuse, forming the right and left atrioventricular canals. The endocardial cushions will serve as the primordium of the atrioventricular valves and the inferior wall of the atria. At this time, the common atria undergoes a complicated process of septation. The *septum primum* grows in a caudal direction toward the endocardial cushions, closing the interatrial communication *(ostium primum)*. As the septum primum reaches its destination, cells in its superior portion undergo apoptosis and coalesce, forming the *ostium secundum*. A muscular *septum secundum* forms to the right of the septum primum and extends to reach the caudal border of the ostium secundum, forming a "flap-like valve" between the atria (Fig. 48-1; Video 48-1).[1] Oxygenated placental blood enters the right atrium from the inferior vena cava and is directed toward the interatrial septum (IAS) by the eustachian valve. The low left atrial pressure, the lack of blood flow through the pulmonary veins, and the preferential flow of the inferior vena cava to the IAS allow oxygenated blood to cross the foramen ovale and enter into the systemic circulation. Blood entering the right atrium from the superior vena cava is directed away from the IAS by the *crista interveniens,* preventing the mixture of nonoxygenated blood in this chamber. The right horn of the

sinus venosus incorporates the superior and inferior venae cavae into the right atrium (Video 48-2).

At birth, the pulmonary vascular resistances and the right cardiac pressures fall, and the left atrial pressure increases, forcing the septum primum against the septum secundum, thus occluding the "valve-like" foramen ovale. Complete occlusion occurs in most people, but the fusion is incomplete in approximately 25% of the population, giving rise to a PFO.[2]

The embryology and other characteristics of PFO and ASD are presented in Table 48-1.

PATENT FORAMEN OVALE

By echocardiography, the incidence of a PFO in the adult population is estimated to be approximately 25%.[2] Autopsy studies revealed the presence of a probe-patent PFO of 0.2 to 0.5 cm in 29%.[3] The frequency of PFO decreases with age but the opening increases in size with each decade of life.[4] Spontaneous PFO closure may occur during adulthood, although recent data suggest that PFOs may recanalize over time.[5] Incidence of PFO is equal across gender and ethnic groups; however, whites and Hispanics have larger PFOs, which are associated with a greater degree of shunt through them.[6]

The presence of a PFO was thought to be inconsequential until 1877, when Cohnheim postulated that a venous thrombosis may paradoxically traverse a PFO and give rise to a systemic embolism.[7] Since that time, PFOs have been associated with various disease processes, including cryptogenic stroke and paradoxical embolization,[8,9] platypnea orthodeoxia syndrome,[10] hypoxemia with normal pulmonary pressures,[11] decompression sickness in divers[6] and in high-altitude pilots,[12] and migraine headaches.[13]

Cryptogenic Stroke

Depending on the age group, the etiology of a cerebrovascular event (CVA) may vary. Atrial fibrillation and small-vessel disease contribute to the majority of strokes in patients older than 50 years of age. In patients younger than 35 years, the most common causes are nonatherosclerotic arteriopathies, arterial dissection, and thromboembolism.[5] However, in 35% to 40% of patients who experience a CVA, the cause remains unknown after a thorough evaluation and is classified as cryptogenic. The term "cryptogenic CVA" may group disparate causes that remain unidentified by current diagnostic modalities. The search for the probable etiologies of cryptogenic stroke has generated conflicting information.

In a retrospective case-control study, PFOs were four times more prevalent in young adults who experienced a stroke without an identifiable cause, compared to others with a stroke of known cause.[9] In a recent meta-analysis, PFOs were found up to six times more frequently in patients younger than 55 years of age with cryptogenic stroke, compared to those

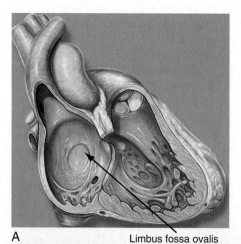

Limbus fossa ovalis

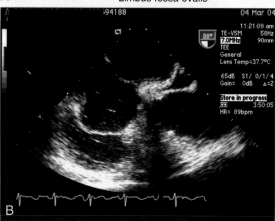

Figure 48-1. Diagram **(A)** and photograph **(B)** of the interatrial septum, depicting the limbus of the fossa ovalis and the anatomic location of the patent foramen ovale. (Courtesy of Patrick J. Lynch, Yale University ITS Web Services, New Haven, CT.)

Table 48-1. Characteristics of Atrial Septal Defect and Patent Foramen Ovale

Patent Foramen Ovale	Atrial Septal Defect
Embryology	
Failure of septum primum and secundum to fuse completely	Failure of septum primum and/or secundum to develop normally
Pathway or channel between tissue flaps	Tissue *defect*
Direction of shunt	
If RA pressure > LA pressure, shunts right to left; if LA pressure > RA pressure, may stay closed or shunt left to right	Usually RA pressure = LA pressure, but shunt is left to right because RV is more compliant; shunt reverses with Eisenmenger physiology
Shunt is dynamic and bidirectional	Same as for PFO
Shunt direction depends on RA-LA pressure difference, RVEDP-LVEDP difference, phase of respiration, and volume status	Same as for PFO

LA, left atrium; LVEDP, left ventricular end-diastolic pressure; PFO, patent foramen ovale; RA, right atrium; RVEDP, right ventricular end-diastolic pressure.

who had a CVA with an identifiable cause.[14] Other researchers have noted a higher frequency of PFO in patients with a cryptogenic stroke irrespective of age (<55 years, 48% vs. 4%; ≥55 years, 38% vs. 8%; $P < .001$), although this finding is not generally accepted.[10] Among patients with cryptogenic stroke, those with PFO were less likely to have traditional cardiovascular risk factors such as hypertension, hypercholesterolemia, or tobacco use, suggesting a different mechanism of CVA in this population subset.[15] The mechanism by which a PFO may participate in the generation of cryptogenic stroke is unclear. In situ thrombosis, paradoxical embolization, and predisposition to atrial arrhythmias have been the proposed as mechanisms for PFO-associated cryptogenic stroke.[16] Paradoxical embolization, the passage of a venous thrombus into the systemic circulation through PFO, has been the predominant theory (Fig. 48-2; Video 48-3).

Evidence that supports the role of a PFO in cryptogenic stroke includes case reports that exemplify thrombus transit across a PFO[17]; the cerebral distribution of cryptogenic CVAs, which suggest an embolic nature[18]; and the increased frequency of deep venous thrombosis in patients with a cryptogenic CVA.[19] The Paradoxical Embolism from Large Veins in Ischemic Stroke (PELVIS) trial noted an increased frequency of positive magnetic resonance venography for pelvic thrombus in patients with PFO and cryptogenic CVA when compared to patients with known causes (20% vs. 4%; $P < .03$).[20] The corollary is also true: patients with a pulmonary embolus have a significantly higher stroke rate in the presence of a PFO (13% vs. 2%; $P = .02$).[21]

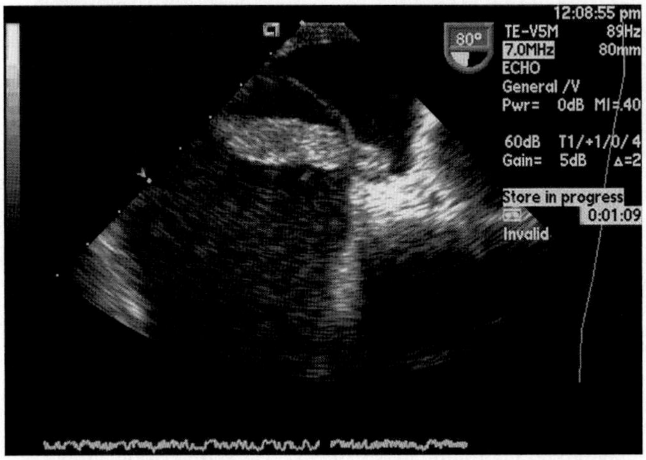

However, this association is still controversial. The majority of the information available on the association of PFOs and cryptogenic stroke originates from small case-control or retrospective studies, which limits the conclusions that can be generated. A large, population-based case-control study that included 1072 participants (random controls, referred controls, patients with noncryptogenic stroke, and patients with cryptogenic stroke) failed to show an association between cryptogenic stroke and the presence of a PFO.[22] The lack of association may have been related to the study design, because case selection included patients without recurrent CVA.

Data from the Stroke Prevention Assessment of Risk in a Community (SPARC) trial,[23] a prospective trial that questioned the veracity of a causal relation between PFO and stroke of unknown etiology, have recently been published. The trial included 588 healthy volunteers who underwent multimodality testing and follow-up in Olmstead County for stroke risk assessment. Over a period of 5 years, 41 patients experienced a stroke. After adjustments for age and other cardiovascular comorbidities, PFO was not an independent predictor of stroke (hazard ratio (HR) = 1.28; 95% confidence interval [CI]: 0.65 to 2.50). The Kaplan-Meier estimate of survival free of CVA was 91% and 93% in patients with and without PFO, respectively. The trial confirmed that the presence of a PFO does not pose an increased risk of stroke in asymptomatic patients. Unfortunately, this trial included an older population (66.9 ± 13 years), whereas most of the other trials have recognized the association with cryptogenic stroke in patients younger than 55 years of age, and had a low prevalence of CVA, which limits its ability to detect a sta-

Figure 48-2. Thrombus in transit from the right atrium through a patent foramen ovale into the left atrium, illustrating the concept of paradoxical embolization.

tistically significant hazard. The HR may be as low as 0.65 or as high as 2.5 and still be consistent with the study's findings.

Stroke Recurrence and Risk Identification

Prospective data from an observational study presented in abstract form have documented the incidence of CVA in patients with PFO as being 1.10/100 person-years, compared with 0.97/100 person-years in patients without PFO.[24] The low incidence does not make primary prevention cost-effective. Additional risk factors that may detect people at risk need to be identified. The reported recurrence rate of cryptogenic stroke varies from 1.2% to greater than 16% but is usually about 2%.[25,26] In retrospective studies, the risk of recurrence has been found to be related to PFO size, patency at rest, shunt severity, and presence of atrial septal aneurysm (ASA).[27-29] A prominent eustachian valve preferentially directs flow to the IAS and has been associated with increased patency of foramen ovale and risk of stroke recurrence (Fig. 48-3; Video 48-4).[30]

It has been postulated that a mobile IAS may increase the size of the PFO, facilitating the passage of thrombi. Recurrence of cryptogenic CVA has been found to be associated with degree of septal protru-

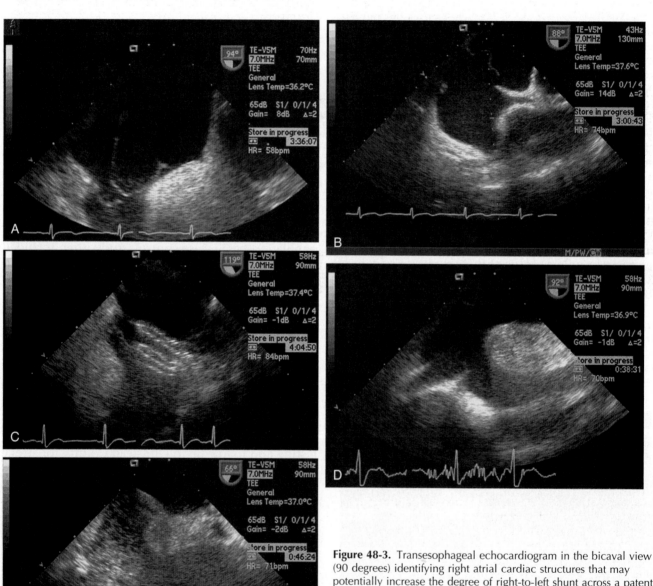

Figure 48-3. Transesophageal echocardiogram in the bicaval view (90 degrees) identifying right atrial cardiac structures that may potentially increase the degree of right-to-left shunt across a patent foramen ovale (PFO) or may complicate the closure procedure: **(A)** prominent eustachian valve; **(B)** atrial septal aneurysm. **C,** A 25-mm AGA foramen occluder successfully captures the septum secundum and primum closing the PFO. **D** and **E,** Lipomatous hypertrophy of the atrial septum also creates a challenge in placing the closure device. Immediately after device deployment (arrow), a saline contrast study is mildly positive.

sion: patients with septum excursion greater than 6.5 mm had a risk of recurrence of 12.3% at 3 years, versus 4.3% for those with lesser septum excursion.[26] The combination of ASA and PFO was associated with an increased risk of recurrence in the French PFO/ASA study (HR = 4.17; 95% CI: 1.47 to 11.84).[31] However, this finding was not supported by the Patent Foramen Ovale in Cryptogenic Stroke Study (PICSS) trial.[32] The PICSS trial was designed to define the rate of recurrent stroke or death in stroke patients with and without PFO who were randomly treated with aspirin or warfarin over a period of 2 years. The study was multicenter and double-blinded; it included 265 patients with cryptogenic stroke and 365 with noncrytpogenic stroke. PFOs were more frequently found in patients with cryptogenic stroke (48% vs. 38%; $P < .02$), and larger PFOs were more frequently associated with the same stroke subtype (20% vs. 9.7%; $P < .001$). There was no statistically significant difference in time to recurrent stroke or death in the cryptogenic stroke group when categorized by PFO status (14.3% vs. 12%). In all stroke patients, there was no difference in stroke recurrence when categorized by the presence of PFO and ASA. However, this study had significant limitations that might alter the generalization of its results. Patients were older and had a higher prevalence of CVA risk factors (diabetes and hypertension); moreover, only 42% of the enrolled patients had a cryptogenic stroke. Because of this, the subgroup analysis of patients with cryptogenic stroke might be underpowered for treatment assumptions in this group.

Because of the inherent limitations of study design, small patient population, and difference in control groups, no conclusion can be made regarding the association of PFO and CVA at the present time. Larger randomized trials are required to answer this question.

Treatment for Cryptogenic Stroke

Medical Treatment

Controversy exists regarding the best method for prevention of recurrent events in patients who have experienced a cryptogenic stroke. Medical treatment with aspirin or oral anticoagulants has been reported. In the PFO/ASA study, 267 patients who experienced a cryptogenic stroke and had a PFO or both PFO and ASA were treated with aspirin, or with aspirin and warfarin if they had a venous thrombosis.[32] After 4 years of follow-up, there were 12 episodes of recurrent strokes and 9 recurrent transient ischemic attacks (TIAs). All episodes occurred in patients treated with aspirin. In the Lausanne study, 140 patients with the same characteristics were followed for 36 months. Treatment was assigned depending on the number of risk factors and included surgical PFO closure (8%), oral anticoagulation with a target international normalized ratio (INR) of 3 to 4 (26%), and aspirin (66%). The yearly event rate was 1.9% for CVA and 3.8% for the combination of CVA and TIA.[33] A meta-analysis

evaluating the benefit of medical therapy versus transcatheter closure of PFO in patients with presumed paradoxical embolization that included 895 patients in the medical therapy arm yielded a 1-year recurrence rate of between 3.8% and 12%.[34] The only prospective, blinded, randomized trail that compared the efficacy of aspirin versus oral anticoagulation in patients with CVA was the PICSS trial.[33] It found no statistically significant difference in stroke recurrence in patients with PFO between those treated with aspirin and those receiving Coumadin treatment (17.9% vs. 9.5%; HR = 0.52; 95% CI: 0.16 to 1.67; $P = .28$). The high recurrence rate suggests other (non-PFO) mechanisms for CVA in the elder population. As expected, there was a slight increase in the rate of minor hemorrhage in patients in the Coumadin arm. Currently, there is no consensus on the superiority of antiplatelet or oral anticoagulation therapy for patients with cryptogenic stroke and PFO.[35]

Surgical Treatment

Surgical closure of PFO in patients with cryptogenic stroke has been reported. The largest series included 91 consecutive patients with a mean age of 44 years and one prior cerebrovascular event. Surgery was evaluated with intraoperative transesophageal echocardiography and was performed by suture or patch closure. Closure was achieved in 98% of cases, and the actuarial freedom from recurrence was 93% at 1 year and 83% at 4 years. The surgical procedure was associated with significant morbidity in 21% of the patients.[36] Other, smaller series reflect similar closure rates with significant morbidity.

Percutaneous Treatment

Percutaneous closure of PFOs has been available for the last decade. There have been no completed randomized trials evaluating the efficacy of percutaneous closure versus medical treatment. The available data reflect single-operator or multiple-center experiences with moderate follow-up. Procedural success has been greater than 90%. Device modifications and a growing experience and familiarity with the technique have greatly reduced the complication rate while maintaining appropriate closure rates. Windeker and colleagues reported on 80 patients with a procedural success rate of 98% and a 2.5% recurrent TIA rate at 5 years.[37] Residual shunt has been identified as a risk for recurrent cerebrovascular events; overall percutaneous closure has recurrent rates similar to those of medical therapy.[38,39] The only series that had compared medical therapy with percutaneous closure in patients with PFO and cryptogenic stroke was published by Windeker and associates.[40] Patients were nonrandomly assigned to percutaneous closure ($n = 150$), medical treatment with aspirin ($n = 78$), or oral anticoagulation ($n = 78$) with an INR of 2 to 3. They were monitored for 2.3 $\pm$ 1.7 years. Groups were comparable in terms of age, gender, and cardiovascular risk factors. Percutaneous closure led to a lower risk of the combined end point of death, recurrent stroke, or TIA (8.5% vs. 24%; $P =$

.05; relative risk [RR] = 0.48; 95% CI: 0.23 to 1.01) Patients with more than one event at baseline and those with complete occlusion of the foramen ovale were at lower risk of recurrent stroke or TIA after percutaneous treatment compared with medical therapy (stroke, 7.3% vs. 33.2%; P = .01; 95% CI: 0.008 to 0.81; and TIA, 6.5% vs. 22%; P = .04; 95% CI: 0.14 to 0.99). With its inherent limitations, this study demonstrates an advantage of percutaneous treatment in high-risk patients (i.e., those with recurrent CVAs).

Percutaneous closure of a PFO in patients who experience a recurrent cerebrovascular event despite being on medical therapy carries a class IIB indication according to the American Heart Association guidelines on stroke prevention.[41] There are insufficient data to make any recommendations regarding PFO closure after a first stroke. The FDA had permitted the use of the Amplatzer and CardioSeal septal occluder device under humanitarian device exemption (HDE) only in patients who have experienced a recurrent cerebrovascular event while receiving conventional medical therapy (oral anticoagulation with a therapeutic INR). Currently, there are two ongoing prospective trials in the United States that are aimed at comparing medical treatment with percutaneous closure of PFO in patients with recurrent cryptogenic stroke. Both CLOSURE-1 (Evaluation of the STARFlex Septal Closure System in Patients with a Stroke or TIA due to the Possible Passage of Clot of Unknown Origin through a Patent Foramen Ovale), and RESPECT (Randomized Evaluation of recurrent Stroke comparing PFO closure to Established Current standard of care Treatment) have faced slow enrollment due to the initial widespread use of the HDE clause and placement of devices in an off-label application. It is strongly recommended that physicians refer patients for enrollment who may be eligible for the trial so that the appropriate questions may be answered. The HDE has been replaced with a registry for the patients who do not meet the criteria for the RESPECT trial (see later discussion).

Migraine Headache

Migraine headaches affect 12% of the population and generate significant morbidity and economic burden. The etiology of migraine headache with aura has remained elusive. People with migraine headaches have a twofold increased risk of experiencing a stroke, and the risk increases to 3.5-fold in patients younger than 35 years of age.[42] Observational studies have also revealed that patients who experience migraines have an increased frequency of silent deep white matter lesions.[43] These, and the growing information obtained from the evaluation of PFO and cryptogenic stroke, prompted researchers to assess the frequency of right-to-left shunt in migraineurs. Anzola and colleagues evaluated the presence of right-to-left shunt by transcranial Doppler ultrasonography in 113 patients with migraine with aura

and compared them to 53 patients with migraine without aura and 25 healthy age-matched controls. The presence of a PFO was significantly higher in migraineurs with aura than in the other two groups: 48%, 23%, and 20%, respectively.[44] Retrospective analyses of patients who underwent PFO closure for cryptogenic stroke have revealed an 80% decreased frequency of attacks of migraine with aura or even complete resolution in 56%.[45,46] However, these studies may have been influenced by recall bias; by the therapeutic effect of aspirin or clopidogrel, which may be used for migraine prophylaxis; by a high placebo effect; and by the fact that the frequency of migraine attacks decreases with age. In addition, retrospective studies do not demonstrate causal association. The high frequency of both PFO and migraine headache in the general population may favor a spurious association. Anzola and colleagues prospectively compared patients with a PFO and cryptogenic stroke who underwent PFO closure (n = 23) with patients who had migraines, peripheral embolic events, or TIA who underwent PFO closure (n = 27) and patients with migraines and PFOs who were treated medically (n = 27). After 12 months, the frequency and intensity of the migraine attacks were significantly decreased in patients who underwent PFO closure.[47]

The association between migraine headache with aura and PFO has generated a new hypothesis on the etiology of migraines. It is now postulated that migraines may be related to microembolic events or the presence of high concentrations of circulating vasoactive substances that are not filtered by the lung because they cross to the systemic circulation via the PFO. To test the association between PFO and migraine headaches with aura, the Evaluate Safety/Effectiveness of PFO Closure With the BioSTAR Septal Repair Implant to Resolve Refractory Migraine with Aura (MIST) trial was designed. Results have been presented but not yet published. The MIST trial was a multicenter, blinded study that randomized 432 patients with migraine to undergo either PFO closure with a STARFlex Septal Repair (NMT Medical, Boston, MA) implant or a sham procedure. The primary end point of cessation of migraines was not met. However, reduction in headache days by at least 50% occurred more frequently in the PFO closure group (42% vs. 23%; P = .038). The U.S.-based trials MIST II (NMT Medical, Boston, MA), PREMERE (St. Jude Medical, Fullerton, CA), and PREMIUM (AGA Medical, Golden Valley, MN) will have longer follow-up and will attempt to answer questions left unanswered on previous attempts. Until these results are available, PFO closure should not be considered for the treatment of migraine headache with aura.

Platypnea-Orthodeoxia and Hypoxia

PFO has also been associated with the rare platypnea-orthodeoxia syndrome. Platypnea refers to the feeling of dyspnea on achieving an upright posture, and orthodeoxia is arterial desaturation on standing. It is postulated that right-to-left shunting occurs across a PFO, particularly if ASA is present. This entity is seen primarily in the elderly and is associated with an event that alters the geometry of the intrathoracic organs, such as a pneumonectomy or an enlarged ascending aorta. Extrinsic compression of the right atrium or decreased compliance of the right ventricle may also predispose to shunting at the atrial level in these patients.[48] Although the mechanism is poorly understood, it is postulated that in patients with an enlarged aorta the heart is shifted laterally, so that the inferior vena cava drains directly toward the atrial septum. This anatomic shift maintains the PFO open throughout the cardiac cycle and generates the physical findings.[49] The diagnosis is made by saline contrast echocardiography in the supine and seated position.[11] Surgical and percutaneous closures have been done successfully with marked improvement in the patients' symptoms.[50,51]

Hypoxia related to a PFO may also be observed in patients with severe pulmonary hypertension. In these patients, the PFO serves as an escape valve that aids the emptying of the right atrium into a lower-pressure circuit (left atrium). In these patients, PFO closure may be fatal.

Decompression Sickness

Decompression sickness is caused by the presence of nitrogen bubbles that come out of solution in the blood as the ambient pressure decreases during ascension from a dive. The amount of nitrogen bubbles generated depends on the total time spent in the dive, the speed of ascent, compliance with decompression stops, and individual factors such as cardiac output. Generally, the nitrogen bubbles stay in the venous circulation and make it to the lungs, where they are rapidly diffused across the lungs. It has been postulated that, in the presence of a PFO, the nitrogen bubbles may enter the systemic circulation and travel superiorly toward the brain, occluding a small arterial branch. Decompression sickness is associated with early onset of cerebral or vestibular symptoms (within 30 minutes after a dive), despite performance of all appropriate rest stops.[52]

The association of PFOs and decompression sickness is relatively new. In a case-control study, Germonpre and coworkers noted a 2.25 odds risk in divers with PFO for development of decompression sickness.[53] In a small case-control study, patients with PFO had an increased odds ratio to develop decompression sickness and were more likely to have silent ischemic lesions in their brain by magnetic resonance imaging.[54] Torti and colleagues noted that divers with PFOs had a higher risk of developing decompression sickness, requiring treatment for decompression sickness, and having decompression sickness that lasted more than 24 hours.[55] Currently, it is unclear whether an invasive treatment such as percutaneous or surgical closure of PFOs may be indicated in these patients, because the avoidance of diving would prevent further recurrence.

Diagnosis

Echocardiography plays an important role in the diagnosis of abnormalities of the atrial septum. Traditionally, transesophageal echocardiography (TEE) has been considered the gold standard to diagnose PFO. It has the advantage of being able to identify all portions of the IAS, allowing for the diagnosis of all subtypes of ASD and fenestrated atrial septum, as well as PFO. TEE also allows the detailed identification of lipomatous hypertrophy of the septum, ASA, prominent eustachian valve, or a long PFO tunnel that may alter the planned closing procedure (see Fig. 48-3; Video 48-5). It also allows the identification of other potential sources of embolization. An ASA is defined as a redundancy of the atrial septum with excursion greater than 10 mm into either atria and a 15-mm base.

The degree and direction of the interatrial shunt depend on the net pressure difference between the atria. The direction of the interatrial shunt changes with the phase of respiration and the cardiac cycle. It can be documented by color Doppler interrogation of the IAS (Fig. 48-4). Color interrogation along the fossa ovalis may lead to erroneous identification of a PFO due to color cross-contamination when lowering the Nyquist limit. Its diagnostic sensitivity is significantly lower than that of a saline contrast study. The addition of saline contrast improves the diagnostic sensitivity of TEE.[56] The injection of saline contrast through the femoral vein has been shown to be superior for the diagnosis of PFO by TEE and for appropriate sizing of ASD.[57] Appropriate provocative measures that transiently increase the right atrial pressure (Valsalva maneuver) may be difficult to perform during a TEE because of the patient's sedation, relative hypovolemia due to fasting state, and inability to close the glottis against the echo probe, limiting its sensitivity (Fig. 48-5; Video 48-7).

Fundamental imaging with transthoracic echocardiography (TTE) has been considered inferior for the diagnosis of a PFO. However, the advent of second harmonic imaging has improved the sensitivity of TTE to 90%.[58] Easier and more effective performance of the provocative maneuver (no sedation, euvolemia, complete glottic closure) during TTE may improve image quality and is associated with a higher sensitivity than that of TEE for the diagnosis of a PFO.[59] In addition, the lack of invasiveness makes TTE a more attractive screening tool for PFO (Fig. 48-6; Video 48-6).

Transcranial Doppler ultrasonography also has a role in the detection and quantification of right-to-left shunt. Transcranial Doppler insonates the middle cerebral artery and detects the presence of high-intensity transient signals when agitated saline is injected through a vein. Its sensitivity is similar to that of TEE, but its major limitation is the inability to detect the origin of the shunt. The number of

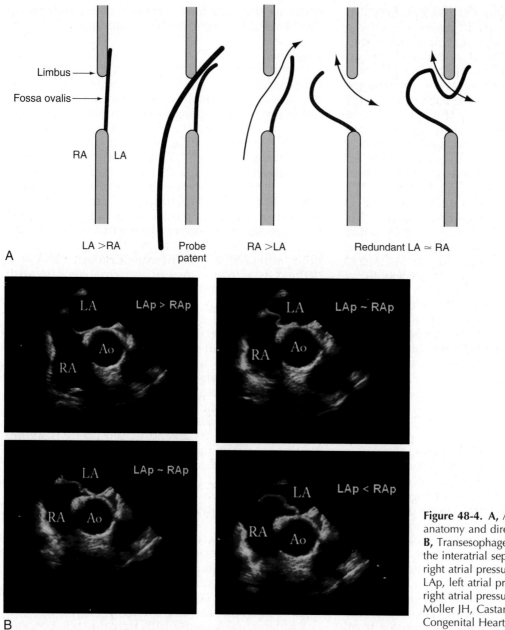

Figure 48-4. **A,** Association of interatrial septal anatomy and direction of interatrial shunt. **B,** Transesophageal echocardiogram depicting the interatrial septal mobility related to left and right atrial pressure. Ao, aorta; LA, left atrium; LAp, left atrial pressure; RA, right atrium; RAp, right atrial pressure. (Modified from Amplate K, Moller JH, Castaneda-Zuniga WR: Radiology of Congenital Heart Disease. St. Louis, Mosby–Year Book, 1993.)

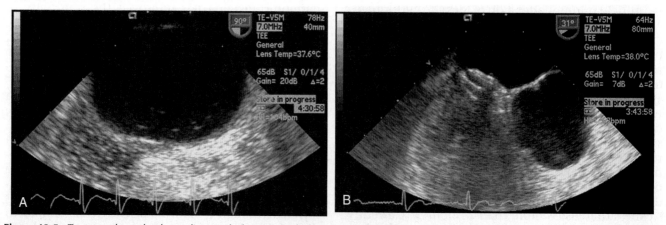

Figure 48-5. Transesophageal echocardiogram before **(A)** and after **(B)** placement of a 25-mm AGA Foramen Occluder. Saline contrast is present in the left atrium before device placement. After device placement, the saline contrast study is negative.

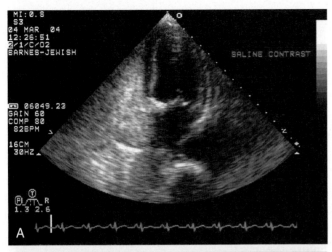

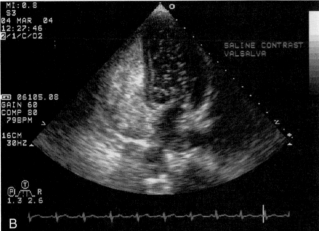

Figure 48-6. Transthoracic echocardiogram with a saline contrast study at rest **(A)** and during Valsalva maneuver **(B).** Transient increase in the right atrial pressure during the release phase of the Valsalva maneuver demonstrates a large right-to-left shunt at the atrial level secondary to a patent foramen ovale.

transient signals has been shown to correlate with PFO size and postprocedure PFO patency.[56,60]

Devices

Currently, two PFO septal occluder devices have been approved by the FDA for use in the United States under a registry and trial basis only: the Amplatzer PFO occluder (AGA Medical) and the STARFlex septal closure device (NMT Medical) for the treatment of recurrent paradoxical embolization in the presence of a therapeutic INR. The Premere PFO closure device by St. Jude Medical is currently under investigation for migraine treatment.

Amplatzer PFO Occluder

The Amplatzer PFO occluder is a self-expanding, double-disk device made from 0.005-inch nitinol wire with a polyester fabric sown into both disks (Fig. 48-7). There are three device sizes based on the right atrial disk diameter: 18, 25, and 35 mm. In contrast

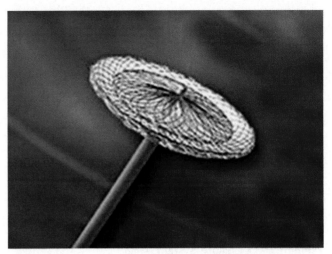

Figure 48-7. Frontal view of the AGA Amplatzer Foramen Occluder.

to the Atrial Septal Occluder, the stem is thin and mobile. The right atrial arm is larger than the left in the 25- and 35-mm sizes, whereas the two arms are equal in the 18-mm device. The right atrial disk appears to stabilize the device, preventing embolization from right to left. The thin stem allows a varying degree of disk mobility, which enables the PFO occluder to seat appropriately in a long tunnel or around a hypertrophied septum. The left atrial disk dimensions are designed to decrease interference with the pulmonary venous drainage or the mitral valve and to minimize the presence of thrombogenic material in the systemic circulation. Device sizing depends on the distance from the PFO to the superior vena cava and from the PFO to the aorta. The right disk radius should not exceed the shortest distance obtained (Table 48-2). The 25-mm device is used in the vast majority of the cases. The AGA Medical device has the advantage of being self-expanding, has a simple deployment, and is placed through a small venous sheath (8 Fr for 18 and 25 mm sizes, 9 Fr for the 35 mm size). It is fully retractable until it is released. Its major disadvantage is that it is bulky within the atrial septum.

STARFlex Septal Occluder

The STARFlex septal occluder is based on the Cardio-Seal device. The CardioSeal device has undergone

Table 48-2. Measurement for AGA PFO Occluder Device Selection

Distance from Defect to Superior Vena Cava or Aorta (mm)	Suggested Device Size (mm)	Delivery Sheath (Fr)
>17.5	35	9
12.5-17.4	25	8
9-12.4	18	8
<9	None	—

significant modifications owing to the presence of hinge rupture and device thrombosis in its original design. It is characterized by a self-centering mechanism made from a single nitinol microspring, which at-taches each arm to the two arms of the opposing umbrella (Fig. 48-8). The change in design decreases arm stress and improves the ability of the device to conform to the atrial septum. Available sizes are 23, 28, and 33 mm and are determined by PFO balloon sizing. The major advantage of the device is its low profile. Although modifications in the delivery system have been made, device retrieval can be cumbersome. Currently, it is available only through participation in the CLOSURE-1 trial.

Premere PFO Closure System

The Premere PFO Closure System is currently available to patients participating in the PFO/Migraine

trial sponsored by St. Jude Medical (Fig. 48-9). It has a very small profile and may be difficult to detect with echocardiography. Placement requires balloon sizing. Its unique design allows the operator to increase tension between the left and right atrial components by pulling a suture linking the two components together until locked, allowing it to conform to various tunnel lengths. Its major disadvantage is the requirement for larger venous sheaths (11 Fr) and the steps required for closure. The operator has to be extremely careful not to tighten excessively the knot that holds the two disks together, because the knot cannot be loosened, and excessively tightened knots may lead to device fracture or malposition.

Future Devices

The next generation of devices will be aimed at reducing the material that persists within the atria after

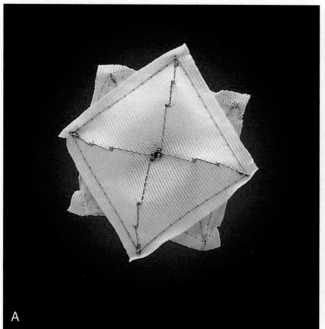

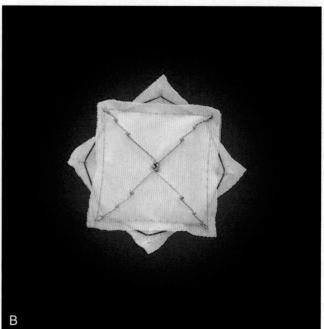

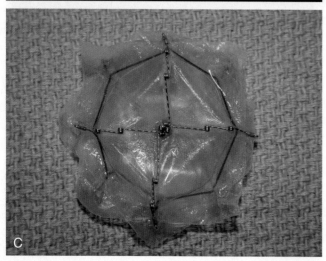

Figure 48-8. Photographs of the CardioSeal (A), STARFlex (B), and BioSTAR (C) septal occluders. (Courtesy of NMT Medical.)

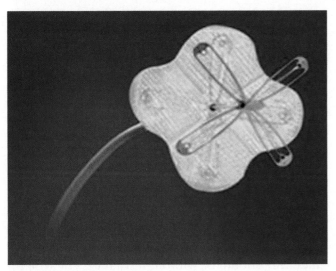

Figure 48-9. Photograph of the St. Jude Premere PFO occluding system. (Courtesy of St. Jude Medical.)

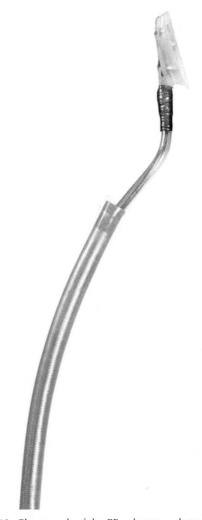

Figure 48-10. Photograph of the PFx closure catheter with radiofrequency ablation. (Courtesy of Cierra Inc.)

closure. Initial trials using a bioabsorbable device, BioSTAR by NMT Medical, are underway (see Fig. 48-8). Alternative methods of closure are also being developed and include suture closure (Sutura [Sutura, Fountain Valley, CA)]) and tissue cauterization with radiofrequency (CoAptus RF [CoAptus Medical Redmond, WA] and PFx [Cierra Redwood City, CA]) (Fig. 48-10); these are expected to be available for research protocols soon. The Helex device (WL Gore and Associates, Flagstaff, AZ) is currently available in Europe and will become available in the United States in the future (Fig. 48-11).

Indications for Closure

There is no indication for PFO closure for primary prevention of a cryptogenic stroke. The American Heart Association and American Academy of Neurology guidelines identify PFO closure after one CVA as a class IIB indication.[42] Currently, PFO closure for cryptogenic stroke is approved for patients who experience recurrent strokes presumed to be paradoxical in nature for whom conventional drug therapy has failed. Conventional drug therapy implies a therapeutic INR achieved with oral anticoagulation.[61] The HDE label is based on demonstration of device safety, not on proven stroke prevention. The only PFO closure devices approved by the FDA under HDE were the CardioSeal Septal Occlusion System and the Amplatzer PFO Occluder. HDE expired for both devices on October 31, 2006. Since that time, PFO closures may be performed only in patients enrolled in ongoing research protocols or registries.

Currently, there is no indication for PFO closure in patients who have migraine with aura and PFO. There are three ongoing trials in the United States (PREMERE, MIST II, and PREMIUM) that are evaluating the efficacy of PFO closure for the treatment of migraines, with many more to follow. Physicians caring for patients who have these findings are

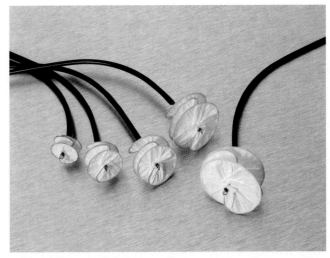

Figure 48-11. Photograph of the Helex septal occluder. (Courtesy of Gore Medical.)

urged to refer them to the study enrollment centers in order to obtain the necessary information to answer whether PFO closure will be part of the therapeutic armamentarium.

Percutaneous treatment for refractory hypoxemia related to right-to-left shunting across a PFO is still available under the HDE.

Technique

Percutaneous closure of PFO is done in the cardiac catheterization laboratory. It is performed under ultrasonographic (TEE or intracardiac echocardiography [ICE]) and fluoroscopic guidance and requires familiarity of the operator with both types of images. Ideally, patients scheduled for PFO closure have the diagnosis confirmed before they arrive at the catheterization laboratory. The general principles described here relate to the procedure as performed in the Cardiac Procedure Center at Barnes Jewish Hospital and focus primarily on the AGA PFO Occluder.

The procedure begins with an explanation to the patient of the risks and benefits of the procedure and obtaining the patient's consent to treatment.

Infection Prophylaxis

PFO occluder devices require the placement of prosthetic material in the IAS. To decrease the risk of prosthetic infection, activities to reduce infection risk are followed. Patients are given intravenous antibiotics (cefazolin or vancomycin) on call to the catheterization laboratory. Indwelling urinary catheters are not recommended, to avoid transient bacteremia or nidus for infection.

Venous Access

Femoral venous access is obtained with an 8 Fr sheath. If intracardiac echocardiography is planned, a second short sheath (9 Fr) is placed in the femoral vein.

Diagnostic Study

A right heart catheterization with oximetry may be performed with determination of the pulmonary artery and pulmonary capillary wedge pressure, although its completion is not critical for the procedure in otherwise healthy young patients with no other contraindications or pulmonary disease.

Crossing the Interatrial Septum

An end-hole multipurpose catheter (MPA) is advanced over a stiff 0.035- or 0.038-inch 1.5-mm "J" tipped guide wire (Amplatzer wire). On arrival at the junction of the right atrium and inferior vena cava, the wire is advanced toward the IAS at the level of the aortic valve. The catheter may be advanced or rotated medially to direct the wire across the PFO. If the guide wire does not cross easily, a Judkins right coronary catheter may be used instead. If the wire still cannot be threaded through the PFO, a hydrophilic coated wire (Glidewire, Terumo Medical Corporation, Tokyo, Japan) may be used to negotiate through the tunnel. If crossing has not been accomplished after a significant amount of time or effort, it is important to confirm or refute the diagnosis of a PFO by repeating a bubble study from the femoral vein. If significant passage of contrast material is seen, one may consider performing a septal puncture and closing the opening of the PFO with a device instead of inserting the device through the tunnel itself.

Once in the left atria, the guide wire is advanced to the proximal portion of the left upper pulmonary vein. It important to remember that passage of the guide wire should be without resistance. The wire tip should be kept in the proximal portion of the pulmonary vein, to avoid perforation of the left atrium or stimulation of a cough reflex. Placing the guide wire in the left atrial appendage is not recommended, because it may lead to perforation. Incorrect location of the wire may be recognized by visualizing the wire coiling within the cardiac silhouette or by the presence of premature atrial depolarizations.

Anticoagulation

Once the guide wire is across the PFO, systemic anticoagulation with heparin to yield an activated clotting time greater that 200 seconds is initiated by administering 30 units of heparin per kilogram of body weight.

Device Selection

Echocardiographic measurements are made to aid in device selection (see Table 48-2). Some operators prefer to measure the PFO diameter with a sizing balloon in order to select the appropriate device (as with the St Jude and CardioSeal devices) or identify a long PFO tunnel. Balloon inflation must be done carefully to avoid tearing of the septum primum. With the use of the Amplatzer PFO occluder, more than 95% of the cases are done using the 25-mm device.

Delivery Sheath Insertion and Device Preparation

Once the device is selected, the short sheath is removed and replaced with a long delivery sheath. The sheath is advanced until the dilator has crossed the IAS. At this time, the dilator is separated and the sheath is advanced slowly into the middle of the left atrium. The dilator and the guide wire are removed, and the sheath connected to the manifold.

The occluder devices are loaded, following the individual instructions. Usually, devices are attached to their delivery cable and then retracted into the delivery catheter. Special care must be placed on flushing the delivery catheter and device aggressively, in order to remove all air bubbles from the device and system. Once flushed, the delivery catheter is introduced into the delivery sheath.

Device Positioning and Release

The device is pushed through the delivery sheath under fluoroscopic guidance, noting the presence of any air bubbles. If air bubbles are present, the device is removed and reprepared while the sheath is allowed to bleed back. Once the device reaches the tip of the delivery sheath, the sheath is withdrawn slowly until the entire left atrial disk is exposed. Echocardiographic confirmation of left disk deployment is required to ensure that the left atrial disk is not in the PFO tunnel. Once the disk is exposed, traction is applied on both the device and the delivery sheath to ensure that the left atrial disk abuts the atrial septum. With the left disk in place, the delivery sheath is withdrawn until the right atrial disk is expanded. As this is confirmed by fluoroscopy and echocardiography, the device is "wiggled" back and forth to ensure appropriate seating (Fig. 48-12). Echocardiographic evaluation of the pulmonary veins, mitral valve, and coronary sinus is then done to avoid device obstruction with these structures. It is normal to see color flow across the center, but not around the Amplatzer PFO occluder device, while it is newly placed and anticoagulation has been started.

If no obstruction exists, the device appears to be properly in place, and it is fully expanded, then release can done according to the manufacturer's recommendations. It is important to retract the delivery cable back into the delivery sheath, to avoid cardiac perforation. After the device is released, its conformation changes slightly. A saline contrast study is then done to assess shunt severity (Video 48-8). Usually, the shunt is absent or at least significantly decreased after the device is released. The bubble study becomes progressively negative as the device reaches its normal conformation and becomes endothelialized (Videos 48-9 through 48-11).

Hemostasis

The venous sheaths are removed once the activated clotting time (ACT) has dropped to a safe level. Bed rest should follow, depending on the size of the sheath placed.

Postprocedure Care

Our preference is to hospitalize patients overnight in a telemetry unit and to administer two more doses of antibiotics. Chest radiography to ensure device position is done the following day. A TTE with bubble study to quantify residual shunt is done 24 hours after the procedure and again in 6 months. Patients are prescribed 75 mg of clopidogrel daily for 1 month, and daily aspirin for 6 months. Standard subacute bacterial endocarditis precautions should be followed for 6 months.

Special Considerations

Transseptal Puncture

Transseptal puncture is only rarely required to close a PFO. It is favored in two instances: (1) when the PFO tunnel is long and passage with a guide wire or

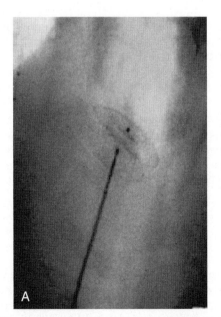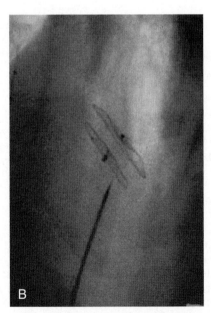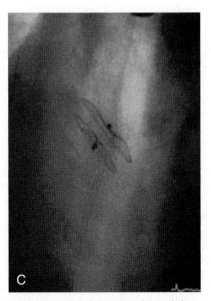

Figure 48-12. Deployment of an AGA septal occluder. **A,** Once in place, the device is "wiggled" to ensure stability. **B,** After stability is confirmed, the device is released by rotating the delivery cable. **C,** Once released, the cable is withdrawn into the delivery sheath to avoid trauma.

delivery sheath is unsuccessful, and (2) when the inferior border of an appropriately measured device interferes with the mitral valve. Some authors favor transseptal puncture when an ASA is encountered, in order to completely grasp it.

Multiple Shunts

If an ASD is seen in association with a PFO, a single septal occluder may be used to minimize the shunt. If there is persistent shunting, then a second device may be placed as long as there is no interaction with the mitral valve or pulmonary veins.

Atrial Septal Aneurysms

The presence of an ASA usually does not necessitate the use of a larger device. Closure of such PFOs is just as successful with a standard technique at 6 months (see Fig. 48-3).[62]

Complications

Percutaneous closure of PFO is a safe procedure. Procedural complications occur in 4% to 7% of cases but are usually mild.[40,63,64] A procedural learning curve and significant device modifications have transformed PFO closure into an effective and safe procedure. Periprocedural complications include air embolism, device migration, cardiac rupture and device erosion, vascular complications, and periprocedural atrial arrhythmias. Complications occurring after discharge include endocarditis, device fracture, and device thrombosis.

Procedure-Related Complications

Air embolus is a potentially devastating complication that is easily recognized and avoided. Air embolus is caused by air entering the delivery sheath as the dilator is removed or during its preparation. It may also be associated with incomplete flushing of the device while introducing it to the delivery catheter or delivery sheath. Air bubbles in the delivery catheter are easily recognized as the device is being pushed through the delivery sheath if done under fluoroscopy. Air embolism can manifest as sudden onset of hypotension, heart block, ventricular tachycardia, inferior ST-segment elevation, and transient neurologic decline.

If air is seen within the delivery sheath, it is important to remove the device slowly in order to reduce the ensuing vacuum, and let the delivery sheath bleed back. If the air bubble has entered the circulation, hypotension or ensuing arrhythmias should be treated with standard Advanced Cardiac Life Support (ACLS) protocol. Supplemental oxygen may influence bubble resolution. Placement of the patient in the Trendelenburg position may decrease the risk of cerebral embolization. Transfer to a hypobaric chamber may be considered if warranted.

Device-Related Complications

Device migration is characterized by loss of the correct position of the device. It may be related to incomplete device exit from the tunnel or to placement of a smaller device in a large PFO or unrecognized ASD. If migration occurs, devices may be removed percutaneously with a snare. If this cannot be done, surgical removal is recommended.

Device arm fracture was seen primarily with the earlier generation of the PFO STAR device, but now it is rarely encountered owing to improved devices.

Although *device erosion* is not seen with PFOs, recent data support that it does occur in patients with closures of large ASDs that lack an appropriate aortic rim of tissue.

Device thrombosis has been seen in patients with concomitant hypercoagulable states who undergo PFO closure. It was also seen in up to 2% of the patients with PFO STAR devices, but newer generations of the device have addressed this limitation.[40] The presence of device thrombus is an indication for surgical removal. It is recommended that every patient who undergoes PFO closure for paradoxical embolization have a workup for hypercoagulable state. If the workup is positive, therapeutic anticoagulation is warranted. There have been no published instances of thrombus detection associated with AGA PFO closure devices.

Transient Arrhythmias

Spontaneous atrial arrhythmias may be observed in the first 6 weeks after treatment and do not usually require treatment.

Nickel Allergy

Brief case reports have noted an increase in headaches after device closure in a patient allergic to nickel. Although allergy is difficult to prove, nickel desensitization should be performed before elective PFO closure.

Endocarditis

Bacterial device infection or colonization can be catastrophic. Strict sterile technique should be followed throughout the procedure, and antibiotic prophylaxis for subacute bacterial endocarditis should be continued for 6 months. Surgical excision is warranted if endocarditis ensues.

Conclusions

Percutaneous closure of PFO is an amenable procedure. Its future will depend on the generation of data that supports its use. Interventional cardiologists should counsel their patients and referring physicians about ongoing trials and registries that will generate the required information to determine who benefits most from PFO closure and under what circumstances is it indicated. Once these questions are answered, this procedure has the potential to benefit a large number of people.

ATRIAL SEPTAL DEFECT

Among the various congenital cardiac anomalies encountered in the adult population, ASD is one of the most commonly seen and most easily treated, with excellent long-term prognosis. Less than a decade ago, surgical repair was considered the standard of care and provided durable long-term results. Since the FDA approved devices for percutaneous ASD closure in December of 2001, there has been a dramatic shift toward catheter-based closure of ASD, which not only provides durable results paralleling those of surgical techniques, but does so with remarkably less morbidity and extremely short recovery time and hospitalization. Both patients and physicians prefer the less invasive percutaneous approach, although no studies to date have directly compared the efficacy and safety of surgical and percutaneous techniques.

The preceding section provided an in-depth discussion of the embryology, physiology, clinical pathophysiology, diagnosis, and catheter-based management of PFO. Because there is a considerable overlap between PFO and ASD, the following discussion highlights the salient characteristics that are specific to ASD.

Embryology

In distinction to a PFO, an ASD occurs when there is absence of a portion of the IAS. Incomplete caudal growth of the septum secundum or excessive resorption of the septum primum give rise to a *secundum ASD*. If the septum primum fails to reach the endocardial cushions, then a *primum ASD* occurs, with its associated abnormalities of cleft mitral valve and inlet ventricular septal defect. A sinus venosus ASD occurs when there is abnormal resorption of atrial septal tissue adjacent to the caval-atrial junction. An "unroofed" coronary sinus or absence of atrial tissue adjacent to the site of coronary sinus drainage into the right atrium results in a coronary sinus ASD (see Table 48-1).[65]

Anatomic and Morphologic Considerations

The secundum ASD is located at the center of the atrial septum involving the fossa ovalis. This is a true tissue defect, in contrast to a PFO. To permit percutaneous closure, there should be adequate tissue margins at the superior and inferior rims of the defect for secure snapping of the closure device to the tissue. Lack of adequate tissue margin predisposes to device prolapse or potential embolization. Furthermore, large defects also predispose to encroachment of the device on the adjacent aortic root and mitral valve, which can result in major complications. Needless to say, real-time assessment of the atrial septum using TEE or ICE is a prerequisite for optimal closure. The choice of imaging depends on operator experience and preferences (Fig. 48-13).

The sinus venosus type of defect is located in the perimeter of the atrial septum, near the entry of the superior vena cava. This defect prevents the normal separation of the pulmonary veins from the right lung and the superior vena cava and right atrium, as a result of which there is anomalous drainage of one or more pulmonary veins.[66] Defects located close to the inferior vena cava are very rare and are termed caval defects; they also can be associated with anomalous pulmonary venous drainage. Ostium primum ASDs, also known as endocardial cushion defects or common atrioventricular canal defects, are accompanied by ventricular septal defects and cleft mitral valve. With the exception of secundum defects, management of other types of ASD requires surgical repair and is not discussed here.

Clinical Presentation

Usually, patients with ASD remain asymptomatic during their childhood. Typically, the pulmonary outflow murmur or a fixed split of the second heart sound detected during a routine physical examination prompts further evaluation, which finally results in the diagnosis. Some may experience recurrent heart failure, predilection for recurrent respiratory infections during childhood, or easy fatigability and exertional dyspnea.[67] In adults, long-standing ASD with significant shunt may manifest with atrial arrhythmias, pulmonary arterial hypertension, and heart failure.

Hemodynamics

The direction and magnitude of the shunt across an ASD depends on the size of the defect, the right and left atrial pressures, right and left ventricular compliance and end-diastolic pressures, vascular resistance in the pulmonary and systemic circuits, the phase of respiration, the intrathoracic pressure, and the intravascular volume status.[68] In most patients who present with moderate to large ASDs, the atria are in open communication, and the mean atrial pressure is equal. But the shunt is directed left to right, because the right ventricle and pulmonary circuit offer lower resistance to the flow. However, in those patients with a very small ASD without equalization of atrial pressures, the gradient across the atria will also play a role in the direction of shunt.

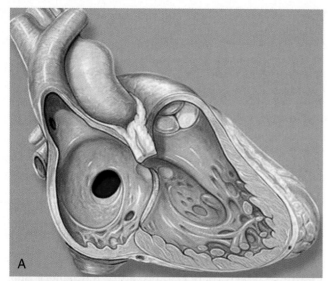

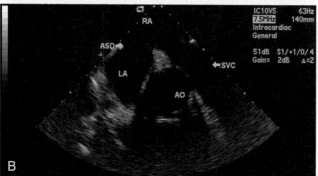

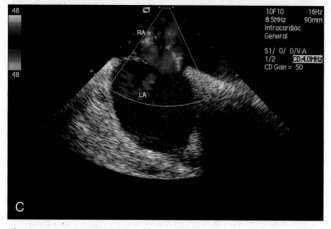

Figure 48-13. A, Diagram of secundum atrial septal defect (ASD). **B,** ASD as seen by intracardiac echocardiogram. **C,** With color Doppler interrogation, a left-to-right shunt is identified. (Courtesy of Patrick J. Lynch, Yale University ITS Web Services, New Haven, CT.)

A close review of the Doppler ultrasonographic study performed across the defect shows that the flow is present during the entire cardiac cycle. Left-to-right shunting occurs mostly during late systole and early diastole, but atrial contraction also provides additional flow augmentation. The shunt results in diastolic overloading of the right ventricle and increased pulmonary blood flow. Depending on the size of the defect, pulmonary blood flow may be as high as five times the systemic flow. In those with

long-standing and untreated ASD, pulmonary hypertension ensues, which may reach suprasystemic levels, reversing the shunt's direction. It should be noted that, even in a uncomplicated ASD, a transient and small right-to-left shunt occurs during the early phase of ventricular systole and is further accentuated by respiration that decreases intrathoracic pressure. This is the rationale behind performing a saline contrast study during echocardiography for detection of the ASD (Video 48-12).

Diagnosis

As noted earlier, physical examination findings usually initiate the evaluation for suspected ASD. This includes a hyperdynamic precordium, a fixed split of the second heart sound without respiratory variation, a loud pulmonic component of the second heart sound, and pulmonary outflow tract murmur. Primum-type defects have associated tricuspid and mitral regurgitation murmurs. Electrocardiography further supports the clinical findings. Right-axis deviation, right ventricular hypertrophy, and rSR'or rsR pattern in the right precordial leads with normal QRS duration are common electrocardiographic findings in ostium secundum defects. Inverted P wave in lead III is seen in sinus venosus defects, whereas left-axis deviation may denote ostium primum defect. Lengthening of the P-R interval secondary to atrial enlargement and conduction delay can be seen in all three types of ASD.[69] Chest radiographic findings include right atrial and ventricular enlargement, prominent pulmonary artery, and increased pulmonary vascular markings.

Echocardiography

Echocardiography has essentially replaced cardiac catheterization techniques for diagnosis of ASD.[70,71] Even the shunt fraction can be reliably calculated using echocardiography. A TTE with saline contrast study should be done first. The defect may be visualized directly by TTE imaging, particularly from a subcostal view of the IAS, but TEE provides much better anatomic characterization of the septum and the adjoining structures.[72,73] Typical echocardiographic findings include right atrial and right ventricular enlargement, increased pulmonary artery pressures, and continuous flow across the atrial septum as documented by Doppler ultrasound.[74] Recently, three-dimensional echocardiography with image reconstruction has been used to plan closure procedural details. ICE can also be used, but its use is mostly restricted to providing imaging guidance for percutaneous closure (see Fig. 48-13).

Cardiac Catheterization

In current clinical practice, use of cardiac catheterization primarily for diagnostic purposes is uncommon but is reserved for when there is discrepancy between clinical and echocardiographic findings. In general, invasive hemodynamic assessment (cardiac catheterization) is performed during a planned percutaneous closure. The presence of a defect in the atrial septum is usually obvious when the guide wire or catheter crosses the midline (atrial septum) into the left atrium. The site at which the catheter crosses provides diagnostic clues for the type of defect. Secundum defects are midseptal, whereas in sinus venosus defects the catheter crosses the IAS at a high level, and in primum defects it crosses at a low level. Angiography (left atrial injection) further demonstrates the presence of shunt and other associated anomalies.[75] An oximetry run and assessment of cardiac output help in estimating the size of the shunt and locating the defect.

Indication for Closure

In clinically stable patients without contraindications for surgery, a pulmonary-to-systemic shunt with flow ratios greater than 1.5 : 1 is widely accepted as an indication for repair. The same criterion holds true for percutaneous closure. However, of late many patients with smaller ASDs (flow ratios <1.5 : 1) are referred for percutaneous closure in the setting of paradoxical embolic manifestations, given the substantially lower morbidity associated with percutaneous technique. Closure, either surgical or percutaneous, is contraindicated in those patients with a pulmonary-to-systemic shunt ratio as low as 0.7 : 1, which signifies severe pulmonary vascular disease.[76]

Devices for Percutaneous Closure of a Secundum Atrial Septal Defect

Percutaneous closure of ASD has proved to be reliable, safe, and effective based on recent available data, but selection of defects with appropriate anatomic characteristics is critical for successful closure. At the present time, only two devices are approved by the FDA for percutaneous closure of ASD, although at least four devices are actively being investigated.[77] Both of the approved devices, the Amplatzer Septal Occluder and the CardioSeal Septal Occlusion System, are in use. The choice of device is dictated by operator experience and preference. A newly revised version of the CardioSeal device, marketed as the STARFlex device in Europe, may be obtained by requesting HDE status from the FDA.

Amplatzer Occlusion Device

The Amplatzer Septal Occluder (AGA Medical) is a self-expandable, double-disk device made from a nitinol wire mesh. The two disks are linked together by a connecting waist, which corresponds to the size of the ASD. To increase its closing ability, the disks and the waist are filled with polyester fabric. The polyester fabric is securely sewn to each disk by a polyester thread. The device is available in various sizes, ranging from 4 to 38 mm (4 to 20 mm at 1-mm increments, 22 to 38 mm at 2-mm increments), and the size refers to the diameter of the waist. Device selection is based on the stretched diameter of the defect (e.g., a 10-mm stretched defect requires a 10-mm device). Devices are generally oversized by 1 mm to ensure an appropriate fit. In distinction to the PFO occluder, the left atrial disk is larger than the right atrial disk. The reported success rate of these devices in closing ASDs is as high as 98%.[78,79] Our own experience using Amplatzer devices is similar. Patient selection and optimal imaging are key to success. Multiple ASDs may be closed with more than one device (Fig. 48-14). Modifications to the basic technique may be used to close very large ASDs (i.e., backstop technique). The proposed advantages of the Amplatzer device include ease of use, ability to deliver using smaller-diameter catheters, and ability to retrieve and reposition the device before complete deployment. Furthermore, the device design permits it to self-center across the defect.

CardioSeal Device

The CardioSeal device has a unique design wherein two self-expanding umbrellas adhere to the atrial septum by spring tension. These umbrellas range in size from 17 to 40 mm. There are four metal arms, attached to each other in the center, that are covered by Dacron patches. Each arm is hinged and spreads from the center of the device to support each umbrella. The hinges are designed to relieve stress during cardiac contraction. Because of the number of device failures, device arm fractures (14%), and pro-

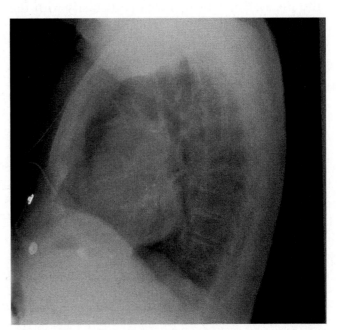

Figure 48-14. Chest radiograph after deployment of two AGA septal occluders.

trusions of one arm through the defect (32%), the original design was revised and an updated version, the STARFlex, is currently being marketed in Europe.[80] The new device sports a self-centering mechanism comprising nitinol springs that join the two umbrellas and a flexible core wire with a pin-pivoting connection. The modified device has been reported to have a lower incidence of arm fractures.[81]

Procedural Details

Patients should be adequately anticoagulated with unfractionated heparin during the entire procedure, and the ACT should be maintained above 200 seconds before device placement. Typically, femoral venous access is used, and the size of the sheath is based on the size of the device and delivery sheath system. A 0.035- or 0.038-inch "J"-tipped guide wire over a 6 Fr multipurpose catheter serves as the best tool to cross the defect. Sizing of the defect is very important for appropriate selection of the occlusion device. The ASD diameter is measured with a balloon specifically designed for sizing atrial communications, such as the Amplatzer Sizing Balloon. Under fluoroscopic and echocardiographic guidance, the balloon catheter is placed across the defect and inflated with diluted contrast medium until the left-to-right shunt ceases, as observed by echocardiography. The maximum stretched diameter of the balloon waist, while occluding flow across the IAS, is measured. Alternatively, determination of the balloon can be established using echocardiographic measurements. Subsequently, the device is deployed under direct fluoroscopic guidance (see Fig. 48-12 and Videos 48-9 through 48-11). The various steps involved in device deployment are summarized in Figure 48-12. Meticulous attention should be paid to avoid suction of air into the system, which is seen particularly with the use of large-caliber delivery sheaths.

Complications

Complications associated with transcatheter closure of a secundum ASD are similar to those associated with PFO closure, discussed earlier. In addition, there are reports of Amplatzer devices' predisposing to erosion of the atrial wall and rupture.[82]

Future Devices

Future devices currently being investigated include the button device, which includes a foam occluder from the left atrium and a counteroccluder from the right atrium[83]; a helix device; angel wings, a self-centering, double-disk device consisting of two square frames made of superelastic nitinol wire and covered by a polyester tissue, each frame with eight eyelets, four in the corners and four at the midpoint of each leg, that function as torsion springs[84]; and the ASD occlusion system (ASDOS),[85] which consists of two self-opening, five-armed umbrellas made of nitinol wire and a thin membrane of polyurethane.

Conclusions

Percutaneous closure of secundum ASDs has changed our approach to structural heart disease. Future improvements in percutaneous technology may provide tools to tackle the other types of ASDs. Percutaneous noncoronary interventions are the new frontier for interventional cardiology.

REFERENCES

1. Moore KL, Persaud TUN: The Developing Human: Clinically Oriented Embryology, 6th ed. Philadelphia, WB Saunders, 1998, pp 349-362.
2. Meissner I, Whissant JP, Khandheria BK, et al: Prevalence of potential risk factors for stroke assessed by TEE and carotid ultrasonography: The SPARC Study. Stroke Prevention Assessment of Risk in a Community. Mayo Clin Proc 1999; 74:862-869.
3. Thompson T, Evans W: Paradoxical embolism. Q J Med 1930;23:135-152.
4. Wu LA, Malouf JF, Dearani JA, et al: Patent foramen ovale in cryptogenic stroke: Current understanding and management options. Arch Intern Med 2004;164:950-956.
5. Germonpre P, Hastir F, Dendale P, et al: Evidence for increasing patency of foramen ovale in divers. Am J Cardiol 2005;95:912-915.
6. Rodriguez CJ, Homma S, Sacco RL, et al: Race-ethnic differences in patent foramen ovale, atrial septal aneurysm, and right atrial anatomy among ischemic stroke patients. Stroke 2003;34:2097-2102.
7. Cohnheim J: Thrombose und Embolie: Vorlesung über allgemeine Pathologie. Berlin, 1877, p 134.
8. Lechat PH, Mas MD, Lascault G, et al: Prevalence of patent foramen ovale in patients with stroke. N Eng J Med 1988;318:1148-1152.
9. Di Tullio M, Sacco RL, Gopal A, et al: Patent foramen ovale as a risk factor for cryptogenic stroke. Ann Intern Med 1992;117:461-465.
10. Seward JB, Hayes DL, Smith HC, et al: Platypnea orthodeoxia: Clinical profile, diagnostic work up, management, and report of seven cases. Mayo Clin Proc 1984;59:221-231.
11. Godart F, Rey C, Prat A, et al: Atrial right to left shunting causing severe hypoxemia despite normal right sided pressures. Eur Heart J 2000;21:483-489.
12. Bason R, Yacavone D: Decompression sickness: US Navy altitude chamber experience 1 October 1981 to 30 September 1988. Aviat Space Environ Med 1991;62:1180-1184.
13. Scherzmann M, Wiher S, Nedeltchev K, et al: Percutaneous closure of patent foramen ovale reduces the frequency of migraine attacks. Neurology 2004;62:1399-1401.
14. Overell JR, Bone I, Lees KR: Interatrial septal abnormalities and stroke: A meta-analysis of case control studies. Neurology 2000;55:1172-1179.
15. Lamy C, Giannesini C, Zuber M, et al: Clinical and imaging findings in cryptogenic stroke patients with and without patent foramen ovale. The PFO-ASA study. Stroke 2002; 33:706-711.
16. Berthet K, Lavergne T, Cohen A, et al: Significant association of atrial vulnerability with atrial septal abnormalities in young patients with ischemic stroke of unknown cause. Stroke 2000;31:298-403.
17. Thanigaraj S, Zajarias A, Lasala J, Perez J: Caught in the act: Serial real time images of a thrombus traversing from the right to left atrium across a patent foramen ovale. Eur J Echo 2006;7:179-181.
18. Sacco RL, Ellenberg JH, Mohr JP, et al: Infarcts of undetermined cause: The NINCDS Stroke Data Bank. Ann Neurol 1989;25:382-390.

19. Cramer SC: Patent foramen ovale and its relationship to stroke. Cardiol Clin 2005;23:7-11.
20. Cramer SC, Rordorf G, Maki JH, et al: Increased pelvic vein thrombi in cryptogenic stroke: Results of the Paradoxical Emboli from Large Veins in Ischemic Stroke (PELVIS) study. Stroke 2004;35:46-50.
21. Konstantinides S, Geibel A, Kapser W, et al: Patent foramen ovale is an important predictor of adverse outcome in patients with major pulmonary embolism. Circulation 1998;97:1946-1951.
22. Petty GW, Mayo K, Khandreia B, et al: Population based study of the relationship between patent foramen ovale and cerebrovascular ischemic events. Mayo Clin Proc 2006;81:602-608.
23. Meissner I, Khandeira B, Heit JA, et al: Patent foramen ovale: Innocent or guilty? J Am Coll Cardiol 2006;47:440-445.
24. Di Tullio MR, Sacco R, Sciacca RR, et al: Patent foramen ovale and risk of ischemic stroke in a community: The northern Manhattan study [abstract]. Stroke 2003;34.
25. Mas JL, Zuber M: Recurrent cerebrovascular events in patients with patent foramen ovale, atrial septal aneurysm or both and cryptogenic stroke or transient ischemic attack. Am Heart J 1995;130:1083-1088.
26. De Castro S, Cartón D, Fiorelli M, et al: Morphological and functional characteristics of patent foramen ovale and their embolic complications. Stroke 2000;31:2407-2413.
27. Cabanes L, Mas JL, Cohen A, et al: Atrial septal aneurysm and patent foramen ovale as risk factors for cryptogenic stroke in patients less than 55 years of age. Stroke 1993;24:1865-1873.
28. Natanzon A, Goldman ME: Patent foramen ovale: Anatomy versus pathophysiology—Which determines stroke risk? J Am Soc Echo 2003;16:71-76.
29. Homma S, Di Tullio MR, Sacco RL, et al: Characteristics of patent foramen ovale associated with cryptogenic stroke: A biplane transesophageal echocardiographic study. Stroke 1994;25:582-586.
30. Schuchlenz HW, Saurer G, Wehis W, Rehak P: Persisting eustachian valve in adults: Relation to patent foramen ovale and cerebrovascular events. J Am Soc Echocardiogr 2004;17:231-233.
31. Mas JL, Aruquizan C, Lamy C, et al: Recurrent cerebrovascular events associated with patent foramen ovale, atrial septal aneurysm or both. N Engl J Med 2001;345:1740-1746.
32. Homma S, Sacco RL, Di Tullio M, et al: Effect of medical therapy in stroke patients with patent foramen ovale: Patent Foramen Ovale in Cryptogenic Stroke Study. Circulation 2002;105:2625-2631.
33. Bogousslavsky J, Garazi S, Jeanrenaud X, et al: Stroke recurrence in patients with patent foramen ovale. Neurology 1996;46:1301-1305.
34. Khairy P, O'Donnell CP, Landzberg MJ: Transcatheter closure versus medical therapy of patent foramen ovale and presumed paradoxical emboli. Ann Intern Med 2003;139:753-760.
35. Messe SR, Silverman IE, Kizer JR, et al: Practice parameter: Recurrent stroke with patent foramen ovale and atrial septal aneurysm. Report of the quality standards subcommittee of the American Academy of Neurology. Neurology 2004;62:1042-1050.
36. Dearani JA, Ugurlu BS, Danielson GK, et al: Surgical patent foramen ovale closure for prevention of paradoxical embolism-related cerebrovascular ischemic events. Circulation 1999;100:II171-II175.
37. Windeker S, Wahl A, Chatterjee T, et al: Percutaneous closure of patent foramen ovale in patients with paradoxical embolism: Long term risk of recurrent thromboembolic events. Circulation 2000;101:893-898.
38. Wahl A, Meier B, Haxel B, et al: Prognosis after percutaneous closure of patent foramen ovale for paradoxical embolism. Neurology 2001;57:1330-1332.
39. Braun M, Fassbender D, Schoen S, et al: Transcatheter closure of patent foramen ovale in patients with cerebral ischemia. J Am Coll Cardiol 2002;39:2019-2025.
40. Windeker S, Wahl A, Nedeltchev K: Comparison of medical treatment with percutaneous closure of patent foramen ovale in patients with cryptogenic stroke. J Am Coll Cardiol 2004;44:750-758.
41. Sacco RL, Adams R, Albers G, et al: Guidelines for the prevention of stroke in patients with ischemic stroke or transient ischemic attack: A statement for healthcare professionals from the American Heart Association/American Stroke Association Council on Stroke. Co-sponsored by the Council on Cardiovascular Radiology and Intervention. The American Academy of Neurology affirms the value of this guideline. Stroke 2006;37:577-617.
42. Piechowski-Jozwiack A, Devuyst G, Bogousslavsky J: Migraine and patent foramen ovale: A residual coincidence or pathophysiological intrigue. Cerebrovasc Dis 2006;22:91-100.
43. Kruit MC, van Buchen MA, Hofman PA, et al: Migraine as a risk factor for subclinical brain lesions. JAMA 2004;291:427-434.
44. Anzola GP, Majuni M, Guindani M: Potential source of cerebral embolism in migraine with aura: A transcranial Doppler study. Neurology 1999;52:1622-1625.
45. Scherzmann M, Wiher S, Nedeltchev K, et al: Percutaneous closure of patent foramen ovale reduces the frequency of migraine attacks. Neurology 2004;62:1399-1401.
46. Resiman M, Christofferson RD, Jesrum J, et al: Migraine headache relief after transcatheter closure of patent foramen ovale. J Am Coll Cardiol 2005;45:493-405.
47. Anzola GP, Morad E, Casilli F, Onorato E: Shunt associated migraine responds favorably to atrial septal repair: A case control study. Stroke 2006;37:430-434.
48. Chen GPW, Goldberg S, Gill EA: Patent foramen ovale and the platypnea orthodeoxia syndrome. Cardiol Clin 2005;2:85-89.
49. Ilkhanoff L, Naidu S, Rohatgi S, et al: Transcatheter device closure of interatrial septal defects in patients with hypoxia. J Interven Cardiol 2005;18:227-232.
50. Waight DJ, Cao QL, Hijazi ZM: Closure of patent foramen ovale in patients with orthodeoxia-platypnea using the Amplatzer devices. Cathet Cardiovasc Intervent 2000;50:195-198.
51. Roxas Timonera M, Larracas C, Gersony D, et al: Patent foramen ovale presenting as platypnea orthodeoxia: Diagnosis by transesophageal echocardiography. J Am Soc Echocardiogr 2001;14:1039-1041.
52. Germonpre P: Patent foramen ovale and diving. Cardiol Clin 2005;23:97-104.
53. Germonpre P, Dendle P, Unger P, et al: Patent foramen ovale and decompression illness in sport divers. J Appl Physiol 1998;84:1622-1626.
54. Scherzmann M, Siller C, Lipp E, et al: Relation between directly detected patent foramen ovale and ischemic brain lesions in sport divers. Ann Intern Med 2001;134:21-28.
55. Torti SR, Billager M, Schwerzmann M, et al: Risk of decompression among 230 divers in relation to the presence and size of PFO. Eur Heart J 2004;25:1014-1020.
56. Kerut EK, Norfleet WT, Plotnick GD, Giles TD: Patent foramen ovale: A review of associated conditions and the impact of physiological size. J Am Coll Cardiol 2001;38:613-623.
57. Hamman GF, Schatzer-Klotz D, Frohlig G, et al: Femoral injection of echo contrast medium may increase the sensitivity of testing for a patent foramen ovale. Neurology 1998;50:1423-1428.
58. Daniels C, Weytjens C, Cosyns B, et al: Second harmonic transthoracic echocardiography: The new reference screening method for the detection of patent foramen ovale. Eur J Echocardiogr 2004;5:449-452.
59. Thanigaraj S, Valika A, Zajarias A, et al: Comparison of transthoracic versus transesophageal echocardiography for the detection of right to left atrial shunting using agitated saline contrast. Am J Cardiol 2005;96:1007-1010.
60. Anzola GP, Mornadi E, Casilli F, Onorato E: Does transcatheter closure of patent foramen ovale really "shut the door?": A prospective study with transcranial Doppler. Stroke 2004;35:2140-2144.
61. U.S. Food and Drug Administration. Humanitarian Device Exemption #H990011. Washington, DC: FDA, 2000.
62. Zajarias A, Thanigaraj S, Lasala J: Predictors and clinical outcomes of residual shunt in patients undergoing percutaneous transcatheter closure of patent foramen ovale. J Invasive Cardiol 2006;18:533-537.
63. Alameddine F, Block PC: Transcatheter patent foramen ovale closure for secondary prevention of paradoxical embolic

events: Acute results from the FORECAST Registry. Catheter Cardiovasc Interv 2004;62:512-516.

64. Braun M, Gliech V, Boscheri A, et al: Transcatheter closure of patent foramen ovale (PFO) in patients with paradoxical embolism: Periprocedural safety and mid-term follow up results of three different device occluder systems. Eur Heart J 2004;25:424-430.

65. Perloff JK: Clinical Recognition of Congenital Heart Disease, 5th ed. Philadelphia, WB Saunders, 2003, pp 232-236.

66. Van Praagh S, Carrera ME, Sanders SP, et al: Sinus venosus defects: Unroofing of the right pulmonary veins—Anatomic and echocardiographic findings and surgical treatment [abstract]. Am Heart J 1994;128:365-379.

67. Hunt CE, Lucas RV Jr: Symptomatic atrial septal defect in infancy. Circulation 1973;42:1042-1048.

68. Levin AR, Spach MS, Boineau JP, et al: Atrial pressure flow dynamics and atrial septal defects (secundum type). Circulation 1968;37:476-488.

69. Clark EB, Kugler JD: Preoperative secundum atrial septal defect with coexisting sinus node and atrioventricular node dysfunction. Circulation 1982;65:976-980.

70. Shub C, Tajik AJ, Seward JB, et al: Surgical repair of uncomplicated atrial septal defect without "routine" preoperative cardiac catheterization. J Am Coll Cardiol 1985;6:49-54.

71. Freed MD, Nadas AS, Norwood WI, Castaneda AR: Is routine preoperative cardiac catheterization necessary before repair of secundum and sinus venosus atrial septal defects? J Am Coll Cardiol 1984;4:333-336.

72. Konstantinides S, Kasper W, Geibel A, et al: Detection of left-to-right shunt in atrial septal defect by negative contrast echocardiography: A comparison of transthoracic and transesophageal approach. Am Heart J 1993;126:909-917.

73. Ishii M, Kato H, Inoue O, et al: Biplane transesophageal echo-Doppler studies of atrial septal defects: Quantitative evaluation and monitoring for transcatheter closure. Am Heart J 1993;125:1363-1368.

74. Silverman NH, Schmidt KG: The current role of Doppler echocardiography in the diagnosis of heart disease in children. Cardiol Clin 1989;7:265-297.

75. Taketa RM, Sahn DJ, Simon AL, et al: Catheter positions in congenital cardiac malformations. Circulation 1975;51:749-757.

76. Steele PM, Fuster V, Cohen M, et al: Isolated atrial septal defect with pulmonary vascular obstructive disease—long term follow up and prediction of outcome after surgical correction. Circulation 1987;76:1037-1042.

77. Schwetz BA: Congenital heart defect devices. From the Food and Drug Administration. JAMA 2002;287:578.

78. Thanopoulos BD, Laskari CV, Tsaousis GS, et al: Closure of atrial septal defects with the Amplatzer occlusion device: Preliminary results. J Am Coll Cardiol 1998;31:1110-1116.

79. Fischer G, Kramer HH, Stieh J, et al: Transcatheter closure of secundum atrial septal defects with the new self-centering Amplatzer septal occluder. Eur Heart J 1999;20:541-549.

80. Pedra CA, Pihkala J, Lee KJ, et al: Transcatheter closure of atrial septal defects using the Cardio-Seal implant. Heart 2000;84:320-326.

81. Carminati M, Chessa M, Butera G, et al: Transcatheter closure of atrial septal defects with the STARFlex device: Early results and follow-up. J Interv Cardiol 2001;14:319.

82. Chessa M, Carminati M, Butera G, et al: Early and late complications associated with transcatheter occlusion of secundum atrial septal defect. J Am Coll Cardiol 2002;39:1061-1065.

83. Aeschbacher BC, Chatterjee T, Meier B: Transesophageal echocardiography to evaluate success of transcatheter closure of large secundum atrial septal defects in adults using the buttoned device. Mayo Clin Proc 2000;75:913-920.

84. Banerjee A, Bengur R, Li JS, et al: Echocardiographic characteristics of successful deployment of the Das Angel-Wings atrial septal defect closure device: Initial multicenter experience in the United States. Am J Cardiol 1999; 83:1236-1241.

85. Sievert H, Babic UU, Hausdorf G; on behalf of ASDOS Study Group. Transcatheter closure of atrial septal defect and patent foramen ovale with the ASDOS device: A multi-institutional European trial. Am J Cardiol 1998;82:1405-1413.

CHAPTER

49 The Left Atrial Appendage: Anatomy, Physiology, and Therapeutic Percutaneous Closure

*Hidehiko Hara, David R. Holmes, Jr.,
Robert A. Van Tassel, and Robert S. Schwartz*

KEY POINTS

- The left atrial appendage (LAA) has traditionally been considered a structure without activity or apparent purpose. Yet evolving evidence suggests quite the contrary. It has a shape and three-dimensional configuration much like a bellows, and it appears to function as a left atrial pressure transducer. It is involved in active neurohormonal release in response to left atrial pressure.

- The LAA is distinct from the left atrium (LA). It is a separate chamber with volume as much as one third or one half that of the atrium. Moreover, it originates embryologically from the pulmonary veins rather than the LA. These facts suggest that it is a fundamentally different biologic structure than the atrium.

- The volume and shape of the LAA make it a chamber with low blood flow, promoting hemostasis that in turn promotes thrombus formation. More than 20% of all strokes are thought to be related to atrial fibrillation and the LA, principally from thrombus embolization, and more than 90% of all emboli originating the heart are from the LAA. The LAA is a principal source of morbidity and mortality in atrial fibrillation.

- Elderly patients have a high rate of stroke from atrial fibrillation but also a high rate of major bleeds while taking warfarin. Mechanical LAA ablation is therefore an attractive therapy. Several implanted devices are under study and are used to close the mouth of this structure at the entrance to the atrium. This permits long-term elimination of warfarin therapy even in patients with chronic atrial fibrillation. Interventional ablation of the LAA in early clinical trials shows early promise to change the clinical approach to patients with chronic atrial fibrillation while simultaneously limiting embolic episodes.

The left atrial appendage (LAA) is a crescent-shaped, tubular, long structure that varies widely across individuals in morphology and size. It lies close to the free wall of the left ventricle (LV), often covering the left main coronary artery and its bifurcation. Although it was traditionally considered a structure with little purpose, recent studies strongly suggest the contrary, because it has anatomic, functional, and physiologic attributes quite different from those of the left atrium (LA) proper. It is a principal source of morbidity in atrial fibrillation and has recently become a therapeutic target for the interventionalist.

LAA closure was first described during mitral valvotomy in the 1930s to 1950s.[1] It was known that almost 50% of all atrial thrombi occurred in the LAA.[2-4] Recent data show an even greater significance for the LAA as a source of cardiac thrombi and emboli, with high prevalence especially in patients with nonrheumatic atrial fibrillation (AF). More than 90% of cardiac emboli appear to originate from the LAA. This includes patients with rheumatic mitral stenosis and atrial fibrillation, in whom 62% of atrial thrombi are LAA in origin. AF is the major cause of cardiogenic stroke, occurring in up to 20% of all cases.[5-7]

Table 49-1. The Stroke Prevention in Atrial Fibrillation (SPAF) Clinical Trials

Trial	Time Interval	Main Findings
SPAF I		
Warfarin vs. placebo	1987-1989	Warfarin substantially reduces stroke
Aspirin vs. placebo	1987-1990	Aspirin reduces stroke
SPAF II		
Warfarin vs. aspirin, age=75 yr	1987-1992	Small absolute reduction in stroke by warfarin over aspirin in unselected patients
Warfarin vs. aspirin, age >75 yr	1989-1992	High rate of intracranial bleeding with warfarin (INR 2-4.5) in patients >75 yr old offset reduction in ischemic stroke
SPAF III		
Warfarin INR 2-3 vs. aspirin plus low-intensity, fixed-dose warfarin in selected high-risk patients	1993-1995	Warfarin INR 2-3 offers large benefits over aspirin plus low-intensity, fixed-dose warfarin for high-risk patients
Aspirin-treated low-risk cohort	1993-1997	Patients whose stroke risk is low when given aspirin can be identified (validation of the SPAF risk stratification scheme)

INR, international normalized ratio.

The gold standard for treating cardiac thrombus has been oral anticoagulation. Many patients cannot or will not take anticoagulants, especially elderly patients. In this group, warfarin (Coumadin) has a narrow therapeutic window and high intracerebral bleeding rates, limiting it as a therapeutic option. The Stroke Prevention in Atrial Fibrillation (SPAF) studies assessed the value of antithrombotic therapies such as warfarin, aspirin, and their combination for preventing stroke in 3950 patients with nonvalvular AF. Table 49-1 summarizes the SPAF trials for cardioembolic events. SPAF II revealed that older patients with AF have a high stroke risk while taking aspirin. Yet the risk of cerebral hemorrhage is unacceptably high with warfarin therapy.[8] It is for this reason that atrial appendage obliteration has attracted recent attention, especially as a percutaneous procedure.

The first percutaneous LAA ablation using a catheter-based closure device was done by Nakai and colleagues, who demonstrated that transcatheter LA obliteration was feasible in an animal study.[9] Benign healing occurred without adverse hemodynamic effects and without residual thrombus or tissue damage around the device. Other trials for stroke prevention in high-risk patients with nonrheumatic AF also used percutaneous LAA transcatheter occlusion devices. The feasibility of this treatment is established, and it suggests that percutaneous therapy is a clear therapeutic strategy for patients with AF and a contraindication to lifelong anticoagulation therapy.[10]

ANATOMY OF THE LEFT ATRIAL APPENDAGE

Embryology

The LAA develops from the primordial LA. Its internal surface arises from the primordial pulmonary vein and is quite uneven compared to the LA.[11] The appendage develops during the third week of gestation, earlier than most smooth portions of the LA cavity.[12] Most of the LA wall originates from primordial pulmonary venous cells. The pulmonary veins form gradually and develop around the dorsal primordial LA wall, forming the four pulmonary veins with separate atrial orifices by about 8 weeks. In contrast, the remainder of the primordial LA wall becomes the LAA, which is tubular and attached to the LA.[11] Fetal echocardiography has recently shown normal and abnormal structures of the developing heart at 16 weeks' gestation, permitting identification of congenital abnormalities such as LA isomerism, which is highly correlated with LAA isomerism found at autopsy or surgery.[13]

Macroscopic and Microscopic Appearance

Many macroscopic LAA features were described from both external and internal vantage points by Sharma and colleagues, who suggested that there was no crest (the "crista terminalis") and that tapered pectinate muscles "spilled" out to the atrial septum. This is unlike the right atrial appendage, and it differentiates the LAA internal surface features from those of the right atrial appendage. Pectinate muscles are confined to the LAA interior, and there is no terminal crest within it. The external LAA morphology is tubular, with a hooked apex in most cases that points downward. By contrast, most of the right atrial appendage had a broad base and a hooked apex that in most cases points upward.[14]

Examination of 500 normal autopsy hearts for LAA lobe count found that two lobes were most often present (54% of cases) (Fig. 49-1). These lobes typically exist in different planes, so that imaging must be done in multiple planes to visualize the entire LAA body.[15] Significant differences were found in mean length, width, and orifice size, which increase with time up to 20 years of age in both sexes. The investigators concluded that LAA dimensions change with individual age and sex.

Ernst and associates described the LAA principal axis course by making casts and measuring minimal and maximal orifice diameters, length, width, and volume. The principal axis was tortuous and spiraled

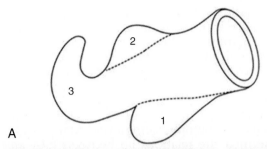

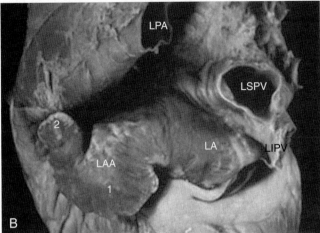

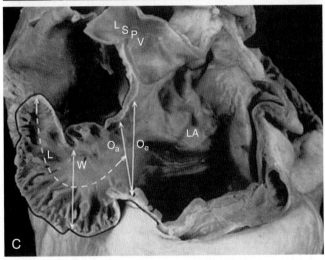

Figure 49-1. A, Drawing of a left atrial appendage (LAA) anatomic specimen consisting of three lobes. Each protrusion from the body comprises a separate lobe. Directional changes or bends in the tail do not usually comprise new lobes. **B,** LAA with two lobes (1 and 2). **C,** Measurements of the LAA in a gross pathologic specimen. The echocardiographic orifice (Oe) is larger than the anatomic orifice (Oa). The length (L) of the appendage is a curvilinear distance (*dashed line*) from Oa to the tip of the tail, whereas the maximal width (W) is a straight-line measurement. Almost all appendages in the adult contain pectinate muscles greater than 1 mm in diameter. Oe is usually measured from the junction of the left superior pulmonary vein (LSPV) as it enters the left atrium (LA) to the junction of the LA and LAA. LIPV, left inferior pulmonary vein; LPA, left pulmonary artery. (From Veinot JP, Harrity PJ, Gentile F, et al: Anatomy of the normal left atrial appendage: A quantitative study of age-related changes in 500 autopsy hearts. Implications for echocardiographic examination. Circulation 1997;96:3112-3115.)

in 42% of hearts, extremely bent and slightly spiraled in 24%, slightly bent and extremely spiraled in 5%, and slightly bent and spiraled in 23%. Fifty-six percent had more than five branches (orifice area, >10 mm^2), and 47% had more than 40 "twigs" (orifice area, 1-10 mm^2). The mean minimal and maximal orifice diameters were 15 and 21 mm, respectively. Mean length (bottom to top) was 30 mm, mean width was 21 mm (at right angles), and mean volume was 5220 mm^3 (5.22 mL).[16] Blood supply to the LAA is typically provided by the left circumflex or right coronary arteries from positions in the left and right atrioventricular sulci.[17]

The microscopic appearance of the LAA in patients with chronic AF has been compared with that in patients with sinus rhythm.[18] Patients with AF generally exhibit marked fibrous endocardial thickening and a much smoother internal LAA surface. It is unclear whether the LAA endocardium resembles the remainder of the heart in structure and function,[19] although LAA myocardial cells are visually similar to those in other parts of the heart.[20] The LAA epicardial thickness is greater for those portions overlying the ventricles.

Morphologic changes occur in the LAA after exposure to ionizing radiation. Generalized collagen (fibrosis) develops in rat hearts exposed to radiation, with reduction of appendage volume and loss of elasticity. These changes appear to negatively influence ventricular function,[21] because evidence suggests that the LAA plays a role in LV filling and contributes to normal cardiac function.[22-25]

PHYSIOLOGY OF THE LEFT ATRIAL APPENDAGE

LAA distensibility is typically higher than that of the atrial body. If the LAA is compressed, LA dimensions and mean atrial pressures are increased, as are transmitral and pulmonary venous flow velocities, as shown by echocardiography.[22] LAA distensibility lowers the LA pressure-volume relationship and augments hemodynamic function. In one preclinical study, LAA distension induced urine output, sodium excretion, and increased heart rate, a reflex presumably due to this diuresis.

The atria and their appendages have a variety of innervations and receptors. Atrial innervation has both sympathetic and parasympathetic fibers. If both appendages are destroyed, parasympathetic afferent reflexes from the cervical vagal nerve and sympathetic efferent pathways are reduced.[23] Myelinated and unmyelinated afferent fibers pass via the vagus to the brainstem or through sympathetic afferents to the spinal cord.[24]

The LAA has prominent muscular ridges. Its contraction is easily visible during open heart surgery,[19] and it has inherent contractions. One case report described a giant LAA that moved more than 3 inches with each systolic beat. The LAA likely contributes to cardiac output. One study found that the cardiac output was halved in ligated compared to intact LAA in a guinea pig model.[25] Such differences in cardiac output suggest that the LAA functions as a contractile cardiac chamber that assists in LV filling. The LAA may stimulate thirst in hypovolemic patients, and it may impair the hemodynamic response to volume overload. Normal LV function in the dog has minimal contribution from the LAA. However, in LV dysfunction, LA and LAA dysfunction reduce cardiac output further.[26]

Another canine study showed that atrial appendectomy decreased cardiac output in experimental high-output heart failure.[27] In patients with LV dysfunction, LAA function is also sometimes depressed. It can improve remarkably after treatment of the heart failure, as measured by LAA size, area, and emptying velocity. LAA size may decrease substantially more than LA size, suggesting that the LAA is more compliant than the LA itself. The LAA may thus be a volume reservoir that limits atrial pressure rise and may help protect against pulmonary congestion.[28]

Another important LAA physiologic function is hormone secretion, making it an endocrine organ. It releases both atrial natriuretic peptide (ANP) and brain natriuretic peptide.[29,30] These have combined natriuretic, diabetic, and vasodilatory properties. In a canine model of experimental high-output heart failure, the atrial appendages contained approximately 30% of the total atrial ANP, and atrial appendectomy decreased the secretory function of ANP.[27] In a human study, ANP concentration was fivefold to tenfold greater than that in the normal functioning heart, particularly the prohormones β-ANP and γ-ANP.[31]

IMAGING AND DETECTION OF THROMBUS

Invasive Studies

Initially, LAA thrombus was detected by invasive angiography, but this procedure required a transseptal approach. Alternatively, pulmonary arteriography was an invasive examination for visualizing the LAA in the levo phase.[32] Since the advent of echocardiography, invasive angiography is rarely performed.

Echocardiography

Transthoracic echocardiography (TTE) is typically not sensitive enough for detecting LAA thrombus, compared with transesophageal echocardiography (TEE).[33,34] New TTE systems may permit detection of LAA thrombi, and accurate determination of LAA function in most patients with neurologic deficits is feasible.[35] Other studies show that several TTE variables are predictive of LAA thrombi, suggesting that TTE may now be useful for detecting LAA thrombi.[36]

TEE remains the gold standard for detecting LAA thrombus and usually provides high-quality images and physiologic information about appendage function. Two-dimensional and three-dimensional (3D) echocardiography and Doppler techniques are widely available. Basic biplane TEE allows the horizontal short-axis view at the base of the heart[37] and the two-chamber longitudinal view of the LA and LV.[38] Figure 49-2 shows multiplane TEE[39] of an LAA with thrombi, before and after percutaneous device–based obliteration. TEE imaging allows great versatility in obtaining views with multiple anatomic planes.[40]

Two-dimensional imaging of the LAA is limited owing to its 3D anatomic complexity. Many reports have examined the relationship between LAA area and ejection fraction and LAA function.[41-50] These studies suggested that functional measurement by LAA cross-sectional area has few advantages over measurement by Doppler echocardiography.[51] Two-dimensional TEE reliably detects spontaneous echocardiographic contrast (SEC) and also semiquantitatively grades SEC.[52,53] Multiplane TEE allows thrombus detection despite complex structural LAA features, although it also may result in misdiagnosis from oversensitivity[54] or undersensitivity.[55]

LAA assessment by 3D echocardiography is now available, and a recent investigation revealed that this modality is promising for evaluating the LAA with or without thrombi. It is important to obtain good-quality images in TTE, because this real-time 3D modality may be used to screen the LAA for better understanding of its complicated 3D anatomy.[56]

Computed Tomography and Magnetic Resonance Imaging

Recent advances in computed tomography (CT) of the cardiovascular system have introduced a new and exciting noninvasive imaging modalities that are complementary to other diagnostic modalities such as echocardiography and invasive methods. Multislice computed tomographic angiography (CTA) provides better image quality for intracardiac thrombus than does conventional CT,[57] and several studies found it to be more sensitive and more specific than TTE in identifying LA thrombus.[58-60] This is especially true for thrombi in the LAA and lateral wall of the LA, which are better detected by multislice CTA than by TTE.[61] The accuracy of multislice CTA is comparable to that of TEE as a semi-invasive diagnostic tool for detecting LAA thrombi. In addition, multislice CTA can reveal the 3D structure of the LAA and its complicated anatomy, which TEE cannot demonstrate (Figs. 49-3 through 49-5).

Electron-beam computed tomography (EBCT) allows high temporal resolution to visualize atrial thrombi in patients with AF better than with TEE.[62] Multislice CT scanning provides higher resolution, better signal-to-noise ratio, and a shorter overall scan time than does EBCT, but at the expense of higher radiation doses. A comparison of the ability to identify LA thrombus by 3D CT scanning versus TEE in patients with persistent AF showed excellent agreement between TEE and CT for LAA size measurement in 31 patients.[63] Multislice CTA may provide excellent image resolution, but it has limitations because of the irregular cycle length in AF.

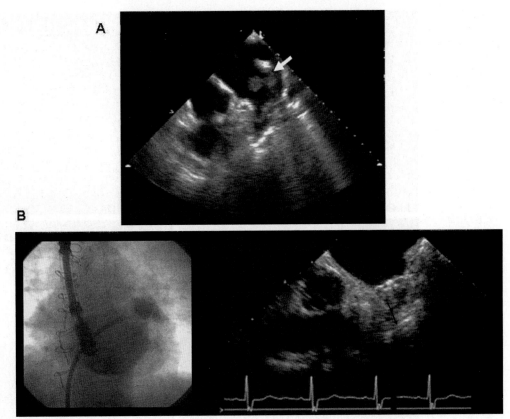

Figure 49-2.
A, Transesophageal echocardiogram (TEE) shows human left atrial appendage (LAA) containing multiple thrombi *(arrow)*. **B,** TEE showing LAA obliteration using the WATCHMAN device after 45 days. The device is well seated in the LAA *(right panel)*. The left panel shows an LAA angiogram from the femoral vein, indicating the location of the LAA and the closure device. The TEE probe in the esophagus is also seen.

Cardiac magnetic resonance imaging (MRI) has satisfactory temporal resolution for LAA imaging (Fig. 49-6), and contrast-enhanced MRI can detect thrombi in the LAA. MRI is also used for planning and follow-up of percutaneous LAA transcatheter occlusion.[64]

Postmortem Studies

Anatomic qualitative and quantitative LAA evaluations of many postmortem hearts were reported in the 1980s and 1990s. LAA morphology was found to be far more complicated than previously thought. Distinct variability was shown for LAA mean orifice size, length, and width. These dimensions increased at an average rate of 0.024, 0.041, and 0.030 cm/yr, respectively, during the first 20 years of life ($P<.01$). Length and width increased more slowly in females. The orifice size and width increased in individuals older than 20 years of age, at average rates of 0.0016 and 0.0019 cm/yr, but the length decreased, at an average rate of 0.0040 cm/yr.[15]

Other studies showed relative enlargement of the LAA volume with AF (7060 mm^3 vs. 4645 mm^3 in sinus rhythm; $P<.01$), LV hypertrophy (5740 mm^3 vs. 4639 mm^3 without hypertrophy; $P<.01$), myocardial scars (5923 mm^3 vs. 4891 mm^3 without scars; $P<.05$), closed foramen ovale (5515 mm^3 vs. 4037 mm^3 with patent foramen ovale; $P<.01$), and LAA thrombi (8566 mm^3 vs. 5027 mm^3 without thrombi; $P<.01$).[16] The authors concluded that LAA configuration varies in volume and shape, and that this variability should be considered when interpreting LAA images, especially when diagnosing LAA thrombi.[16] Better morphologic understanding is needed for future treatments that may use these new modalities.

PATHOPHYSIOLOGY AND RELATED DISORDERS

Isomerism

LAA isomerism is a rare condition that is often associated with other congenital anomalies and is known for its dire prognosis. The diagnosis is confirmed at surgery or autopsy and is defined by bilateral LAA and bilateral, bilobed lungs. The LAA arises from a narrow base, with a long, finger-like appearance compared with the right atrial appendage, which has a broad base and triangular shape. In isomerism, the LAA pectinate muscles are confined to only the appendage itself. It is often complicated by ventricular noncompaction. The echocardiographic diagnosis of LAA isomerism is made by concomitant findings of atrioventricular canal defects, interrupted inferior vena cava with azygos vein continuation, and heart block, usually in the presence of abdominal situs.[65] LAA isomerism is also a diagnostic feature of LA isomerism, called the polysplenia syndrome. It may necessitate eventual cardiac transplantation because of the high mortality rate due to other cardiac and noncardiac anomalies.[66,67]

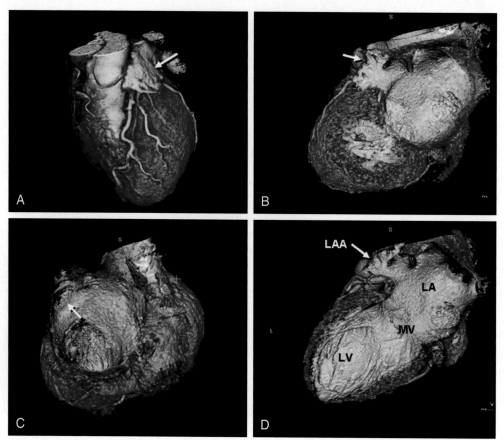

Figure 49-3. Multislice computed tomographic angiography. Images were obtained with the volume-rendered technique (VRT) and show the location of the left atrial appendage (LAA) above the left main coronary artery. Multislice computed tomography allows three-dimensional (3D) visualization of the LAA in living patients. These VRT images were reconstructed with the use of a 3D workstation (Vitrea2, Vital Images Inc., Minnetonka, MN). **A,** Exterior anterior view of the heart including the LAA (*arrow*), typically situated above and covering the left main coronary artery and its bifurcation. The coronary artery emerging from under the LAA is the left anterior descending, with several diagonal branches easily seen. **B,** Lateral view from left side of the heart after digital trimming of the left atrium (LA) and sectioning of the LAA in half. The LAA is located in the anterior portion of this image (*arrow*), and its orifice is separated from left superior pulmonary vein. Pectinate muscles can be seen inside the LAA. **C,** Cranial view from the heart after digital removal of the superior portion of the LA, pulmonary arteries, and veins. The ostium of the LAA is seen (*arrow*), and the pectinate muscles inside the LAA orifice are seen. **D,** After trimming of the left side of the LA and left ventricle (LV), the location of the LAA is easily visible. MV, mitral valve.

Juxtaposition

The first case of levojuxtaposition of the right atrial appendage was reported by Birmingham.[68] Since then, many cases of this abnormality have been described, often in association with other anomalies such as abnormal ventricular looping and abnormalities of the conus. In the 1950s, the term "atrial appendage juxtaposition" was introduced, describing its positional analysis. In atrial appendage positional right-sided juxtaposition, the right-sided structure is morphologically the LAA; this is the opposite of the more familiar situation of left-sided juxtaposition, in which the morphologically right atrial appendage is malpositioned.[69] It is usually associated with other cardiac anomalies including hypoplastic LV and normal sinus. Juxtaposition of the right atrial appendage typically has a hypoplastic right ventricle and abnormal conus.[70,71] Recently, fetal echocardiography has provided clues to its diagnosis before

birth. Abnormal vascular spaces are seen on the left side of the cross-sections and in the great arterial trunks in the case of atrial appendage juxtaposition.[72] A preclinical model for left juxtaposition of the atrial appendage in chicks has been investigated to resolve several morphogenetic questions of human congenital cardiac malformations.[73]

Left Atrial Appendage Dysfunction and Myopathy

AF is the most significant cause of emboli from the LAA. Poor LAA contraction causes thrombus formation not only in AF but also in sinus rhythm on occasion.[74] LAA contraction is absent, comparable to LAA stunning, and produces an "acute LAA myopathy" that results in thrombus formation. On occasion, the cardiac musculature of some patients may gradually fatigue and develop a "delayed myopathy," which creates susceptible environments for

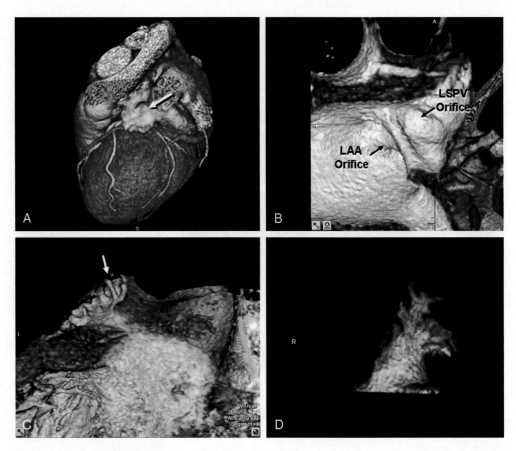

Figure 49-4. A, Multislice computed tomographic angiography was used with volume-rendered technique (VRT) to derive this left anterior oblique view of the heart of a living patient. The complex structure of the left atrial appendage (LAA) is visualized (*arrow*). **B,** View of the LAA orifice from the left atrium, showing the orifice location next to the opening of left superior pulmonary vein (LSPV). **C,** Magnified lateral view of LAA internal anatomy, illustrating the complicated pectinate muscle anatomy (*arrow*). **D,** Isolated VRT image showing the structure of the LAA in a different patient. This LAA is smaller, but its complex three-dimensional structure can again be seen.

thrombus formation. TEE should be performed for patients with AF in whom there is a question of LAA myopathy and thrombus, to measure flow velocity and magnitude. It may allow early anticoagulation therapy even in patients with sinus rhythm. In such LAA dysfunction related to AF, atrial pacing at increased rates and isoproterenol may reverse mechanical atrial stunning associated with short-duration AF. In contrast, long-duration AF has an attenuated response to this therapy.[75]

Other Conditions: Aneurysm, Infarction, Cardiomyopathy, Amyloidosis

Many LAA dysfunctional conditions and related syndromes have been described. LAA aneurysms are rare but are commonly associated with atrial tachyarrhythmias and thromboembolism.[76] Aneurysm resection is the only reported curative strategy, but percutaneous LAA closure may become an alternative, similar to aortic aneurysms that are treated with percutaneous endovascular grafts.[77]

LAA infarction is also rare, but one report indicated appendiceal thrombosis in an infant after twisting of the appendage base with subsequent thrombosis within myocardial vessels.[78] Isolated atrial amyloidosis is a cause of AF, and there is an inverse correlation with atrial fibrosis.[79] In the setting of the hypertrophic and dilated cardiomyopathy, LAA function as a

means to measure pulmonary venous flow patterns may be useful to predict clinical outcomes.[50,80]

Cardiovascular and Cerebrovascular Events

Several studies have suggested that measuring LAA function allows prediction of thrombotic or thromboembolic risk in patients with AF or atrial flutter. LAA function is often unrelated to global LA function.[51] Reasons for this difference may be that the LAA and the main LA cavity originate from different embryologic sources. The trabecular LAA is a remnant of the embryonic LA, whereas the smooth LA cavity originates from an outgrowth of the pulmonary veins, as noted previously. Dissociation of LA and LAA mechanical activity typically occurs in patients who have undergone cardioversion, in whom organized LA mechanical activity may be present along with disorganized LAA contraction.[81] High-velocity blood flow in the LAA is sometimes observed in patients with AF. Apparent differences between LA and LAA function may result from the multiple determinants of mitral inflow velocities that are independent of LA contractility, such as LV diastolic characteristics and loading conditions. In spite of these dissociations, LAA function may be a clinically applicable surrogate for overall LA function.[51] In addition, many studies have revealed an association between LAA dysfunction and previous systemic embolic events, primarily cerebral emboli.[82-86]

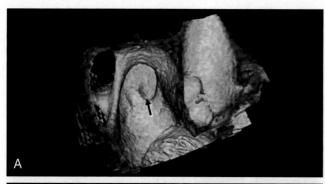

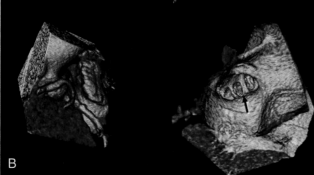

Figure 49-5. **A,** Multislice computed tomographic angiography (CTA) image derived with volume-rendered technique (VRT) showing a magnified view of the left atrial appendage (LAA) orifice from the left atrium (*arrow*). The orifice forms a three-dimensional spiral configuration rather than a single circular ostium. **B,** Magnified multislice CTA VRT image of the LAA from the external (*left*) and internal (*right*) views. Pectinate muscles appear as columns and can be seen in the inner portion of the LAA (*arrow*).

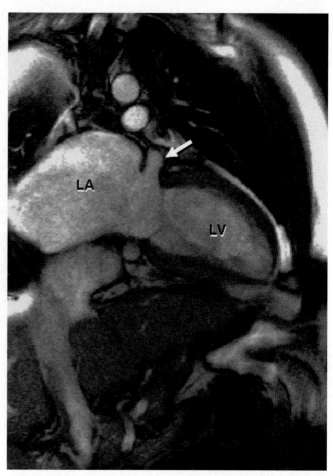

Figure 49-6. Still frame from cine cardiac magnetic resonance imaging study showing the left atrial appendage (*arrow*) and its relation to the left atrium (LA). LV, left ventricle. (Courtesy Dr. John Lesser, Minneapolis Heart Institute Advanced Imaging Center.)

Left Ventricular Dysfunction and the Left Atrial Appendage

Atrial function, including LAA emptying, is closely related to LV dysfunction[87] in canine models. Atrial failure has little effect on cardiac output and right-sided heart pressures in normal LV function because of compensatory conduit function. If early LV dysfunction coexists, however, reservoir and conduit functions became insufficient to compensate for impaired atrial contraction. AF impairs LV cardiac function, a fact that has been known for a century. This includes not only diastolic dysfunction but also AF-mediated systolic dysfunction. Therefore, LAA function should always be checked in patients with AF.

Mitral Valve Disease

Mitral stenosis is well known to increase resistance to LAA emptying, both actively and passively, resulting in lower LAA flow velocities despite normal cardiac rhythms. It is hemodynamically very important: one investigation suggested that LAA contraction velocity is significantly lower in patients with mitral stenosis compared to patients without rheu-

matic heart disease. This is true both in sinus and AF rhythms.[88] Mitral stenosis especially limits normal augmentation of LAA flow during diastole in patients with AF, according to stenosis severity.[89] Rheumatic AF with severe mitral stenosis demonstrates low-to-absent LAA velocity, in contrast to nonrheumatic AF, which shows a wide spectrum of flow velocities.[82] Direct LA and LAA involvement in the rheumatic inflammatory process may elevate LAA pressure. Also, severe hemodynamic impairment from mitral stenosis occurs and also may elevate LA pressure. Atrial myopathy is a frequent cause of chronic LA pressure elevation. Similar phenomena have been noted in patients with mitral valve prostheses.[90]

PATHOGENESIS OF STROKE AND TRANSIENT ISCHEMIC ATTACK

Left Atrial Appendage Flow and Thrombus Formation in Atrial Fibrillation and Atrial Flutter

Blood flow patterns in the LAA have been studied by TEE, and thromboembolism risk is greater with slower flow velocity. Low velocity in AF correlates well with thrombi in the appendage. It is often found in atrial stunning, such as after cardioversion, and in spontaneous recovery from AF. The magnitude of LAA filling and emptying in AF may not relate to ventricular rate and may be of limited relevance for preventing thromboembolism. LAA contraction velocities less than 20 cm/sec are associated with SEC in 75% of patients, significantly more than the 58% frequency observed in patient groups with higher-velocity flow, as was shown in the SPAF III TEE substudy. Significant LAA dysfunction is correlated with LAA thrombus formation,[53,91] and anticoagulation decreases the chances of thrombus formation. LAA flow velocities independently predict thrombus formation even in various clinical hemostatic settings.[92]

The SPAF III trial showed a relationship between thrombus formation and LAA flow velocity. Namely, low-to-absent flow velocities in the LAA (≤20 cm/sec) indicated higher thrombus prevalence than in patients with high LAA velocity (17% vs. 5%, respectively).[93] This study prospectively confirmed that LAA dysfunction is a risk factor for future embolic events. Patients with low flow velocities in the LAA (≤20 cm/s) have 2.6 times greater ischemic stroke risk than patients with higher LAA velocities. Decreased LAA velocities indicate increased clinical risk for thromboembolization.[94] SEC and LAA dysfunction are strongly correlated with thrombus formation and thromboembolism in rheumatic heart disease, and more so in AF than in atrial flutter,[43,82] because there is less LAA dysfunction in flutter. Decreased LAA flow velocities after catheter ablation of chronic atrial flutter recover slowly, and SEC typically resolves within 2 weeks in patients with preserved LV function.[95]

Imaging of Low-Flow "Smoke"

SEC results from blood stagnation in the LA and LAA and carries a high incidence of thrombus and thrombogenic events. "Smoke-like" formation visualized by TTE has been known for more than 20 years. TTE remains the standard method used to detect SEC and evaluate the LAA. EBCT and multislice CT scanners are becoming widely available and have sufficient spatial resolution to assess fine LAA anatomic structure. LAA thrombus, even without AF, can be detected. TEE remains the gold standard for LAA evaluation, because multislice CT requires exposure to contrast agent and radiation. TEE is a semi-invasive tool, however, and it is not feasible in certain situations in which multislice CTA may be a reliable alternative because of shorter overall examination times and better images with less contrast utilization.[96]

MRI visualizes the LAA and thrombus even in patients with nonrheumatic AF.[97] One study evaluated 50 subjects with nonrheumatic AF and a history of cardioembolic stroke with MRI and TEE. In all subjects, MRI allowed visualization of high-intensity masses in the LAA and clearly distinguished thrombus from LAA wall structure using triple-inversion recovery sequences. In the severe SEC cases, the LAA lumen was seen in great detail. With thrombus in SEC, a high-intensity mass was seen. Compared with TEE, MRI does not require esophageal intubation, and the detection of high-intensity masses between these two modalities is concordant.

CLOSURE OF THE LEFT ATRIAL APPENDAGE

Concepts

LAA obliteration is both theoretically and practically feasible, and it is commonly performed during cardiac surgery, because the LAA is generally responsible for thrombi.[1] Anticoagulation is underused, has poor patient compliance, and is often contraindicated, so that prevention of LAA thrombus without warfarin therapy is of great interest for patients without other options. The concept of LAA obliteration has received increased attention as evidence has accumulated for its use as a replacement for anticoagulation. Studies to answer this question are currently underway.[98]

Surgical Closure and Results

Patients undergoing surgical LAA closure have not been systematically evaluated. Nevertheless, surgical closure is universal during mitral valve surgery, presumably to decrease the risk of embolic events.[4,99-102] Several investigations have suggested that surgical obliteration may fail to completely close the LAA.[103,104] One study revealed that incomplete surgical LAA ligation was frequent, because the investigators found patent flow between LAA and LA by TEE in 50 patients undergoing concurrent mitral valve surgery. In their study, 18 (36%) of 50 patients had incomplete LAA ligation, and the incidence was no different between patients studied immediately or later after surgery. In addition, LA size, degree of mitral regurgitation, operative approach (sternotomy or port access), and type of surgery (replacement or plasty) did not correlate with these results. The important fact is that SEC or thrombus was detected within the appendages in 9 (50%) of 18 patients with insufficient closure, and 4 (22%) of the 18 patients had thromboembolic events after the procedure. The authors suggested that residual communication between the insufficiently ligated appendage and the LA body might produce an enhanced prothrombotic environment because of stagnant LAA blood flow and be a potential source of increased embolic events.[104]

A recent study suggested that better results were obtained with a stapling device than with sutures during coronary artery bypass grafting (CABG) in 77 patients. Only 45% (5/11) of patients demonstrated complete occlusion with the use of sutures, compared with 72% (24/33) when the surgical stapler was used. The rate of LAA occlusion by individual surgeons increased from 43% (9/21) to 87% (20/23) after performing at least four cases (*P*=.0001). Stapling can be safely undertaken during CABG, although two patients (2.6%) had perioperative thromboembolic events: one was an intraoperative stroke and the other a TIA occurring on the third postoperative day.[105]

Thoracoscopic Extracardiac Closure

Ligation of the LAA with an automatic surgical stapler makes LAA obliteration possible in open-chest procedures.[101] This was accomplished in combination with a technique dealing with the pericardium, such as pericardiectomy, pericardiocentesis, or resection of pericardial cysts. This method allowed LAA obliteration via thoracoscopy in an animal study. Thoracoscopy showed rapid (21.3±7.6 minutes) and successful obliteration in all cases, but with bleeding, pneumothorax, and fibrinous pericarditis as complications.[106] A human study entitled Thoracoscopic Left Appendage Total Obliteration No cardiac Invasion (LAPTONI) revealed that 14 of 15 patients had successful procedures, although 1 patient required urgent open thoracotomy because of bleeding. Patients had a history of prior thromboembolism and were observed for 8 to 60 months (mean, 42±14 months). One fatal stroke occurred at 55 months, and one disabling stroke occurred 3 months after the procedure. Two non–procedure-related deaths were observed, one after CABG and the other from hepatic failure. The annual rate of stroke was 5.2% per year (95% confidential interval [CI]: 1.3 to 21), compared with 13% per year for similar, aspirin-treated patients from the SPAF trials (*P*=.15). The authors concluded the LAPTONI procedure was technically feasible without immediate neurologic morbidity or mortality.[107]

Percutaneous Transcatheter Occlusion: WATCHMAN, PLAATO, and the Amplatzer Septal Occluder

WATCHMAN

The WATCHMAN LAA closure system (Atritech Inc., Plymouth, MN) is a device that is designed to seal the LAA orifice and allow endothelialization (Figs. 49-7 and 49-8). A self-expanding nitinol frame contains a porous 160-μm polyethylene terephthalate (PET) membrane on its proximal face that filters LAA blood entering and leaving the appendage. Fixation barbs surround the midportion of the device to engage the LAA wall. It is available in diameters from 21 to 33 mm according to the diameter of the LAA orifice.

PLAATO

The PLAATO device (ev3, Inc., Plymouth, MN) was the first percutaneously implanted occluder to find human use (see Fig. 49-8). Its framework is a nitinol basket with a tissue anchoring system on the struts designed to maintain position. A minimally thrombogenic expanded polytetrafluoroethylene (ePTFE) membrane covers the basket and is designed to seal the LAA orifice and allow endothelialization.

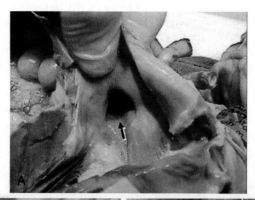

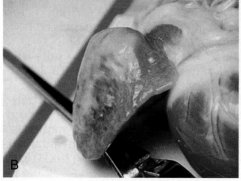

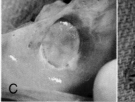

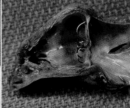

Figure 49-7. A, Postmortem human heart reveals the three-dimensional internal anatomy of the left atrial appendage (LAA) orifice (*arrow*). **B,** Photograph of the LAA after deployment of the WATCHMAN device into a canine heart. This image reveals no injury as seen from external observation. **C,** Internal view of canine LAA orifice, showing complete neointimal covering on the surface of this canine device (*left panel*). Formalin-fixed LAA reveals device attachment to the LAA from a longitudinal section (*right panel*).

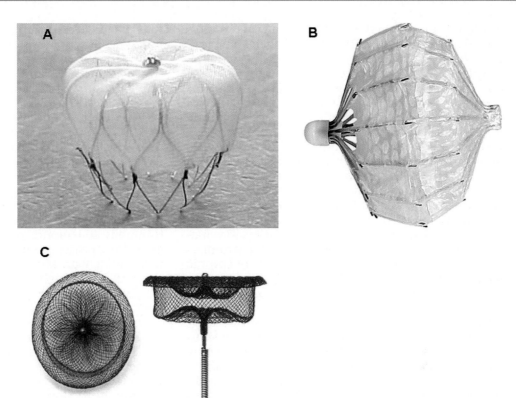

Figure 49-8. Examples of percutaneous left atrial appendage obliteration systems in development. **A,** WATCHMAN Filter System, showing nitinol frame and a permeable 160-μm membrane covering the proximal atrial facing surface of the device. Fixation barbs are located around the midperimeter of the device. **B,** PLAATO system, showing the self-expandable nitinol cage with nonthrombogenic expanded polytetrafluoroethylene membrane covering. Each strut has three fixation anchors for stabilization. **C,** The Amplatzer Septal Occluder, showing nitinol wire frame mesh with incorporated Dacron patches to enhance occlusion.

Amplatzer Septal Occluder

The Amplatzer septal occluder (AGA Medical Corporation) has also been used for LAA closure (see Fig. 49-8), although it too appears to have been suspended in favor of newer device designs. This device is a double-disk with a short, broad waist and is designed for closing atrial septal defects.[108]

Implantation Techniques

Most percutaneous LAA device implant procedures have been performed with an international normalized ratio (INR) of less than 2.0. Antiplatelet therapy with aspirin and clopidogrel is typically begun at least 1 day before procedure. Aspirin is generally continued indefinitely, and clopidogrel is used for several months to prevent thrombosis around the device. Aspirin and warfarin also are often used for several months after implantation. The implant procedure is performed using femoral vein access, so that general anesthesia is not needed. Conventional transseptal catheterization should be performed unless a patent foramen ovale or atrial septal defect is present. A heparin bolus is usually administered after transseptal puncture, and the activated clotting time (ACT) generally is maintained at 200 seconds or longer during the procedure. A contrast "appendogram" is performed in at least two views as a hand injection of contrast medium after the catheter is advanced. TEE or intracardiac echocardiography (ICE) is also recommended to assess the possibility of mobile thrombi and to size the LAA orifice diameter and

length. These echocardiographic tools allow visualization of complicated structures, especially LAA neck anatomy, number of lobes, the anatomic relationship between the pulmonary veins and the LAA, and device position including leakage around the device after implantation. Endocarditis antibiotic prophylaxis is sometimes given and continued until echocardiographic follow-up.

Preclinical Studies

A preclinical study using the PLAATO device for percutaneous transcatheter LAA closure was performed in 25 dogs.[9] The device was implanted, and LAA sealing was confirmed by ICE and contrast fluoroscopy. The device could be replaced or recaptured if it did not fit properly in the LAA. After the procedure, the LAA was examined from 2 days to 6 months later for healing, migration, perforation, and any thrombus, both grossly and histologically. Healing occurred by 1 month in 90% and was complete by 3 months. The atrial-facing surface was studied, and no mobile thrombi around the device were observed; neither were embolic events found in other organs. The investigators concluded that benign healing without new thrombus or damage was seen around the structures.

Human Clinical Studies

A clinical study using PLAATO was carried out in nonrheumatic AF patients who had contraindications to long-term anticoagulation therapy and were at high risk for thromboembolism. Their risk factors included congestive heart failure, diabetes mellitus, hypertension, history of TIA or stroke, and SEC in the LAA by TEE.[109] Fifteen patients were recruited, and the PLAATO device was implanted. All implants were successful, although one patient had hemopericardium associated with LAA access before implantation, diagnosed with intraprocedure TEE. Pericardiocentesis was performed without sequelae, and the LAA was successfully occluded 4 weeks later. One month follow-up was performed by TEE and fluoroscopy, and no adverse events observed. Conclusions were that this technology was appropriate for patients with AF who could not have long-term anticoagulation therapy. Contraindications to warfarin were defined as cerebral hemorrhage, gastrointestinal bleeding, an unstable INR, and severe chronic liver disease.

Another study reported LAA occlusion using the Amplatzer device. Sixteen patients were enrolled, ranging from 58 to 63 years of age. All were diagnosed with AF, although eight patients were in sinus rhythm at the time of implantation. There was one technical failure (device embolization) requiring surgery. No other complications occurred during an overall follow-up of 5 patient-years. The study concluded that the Amplatzer device could be delivered percutaneously by venous puncture under local anesthesia without echocardiographic guidance.[110]

A recent investigation of LAA occlusion by PLAATO reported on mitral valve and left upper pulmonary vein (LUPV) function. Eleven patients (mean age, 72±7 years) were enrolled in the study. There were no significant changes in LUPV diameter at baseline, 1 month, and 6 months (mean: 1.55, 1.61, and 1.54 cm, respectively; P=.13), nor in peak systolic flow velocity (mean: 0.38, 0.34, and 0.31 m/sec; P=.72) or peak diastolic flow velocity (mean: 0.39, 0.40, and 0.42 m/sec; P=.46). The devices remained stable at the deployment site, with minimal residual flow around them. The authors concluded that the PLAATO device could achieve a satisfactory seal of the LAA neck without significant effects on LA or LUPV structure or function.[111]

Ostermayer and colleagues[10] evaluated the feasibility of LAA percutaneous occlusion in two previously described prospective, multicenter trials[109,111] using the PLAATO system. They showed that LAA obliteration was successful in 111 patients (mean age, 71±9 years).[10] Indications for the PLAATO device were at least one stroke risk factor, such as history of TIA or stroke, presence of congestive heart failure, low LV ejection fraction, hypertension, diabetes mellitus, age greater than 65 years, coronary artery disease, moderate or dense SEC, or less than or equal to 20 cm/sec blood flow velocity within LAA. The patients had nonrheumatic AF of at least 3 months' duration and a contraindication for anticoagulation therapy. Patients were administered aspirin (300-325 mg) and clopidogrel (75 mg) twice daily, starting 48 hours before the procedure. Antibiotics were given 1 hour before the intervention. The exclusion criteria

were LA or LAA thrombus, complex aortic plaque, mitral or aortic stenosis or regurgitation, LA diameter greater than 6.5 cm, acute coronary syndrome, recent stroke (<2 months), and symptomatic carotid disease. Implantation was successful in 18 of 111 patients (97.3%; 95% CI: 92.3% to 99.4%) who underwent 113 procedures. One patient (0.9%; 95% CI: 0.02% to 4.9%) had two major adverse events in the first 30 days. This patient needed surgical treatment and suffered neurologically confirmed death in-hospital. Three patients received pericardiocentesis because of hemopericardium. Average follow-up was 9.8 months. Two patients had strokes during this period. The implanted device showed no migration or mobile thrombus at 1 month or 6 months after the procedure. Conclusions were that PLAATO implantation was feasible with acceptable risk. The possibility was raised that this might become an alternative method for patients with AF and contraindications for lifelong anticoagulation therapy.[10]

The WATCHMAN LAA isolation device is a nitinol structure that is designed to fit securely in the LAA and has a PET porous filter membrane on its atrial surface to prevent thrombus from exiting the LAA. This membrane typically develops a healthy intimal covering in the long term. The PROTECT AF Trial is a human clinical study using the WATCHMAN device in patients with AF. The design of this multicenter, prospective randomized study was published in May 2006,[112] and recruitment is proceeding well. Patients are enrolled according to their CHADS score (≥1), and those with paroxysmal, persistent, or permanent nonvalvular AF are also included. Criteria for the CHADS score are shown in Table 49-2. The INR of control patients should be kept between 2.0 and 3.0 and is monitored at least once monthly. Follow-up is planned at 45 days; then at 6, 9, and 12 months; and then annually up 60 months after the procedure. Results of this study are pending. This trial is focused on the relative benefits of the WATCHMAN device versus standard anticoagulation therapy.

Concerns About Left Atrial Appendage Obliteration

Device-based LAA closure appears to be successful in reducing embolic events in patients with AF, although the data are preliminary. Early concerns about adverse effects (hemodynamic or neurohumoral) appear unfounded, as evidenced by several years' experience with surgical closure and now two clinical trials of percutaneous closure.

Table 49-2. CHADS Score

Risk Factor	Points
Recent CHF	1
Hypertension	1
Age ≥75 yr	1
Diabetes mellitus	1
History of stroke or TIA	2

CHADS, congestive heart failure, hypertension, age, diabetes, and stroke; CHF, congestive heart failure; TIA, transient ischemic attack.

Elimination of warfarin therapy also appears possible using device-based or surgical LAA closure. This is key, because, when a clopidogrel-aspirin combination was recently tested as an alternative to warfarin (in the ACTIVE-W trial, a subset of the Atrial fibrillation Clopidogrel Trial with Irbesartan for prevention of Vascular Events [ACTIVE] trial), the study was discontinued prematurely after a significant difference showed that the clopidogrel-aspirin combination was clearly inferior to warfarin in preventing events.[113]

The ability to eliminate anticoagulation in AF is considered a "Holy Grail" for clinical cardiology, and data for this possibility are forthcoming. The risk of AF and thromboembolism is markedly increasing as the population ages and as AF becomes increasingly prevalent.

CONCLUSIONS

The LAA is a structure remarkable for its anatomic and functional features, and some cardiologists are now suggesting the heart actually has six chambers (two atria, two ventricles, and two atrial appendages). Increasingly, it appears that the LAA is significantly more than a simple chamber appended to the atrium without function. It differs from the LA proper in embryology, structure, function, and neurohormonal function. It is the source of more than 90% of all cardiac-based emboli, especially in AF and atrial flutter, mandating lifelong anticoagulation therapy to limit the likelihood of stroke. At present, only limited data exist regarding the feasibility and safety of these devices, yet the evidence is increasingly positive. Percutaneous LAA closure appears to be safe, practical, and possibly effective to simultaneously eliminate the need for warfarin therapy and significantly reduce cardioembolic events.

REFERENCES

1. Blackshear JL, Odell JA: Appendage obliteration to reduce stroke in cardiac surgical patients with atrial fibrillation. Ann Thorac Surg 1996;61:755-759.
2. Madden J: Resection of the left auricular appendix. JAMA 1948;140:769-772.
3. Bailey CP, Olsen AK, Keown KK, et al: Commissurotomy for mitral stenosis: Technique for prevention of cerebral complications. JAMA 1952;149:1085-1091.
4. Belcher JR, Somerville W: Systemic embolism and left auricular thrombosis in relation to mitral valvotomy. Br Med J 1955;2(4946):1000-1003.
5. Wolf PA, Dawber TR, Thomas HE Jr, et al: Epidemiologic assessment of chronic atrial fibrillation and risk of stroke: The Framingham study. Neurology 1978;28:973-977.
6. Wolf PA, Benjamin EJ, Belanger AJ, et al: Secular trends in the prevalence of atrial fibrillation: The Framingham Study. Am Heart J 1996;131:790-795.
7. Kannel WB, Wolf PA, Benjamin EJ, et al: Prevalence, incidence, prognosis, and predisposing conditions for atrial fibrillation: Population-based estimates. Am J Cardiol 1998;82:2N-9N.
8. Hart RG, Halperin JL, Pearce LA, et al: Lessons from the Stroke Prevention in Atrial Fibrillation trials. Ann Intern Med 2003;138:831-838.
9. Nakai T, Lesh MD, Gerstenfeld EP, et al: Percutaneous left atrial appendage occlusion (PLAATO) for preventing cardioembolism: First experience in canine model. Circulation 2002;105:2217-2222.
10. Ostermayer SH, Reisman M, Kramer PH, et al: Percutaneous left atrial appendage transcatheter occlusion (PLAATO system) to prevent stroke in high-risk patients with non-rheumatic atrial fibrillation: Results from the international multi-center feasibility trials. J Am Coll Cardiol 2005;46:9-14.
11. Moore KL: The Developing Human: Clinically Oriented Embryology, 6th ed. Philadelphia, WB Saunders, 1998.
12. Sadler TW: Cardiovascular system. In Sadler TW (ed): Langman's Medical Embryology, 6th ed. Philadelphia, Williams & Wilkins, 1990, pp 179-227.
13. Phoon CK, Villegas MD, Ursell PC, et al: Left atrial isomerism detected in fetal life. Am J Cardiol 1996;77:1083-1088.
14. Sharma S, Devine W, Anderson RH, et al: The determination of atrial arrangement by examination of appendage morphology in 1842 heart specimens. Br Heart J 1988;60:227-231.
15. Veinot JP, Harrity PJ, Gentile F, et al: Anatomy of the normal left atrial appendage: A quantitative study of age-related changes in 500 autopsy hearts—Implications for echocardiographic examination. Circulation 1997;96:3112-3115.
16. Ernst G, Stollberger C, Abzieher F, et al: Morphology of the left atrial appendage. Anat Rec 1995;242:553-561.
17. James TN: Small arteries of the heart. Circulation 1977;56:2-14.
18. Shirani J, Alaeddini J: Structural remodeling of the left atrial appendage in patients with chronic non-valvular atrial fibrillation: Implications for thrombus formation, systemic embolism, and assessment by transesophageal echocardiography. Cardiovasc Pathol 2000;9:95-101.
19. Al-Saady NM, Obel OA, Camm AJ: Left atrial appendage: Structure, function, and role in thromboembolism. Heart 1999;82:547-554.
20. Lannigan RA, Zaki SA: Ultrastructure of the myocardium of the atrial appendage. Br Heart J 1966;28:796-807.
21. Kruse JJ, Zurcher C, Strootman EG, et al: Structural changes in the auricles of the rat heart after local ionizing irradiation. Radiother Oncol 2001;58:303-311.
22. Tabata T, Oki T, Yamada H, et al: Role of left atrial appendage in left atrial reservoir function as evaluated by left atrial appendage clamping during cardiac surgery. Am J Cardiol 1998;81:327-332.
23. Kappagoda CT, Linden RJ, Scott EM, et al: Atrial receptors and heart rate: The efferent pathway. J Physiol 1975;249:581-590.
24. Bishop VS: Handbook of Physiology. Bethesda, MD, American Physiological Society 1983, pp 497-555.
25. Massoudy P, Beblo S, Raschke P, et al: Influence of intact left atrial appendage on hemodynamic parameters of isolated guinea pig heart. Eur J Med Res 1998;3:470-474.
26. Hoit BD, Gabel M: Influence of left ventricular dysfunction on the role of atrial contraction. J Am Coll Cardiol 2000;36:1713-1719.
27. Nishimura K: Does atrial appendectomy aggravate secretory function of atrial natriuretic polypeptide? J Thorac Cardiovasc Surg 1991;101:502.
28. Ito T, Suwa M, Kobashi A, et al: Influence of altered loading conditions on left atrial appendage function in vivo. Am J Cardiol 1998;81:1056-1059.
29. Rodeheffer RJ, Naruse M, Atkinson JB, et al: Molecular forms of atrial natriuretic factor in normal and failing human myocardium. Circulation 1993;88:364-371.
30. Inoue S, Murakami Y, Sano K, et al: Atrium as a source of brain natriuretic polypeptide in patients with atrial fibrillation. J Card Fail 2000;6:92-96.
31. Rodeheffer RJ, Naruse M, Atkinson JB, et al: Molecular forms of atrial natriuretic factor in normal and failing human myocardium. Circulation 1993;88:364-371.
32. Furuse A, Mizuno A, Inoue H, et al: Echocardiography and angiocardiography for detection of left atrial thrombosis. Jpn Heart J 1976;17:163-171.

33. Aschenberg W, Schluter M, Kremer P, et al: Transesophageal two-dimensional echocardiography for the detection of left atrial appendage thrombus. J Am Coll Cardiol 1986;7: 163-166.

34. Black IW, Hopkins AP, Lee LC, et al: Role of transoesophageal echocardiography in evaluation of cardiogenic embolism. Br Heart J 1991;66:302-307.

35. Omran H, Jung W, Rabahieh R, et al: Imaging of thrombi and assessment of left atrial appendage function: A prospective study comparing transthoracic and transoesophageal echocardiography. Heart 1999;81:192-198.

36. Ellis K, Ziada KM, Vivekananthan D, et al: Transthoracic echocardiographic predictors of left atrial appendage thrombus. Am J Cardiol 2006;97:421-425.

37. Seward JB, Khandheria BK, Oh JK, et al: Transesophageal echocardiography: Technique, anatomic correlations, implementation, and clinical applications. Mayo Clin Proc 1988;63:649-680.

38. Seward JB, Khandheria BK, Edwards WD, et al: Biplanar transesophageal echocardiography: Anatomic correlations, image orientation, and clinical applications. Mayo Clin Proc 1990;65:1193-1213.

39. Seward JB, Khandheria BK, Freeman WK, et al: Multiplane transesophageal echocardiography: Image orientation, examination technique, anatomic correlations, and clinical applications. Mayo Clin Proc 1993;68:523-551.

40. Chan SK, Kannam JP, Douglas PS, et al: Multiplane transesophageal echocardiographic assessment of left atrial appendage anatomy and function. Am J Cardiol 1995;76: 528-530.

41. Pollick C, Taylor D: Assessment of left atrial appendage function by transesophageal echocardiography: Implications for the development of thrombus. Circulation 1991;84: 223-231.

42. Li YH, Lai LP, Shyu KG, et al: Clinical implications of left atrial appendage function: Its influence on thrombus formation. Int J Cardiol 1994;43:61-66.

43. Hwang JJ, Li YH, Lin JM, et al: Left atrial appendage function determined by transesophageal echocardiography in patients with rheumatic mitral valve disease. Cardiology 1994;85: 121-128.

44. Fatkin D, Feneley MP: Patterns of Doppler-measured blood flow velocity in the normal and fibrillating human left atrial appendage. Am Heart J 1996;132:995-1003.

45. Tabata T, Oki T, Fukuda N, et al: Influence of aging on left atrial appendage flow velocity patterns in normal subjects. J Am Soc Echocardiogr 1996;9:274-280.

46. Tabata T, Oki T, Fukuda N, et al: Influence of left atrial pressure on left atrial appendage flow velocity patterns in patients in sinus rhythm. J Am Soc Echocardiogr 1996;9:857-864.

47. Porte JM, Cormier B, Iung B, et al: Early assessment by transesophageal echocardiography of left atrial appendage function after percutaneous mitral commissurotomy. Am J Cardiol 1996;77:72-76.

48. Tabata T, Oki T, Iuchi A, et al: Evaluation of left atrial appendage function by measurement of changes in flow velocity patterns after electrical cardioversion in patients with isolated atrial fibrillation. Am J Cardiol 1997;79: 615-620.

49. Ito T, Suwa M, Kobashi A, et al: Influence of altered loading conditions on left atrial appendage function in vivo. Am J Cardiol 1998;81:1056-1059.

50. Ito T, Suwa M, Hirota Y, et al: Influence of left atrial function on Doppler transmitral and pulmonary venous flow patterns in dilated and hypertrophic cardiomyopathy: Evaluation of left atrial appendage function by transesophageal echocardiography. Am Heart J 1996;131:122-130.

51. Agmon Y, Khandheria BK, Gentile F, et al: Echocardiographic assessment of the left atrial appendage. J Am Coll Cardiol 1999;34:1867-1877.

52. Black IW, Hopkins AP, Lee LC, et al: Left atrial spontaneous echo contrast: A clinical and echocardiographic analysis. J Am Coll Cardiol 1991;18:398-404.

53. Fatkin D, Kelly RP, Feneley MP: Relations between left atrial appendage blood flow velocity, spontaneous echocardio-

54. Seward JB, Khandheria BK, Oh JK, et al: Critical appraisal of transesophageal echocardiography: Limitations, pitfalls, and complications. J Am Soc Echocardiogr 1992;5:288-305.

55. Herzog E, Sherrid M: Bifid left atrial appendage with thrombus: Source of thromboembolism. J Am Soc Echocardiogr 1998;11:910-915.

56. Agoston I, Xie T, Tiller FL, et al: Assessment of left atrial appendage by live three-dimensional echocardiography: Early experience and comparison with transesophageal echocardiography. Echocardiography 2006;23:127-132.

57. Alam G, Addo F, Malik M, et al: Detection of left atrial appendage thrombus by spiral CT scan. Echocardiography 2003;20:99-100.

58. Kitayama H, Kiuchi K, Endo T, et al: Value of cardiac ultrafast computed tomography for detecting right atrial thrombi in chronic atrial fibrillation. Am J Cardiol 1997;79: 1292-1295.

59. Love BB, Struck LK, Stanford W, et al: Comparison of two-dimensional echocardiography and ultrafast cardiac computed tomography for evaluating intracardiac thrombi in cerebral ischemia. Stroke 1990;21:1033-1038.

60. Helgason CM, Chomka E, Louie E, et al: The potential role for ultrafast cardiac computed tomography in patients with stroke. Stroke 1989;20:465-472.

61. Tomoda H, Hoshiai M, Tagawa R, et al: Evaluation of left atrial thrombus with computed tomography. Am Heart J 1980;100:306-310.

62. Achenbach S, Sacher D, Ropers D, et al: Electron beam computed tomography for the detection of left atrial thrombi in patients with atrial fibrillation. Heart 2004;90: 1477-1478.

63. Jaber WA, White RD, Kuzmiak SA, et al: Comparison of ability to identify left atrial thrombus by three-dimensional tomography versus transesophageal echocardiography in patients with atrial fibrillation. Am J Cardiol 2004;93: 486-489.

64. Mohrs OK, Schraeder R, Petersen SE, et al: Percutaneous left atrial appendage transcatheter occlusion (PLAATO): Planning and follow-up using contrast-enhanced MRI. AJR Am J Roentgenol 2006;186:361-364.

65. Friedberg MK, Ursell PC, Silverman NH: Isomerism of the left atrial appendage associated with ventricular noncompaction. Am J Cardiol 2005;96:985-990.

66. Gilljam T, McCrindle BW, Smallhorn JF, et al: Outcomes of left atrial isomerism over a 28-year period at a single institution. J Am Coll Cardiol 2000;36:908-916.

67. Phoon CK, Villegas MD, Ursell PC, et al: Left atrial isomerism detected in fetal life. Am J Cardiol 1996;77:1083-1088.

68. Birmingham A: Extreme anomaly of the heart and great vessels. J Anat Physiol 1893;27:139-150.

69. Van Praagh S, O'Sullivan J, Brili S, et al: Juxtaposition of the morphologically left atrial appendage in solitus and inversus atria: A study of 18 postmortem cases. Am Heart J 1996;132(2 Pt 1):391-402.

70. Van Praagh S, O'Sullivan J, Brili S, et al: Juxtaposition of the morphologically right atrial appendage in solitus and inversus atria: A study of 35 postmortem cases. Am Heart J 1996;132(2 Pt 1):382-390.

71. Lai WW: Juxtaposition of the atrial appendages: A clinical series of 22 patients. Pediatr Cardiol 2001;22:121-127.

72. Abduullah M: Diagnosis of left juxtaposition of the atrial appendages in the fetus. Cardiol Young 2000;10:220-224.

73. Manner J: A model for left juxtaposition of the atrial appendages in the chick. Cardiol Young 2003;13:152-160.

74. Pollick C: Left atrial appendage myopathy. Chest 2000; 117:297-298.

75. Sanders P, Morton JB, Kistler PM, et al: Reversal of atrial mechanical dysfunction after cardioversion of atrial fibrillation: Implications for the mechanisms of tachycardia-mediated atrial cardiomyopathy. Circulation 2003;108: 1976-1984.

76. Mathur A, Zehr KJ, Sinak LJ, et al: Left atrial appendage aneurysm. Ann Thorac Surg 2005;79:1392-1393.

77. Ince H, Petzsch M, Rehders T, et al: Percutaneous endovascular repair of aneurysm after previous coarctation surgery. Circulation 2003;108:2967-2970.

78. Spigel J, Key C: Thrombosis and infarction of the left atrial appendage in an infant: A case report. Am J Cardiovasc Pathol 1988;2:87-90.

79. Rocken C, Peters B, Juenemann G, et al: Atrial amyloidosis: An arrhythmogenic substrate for persistent atrial fibrillation. Circulation 2002;106:2091-2097.

80. Ito T, Suwa M, Kobashi A, et al: Prognostic value of left atrial appendage function in patients with dilated cardiomyopathy. Jpn Circ J 2000;64:340-344.

81. Bellotti P, Spirito P, Lupi G, et al: Left atrial appendage function assessed by transesophageal echocardiography before and on the day after elective cardioversion for nonvalvular atrial fibrillation. Am J Cardiol 1998;81:1199-1202.

82. Mugge A, Kuhn H, Nikutta P, et al: Assessment of left atrial appendage function by biplane transesophageal echocardiography in patients with nonrheumatic atrial fibrillation: Identification of a subgroup of patients at increased embolic risk. J Am Coll Cardiol 1994;23:599-607.

83. Verhorst PM, Kamp O, Visser CA, et al: Left atrial appendage flow velocity assessment using transesophageal echocardiography in nonrheumatic atrial fibrillation and systemic embolism. Am J Cardiol 1993;71:192-196.

84. Mitusch R, Garbe M, Schmucker G, et al: Relation of left atrial appendage function to the duration and reversibility of nonvalvular atrial fibrillation. Am J Cardiol 1995;75:944-947.

85. Shively BK, Gelgand EA, Crawford MH: Regional left atrial stasis during atrial fibrillation and flutter: Determinants and relation to stroke. J Am Coll Cardiol 1996;27:1722-1729.

86. Li YH, Hwang JJ, Lin JL, et al: Importance of left atrial appendage function as a risk factor for systemic thromboembolism in patients with rheumatic mitral valve disease. Am J Cardiol 1996;78:844-847.

87. Hoit BD, Gabel M: Influence of left ventricular dysfunction on the role of atrial contraction: an echocardiographic-hemodynamic study in dogs. J Am Coll Cardiol 2000;36:1713-1719.

88. Hwang JJ, Li YH, Lin JM, et al: Left atrial appendage function determined by transesophageal echocardiography in patients with rheumatic mitral valve disease. Cardiology 1994;85:121-128.

89. Lin JM, Hsu KL, Hwang JJ, et al: Interference of mitral valve stenosis with left ventricular diastole and left atrial appendage flow. Cardiology 1996;87:537-544.

90. Lee TM, Chou NK, Su SF, et al: Left atrial spontaneous echo contrast in asymptomatic patients with a mechanical valve prosthesis. Ann Thorac Surg 1996;62:1790-1795.

91. Garcia-Fernandez MA, Torrecilla EG, San Roman D, et al: Left atrial appendage Doppler flow patterns: Implications on thrombus formation. Am Heart J 1992;124:955-961.

92. Heppell RM, Berkin KE, McLenachan JM, et al: Haemostatic and haemodynamic abnormalities associated with left atrial thrombosis in non-rheumatic atrial fibrillation. Heart 1997;77:407-411.

93. The Stroke Prevention in Atrial Fibrillation Investigators Committee on Echocardiography: Transesophageal echocardiographic correlates of thromboembolism in high-risk patients with nonvalvular atrial fibrillation. Ann Intern Med 1998;128:639-647.

94. Zabalgoitia M, Halperin JL, Pearce LA, et al: Transesophageal echocardiographic correlates of clinical risk of thromboembolism in nonvalvular atrial fibrillation. Stroke Prevention in Atrial Fibrillation III Investigators. J Am Coll Cardiol 1998;31:1622-1626.

95. Takami M, Suzuki M, Sugi K, et al: Time course for resolution of left atrial appendage stunning after catheter ablation of chronic atrial flutter. J Am Coll Cardiol 2003;41:2207-2211.

96. Achenbach S, Sacher D, Ropers D, et al: Electron beam computed tomography for the detection of left atrial thrombi in patients with atrial fibrillation. Heart 2004;90:1477-1478.

97. Ohyama H, Hosomi N, Takahashi T, et al: Comparison of magnetic resonance imaging and transesophageal echocardiography in detection of thrombus in the left atrial appendage. Stroke 2003;34:2436-2439.

98. Lindsay BD: Obliteration of the left atrial appendage: A concept worth testing. Ann Thorac Surg 1996;61:515.

99. Thomas TV: Left atrial appendage and valve replacement. Am Heart J 1972;84:838-839.

100. Landymore R, Kinley CE: Staple closure of the left atrial appendage. Can J Surg 1984;27:144-145.

101. DiSesa VJ, Tam S, Cohn LH: Ligation of the left atrial appendage using an automatic surgical stapler. Ann Thorac Surg 1988;46:652-653.

102. Lynch M, Shanewise JS, Chang GL, et al: Recanalization of the left atrial appendage demonstrated by transesophageal echocardiography. Ann Thorac Surg 1997;63:1774-1775.

103. Schneider B, Stollberger C, Sievers HH: Surgical closure of the left atrial appendage: A beneficial procedure? Cardiology 2005;104:127-132.

104. Katz ES, Tsiamtsiouris T, Applebaum RM, et al: Surgical left atrial appendage ligation is frequently incomplete: A transesophageal echocardiograhic study. J Am Coll Cardiol 2000;36:468-471.

105. Healey JS, Crystal E, Lamy A, et al: Left Atrial Appendage Occlusion Study (LAAOS): Results of a randomized controlled pilot study of left atrial appendage occlusion during coronary bypass surgery in patients at risk for stroke. Am Heart J 2005;150:288-293.

106. Odell JA, Blackshear JL, Davies E, et al: Thoracoscopic obliteration of the left atrial appendage: Potential for stroke reduction? Ann Thorac Surg 1996;61:565-569.

107. Blackshear JL, Johnson WD, Odell JA, et al: Thoracoscopic extracardiac obliteration of the left atrial appendage for stroke risk reduction in atrial fibrillation. J Am Coll Cardiol 2003;42:1249-1252.

108. Hein R, Bayard Y, Taaffe M, et al: Patent foramen ovale and left atrial appendage: New devices and methods for closure. Pediatr Cardiol 2005;26:234-240.

109. Sievert H, Lesh MD, Trepels T, et al: Percutaneous left atrial appendage transcatheter occlusion to prevent stroke in high-risk patients with atrial fibrillation: Early clinical experience. Circulation 2002;105:1887-1889.

110. Meier B, Palacios I, Windecker S, et al: Transcatheter left atrial appendage occlusion with Amplatzer devices to obviate anticoagulation in patients with atrial fibrillation. Catheter Cardiovasc Interv 2003;60:417-422.

111. Hanna IR, Kolm P, Martin R, et al: Left atrial structure and function after percutaneous left atrial appendage transcatheter occlusion (PLAATO): Six-month echocardiographic follow-up. J Am Coll Cardiol 2004;43:1868-1872.

112. Fountain RB, Holmes DR, Chandrasekaran K, et al: The PROTECT AF (WATCHMAN Left Atrial Appendage System for Embolic PROTECTion in Patients with Atrial Fibrillation) trial. Am Heart J 2006;151:956-961.

113. Connolly S, Pogue J, Hart R, et al: Clopidogrel plus aspirin versus oral anticoagulation for atrial fibrillation in the Atrial fibrillation Clopidogrel Trial with Irbesartan for prevention of Vascular Events (ACTIVE W): A randomised controlled trial. Lancet 2006;367:1903-1912.

50 Mitral Valvuloplasty

Alec Vahanian, Bertrand Cormier, and Bernard Iung

KEY POINTS

- The efficacy, safety, and applicability of the Inoue balloon technique are clearly established worldwide, and this technique is currently the point of reference for percutaneous mitral commissurotomy (PMC).
- Echocardiography is essential for monitoring the procedure and for assessment of the immediate results.
- The importance of experience cannot be stressed enough for the safety of the procedure and the selection of patients.
- PMC shows good immediate and long-term clinical results and carries a low risk when performed by experienced teams.

- The prediction of results is multifactorial; therefore, patient selection must be based on anatomy as well as other characteristics.
- PMC is the treatment of choice in patients with favorable characteristics.
- For other patients, the decision must be individualized, and PMC and valve replacement should be considered complementary techniques.

Until the first publication by Inoue and coworkers[1] describing percutaneous mitral commissurotomy (PMC) in 1984, surgery was the only treatment for patients with mitral stenosis. Most reports concerning PMC have been published since 1986. Since then, a considerable evolution in the technique has occurred. A large number of patients have now been treated, enabling efficacy and risk to be assessed, and midterm results are available, so we are better able to select the most appropriate candidates for treatment by this method.

As expected from the earlier experience with closed surgical commissurotomy, the good immediate and midterm results obtained during this period have led to increased worldwide use of the technique in several thousand patients. This chapter begins with a report of our own experience and then reviews the data available in the literature.

PERSONAL EXPERIENCE

Patients

We have attempted PMC in 2773 patients, whose mean age was 47 ± 15 years (range, 9-86 years).[2,3] Altogether, 71% were in class III or IV according to the classification system of the New York Heart Association (NYHA), and 31% were in atrial fibrillation. After fluoroscopic examination and echocardiography, the patients were divided into the following anatomic groups for selection of the most adequate treatment alternative[2]:

- The first group (11%) had flexible valves and mild subvalvular disease.
- The second group (62%) had flexible valves but extensive subvalvular disease (length of chordae <1 cm).
- The third group (27%) had calcified valves, as determined by echocardiography and confirmed by fluoroscopy.

Mild mitral regurgitation (grade 1/4) was present in 39% of patients. Regurgitation was moderate (grade 2/4) in only 2%.

Procedure

The antegrade approach was used in all cases. Transseptal catheterization was performed via the right femoral vein, using a standard Brockenbrough needle and a dilator (Cook). The atrial puncture was carried out using anteroposterior and 30-degree right anterior oblique views under continuous pressure monitoring. At this stage, heparin was given (3000 to 4000 U when using the Inoue technique).

In the early cases, we used a single-balloon technique ($n = 30$). We have also used the combination of a trefoil and a conventional balloon ($n = 586$). Since 1990, we have used the stepwise Inoue technique ($n = 2125$). No left heart catheterization was performed in the last 500 cases.

Patients were usually discharged 1 to 2 days after the procedure. Oral anticoagulation was continued in cases of atrial fibrillation or previous embolism.

Results

Immediate Hemodynamic and Echocardiographic Results

Successful PMC brought immediate hemodynamic improvement, as shown in Table 50-1. Echocardiographic techniques confirmed the results obtained by hemodynamics. The valve area increased from 1.0 ± 0.2 to 1.9 ± 0.3 cm^2, as assessed by two-dimensional echocardiography.

Poor results, as defined by a valve area less than 1.5 cm^2 or mitral regurgitation greater than 2/4 (or both), occurred in 11.5% of patients.

Technical Failures and Complications

We attempted PMC in 2773 patients, but the procedure was discontinued in 32 patients (1.2%) because of complications that occurred before PMC or technical failure.

The major adverse events were in-hospital death in 11 patients (0.4%), tamponade in 6 (0.2%), embolism with sequelae in 11 (0.4%), and severe mitral regurgitation ($\geq$3/4) in 113 (4.1%). Among the last group of patients, 84% were operated on, and valve repair was performed in 48% with good results. Other adverse events included local complications leading to urgent surgery in 17 patients (0.7%). Finally, 5% of patients had one or more major complications, and 130 (4.7%) underwent surgery within 1 month.

Midterm Results

The midterm results were obtained from a series of 1024 consecutive patients residing in France who underwent PMC.[4] Altogether, 96% of these patients were monitored for a mean of 52 months (range, 1-132 months). The follow-up evaluation consisted of a clinical examination with three major end points: survival, need for secondary surgery, and quality of the functional results. At 10 years, the midterm results were good: $85\% \pm 4\%$ of patients were alive, $61\% \pm 4\%$ were free from reoperation, and $56\% \pm 4\%$ were in good functional condition (i.e., NYHA class I or II).

Among patients with *poor initial results* ($n = 112$) due to severe mitral regurgitation or insufficient initial opening, 16 died (cardiac causes in 12); 74 were operated on (valve replacement in 60, conservative surgery in 14), and 6 were in NYHA class III or IV but were not operated on because of contraindications to surgery. In the remaining patients, the moderate improvement in valve function nevertheless provided transient symptomatic improvement.

In the group of patients with *initially successful PMC* ($n = 912$), the midterm results were good. The 10-year actuarial rates for (1) global survival (i.e., survival with no cardiac-related death), (2) survival with no cardiac-related death and no need for surgery or repeat dilation, and (3) the composite end point of good functional results were, respectively, $87\% \pm 4\%$, $67\% \pm 4\%$, and $61\% \pm 5\%$. A total of 46 patients died during follow-up (23 of cardiac-related causes). A repeat mitral valve procedure was required in 109 patients: repeat dilation in 21, open-heart commissurotomy in 13, and mitral valve replacement in 75. Surgical findings during the operations were restenosis in 97% of patients.

DEVICES AND TECHNIQUE

PMC acts in the same way as surgical commissurotomy, by opening the fused commissures (Fig. 50-1). PMC is of little or no help in cases of restricted valvular mobility caused by valve fibrosis or severe subvalvular disease. The techniques and devices used for PMC have varied over time and from group to group. At the present time, there are two approaches: transarterial and transvenous.

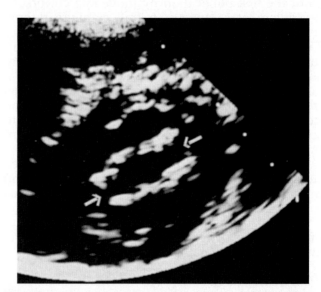

Figure 50-1. Transthoracic echocardiography (parasternal short-axis view) showing bicommissural opening *(arrows)*.

Table 50-1.   Immediate Results of Percutaneous Mitral Commissurotomy

Condition	Mean Pulmonary Artery Pressure (mm Hg)	Mean Left Atrial Pressure (mm Hg)	Cardiac Index (mm Hg)	Valve Area (cm^2)	Mean Gradient (mm Hg)
Before PMC	35 ± 13	22 ± 7	2.9 ± 0.7	1.04 ± 0.23	10.8 ± 4.8
After PMC	26 ± 10	13 ± 5	3.1 ± 5	1.92 ± 0.31	4.8 ± 2.1

PMC, percutaneous mitral commissurotomy.

Transarterial or Retrograde Approach

The transarterial approach has the advantage of minimizing or eliminating the risk of atrial septal defect and the disadvantage of potential arterial damage. The retrograde transarterial technique has now been abandoned because of its complexity. The retrograde technique without transseptal catheterization[5] has been used with good results and no serious complications, but its use is not widespread.

Transvenous or Antegrade Approach

The transvenous or antegrade approach is more widely used. It is performed through the femoral vein or, exceptionally, through the jugular vein.[6] Transseptal catheterization is the first step of the procedure and one of the most crucial steps. The conditions necessary for safe and successful transseptal catheterization are (1) knowledge of the anatomy, which may be modified in patients with mitral stenosis in whom normal geometry has been lost because both atria are enlarged and the convexity of the septum is exaggerated; (2) knowledge of the contraindications; and (3) experience of the operators with continuing performance of the technique. Usually, transseptal catheterization is performed under fluoroscopic guidance using one or several views. Continuous pressure monitoring is recommended.

Double-Balloon Technique

The double-balloon technique is one of the two main balloon techniques in current use; it has been described extensively.[2,7] Briefly, the technique is as follows. After transseptal catheterization, the left ventricle is catheterized with the use of a floating balloon catheter. One or two long exchange guide wires are positioned in the apex of the left ventricle or, less frequently, in the ascending aorta. The interatrial septum is dilated with the use of a peripheral angioplasty balloon (8 or 6 mm in diameter). Finally, the balloons (15 to 20 mm in diameter) are positioned across the mitral valve.

The Multi-Track system is a recent refinement of the double-balloon technique that uses a monorail system, requiring the presence of only one guide wire and easing the performance of the dilation compared with the standard double-balloon technique. Clinical experience with this device is still limited.[8]

Inoue Technique

The Inoue technique was the first one described,[1] and wide experience has now been acquired by a number of groups worldwide. The Inoue balloon, composed of nylon and rubber micromesh, is self-positioning and pressure-extensible. It is large (24 to 30 mm in diameter) and has a low profile (4.5 mm). The balloon has three distinct parts, each with a specific elasticity, enabling them to be inflated sequentially. This sequence allows fast, stable positioning across the valve. There are four sizes of the Inoue balloon (24, 26, 28, and 30 mm); each is pressure-dependent, so its diameter can be varied by up to 4 mm as required by circumstances. The main steps are as follows. After transseptal catheterization, a stiff guide wire is introduced into the left atrium. The femoral entry site and the atrial septum are dilated using a rigid dilator (14 Fr), and the balloon is introduced into the left atrium.

Inoue recommended the use of a stepwise dilation technique under echocardiographic guidance. Balloon size is chosen in accordance with the patient's height (26 mm in very small patients or infants, 28 mm in patients shorter than 1.60 m, and 30 mm in patients taller than 1.60 m). The balloon is inflated sequentially. First, the distal portion is inflated with 1 or 2 mL of a diluted contrast medium; it acts as floating balloon catheter when crossing the mitral valve. Second, the distal part is further inflated, and the balloon is pulled back into the mitral orifice. Inflation then occurs at the level of the proximal part and finally in the central portion, with the disappearance of the central waist at full inflation (Fig. 50-2; Videos 50-1 and 50-2).

The first inflation is performed 4 mm below the maximal balloon size, and the balloon size is increased in steps of 1 mm each. The balloon is then deflated and withdrawn into the left atrium. If mitral regurgitation (assessed by color Doppler echocardiography) has not increased by more than 1/4 and the valve area is less than $1 \text{ cm}^2/\text{m}^2$ of body surface area, the balloon is readvanced across the valve,[5] and PMC is repeated with a balloon diameter increased by 1 mm (Fig. 50-3). The criteria for ending are an adequate valve area or an increase in the degree of mitral regurgitation.

Data currently available comparing the double-balloon and Inoue techniques suggest that the Inoue technique eases the procedure and has equivalent efficacy and lower risk.[9] In fact, the Inoue technique has already become the most popular in the world, having been used in more than 10,000 patients. Finally, even though randomized studies are lacking and intraprocedural echocardiography lacks practicality, the stepwise technique under echocardiographic guidance certainly allows the best use of the mechanical properties of the Inoue balloon and therefore optimizes the results.

Metallic Commissurotome

During the late 1990s, Cribier and colleagues introduced the metallic commissurotome, which uses a device similar to the Tubb dilator used during closed commissurotomy.[10] Experience with this device comprises about 1000 cases, mainly from developing countries. The initial results suggest that the technique has efficacy similar to that of balloon commissurotomy, but the risk of hemopericardium seems higher owing to the presence of a stiff guide wire in the left ventricle. In addition, this technique is more demanding on the operator than the Inoue

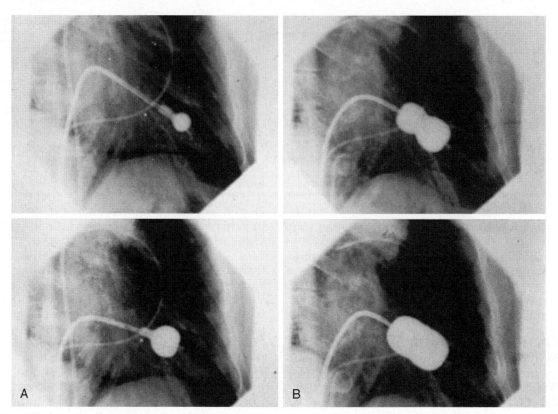

Figure 50-2. Inoue's percutaneous mitral commissurotomy technique. **A,** Inflation of the distal portion of the balloon, which is thereafter pulled back and anchored at the mitral valve. **B,** Subsequent inflation of the proximal and middle portions of the balloon. At full inflation, the waist of the balloon in its midportion has disappeared.

technique. The potential advantage is that the dilator is reusable, which reduces the cost of the procedure.

MONITORING AND EVALUATION OF IMMEDIATE RESULTS

There are two ways to assess immediate results in the catheterization laboratory: hemodynamics and echocardiography. Although echocardiography may be difficult to perform in the catheterization laboratory for logistic reasons, it provides essential information. First, echocardiography may facilitate puncture of the interatrial septum and perhaps crossing of the valve. This has been done primarily with the transesophageal approach,[11] which is superior to the transthoracic approach for imaging the interatrial septum. Nevertheless, the transesophageal approach is not easy in the catheterization laboratory and should probably be restricted to cases in which technical difficulties are encountered (e.g., severe anatomic distortion) (Video 50-3). More recently, intracardiac echocardiography has been used, although the price of the device is a serious limitation in most places.[12] Second, echocardiography provides essential information on the course of the mitral opening, which is of utmost importance when using the stepwise Inoue technique. Third, echocardiography enables detection of early complications such as a pericardial hemorrhage or severe mitral regurgitation.

The following guidelines have been suggested for the procedure. First, use of the mean left atrial pressure and mean valve gradient can be criticized because of variations that may occur, particularly with respect to changes in the heart rate or cardiac output. Second, repeated evaluation of the valve area during the procedure by hemodynamic measurements lacks practicality and may be subject to error because of the instability of the patient's condition and the inaccuracy of Gorlin's formula in the presence of atrial shunts or mitral regurgitation. The accuracy of Doppler measurements during valvuloplasty is low, so planimetry from two-dimensional echocardiography appears to be the method of choice if it is technically feasible.[13] Third, color Doppler assessment is the method of choice for sequential evaluation of the changes in the degree of regurgitation. Fourth, the commissural opening can be assessed by two-dimensional echocardiography using the short-axis view (Video 50-4).

The following criteria have been proposed for the desired end point of the procedure: (1) mitral valve area of more than 1 cm²/m² of the body surface area; (2) complete opening of at least one commissure; or (3) appearance or increment of regurgitation greater than 1/4. It is vital that the strategy be tailored to the individual circumstances, taking into account clinical factors together with anatomic factors and the cumulative data of periprocedural monitoring.

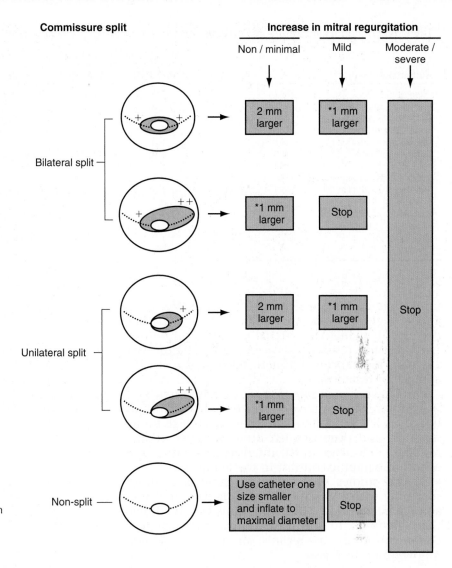

Figure 50-3. Decision-making during the stepwise dilation technique based on echocardiographic findings after each balloon dilation. +, incomplete split; + +, complete split; *, stop in cases of severely diseased valve or age older than 65 years.

For example, balloon size, increments of size, and expected final valve area are smaller in elderly patients and in the presence of tight mitral stenosis, extensive valve or subvalvular disease, or nodular commissural calcification.

After the procedure, the most accurate evaluation of valve area is achieved by echocardiography. To allow for the slight loss during the first 24 hours, this should be performed 1 to 2 days after mitral valvuloplasty, when the valve area may be calculated by planimetry or by the half-pressure time or continuity equation method. The degree of regurgitation may be finally assessed by angiography or color Doppler flow. The most sensitive method for assessing shunting is color Doppler flow, especially when transesophageal echocardiography (TEE) is used; this modality shows the importance of the defect and detects shunting in a more sensitive way than hemodynamic measurements. In current practice, we restrict the use of postvalvuloplasty TEE to patients with severe mitral regurgitation to evaluate the mechanisms or, in case of doubt, the degree of postprocedural mitral regurgitation.

In practice, in experienced centers, the procedure can be performed using a single venous approach and noninvasive monitoring, which diminishes the risk, discomfort, and costs.

Failures

The failure rate ranges from 1% to 17%.[2,3,14-17] Failure is often caused by an inability to puncture the atrial septum or position the balloon correctly across the valve. Most failures occur early in the investigator's experience. Failures can also result from unfavorable anatomy, such as severe atrial or predominant subvalvular stenosis.

Immediate Results

Hemodynamics

Our results, like those of others, demonstrate the efficacy of PMC, which usually provides an increase of more than 100% in the valve area (Table 50-2). The improvement in valve function results in an

Table 50-2. Immediate Results of Percutaneous Commissurotomy (PMC): Increase in Mitral Valve Area

Author (Ref. No.)	N	Age (Yr)	Mitral Valve Area (cm²)		Technique
			Before PMC	After PMC	
Chen et al. (16)	4832	37	1.1	2.1	Inoue balloon
Meneveau et al. (34)	532	54	1.0	1.7	Double- or Inoue ballon
Stefanadis et al. (5)	441	44	1.0	2.1	Modified single-, double-, or Inoue ballon (retrograde)
Bonhoeffer et al. (8)	100	31	0.8	2.0	Multitrack balloon
Hernandez et al. (35)	561	53	1.0	1.8	Inoue balloon
Cribier et al. (10)	500	34	0.9	2.1	Metallic commissurotome
Kang et al. (9)	152	42	0.9	1.8	Inoue balloon
(randomized comparison)	150	40	0.9	1.9	Double-balloon
Ben Farhat et al. (14)	654	33	1.0	2.1	Inoue or double-balloon
Arora et al. (15)	4850	27	0.7	1.9	Inoue or double-balloon or metallic commissurotome
Palacios et al. (7)	879	55	0.9	1.9	Inoue or double-balloon
Neumayer et al. (29)	1123	57	1.1	1.8	Inoue balloon
Iung et al. (3)	2773	47	1.0	1.9	Inoue, single-, or double-balloon
Fawzy et al. (37)	493	31	0.9	2.0	Inoue balloon

immediate decrease in left atrial pressure (Fig. 50-4) and a slight increase in cardiac index. A gradual decrease in pulmonary arterial pressure and pulmonary vascular resistance is seen.[18] High pulmonary vascular resistance continues to decrease in the absence of restenosis.

PMC has a beneficial effect on exercise capacity.[19] In addition, studies have shown that this technique improves left atrial and left atrial appendage pump function and decreases left atrial stiffness. It also results in a decrease in the intensity of spontaneous echocardiographic contrast in the left atrium.[20]

Several studies have compared surgical commissurotomy with PMC, mostly in patients with favorable characteristics. They have consistently shown that valvuloplasty is at least comparable to surgical commissurotomy as regards short and midterm follow-up up to 7 years.[21,22]

Complications

Large series[2,3,7,14-17] enable assessment of the risks in the technique (Table 50-3). Procedural *mortality* has ranged from 0% to 3% in most series. The main causes of death are left ventricular perforation and poor general condition of the patient.

The incidence of *hemopericardium* has varied from 0.5% to 12.0%. Pericardial hemorrhage may be related to transseptal catheterization or to apex perforation by the guide wires or the balloon itself when exaggerated movement occurs. If hemopericardium occurs, pericardiocentesis in the catheterization laboratory usually allows stabilization of the patient's condition and secondary transfer for cardiac surgery.

Embolism is encountered in 0.5% to 5.0% of cases. It is seldom the cause of permanent incapacitation and even more seldom the cause of death. It can be caused by gas if it occurs immediately after balloon rupture, by fibrinothrombotic material, or, on occasion, by calcium accumulation. Although the incidence of embolism is low, its potential consequences

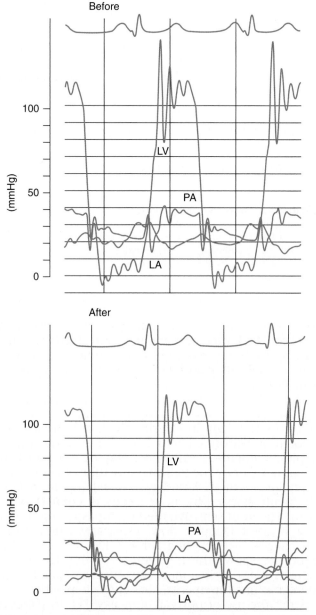

Figure 50-4. Hemodynamic changes after percutaneous mitral commissurotomy. LA, left atrium; LV, left ventricle; PA, pulmonary artery pressure.

Table 50-3. Severe Complications of Percutaneous Mitral Commissurotomy

Author (Ref. No.)	N	Age (Yr)	In-hospital Death (%)	Tamponade (%)	Embolic Events (%)	Severe Mitral Regurgitation (%)
NHLBI Registry* (31)	738	54				
n < 25			2	6	4	4
25 ≤ *n* < 100			1	4	2	3
n ≥ 100			0.3	2	1	3
Chen et al.* (16)	4832	37	0.1	0.8	0.5	1.4
Meneveau et al. (34)	532	54	0.2	1.1	—	3.9
Stefanadis et al.* (5)	441	44	0.2	0	0	3.4
Hernandez et al. (35)	620	53	0.5	0.6	—	4.0
Ben Farhat et al. (14)	654	33	0.5	0.6	1.5	4.6
Arora et al. (15)	4850	27	0.2	0.2	0.1	1.4
Palacios et al. (7)	879	55	0.6	1.0	1.8	9.4
Neumayer et al. (29)	1123	57	0.4	0.9	0.9	6.0
Iung et al. (3)	2773	47	0.4	0.2	0.4	4.1
Fawzy et al. (37)	504	31	0	0.8	0.6	1.8

*Multicenter series.
NHLBI, National Heart, Lung and Blood Institute.

are severe, and all possible precautions must be taken to prevent it.

In most cases, the degree of *mitral regurgitation* remains stable or, more often, slightly increases after PMC (Fig. 50-5). Conversely, in a few cases the degree of mitral regurgitation decreases, probably because of increased mobility of the leaflets.

Severe mitral regurgitation is rare, its frequency ranging from 2% to 19%.[2,3,14-17,23] Surgical findings[24] have shown that it is related to noncommissural tearing of the posterior or anterior leaflet. In these cases, one or both commissures are too tightly fused to be split. It may also be caused by excessive commissural splitting or, in rare cases, by rupture of a papillary muscle. In our experience, anatomic findings on surgery showed that severe mitral regurgitation occurred in patients with unfavorable anatomy: all had extensive subvalvular disease, and half had valve calcification. It has been suggested that the development of severe regurgitation depends more on the distribution of morphologic changes than on their severity.[25,26] Severe mitral regurgitation may be well tolerated; more often in our experience it is not, and surgery must be scheduled. In most cases, valve replacement is necessary because of the severity of the underlying valve disease. Conservative surgery, combining suture of the tear and commissurotomy, has been performed successfully in patients with a less severe valve deformity. In groups with good experience of mitral valve reconstruction, the need for valve replacement is more closely related to the extent of valve disease than to the tear itself. Overall, the occurrence of mitral regurgitation remains largely unpredictable in an individual patient.

The frequency of *atrial septal defect*[27] after PMC varies from 10% to 90% according to the technique used for its detection (Fig. 50-6; Video 50-5). These shunts are usually small and restrictive, with high-velocity flow. Right-to-left shunts occur on rare occasion in patients with elevated right-sided heart pressures and pulmonary hypertension.

The incidence of transient, complete *heart block* is 1.5%, and it seldom requires a permanent pacemaker. After the transvenous approach, *vascular complications* are the exception. *Urgent surgery* (within 24 hours) is seldom needed for complications resulting from PMC. It may be required, however, for massive hemopericardium resulting from left ventricular perforation unresponsive to pericardiocentesis or, less frequently, for severe mitral regurgitation leading to hemodynamic collapse or refractory pulmonary edema.

Overall, the incidence of failures and serious complications such as tamponade is clearly related to experience. When performed by experienced teams

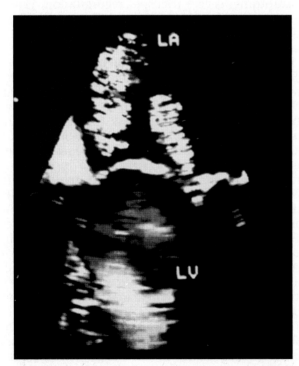

Figure 50-5. Transesophageal echocardiography (apical four-chamber view) showing two small jets of mitral regurgitation. LA, left atrium; LV, left ventricle.

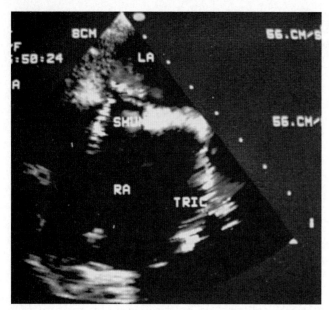

Figure 50-6. Transesophageal echocardiographic view of the atrial septum showing a small left-to-right shunt across the foramen ovale. LA, left atrium; RA, right atrium; TRIC, tricuspid valve.

Table 50-4. Late Results after Percutaneous Mitral Commissurotomy

Author (Ref. No.)	N	Age (Yr)	Follow-up (Yr)	Event-Free Survival (%)
Cohen et al. (30)	146	59	5	51*
Dean et al. NHLBI registry (31)	736	54	4	60*
Orrange et al. (32)	132	44	7	65*
Meneveau et al. (34)	532	54	7.5	52†
Stefanadis et al. (5)	441	44	9	75†
Hernandez et al. (35)	561	53	7	69†
Iung et al. (4)	1024	49	10	56†
Ben Farhat et al. (14)	654	34	10	72†
Palacios et al. (7)	879	55	12	33†
Fawzy et al. (37)	493	31	13	74†

*Survival without intervention.
†Survival without intervention and in New York Heart Association class I or II.

on properly selected patients, PMC is a relatively low-risk procedure.

Predictors of Immediate Results

Evaluation of immediate results is mainly based on hemodynamic criteria. The definition of good immediate results varies from series to series. The two definitions frequently employed are (1) a final valve area larger than 1.5 cm^2 and an increase in valve area of at least 25%, and (2) a final valve area larger than 1.5 cm^2 without mitral regurgitation greater than 2/4.

Many studies using different techniques of valvuloplasty have identified anatomy as a predictive factor of mitral valve area after the procedure. It was initially[28] thought to be the main predictor of the results, but it later appeared to be only a relative predictor. In fact, prediction of results is multifactorial.[2,7] Several studies have shown that, in addition to morphologic factors, preoperative variables such as age,[29] history of surgical commissurotomy, functional class, small mitral valve area, presence of mitral regurgitation before valvuloplasty, sinus rhythm, pulmonary artery pressure, and presence of severe tricuspid regurgitation, as well as procedural factors such as balloon size, are all independent predictors of the immediate results.

Identification of these variables linked to outcome has enabled models to be developed with a high sensitivity of prediction. Nevertheless, the specificity is low, indicating insufficient prediction of poor immediate results. This low specificity is particularly true in regard to the lack of accurate prediction of severe mitral regurgitation.

Midterm Results

We are now able to analyze follow-up data up to 15 years, which represents midterm results.[4,7,14,30-37] However, these data cover a relatively short period compared with surgical results.

In clinical terms, which are the most widely used, the overall midterm results of valvuloplasty are encouraging, as shown in Table 50-4. Prediction of long-term results is also multifactorial, based on clinical variables such as age, valve anatomy as assessed by echocardiography scores, factors related to the evolutionary stage of the disease (i.e., higher NYHA class before valvuloplasty), history of previous commissurotomy, severe tricuspid regurgitation, cardiomegaly, atrial fibrillation, high pulmonary vascular resistance, and the results of the procedure. The quality of the late results is generally considered to be independent of the technique used.[9]

Identification of these predictors provides important information for patient selection and is relevant to follow-up: Patients who have good immediate results but who are at high risk for further events must be carefully monitored to detect deterioration and allow timely intervention. Awareness of these predictors explains the discrepancies in follow-up results from reports that included patients with different characteristics: late results are clearly less satisfactory in North American and European series, where patients are older and frequently have severe valve deformities, than in studies from developing countries, where the patients studied have more favorable characteristics. Interpretation of the results must also take into account the regular inclusion of patients with poor immediate results in several series.

If PMC is *initially successful,* survival rates are excellent, the need for secondary surgery is infrequent, and functional improvement occurs in most cases. Ultrasound techniques are ideally suited for serially assessing the results of the procedure, whereas serial hemodynamic data are more difficult to obtain and

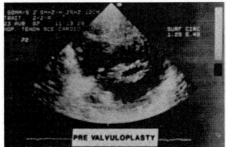
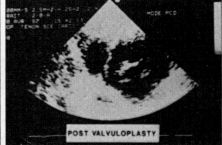
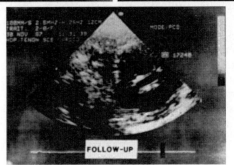

Figure 50-7. Transthoracic echocardiography (parasternal short-axis view) showing stable improvement in valve area after percutaneous mitral commissurotomy with a persistent bicommissural opening on follow-up.

less satisfactory because of overestimation of the valve area immediately after the procedure. With two-dimensional echocardiography or the Doppler technique, in most cases the improvement in valve function is stable (Fig. 50-7).

Determining the incidence of restenosis is compromised by the absence of a uniform definition. Restenosis after PMC has generally been defined as a loss of more than 50% of the initial gain with a valve area less than 1.5 cm^2. After successful PMC, the incidence of restenosis is usually low, between 2% and 40%,[4,7,14,33,37,38] at time intervals ranging from 3 to 10 years. Age, mitral valve area after PMC, and anatomy are considered predictors of restenosis, but the small number of series reporting patients with restenosis and the limited duration of follow-up preclude any definite conclusion in this regard. The ability to perform repeat valvuloplasty in cases of recurrent mitral stenosis is one of the potentials of this non-surgical procedure. Repeat valvuloplasty can be proposed if recurrent stenosis leads to symptoms, if it occurs several years after an initially successful procedure, and if the predominant mechanism of restenosis is commissural refusion. At the moment, despite the fact that repeat PMC represents 10% to 30% of the total number of balloon commissurotomies, only a few series are available on revalvuloplasty[39-41]; they report good immediate and midterm outcomes in patients with favorable characteristics. In our personal experience of 53 patients with favorable presenting characteristics who underwent repeat PMC,[39] the 5-year rates of continuing good functional results were 69% for the total population and 76% after a successful procedure.[39] Although the results are less favorable in patients presenting with worse characteristics, repeat valvuloplasty has a palliative role in patients who are not surgical candidates.[40] These preliminary results are encouraging, but the exact role

of revalvuloplasty must await larger series with longer follow-up to be defined.

If the immediate results are *unsatisfactory*, midterm functional results are usually poor. The prognosis of patients with severe mitral regurgitation after surgical commissurotomy or PMC is usually poor, with a lack of symptom alleviation and secondary objective deterioration. Surgical treatment is usually necessary during the following months.

In cases of an insufficient initial opening, delayed surgery is usually performed when the extracardiac conditions allow it. Here, valve replacement is necessary in almost all cases because of the unfavorable valve anatomy that was responsible for the poor initial results.

Follow-up studies using sequential TEE have shown that, despite numerous individual variations, the degree of mitral regurgitation, on the whole, remains stable or slightly decreases during follow-up. Atrial septal defects are likely to close later in most cases because of a reduced interatrial pressure gradient. The persistence of shunts is related to their magnitude (diameter of the defect > 0.5 cm or QP [pulmonary blood flow]/QS [systemic blood flow] ratio >1.5) or to unsatisfactory relief of the valve obstruction.

The low incidence of embolism during follow-up, the progressive decrease in intensity or disappearance of spontaneous echocardiographic contrast, and the improved left atrial function after PMC suggest a beneficial effect of the procedure on left atrial blood stasis, from which a lower risk of thromboembolism may be expected.[42] Finally, there is no direct evidence that PMC reduces the incidence of atrial fibrillation, even though it has a favorable influence on the predictors of atrial fibrillation (e.g., atrial size, degree of obstruction).[43]

To summarize the current experience, midterm follow-up data obtained after PMC are comparable to those from closed commissurotomy, which was to be expected from the similar mechanisms of these two techniques.

PARTICULAR APPLICATIONS OF PERCUTANEOUS MITRAL COMMISSUROTOMY

PMC after Surgical Commissurotomy

Several series have reported the results of PMC in patients with previous surgical commissurotomy.[44,45] This category of patients is of interest, because in Western countries recurrent mitral stenosis is becoming more frequent than primary mitral stenosis. Reoperation in this context is associated with a higher risk of morbidity and mortality and requires valve replacement in most cases.

All of the series reported to date show that PMC is feasible in this setting, although the procedure may be technically difficult in the case of "funnel-shaped" stenosis, which is frequent in these circumstances. PMC significantly improves valve function. The risks appear to be low, on a par with those of initial procedures. Midterm results are also satisfactory. As illustrated in our series of 232 patients who underwent PMC a mean of 16 years after surgical commissurotomy, the 8-year survival rate without intervention and without symptoms was 48% for the total series and 58% after good initial results.[44] On the whole, the results are good, even if slightly less satisfactory than those obtained in patients without previous commissurotomy; this probably can be attributed to less favorable characteristics observed in patients previously subjected to operation.

These encouraging preliminary data suggest that PMC may well postpone reoperation in selected patients with restenosis after commissurotomy. The indications for PMC in this subgroup of patients are similar to those for "primary PMC," but echocardiographic examination must be conducted with great care to exclude any patients in whom restenosis is due mainly to valve rigidity without significant commissural refusion. The latter mechanism could be responsible for the exceptional cases of mitral stenosis that develop in patients who have undergone mitral ring annuloplasty for correction of mitral regurgitation.

PMC in Patients with High Surgical Risk

Valvuloplasty is the only solution when surgery is contraindicated. It is also preferable to surgery, at least as the first attempt, in patients with an increased risk for surgery of cardiac origin, as in the following situations.

Preliminary reports have suggested that valvuloplasty can be performed safely and effectively in patients with *severe pulmonary hypertension*.[46] These results are encouraging even though they concern a limited number of patients.

In Western countries, many patients with mitral stenosis have concomitant noncardiac disease, which may also increase the risk of surgery.[38] Valvuloplasty can be performed as a life-saving procedure in *critically ill* patients,[47] as the sole treatment when there is an absolute contraindication to surgery, or as a "bridge" to surgery in other cases. In this context, dramatic improvement has been observed in young patients; on other hand, the outcome is very bad in elderly patients presenting with "end-stage" disease, who should probably be better treated conservatively.

In *elderly* patients, valvuloplasty results in moderate but significant improvement in valve function at an acceptable risk, although subsequent functional deterioration is frequent.[29,38] Therefore, valvuloplasty is a valid, if only a palliative, treatment for these patients.

During *pregnancy,* surgery carries a substantial risk of fetal mortality and morbidity, especially if extracorporeal circulation is required. The experience of PMC during pregnancy is still limited[48,49] but suggests the following. From a technical point of view, during the last weeks of pregnancy (which was the time of PMC in most cases), the procedure may be more difficult because of the enlarged uterus. The Inoue technique seems to be particularly attractive in this setting, because the fluoroscopy time is reduced and the short inflation-deflation cycle probably reduces the hemodynamic compromise. The procedure is effective and results in normal delivery in most cases. Regarding radiation exposure, PMC is safe for the fetus, provided that protection is provided by a shield that completely surrounds the patient's abdomen and the procedure is performed after the 20th week. In addition to radiation, PMC carries the potential risk of related hypotension and the always-present risk of complications that require urgent surgery. These preliminary data, which now represent several hundreds of cases, suggest that PMC can be a useful technique in the treatment of pregnant patients with mitral stenosis and refractory heart failure despite medical treatment.

PMC and Left Atrial Thrombosis

Left atrial thrombosis is generally considered a contraindication to PMC. However, a few limited series have shown that PMC using the Inoue balloon is feasible and is not a cause of systemic embolization.[50] In cases of left atrial thrombosis, if the clinical condition of the patient requires urgent treatment, the limited number of patients in these series does not allow us to recommend PMC if the patient is a candidate for surgery.[51,52] This recommendation is self-evident if the thrombus is free-floating or is situated in the left atrial cavity; it also applies when the thrombus is located on the interatrial septum. If the thrombus is located in the left atrial appendage, it has not been shown to our satisfaction that the Inoue technique under transesophageal guidance precludes a risk of embolism. If the patient is clinically stable, as is the case for most patients with mitral stenosis, anticoagulant therapy can be given for 2 to 6 months[53]; then, if a new transesophageal examination shows that the thrombus has disappeared, PMC can be attempted.

SELECTION OF PATIENTS

The application of PMC depends on four major factors: the patient's clinical condition; the valve anatomy; the experience of the medical and surgical teams of the institution concerned; and the financial aspect.[51,52]

Evaluation of Patient's Clinical Condition

Evaluation must take into account the degree of functional disability, the presence of contraindications to transseptal catheterization, and the alternative risk of surgery as a function of the underlying cardiac and noncardiac status. Because of the small but definite risk inherent in the technique, truly asymptomatic patients with severe mitral stenosis (i.e., patients with normal physical working capacity on exercise testing) usually are not candidates for PMC, except in cases of urgent need for extracardiac surgery, to allow pregnancy in young women, or in patients with an increased risk of embolism, such as those with a previous history of embolism, heavy spontaneous contrast in the left atrium, or recurrent atrial arrhythmias. Finally, PMC can be proposed in patients who declare to be asymptomatic but who have pulmonary hypertension either at rest (systolic pulmonary pressure >50 mm Hg) or on exercise (>60 mm Hg), the thresholds of which should be refined by the increasing experience gained in exercise echocardiography. Under these conditions, PMC should be performed only by experienced interventionists when the anatomy is suitable, leading to a safe, effective procedure.

Contraindications to transseptal catheterization include suspected left atrial thrombosis (Video 50-6), severe hemorrhagic disorder, and severe cardiothoracic deformity. Increased surgical risk of cardiac origin (previous surgical commissurotomy or aortic valve replacement) or extracardiac origin (respiratory insufficiency, old age) makes balloon valvuloplasty preferable to surgery, at least as the first attempt, or even as the only solution in case of a strict contraindication to surgery. The coexistence of moderate aortic valve disease and severe mitral stenosis is another situation in which PMC is preferable to postpone the inevitable later surgical treatment of both valves.

Valve Anatomy

The assessment of anatomy has several aims when establishing indications and prognostic considerations. It is critical to ensure that there are no anatomic contraindications to the technique (Table 50-5). The first of these is the presence of left atrial thrombosis, which must be excluded by systematic performance of TEE a few days before the procedure.

Table 50-5. Contraindications to Mitral Valvuloplasty

Left atrial thrombosis
Mitral regurgitation >2/4
Massive or bicommissural calcification
Severe aortic valve disease, or severe tricuspid stenosis + regurgitation, associated with mitral stenosis
Severe concomitant coronary artery disease requiring bypass surgery

The second is mitral regurgitation greater than grade 2/4, which contraindicates valvuloplasty. Third, in cases of combined mitral stenosis and severe aortic disease, the indication for surgery is obvious in the absence of contraindications. Fourth, the presence of combined severe tricuspid stenosis and tricuspid regurgitation with clinical signs of heart failure is an indication for surgery on both valves. On the other hand, the existence of tricuspid regurgitation is not a contraindication to the procedure even though it represents a negative prognostic factor.[54]

Our view on the performance of PMC in patients with only mild mitral stenosis (valve area >1.5 cm^2) is that the risks probably outweigh the benefits, and these patients are usually well managed by medical treatment.[51,52]

For prognostic considerations, echocardiographic assessment allows the classification of patients into anatomic groups with a view to predicting the results. Most investigators use the Wilkins score (Table 50-6),[28] whereas others, such as Cormier and colleagues,[2] use a more general assessment of valve anatomy (Table 50-7). Controversy exists regarding the most effective echocardiography scoring system in the prediction of results of mitral valvuloplasty. In

Table 50-6. Anatomic Classification of the Mitral Valve (Massachusetts General Hospital, Boston)

Leaflet Mobility
Highly mobile valve with restriction of only the leaflet tips
Midportion and base of leaflets have reduced mobility
Valve leaflets move forward during diastole, mainly at the base
No or minimal forward movement of the leaflets during diastole

Valvular Thickening
Leaflets near normal (4-5 mm)
Midleaflet thickening, marked thickening of the margins
Thickening extends through the entire leaflets (5-8 mm)
Marked thickening of all leaflet tissue (>8-10 mm)

Subvalvular Thickening
Minimal thickening of chordal structures just below the valve
Thickening of chordae extending up to one third of chordal length
Thickening extending to the distal third of the chordae
Extensive thickening and shortening of all chordae extending down to the papillary muscle

Valvular Calcification
Single area of increased echocardiographic brightness
Scattered areas of brightness confined to leaflet margins
Brightness extending into the midportion of leaflets
Extensive brightness through most of the leaflet tissue

Adapted from Abascal V, Wilkins GT, O'Shea JP, et al: Prediction of successful outcome in 130 patients undergoing percutaneous balloon mitral valvotomy. Circulation 1990;82:448-456.

Table 50-7. Anatomic Classification of the Mitral Valve (Bichat Hospital, Paris)

Echocardiographic Group	Mitral Valve Anatomy
1	Pliable noncalcified anterior mitral leaflet and mild subvalvular disease (i.e., thin chordae ≥10 mm long)
2	Pliable noncalcified anterior mitral leaflet and severe subvalvular disease (i.e., thickened chordae <10 mm long)
3	Calcification of mitral valve of any extent, as assessed by fluoroscopy, whatever the state of subvalvular apparatus

Adapted from Iung B, Cormier B, Ducimetiere P, et al: Immediate results of percutaneous mitral commissurotomy. Circulation 1996;94:2124-2130.

fact, none of the scores available today has been shown to be superior to the others, and all echocardiographic classifications have the same limitations: (1) reproducibility is difficult, because the scores are only semiquantitative; (2) lesions may be underestimated, especially with regard to the assessment of subvalvular disease; and (3) the use of scores describing the degree of overall valve deformity may not identify localized changes in specific portions of the valve apparatus (leaflets, commissures), which may increase the risk of severe mitral regurgitation (Table 50-8).[26] Therefore, we can only recommend the use of the system with which one is most familiar and at ease. More recently, scores that take into account the uneven distribution of the anatomic deformities of the leaflets or the commissural area have been developed[55]; their preliminary results are promising but disputed, so further studies are needed to determine their exact value.[56]

Table 50-8. Calculation of Echocardiography Score to Predict Mitral Regurgitation after PMC

A/B: Calcification/fibrosis of leaflets
(Score anterior and posterior leaflets)
Thickening normal (4-5 mm) or only one thick segment
Evenly fibrotic/calcified without thin areas
Uneven distribution of Ca^{2+} thickening; thinner segments are mildly thickened (5-8 mm)
Uneven distribution of Ca^{2+} thickening; thinner segments are near normal (4-5 mm)

C: Fibrosis/Ca^{2+} of commissures
Only one commissure affected
Both commissures mildly affected
Ca^{2+} both commissures: one severely affected
Marked Ca^{2+} both commissures

D: Subvalvular disease
Minimal chordal thickening just below valve
Chordal thickening to one third of length
Thickening to distal one third of chordae
Shortening/fibrosis of all chordae to papillary muscle

Adapted from Padial LR, Freitas N, Sagie A, et al: Echocardiography can predict which patients will develop severe mitral regurgitation after percutaneous mitral valvulotomy. J Am Coll Cardiol 1996;27:1225-1231.

Experience of the Medical and Surgical Teams

The importance of training for PMC is demonstrated by the comparison of early and late experience in the same groups or of large-volume center reports and multicenter studies, including centers with variable experience. The incidence of technical failures and complications, particularly those related to transseptal catheterization, is clearly related to the operator's experience. In addition to improvements in the management of the interventional procedure, experience improves the selection of patients by means of clinical evaluation and echocardiographic assessment.[3]

Even though the considerable simplification resulting from use of the Inoue balloon may lead to a false sense of security when applying the technique, PMC clearly should be restricted to teams that have extensive experience with transseptal catheterization and are able to perform an adequate number of procedures. The interventionists who perform PMC must also be able to perform emergency pericardiocentesis. Immediate surgical backup does not seem to be compulsory. The exact arrangement for surgical backup varies from institution to institution, according to the severity of the condition being treated and the experience of the cardiologic and surgical teams.

Potential Indications

The selection of an individual candidate for PMC must be based on both clinical and anatomic variables, bearing in mind that anatomy is a simple, practical way to select patients for PMC even though it is not the sole criterion. No problem of indication is presented in cases in which surgery is contraindicated or with "ideal candidates," such as young adults with good anatomy: pliable valves and only moderate subvalvular disease (echocardiography score <8 [see Table 50-6]). Randomized studies comparing valvuloplasty with surgical commissurotomy showed that valvuloplasty is at least comparable to surgical commissurotomy in terms of efficacy and is no doubt more comfortable for the patient.[51,52] In practice, in Europe PMC has virtually replaced surgical commissurotomy.[57] Hence, PMC appears to be the procedure of choice for these patients, provided that it is affordable. In addition, if restenosis occurs, patients treated by valvuloplasty can undergo repeat balloon catheterization or surgery without the difficulties and inherent risk resulting from pericardial adhesions and chest wall scarring.[58]

On the other hand, much remains to be done to refine the indications for other patients, especially those with unfavorable anatomy, who are more common in Western countries. For this group, some advocate immediate surgery because of the less satisfying results of valvuloplasty, whereas others prefer valvuloplasty as an initial treatment for selected candidates, reserving the use of surgery for cases of failure or late deterioration.[59,60]

Unfortunately, no randomized studies are available for these patients, and a comparison of the results of balloon commissurotomy with those of surgical series is difficult because of differences in the patients involved and the fact that the surgical alternative is valve replacement in most cases (since open commissurotomy is now very seldom performed). Valve replacement has its drawbacks: operative mortality, particularly in the elderly, and prosthesis-related complications whose cumulative incidence compromises the late outcome, particularly in young patients who are most exposed to the risk of long-term deterioration.[61] The indications in this subgroup of patients must take into account its heterogeneity with respect to anatomy, especially the extent and location of calcification. Clinical status is even more vital, because this group includes both patients in good clinical condition and others who are not surgical candidates because of an associated comorbid condition. In this group of patients, we favor an individualistic approach that allows for the multifactorial nature of prediction. It is not possible to exclude the possibility of good results in poor candidates; consequently, we are led to propose wider indications for valvuloplasty as an initial treatment in selected patients.

As an illustration of what can be obtained by PMC in this setting, we analyzed the outcome of 432 patients who underwent PMC for mitral stenosis with mild to moderate calcification. At 8 years, the rate of continuing good functional results was 36%. The predictors were a young age, a low NYHA class, and sinus rhythm.[60] With other presenting characteristics, the 5-year rate of good functional results varied from 15% to 90% (Fig. 50-8).

Current opinion is that surgery can be considered the treatment of choice in patients with bicommissural or heavy calcification. On the other hand, in our opinion, balloon valvuloplasty can be attempted as a first approach in patients with extensive lesions of the subvalvular apparatus or moderate or unicommissural calcification, the more so because their clinical status argues in favor of it. Surgery should be considered reasonably early if the results are unsatisfactory or there is secondary deterioration.

The option of PMC in patients who are candidates for surgical commissurotomy depends on the results previously obtained by surgery and PMC in the given institution.

In our 15-year experience, candidates for PMC have become older and have less favorable anatomy; however, they undergo the procedure at an earlier functional stage. The stability of the results, despite the less favorable characteristics, may be related to the role of experience in improving the technique and patient selection.[3]

FUTURE PROSPECTS

Large-scale use of the technique would be beneficial in developing countries, where mitral stenosis occurs frequently[62] in patients with anatomy favorable for PMC. However, this fundamentally depends on the solution of logistic and economic problems.

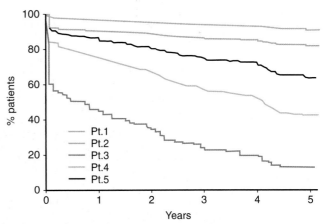

Figure 50-8. Predicted probability of good immediate results (valve area ≥ 1.5 cm^2 without regurgitation, Sellers' grade >2) and good late functional results (survival with no intervention and in New York Hearth Association [NYHA] class I or II) according to patient characteristics. Values are given for a procedure using an Inoue balloon with an effective balloon dilating area of 5.5 cm^2 or more (i.e., final diameter ≥ 27 mm). Pt. 1: <50 years of age, NYHA class II, sinus rhythm, calcium grade 1, valve area 1.25-1.50 cm^2. Pt. 2: age <50, class II, sinus rhythm, grade 2, area 1.00-1.25 cm^2. Pt. 3: age 50-70, class III, sinus rhythm, grade 2, area 1.25-1.50 cm^2. Pt. 4: age 50-70, class III, atrial fibrillation, grade 2, area 1.25-1.50 cm^2. Pt. 5: ≥ 70 years, class III, atrial fibrillation, grade 3, area 0.75-1.00 cm^2. (From Iung B, Garbarz E, Doutrelant L, et al: Late results of percutaneous mitral commissurotomy for calcific mitral stenosis. Am J Cardiol 2000;85:1308-1314.)

In industrialized countries, the problems are different because most candidates are older, with somewhat less favorable anatomy. Careful evaluation of immediate and long-term results in this population is still needed to define clearly the respective indications for PMC and valve replacement. This process will be improved through better imaging.[63] Further improvement may be achieved through combining PMC with other interventional procedures such as closure of left atrial appendage or ablation of the pulmonary veins,[64] or even percutaneous mitral valve repair or replacement[65] in case of failure or deterioration after PMC.

The good results that have been obtained with PMC enable us to say that, currently, this technique has an important place in the treatment of mitral stenosis and has virtually replaced surgical commissurotomy. Finally, in our opinion, when treating mitral stenosis, PMC and valve replacement must be considered not as rivals but complementary techniques, each applicable at the appropriate stage of the disease.

REFERENCES

1. Inoue K, Owaki T, Nakamura T, et al: Clinical application of transvenous mitral commissurotomy by a new balloon catheter. J Thorac Cardiovasc Surg 1984;87:394-402.
2. Iung B, Cormier B, Ducimetiere P, et al: Immediate results of percutaneous mitral commissurotomy. Circulation 1996;94: 2124-2130.

3. Iung B, Nicoud-Houel A, Fondard O, et al: Temporal trends in percutaneous mitral commissurotomy over a 15-year period. Eur Heart J 2004;25:701-707.

4. Iung B, Garbarz E, Michaud P, et al: Late results of percutaneous mitral commissurotomy in a series of 1024 patients: Analysis of late clinical deterioration—Frequency, anatomic findings, and predictive factors. Circulation 1999;99:3272-3278.

5. Stefanadis C, Stratos C, Lambrou S, et al: Retrograde nontransseptal balloon mitral valvuloplasty: Immediate results and intermediate long-term outcome in 441 cases. A multi-center experience. J Am Coll Cardiol 1998;32:1009-1016.

6. Joseph G, Chandy S, George P, et al: Evaluation of a simplified transseptal mitral valvuloplasty technique using over-the-wire single balloons and complementary femoral and jugular venous approaches in 1,407 consecutive patients. J Invasive Cardiol 2005;17:132-138.

7. Palacios IF, Sanchez PL, Harrell LC, et al: Which patients benefit from percutaneous mitral balloon valvuloplasty? Prevalvuloplasty and postvalvuloplasty variables that predict long-term outcome. Circulation 2002;105:1465-1471.

8. Bonhoeffer P, Hausse A, Yonga G, et al: Technique and results of percutaneous mitral valvuloplasty with the multi-track system. J Interv Cardiol 2000;13:263-269.

9. Kang DH, Park SW, Song JK, et al: Long-term clinical and echocardiographic outcome of percutaneous mitral valvuloplasty: Randomized comparison of Inoue and double-balloon techniques. J Am Coll Cardiol 2000;35:169-175.

10. Cribier A, Eltchaninoff H, Carlot R: Percutaneous mechanical mitral commissurotomy with the metallic valvotome: Detailed technical aspect and overview of the results of the multi-center registry 882 patients. J Interv Cardiol 2000;13:255-256.

11. Park SH, Kim MA, Hyon MS: The advantages of on-line transesophageal echocardiography guide during percutaneous balloon mitral valvuloplasty. J Am Soc Echocardiogr 2000;13:26-34.

12. Green NE, Hansgen AR, Carroll JD: Initial clinical experience with intracardiac echocardiography in guiding balloon mitral valvuloplasty: Technique, safety, utility, and limitations. Catheter Cardiovasc Interv 2004;63:385-394.

13. Palacios IG: What is the gold standard to measure mitral valve area post-mitral balloon valvuloplasty? Catheter Cardiovasc Diagn 1994;33:315-316.

14. Ben Farhat M, Betbout F, Gamra H, et al: Predictors of long-term event-free survival and of freedom from restenosis after percutaneous balloon mitral commissurotomy. Am Heart J 2001;142:1072-1079.

15. Arora R, Kalra G, Murty GS, et al: Percutaneous transatrial mitral commissurotomy: Immediate and intermediate results. J Am Coll Cardiol 1994;23:1327-1332.

16. Chen CR, Cheng TO: Percutaneous balloon mitral valvuloplasty by the Inoue technique: A multicenter study of 4832 patients in China. Am Heart J 1995;129:1197-1202.

17. National Heart, Lung, and Blood Institute Balloon Valvuloplasty Registry: Complications and mortality of percutaneous balloon mitral commissurotomy. Circulation 1992;85:2014-2024.

18. Krishnamoorthy KM, Dash PK, Radhakrishnan S, Shrivastava S: Response of different grades of pulmonary artery hypertension to balloon mitral valvuloplasty. Am J Cardiol 2002;90:1170-1173.

19. Tanabe Y, Oshima M, Suzuki M, et al: Determinants of delayed improvement in exercise capacity after percutaneous transvenous mitral commissurotomy. Am Heart J 2000;139:889-894.

20. Cormier B, Vahanian A, Iung B, et al: Influence of percutaneous mitral commissurotomy on left atrial spontaneous contrast of mitral stenosis. Am J Cardiol 1993;71:842-847.

21. Ben Fahrat M, Ayari M, Maatouk F: Percutaneous balloon versus surgical closed and open mitral commissurotomy: Seven-year follow-up results of a randomized trial. Circulation 1998;97:245-250.

22. Cardoso LF, Grinberg M, Pomerantzeff PM, et al: Comparison of open commissurotomy and balloon valvuloplasty in mitral stenosis: A five-year follow-up. Arq Bras Cardiol 2004;83:248-252.

23. Varma PK, Theodore S, Neema PK, et al: Emergency surgery after percutaneous transmitral commissurotomy: Operative versus echocardiographic findings, mechanisms of complications, and outcomes. J Thorac Cardiovasc Surg 2005;130:772-776.

24. Choudhary SK, Talwar S, Venugopal P: Severe mitral regurgitation after percutaneous transmitral commissurotomy: Underestimated subvalvular disease. J Thorac Cardiovasc Surg 2006;131:927-928.

25. Hernandez R, Macaya C, Benuelos C, et al: Predictors, mechanisms, and outcome of severe mitral regurgitation complicating percutaneous mitral valvotomy with the Inoue balloon. Am J Cardiol 1993;70:1169-1174.

26. Sutaria N, Shaw TR, Prendergast B, Northridge D: Transoesophageal echocardiographic assessment of mitral valve commissural morphology predicts outcome after balloon mitral valvotomy. Heart 2006;92:52-57.

27. Cequier A, Bonan R, Dyrda I, et al: Atrial shunting after percutaneous mitral valvuloplasty. Circulation 1990;81:1190-1197.

28. Abascal V, Wilkins GT, O'Shea JP, et al: Prediction of successful outcome in 130 patients undergoing percutaneous balloon mitral valvotomy. Circulation 1990;82:448-456.

29. Neumayer U, Schmidt HK, Fassbender D, et al: Early (three-month) results of percutaneous mitral valvotomy with the Inoue balloon in 1123 consecutive patients comparing various age groups. Am J Cardiol 2002;90:190-193.

30. Cohen DJ, Kuntz RE, Gordon SPF, et al: Predictors of long-term outcome after percutaneous balloon mitral valvuloplasty. N Engl J Med 1992;327:1329-1335.

31. Dean L, Mickel M, Bonan R, et al: Four-year follow-up of patients undergoing percutaneous balloon commissurotomy: A report from the National Heart, Lung and Blood Institute Balloon Valvuloplasty Registry. J Am Coll Cardiol 1996;28:1452-1457.

32. Orrange SE, Kawanishi DT, Lopez BM, et al: Actuarial outcome after catheter balloon commissurotomy in patients with mitral stenosis. Circulation 1997;95:382-389.

33. Wang A, Krasuski RA, Warner JJ, et al: Serial echocardiographic evaluation of restenosis after successful percutaneous mitral commissurotomy. J Am Coll Cardiol 2002;39:328-334.

34. Meneveau N, Schiele F, Seronde MF, et al: Predictors of event-free survival after percutaneous mitral commissurotomy. Heart 1998;80:359-364.

35. Hernandez R, Bañuelos C, Alfonso F, et al: Long-term clinical and echocardiographic follow-up after percutaneous mitral valvuloplasty with the Inoue balloon. Circulation 1999;99:1580-1586.

36. Chen CR, Cheng T, Chen JY, et al: Long-term results of percutaneous balloon mitral valvuloplasty for mitral stenosis: A follow-up study to 11 years in 202 patients. Catheter Cardiovasc Diagn 1998;43:132-139.

37. Fawzy ME, Hegazy H, Shoukri M, et al: Long-term clinical and echocardiographic results after successful mitral balloon valvotomy and predictors of long-term outcome. Eur Heart J 2005;26:1647-1652.

38. Hildick-Smith DJR, Taylor GJ, Shapiro LN: Inoue balloon mitral valvuloplasty: Long-term clinical and echocardiographic follow-up of a predominantly unfavorable population. Eur Heart J 2000;21:1691-1698.

39. Iung B, Garbarz E, Michaud P, et al: Immediate and mid-term results of repeat percutaneous mitral commissurotomy for restenosis following earlier percutaneous mitral commissurotomy. Eur Heart J 2000;21:1683-1690.

40. Pathan AZ, Mahdi NA, Leon MN, et al: Is redo percutaneous mitral balloon valvuloplasty (PMV) indicated in patients with post-PMV mitral restenosis? J Am Coll Cardiol 1999;34:49-54.

41. Turgeman Y, Atar S, Suleiman K, et al: Feasibility, safety, and morphologic predictors of outcome of repeat percutaneous balloon mitral commissurotomy. Am J Cardiol 2005;95:989-991.

42. Chiang C-W, Lo S-K, Ko Y-S, et al: Predictors of systemic embolism in patients with mitral stenosis: A prospective study. Ann Intern Med 1998;128:885-889.

43. Krasuski RA, Assar MD, Wang A, et al: Usefulness of percutaneous balloon mitral commissurotomy in preventing the development of atrial fibrillation in patients with mitral stenosis. Am J Cardiol 2004;93:936-939.

44. Iung B, Garbarz E, Michaud P: Percutaneous mitral commissurotomy for restenosis after surgical commissurotomy. J Am Coll Cardiol 2000;35:1295-1302.

45. Fawzy ME, Hassan W, Shoukri M, et al: Immediate and long-term results of mitral balloon valvotomy for restenosis following previous surgical or balloon mitral commissurotomy. Am J Cardiol 2005;96:971-975.

46. Maoqin S, Guoxiang H, Zhiyuan S, et al: The clinical and hemodynamic results of mitral balloon valvuloplasty for patients with mitral stenosis complicated by severe pulmonary hypertension. Eur J Intern Med 2005;16:413-418.

47. Vahanian A, Iung B, Nallet O: Percutaneous valvuloplasty in cardiogenic shock. In Hasdai D, Berger P, Battler A, Holmes D (eds): Cardiogenic Shock: Diagnosis and Treatment. Totowa, New Jersey, Humana Press, 2002, pp 181-193.

48. Weiss BM: Managing severe mitral valve stenosis in pregnant patients: Percutaneous balloon valvuloplasty, not surgery, is the treatment of choice. J Cardiothorac Vasc Anesth 2005;19:277-278.

49. Sivadasanpillai H, Srinivasan A, Sivasubramoniam S, et al: Long-term outcome of patients undergoing balloon mitral valvotomy in pregnancy. Am J Cardiol 2005;95:1504-1506.

50. Chen WJ, Chen MF, Liau CS, et al: Safety of percutaneous transvenous balloon mitral commissurotomy in patients with mitral stenosis and thrombus in the left atrial appendage. Am J Cardiol 1992;70:117-119.

51. Iung B, Gohlke-Bärwolf C, Tornos P, et al: Recommendations on the management of the asymptomatic patient with valvular heart disease. Eur Heart J 2002;23:1253-1266.

52. Bonow RO, Carabello BA, Chatterjee K, et al: ACC/AHA 2006 guidelines for the management of patients with valvular heart disease: A report of the American College of Cardiology/American Heart Association Task Force on Practice Guidelines. J Am Coll Cardiol 2006;48:e1-e148.

53. Silaruks S, Thinkhamrop B, Kiatchoosakun S, et al: Resolution of left atrial thrombus after 6 months of anticoagulation in candidates for percutaneous transvenous mitral commissurotomy. Ann Intern Med 2004;140:101-105.

54. Song JM, Kang DH, Song JK, et al: Outcome of significant functional tricuspid regurgitation after percutaneous mitral valvuloplasty. Am Heart J 2003;145:371-376.

55. Padial LR, Abascal VM, Moreno PR, et al: Echocardiography can predict the development of severe mitral regurgitation after percutaneous mitral valvuloplasty by the Inoue technique. Am J Cardiol 1999;83:1210-1213.

56. Mezilis ME, Salame MY, Oakly DG: Predicting mitral regurgitation following percutaneous mitral valvotomy with the Inoue balloon: Comparison of two echocardiographic scoring systems. Clin Cardiol 1999;22:453-458.

57. Iung B, Baron G, Butchart EG, et al: A prospective survey of patients with valvular heart disease in Europe: The Euro Heart Survey on valvular heart disease. Eur Heart J 2003;13:1231-1243.

58. Gamra H, Betbout F, Ben Hamda K, et al: Balloon mitral commissurotomy in juvenile rheumatic mitral stenosis: A ten-year clinical and echocardiographic actuarial results. Eur Heart J 2003;24:1349-1356.

59. Post JR, Feldman T, Isner J, et al: Inoue balloon mitral valvotomy in patients with severe valvular and subvalvular deformity. J Am Coll Cardiol 1995;25:1129-1136.

60. Iung B, Garbarz E, Doutrelant L, et al: Late results of percutaneous mitral commissurotomy for calcific mitral stenosis. Am J Cardiol 2000;85:1308-1314.

61. Hammermeister K, Seth GK, Henderson WG, et al: Outcomes 15 years after valve replacement with a mechanical versus a bioprosthetic valve: Final report of the veterans affairs randomized trial. J Am Coll Cardiol 2000;36:1152-1158.

62. Bahadur KC, Sharma D, Shresta MP, et al: Prevalence of rheumatic and congenital heart disease in schoolchildren of Kathmandu valley in Nepal. Indian Heart J 2003;55:615-618.

63. Zamorano J, Perez de Isla L, Sugeng L, et al: Non-invasive assessment of mitral valve area during percutaneous balloon mitral valvuloplasty: Role of real-time 3D echocardiography. Eur Heart J 2004;25:2086-2091.

64. Adragao P, Machado FP, Aguiar C, et al: Ablation of atrial fibrillation in mitral valve disease patients: Five year follow-up after percutaneous pulmonary vein isolation and mitral balloon valvuloplasty. Rev Port Cardiol 2003;22:1025-1036.

65. Vahanian A, Palacios IF: Percutaneous approaches to valvular disease. Circulation 2004;109:1572-1579.

51 Percutaneous Mitral Valve Repair

Ryan D. Christofferson and Samir R. Kapadia

KEY POINTS

- Mitral regurgitation (MR) is a significant problem, and the number of patients with MR is growing because of an increase in congestive heart failure. Surgical correction of MR with repair techniques yields better results than valve replacement; however, a significant number of patients undergo valve replacement even in the current era.

- Various percutaneous approaches to mitral valve repair are under preclinical and clinical investigation and show great promise for the future. These approaches are predominantly based on established surgical strategies.

- Different percutaneous techniques provide specific advantages depending on the anatomical and functional characteristics of mitral regurgitation. Selection of the appropriate technique for each individual patient will ultimately determine the success of these emerging technologies.

- Integration of established imaging modalities both in and out of the catheterization laboratory is critical for safety and efficacy of percutaneous repair technologies. The development of emerging imaging modalities will likely play a role in the future of percutaneous technologies.

- Evaluation of new percutaneous devices poses a significant challenge because these devices have to be compared to surgical options that may have different expectations in the overall management of the patient. It is likely that percutaneous techniques will have a complementary role to surgery.

New percutaneous technology is poised to significantly alter the treatment paradigm for chronic mitral regurgitation (MR). Percutaneous mitral valve repair offers the potential benefit of decreased morbidity, improved recovery time and shorter hospital stays compared to open-heart surgery. However, before widespread adoption, percutaneous repair faces a number of challenges, namely the accomplishment of reasonably equivalent long-term results compared to surgical repair. The bar is set high, given that surgical mitral valve repair, when feasible, and performed in an experienced center, carries a high success rate and low rate of morbidity and mortality Additionally, current iterations of percutaneous techniques cannot completely approximate the current surgical options, given that no single device can perform both an annuloplasty and a leaflet repair.

There are several mechanisms of chronic MR and it is unlikely for a "one-size-fits-all" device to be created that is capable of addressing all these different forms. In fact, it is likely that percutaneous techniques will be more specific to the particular type of MR and to a patient's anatomical characteristics than surgical mitral valve repair. Therefore, a thorough understanding of the mechanisms of MR and the imaging studies necessary to characterize a patient's anatomy are necessary for proper patient selection. In addition, an understanding of the indications for surgery and outcomes of surgery are necessary to properly advise a patient considering percutaneous mitral valve repair.

Current percutaneous options are loosely based on surgical repair techniques, with four primary methods to accomplish a reduction in MR. Edge-to-edge leaflet repair, indirect coronary sinus annuloplasty, direct annuloplasty and septal-lateral annular cinching are the predominant device design concepts. It remains to be seen if percutaneous techniques must be equivalent to surgery in order to be successful, given the potentially low rate of morbidity associated with percutaneous procedures. The future of percutaneous mitral valve repair may actually be in treatment of less symptomatic or less advanced MR prior to the development of left ventricular dysfunction, with preservation of surgical options for more advanced disease. The use of percutaneous devices for acute MR remains to be explored. Regardless, it appears that percutaneous valve intervention will remain a hot topic for the foreseeable future.

MITRAL VALVE DISEASE

Mitral Valve Anatomy

The mitral valve complex is composed of the mitral annulus, anterior and posterior leaflet, chordae tendineae, and papillary muscles.[1] The mitral annulus is the elliptical area of attachment of the mitral valve to the base of the left atrium (Fig. 51-1). The posterior leaflet is attached to the posterior annulus and has three lobes or scallops, the lateral (P1), central (P2), and medial scallop (P3), respectively. The anterior leaflet does not have scallops per se but has named segments that correspond to the posterior leaflet scallops, namely A1, A2, and A3. The valve leaflets meet at each end of the annulus, called the lateral (anterolateral) and medial (posteromedial) commissure, respectively. The chordae connect each leaflet to both the lateral (anterolateral) and medial (posteromedial) papillary muscles. The primary chordae connect to the free edge of the leaflet. The secondary chordae, known as "strut" chords, are thicker and connect to the rough zone of the leaflet. The tertiary chordae are short and connect the basal zone of the leaflet to the ventricular free wall.

Normal mitral valve closure is dependent on the appropriate anatomy and function of each component of the mitral valve.[2] Closure of the mitral valve occurs because of traction of the papillary muscles at the onset of systole, moving the leaflets into apposition. In addition, contraction of the myocardium underlying the annulus results in a decrease in annular area, mainly due to the posterior flexible portion of the leaflet, aiding leaflet coaptation. Elevation in left ventricular pressure, combined with vortices produced on the ventricular side as a result of flow deceleration across the valve, forces the leaflets into apposition. Systolic left ventricular contraction combined with papillary muscle traction on the leaflets produces a billowing but not eversion of the leaflets. The significant redundancy of the leaflets allows the force generated by ventricular contraction to be transmitted to the area of leaflet contact, maintaining valve competence.

Etiology and Mechanism of Mitral Regurgitation

Anatomic or functional abnormalities of any of the structures in the mitral valve apparatus may lead to MR.[3,4] The disease process leading to MR may be a primary mitral valve disease, secondary regurgitation resulting from another cardiac disease, or mitral valve involvement in a systemic inflammatory disease (Table 51-1). Primary mitral valve diseases include myxomatous degeneration of the leaflets and chordae, with resulting chordae elongation or rupture, flail leaflet or mitral valve prolapse, rheumatic heart disease with leaflet and chordal thickening and fusion, and infective endocarditis leading to leaflet and annular disruption. Secondary valve disease is generally caused by structural disruption of the geometric arrangement of the mitral apparatus. Cardiomyopathy, either due to ischemic or non-ischemic etiology, leads to ventricular dilatation, resulting in mitral annular dilation and altered papillary muscle-leaflet interaction. In addition, ischemic cardiac disease can result in a papillary muscle dysfunction or rupture. In hypertrophic cardiomyopathy the anterior mitral leaflet motion is altered by left ventricular outflow tract obstruction, resulting in systolic anterior motion and mitral regurgitation. Systemic inflammatory diseases, such as systemic lupus erythematosus, rheumatoid arthritis, and scleroderma are less commonly encountered and even less frequently managed with valve repair, as the condition frequently improves with treatment of the underlying systemic disorder.

Various terminology is used to characterize the mechanisms of mitral regurgitation. The morphologic description, proposed by Carpentier,[5] classifies the mechanism of regurgitation according to leaflet pathophysiology (Fig. 51-2). In this characterization,

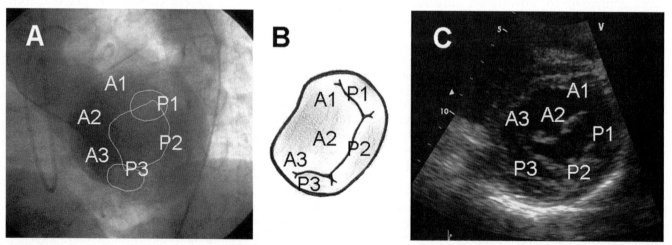

Figure 51-1. Mitral valve anatomy: **A,** left ventriculogram in the left anterior oblique projection showing the mitral valve in short axis, with labeled leaflet segments; **B,** a schematic of the mitral valve in short axis; **C,** a transthoracic echocardiographic image of the mitral valve in the parasternal short axis projection.

Type I regurgitation occurs in the presence of normal leaflet motion and is usually caused by annular dilatation or leaflet perforation. Type II is caused by leaflet prolapse, which is commonly the result of degenerative (myxomatous) disease, chordal elongation or rupture, and papillary muscle elongation or rupture. Type III is due to restricted leaflet motion, which may be due to posterior wall motion abnormality or papillary muscle dysfunction from ischemic cardiac disease, and commissural fusion and/or leaflet or chordal thickening from rheumatic heart disease. This simplification has utility in terms

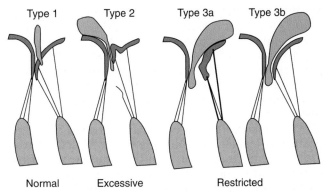

Figure 51-2. Carpentier classification of mitral regurgitation according to function leaflet mobility. Type 1 exhibits normal leaflet mobility as with endocarditis. Type 2 exhibits excessive leaflet mobility as in degenerative disease or mitral valve prolapse. Type 3a exhibits restricted leaflet motion due to chordal and leaflet thickening from rheumatic heart disease. Type 3b exhibits restricted leaflet motion due to ventricular wall motion abnormality from dilated or ischemic cardiomyopathy.

Table 51-1. Causes of Chronic Mitral Regurgitation

Primary mitral valve disorder
Degenerative valve disease
  Myxomatous degeneration
  Mitral valve prolapse
  Mitral annular calcification
Rheumatic valve disease
Infective endocarditis
Chordal rupture
  Idiopathic
  Traumatic
Congenital lesions
  Cleft anterior mitral leaflet or fenestration
  Parachute mitral valve abnormality
Prosthetic valve disorder
  Paravalvular regurgitation
  Prosthetic valve degeneration
  Prosthetic valve endocarditis

Secondary mitral valve disorder (cardiac cause)
Ischemic mitral regurgitation (coronary artery disease)
  Papillary muscle dysfunction or rupture
  Mitral valve annular dilation
  Global or regional ventricular dysfunction
  Left ventricular dilation
Dilated (nonischemic) cardiomyopathy
Hypertrophic cardiomyopathy

Systemic/inflammatory disease
Systemic lupus erythematosus
Amyloidosis
Connective tissue disorder
Rheumatoid arthritis

of surgical and percutaneous approach, as the goal of therapy may be to restore normal leaflet function, but not necessarily normal valve anatomy.

Another common method of categorizing MR is based on the etiology and mechanism of MR. This classification is commonly used in literature to study the clinical outcomes of patients (Table 51-2). In this classification scheme, MR is divided loosely into four categories: degenerative, functional, ischemic, and rheumatic.

Degenerative disease includes mitral valve prolapse, Barlow's syndrome, and myxomatous degeneration, and the mechanism of MR is leaflet prolapse or flail. This is the most common etiology to present for surgical mitral valve repair, representing approximately 70% of the US surgical population. Functional MR occurs in the setting of severe left ventricular dysfunction accompanied by annular dilation, with an increase in interpapillary muscle distance,

Table 51-2. Mechanisms and Classification of Mitral Regurgitation (MR)

Carpentier's Morphologic Classification	**Etiologic Classification**
Type I: Normal leaflet motion Annular dilation Dilated cardiomyopathy Leaflet perforation Annular calcification	Functional MR*
Type II: Leaflet prolapse Chordal rupture/flail leaflet Chordal elongation Papillary muscle elongation Papillary muscle rupture	Degenerative MR
Type III: Restricted leaflet motion IIIA: Fibrosis of the subvalvular apparatus IIIB: Regional LV remodeling/wall motion abnormality	Rheumatic MR Ischemic MR

*"Functional MR" is sometimes used to describe both ischemic and nonischemic MR, because they share a common characteristic of left ventricular geometric remodeling and annular dilation with normal leaflet morphology.

amplified leaflet tethering, and decreased mitral closing forces. It is estimated that 20% of all congestive heart failure patients have MR, representing approximately 3 million patients worldwide. The development of MR portends a worse prognosis in congestive heart failure, and can initiate a cascade of worsening left ventricular dilation, dysfunction, and regurgitation.

When functional MR occurs as a result of restricted posterior leaflet motion due to ventricular wall motion abnormality or papillary muscle tethering, typically after inferior myocardial infarction, it is termed functional ischemic MR or simply ischemic MR.[6] In this condition, changes in left ventricular geometry lead to leaflet "tenting" and anterior leaflet override, which prevents proper coaptation (Fig. 51-3).[7] Around 30% of all patients undergoing revascularization have moderate to severe mitral regurgitation. Finally, MR in rheumatic disease is a result of leaflet deformity due to severe calcification and apical leaflet doming. Although this is a common cause of MR worldwide, it is less frequently encountered in the United States and even less frequently managed surgically. Regardless of the mechanism of MR, mitral annular remodeling and dilation appear to play a significant role.[8,9]

Pathophysiology

Mitral regurgitation leads to ventricular volume overload. In the setting of acute severe MR, such as with papillary muscle rupture, the acute volume overload leads to elevated left ventricular filling pressure,

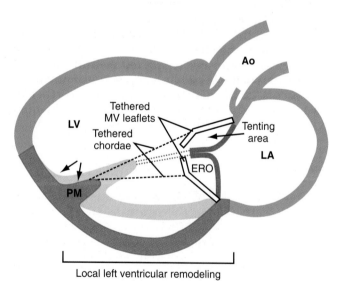

Figure 51-3. The mechanism of ischemic MR is posterior wall remodeling and wall motion abnormality due to myocardial ischemia and infarction, leading to altered left ventricular geometry and tethering of the mitral valve leaflets. Proper coaptation of the leaflets is prevented, leading to mitral regurgitation. The area under the leaflets is termed the tenting area, and ERO represents effective regurgitant orifice. (Adapted from Bursi F, Enriquez-Sarano M, Jacobsen SJ, Roger VL: Mitral regurgitation after myocardial infarction: A review. Am J Med 2006;119:103-112.)

causing severe left heart failure. However, in chronic severe MR, elevated left ventricular filling pressure is compensated by left ventricular enlargement and eccentric hypertrophy, restoring normal filling pressure.[10] The ejection fraction is actually supranormal, as the ejection fraction reflects both antegrade aortic stroke volume and regurgitant volume. Left atrial pressure may be mildly elevated. Compensation may be maintained for many years; however, myocardial contractile dysfunction ensues in some patients, potentially due to molecular mechanisms. The left ventricle becomes dilated and end-diastolic volume increases, leading to mitral annular dilation and further worsening of the severe MR. The stroke volume decreases and the ejection fraction falls below normal, with an increase in ventricular preload and left atrial pressure, resulting in pulmonary hypertension.

Patients with chronic severe MR often complain of gradual and progressive dyspnea on exertion. They may also experience chronic fatigue and weakness due to a low cardiac output. On exam, patients with MR often demonstrate a harsh, pansystolic murmur, predominantly at the apex, but frequently radiating to the axilla or neck. A systolic click may be present in patients with mitral valve prolapse. A thrill may occasionally be palpated at the apex. The murmur should not change with inspiration, but may increase with Valsalva maneuver. The apical impulse may be hyperkinetic. Lung exam is frequently normal in chronic MR, while the chest roentgenogram shows cardiomegaly and left atrial enlargement. The electrocardiogram often demonstrates left ventricular hypertrophy, left atrial enlargement, and frequently the rhythm is atrial fibrillation.

Natural History

The natural history of patients with chronic MR depends on the degree of regurgitation,[11] the cause of the underlying disorder,[12] and the degree of left ventricular dysfunction.[13] Available data on the natural history of the disease is limited by small sample size, selection bias, inconsistent measures of MR severity, and the inclusion of disparate etiologies of regurgitation. However, it appears that many patients with chronic MR may remain asymptomatic for many years.[14] Among patients with mild MR, there is an inconsistent rate of progression to severe MR that appears to be independent of medical treatment.[15] When chronic severe MR is present, there is a consistent rate of decline in clinical status, such that approximately 5-10% of patients per year develop significant symptoms, clinical indication for surgery, and/or death.[14,16] This may occur in the absence of prognostically important endpoints such as left ventricular dysfunction, indicating that earlier intervention, prior to the development of overt structural changes, may influence the natural history of the disease.[16]

The importance of symptoms on long-term prognosis is demonstrated by the high mortality rate reported for patients with New York Heart Association class III or IV symptoms and flail mitral leaflet (Fig. 51-4). Left ventricular ejection fraction, however, remains an important independent predictor of outcome in patients with chronic severe MR due to degenerative disease.[13]

The management of asymptomatic patients with severe MR remains controversial, with recent opinion in favor or earlier intervention when valve repair can be undertaken successfully.[17] Patients with degenerative valve disease have a favorable long-term prognosis whether treated medically, or when indicated, surgically. However, patients with degenerative valve disease and coronary disease are fundamentally different than those with degenerative disease alone, and have a worse prognosis that is dominated by the contribution of coronary disease.[12] In addition, ischemic MR actually worsens the long-term prognosis of patients with MR of any degree after a myocardial infarction. The presence and degree of mitral regurgitation is an independent predictor of mortality in this group,[18] emphasizing the importance of accurately quantifying MR after myocardial infarction.

IMAGING

Echocardiography

Echocardiography is the dominant modality for imaging the mitral valve and assessment of MR severity. Two-dimensional echocardiography is useful to evaluate valvular structure and the consequences of volume overload on the left ventricle. Additional information may include the presence of calcification, leaflet tethering, flail leaflet, or wall motion abnormalities. The severity of the regurgitation can be accurately quantified, as well as the specific hemodynamic consequences of the regurgitation. In most cases, a combination of clinical information and echocardiographic data will establish the etiology of mitral regurgitation and the particular anatomy of the mitral valve, which is important in assessing candidacy for surgical or percutaneous intervention. Longitudinal data collected by serial echocardiography is used to determine timing of intervention and to follow-up the results. If transthoracic images are not adequate, transesophageal echocardiography provides an excellent assessment of mitral valve anatomy and severity of regurgitation. This can be particular useful to determine if valve repair is feasible.

The evaluation of the severity of valvular regurgitation by echocardiography relies heavily on Doppler methods, including Color Doppler, Pulsed wave (PW) and Continuous wave (CW) Doppler. The American Society of Echocardiography has determined the qualitative and quantitative echocardiographic parameters that are useful in grading MR (Table 51-3).[19] The assessment of severity should rely on the integration of both quantitative and qualitative measures obtained by Doppler techniques.[20] In addition, structural findings such as flail leaflet or enlarged left atrium can add useful information with regards to regurgitation severity.

Color Doppler provides qualitative visualization of the origin and width of the regurgitant jet, the spatial orientation of the jet, and the area of the left atrium occupied by regurgitant flow. A proximal flow convergence on color Doppler is present in severe regurgitation. The proximal isovelocity surface area (PISA) of this flow convergence can be utilized to accurately quantitate effective regurgitant orifice area (ERO) (see Fig. 51-8).[21] The width of the regurgitant jet at or just downstream from the regurgitant orifice is known as the vena contracta, and is slightly smaller than the anatomic regurgitant orifice.[22] The jet area can provide a rapid semi-quantitative assessment of regurgitation severity. However, jet area is influenced by instrument factors including instrument gain, and jet orientation, as a central jet may appear more severe than an equally large jet that impinges on the atrial wall. The direction of the regurgitant jet, if eccentric, can indicate a possible structural problem such as prolapse or flail with the leaflet opposite of the color jet. In addition, the color jet area is influenced by the driving pressure across the valve, and can be enhanced by elevated blood pressure.

Regurgitant volume can be assessed by continuous wave Doppler data. Regurgitant volume is calculated by applying the continuity equation (conservation of mass), where left-sided regurgitant volume is calculated as the difference between Doppler-derived flow across the aortic and mitral valves.[23] The stroke volume equals the cross-sectional area of the valve annulus, multiplied by the velocity-time integral of flow across the annulus. The regurgitant volume at the mitral valve is calculated as the difference between the stroke volume across the mitral valve and the aortic valve. This can also be expressed as a regurgitant fraction.

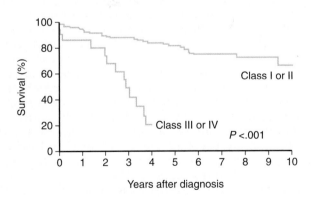

No. at risk

Class I or II	162	117	102	95	80	69	50	33	20	12	7
Class III or IV	66	15	12	7	3						

Figure 51-4. Long-term survival of patients with flail leaflet according to New York Heart Association functional class. Survival is significantly less in patients with Class III or IV heart failure. (From Ling LH, Enriquez-Sarano M, Seward JB, et al: Clinical outcome of mitral regurgitation due to flail leaflet. N Engl J Med 1996;335:1417-1423.)

Table 51-3. Qualitative and Quantitative Parameters for Grading the Severity of Mitral Regurgitation

Parameter	Mild	Moderate	Severe
Structural			
Size of LA	Normal	Normal or dilated	Usually dilated
Size of LV	Normal	Normal or dilated	Usually dilated
Mitral leaflets or support apparatus	Normal or abnormal	Normal or abnormal	Abnormal/flail leaflet/ruptured papillary muscle
Doppler			
Color flow jet area	Small, central jet (usually <4 cm² or <20% of LA area)	Variable	Large central jet (usually >10 cm² or >40% of LA area) or variable-size wall-impinging jet swirling in LA
Mitral inflow—PW	A-wave dominant	Variable	E-wave dominant
Jet density—CW	Incomplete or faint	Dense	Dense
Jet contour—CW	Parabolic	Usually parabolic	Early-peaking to triangular
Pulmonary vein flow	Systolic dominance	Systolic blunting	Systolic flow reversal
Quantitative			
Width of vena contracta (cm)	<0.3	0.3-0.69	≥0.7
Regurgitant volume (mL/beat)	<30	30-59	≥60
Regurgitant fraction (%)	<30	30-49	≥50
ERO (cm²)	<0.20	0.20-0.39	≥0.40

CW, continuous wave; ERO, effective regurgitant orifice; LA, left atrium; LV, left ventricle; PW, pulse wave.
From Zoghbi WA, Enriquez-Sarano M, Foster E, et al: Recommendations for evaluation of the severity of native valvular regurgitation with two-dimensional and Doppler echocardiography. J Am Soc Echocardiogr 2003;16:777-802.

Pulsed wave Doppler is useful to assess the effect of regurgitation on the pulmonary venous flow. If the pulmonary venous flow is blunted or reversed in systole, this can give an indication of severe regurgitation.[24,25] The contour and density of the regurgitant envelope on Continuous wave Doppler is also useful, as dense, early peaking or triangular envelope is most consistent with severe regurgitation. In addition, on Pulsed wave Doppler, the mitral inflow pattern is typically E wave dominant in severe regurgitation, reflecting increased flow across the valve.

Alternate Imaging Modalities

While echocardiography remains the dominant imaging modality in assessment of MR, cardiac computed tomography (CT),[26] cardiac magnetic resonance (CVMR),[27] and three-dimensional (3D) echocardiography[20] are likely to play a more important role in the future. As coronary sinus devices are under development to indirectly alter annular geometry, the proximity of the coronary sinus to the mitral annulus is increasingly important information (Fig. 51-5). In addition, the coronary sinus and left circumflex artery are in close proximity and at times overlap, creating the potential for cinching devices to hinder coronary blood flow. It remains to be seen how this technology may be used to select patients for percutaneous repair.

With CVMR it is possible to obtain significant structural information regarding the geometry of the left ventricle, mitral annulus and leaflets, and quantitative regurgitant volumes (Fig. 51-6).[27] It is likely that the regurgitant volumes calculated with CVMR may be more accurate and operator/reader independent than with transthoracic echocardiography.

However, limited experience with this modality currently limits its utility to research purposes. Finally, 3D echocardiography may become important in assessing valve characteristics and geometry, in addition to the possibility of providing "real time" guidance of percutaneous valve interventions, an application limited by current technological capabilities.

SURGICAL MITRAL VALVE REPAIR

Mitral valve repair is the preferred method of surgical management of MR.[28] When compared to mitral valve replacement, the major advantages of mitral valve repair are improved survival, preservation of left ventricular function, freedom from anticoagulation, and fewer complications.[29,30] Despite the advantages of repair, this technique appears to be underutilized, as less than half of patients undergoing mitral valve surgery currently get a repair procedure although about 90% of patients are candidates for repair.[31,32] In the United States, the most commonly encountered categories of mitral valve dysfunction are degenerative, functional, and ischemic MR, which represent the conditions for which repair is likely to succeed. The goal of mitral valve repair is to restore normal leaflet function and annular size.

The American College of Cardiology and American Heart Association recently released new guidelines for patient selection and timing of mitral valve surgery.[28] Any patient with acute severe MR should undergo valve surgery. In addition, any patient with symptomatic chronic severe MR should have surgery, even if there is normal left ventricular systolic function (New York Heart Association heart failure class

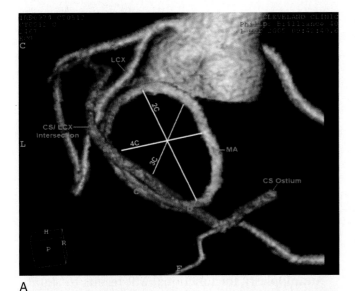

A

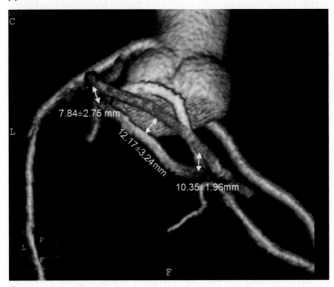

B

Figure 51-5. Computed tomography images of the relationship between the mitral annulus (MA), coronary sinus (CS) and left circumflex coronary artery (LCX). Panel A shows the coronary sinus traveling along the posterior mitral annulus, and crossing over the left circumflex artery. Panel B shows that the distance between the annulus and the coronary sinus varies depending on the location along the annulus.

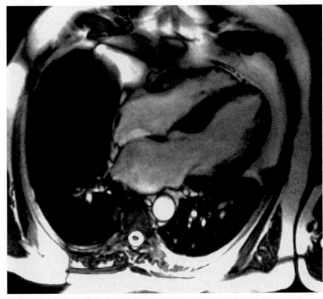

A

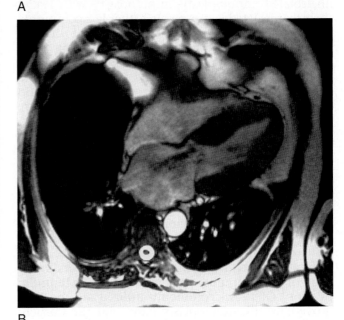

B

Figure 51-6. Magnetic resonance images of the mitral valve in systole (Panel A) and diastole (Panel B), demonstrating significant mitral regurgitation as a result of hypertrophic cardiomyopathy and systolic anterior motion of the mitral leaflet. (Courtesy of Dr. Sri Sola).

II-IV). If the patient is asymptomatic with chronic severe MR, the development of left ventricular dysfunction (ejection fraction <60%) or dilation of the left ventricle (end-systolic dimension = 40 mm) should mandate surgical intervention. It is acceptable to attempt mitral valve repair in asymptomatic patients with preserved left ventricular size and systolic function, if the surgical center is experienced in repair techniques, and repair is deemed to be likely (>90% chance of success).

The onset of atrial fibrillation, or the development of significant pulmonary hypertension (pulmonary artery systolic pressure >50 mm Hg at rest or >60 mm Hg with exercise) in an asymptomatic patient with normal left ventricular size and systolic function can also be an indication for surgery. In patients with primary valve disease and severe left ventricular dilation (end-systolic dimension >55 mm) or severe left ventricular dysfunction (ejection fraction <30%), mitral valve surgery is reasonable if repair is likely. If there is secondary valve dysfunction (functional MR) and severely decreased left ventricular function (ejection fraction <30%), repair may be considered after medical optimization and biventricular pacing, if indicated.

Surgical Approach

Mitral valve surgery can be perfomed by median sternotomy or minimally invasive approach, utilizing the partial upper sternotomy or small right thoracotomy. Median sternotomy is required if concomitant coronary bypass is undertaken. Cardioplegic arrest and cardiopulmonary bypass are necessary regardless of the type of chest wall incision, although typically less than one hour is required for a valve repair. After exposure of the mitral valve is obtained, the valve is interrogated with a nerve hook to determine the site of prolapse or flail and to assess for candidacy of repair.[5] The most frequently utilized methods of repair address the annulus, including annuloplasty (with or without a rigid or flexible ring), decalcification and debridement; or the leaflets, including triangular resection, quadrangular resection, sliding annuloplasty, patch enlargement, decalcification, or edge-to-edge repair. This can be done as an isolated annuloplasty, annuloplasty with leaflet repair, or isolated leaflet repair. Other less commonly utilized repair methods have been applied to address abnormalities of the commissures, including commissurotomy or sliding annuloplasty; the chordae, including chordal resection, division, transposition, shortening, or artificial chordae implantation; and the papillary muscles with papillary muscle division, reimplantation, shortening, or lengthening.

Isolated Annuloplasty

Available annuloplasty techniques include suture alone, suture with buttressing material, or prosthetic annuloplasty devices. The choice of annuloplasty technique is debated among surgeons. The placement of a prosthetic annuloplasty band or ring is utilized to correct annular dilation, increase leaflet coaptation by reducing the anterior-posterior dimension of the annulus, and prevent future annular dilation. Of these, commonly utilized are the Cosgrove-Edwards annuloplasty band and the Carpentier-Edwards annuloplasty ring. The major difference in the above devices is that the Cosgrove-Edwards device is a located along the posterior annulus, which has been shown to be the area of greatest annular dilation in degenerative and functional mitral regurgitation. The location and flexibility of this band may allow preservation of normal annular motion, although this has not been demonstrated to influence clinical outcome.[33] Functionally, the annuloplasty ring has the effect of transforming the mitral valve into a monocuspid valve, as frequently posterior leaflet motion is restricted after the repair.

To perform an annuloplasty, sutures are passed through the mitral annulus, then through the valvuloplasty band or ring. In suture-only annuloplasty, the suture is placed in a double semi-circular configuration around the posterior annulus and reinforced with pledgets at the commissures. As the sutures are tied, the annulus is effectively plicated and the annular size is reduced, with the intent of improving leaflet coaptation and reducing mitral regurgitation. There is considerable debate regarding the optimal type of annuloplasty and size of the annuloplasty ring. It is common practice to undersize the annuloplasty ring for functional MR.

Isolated ring annuloplasty without leaflet repair is the dominant strategy for MR resulting from functional or ischemic cardiomyopathy. It can be performed safely in patients with severe left ventricular dysfunction, resulting in a low operative mortality (~2%) and favorable perioperative morbidity.[34,35] Direct comparisons of repair versus replacement in this setting favor repair owing to lower operative morbidity and mortality.[36] Although suture-only annuloplasty is less expensive and has been shown to provide reasonable results,[37,38] ring annuloplasty may have better durability and survival[39] and remains the dominant strategy.

Annuloplasty for functional MR results in significant improvement in NYHA class, decreased admissions for heart failure, and modest survival rates of 71-82% at 2 years and 58% at 5 years. Although favorable changes in left ventricular size, shape and function have been demonstrated after successful mitral valve repair,[35] a propensity analysis failed to demonstrate a mortality benefit compared to matched patients not undergoing valve surgery.[40] The recurrence rate of functional MR after isolated annuloplasty is disappointing (28% at one year), and remains a limitation to widespread utilization of the procedure.[41] It appears that in ischemic cardiomyopathy, severe posterior papillary muscle displacement is one mechanism of recurrence,[42] in addition to increasing annular diameter and higher tethering height.[43]

Annuloplasty with Leaflet Repair

The combination of annuloplasty and leaflet repair, often referred to as Carpentier's techniques, is most frequently performed for degenerative mitral valve disease. Of the surgical methods of mitral leaflet repair, correction of posterior leaflet or bileaflet prolapse is the most common. Posterior leaflet prolapse occurs in the majority of cases of degenerative mitral valve disease, and is the primary cause of regurgitation in approximately one half of patients. Prolapse is a result of chordal elongation or rupture, and affects the P2 segment most frequently. This type of problem is most frequently corrected by posterior leaflet quadrangular resection and plication of the valve annulus.[5] It is generally accompanied by the placement of a prosthetic annuloplasty ring, except in cases of severe calcification of the annulus.

Anterior leaflet prolapse, although less common than posterior leaflet prolapse, is a more challenging problem, and is commonly treated with initial valve replacement. However, several methods have been developed to treat anterior leaflet prolapse by leaflet repair. The most common are chordal transfer, artificial chordae creation, and the Alfieri edge-to-edge repair. Chordal transfer is performed by resection of a segment of the posterior leaflet that is then trans-

Table 51-4. Recurrence Rates for 3+ or Greater Mitral Regurgitation (MR) and Reoperation Rates with Standard Carpentier Surgical Repair Techniques

Study	N	Reoperation Rate at Latest Follow-up	MR≥3+ at Latest Follow-up
Gillinov et al. (Ann Thorac Surg, 2000)	197	5% at 5 yr	9% at 1.5 yr
Flameng et al. (Circulation, 2003)	242	5.8% at 7 yr	29% at 7 yr

ferred and sewn to the prolapsing segment of the anterior leaflet. A quadrangular repair of the anterior leaflet completes this procedure. Another method of anterior leaflet repair involves the creation of artificial chordae from Gore-Tex sutures. These artificial chordae are attached to the prolapsing leaflet and the papillary muscle by pledgeted sutures.

The long-term results for mortality, recurrent MR, and reoperation with Carpentier's repair in experienced centers are better than with mitral valve replacement,[44] and with a mortality rate similar to that of the general population (86-93% survival at 5 years).[33,44-46] The long-term recurrance rates are favorable with Carpentier's repair (Table 51-4).[45,46] The Cleveland Clinic has achieved excellent results, including a 0.3% operative mortality rate, and ten year freedom from reoperation of 93% (Fig. 51-7).[45] The majority of reoperations were for progression of degenerative disease. The recurrence rate of severe MR (grade 3+ or 4+) after repair is 3.7% per year.[46]

Isolated Leaflet Repair with Edge-to-Edge Technique

Alfieri has pioneered a creative repair initially developed for anterior leaflet prolapse, where the free edge of the anterior and the posterior leaflets are sewn together in an attempt to increase leaflet contact and coaptation, and reduce regurgitation.[47] This technique also works for posterior leaflet and bileaflet prolapse. It is useful in preventing systolic anterior motion of the anterior mitral leaflet following tradi-

tional mitral valve repair techniques.[48] The resulting double-orifice mitral valve does not generally cause stenosis, even when combined with an annuloplasty ring.

The first report of this technique was published in 1998 by Dr. Alfieri's group in Milan, Italy.[47] From a total of 432 patients undergoing valve repair at their institution between January of 1991 to September of 1997, 121 patients underwent edge-to-edge correction. The indication was anterior prolapse in 61% of patients. The majority of patients had a double-orifice repair (60%) with the remainder undergoing a paracommissural repair. There was a low rate of in-hospital mortality (1.6%) and overall survival was good (92% at 6 years) with 95% freedom from reoperation (Fig. 51-8). The majority of patients were NYHA class I or II (>80%).

Following Dr. Alfieri's lead, the technique was adopted into practice at many prominent institutions performing mitral valve repair, although generally as a specialized technique and not a primary method. The introduction of percutaneous edge-to-edge repair has fueled interest in the surgical outcomes of this procedure, leading to the publication of a number of single-center case series (Table 51-5).[48-53] The procedure has been applied to both degenerative and ischemic MR with favorable results.

PERCUTANEOUS MITRAL VALVE REPAIR

The advantage of percutaneous valve repair technology is its promise to reduce the morbidity and

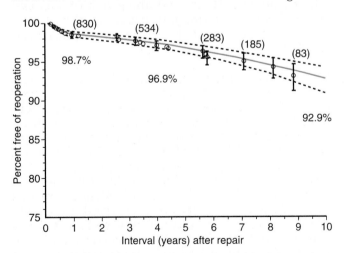

Figure 51-7. Freedom from reoperation after standard Carpentier repair for degenerative disease. (From Gillinov AM, Cosgrove DM, Blackstone EH, et al: Durability of mitral valve repair for degenerative disease. J Thorac Cardiovasc Surg 1998;116:734-743.)

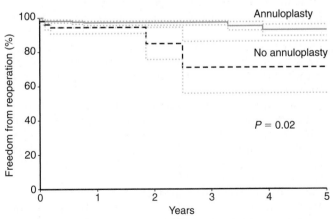

Figure 51-8. Long-term mortality results from the initial surgical edge-to-edge repair cohort from Milan, Italy. (From Alfieri O, Maisano F, De Bonis M, et al: The double-orifice technique in mitral valve repair: A simple solution for complex problems. J Thorac Cardiovasc Surg 2001;122:674-681.)

Table 51-5. Published Reports of Surgical Edge-to-Edge Repair for Mitral Insufficiency: Etiology, Prevalence of Associated Annuloplasty, and Outcomes

Parameter	Alfieri (2001)	Lorusso (2001)	Kherani (2004)	Bhudia (2004)	De Bonis (2005)	Kuduvalli (2006)
No. patients	260	75	71	224	54	41
Pathology (%)						
Degenerative	81	49	N/R	14	—	73
Ischemic	2	3	N/R	64	66	12
Rheumatic	10	24	N/R	—	—	5
Endocarditis	6	21	N/R	3	—	2
Other	1	3	N/R	19	33	8
Associated annuloplasty (%)	80	82	56	84	100	80
In-hospital mortality (%)	0.7	3.7	4.2*	2	4.3	4.8
Long-term outcome						
Years of follow-up	5	8	5	5	2.7	5
Survival (%)	94.4	92	58.3	65	90.7	95.1
Freedom from reoperation (%)	90	80	—†	—‡	—§	86
MR≥3+ (%)	N/R	14	N/R	24	9	0

*30-day mortality.
†3 reoperations.
‡21 reoperations including 7 transplantations.
§2 reoperations.
MR, mitral regurgitation; N/R, not reported.

mortality associated with traditional invasive surgical repair. However, the results of such a procedure should be comparable to the surgical standard. To accomplish this goal, new valve technology must overcome, some of the limitations inherent in percutaneous procedures, namely vascular access, decreased visualization, and reduced tactile feedback. This is counterbalanced by the ability to perform percutaneous procedures under echocardiographic and fluoroscopic guidance without the need for cardioplegia and cardiopulmonary bypass. In addition, percutaneous repair offers the ability to assess the results of the repair on a beating heart, making it possible to adjust or reposition the device to achieve optimal results. However, there is currently no device capable of combining an annuloplasty and leaflet repair. If percutaneous and minimally invasive cardiac valve technologies can be made simple, relatively fail-safe, and preserve surgical options, they represent the future of valve intervention. Critical to successful percutaneous repair are improved imaging techniques, such as cardiac CT, MRI, and 3-D echocardiography. In addition, interventionalists should understand the valve pathology and indications for intervention.

There are currently four major approaches to percutaneous repair. The best-studied approach is the edge-to-edge repair, based loosely on the surgical repair championed by Dr. Alfieri. One such device (MitraClip) is currently in phase II clinical trials. The second approach utilizes the proximity of the coronary sinus to the mitral annulus to accomplish favorable changes in annular geometry, bringing the posterior leaflet towards the anterior leaflet, improving coaptation. Several devices are under investigation in early clinical trials. Next, left ventricular reshaping, accomplishing a reduction in septal-to-lateral diameter and improving leaflet coaptation,

can reduce mitral regurgitation. There is a minimally invasive surgical device with early clinical results (Coapsys), currently under modification to be used percutaneously. Finally, mitral annuloplasty can be performed by a transventricular (direct) approach using different approaches, including a suture-based annular cinching device, radiofrequency ablation catheter to shrink the annulus, and placement of shape-modifying annular devices that can be subsequently adjusted percutaneously. This area is less well developed, and pre-clinical studies are underway.

This chapter will focus on the procedural description, preclinical and clinical results, and the advantages and disadvantages of each approach (Table 51-6). The devices included in this review were selected primarily because of the extent of data and availability of information regarding the device. There are many other devices in development not selected for this chapter.

Edge-to-edge (Double-Orifice) Leaflet Repair

One of the early applications of surgical repair techniques to the problem of percutaneous valve intervention is the use of the edge-to-edge repair as conceived by Alfieri. While the surgical double orifice mitral valve repair has been shown to be effective as a treatment for structural or functional mitral valve disease, application of the surgical literature in this case is limited by the lack of data regarding isolated edge-to-edge repair, as most of the cases reported also had annuloplasty. However, an isolated edge-to-edge repair has been shown in a small series to have reasonable long-term results.[54] When successful, it appears that the percutaneous edge-to-edge procedure does produce the same double-orifice and fibrosing bridge segment as the surgical procedure, without

Table 51-6. Percutaneous or Minimally Invasive Mitral Valve Repair Devices under Development

Device Design	Developmental Phase
Edge-to-edge leaflet repair (edge-to-edge)	
MitraClip (Evalve, Menlo Park, CA)	Human phase II trial
MOBIUS (Edwards Lifesciences, Irvine, CA)	Human phase I trial
Indirect annuloplasty via coronary sinus	
Viacor PTMA (Viacor, Wilmington, MA)	Human phase I trial
CARILLON Mitral Contour System (Cardiac Dimensions, Kirkland, WA)	Human phase I trial
MONARC PTMA (Edwards Lifesciences, Irvine, CA)	Human phase I trial
Asymmetric sinus annuloplasty (St. Jude Medical, St. Paul, MN)	Preclinical phase
Septal-to-lateral diameter reduction	
iCoapsys (Myocor, Maple Grove, MN)	Preclinical phase
PS³ System (Ample Medical Inc., Foster City, CA)	Human phase I trial
Transventricular (retrograde) direct annuloplasty	
Mitralign Direct Annuloplasty System (Mitralign, Salem, NH)	Human phase I trial
GDS Accucinch Annuloplasty system (Guided Delivery Systems, Santa Clara, CA)	Preclinical phase
Other	
QuantumCor RF Annuloplasty (QuantumCor, Lake Forest, CA)	Preclinical phase
Micardia Dynamic Annuloplasty Ring (Micardia, Irvine, CA)	Preclinical phase

Phase I trial, feasibility and safety; phase II trial, pivotal clinical trial; preclinical, animal models or bench testing; PTMA, percutaneous transvenous mitral annuloplasty.

significant mitral stenosis.[55] There are two major devices in this class with significant preclinical and clinical data to evaluate their safety and efficacy.

Endovascular Cardiovascular Valve Repair System (CVRS)

In terms of clinical data, the best characterised of the percutaneous mitral valve repair technologies is that of St. Goar and Evalve Inc. (Menlo Park, CA), entitled the endovascular Cardiovascular Valve Repair System (CVRS), which utilizes a 24F steerable delivery guide catheter and a transseptal approach to place a v-shaped clip (MitraClip) on the mitral leaflets (Fig. 51-9).[56] The clip is designed to grasp the leaflets from beneath the valve, creating an effective double-orifice repair. The procedure is performed with transesophageal echocardiographic and fluoroscopic guidance. The clip is introduced via guide catheter into the left atrium, where the arms are deployed when the clip

is aligned with the long axis of the heart. The arms of the clip are then rotated until they are perpendicular to the line of coaptation of the valve leaflets. The open clip is advanced into the left ventricle, and retracted during systole to grasp the middle scallops of the anterior and posterior valve leaflets in the gripper arms. The positioning is confirmed by echo and the clip is locked into position. If needed, the clip is reopened, detaching from the leaflets, withdrawn into the left atrium, and the process is repeated until a functional double orifice is created. When the positioning is considered adequate, the clip is released from the guide and remains attached to the mitral valve leaflets. Eventually, fibrosis and scarring occur in the bridging segment, similar to that seen with the surgical edge-to-edge repair.[55]

Data from a porcine model was published in 2003, showing that in adult pigs with no mitral regurgitation (N=14), a functional double-orifice could be successfully created by endovascular placement of a mitral valve clip.[56] However, in two animals the

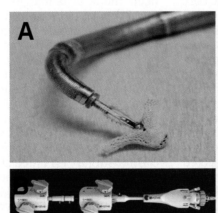

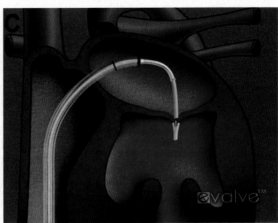

Figure 51-9. The Evalve MitraClip and delivery system. Panel A shows the device with gripper arms open, attached to the delivery catheter. Panel B shows the device delivery manipulation system. Panel C is a schematic of the delivery catheter and device across the septum and in place on the mitral valve, prior to device release.

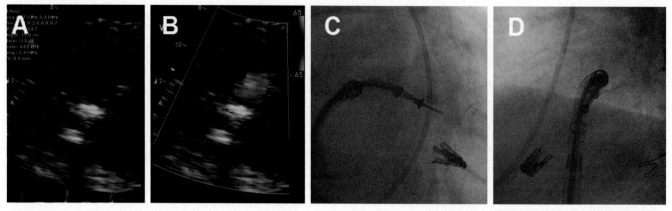

Figure 51-10. A demonstration of two clips on the mitral valve to prevent residual regurgitation after the placement of a single clip. Panel **A** shows a transthoracic image of the mitral valve in short axis, with two clips visible as echodense signals. Panel **B** shows the same image with color Doppler added. Panel **C** is a fluoroscopic image from the right anterior oblique projection, showing the two clips and a single delivery catheter, after the second clip has been released. Panel **D** shows the same image from a left anterior oblique projection.

anterior leaflet was incompletely grasped, resulting in clip detachment from the anterior leaflet after the device was released. No hemodynamic instability or mitral stenosis was seen. After clip placement, the animals were sacrificed and examined, post-mortem, revealing no trauma to any cardiac or vascular structure. In a separate follow-up study (4-52 weeks) in adult pigs (N=21), one clip separated from the posterior leaflet at four weeks without affecting valve function. The friction element on the clip was subsequently modified to address this problem.[55] Two animals developed endocarditis at 12 and 17 weeks, respectively. In the remainder of the animals, progressive healing was observed in follow-up, such that a mature, continuous bridge of tissue developed between the anterior and posterior leaflets at the site of the clip. In three animals where scanning electron microscopy was performed, there was complete endothelialization and encapsulation of the clip. No clip embolization or thromboembolism was seen.

A phase I prospective, multi-center safety and feasibility trial (EVEREST: Endovascular Valve Edge-to-Edge Repair Study) has been completed, with short-term and six-month results in the first 27 patients published in 2005.[57] All patients had moderate to severe MR (3+ or 4+) by echocardiographic core lab criteria and were candidates for mitral valve surgery in the event of complications. Patients with rheumatic or infectious MR were excluded, as were patients with recent surgical or interventional procedure and those with a dilated ventricle (end-systolic dimension >55 mm), severe (<30%) left ventricular dysfunction, severe mitral annular calcification, or mitral orifice area <4 cm^2. The regurgitation had to be centered between A2 and P2, and meet prespecified parameters for flail dimensions or leaflet tethering such that the device could reasonably be expected to capture the leaflets adequately.

The majority of the patients enrolled had degenerative valve disease (93%) with the remainder of ischemic etiology (7%). The clip was successfully deployed in 24 (89%) patients. The three patients not receiving a clip had inadequate intraprocedural reduction of MR and the device was removed, with the patients going on to successful surgical repair (2) or replacement (1). There was no prolonged mechanical ventilation (>24 hours) or access site complications requiring surgery. All patients were discharged home without home health. The average hospital stay was 2.5 days. Of the 24 receiving a clip, there was partial clip detachment in 3 patients (13%), all of whom went on to successful elective repair. At 30-day follow-up, there were 6 patients (25%) with MR severity=3+. Two of these 6 patients went on to successful repair (1) or replacement (1). Of the 27 original patients, thirteen patients (48%) received a clip successfully and remained with MR severity=2+ at six months follow-up. A total of 8 patients (30%) had successful elective repair or replacement subsequent to enrollment. A modification in the protocol at the midway point of the study allowed for two clips (Fig. 51-10) to be placed if the MR reduction was inadequate with one clip, a change that could be speculated to have improved the results for MR reduction if this practice had been allowed from the beginning of the study. Subsequent one-year follow-up has been made available in abstract form,[58] showing a durability of reduction in MR up to one year if acute procedural success was achieved (Fig. 51-11). The two-year results of the first human implant have also been reported, showing only mild regurgitation and positive ventricular remodeling with a left ventricular internal diameter at end-diastole of 5.77 cm before the procedure, down to 5.16 cm at two years.[59]

The primary endpoint of EVEREST I was acute safety at 30 days, which is defined as freedom from death, myocardial infarction, cardiac tamponade, cardiac surgery for failed clip, clip detachment, stroke, or septicemia. The endpoint was met if the major adverse event rate was=34.4%, prespecified based on comparison to surgical event rates. Indeed, the study endpoint was met, as only 15% of patients had expe-

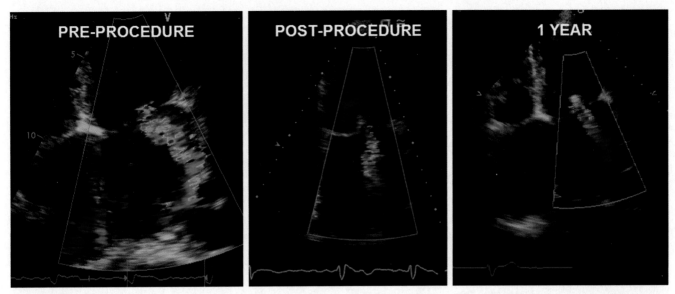

Figure 51-11. Transthoracic echocardiographic images of a patient before (pre-procedure), after (post-procedure), and 1year after percutaneous mitral valve repair with the Evalve MitraClip.

rienced a major adverse event (3 clip detachments and 1 permanent stroke). Additional unpublished results have been presented at national meetings with respect to safety and efficacy now in 70 patients, showing similar findings to the first 27 patients.[60]

The pivotal phase II trial has been initiated (EVEREST II), comparing the endovascular CVRS approach to standard cardiac surgery. The study design is a prospective, multicenter, randomized, controlled trial with a 2:1 randomization to study and control arms, respectively. There is also an allowance for roll-ins from EVEREST I and the inclusion of non-randomized patients. The study has two primary endpoints. The primary efficacy endpoint is designed to determine non-inferiority to cardiac surgery with respect to a composite endpoint of freedom from surgery for valve dysfunction, death, and MR=2+. The second primary endpoint is a safety endpoint, with the expectation to show superiority of safety of an endovascular treatment strategy versus surgical mitral valve repair or replacement defined as freedom from major adverse events at 30 days.

In addition to the determination of safety and efficacy as defined in the pivotal trial, there are additional questions to be answered with the Evalve CVRS prior to widespread adoption of this procedure. One important issue is the prolonged procedure time (204±116 min) and steep learning curve for device implantation. It does appear from unpublished EVEREST I data that compared to first procedures (device time for one clip=181 min), subsequent procedures for an individual operator have a much shorter duration (134 min).[60] A second issue is whether the clip will eliminate subsequent surgical options, thus failing the "nothing to lose" standard. This question was addressed in a publication detailing the initial experience in the first 6 patients undergoing surgery after clip placement, showing that in all cases the clip was uneventfully removed and the

surgical options were not limited (5 repairs and 1 replacement).[61] Finally, it remains to be seen if this device is useful only for degenerative disease, or whether this device can also be used for functional mitral regurgitation. In an abstract presented at the scientific meeting of the American College of Cardiology in 2006, the first six patients with functional MR showed promising results, with 5/6 patients obtaining a result of MR=2+ at 30 days.[62]

MOBIUS Leaflet Repair System

A second device in this class is under development by Edwards Lifesciences, Inc. (Irvine, CA) named the MOBIUS. This device uses a deflectable 16F transseptal delivery catheter to bring a therapy catheter into position to place a suture between the anterior and posterior leaflets, creating a double-orifice repair (Fig. 51-12). Through the delivery catheter is introduced a 10F therapy catheter with a vacuum port, needles, and suture. The therapy catheter is brought adjacent to the valve leaflet, and the leaflet is engaged in the port by vacuum suction. A suture is delivered into the engaged leaflet, the vacuum released, and the device is rotated to the opposing leaflet, where the process is repeated. A 6F internal fastener catheter is advanced over the suture, and a nitinol fastener is placed on the suture, following which the suture is cut. From one to three sutures may be placed.

The results of animal experiments for an earlier iteration of the device have been presented.[63] In a sheep beating-heart model (N=8), it was shown to be feasible to place a suture on the mitral valve using a trocar-type device through an access cannula port in the left atrium, guided by epicardial echocardiography. The current iteration of the device is at present enrolling in a phase I feasibility study called Milano II in Europe and Canada. The purpose of the study

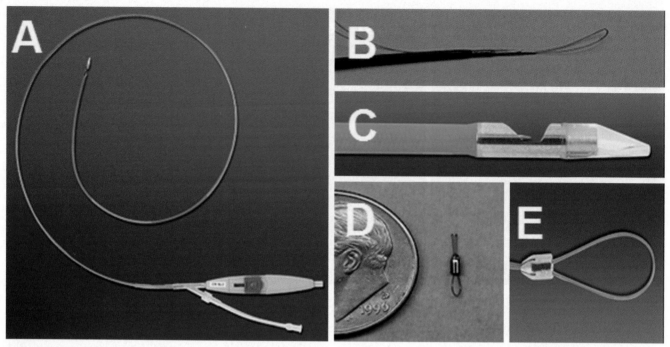

Figure 51-12. The Edwards MOBIUS device (used with permission from Edwards, Inc). Panel **A** shows the steerable delivery catheter. Panel **B** shows the needle and suture delivery device. Panel **C** shows the needle and suture delivery device within the steerable delivery catheter. Panel **D** demonstrates the size of the suture with locking element after it is deployed. Panel **E** is the suture and locking element, magnified to show detail.

is to demonstrate safety and efficacy. The study is actively enrolling, and data from the first seven patients have been presented informally and are available online at *www.tctmd.com*. As presented by Dr. Maurice Buchbinder, technical success was achieved in 5 of 7 patients. Subsequent to a successful procedure, there was one fastener clip failure, leading to 4+ MR. There were 2 additional recurrences of 3+ MR. All three of these patients, as well as one initial failure, went on to surgical repair. It is likely too early in the experience for this device to tell if it will be safe or efficacious.

Indirect Annuloplasty Via Coronary Sinus

This approach utilizes anatomic proximity of coronary sinus to the mitral annulus for modulating the shape and size of the annulus through device placement in the coronary sinus. As detailed above, annuloplasty is the integral part of mitral valve repair in the majority of surgical approaches. In many patients without degenerative disease, this is the only intervention necessary to reduce mitral regurgitation. Therefore, this approach is very promising with regards to its scope if accomplished safely and efficaciously. However, there are several challenges that need to be tackled. Proximity of coronary sinus to the annulus may be variable in different individuals and in different locations along the length of the annulus (see Fig. 51-5).[64] The coronary sinus covers about 50% of the mitral annulus perimeter and 80% of the posterior intertrigonal distance.[65] In addition, the left circumflex artery crosses below the coronary

sinus in nearly half of cases.[64,65] Proper definition of these relationships with different imaging techniques including cardiac CT, angiography, and echocardiography may be helpful in matching appropriate approach to the anatomy. Ultimate success of this approach will also depend on long-term safety of instrumenting the coronary sinus (e.g. displacement of device or forces, thrombosis, perforation) and the need for other devices in the coronary sinus (e.g. biventricular pacing).

Viacor Percutaneous Transvenous Mitral Annuloplasty

Developed by Viacor, Inc. (Wilmington, MA), the percutaneous transvenous mitral annuloplasty (PTMA) system utilizes the relationship between the coronary sinus and the mitral valve to decrease the septal-lateral mitral annular diameter. This reduction in annular dimension increases leaflet coaptation, and reduces or eliminates MR. The device is composed of two major elements, a diagnostic system and a permanent implant. Both systems employ the same therapeutic principles. The diagnostic system is designed to establish a temporary correction that acutely simulates the effect of the permanent implant with a fully removable device. With both devices a dedicated multi-lumen access catheter is placed into the target venous continuity via the subclavian vein, and then nitinol treatment devices of various length and stiffness patterns are delivered internal to the access catheter to effect remodeling of the coronary sinus–great cardiac vein. The result is an increase in leaflet coaptation (Fig. 51-13).

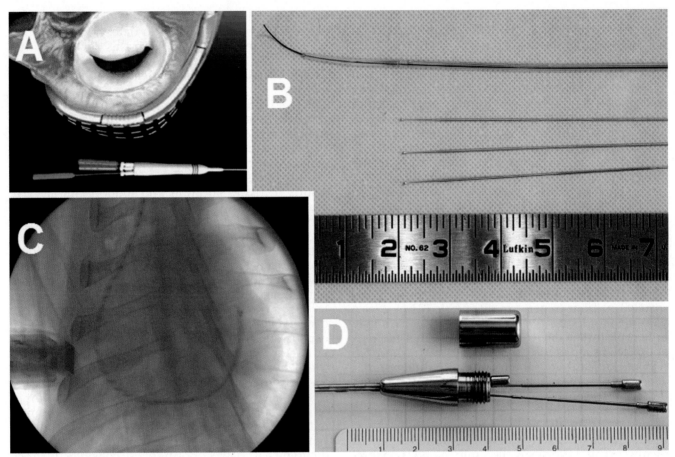

Figure 51-13. The Viacor Percutaneous Transvenous Mitral Annuloplasty (PTMA) device (used with permission from Viacor, Inc). Panel **A** is a representation of the device concept, with the multilumen delivery catheter in the coronary sinus. The dashed lines represent progressive remodeling of the coronary sinus with each device placed in the multilumen catheter. Panel **B** shows the custom PTMA devices, and the multilumen delivery catheter. The custom devices come in various lengths and stiffness. Panel **C** is a fluoroscopic image of the device in the coronary sinus. Panel **D** is a close-up view of the multilumen delivery catheter hub, which is implanted subcutaneously post-procedure.

Access is obtained in the right or left subclavian vein and a balloon-tipped catheter is advanced to the ostium of the coronary sinus. The balloon is inflated and a coronary venogram is performed to identify the anterior interventricular branch of the great cardiac vein. This vein is then engaged by a standard hydrophilic wire, after which a standard 8F coronary sinus access sheath is introduced into the coronary sinus. The multi-lumen PTMA diagnostic catheter is then advanced until the distal tip is within the proximal descending anterior interventricular vein. PTMA devices are then introduced into the lumens of the delivery catheter and advanced into portion within the target venous continuity. Under fluoroscopic and echo guidance, devices of increasing length and stiffness are added while treatment effect is continuously evaluated. The first iteration of the device had only one rod implanted into the coronary sinus delivery catheter during the procedure; now up to three devices can be implanted and the stiffness and length of each device can be modified until the optimal combination is determined. The delivery catheter is exchanged for a proprietary multi-lumen implant catheter, which is filled with the optimal combination of device rods, after which it is capped and implanted subcutaneously. The device can be reaccessed subsequently and the number and stiffness of devices revised if needed.

Early device results were reported in a sheep model of ischemic mitral regurgitation, induced by experimental snaring or balloon occlusion of the circumflex artery or its branches.[66] Within 1 min of circumflex occlusion, all animals developed 3-4+ ischemic MR. A single annuloplasty rod was placed, its impact on the MR assessed, then circumflex flow was reestablished and the device removed. This cycle was repeated up to five times in each animal, using devices of increasing length of the stiff distal segment to find the optimal device. The results were reported only for the optimal device placed in each animal. Device placement resulted in reduction of MR to 1-2+ in all animals. In addition, the MR jet area decreased from 6.5 ± 2.2 to 0.4 ± 0.5 cm^2 (P<0.03), and the vena contracta width was reduced from 8.2 ± 4.7 to 2.6 ± 0.9 cm^2 (P=0.03). The mitral annular diameter went from 30 ± 2.1 to 24 ± 1.7 mm (P=0.03) following device placement. There was no mitral stenosis induced by the device, and left ventricular ejection fraction was improved.

A subsequent sheep experiment using three-dimensional echocardiography assessed the effect of percutaneous placement of up to three annuloplasty devices of varying size and stiffness in the custom multi-lumen coronary sinus catheter.[67] At 8 weeks following experimental induced posterior myocardial infarction, the annuloplasty device significantly reduced the MR jet area, the mitral annular A-P dimension in systole, and diastole and mitral valve tenting area in all three planes.

On the basis of these publications, as well as experience with more than 300 sheep in chronic diagnostic and implant studies, pilot studies of human implantation have begun. The first phase of work was performed in 2003-2005 on a total of 10 patients undergoing conventional annuloplasty surgery for functional MR.[68] Investigators were given approximately one hour to perform diagnostic PTMA device placement prior to open heart surgery. The single lumen prototype device was attempted in 4 patients and placed successfully in 3 patients, with confirmation of the feasibility of alteration of mitral annular geometry. In the next 6 patients the multi-lumen device was evaluated, with successful delivery in 5 patients. The MR was reduced by a maximum of 2 grades in 2 patients, had no effect in 1 patient, and could not be accurately assessed in the final patient owing to alterations in systemic blood pressure. During 2006, initial cases of pilot implantation of the device were initiated.

Advantages of the Viacor PTMA device include the ease of placement, the number of combinations of devices of varying lengths and strengths that can be used to optimize the reduction in MR, and the ability to return later and change the device to further reduce MR if it recurs. The major drawback to the device includes the limitations inherent to a coronary sinus device, including coronary sinus proximity to the mitral annulus and left circumflex artery. There have been no reports to date, however, of left circumflex artery ischemia with this device.

CARILLON Mitral Contour System

The CARILLON Mitral Contour System developed by Cardiac Dimensions (Kirkland, WA) is a fixed length, double anchor device (Fig. 51-14) that is advanced through a catheter and positioned in the coronary sinus. After the device is deployed and locked into position, tension applied to the anchors of the device results in tissue plication and reduces mitral valve annular diameter, resulting in decreased MR. The procedure is performed percutaneously via internal jugular vein access, followed by distal coronary sinus cannulation with a 9F catheter. A measuring catheter is used to determine the optimal positioning of the distal anchor in the coronary sinus. The nitinol annuloplasty device is advanced down the catheter to the target position in the coronary sinus. The distal anchor of the device is deployed by passive expansion, and locks into fully expanded position by use of the delivery catheter. Tension is placed on the delivery system, bringing the proximal anchor towards the coronary sinus ostium, and creating tissue plication between the anchors. The amount of tension can be manipulated as needed to optimize reduction in annular dimension (~125%) and reduction in MR, which is verified by real-time echocardiograpy. If device position is considered to be optimal, the proximal anchor is deployed and locked into position in a similar fashion to the distal anchor. If there is a concern for safety or efficacy, the device can be recaptured by advancing the delivery catheter over the device, collapsing the device anchors.

The earliest preclinical testing with this device was done in a canine tachycardia-induced cardiomyopathy model, with both acute and chronic (4 week) hemodynamic evaluation of the device.[69] The early canine experience highlighted some of the anatomi-

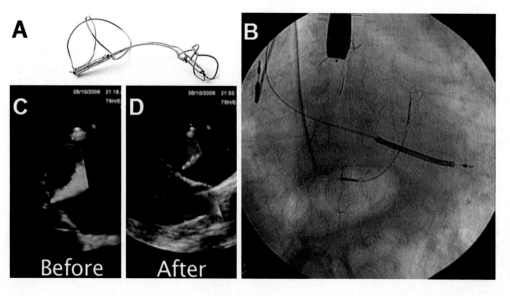

Figure 51-14. The CARILLON device from Cardiac Dimensions (used with permission from Cardiac Dimensions, Inc.). Panel **A** shows the device with proximal and distal anchors, with tension element. Panel **B** is a fluoroscopic image of the device in place in the coronary sinus. Panel **C** is an echocardiographic image mitral regurgitation before device placement. Panel **D** shows the same view after device placement, with a significant reduction in the color jet of mitral regurgitation.

cal, design, and safety issues with the device, as 3 of 12 dogs had coronary anatomy that precluded placement of the device without left circumflex ischemia (including 2 fatalities), and 2 of 12 dogs could not get a device owing to inadequate size of the early prototype. Of the seven dogs with a successful implant, at 4 weeks there was a reduction in mitral annular size (cm) compared to those with unsuccessful implant, respectively (3.37±0.23 vs. 3.73±0.11), as well as MR jet area to left atrial area (MR:LA%; 0.11±0.04 vs. 0.39±0.05, P<0.05). A subsequent ovine model of experimental tachycardia-induced heart failure demonstrated the acute hemodynamic effects of the device.[70] Each animal (N=9) was paced in the ventricle for five to eight weeks at 190 beats per minute, following which MR of moderate severity was confirmed by echocardiography. The device was successfully placed in all animals, with a significant reduction in mitral annular diameter (cm) from 4.17±0.14 to 3.24±0.11 (P<0.001) and MR jet area to left atrial area (MR:LA%) from 41.9±6.4 to 4.1±2.8 (P=0.003). Mitral regurgitation was essentially absent in 7 of 9 animals after device placement. The cardiac output increased and pulmonary capillary wedge pressure and mean pulmonary artery pressure were reduced. The chronic effect of the device was also studied in the ovine tachycardia-induced cardiomyopathy model,[71] showing similar one-month results to the canine model, with respect to mitral annular diameter percent reduction (23.7±1.45) and MR:LA% (27.84±1.96 pre-procedure, decreased to 2.40±0.98 post procedure; P<0.05). There were no premature deaths in the ovine study; however, in sheep the left circumflex artery does not run in the atrioventricular groove, precluding an assessment of safety with respect to ischemia.

The CARILLON device is advantageous in that it is simple, adjustable, and has easy deliverability. The major disadvantages of the device include the same anatomic disadvantages to any device using the coronary sinus, namely the lack of consistent proximity of the coronary sinus to the mitral annulus, and the variability in the relation of the left circumflex artery with potential to induce ischemia. A subtle modification in the shape of the distal anchor with interlocking wires has enabled reliable anchoring in the early clinical experience. A multi-center human safety and feasibility study is currently underway in Europe entitled AMADEUS. This trial is enrolling patients with 2-4+ functional MR and NYHA Classes II-IV. The Phase I IDE "COMPETENT" study in the United States targeting a similar patient population is designed to assess clinical efficacy utilizing hemodynamics, quality of life, and both sub-maximal and maximal exercise testing.

MONARC Percutaneous Transvenous Mitral Annuloplasty System

Originally developed as the VIKING system (Edwards Lifesciences Inc., Irvine, CA), the first iteration of this device consisted of a distal self-expanding anchor, a spring-like "bridge" segment, and a proximal self-expanding anchor. The distal anchor is deployed in the great cardiac vein, and the proximal anchor deployed in the proximal coronary sinus. The bridge segment was designed with shape-memory properties that lead to shortening of the device at body temperature. A new iteration of the device is now in use. Implantation is performed by internal jugular venous access with a large diameter sheath. The coronary sinus is cannulated with a standard 6F catheter, and a hydrophilic wire advanced into the distal great cardiac vein. A measurement catheter is used to select the proper device size. A 12F device delivery catheter is advanced over the guidewire into the coronary venous system. Left coronary injections are used to verify proper device positioning, and the distal anchor released by retracting the outer restraining sheath. The intended location of the distal anchor of the device is on the inner curve of the coronary sinus. Slack is removed from the bridge element by placing tension on the delivery catheter, and the proximal anchor is released just within the proximal edge of the coronary sinus by further retraction of the outer restraining sheath of the delivery catheter. The device cannot be recaptured after the anchor has been deployed.

Initial results in humans were reported for five patients with chronic ischemic mitral regurgitation.[72] Implantation of the device was successful in four patients, with one failure due to difficulty in advancing the device, leading to perforation of the anterior interventricular vein and pericardial effusion. A subsequent reattempt was also unsuccessful. The patients were followed for 180 days with serial exam, chest x-ray and echocardiogram. There was one late death (day 148) due to progressive heart failure, and not related to the device. Coronary angiogram at 90 days showed no evidence of circumflex artery compromise and the coronary sinus remained patent in all three surviving patients. Separation of the device bridge element was documented on follow-up chest x-ray in three patients (day 22, 28, and 81). Although migration of the anchors was not observed and there were no adverse clinical events in these patients, the feasibility study enrollment was discontinued. There was no significant change in the mitral annulus diameter, NYHA failure class, or MR grade at follow-up.

Because of this experience, the device has been redesigned, and is now called the MONARC system (Fig. 51-15). The nitinol bridging segment has been replaced with a "delayed-release system" that utilizes a slow conformational change in the bridge element to shorten the distance between the proximal and distal anchors. The shape change occurs because of the delayed breakdown of a biodegradable polymer in the bridge segment. In the primary device configuration, the polymer is interposed between bridge segment links, elongating the device. When the polymer is degraded in vivo, the device shortens, occurring over 3-6 weeks. This shortening is intended to induce a conformational change in the coronary

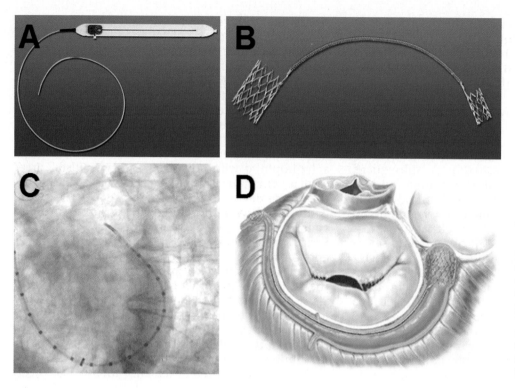

Figure 51-15. The Edwards MONARC annuloplasty system (used with permission from Edwards, Inc.). Panel **A** shows the delivery catheter. Panel **B** is the device, with proximal (smaller) and distal (larger) anchoring elements, as well as the bridge element, that shortens over time post-procedure. Panel **C** is a fluoroscopic image of the measuring device used to size the device. Panel **D** is a schematic of the device within the coronary sinus.

sinus, extending to the mitral annulus, further reducing any post-procedural MR.

The EVOLUTION trial is a multicenter feasibility and safety study in Europe and Canada, intended to evaluate the MONARC device using an echocardiographic core lab. The study enrolls patients with functional MR, grade 2+ to 4+, with proper coronary sinus dimensions to fit device specifications. Patients with recent ischemia or planned intervention are excluded, as are patients with an implanted cardiac defibrillator (ICD) or pacing leads in the coronary sinus. Other exclusions include patients with a low ejection fraction (<25%), mitral valve prolapse, or moderate to severe mitral annular calcification. The primary safety objective of the study is procedural success and 30-day safety. Acute procedural success is defined as device implantation without occurrence of in-hospital death, tamponade or myocardial infarction. The 30-day safety endpoint defined as freedom from death, tamponade or myocardial infarction. The 90-day efficacy endpoint is reduction in MR by one grade.

Preliminary results of the EVOLUTION study were presented at Transcatheter Therapeutics (TCT) 2006, showing successful implantation (device placed with no complications) in 32 of 36 patients (89%).[73] In two patients, the device could not be placed owing to venous tortuosity, and in 2 patients implantation was not attempted as coronary sinus length or diameter was not appropriate for the currently available device. There were two patients who developed cardiac tamponade after the device was implanted, but no other complications prior to discharge. The primary 30-day safety endpoint was met in 28 of 32 patients (87.5%), including a single myocardial

infarction in the diagonal artery due to device misplacement (occurring at 17 days), and death in one patient from recurrent ventricular tachycardia unrelated to the device. The 90-day safety data has been analyzed in 19 patients, with 16 of 19 patients (84.2%) meeting this safety endpoint. An additional death unrelated to the device occurred in this time interval.

The preliminary efficacy data from this study indicates the efficacy endpoint (MR reduction by 1 grade at 90 days) has been met in 9 of 17 patients analyzed (53% response rate). The mean MR grade went from 2.8 to 1.9 ($P=0.004$). When divided into two groups, including patients with MR grade 2+ ($N=7$) and those with 3+ to 4+ MR ($N=10$), the 90-day results are more striking. There was essentially no change in MR grade at 90 days among the patients with baseline MR grade 2+ (2.0 to 2.0; $P=NS$), but a significant change in 10 patients with baseline MR grade 3-4+ (3.3 to 1.9; $P=0.001$). These data should be considered preliminary owing to the limited number of patients and limited long-term follow-up.

The EVOLUTION study is the largest human cohort of coronary sinus implants, and interim results from this study indicate acceptable device safety. The procedure is straightforward and reproducible, and early efficacy data suggests that moderate to severe MR patients are the most likely to benefit from this device. The lack of efficacy in the preliminary experience with mild to moderate MR (grade 2+) is intriguing given the interest in the use of percutaneous devices for less severe MR to prevent adverse remodeling of the LV. Data regarding left ventricular parameters is not yet available, and it remains to be seen if there is still some long-term clinical benefit to early implantation of the device long-term due to prevention of MR progression.

Asymmetric Sinus Annuloplasty

Another coronary sinus annuloplasty device is under development by St. Jude Medical (St. Paul, MN), with a unique device design that will make it a niche product for asymmetric MR located around P2 and P3 scallops of the mitral valve. The device accomplishes an asymmetric annuloplasty by reducing and fixing the distance between two anchors deployed in the left ventricular myocardium via the coronary sinus. The device is placed via venous access and cannulation of the coronary sinus. The first anchor is placed in the myocardium at the level of the P2 scallop. The second anchor is placed near the posteromedial trigone, and the device is cinched to create a plication annuloplasty. This device is currently under investigation in an animal model.

Septal-to-Lateral Annular Cinching

Functional MR due to dilated cardiomyopathy (or ischemic MR) is caused by geometric alterations that are the result of left ventricular enlargement and mitral annular dilation. The observation that the septal-to-lateral (SL or anteroposterior) mitral annular diameter is increased in a tachycardia-induced model of functional MR[74] has led to the development of a new surgical technique for prevention of MR known as septal-to-lateral annular cinching (SLAC). This technique is based on reduction in the SL annular diameter, with initial data regarding the feasibility of this concept obtained in a sheep model using suture devices.[75,76] One potential limitation of the typical ring annuloplasty is the fact that the intertrigonal distance, thought to be fixed in size, may not actually be constant and can increase with rest of the annulus.[77] Therefore, a ring that does not address this part of the annulus may be only partially successful, especially in ischemic patients. The SLAC approach overcomes this problem because it remodels the ventricular apparatus.

Coapsys and iCoapsys

The current iteration of this technology, termed Coapsys (Myocor, Maple Grove, MN) annuloplasty, involves surgical placement of pericardial implants off-pump. These implants are placed on each side of the heart, with a tethering subvalvular cord that crosses the ventricle directly. This cord is then cinched up to decrease the SL diameter and eliminate MR (Fig. 51-16). In initial animal studies using a canine tachycardia model of functional MR ($N=10$), this device reduced the mean MR grade from 2.9 ± 0.7 to 0.6 ± 0.7 ($P<.001$), without adverse consequence on ventricular function.[78,79] The initial feasibility trial was conducted in India where 34 patients underwent surgical implantation for functional mitral regurgitation at the time of bypass surgery.[80] The data from 11 out of 34 patients completing one-year follow up were reported recently. In this initial experience, there was a significant reduction in MR, which was sustained over 1 year, with improvement in functional class. There were no deaths, device failures or valve reoperations on follow-up. A US randomized trial (RESTORE-MV) is enrolling patients with coronary artery disease and ischemic MR, comparing traditional open CABG and mitral repair to CABG and Coapsys device placement. Intraoperative results from this trial have been reported in the first 19 patients receiving the implant, showing a reduction in MR grade from 2.7 ± 0.8 to 0.4 ± 0.7 after implantation ($P<.0001$).[81] All implants were performed successfully without cardiopulmonary bypass and no hemodynamic compromise or structural damage to the mitral apparatus.

This system is currently under development for percutaneous use (iCoapsys). The initial device design of the iCoapsys differed from that of the Coapsys device, in that it had three extracardiac components, namely, a posterior securement pad, a septal-lateral (SL) deflector, and an anterior securement pad, all connected in series by a sizing chord. The device was implanted percutaneously through a pericardial access sheath. The device was initially tested in a canine model ($N=8$), achieving a reduction in MR grade from 3.2 to 0.7.[82] However, device design has been subsequently significantly modified to more closely mimic the surgically-placed device.

For iCoapsys (Fig. 51-17), a specifically designed needle, guidewire and sheath are used to obtain controlled access in to the pericardial space. Steerable suction-based catheters with intracardiac echo capability are positioned on the anterior and posterior ventricular wall. The posterior target zone is between the papillary muscle and the P2 segment of the mitral

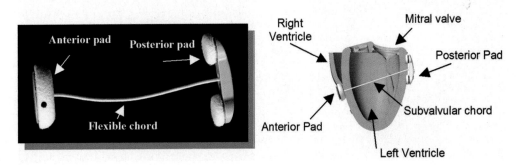

Figure 51-16. The Coapsys device (used with permission from Myocor, Inc.).

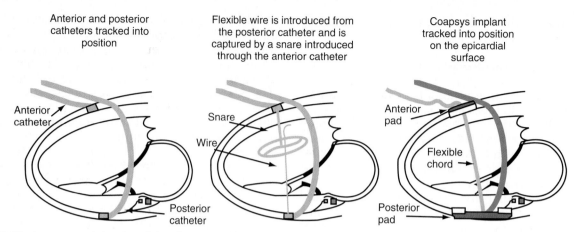

Anterior and posterior catheters tracked into position

Flexible wire is introduced from the posterior catheter and is captured by a snare introduced through the anterior catheter

Coapsys implant tracked into position on the epicardial surface

Figure 51-17. A conceptual drawing of the placement of the iCoapsys device (used with permission from Myocor, Inc.)

annulus, about 2 cm apical to the atrioventricular groove. Once proper alignment is achieved, a needle is passed from each catheter into the ventricle. A flexible wire introduced through the posterior catheter is captured by a snare from the anterior catheter. The flexible wire is used to place the transventricular cord, which is exteriorized through the delivery sheath. Then permanent implant device is placed over the cord, posterior pad first. The cord is tightened to achieve the desired effect, trimmed, and the catheters are removed leaving the device in place. This procedure will be guided by epicardial echocardiography, transesophageal echocardiography, and fluoroscopy.

Advantages of the Coapsys system include the ability to treat functional mitral regurgitation off-pump, allowing the combination of off-pump bypass and mitral valve repair. The percutaneous iteration of the device will offer the ability to intervene in functional MR especially in those patients that have been percutaneously revascularized. Both versions of the device conceptually provide a more comprehensive mechanism of action, preserving normal valve dynamics, and addressing both the mitral annulus as well as the subvalvular space and abnormal left ventricular geometry. This geometric reshaping of the ventricle may be advantageous to ventricular func-

tion and remodeling and is unique to this device. Percutaneous pericardial access is the primary requirement for the iCoapsys device, which will limit this device to patients without prior bypass surgery or thoracotomy. Current human data of surgical implant are only in patients with ischemic functional MR. Safety and efficacy of the iCoapsys device in humans needs to be proven.

PS³ System

An additional percutaneous device is under development, based on the same concept of SLAC, although this device utilizes the coronary sinus and a septal closure device to place a cord across the atrium, create tension on the annulus, and reduce the septal-to-lateral dimension (Fig. 51-18). The percutaneous septal sinus shortening (PS³) system, developed by Ample Medical Inc. (Foster City, CA) differs from the Coapsys system in that it creates a transatrial bridge as opposed to a transventricular bridge.

Using a 12F sheath in the right internal jugular vein, a proprietary catheter called the great cardiac vein (GCV) MagneCath is advanced into the coronary sinus over a hydrophilic wire. This catheter, incorporating a shaped permanent magnet on its tip,

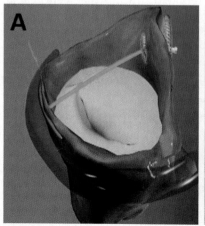

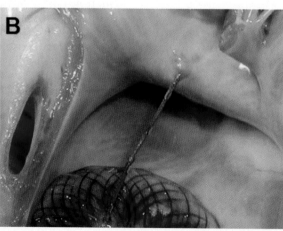

Figure 51-18. The Percutaneous Septal Sinus Shortening (PS³) device, from Ample Medical, Inc. Panel **A** is a schematic of the device showing the septal occluder device, tensioning element, and coronary sinus anchoring element in place. Panel **B** is a photograph of the device in vivo.

is positioned behind the posterior mitral leaflet. Following standard transseptal puncture and placement of a right common femoral 12F Mullins catheter in the left atrium, the left atrial (LA) MagneCath is advanced and manipulated in the left atrium until the tips of both catheters are magnetically mated. A crossing catheter, introduced via the LA MagneCath, is advanced into the GCV MagneCath, making a small hole in the left atrial wall. A glide wire is then advanced from the LA MagneCath into the coronary sinus and remains as a continuous externalized loop across the left atrium after both MagneCaths are removed. A T-bar element is placed over the wire into the coronary sinus, and an attached suture is pulled across the left atrium and externalized at the right common femoral vein. Advanced over the suture element, the septal anchor (an Amplatzer patent foramen ovale occluder, Golden Valley, MN) is deployed in standard fashion. Tension is applied on the suture to cause septal-lateral shortening, improving leaflet coaptation and reducing mitral regurgitation. The suture is locked into place with tension element, completing the procedure.

This device has been applied to an ovine model of tachycardia-induced cardiomyopathy created by rapid right ventricular pacing.[83] The degree of reduction in functional MR, and in the septal-lateral systolic distance, was the primary efficacy measure of this study. Sheep in this experiment underwent short-term ($n=19$) and long-term ($n=4$) evaluation. The device was successfully placed in all animals with no evidence of circumflex coronary artery impingement or coronary sinus occlusion. The short-term results indicated a significant reduction in septal-lateral diameter from 32.5 ± 3.5 mm pre-procedure to 24.6 ± 2.4 mm post-procedure ($P<.001$). This was maintained at 30 days in the long-term animals where the septal-lateral diameter was 30.4 ± 1.9 mm preprocedure and 25.3 ± 0.8 mm after 30 days (P value not given). The results for reduction in MR in the short-term were similar, with an MR grade of 2.1 ± 0.6 pre-procedure versus 0.4 ± 0.4 post-procedure ($P<.001$). This result was maintained at thirty days (MR grade 0.2 ± 0.1). Additional hemodynamic and laboratory data were consistent with improved cardiac function.

The first human implant was recently performed without complication and the case was presented at TCT 2006.[84] The advantages of the PS[3] system include relative ease of placement, avoidance of circumflex coronary artery impingement, and potentially safer use of transseptal puncture when compared to the similar transventricular cinching device, to be discussed below. However, the transventricular device may have additional advantages in terms of left ventricular remodeling that may not be afforded by a transatrial approach.

Transventricular (Retrograde) Direct Annuloplasty

Devices that are placed on the valve annulus by retrograde transventricular approach will soon achieve the milestone of clinical testing, although little published data is currently available to evaluate this class of devices. The obvious advantage to this approach is the ability to apply a repair directly to the annulus, where the pathologic mechanism of MR is frequently located. This approach eliminates the anatomic uncertainty regarding circumflex artery anatomy and coronary sinus proximity to the annulus that plagues coronary sinus approaches.

Mitralign Direct Annuloplasty System

Surgical suture annuloplasty has been shown to have good long-term results, comparable to ring annuloplasty, with the possible advantage of preservation of annular contraction, usually impaired by the ring implant.[37,38] Based loosely on the concept of direct suture annuloplasty, the Mitralign Direct Annuloplasty System (Mitralign, Salem, NH) uses a device composed of three metal anchors, connected by standard suture material. The anchors are placed in the mitral annulus and the suture is cinched to perform the annuloplasty (Fig. 51-19).

The device is placed via arterial access, using direct ventricular access with a unique translation catheter of trident design for device delivery. The initial device design used a magnetic guiding catheter placed in the coronary sinus; however, the new device design is guided by standard imaging techniques. The translation catheter is advanced across the aortic valve and into position in the ventricle just below the valve by magnetic attraction to the coronary sinus catheter. After proper positioning of the translation catheter is verified, the arms are expanded out from the center, spanning from 3-5 cm beneath the valve to create a trident shape. The three anchors are positioned below the valve at the level of each posterior leaflet scallop and then deployed directly through

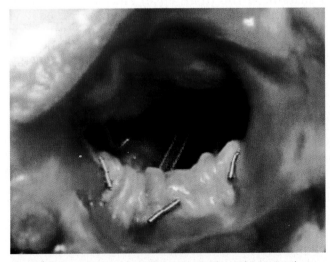

Figure 51-19. The Mitralign direct annuloplasty device in place along the mitral annulus (used with permission from Mitralign, Inc.).

the mitral annulus, remaining connected by suture material. The suture is then cinched, directly plicating the annulus, emulating the results of a surgical, suture-based annuloplasty.

Advantages of this device include direct placement on the mitral valve annulus, avoiding the concern for left circumflex artery compromise. The device is adjustable to deliver the appropriate amount of tension to the annulus, and because of its design, there are no sizing issues, as a single device is intended for use with all patients. The coronary sinus remains free of permanent implant, allowing for subsequent placement of coronary sinus leads for biventricular pacing. Long-term durability will be an issue to follow with this device. The Mitralign pilot study in humans is currently enrolling patients in Germany and Canada.

GDS AccuCinch Annuloplasty System

Another device is under development, similar to the Mitralign device described above, using a catheter-based transventricular approach to place anchors in the myocardium directly beneath the mitral annulus, performing a plication annuloplasty. A startup company called Guided Delivery Systems (GDS, Santa Clara, CA) has begun preclinical studies using the device, termed the GDS Accucinch Annuloplasty System. Preliminary data on this device is expected to be available soon.

Other Annuloplasty Devices

The application of radio frequency (RF) to remodel the mitral annulus is under development by QuantumCor (Lake Forest, CA). The concept is termed transventricular annulus remodeling, and relies on scarring and shrinkage of the mitral annulus after application of RF energy directly to the annulus. The device is intended both for surgical and transcatheter use (transseptal) and has a malleable tip with eight electrodes to deliver RF energy. The catheter is connected to a pulse generator that is modulated by temperature sensors in the electrodes to regulate the amount and time of energy delivered. The catheter can be manipulated to deliver energy to specific locations on the annulus, allowing for adjustment of the procedure to individual anatomy. This device is currently under study in an animal model.

Another device developed by Micardia uses an adjustable annuloplasty ring, implanted surgically during conventional repair procedures. The ring responds to electrical stimulation by RF wires placed directly against the ring in the activation zones of the ring. In vivo activation of the ring by direct RF application causes the ring to change configuration, allowing the ring to take a favorable shape to eliminate mitral regurgitation. The ring may be reshaped intraoperatively or subsequently via transseptal approach if MR recurs. This device is in the early phases of development and has not yet been used in humans.

PATIENT SELECTION

Currently all of the percutaneous and endovascular mitral repair devices are available only as investigational devices, and as such, patients would need to meet inclusion criteria for each individual device study. To be evaluated for device placement, patients may be referred to study centers, many of which are currently available only outside of the United States. Unlike the percutaneous aortic valve arena, many patients enrolling in mitral valve repair trials are in fact surgical candidates, as this technology is viewed as less prohibitive of future surgical intervention and the efficacy of surgical repair is not as clear, particularly in functional mitral regurgitation.

A broader categorization can be made with respect to patient selection based on device category. The edge-to-edge devices are currently implanted mainly in patients with degenerative valve disease, with a small percentage of patients with functional/ischemic mitral regurgitation. However, their use may be limited in patients with functional regurgitation associated with a severely dilated annulus or exaggerated leaflet tenting. The coronary sinus devices are targeted at the population of patients with functional mitral regurgitation (ischemic or non-ischemic) and may be most useful in patients with a dilated annulus. The septal-lateral annular cinching (SLAC) and direct annuloplasty devices are also targeted at patients with functional MR and dilated annulus. Combining an annuloplasty with leaflet repair, which would be useful for patients with degenerative disease and severely dilated annulus, may be a useful approach when these devices are available outside of research constraints.

SUMMARY/FUTURE DIRECTIONS

Percutaneous mitral repair is an exciting new field with many devices at early stages of preclinical and clinical evaluation. The majority of strategies are based on principles learned from surgical mitral valve repair techniques. The most advanced technique to date is the edge-to-edge repair, where a phase II clinical trial is underway, comparing percutaneous repair directly with surgical repair.

As the majority of percutaneous mitral valve repair devices are at early developmental stages, there are many issues remaining to be resolved before widespread application of this technology. Percutaneous mitral repair has the potential to be considered a "preventive" technology, as it may be applied early in the disease course to alter the natural history of MR by disrupting the pathologic feedback loop of MR and left ventricular dysfunction. In addition, it is unclear if percutaneous devices will need to eliminate all MR to be effective. If a percutaneous repair can achieve a significant and durable reduction but not elimination of MR, this may be a worthy goal if this prevents clinical events. However, it remains important for percutaneous devices to preserve future surgical options. If the procedure is safe, relatively free of complications, and preserves surgical options, then it meets the "nothing to lose" standard that may be applied to these devices.

There remains a need to determine which patients should be allowed in clinical trials. Is it ethical to allow patients who are good surgical candidates to undergo a developmental percutaneous procedure, or should the clinical trials focus mainly on non-surgical candidates as with the aortic valve technology? Surgical technique is tailored to the specific valve anatomy, but percutaneous techniques currently use only a single approach. It seems likely that the future of percutaneous repair will be in a combination of techniques. However, this poses significant limitations to the device development process with current regulations.

As percutaneous devices may be more specifically tailored to etiology of MR and anatomy of the individual patient, we will have to learn for each device the proper imaging and patient selection criteria. Improvement of imaging techniques will be necessary to aid in percutaneous repair, both during the procedure and in following the results. Finally, it will be critical for collegial interaction to develop between the specialties of cardiac imaging, interventional cardiology, and cardiothoracic surgery to facilitate advancement in this burgeoning field.

REFERENCES

1. Ho SY: Anatomy of the mitral valve. Heart 2002;88(Suppl 4): iv5-iv10.
2. Perloff JK, Roberts WC: The mitral apparatus: Functional anatomy of mitral regurgitation. Circulation 1972;46: 227-239.
3. Roberts WC, Perloff JK: Mitral valvular disease: A clinicopathologic survey of the conditions causing the mitral valve to function abnormally. Ann Intern Med 1972;77:939-975.
4. Braunwald E: Valvular heart disease. In Zipes DP, Braunwald E (eds): Braunwald's Heart Disease: A Textbook of Cardiovascular Medicine. Philadelphia, WB Saunders, 2005.
5. Carpentier A: Cardiac valve surgery: The "French correction." J Thorac Cardiovasc Surg 1983;86:323-337.
6. Kumanohoso T, Otsuji Y, Yoshifuku S, et al: Mechanism of higher incidence of ischemic mitral regurgitation in patients with inferior myocardial infarction: Quantitative analysis of left ventricular and mitral valve geometry in 103 patients with prior myocardial infarction. J Thorac Cardiovasc Surg 2003;125:135-143.
7. Srichai MB, Grimm RA, Stillman AE, et al: Ischemic mitral regurgitation: Impact of the left ventricle and mitral valve in patients with left ventricular systolic dysfunction. Ann Thorac Surg 2005;80:170-178.
8. Mihalatos DG, Mathew ST, Gopal AS, et al: Relationship of mitral annular remodeling to severity of chronic mitral regurgitation. J Am Soc Echocardiogr 2006;19:76-82.
9. De Simone R, Wolf I, Hoda R, et al: Three-dimensional assessment of left ventricular geometry and annular dilatation provides new mechanistic insights into the surgical correction of ischemic mitral regurgitation. Thorac Cardiovasc Surg 2006;54:452-458.
10. Carabello BA, Crawford FA Jr: Valvular heart disease. N Engl J Med 1997;337:32-41.
11. Enriquez-Sarano M, Avierinos JF, Messika-Zeitoun D, et al: Quantitative determinants of the outcome of asymptomatic mitral regurgitation. N Engl J Med 2005;352:875-883.
12. Gillinov AM, Blackstone EH, Rajeswaran J, et al: Ischemic versus degenerative mitral regurgitation: Does etiology affect survival? Ann Thorac Surg 2005;80:811-819.
13. Ling LH, Enriquez-Sarano M, Seward JB, et al: Clinical outcome of mitral regurgitation due to flail leaflet. N Engl J Med 1996;335:1417-1423.
14. Rosenhek R, Rader F, Klaar U, et al: Outcome of watchful waiting in asymptomatic severe mitral regurgitation. Circulation 2006;113:2238-2244.
15. Enriquez-Sarano M, Basmadjian AJ, Rossi A, et al: Progression of mitral regurgitation: A prospective Doppler echocardiographic study. J Am Coll Cardiol 1999;34:1137-1144.
16. Rosen SE, Borer JS, Hochreiter C, et al: Natural history of the asymptomatic/minimally symptomatic patient with severe mitral regurgitation secondary to mitral valve prolapse and normal right and left ventricular performance. Am J Cardiol 1994;74:374-380.
17. Griffin BP: Timing of surgical intervention in chronic mitral regurgitation: Is vigilance enough? Circulation 2006;113: 2169-2172.
18. Grigioni F, Enriquez-Sarano M, Zehr KJ, et al: Ischemic mitral regurgitation: Long-term outcome and prognostic implications with quantitative Doppler assessment. Circulation 2001;103:1759-1764.
19. Zoghbi WA, Enriquez-Sarano M, Foster E, et al: Recommendations for evaluation of the severity of native valvular regurgitation with two-dimensional and Doppler echocardiography. J Am Soc Echocardiogr 2003;16:777-802.
20. Khanna D, Miller AP, Nanda NC, et al: Transthoracic and transesophageal echocardiographic assessment of mitral regurgitation severity: Usefulness of qualitative and semiquantitative techniques. Echocardiography 2005;22: 748-769.
21. Enriquez-Sarano M, Miller FA Jr, Hayes SN, et al: Effective mitral regurgitant orifice area: Clinical use and pitfalls of the proximal isovelocity surface area method. J Am Coll Cardiol 1995;25:703-709.
22. Fehske W, Omran H, Manz M, et al: Color-coded Doppler imaging of the vena contracta as a basis for quantification of pure mitral regurgitation. Am J Cardiol 1994;73: 268-274.
23. Enriquez-Sarano M, Seward JB, Bailey KR, Tajik AJ: Effective regurgitant orifice area: A noninvasive Doppler development of an old hemodynamic concept. J Am Coll Cardiol 1994;23:443-451.
24. Klein AL, Stewart WJ, Bartlett J, et al: Effects of mitral regurgitation on pulmonary venous flow and left atrial pressure: An intraoperative transesophageal echocardiographic study. J Am Coll Cardiol 1992;20:1345-1352.
25. Pu M, Griffin BP, Vandervoort PM, et al: The value of assessing pulmonary venous flow velocity for predicting severity of mitral regurgitation: A quantitative assessment integrating left ventricular function. J Am Soc Echocardiogr 1999;12: 736-743.
26. Alkadhi H, Bettex D, Wildermuth S, et al: Dynamic cine imaging of the mitral valve with 16-MDCT: A feasibility study. AJR Am J Roentgenol 2005;185:636-646.
27. Fujita N, Chazouilleres AF, Hartiala JJ, et al: Quantification of mitral regurgitation by velocity-encoded cine nuclear magnetic resonance imaging. J Am Coll Cardiol 1994;23: 951-958.
28. Bonow RO, Carabello BA, Chatterjee K, et al: ACC/AHA 2006 Guidelines for the management of patients with valvular heart disease: A report of the American College of Cardiology/ American Heart Association Task Force on Practice Guidelines (Writing Committee to Revise the 1998 Guidelines for the management of patients with valvular heart disease) developed in collaboration with the Society of Cardiovascular Anesthesiologists endorsed by the Society for Cardiovascular Angiography and Interventions and the Society of Thoracic Surgeons. J Am Coll Cardiol 2006;48:e1-e148.
29. Enriquez-Sarano M, Schaff HV, Orszulak TA, et al: Valve repair improves the outcome of surgery for mitral regurgitation: A multivariate analysis. Circulation 1995;91:1022-1028.
30. Grossi EA, Goldberg JD, LaPietra A, et al: Ischemic mitral valve reconstruction and replacement: Comparison of long-term

survival and complications. J Thorac Cardiovasc Surg 2001;122:1107-1124.

31. Savage EB, Ferguson TB Jr, DiSesa VJ: Use of mitral valve repair: Analysis of contemporary United States experience reported to the Society of Thoracic Surgeons National Cardiac Database. Ann Thorac Surg 2003;75:820-825.

32. Oliveira JM, Antunes MJ: Mitral valve repair: Better than replacement. Heart 2006;92:275-281.

33. Braunberger E, Deloche A, Berrebi A, et al: Very long-term results (more than 20 years) of valve repair with Carpentier's techniques in nonrheumatic mitral valve insufficiency. Circulation 2001;104:I8-I11.

34. Bolling SF, Pagani FD, Deeb GM, Bach DS: Intermediate-term outcome of mitral reconstruction in cardiomyopathy. J Thorac Cardiovasc Surg 1998;115:381-386; discussion 387-388.

35. Bishay ES, McCarthy PM, Cosgrove DM, et al: Mitral valve surgery in patients with severe left ventricular dysfunction. Eur J Cardiothorac Surg 2000;17:213-221.

36. Gillinov AM, Wierup PN, Blackstone EH, et al: Is repair preferable to replacement for ischemic mitral regurgitation? J Thorac Cardiovasc Surg 2001;122:1125-1141.

37. Nagy ZL, Bodi A, Vaszily M, et al: Five-year experience with a suture annuloplasty for mitral valve repair. Scand Cardiovasc J 2000;34:528-532.

38. Aybek T, Risteski P, Miskovic A, et al: Seven years' experience with suture annuloplasty for mitral valve repair. J Thorac Cardiovasc Surg 2006;131:99-106.

39. Grossi EA, Bizekis CS, LaPietra A, et al: Late results of isolated mitral annuloplasty for "functional" ischemic mitral insufficiency. J Card Surg 2001;16:328-332.

40. Wu AH, Aaronson KD, Bolling SF, et al: Impact of mitral valve annuloplasty on mortality risk in patients with mitral regurgitation and left ventricular systolic dysfunction. J Am Coll Cardiol 2005;45:381-387.

41. McGee EC, Gillinov AM, Blackstone EH, et al: Recurrent mitral regurgitation after annuloplasty for functional ischemic mitral regurgitation. J Thorac Cardiovasc Surg 2004;128:916-924.

42. Matsunaga A, Tahta SA, Duran CM: Failure of reduction annuloplasty for functional ischemic mitral regurgitation. J Heart Valve Dis 2004;13:390-397; discussion 397-398.

43. Kongsaerepong V, Shiota M, Gillinov AM, et al: Echocardiographic predictors of successful versus unsuccessful mitral valve repair in ischemic mitral regurgitation. Am J Cardiol 2006;98:504-508.

44. Mohty D, Orszulak TA, Schaff HV, et al: Very long-term survival and durability of mitral valve repair for mitral valve prolapse. Circulation 2001;104:I-1-I-7.

45. Gillinov AM, Cosgrove DM, Blackstone EH, et al: Durability of mitral valve repair for degenerative disease. J Thorac Cardiovasc Surg 1998;116:734-743.

46. Flameng W, Herijgers P, Bogaerts K: Recurrence of mitral valve regurgitation after mitral valve repair in degenerative valve disease. Circulation 2003;107:1609-1613.

47. Maisano F, Torracca L, Oppizzi M, et al: The edge-to-edge technique: A simplified method to correct mitral insufficiency. Eur J Cardiothorac Surg 1998;13:240-245; discussion 245-246.

48. Bhudia SK, McCarthy PM, Smedira NG, et al: Edge-to-edge (Alfieri) mitral repair: Results in diverse clinical settings. Ann Thorac Surg 2004;77:1598-1606.

49. Alfieri O, Maisano F, De Bonis M, et al: The double-orifice technique in mitral valve repair: A simple solution for complex problems. J Thorac Cardiovasc Surg 2001;122:674-681.

50. Lorusso R, Borghetti V, Totaro P, et al: The double-orifice technique for mitral valve reconstruction: Predictors of postoperative outcome. Eur J Cardiothorac Surg 2001;20:583-589.

51. Kherani AR, Cheema FH, Casher J, et al: Edge-to-edge mitral valve repair: The Columbia Presbyterian experience. Ann Thorac Surg 2004;78:73-76.

52. De Bonis M, Lapenna E, La Canna G, et al: Mitral valve repair for functional mitral regurgitation in end-stage dilated cardiomyopathy: Role of the "edge-to-edge" technique. Circulation 2005;112:I402-I408.

53. Kuduvalli M, Ghotkar SV, Grayson AD, Fabri BM: Edge-to-edge technique for mitral valve repair: Medium-term results with echocardiographic follow-up. Ann Thorac Surg 2006;82:1356-1361.

54. Maisano F, Vigano G, Blasio A, et al: Surgical isolated edge-to-edge mitral valve repair without annuloplasty: Clinical proof of the principle for an endovascular approach. EuroIntervention 2006;2:181-186.

55. Fann JI, St Goar FG, Komtebedde J, et al: Beating heart catheter-based edge-to-edge mitral valve procedure in a porcine model: Efficacy and healing response. Circulation 2004;110:988-993.

56. St Goar FG, Fann JI, Komtebedde J, et al: Endovascular edge-to-edge mitral valve repair: Short-term results in a porcine model. Circulation 2003;108:1990-1993.

57. Feldman T, Wasserman HS, Herrmann HC, et al: Percutaneous mitral valve repair using the edge-to-edge technique: Six-month results of the EVEREST phase I clinical trial. J Am Coll Cardiol 2005;46:2134-2140.

58. Feldman T, Wasserman HS, Herrmann HC, et al: Edge-to-edge mitral valve repair using the percutaneous Evalve Mitraclip: One-year results of the EVEREST phase I clinical trial. Am J Cardiol 2005;96(Suppl 7A):49H.

59. Condado JA, Acquatella H, Rodriguez L, et al: Percutaneous edge-to-edge mitral valve repair: 2-Year follow-up in the first human case. Catheter Cardiovasc Interv 2006;67:323-325.

60. Leon M: The Evalve concept for mitral valve repair: Results of the EVEREST trial. Presented at the Transcatheter Cardiovascular Therapeutics Meeting, Washington, DC, 2006.

61. Dang NC, Aboodi MS, Sakaguchi T, et al: Surgical revision after percutaneous mitral valve repair with a clip: Initial multicenter experience. Ann Thorac Surg 2005;80:2338-2342.

62. Block PC, Herrmann HC, Whitlow P, et al: Percutaneous edge-to-edge mitral valve repair using the Evalve MitraClip: Initial experience with functional mitral regurgitation in the EVEREST I trial. J Am Coll Cardiol 2006;47:283A.

63. Alfieri O, Elefteriades JA, Chapolini RJ, et al: Novel suture device for beating-heart mitral leaflet approximation. Ann Thorac Surg 2002;74:1488-1493.

64. Choure AJ, Garcia MJ, Hesse B, et al: In vivo analysis of the anatomical relationship of coronary sinus to mitral annulus and left circumflex coronary artery using cardiac multidetector computed tomography: Implications for percutaneous coronary sinus annuloplasty. J Am Coll Cardiol 2006;48:1938-1945.

65. Iansac E, Di Centa I, Al Attar N, et al: Percutaneous mitral annuloplasty through the coronary sinus: An anatomical point of view. Circulation 2006;114:II-565.

66. Liddicoat JR, Mac Neill BD, Gillinov AM, et al: Percutaneous mitral valve repair: A feasibility study in an ovine model of acute ischemic mitral regurgitation. Catheter Cardiovasc Interv 2003;60:410-416.

67. Daimon M, Fukuda S, Adams DH, et al: Mitral valve repair with Carpentier-McCarthy-Adams IMR ETlogix annuloplasty ring for ischemic mitral regurgitation: Early echocardiographic results from a multi-center study. Circulation 2006;114:I588-I593.

68. Gillinov AM, Liddicoat JR: Percutaneous transvenous mitral annuloplasty. EuroIntervention 2006;1(Suppl A):A40-A43.

69. Maniu CV, Patel JB, Reuter DG, et al: Acute and chronic reduction of functional mitral regurgitation in experimental heart failure by percutaneous mitral annuloplasty. J Am Coll Cardiol 2004;44:1652-1661.

70. Kaye DM, Byrne M, Alferness C, Power J: Feasibility and short-term efficacy of percutaneous mitral annular reduction for the therapy of heart failure-induced mitral regurgitation. Circulation 2003;108:1795-1797.

71. Byrne MJ, Kaye DM, Mathis M, et al: Percutaneous mitral annular reduction provides continued benefit in an ovine model of dilated cardiomyopathy. Circulation 2004;110:3088-3092.

72. Webb JG, Harnek J, Munt BI, et al: Percutaneous transvenous mitral annuloplasty: Initial human experience with device implantation in the coronary sinus. Circulation 2006;113:851-855.

73. Webb JG, Kuck K, Stone G, et al: Percutaneous mitral annuloplasty with the MONARC system: Preliminary results from the EVOLUTION trial. Am J Cardiol 2006;98:49M.

74. Timek TA, Dagum P, Lai DT, et al: Pathogenesis of mitral regurgitation in tachycardia-induced cardiomyopathy. Circulation 2001;104:I47-I53.

75. Timek TA, Lai DT, Tibayan F, et al: Septal-lateral annular cinching abolishes acute ischemic mitral regurgitation. J Thorac Cardiovasc Surg 2002;123:881-888.

76. Tibayan FA, Rodriguez F, Langer F, et al: Does septal-lateral annular cinching work for chronic ischemic mitral regurgitation? J Thorac Cardiovasc Surg 2004;127:654-663.

77. Ahmad RM, Gillinov AM, McCarthy PM, et al: Annular geometry and motion in human ischemic mitral regurgitation: Novel assessment with three-dimensional echocardiography and computer reconstruction. Ann Thorac Surg 2004;78:2063-2068; discussion 2068.

78. Fukamachi K, Inoue M, Popovic ZB, et al: Off-pump mitral valve repair using the Coapsys device: A pilot study in a pacing-induced mitral regurgitation model. Ann Thorac Surg 2004;77:688-692; discussion 692-693.

79. Fukamachi K, Popovic ZB, Inoue M, et al: Changes in mitral annular and left ventricular dimensions and left ventricular pressure-volume relations after off-pump treatment of mitral regurgitation with the Coapsys device. Eur J Cardiothorac Surg 2004;25:352-357.

80. Mishra YK, Mittal S, Jaguri P, Trehan N: Coapsys mitral annuloplasty for chronic functional ischemic mitral regurgitation: 1-Year results. Ann Thorac Surg 2006;81:42-46.

81. Grossi EA, Saunders PC, Woo YJ, et al: Intraoperative effects of the Coapsys annuloplasty system in a randomized evaluation (RESTOR-MV) of functional ischemic mitral regurgitation. Ann Thorac Surg 2005;80:1706-1711.

82. Pederson WR, Block PC, Feldman T: The iCoapsys Repair System for the percutaneous treatment of functional mitral insufficiency. EuroIntervention 2006;1(Suppl A):A44-A48.

83. Rogers JH, Macoviak JA, Rahdert DA, et al: Percutaneous septal sinus shortening: A novel procedure for the treatment of functional mitral regurgitation. Circulation 2006;113:2329-2334.

84. Palacios IF, Condado JA, Brandi S, et al: First-in-man: Percutaneous septal sinus shortening (the PS[3] system) for functional mitral regurgitation. Am J Cardiol 2006;98:49M.

CHAPTER

52 Percutaneous Aortic Valvular Approaches: Balloon Aortic Valvuloplasty and Percutaneous Valve Replacement with the Cribier-Edwards Bioprosthesis

Alain Cribier, Helene Eltchaninoff, Christophe Tron, and Lowell Gerber

KEY POINTS

- Aortic stenosis is the most common form of adult valvular heart disease, and it has become more prevalent in the aging population. Surgical aortic valve replacement is the treatment of choice, and it is the only definitive treatment to relieve symptoms and improve survival. Despite guidelines and recommendations, one third of patients are not referred to surgery, often because of old age, left ventricular dysfunction, and comorbidities.

- Balloon aortic valvuloplasty (BAV) is a palliative procedure that can provide immediate relief of symptoms. Advanced technologies have made the procedure safer, faster, and more efficient. However, the possibility of improved survival is limited to patients who can be bridged to surgery or can undergo serial dilatations. With the aging population, there is a renewed interest in BAV, which offers the only therapeutic option to palliate the symptoms of inoperable or high-surgical-risk patients until approval of the percutaneous valve implantation techniques.

- Percutaneous aortic valve implantation is a promising new technique, still under investigation, with ongoing technical improvements in devices, materials, and protocols for delivery. It offers durable improvement in valve area asso-

ciated with improved left ventricular function and long-lasting (up to 3 years) alleviation of symptoms. Valve implantation has been restricted to patients who have been determined to be inoperable or for whom surgery is considered inappropriate because of age, poor left ventricular function, and/or cardiac or noncardiac comorbidities.

- The percutaneous aortic valve was initially implanted using the antegrade-transseptal approach. The retrograde approach, using an advanced technology, is less demanding and is currently receiving the most interest. The transapical approach (through the apex of the left ventricle after a small chest opening) is beginning clinical trials. In the future, these various methods for valve implantation should be considered according to the patient's clinical status and the quality of vascular access.

- With the onset of non–surgically implantable heart valves, a multidisciplinary approach is required. It is time for a close collaboration between noninvasive and interventional cardiologists, cardiac and vascular surgeons, internists and geriatricians, along with engineers and representatives from industry and government, to bring the potential of this new treatment modality into reality.

With the development of nonsurgical heart valve replacement, the treatment of aortic valve stenosis (AS) for adult patients who are considered inoperable or have too high a risk for surgical valve replacement has entered a new era.

AS remains the most common form of adult acquired valvular heart disease in developed countries, increasing in prevalence with age.[1] Because of the aging demographics, the management of AS in elderly patients, particularly when associated with more complex comorbidities, is becoming an important problem for geriatricians and cardiologists. The only proven therapy for definitive relief of symptoms and improved survival is surgical valve replacement. The operative mortality and incidence of postoperative morbidity increase with age, and they are significantly higher when surgery is done urgently or emergently or when preexisting comorbidities are present, such as coronary artery disease, poor left ventricular (LV) function, renal insufficiency, pulmonary disease, and diabetes.[2,3]

Before the advent of balloon aortic valvuloplasty (BAV) in 1986,[4] surgical valve replacement was the only recommended therapy for patients with symptomatic severe AS, and the only alternative was expectant observation if they were thought to be "too old" or "high risk".[5] The onset of "old age" has continued to be redefined, resulting in a moving target for comparison as these techniques have been evolving and the population has been aging. At this date, age is no longer considered a contraindication, and very old patients, including octogenarians and older, are offered the option if they do not have significant physical or psychological comorbidities.[6-8] The percentage of patients 90 years of age and older undergoing heart surgery doubled from 1994 to 2001.[7] Patients with poor LV function are also more aggressively managed surgically.[9-11] Still, there are a large number of patients with severe AS who, because of age, high-risk cardiac disease, or other comorbidities are not offered valve replacement, amounting to almost one third of potential patients, as reported in the Euro Heart Survey on Valvular Heart Disease.[12] Likewise, a significant percentage of patients with severe AS living in the United States and not referred for aortic valve replacement (AVR) has also been reported.[13]

In the 1990s, the early enthusiasm for BAV in adult patients as a possible alternative to surgical AVR was annihilated after the recognition of the problem of restenosis. The procedure appeared to provide only temporary benefit in symptoms and, at best, a modest survival benefit with a relatively high rate of complications.[14,15] As more experience was reported, there were discrepancies in outcome regarding both results and complication rates. Whereas the benefit of the procedure in neonates, infants, and young patients has been agreed upon, the role of BAV in adults remains controversial, as reflected in the updated American College of Cardiology/American Heart Association (ACC/AHA) guidelines for management of patients with valvular heart disease.[16]

For the high-risk elderly patient with severe calcific AS, the response by the cardiologist has been to limit the recommendation for BAV and for the cardiac surgeon to continue to broaden the inclusion of patients for surgery, regardless of age or LV function. A large number of patients with severe AS and comorbidities that render them inoperable or with very high risk still remain untreated, particularly when the risk assessment by the Parsonnet score or the EuroSCORE appears unfavorable.[17] Although they are too sick for surgery, BAV is not offered to them in most centers because of its perceived limitations.[12]

Percutaneous AVR has been recently introduced for that subset of patients[18] and might offer in the near future a new therapeutic option. However, because the percutaneous heart valve (PHV) is still in the early development stages and not ready for clinical application outside of well-designed trials, BAV has continued to evolve as a palliative, albeit temporary, therapy for the same high-risk patients. There have been significant changes and advances in materials, techniques, and clinical applications, making the procedure easier, safer, and quicker to perform.

Because the population is aging and also because it is an integral technical step of PHV placement, there is increased interest in learning the percutaneous AVR technique by interventional cardiologists as well as by cardiac surgeons.

The objectives of this chapter are as follows:
1. Present our current technique of BAV, highlighting the new materials and technical changes, to review our recent results, to discuss the role of BAV in today's practice, and to provide a perspective of BAV in the PHV era.
2. Review the development of PHV for calcific AS in adults, describe the current device and techniques for implantation, present our early experience and trial results, and provide insight into the future advances and clinical applications.

BALLOON AORTIC VALVULOPLASTY

Since our first reported cases,[4] we have published our continuing experience, which now exceeds 1000 cases.[19-25] Like others,[14,15] we could obtain immediate improvement in symptoms, hemodynamics, and LV function, but with disappointing midterm and long-term results. In our hands, BAV remains a valuable palliative procedure for frail patients who are extremely old, often with compromised clinical status due to concomitant coronary artery disease and other extracardiac comorbidities. Most of our patients have been turned down by the surgeons before being referred to us, and BAV is attempted as a "bridge to surgery" in about one third of the cases. The technique used now allows us to obtain improved hemodynamic results and reduced complications in this high-risk subset of patients.[25]

The goal of the procedure is to achieve a 100% increase in aortic valve area. This requires attention to obtaining the maximum pressure exerted on the valve leaflets during balloon inflation, proper balloon sizing, and optimal contact with the valve structures. Improper techniques may explain the disparity of the results in the literature. In some reported series, the increase in aortic valve area after the procedure was very modest,[26,27] whereas final valve area is a determinant of prognosis.[14]

The results of BAV are limited by the pathology involved in the disease. The "degenerative" process has become over time the main cause of AS.[28-30] In contrast to mitral stenosis, which is rheumatic in origin, commissural fusion is not the predominant feature in most elderly patients with calcific AS, which is more similar to the chronic inflammatory atherosclerotic process.[31] Whereas commissural splitting may play a role, it is not the major factor in balloon dilation of calcific AS in the adult, in contrast to its being the major therapeutic mechanism in rheumatic mitral stenosis.[32] The primary mechanism of the balloon action in AS is fracture of the nodular calcium deposits, which improves leaflet mobility, allowing increased valve opening and blood flow during LV contraction.[33] The rigidly inflated balloon at full inflation is also able to stretch the elastic component of the valve structures and annulus. These elastic properties can result in immediate or early recoil, which can be one of the causes of an unsuccessful or suboptimal procedure. Overstretching can result in tearing or rupture of the elastic and fibrocalcific components of the leaflets, annulus, or adjacent myocardium.[34]

Despite improvement in technique and materials, restenosis remains the nemesis of BAV,[15,35-37] and it is probably multifactorial. Early restenosis occurring within hours or days, as mentioned earlier, is probably a phenomenon of early recoil resulting from stretching of valve structures by the balloon. This could be related to the pathology of the valve structures, a balloon diameter that is too small, or a balloon that is not inflated sufficiently to be effective.

When the restenosis occurs later, within several months, the process may be multifactorial, including the original degenerative process and an altered healing process with fibrosis and bone formation.[37,38] When patients develop recurrent symptoms, BAV can be repeated, usually after an interval of 12 to 24 months, and the dilations can be done serially.[23-25,39,40] In some cases, the patient may be "bridged" to AVR.[16] Despite its limitations, BAV can provide symptomatic relief and a modest survival benefit for selected patients who are very old or who have comorbidities and may have no other option.[14-16,24]

BAV can be done using either a retrograde or an antegrade approach. The retrograde approach was first described by Lababidi and colleagues in infants and children,[41] and then by our group in adults.[4] The antegrade approach was reported by Block and Palacios,[42] and comparisons between the techniques have been reported.[43,44] There has been no significant benefit of the antegrade approach over the retrograde

approach except in the case of deficient arterial access due to peripheral vascular disease or small-caliber, diffusely diseased femoral and iliac vessels, which is present in almost 20% of the elderly patients.[45] For both approaches, we typically perform the baseline hemodynamic study to confirm the presence of severe AS at the same setting as the planned BAV intervention.

The Retrograde Approach

Using our current technique for the retrograde approach, the procedure is usually performed in less than 1 hour with few complications. Understanding and applying the technical "tips and tricks" that we have learned is helpful to make the procedure faster and safer in this critically ill, fragile, elderly population of patients.

Patient Preparation

We use mild sedation with intravenous midazolam and local anesthesia. Unfractionated heparin is given intravenously (50 IU/kg) at the start of the procedure. All of the anticipated supplies are brought to the catheterization laboratory table to reduce procedure time.

Femoral arterial and venous access is obtained with 8-Fr sheaths. Coronary angiography is obtained, and, if indicated, coronary intervention is performed in the same setting, but usually after the BAV is completed. Right-sided heart catheterization is performed using a Swan-Ganz thermodilution catheter.

Technique for Retrograde Crossing of the Native Aortic Valve

With the appropriate technique, the stenotic aortic valve can be crossed within a few minutes in most cases. We use either a 7-Fr Sones type B catheter or an Amplatz left coronary catheter, more particularly when the ascending aorta is enlarged. The central aortic pressure is recorded from the catheter that is intended to cross the valve, and this pressure wave form is superimposed and compared to the aortic pressure from the femoral artery recorded from the side arm of the sheath. In the elderly, it is not uncommon to find a baseline "gradient" between the two pressures resulting from obstructive peripheral vascular disease.

A straight-tip, fixed-core, 0.035-inch guidewire is positioned at the tip of the catheter. In the 40-degree left anterior oblique (LAO) projection, the catheter tip is positioned at the rim of the valve. The catheter is slowly pulled back while firm clockwise rotation is maintained, to direct the catheter tip toward the center of the valve plane (Fig. 52-1A). The guidewire is carefully moved in and out of the catheter tip, sequentially mapping the valve surface and exploring for the valve orifice. Once the wire crosses the

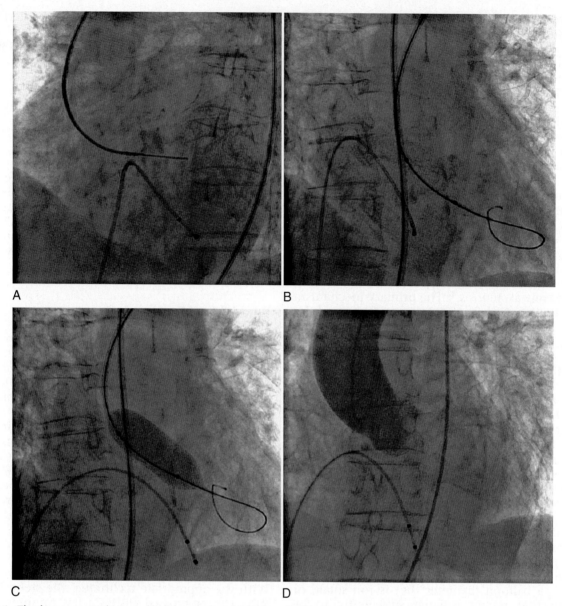

Figure 52-1. The four sequential steps of balloon aortic valvuloplasty (BAV). **A,** Crossing the valve with a straight guidewire within a 7-Fr Sones catheter (type B) in the left anterior oblique view. **B,** The 260-cm long, extra-stiff guidewire with its preshaped distal end placed in the left ventricle. **C,** The 23-mm balloon is fully inflated within the native aortic valve during rapid pacing. **D,** Post-BAV supra-aortic angiography showing no residual aortic regurgitation.

valve, the catheter is advanced over the wire and positioned in the middle of the LV.

The transvalvular gradient is obtained using the sidearm of the femoral sheath to record aortic pressure. Ice-cold saline is used to obtain thermodilution cardiac output using a Swan-Ganz catheter positioned in the pulmonary artery. The aortic valve area is calculated using Gorlin's formula.[46]

In the presence of adequate renal function, left ventriculography is obtained in the 30-degree right anterior oblique (RAO) projection. If the patient could be considered for PHV placement in the future, then, before crossing, or at completion after the pull-back pressure recording, supra-aortic angiography is obtained in a posteroanterior or shallow LAO projec-tion, followed by abdominal aortic and pelvic vessel angiography.

Hardware Required for Balloon Aortic Valvuloplasty

Guidewire

An extra-stiff Amplatz 0.035-inch, 270-cm guidewire (Cook, Bjaeverskov, Denmark) is used to replace the crossing catheter with the pigtail catheter, and then to facilitate passage of the balloon catheter to and across the aortic valve; it also assists in controlling and stabilizing the balloon during positioning for inflation and in withdrawal during deflation. Before use, a large, pigtail-shaped curve is formed at the

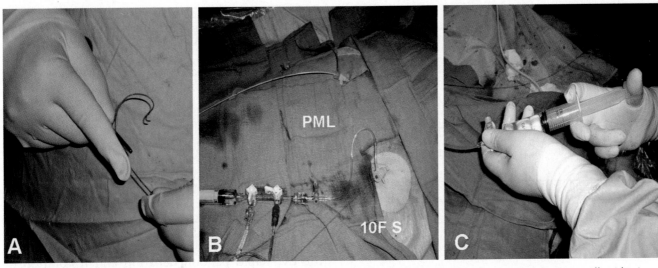

Figure 52-2. Basic technical aspects of balloon aortic valvuloplasty. **A,** Method of preshaping the distal end of the extra-stiff guidewire. **B,** A view of the two entry sites, with the 8-Fr sheath in the right femoral vein for Swan-Ganz catheterization and pacemaker lead (PML) placement and a 10-Fr sheath in the femoral artery; the left femoral artery was preferred in this patient. **C,** Balloon inflation using a 30-mL syringe with 30:70 contrast/saline solution.

distal end of the wire, using a dull instrument (Fig. 52-2A).

Sheaths

For arterial access, the 8-Fr sheath is replaced over the extra-stiff wire with a 10-, 12-, or 14-Fr sheath, depending on the balloon catheters used. As the technique has evolved, the profile of the access devices has been reduced, decreasing the incidence of local complications at the femoral artery puncture site, which had been the most frequent of the complications reported.[47] Until recently, we used 12- to 14-Fr sheaths, facilitating hemostasis by "preclosing" with a 10-Fr Perclose device (Prostar, Abbott Vascular, Redwood City, CA). Currently, because a 10-Fr sheath is generally required, we are able to close the femoral access using an 8-Fr Angioseal vascular closure device (St. Jude Medical, Belgium) at the end of the procedure.

Balloon Catheters

The majority of our experience was obtained with balloon catheters that were specifically designed for BAV. The Cribier-Letac catheters were double-sized balloons mounted on a 9-Fr triple-lumen, pigtail-tipped catheter, which facilitated the procedure by allowing sequentially larger dilations followed by assessment of gradients and valve areas without the need to exchange catheters. The disadvantage was that the profile required a 14-Fr sheath to access the artery. When the production of those catheters was discontinued, we chose the Z-Med II balloon catheter (NuMed, Canada), compatible with a 12- or 14-Fr sheath, and currently the lower-profile Cristal balloons (Balt Extrusion, Montmorency, France), which are compatible with a 10-Fr sheath. The 20-mm and 23-mm diameter balloons are 45 mm in length, and the 25-mm balloon is 50 mm in length. The catheter

shaft is 7 Fr (20- and 23-mm balloons) or 9 Fr (25-mm balloon).

The first chosen balloon diameter is usually 23 mm. The 20-mm balloon is used in those patients who have densely calcified valves and/or a small annulus diameter (<19 mm by echocardiographic measurement). In up to 25% of the cases, the 25-mm balloon may be required to achieve better results if the aortic annulus diameter is larger than 24 mm. In our earlier experience, we started out with smaller (15- and 18-mm) balloon sizes, but this is not routinely done now.

Initial Steps of the Procedure

A 5-Fr temporary bipolar pacing lead is positioned in the right ventricular apex and connected to a pulse generator capable of pacing at up to 220 beats/min. Pacing and sensing parameters are determined, and then the blood pressure response to pacing at 200 to 220 beats/min is evaluated. The rapid ventricular pacing must cause a precipitous fall of blood pressure to at least 50 mm Hg to be effective (Fig. 52-3). If this is not achieved at a rate of 200 beats/min, then the response is checked again at 220 beats/min, which is required in most cases. The pacer is set on demand mode at 80 beats/min, serving as a backup in the event that a vagal episode or interruption of atrioventricular conduction occurs, resulting in bradycardia or asystole in response to balloon inflations.

The diagnostic catheter is removed from the LV over the extra-stiff wire while the looped flexible segment of wire is carefully maintained in the LV cavity (see Fig. 52-1B). The 8-Fr sheath is replaced by the 10-Fr sheath over the extra-stiff wire (see Fig. 52-2B).

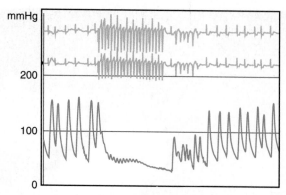

Figure 52-3. Electrocardiogram and aortic pressure curves showing the effect of rapid pacing of the right ventricle (220 beats/min).

A short extension tubing with a three-way stopcock attached is connected to a hand-held 30-mL syringe filled with diluted contrast material. The contrast is diluted 15:85 with saline to reduce viscosity in order to facilitate the inflation/deflation cycles. The ability to obtain adequate visualization of the balloon can be tested by observing the syringe on fluoroscopy.

After flushing of the distal lumen and application of negative pressure on the balloon port, the balloon catheter is mounted on the extra-stiff wire and advanced into the aorta, letting it rest just above the aortic valve. At this time, the balloon is partially inflated and then completely deflated one or more times to completely purge it of air bubbles, which can be observed on fluoroscopy. Accumulated air is discharged from the syringe, which is then topped off to 30 mL if necessary, using the three-way stopcock. If on subsequent balloon inflations air bubbles are noted, it is imperative to stop the inflation and repurge the air completely, to avoid the possibility of air embolization in the event of balloon rupture.

The balloon catheter is advanced across the aortic valve, positioning it with the aortic calcifications midway between the two markers. Before the use of rapid ventricular pacing, it was always challenging to maintain the balloon in optimal position during balloon inflation. The inflated balloon would tend to "pop" into the LV, abruptly striking the apex, or it would "eject" itself back into the aorta, with the possibility of disrupting atheromatous plaque, which could then embolize.

Rapid Ventricular Pacing and Balloon Inflation

Simultaneous forward pressure on the balloon catheter and forward pressure on the extra-stiff wire help to stabilize the balloon while it is being partially filled with dilute contrast solution. It is necessary to quickly "lock" the balloon in place by suddenly expanding the partially filled balloon when it is in the optimal position, using a full inflation with a 30-mL syringe (see Fig. 52-2C). This has been made much easier by the use of rapid ventricular pacing to arrest the forceful contractions of the heart, thereby allowing the operator to stabilize the balloon in the optimal position.

There must be clear communication between the operator manipulating the balloon catheter and the one managing the pacing device. Rapid ventricular pacing is turned on, and balloon inflation is started quickly and with enough pressure to rapidly inflate the balloon (see Fig. 52-1C) as soon as the blood pressure falls. Rapid ventricular pacing is continued for a few seconds after the balloon reaches maximal inflation. Balloon deflation is rapidly performed, the pacer is turned off, and the balloon is withdrawn from the valve. This step requires coordination of the two operators to quickly allow restoration of antegrade flow while maintaining safe wire position in the LV. Rapid balloon deflation and restoration of blood flow is important to minimize the duration of hypotension and hypoperfusion in these hemodynamically compromised patients. We allow time for the heart rate and blood pressure to return to preinflation parameters before deciding to inflate the balloon again.

Because the pressure gradient cannot be measured through the current generation of balloon catheters, it is important to assess the effects of the balloon dilation and the hemodynamic consequences by observation of the wave form of the aortic pressure tracing as well as the heart rate response, rhythm, and blood pressure recovery. For example, a sudden change in wave form with loss of the dicrotic notch or falling diastolic blood pressure could indicate the presence of severe aortic regurgitation.

One or more inflations are usually carried out, using the profile of the expanded balloon on fluoroscopy as a guide and assessing the hemodynamic results before remeasuring the transaortic gradient. The balloon catheter is removed while strong negative pressure is applied with a 60-mL syringe on the balloon port, maintaining guidewire position in the LV. Particular care must be taken as the deflated balloon is drawn through the sheath. If resistance is encountered, it may be necessary to remove the catheter and sheath together as a single unit.

The residual gradient is then obtained by simultaneous measurement of the pressure using a pigtail catheter placed over the extra-stiff wire in the LV, with the pressure recorded from the sidearm of the sheath (Fig. 52-4). If there is a significant gradient, the next larger size balloon may be chosen and the sequence repeated. A pullback gradient is also obtained after the final balloon inflation. For the final results, the pacemaker is removed and replaced with the thermodilution Swan-Ganz catheter. Gorlin's formula is used to determine the final aortic valve area, and an optimal result is considered to be doubling of the valve area compared with the baseline value.

As mentioned previously, at this time supra-aortic angiography may be performed to determine the presence and/or severity of aortic regurgitation (see

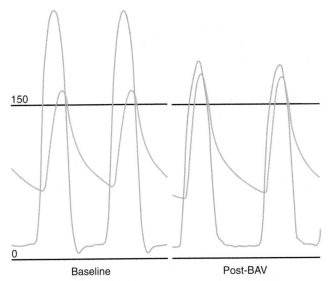

150

0

Baseline   Post-BAV

Figure 52-4. Example of the improvement in transvalvular gradient obtained after inflations of a 23-mm balloon. In this case, the mean transvalvular gradient decreased from 86 mm Hg (baseline) to 22 mm Hg (post-BAV), and the valve area increased from 0.48 to 1.04 cm².

Fig. 52-1D). This may be followed by abdominal and pelvic angiography, depending on the patient's renal status, to determine the strategy regarding future PHV placement.

Immediate Management after Balloon Inflation

After the final result is obtained, the balloon catheter, Swan-Ganz catheter, and sheaths are removed. Manual compression is used for hemostasis at the venous entry site. With the use of the 14-Fr sheath, the previously placed Perclose sutures are used to close the arterial puncture. Now, the femoral artery access site is closed using an 8-Fr Angioseal device whenever the 10-Fr sheath has been used. This has been successful in the vast majority of the cases in which it has been attempted. If a technical failure occurs, a pneumatic pressure device is used (Femo-Stop II Plus, Radi Medical Systems AB, Uppsala, Sweden). If the case is uncomplicated, the patient is usually discharged within 2 days. However, if BAV is performed in patients with severely impaired LV function, or for rescue of a premortem patient from cardiogenic shock, hemodynamic monitoring with inotropic support is usually required. Vagal reactions are the most common cause of hypotension associated with BAV. There must be a low threshold for ruling out the occurrence of pericardial tamponade or retroperitoneal bleed when evaluating the hypotensive patient after BAV.

The Antegrade Transseptal Approach

We reserve the use of the antegrade transseptal approach for BAV for those patients who have severe peripheral vascular disease that precludes femoral arterial access or would increase complications using the retrograde approach.

Patient Preparation

The patient is given mild intravenous sedation and local anesthesia at the access sites. Femoral venous access is obtained bilaterally, with an 8-Fr sheath in the right femoral vein and a 6-Fr sheath in the left femoral vein. Through a 6-Fr sheath in the femoral artery, if possible, or in the brachial (or radial) artery, a coronary angiography is performed if indicated, and a pigtail catheter is placed above the aortic valve. Right-sided heart catheterization and baseline hemodynamic measurements are recorded. Using the left femoral vein access, a bipolar pacing catheter is positioned in the right ventricular apex. Pacing parameters are determined, and rapid ventricular stimulation is assessed, as described earlier.

Transseptal Catheterization

Transseptal catheterization is performed using an 8-Fr Mullins sheath and Brockenbrough needle via the right femoral vein. In our method, we cross the septum in the left lateral view. A pigtail catheter is positioned in the ascending aorta throughout the procedure for monitoring of blood pressure, and at this stage it serves as a reference marker for the transseptal puncture. The puncture is made in the middle third of a virtual line connecting the distal tip of the pigtail catheter adjacent to the aortic calcification and the posterior border of the heart. After entry into the left atrium is confirmed, heparin (50 IU/kg) is administered intravenously.

The Mullins sheath is then used to direct a 7-Fr Swan-Ganz catheter that has an inner lumen compatible with a 0.035-inch guidewire (Edwards Lifesciences, Irvine, CA) across the mitral valve into the LV under fluoroscopic guidance in the 40-degree RAO projection. The transaortic gradient is determined with the Swan-Ganz catheter in the LV and the pigtail catheter in the aorta. The aortic valve area is calculated using Gorlin's formula, the cardiac output having been previously measured.

Crossing the Aortic Valve

The Mullins sheath is advanced approximately 2 cm beyond the mitral valve. The balloon of the Swan-Ganz catheter is inflated and directed into the LV outflow, approaching the native aortic valve. A 0.035-inch straight wire may facilitate crossing of the aortic valve with the balloon deflated, as the catheter is pushed over the wire into the ascending aorta. The wire is removed, and the balloon is reinflated. The catheter is advanced into the descending aorta and positioned at the level of the distal aortic bifurcation with an Amplatz 0.035-inch, 360-cm long Extra-Stiff Guidewire (Cook). The balloon is deflated, and the Swan-Ganz catheter is removed.

The "Essential" Guidewire Loop in the Left Ventricle

We have learned that, during this step of the procedure, it is very important to keep a large loop in the guidewire within the LV. Straightening of the guidewire between the mitral valve and the aortic valve can keep the mitral valve open, resulting in severe mitral regurgitation with hemodynamic deterioration. The loop within the LV is maintained with continuous monitoring at each step of the procedure.

The 8-Fr venous sheath is replaced with a 10-Fr sheath for the subsequent balloon dilations using the Cristal balloon catheter (12- or 14 Fr if NuMed balloons are used).

Atrial Septostomy

The atrial septum is dilated with an 8-mm diameter balloon septostomy catheter through the 10-Fr sheath in the right femoral vein. Diluted solution of contrast medium in saline (30:70) is used with a 10-mL syringe for at least two balloon inflations of 30 seconds each.

Antegrade Balloon Aortic Valvuloplasty

The same balloon catheters are used for antegrade BAV as for the retrograde approach. Dilation of the aortic valve is done preferentially with the 23-mm diameter balloon, which is advanced through the 10-Fr sheath and positioned across the aortic valve while the loop in the LV is maintained carefully. The balloon is purged of air after it is positioned in the LV, before crossing the valve, and then BAV is performed as described earlier, using rapid ventricular pacing for stabilization during balloon inflations. Again, the loop in the LV must be carefully monitored during this step, particularly as the balloon is withdrawn from the valve quickly during balloon deflation.

It is not feasible to measure the gradient after inflations of each diameter of balloon with this technique. After the initial balloon inflations are completed, the hemodynamic result is assessed by observing the aortic pressure waveform. If a significant fall of the diastolic pressure is not present, then the next larger balloon size may be chosen.

After the inflations using the largest selected balloon size are completed, usually after two or three inflations, the balloon catheter is removed. A 5-Fr pigtail catheter is advanced over the extra-stiff wire and positioned over the arch so that the wire can be removed shielded by the catheter, avoiding cutting injury to the aorta or mitral valve. The final gradient is obtained with the pigtail catheter in the LV, and another 4- or 5-Fr catheter in the aorta. Supra-aortic and LV angiograms can be obtained.

If there is no atrioventricular conduction defect, the pacing catheter is removed and replaced with the Swan-Ganz catheter for final hemodynamic measurements. Hemostasis is obtained with manual compression of the femoral artery and vein after sheath removal. Bed rest is recommended for 24 hours. Observation in the intensive care unit with inotropic support and prolonged hemodynamic monitoring is required in rare instances for hemodynamically unstable patients, typically those presenting with poor LV function or in cardiogenic shock.

Results Using Contemporary Techniques

We recently published the results of our most recent series of 141 patients with severe AS whose BAV procedures were done consecutively (with the exception of patients undergoing PHV implantation) between January 2002 and April 2005.[25] In this group of patients, the average age was 80.3±10 years; 45% were women, and all patients were high risk for surgery or considered inoperable. The Parsonnet score was 41±8. Eighty percent were in New York Heart Association (NYHA) functional class IV, with 28% of patients having poor LV function (ejection fraction <30%). The procedure was done emergently for patients in cardiogenic shock in 5.6% of cases. The retrograde approach was used in 95% of the cases. The largest balloon used was 23 mm in 84% of the procedures.

The immediate results showed an increase in aortic valve area, from 0.59±0.19 to 1.02±0.34 cm^2 ($P<.001$), and a decrease in transvalvular gradient, from 49.3±21.2 to 22.2±11.8 mm Hg ($P<.001$). Post-BAV aortic regurgitation was grade 2 in 14%, grade 3 in 3.5%, and grade 4 in 1.4% of the cases.

Six patients (4%) died, three during aortic valve dilation. Nonfatal severe complications occurred in nine patients (6%) and included two transient strokes, five episodes of complete atrioventricular block, and two instances of severe aortic regurgitation. There were eight vascular complications not requiring surgical repair. Discharge from the hospital was at 5.6±3 days.

In our series, the frequency of clinically apparent neurologic events was less than 2%, and this result is favorable compared with the reported incidence in a series of retrograde catheterizations of the aortic valve without intervention.[48] We give heparin before crossing the valve and then use a technique that minimizes trauma to the aortic valve structure during attempted crossing. Although feared as a potentially fatal and disabling complication, embolization of atheromatous debris, which can be broken loose during the balloon's impact on the valve, is actually quite uncommon. Because many of these patients have concomitant cerebrovascular disease, hypotension and hypoperfusion during balloon inflation can also result in a neurologic event. Minimizing the

Table 52-1. Comparison of Complication Rates in the Rouen Series and in an Early Registry

Complications Reported	Mansfield Scientific Aortic Valvuloplasty Registry, 1986-1988 (*N*=492)	Rouen Series, 2002-2005 (*N*=141)
Procedural deaths	2 (4.9%)	3 (2.1%)
Postprocedural deaths (<7 days)	13 (2.6%)	3 (2.1%)
Cerebral embolic events	11 (2.2%)	2 (1.4%)
Transient ischemic attacks	5 (1.1%)	0 (0%)
Ventricular perforation with tamponade	11 (2.2%)	0 (0%)
Severe aortic insufficiency	5 (1.1%)	2 (1.4%)
Vascular complications (surgical repair)	27 (5.5%)	0 (0%)
Nonfatal arrhythmias	5 (1.1%)	5 (3.5%)
Other: myocardial infarction, sepsis, renal failure	8 (1.6%)	1 (1%)

duration of rapid ventricular pacing and balloon inflation are important technical issues, and maintaining optimal heart rate and blood pressure during the procedure is crucial. Preventing, recognizing, and treating vagal reactions expeditiously is also important to avoid the possible neurologic consequences of hypotension.

Improvements in the procedure, such as rapid ventricular pacing and vascular closure devices, as well as continued experience have resulted in decreased complications despite an increasingly aged and sicker population of patients. The large registries have reported higher complication rates, possibly related to the multiple participating centers, many of whose operators were reporting their first experience.[15,47] The reduction of complications in our series, compared with the results of an early registry, is notable (Table 52-1).

Current Perspectives of Balloon Aortic Valvuloplasty

The recently updated ACC/AHA Guidelines for the management of patients with valvular heart disease continue to regard the role of BAV as controversial.[16] They have no class I or IIa recommendations for BAV. The class IIb indications for adult patients with severe AS are for patients who are at high risk for AVR because they are hemodynamically unstable and who would be candidates for "a bridge to surgery" or for BAV as a palliative procedure because they have a serious comorbid condition that precludes AVR.

It is clear that BAV should not be considered a substitute for AVR, even in the elderly.[16] All of those patients who are suitable candidates should have surgical AVR. However, in elderly patients, particularly those of very old age with comorbidities, the perioperative complications must be kept in mind, along with the individual desires of the patient, as well as ethical and economic considerations.

Another potential indication for BAV is for the management of patients who present with critical AS and the need for noncardiac emergency surgery. The hemodynamic improvement of BAV is immediate and may decrease the risk of general anesthesia. In these situations, the BAV should be reserved for those patients with severe AS who have the potential for hemodynamic compromise.

Very Old Age

Because of improvements in surgical techniques, age alone is no longer considered a contraindication to surgery, and there are increasing reports of octogenarians and nonagenarians who benefit from cardiac surgery.[6,7,49,50] However, we see more frequently the frail elderly, who often have been hospitalized for congestive heart failure and who have been dissuaded from surgery because of their age, comorbidities, risks for general anesthesia, concern about loss of cognitive function, and likelihood for a prolonged postsurgical recovery. Because patients such as these are often excluded from surgical series of the elderly, and because of the selection of these patients preferentially for BAV, it has never been possible to compare the results of the two treatment modalities, and no randomized trial has been done.

Many such patients are seeking relief of symptoms and improved quality of remaining life and are less concerned about prolonging their life, particularly if they are debilitated by recurrent symptoms of heart failure, angina, syncope, and weakness from reduced cardiac output. In the high-risk population, the operative mortality is increased. Although this risk has been evaluated very subjectively in the past, it can now be assessed using the STS and EuroSCORE calculators, which are available on the Internet.[2,51,52] In these high-risk patients, significant postoperative complications can be anticipated in 37% of the survivors, with hospital stays of 25±17 days; after discharge, they are more likely to require supervised medical care.[53] When given the choice of open heart surgery with its associated potential risks or BAV with its palliative role, the very-high-risk elderly often chose the latter, preferring the possibility of more immediate relief of symptoms and a shorter hospital stay.

For the truly inoperable patient (who still remains difficult to characterize), medical therapy is acceptance of the inevitable deterioration of functional status, recurrent hospitalization, bedridden care, and eventual demise. The decision to prolong the life or the suffering, with the possible risk of shortening the remaining life span with surgery, is a difficult and personal choice for each patient and is also influenced by the counseling physician.[54-56] For many of these patients, sudden death is not a feared outcome, whereas life after a stroke or with loss of cognitive function is a major concern.[57] For most of these patients, particularly those with intact mental acuity, BAV offers symptomatic relief. Some consider the possibility of AVR later, with the BAV as a "bridge to surgery" if it can improve their operative suitability, or they may consider serial dilations if symptoms recur.

In 1995, we reported our results of BAV in a series of 148 such patients who were older than 80 years of age (mean, 85±4 years) and severely symptomatic.[24] Hemodynamic improvement was obtained, with a decrease of the mean gradient from 72 to 26 mm Hg, associated with an increased aortic valve area, from 0.54 to 0.96 cm². The total complication rate was 12%, which included four deaths (2.7%), three strokes (2.0%), one ventricular fibrillation (1.0%), two persistent atrioventricular blocks (1.4%), and eight complications at the femoral entry site requiring surgery (5.0%). There were no events of myocardial infarction or tamponade.

The duration of the hospitalization was 6±5 days. At a follow-up of 13±9 months (range, 4 to 32 months) eight patients had AVR and four patients had repeat BAV because of recurrent symptoms. There were 27 deaths (mean age, 86±3 years), resulting in an actuarial survival rate of 73% at 1 year, and 78% of the patients reported improvement of symptoms.

These elderly patients who are not good surgical candidates can have BAV with meaningful improvement in their quality of life, with an acceptable mortality rate and complications that are favorable (and now lower with the updated techniques used) compared to those of surgery in a lower-risk population.

What is more controversial is the question of the ability of BAV to affect survival. This has been difficult to tease out of the data, and is not possible to know definitively without a randomized trial. We reported a 27% mortality rate at 13 months in our series of very old patients. This actually compares favorably with the mortality rate in other series of patients with severe AS who did not undergo intervention.[58] There have been conflicting results reported regarding any survival benefit, most likely related to early operator experience and technique when the procedure was first introduced.

Although the purpose of BAV in this population of very old patients with severe disease is to relieve suffering, palliate symptoms, and improve the quality of the last remaining months of life, the data suggest that, at least for some patients, survival is also improved. Striving for a larger reduction in gradient and a larger increase in valve area, and the strategy of serial BAV (up to five times in our practice) performed for recurrent symptoms, as well as "bridging to surgery," have contributed to the improved survival in some patients in our series and others.[25,40]

Left Ventricular Dysfunction

Left ventricular function is a major determinant of acute and long-term results of AVR.[9-11,59,60] The risk is particularly elevated when the patient with severe AS presents with severe congestive heart failure or cardiogenic shock. Results of BAV show that improvement of LV function can be obtained in these critically ill subsets of patients whose risk of surgery would be extremely high.[61-63] Recognizing the temporary benefit of BAV, the procedure should be considered as a "bridge to surgery.[16] AVR should be carried out as soon as the patient is clinically stabilized and LV function is optimal as determined by noninvasive imaging. In our experience, this should not be delayed more than 2 to 3 months after BAV.

Patients with poor LV function and low-gradient AS are offered surgery despite an increased perioperative mortality rate as high as 30%.[59,60] The benefit of long-term survival in these patients with low-gradient AS is improved by ensuring an effective prosthetic aortic valve size to minimize the effects of patient prosthetic mismatch.[64] The patients with no demonstrated contractile reserve can have a perioperative mortality as high as 62%.[65] However, AVR is recommended for those patients, because almost two thirds of them may still recover LV function, as was shown by Quere and associates.[66] BAV may be considered an alternative therapy in this subset. A lower subsequent operative mortality rate and improved prognosis could be anticipated in those patients without contractile reserve who do show improved LV function after BAV. For patients who are refused by the surgeon, the result is likened to a death sentence,[67] with a 4-year survival rate as low as 15%.[13,68] For these patients, PHV might become a new therapeutic option.

Until PHV becomes a clinical reality, BAV remains a viable alternative for the management of selected patients with severe AS who are elderly or have comorbidities that make them unlikely or unacceptable candidates for AVR. The ACC/AHA Guidelines should not be interpreted as recommendations to avoid using BAV. In Europe and in the United States, there are significant proportions of patients with severe AS who are not treated at all according to the guidelines. BAV continues to have an important role in the management of AS, particularly as a palliative modality for our increasing population of elderly patients for whom the risk of surgery is too high or not appropriate.[24,25,40,55,56] This technique should again become familiar to the interventional cardiologist and should be learned by the cardiac surgeon who is interested in the percutaneous or transapical approach to implantation of an aortic valve.

THE PERCUTANEOUS HEART VALVE

A definitive nonsurgical answer to the problem of restenosis after BAV is under intense investigation with the development of the PHV, which, if its promise is met, may become a primary therapeutic modality for high-risk and inoperable patients with critical AS.

The development of percutaneous catheter-based systems for the treatment of patients with valvular disease has been an exciting area for research since the mid-1960s. The initial animal investigations were performed by Davies in 1965,[69] followed by Moulopoulos and associates in 1971,[70] Phillips and colleagues in 1976,[71] and Matsubara and colleagues in 1992.[72] These investigators reported various catheter-based systems for temporary relief of aortic insufficiency, but no further human application was possible due to unsolved major limitations. A new era of investigations started with the development of endovascular stents, raising the concept of a balloon-expandable valvular prosthesis. In 1992, Andersen and associates[73] reported their work in a porcine model in which they evaluated a transluminal stented heart valve. Here again, despite encouraging experimental results, several important limitations precluded human application. Subsequently, in 2000, Bonhoeffer and coworkers, using a valve from a bovine jugular vein mounted within an expandable stent, reported the feasibility of delivering such a device inside the native pulmonary valve of lambs[74]; thereafter, they were able to perform the first successful human percutaneous replacement of a pulmonary valve in a right ventricle-to-pulmonary prosthetic conduit with valve dysfunction.[75] They have had to date satisfactory midterm results and no mortality in more than 100 patients (personal communication, P. Banhoeffer, May 2006).

As far as our team is concerned, the concept of catheter-based valve replacement emerged during the early 1990s as a potential therapeutic solution for patients with nonsurgical calcific AS and as a potential way to overcome the high restenosis rate observed after balloon valvuloplasty. A non–surgically implantable valve might offer an ideal therapeutic option to these patients. In 1994, we did a series of stent implantations in human cadavers with AS. This gave us information regarding the ability of the calcified and fibrotic aortic annulus to anchor a stent and provided the initial requirements for stent length and diameter. After 5 years of searching for a company interested in this project, one was finally identified in 1999. With the help of Percutaneous Valve Technologies (PVT, Fort Lee, NJ), an original PHV has been developed and tested in the sheep model.[76] Hemodynamic characteristics and durability of the valve were extensively tested in vitro. However, chronic interactions in a living system to evaluate thrombogenicity, biocompatibility, degeneration, and calcification required in vivo testing. The proximity of the coronary ostia to the mitral valve insertions resulted in difficulty positioning the device in the animal model. When the device was implanted in the aorta, valve leaflet motion was not reliably reproduced. We subsequently devised an original animal model of chronic aortic regurgitation that allows for long-term evaluation of the PHV in the systemic circulation of experimental animals.[77] By causing controlled aortic regurgitation percutaneously, a closing gradient is created that allows for a more reliable means of testing artificial valve function, performance, and durability.

The first percutaneous aortic valve implant in a human was performed by our group in April 2002[18] and was followed by an initial series of human implantations for compassionate use that were serially reported.[78-80] After the acquisition of PVT by Edwards Lifesciences in 2003, further modifications of the device (Cribier-Edwards Percutaneous Heart Valve) preceded multicenter clinical trials. Results from other centers have been published[81-82] that confirm the feasibility of the PHV. To date, more than 150 PHVs have been implanted worldwide.

This chapter provides a view of the current procedural techniques, results, and future strategies with the Cribier-Edwards device.

Percutaneous Heart Valve Implantation using the Cribier-Edwards Bioprosthetic Valve

The first percutaneously implanted aortic valve in a human was done in 2002 using the antegrade approach because the patient had severe occlusive peripheral vascular disease and no arterial vascular access.[18] Since then, there have already been continued refinements in the device and, with continuing experience, changes in the protocols for device delivery, including the retrograde approach.

Percutaneous Valve and Delivery Systems: Current Generation and Innovations

The Cribier-Edwards PHV (Edwards Lifesciences) consists of a bioprosthetic valve, which is now available in two sizes; the balloon catheter on which it is mounted; and the device for crimping the balloon onto the delivery catheter.

The Percutaneous Heart Valve
The bioprosthetic valve (Fig. 52-5), composed of a stainless steel balloon-expandable stent with an integrated unidirectional trileaflet valve, was initially composed of three equal sections of equine pericardium, now converted to bovine tissue. A fabric cuff is sewn onto the frame covering one third of the device, which is oriented toward the LV when deployed. The original stent, 14.5 mm in length, was designed for a maximal expansion to 23 mm diameter. Because of the undesirable rate of perivalvular leaks observed in the initial trials, a larger stent was produced, 26 mm in diameter and 16 mm in length. Durability of greater than 10 years has been established for the PHV in bench testing.

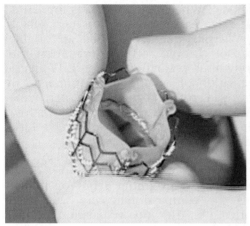

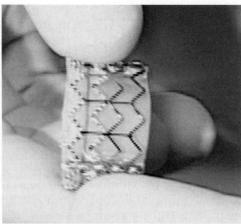

Figure 52-5. Top (*left*) and lateral (*right*) views of the Cribier-Edwards Percutaneous Heart Valve showing the three pericardial leaflets sutured to the stainless steel stent and the fabric cuff covering one third of the device, which is oriented toward the left ventricle when deployed.

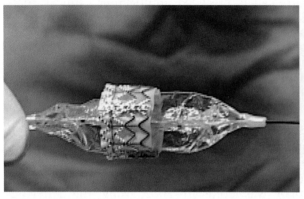

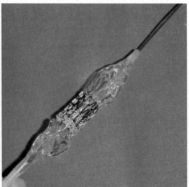

Figure 52-6. View of the Percutaneous Heart Valve in position over a 3×22 mm Z-Med II balloon catheter before (*left*) and after (*right*) crimping.

The Balloon Catheter

To deliver and deploy the PHV, a balloon mounted on a catheter (Z-Med) that is custom manufactured by NuMed is used. The 9-Fr catheter is 120 cm long. The balloon dimensions are 30 mm in length, with diameters at full inflation of either 22 mm or 25 mm for the new, larger device. The 23-mm PHV, when crimped onto its delivery balloon (Fig. 52-6), is compatible with a 22-Fr sheath, and the 26-mm PHV with a 24-Fr sheath.

The Crimping Tool

An original crimping device (Fig. 52-7) is used to symmetrically compress the overall diameter of the PHV from its expanded size to its minimal delivery profile. The mechanism is manual and is activated by a rotary knob on the housing. A cylindrical gauge is used to confirm the collapsed profile of the delivery system, to ensure that it will move smoothly through the introducer sheath. A measuring ring is used to calibrate the balloon inflation to its desired size and to determine the amount of diluted contrast mixture in the syringe that will be necessary for proper inflation at the time of deployment.

The Flex Guiding Catheter

An innovation to facilitate the retrograde approach for deploying the PHV that has been evaluated by Webb and colleagues[82] is the use of the Flex catheter

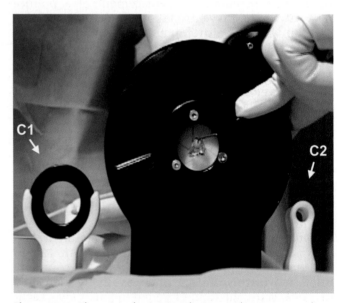

Figure 52-7. The original crimping device used to compress the Percutaneous Heart Valve to its minimal profile. Cylindrical calibers are used to confirm the inflated size of the delivery balloon (C1) and the collapsed profile of the delivery system (C2) to be sure that it can pass through the selected sheath.

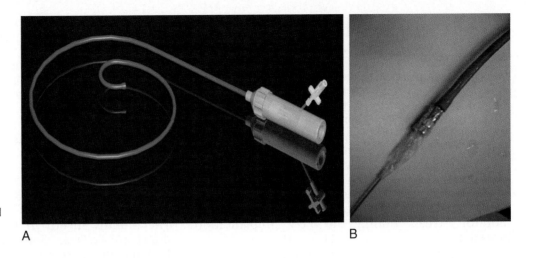

Figure 52-8. A, The Flex catheter currently used for implantation of the Percutaneous Heart Valve (PHV) retrograde from the femoral artery. This active deflection catheter facilitates redirection within the iliofemoral arteries, the aortic arch, and the center of the aortic valve. **B,** The PHV assembly protrudes distally and is not covered by the guide catheter.

(Edwards Lifesciences). This catheter (Fig. 52-8A) has an 18-Fr diameter that increases to 22-Fr distally, where it has a deflectable tip. The tip changes direction when activated by rotation of an external hub incorporated into the handle on the proximal end of the shaft. The PHV assembly and deflecting guiding catheter are introduced through a 25-cm, hydrophilic-coated femoral sheath, facilitated with a hemostatic loading device. The PHV assembly protrudes distally and is not covered by the guide catheter (see Fig. 52-8B). The guide catheter is then used to direct the PHV assembly through the arterial system, around the aortic arch, and across the aortic valve. This provides a less traumatic passage of the PHV through tortuous iliac arteries and diseased abdominal aorta and arch. There is also improved ability to center and push the PHV assembly across the calcified and stenotic native valve. This system also provides precise positioning of the PHV at the aortic annulus. Retrograde delivery of the larger, 26-mm diameter PHV, is possible and has decreased paravalvular leaks, reduced PHV embolization, and improved the final aortic valve area.

Techniques of Implantation of the Cribier-Edwards Valve in the Rouen Series

The techniques described here include the antegrade transseptal approach and the retrograde approach, as used at the University Hospital of Rouen.

Preprocedural Evaluation and Baseline Measurements

The patient's clinical status is determined to be very high risk or inoperable. This is a prerequisite for inclusion into one of the approved PHV trials. For a patient to be considered, severe AS ($\leq$0.7 cm^2) and associated symptoms (dyspnea class IV by NYHA classification) must be present and expected to benefit from isolated valve replacement. Patients must have been refused for standard AVR by two independent cardiac surgeons and classified as having a high operative risk by a Parsonnet score of 30 or higher. Exclusion criteria include the following: intracardiac thrombus, unprotected stenosis of the left main coronary artery not amenable to percutaneous intervention, myocardial infarction within the previous 7 days, prosthetic heart valve, active infection, active bleeding, coagulopathy, or significant vascular disease that precludes access. Patients who cannot be fully dilated with a 23-mm aortic valvuloplasty balloon (notable waist) and patients with a native aortic valve annulus size greater than 25 mm or smaller than 19 mm are also excluded.

Appropriate informed consent is obtained from the patient. Baseline transthoracic echocardiography (TTE), transesophageal echocardiography (TEE), right- and left-sided heart catheterization, left ventriculography, supra-aortic angiography, and coronary angiography are obtained before the planned PHV implantation. This is necessary to determine the severity of the AS and the amount and distribution of calcification, the diameter of the annulus, LV function, and associated coronary artery disease. Aortography with angiography of the iliac and femoral arteries before the procedure, computed tomographic angiography, or magnetic resonance angiography of the aorta and pelvic vessels is necessary to plan the strategy for a retrograde femoral artery approach or an antegrade femoral venous transseptal approach.

Predilatation of the Native Valve

Common to each technique is BAV before PHV deployment, to prepare the native aortic valve and to facilitate crossing, usually with a 23-mm diameter balloon (or a 20-mm diameter balloon in the case of a small calcified annulus) and rapid ventricular pacing during balloon inflation, as described in detail earlier in this chapter. In our center, BAV is carried out often in advance of the procedure and then repeated at the beginning of the PHV implantation session. The retrograde approach, which is simpler and quicker, is used for the predilatation step in all possible cases, as described earlier.

Baseline Measurements

At the time of PHV implantation, baseline hemodynamic measurements and cardiac output, using the thermodilution technique, are obtained. A temporary transvenous pacemaker lead is positioned in the right ventricle, pacing and sensing parameters are determined, the response to pacing at 200 to 220 beats/min is evaluated, and the pacer is set on demand mode at 80 beats/min. Supra-aortic angiography is performed to determine the optimal projection for PHV deployment. This view (usually anteroposterior) shows the aortic valve and annulus perpendicular to the screen, with the coronary artery ostia easily visible. A frame is stored for display on an adjacent monitor screen during the PHV implantation procedure.

Medical Management

Aspirin (160 mg) and clopidogrel (300 mg) are given orally at least 24 hours before the procedure. Antibiotics are given for up to 48 hours after the procedure. Subcutaneous enoxaparin (40 mg/day) is administered until the day of discharge. Clopidogrel (75 mg/day) is continued for 1 month, and aspirin (160 mg/day) is continued indefinitely.

The Antegrade Transseptal Approach

Transseptal Catheterization

As previously described, transseptal catheterization is performed using an 8-Fr Mullins sheath and Brockenbrough needle from the right femoral vein, using standard technique. We use fluoroscopy in the left lateral view and perform the puncture in the middle of a virtual line connecting the distal tip of the pigtail catheter adjacent to the aortic calcification and the posterior border of the heart. A slightly low puncture may facilitate subsequent catheter and device passage across the mitral valve and into the aorta. Heparin (5000 IU) is then administered.

Crossing the Aortic Valve and Externalization of the Guidewire

The Mullins sheath in the left atrium is used to direct a 7-Fr Swan-Ganz catheter with an internal lumen diameter that is compatible with a 0.035-inch guidewire (Edwards Lifesciences) across the mitral valve into the LV under fluoroscopic guidance in the 40-degree RAO projection (Fig. 52-9A). A 0.035-inch straight wire can be used to facilitate crossing of the aortic valve. The catheter is advanced over the wire into the descending aorta, where it is replaced with a 6-Fr pigtail catheter. Through this catheter, an Amplatz 0.035-inch, 360-cm long Extra Stiff Guidewire (Cook) is placed in the descending aorta. It is snared with a 7-Fr catheter snare (Fig. 52-10) with an 18- to 30-mm diameter range and 12 cm length (Entrio Snare, SN18307, Bard Peripheral Vascular, Olen, Belgium) and then externalized through the 10-Fr sheath in the left femoral artery.

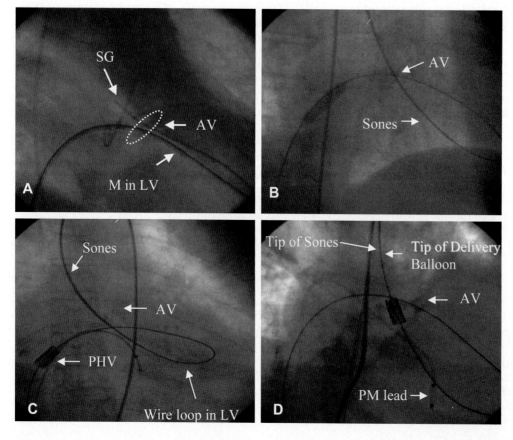

Figure 52-9. Four sequential steps in implantation of the Percutaneous Heart Valve (PHV) in the antegrade approach. **A,** After transseptal catheterization, the Mullins sheath (M) is advanced into the left ventricle (LV) across the mitral valve, and a Swan-Ganz (SG) catheter is used to cross the native aortic valve (AV). **B,** The intra-atrial septum is dilated with a 10-mm septostomy balloon; a Sones (type B) catheter has been previously advanced from the femoral artery into the LV to help maintain the wire loop in the LV during the procedure. **C,** During advancement of the PHV over the wire, special attention is given to preserve the wire loop in the LV. **D,** Accurate positioning of the PHV at the midsegment of the native valve using counterpressure with the Sones catheter on the tip of the PHV assembly. PM leaf, posterior mitral leaf.

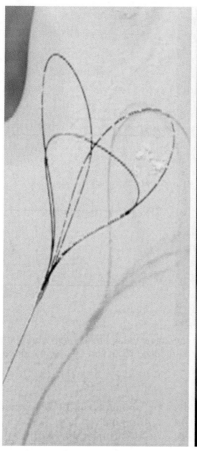
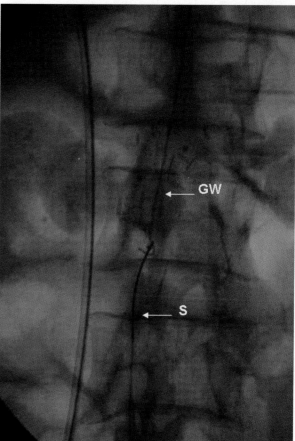

Figure 52-10. Implantation of the Percutaneous Heart Valve in the antegrade approach. The 7-Fr catheter snare (S), shown on the *left panel,* is advanced in the descending aorta *(right panel)* and used to externalize the extra-stiff guidewire (GW) through the 10-Fr sheath in the left femoral artery.

The "Essential" Guidewire Loop in the Left Ventricle

As explained in the discussion of the BAV procedure, when the antegrade approach is used, continuous maintenance of a large guidewire loop within the LV during the procedure is crucial to avoid the severe mitral regurgitation with hemodynamic deterioration that can be induced by guidewire traction on the mitral valve apparatus. During the PHV implantation procedure, this maneuver is facilitated by use of a 7-Fr Sones catheter (type B), which is introduced from the femoral artery and advanced across the aortic valve into the middle part of the LV. This position of the Sones catheter is maintained until the PHV is advanced to the native aortic valve.

Atrial Septostomy

The atrial septum is dilated with a 10-mm balloon septostomy catheter (Owens, Boston-Scientific Scimed, Inc., Maple Grove, MN) through a 10-Fr sheath in the right femoral vein (see Fig. 52-9B). Diluted solution of contrast medium in saline (30:70) is used with a 10-mL syringe for at least two balloon inflations at maximal pressure of 30 seconds each. Passage of the partially deflated septostomy balloon across the septal puncture without resistance is a good sign that the PHV assembly will be able to cross easily.

Delivery and Stabilization of the Percutaneous Heart Valve Assembly

The PHV is crimped onto its delivery balloon catheter and assembled as previously described. A 24-Fr sheath (Cook) is introduced into the right femoral vein. The PHV assembly is then pushed over the wire into the LV (see Fig. 52-9C) and advanced to the native aortic valve. It is emphasized again that it is necessary to maintain the loop of the guidewire in the body of the LV during this maneuver, by tracking back on the guidewire from the femoral vein or applying forward pressure on the Sones catheter through the femoral artery. The Sones catheter is withdrawn to approximately 2 cm above the aortic valve calcifications just as the PHV assembly approaches the native valve from below. With this technique, we have almost eliminated the problems of guidewire-induced hemodynamic compromise.

The valve calcifications and stored images of supra-aortic contrast injections serve as markers for accurate positioning of the PHV at the midsegment of the native valve, or slightly toward the LV in anticipation of upward creep of the apparatus during balloon inflation. Counterpressure with the Sones catheter on the tip of the PHV assembly and test injections help to provide the critical precise positioning required (see Fig. 52-9D). Rapid ventricular pacing is started, and quick and complete inflation of the

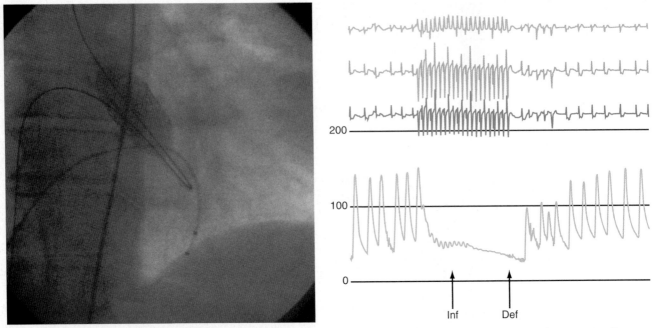

Figure 52-11. Deployment of the Percutaneous Heart Valve in the antegrade approach (*left*) during rapid ventricular pacing. Balloon inflation (Inf) and deflation (Def) are performed during the pacing-induced reduction of systemic pressure (*right*).

delivery balloon is performed when the pressure falls with the rapid heart rate (Fig. 52-11). As soon as the PHV is fully deployed, the balloon is completely deflated. Care must be taken to discontinue pacing after balloon deflation, to avoid ejection of the partially inflated balloon and subsequent device malposition or migration. If a significant perivalvular leak is detected on a supra-aortic injection, a repeat balloon inflation can be carried out with an additional 1 mL of contrast solution in the syringe. The delivery balloon is removed and replaced with a pigtail catheter, which is advanced around the arch. The Amplatz wire can then be safely removed through the femoral vein via the catheter, which prevents injury to the PHV leaflets or the mitral valve apparatus. The pigtail catheter is positioned in the middle of the LV to obtain final hemodynamic measurements.

Immediate Assessment after Deployment

The trans-PHV pressure gradient is measured through the pigtail catheter in the LV (Fig. 52-12), and either the pigtail monitoring catheter or the Sones positioning catheter remains in the ascending aorta. Oximetry is obtained, and calculations for intra-atrial shunting are done. Supra-aortic angiography is done to assess the degree of perivalvular aortic insufficiency and to evaluate the patency of the coronary arteries (see Fig. 52-12). TTE and/or TEE is obtained at the conclusion of the procedure. Typically, the gradient is less than 5 mm Hg, and the valve area is expected to be at least 1.7 cm^2.

The arterial entry sites are closed with a mechanical device (Angioseal), and manual compression is used for venous hemostasis (Fig. 52-13).

Comments on the Antegrade Approach to the Aortic Valve

The advantage of the antegrade approach is that it is truly percutaneous and performed under local anesthesia. This technique avoids the potential complications related to small-caliber, diffusely diseased, and tortuous iliac and femoral arteries of the elderly and to local complications at the puncture site. The PHV assembly is positioned and deployed in the direction of blood flow across the surface of the valve, which is usually less diseased, resulting in smoother passage and more stability. Actually, we have never failed to cross the native valve using the antegrade approach. Although the septum is crossed with a large-profile device, there has been no problem with residual shunting.

The disadvantage of this technique is that the procedure is more complex and more technically demanding than the retrograde approach, which is similar to routine BAV and is more familiar to the interventional cardiologist. The antegrade technique requires a significant learning curve, which definitely limits its widespread use. Because of the complexity of the antegrade approach and the hemodynamic instability that can arise from interference or injury to the mitral valve if the guidewire is not handled properly, there has been renewed emphasis on refining the retrograde approach. However, there will always be patients with small-caliber vessels, severe tortuosities, obstructions of the femoral and iliac arteries, or extensive atherosclerotic disease of the abdominal or aortic arch.[45,83]

Thus, for the foreseeable future, there will be a role for the antegrade approach, more particularly for patients with peripheral vascular disease and contra-

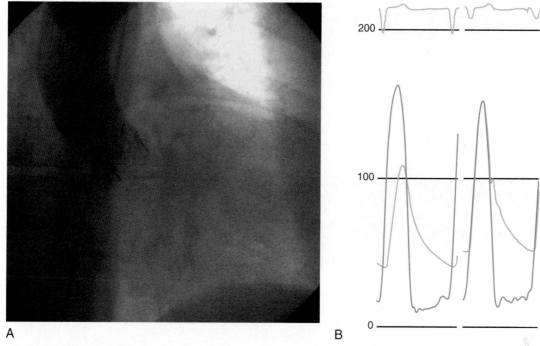

Figure 52-12. Evaluation of results of Percutaneous Heart Valve (PHV) placement. **A,** Supra-aortic angiogram shows no aortic regurgitation and the subcoronary position of the PHV. **B,** Simultaneous recordings of left ventricular and aortic pressure show no residual transvalvular gradient.

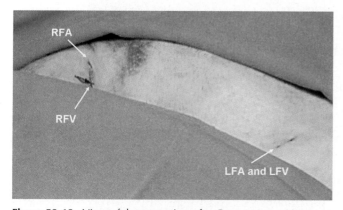

Figure 52-13. View of the entry sites after Percutaneous Heart Valve implantation in the antegrade approach. The right femoral (RFA) and left femoral (LFA) arteries are closed with Angioseal closing devices. Manual or mechanical compression is used to close the right and left femoral veins (RFV and LFV, respectively).

indication to the general anesthesia that is recommended for the retrograde approach and is necessary for the new transapical approach (discussed later).

The Retrograde Approach

Valve Crossing and Predilation of Valve and Femoral Artery

The patient is prepared, and baseline measurements are obtained as described previously. In four patients, we performed preclosure of the common femoral artery puncture site before introduction of the 24-Fr sheath, using two 10-Fr Prostar XL devices (Abbott Vascular Devices, Redwood City, California).

After retrograde catheterization of the aortic valve, the crossing catheter is exchanged for an extra-stiff guidewire, and predilation of the aortic valve is done as described previously. The femoral artery is then predilated with a series of dilators of increasing size (18, 20, and 22 Fr) to facilitate entry of the 24-Fr sheath.

Delivery and Deployment of the Percutaneous Heart Valve

The PHV is advanced over the extra-stiff guidewire, placed within the native valve, and deployed using rapid ventricular pacing, as previously described (Fig. 52-14). Postimplantation hemodynamic and angiographic measurements are similar to those obtained in the antegrade approach. Arterial access is managed by using closure devices or by surgical repair in case of device failure or if preclosing was not done. The use of vascular closure devices has resulted in decreased complications at the access sites when large sheaths are used.[84]

Comments on the Retrograde Approach to the Aortic Valve

In our institution, familiarity with retrograde BAV bred enthusiasm for a method of retrograde delivery of the PHV. However, our first patient had severe peripheral vascular disease that precluded the retrograde femoral approach. Because of the profile and rigidity of the first-generation PHV assembly hardware, the status of the patient's vascular system

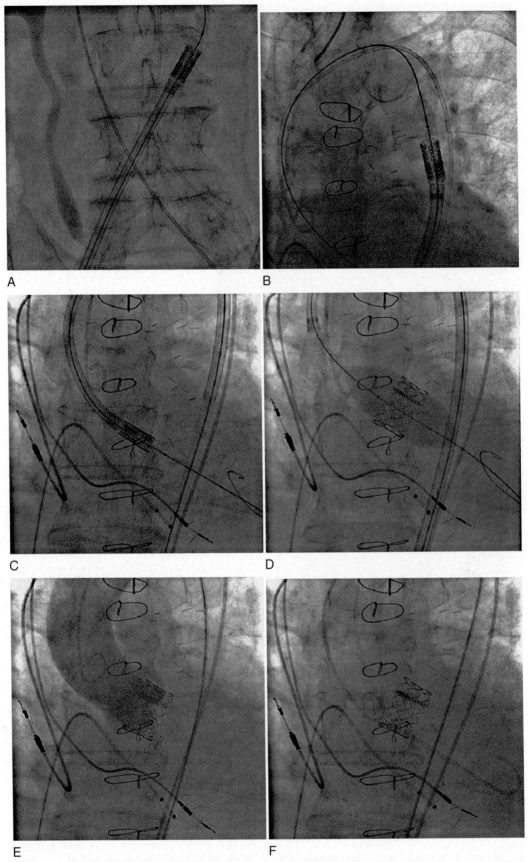

Figure 52-14. The steps of Percutaneous Heart Valve (PHV) implantation in the updated retrograde approach using the Flex catheter. **A,** The PHV is advanced over the extra-stiff guidewire after sequential dilatation of the iliofemoral arteries using 14- to 22-Fr polyethylene dilators. **B,** Deflection of the Flex catheter facilitates redirection within the aortic arch. **C,** The PHV is positioned within the native aortic valve. **D,** Balloon inflation is performed during rapid ventricular pacing. **E,** Supra-aortic angiogram showing mild residual aortic regurgitation and patency of the coronary arteries. **F,** Two pigtail catheters are positioned, one beyond and one beneath the PHV, to measure the transvalvular gradient.

remains a significant determinant for success using the retrograde technique.

An additional significant limitation is entrapment of the guidewire eccentrically between the valve cusps, which interferes with crossing of the native valve. This problem occurred in three of seven attempted cases using the retrograde approach in our series. Because of these limitations, we temporarily abandoned this approach, pending technical improvements. Following improvements, the retrograde approach subsequently became our preferred method, as described later.

Clinical Results of the Rouen Series

Following the report of our first PHV implant,[18] it was necessary to show that the procedure could be reproducibly performed with acceptable results in a similar subset of very-high-risk patients. In this series of procedures done between April 2002 and April 2005, all patients had critical end-stage AS and were selected on a compassionate basis. To be included in the study, they had individual review by the institutional review committee after being formally declined for valve replacement by two independent cardiac surgeons. The series included patients who were treated with either the antegrade or the retrograde approach (I-REVIVE trial) and those treated with the antegrade approach only (RECAST trial). The results of these studies have been reported.[78,80]

Patient Selection

There were 36 patients in the combined trials, with a mean age of 80 ± 7 years and a valve area of less than 0.7 cm²; all were in NYHA functional class IV and had multiple comorbidities with a Parsonnet score of 47 ± 9. One patient died after enrollment but before the procedure, and the remaining 35 patients were taken to the catheterization laboratory. The severity of illness in these patients is highlighted by the fact that, during the recruitment phase, 31 other screened patients died while waiting for enrollment for the procedure.

Percutaneous Heart Valve Implantation

PHV implantation was not performed in 2 of the 35 patients. One procedure was cancelled because the annulus size was inappropriately large for a 23-mm PHV. The second patient, who was in cardiogenic shock, had a cardiac arrest during predilation of the aortic valve and could not be resuscitated. PHV implantation was subsequently attempted in 33 patients. The antegrade transseptal approach was used as the primary intention in 26 cases, and the retrograde approach in 7 cases.

Implantations were successful in 22 (85%) of the 26 patients using the antegrade technique. Of the four unsuccessful cases, two procedures were aborted when the patient became hemodynamically unstable due to the presence of the guidewire across the mitral valve. In the other two cases, PHV migration occurred

immediately after the PHV was deployed. In one case, the PHV was positioned too high, and in the other there was only mild calcification of the valve, a factor that resulted in insufficient anchoring. In both of these cases, the PHVs were deployed safely and without sequelae at alternative sites in the thoracic aorta.

There were seven attempts at PHV deployment using the retrograde approach, and four were successful. One of the failures was converted to the antegrade approach during the same session and was successful.

There is a definite learning curve for the antegrade approach, as demonstrated by a decrease of procedural time from 164 ± 38 minutes during I-REVIVE to 130 ± 30 minutes during RECAST. The retrograde approach, which is a more familiar and less complex technique, had a shorter average procedure time of 96 ± 23 minutes.

Hemodynamic and Angiographic Results

PHV implantation was successful in 27 (75%) of the 36 patients enrolled (Fig. 52-15). Success was obtained in 23 patients using the antegrade approach (85%) and in 4 of 7 patients using the retrograde technique (57%). From baseline hemodynamic measurements and by TTE, the valve area improved at day 1 from 0.60 ± 0.09 cm² to 1.70 ± 0.11 cm² ($P<.0001$), and the mean gradient decreased from 37 ± 13 to 9 ± 2 mm Hg ($P<.0001$). PHV was implanted in the subcoronary position in all cases.

Aortic regurgitation due to paravalvular leak was grade 0 to 1 in 10 patients, grade 2 in 12 patients, and grade 3 in 5 patients. Improvement of LV function in 12 patients was noted as early as 1 week after the procedure (from $45\%\pm18\%$ to $53\%\pm14\%$; $P=.02$) and was most pronounced in patients with an abnormal baseline LV ejection fraction of less than 50% (from $35\%\pm10\%$ to $50\%\pm16\%$; $P<.0001$).

Complications

During the first 30 days, major adverse cardiac events (MACE) occurred in 7 patients (26%) (Table 52-2). There were six fatal in hospital complications. Two patients died as a result of pericardial tamponade. One death resulted from a difficult transseptal puncture in a patient with severe dextrorotation, and the other from perforation of the right ventricle by a pacing lead. Other major procedural complications and deaths were due to stroke (during retrograde crossing of the aortic valve, leading to death on day 33), complete heart block with temporary loss of pacing resulting in anoxic brain damage after prolonged resuscitation, urosepsis, and irreversible hypotension after the 24-Fr sheath was removed (crushing syndrome). A patient with a severe cardiomyopathy died at day 18 from arrhythmia.

Midterm Clinical Follow-up

Among the surviving patients, there was remarkable improvement of symptoms and functional class. Nineteen patients improved to NYHA class I or II

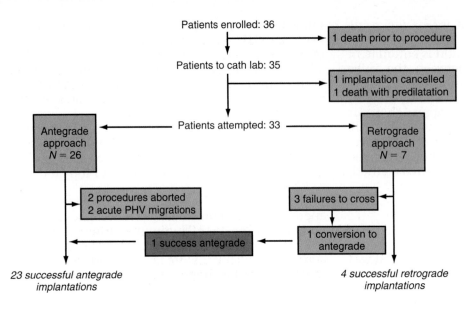

Figure 52-15. Combined I-REVIVE and RECAST series of Percutaneous Heart Valve implantations on a compassionate basis. Schematic representation of patient enrollment and procedural success.

after the procedure. However, long-term survival was limited by their severe comorbidities. Three patients died from renal failure, three from postoperative complications (two vascular, one orthopedic), and one patient each from pulmonary embolus, pneumonia, and metastatic cancer.

Eleven patients were still alive as of March 2006, at a follow-up of 16 to 30 months. Symptoms improved in all patients (>90% NYHA to functional class I to II), and all returned to a normal life. The valve area by TTE of 1.69 ± 0.10 cm^2 measured 3 to 24 months after PHV implantation remained unchanged at follow-up. Aortic regurgitation due to paravalvular leaks was mild and well tolerated (grade 0/1 in seven patients and grade 2 in four patients). Left ventricular ejection fraction in this group was $53\% \pm 12\%$ at follow-up. When compared to the temporary beneficial results of BAV, the improvements in valve area, symptoms, and functional class after PHV appeared durable.

Importantly, during follow-up there was no evidence of device dysfunction or migration, there was no evidence of device-related compromise of coronary perfusion, and no device-related deaths occurred.

Discussion

The results of this "first in man" series of patients demonstrated that PHV implantation for AS is feasible. Although the MACE incidence of 26% at 30 days and 37% at 6 months appears high, this was an extremely high-risk group of patients who were considered for inclusion in these early trials, during which time all of the procedural and technical features were developed and learned.

The Parsonnet score of 47 and EuroSCORE of 12 are associated with a very high 30-day mortality risk for cardiac surgery, 25% and more than 20%, respectively.[17] We successfully implanted the PHV in patients who were deemed not suitable for surgery, and therefore it is difficult to compare our outcomes with those of surgical series. Only 1 (2.8%) of 35 patients in our series of high-risk patients had a stroke, which occurred at the time of predilatation of

Table 52-2. Major Adverse Cardiac Events (MACE) after Percutaneous Heart Valve Implantation on a Compassionate Basis (N=27)

MACE at 30 Days		MACE at 6 Months	
Event	**n**	**Event**	**n**
Death—Total	6	Death—Total	10
Tamponade	2	Renal failure	3
Sepsis	1	Postoperative death	3
Brain death after resuscitation	1	Pulmonary embolus	1
Crush syndrome	1	Pneumonia	1
Multiorgan failure VT	1	Cancer	1
		Multiorgan failure	1
Stroke	1	Stroke	0
Myocardial infarction	0	Myocardial infarction	0
Emergent cardiac surgery	0	Emergent cardiac surgery	0
Total MACE	7	Total MACE	10

VT, ventricular tachyarrhythmia.

the native valve, and this is comparable to the rate of stroke in patients undergoing surgical valve replacement in a lower-risk population.[85]

The mortality rate at 6 months was related to the extensive comorbidities of these patients, and no subsequent mortality was related to the PHV procedure or to PHV failure. A stable valve area, improved LV function in patients who had a lower baseline ejection fraction, and amelioration of symptoms up to 2.5 years later show that, at midterm evaluation, the results are durable.

The balloon-expandable stent frame has demonstrated the necessary radial force and ability to reliably anchor the valve in the subcoronary position. The valve leaflet design results in a stable effective orifice area that is as good as, or better than, that of surgically implanted valves of the same diameter.

The success rate of implantation with the antegrade approach in our series was 85%. However, technical issues and the learning curve described earlier may limit applicability at many centers. Although the retrograde approach was faster and simpler to perform, the success rate was only 57% with the first-generation devices. Many patients could not be considered for this technique because of peripheral vessel size and atherosclerotic disease. Of those selected, there was difficulty crossing the valve because of lack of centering due to guidewire bias and insufficient ability to push the PHV through the stenotic valve.

Technical and Procedural Improvements

To enhance the retrograde approach, a lower-profile system with better ability to traverse the vascular system and aortic arch and with the ability to overcome wire bias and resistance to crossing the native valve was needed. Furthermore, because of concern about PHV migration and paravalvular leaks, a larger-diameter PHV was designed and produced.

The percutaneous retrograde approach using the lower-profile, steerable Flex catheter, an innovation first used by Webb and colleagues, is a step forward in overcoming the described limitations. This technique has become the preferred approach in the ongoing multicenter studies. Webb's group has already published their preliminary results in 18 patients.[82] In this initial series, the mean age was 81±6 years, and all patients were at high surgical risk (EuroSCORE of 26). The 23-mm diameter PHV was deployed in 7 patients, and the 26-mm PHV, after it became available, was implanted in 7 patients successfully, with no procedural deaths. The aortic valve area improved from 0.6 cm² to 1.6 cm². When the angiographic results of the 23-mm PHV were compared with those of the 26-mm device, there was a decreased frequency and severity of paravalvular aortic regurgitation with the larger PHV diameter. All of the cases had planned open surgical closures of the femoral artery. There were four cases in which valve deployment was unsuccessful. There were two valve embolizations, both with the smaller (23-mm)

PHV; those devices were subsequently deployed in the transverse or descending aorta. One of these patients subsequently had surgical AVR. Two valves were removed, one because of inability to traverse a diseased iliac artery and one because of inability to cross the native valve; both of these PHVs were removed. At a follow-up of 75±55 days, 16 patients (89%) were alive. Two patients died before 30 days, one of multiorgan failure and the other with obstruction of the left main coronary artery by a calcified nodule.

Webb and colleagues recently reported their updated series of 50 patients (EuroPCR, Paris, May 2006), showing similarly good results. Mortality at 30 days was 12% (6 patients). The data also showed improvement after a learning curve of 25 procedures. There is no doubt that transarterial, retrograde PHV implantation does represent a significant enhancement with respect to delivery and procedural simplicity.

The Transapical Approach

The transapical approach for PHV implantation has been recently described. In this approach, the same Cribier-Edwards PHV and delivery catheter are introduced under direct vision into the LV via a minithoracotomy and ventricular puncture and directed across the aortic valve under guidance by TEE and fluoroscopy. This obviates the concerns of access sites in the presence of small-caliber vessels and/or vascular occlusive disease. It also reduces the risk for stroke, which could be related to passage of a stiff device through a diseased and tortuous aorta. This technique may also have a future role in patients with a "porcelain aorta," previous cardiac surgery, or a history of mediastinal irradiation. Currently, general anesthesia and mechanical ventilation are required, limiting applicability of the procedure in patients with chronic lung disease or other disorders that would contraindicate general anesthesia. The feasibility of this technique was shown in animal experiments,[86] and its application has been recently reported in humans.[87,88]

In the future, the interventional cardiologist should have several technical alternatives to ensure the procedural success of PHV implantation, depending on various anatomic and clinical features, as summarized in Table 56-3.

Future Strategies

Pulmonary Valve and Degenerated Bioprosthetic Valve

There is one experimental animal report of this PHV in the pulmonary position,[89] and there is one report of implantation in an adolescent who had a prior Ross procedure and subsequent replacement of a homograft in the pulmonary position.[90] When the homograft became stenotic, the patient had stenting

Table 52-3. Alternative Approaches for Percutaneous Heart Valve Implantation

I. Preliminary evaluation
A. Peripheral arteries, abdominal and thoracic aorta for patency, diameter, tortuosity, atheroma, and calcification
B. Contrast angiography at the time of diagnostic cardiac catheterization, computed tomography, and/or magnetic resonance angiography

II. Selection of approach
A. Retrograde approach via femoral artery (preferred)
B. Transapical route via thoracotomy
  1. If there is significant femoral-iliac or aortic disease or lack of arterial access or contraindication to general anesthesia
  2. In an experienced center
C. Antegrade transseptal approach via femoral vein
  1. If any of the following are present:
    a. Porcelain aorta (calcified ascending aorta)
    b. Transseptal approach contraindicated or anticipated to be difficult (e.g., IVC filter)
    c. Patient did not tolerate antegrade transseptal BAV, hemodynamic instability
  2. Patient is able to tolerate general anesthesia and thoracotomy

BAV, balloon aortic valvuloplasty; IVC, inferior vena cava.

of the pulmonary valve followed by deployment of the Cribier-Edwards valve with a successful result.

Balloon valvuloplasty has been carried out on bioprosthetic valves also in the aortic, tricuspid, and mitral positions.[91-94] Because the bioprosthetic "stent" can provide a means of anchoring the PHV, there is future potential for nonsurgical management of bioprosthetic valve failure with this balloon-expandable device.[95] A surgical valve-in-valve procedure has been performed in a patient with a failed bioprosthetic mitral valve, suggesting the feasibility of this approach.[96]

The broader application of the PHV, to include clinical scenarios such as endocarditis, aortic dilation, or dissection, depends on the imagination of the engineers. A limitation of the balloon-expandable stent is the need for an anchoring substrate, which is not present in many cases of aortic regurgitation; however, different-sized valves with configurations to provide an anchor are possible. An antibiotic coated cuff around the stent might be of benefit for patients with endocarditis and acute aortic regurgitation who would be at very high risk for surgery.

Competing Technologies

There is intense interest in PHV technology, and there are multiple devices at various stages of development in animals and humans. The CoreValve is a self-expanding, stented valve that is being developed for the treatment of aortic regurgitation as well as AS. The immediate and midterm results with this device are promising.[97,98]

Surgical approaches include the transapical technique, as described earlier, and in addition the technique of aortic valve "bypass" using conduits from the LV apex to the thoracic aorta, which is already established in cardiac surgical practice.[99-101] The patients must be able to tolerate general anesthesia and thoracotomy, and this excludes many of the "inoperable" patients. The technique may have a role for patients with calcified ascending aorta and prior thoracic surgery or irradiation. The transapical approach has the potential to accomplish the same relief in this set of patients, although with less trauma to the patient who may have compromised cardiopulmonary reserve.

An interesting concept is the use of external beam irradiation to delay the onset or modify the course of restenosis after BAV.[102] The results are limited to a very small number of patients, and the technique deserves further study. It is possible that it may provide some temporary relief to the subset of patients with critical AS for whom, because of comorbidities or lack of vascular access, neither surgical valve replacement nor PHV is considered appropriate. Given the uncertainty of the time required to bring the PHV into general clinical practice, the concept of using external irradiation to delay restenosis, if proven to be valid in a randomized multicenter trial, could serve as a temporizing measure until PHV is available, as a "bridge to PHV."

Conclusions

Patients who were in the premortem stage of severe AS, with severe comorbidities, low ejection fraction, and/or advanced age were the first population of patients included in our series. Technological improvements that will continue to make the procedures safer and more effective, along with anticipated continued good immediate and long-term results in the ongoing multicenter European/Canadian (REVIVE) and U.S. (REVIVAL) trials, will determine the future expansion of the technique to include patients at lower surgical risk. After approval by the U.S. Food and Drug Administration, the indications for PHV implantation should expand as clinical experience increases.

If subsequent trials show comparable morbidity and mortality to conventional open-chest AVR, PHV may well become the preferred therapeutic option for a large number of high-surgical-risk patients with aortic valve disease.

The future of this technology and its application depends on the continued collaboration of clinicians, cardiologists, surgeons, engineers, and industry.[103] Because there is a substantial learning curve with each of the techniques and for each device, there must be collaboration between physicians of the same discipline (cardiology, surgery) at different centers in order to disseminate the necessary knowledge and skills. Only a portion of this can be taught in a lecture hall or on a simulator. Fundamental knowledge, skill sets, and practice wisdom of clinicians, imagers, interventionalists, and surgeons must be shared, coordinated, and in fact synchronized for the successful outcome of each procedure and to ensure the future development of the techniques.

It is very important to include primary care physicians and geriatricians with an interest in valvular heart disease of the elderly in the development and implementation process of this new therapy for it to realize its potential. These clinicians have a very profound role in reducing the burden of unrecognized and untreated patients with AS, a burden that is likely to increase as the population ages over the next decades. Octogenarians, nonagenarians, and even centenarians will become a rapidly growing minority in our patient population.

Selection of the appropriate patients for surgical AVR, PHV, BAV, or palliative hospice care is becoming more complex. It demands attention to each individual patient's desires regarding the quality versus quantity of life. A broader array of therapeutic options, including PHV implantation for treatment of severe calcific AS in high-risk and inoperable patients, is within reach.

REFERENCES

1. Lindroos M, Kupari M, Heikkila J, et al: Prevalence of aortic valve abnormalities in the elderly: An echocardiographic study of a random population sample. J Am Coll Cardiol 1993;21:1220-1225.
2. Society of Thoracic Surgeons: STS national database: STS U.S. Cardiac Surgery Database—1997. Aortic valve replacement patients: Preoperative risk variables. Chicago: Society of Thoracic Surgeons, 2000. Available at http://www.ctsnet.org/doc/3031 (accessed April 30, 2007).
3. Otto C: Valvular aortic stenosis: Disease severity and timing of intervention. J Am Coll Cardiol 2006;47:2141-2151.
4. Cribier A, Savin T, Saoudi N, et al: Percutaneous transluminal valvuloplasty in acquired aortic stenosis in elderly patients: An alternative to valve replacement? Lancet 1986;1:63-67.
5. Schwarz F, Baumann P, Manthey J, et al: The effect of aortic valve replacement on survival. Circulation 1982;66:1105-1110.
6. Kohl P, Kerzman A, Lahaye L: Cardiac surgery in octogenarians: Peri-operative outcome and long-term results. Eur Heart J 2001;22:1235-1243.
7. Bridges CR, Edwards FH, Peterson ED: Cardiac surgery in nonagenarians and centenarians. J Am Coll Surg 2003;197:347-357.
8. Chukwuemeka A, Borger MA, Ivanov J, et al: Valve surgery in octogenarians: A safe option with good medium-term results. J Heart Valve Dis 2006;15:191-196.
9. Connolly HM, Oh JK, Schaff HV, et al: Severe aortic stenosis with low transvalvular gradient and severe left ventricular dysfunction: Result of aortic valve replacement in 52 patients. Circulation 2000;101:1940-1946.
10. Tarantini G, Buja P, Scognamiglio R, et al: Aortic valve replacement in severe aortic stenosis with left ventricular dysfunction: Determinants of cardiac mortality and ventricular function recovery. Eur J Cardiothorac Surg 2003;24:879-885.
11. Vaquette B, Corbineau H, Laurent M, et al: Valve replacement in patients with critical aortic stenosis and depressed left ventricular function: Predictors of operative risk, left ventricular function recovery, and long term outcome. Heart 2005;91:1324-1329.
12. Iung B, Baron G, Butchart E: A prospective survey of patients with valvular heart disease in Europe: The Euro Heart Survey on Valvular Heart Disease. Eur Heart J 2003;24:1231-1243.
13. Kapoor N, Varadajan P, Pai R: Survival patterns in conservatively treated patients with severe aortic stenosis: Prognostic

14. variables in 457 patients. Circulation 2004;110(Suppl III):548.
14. O'Neill WW: Predictors of long term survival after percutaneous aortic valvuloplasty: Report of the Mansfield scientific balloon aortic valvuloplasty registry. J Am Coll Cardiol 1991;17:193-198.
15. NHLBI Balloon Valvuloplasty Registry: Percutaneous balloon aortic valvuloplasty: Acute and 30-day follow-up results in 674 patients from the NHLBI Balloon Valvuloplasty Registry. Circulation 1991;84:2383-2397.
16. Bonow RO, Carabello BA, Chatterjee K, et al: ACC/AHA 2006 Guidelines for the management of patients with valvular heart disease: A report of the American College of Cardiology/American Heart Association Task Force on Practice Guidelines (Writing Committee to Develop Guidelines for the Management of Patients with Valvular Heart Disease). American College of Cardiology Web Site. Available at: http://content.onlinejacc.org/cgi/content/full/48/3/e1?ct (accessed April 30, 2007).
17. Kawachi Y, Nakashima A, Toshima Y, et al: Risk stratification analysis of operative mortality in heart and thoracic aorta surgery: Comparison between Parsonnet and Euro-SCORE additive model. Eur J Cardiothorac Surg 2001;20:961-966.
18. Cribier A, Eltchaninoff H, Bash A, et al: Percutaneous transcatheter implantation of an aortic valve prosthesis for calcific aortic stenosis: First human case description. Circulation 2002;106:3006-3008.
19. Letac B, Cribier A, Koning R, et al: Results of percutaneous transluminal valvuloplasty in 218 patients with valvular aortic stenosis. Am J Cardiol 1988;62:1241-1247.
20. Letac B, Cribier A, Koning R, et al: Aortic stenosis in elderly patients aged 80 or older: Treatment by percutaneous balloon valvuloplasty in a series of 92 cases. Circulation 1989;80:1514-1520.
21. Berland J, Cribier A, Savin T, et al: Percutaneous balloon valvuloplasty in patients with severe aortic stenosis and low ejection fraction: Immediate results and 1-year follow-up. Circulation 1989;79:1189-1196.
22. Letac B, Cribier A, Eltchaninoff H, et al: Evaluation of restenosis after balloon dilation in adult aortic stenosis by repeat catheterization. Am Heart J 1991;122:55-60.
23. Koning R, Cribier A, Asselin C, et al: Repeat balloon aortic valvuloplasty. Catheter Cardiovasc Diagn 1992;26:249-254.
24. Eltchaninoff H, Cribier A, Tron C, et al: Balloon aortic valvuloplasty in elderly patients at high risk for surgery, or inoperable: Immediate and mid-term results. Eur Heart J 1995;16:1079-1084.
25. Agatiello C, Eltchaninoff H, Tron C, et al: Balloon aortic valvuloplasty in the adult: Immediate results and in-hospital complications in the latest series of 141 consecutive patients at the University Hospital of Rouen (2002-2005). Arch Mal Coeur. 2006;99:195-200.
26. Litvack F, Jakubowski AT, Butchbinder NA, et al: Lack of sustained clinical improvement in an elderly population after percutaneous aortic valvuloplasty. Am J Cardiol 1988;62:270-275.
27. Lieberman EB, Bashore TM, Hermiller JB, et al: Balloon aortic valvuloplasty in adults: Failure of procedure to improve long term survival. J Am Coll Cardiol 1995;26:1522-1528.
28. Dare AJ, Veinot JP, Edwards WD, et al: New observations on the etiology of aortic valve disease: A surgical pathologic study of 236 cases from 1990. Hum Pathol 1993;24:1330-1338.
29. Roberts WC, Ko JM: Frequency by decades of unicuspid, bicuspid, and tricuspid aortic valves in adults having isolated aortic valve replacement for aortic stenosis, with or without associated aortic regurgitation. Circulation 2005;111:920-925.
30. Freeman R, Otto C: Spectrum of calcific aortic valve disease: Pathogenesis, disease progression, and treatment strategies. Circulation 2005;111:3316-3326.
31. O'Brien KD: Pathogenesis of calcific aortic valve disease: A disease process comes of age (and a good deal more). Arterioscler Thromb Vasc Biol 2006;26:1721-1728.

32. Inoue K, Owaki T, Nakamura T, et al: Clinical application of transvenous mitral commisurotomy by a new balloon catheter. J Thorac Cardiovasc Surg 1984;87:394-402.

33. Letac B, Gerber L, Koning R: Insight in the mechanism of balloon aortic valvuloplasty of aortic stenosis. Am J Cardiol 1988;62:1241-1247.

34. Lembo NJ, King SB, Roubin GS: Fatal aortic rupture during percutaneous balloon valvuloplasty for valvular aortic stenosis. Am J Cardiol 1987;60:733-737.

35. Letac B, Cribier A, Eltchaninoff H, et al: Evaluation of restenosis after balloon dilation in adult aortic stenosis by repeat catheterization. Am Heart J 1991;122:55-60.

36. Bashore TM, Davidson CJ, and the Mansfield Scientific Aortic Valvuloplasty Registry Investigators: Follow-up recatheterization after balloon aortic valvuloplasty. J Am Coll Cardiol 1991;17:1181-1195.

37. Feldman T, Glagov S, Caroll J: Restenosis following successful balloon valvuloplasty: Bone formation in aortic valve leaflets. Catheter Cardiovasc Interv 1993;29:1-7.

38. van den Brand M, Essed CE, Di Mario C, et al: Histological changes in the aortic valve after balloon dilation: Evidence for a delayed healing process. Br Heart J 1992;67:445-449.

39. Soyer R, Bouchart F, Bessou JP, et al: Aortic valve replacement after aortic valvuloplasty for calcified aortic stenosis. Eur J Cardiothorac Surg 1996;10:977-982.

40. Agarwal A, Kini AS, Attani S, et al: Results of repeat balloon valvuloplasty for treatment of aortic stenosis in patients aged 59 to 104 years. Am J Cardiol 2005;95:43-47.

41. Lababidi Z, Wu JR, Walls JT: Percutaneous balloon aortic valvuloplasty: Results in 23 patients. Am J Cardiol 1984;53:194-197.

42. Block PC, Palacios IF: Comparison of hemodynamic results of antegrade versus retrograde percutaneous balloon aortic valvuloplasty. Am J Cardiol 1987;60:659-662.

43. Orme EC, Wray RB, Barry WH, et al: Comparison of three techniques for percutaneous balloon aortic valvuloplasty of aortic stenosis in adults. Am Heart J 1989;117:11-17.

44. Sakata,Y, Syed Z, Salinger M, et al: Percutaneous balloon aortic valvuloplasty: Antegrade transeptal vs conventional retrograde transarterial approach. Catheter Cardiovasc Interv 2005;64:314-321.

45. Rutgers D, Bots ML, Hofman A, et al: Peripheral arterial disease in the elderly, the Rotterdam study. Arterioscler Thromb Vasc Biol 1998;18:185-192.

46. Gorlin R, Gorlin SG: Hydraulic formula for calculations of the area of the stenotic mitral valve, other cardiac valves, and central circulatory shunts. Am Heart J 1951;41:1-29.

47. McKay RG: The Mansfield Scientific Aortic Valvuloplasty Registry: Overview of acute hemodynamic results and procedural complications. J Am Coll Cardiol 1991;17:485-491.

48. Omram H, Schmidt H, Hackenbroch M, et al: Silent and apparent cerebral embolism after retrograde catheterization of the aortic valve in valvular stenosis: A prospective, randomized study. Lancet 2003;361:1241-1244.

49. Rosengart TK, Finnin EB, Kim DY, et al: Open heart surgery in the elderly: Results from a consecutive series of 100 patients aged 85 years or older. Am J Med 2002;112:143-147.

50. Conti V, Lick S: Cardiac surgery in the elderly: Indications and management options to optimize outcomes. Clin Geriatr Med 2006;22:559-574.

51. Roques F, Nashef SA, Michel P, et al: Risk factors and outcome in European cardiac surgery: Analysis of the EuroSCORE multinational database of 19030 patients. Eur J Cardiothorac Surg 1999;15:816-822.

52. Roques F, Michel P, Goldstone AR, Nashef SA: The logistic EuroSCORE. Eur Heart J. 2003;24:881-882. Available at: http://euroscore.org/calc.html (accessed April 30, 2007).

53. Khan JH, McElhinney DB, Hall TS, et al: Cardiac surgery in octogenarians: Improving quality of life and functional status. Arch Surg 1998;133:887-893.

54. Wong JB, Salem DN, Pauker SG: Occasional notes: You're never too old. N Engl J Med 1993;328:972-975.

55. Dauterman KW, Michaels AD, Ports TA: Is there any indication for aortic valvuloplasty in the elderly? Am J Geriatr Cardiol 2003;12:190-196.

56. Feldman T: Proceedings of the TCT: Balloon aortic valvuloplasty appropriate for elderly valve patients. J Interven Cardiol 2006;19:276-279.

57. Zimpfe D, Czerny M, Kilo J, et al: Cognitive deficit after aortic valve replacement. Ann Thorac Surg 2002;74:407-412.

58. O'Keefe JH Jr, Vlietstra RE, Baily KR, et al: Natural history of candidates for balloon aortic valvuloplasty. Mayo Clin Proc 1987;62:986-991.

59. Connolly HM, Oh JK, Orszulak TA, et al: Aortic valve replacement for aortic stenosis with severe left ventricular dysfunction: Prognostic indicators. Circulation 1997;95:2395-2400.

60. Powell DE, Tunick PA, Rosenzweig BP, et al: Aortic valve replacement in patients with aortic stenosis and severe left ventricular dysfunction. Arch Intern Med 2000;160:1337-1341.

61. Desnoyers MR, Salem DN, Rosenfield K, et al: Treatment of cardiogenic shock by emergency aortic balloon valvuloplasty. Ann Intern Med 1988;108:833-835.

62. Cribier A, Remadi F, Koning R, et al: Emergency aortic balloon valvuloplasty as initial treatment of patients with aortic stenosis and cardiogenic shock. N Engl J Med 1992;323:646.

63. Moreno PR, Jang IK, Newell JB, et al: The role of percutaneous aortic balloon valvuloplasty in patients with cardiogenic shock and critical aortic stenosis. J Am Coll Cardiol 1994;23:1071-1075.

64. Kulik A, Burwash IG, Kapila V, et al: Long-term outcomes after valve replacement for low-gradient aortic stenosis: Impact of prosthesis-patient mismatch. Circulation 2006;114(Suppl I):I-553-I-558.

65. Monin JL, Quere JPM, Monchi M, et al: Low-gradient aortic stenosis: Operative risk stratification and predictors for long-term outcome. A multicenter study using dobutamine stress hemodynamics. Circulation 2003;108:319-324.

66. Quere J-P, Monin J-L, Levy F, et al: Influence of preoperative left ventricular contractile reserve on postoperative ejection fraction in low-gradient aortic stenosis. Circulation 2006;113:1738-1744.

67. Bauer F, Cribier A: Percutaneous aortic valve implantation, helping the failing heart. Future Cardiol 2006;2:381-385.

68. Pereira JJ, Lauer MS, Bashir M, et al: Survival after aortic valve replacement for severe aortic stenosis with low transvalvular gradients and severe left ventricular dysfunction. J Am Coll Cardiol 2002;39:1356-1363.

69. Davies H: Catheter mounted valve for temporary relief of aortic insufficiency. Lancet 1965;1:250.

70. Moulopoulos SD, Anthopoulos L, Stamatelopoulos S, et al: Catheter mounted aortic valves. Ann Thorac Surg 1971;11:423-430.

71. Phillips SJ, Ciborski M, Freed PS, et al: A temporary catheter-tip aortic valve: Hemodynamic effects for experimental relief of acute aortic insufficiency. Ann Thorac Surg 1976;21:134-137.

72. Matsubara T, Yamazoe M, Tamura Y, et al: Balloon catheter with check valves for experimental relief of acute aortic regurgitation. Am Heart J 1992;124:134-137.

73. Andersen HR, Knudsen LL, Hasenkam JM: Transluminal implantation of artificial heart valves: Description of a new expandable aortic valve and initial results with implantation by catheter technique in closed chest pigs. Eur Heart J 1992;13:704-708.

74. Bonhoeffer P, Boudjemline Y, Saliba Z, et al: Transcatheter implantation of a bovine valve in a pulmonary position: A lamb study. Circulation 2000;102:813-816.

75. Bonhoeffer P, Boudjemline Y, Saliba Z, et al: Percutaneous replacement of pulmonary valve in a right-ventricle to pulmonary-artery conduit with valve dysfunction. Lancet 2000;356:1403-1405.

76. Cribier A, Eltchaninoff H, Letac B: Advances in percutaneous techniques for the treatment of aortic and mitral stenosis. In Topol EJ (ed): Textbook of Interventional Cardiology, 4th ed. Philadelphia, WB Saunders, 2003, pp 941-953.

77. Eltchaninoff H, Nusimovici-Avadis D, Babaliaros V, et al: Five month study of percutaneous heart valves in the systemic circulation of sheep using a novel model of aortic insufficiency. Eurointervention 2006;1:438-444.

78. Cribier A, Eltchaninoff H, Tron C, et al: Early experience with percutaneous transcatheter implantation of heart valve prosthesis for the treatment of end-stage inoperable patients with calcific aortic stenosis. J Am Coll Cardiol 2004;43:698-703.
79. Bauer F, Eltchaninoff H, Tron C, et al: Acute improvement in global and regional left ventricular systolic function after percutaneous heart valve implantation in patients with symptomatic aortic stenosis. Circulation 2004;110: 1473-1476.
80. Cribier A, Eltchaninoff H, Tron C, et al: Treatment of calcific aortic stenosis with the percutaneous heart valve: Mid-term follow-up from the initial feasibility studies. The French experience. J Am Coll Cardiol 2006;47:1214-1223.
81. Hanzel GS, Harrity PJ, Schreiber TL, et al: Retrograde percutaneous aortic valve implantation for critical aortic stenosis. Catheter Cardiovasc Interv 2005;64:322-326.
82. Webb GW, Chandavimol M, Thompson CR, et al: Percutaneous aortic valve implantation retrograde from the femoral artery. Circulation 2006;113:842-850.
83. Weisenberg D, Sahar Y, Sahar G, et al: Atherosclerosis of the aorta is common in patients with severe aortic stenosis: An intra-operative transesophageal echocardiographic study. J Thorac Cardiovasc Surg 2005;130:29-32.
84. Solomon LW, Fusman B, Jolly N, et al: Percutaneous suture closure for management of large French size arterial puncture in aortic valvuloplasty. J Invasive Cardiol 2001;13:592-596.
85. Kolh P, Kerzmann A, Lahaye L, et al: Cardiac surgery in octogenarians: Peri-operative outcome and long-term results. Eur Heart J 2001;22:1235-1243.
86. Waither T, Dewey T, Wimmer-Greinecker G, et al:. Transapical approach for sutureless stent-fixed aortic valve implantation: Experimental results. Eur J Cardiothorac Surg 2006; 29:703-708.
87. Ye J, Cheung A, Lichtenstein SV, et al: Transapical aortic valve implantation in humans. J Thorac Cardiovasc Surg 2006;13:1194-1196.
88. Lichtenstein SV, Cheung A, Ye J, et al: Transapical transcatheter aortic valve implantation in humans: Initial clinical experience. Circulation 2006;114:591-596.
89. Garay F, Cao Q-L, Olin J, et al: The Edwards-Cribier percutaneous heart valve in the pulmonic position: Initial animal experience. Eurointervention 2006;1(Suppl A):A32-A35.
90. Garay F, Webb J, Hijazi Z: Percutaneous replacement of pulmonary valve using the Edwards-Cribier percutaneous heart valve: First report in a human patient. Catheter Cardiovasc Interv 2006;67:659-662.
91. Calvo OL, Sobrino N, Gamallo C: Balloon percutaneous valvuloplasty for stenotic bioprosthetic valves in the mitral position. Am J Cardiol 1987;60:736-737.
92. Fert F, Stecy PJ, Nachaime MS: Percutaneous balloon valvuloplasty for stenosis of a porcine bioprosthesis in the tricuspid valve position. Am J Cardiol 1986;58:363-364.
93. Waller BF, McKay C, VanTassel J, et al: Catheter balloon valvuloplasty of stenotic porcine bioprosthetic valves: Part II. Mechanisms, complications, and recommendations for clinical use. Clin Cardiol 1991;14:764-772.
94. Kirwan C, Richardson G, Rothman MT, et al: Is there a role for balloon-valvuloplasty in patients with stenotic bioprosthetic valves? Catheter Cardiovasc Interv 2004;63:251-253.
95. Bonan R: Aortic valve: The new challenge for interventional cardiology. Catheter Cardiovasc Interv 2004;63:254.
96. Tateishi M: Valve-in-valve replacement of primary tissue valve failure of bovine pericardial valve. Kyobu Geka 2006;59:61-64.
97. Grube E, Laborde JC, Zickermann B, et al: First report on a human percutaneous transluminal implantation of a self expanding valve prosthesis for interventional treatment of aortic valve stenosis. Catheter Cardiovasc Interv 2005;66: 465-469.
98. Laborde JC, Borenstein N, Behr L, et al: Percutaneous implantation of the Corevalve aortic valve prosthesis for patients presenting high risk for surgical valve replacement. Eurointervention 2006;1:472-474.
99. Miyatake T, Murashita T, Oyama N, et al: Apicoaortic valved conduit for a patient with porcelain aorta. Asian Cardiovasc Thorac Ann 2006;14:76-79.
100. Gammie JS, Brown JW, Brown JM: Aortic valve bypass for the high-risk patient with aortic stenosis. Ann Thorac Surg 2006;81:1605-1610.
101. Crestanello JA, Zehr KJ, Daly RC, et al: Is there a role for the left ventricle apical-aortic conduit for acquired aortic stenosis? J Heart Valve Dis 2004;13:57-63.
102. Pedersen WR, Van Tassel RA, Pierce TA, et al: Radiation following percutaneous aortic valvuloplasty to prevent restenosis (RADAR Pilot Trial). Catheter Cardiovasc Interv 2006;68:183-192.
103. Vassiliades TA Jr, Block PC, Cohn LH, et al: The clinical development of percutaneous heart valve technology: A position statement of the Society of Thoracic Surgeons (STS), the American Association for Thoracic Surgery (AATS), and the Society for Cardiac Angiography and Interventions (SCAI). J Am Coll Cardiol 2005;45:1554-1560.

53 Pulmonary and Tricuspid Valve Interventions

Louise Coats and Philipp Bonhoeffer

KEY POINTS

- Percutaneous pulmonary valve implantation (PPVI) is suitable for patients with dysfunctional right ventricle-to-pulmonary artery conduits that measure less than 22 mm in diameter.
- PPVI is performed under general anesthesia from a femoral approach.
- PPVI results in an early symptomatic improvement and reduction in right ventricular volumes.
- PPVI can be complicated by device displacement, homograft rupture, or coronary artery compression at the time of implantation.
- PPVI requires careful radiographic and echocardiographic follow-up for early detection and treatment of stent fractures.

- PPVI is less invasive than surgery and compares well in terms of safety.
- PPVI prolongs conduit life and may reduce the number of operations required by patients with congenital heart disease during their lifetime.
- PPVI is likely to become clinical practice in the near future.
- Percutaneous tricuspid valve replacement is experimental and has not been tested in the clinical setting; it may be superseded by percutaneous repair techniques.

Acquired pulmonary and tricuspid valve disease in the adult population is unusual and mostly relates to rarities such as carcinoid disease, rheumatic fever and infective endocarditis, typically in the context of intravenous drug use. For those with congenital heart disease, however, dysfunction of these valves is a primary component of many conditions and, in the case of the pulmonary valve, is also a common consequence of several early repair strategies. With growing information regarding the harmful effects of chronic pulmonary regurgitation, surgical revision of the right ventricular outflow tract (RVOT) is now a commonly performed operation in this population, with some patients requiring several reoperations during a lifetime to maintain valvar function.

Percutaneous pulmonary valve implantation (PPVI) was first proposed and tested experimentally by one of us in 2000.[1] This procedure is now on the verge of widespread clinical use and has the potential to significantly reduce surgical reintervention in the growing population of adults with repaired congenital heart disease. Percutaneous tricuspid valve replacement, on the other hand, is currently remote from clinical application, although early experimental work has been carried out.[2] This chapter reviews these novel interventional techniques, discusses indications and patient selection, reports current results, and contemplates future directions.

PERCUTANEOUS PULMONARY VALVE IMPLANTATION

Background and Clinical Indications

Progress in surgery for congenital heart disease over the last 60 years has led to a considerable improvement in survival, with more than 85% of babies now reaching adulthood.[3] Consequently, focus has shifted toward the management of late morbidity in this growing population, with repeated surgery often employed to treat various residual lesions or complications.

Pulmonary regurgitation, which is common after transannular patch repair of tetralogy of Fallot, is a major cause of morbidity and may cause right ventricular (RV) dysfunction, impaired exercise capacity, and an increased risk of ventricular arrhythmia and sudden death.[4-6] Surgical pulmonary valve replacement can halt and may reverse these detrimental outcomes.[7,8] Current indications for surgery include free pulmonary regurgitation in association with moderate to severe RV enlargement, important tricuspid regurgitation, sustained atrial or ventricular arrhythmias, or deteriorating exercise performance.[9] It has been suggested that intervention is being performed too late, because the ability of the RV to remodel after surgery may be limited.[10] However, implanted biologic valves have a limited life span, and the desire to avoid progressive RV dysfunction has been moderated by the risks associated with repeat surgery and cardiopulmonary bypass.[11,12] RVOT obstruction may also cause symptoms in patients with conduits or after the arterial switch operation.[13-15] Although percutaneous placement of bare stents can treat this situation and is usually recommended in those with RV pressures greater than two-thirds of the systemic pressure, it is complicated by inevitable pulmonary regurgitation.[9,16-18]

PPVI is a novel transcatheter approach that can treat both pulmonary regurgitation and stenosis in patients with suitable RVOT anatomy. Traditional criteria for surgery have provided the baseline clinical indications for trials of this new technique. However, in the future, its less invasive nature is likely to support the trend toward earlier intervention while also offering a treatment option for those who are not surgical candidates. Importantly, PPVI does not affect subsequent suitability for surgery. Careful investigation will be required to redefine the indications clearly and determine the optimal timing for treatment in this growing patient population. In some rare cases of acquired pulmonary valvular disease (e.g., carcinoid disease), PPVI may also be considered as a treatment option.

The Device

The Melody transcatheter pulmonary valve (Medtronic, Minneapolis, MN) is composed of a segment of bovine jugular vein with a thinned-down wall and a central valve (Fig. 53-1). The vein is sutured inside an expanded platinum-iridium stent with a length of 34 mm that can be crimped to a size of 6 mm and re-expanded up to 24 mm. The current stent design, which has an eight-crown zigzag pattern with six segments along its length, is reinforced at each strut intersection with gold weld. The venous segment is attached to the stent by continuous 5-0 polypropylene sutures around the entire circumference at the inflow and outflow and also discretely at each strut intersection. The suture is clear for all points except the outflow line, which is blue to signify the outflow end of the device. The venous segment is fixed in a buffered glutaraldehyde solution in a concentration low enough to preserve the flexibility of the venous valve leaflets. A final sterilization step is performed on the combined device using a proprietary sterilant containing glutaraldehyde and isopropyl alcohol, in which it is then packaged.

The Delivery System

The delivery system (Ensemble), also manufactured by Medtronic, comprises a balloon-in-balloon (BiB)

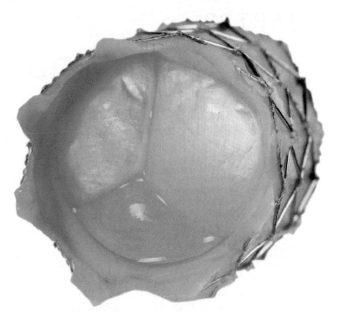

Figure 53-1. The Melody percutaneous pulmonary valve device. (Courtesy of Medtronic, Inc.)

deployment design at its distal end, onto which the valved stent is front-loaded and crimped (Fig. 53-2). The system is available with three outer balloon diameters: 18, 20, and 22 mm. The tip of the system is blue to correspond with the outflow suture of the device and encourage correct orientation. The body of the system is composed of a one-piece Teflon sheath containing a braided-wire reinforced elastomer lumen. This design minimizes the risk of kinking while optimizing flexibility and retaining the necessary pushability required for the procedure. A retractable sheath covers the stented valve during delivery

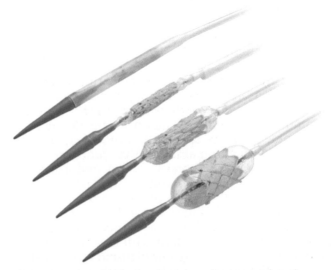

Figure 53-2. Percutaneous pulmonary valve mounted on the Ensemble balloon-in-balloon delivery system (*left to right:* sheathed, unsheathed, inner balloon inflation, outer balloon inflation). (Courtesy of Medtronic, Inc.)

and is pulled back just before deployment. Contrast solution can be delivered via the retracted sheath from a side port to confirm positioning of the device before deployment. Proximally, there are three ports, one for the **g**uidewire (**g**reen), one to deploy the **i**nner balloon (**i**ndigo), and one to deploy the **o**uter balloon (**o**range).

Animal Studies

Feasibility of PPVI was first demonstrated in 11 lambs weighing between 16 and 18 kg.[1] The device, which was a precursor of that described earlier, was developed from commercially available products (Contegra [Medtronic] and CP stent [NuMed, Inc., Hopkinton, NY]) that have proven utility in the clinical setting.[19,20] Bench testing confirmed that crimping and re-expansion of the device by balloon catheter would not affect valvar competence. Anesthesia was induced with 10 mg/kg thiopental sodium and maintained with halothane during mechanical ventilation. Heparin (100 IU/kg) and penicillin were administered prophylactically. Catheterization was performed from a right internal jugular approach. A guidewire was placed in a distal pulmonary artery, and the device, front-loaded onto the delivery system, was then introduced and tracked under fluoroscopy as it was advanced into position. The delivery system was selected according to the size of the pulmonary artery (18-, 20-, or 22-mm balloon). The valved stent was deployed in the native pulmonary artery of 7 of the 11 lambs. The procedure failed in 4 animals owing to an inability to cross the tricuspid valve. In humans, the femoral vessel, which is relatively larger, can be used and promotes a straighter catheter course, overcoming this technical difficulty. In the seven lambs that received implants, five stents were in the desired position, impinging on the function of the native valve. In the remaining two animals, one stent was implanted proximal to the valve and the other distal. No complications occurred during the procedure or follow-up. Mild fever occurred in two animals but disappeared within 48 hours without intervention. During the 2-month period of the study, the lambs were completely asymptomatic and almost doubled their body weight. At the end of the protocol, hemodynamic evaluation showed normal pulmonary pressure in all lambs with stents implanted. One of the seven stents was mildly stenotic, with a gradient of 15 mm Hg across it. At autopsy, fibrosis of the valve leaflets was observed in the two devices that had not been implanted in the desired position.

Despite technical difficulties of valve implantation in lambs, this work demonstrated feasibility of the concept of PPVI and set the scene for application in humans. Bare stent implantation in the RVOT was already common clinical practice, and the catheterization technique did not fundamentally differ. Moreover, the function of the implanted heterografts appeared to be identical to that of biologic valves implanted surgically.

Subsequently, other valved stent designs have been tested in the pulmonary position in animal trials with positive results.[21-23]

Clinical Studies

The first human application of transcatheter PPVI was reported in 2000. A 12-year-old boy, with an original diagnosis of pulmonary atresia and ventricular septal defect, underwent PPVI to treat stenosis and insufficiency of an 18-mm Carpentier-Edwards conduit that had been placed between the RV and pulmonary artery 8 years earlier.[24] The procedure was uncomplicated and resulted in complete relief of the insufficiency and partial relief of the stenosis. Further patient series have also been reported in the literature.[25,26] Our centers' current experience of 147 valve implantations performed in 133 patients, the results of which are described in the following sections, is the largest clinical experience of this technique worldwide. At present, PPVI has full regulatory approval in Europe and Canada. In the United States, implantations are being performed as part of a Food and Drug Administration feasibility study.

Patient Cohort

Dysfunctional conduits, especially homografts, provide the most suitable RVOT morphology for treatment with PPVI. Most patients in our series had undergone at least one surgical RVOT revision with conduit placement, usually after transannular patch repair of tetralogy of Fallot. Some, however, had had their conduit placed as part of the primary repair strategy (truncus arteriosus, Rastelli repair for transposition of the great arteries, or Ross operation for aortic valve disease). PPVI has been attempted in a few patients with native outflow tracts or transannular patches, but these cases were exceptional and some were complicated. Characteristics of the patient population treated to date are shown in Table 53-1.

The Procedure

PPVI is performed with the patient under general anesthesia, predominantly via a right femoral venous approach, with invasive blood pressure monitoring. A full aseptic technique to surgical standards is used, and a single dose of broad-spectrum intravenous antibiotics is given for endocarditis prophylaxis. In addition, 50 IU/kg heparin, or a standard dose of 5000 IU in adults, is administered routinely at the beginning of the procedure and repeated hourly thereafter, as required. Right-sided heart catheterization is performed according to standard techniques to assess pressures and saturations. Routinely, measurements are made in the RV, pulmonary artery, and aorta, with additional measurements (e.g., in the branch pulmonary arteries) made as appropriate. A

Table 53-1. Patient Characteristics at Implantation (N=133)

Characteristic	Category	n	%
Gender	Male	78	58.6
Age (Yr)	Median, 18 (range, 7-59)		
NYHA class	I	21	15.8
	II	65	48.9
	III	34	25.6
	IV	10	7.5
	Unable to assess	3	2.3
Diagnosis	Tetralogy of Fallot	79	59.5
	Transposition of great arteries	14	10.5
	Aortic valve disease (Ross)	10	7.5
	Truncus arteriosus	14	10.5
	Isolated pulmonic stenosis	2	1.5
	Other	14	10.5
Previous surgeries	<2	65	48.9
	3-4	60	45.1
	>4	8	6.0
Outflow tract	Homograft	108	81.2
	Biologic valved conduit	16	12.0
	Native or transannular patch	6	4.5
	Other	3	2.3
RVOT lesion	Stenosis	37	27.8
	Regurgitation	51	38.3
	Mixed	45	33.9

NYHA, New York Heart Association; RVOT, right ventricular outflow tract.

stiff guidewire (0.035 Amplatz Ultrastiff, Cook Inc., Bloomington, IN) is then positioned into a distal branch pulmonary artery to provide an anchor from which to advance the delivery system.

First, biplane angiography is performed using a Multi-Track catheter (NuMed) with the tip placed just beyond the expected position of the pulmonary valve, to allow assessment of the proposed site for device implantation and quantification of pulmonary regurgitation. Concurrently, the valved stent is prepared in three sequential saline baths (5 minutes in each) to wash off the glutaraldehyde in which it is stored. The valved stent is then hand-crimped over the barrel of a sterile 2-mL syringe before being front-loaded onto the delivery system. The blue stitching on the distal portion of the device is matched to the blue portion of the delivery system and verified by an independent observer to guarantee correct orientation. Further hand-crimping is performed, after which the sheath is retracted over the device while a saline flush is administered via the side port to exclude air bubbles from the system. After removal of the Multi-Track catheter, the femoral vein is dilated to 24 Fr and the front-loaded delivery system is advanced into the RVOT, under fluoroscopic guidance. The sheath is retracted from the valved stent, and contrast is injected via the side port to confirm position. Partial deployment is achieved by hand-inflation of the inner balloon, and, after final confirmation of position, the outer balloon is also hand-inflated to complete deployment. The balloons are deflated and the delivery system withdrawn. Repeat angiography and pressure measurements are made to confirm a positive outcome.

Modification of the Technique

Because the nature and position of RV-to-pulmonary artery conduits are heterogenous, cannulation with a large delivery system can be challenging. It is our practice to predilate (Mullins balloon [NuMed] and indeflator) and in some cases to place a bare stent (Max LD, ev3, Plymouth, MN) in conduits that are heavily calcified or tortuous. to facilitate passage of the system and optimize the final result. Further maneuvers that can be used to advance the delivery system, when it is at the entrance to the conduit, include looping the system within the right atrium and partially retracting the sheath. Both actions generate a forward force, often overcoming any resistance the system is experiencing, and aid passage into the conduit. Once deflated, the delivery system is withdrawn. If further dilation of the valved stent is required, this is done using a high-pressure Mullins balloon (NuMed) and indeflator. Care is taken not to dilate conduits beyond their original documented size, to minimize the risk of rupture. Postdilation of the device has not been observed to cause any damage to valve leaflets or to affect valve competency. Although our preferred approach is via the right femoral vein, mainly for practical and logistic reasons, we have successfully implanted valves via left femoral vein and via both right and left internal jugular veins. We do not practice or recommend a transhepatic route in view of the size of the delivery system.

Results

Procedural Results

A total of 133 patients underwent PPVI at our centers between September 2000 and July 2006. Mean procedure time was 101.0±46.7 minutes, and mean fluoroscopy time was 26.3±22.1 minutes. Failure to deliver the valved stent occurred on three occasions; two patients subsequently underwent successful implantations after a design change in the delivery system, and the third was referred for surgery. Twelve patients underwent prestenting of the conduit/pulmonary artery before percutaneous valve implantation. Additional procedures performed concurrently included stenting of a branch pulmonary artery in nine patients, ventricular septal defect closure in two, paravalvular leak closure in one, and coarctation stenting in one. Fourteen patients subsequently had repeat PPVI for a variety of indications that are discussed later.

Hemodynamic Results

After PPVI, angiography showed a significant improvement in regurgitation, with no patient having more than trivial to mild regurgitation (Fig. 53-3). The gradient across the RVOT fell (from 36.5±20.4 to 17.6±10.5 mm Hg; $P<.001$) and was

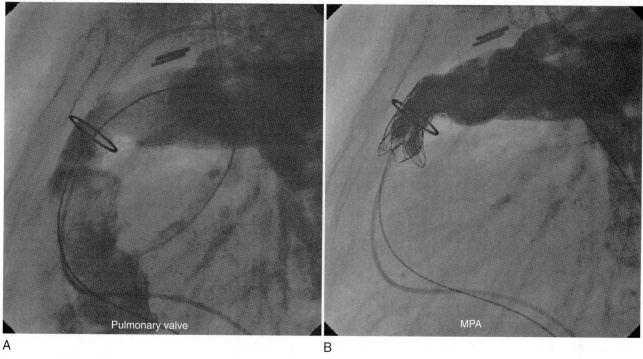

A   B

Figure 53-3. Lateral angiograms taken before (**A**) and after (**B**) percutaneous pulmonary valve implantation into a Hancock conduit, demonstrating complete relief of pulmonary regurgitation.

associated with falls in RV systolic pressure (from 62.8±18.3 to 46.1±13.6 mm Hg; $P<.001$) and end-diastolic pressure (from 11.5±4.0 to 9.9±4 mm Hg; $P<.001$). Pulmonary artery diastolic pressure increased (from 9.9±4.0 to 14.1±10.2 mm Hg; $P<.001$), reflecting the restoration of a competent pulmonary valve. These findings occurred in the context of a small rise in systemic pressure (from 93.9±15.7 to 101.5±17.8 mm Hg; $P<.001$) that may reflect improved cardiac output but could also indicate lightening of the anesthesia toward the end of the procedure. Subsequent investigation has suggested that different patterns of hemodynamic change can be expected depending on the nature of the RVOT dysfunction being treated.[27,28]

Procedural Complications

Six patients experienced major procedural complications that necessitated conversion to surgery. In two patients, this was caused by device instability in dilated regurgitant outflow tracts. In two patients, homograft rupture occurred after deployment of the valved stent and led to hemothorax and hemodynamic compromise. In one patient, who had previously undergone bare stenting of her conduit, PPVI was complicated by compression of the left coronary artery (Fig. 53-4A). Manual chest compressions had the fortuitous effect of compressing the device and permitting reperfusion and hemodynamic recovery (see Fig. 53-4B). In the final case, deployment of the percutaneous valve obstructed the right pulmonary artery.

Three minor complications also occurred: perforation of a distal pulmonary artery by the guidewire; damage to the tricuspid valve, probably from entrapment of the delivery system in the chordae; and a limited homograft rupture. All three patients responded to conservative management.

Follow-Up and Clinical Consequences

Mean follow-up was 19.6±15.6 months and was 100% complete for mortality and freedom from explantation. Patients were subject to clinical review, electrocardiography, anteroposterior and lateral chest radiography, and transthoracic echocardiography at 1, 3, 6, and 12 months after the procedure and at yearly intervals thereafter.

Patients reported an early symptomatic improvement, with 57.1% in NYHA functional class I within 1 month after the procedure, compared with 15.8% before ($P<.001$). This was associated with an early improvement in objective exercise capacity (oxygen consumption [VO_2 max] and anaerobic threshold) in the overall group.[26] Subset analysis suggested that this finding was more prominent in those being treated for RVOT obstruction rather than pulmonary regurgitation.[27,28] Early assessment with magnetic resonance imaging (MRI) showed a reduction in RV volume, an increase in left ventricular volume, and improvements in stroke volume and cardiac output.[26] Again, the mechanism appeared to be different in pressure- and volume-overload RVs, but the results suggested, overall, that these hearts tolerate load poorly.

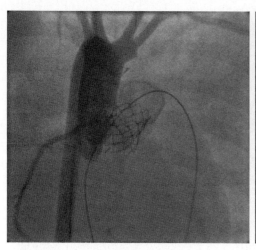
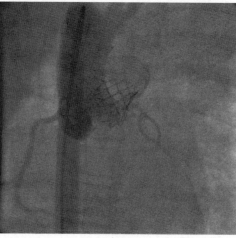

Figure 53-4. *Left,* Angiogram (left anterior oblique projection) showing compression of the left main stem coronary artery after deployment of the percutaneous pulmonary valve. *Right,* Reperfusion after compression of the device during cardiac massage.

Valvar competency was well maintained, with the rate of freedom from moderate or severe pulmonary regurgitation on echocardiography being 98.9% at 1 year (number at risk, 86) and 96.2% at 5 years (number at risk, 5). Significant regurgitation was predominantly associated with endocarditis. Device-related complications more often occurred in the setting of RVOT obstruction.

Device-Related Complications

The "Hammock" Effect
The "hammock" effect became apparent in the early cohort of patients undergoing valve implantation, when a high incidence of in-stent stenosis was noted (7/22 patients, 31.8%). Originally, the venous segment of the bovine valve was sutured to the stent only at its distal extremities. This permitted passage of blood between the wall of the vein and the recipient outflow tract, resulting in an effective stenosis. Recognition of this problem led to additional sutures being placed at all strut intersections, which resolved the issue with no further cases being seen. In theory, the "hammock" effect could still occur in the context of stent fracture or suture rupture, if adherence of the venous wall to the stent becomes disrupted.

Stent Fractures
Stent fractures are a well recognized sequela of stent implantation for all cardiovascular applications. The etiology is likely to be multifactorial and depends both on the nature of the stent and the characteristics of the implantation site. Prevalence of stent fracture in bare stenting of the RVOT has been reported to be as high as 43%, with embolization occurring in 11%, although without death or acute hemodynamic compromise.[29]

After PPVI, stent fracture has been detected in 27 patients (20.3%) at varying intervals. In most cases (*n*=21), this has been an incidental finding detected on routine chest radiography (Fig. 53-5). RVOT obstruction developed in five patients, however, and in one patient device embolization occurred. In these cases, further percutaneous or surgical intervention was required.[29a]

Serial radiographic and echocardiographic follow-up is essential to detect stent fractures and allow early treatment in those with hemodynamic consequences before device embolization occurs. Fluoroscopy provides a useful adjunct to assess stent stability in this situation and to aid decisions regarding the need for reintervention.

Hemolysis
Hemolysis has occurred in one patient (0.8%), in whom sequential balloon dilatation and PPVI failed to adequately relieve RVOT obstruction in a small conduit (15-mm homograft). On the first day after the procedure, the patient developed dark urine containing free hemoglobin on dipstick, and his serum

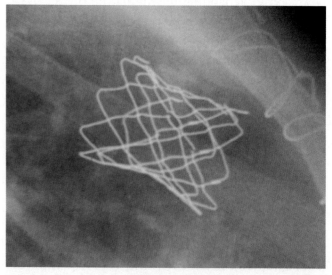

Figure 53-5. Incidental stent fractures detected on routine chest radiography in a percutaneous pulmonary valve device.

hemoglobin dropped from 13 to 9 g/dL. After transfusion, the patient went to surgery at 21 days and made an uneventful recovery. Screening for hemolysis after PPVI is not routinely performed.

Endocarditis

Endocarditis of the valved stent has been seen in five patients (3.8%) and can occur either on the venous wall or on the valve itself. Three patients developed pulmonary regurgitation, one developed RVOT obstruction, and one had no consequences for device function. Two cases occurred after failure to take prophylactic antibiotics before dental procedures, and one patient required explantation of the device. One further patient, who was immunologically compromised, developed candidal endocarditis of the aortic valve and underwent aortic valve replacement with a 21-mm St Jude prosthesis. The valved stent was also removed by necessity and replaced with a 19-mm aortic homograft.

Thromboembolism

Thromboembolism has not been documented after PPVI. Patients are advised to take aspirin (75 mg) daily for life.

Treatment of Device-Related Complications

Experience with bare stenting[17-19,21] has shown that repeat intervention using a stent-in-stent technique is both a feasible and an effective treatment for suboptimal results. After PPVI, 14 patients underwent implantation of a second valve stent (12 with a stent-in-stent technique and 2 after interim surgery). Indications included the "hammock" effect, stent fracture, residual stenosis, and, in the surgical cases, early homograft stenosis. Procedural technique is unchanged for stent-in-stent PPVI, and hemodynamic results have been both excellent and sustained. In the future, issues such as the "hammock" effect will become irrelevant, and indications may shift toward the treatment of late valvar degeneration.

Repeat PPVI is not suitable for all suboptimal or complicated outcomes. Clearly, infection, external conduit compression, and conduit outgrowth will still require surgical revision of the pulmonary valve. Nevertheless, this approach should be considered, if appropriate, before proceeding to surgery, because adopting such a management strategy could defer the need for surgical reintervention indefinitely.

Mid-term Follow-Up and Mortality

Actuarial freedom from device explantation after PPVI is currently 91% at 1 year (number at risk, 86), 76% at 3 years (number at risk, 20) and 72% at 5 years (number at risk, 5) (Fig. 53-6).

Mortality after PPVI is 1.5%, but this represents two patients who were in cardiogenic shock at presentation and underwent PPVI as a palliative procedure. The first, who had undergone five previous surgeries, was in chronic atrial fibrillation with ascites and pleural effusions. Despite a successful procedure,

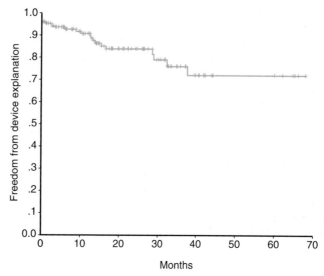

Figure 53-6. Kaplan-Meier survival plot depicting freedom from device explantation.

the patient's condition deteriorated 6 weeks later, after a chest infection, and the patient died. The second patient presented in a coma with severe fluid overload and renal and hepatic impairment. Despite technically successful transcatheter treatment of recoarctation and RVOT homograft obstruction, the patient died some hours later from intractable pulmonary edema. There have been no other deaths during early or late follow-up.

Comparison with Surgery

At present, PPVI cannot be directly compared with surgery, because it is not available to the same patient population. In addition, surgery permits resection of patch aneurysms or hypertrophied muscle bundles and remodeling of the RVOT. Nevertheless, early safety and efficacy data are encouraging, and the technique should be regarded as an important complementary therapy in the lifetime management of congenital heart disease.[30] Treatment of residual lesions such as ventricular septal defects can also now be carried out by catheter techniques. The aim of PPVI should be to prolong conduit life, without the complication of pulmonary regurgitation associated with bare stenting, and to reduce the number of surgical interventions a patient will require. Perhaps evolving device design and procedural technique will allow direct comparison with surgical results in the future.

Patient Selection

The main limitation of the currently available transcatheter valve device is the maximum diameter to which it can be deployed (22 mm) before compromising valvar competence. Selection of patients with suitable anatomy for PPVI is critical, both to ensure procedural success and to optimize long-term outcome. We employ a stepwise approach with a particular emphasis on three-dimensional noninvasive imaging.

In the first instance, the surgical history and nature of the RVOT must be clearly understood before a patient is accepted for further assessment. We have found that homografts or other circumferential conduits (Hancock, Carpentier-Edwards, Shellhigh) provide the optimal implantation target because of their tendency to deform in a predictable manner. Transannular patches and native outflow tracts are rarely suitable, because they deform asymmetrically and thus risk device stability. One exception occurs after the arterial switch operation: the obstructed native RVOT, in our experience, does offer a safe environment for PPVI. Even when the predominant indication for intervention is pulmonary regurgitation, the presence of some level of obstruction or at least calcification of the conduit is essential to achieve device stability. We perform anteroposterior and lateral chest radiography to identify conduit calcification and transthoracic echocardiography to assess the gradient across the RVOT. The absence of calcification or a measurable gradient should raise concern, particularly in larger homografts or conduits.

Establishing the precise morphology of the proposed implantation site by echocardiography is often difficult because of limited echo windows and two-dimensional imaging planes. Assessment of these patients with MRI (or with computed tomography if MRI is contraindicated) is extremely valuable. Measurement of the RVOT dimensions is best made on two perpendicular gradient-echo cine images (Fig. 53-7A,B), because this permits measurement of the maximum (systolic) diameter at the potential site of implantation. Reliance on "black-blood" spin-echo measurements (usually acquired in middle to late diastole) or on angiographic images (nongated image acquisition) may underestimate the maximum size of the RVOT. However, gadolinium contrast-enhanced angiography, although it should not be used for measurements, allows three-dimensional reconstruction of the entire RVOT and a more complete appreciation of the overall morphology (see Fig. 53-7C). MRI is also used to quantify the pulmonary regurgitation, assess the right and left ventricular dimensions and function, and determine the presence of distal pulmonary artery stenoses or other intracardiac defects.[31]

Finally, there are two important considerations at the time of catheterization. First, those patients who have borderline RVOT dimensions on MRI (20-24 mm) should undergo balloon sizing (PTS sizing balloon [NuMed]) before proceeding to PPVI. In addition to providing further measurement, this permits assessment of the distensibility of the conduit wall and the likelihood of device stability. Second, the course of the coronary circulation with respect to the RVOT should be defined if this is not known. An aortogram, with or without simultaneous injection into the RVOT depending on the degree of conduit calcification, is usually sufficient to alleviate uncertainty. If concern remains with regard to the proximity of these structures, selective coronary angiography with simultaneous balloon inflation (18-20 mm Mullins balloon [NuMed]) in the RVOT, designed to mimic PPVI, should be carried out. Potential compression of the coronary artery can thus be identified prospectively (Fig. 53-8), allowing safe termination of the procedure and referral for surgery.

Extending the Indications

Many patients, particularly those who have undergone transannular patch repair of tetralogy of Fallot, have RVOTs that are greater than 30 mm in diameter. PPVI is therefore technically impossible with the current device. To broaden the application of PPVI to all RVOT morphologies, a number of strategies have been proposed.

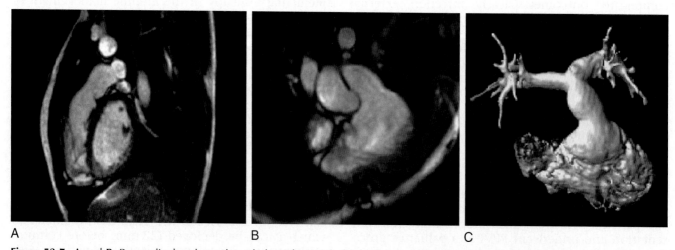

Figure 53-7. A and **B,** Perpendicular planes through the right ventricular outflow tract (gradient-echo cine sequences). **C,** Three-dimensional reconstruction of the right ventricular outflow tract from gadolinium contrast enhanced angiography. (Courtesy of Dr. Andrew Taylor, Cardiac Magnetic Resonance Unit, UCL Institute of Child Health, London.)

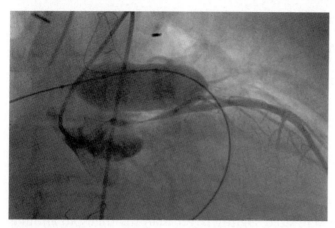

Figure 53-8. Angiogram (left anterior oblique projection with 20 degrees of cranial angulation) showing compression of the left anterior descending coronary artery during balloon inflation in the conduit. (From Sridharan S, Coats L, Khambadkone S, et al: Transcatheter right ventricular outflow tract intervention: The risk to the coronary circulation. Circulation 2006;113:e934-e935.)

Stent Design

The limiting factor of the current device is the bovine jugular venous valve, which is available only up to 22 mm. The Cribier-Edwards valve (Edwards Lifesciences, Irvine, CA), an equine pericardial valve mounted inside a balloon-expandable stainless steel stent, has been proposed for use in the pulmonary position and is available in a diameter of 26 mm.[32,33] However, a degree of obstruction is still required for anchorage of the device, making it unsuitable for patients with transannular patches.

To implant valves into dilated unobstructed outflow tracts, a new type of stent that downsizes the implantation site has been proposed and tested experimentally.[34] This self-expandable nitinol stent has an outer diameter consistent with the outflow tract (30 mm) but a central restriction (18 mm) that is designed to contain the valve. To guarantee sealing, a polytetrafluoroethylene (PTFE) membrane is sutured to the outside of the stent. Experimental work carried out in ewes with RVOTs larger than 25 mm confirmed the feasibility, both of implanting this novel device as a one-step procedure, and also of implanting the nitinol stent first and a conventional balloon-expandable valved stent later, in a two-step procedure. The two-step procedure would permit a more cautious approach in those with asymmetric anatomy, in whom partial deployment of the device may pose a risk. Paravalvular leak, stent migration, and thromboembolism did not occur, and the stents became integrated into the wall of the pulmonary artery by 3 months.

Further work is required to develop a downsizing self-expandable valved stent device for application in humans. Development of rapid prototype models from MRI datasets highlights the heterogeneous RVOT morphology present in this patient population but also offers an opportunity to tailor device construction to patient anatomy.[35] It is hoped that devices for transcatheter implantation will become available in the near future.

Hybrid Procedures

One limitation of animal experiments, already alluded to, is the uniform RVOT morphology that is encountered. In fact, pulmonary anatomy is commonly tortuous after repair of complex congenital heart disease. For this reason, deployment of self-expandable valved stents, as described previously, could be problematic. Insertion of the present device into a dilated outflow tract may, however, be facilitated by a simple surgical modification. Experimental work has demonstrated the feasibility of a hybrid procedure that combines banding of the RVOT via a left thoracotomy with subsequent valve implantation.[36] Two 18-mm radiopaque rings are placed around the RVOT to reduce its size. These rings also act as guides to aid placement and provide support for the subsequent percutaneous valve device. Either percutaneous or transventricular valve implantation is then possible; in human applications, the transventricular approach may be preferred, because stitches can be placed to secure the valved stent and access to cardiopulmonary bypass, if needed, is more easily achieved.

Recently, implantation of the Shellhigh Injectable Stented Pulmonic Valve has been reported in humans.[37,38] The device consists of a porcine pulmonic valve mounted inside a self-expandable stent and covered by No-React–treated pericardium. It is available in sizes 17 to 29 mm and is delivered, via a standard median sternotomy, with a trocar that is introduced through a small incision in the distal RVOT. After deployment, the valve is secured in position with several transmural sutures placed at the proximal and distal rims. Although this approach avoids cardiopulmonary bypass and its adverse effects, it still requires resternotomy, which is itself associated with substantial risk. Although not strictly in the realm of interventional cardiology, the development of such procedures underlines the impact that advances in percutaneous valve technology are having on conventional surgical practice.

Rethinking the Substrate

The deleterious effects of pulmonary regurgitation on RV function are now well documented. In an attempt to minimize this complication, surgeons have moved toward placing smaller transannular patches and, where possible, valved conduits as part of the primary repair. The development of percutaneous valve technology places an additional responsibility on the surgeon, who must now try to prepare the patient for percutaneous rather than surgical intervention in the future. At present, the size of the delivery system precludes PPVI in those younger than 5 years of age or less than 20 kg in weight. Although a smaller, tailor-made device that can be implanted on a 16-Fr system has been described,[39] implantation is technically difficult and does not address the impact of somatic growth on conduit function. A novel concept that has been tested in the experimental setting is the insertion of an expandable, valved conduit for reconstruction of the RVOT.[40] The principle of this approach is that the conduit could be balloon-dilated in accordance with somatic growth, and, when valve failure occurs, percutaneous valve implantation could be safely performed.

Future Directions

Despite the potential for repeat percutaneous valve implantations with the currently available device, the endurance of biologic valves remains an important issue for both surgeons and interventionalists. The mechanisms of degradation are multifactorial and include immunologic rejection, mechanical deterioration, calcification, and enzymatic digestion. There is much interest in developing valves that would have infinite durability but comparable function and no need for anticoagulation. In the percutaneous field, low-profile biodegradable pulmonary valves made of small intestinal submucosa have been tested experimentally.[41] These valves provide a decellularized matrix that is repopulated after implantation by the adjacent host tissue and does not invoke significant immunologic rejection. However, the development of progressive leaflet thickening in the animal model currently precludes human application. An alternative approach is preimplantation seeding of the matrix by means of tissue engineering. Transcatheter implantation of such valves in the pulmonary position has recently been reported.[42]

PERCUTANEOUS TRICUSPID VALVE IMPLANTATION

Background and Clinical Indications

Disease of the tricuspid valve is often regarded as being of lesser clinical consequence than that of the other heart valves. Nevertheless, dysfunction is common, particularly in the setting of congestive heart failure, and can lead to atrial arrhythmias, hepatic congestion, ascites, and peripheral edema. Other etiologies include rheumatic heart disease, pulmonary hypertension, infective endocarditis, and congenital conditions such as Ebstein's anomaly.[43]

At present, tricuspid valve replacement represents the last treatment option for patients with tricuspid regurgitation or stenosis for whom medical management has failed and repair of the valve is not feasible. Mortality and morbidity are high, reflecting the poor preoperative condition of these patients, and the decision to intervene requires the presence of symptoms or an indication for concomitant mitral valve surgery.[44,45] A percutaneous approach to replacing

the tricuspid valve may therefore have significant benefits for this high-risk population.

Animal Studies

To date, there has been only one published study examining the feasibility of percutaneous tricuspid valve replacement.[46] The work, carried out in eight ewes weighing 60 to 70 kg, reported on a new type of device tailored to the nature of the implantation site. The device comprised a self-expandable nitinol stent with two flat disks (diameter, 40 mm) and a tubular portion (diameter, 18 mm) that supported a bovine jugular venous valve (Fig. 53-9). The devices were sized slightly larger than the tricuspid annulus to ensure secure anchorage. The ventricular disk was covered with PTFE to ensure sealing, whereas the atrial disk was uncovered to limit the risk of coronary sinus occlusion. The delivery system consisted of a "homemade" front-loading device (Cook Inc., Charenton le Pont, France).

Anesthesia was induced with 10 mg/kg thiopental sodium and maintained with isoflurane during mechanical ventilation. Catheterization was performed from a right internal jugular approach. A guidewire was placed in a distal pulmonary artery, and the device, front-loaded onto an 18-Fr delivery system, was then introduced and guided into position. As with percutaneous atrial septal defect closure, the distal disk was deployed first in the RV by pulling on the external sheath while maintaining the delivery system in position. This disk was then applied to

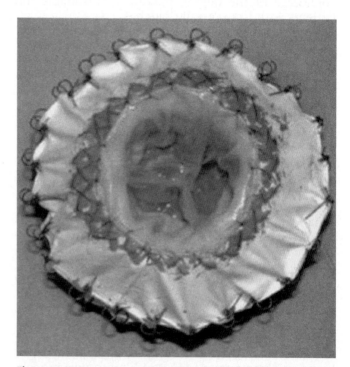

Figure 53-9. Percutaneous tricuspid valve device. (From Boudjemline Y, Agnoletti G, Bonnet D, et al: Steps toward the percutaneous replacement of atrioventricular valves: An experimental study. J Am Coll Cardiol 2005;46:360-365.)

the tricuspid annulus by pulling on the system. After deployment of the tubular part containing the valve, the second disk was delivered similarly in the right atrium, thus sandwiching the annulus between the disks. The percutaneous valves were successfully implanted in seven of eight animals, with one device being misdeployed owing to entrapment in the tricuspid chordae. Despite frequent ectopy during wire placement and device deployment, there was no sustained arrhythmia. Mean right atrial pressure increased acutely after valve implantation and then remained stable. There were no early or late stent migrations. A significant paravalvular leak was found at 1 month in one case and was caused by a tear in the PTFE membrane resulting from a weld fracture. At autopsy, the devices were found to be partially covered by fibrous tissue and had become integrated into the walls of the right atrial and ventricular cavities. The native tricuspid valves were completely inactivated by the stent and partially retracted.

Although this work established the feasibility of percutaneous tricuspid valve replacement, application in humans remains remote. The pathologic tricuspid valve is likely to present a number of difficulties for this technique not addressed here. In Ebstein's anomaly, for example, the deployment of this device would be problematic because of the lack of an identifiable annulus. Further, the dynamic nature of the tricuspid annulus raises major concerns regarding the long-term stability of such devices, the risk of stent fracture, and the potential for myocardial trauma.

Future Directions

Percutaneous repair strategies have demonstrated much promise for the treatment of mitral valve disease.[47,48] In particular the edge-to-edge repair, which opposes the valve leaflets with a stitch or clip to reduce valve excursion and thus regurgitation, could be applied in the right heart. This repair technique, which has been used surgically for tricuspid valve repair, may overcome some of the problems encountered when trying to replace the valve by catheter.[49]

SUMMARY

Percutaneous valve therapies are currently one of the most exciting areas of interventional cardiology. Their application in the right heart covers the spectrum from clinically applicable devices to purely experimental models. The next few years are likely to see rapid advances in this field, but creative thought will be required to optimize device design, and cooperation between cardiologists and surgeons will be essential for safe introduction of the technology.

REFERENCES

1. Bonhoeffer P, Boudjemline Y, Saliba Z, et al: Transcatheter implantation of a bovine valve in pulmonary position: A lamb study. Circulation 2000;102:813-816.

2. Boudjemline Y, Agnoletti G, Bonnet D, et al: Steps toward the percutaneous replacement of atrioventricular valves: An experimental study. J Am Coll Cardiol 2005;46:360-365.

3. Warnes CA, Liberthson R, Danielson GK, et al: Task force 1: The changing profile of congenital heart disease in adult life. J Am Coll Cardiol 2001;37:1170-1175.

4. Frigiola A, Redington AN, Cullen S, Vogel M: Pulmonary regurgitation is an important determinant of right ventricular contractile dysfunction in patients with surgically repaired tetralogy of Fallot. Circulation 2004;110(Suppl I):II-153-II-157.

5. Carvalho JS, Shinebourne EA, Busst C, et al: Exercise capacity after complete repair of tetralogy of Fallot: Deleterious effects of residual pulmonary regurgitation. Br Heart J 1992;67:470-473.

6. Gatzoulis MA, Balaji S, Webber SA, et al: Risk factors for arrhythmia and sudden cardiac death late after repair of tetralogy of Fallot: A multicentre study. Lancet 2000;356:975-981.

7. Eyskens B, Reybrouck T, Bogaert J, et al: Homograft insertion for pulmonary regurgitation after repair of tetralogy of Fallot improves cardio-respiratory exercise performance. Am J Cardiol 2000;85:221-225.

8. Therrien J, Siu SC, Harris L, et al: Impact of pulmonary valve replacement on arrhythmia propensity late after repair of tetralogy of Fallot. Circulation 2001;103:2489-2494.

9. Canadian Cardiovascular Society Consensus Conference: 2001 Update: Recommendations for the Management of Adults with Congenital Heart Disease. Part II. Can J Cardiol 2001;17:1029-1050.

10. Therrien J, Siu SC, McLaughlin PR, et al: Pulmonary valve replacement in adults late after repair of tetralogy of Fallot: Are we operating too late? J Am Coll Cardiol 2000;36:1670-1675.

11. Stark J, Bull C, Stajevic M, et al: Fate of subpulmonary homograft conduits: Determinants of late homograft failure. J Thorac Cardiovasc Surg 1998;115:506-516.

12. Meyns B, Jashari R, Gewillig M, et al: Factors influencing the survival of cryopreserved homografts: The second homograft performs as well as the first. Eur J Cardiothorac Surg 2005;28:211-216.

13. Cleveland DC, Williams WG, Razzouk AJ, et al: Failure of cryopreserved homograft valved conduits in the pulmonary circulation. Circulation 1992;86(5 Suppl):II-150-II-153.

14. Bando K, Danielson GK, Schaff HV, et al: Outcome of pulmonary and aortic homografts for right ventricular outflow tract reconstruction. J Thorac Cardiovasc Surg 1995;109:509-517.

15. Williams WG, Quaegebeur JM, Kirklin JW, Blackstone EH: Outflow obstruction after the arterial switch operation: A multiinstitutional study. J Thorac Cardiovasc Surg 1997;114:975-987.

16. Powell AJ, Lock JE, Keane JF, Perry SB: Prolongation of RV-PA conduit life span by percutaneous stent implantation: Intermediate-term results. Circulation 1995;92:3282-3288.

17. Fogelman R, Nykanen D, Smallhorn JF, et al: Endovascular stents in the pulmonary circulation: Clinical impact on management and medium-term follow-up. Circulation 1995;92:881-885.

18. Sugiyama H, Williams W, Benson LN: Implantation of endovascular stents for the obstructive right ventricular outflow tract. Heart 2005;91:1058-1063.

19. Boethig D, Thies WR, Hecker H, Breymann T: Mid term course after pediatric right ventricular outflow tract reconstruction: A comparison of homografts, porcine xenografts and Contegras. Eur J Cardiothorac Surg 2005;27:58-66.

20. Ewert P, Schubert S, Peters B, et al: The CP stent—short, long, covered—for the treatment of aortic coarctation, stenosis of pulmonary arteries and caval veins, and Fontan anastomosis in children and adults: An evaluation of 60 stents in 53 patients. Heart 2005;91:948-953.

21. Webb JG, Munt B, Makkar RR, et al: Percutaneous stent-mounted valve for treatment of aortic or pulmonary valve disease. Catheter Cardiovasc Interv 2004;63:89-93.

22. Attmann T, Jahnke T, Quaden R, et al: Advances in experimental percutaneous pulmonary valve replacement. Ann Thorac Surg 2005;80:969-975.

23. Attmann T, Quaden R, Jahnke T, et al: Percutaneous pulmonary valve replacement: 3-Month evaluation of self-expanding valved stents. Ann Thorac Surg 2006;82:708-713.

24. Bonhoeffer P, Boudjemline Y, Saliba Z, et al: Percutaneous replacement of pulmonary valve in a right-ventricle to pulmonary-artery prosthetic conduit with valve dysfunction. Lancet 2000;356:1403-1405.

25. Bonhoeffer P, Boudjemline Y, Qureshi SA, et al: Percutaneous insertion of the pulmonary valve. J Am Coll Cardiol 2002;39:1664-1669.

26. Khambadkone S, Coats L, Taylor A, et al: Percutaneous pulmonary valve implantation in humans: Results in 59 consecutive patients. Circulation 2005;112:1189-1197.

27. Coats L, Khambadkone S, Derrick G, et al: Physiological and clinical consequences of relief of right ventricular outflow tract obstruction late after repair of congenital heart defects. Circulation 2006;113:2037-2044.

28. Coats L, Khambakone S, Derrick, G, et al: Physiological consequences of percutaneous pulmonary valve implantation: The different behaviour of volume- and pressure-overloaded ventricles. Eur Heart J 2007;26 [Epub ahead of print].

29. Peng LF, McElhinney DB, Nugent AW, et al: Endovascular stenting of obstructed right ventricle-to-pulmonary artery conduits: A 15-year experience. Circulation 2006;113: 2598-2605.

29a. Noromeyer J, Khambadkone S, Coats L, et al: Risk strantication, systematic classification, and anticipatory management strategies for stent fracture after percutaneous pulmonary valve implantation. Circulation 2007;115:1392-1397.

30. Coats L, Tsang V, Khambadkone S, et al: The potential impact of percutaneous pulmonary valve stent implantation on right ventricular outflow tract re-intervention. Eur J Cardiothorac Surg 2005;27:536-543.

31. Taylor AM: Assessment of the pulmonary valve with magnetic resonance imaging. In Hijazi ZM, Bonhoeffer P, Feldman T, Ruiz CE (eds): Transcatheter Valve Repair. London, Taylor Francis, 2006, pp 25-44.

32. Garay F, Cao Q, Olin J, Hijazi ZM: The Cribier-Edwards percutaneous heart valve in the pulmonic position: Initial animal experience. Eurointervention 2006;1(Suppl A):32-35.

33. Garay F, Webb J, Hijazi ZM: Percutaneous replacement of pulmonary valve using the Edwards-Cribier percutaneous heart valve: First report in a human patient. Catheter Cardiovasc Interv 2006;67:659-662.

34. Boudjemline Y, Agnoletti G, Bonnet D, et al: Percutaneous pulmonary valve replacement in a large right ventricular outflow tract: An experimental study. J Am Coll Cardiol 2004;43:1082-1087.

35. Schievano S, Migliavacca F, Coats L, et al: Percutaneous pulmonary valve implantation based on rapid prototyping of right ventricular outflow tract and pulmonary trunk from MR data. Radiology 2006;242:490-497.

36. Boudjemline Y, Schievano S, Bonnet C, et al: Off-pump replacement of the pulmonary valve in large right ventricular outflow tracts: A hybrid approach. J Thorac Cardiovasc Surg 2005;129:831-837.

37. Schreiber C, Bauernschmitt R, Augustin N, et al: Implantation of a prosthesis mounted inside a self-expandable stent in the pulmonary valvar area without use of cardiopulmonary bypass. Ann Thorac Surg 2006;81:e1-e3.

38. Berdat PA, Carrel T: Off-pump pulmonary valve replacement with the new Shelhigh Injectable Stented Pulmonic Valve. J Thorac Cardiovasc Surg 2006;131:1192-1193.

39. Feinstein JA, Kim N, Reddy VM, Perry SB: Percutaneous pulmonary valve placement in a 10-month-old patient using a hand crafted stent-mounted porcine valve. Catheter Cardiovasc Interv 2006;67:644-649.

40. Boudjemline Y, Laborde F, Pineau E, et al: Expandable right ventricular-to-pulmonary artery conduit: An animal study. Pediatr Res 2006;59:773-777.

41. Ruiz CE, Iemura M, Medie S, et al: Transcatheter placement of a low-profile biodegradable pulmonary valve made of small intestinal submucosa: A long-term study in a swine model. J Thorac Cardiovasc Surg 2005;130:477-484.

42. Stock UA, Degenkolbe I, Attmann T, et al: Prevention of device-related tissue damage during percutaneous deployment of tissue-engineered heart valves. J Thorac Cardiovasc Surg 2006;131:1323-1330.

43. Hauck AJ, Freeman DP, Ackermann DM, et al: Surgical pathology of the tricuspid valve: A study of 363 cases spanning 25 years. Mayo Clin Proc 1988;63:851-863.

44. Carrier M, Hébert Y, Pellerin M, et al: Tricuspid valve replacement: An analysis of 25 years of experience at a single center. Ann Thorac Surg 2003;75:47-50.

45. Bonow RO, Carabello BA, Kanu C, et al: ACC/AHA 2006 Guidelines for the management of patients with valvular heart disease: A report of the American College of Cardiology/American Heart Association Task Force on Practice Guidelines (Writing Committee to Revise the 1998 Guidelines for the Management of Patients with Valvular Heart Disease). Developed in collaboration with the Society of Cardiovascular Anesthesiologists: Endorsed by the Society for Cardiovascular Angiography and Interventions and the Society of Thoracic Surgeons. Circulation 2006;114:e84-e231.

46. Boudjemline Y, Agnoletti G, Bonnet D, et al: Steps toward the percutaneous replacement of atrioventricular valves: An experimental study. J Am Coll Cardiol 2005;46:360-365.

47. Feldman T, Wasserman HS, Herrmann HC, et al: Percutaneous mitral valve repair using the edge-to-edge technique: Six-month results of the EVEREST Phase I Clinical Trial. J Am Coll Cardiol 2005;46:2134-2140.

48. Webb JG, Harnek J, Munt BI, et al: Percutaneous transvenous mitral annuloplasty: Initial human experience with device implantation in the coronary sinus. Circulation 2006;113: 851-855.

49. De Bonis M, Lapenna E, La Canna G, et al: A novel technique for correction of severe tricuspid valve regurgitation due to complex lesions. Eur J Cardiothorac Surg 2004;25:760-765.

54 Hypertrophic Cardiomyopathy

Matthew C. Becker and Samir R. Kapadia

KEY POINTS

- Hypertrophic cardiomyopathy is a disease process that varies broadly in its clinical presentation and has been associated with many different genetic mutations.
- Obstructive disease is present in a small proportion of patients; severity of obstruction varies depending on loading conditions and adrenergic state in an individual patient.
- Echocardiography and magnetic resonance imaging are primarily used to make this diagnosis.
- Medical management is indicated in symptomatic patients as an initial intervention; patients who are at high risk for

sudden cardiac death should be considered for implantable cardioverter-defibrillator therapy.
- Myectomy is considered to be the treatment of choice when symptoms persist despite optimal medical therapy in good surgical candidates, if an experienced surgical team is available.
- Alcohol septal ablation provides an excellent treatment option when surgical myectomy is not thought to be optimal for an individual patient. Targeted ablation with careful attention to anatomic details and appropriate selection of patients is necessary for procedural success.

By virtue of the broad variability in its phenotypic expression, hypertrophic cardiomyopathy (HCM) is a unique cardiovascular condition with the potential for the development of clinical symptoms during any phase of life, from infancy to old age.[1-7] The genetic foundation of HCM has been directly related to abnormalities of the genes encoding the cardiac sarcomere unit and may result in a complex disease phenotype that encompasses a spectrum of clinical and pathologic presentations. In the past, the nomenclature regarding HCM was often misleading. Idiopathic hypertrophic subaortic stenosis, or hypertrophic obstructive cardiomyopathy (HOCM), typically described only a subset of patients with this disorder. With an improved understanding of the clinical heterogeneity of this process, HCM appears to be a more appropriate descriptive term.

The rapid demystification of the genetic underpinnings of HCM has greatly expanded understanding of this entity. HCM is inherited in an autosomal dominant fashion, with more than 12 genes identified as being involved in the phenotypic manifestation.[1,7-10] Three of those genes account for more than 50% of the known cases of HCM.[1,9,11] Traditionally, the diagnosis of HCM has been primarily clinical, involving the use of echocardiography to evaluate for certain characteristic features, such as asymmetric septal hypertrophy and systolic anterior motion (SAM) of the mitral valve with left ventricular outflow

tract (LVOT) obstruction. Although there have been dramatic advances in understanding of the genetic predisposition for this disease state, the utility of genetic study for the absolute diagnosis remains preliminary at this time. However, the future holds promise that genetics will become a more reliable tool for establishing and confirming this diagnosis.

Given the heterogeneity of the disease process, even within the same family, clinical course and long-term outcomes differ significantly. Therefore, management strategies span the range from close outpatient follow-up to surgical remodeling of the myocardium. HCM appears to be an evolving process in some patients, with a change in the phenotype with age. This presents a challenging dilemma in terms of grasping the clinical course of this disorder. Consequently, therapeutic strategies need to be individualized based on the specific patient.

EPIDEMIOLOGY

With a prevalence on the order of 1:500 in the general adult population, this is one of the more common cardiac genetic disorders known.[1,6,9] Although it is not routinely accounted for in general practice, it is not uncommon to see these patients in tertiary referral centers. The clinical heterogeneity of this disorder plays into the difficulty in establishing a diagnosis. Often, the presentation lacks the classic features noted on echocardiography. HCM is a disease process that is known to evolve with age, and the development of left ventricular hypertrophy (LVH) has been observed to occur in children after full growth is attained.[12-14] This can make diagnosis of HCM challenging and suggests that repeat evaluation may be required to establish a diagnosis.

NATURAL HISTORY OF THE DISEASE

The heterogeneity of HCM lies not only in its varied manifestations but also in the natural history of disease in the patient population. Attempts to understand any link between genotype, phenotype, and natural history have as yet yielded only limited clinical associations. One of the most interesting aspects regarding the study of the natural history of HCM is how selection bias has played a significant role in initial attempts to characterize patient outcomes. Earlier studies from tertiary referral centers implied ominously high annual mortality rates of 3% to 6%; however, this work was limited by a significant referral bias.[1] More recent data from regional and community-based centers suggest an annual mortality rate of approximately 1%.[3,4] However, in selected populations, the annual mortality rate may be as high as 5% to 6%, particularly in those symptomatic patients who eventually present at larger referral centers.[1,15,16]

The clinical course of HCM is often difficult to predict and poses a challenge to clinicians. However, the options in terms of disease progression remain limited. The most feared and least predictable of the entities is sudden cardiac death (SCD), particularly in the younger population. More commonly, patients develop symptoms such as angina, syncope, or exertional dyspnea. These symptoms can become progressively worse over time. These patients can progress toward end-stage heart failure with left ventricular failure. HCM patients also develop atrial fibrillation and are at risk for embolic strokes. A certain percentage of HCM patients remain asymptomatic and have a comparably normal life expectancy. However, at some point even these patients are at risk for SCD or development of atrial fibrillation. The challenge for clinicians is to closely monitor those who may eventually develop symptoms and offer timely therapy when indicated.

CLINICAL PRESENTATION

Although the spectrum of clinical presentation in HCM is large, most patients are asymptomatic and are diagnosed as the result of a murmur on examination, an abnormal electrocardiogram (ECG), or unexplained LVH discovered by echocardiography. The complex pathophysiologic interplay between LVOT obstruction, diastolic dysfunction, myocardial ischemia, and mitral regurgitation usually results in the presenting complaints of exertional dyspnea, chest discomfort, syncope or near-syncope, and SCD. Symptomatic patients who have an adverse clinical

course typically follow along one of several pathways: (1) high risk for SCD, (2) progressive symptoms of exertional dyspnea and chest pain associated with presyncope or syncope in the setting of preserved left ventricular function, (3) development of progressive congestive heart failure due to severe left ventricular remodeling resulting in systolic dysfunction, and (4) consequences of supraventricular or ventricular arrhythmias such as atrial fibrillation or ventricular tachycardia.[1,7,17-19]

SCD is the most common presentation and cause of mortality in patients with HCM.[1,7,18,20,21] In addition, SCD is the single largest cause of cardiovascular death among young people, as well as the most common cause of mortality in competitive athletes.[1,22] Although SCD is most commonly observed in asymptomatic children and young adults, it appears that there is no advanced age at which the risk of SCD becomes negligible.[23] SCD is obviously the most fearsome and dramatic complication of HCM, but those at high risk for SCD actually constitute only a small fraction of the disease spectrum,[1,6,7,24,25] and much effort has been devoted to the premorbid identification of this subset of patients. Currently identified risk factors for SCD include prior cardiac arrest, family history of SCD, unexplained syncope or near-syncope, left ventricular thickness greater than 30 mm, a high-risk genetic mutation (e.g., beta-myosin heavy chain mutations Arg403Gln and Arg719Gln), hypotensive response during exercise stress testing, and nonsustained ventricular tachycardia (NSVT) on Holter monitoring.[1,7,14,24,26-31] In addition, an LVOT gradient greater than 30 mm Hg has been associated with an increased risk of SCD, progression to heart failure, and morbidity related to arrhythmia including stroke.[32,33] However, incremental increase in the subaortic gradient above 30 mm Hg has not been demonstrated to impart any additional risk. It is uncommon that HCM patients suffer SCD without at least one of the aforementioned risk factors (<3%).[24] It has been suggested that the etiology of SCD in this population is related to the development of complex ventricular tachyarrhythmia,[7,34,35] often during mild to moderate physical exertion and with a circadian predilection for the early morning hours (Table 54-1).[36]

Chest pain, both typical and atypical in character, is a common feature in HCM and has been reported in up to 80% of patients in this population.[37] In many cases, angiography reveals normal coronary arteries. Despite this finding, numerous studies incorporating nuclear single-photon emission computed tomography (SPECT), positron emission tomography (PET), and magnetic resonance imaging (MRI) technologies have demonstrated significant reversible and nonreversible myocardial perfusion defects in this subset of patients, including autopsy data that reported findings of myocardial infarction in up to 15% of such patients.[1,7,37-41] Collectively, these data have led to a mounting body of evidence suggesting that microvascular dysfunction may have a pivotal role in the development of myocardial ischemia and

Table 54-1. Risk Factors for Sudden Cardiac Death

Spontaneous sustained VT
Nonsustained VT (>3 beats at a rate of >120 beats/min) on ambulatory monitoring
Family history of cardiac arrest or SCD
Prior personal history of cardiac arrest
Unexplained syncope (especially if exertional)
Abnormal response to exercise stress testing (especially hypotension)
LV thickness >30 mm
High-risk genetic mutation (see Table 54-2)
LVOT gradient >30 mm Hg*
Atrial fibrillation*
Near-syncope*

*Direct relationship with SCD less well established.
LV, left ventricular; LVOT, left ventricular outflow tract; SCD, sudden cardiac death; VT, ventricular tachycardia.

infarction in this group. The etiology of microvascular dysfunction is probably multifactorial and caused, in part, by arteriolar medial hypertrophy resulting in reduced luminal diameter, impaired coronary vasodilatory response, and a supply-demand mismatch due to an abnormally thickened ventricle.[1,7,38,42] In addition, early work has suggested that evidence of microvascular dysfunction, as demonstrated by PET, is an independent predictor of increased mortality and may portend a worse prognosis years before the development of clinical deterioration.[43]

Syncope in patients with HCM is not an uncommon phenomenon and has a diverse array of possible causes, making the exact determination of mechanism challenging. Although it is regarded as an ominous prognostic sign and a known risk factor for SCD in the younger population, syncope in the adult population has not been independently associated with premature death, and recurrent episodes are rarely reported in patients with SCD.[44-46] Arrhythmic sources of syncope may be supraventricular, such as atrial fibrillation or flutter, or ventricular, such as ventricular tachycardia or fibrillation. Hemodynamic mechanisms of syncope all result in a sudden and severe reduction in cardiac output that may involve ischemia, outflow tract obstruction, or severe diastolic dysfunction. Additionally, it has been suggested that activation of left ventricular baroreceptors due to elevated intracavity pressures may induce reflex hypotension and consequent syncopal episode in a select subgroup of patients.[47]

Heart failure, as manifested by a symptom complex of exertional dyspnea, orthopnea, and progressive fatigue, is most commonly encountered in adult patients with HCM but has been described in the juvenile population as well.[1] It usually occurs in the setting of preserved systolic function, and symptoms are most commonly the consequence of diastolic dysfunction resulting from an abnormally thickened and noncompliant ventricle.[7] The combined influence of other variables, such as ischemia, atrial fibrillation, and mitral regurgitation, may also play a significant role in the development of hemodynamic

decompensation in this population. A smaller number of patients with HCM and heart failure may have significantly reduced left ventricular systolic function and chamber enlargement. It is important to recognize this subset of patients, given the potential alteration in therapeutic strategy.[45]

Atrial fibrillation complicates the course of approximately 20% of patients with HCM and is associated with an increased risk of heart failure–related death.[21,28] The risk seems to be substantially greater in the subset of patients with outflow tract obstruction or an earlier onset of arrhythmia (<50 years of age). Advancing age, left atrial enlargement, and congestive symptoms are independently linked to the development of atrial fibrillation. Although atrial fibrillation is strongly associated with an increased risk of fatal and nonfatal stroke, it does not appear to be a risk factor for the development of SCD, and approximately one third of patients have no long-term sequelae from this arrhythmia.[28] Severe functional deterioration due to dyspnea, chest pain, palpitations, or pulmonary edema may complicate the course of the chronically affected. These symptoms are most likely caused by the loss of atrial contraction, reduction in diastolic filling time, and exacerbation of underlying ischemia.[7,28]

The nature of clinical presentation may also be affected by a particular patient's age or gender. In contrast to their younger counterparts, elderly patients with HCM often develop marked symptomatology at an advanced age (>55 years), have lesser degrees of LVH (usually confined to the septum), and have a dynamic subaortic gradient caused by restricted excursion of the often anteriorly displaced mitral leaflets and posteriorly directed septal motion.[48] Whereas HCM seems to have a male predominance, female patients often present at a later age, are more symptomatic, and are at a greater risk of death due to heart failure or stroke.[49]

DIAGNOSIS

Echocardiography

Given its safety and ubiquity, two-dimensional echocardiography is the most common method for establishing the clinical diagnosis of HCM via the identification of a thickened, nondilated left ventricle in the absence of comorbidities known to cause such a degree of LVH (i.e., hypertension or aortic stenosis).[1,7,50] Classically thought to involve primarily the ventricular septum, the morphologic expression of LVH is extremely heterogeneous, and virtually any pattern of thickening may be observed.[1,7,51] In addition, there are significant differences in the pattern of hypertrophy between young and elderly patients. Elderly patients are often found to have an *elliptical* ventricular cavity, with hypertrophy predominantly of the basal septum. In contrast, younger patients (<55 years) often have a "crescent-shaped" ventricular cavity associated with diffuse hypertrophy of the interventricular septum.[52] Whereas a maximal wall

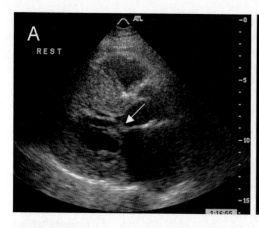
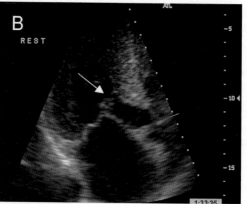

Figure 54-1. Echocardiograms in the parasternal long view (**A**) and the apical three-chamber view (**B**) demonstrate systolic anterior motion (SAM, *arrow*) at rest, resulting in severe left ventricular outflow tract obstruction in a patient with severe, symptomatic hypertrophic obstructive cardiomyopathy.

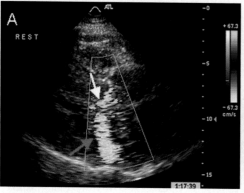
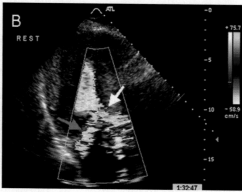

Figure 54-2. Color Doppler images display flow acceleration in the left ventricular outflow tract (*white arrow*) and resulting posteriorly directed mitral regurgitation (*orange arrow*) in the parasternal long view (**A**) and apical three-chamber view (**B**).

thickness greater than 15 mm is the traditional echocardiographic benchmark for HCM, the degree of hypertrophy may demonstrate considerable variability (with a mean thickness of approximately 22 mm).[51] It is import to realize, however, that the paucity of characteristic LVH (>15 mm) on echocardiographic examination *does not* exclude the presence of an HCM gene mutation.[7,9,53-55] Serial echocardiographic assessment may be necessary for adequate identification of suspected carriers, especially in the younger population, in whom development of LVH may be delayed until after puberty.[1,18,55]

LVOT obstruction is observed in approximately 20% of patients with HCM and is usually dynamic in nature.[21,32] Subaortic obstruction is caused by SAM of the anterior mitral leaflet resulting in mitral-septal contact during midsystole (Fig. 54-1).[7] Obstruction may not be present under resting conditions but is provoked by pharmacologic agents (i.e., amyl nitrite) or physiologic maneuvers (i.e., Valsalva). Significant mitral regurgitation frequently accompanies SAM because of distortion of the valvular apparatus and malcoaptation of the anterior and posterior leaflets (Fig. 54-2). Mitral regurgitation is also observed in up to 30% of patients who do not demonstrate obstructive physiology, primarily due to leaflet prolapse, chordal rupture, or trauma resulting in calcification or fibrosis.[12] Less commonly, a midcavity gradient is formed as a result of the anomalous insertion of the anterolateral papillary muscle directly onto the anterior mitral leaflet or an exaggerated proliferation of

midventricular papillary musculature coming into apposition with the ventricular septum.[7,13,56] Although the threshold for therapeutic intervention has traditionally been a gradient greater than 50 mm Hg, it has been demonstrated that the presence of a resting LVOT obstruction greater than 30 mm Hg is independently predictive of death from heart failure or stroke, progression of heart failure symptoms, and reduced functional capacity, as well as SCD.[32] It is important not to misinterpret the Doppler spectral display of mitral regurgitation for LVOT gradient, given its frequent presence in the setting of obstruction and its close spatial relation to the LVOT. In the setting of SAM, mitral regurgitation is usually posteriorly directed into the left atrium and is often difficult to distinguish from LVOT flow. It is most useful to sweep anterior to posterior with continuous Doppler to distinguish these two flows.

Given the magnitude of LVH consummate with HCM, it is not surprising that more than 80% of patients have evidence of diastolic dysfunction by echocardiography. This is manifested by reduced maximal flow velocity in early diastole, an increase in isovolumic relaxation time, and increased atrial contribution to ventricular filling.[50,57] These findings are similar in patients both with and without an LVOT gradient or cardiac symptoms, suggesting that diastolic dysfunction may be an earlier clinical manifestation in the spectrum of this disease process. Several studies have suggested that the presence of significant diastolic dysfunction by transthoracic or tissue Doppler echocardiography may imply an increased risk of cardiac arrest, ventricular tachycardia, or progression to significant cardiac symptoms.[58]

Electrocardiography

ECG findings in HCM are extremely heterogeneous, and more than 90% of patients have demonstrable abnormalities.[1,7,11,59] However, no pattern is highly specific for the condition, and the presence of a normal tracing does not imply absence of the disease state.[11,60] Increased voltages consistent with LVH and early repolarization abnormalities are most commonly encountered, and left axis deviation, left atrial enlargement, T-wave inversion, and nonspecific ST-segment abnormalities are also frequently noted. The degree of LVH by ECG does not appear to correlate with the magnitude of hypertrophy as assessed by echocardiography.[14] In a subset of Japanese patients with hypertrophy primarily limited to the ventricular apex, giant T-wave inversions were frequently noted in the anterior leads; this was often termed "Yamaguchi's disease."[61] Pathologic Q waves, often in the inferolateral leads, may be observed in up to 50% of patients with known HCM. Although it is not apparent on surface ECG, approximately one third of patients have delayed His-Purkinje conduction on formal electrophysiologic studies, possibly due to strain of the anterior fasciculus that overlies the hypertrophied ventricle.[59]

Magnetic Resonance Imaging

In comparison to traditional echocardiography, cardiac MRI offers the advantages of superior resolution with precise morphologic characterization, enhanced tissue contrast capability, reduced exposure to ionizing radiation, and production of three-dimensional images.[62] These advantages result in the ability of cardiac MRI to better detect areas of hypertrophy that are not well visualized or are missed by traditional echocardiography. Particularly in patients with atypical hypertrophy of the anterolateral free wall, cardiac MRI is a powerful adjunctive tool in the diagnosis of HCM.[62]

Through delayed hyperenhancement techniques, cardiac MRI has demonstrated that asymptomatic patients with HCM frequently have patchy foci of myocardial scarring at the junction of the interventricular septum and the right ventricular free wall. Furthermore, scarring was limited to the areas of abnormal hypertrophy, and the degree of scarring was proportional to the magnitude of hypertrophy, whereas wall thickening was inversely related.[39] In addition, a greater extent of hyperenhancement was positively associated with high risk for SCD and with progressive disease.[63] Cardiac MRI also allows for better characterization of papillary muscle insertion and orientation. It is not uncommon to see hypertrophic, displaced, or distorted papillary muscles contributing to the obstruction and/or mitral valve

dysfunction. Considering all of these advantages, cardiac MRI is a valuable adjunctive imaging modality for the diagnosis of HCM.

Catheterization and Hemodynamics

Given the wealth of hemodynamic and anatomic data that can be derived noninvasively by echocardiography, cardiac catheterization is not required for the diagnosis of HCM. Catheterization is often employed, however, if noninvasive imaging is of insufficient quality to quantify the degree or location of obstruction, to evaluate for coronary disease before a planned surgical therapy (i.e., myectomy or pacemaker), or if anginal symptoms are present in older patients that may be attributable to ischemia. The coronary arteries in patients with HCM are usually normal and typically of large caliber. Quite different from intramyocardial "bridging," compression of the left anterior descending coronary artery (LAD) may be observed during systole due to contraction of the hypertrophied ventricle, resulting in a "sawfish" appearance.[64] Ventriculography may demonstrate systolic cavity obliteration, varying degrees of mitral regurgitation, and occasionally the hypertrophied septum prolapsing into the LVOT.

Direct measurement and localization of the gradient is easily obtained by passing a multipurpose catheter into the apical portion of the left ventricle and then slowly withdrawing it while continuously monitoring the pressure waveform. Use of a wire via a guide catheter often results in increased control during the pullback and a more accurate determination of the level of obstruction. As opposed to what is observed in aortic stenosis, the gradient is reduced before crossing of the aortic valve. This same technique can be performed using simultaneous aortic and left ventricular pressure waveforms to allow side-by-side comparison. The gradient in HCM is characteristically labile, and various pharmacologic and physiologic maneuvers similar to those used in echocardiography may be employed to accentuate the obstruction in the catheterization laboratory.

Post-extrasystolic potentiation (as first described in 1961 by Brockenbrough, Braunwald, and Morrow[64a]) refers to the augmentation of left ventricular pressure with a concomitant decrement in the aortic systolic and pulse pressures, as a result of increased LVOT obstruction in the cardiac cycle, that follows a premature ventricular contraction. A post-extrasystolic increase in gradient between the left ventricle and the aorta is seen even with aortic stenosis, but, unlike HCM, the pulse pressure (stroke volume) does not decrease, because in aortic stenosis the larger stroke volume of the post-extrasystolic beat leads to a higher gradient with no change in severity of obstruction (Fig. 54-3).

Genetic Overview

HCM is the result of mutations to genes primarily encoding sarcomeric proteins that regulate

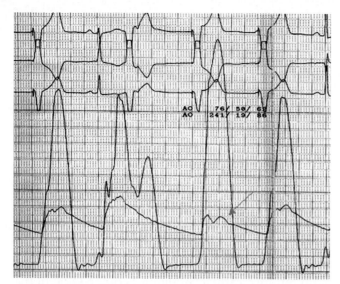

Figure 54-3. Brockenbrough-Braunwald-Morrow sign (post-extrasystolic potentiation). Simultaneous left ventricular and aortic pressure tracing demonstrates the augmentation in left ventricular pressure with concomitant decrement in the aortic systolic and pulse pressures as a result of increased left ventricular outlet tract obstruction after premature ventricular contraction (*arrow*).

Table 54-2. Sarcomeric Gene Mutations of Hypertrophic Cardiomyopathy

Gene	Locus	Symbol	Frequency (%)
Beta-myosin heavy chain	14q12	*MYH7*	30-40
Myosin binding protein C	11q1	*MYBP3*	30-40
Cardiac troponin T	1q32	*TNNTT2*	15-20
Cardiac troponin I	19q13.4	*TNNI3*	1-5
Alpha-tropomyosin	15q22.1	*TPM1*	1-5
Myosin essential light chain	3p21	*MYL3*	<1
Myosin regulatory light chain	12q24.3	*MYL2*	<1
Cardiac troponin C	3p	*TNNC1*	Rare
Alpha-myosin heavy chain	14q12	*MYHH6*	Rare
Actin	15q14	*ACTC*	Rare
Titin	2q24.3	*TTN*	Rare

Modified from Tsoutsman T, Lam L, Semsarian C: Genes, calcium and modifying factors in hypertrophic cardiomyopathy. Clin Exp Pharmacol Physiol 2006;33:139-145; and Ho CY, Seidman CE: A contemporary approach to hypertrophic cardiomyopathy. Circulation 2006;113: e858-e862.

contractile, regulatory, and structural functions that are inherited in an autosomal dominant manner.[1,7-10] To date, more than 400 mutations have been described involving 12 genes, the most common of which include cardiac troponins T, C, and I; cardiac myosin binding protein C; cardiac beta- and alpha-myosin heavy chains; myosin ventricular essential and regulatory light chains; cardiac alpha actin; and titin.[8,10] Although most of these mutations are missense with resultant substitution of the correct amino acid for another, deletions, insertions, and splice-site mutations are also well described.[65] Several nonsarcomeric mutations that produce phenotypes similar to HCM have recently been identified. *PRKAG2* affects the regulatory subunit of the adenosine monophosphate (AMP)-activated protein kinase and may result in pre-excitation, progressive conduction system abnormalities, and mild ventricular hypertrophy due to aberrant accumulation of glycogen within the myocyte.[65-67] Mutation to 2-α-galactosidase or acid α-1,4-glucosidase (both lysosome-associated membrane proteins) frequently results in multisystem glycogen storage disease and may also manifest with extreme LVH associated with ventricular pre-excitation and mental retardation.[65,66,68]

There exists great phenotypic heterogeneity among carriers of the same mutations, in part because of the effects of modifier genes and environmental factors.[7,69] It is known that many young carriers do not demonstrate the morphologic characteristics of the disease state until after adolescence, and it has now been demonstrated that phenotypic expression of LVH can be delayed into late adulthood due to incomplete penetrance of mutations involving cardiac myosin-binding protein C or troponin T.[7,53,54,60,70] Whereas

the majority of studied HCM cases involve familial mutations, sporadic cases are also well described and may constitute a significant proportion of the population. Recent work involving the systematic molecular screening of known HCM cases demonstrated that two mutations (*MYBPC3* and *MYH7*) accounted for 82% of familial cases and also detected mutations in up to 60% of "sporadic cases."[10] These data imply that a relatively limited screening process may be sufficient to identify the culprit gene in most familial cases and that identifiable mutations are responsible for the majority of "sporadic cases."

Because a number of studies have identified specific genetic mutations seemingly associated with a worse clinical prognosis and higher rates of SCD, there was initial enthusiasm that genetic testing could prospectively identify patients at higher risk for premature death.[1,9,18,31,53,54,71] However, significant limitations, including selection bias, the small number of included familial cohorts, low frequency of specific gene mutations, and variability of the phenotypic product, have hindered most genotype-phenotype correlation studies.[71-73] Therefore, because of the numerous genetic and environmental influences affecting the phenotypic product, there remains a great deal of clinical heterogeneity associated with specific mutations, making accurate risk stratification based on genetic analysis alone impractical at this time (Table 54-2).

TREATMENT

Medical Therapy

Medical therapy should be considered the initial therapeutic approach for the treatment of symptoms arising from the numerous pathophysiologic processes constituting HCM. Because of the relatively small number of cases, pharmacologic therapy for HCM is largely based on expert opinion, clinical experience, and retrospective, observational analyses. Although patients with LVOT obstruction make up the greatest proportion of the symptomatic population, a significant number of patients without obstruction may also suffer the consequences of diastolic dysfunction, such as heart failure, angina, and atrial fibrillation.[1,7,18] With the increasing use of early genetic and echocardiographic screening of athletes and affected families, it has become apparent that a significant percentage of phenotypically affected patients are entirely asymptomatic for an extended period. Moreover, although this conclusion is somewhat controversial, the available data suggest that this population does not warrant empiric therapy until symptoms develop (if ever).[1,5,7,21] Historically, the pharmacologic treatment of HCM has been limited to β-blockers, verapamil, and disopyramide.

Pharmacotherapy

β-Adrenergic Receptor Blocking Agents

β-Blockers have traditionally been the drug of choice for the treatment of HCM. This may stem from the fact that the physiologic effects of these agents are well suited to address much of the problematic pathophysiology encountered in this population. Their negative chronotropic effect results in increased diastolic filling time, which reduces left atrial pressure and may improve congestive symptoms related to diastolic dysfunction. This is especially true in cases complicated by supraventricular arrhythmias such as atrial fibrillation. The negative inotropic effect of these agents results in reduced myocardial oxygen consumption, with a resultant decrease in anginal symptoms. Although there is no convincing evidence that β-blockers effectively reduce *resting* LVOT gradients, previous work and a large amount of clinical experience suggest that these agents reduce provocable gradients in addition to substantially improving disabling symptoms related to exertion.[1,2,7,74] This is supported by data demonstrating an inverse relation between peak oxygen consumption (VO₂) and degree of LVOT obstruction during cardiopulmonary exercise testing.[7,75] As a result, β-blockers as a class are the favored agents for patients with *latent* LVOT obstruction.

Propranolol, the first agent used for the treatment of HCM, has largely been replaced by newer-generation, longer-acting, and nonselective β-blocking agents, including atenolol and metoprolol.[7,16,74] Given the significant heterogeneity in clinical symptomatology, even within the same patient at different times in the disease course, it is important to individually titrate the therapy based on current symptoms, resting heart rate (goal of 60 beats/min), exertional capacity, and the presence of potential untoward side effects.

Verapamil

Functioning both as a negative inotrope and a chronotrope by blocking the intracellular migration of calcium ions, the non-dihydropyridine calcium channel blocking agent, verapamil, produces symptomatic improvement in patients with HCM as a result of increased diastolic filling time, enhanced diastolic ventricular relaxation without negative impact on systolic function, and reduced myocardial oxygen consumption.[7,76,77] In addition, verapamil has been shown to increase the absolute myocardial blood flow during pharmacologic stress testing and to reduce the ischemic burden and improve exercise tolerance in the asymptomatic patient population.[78,79] These observations may be related to verapamil's enhanced vasodilatory properties, which are more pronounced than those seen with β-blockade, and may well explain this agent's superior efficacy in patients with chest pain. Although verapamil has classically been used in both obstructing and nonobstructing patients, caution should be exercised when initiating this agent in symptomatic patients with large resting gradients, because of the well-documented reports of severe hemodynamic decompensation resulting in cardiogenic shock and pulmonary edema.[7] In addition, verapamil should not be used in infants with HCM because of a well-established increased risk of SCD when it is administered in the intravenous formulation.[7]

Approximately 5% of patients with HCM progress to an "end stage" characterized by impaired systolic function and symptoms of heart failure. Standard therapy for congestive heart failure, including diuretics, cautious use of vasodilators, β-blockers, avoidance of calcium channel blockers, and possibly digoxin should constitute the pharmacologic regimen in these patients.[1]

In symptomatic patients, it is common clinical practice to initiate therapy using β-blockers rather than verapamil. Should the patient be intolerant of side effects (i.e., fatigue, depression, impotence), or if symptoms persist despite adequate titration of the medication, consideration should be given to substituting (or adding) verapamil.[1,7,45] At present, there are no data to suggest that combination therapy is more effective than either agent alone.

Disopyramide

A class IA antiarrhythmic agent, disopyramide, has a side effect profile that includes a negative inotropic effect with reduced contractility and a reflexive increase in systemic vascular resistance, both of which have made it an attractive agent for the treatment of HCM for more than 30 years. Although disopyramide appears to have little or no effect on diastolic function, it has been shown to effectively reduce the outflow obstruction caused by SAM, with improved symptomatic control in patients with resting gradients that have failed to improve with other forms of therapy.[7,80-82] Because of the possible potentiation of supraventricular arrhythmias such as atrial fibrillation and case reports of QT prolongation leading to torsades de pointes, close supervision and monitoring are essential during the initiation of this therapy.[83] Other side effects of disopyramide are primarily related to its anticholinergic properties and include dry mouth (32%), urinary retention (14%), constipation (11%), and, rarely, hypoglycemia.

Amiodarone

Although current data is somewhat conflicting and conclusive evidence is lacking, it has been suggested that amiodarone may reduce the risk of SCD and improve survival in selected high-risk patients noted to have NSVT on Holter monitering.[84] However, some reports suggest that amiodarone may improve a patient's symptom score and functional status but be proarrhythmic, leading to an *increased* risk of SCD due to ventricular arrhythmia.[85,86] In contrast, more recent data have found that lower-dose amiodarone (200 mg/day) in high-risk patients with recurrent NSVT is not associated with any increase in cardiovascular mortality.[29] Amiodarone has been demonstrated to be effective therapy for treatment and prevention of supraventricular tachyarrhythmias in patients with HCM.[87] Selection of which patients are appropriate for chronic, long-term empiric therapy with this agent, especially considering its attendant side-effect profile, may be impossible until more definitive trial data become available.

Dual-Chamber Pacing

Dual-chamber pacing, as a less invasive alternative to the surgical septal myectomy, was met with initial enthusiasm in the early 1990s when several observational and uncontrolled studies demonstrated that dual-chamber pacing resulted in a significant decrease in outflow gradient, reduced symptomatology with improved quality of life, and homogenous redistribution of myocardial perfusion reserve.[88,89] Although the exact mechanism is unclear, it has been proposed that activation of the right ventricular apex results in a dyssynchronous contraction of the septum, with a reduction in outflow tract obstruction in the short term and a positive ventricular remodeling effect in the long term.[88,90] However, subsequent randomized, controlled, crossover trials comparing DDD to AAI mode pacing demonstrated a significant placebo effect in regard to sustained symptomatic relief and quality of life assessment, little improvement in functional capacity, and a more modest reduction in outflow gradient in most patients, compared with the earlier, uncontrolled trials.[1,7,90-92] Of importance, a subpopulation of elderly patients (age >65 years) were objectively measured to have both symptomatic and clinical benefit as a result of DDD pacing.[91] In the same period, however, a randomized trial demonstrated significant improvement in exercise tolerance, symptom score, and LVOT gradient in patients with symptoms refractory to drug therapy and resting gradients greater than 30 mm Hg.[92] Therefore, there may exist subsets of patients for whom dual-chamber pacing may be of some symptomatic or clinical benefit. However, there are no data to suggest that

dual-chamber pacing effectively reduces risk of SCD in this patient population.[7,88,91]

Further work has suggested that the reduction in LVOT gradient is dependent on optimal timing of the atrioventricular interval: too short an interval interferes with diastolic filling and left atrial emptying, whereas too long an interval results in ineffective reduction of outflow obstruction.[93] Taking this into account, recent nonrandomized, observational data have demonstrated a significant reduction in symptoms, improved functional capacity, and consistent reduction in LVOT gradient when serial echocardiographic assessment was used to optimize the atrioventricular interval, pacing rate, and mode settings in patients treated with DDD pacemakers.[94] This may constitute the foundation for further randomized trials in this area.

Whereas data comparing dual-chamber pacing with surgical septal myectomy demonstrated improvement in both groups in regard to functional status, a significantly greater reduction in LVOT gradient, improved subjective symptom status, and increased overall exercise duration were reported in patients who underwent myectomy.[95] Therefore, although dual-chamber pacing is not considered a primary therapeutic modality for most patients with symptomatic HCM, it has been suggested that its use may be reasonable in certain subsets of patients, including elderly patients averse to more invasive therapies and those in whom pharmacotherapy is limited due to bradycardia.[7]

Cardioverter-Defibrillator Implantation

Ventricular fibrillation or tachycardia is the primary mode of SCD in patients with HCM. Given the success of the implantable cardioverter-defibrillator (ICD) in reducing arrhythmic mortality in patients with coronary artery disease and a reduced ejection fraction, there has been increasing interest in using the ICD for the prevention and treatment of HOCM-related arrhythmic death.[96] Although randomized data are lacking, a multicenter, retrospective trial demonstrated that implantation of an ICD in patients classically considered to be at high risk for SCD resulted in appropriate device intervention and aborted SCD in almost 25% of the enrolled patients over a 3-year period.[35] Patients in whom the device was implanted for primary prevention purposes experienced appropriate intervention at a rate of 5% annually; in contrast, patients who received the device after cardiac arrest or sustained ventricular tachycardia had appropriate intervention at a rate of 11% annually.[1,7,35,97] Based on these results, it has been suggested that ICD implantation is reasonable, should be considered in patients with one or more risk factors for SCD, and is warranted in patients with a prior history of cardiac arrest or sustained ventricular tachycardia.[1,7] Device selection should be based primarily on individual patient preference and characteristics. Dual-chamber devices have the advantage of atrial sensing and pacing functions, as well as the ability to discriminate supraventricular from ventricular arrhythmias, which results in a reduction in the number of inappropriate interventions. Unfortunately, the dual-chamber devices have a higher potential for complications (usually related to the transvenous lead systems) than do single-chamber devices.[97] The 2002 American College of Cardiology/ American Heart Association/North American Society of Pacing and Electrophysiology (ACC/AHA/NASPE) consensus guidelines designated implantation of an ICD as a prophylactic measure in selected high-risk patients as a class IIb intervention (i.e., usefulness and/or efficacy is less well established), whereas implantation of an ICD for secondary prevention was designated a class I intervention (i.e., evidence or consensus that the given procedure or treatment is useful and effective).[98]

Surgery

Patients with resting or provocable gradients of greater than 50 mm Hg who continue to experience significant functional limitation (i.e., New York Heart Association [NYHA] class III-IV) because of limiting symptoms of exertional dyspnea, chest pain, or recurrent syncope despite maximal medical therapy may be considered candidates for surgical therapy.[1,7,18] Surgical therapy is not currently recommended for patients *without* significant LVOT obstruction, nor for patients with relatively *mild* symptoms with obstruction, nor to treat associated complications of this condition, such as atrial fibrillation or syncope, alone.[7]

Surgical therapy for HOCM was originally designed to effectively reduce LVOT obstruction but has undergone significant evolution, from the original isolated septal myotomy performed by Cleland in the 1960s[98a] to the more modern and widely employed Morrow myectomy[99] in combination with mitral valve repair or even replacement in selected patients.[100,101] The "gold standard" septal myectomy, described by Morrow, is performed via an aortotomy so that the proximal septum is approachable via the aortic valve. Between 5 and 15 g of myocardial tissue is resected from the base of the aortic valve to a region distal to the mitral leaflets, such that the area of mitral-septal contact that results in SAM is removed and the LVOT is enlarged.[7,99,100] Because it is critically important to correctly identify the involved portion of the ventricular septum and to resect enough myocardium to relieve the outflow tract gradient, most experienced centers employ transesophageal echocardiography (TEE) to assist in localizing the desired region for resection, as well as to monitor the effect of resection on the gradient intraoperatively.[100] Despite its more aggressive nature, an alteration of the classic Morrow procedure has been described in which an extended myectomy is combined with partial excision and mobilization of the papillary muscles to result in amelioration of the outflow tract obstruction, reduced tethering of the subvalvular mitral structures, and a more individualized surgical resection depending on

the extent and location of the patient's LVH.[100-102] In patients with specific comorbidities, such as atrial fibrillation or coronary artery disease, myectomy may be combined with adjunctive surgical procedures such as the MAZE procedure or coronary bypass grafting in a single, efficient procedure.

Mitral valvular abnormalities, such as elongated and flexible leaflets, may substantially contribute to the degree of LVOT obstruction in an important minority of patients. These patients often benefit from mitral valve plication at the time of myectomy, to more effectively reduce the degree of obstruction that results from SAM and to reduce the associated mitral regurgitation.[12,100,103,104] Mitral valve replacement is usually reserved for patients with significant primary valvular abnormalities, such as myxomatous degeneration leading to mitral valve prolapse or regurgitation.[7,105]

The modern-day septal myectomy procedure carries a relatively low operative risk owing to continued technical refinement, with a cumulative operative mortality rate of approximately 1% to 3% overall, and more recent data reporting rates of less than 1% in very experienced centers.[1,7,45,106,107] Left bundle branch block (LBBB) after myectomy is understandably very common due to the location of the procedure. Complete heart block requiring implantation of a permanent pacemaker is more recently a rare complication, as is iatrogenic formation of a ventricular septal defect.[7,105,108]

Whereas a conclusive reduction in long-term mortality after myectomy has yet to be demonstrated in a randomized controlled fashion, nonrandomized, multicenter, observational data (as well as a wealth of clinical experience) suggest that this procedure results in significant improvement in a patient's functional capacity, heart failure symptoms, and quality of life and may even extend life expectancy.[1,7,18,100] In addition, reduction of the outflow tract gradient usually results in amelioration of SAM of the mitral apparatus and the resultant mitral regurgitation.[7,100,109,110] In fact, a recent clinical surgical series suggested that patients treated with surgical myectomy have an excellent prognosis, with a life expectancy similar to that of the general population, which may be partly due to a reduction in the rate of SCD.[111]

Septal Ablation

In an effort to provide an alternative treatment strategy to relieve outflow tract obstruction in symptomatic patients who do not desire the more invasive surgical myectomy are suboptimal surgical candidates because of comorbidities, or who are located in areas without sufficient surgical expertise, the percutaneous septal ablation was introduced by Sigwart in 1995.[112] Through the selective infusion of 100% ethanol into either the first or second septal perforator arteries, the septal ablation technique attempts to mimic the effect of the more traditional Morrow myectomy by inducing a controlled infarct in the basal portion of the hypertrophied septum; this causes scarring, thinning, and akinesis, resulting in a significant reduction in the LVOT gradient and SAM of the mitral valvular apparatus.[1,7,45,112-115] Despite the paucity of large-scale randomized, controlled trials documenting the long-term outcome of these patients, short-term observational studies have demonstrated a significant reduction in LVOT gradient, often a rapid reduction in limiting symptoms, and improved exercise tolerance after ablation, with a reported mortality rate similar to or less than that of surgery at 1% to 4%.[7,113-118] The short-term success of this procedure, combined with its obviously less invasive nature, has led to a dramatic increase in its use over the past 10 years, with ablation estimated to be 15 to 20 times more common than surgical myectomy and more than 4000 ablations performed worldwide to date.[7,119,120]

It is very important to carefully screen all patients being considered for septal ablation and to select for patients who can realize maximum benefit from the intervention. As with patients recommended for the traditional myectomy, the updated American College of Cardiology/European Society of Cardiology (ACC/ESC) consensus statement recommends that selection criteria include septal hypertrophy greater than 18 mm, dynamic LVOT obstruction with a gradient greater than 50 mm Hg (either at rest or with provocation), and severely limiting heart failure symptoms (i.e., NYHA functional class III-IV) despite maximal medical therapy (Table 54-3).[7,121]

A thorough search for abnormalities that are better addressed surgically is essential before proceeding with catheter-based septal ablation. Such abnormalities include anomalous papillary muscle insertion into the mitral valve, anatomically abnormal mitral valve with a long anterior/posterior leaflet, coexistent coronary artery disease, primary valvular disease (aortic or mitral), and subaortic membrane or pannus—all of which are not adequately addressed by septal ablation.[7,121] In addition, abnormally elongated and flexible anterior mitral leaflets resulting in an anterior location of the coaptation line and outflow tract obstruction are not correctable via catheter-based techniques and require surgical myectomy with plication.[12] In addition, many experienced

centers refer patients with a septal thickness greater than 2.5 cm for surgical correction.

Procedural Technique

Given the fact that most patients with HOCM are diagnosed noninvasively with echocardiography and many have not had invasive hemodynamic studies performed before presenting for ablation, many operators reconfirm the presence of significant LVOT obstruction by positioning an end-hole catheter in the ventricular apex and recording a slow pullback under fluoroscopy. Alternatively, simultaneous measurement of the ascending aortic and intracavity pressures may be obtained via placement of an ascending aortic catheter and an end-hole catheter as described earlier. If an LVOT gradient is not confirmed under basal/resting conditions, provocation with amyl nitrate or the Valsalva maneuver may be attempted.[121] Failure to confirm a significant gradient after these maneuvers should prompt the operator to further pursue alternative causes for the patient's symptom complex.

Standard diagnostic coronary cineangiography is performed as a first step to clearly define the patient's anatomy and evaluate for concomitant atherosclerotic disease. Once this is completed, attention is turned toward selection of the appropriate septal perforator branch through which the ablation will be performed. To best view the anatomic course of the septal branches as they course through the basal interventricular septum, the camera should be positioned in the right anterior oblique (RAO) or posteroanterior (PA) cranial view. It is also important to determine the septal vessel's course along the septum (i.e., on the right or left side), using the left anterior oblique projection. At times, septal anatomy may vary such that one subdivision runs along the left side of the septum while another runs along the right. Selection of the left-sided subdivision is optimal for ablation, because there is a reduced likelihood of inducing complete heart block during ethanol infusion when the left side is used. Whereas the vast majority of septal perforators arise from the LAD, substantial anatomic variation has been described, and vessels may arise from the left main trunk, ramus intermedius, left circumflex, or diagonal branches, or even from a branch of the right coronary artery.[121]

A temporary transvenous pacemaker is placed in advance as a prophylactic measure, in case of the development of complete heart block during the ablation, or in the early days after the procedure. Given that heparin will be used for anticoagulation, care should be taken to minimize the risk of bleeding during pacemaker insertion. Most experienced operators prefer access via the right internal jugular vein, using a micropuncture needle kit. Because many of the commercially available blunt-tip transvenous pacing wires have a proclivity for movement after placement, it is common practice to place screw-in

---

Table 54-3. Patient Selection Criteria for Alcohol Septal Ablation

Severe heart failure symptoms (i.e., NYHA class III-IV) despite maximal medical therapy
Septal thickness >18 mm
Subaortic gradient >50 mm Hg (resting or with provocation) due to mitral-septal contact
Absence of papillary muscle or mitral valvular anomalies (i.e., anomalous papillary muscle insertion)
Absence of significant coronary arterial disease
Compatible septal perforator branch arterial anatomy
Relative contraindications to surgical myectomy (i.e., age, comorbidity)

NYHA, New York Heart Association.

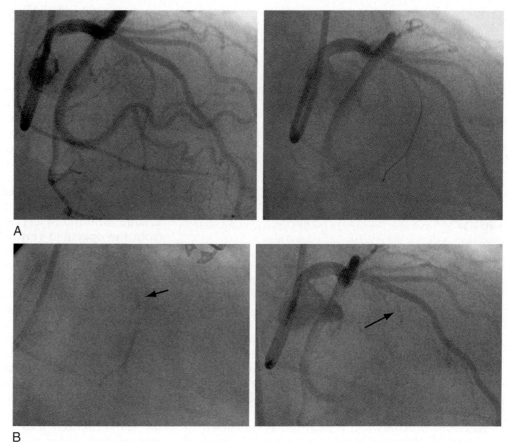

Figure 54-4. A, Coronary digital subtraction angiogram demonstrating introduction of a 0.014-inch guidewire (*right panel*) into a septal perforator branch with anatomic characteristics ideal for septal ablation. **B,** Coronary angiogram demonstrating introduction of a 1.5×10 mm balloon (*arrow*) into the selected septal vessel (*left panel*). Injection of contrast into the balloon and left anterior descending coronary artery confirms correct positioning (*right panel*).

type pacing leads into the right ventricular apex. After successful placement of both the temporary pacemaker and the arterial sheath, heparin is administered to achieve an activated clotting time of 250 to 300, to prevent thrombosis in guide catheters and on wires.

After angiographic identification of the septal arteries, close attention must be given to vessel size, angulation, and the distribution of myocardial territories served by the given vessel. Because arteries with a diameter greater than 2.0 mm often subtend a larger myocardial distribution than is desired, injection of ethanol into a vessel of this caliber is avoided to prevent induction of an overly generous infarct. Angulation of the septal vessels, either at the origin from the primary vessel (e.g., LAD) or at the bifurcation of a larger septal artery, is an important consideration in vessel selection. Vessels with angulation greater than 90 degrees are often technically challenging and result in difficulty passing the balloon into the selected vessel, with frequent prolapse of the wire into the mid-LAD.[121]

Substantial variation exists in the distribution of blood flow supplied by the septal perforators in patients with HOCM, compared to the unaffected population. In both autopsy and angiography studies, it has been demonstrated that the first septal artery may provide blood flow to regions other than the targeted basal septum (including the right ventricle);

it may supply the basal septum incompletely and share this responsibility with a second septal branch, or it may subtend a substantially larger distribution of myocardium than would be expected.[121,122] Therefore, an intimate knowledge of the myocardial distribution of blood flow supplied by the selected septal branch is essential to accurately target the correct area for ablation and to avoid infarction of an unanticipated region or an oversized infarction of the septum itself. This is most commonly accomplished during the procedure by selective injection of dye under cine guidance and the concomitant use of transthoracic echocardiography (TTE), using injectable contrast material.

After angiographic assessment of the septal anatomy, a guide catheter providing extra support (such as a 6- or 7-Fr XB catheter) is used to engage the left main trunk. Subsequently, a 0.014-inch extra-support wire with a soft tip is passed into the selected septal perforator branch, most commonly the first septal perforator (Fig. 54-4). A short angioplasty balloon, usually 1.5 to 2 mm in diameter and 10 mm in length, is passed over the guidewire and into the septal branch. Difficulty in passing the balloon may be resolved by using a stiffer guidewire to provide greater support for balloon placement.[121] Care must be taken that the balloon is seated deeply enough into the septal artery to ensure that the injected ethanol is not refluxed into the LAD. Conversely, if

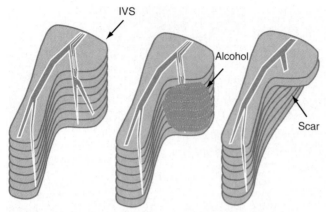

IVS

Alcohol

Scar

Figure 54-5. Schematic overview of the alcohol septal ablation procedure depicting the resultant basal septal scar and enlargement of the left ventricular outflow tract. If the balloon is placed distally, the anterior septum is not ablated, which can produce a suboptimal result. IVS, interventricular septum.

the balloon is placed too deeply into the septal vessel, the injected ethanol may spare the basal-most portion of the septum, resulting in an unsuccessful procedure (Fig. 54-5). After successful placement, the balloon is inflated to occlude the perforator (typically to 10 to 12 atmospheres).

As noted previously, it is essential at this point to verify the distribution of myocardium being supplied by the selected vessel, given the substantial degree of variability in the anatomy of this patient population. This is accomplished with the use of both traditional angiography and TEE. After correct positioning of the balloon, as noted earlier, the operator inflates the balloon, and 1 to 2 mL of contrast solution is injected to assess the full extent of myocardium supplied by the chosen vessel. Contrast should be slowly injected so as to mimic the anticipated alcohol infusion. Extreme caution should be taken to verify that the infused contrast does not reflux into the LAD or into other coronary arteries (e.g., posterior descending artery), which could possibly expose a large amount

of unintended myocardium to damage when the ethanol is infused.

After angiographic confirmation, further assessment of the septal distribution is obtained via contrast echocardiography (Fig. 54-6). After careful inspection of the septum in the apical long-axis, four-chamber, and parasternal long-axis views, 1 to 2 mL of Albunex contrast is injected into the septal branch through a tuberculin-type syringe. Albumex, a first-generation echocardiographic contrast agent, is no longer available in many countries, so second- and third-generation agents are currently employed. These agents have proved to be suboptimal because they rapidly traverse the capillary beds and produce a large amount of echocardiographic "shadowing" from the opacified ventricles. Therefore, it is important to dilute these agents before injection. In our laboratory, the contrast vials are typically opened 10 to 15 minutes before the time of expected use, to decrease their potency. The contrast is then further diluted with sterile saline in a 1:5 or 1:10 mixture at the time of injection. Pulsed-wave Doppler is the imaging method of choice when using the diluted contrast, so as to avoid destruction of the microbubbles with the higher-frequency continuous-wave ultrasound. This procedure allows the operator to verify that the chosen vessel primarily supplies the proximal interventricular septum and not portions of the inferior wall, left ventricular papillary musculature, or the right ventricular free wall via the moderator band.[121,123]

Ideally, contrast material will appear in the basal portion of the septum that is responsible for the greatest extent of septal-mitral contact. Appearance of contrast in the distal septum or in other regions of myocardium is a contraindication to ethanol infusion, because this could result in infarction of an undesired territory or of unanticipated size. As a final method of documenting that the desired area of myocardium has been selected, it is recommended that the operator document a greater than 30% reduction in the LVOT gradient during balloon inflation. A rather rapid reduction in gradient can be

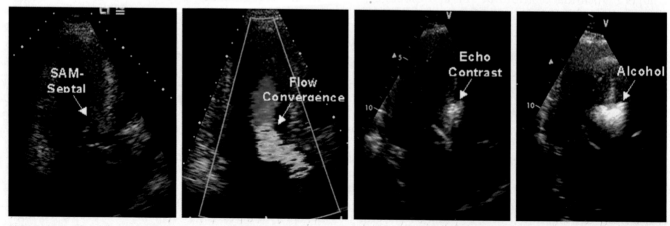

SAM-Septal

Flow Convergence

Echo Contrast

Alcohol

Figure 54-6. Contrast echocardiography (apical three-chamber view) confirming the desired distribution of myocardial blood flow through the injection of an appropriately selected septal perforator artery before ethanol infusion.

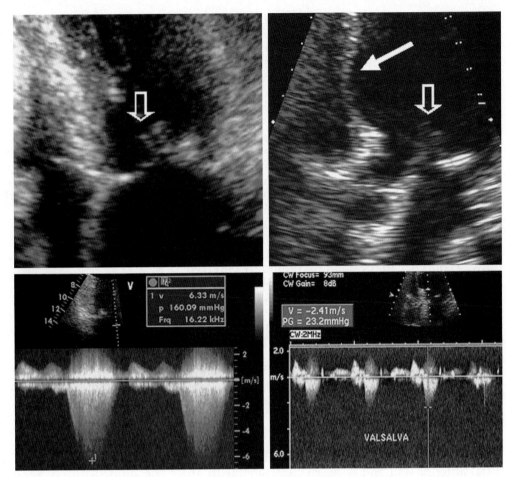

Figure 54-7. Contrast echocardiography. The images on the left were taken before alcohol ablation. The images on the right were acquired from the same patient 6 months after successful ablation and clearly demonstrate scarring (*white arrow*) in the basal septum, with a resultant increase in the area of the left ventricular outflow tract and a decrease in the outflow tract obstruction. Systolic anterior motion (*open arrow*) is present at baseline and is absent on follow-up.

observed with prolonged balloon occlusion of a septal perforator branch. Such an observation suggests that the correct septal distribution has been targeted for ablation.[121,124]

Before proceeding with ethanol injection, it is essential to confirm that the balloon has not migrated during the testing process and that the previously placed temporary pacemaker continues to have a suitable pacing threshold. This is easily done by fluoroscopic verification and injection of another 1 to 2 mL of contrast material through the guide catheter. With confirmation of proper balloon positioning, the operator may proceed with ethanol injection. Although most experienced centers use between 1 and 3 mL of desiccated ethanol, this volume may be adjusted based on the appearance of the septal anatomy and the degree of contrast washout.[7,114,121,125-127] Recent work has documented similar midterm hemodynamic outcomes with reduced complication rates when smaller amounts of ethanol (1-2 mL) are used.[128]

In situations where there is rapid contrast washout due to collateralization of the septal branch, the rate and volume of ethanol infusion should be reduced to prevent escape of the alcohol to undesirable areas of myocardium via the collaterals.[113,114,121] At this point, the ethanol is injected into the vessel over a 1- to 5-minute period with the balloon remaining inflated. After alcohol injection, 0.3 to 0.5 mL of normal saline is injected into the septal vessel to flush through any residual alcohol and to prevent reflux of ethanol into the LAD after the septal branch is no longer occluded. The balloon should remain inflated for another 10 minutes to prevent reflux of ethanol into the LAD and to allow prolonged ethanol-tissue contact. During the initial infusion, continued monitoring of the resting gradient is essential to judge the efficacy of the procedure. In general, a reduction in the LVOT gradient to less than 30 mm Hg in the setting of a resting gradient greater than 50 mm Hg, or a greater than 50% reduction of a provocable gradient, is considered indicative of a successful procedure in the catheterization laboratory (Fig. 54-7).[114,121]

Before the balloon is disengaged from the septal vessel, it is recommended that the guidewire be replaced into the septal branch for smooth removal of the balloon and maintenance of access across the left main trunk and LAD. As a final step, angiography of the LAD and septal vessels is performed to verify the integrity of the coronary circulation. Phasic flow may be observed in the injected septal branch immediately after the ablation, although total occlusion is frequently observed.

Postprocedural care should take place in a coronary intensive care unit for 48 hours after ablation, to allow for the rapid identification and treatment of possible complications. The amount of induced myocardial tissue destruction often results in elevation of the creatine phosphokinase (CPK) to levels between 800 and 1200 U/L, although this is variable depending on the amount of alcohol injected, vessel size, and the method of enzyme measurement.[7,113,120,127,128] The transvenous pacing wire may be discontinued 48 hours after the procedure if there is an absence of bradyarrhythmia or heart block that would require continued observation or a permanent pacemaker. In most centers, the patient is transferred to a regular nursing floor for another 48 to 72 hours to observe for postprocedural complications before discharge.

The complication rate after septal ablation is relatively low and is comparable to that of septal myectomy. As opposed to the LBBB so commonly observed after septal myectomy, a right bundle branch block is observed in up to 80% of patients after ablation.[7,114,121] The incidence of complete heart block has decreased in recent years and ranges from 5% to 40%, with an average value of 12% to 15% at experienced centers.[7,107,114,115,121,129] The presence of a preexisting LBBB and a rapid bolus injection of ethanol during ablation have both been positively correlated with an increased incidence of high-degree atrioventricular block requiring permanent pacemaker implantation.[129] Extravasation of alcohol into the LAD during infusion is a rare but catastrophic complication that often results in a large infarction of the middle to distal anterior wall and is clearly associated with an increased mortality. Coronary dissection from either the extra-support guidewire or the catheter has been reported in rare instances. Tamponade due to perforation of the right ventricular apex during transvenous pacing wire insertion or during interatrial septal puncture for hemodynamic monitoring during the procedure have also been reported. Overly extensive infarction of the interventricular septum as a result of too generous a quantity of infused alcohol or too rapid an infusion rate during ablation can result in a ventricular septal rupture.[121] Ventricular arrhythmias can be seen, both during the procedure and up to 48 hours afterward, but this is rare and usually does not require prolonged therapy. Unlike myectomy, septal ablation results in the formation of a large intramyocardial scar that may serve as substrate for future malignant ventricular arrhythmias. There has been some conjecture that this could result in an increased risk of late arrhythmic mortality, especially in younger patients undergoing ablation.[7,35,114,126] However, this hypothesis has yet to garner substantial evidentiary support.

Patients should be monitored closely for recurrence of symptoms or any arrhythmia. ICD implantation should be considered if there is evidence of NSVT. Objective assessment of functional capacity using exercise testing is appropriate for monitoring these patients. Repeat alcohol ablation can be considered if symptoms recur and an appropriate septal perforator is available for injection. If repeat ablation

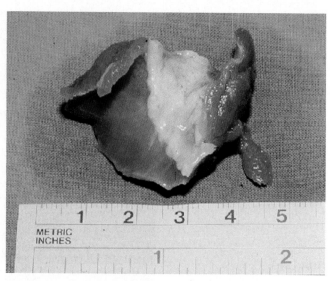

Figure 54-8. Pathology specimen of the basal interventricular septum in a patient with hypertrophic cardiomyopathy several years after an ethanol ablation, demonstrating fibrosis and scarring.

is not feasible, surgical myectomy may need to be considered in this group (Fig. 54-8).[130]

Although randomized, controlled trials have yet to be conducted, existing data suggest that septal ablation and surgical myectomy have a similar success rate on both short-term and midterm follow-up. In the immediate postprocedural period (3-72 hours), both modalities of septal reduction resulted in similar degrees of LVOT gradient reduction, and this improvement appeared to be maintained up to 1 year after either procedure.[1,7,107,114,118,127,130-132] In addition, improvements in NYHA functional class and Canadian Cardiovascular angina class were observed and the number of syncopal and presyncopal events was significantly reduced to a similar degree in both groups at both 6- and 12-months' follow-up.[107,118,131] Both procedures have advantages as well as associated complications, and this underscores the importance of careful patient selection and consideration of comorbidities before selection of an intervention. Complete heart block requiring implantation of a permanent pacemaker has been reported in up to 25% of patients undergoing alcohol ablation, compared with only 5% to 10% of those undergoing myectomy.[107,131] Given that ablation commonly produces a right bundle branch block pattern, patients with a preexisting LBBB are at very high risk of complete heart block after the procedure. In addition, it has been suggested that female gender, first-degree atrioventricular block, and an increased volume of injected alcohol are also risk factors for postprocedural complete heart block.[133] In contrast, myectomy produces an LBBB and less commonly requires permanent pacing. Myectomy can result in mild to moderate aortic insufficiency in up to 10% to 20% of patients but rarely leads to an adverse outcome.[131] By the nature of the procedure, ablation results in a permanent scar in the interventricular septum, and there remains some concern that this may serve as substrate for future ventricular arrhythmias, although this has not been objectively documented. Expectedly, ablation results in a reduced length of hospital stay compared with myectomy and substantially contributes to an overall reduction in cost. Mortality is relatively low with both interventions and approaches approximately 1% in experienced centers.[7,45,107,131] In summary, either surgical myectomy or alcohol ablation may be selected as treatment option in symptomatic patients with LVOT obstruction after taking into consideration the patient's clinical situation and anatomic characteristics and the institutional expertise.

REFERENCES

1. Maron BJ: Hypertrophic cardiomyopathy: A systematic review. JAMA 2002;287:1308-1320.
2. Braunwald E, Lambrew CT, Rockoff SD, et al: Idiopathic hypertrophic subaortic stenosis: I. A description of the disease based upon an analysis of 64 patients. Circulation 1964;30(Suppl 4):3-119.
3. Maron BJ, Spirito P: Impact of patient selection biases on the perception of hypertrophic cardiomyopathy and its natural history. Am J Cardiol 1993;72:970-972.
4. Maron BJ, Casey SA, Poliac LC, et al: Clinical course of hypertrophic cardiomyopathy in a regional United States cohort. JAMA 1999;281:650-655.
5. Spirito P, Chiarella F, Carratino L, et al: Clinical course and prognosis of hypertrophic cardiomyopathy in an outpatient population. N Engl J Med 1989;320:749-755.
6. Elliott P: Relation between the severity of left ventricular hypertrophy and prognosis in patients with hypertrophic cardiomyopathy. Lancet 2001;357:420-424.
7. Maron BJ, McKenna WJ, et al:: ACC/ESC Expert Consensus Document on Hypertrophic Cardiomyopathy. J Am Coll Cardiol 2003;42:1687-1713.
8. Ho CY, Seidman CE: A contemporary approach to hypertrophic cardiomyopathy. Circulation 2006;113:e858-e862.
9. Maron BJ, Moller JH, Seidman CE, et al: Impact of laboratory molecular diagnosis on contemporary diagnostic criteria for genetically transmitted cardiovascular diseases: Hypertrophic cardiomyopathy, long-QT syndrome, and Marfan syndrome. A statement for healthcare professionals from the Councils on Clinical Cardiology, Cardiovascular Disease in the Young, and Basic Science, American Heart Association. Circulation 1998;98:1460-1471.
10. Richard P, Charron P, Carrier L, et al: Hypertrophic cardiomyopathy: Distribution of disease genes, spectrum of mutations, and implications for a molecular diagnosis strategy. Circulation 2003;107:2227-2232.
11. Maron BJ: The electrocardiogram as a diagnostic tool for hypertrophic cardiomyopathy: Revisited. Ann Noninvasive Electrocardiol 2001;6:277-279.
12. Klues HG, Maron BJ, Dollar AL, et al: Diversity of structural mitral valve alterations in hypertrophic cardiomyopathy. Circulation 1992;85:1651-1660.
13. Wigle ED, Sasson Z, Henderson MA, et al: Hypertrophic cardiomyopathy: The importance of the site and the extent of hypertrophy. A review. Prog Cardiovasc Dis 1985;28:1-83.
14. Maron BJ, Wolfson JK, Ciro E, et al: Relation of electrocardiographic abnormalities and patterns of left ventricular hypertrophy identified by 2-dimensional echocardiography in patients with hypertrophic cardiomyopathy. Am J Cardiol 1983;51:189-194.
15. McKenna WJ, Deanfield JE: Hypertrophic cardiomyopathy: An important cause of sudden death. Arch Dis Child 1984;59:971-975.
16. Shah PM, Adelman AG, Wigle ED, et al: The natural (and unnatural) history of hypertrophic obstructive cardiomyopathy. Circ Res 1974;35(Suppl II):179-195.
17. Maron BJ: Hypertrophic cardiomyopathy. Lancet 1997;350:127-133.
18. Spirito P: The management of hypertrophic cardiomyopathy. N Engl J Med 1997;336:775-785.
19. Maron BJ: Clinical profile of stroke in 900 patients with hypertrophic cardiomyopathy. J Am Coll Cardiol 2002;39:301-307.
20. Elliott P, McKenna WJ: Hypertrophic cardiomyopathy. Lancet 2004;363:1881-1891.
21. Spirito P, Autore C: Management of hypertrophic cardiomyopathy. BMJ 2006;332:1251-1255.
22. Maron BJ, Shirani J, Poliac LC, et al: Sudden death in young competitive athletes: Clinical, demographic, and pathological profiles. JAMA 1996;276:199-204.
23. Maron BJ, Olivotto I, Spirito P, et al: Epidemiology of hypertrophic cardiomyopathy-related death: Revisited in a large non-referral-based patient population. Circulation 2000;102:858-864.
24. Elliott PM, Poloniecki J, Dickie S, et al: Sudden death in hypertrophic cardiomyopathy: Identification of high risk patients. J Am Coll Cardiol 2000;36:2212-2218.
25. Spirito P, Bellone P, Harris KM, et al: Magnitude of left ventricular hypertrophy and risk of sudden death in hypertrophic cardiomyopathy. N Engl J Med 2000;342:1778-1785.
26. Monserrat L, Elliott PM, Gimeno JR, et al: Non-sustained ventricular tachycardia in hypertrophic cardiomyopathy: An independent marker of sudden death risk in young patients. J Am Coll Cardiol 2003;42:873-879.
27. Yoshida N, Ikeda H, Wada T, et al: Exercise-induced abnormal blood pressure responses are related to subendocardial ischemia in hypertrophic cardiomyopathy. J Am Coll Cardiol 1998;32:1938-1942.
28. Olivotto I, Cecchi F, Casey SA, et al: Impact of atrial fibrillation on the clinical course of hypertrophic cardiomyopathy. Circulation 2001;104:2517-2524.
29. Cecchi F, Olivotto I, Montereggi A, et al: Prognostic value of non-sustained ventricular tachycardia and the potential role of amiodarone treatment in hypertrophic cardiomyopathy: Assessment in an unselected non-referral based patient population. Heart 1998;79:331-336.
30. Moolman JC, Corfield VA, Posen B, et al: Sudden death due to troponin T mutations. J Am Coll Cardiol 1997;29:549-555.
31. Watkins H: Sudden death in hypertrophic cardiomyopathy. N Engl J Med 2000;342:422-424.
32. Maron MS, Olivotto I, Betocchi S, et al: Effect of left ventricular outflow tract obstruction on clinical outcome in hypertrophic cardiomyopathy. N Engl J Med 2003;348:295-303.
33. Kofflard MJ, Ten Cate FJ, van der Lee C, et al: Hypertrophic cardiomyopathy in a large community-based population: Clinical outcome and identification of risk factors for sudden cardiac death and clinical deterioration. J Am Coll Cardiol 2003;41:987-993.
34. Elliott PM, Sharma S, Varnava A, et al: Survival after cardiac arrest or sustained ventricular tachycardia in patients with hypertrophic cardiomyopathy. J Am Coll Cardiol 1999;33:1596-1601.
35. Maron BJ, Shen WK, Link MS, et al: Efficacy of implantable cardioverter-defibrillators for the prevention of sudden death in patients with hypertrophic cardiomyopathy. N Engl J Med 2000;342:365-373.
36. Maron BJ, Kogan J, Proschan MA, et al: Circadian variability in the occurrence of sudden cardiac death in patients with hypertrophic cardiomyopathy. J Am Coll Cardiol 1994;23:1405-1409.
37. Maron BJ, Epstein SE, Roberts WC: Hypertrophic cardiomyopathy and transmural myocardial infarction without significant atherosclerosis of the extramural coronary arteries. Am J Cardiol 1979;43:1086-1102.
38. Dilsizian V, Bonow RO, Epstein SE, et al: Myocardial ischemia detected by thallium scintigraphy is frequently related to cardiac arrest and syncope in young patients with hypertrophic cardiomyopathy. J Am Coll Cardiol 1993;22:796-804.

39. Choudhury L, Mahrholdt H, Wagner A, et al: Myocardial scarring in asymptomatic or mildly symptomatic patients with hypertrophic cardiomyopathy. J Am Coll Cardiol 2002;40:2156-2164.

40. Basso C, Thiene G, Corrado D, et al: Hypertrophic cardiomyopathy and sudden death in the young: Pathologic evidence of myocardial ischemia. Hum Pathol 2000;31:988-998.

41. Schwartzkopff B, Mundhenke M, Strauer BE: Alterations of the architecture of subendocardial arterioles in patients with hypertrophic cardiomyopathy and impaired coronary vasodilator reserve: A possible cause for myocardial ischemia. J Am Coll Cardiol 1998;31:1089-1096.

42. Schwartzkopff B, Mundhenke M, Strauer BE: Remodelling of intramyocardial arterioles and extracellular matrix in patients with arterial hypertension and impaired coronary reserve. Eur Heart J 1995;16(Suppl I):82-86.

43. Cecchi F, Olivotto I, Gistri R, et al: Coronary microvascular dysfunction and prognosis in hypertrophic cardiomyopathy. N Engl J Med 2003;349:1027-1035.

44. Maron BJ, Roberts WC, Epstein SE: Sudden death in hypertrophic cardiomyopathy: A profile of 78 patients. Circulation 1982;65:1388-1394.

45. Spirito P, Seidman CE, McKenna WJ, et al: The management of hypertrophic cardiomyopathy. N Engl J Med 1997;336:775-785.

46. Nienaber CA, Hiller S, Spielmann RP, et al: [Risk of syncope in hypertrophic cardiomyopathy: A multivariate analysis of prognostic variables]. Z Kardiol 1990;79:286-296.

47. Gilligan D: Investigation of a hemodynamic basis for syncope in hypertrophic cardiomyopathy: Use of a head-up tilt test. Circulation 1992;85:2140-2148.

48. Lewis JF, Maron BJ: Clinical and morphologic expression of hypertrophic cardiomyopathy in patients > or =65 years of age. Am J Cardiol 1994;73:1105-1111.

49. Olivotto I, Maron MS, Adabag AS, et al: Gender-related differences in the clinical presentation and outcome of hypertrophic cardiomyopathy. J Am Coll Cardiol 2005;46:480-487.

50. Poliac LC, Barron ME, Maron BJ: Hypertrophic cardiomyopathy. Anesthesiology 2006;104:183-192.

51. Klues HG, Schiffers A, Maron BJ: Phenotypic spectrum and patterns of left ventricular hypertrophy in hypertrophic cardiomyopathy: Morphologic observations and significance as assessed by two-dimensional echocardiography in 600 patients. J Am Coll Cardiol 1995;26:1699-1708.

52. Lever HM, Karam RF, Currie PJ, et al: Hypertrophic cardiomyopathy in the elderly: Distinctions from the young based on cardiac shape. Circulation 1989;79:580-589.

53. Watkins H, McKenna WJ, Thierfelder L, et al: Mutations in the genes for cardiac troponin T and alpha-tropomyosin in hypertrophic cardiomyopathy. N Engl J Med 1995;332:1058-1064.

54. Niimura H, Bachinski LL, Sangwatanaroj S, et al: Mutations in the gene for cardiac myosin-binding protein C and late-onset familial hypertrophic cardiomyopathy. N Engl J Med 1998;338:1248-1257.

55. Spirito P, Maron BJ: Absence of progression of left ventricular hypertrophy in adult patients with hypertrophic cardiomyopathy. J Am Coll Cardiol 1987;9:1013-1017.

56. Klues HG, Roberts WC, Maron BJ: Anomalous insertion of papillary muscle directly into anterior mitral leaflet in hypertrophic cardiomyopathy: Significance in producing left ventricular outflow obstruction. Circulation 1991;84:1188-1197.

57. Maron BJ, Spirito P, Green KJ, et al: Noninvasive assessment of left ventricular diastolic function by pulsed Doppler echocardiography in patients with hypertrophic cardiomyopathy. J Am Coll Cardiol 1987;10:733-742.

58. Chikamori T, Dickie S, Poloniecki JD, et al: Prognostic significance of radionuclide-assessed diastolic function in hypertrophic cardiomyopathy. Am J Cardiol 1990;65:478-482.

59. Fananapazir L, Tracy CM, Leon MB, et al: Electrophysiologic abnormalities in patients with hypertrophic cardiomyopathy: A consecutive analysis in 155 patients. Circulation 1989;80:1259-1268.

60. Maron BJ, Niimura H, Casey SA, et al: Development of left ventricular hypertrophy in adults in hypertrophic cardiomyopathy caused by cardiac myosin-binding protein C gene mutations. J Am Coll Cardiol 2001;38:315-321.

61. Yamaguchi H, Ishimura T, Nishiyama S, et al: Hypertrophic nonobstructive cardiomyopathy with giant negative T waves (apical hypertrophy): Ventriculographic and echocardiographic features in 30 patients. Am J Cardiol 1979;44:401-412.

62. Rickers C, Wilke NM, Jerosch-Herold M, et al: Utility of cardiac magnetic resonance imaging in the diagnosis of hypertrophic cardiomyopathy. Circulation 2005;112:855-861.

63. Moon JC, McKenna WJ, McCrohon JA, et al: Toward clinical risk assessment in hypertrophic cardiomyopathy with gadolinium cardiovascular magnetic resonance. J Am Coll Cardiol 2003;41:1561-1567.

64. Brugada P, Bar FW, de Zwaan C, et al: "Sawfish" systolic narrowing of the left anterior descending artery: An angiographic sign of hypertrophic cardiomyopathy. Circulation 1982;66:800-803.

64a. Brockenbrough EC, Braunwald E, Morrow AG: A hemodynamic technic for the detection of hypertrophic subaortic stenosis. Circulation 1961;23:189-194.

65. Maron BJ, Seidman JG, Seidman CE: Proposal for contemporary screening strategies in families with hypertrophic cardiomyopathy. J Am Coll Cardiol 2004;44:2125-2132.

66. Arad M, Benson DW, Perez-Atayde AR, et al: Constitutively active AMP kinase mutations cause glycogen storage disease mimicking hypertrophic cardiomyopathy. J Clin Invest 2002;109:357-362.

67. Gollob MH, Green MS, Tang AS, et al: Identification of a gene responsible for familial Wolff-Parkinson-White syndrome. N Engl J Med 2001;344:1823-1831.

68. Arad M, Maron BJ, Gorham JM, et al: Glycogen storage diseases presenting as hypertrophic cardiomyopathy. N Engl J Med 2005;352:362-372.

69. Osterop AP, Kofflard MJ, Sandkuijl LA, et al: AT1 receptor A/C1166 polymorphism contributes to cardiac hypertrophy in subjects with hypertrophic cardiomyopathy. Hypertension 1998;32:825-830.

70. Erdmann J, Raible J, Maki-Abadi J, et al: Spectrum of clinical phenotypes and gene variants in cardiac myosin-binding protein C mutation carriers with hypertrophic cardiomyopathy. J Am Coll Cardiol 2001;38:322-330.

71. Anan R, Shono H, Kisanuki A, et al: Patients with familial hypertrophic cardiomyopathy caused by a Phe110Ile missense mutation in the cardiac troponin T gene have variable cardiac morphologies and a favorable prognosis. Circulation 1998;98:391-397.

72. Marian AJ: On genetic and phenotypic variability of hypertrophic cardiomyopathy: Nature versus nurture. J Am Coll Cardiol 2001;38:331-334.

73. Tsoutsman T, Lam L, Semsarian C: Genes, calcium and modifying factors in hypertrophic cardiomyopathy. Clin Exp Pharmacol Physiol 2006;33:139-145.

74. Flamm MD, Harrison DC, Hancock EW: Muscular subaortic stenosis: Prevention of outflow obstruction with propranolol. Circulation 1968;38:846-858.

75. Sharma S, Elliott P, Whyte G, et al: Utility of cardiopulmonary exercise in the assessment of clinical determinants of functional capacity in hypertrophic cardiomyopathy. Am J Cardiol 2000;86:162-168.

76. Bonow RO, Dilsizian V, Rosing DR, et al: Verapamil-induced improvement in left ventricular diastolic filling and increased exercise tolerance in patients with hypertrophic cardiomyopathy: Short- and long-term effects. Circulation 1985;72:853-864.

77. Bonow RO, Rosing DR, Bacharach SL, et al: Effects of verapamil on left ventricular systolic function and diastolic filling in patients with hypertrophic cardiomyopathy. Circulation 1981;64:787-796.

78. Gistri R, Cecchi F, Choudhury L, et al: Effect of verapamil on absolute myocardial blood flow in hypertrophic cardiomyopathy. Am J Cardiol 1994;74:363-368.

79. Udelson JE, Bonow RO, O'Gara PT, et al: Verapamil prevents silent myocardial perfusion abnormalities during exercise in

asymptomatic patients with hypertrophic cardiomyopathy. Circulation 1989;79:1052-1060.

80. Pollick C: Muscular subaortic stenosis: Hemodynamic and clinical improvement after disopyramide. N Engl J Med 1982;307:997-999.

81. Matsubara H, Nakatani S, Nagata S, et al: Salutary effect of disopyramide on left ventricular diastolic function in hypertrophic obstructive cardiomyopathy. J Am Coll Cardiol 1995;26:768-775.

82. Sherrid M, Delia E, Dwyer E: Oral disopyramide therapy for obstructive hypertrophic cardiomyopathy. Am J Cardiol 1988;62:1085-1088.

83. Podrid PJ, Lampert S, Graboys TB, et al: Aggravation of arrhythmia by antiarrhythmic drugs: Incidence and predictors. Am J Cardiol 1987;59:38E-44E.

84. McKenna WJ, Oakley CM, Krikler DM, et al: Improved survival with amiodarone in patients with hypertrophic cardiomyopathy and ventricular tachycardia. Br Heart J 1985;53:412-416.

85. Fananapazir L, Leon MB, Bonow RO, et al: Sudden death during empiric amiodarone therapy in symptomatic hypertrophic cardiomyopathy. Am J Cardiol 1991;67:169-174.

86. Prasad K, Frenneaux MP: Hypertrophic cardiomyopathy: Is there a role for amiodarone? Heart 1998;79:317-318.

87. Almendral JM, Ormaetxe J, Martinez-Alday JD, et al: Treatment of ventricular arrhythmias in patients with hypertrophic cardiomyopathy. Eur Heart J 1993;14(Suppl J): 71-72.

88. Fananapazir L, Epstein ND, Curiel RV, et al: Long-term results of dual-chamber (DDD) pacing in obstructive hypertrophic cardiomyopathy: Evidence for progressive symptomatic and hemodynamic improvement and reduction of left ventricular hypertrophy. Circulation 1994;90:2731-2742.

89. Posma JL, Blanksma PK, Van Der Wall EE, et al: Effects of permanent dual chamber pacing on myocardial perfusion in symptomatic hypertrophic cardiomyopathy. Heart 1996;76: 358-362.

90. Nishimura RA, Trusty JM, Hayes DL, et al: Dual-chamber pacing for hypertrophic cardiomyopathy: A randomized, double-blind, crossover trial. J Am Coll Cardiol 1997; 29:435-441.

91. Maron BJ, Nishimura RA, McKenna WJ, et al: Assessment of permanent dual-chamber pacing as a treatment for drug-refractory symptomatic patients with obstructive hypertrophic cardiomyopathy: A randomized, double-blind, crossover study (M-PATHY). Circulation 1999;99:2927-2933.

92. Kappenberger L, Linde C, Daubert C, et al: Pacing in hypertrophic obstructive cardiomyopathy: A randomized crossover study. PIC Study Group. Eur Heart J 1997;18: 1249-1256.

93. Betocchi S, Elliott PM, Briguori C, et al: Dual chamber pacing in hypertrophic cardiomyopathy: Long-term effects on diastolic function. Pacing Clin Electrophysiol 2002;25: 1433-1440.

94. Topilski I, Sherez J, Keren G, et al: Long-term effects of dual-chamber pacing with periodic echocardiographic evaluation of optimal atrioventricular delay in patients with hypertrophic cardiomyopathy >50 years of age. Am J Cardiol 2006;97: 1769-1775.

95. Ommen SR, Nishimura RA, Squires RW, et al: Comparison of dual-chamber pacing versus septal myectomy for the treatment of patients with hypertropic obstructive cardiomyopathy: A comparison of objective hemodynamic and exercise end points. J Am Coll Cardiol 1999;34:191-196.

96. Moss AJ, Zareba W, Hall WJ, et al: Prophylactic implantation of a defibrillator in patients with myocardial infarction and reduced ejection fraction. N Engl J Med 2002;346:877-883.

97. Boriani G, Maron BJ, Shen WK, et al: Prevention of sudden death in hypertrophic cardiomyopathy: But which defibrillator for which patient? Circulation 2004;110: e438-e442.

98. Gregoratos G, Abrams J, Epstein AE, et al: ACC/AHA/NASPE 2002 Guideline Update for Implantation of Cardiac Pacemakers and Antiarrhythmia Devices: Summary article. A report of the American College of Cardiology/American Heart Association Task Force on Practice Guidelines (ACC/ AHA/NASPE Committee to Update the 1998 Pacemaker Guidelines). J Am Coll Cardiol 2002;40:1703-1719.

98a. Cleland WP: The surgical managment of obstructive cardiomyopathy. J Cardiovasc Surg (Torino) 1963;4:489-491.

99. Morrow AG: Hypertrophic subaortic stenosis: Operative methods utilized to relieve left ventricular outflow obstruction. J Thorac Cardiovasc Surg 1978;76:423-430.

100. Maron BJ, Dearani JA, Ommen SR, et al: The case for surgery in obstructive hypertrophic cardiomyopathy. J Am Coll Cardiol 2004;44:2044-2053.

101. Schoendube FA, Klues HG, Reith S, et al: Long-term clinical and echocardiographic follow-up after surgical correction of hypertrophic obstructive cardiomyopathy with extended myectomy and reconstruction of the subvalvular mitral apparatus. Circulation 1995;92(9 Suppl):II-122-II-127.

102. Maron BJ, Nishimura RA, Danielson GK: Pitfalls in clinical recognition and a novel operative approach for hypertrophic cardiomyopathy with severe outflow obstruction due to anomalous papillary muscle. Circulation 1998;98: 2505-2508.

103. McIntosh CL, Maron BJ, Cannon RO 3rd, et al: Initial results of combined anterior mitral leaflet plication and ventricular septal myotomy-myectomy for relief of left ventricular outflow tract obstruction in patients with hypertrophic cardiomyopathy. Circulation 1992;86(5 Suppl): II-60-II-67.

104. van der Lee C, Kofflard MJ, van Herwerden LA, et al: Sustained improvement after combined anterior mitral leaflet extension and myectomy in hypertrophic obstructive cardiomyopathy. Circulation 2003;108:2088-2092.

105. Krajcer Z, Leachman RD, Cooley DA, et al: Mitral valve replacement and septal myomectomy in hypertrophic cardiomyopathy: Ten-year follow-up in 80 patients. Circulation 1988;78(3 Pt 2):I-35-I-43.

106. Merrill WH, Friesinger GC, Graham TP Jr, et al: Long-lasting improvement after septal myectomy for hypertrophic obstructive cardiomyopathy. Ann Thorac Surg 2000;69:1732-1735; discussion 1735-1736.

107. Qin JX, Shiota T, Lever HM, et al: Outcome of patients with hypertrophic obstructive cardiomyopathy after percutaneous transluminal septal myocardial ablation and septal myectomy surgery. J Am Coll Cardiol 2001;38:1994-2000.

108. McCully RB, Nishimura RA, Tajik AJ, et al: Extent of clinical improvement after surgical treatment of hypertrophic obstructive cardiomyopathy. Circulation 1996;94:467-471.

109. Sherrid MV, Chaudhry FA, Swistel DG: Obstructive hypertrophic cardiomyopathy: Echocardiography, pathophysiology, and the continuing evolution of surgery for obstruction. Ann Thorac Surg 2003;75:620-632.

110. Nishimura RA, Holmes DR Jr: Clinical practice: Hypertrophic obstructive cardiomyopathy. N Engl J Med 2004;350: 1320-1327.

111. Ommen SR: The effect of surgical myectomy on survival in patients with hypertrophic cardiomyopathy. J Am Coll Cardiol 2004;43(Suppl A):215A.

112. Sigwart U: Non-surgical myocardial reduction for hypertrophic obstructive cardiomyopathy. Lancet 1995;346: 211-214.

113. Faber L, Meissner A, Ziemssen P, et al: Percutaneous transluminal septal myocardial ablation for hypertrophic obstructive cardiomyopathy: Long term follow up of the first series of 25 patients. Heart 2000;83:326-331.

114. Gietzen FH, Leuner CJ, Raute-Kreinsen U, et al: Acute and long-term results after transcoronary ablation of septal hypertrophy (TASH): Catheter interventional treatment for hypertrophic obstructive cardiomyopathy. Eur Heart J 1999; 20:1342-1354.

115. Lakkis NM, Nagueh SF, Dunn JK, et al: Nonsurgical septal reduction therapy for hypertrophic obstructive cardiomyopathy: One-year follow-up. J Am Coll Cardiol 2000;36: 852-855.

116. Knight C, Kurbaan AS, Seggewiss H, et al: Nonsurgical septal reduction for hypertrophic obstructive cardiomyopathy: Outcome in the first series of patients. Circulation 1997; 95:2075-2081.

117. Ruzyllo W, Chojnowska L, Demkow M, et al: Left ventricular outflow tract gradient decrease with non-surgical myocardial reduction improves exercise capacity in patients with hypertrophic obstructive cardiomyopathy. Eur Heart J 2000;21:770-777.

118. Firoozi S, Elliott PM, Sharma S, et al: Septal myotomy-myectomy and transcoronary septal alcohol ablation in hypertrophic obstructive cardiomyopathy: A comparison of clinical, haemodynamic and exercise outcomes. Eur Heart J 2002;23:1617-1624.

119. Maron BJ: Role of alcohol septal ablation in treatment of obstructive hypertrophic cardiomyopathy. Lancet 2000;355:425-426.

120. Roberts R, Sigwart U: Current concepts of the pathogenesis and treatment of hypertrophic cardiomyopathy. Circulation 2005;112:293-296.

121. Holmes DR Jr, Valeti US, Nishimura RA: Alcohol septal ablation for hypertrophic cardiomyopathy: Indications and technique. Catheter Cardiovasc Interv 2005;66:375-389.

122. Singh M, Edwards WD, Holmes DR Jr, et al: Anatomy of the first septal perforating artery: A study with implications for ablation therapy for hypertrophic cardiomyopathy. Mayo Clin Proc 2001;76:799-802.

123. Nagueh SF, Lakkis NM, He ZX, et al: Role of myocardial contrast echocardiography during nonsurgical septal reduction therapy for hypertrophic obstructive cardiomyopathy. J Am Coll Cardiol 1998;32:225-229.

124. Bhagwandeen R, Woo A, Ross J, et al: Septal ethanol ablation for hypertrophic obstructive cardiomyopathy: Early and intermediate results of a Canadian referral centre. Can J Cardiol 2003;19:912-917.

125. Faber L, Seggewiss H, Gleichmann U: Percutaneous transluminal septal myocardial ablation in hypertrophic obstructive cardiomyopathy: Results with respect to intraprocedural myocardial contrast echocardiography. Circulation 1998;98:2415-2421.

126. Kuhn H, Gietzen FH, Leuner C, et al: Transcoronary ablation of septal hypertrophy (TASH): A new treatment option for hypertrophic obstructive cardiomyopathy. Z Kardiol 2000;89(Suppl 4):IV-41-I-54.

127. Boekstegers P, Steinbigler P, Molnar A, et al: Pressure-guided nonsurgical myocardial reduction induced by small septal infarctions in hypertrophic obstructive cardiomyopathy. J Am Coll Cardiol 2001;38:846-853.

128. Veselka J, Duchonova R, Prochazkova S, et al: Effects of varying ethanol dosing in percutaneous septal ablation for obstructive hypertrophic cardiomyopathy on early hemodynamic changes. Am J Cardiol 2005;95:675-678.

129. Chang SM, Nagueh SF, Spencer WH 3rd, et al: Complete heart block: Determinants and clinical impact in patients with hypertrophic obstructive cardiomyopathy undergoing nonsurgical septal reduction therapy. J Am Coll Cardiol 2003;42:296-300.

130. Ralph-Edwards A, Woo A, McCrindle BW, et al: Hypertrophic obstructive cardiomyopathy: Comparison of outcomes after myectomy or alcohol ablation adjusted by propensity score. J Thorac Cardiovasc Surg 2005;129:351-358.

131. Nagueh SF, Ommen SR, Lakkis NM, et al: Comparison of ethanol septal reduction therapy with surgical myectomy for the treatment of hypertrophic obstructive cardiomyopathy. J Am Coll Cardiol 2001;38:1701-1706.

132. van Dockum WG, Beek AM, ten Cate FJ, et al: Early onset and progression of left ventricular remodeling after alcohol septal ablation in hypertrophic obstructive cardiomyopathy. Circulation 2005;111:2503-2508.

133. Talreja DR, Nishimura RA, Edwards WD, et al: Alcohol septal ablation versus surgical septal myectomy: Comparison of effects on atrioventricular conduction tissue. J Am Coll Cardiol 2004;44:2329-2332.

55 Percutaneous Balloon Pericardiotomy for Patients with Pericardial Effusion and Tamponade

Andrew A. Ziskind, Hani Jneid, and Igor F. Palacios

KEY POINTS

■ Percutaneous balloon pericardiotomy (PBP) is an effective therapy for recurrent, free-flowing and hemodynamically significant pericardial effusions, especially if associated with neoplastic disease.

■ PBP consists of creating a parietal pericardial window with a balloon dilating catheter under fluoroscopic guidance in the cardiac catheterization laboratory.

■ PBP is a less invasive alternative to surgical pericardial window and avoids its perioperative risks.

■ PBP should be avoided if possible in patients with large pleural effusions or marginal pulmonary reserve to avoid further pulmonary compromise.

■ The pericardial space can be safely entered with a blunt-tip needle via a subxiphoid approach under fluoroscopic guidance, even in the absence of significant pericardial effusion.

■ Catheter-based diagnostic and interventional techniques in the pericardial space have become increasingly common and include epicardial mapping and ablation, intrapericardial delivery of therapies, intrapericardial echocardiography, pericardioscopy-guided biopsy, and potentially other advanced techniques.

Pericardial effusion may result from a variety of clinical conditions, including malignancy, renal failure, infectious processes, radiation damage, aortic dissection, hypothyroidism, and collagen vascular diseases. It can also occur after trauma or acute myocardial infarction, as a postpericardiotomy syndrome after cardiac or thoracic surgery, and as an idiopathic pericardial effusion. The clinical presentation varies, from patients who are completely asymptomatic to those presenting with cardiac tamponade. Among medical patients, malignant disease is the most common cause of pericardial effusion with tamponade.[1] In all cases of cardiac tamponade, the initial treatment consists of removing pericardial fluid by prompt pericardiocentesis and drainage. Reaccumulation of fluid with recurrence of cardiac tamponade may be an indication for a surgical intervention.[2] Autopsy and surgical studies have shown that myocardial or pericardial metastases are found in approximately 50% of patients who present with cardiac tamponade due to malignancy.[3-7] Although the short-term survival of patients with cardiac tamponade

depends primarily on its early diagnosis and relief, long-term survival depends on the prognosis of the primary illness, regardless of the intervention performed.[4,5,8]

The management of cardiac tamponade or large pericardial effusions at risk for progression to tamponade remains controversial and is dictated to a large extent by local institutional practices. Life-threatening cardiac tamponade requires immediate removal of pericardial fluid to relieve the hemodynamic compromise. Furthermore, it is desirable to prevent recurrence. For many patients with a pericardial effusion and tamponade, standard percutaneous pericardial drainage with an indwelling pericardial catheter is sufficient to avoid recurrence. Recurrences after catheter drainage have been reported in 14% to 50% of patients with pericardial effusion and tamponade.[5,9-11] Patients who continue to drain more than 100 mL/24 hours three days after standard catheter drainage have been considered for more aggressive therapy.

Several additional approaches are available to prevent reaccumulation of pericardial fluid, including intrapericardial instillation of sclerosing agents, use of chemotherapy, and radiation therapy.[12,13] With tetracycline sclerosis, a failure rate of 17% has been described.[12] A surgically created pericardial window may provide an alternative for the treatment of pericardial effusions,[14,15] but morbidity and late recurrence of symptoms are not uncommon.[8,16,17] The use of subxiphoid pericardial windowing has been advocated by some as primary therapy for malignant pericardial tamponade based on the high initial success in relieving tamponade[16-21] and an acceptable rate of recurrence.[17] Although open transthoracic surgical approaches offer a lower recurrence rate, they are associated with high morbidity rates.[8,14-21] Therefore, extensive pericardial resection is usually reserved for patients in whom a longer survival can be anticipated.

Patients with advanced malignancy and cardiac tamponade are often poor candidates for surgical therapy. Their life expectancy is limited to the point that the increased length of hospital stay associated with a surgical procedure may make up a significant portion of their remaining life span. In addition, the malnutrition and chemotherapy associated with advanced malignant disease increase the risk of infection and other perioperative complications. Because subxiphoid surgical windowing does not appear to improve survival and carries a modest perioperative risk,[4] it is preferable to offer a less invasive alternative. Palacios and colleagues[22] proposed the technique of percutaneous balloon pericardiotomy (PBP) as a less invasive alternative to surgical windowing. With this technique, a pericardial window and adequate drainage of pericardial effusion can be done percutaneously with a balloon dilating catheter (Fig. 55-1). Since this initial report on eight patients, the multicenter PBP registry has reported data on 130 patients.[23,24]

TECHNIQUE

The PBP technique is relatively simple and safe. It is performed in the catheterization laboratory with the patient under local anesthesia and mild sedation with intravenous narcotics and a short-acting benzodiazepine. There is minimal discomfort. Patients may be candidates for PBP if they have undergone prior pericardiocentesis and have persistent catheter drainage, or PBP may be done as primary therapy at the time of initial pericardiocentesis.

For those who have previously undergone standard pericardiocentesis using the subxiphoid approach, a pigtail catheter has typically been left in the pericardial space for drainage. For patients who after 3 days continue to drain more than 100 mL/24 hours, PBP is offered as an alternative to a surgical procedure. The subxiphoid area around the indwelling pigtail pericardial catheter is infiltrated with 1% lidocaine. A 0.038-inch guidewire with a preshaped curve at the tip is advanced through the pigtail catheter into the pericardial space (Fig. 55-2A). The catheter is then removed, leaving the guidewire in the

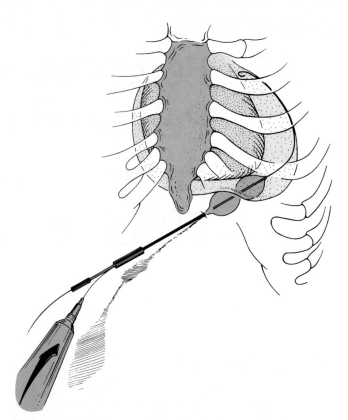

Figure 55-1. Percutaneous balloon pericardiotomy technique. (From Ziskind AA, Pearce AC, Lemmon CC, et al: Percutaneous balloon pericardiotomy for the treatment of cardiac tamponade and large pericardial effusions: Description of technique and report of the first fifty cases. J Am Coll Cardiol 1993;21:1-5.)

pericardial space. The location of the wire should be confirmed by its looping within the pericardium. After predilation along the track of the wire with a 10-Fr dilator, a 20-mm diameter, 3-cm long balloon dilating catheter (Boston Scientific, Watertown, MA) is advanced over the guidewire and positioned to straddle the parietal pericardium. Care should be taken to advance the proximal end of the balloon beyond the skin and subcutaneous tissue. Precise localization of the balloon is accomplished by gentle inflation to identify the waist at the pericardial margin. The balloon is inflated manually until the waist produced by the parietal pericardium disappears (see Fig. 55-2B,C). If the pericardium is apposed to the chest wall, as indicated by failure of the proximal portion of the balloon to expand, a countertraction technique should be used in which the catheter is withdrawn slightly, then gently advanced while the skin and soft tissues are pulled in the opposite direction. This maneuver isolates the pericardium for dilation (Fig. 55-3). Biplane fluoroscopy is helpful to ensure correct positioning of the balloon, which should be straddling the parietal pericardium (Fig. 55-4). At the operator's discretion, 5 to 10 mL of radiographic contrast material may be instilled into the pericardial space to help identify the pericardial margin. Two or three balloon inflations are then

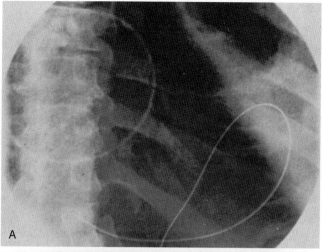

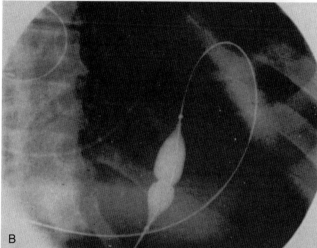

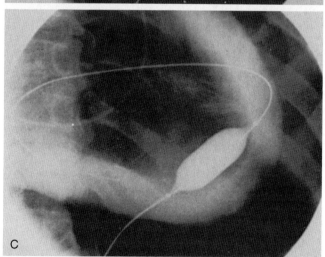

Figure 55-2. Anteroposterior fluoroscopic images. **A,** The guidewire (0.038-inch) has been advanced through the pigtail catheter and can be seen looping freely in the pericardial space. **B,** As the balloon is inflated manually, a waist is seen at the pericardial margin. **C,** The waist disappears with full inflation of the balloon as the pericardial window is created.

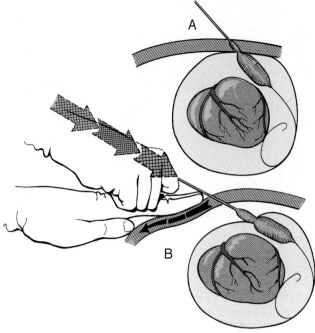

Figure 55-3. Countertraction technique to separate the pericardium from the adjacent chest wall (transverse view from below). **A,** Initial trial inflation of the balloon demonstrates trapping of the proximal portion of the balloon in the chest wall structures. **B,** Simultaneous traction on the skin and pushing of the balloon catheter results in displacement of the pericardium away from the chest wall, allowing proper inflation to occur. (Redrawn from Ziskind AA, Burstein S: Echocardiography vs. fluoroscopic imaging [letter]. Catheter Cardiovasc Diagn 1992;27:86.)

performed to ensure creation of an adequate opening of the pericardium. The use of at least single-plane fluoroscopy to localize the dilating balloon is mandatory. Our experience with transthoracic and transesophageal echocardiography has shown that the balloon cannot be imaged with adequate detail to identify the waist at the site of the pericardial margin.[25] The balloon dilating catheter is then removed, leaving the 0.038-inch guidewire in the pericardial space. A new pigtail catheter is then advanced over this guidewire and placed in the pericardial space.

If PBP is being performed at the time of primary pericardiocentesis, the pericardium is entered by a standard subxiphoid approach, and a drainage catheter is inserted into the pericardial space. After the pericardial pressure has been measured, most of the pericardial fluid should be withdrawn. This reduces the volume remaining to pass into the pleural space. However, it is important to leave a small amount of fluid in the pericardial space to provide a measure of safety in the event that the catheter is displaced and repeat needle entry of the pericardial space is necessary.

Technical variations of the subxiphoid technique have included dilation of two adjacent pericardial sites, use of the apical approach,[26] use of an Inoue balloon catheter,[26-28] use of double balloons,[29] use of

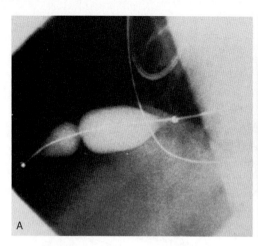

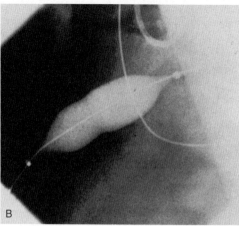

Figure 55-4. Lateral fluoroscopic image of balloon inflation. A waist is seen at the pericardial margin (**A**); it disappears with full inflation (**B**).

a combination of one long and one short balloon,[30] and use of an 18-mm dilating balloon to facilitate introduction of a 16-Fr chest tube into the pericardial space.[31] Other investigators have attempted laparoscopic pericardial fenestration,[32,33] used a cutting pericardiotome,[34] or implanted a pericardioperitoneal shunt.[35] Thoracoscopic techniques have been developed to create a larger pericardial window with low morbidity compared with open surgical techniques.[36] With this technique, adequate long-term drainage may be provided, and specimens for pathologic study may be obtained.[32,37]

POSTPROCEDURE MANAGEMENT AND FOLLOW-UP

After PBP, patients are returned to a telemetry floor. The pericardial catheter should be aspirated every 6 hours and flushed with heparin (5 mL, 100 U/mL). Pericardial drainage volumes should be recorded, and the catheter should be removed after there is no significant pericardial drainage (<75 mL) for 24 hours. Frequently, at the time of catheter removal, there is evidence on the chest radiograph of a new or increasing pleural effusion. Follow-up two-dimensional echocardiography is performed approximately 48 hours after removal of the pericardial catheter. Data are being collected on immediate removal of the pericardial catheter after PBP to facilitate early discharge. However, leaving the pericardial catheter in place may provide a measure of safety by allowing monitoring to determine whether the window is effective and whether bleeding is occurring. Periodic postprocedure echocardiography can be used to check for reaccumulation of pericardial fluid. Chest radiography should be performed to monitor the possible development of a pleural effusion (usually left) caused by drainage of the pericardial fluid.

MECHANISM OF PERCUTANEOUS BALLOON PERICARDIOTOMY

The precise mechanism by which PBP works remains unclear. We assume that balloon inflation results in

localized tearing of the parietal pericardial tissues, leading to a communication of the pericardial space with the pleural space and possibly with the abdominal cavity.[38,39] The use of a flexible fiberoptic pericardioscope introduced over the guidewire after PBP has demonstrated a pericardial window that freely communicates with the left pleural space (Fig. 55-5).[40] Chow and Chow supported this finding with their postmortem studies of balloon dilation in which they used an Inoue balloon inflated to a maximum diameter of 23 mm. Balloon dilation produced, without tearing, a smooth, oval pericardial

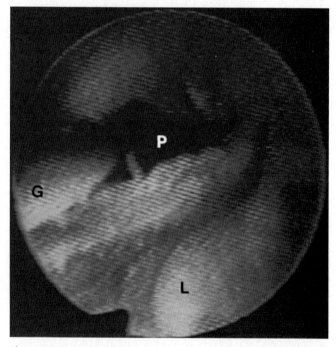

Figure 55-5. Pericardioscopic view of the balloon pericardiotomy site. The scope has been withdrawn over a guidewire to visualize the external pericardial surface. This figure demonstrates direct communication of the pericardial window with the left pleural space. G, guidewire; L, lung in left pleural space immediately outside the pericardium; P, pericardial window created by balloon dilation.

window measuring 18.8×16.4 mm. Histologic analysis revealed fragmentation and breakage of elastic and collagenous fibers in the connective tissues bordering the pericardial sites.[41] We have demonstrated passage of pericardial fluid from the pericardial space to the pleural space in some patients after PBP by manually injecting 10 mL of radiographic contrast material through the pericardial catheter. However, the ability to visualize free exit of contrast from the pericardial space does not appear to correlate with procedural success.

Based on the experience with subxiphoid surgical pericardial windowing, it is unlikely that a long-term communication persists between the pericardium and the pleural cavity or subcutaneous tissues. Sugimoto and colleagues studied 28 patients who underwent surgical subxiphoid pericardial windowing followed by tube decompression, 93% of whom had permanent relief.[42] Postoperative echocardiograms demonstrated thickening of the pericardium-epicardium with obliteration of the pericardial space. Autopsy data that confirmed this fusion were available for four patients. These authors concluded that the success of subxiphoid pericardial windowing depends on the inflammatory fusion of the epicardium to the pericardium, not on maintenance of a window.[42] Based on this surgical experience, it is unlikely that percutaneous balloon windows remain open indefinitely. It is also possible that PBP, by leading to more effective pericardial drainage and maintaining a fluid-free pericardial space for a prolonged time, may permit autosclerosis to occur.

RESULTS

Palacios and coworkers reported the initial results of PBP windowing in eight patients with malignant pericardial effusion and tamponade.[22] The technique was successful in all patients. There were no immediate or late complications related to the procedure. The mean time to radiologic development of a new or a significantly increased pleural effusion was 2.9 ± 0.4 days (range, 2 to 5 days). The mean follow-up in this initial report was 6 ± 2 months (range, 1 to 11 months). No patients had recurrence of pericardial tamponade or pericardial effusion. Death occurred in five patients at 1, 4, 9, 10, and 11 months after PBP. In all cases, the cause of death was the patient's primary malignant disease. The remaining three patients were alive and free of cardiac symptoms at the time of the report. After the initial favorable experience, the multicenter PBP registry was developed to collect additional data in a larger group of patients.

MULTICENTER REGISTRY EXPERIENCE

The PBP technique has been studied in a multicenter registry to evaluate the therapeutic efficacy and risks

Table 55-1. Clinical Characteristics of 130 Patients Undergoing Percutaneous Balloon Pericardotomy

Parameter	Result
Age (yr), mean±SD	59±13 (range 25-87)
Male/female (no.)	68/62
Tamponade present	90 (69%)
Prior pericardiocentesis	75 (58%)
Clinical history	
Known malignancy	110 (85%)
Lung	55
Breast	21
Other	34
Nonmalignant	20 (15%)
Idiopathic	5
HIV disease	4
Postoperative/trauma	4
Uremia	2
Renal transplant	1
Hypothyroidism	1
Congestive heart failure	1
Viral infection	1
Autoimmune disease	1

HIV, human immunodeficiency virus; SD, standard deviation.

systematically. Data on 130 patients undergoing PBP from 1987 to 1994 in 16 centers have been presented.[23,24] The clinical characteristics of the 130 patients are shown in Table 55-1.

PBP was defined as successful if there was no recurrence of pericardial effusion on echocardiographic follow-up and if no complications occurred that required surgical exploration or a surgical pericardial window. PBP was successful in 111 (85%) of 130 patients, with no recurrences of pericardial effusion/tamponade during a mean follow-up of 5.0 ± 5.8 months. Five cases were considered failures because of pericardial bleeding, and those patients underwent surgical windowing. Thirteen patients had recurrence of pericardial effusion (mean time to recurrence, 54 ± 65 days). Twelve of those 13 patients underwent surgical windowing, but 6 again had a recurrence. Minor complications occurred in 11 patients (13%), the most frequent being fever. No patient had documented bacteremia or positive pericardial fluid cultures. After PBP, thoracentesis or chest tube placement was required in 15% of patients with preexisting pleural effusions, compared with 9% of patients without preexisting pleural effusions.

Of the 104 patients with a history of malignancy, 86 died, compared with 2 of 16 patients with nonmalignant disease. The mean survival time for patients with a history of malignancy was 3.8 ± 3.3 months. No procedure-related variables were found to influence either survival or freedom from recurrence (e.g., number of sites dilated, visualization of free fluid exit, duration of catheter placement). There was no significant difference in recurrence rate if PBP was performed as primary treatment or after failed pericardiocentesis.

TECHNICAL CONSIDERATIONS

Echocardiographic and Chest Radiographic Qualifications

Echocardiography should be performed before PBP to rule out the presence of loculated pericardial fluid. If pericardial fluid is not free-flowing, a surgical approach should be considered. If the chest radiograph reveals evidence of a large pleural effusion before PBP, this issue is less clear. If a left effusion is moderate or large before PBP, the chance of needing thoracentesis is high, and PBP should be performed only if the cardiac benefits outweigh the risks of thoracentesis or chest tube placement. Patients with marginal pulmonary mechanics, such as those who have undergone pneumonectomy, should be evaluated with caution, because the development of a left pleural effusion may compromise their remaining lung function.

Prophylactic Antibiotics

Febrile episodes were seen six times in the first 37 patients, although no patient had documented bacteremia or positive pericardial drainage cultures. Beginning with the 38th patient, prophylactic antibiotic therapy was initiated and continued until the catheter was removed. No febrile episodes were seen in 49 subsequent patients. It is unclear whether this represents efficacy of prophylactic antibiotics for preventing infection, a random effect, or more extensive operator experience with a concomitant decrease in procedural time and catheter manipulation.

Patients with Bleeding Risk

The risk of bleeding from the pericardiotomy site appears to be increased in patients with platelet or coagulation abnormalities. For this reason, we do not recommend performing PBP on patients with uremic pericardial effusions or when coagulation parameters cannot be normalized (refractory coagulopathy or thrombocytopenia). In those patients at high risk for bleeding, a surgical procedure under direct visualization may be safer.

Fluoroscopic Guidance

Attempts to guide balloon placement by transthoracic or transesophageal echocardiography have been disappointing. Although the dilating balloon can be visualized, it is not possible to distinguish proper placement (with a discrete waist) from entrapment of the proximal balloon in the soft tissues and ineffective pericardial dilation. We have found fluoroscopic guidance to be particularly essential to the countertraction technique and believe it is mandatory for PBP.[25]

Risks of Cardiac and Pulmonary Injury

Because PBP is not performed until successful access to the pericardial space is obtained and the guidewire is seen to be freely looping within the pericardium, the risks of cardiac injury should be small. If the right ventricle were inadvertently entered and the balloon advanced, the results would be catastrophic. For this reason, PBP should be performed only by operators who have extensive experience with pericardiocentesis. In the emergency setting, it may be prudent to stabilize the patient with pericardiocentesis and leave a catheter in place for elective PBP under more controlled conditions.

Pleural Effusion

A significant concern after PBP is the development of a large pleural effusion. A left pleural effusion develops in most patients within 24 to 48 hours of the procedure (Fig. 55-6). In most cases this resolves, presumably because of the greater resorptive capacity of the pleural surfaces. As noted earlier, thoracentesis or chest tube placement was required in 15% of patients with preexisting pleural effusions, compared with 9% of those without preexisting pleural effusions. It is likely that some patients have a large volume of fluid flow from the pericardial to the pleural space; however, in many cases it is difficult to determine whether the effusion results from drainage of fluid from the pericardial space or from the progression of concomitant pleural disease. For this reason, it is desirable to remove most of the pericardial fluid before creating the balloon window, to limit the potential volume of fluid that can immediately move to the pleural space.

Duration of Catheter Placement

Most patients have had a drainage catheter left in the pericardial space to monitor fluid output after the procedure. This is typically removed after flows are less than 75 mL/24 hours. It may be possible to perform PBP without leaving a pericardial catheter in place, permitting an even shorter hospital stay and further decreasing the risk of infection.

Management of Balloon Rupture

Balloon rupture at the time of PBP can occur as a result of the combination of a large balloon, excessive inflation pressure, and an inelastic pericardium. Uncommonly, balloon rupture is accompanied by catheter fracture, because excessive resistance limits withdrawal. Our experience suggests that the frequency of balloon rupture can be minimized with proper technique, particularly the use of countertraction to isolate the pericardium, thereby avoiding dilation of the adjacent nonpericardial tissues.[25] Hemiballoon dislodgement sometimes occurs, and Block and Wilson have described a technique to retrieve it. They place a second pericardial catheter,

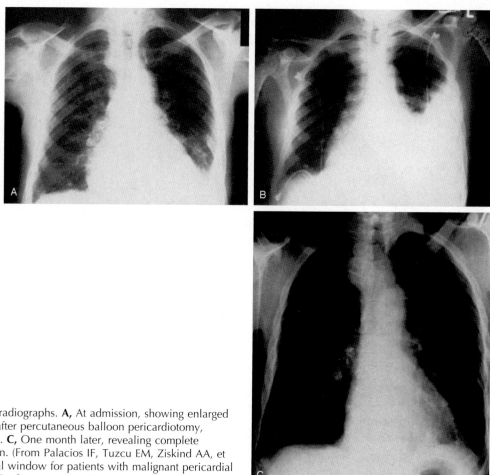

Figure 55-6. Posteroanterior chest radiographs. **A,** At admission, showing enlarged cardiac silhouette. **B,** At 24 hours after percutaneous balloon pericardiotomy, showing a new left pleural effusion. **C,** One month later, revealing complete resolution of the left pleural effusion. (From Palacios IF, Tuzcu EM, Ziskind AA, et al: Percutaneous balloon pericardial window for patients with malignant pericardial effusion and tamponade. Catheter Cardiovasc Diagn 1991;22:244-249.)

snare the guidewire, and use a second catheter to push the balloon fragment back through the pericardium and out to the skin.[43]

ADJUNCTIVE DIAGNOSTIC APPROACHES

Although patients with a pericardial effusion may have a history of malignancy, in only 50% of such patients is malignancy the cause of their pericardial effusion.[4,44,45] Although pericardial fluid cytologic analysis may aid in the diagnosis, pericardial tissue is not obtained by PBP for pathologic analysis (as it would be if surgical pericardial windowing were performed.) To address this need, a percutaneously introduced pericardial bioptome has been successful in providing diagnostic-quality tissue.[40] With the use of an aggressive, serrated-jaw bioptome (Boston Scientific) (Fig. 55-7A) that is advanced though an 8-Fr vascular introducer, multiple samples can be obtained from the posterolateral aspect of the parietal pericardium (see Fig. 55-7B). This technique remains investigational.

CONCLUSIONS

PBP offers a nonsurgical alternative for the management of pericardial effusion. PBP is particularly useful for critically ill patients with advanced malignancy and limited survival in whom it is desirable to avoid the risks and discomfort of anesthesia and surgery. For such patients, PBP appears to palliate malignant pericardial disease successfully for the duration of their survival.

The decision of whether to perform PBP, rather than pericardiocentesis with or without sclerotherapy, may depend on patient and institutional variables. PBP should be considered if pericardial fluid recurs after primary pericardiocentesis. In institutions with an aggressive surgical approach toward malignant pericardial disease, this "less invasive" alternative to a surgical pericardial window may be considered for the primary treatment of malignant cardiac tamponade.

In contrast, pericardiocentesis alone, without PBP at that time, is preferred if the cause of the pericardial fluid is unknown. Samples of pericardial fluid should be sent for cell counts, cytologic analysis, culture, and special stains to assist with the diagnosis. Simple pericardiocentesis is also preferred if uremic platelet dysfunction or other coagulation abnormalities are present or if there is the possibility of bacterial or fungal infection that could be spread to the pleural space.

The immediate and late results of PBP for patients with malignant pericardial effusion appear to be

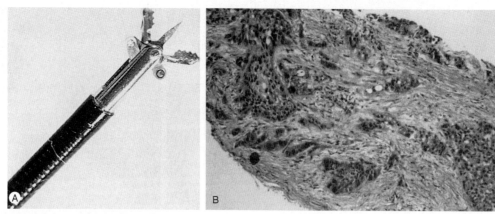

Figure 55-7. A, Pericardial bioptome with center needle and aggressive serrated-jaw configuration. **B,** Percutaneous pericardial biopsy specimen from a patient with newly diagnosed lung cancer. It contains sheets of squamous cell carcinoma. Malignant cells are seen trapped in the fibrin of the inflammatory exudate. (From Ziskind AA, Rodriguez S, Lemmon C, Burstein S: Percutaneous pericardial biopsy as an adjunctive technique for the diagnosis of pericardial disease. Am J Cardiol 1994;74:288-291.)

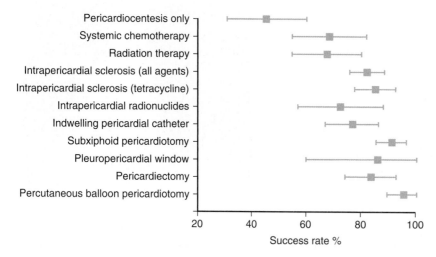

Figure 55-8. Success rates with 95% confidence intervals (indicated by bars) for various treatment modalities of malignant pericardial effusions. (From Vaitkus PT, Herrmann HC, Le Winter MM: Treatment of malignant pericardial effusion. JAMA 1994;272:272.)

similar to those of surgical pericardiotomy. However, the role of PBP in the management of nonmalignant pericardial disease remains unclear. It is possible that PBP could be used for the treatment of pericardial effusions caused by viral infection, human immunodeficiency virus (HIV)-related disease, hypothyroidism, collagen vascular disease, and idiopathic effusions. PBP was reported with favorable results in a series of pediatric patients with nonmalignant effusions.[46] Additional long-term follow-up is needed on larger numbers of patients to clarify more fully the role of this procedure in nonmalignant pericardial disease.

The application of PBP to patients with malignant pericardial disease is likely to increase in the future. It may potentially expand to the treatment of patients without malignancy,[46] especially those with limited survival time (e.g., advanced HIV infection). PBP need not be limited to tertiary-care hospitals, although it should be performed in centers that routinely perform pericardiocentesis.

The infrequency of effusive pericardial disease and the larger number of patients required limit the feasibility of randomized studies to compare the effectiveness of various treatment strategies. Vaitkus and colleagues did a meta-analysis of prior studies in which treatment of malignant pericardial effusions was defined as successful if the patient survived the procedure, the symptoms did not recur, and no other interventions directed at the pericardium were required, regardless of the length of survival.[47] Success rates for the various treatments are shown in Figure 55-8. Because no randomized data are available comparing the efficacy of PBP with that of a surgical or thoracoscopic pericardial window, or with catheter drainage and sclerotherapy, the combined use of PBP with sclerotherapy has not been done.

NOVEL CATHETER-BASED INTERVENTION TECHNIQUES IN THE PERICARDIAL SPACE

The use of percutaneous intervention techniques in the pericardial space has been progressively increasing and now encompasses multiple disciplines in cardiology.

A multitude of reasons have contributed to the emergence of these techniques. On the one hand, epicardial scar-related reentry has been recognized as an important cause of ventricular tachycardia, especially in patients with nonischemic cardiomyopathy. Other infrequent but clinically significant arrhythmias, such as supraventricular tachycardias and idiopathic ventricular tachycardia, were also found to possess epicardial foci that cannot be ablated but from the epicardium. Epicardial catheter mapping and ablation in the electrophysiology laboratory have thus opened a new perspective in cardiac electrophysiology, which was previously limited largely to the operating room. On the other hand, the pericardial space is recognized as a natural drug receptacle that can restrict drug delivery to the heart, with many investigators attempting to exploit it as a reservoir to deliver therapeutic substances to the heart and coronary arteries.[48] In addition, there has been increasing need to replace the standard pericardiocentesis with a safer technique, particularly in patients with small pericardial effusions who are at high risk for complications.

Catheter-based intervention techniques in the pericardial space gained momentum after invasive cardiologists realized that the presence of pericardial fluid is not a prerequisite for a safe percutaneous entry into the pericardial space. Sosa and colleagues[49] were the first to show that the pericardial space can be safely entered with a blunt-tip needle via a subxiphoid approach under fluoroscopic guidance. In their seminal work in 1996 in patients with Chagas disease,[49] they advanced an epidural needle toward the right ventricle apex until a slight negative pressure was felt and confirmed the needle position by small injections of contrast medium to delineate the cardiac silhouette. They thus established the feasibility and safety of epicardial mapping in patients with Chagas disease and recurrent ventricular tachycardia, one of whom underwent a successful epicardial circuit ablation.[49] Laham and colleagues[50] subsequently confirmed the safety of subxiphoid access of the normal pericardium in a large animal model, using, in addition to fluoroscopy, continuous positive pressure of 20 to 30 mm Hg (achieved by saline infusion using an intraflow system) to push the right ventricle away from the needle's path. Access of the pericardial space was achieved in all 49 Yorkshire pigs with no adverse events, and histologic examination in 15 animals 1 month after the procedure showed no evidence of myocardial damage.[50] Many interventional cardiologists argue that needle advancement under continuous positive pressure by saline infusion may not be necessary for a successful technique.

Epicardial mapping and ablation were thereafter adopted by several interventional electrophysiologists.[51] Sosa and colleagues[52] performed epicardial mapping to guide endocardial and epicardial ablation in a series of 10 consecutive patients with ventricular tachycardia and Chagas disease. Epicardial mapping in that study enabled the detection of an epicardial circuit in 14 of 18 mappable ventricular tachycardias and helped guide endocardial ablation

in four patients, and epicardial ablation in six. The same approach was also attempted successfully in patients with recurrent ventricular tachycardia after myocardial infarction, demonstrating that postinfarction pericardial adherence does not preclude epicardial mapping and ablation.[53] It has since become clear that failure of endocardial ablation can reflect the presence of an epicardial arrhythmia substrate, which can be safely treated by epicardial mapping and ablation using the percutaneous pericardial technique. In one series of 48 patients with prior unsuccessful endocardial ablation, for example, Schweikert et al.[54] showed that epicardial instrumentation and ablation was a safe and effective alternative strategy.

In addition to the subxiphoid approach for pericardial puncture (i.e., from the epicardial surface of the heart), other investigational approaches have been studied. Mickelsen and colleagues examined transvenous access to the pericardial space for epicardial lead implantation for cardiac resynchronization therapy.[55] This approach was feasible in eight pigs, which underwent puncture of the terminal anterior superior vena cava or the right atrial appendage to access the pericardial space; however, it resulted in a hemodynamically significant pericardial effusion in four of the eight animals.[55] Intrapericardial echocardiography is currently being investigated at the Massachusetts General Hospital[56] and represents yet another example of a promising catheter-based technique in the pericardial space. Rodrigues and coworkers[56] introduced phased-array ultrasound transducers into the pericardial space of seven goats (using 10-Fr steerable catheters advanced via the transthoracic subxiphoid approach) and obtained detailed imaging of cardiac structures. This promising approach may help establish the relative positions of the ablation catheters and may facilitate epicardial ablation in the electrophysiology laboratory. Several devices are currently under study for safe and effective percutaneous access of the pericardial space. An example of these devices is the PerDUCER (Comedicus Inc., Columbia Heights, MN), which was proven to provide efficient, safe, and effective pericardial access in the normal or minimally abnormal pericardial space.[57,58]

Percutaneous access to the pericardial space and the use of pericardioscopy opened also other opportunities for the use of this space in diagnostic and interventional techniques. For example, Seferovic and associates[59] reported on the use of pericardioscopy to assist pericardial biopsy. Their study included 49 patients with a large pericardial effusion undergoing parietal pericardial biopsy. In 12 patients (group 1), pericardial biopsy was guided by fluoroscopy (three to six samples per patient). In 22 patients (group 2), four to six pericardial biopsies per patient were obtained by pericardioscopy guidance using a 16-Fr flexible endoscope. In group 3, extensive pericardial sampling (18 to 20 samples per patient) was performed, guided by pericardioscopy in 15 patients. Sampling efficiency was better with pericardioscopy (group 2, 84.9%; group 3, 84.2%) compared with fluoroscopic guidance (group 1, 43.7%; $P<.01$). Pericardial biopsy in group 3 had higher diagnostic value than in group 1 for revealing new diagnosis (40% versus 8.3%, $P<.05$) and etiology (53.3% versus 8.3%, $P<.05$). In group 2, pericardial biopsy had a higher yield in establishing etiology than in group 1 (40.9% versus 8.3%; $P<.05$). Pericardial biopsy was falsely negative in 58.3% of group 1 patients, compared with 6.7% of those in group 3 ($P<.01$). There were no major complications in the study.

Adequate visualization of the space and the epicardial surface allows identification of scarred areas in the ventricles that could be treated by intrascar administration of vascular growth factors and/or cultured myocardial cells. Furthermore, techniques such as left atrial appendage exclusion could be attempted using this approach and imaging. Finally, we anticipate the use of this space for successful percutaneous treatment of valvular heart disease, alone or in combination with endovascular techniques.

REFERENCES

1. Guberman B, Fowler N, Engel P, et al: Cardiac tamponade in medical patients. Circulation 1981;64:633-640.
2. Fowler N: Cardiac tamponade. In No F (ed): The Pericardium in Health and Disease. New York, Futura, 1985, pp 247-280.
3. Cohen G, Perry T, Evans JM: Neoplastic invasion of the heart and pericardium. Ann Intern Med 1955;43:1238-1245.
4. Mills SA, Julian S, Holliday RH, et al: Subxiphoid pericardial window for pericardial disease. Cardiovasc Surg 1989;30:768-773.
5. Markiewicz W, Borovik R, Ecker S: Cardiac tamponade in medical patients: Treatment and prognosis in the echocardiographic era. Am Heart J 1986;111:1138-1142.
6. Bisel HF, Wroblewski F, LaDue JS: Incidence and clinical manifestations of cardiac metastases. JAMA 1953;153:712-715.
7. Goldman BS, Pearson F: Malignant pericardial effusion: Review of hospital experience and report of a case successfully treated by talc poudrage. Can J Surg 1965;8:157-161.
8. Piehler JM, Pluth JR, Schaff HV, et al: Surgical management of effusive pericardial disease: Influence of extent of pericardial resection on clinical course. J Thorac Cardiovasc Surg 1985;90:506-516.
9. Flannery EP, Gregoratos G, Corder MP: Pericardial effusions in patients with malignant diseases. Arch Intern Med 1975;135:976-977.
10. Kopecky SL, Callahan JA, Tajik AJ, Seward JB: Percutaneous pericardial catheter drainage: Report of 42 consecutive cases. Am J Cardiol 1986;58:633-635.
11. Patel AK, Kosolcharoen PK, Nallasivan M, et al: Catheter drainage of the pericardium: Practical method to maintain long-term patency. Chest 1987;92:1018-1021.
12. Shepherd FA, Morgan C, Evans WK, et al: Medical management of malignant pericardial effusion by tetracycline sclerosis. Am J Cardiol 1987;60:1161-1166.
13. Davis S, Sharma SM, Blumberg ED, Kim CS: Intrapericardial tetracycline for the management of cardiac tamponade secondary to malignant pericardial effusion. N Engl J Med 1978;299:1113-1114.
14. Fontanelle LJ, Cuello L, Dooley BN: Subxyphoid pericardial window: A simple and safe method for diagnosing and treating acute and chronic pericardial effusions. J Thorac Cardiovasc Surg 1971;62:95-97.
15. Santos GH, Frater RWM: The subxiphoid approach in the treatment of pericardial effusion. Ann Thorac Surg 1977;23:467-470.
16. Palatianos GM, Thurer RJ, Kaiser GA: Comparison of effectiveness and safety of operations on the pericardium. Chest 1985;88:30-33.
17. Palatianos GM, Thurer RJ, Pompeo MQ, Kaiser GA: Clinical experience with subxiphoid drainage of pericardial effusions. Ann Thorac Surg 1989;48:381-385.
18. Hankins JR, Satterfield JR, Aisner J, et al: Pericardial window for malignant pericardial effusion. Ann Thorac Surg 1980;30:465-469.
19. Levin BH, Aaron BL: The subxiphoid pericardial window. Surg Gynecol Obstet 1982;155:804-806.
20. Alcan KE, Zabetakis PM, Marino ND, et al: Management of acute cardiac tamponade by subxiphoid pericardiotomy. JAMA 1982;247:1143-1148.
21. Little AG, Kremser PC, Wade JL, et al: Operation for diagnosis and treatment of pericardial effusions. Surgery 1984;96:738-744.
22. Palacios IF, Tuzcu EM, Ziskind AA, et al: Percutaneous balloon pericardial window for patients with malignant pericardial effusion and tamponade. Catheter Cardiovasc Diagn 1991;22:244-249.
23. Ziskind AA, Rodriguez S, Lemmon CC, et al: Percutaneous balloon pericardiotomy for the treatment of effusive pericardial disease: 104 Patient follow-up. J Am Coll Cardiol 1994;23:274A.
24. Ziskind A, Lemmon C, Rodriguez S, et al: Final report of the percutaneous balloon pericardiotomy registry for the treatment of effusive pericardial disease. Circulation 1994;90(Suppl I):I-121.
25. Ziskind AA, Burstein S: Echocardiography vs. fluoroscopic imaging. Catheter Cardiovasc Diagn 1992;27:86-88.
26. Chow WH, Chow TC, Cheung KL: Nonsurgical creation of a pericardial window using the Inoue balloon catheter. Am Heart J 1992;124:1100-1102.
27. Chow WH, Chow TC, Yip AS, Cheung KL: Inoue balloon pericardiotomy for patients with recurrent pericardial effusion. Angiology 1996;47:57-60.
28. Ohke M, Bessho A, Haraoka K, et al: Percutaneous balloon pericardiotomy by the use of the Inoue balloon for the management of recurrent cardiac tamponade in a patient with lung cancer. Intern Med 2000;39:1071-1074.
29. Iaffaldano RA, Jones P, Lewis BE, et al: Percutaneous balloon pericardiotomy: A double-balloon technique. Catheter Cardiovasc Diagn 1995;36:79-81.
30. Hsu KL, Tsai CH, Chiang FT, et al: Percutaneous balloon pericardiotomy for patients with recurrent pericardial effusion using a novel double-balloon technique with one long and one short balloon. Am J Cardiol 1997;80:1635-1637.
31. Hajduczok ZD, Ferguson DW: Percutaneous balloon pericardiostomy for non-surgical management of recurrent pericardial tamponade: A case report. Intensive Care Med 1991;17:299-301.
32. Ready A, Black J, Lewis R, Roscoe B: Laparoscopic pericardial fenestration for malignant pericardial effusion. Lancet 1992;339:1609.
33. Hartnell GG: Laparoscopic pericardial fenestration. Lancet 1992;340:737.
34. Sochman J, Peregrin J, Pavcnik D: The cutting pericardiotome: Another option for pericardiopleural draining in recurrent pericardial effusion. Initial experience. Int J Cardiol 2001;77:69-74.
35. Wang N, Feikes R, Morgansen T, et al: Pericardioperitoneal shunt: An alternative treatment for malignant pericardial effusions. Ann Thorac Surg 1994;57:289-292.
36. Ozuner G, Davidson PG, Isenberg JS, McGinn JTJ: Creation of a pericardial window using thorascopic techniques. Surg Gynecol Obstet 1992;175:69-71.
37. Fiocco M, Krasna MJ: Thoracoscopic pericardiectomy. Surg Laparosc Endosc 1995;5:202-204.
38. Bertrand O, Legrand V, Kulbertus H: Percutaneous balloon pericardiotomy: A case report and analysis of mechanism of action. Catheter Cardiovasc Diagn 1996;38:180-182.
39. Block PC: Whither pericardial fluid? [editorial; comment]. Catheter Cardiovasc Diagn 1996;38:183.
40. Ziskind AA, Pearce AC, Lemmon CC, et al: Feasibility of percutaneous pericardial biopsy and pericardioscopy as an adjunct to balloon pericardiotomy for the diagnosis and treatment of pericardial disease. J Am Coll Cardiol 1992;19:267A.

41. Chow LT, Chow WH: Mechanism of pericardial window creation by balloon pericardiotomy. Am J Cardiol 1993;72:1321-1322.
42. Sugimoto JT, Little AG, Ferguson MK, et al: Pericardial window: Mechanisms of efficacy. Ann Thorac Surg 1990;50:442-445.
43. Block PC, Wilson MA: Hemi-balloon dislodgement during a percutaneous balloon pericardial window procedure: Removal using a second pericardial catheter. Catheter Cardiovasc Diagn 1993;29:289-291.
44. Goudie RB: Secondary tumors of the heart and pericardium. Br Heart J 1955;17:183-188.
45. Krikorian JG, Hancock EW: Pericardiocentesis. Am J Med 1978;65:808-814.
46. Thanopoulos BD, Georgakopoulos D, Tsaousis GS, et al: Percutaneous balloon pericardiotomy for the treatment of large, nonmalignant pericardial effusions in children: Immediate and medium-term results. Catheter Cardiovasc Diagn 1997;40:97-100.
47. Vaitkus PT, Herrmann HC, LeWinter MM: Treatment of malignant pericardial effusion. JAMA 1994;272:59-64.
48. Stoll HP, Carlson K, Keefer LK, et al: Pharmacokinetics and consistency of pericardial delivery directed to coronary arteries: Direct comparison with endoluminal delivery. Clin Cardiol 1999;22(1 Suppl 1):I-10-I-16.
49. Sosa E, Scanavacca M, d'Avila A, et al: A new technique to perform epicardial mapping in the electrophysiology laboratory. J Cardiovasc Electrophysiol 1996;7:531-536.
50. Laham RJ, Simons M, Hung D: Subxyphoid access of the normal pericardium: A novel drug delivery technique. Catheter Cardiovasc Interv 1999;47:109-111.
51. Strickberger SA: Pericardial space exploration for ventricular tachycardia mapping: Should the countdown begin? J Cardiovasc Electrophysiol 1996;7:537-538.
52. Sosa E, Scanavacca M, D'Avila A, et al: Endocardial and epicardial ablation guided by nonsurgical transthoracic epicardial mapping to treat recurrent ventricular tachycardia. J Cardiovasc Electrophysiol 1998;9:229-239.
53. Sosa E, Scanavacca M, d'Avila A, et al: Nonsurgical transthoracic epicardial catheter ablation to treat recurrent ventricular tachycardia occurring late after myocardial infarction. J Am Coll Cardiol 2000;35:1442-1449.
54. Schweikert RA, Saliba WI, Tomassoni G, et al: Percutaneous pericardial instrumentation for endo-epicardial mapping of previously failed ablations. Circulation 2003;108:1329-1335.
55. Mickelsen SR, Ashikaga H, DeSilva R, et al: Transvenous access to the pericardial space: An approach to epicardial lead implantation for cardiac resynchronization therapy. Pacing Clin Electrophysiol 2005;28:1018-1024.
56. Rodrigues AC, d'Avila A, Houghtaling C, et al: Intrapericardial echocardiography: A novel catheter-based approach to cardiac imaging. J Am Soc Echocardiogr 2004;17:269-274.
57. Macris MP, Igo SR: Minimally invasive access of the normal pericardium: Initial clinical experience with a novel device. Clin Cardiol 1999;22(1 Suppl 1):I-36-I-39.
58. Hou D, March KL: A novel percutaneous technique for accessing the normal pericardium: A single-center successful experience of 53 porcine procedures. J Invasive Cardiol 2003;15:13-17.
59. Seferovic PM, Risti AD, Maksimovi R, et al: Diagnostic value of pericardial biopsy: Improvement with extensive sampling enabled by pericardioscopy. Circulation 2003;107:978-983.

56 Transcatheter Therapies for Congenital Heart Disease

Robert H. Beekman III, Thomas R. Lloyd, and Russel Hirsch

KEY POINTS

- Catheter-based therapies are available for a wide variety of congenital cardiovascular defects.
- Balloon dilation provides effective relief of obstruction for patients with congenital pulmonary or aortic valve stenosis. This therapy may not be adequate if the valve is hypoplastic or calcified.
- Congenital pulmonary artery stenosis can be very effectively relieved with balloon-expandable stents; late stent redilation may be necessary in a growing child.

- Coarctation of the aorta can be treated with balloon-expandable stenting; the technique is generally restricted to patients large enough to safely accept an 8- to 9-Fr arterial sheath.
- Transcatheter occlusion devices are available to safely and effectively treat patients with a secundum type atrial septal defect or a patent ductus arteriosus.

This chapter summarizes the current state of the art of transcatheter therapy for patients with congenital heart disease. It discusses catheter-based therapies available for some of the most common congenital defects, including semilunar valve stenosis, pulmonary artery stenosis, coarctation of the aorta, secundum atrial septal defect (ASD), and patent ductus arteriosus (PDA). Percutaneous balloon valvuloplasty provides effective treatment in patients with congenital pulmonary or aortic valve stenosis. For patients of all age, surgical valvotomy for congenital semilunar valve stenosis has been replaced by these interventional catheterization techniques. Balloon-expandable stenting is currently regarded as standard therapy for most patients with pulmonary artery stenosis. These lesions are often elastic in nature, a characteristic that makes balloon angioplasty alone a less successful intervention. More recently, coarctation stenting has also emerged as an effective therapeutic intervention for selected patients with coarctation of the aorta. Finally, transcatheter occlusion devices provide a safe, highly-effective therapy for patients with a secundum ASD or a PDA.

PULMONARY BALLOON VALVULOPLASTY

Pulmonary valve stenosis is a common disorder, accounting for approximately 8% of all congenital heart disease.[1] Except for neonates with critical pulmonary stenosis, untreated patients often survive well into adulthood.[2] However, when more than mild obstruction to right ventricular (RV) outflow is present, pulmonary valve stenosis should be relieved to prevent progression of obstruction,[3] progressive RV hypertrophy, and RV myocardial fibrosis and dysfunction. If left untreated, significant pulmonary valve stenosis eventually produces clinical symptoms such as fatigue, dyspnea, and exercise intolerance. These long-term sequelae are more likely to be avoided if pulmonary valve stenosis is treated in childhood. Nevertheless, treatment is indicated at any age if hemodynamically significant pulmonary stenosis is documented. Since its introduction in 1982 by Kan and associaes,[4] percutaneous balloon valvuloplasty has been shown to provide substantial relief of right ventricular outflow tract (RVOT) obstruction in patients with valvar pulmonary stenosis. Balloon pulmonary valvuloplasty can be performed safely and is obviously much less invasive than a surgical procedure. It is therefore regarded as the treatment of choice for patients with moderate to severe isolated pulmonary valve stenosis.

In congenital pulmonary valve stenosis, the valve leaflets are thickened and the commissures are fused to a varying degree. The lines of commissural fusion may appear as two or three raphes extending from

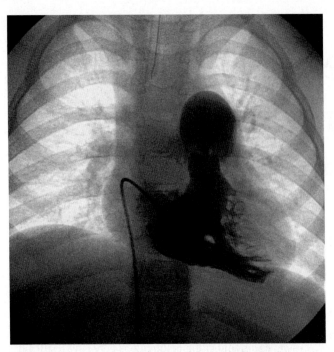

Figure 56-1. Anteroposterior right ventricular angiogram in a child with severe valvar pulmonary stenosis. The valve is thickened, and a systolic jet of contrast material is seen entering the dilated main pulmonary artery.

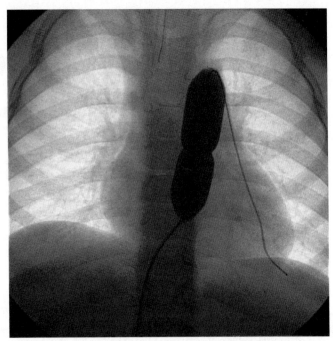

Figure 56-2. Anteroposterior view during pulmonary balloon valvuloplasty in a child with severe pulmonary stenosis. The dilation balloon is inflated across the valve, and the impression of the valve annulus is clearly evident near the middle of the balloon.

the valve annulus to a small central orifice.[5] During childhood and young adulthood, the pulmonary valve leaflets are typically supple, doming upward during systole (Fig. 56-1). In older adults, pulmonary valve calcification may occur and may lead to diminished leaflet mobility. A much less common form of pulmonary stenosis has been referred to as "pulmonary valve dysplasia."[5,6] It often occurs as a familial trait or as part of Noonan syndrome. A dysplastic pulmonary valve is characterized by thick, cartilaginous valve leaflets with poor mobility. The pulmonary valve annulus is often hypoplastic, and there may be little or no commissural fusion. In isolated pulmonary valve stenosis, balloon dilation reduces the degree of valvar obstruction by separating fused commissures or by tearing the valve leaflets themselves.[7,8] Patients who have severe pulmonary valve dysplasia, with marked hypoplasia of the annulus and absence of commissural fusion, may have minimal improvement after balloon valvuloplasty.[9] However, because a spectrum of pulmonary valve dysplasia exists, some patients with this disorder may derive substantial benefit from the balloon valvuloplasty procedure.[10]

Technique

Balloon pulmonary valvuloplasty is technically less challenging than balloon mitral or aortic valvuloplasty procedures. It is performed entirely transvenously and without the need for a transseptal left-sided heart catheterization. The procedure also differs from aortic valvuloplasty in that use of an oversized balloon, approximately 25% larger than the valve annulus diameter, is required for the most effective relief of obstruction. In general, we believe that pulmonary valvuloplasty is indicated for isolated pulmonary valve stenosis if the resting peak systolic pressure gradient exceeds 40 mm Hg in the presence of a normal cardiac output. In an infant with critical pulmonary stenosis, a right-to-left atrial shunt, and a PDA, valvuloplasty is indicated even if the measured transvalvar gradient is less than 40 mm Hg.

Balloon pulmonary valvuloplasty is usually performed via a percutaneous transfemoral approach. Right-sided heart catheterization documents the severity of the lesion. RV angiocardiography is performed to confirm the nature of the lesion and to measure the pulmonary valve annulus diameter. Typically, the lateral projection is best suited to this purpose. Once the decision is made to proceed with valvuloplasty, an end-hole catheter is advanced to the left pulmonary artery. The left pulmonary artery provides better wire and balloon stability than a right pulmonary artery position. An exchange-length guidewire is advanced to the distal left pulmonary artery, and the end-hole catheter is removed. The balloon valvuloplasty catheter is then inserted over the exchange wire. A balloon valvuloplasty catheter is used whose inflated balloon diameter is approximately 25% larger than the pulmonary valve annulus diameter (Fig. 56-2). Balloon oversizing improves valvuloplasty effectiveness, and injury to the pulmonary valve annulus is unlikely when balloons smaller

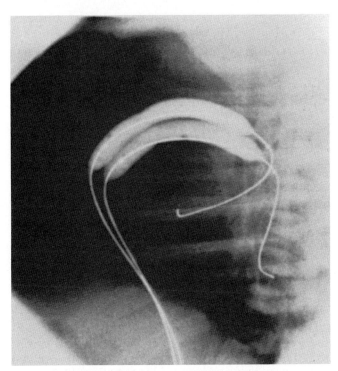

Figure 56-3. Double-balloon pulmonary valve dilation in a child with severe pulmonary valve stenosis. Two balloons may be used if a single-balloon catheter requires a sheath thought to be too large for the child's femoral vein.

than 140% of the annulus diameter are used.[11,12] We recommend a double-balloon technique, with two balloons positioned across the valve and inflated simultaneously, if the pulmonary valve annulus exceeds 18 to 19 mm or if the single balloon catheter required is too large for safe introduction into a patient's femoral vein (Fig. 56-3). With the double-balloon technique, two similar-sized balloons are chosen whose balloon diameter sum is approximately 60% greater than the valve annulus diameter. This yields an effective dilating cross-sectional area approximately equal to the cross-sectional area of the single balloon that would be used for the same valve annulus size.

Once inserted, the balloon valvuloplasty catheter is advanced across the valve and is positioned with the valve at the midportion of the balloon. Partial balloon inflation, with a mixture of saline and contrast, is helpful to determine the precise location of the valve on the balloon. The valvuloplasty balloon (or balloons) is then inflated by hand until the waist produced by the valve on the balloon disappears. The period of balloon inflation is kept as brief as possible, to minimize the obstruction to RV outflow. Typically, three or four balloon inflations are performed, with minor adjustments in balloon position to ensure adequate dilation of the pulmonary valve. After the dilation is completed, the valvuloplasty catheter is withdrawn and is replaced with a diagnostic catheter. The residual RVOT gradient and cardiac output are measured to document the effectiveness of the procedure. We perform a repeat RV angiogram if we believe it necessary to document the degree of subvalvar infundibular narrowing (which may be increased immediately after valvuloplasty) (Fig. 56-4).

Acute Results

In patients with isolated pulmonary valve stenosis, percutaneous balloon valvuloplasty can be expected to provide excellent relief of RVOT obstruction (Fig. 56-5). Numerous studies have clearly documented significant acute reduction in the peak systolic pulmonary valve gradient to 30 mm Hg or less (i.e., mild residual stenosis). In their landmark article, Kan and associates reported the acute effects of valvuloplasty in an 8-year-old child with pulmonary stenosis.[4] The procedure decreased the peak transvalvar gradient from 48 to 14 mm Hg and was performed without significant complications. Other studies subsequently confirmed Kan's initial observation that valvuloplasty provides impressive gradient relief

Figure 56-4. Lateral right ventricular angiogram before (**A**) and immediately after (**B**) valvuloplasty in an infant with pulmonary stenosis. Note the marked systolic narrowing of the right ventricular infundibulum after valvuloplasty, which was not present before the procedure. Such dynamic infundibular narrowing may account for some residual gradient that is often measured immediately after the procedure and is expected to improve with time.

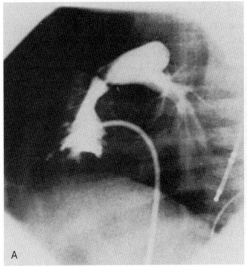

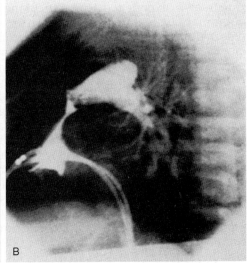

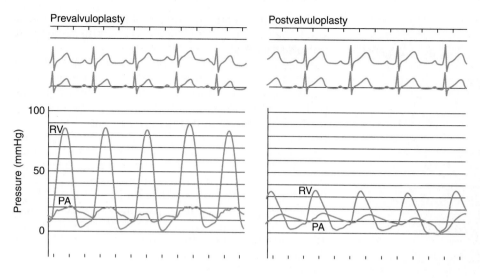

Figure 56-5. Simultaneous right ventricular and pulmonary artery pressure recordings (made on the same scale) before and immediately after pulmonary valve dilation in a 15-month-old boy with severe pulmonary stenosis. The right ventricular systolic pressure was reduced from 86 to 36 mm Hg. The pulmonary valve systolic gradient decreased from 66 to 20 mm Hg.

acutely.[11,13-19] The largest published clinical series of balloon pulmonary valvuloplasty was reported by the Pediatric Valvuloplasty Registry.[13] The Registry reported the acute results of pulmonary valvuloplasty performed in 784 patients between 1981 and 1986. Overall, balloon dilation resulted in an acute decrease in the peak systolic pressure gradient from 71 to 28 mm Hg. The residual pressure gradients immediately after valvuloplasty were, in part, ascribed to subvalvar infundibular obstruction related to RV hypertrophy. Effectiveness of the procedure was not related to age (the series included 35 adults older than age 21 years), but a larger residual gradient was observed in patients with a dysplastic pulmonary valve. The Pediatric Valvuloplasty Registry described five major complications (0.6%), primarily confined to infancy. There were two procedure-related deaths (0.2%), both two infants, and in one neonate RVOT perforation and tamponade occurred. In two children, severe tricuspid regurgitation developed related to injury to the tricuspid valve apparatus. Minor complications reported included femoral venous thrombosis, hemorrhage, and transient arrhythmias.

Our own experience with percutaneous balloon pulmonary valvuloplasty is consistent with that reported from other centers. During our first 10 years of experience, from 1982 to 1992, balloon valvuloplasty was performed in 90 patients with isolated pulmonary valve stenosis (Table 56-1). These patients ranged in age from 1 day to 34 years (mean±standard deviation [SD], 4.2±5.2 years) and in weight from 3.2 to 89 kg (mean±SD, 18.4±17.2 kg). Valvuloplasty was performed with balloons ranging in diameter from 5 to 20 mm, and the double-balloon technique was used in 16 instances. Overall, valvuloplasty decreased the peak systolic valve gradient acutely by 57%. The peak pulmonary stenosis gradient decreased from 70±24 to 30±17 mm Hg after valvuloplasty (P<.0001). RV systolic pressure decreased from 91±24 to 50±17 mm Hg (P<.0001), and RV end-diastolic pressure decreased from 9.8±3.2 mm Hg

to 8.5±2.5 mm Hg (P<.01). There was no significant change in heart rate or cardiac output after the procedure. In our experience, there has been no relationship between patient age or size and the residual pulmonary valve gradient after valvuloplasty.

Infants

Newborns and infants with critical pulmonary stenosis are frequently critically ill and hypoxemic (because of a right-to-left atrial shunt) and may have associated hypoplasia of the RV and tricuspid valve (Fig. 56-6). Because of these factors, in addition to the presence of severe RVOT obstruction, it is a technical challenge to successfully catheterize the pulmonary artery and properly position a valvuloplasty balloon across the RVOT in these infants.[16,17,19-21] In infants with critical pulmonary stenosis, we prefer to perform the procedure with the child receiving prostaglandin E_1 infusion, for three reasons. First, the infant is in a more stable hemodynamic state during the

Table 56-1. Characteristics of 90 Patients Before and After Balloon Pulmonary Valvuloplasty

Parameter	Result
Age (yr)	
Mean±SD	4.2±5.2
Range	1 day to 34 yr
Weight (kg)	
Mean±SD	18.4±17.2
Range	3.2-89
Systolic gradient (mm Hg)	
Before	70±24
Immediately after	30±17
Right ventricle systolic pressure (mm Hg)	
Before	91±24
Immediately after	50±17
Cardiac index (L/min/m²)	
Before	3.55±0.91
Immediately after	3.69±0.81

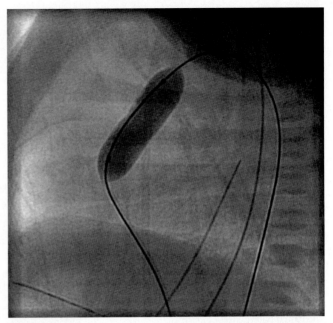

Figure 56-7. Lateral image during balloon dilation in a newborn with critical pulmonary stenosis (same patient as Fig. 56-6). The balloon is stabilized by a wire course through the patent ductus arteriosus and into the descending aorta.

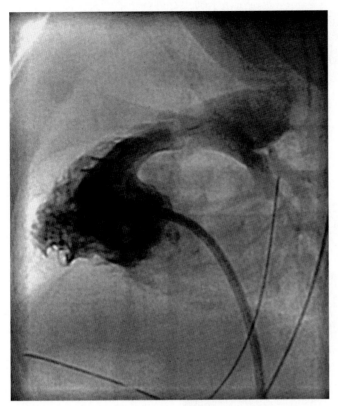

Figure 56-6. Lateral right ventricular angiogram in a newborn with critical pulmonary valve stenosis. The right ventricle is coarsely trabeculated, and there was mild tricuspid valve hypoplasia.

procedure. Second, a left-to-right ductal shunt maintains pulmonary blood flow during balloon occlusion of the RVOT. Finally, the presence of a PDA permits the exchange guidewire to be positioned across the pulmonary valve and into the descending aorta, a course that facilitates catheter exchanges and subsequent valve dilation (Fig. 56-7).

We have reported the results of balloon valvuloplasty attempted in 12 infants with critical pulmonary stenosis ($n=10$) or membranous pulmonary atresia with intact ventricular septum ($n=2$).[20] These infants ranged in age from 1 to 38 days and in weight from 2.9 to 4.5 kg. Nine were receiving a prostaglandin E_1 infusion. In one child with critical pulmonary stenosis and a diminutive RV, the RVOT was perforated during an attempt to cross the valve. This child was taken to the operating room, where the perforation was oversewn and a Blalock-Taussig shunt performed. In the remaining 11 infants, balloon valvuloplasty was successfully performed using balloons ranging in diameter from 2.5 to 12 mm. In the two patients with membranous pulmonary atresia (Fig. 56-8), a 5-Fr right coronary catheter was positioned immediately below the atretic valve, and the membrane was perforated with the stiff end of a 0.021-inch guidewire. In the 11 infants who underwent successful valvuloplasty, the procedure acutely reduced the peak systolic transvalvar pressure gradient from 86 to 16 mm Hg. Similarly, the RV systolic

pressure, which was suprasystemic in all children, decreased acutely from 112 to 50 mm Hg. Seven of these 11 children (including 1 with pulmonary atresia) have required no further intervention. The remaining children required surgical intervention for persistent severe hypoxemia despite having undergone a successful pulmonary valvuloplasty (residual gradient, 16 mm Hg). In these children, hypoxemia (due to a right-to-left atrial shunt) persisted because of relative hypoplasia of the right-sided heart structures (tricuspid valve, pulmonary valve, and the RV chamber itself).

Adults

Several reports have described the successful application of percutaneous balloon valvuloplasty for treatment of adults with pulmonary valve stenosis.[14,18,22-32] Table 56-2 summarizes the pertinent clinical and hemodynamic data from 14 publications (including this report) describing the acute results of pulmonary valvuloplasty in adolescents and adults. Pulmonary valvuloplasty has been performed successfully in patients as old as 84 years of age. In most published cases, a single-balloon technique was used. If a 20-mm diameter balloon was insufficient, the double-balloon technique was usually necessary. In these reports, balloon valvuloplasty acutely reduced the peak systolic gradient by an average of 60% to 65%, from a range of 53 to 260 mm Hg before the procedure to 2 to 90 mm Hg after valvuloplasty. In most cases, the peak systolic gradient immediately after valvuloplasty was in the mild range (20 to 40 mm Hg). For example, Al Kasab and colleagues[18] reported the

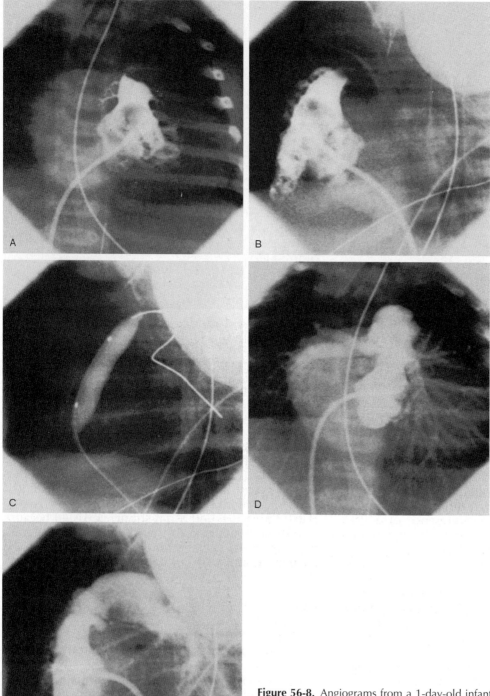

Figure 56-8. Angiograms from a 1-day-old infant with pulmonary atresia and intact ventricular septum. Before valvuloplasty, the anteroposterior (**A**) and lateral (**B**) right ventricular angiograms demonstrated membranous pulmonary atresia. After the atretic membrane was perforated, balloon dilation was performed with a 10-mm balloon (**C**). Repeat right ventricular angiography in the anteroposterior (**D**) and lateral (**E**) projections revealed unobstructed outflow from the right ventricle. The residual pulmonary stenosis gradient was 10 mm Hg.

Table 56-2. Summary of Published Reports of Pulmonary Valvuloplasty in Adults

| Study (Ref. No.) | N | Age Range (Yr) | Balloon Technique | Peak Systolic Gradient (mm Hg) | |
				Before	After
Beekman*	4	21-35	Double	53	15
Tentolouris (22)	1	84	Double	70	34
Herrmann (23)	8	23-66	Single	66	22
Sherman (24)	4	48-67	Single (3) and double (1)	109	38
Al Kasab (18)	2	21-37	Double	86	28
Fawzy (25)	8	21-45	Double	107	36
Flugelman (26)	1	62	Single	260	90
Presbitero (27)	3	21-45	Single	130	29
Park (28)	3	24-40	Double	108	51
Cooke (29)	1	61	Single	105	13
Leisch (30)	6	21-59	Single	78	38
Shuck (31)	1	23	Single	30	2
Pepine (14)	1	59	Single	130	30
Chen (32)	53	13-55	Single	191	38

*This report.

effects of valvuloplasty in 12 adults with valvar pulmonary stenosis, ranging in age from 21 to 37 years. In these patients, valvuloplasty acutely reduced the peak systolic gradient from 86 to 28 mm Hg. Transient ventricular arrhythmias were noted in 30% of patients, but no serious complications were described. Similarly, Fawzy and colleagues[25] described eight adult patients with valvar pulmonary stenosis in whom percutaneous balloon valvuloplasty reduced the peak systolic gradient from 107 to 36 mm Hg. Thus, available data clearly indicate that percutaneous balloon valvuloplasty provides effective therapy in adults, as well as in children, with congenital pulmonary valve stenosis. Balloon valvuloplasty appears to be effective even in the oldest patients, in whom valve calcification may be present.[22]

Long-Term Studies

Long-term studies of balloon pulmonary valvuloplasty have confirmed that the benefits of this procedure are durable and comparable to those of surgical valvotomy. McCrindle and Kan[33] reported the long-term results of balloon valvuloplasty performed between 1981 and 1986 in 42 patients (median age, 4.6 years), for whom follow-up data beyond 2 years were available. Balloon valvuloplasty acutely reduced the peak systolic gradient from 70 to 23 mm Hg, and at long-term follow-up more than 2 years after the procedure the Doppler-predicted gradient was 20 mm Hg. Doppler peak instantaneous gradients were less than 36 mm Hg at long-term follow-up in 86% of patients. The authors found age younger than 2 years at time of balloon valvuloplasty to be a risk factor for late follow-up gradients exceeding 36 mm Hg. Long-term data from the Pediatric Valvuloplasty Registry were reported on 533 patients up to 8.7 years after balloon pulmonary valvuloplasty.[34] Eighty-four patients (16%) required either a surgical valvotomy or a repeat balloon dilation for suboptimal results. Of the remaining 449 patients who had

not undergone a repeat procedure, 399 had mild residual stenosis (<36 mm Hg), 36 had residual stenosis exceeding 36 mm Hg, and the late gradient was unknown in 14. Independent risk factors for a suboptimal late outcome included small valve annulus diameter, higher early residual gradient, smaller balloon-to-annulus diameter ratio, and younger age at initial intervention.

We assessed the long-term (4 to 5 years) outcome after balloon pulmonary valvuloplasty in childhood and compared the results with those of a matched surgical control group.[35] Follow-up data obtained in 20 children at 4 to 7.8 years after balloon valvuloplasty documented excellent late results without significant restenosis. The peak systolic gradient measured at cardiac catheterization in these children averaged 76 mm Hg before and 35 mm Hg immediately after balloon valvuloplasty. At long-term follow-up, the Doppler peak instantaneous gradient was 24 mm Hg, significantly less than that measured by catheterization immediately after the procedure (Fig. 56-9). Pulmonary valve insufficiency was mild in 9 of 20 patients and absent in the remainder. Twenty-four-hour Holter monitoring documented only grade 1 ventricular ectopic activity in 1 patient and none in the remaining 19 patients. Comparison to the matched surgical control group demonstrated that, although their residual gradient was slightly less after surgery (16 versus 24 mm Hg; P=.01), the surgical group had significantly more pulmonary valve insufficiency and late ventricular arrhythmias. Late follow-up data, therefore, document excellent long-term results after percutaneous pulmonary balloon valvuloplasty and support the use of this procedure as treatment of choice for patients with isolated valvar pulmonary stenosis.

Complications

Beyond infancy, percutaneous balloon pulmonary valvuloplasty is a very safe procedure. In the Pediatric

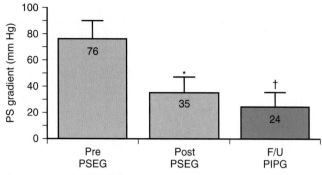

Figure 56-9. Serial pulmonary stenosis (PS) gradients in 20 children before and immediately after valvuloplasty and at follow-up (F/U) an average of 5.4 years later. PIPG, peak instantaneous pressure gradient; PSEG, peak systolic ejection gradient (From O'Connor EK, Beekman RH, Lindauer A, Rocchini A: Intermediate-term outcome after pulmonary balloon valvuloplasty: Comparison to a matched surgical control group. J Am Coll Cardiol 1992;20:169-173.)

Valvuloplasty Registry, the only two deaths occurred in infants with critical pulmonary stenosis, and the single case of perforation and tamponade occurred in an 8-day-old neonate.[13] Minor complications were primarily related to vascular injury or hemorrhage and were also much more common during the first 12 months of life. Overall, the Pediatric Valvuloplasty Registry noted a 1.2% to 1.8% frequency of major complications and a 4.8% frequency of minor complications in 168 infants. In contrast, among the 656 children and adults, these frequencies were 0.8% and 1.7%, respectively. Premature ventricular beats and right bundle-branch block occur commonly during the procedure, owing to catheter and wire manipulation within the RV, but there have been no reports of long-term arrhythmias after valvuloplasty. Valvuloplasty may cause injury to the femoral vein, especially when the procedure is performed in infancy. Finally, the mild pulmonary valve insufficiency commonly seen after pulmonary valvuloplasty is rarely of clinical importance and may be less severe than after surgical valvotomy.[35]

Conclusions and Recommendations

Percutaneous balloon pulmonary valvuloplasty is the treatment of choice for children and adults with isolated congenital valvar pulmonary stenosis. Valvuloplasty successfully reduces significant RVOT obstruction, with a residual gradient that is usually in the trivial to mild range (i.e., <30 mm Hg). Follow-up studies have documented long-term effectiveness, with little restenosis as late as 9 years after the procedure. In our opinion, pulmonary valvuloplasty is indicated in patients with isolated pulmonary valve stenosis whose resting peak systolic pressure gradient exceeds 40 mm Hg in the presence of a normal cardiac output. The procedure is effective in neonates, children, and adults as old as 84 years.[22] Patients with a calcified or dysplastic pulmonary valve, unless the valve annulus is severely hypoplastic, may also derive significant hemodynamic benefit from balloon valvuloplasty.

AORTIC BALLOON VALVULOPLASTY

Aortic valve stenosis accounts for 4% to 6% of all cases of congenital heart disease.[36] Left ventricular outflow tract obstruction elicits left ventricular hypertrophy and myocardial fibrosis, which may eventually lead to left ventricular dysfunction and congestive heart failure. Unlike most cases of congenital pulmonary valve stenosis, congenital aortic stenosis tends to progress over time.[37] Nevertheless, intervention usually is not indicated unless the degree of left ventricular outflow tract obstruction is severe (catheter gradient >65 mm Hg) or there is associated left ventricular dysfunction, heart failure, ischemia, or symptoms of angina, syncope, or presyncope. This recommendation is based on the fact that all current forms of therapy for aortic valve stenosis are palliative in nature. Surgical valvotomy, widely regarded in the past as the initial treatment of choice for congenital aortic valve stenosis, is associated with a high incidence of late (5 to 20 years) restenosis.[38] Prosthetic aortic valve replacement is associated with risks of thromboembolic complications and risks associated with anticoagulation therapy that may be considerable in young, active patients. Therefore, because current treatment options are not curative, intervention for congenital aortic valve stenosis is usually delayed until clear indications exist.

Percutaneous balloon valvuloplasty for treatment of congenital valvar aortic stenosis in children was first described in 1984.[39] Balloon valvuloplasty typically reduces the left ventricular outflow obstruction to the mild range and is the treatment of choice for children with congenital aortic stenosis who require intervention. The effectiveness of balloon dilation relates to the underlying morphologic substrate. Most congenitally stenotic aortic valves are bicuspid, with a single central or eccentric commissure with a variable degree of fusion of its edges. The valve leaflets themselves are thickened but are rarely calcified in childhood (Fig. 56-10). In older patients and in children with prior valve surgery, the leaflets may calcify, becoming less mobile and less amenable to balloon dilation.

In congenital aortic valve stenosis, as in pulmonary valve stenosis, balloon valvuloplasty reduces the degree of stenosis by separating valve leaflets along the lines of commissural fusion (Fig. 56-11). Because the valve leaflets are typically supple in younger patients, and the obstruction to ventricular outflow relates primarily to incomplete cusp separation during systole, balloon dilation provides substantial hemodynamic improvement in these cases. This is in marked contrast to older patients with calcific aortic stenosis, in whom balloon valvuloplasty has proved to be much less successful.[40] In these patients, the aortic valve stenosis is acquired, primarily as a result of calcium deposition within the leaflets, and little or no commissural fusion is present.[41,42]

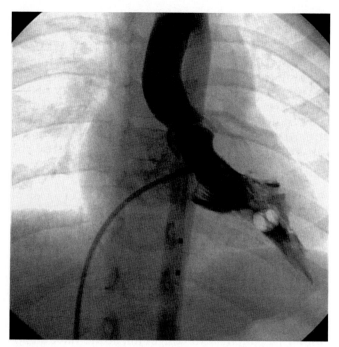

Figure 56-10. Anteroposterior left ventricular angiogram in a child with severe valvar aortic stenosis. The valve is thickened and domes in systole. There is left ventricular hypertrophy.

Therefore, differences in valve morphology, and thus in the mechanism by which balloon dilation improves valve function, explain the observation that balloon valvuloplasty is effective in younger patients with congenital aortic stenosis but is typically ineffective in adults with calcific aortic stenosis.

Successful percutaneous balloon valvuloplasty in children with congenital aortic valve stenosis was first reported in 1984 by Lababidi, Walls, and colleagues.[39,43] Subsequently, the effectiveness of balloon valvuloplasty in children and adolescents with congenital aortic valve stenosis was clearly demonstrated.[44-52] The procedure usually reduces the peak systolic gradient by approximately 60%, and severe aortic regurgitation is uncommon. Vascular complications have been limited primarily to neonates and young infants and have diminished in recent years with the development of smaller-profile valvuloplasty catheters.

Technique

Percutaneous aortic valvuloplasty usually is performed from a retrograde transarterial approach, although the antegrade, transseptal approach can also be used. We prefer the retrograde approach, using a transseptal catheter for continuous left ventricular pressure monitoring throughout the procedure. After the transseptal puncture is accomplished, heparin is administered to increase the activated clotting time to approximately 250 to 300 seconds. The aortic stenosis gradient is measured before angiography from simultaneous ventricular and aortic pressure recordings. In our center, the criteria for performing aortic balloon dilation include (1) a

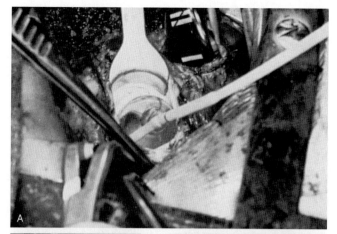

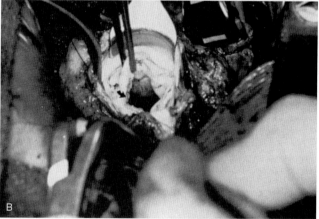

Figure 56-11. Mechanism of balloon aortic valvuloplasty demonstrated during surgery in an 18-year-old woman with congenital aortic valve stenosis. A 20-mm balloon was inflated across the valve (**A**) and produced a 3- to 4-mm tear across the line of commissural fusion (*arrowhead*) (**B**). The valve leaflets are thick and dysplastic.

peak systolic pressure gradient at rest of 65 mm Hg or more, (2) a peak systolic gradient of 50 to 64 mm Hg in association with symptoms or ischemic changes on the electrocardiogram, or (3) low cardiac output regardless of measured pressure gradient. A modest aortic stenosis gradient is typical in infants with critically severe aortic stenosis in whom left ventricular failure and shock are present.

Once the decision to proceed with balloon valvuloplasty has been made, the correct balloon diameter must be selected. Proper balloon size depends on aortic valve annulus diameter, which can be measured by echocardiography or angiocardiography. If a single-balloon technique is used, a balloon is chosen whose diameter is equal to, or 1 mm smaller than, the diameter of the aortic valve annulus. If a double-balloon technique is used, we use two balloons of similar diameter whose sum is approximately 1.3 times the diameter of the aortic annulus.[45] We prefer the double-balloon technique in patients whose aortic valve annulus exceeds 25 mm and in those whose aortic valve annulus is large for their body size, to minimize the size of the balloon catheter and

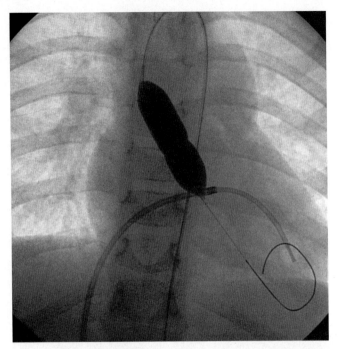

Figure 56-12. Balloon dilation in a child with severe aortic valve stenosis (same case as Fig. 56-10). The waist produced by the valve annulus on the balloon is evident. Ventricular pressure was monitored throughout the procedure by a catheter placed in the left ventricle through a transseptal puncture.

arterial sheath required for the procedure. Unlike pulmonary balloon valvuloplasty, oversized balloons are not used for aortic valvuloplasty, because they have been shown to increase the risk of injury to the aortic valve and annulus.[46] The balloon (or balloons) is inflated by hand (i.e., a manometer is not used) until the waist produced on the balloon by the valve is relieved (Fig. 56-12). Balloon inflation is kept as

brief as possible to minimize arterial hypotension during the procedure. Because the inflated balloon may be ejected across the aortic valve, several balloon inflations may be required, with minor adjustments in position to ensure that the valve is adequately dilated. Repeat simultaneous measurements of left ventricular and aortic pressures are made to quantify the residual aortic stenosis gradient. An aortic root angiogram is performed to detect any aortic insufficiency that may have been produced by the procedure.

Acute Results

In most patients with congenital aortic valve stenosis, balloon valvuloplasty provides relief of left ventricular outflow tract obstruction (Fig. 56-13) that is comparable to the results of surgical valvotomy.[37,53] The expected peak systolic ejection gradient across the aortic valve after the procedure is approximately 20 to 40 mm Hg.[44-51] If a technically adequate balloon dilation fails to achieve a satisfactory hemodynamic result in a patient with congenital aortic valve stenosis, then a more complex diagnosis is suggested. Such patients may be found to have annular hypoplasia or valve leaflet calcification.

The largest series of balloon aortic valvuloplasty procedures for congenital aortic stenosis was reported by the Pediatric Valvuloplasty Registry.[44,51] The acute results of 630 balloon valvuloplasty procedures were reported in 606 children ranging in age from 1 day to 18 years, who underwent the procedure at 23 institutions between 1984 and 1992. Overall, the procedure resulted in an immediate decrease in peak systolic pressure gradient across the aortic valve by 60%. In the initial Registry report of 204 children,[44] most of the acute complications and deaths occurred in newborns. Five deaths were reported (mortality

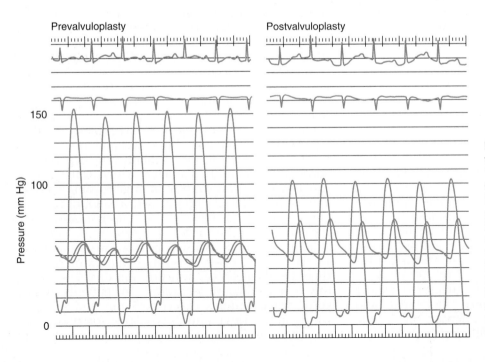

Figure 56-13. Aortic and left ventricular pressure tracings in an 11-day-old infant with critical aortic stenosis, measured before and immediately after balloon dilation. The peak systolic gradient decreased from 96 to 29 mm Hg. Note the improved aortic pulse pressure after valvuloplasty, which is indicative of an improved cardiac output. (From Beekman RH, Rocchini AP, Andes A: Balloon valvuloplasty for critical aortic stenosis in the newborn: Influence of new catheter technology. J Am Coll Cardiol 1991;17:1172-1176.)

rate, 2.4%), four of which occurred in newborns and one in a 3-month-old child. Two deaths were related to aortic rupture, two to aortic valve trauma, and one to a torn iliofemoral artery. There was no mortality in patients older than 3 months of age. The larger report[51] evaluated predictors of a suboptimal outcome, which was defined as failure to perform the valvuloplasty (which occurred in 4.1%), an immediate residual gradient of 60 mm Hg or more, a left ventricular systolic pressure exceeding the aortic systolic pressure by 60% or more, mortality, or major morbidity. Overall, a suboptimal outcome was reported for 17% of the 630 valvuloplasty procedures. The identified independent predictors for a suboptimal outcome included age younger than 3 months, a greater predilation systolic gradient, a balloon-to-annulus diameter ratio of less than 0.9, the coexistence of an unrepaired coarctation, and an earlier date of procedure. Three months appeared to be a significant threshold below which procedure outcome was significantly affected. Patients younger than 3 months of age were more likely to experience failure to perform the procedure (15.7% versus 1.7%), suboptimal residual stenosis (17.8% versus 7.5%), major morbidity (16.7% versus 4.1%), and mortality (8.3% versus 0.6%). The effect of the balloon-to-annulus diameter ratio was thoroughly evaluated, and the optimal ratio was found to be between 0.90 and 0.99. Smaller ratios were associated with an increased risk of suboptimal gradient relief. Larger ratios were associated with a greater risk of aortic insufficiency after valvuloplasty.

Our own experience with percutaneous balloon aortic valvuloplasty is similar. Between 1985 and 1992, balloon aortic dilation was performed in 68 children, adolescents, and young adults with congenital aortic valve stenosis (Table 56-3). Patients ranged in age from 1 day to 24 years (8.7±6.9 years) and in weight from 2.1 to 120 kg (35.7±27.7 kg). The valvuloplasty procedure was performed with balloon diameters ranging from 5 to 20 mm, and the double-balloon technique was used in 36 patients. Percutaneous balloon valvuloplasty acutely decreased the peak systolic aortic stenosis gradient by 56%, from 77±22 to 34±16 mm Hg. Left ventricular systolic pressure decreased acutely from 171±31 to 133±25 mm Hg, and left ventricular end-diastolic pressure decreased slightly from 14.5±4.3 to 11.9±5.7 mm Hg. There was no change in cardiac output or heart rate after the dilation procedure. In 52 (76%) of 68 patients, there was no increase in the degree of aortic insufficiency from that present before balloon valvuloplasty. An increase of one grade (on a scale of 0 to 4+) occurred acutely in 10 patients (15%), and a two-grade increase occurred in six patients (9%). No patient required emergent or urgent surgical intervention because of valvuloplasty-induced aortic insufficiency.

In our series, we found no relationship between the effectiveness of balloon valvuloplasty and patient age or size. We noted, however, that patients with an unsatisfactory degree of gradient relief (residual gradient >45 mm Hg) had more complex disease, including annulus hypoplasia or valve leaflet calcification. In this series, there was no patient with unsatisfactory gradient relief from balloon valvuloplasty who subsequently underwent a successful surgical valvotomy. Such patients, instead, required more complex surgical intervention, including prosthetic aortic valve replacement or the Konno operation.

Infants

Infants with critical aortic stenosis typically present in severe congestive heart failure and shock, with profound left ventricular dysfunction (Fig. 56-14). At times it can be difficult to distinguish neonatal critical aortic stenosis from hypoplastic left heart syndrome, because the aortic valve annulus, the mitral valve annulus, and even the left ventricular length can be undersized. In addition, the aortic valve leaflets (or leaflet) often exhibit a markedly dysplastic appearance on echocardiography, which in an older child would indicate a low likelihood of successful balloon valvuloplasty. Despite these real or apparent obstacles to success, balloon aortic valvuloplasty has proved to be remarkably successful, with results comparable to those of surgical intervention at several premier institutions.[54-57] The clinical status of these patients generally leaves little room for doubt that urgent intervention is required, but the choice between relief of aortic stenosis and univentricular palliation is not always obvious. Unlike critical pulmonary stenosis, in which placement of a systemic-to-pulmonary artery shunt can compensate for inadequate support of the pulmonary circulation by hypoplasia of right heart structures, patients with left-sided heart structures that are inadequate to support the systemic circulation face death unless a successful Norwood palliation can be performed. Several systems have been developed for predicting which neonates have the potential for adequate systemic perfusion after relief of aortic valve stenosis,

Table 56-3. Characteristics of 68 Patients Before and After Balloon Aortic Valvuloplasty

Parameter	Result
Age (yr)	
Mean±SD	8.7±6.9
Range	1 day to 24 yr
Weight (kg)	
Mean±SD	35.7±27.7
Range	2.1-120
Systolic gradient (mm Hg)	
Before	77±21
Immediately after	34±16
Left ventricle systolic pressure (mm Hg)	
Before	171±31
Immediately after	133±25
Cardiac index (L/min/m²)	
Before	3.64±0.95
Immediately after	3.35±0.80

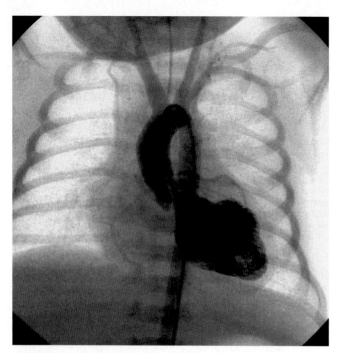

Figure 56-14. Anteroposterior left ventricular angiogram in a newborn with critical aortic valve stenosis. The aortic valve leaflets are thickened, and there was severe left ventricular dysfunction.

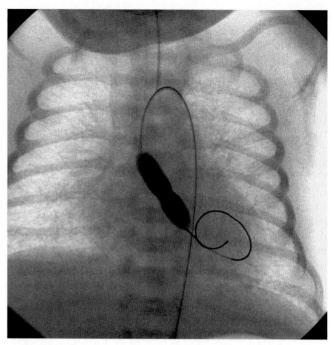

Figure 56-15. Balloon dilation in a newborn with critical aortic stenosis (same patient as Fig. 56-14). The catheter was introduced through the umbilical artery, thereby avoiding potential femoral artery injury in a newborn with low cardiac output.

the most popular of which was reported by Rhodes and colleagues.[58]

The child should be stabilized with prostaglandin E_1 infusion and intravenous inotropic support before the procedure, with extracorporeal life support if necessary. If possible, we use the transumbilical approach (Fig. 56-15) to spare the infant's femoral artery (which may be required for future percutaneous valve dilation procedures). Carotid artery[59] and transvenous antegrade[60] approaches have also been reported as means to avoid femoral artery injury in newborn infants. We have tended to employ a single balloon, typically 6 to 7 mm in diameter, aiming for a single inflation. In contrast, McElhinney and colleagues[56] begin with smaller balloons and perform serial dilations with progressively larger balloons until the desired degree of relief is obtained.

The Congenital Heart Surgeons Society reported the results of intervention in 110 neonates with critical aortic stenosis from 18 institutions.[55] Balloon aortic valvuloplasty was the initial procedure in 82 patients and surgical valvotomy in the remaining 28. Relief of aortic stenosis was significantly better in the balloon valvuloplasty group (gradient reduction of $65 \pm 17\%$ and median residual gradient of 20 mm Hg, versus $41 \pm 32\%$ and 36 mm Hg with surgery), although there was also a trend toward more aortic insufficiency in this group. Early mortality was 18%, with no difference between groups. In our own study,[54] 30 neonates were assigned to balloon valvuloplasty and 17 to surgical intervention on an intent-to-treat basis; early mortality was 13% in both groups. Early mortality was 14% in a series of 113 neonates

treated with balloon aortic valvuloplasty, with about one third of the survivors requiring repeat intervention within 1 year.[56] Echocardiographic estimates of valve thickness or mobility have not correlated with valvuloplasty success in neonates.

Young Adults

Balloon aortic valvuloplasty in young adults with congenital aortic valve stenosis yields results similar to those in children with the same disease and in patients with rheumatic aortic stenosis, all of whom exhibit commissural fusion to a significant degree. In contrast, balloon valvuloplasty is of limited utility in patients with degenerative or calcific aortic stenosis.[40,61-63] We have reported our experience with balloon valvuloplasty in 15 young adult patients, aged 15 to 24 years, all of whom were judged to have severe congenital aortic valve stenosis.[52] The valve annulus ranged from 18.5 to 30 mm in diameter. Balloons were used ranging in diameter from 10 to 20 mm, and the double-balloon technique was used in 12 patients. In one patient with access available to only one femoral artery, the double-balloon technique was performed using a single retrograde balloon together with a balloon placed anterograde through a transseptal puncture. In these 15 young adults, balloon valvuloplasty acutely reduced the peak systolic aortic valve gradient from 73 to 35 mm Hg. Left ventricular systolic pressure decreased from 179 to 147 mm Hg, without an associated change in cardiac output. Aortic insufficiency was unchanged by the procedure in nine patients, increased by one grade in four patients, and increased by two grades in two patients. An unsatisfactory result was obtained in three patients, in whom the residual systolic gradient was 70 mm Hg or higher. Two of these patients had mild annular hypoplasia (18.5 and 19 mm), and the third had moderate valve leaflet calcification (related to prior surgical valvotomy in childhood). All three patients required prosthetic aortic valve replacement. The remaining 12 patients have done well during intermediate-term follow-up. Eight of them underwent elective follow-up cardiac catheterization, 1 to 2.5 years after balloon valvuloplasty, which documented no restenosis. In these patients, the follow-up peak systolic gradient at cardiac catheterization was 30 mm Hg, and there was no change in the degree of aortic regurgitation. Although this is a small series, the data lead us to believe that percutaneous balloon valvuloplasty should be attempted in young adults with congenital aortic valve stenosis, unless the valve annulus is hypoplastic or the valve is calcified.

Long-Term Studies

Percutaneous balloon valvuloplasty for congenital aortic stenosis should be regarded as a palliative therapeutic procedure. As is the case after surgical aortic valvotomy,[38] late restenosis (5 to 20 years) should be expected after a successful balloon dilation procedure. We would warn, however, against comparing follow-up peak instantaneous gradients determined by Doppler echocardiography against catheter-based measurements of peak systolic gradient obtained immediately after valvuloplasty.[64] Because Doppler peak instantaneous and catheter peak systolic gradients can differ substantially, particularly in patients with aortic insufficiency, a false impression of restenosis may be obtained.

The intermediate-term effectiveness of balloon valvuloplasty in children with congenital aortic stenosis was prospectively evaluated in our center.[65] A follow-up cardiac catheterization was performed in 27 of the first 30 children to undergo successful percutaneous balloon dilation at our institution between 1985 and 1988, at an average of 1.7 years (0.8 to 3.8 years) after balloon valvuloplasty. No restenosis was documented in these patients, and the greatest increase in peak systolic gradient at recatheterization was 14 mm Hg. In this group of 27 children (mean age, 8.6 years), balloon valvuloplasty acutely decreased the peak systolic gradient from 76 to 31 mm Hg. At follow-up 1.7 years later, the peak systolic gradient remained 29 mm Hg (Fig. 56-16). At the follow-up cardiac catheterization, 20 (74%) of 27 patients had no increase in the degree of aortic insufficiency that had been present before balloon valvuloplasty. In the seven patients in whom balloon dilation resulted in increased valve insufficiency, five had a 2+ increase in aortic insufficiency and two had a 1+ increase in aortic insufficiency at the follow-up study (compared with prevalvuloplasty insufficiency). The degree of

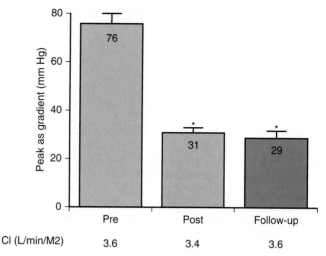

Figure 56-16. Peak systolic pressure gradient determined at cardiac catheterization before (PRE) and immediately after (POST) valvuloplasty and at follow-up catheterization 1.7 years later in 27 children who underwent balloon dilation for congenital aortic stenosis. (From O'Connor BK, Beekman RH, Rocchini AP, Rosenthal A: Intermediate-term effectiveness of balloon valvuloplasty for congenital aortic stenosis: A prospective follow-up study. Circulation 1991;84:732-738.)

the aortic insufficiency after valvuloplasty remained stable during the follow-up period in four of these seven patients and increased by one to two grades in the remaining three patients.

Galal and colleagues reported the results of 3- to 9-year follow-up of 26 patients who had balloon aortic valvuloplasty at ages ranging from 6 weeks to 20 years.[60] Restenosis requiring reintervention occurred within 2 years in 23% of the group, and actuarial reintervention-free survival was 76%. Neonates with critical aortic stenosis appear to have a substantially higher risk of restenosis and progressive aortic insufficiency after balloon valvuloplasty: Reintervention-free survival has been approximately 50% at 5 years,[54-56] with aortic valve replacement or surgical repair of aortic insufficiency required in approximately 50% of patients by 10 years.[54,56]

Complications

Percutaneous balloon aortic valvuloplasty is a relatively safe procedure, with rare mortality outside of early infancy. The Pediatric Valvuloplasty Registry[35] described five deaths, four in the neonatal period and one in a critically ill 3-month-old. Early mortality after balloon valvuloplasty in neonates has ranged from 13% to 18%; appreciable late mortality has also been observed in these series, with 5-year survival rates of 72% to 83%.[54-56] These data compare favorably with the surgical experience, in which morbidity and mortality rates have been relatively high in neonates with critical aortic stenosis. Other complications reported in the Pediatric Valvuloplasty Registry included potentially life-threatening arrhythmias in three infants, perforation of the left ventricle requiring surgery, and a mitral valve tear also requiring surgical repair.

Valvuloplasty-induced aortic valve insufficiency may be the most significant complication of the procedure. In our experience, valve insufficiency occurs in approximately 24% of patients and is mild in most. Moderate to severe aortic insufficiency may be induced by balloon valvuloplasty in approximately 3% to 6% of patients and is more common if the balloon-to-annulus diameter ratio exceeds 1.0. Surgical techniques allowing repair rather than replacement of balloon-damaged valves have been a welcome development.[66] Femoral artery injury, thrombosis, or occlusion has been relatively common in the past, particularly in infants. In the Pediatric Valvuloplasty Registry, femoral artery injury was reported in 12% of children, most of whom were younger than 12 months of age.[44] In our follow-up evaluation,[65] femoral artery occlusion or stenosis was observed in 3 of 5 children younger than 12 months of age, compared with only 1 of 22 children older than 12 months of age at the time of the valvuloplasty procedure ($P=.01$). Since 1988, when lower-profile catheters became available, femoral artery injury has become much less common.[67] We prefer not to exceed a 4-Fr exit profile in neonatal femoral arteries and to use the transumbilical approach for neonatal critical aortic stenosis if possible. Because future transfemoral valvuloplasty procedures (for restenosis) are likely to be necessary in these patients, femoral artery access should be preserved if at all possible.

Conclusions and Recommendations

Percutaneous balloon aortic valvuloplasty provides effective palliative treatment for children and young adults with congenital valvar aortic stenosis. Valvuloplasty successfully reduces the peak systolic aortic stenosis gradient to the range of 20 to 40 mm Hg, which compares favorably with open surgical valvotomy. Aortic insufficiency is not increased from its prevalvuloplasty status in most patients. Aortic insufficiency is produced in approximately 20% to 25% of patients but is mild in most of these cases. Mortality has been limited to critically ill neonates and young infants. Follow-up studies have documented early restenosis to be uncommon, but long-term investigations are lacking.

Balloon valvuloplasty is an excellent therapeutic option for most patients with congenital aortic valve stenosis. At most pediatric cardiology centers, it is the treatment of choice. We recommend balloon valvuloplasty for patients whose resting peak systolic pressure gradient exceeds 65 mm Hg, for those with a resting peak gradient of 50 to 65 mm Hg in association with ischemic changes or symptoms, and for those patients with heart failure and low cardiac output regardless of gradient. Balloon valvuloplasty is effective in neonates, children, and young adults with congenital aortic valve stenosis in whom commissural fusion is the primary anatomic cause of outflow obstruction. The procedure is less likely to be effective in patients with a hypoplastic valve annulus or with valve leaflet calcification.

BALLOON-EXPANDABLE STENTING FOR PULMONARY ARTERY STENOSIS

Pulmonary artery stenosis occurs commonly in patients with congenital heart disease. It is encountered as an isolated lesion in patients with the Williams or Alagille syndrome or as a feature of complex congenital heart disease such as tetralogy of Fallot with or without pulmonary atresia. Balloon angioplasty of pulmonary artery stenosis or hypoplasia has yielded mixed results. Numerous reports have documented an immediate success rate of only 50% to 60% after balloon angioplasty of this lesion.[68,69] Failure of angioplasty is often related to elastic recoil of the pulmonary artery. Follow-up studies show that the long-term success rate is even lower after angioplasty alone.[70] These observations led to the evaluation of balloon-expandable stents to treat peripheral pulmonary artery stenosis or hypoplasia. During the past decade, stenting has become the initial treatment of choice for many patients with pulmonary artery stenosis, and numerous reports have documented a substantial therapeutic advantage compared with angioplasty alone.

Animal Studies

Balloon-expandable stents have been evaluated in experimental animal models of pulmonary artery stenosis. Benson and coworkers[71,72] implanted a balloon-expandable stent (Palmaz P-308; Johnson & Johnson, Warren, NJ) into the left pulmonary artery of nine pigs with a surgically created pulmonary artery stenosis. The diameter of the pulmonary artery stenosis increased from an average of 3.9 to 8.3 mm, and the mean pressure gradient decreased from 7 to 1 mm Hg. Follow-up catheterization studies 3 weeks and 3.5 months later documented no restenosis and no thrombosis, aneurysm formation, or obstruction to arterial side-branch vessels. Histologic evaluation (approximately 3 months after implantation) documented virtually complete stent coverage with a neointima composed of fibroblasts, and medial compression with mild fibrosis beneath the stent wires. Scanning electron microscopy disclosed the presence of a thin layer of neoendothelial cells covering the stent arms, with the exception of areas overlying arterial side branches, where stents remain uncovered and side-branch vessels patent.

Our animal studies also documented the effectiveness of balloon-expandable stainless-steel stents (Palmaz P-308) in dogs with experimental pulmonary artery stenosis.[73] Follow-up cardiac catheterization 6 months after stent placement documented persistent relief of stenosis, with no thrombosis, aneurysm formation, or compromise of flow to arterial side-branch vessels. We also evaluated the feasibility and effectiveness of stent redilation in an experimental model of left pulmonary artery stenosis.[74] Six 3- to 4-month-

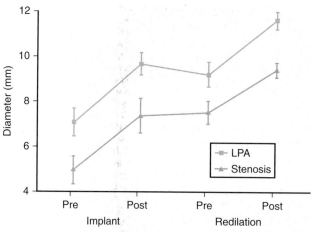

Figure 56-17. Effectiveness of stent redilation for experimental left pulmonary artery (LPA) stenosis in six puppies. Diameters were measured before (PRE) and after (POST) implantation of a Palmaz P-308 stent, and before and after stent redilation 4 months later. The stenosis increased initially from 4.8 to 7.4 mm and increased further on redilation to 9.2 mm. The more proximal LPA increased initially from 7.3 to 9.6 mm and increased further on redilation to 11.5 mm. Values shown represent means ±1 standard error.

old puppies underwent stent implantation (Palmaz P-308), using an 8- to 10-mm balloon, at the site of a surgically created stenosis in the left pulmonary artery. The vessel diameter at the stenosis increased from 4.8 to 7.4 mm, and the diameter of the proximal stented left pulmonary artery increased from 7.3 to 9.6 mm (Fig. 56-17). Four months after stent implantation, when the puppies had increased in weight by 54%, each stent was redilated to a larger diameter using a 12-mm angioplasty balloon. Redilation was effective, with the stenosis diameter increasing from 7.4 to 9.2 mm and the proximal stented portion of the vessel enlarging from 9.2 to 11.5 mm. Redilation caused the stents to shorten from 27.4 to 25.7 mm (initial preimplantation length was 30 mm). Acute examination of two redilated stents documented small, 1- to 3-mm linear tears in the neointima. Gross examination of specimens 1 month after redilation in the four remaining animals revealed an intact neointima without restenosis, intimal tears, aneurysm formation, or obstruction of side-branch arteries. In one specimen, a small organized thrombus was found on the proximal portion of a stent that protruded freely into the main pulmonary artery. These experimental data suggest that pulmonary artery stents can be safely and effectively redilated after they have been in place for up to 4 months.

Clinical Studies

Most clinical studies of pulmonary artery stenting have used the Palmaz or Palmaz-Genesis (Johnson & Johnson) stainless-steel balloon-expandable stents (Figs. 56-18 and 56-19).[75-79] In their 1991 landmark study, O'Laughlin and colleagues reported the acute

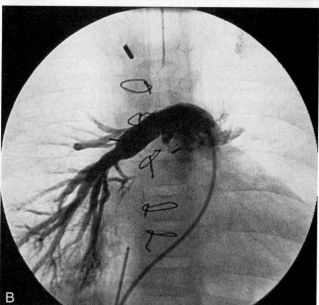

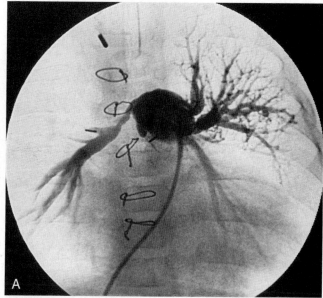

Figure 56-18. Anteroposterior pulmonary artery angiograms before (**A**) and after (**B**) right pulmonary artery stenting in a 6-month-old infant after repair of pulmonary atresia and ventricular septal defect. There is severe proximal right pulmonary artery stenosis before stenting. After stent implantation, the stenosis is relieved and distal pulmonary artery flow is improved.

and short-term follow-up results of 31 stent implantations in 23 patients with pulmonary artery stenosis.[75] Stenoses and vessels were documented to be dilatable by balloon inflation before stent implantation. The stent was then delivered through an 11- or 12-Fr sheath and implanted with a 10- to 12-mm diameter balloon. Stent implantation increased pulmonary artery diameter from 4.6 to 10.9 mm acutely, with a decrease in the stenosis gradient from 51 to 16 mm Hg. Follow-up catheterization in six patients, 3 to 9 months after stent implantation, demonstrated no change in the appearance of the stented vessel

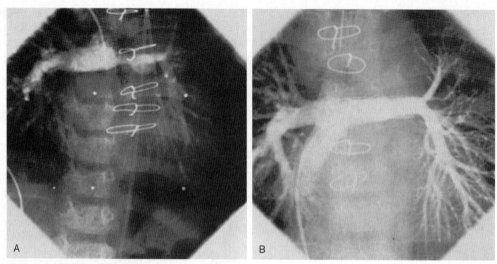

Figure 56-19. Anteroposterior pulmonary artery angiograms from a 1-year-old child with hypoplastic left heart syndrome and left pulmonary artery hypoplasia. Angiography before stenting (**A**) demonstrates diffuse hypoplasia of the proximal left and central pulmonary artery, which measured 4 mm in diameter. Intraoperative stenting of the left pulmonary artery was performed in conjunction with a Fontan operation. Angiography 6 months later (**B**) documents patency of the left pulmonary artery, which now measures 10 to 11 mm in diameter. There is a thin neointima within the stent.

and no restenosis or late thrombus formation. A multi-institutional study of percutaneous stenting in the pediatric population was reported by the same investigators in 1993.[78] A total of 121 Palmaz stents, 80 for branch pulmonary artery stenosis, were implanted in 85 patients, in whom the most common diagnosis was postoperative tetralogy of Fallot. In this series, stenting resulted in an increase in pulmonary artery diameter, from 4.6 to 11.3 mm, with immediate hemodynamic improvement with a decrease in RV systolic pressure. A follow-up cardiac catheterization was performed in 25 patients 8 months after stenting, and restenosis was identified in only 1 patient. These data indicated that pulmonary artery stenting was more effective than balloon angioplasty alone for most cases of pulmonary artery stenosis or hypoplasia.

In 1995, Fogelman and colleagues[79] demonstrated the clinical benefits derived from pulmonary artery stenting in children with pulmonary artery stenosis. In this large, single-institution series, the pulmonary artery stenting was shown to result in important hemodynamic improvement, alleviation of symptoms, and deferral of surgical reintervention in many patients. The largest series of pulmonary artery stenting in children was reported by McMahon and colleagues in 2002.[80] Over a 12-year period, 664 Palmaz stents were implanted in 338 patients, most of whom had undergone tetralogy of Fallot repair. The mean systolic pressure gradient across the stenosis decreased from 41 to 9 mm Hg, and the mean pulmonary artery diameter of the stented vessel increased from 5.4 to 11.2 mm. At a follow-up of 5.6 years, the pulmonary artery systolic gradient averaged 20 mm Hg and the vessel diameter was 9.3 mm. Morbidity and mortality decreased significantly during the second half of this

series, with improved techniques and increased experience.

When pulmonary artery stents are implanted in growing children, it is important that they can be safely and effectively redilated to a larger diameter as the child grows. Reports from several institutions have confirmed the experimental observations that pulmonary artery stents can be safely redilated to a larger diameter when required because of somatic growth.[78,79,81-83] In 2003, Duke and colleagues[83] reported safe and effective stent redilation in 12 children with branch pulmonary artery stenosis. Redilation was required because of a combination of patient growth and neointimal ingrowth within the stents. Redilation increased pulmonary artery stent diameter from 6.9 to 8.8 mm, with an associated decrease in systolic gradient from 24 to 12 mm Hg. A significant tear occurred in one distal pulmonary artery vessel. The authors concluded that redilation of pulmonary artery stents is effective and relatively safe.[83]

Conclusions and Recommendations

Experimental and clinical data from several centers indicate that balloon-expandable stenting provides an effective form of therapy for many patients with pulmonary artery hypoplasia or stenosis. Because balloon angioplasty alone is unsuccessful in as many as 50% to 60% of patients, stenting is now considered standard first-line therapy for most children with pulmonary artery stenosis. For infants and small children, in whom larger stents are difficult to implant, we often prefer balloon angioplasty alone in an attempt to avoid implanting smaller stents that have limited potential for increasing the diameter with growth.

BALLOON-EXPANDABLE STENTING FOR COARCTATION OF THE AORTA

Coarctation of the aorta accounts for 8% to 10% of all congenital heart disease. Since the 1940s, surgical repair has been a conventional therapy for patients with a native (unoperated) or recurrent postoperative coarctation. Balloon angioplasty of native and recurrent coarctation has been available since the mid-1980s, but its effectiveness has been diminished by restenosis (15% to 20% of patients) and aneurysm formation (approximately 5% of patients). Therefore, balloon-expandable stenting has emerged as a promising transcatheter therapy for coarctation. The stent's radial strength opposes elastic aortic wall recoil and may improve vessel integrity, thereby decreasing the risk of aneurysm formation at the dilation site.

Animal Studies

In 1993, we reported the acute effectiveness of balloon-expandable stenting in six dogs with an experimental coarctation.[84] Transcatheter stenting was performed successfully in six animals 2 months after surgical creation of a discrete thoracic coarctation. A follow-up study 1 to 1.5 months after stent implantation documented an excellent early result. There was no restenosis, stent thrombosis, aneurysm formation, or stent migration. Evaluation of explanted segments of the stented aorta demonstrated that the stents were thoroughly covered by a neointima composed of intimal cells with fibrosis and an endothelial cell surface (Fig. 56-20). Neointima coverage was absent only where side-branch arteries, such as intercostals, arose from the aorta. Morrow and colleagues[85] reported similar data in a study of stent implantation for experimental coarctation in 10 juvenile swine. Specimens were examined by light microscopy and scanning electron microscopy approximately 2 months after stent implantation. A neointima was observed covering the stent wherever the stent struts were in contact with the aortic wall. Compression of the underlying media was observed immediately under the struts, but without dissection.

As is the case with stent implantation in pulmonary arteries of children, stents implanted in the aorta of growing children may require redilation after a period of somatic growth. There are limited animal data to document effectiveness and safety of coarctation stent redilation. In 1996, our group[74] reported data in a small experimental study of coarctation stent redilation. An experimental coarctation was surgically created in eight puppies, and stent implantation (Palmaz P-308) was performed at 2 to 3 months. Stent redilation was subsequently performed after 6 to 10 months in seven animals, increasing the stenosis diameter from 9.8 to 13.5 mm. Redilation was effective in five animals, but aortic rupture through the stent resulted in death of two animals. In contrast, Morrow's group reported data on aortic stent redilation in two experimental studies with relative safety and no acute animal deaths.[85,86]

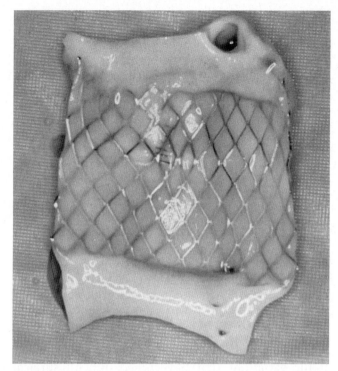

Figure 56-20. Aortic stent explanted 6 weeks after stenting of an experimental coarctation in a canine model. The Palmaz P-308 stent is almost completely covered with a thin layer of neointima. The sutures used to create the experimental coarctation are evident.

Clinical Studies

Clinical studies documenting the effectiveness of transcatheter stenting in patients with coarctation of the aorta are relatively recent and limited in number.[87-93] Nevertheless, the technique appears to be quite effective and has been applied with increasing frequency in recent years in many centers. Stent therapy can be applied to patients with a native unoperated coarctation or to those with a recurrent postoperative coarctation with equal effectiveness. Most interventionalists have attempted to limit stenting to older children and adolescents, to minimize the need for later stent redilation after somatic growth has occurred. In most reported series, the Palmaz or Palmaz-Genesis stainless steel balloon-expandable stent has been used. More recently, use of the covered CP platinum stent has been reported; it may be particularly effective for stenting of complex coarctation anatomy or in patients with advanced age, in whom the aortic wall may be more fragile.[94]

Suarez deLezo and colleagues reported one of the larger early clinical series of coarctation stenting.[88] In their series, stainless steel Palmaz balloon-expandable stents were implanted in 48 patients with a coarctation of the aorta. The average patient age at implantation was 14 years. Follow-up cardiac catheterization was performed in 30 patients 2 years after stent implantation. The authors documented excellent relief of stenosis, with a residual systolic coarctation gradient of 3 mm Hg at follow-up. Twenty-seven percent of patients had a mild degree of neointimal ingrowth within the stent noted by angiography, but there was no clinical need for stent redilation at the 2-year follow-up study. A small aneurysm at the stent site was identified in two patients (7%), and in both cases the aneurysm was occluded by coil implantation through the stent. More recently, Harrison and colleagues[91] reported outcomes after coarctation stenting in 27 adolescent and adult patients. At follow-up evaluation 1.8 years after stent implantation, the clinical systolic gradient was 4 mm Hg, and nine patients had been weaned from antihypertension drugs. In this series, stenting complications included a cerebrovascular accident in one patient and an aortic aneurysm at the stent site in three patients (11%). Aortic dissection has also been reported as a rare complication of coarctation stenting, and it appears to be more common when coarctation is stented in elderly patients.[95]

Transcatheter stent therapy for coarctation may also provide a reasonable treatment strategy for anatomic variations that have posed difficult surgical dilemmas in the past. For example, hypoplasia of the transverse aortic arch is responsible for residual obstruction in a small proportion of patients after surgical repair of coarctation. These lesions may be difficult to manage surgically, because the operative procedure often requires a period of hypothermic circulatory arrest. Pihkala and colleagues[96] reported the successful use of stent therapy in four children with transverse arch hypoplasia after surgical coarctation repair. The procedure was successful in all four children, with anatomic and hemodynamic relief of arch obstruction. We have also used stenting in several infants with complex aortic arch obstruction after the Norwood operation for hypoplastic left heart syndrome (Fig. 56-21). In these infants, a relatively large stent (Palmaz P-188, Palmaz P-308, or Palmaz-Genesis 1910) was implanted via a right carotid cutdown and successfully relieved important arch obstruction. The carotid cutdown approach was used to avoid potential femoral artery injury associated with the relatively large sheath (8 Fr) required to deliver such stents.

Mild coarctation (i.e., resting systolic gradient <20 mm Hg) also posed a therapeutic dilemma in the past, because it was often thought that the benefits did not outweigh the risks of surgery, which may require partial bypass because of poorly developed collateral circulation with mild coarctation. Nevertheless, more recent data suggest that mild coarctation (Fig. 56-22) may be associated with long-term rest and exercise hypertension and perhaps left ventricular hypertrophy and diastolic dysfunction. Marshall and colleagues[89] reported the results of stent treatment in 33 patients, many of whom had a mild coarctation by traditional criteria. Stent implantation decreased the systolic gradient from 25 mm Hg to 5 mm Hg. At follow-up catheterization, left

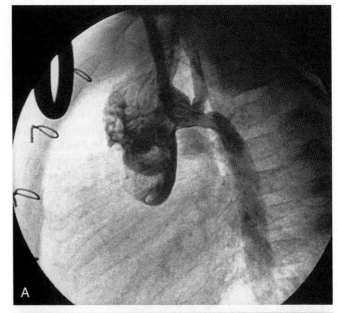

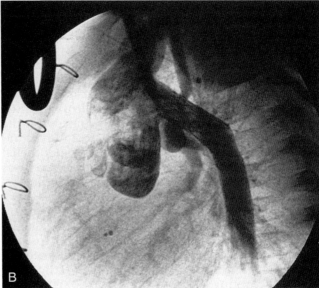

Figure 56-21. Lateral aortic angiogram in a 3-month-old infant with hypoplastic left heart syndrome and aortic arch obstruction after a Norwood procedure. Angiography before stenting (**A**) demonstrates moderate arch stenosis adjacent to the origin of the left subclavian artery. The systolic pressure gradient was 34 mm Hg. Angiography after stenting (**B**) through a right carotid cutdown demonstrates resolution of the stenosis, with maintenance of flow to the left subclavian artery. The pressure gradient was eliminated.

ventricular end-diastolic pressure had decreased from 17 mm Hg to 14 mm Hg, suggesting an improvement in diastolic function. These data suggest that nonsurgical intervention for even mild degrees of coarctation may have beneficial effects on cardiovascular function. Larger clinical studies, with longer follow-up and more sensitive measures of ventricular function, are required to determine the true benefit of coarctation stenting for such patients.

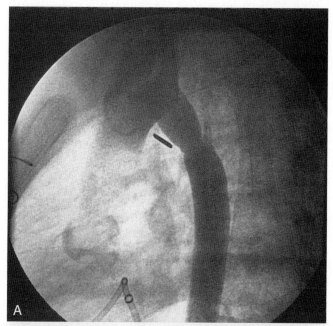

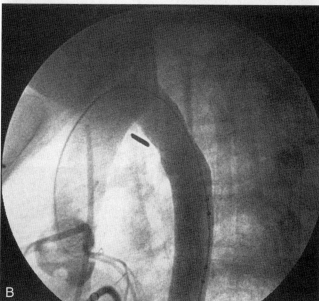

Figure 56-22. Lateral aortic angiograms in a 13-year-old child with mild residual coarctation after surgical repair during infancy. A 15 mm Hg resting systolic gradient was present before stenting (**A**), and there was an elevated left ventricular end-diastolic pressure. After percutaneous stenting with a Palmaz P-308 stent (**B**), the systolic pressure gradient was eliminated.

Conclusions and Recommendations

Coarctation stenting is a relatively new nonsurgical approach to native and postoperative recurrent coarctation of the aorta. Most pediatric interventionalists limit stent implantation to large children and adolescents, to avoid the need for aortic stent redilation as a smaller child grows. Stent implantation is a promising intervention for more difficult variations on coarctation anatomy, particularly transverse arch

hypoplasia, arch obstruction after the Norwood operation, and mild degrees of coarctation that have not warranted surgery in the past. In older adults in whom the aortic wall is friable, covered stents may provide a safer alternative because of the risk of aortic dissection with coarctation dilation. Longer-term follow-up studies are necessary to more precisely define the late risks of stent restenosis, aortic aneurysm formation, safety of late stent redilation after somatic growth in children, and blood pressure response to exercise in the face of a rigid, stented aortic segment.

TRANSCATHETER CLOSURE OF SECUNDUM ATRIAL SEPTAL DEFECTS

ASDs result from deficient development of the intra-atrial septum. The exact position of the defect is determined by the specific area that fails to develop and is traditionally described in anatomic terms. Sinus venosus defects result from abnormal development of either the superior or the inferior horns of the sinus venosus and are located superiorly or inferiorly along the posterior margin of the atrial septum. Superior sinus venosus defects frequently have associated anomalous drainage of the right upper pulmonary vein. Primum ASDs result from deficiencies of the septum secundum, frequently as part of the complex of maldevelopment of the endocardial cushions (atrioventricular canal [AVC] defects). In the most severe form (complete AVC), the primum defect is part of a complex that also includes an inlet ventricular septal defect (VSD) and a common atrioventricular valve. In the least severe form, the primum ASD defect is associated with a cleft in the anterior mitral valve leaflet. Secundum ASDs result from deficiencies of the central portion of the atrial septum, the septum primum. These defects, usually in the region of the fossa ovalis, may be extensive in size, are varied in shape, and are often multiple in number (fenestrated atrial septum). It is secundum-type defects, often with substantial peridefect margins and positioned some distance from other vital structures, that lend themselves well to percutaneous device closure. Further discussion in this section focuses on secundum ASDs.

Physiology

ASDs represent one of the most common forms of isolated acyanotic congenital heart disease.[97] Whereas the left atrial pressure is typically higher than that in the right atrium, flow across the atrial septum is determined in large part by the end-diastolic pressure within each ventricle, which in turn is reflective of relative ventricular compliance. The net size of the atrial-level shunt is therefore only in part dependent on the size of the ASD. It is also important to realize that abnormal elevation of either left or RV systolic pressure in the face of ventricular outflow tract obstruction will not affect atrial-level shunting if ventricular relaxation is not adversely affected.

With persistence of atrial-level shunting, the right atrial and ventricular end-diastolic volumes are chronically increased. The atrial and ventricular dimensions increase to accommodate the additional atrial-level shunt, adding to the normal atrial volume resulting from systemic venous return.[97] Additional RV volume results, first, in delayed pulmonary valve closure compared with the aortic valve (causing the clinical sign of the fixed, split second heart sound) and a flow murmur across a normal pulmonary valve (identical to that of pathologic pulmonary valve stenosis, but without an ejection click).[98] The additional pulmonary blood flow is well tolerated in most cases, but can lead to pulmonary hypertension and pulmonary vascular occlusive disease in rare cases. Ultimately, Eisenmenger-type physiology prevails, at which point shunt flow is right-to-left, and the patient becomes cyanotic.[99-101] That pathologic end point should not be confused with right-to-left shunting that results from a decrease in RV compliance with long-standing RV dilation. This latter scenario carries a substantially better prognosis than pulmonary vascular occlusive disease, and it can be diagnosed either on the basis of relatively normal RV and pulmonary artery pressures, as determined by echocardiography, or at cardiac catheterization.

Clinical Presentation and Diagnosis

ASDs typically cause no symptoms during the first 2 decades of life. Diagnosis is most often made after detection of a murmur, indistinguishable from that of pulmonary valve stenosis, or with auscultation of a fixed, split second heart sound.[98] Infrequently, infants or children present with failure to thrive or other more overt signs of congestive heart failure, or with recurrent lower respiratory tract infections. Later, in the third and fourth decades, if previously undiagnosed, symptoms may include undue fatigue, increased dyspnea on exertion, and a frequent sensation of palpitations.[97,101]

The electrocardiogram (ECG) may be normal early in childhood, or at any age if right atrial enlargement or RV dilation has not yet occurred. As those changes progress over time, typical ECG changes with right axis deviation, right atrial enlargement and RV dilation become more clearly apparent. Echocardiography, either transthoracic (TTE) or transesophageal (TEE), remains the mainstay of diagnosis.[102] In standard long-axis views, the first evidence of an ASD may be dilation of the anteriorly located RV. In short-axis views, that dilation may again be noted, especially in the region of the infundibulum. In four-chamber views, both the right atrium and the RV are seen to be dilated. However, the ASD is best seen and evaluated from the subcostal views, in both long and short axis. These views allow for complete evaluation of the total septal length and provide excellent visualization of the defect margins. Color flow mapping is of great importance. This allows determination of the direction of flow across the defect (left-to-right versus right-to-left) and provides further assessment to exclude the possibility of multiple defects (Fig. 56-23). Occasionally, poor acoustic windows may preclude clear TTE images. This is more likely in the adult patient or in the presence of obesity. At those times, elective TEE can be performed to confirm the diagnosis of an ASD, before further discussion regarding possible defect closure and repair.[103]

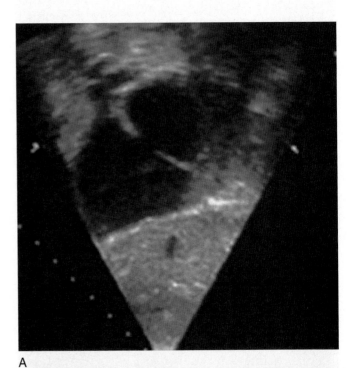

A

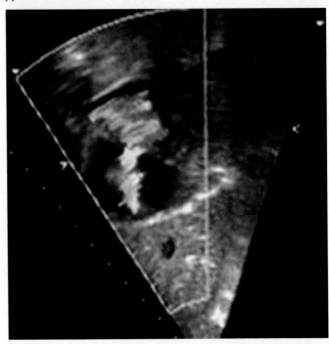

B

Figure 56-23. Subcostal short-axis transthoracic echocardiographic images showing a secundum atrial septal defect in two dimensions (**A**) and with color-flow mapping (**B**). The defect is central in the septum and has excellent margins for device support.

Echocardiography is also invaluable in achieving a noninvasive measure of RV and pulmonary artery pressures. Excessive elevation of right-sided pressures should introduce some caution before proceeding with defect repair, especially if there is color flow evidence of right-to-left shunting across the ASD.

Treatment and Outcomes

Surgical repair has long been the mainstay of treatment for ASDs.[100,101,104] However, over the last decade, substantial advances have been made with percutaneous closure devices. At this time, percutaneous closure of secundum ASDs is considered the standard of care.[105-107] Currently in the United States, two devices are approved for use by the Food and Drug Administration (FDA): the Amplatzer Septal Occluder (AGA Medical, Golden Valley, MN) and the Helix Septal Occluder (W. L. Gore and Associates, Flagstaff, AZ).[108,109] Although the two devices are different in design and construction, the principles of function, deployment, and follow-up are similar (Figs. 56-24 and 56-25). After deployment, both devices are designed to have two discs separated by a central core or waist. One disc is positioned on the left atrial side of the defect, with the core or waist straddling the defect, and the other disc is opposed to the atrial membrane from the right atrial side of the atrial septum. The devices have intrinsic recoil that opposes both discs to each other, holding the devices in place on the atrial septum.

Irrespective of the device used, defect sizing is required before deployment. Reliance may be made on the TTE measurements with an empiric factor adjustment (e.g., 115% of the TTE measurement).

However, most operators continue to rely on balloon sizing of the defect before choosing a particular sized device.[106,107] That is accomplished with a large, compliant balloon inflated across the atrial septum, with the narrowest area ("stretched diameter" or "waist") measured with angiographic calibration (Fig. 56-26). A device is then chosen accordingly. Irrespective of the measurements, it is imperative to ensure that the margins of both the left and right atrial discs are sufficiently large that, once deployed, the device will remain stable on the atrial septum, but not so large that other vital cardiac structures (e.g., pulmonary veins, coronary sinus, atrioventricular valves) are impinged upon.

Both devices are deployed though a delivery sheath that typically extends from the femoral region, although other access sites have been used. The left atrial disc is initially deployed, and the device is retracted back onto the atrial septum. The remainder of the device is then deployed within the right atrium, so that the waist or core of the device straddles the defect. The delivery cable remains attached to the device until the time of release and can be used to retract the device if positioning is not acceptable (Figs. 56-27). Even after release, the devices can be retrieved with various intravascular snares if necessary.

To ensure adequate device deployment, echocardiographic imaging is used in addition to fluoroscopy.[102] The majority of pediatric institutions continue to use TEE, but intracardiac echocardiog-

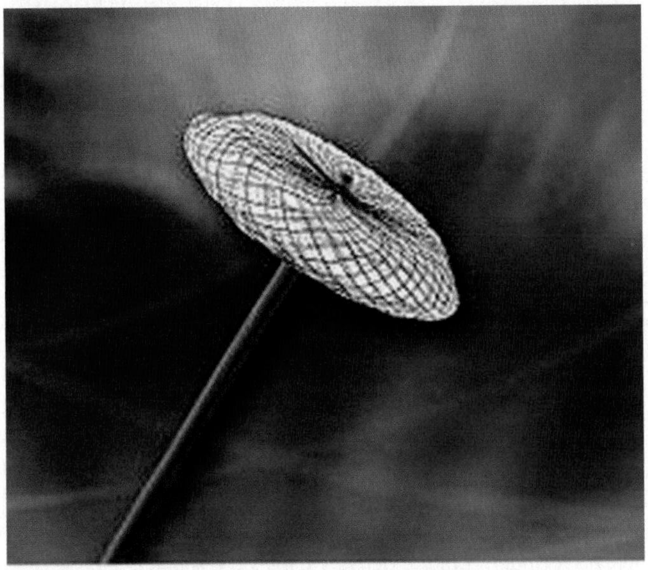

Figure 56-24. Amplatzer Septal Occluder. The device is constructed from an alloy of nickel and titanium. The two atrial discs are separated by the central waist. In this photograph, the tethering cable, covered by the delivery sheath, remains attached to the device. (Courtesy of AGA Medical.)

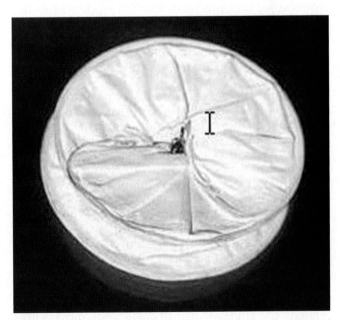

Figure 56-25. The Helix Septal Occluder. The device is composed of a nickel-titanium wire with a patch of microporous expanded polytetrafluoroethylene attached along its length. The elastic properties of the wire form the device into two equal-size opposing disks that reside on either side of the atrial septum after deployment, thus occluding the defect. (Courtesy of W. L. Gore and Associates.)

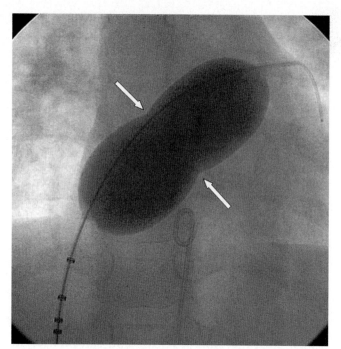

Figure 56-26. Still frame of an angiogram demonstrating inflation of the balloon sizing catheter across the atrial septum. The indentations on the balloon (*white arrows*) indicate the stretched margin of the atrial septal defect. That diameter is measured, and an appropriate-sized septal occluder is chosen accordingly.

raphy (ICE) has increased in popularity. This avoids the necessity of general anesthesia in most patients, but an additional 9-Fr femoral venous access site is required for positioning of the ICE probe within the right atrium. Deployment of the devices using echocardiography alone has also been described.[103] Three-dimensional echocardiographic evaluation has been used, but the advantage of this modality is still unclear.

Percutaneous device closure has proved effective in the repair of ASDs, with minimal morbidity and essentially no mortality. Closure rates are comparable to those of surgery over similar time periods (97% to 99% at 12 months), but procedural morbidity is considerably lower.[105,110] Percutaneous closure avoids the necessity of a sternotomy, cardiopulmonary bypass, and mediastinal and chest-tube drainage, but it does have the disadvantage of limited exposure to ionizing radiation. Fluoroscopy times are brief (<4 minutes), and low-dose adjustments can be used. The risk of device embolization is small and in most cases is related to operator inexperience. The incidence of this complication is approximately 0.1%.[106,107] The majority of acute complications have been related to rhythm disturbances, in most cases atrial flutter or intermittent supraventricular tachyarrhythmia. However, these complications are also rare, occurring less than 1% of the time. Thrombus formation on the device, with subsequent distal embolization, is of great concern, justifying the recommendation for aspirin therapy until device

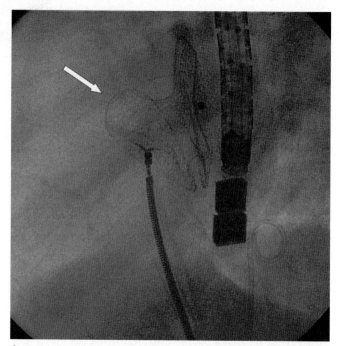

A

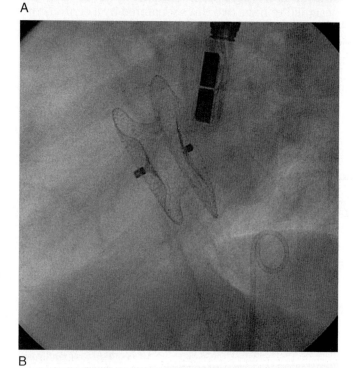

B

Figure 56-27. A, Still frame from an angiogram demonstrates full deployment of an Amplatzer Septal Occluder with the tethering cable still attached. Distortion of the superior margin of the right atrial disc of the device (*solid white arrow*), resulting from downward tension by the delivery cable, is typical at this point of deployment. Retraction and redeployment of the device is easily achieved while it is still attached to the delivery cable. A transesophageal echocardiographic probe is noted in the image. **B,** Still frame from an angiogram after release of the Amplatzer Septal Occluder from the delivery cable. The septal occluder immediately assumes the typical position, with the right and left atrial discs parallel to each other.

endothelialization has occurred.[111] Collective review of this potential problem, including evaluation of various generations of early septal occluder devices, reveals a low incidence (54 patients over a 14-year period).

Cardiac erosion with possible hemodynamic compromise, particularly by the Amplatzer Septal Occluder, is the most significant short- and long-term complication of percutaneous ASD closure.[112,113] The incidence appears to be low (<0.11%), according to both the manufacturer and published data, and in most cases is related to device oversizing. An oversized device causes aortic compression of the waist at the superior rim, which in turn stretches the atrial free wall over the device discs, causing erosion at the superior/aortic rim area. The presence of this complication has altered follow-up, with the general recommendation to obtain an echocardiogram within 24 hours of implantation to rule out the presence of a pericardial effusion.

Follow-Up

After device implantation, patients should remain on aspirin therapy for at least 6 months, during which time complete device endothelialization occurs. Subacute bacterial endocarditis prophylaxis is also recommended during that period and should be continued if residual atrial-level shunting is apparent at the time of the echocardiogram at 6 months. After that, follow-up should be at least on an annual basis, with echocardiography obtained during those visits. The right atrial and RV dimensions return to normal within 6 months if no significant atrial-level shunting remains.[114]

TRANSCATHETER CLOSURE OF PATENT DUCTUS ARTERIOSUS

The ductus arteriosus is a muscular artery that extends from the roof of the main pulmonary artery to the undersurface of the aortic arch. Although some degree of anatomic variation does occur (such as with a right aortic arch, where the ductus passes from the main pulmonary artery to the base of the left innominate artery), the relationship is generally consistent. It provides a vital function during fetal life, allowing blood that has entered the main pulmonary artery via the RV to be redirected away from the lungs and into the aorta. At birth, with an increase in arterial oxygen content and a decrease in circulating prostaglandins, the ductus arteriosus spasms and later becomes fibrotic, with permanent closure. This occurs usually by 5 to 7 days in full-term infants. Persistence of the ductus arteriosus after that time occurs in 1 of every 2500 to 5000 live births.[115,116] After closure, the ductus arteriosus has no further significance, unless a right aortic arch with an aberrant left subclavian artery is present, in which case a vascular ring could prove clinically significant.

Physiology

Discussion regarding the influence of the PDA on the physiology of the neonate, particularly with regard to prematurity and hyaline membrane disease, is beyond the scope of this text. This discussion here is confined to the effect of the PDA on older children and adults, in whom the impact is similar.

The main factors contributing to the effects of a PDA are the size of the vessel and the relative resistance between the systemic and pulmonary vascular beds. If the PDA is small, the hemodynamic effect is negligible, with flow occurring only during systole, and is limited by the resistance of flow through the narrow ductus. As the PDA increases in size, flow through the PDA continues to be left-to-right as long as the pulmonary vascular resistance is lower than that of the systemic vascular bed, even in the presence of a completely unrestrictive vessel. Under those circumstances, pulmonary artery pressures are equal to aortic, and the flow is left-to-right during both systole and diastole. With persistent shunting through a large ductus, the left atrium and ventricle become increasingly volume loaded and dilated. Further, because of this increased runoff into a lower-resistance pulmonary vascular bed, the aortic pulse pressure (difference between aortic systolic and diastolic pressures) widens considerably. With continued left ventricular dilation, wall stress and end-diastolic pressures continue to increase, in turn increasing myocardial oxygen requirement. With the decrease in aortic diastolic pressure, coronary perfusion pressure can at times become narrowed. However, although this is theoretically important, it is usually of little clinical concern, and the presence of coronary ischemia with only an isolated PDA has not been described.

Similar to other shunt lesions that expose the pulmonary vascular bed to persistently high pressure and flow situations, large PDAs ultimately result in the development of pulmonary vascular occlusive disease.[117] At that time, the flow direction across the PDA reverses, and Eisenmenger physiology prevails.[118] Development of those changes depends on the size of the duct and the duration of its presence, resistance to flow across the vessel, and individual patient susceptibility.

Clinical Presentation and Diagnosis

In infancy and childhood, the clinical presentation of PDA varies, from completely asymptomatic through to the full spectrum of congestive heart failure. Symptoms may be completely absent, but could include failure to thrive, dyspnea, poor feeding, and excessive perspiration. In older children, adolescents, and adults, congestive symptoms are less likely. It is not uncommon for the diagnosis to be suspected when an incidental murmur is heard during a well-child examination. Rarely, patients who have not been diagnosed in infancy may present with symptoms of endocarditis or pulmonary vascular occlusive disease if the PDA is sufficiently unrestrictive.[119]

Clinical signs may be absent if the PDA is small and hemodynamically insignificant. However, with increasing size of the PDA, more typical clinical features become apparent. The pulse pressure may be wider than expected (by palpation and blood pressure measurement), and a murmur of variable grade and duration may be auscultated. If the PDA is small, flow may occur only during systole, and a systolic regurgitant murmur is present. In the larger PDA, flow occurs throughout the entire cardiac cycle, and the more typical multiphasic continuous machinery murmur is present. As with all left-to-right shunt lesions, if flow is substantial, a mid-diastolic tricuspid flow murmur may also be audible. These clinical features remain the same if the PDA is sufficiently stenotic. However, if the PDA offers little resistance to flow and pulmonary artery pressures remain significantly elevated over time, the murmur may become diminished and disappear altogether as pulmonary vascular resistance increases to systemic levels. At that point, with Eisenmenger physiology present, flow across the PDA becomes right-to-left, and measured oxygen saturations in the lower extremities are lower than those in the upper extremities.[120]

Confirmation of the diagnosis relies on echocardiography. The PDA is well seen in many different views, but the parasternal short-axis view, immediately above the level of the pulmonary valve, is ideal. If the PDA is small, two-dimensional imaging may not be helpful; in those cases, color-flow mapping in the main pulmonary artery reveals the flow occurring in an opposite direction to the antegrade pulmonary artery flow. Caution should be used to avoid confusing a pulmonary insufficiency color jet from that of the PDA. Doppler interrogation of the ductal flow can also help in determining the degree of stenosis across the PDA and in estimating the pulmonary artery pressure.

Treatment and Outcomes

During the past 2 decades, percutaneous therapy for the patient with an isolated PDA has become the standard of care at most institutions in the United States.[121] The exception to this is in premature neonates or in those patients in early infancy with particularly large, hemodynamically significant lesions. In those cases, surgical therapy is still regarded as routine. Surgical PDA repair is performed in most cases via the left lateral thoracotomy approach. Usually, the PDA is identified and ligated or divided. A left-sided chest tube drain remains in place for a brief period after surgery, and hospitalization lasts for 3 to 4 days. The most significant, albeit rare, complications involve inadvertent ligation of the left pulmonary artery or descending aorta, often with catastrophic effects if not immediately identified.

There is low, but not unexpected, morbidity from wound and skin infections. Pain and discomfort are not insignificant, and in most cases opioid analgesics are required in the first 24 hours. There is also a low incidence of recanalization, but that may be dependent on surgical technique.

Transcatheter device closure of the PDA has now been available for almost 20 years. Different methods have been available during this time, but with evolution of device technology and operator technique, two categories of devices are currently in use: coils and occluder devices. Given the differences in their design and delivery, these are discussed separately.

Coils

Stainless steel Gianturco coils (Cook, Bloomington, IN) of various thicknesses, lengths, and loop diameters were initially available for occlusion of peripheral vascular malformations (Fig. 56-28).[122-124] The application of these coils for small PDA closure began in the early 1990s, and since then, several techniques for their safe delivery and variations on the initial design and delivery have been developed. Generally, after basic angiography of the PDA is complete, an appropriately sized coil is chosen. The PDA deemed ideal for coil closure should narrow significantly along its course (to <2 mm), should be sufficiently long to accommodate the multiple loops of the coil, and should have a sufficient aortic ductal diverticulum. In that way, the loops of the coil on the aortic end of the PDA do not cause flow disturbance in the proximal descending aorta once deployed. Gianturco coils are delivered in a retrograde manner from the aortic end. Once the delivery catheter (typically a right coronary artery catheter) has crossed the PDA, approximately two thirds of the coil is extruded beyond the catheter tip (within the main pulmonary artery) by an appropriate-diameter pusher wire. The entire catheter-coil complex is then slowly withdrawn until the partially extruded coil is seen to "catch" on the pulmonary artery wall. At that point, the catheter is retracted back over the pusher wire into the aorta, with the coil held statically in place. As the catheter is withdrawn, the body of the coil straddles the length of the PDA, until it is completely extruded from the delivery catheter, when it springs back into the aortic ductal diverticulum and coils appropriately (Fig. 56-29). With correct delivery, approximately two thirds of the coil should remain on the pulmonary end of the PDA, with a portion of the coil straddling the narrow section and the remainder of the coil is tightly looped within the aortic ampulla. Repeat angiography is performed about 10 to 15 minutes after delivery to confirm appropriate placement and complete closure.

The risk of coil embolization has resulted in modifications of both the coil design and the delivery method. Detachable coils (Cook) used a screw mechanism on a modified Gianturco coil that allowed repositioning and retrieval if initial positioning was incorrect.[125,126] However, that modification did not

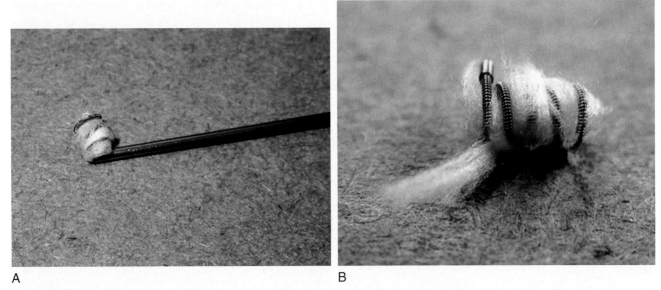

Figure 56-28. Partial (**A**) and full (**B**) extrusion of a Gianturco coil from the delivery sleeve. The coil has polyester fibers attached that promote stasis and thrombosis once deployed.

completely alleviate the risk of coil embolization after deployment. Snare techniques to control coil delivery have also been described.[127] Once the initial loop of coil is advanced into the main pulmonary artery, and before the retraction of the delivery catheter back into the aorta, a goose neck–type snare is positioned on the coil to maintain control at the time of delivery. Although this is successful in experienced hands, greater coordination between the primary catheterizer and the assistant is necessary. Some difficulty loosening the snare from the coil after complete delivery may also result in displacement after an initial apparently successful coil deployment. Multiple, simultaneous coil deployment has

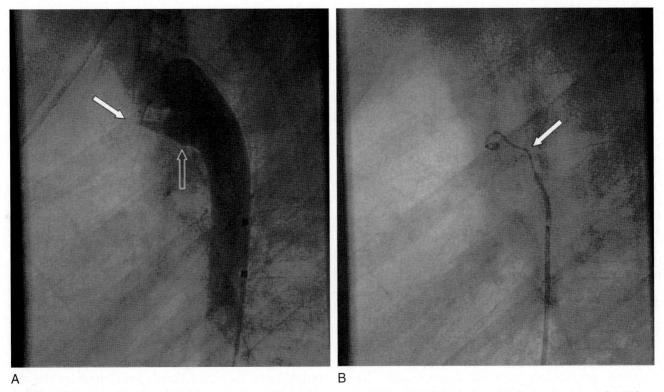

Figure 56-29. A, Still frame from an angiogram of a small patent ductus arteriosus (PDA). The narrowed pulmonary artery end (*solid white arrow*) and the aortic ductal diverticulum are clearly shown. **B,** The coil has been partially deployed, with the initial loop placed within the pulmonary artery end. The body of the coil (*solid white arrow*) elongates as the delivery catheter is retracted back into the proximal descending aorta.

Continued

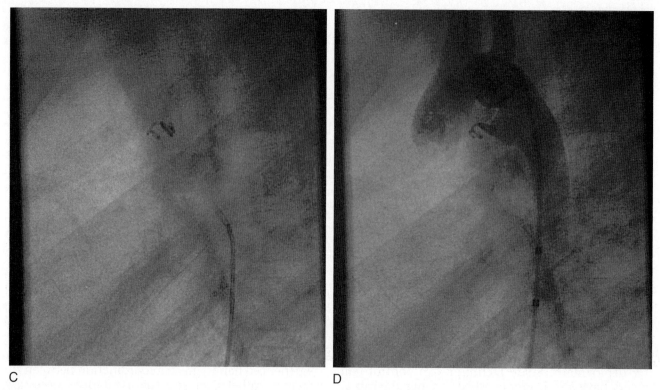

C

D

Figure 56-29, cont'd C, The entire coil has been released. The body of the coil has sprung back and is looped within the aortic ductal diverticulum. **D,** Still frame from an angiogram after coil occlusion of the PDA. No further shunting is seen across the coiled PDA.

also been used for closure of large PDAs.[128,129] However, with the advent of the duct occluder devices, this has become largely unnecessary.

Generally, coil occlusion has been successful in occluding small PDAs, with closure rates between 95% and 100% at 2 years.[130,131] Duct size has been shown to be the single most important factor in predicting complete early and late closure. The presence of small, residual shunts early after attempted closure raises the prospect of persistent hemolysis with resulting anemia.[132] In most cases, this resolves within 72 hours; if not, a repeat catheterization with further coil placement may be necessary. Early experience with coil occlusion was also associated with the concern for mild stenosis of the left pulmonary artery or descending aorta.[133] However, with refinement of technique and appropriate patient selection for coil placement, this is less of a clinical concern in the current era of PDA closure.

Two further modifications of PDA coil closure devices bear mention. The first is the Gianturco-Grifka Vascular Occlusion Device (GGVOD; Cook).[134] This device allows delivery of a large Gianturco coil into a previously extruded bag. This is of use in selected instances, such as when the PDA is unusually large or tubular, with no stenotic areas. The GGVOD has the theoretical advantages of conforming to the shape of the vessel, but it can also be retracted and repositioned if necessary. The second device is the Nit-Occlud PDA occluder (pFm

Corporation).[135] This is a preloaded coil that is positioned across the PDA. It is designed for occlusion of larger vessels and will conform to various PDA shapes. As it is deployed, it assumes a tight, conical shape that straddles the PDA and results in obstruction to flow. Closure rates with this device have been similar to those obtained with other coil and device closure options.

Duct Occluder Devices

Currently, the only noncoil device approved in the United States by the FDA is the Amplatzer Ductal Occluder (AGA Medical).[136,137] This is a cone-shaped device that tapers from a larger-circumference rimmed edge ("cap"). This device is designed to deliver through a sheath via the antegrade venous approach, and the delivery cable remains attached until release (Fig. 56-30). The cable can also be used for retraction and repositioning of the device if necessary. Once the delivery sheath has been placed across the PDA and in the proximal descending aorta, the larger, aortic end with the "cap" is advanced out of the aortic end of the sheath. The device and sheath complex is then pulled back with the "cap" positioned on the side wall of the aorta or within the ductal diverticulum. At that point, the delivery cable and device are kept exactly in place, and the sheath is pulled back to deploy the remainder of the device within the body

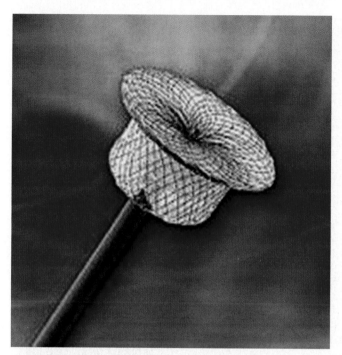

Figure 56-30. Amplatzer Duct Occluder. The device is constructed from an alloy of nickel and titanium. The larger end with the cap is designed to be placed on the aortic end of the PDA, within the ductal diverticulum. The other end tapers slightly and houses the screw thread for placement of the delivery cable. This image shows the device attached to the delivery cable and the delivery sheath. (Courtesy of AGA Medical.)

of the PDA. Repeat angiography can then be performed to ensure adequate positioning of the device, before final release is obtained with unscrewing of the delivery cable (Fig. 56-31).

This device has proved to be highly effective in closing larger PDAs, with rates exceeding 98% at 6 to 12 months after closure.[137] The complication profile for this device has also been low, with few serious side effects. Similar concerns regarding left pulmonary artery or aortic coarctation apply, but in practice this has not been of particularly large concern.[137] Patient selection is important in avoiding those complications, and this device should be avoided if the PDA is less than 1 to 1.5 mm in the narrowest diameter, or if the PDA is an aortopulmonary window–type defect with no obvious ampulla. Under those circumstances, a modification of device delivery can be employed, with positioning of the aortic cap within the PDA itself, and not against the side wall of the aorta. Hemolysis occurring immediately after delivery of Amplatzer occluder devices has also been described rarely, but it has either been self-limited or resolved with coil placement within the device.[138]

Follow-Up

Anticoagulation is not required after PDA occlusion with either coils or other devices. Subacute bacterial endocarditis prophylaxis remains indicated for at least the first 6 months, and as long as residual PDA

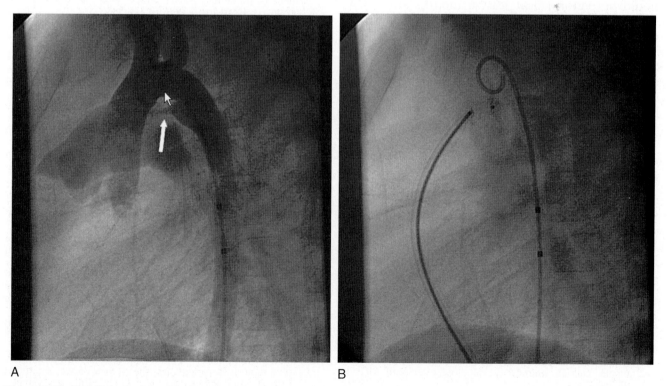

A   B

Figure 56-31. A, Still frame from an angiogram of a moderate-sized patent ductus arteriosus (PDA). The moderate PDA (*solid white arrow*) with a well-formed ductal diverticulum is noted. **B,** The Amplatzer Duct Occluder device has been deployed within the PDA but remains attached to the delivery cable. Retraction and redeployment are still possible at this point.

Continued

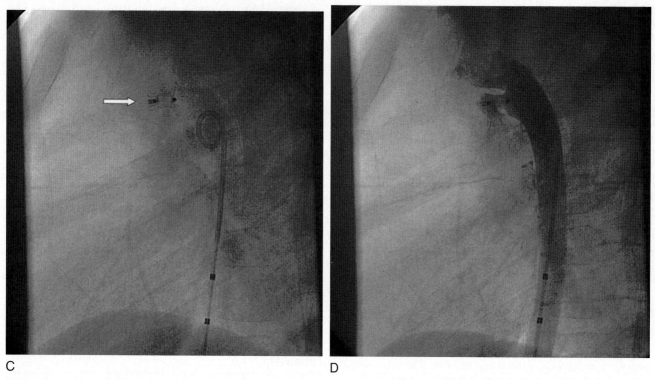

C   D

Figure 56-31, cont'd C, The delivery cable has been removed, and the device remains stable in position across the ductus arteriosus (*solid white arrow*). **D,** Still frame from an angiogram demonstrating a small amount of residual flow passing through the device. This resolves within the first 24 hours after deployment as thrombosis occurs within the ductal occluder.

shunting is present. Follow-up echocardiography should be performed at least 6 months after PDA closure; thereafter, if no murmur is present, further testing is no longer necessary.

REFERENCES

1. Emmanouilides GC, Baylen BG: Pulmonary stenosis. In Adams FH, Emmanouilides GC (eds): Heart Disease in Infants, Children, and Adolescents, 3rd ed. Baltimore, Williams & Wilkins, 1983, p 234.
2. Perloff JK: Postpediatric congenital heart disease: Natural survival patterns. In Roberts WC (ed): Congenital Heart Disease in Adults. Philadelphia, FA Davis, 1979, pp 27-51.
3. Nugent EW, Freedom RM, Nora JJ, et al: Clinical course in pulmonary stenosis. Circulation 1977;56(Suppl I): I-38-I-47.
4. Kan JS, White RI, Mitchell SE, Gardner TJ: Percutaneous balloon valvuloplasty: A new method for treatment of congenital pulmonary-valve stenosis. N Engl J Med 1982;307:540-542.
5. Becker AE, Anderson AH: Anomalies of the ventricular outflow tracts. In Becker AE, Anderson AH (eds): Cardiac Pathology. New York, Raven, 1983, pp 13.1-13.22.
6. Jeffery RF, Moller JH, Amplatz K: The dysplastic pulmonary valve: A new roentgenographic entity. Am J Roentgenol Ther Radium Nucl Med 1972;114:322-339.
7. Lababidi Z, Wu JR: Percutaneous balloon pulmonary valvuloplasty. Am J Cardiol 1983;52:560-562.
8. Walls JT, Lababidi Z, Curtis JJ: Morphologic effects of percutaneous balloon pulmonary valvuloplasty. South Med J 1987;80:475-477.
9. DiSessa TG, Alpert BS, Chase NA, et al: Balloon valvuloplasty in children with dysplastic pulmonary valves. Am J Cardiol 1987;60:405-407.
10. Rocchini AP, Beekman RH: Balloon angioplasty in the treatment of pulmonary valve stenosis and coarctation of the aorta. Tex Heart Inst J 1986;13:377-385.
11. Radtke W, Keane JF, Fellows KE, et al: Percutaneous balloon valvotomy of congenital pulmonary stenosis using oversized balloons. J Am Coll Cardiol 1986;8:909-915.
12. Ring JC, Kulik TJ, Burke BA, Lock JE: Morphologic changes induced by dilation of the pulmonary valve annulus with overlarge balloons in normal newborn lambs. Am J Cardiol 1985;55:210-214.
13. Stanger P, Cassidy SC, Girod DA, et al: Balloon pulmonary valvuloplasty: Results of the Valvuloplasty and Angioplasty of Congenital Anomalies Registry. Am J Cardiol 1990;65: 775-783.
14. Pepine CJ, Gessner IH, Feldman RL: Percutaneous balloon valvuloplasty for pulmonary valve stenosis in the adult. Am J Cardiol 1982;50:1442-1445.
15. Rocchini AP, Kveselis DA, Crowley D, et al: Percutaneous balloon valvuloplasty for treatment of congenital pulmonary valvular stenosis in children. J Am Coll Cardiol 1984; 3:1005-1012.
16. Zeevi B, Keane JF, Fellows K, Lock JE: Balloon dilation of critical pulmonary stenosis in the first week of life. J Am Coll Cardiol 1988;11:821-824.
17. Rey C, Marache P, Francart C, Dupuis C: Percutaneous transluminal balloon valvuloplasty of congenital pulmonary valve stenosis, with a special report on infants and neonates. J Am Coll Cardiol 1988;11:815-820.
18. Al Kasab S, Ribeiro PA, al Raibag M, et al: Percutaneous double balloon pulmonary valvotomy in adults. Am J Cardiol 1988;62:822-824.
19. Khan MAA, Al-Yousef S, Huhta JC, et al: Critical pulmonary valve stenosis in patients less than 1 year of age: Treatment with percutaneous gradational balloon pulmonary valvuloplasty. Am Heart J 1989;117:1008-1014.
20. Fedderly RT, Lloyd TR, Mendelsohn AM, Beekman RH: Determinants of successful balloon valvotomy in infants

with critical pulmonary stenosis or membranous pulmonary atresia with intact ventricular septum. J Am Coll Cardiol 1995;25:460-465.

21. Colli AM, Perry SB, Lock JE, Keane JF: Balloon dilation of critical valvar pulmonary stenosis in the first month of life. Cathet Cardiovasc Diagn 1995;34:23-28.

22. Tentolouris CA, Kyriakidis MK, Gaualiatsis IP, et al: Percutaneous pulmonary valvuloplasty in an octogenarian with calcific pulmonary stenosis. Chest 1992;101:1456-1458.

23. Herrmann HC, Hill JA, Krol J, et al: Effectiveness of percutaneous balloon valvuloplasty in adults with pulmonic valve stenosis. Am J Cardiol 1991;68:1111-1113.

24. Sherman W, Hershman R, Alexopoulos D, et al: Pulmonic balloon valvuloplasty in adults. Am Heart J 1990;119: 186-190.

25. Fawzy ME, Mercer EN, Dunn B: Late results of pulmonary balloon valvuloplasty in adults using double balloon technique. J Intervent Cardiol 1988;1:35-42.

26. Flugelman MY, Halon DA, Lewis BS: Pulmonary balloon valvuloplasty in the seventh decade of life. Isr J Med Sci 1988;24:112-113.

27. Presbitero P, Orzan F, Defilippi G, et al: Percutaneous pulmonary valvuloplasty in adults. G Ital Cardiol 1988;18: 155-159.

28. Park JH, Yoon YS, Yeon KM, et al: Percutaneous pulmonary valvuloplasty with a double-balloon technique. Radiology 1987;164:715-718.

29. Cooke JP, Seward JB, Holmes DR: Transluminal balloon valvotomy for pulmonic stenosis in an adult. Mayo Clin Proc 1987;62:306-311.

30. Leisch F, Schutzenberger W, Kerschner K, et al: Percutaneous pulmonary valvuloplasty in adults. Z Kardiol 1986;75: 426-430.

31. Shuck JW, McCormick DJ, Cohen IS, et al: Percutaneous balloon valvuloplasty of the pulmonary valve: Role of right to left shunting through a patent foramen ovale. J Am Coll Cardiol 1984;4:132-135.

32. Chen CR, Cheng TO, Huang T, et al: Percutaneous balloon valvuloplasty for pulmonary stenosis in adolescents and adults. N Engl J Med 1996;335:21-25.

33. McCrindle BW, Kan JS: Long-term results after balloon pulmonary valvuloplasty. Circulation 1991;83:1915-1922.

34. McCrindle BW: Independent predictors of long-term results after balloon pulmonary valvuloplasty. Circulation 1994;89:1751-1759.

35. O'Connor BK, Beekman RH, Lindauer A, Rocchini A: Intermediate-term outcome after pulmonary balloon valvuloplasty: Comparison to a matched surgical control group. J Am Coll Cardiol 1992;20:169-173.

36. Friedman WF: Aortic stenosis. In Adams FH, Emmanouilides GC (eds): Heart Disease in Infants, Children, and Adolescents, 3rd ed. Baltimore, Williams & Wilkins, 1983, p 224.

37. Wagner HR, Ellison RC, Keane JF, et al: Clinical course in aortic stenosis. Circulation 1977;56(Suppl I):I-47-I-56.

38. Hsieh K, Keane JF, Nadas AS, et al: Long-term follow-up of valvotomy before 1968 for congenital aortic stenosis. Am J Cardiol 1986;58:338-341.

39. Lababidi Z, Wu J, Walls JT: Percutaneous balloon aortic valvuloplasty: Results in 23 patients. Am J Cardiol 1984;53: 194-197.

40. NHLBI Balloon Valvuloplasty Registry Participants: Percutaneous balloon aortic valvuloplasty: Acute and 30-day follow-up results in 674 patients from NHLBI Balloon Valvuloplasty Registry. Circulation 1991;84:2383-2397.

41. McKay RG, Safian RD, Lock JE, et al: Balloon dilation of calcific aortic stenosis in elderly patients: Postmortem, intraoperative, and percutaneous valvuloplasty studies. Circulation 1986;74:119-125.

42. Berdoff RL, Strain J, Crandall C, et al: Pathology of aortic valvuloplasty: Findings after postmortem successful and failed dilatations. Am Heart J 1989;117:688-690.

43. Walls JT, Lababidi Z, Curtis JJ, Silver D: Assessment of percutaneous balloon pulmonary and aortic valvuloplasty. J Thorac Cardiovasc Surg 1984;88:352-356.

44. Rocchini AP, Beekman RH, Ben Shachar G, et al: Balloon aortic valvuloplasty: Results of the valvuloplasty and angioplasty of congenital anomalies registry. Am J Cardiol 1990;65:784-789.

45. Beekman RH, Rocchini AP, Crowley DC, et al: Aortic balloon valvuloplasty: Two balloons are better than one. Circulation 1987;76:266-271.

46. Helgason H, Keane JF, Fellows KE, et al: Balloon dilation of the aortic valve: Studies in normal lambs and in children with aortic stenosis. J Am Coll Cardiol 1987;9:816-822.

47. Sholler GF, Keane JF, Perry SB, et al: Balloon dilation of congenital aortic valve stenosis: Results and influences of technical and morphological features on outcome. Circulation 1988;78:351-360.

48. Meliones JN, Beekman RH, Rocchini AP, Lacina SJ: Balloon valvuloplasty for recurrent aortic stenosis after surgical valvotomy in childhood: Immediate and follow-up studies. J Am Coll Cardiol 1989;13:1106-1110.

49. Vogel M, Benson LN, Burrows P, et al: Balloon dilatation of congenital aortic valve stenosis in infants and children: Short term and intermediate results. Br Heart J 1989;62: 148-153.

50. Keane JF, Perry SB, Lock JE: Balloon dilation of congenital valvular aortic stenosis. J Am Coll Cardiol 1990;16: 457-458.

51. McCrindle BW: Independent predictors of immediate results of percutaneous balloon aortic valvotomy in childhood. Am J Cardiol 1996;77:286-293.

52. Sandhu SK, Lloyd TR, Crowley DC, Beekman RH: Effectiveness of balloon valvuloplasty in the young adult with congenital aortic stenosis. Cathet Cardiovasc Diagn 1995;36: 122-127.

53. Jones M, Barnhart GR, Morrow AG: Late results after operations for left ventricular outflow tract obstruction. Am J Cardiol 1982;50:569-579.

54. Cowley CG, Dietrich M, Mosca RS, et al: Balloon valvuloplasty versus transventricular dilation for neonatal critical aortic stenosis. Am J Cardiol 2001;87:1125-1127.

55. McCrindle BW, Blackstone EH, Williams WG, et al: Are outcomes of surgical versus transcatheter balloon valvotomy equivalent in neonatal critical aortic stenosis? Circulation 2001;104(Suppl I):I-152-I-158.

56. McElhinney DB, Lock JE, Keane JF, et al: Left heart growth, function, and reintervention after balloon aortic valvuloplasty for neonatal aortic stenosis. Circulation 2005;111: 451-458.

57. Magee AG, Nykanen D, McCrindle BW, et al: Balloon dilation of severe aortic stenosis in the neonate: Comparison of anterograde and retrograde catheter approaches. J Am Coll Cardiol 1997;30:1061-1066.

58. Rhodes LA, Colan SD, Perry SB, et al: Predictors of survival in neonates with critical aortic stenosis. Circulation 1991;84:2325-2335.

59. Fischer DR, Ettedgui JA, Park SC, et al: Carotid artery approach for balloon dilation of aortic valve stenosis in the neonate: A preliminary report. J Am Coll Cardiol 1990;15: 1633-1636.

60. Galal O, Rao PS, Al-Fadley F, Wilson AD: Follow-up results of balloon aortic valvuloplasty in children with special reference to causes of late aortic insufficiency. Am Heart J 1997;133:418-427.

61. Safian RD, Berman AD, Diver DJ, et al: Balloon aortic valvuloplasty in 170 consecutive patients. N Engl J Med 1988;319:125-130.

62. Block PC, Palacios IF: Clinical and hemodynamic follow-up after percutaneous aortic valvuloplasty in the elderly. Am J Cardiol 1988;62:760-763.

63. Del Core MG, Nair CK, Peetz D Jr, et al: Early restenosis following successful percutaneous balloon valvuloplasty for calcific valvular aortic stenosis. Am Heart J 1989;118: 181-182.

64. Beekman RH, Rocchini AP, Gillon JH, Mancini GBJ: Hemodynamic determinants of the peak systolic pressure gradient in children with valvar aortic stenosis. Am J Cardiol 1992;69: 813-815.

65. O'Connor BK, Beekman RH, Rocchini AP, Rosenthal A: Intermediate-term effectiveness of balloon valvuloplasty for

congenital aortic stenosis: A prospective follow-up study. Circulation 1991;84:732-738.

66. Bacha EA, Satou GM, Moran AM, et al: Valve-sparing operation for balloon-induced aortic regurgitation in congenital aortic stenosis. J Thorac Cardiovasc Surg 2001;122:162-168.

67. Beekman RH, Rocchini AP, Andes A: Balloon valvuloplasty for critical aortic stenosis in the newborn: Influence of new catheter technology. J Am Coll Cardiol 1991;17:1172-1176.

68. Kan JS, Marvin WJ, Bass JL, et al: Balloon angioplasty for branch pulmonary artery stenosis: Results from the valvuloplasty and angioplasty of congenital anomalies registry. Am J Cardiol 1990;65:798-801.

69. Lock JE, Castaneda-Zuniga WR, Fuhrman BP, Bass JL: Balloon dilation angioplasty of hypoplastic and stenotic pulmonary arteries. Circulation 1983;67:962-967.

70. Rothman A, Perry SB, Keane JF, Lock JE: Early results and follow-up of balloon angioplasty for branch pulmonary artery stenoses. J Am Coll Cardiol 1990;15:1109-1117.

71. Benson LN, Hamilton F, Dasmahapatra HK, Coles JG: Implantable stent dilation of the pulmonary artery: Early experience [abstract]. Circulation 1988;78(Suppl II):II-100.

72. Benson LN, Hamilton F, Dasmahapatra HK, et al: Percutaneous implantations of a balloon-expandable endoprosthesis for pulmonary artery stenosis: An experimental study. J Am Coll Cardiol 1991;18:1303-1308.

73. Rocchini AP, Meliones JP, Beekman RH, et al: Use of balloon-expandable stents to treat experimental pulmonary artery and superior vena caval stenosis: Preliminary experience. Pediatr Cardiol 1992;13:92-96.

74. Mendelsohn AM, Dorostkar PC, Moorehead CP, et al: Stent redilation in models of congenital heart disease: Pulmonary artery stenosis and coarctation. Cathet Cardiovasc Diagn 1996;38:430-440.

75. O'Laughlin MP, Perry SB, Lock JE, Mullins CE: Use of endovascular stents in congenital heart disease. Circulation 1991;83:1923-1939.

76. Hosking MC, Benson LN, Nakanishi T, et al: Intravascular stent prosthesis for right ventricular outflow obstruction. J Am Coll Cardiol 1992;20:373-380.

77. Mendelsohn AM, Bove EL, Lupinetti FM, et al: Intraoperative and percutaneous stenting of congenital pulmonary artery and vein stenosis. Circulation 1993;88:210-217.

78. O'Laughlin MP, Slack MC, Grifka RG, et al: Implantation and intermediate term follow-up of stents in congenital heart disease. Circulation 1993;88:605-614.

79. Fogelman R, Nykanen D, Smallhorn JF, et al: Endovascular stents in the pulmonary circulation: Clinical impact on management and medium-term follow-up. Circulation 1995;92:881-885.

80. McMahon CJ, El Said HG, Vincent JA, et al: Refinements in the implementation of pulmonary arterial stents. Cardiol Young 2002;12:445-452.

81. Shaffer KM, Mullins CE, Grifka RG, et al: Intravascular stents in congenital heart disease: Short and long-term results from a large single-center experience. J Am Coll Cardiol 1998;31:661-667.

82. Ing FF, Grifka RG, Nihill MR, Mullins CE: Repeat dilation of intravascular stents in congenital heart defects. Circulation 1995;92:893-897.

83. Duke C, Rosenthal E, Qureshi SA: The efficacy and safety of stent redilation in congenital heart disease. Heart 2003;89:905-912.

84. Beekman RH, Muller DW, Reynolds PI, et al: Balloon-expandable stent treatment of experimental coarctation of the aorta: Early hemodynamic and pathological evaluation. J Intervent Cardiol 1993;6:113-123.

85. Morrow WR, Smith VC, Ehler WJ, et al: Balloon angioplasty with stent implantation in experimental coarctation of the aorta. Circulation 1994;89:2677-2683.

86. Morrow WR, Palmaz JC, Tio FO, et al: Re-expansion of balloon-expandable stents after growth. J Am Coll Cardiol 1993;22:2007-2013.

87. Ebeid MR, Prieto LR, Latson LA: Use of balloon expandable stents for coarctation of the aorta. J Am Coll Cardiol 1997;30:1847-1852.

88. Suarez de Lezo J, Pan M, Romero M, et al: Immediate and follow-up findings after stent treatment for severe coarctation of the aorta. Am J Cardiol 1999;83:400-406.

89. Marshall AC, Perry SB, Keane JF, Lock JE: Early results and medium-term follow-up of stent implantation for residual aortic coarctation. Am Heart J 2000;139:1054-1060.

90. Transpoulous BD, Hadjinikolaou L, Konstadopoulou GN, et al: Stent treatment for coarctation of the arota: Intermediate term follow-up and technical considerations. Heart 2000;84:65-70.

91. Harrison DA, McLaughlin PR, Lazzam C, et al: Endovascular stents in the management of coarctation of the aorta in the adolescent and adult: One year follow-up. Heart 2001;85:561-566.

92. Johnston TA, Grifka RG, Jones TK: Endovascular stents for treatment of coarctation of the aorta: Acute results and follow-up experience. Catheter Cardiovasc Interv 2004;62:499-505.

93. Shah L, Hijazi Z, Sandhu S, et al: Use of endovascular stents for the treatment of coarctation of the aorta in children and adults: Immediate and midterm results. J Envasive Cardiol 2005;17:614-618.

94. Tzifa A, Ewert T, Brzezinska-Rajszys G, et al: Covered Cheatham-platinum stents for aortic coarctation. J Am Coll Cardiol 2006;47:1457-1463.

95. Varma C, Benson LN, Butany J, McLaughlin PR: Aortic dissection after stent dilatation for coarctation of the aorta: A case report and literature review. Catheter Cardiovasc Interv 2003;59:528-535.

96. Pihkala J, Pedra CA, Nykanen D, Benson LN: Implantation of endovascular stents for hypoplasia of the transverse arch. Cardiol Young 2000;10:3-7.

97. Brassard M, Fouron JC, van Doesburg NH, et al: Outcome of children with atrial septal defect considered too small for surgical closure. Am J Cardiol 1999;83:1552-1555.

98. Tabery S, Daniels O: How classical are the clinical features of the "ostium secundum" atrial septal defect? Cardiol Young 1997;7:294-301.

99. Andrews R, Tulloh R, Magee A, Anderson D: Atrial septal defect with failure to thrive in infancy: Hidden pulmonary vascular disease? Pediatr Cardiol 2002;23:528-530.

100. Shah D, Azhar M, Oakley CM, et al: Natural history of secundum atrial septal defect in adults after medical or surgical treatment: A historical prospective study. Br Heart J 1994;71:224-228.

101. Konstantinides S, Geibel A, Olschewski M, et al: A comparison of surgical and medical therapy for atrial septal defect in adults. N Engl J Med 1995;333:469-514.

102. Salaymeh K, Taeed R, Michelfelder EC, et al: Unique echocardiographic features associated with deployment of the Amplatzer atrial septal defect device. J Am Soc Echocardiogr 2001;14:128-137.

103. Ewert P, Daehnert I, Berger F, et al: Transcatheter closure of atrial septal defects under echocardiographic guidance without x-ray: Initial experiences. Cardiol Young 1999;9:136-140.

104. Formigari R, Di Donato RM, Mazzera E, et al: Minimally invasive or interventional repair of atrial septal defects in children: Experience in 171 cases and comparison with conventional strategies. J Am Coll Cardiol 2001;37:1707-1712.

105. Cowley CG, Lloyd TR, Bove EL, et al: Comparison of results of closure of secundum atrial septal defect by surgery versus Amplatzer Septal Occluder. Am J Cardiol 2001;88:589-591.

106. Berger F, Ewett P, Björnstad PG, et al: Transcatheter closure as standard treatment for most interatrial defects: Experience in 200 patients treated with the Amplatzer™ Septal Occluder. Cardiol Young 1999;9:468-473.

107. Bilkis AA, Alwi, M, Hasri S, et al: The Amplatzer Duct Occluder: Experience in 209 patients. J Am Coll Cardiol 2001;37:258-261.

108. Chan KC, Godman MJ, Walsh K, et al: Transcatheter closure of atrial septal defect and interatrial communications with a new self expanding nitinol double disc device (Amplatzer Septal Occluder): Multicentre UK experience. Heart 1999;82:300-306.

109. Zahn EM, Wilson N, Cutright W, Latson LA: Development and testing of the Helex Septal Occluder, a new expanded polytetrafluoroethylene atrial septal defect occlusion system. Circulation 2001;104:711-716.

110. Berger F, Vogel M, Alexi-Meskishvili V, Lange PE: Comparison of results and complications of surgical and Amplatzer device closure of atrial septal defects. J Thorac Cardiovasc Surg 1999;118:674-680.

111. Sherman JM, Hagler DJ, Cetta F: Thrombosis after septal closure device placement: A review of the current literature. Cathet Cardiovasc Interv 2004;63:486-489.

112. Amin Z, Hijazi ZM, Bass JL, et al: Erosion of Amplatzer Septal Occluder device after closure of secundum atrial septal defects: Review of registry of complications and recommendations to minimize future risk. Cathet Cardiovasc Interv 2004;63:496-502.

113. Divekar A, Gaamangwe, T, Shaikh N, et al: Cardiac perforation after device closure of atrial septal defects with the Amplatzer Septal Occluder. J Am Coll Cardiol 2005;45:1213-1218.

114. Veldtman GR, Razack V, Siu S, et al: Right ventricular form and function after percutaneous atrial septal defect device closure. J Am Coll Cardiol 2001;37:2108-2113.

115. Arlettaz R, Archer N , Wilkinson AR: Natural history of innocent murmurs in newborn babies: Controlled echocardiography study. Arch Dis Child Fetal Neonatal Ed 1998;78:F166-F170.

116. Jan SL, Hwang B, Fu YC, Chi CS: Prediction of ductus arteriosus closure by neonatal screening echocardiography. Int J Cardiovasc Imaging 2004;20:349-356.

117. Waddell TK, Bennett L, Kennedy R, et al: Heart-lung or lung transplantation for Eisenmenger syndrome. J Heart Lung Transplant 2002;21:731-737.

118. Sohn DW, Kim YJ, ZO JH, et al: The value of contrast echocardiography in the diagnosis of patent ductus arteriosus with Eisenmenger's syndrome. J Am Soc Echocardiogr 2001;14:57-59.

119. Bilge M, Uner A, Ozeren A, et al: Pulmonary endarteritis and subsequent embolization to the lung as a complication of a patent ductus arteriosus: A case report. Angiology 2004;55:99-102.

120. Panetta G, Schiller N: Evidence of patent ductus arteriosus and right-to-left shunt by finger pulse oximetry and Doppler signals of agitated saline in abdominal aorta. J Am Soc Echocardiogr 1999;12:763-765.

121. Moore JW, Levi DS, Moore SD, et al: Interventional treatment of patent ductus arteriosus in 2004. Cathet Cardiovasc Interv 2005;64:91-101.

122. Rothman A, Lucas VW, Sklansky MS, et al: Percutaneous coil occlusion of patent ductus arteriosus. J Pediatr 1997;130:447-454.

123. Wang J-K, Liau C-S, Huang J-J, et al: Transcatheter closure of patent ductus arteriosus using Gianturco coils in adolescents and adults. Cathet Cardiovasc Interv 2002;55:513-518.

124. Alwi M, Kang LM, Samion H, et al: Transcatheter occlusion of native persistent ductus arteriosus using conventional Gianturco coils. Am J Cardiol 1997;79:1430-1432.

125. Uzun O, Hancock S, Parsons JM, et al: Transcatheter occlusion of the arterial duct with Cook detachable coils: Early experience. Heart 1996;76:269-273.

126. Bermudez-Canete R, Santoro G, Bialkowsky J, et al: Patent ductus arteriosus occlusion using detachable coils. Am J Cardiol 1998;82:1547-1549.

127. Ing FF, Sommer RJ: The snare-assisted technique for transcatheter coil occlusion of moderate to large patent ductus arteriosus: Immediate and intermediate results. J Am Coll Cardiol 1999;33:1710-1718.

128. Hijazi ZM, Lloyd TR, Beekman RH III, Geggel RL: Transcatheter closure with single or multiple Gianturco coils of patent ductus arteriosus in infants weighing ≤8 kg: Retrograde versus antegrade approach. Am Heart J 1996;132:827-835.

129. Hijazi ZM, Geggel RL: Transcatheter closure of large patent ductus arteriosus (≥4 mm) with multiple Gianturco coils: Immediate and mid-term results. Heart 1996;76:536-540.

130. Goyal VS, Fulwant MC, Ramakantan R, et al: Follow-up after coil closure of patent ductus arteriosus. Am J Cardiol 1999;83:463-466.

131. Shim, D, Fedderly RT, Beekman RH III, et al: Follow-up of coil occlusion of patent ductus arteriosus. J Am Coll Cardiol 1996;28:207-211.

132. Radha S, Sivakumar K, Philip AK, et al: Clinical course and management strategies for hemolysis after transcatheter closure of patent arterial ducts. Cathet Cardiovasc Interv 2003;59:538-543.

133. Carey LM, Vermilion RKP, Shim D, et al: Pulmonary artery size and flow disturbances after patent ductus arteriosus coil occlusion. Am J Cardiol 1996;78:1307-1309.

134. Grifka RG, Vincent JA, Nihill MR, et al: Transcatheter patent ductus arteriosus closure in an infant using the Gianturco-Grifka Vascular Occlusion Device. Am J Cardiol 1996;78:721-723.

135. Tometzki A, Chan K, De Giovanni J, et al: Total UK multicentre experience with a novel arterial occlusion device (Duct Occlud pfm). Heart 1996;76:520-524.

136. Masura J, Tittel P, Gavora P, Podnar T: Long-term outcome of transcatheter patent ductus arteriosus closure using Amplatzer Duct Occluders. Am Heart J 2006;151:755.e7-755.e10.

137. Pass RH, Hijazi Z, Hsu DT, et al: Multicenter USA Amplatzer Patent Ductus Arteriosus Occlusion Device Trial: Initial and one-year results. J Am Coll Cardiol 2004;44:513-519.

138. Joseph G, Mandalay A, Zacharias TU, George B: Severe intravascular hemolysis after transcatheter closure of a large patent ductus arteriosus using the Amplatzer Duct Occluder: Successful resolution by intradevice coil deployment. Cathet Cardiovasc Interv 2002;55:245-249.

57 Percutaneous Transmyocardial Revascularization: Lasers and Biologic Compounds

Ran Kornowski and Shmuel Fuchs

KEY POINTS

- A growing population of patients suffer severe cardiac disease that cannot be treated effectively using conventional modalities such as pharmacotherapy, coronary angioplasty, and/or coronary bypass surgery. This is the "target" population for transmyocardial therapeutic approaches.

- The effect of surgical laser transmyocardial revascularization (TMR) on vascular and myocardial functions was studied and growing clinical experiences were derived from surgical TMR procedures indicating symptomatic benefit among treated patients.

- The results of pivotal randomized efficacy studies comparing percutaneous TMR to best medical treatment or sham controls were reported. Altogether these studies dictated the doubtful fate of this technique as an alterna-

- tive mode of myocardial revascularization that is no longer in routine clinical use.

- Currently, it is unknown whether dissimilarities among TMR devices may account for the differences in clinical outcomes observed among the clinical trials.

- The delivery of biologic compounds (e.g., genetic or progenitor cell experimental compounds) has been considered as an alternative and more "natural" approach for restoration of myocardial perfusion and/or mechanical function in the diseased ischemic heart.

- It remains to be seen to what extent transmyocardial delivery of biologic agents can diminish myocardial damage and/or restore blood flow in ischemic cardiomyopathy syndromes.

Despite the great achievements in preventing and treating coronary artery disease and cardiovascular disorders over the last decade, there is still a wide-scale population of patients who suffer severe cardiac disease that cannot be treated effectively using conventional treatment modalities such as pharmacotherapy, coronary angioplasty, and/or coronary artery bypass grafting (CABG). This population, which has been estimated as 3% to 15% of patients referred for invasive cardiac evaluation, may suffer from significant morbidity and mortality throughout the years after diagnosis.[1,2]

In recent years, alternative therapeutic options (e.g., enhanced external counterpulsation, spinal cord stimulation, and novel antiangina pectoris medications) have been used to alleviate angina symptoms and improve quality of life in patients with refractory myocardial ischemia. Moreover, a variety

of mechanical devices and energy sources have been investigated, aiming at improving angina pectoris symptoms and enhancing myocardial perfusion by creating intramyocardial penetrating channels.[3-5] Most mechanical strategies for transmyocardial revascularization (TMR) have employed a laser energy source via either surgical (transepicardial) or catheter-based (transendocardial) techniques. However, none of these techniques has become the "gold standard" of medical care in this challenging clinical scenario. Experimental strategies such as gene transfer and progenitor cell transplantation approaches have been explored to enrich collateral perfusion and improve contractility in the severely ischemic myocardium; these procedures are still considered purely investigational. This chapter describes these various therapeutic strategies and discusses the evolution of the field defined as "transmyocardial therapeutics" using either laser energy or biologic compounds delivered into the ischemic or infarcted myocardium.

CANDIDATES FOR TREATMENT

The patients under discussion are those who continue to suffer severe refractory angina pectoris despite maximal medical (i.e., pharmacologic) treatment, and in whom most invasive treatments such as coronary angioplasty or CABG have been used multiple times with temporary or only limited success. In addition, there is a population of patients with cardiac insufficiency and a combination of symptoms such as chest pain and shortness of breath. These patients are also frequently hospitalized, and the treatments presently suggested can only slightly improve the suffering bound to their disease.[6]

We propose herein clinical criteria for defining those patients who are candidates for "alternative" revascularization procedures[7]:

1. Patients with symptomatic coronary artery disease that cannot be treated effectively using percutaneous and/or surgical approaches, agreed by both the cardiologist and the surgeon
2. Patients with symptomatic chronic myocardial ischemia (either moderate to severe angina pectoris of Canadian Cardiovascular Society [CCS] class II, III, or IV or angina equivalent symptoms) while on best attempted medical treatment, defined as the administration of antiangina medications (e.g., β-blockers, nitrates, calcium channel blockers, angiotensin blockers, antiplatelet agents, and statin medications), other risk factors modifiers, and heart failure management if indicated
3. Patients with limited exercise capacity due to typical effort-related symptoms (e.g., <8 minutes on modified Bruce or equivalent exercise protocol) or, if exercise treadmill testing (ETT) is the only objective test for assessing myocardial ischemia, then transient ST-segment depression >1 mm at 80 msec after the J point present during and/or immediately after the test
4. Unequivocal reversible perfusion defects (either partial or complete) on single-photon emission computed tomography (SPECT) nuclear imaging study (either single- or dual-isotope study), positron emission tomography (PET), or magnetic resonance imaging (MRI) and/or with stress-induced functional impairment findings using dobutamine echocardiography
5. A target region for experimental intervention that is defined upfront and regional left ventricular dysfunctional myocardium that is categorized as a viable or nonviable territory.

For the viable myocardium, the main endeavor is to restore perfusion and, in case of impaired contractility, to improve function. For the nonviable myocardium, restoration of function (i.e., myocardial "regeneration") is the primary end point, and enhancing perfusion may be necessary to allow survival

support of the implanted compound (e.g., cells, grafted tissue). For transmyocardial interventions, identification of potential sources of collateral vessels is imperative, because the absence of *any* collateral source (i.e., no vascular conduit without a significant narrowing) compromises the ability to achieve a meaningful clinical response. Data have indeed suggested that patients with good blood flow to at least one region of the heart through a native artery or a patent vascular graft have a markedly better clinical outcome after TMR treatment.[8]

A typical profile of patients with chronic refractory myocardial ischemia includes the following characteristics: (1) age between 55 and 70 years and relatively early initial clinical onset of coronary artery disease, (2) long-standing history (e.g., >10 years) of coronary artery disease, (3) multivessel coronary artery disease, (4) previous CABG and/or multiple angioplasty procedures, (5) previous myocardial infarction, (6) at least one viable myocardial territory that is supplied by an occluded vessel and has a compromised collateral-dependent perfusion, (7) relatively preserved left ventricular function (e.g., left ventricular ejection fraction [LVEF] >40%), (8) high prevalence of diabetes mellitus (~40%) along with other multiple cardiovascular risk factors, and (9) predominantly male patients.

TRANSMYOCARDIAL LASER REVASCULARIZATION

The effect of surgical laser TMR on myocardial tissue and on microvascular and myocardial nerve functions was studied in numerous experimental models.[9] In addition, growing clinical experiences were derived from surgical TMR procedures indicating symptomatic benefit among treated patients.[10,11] The clinical experience with surgical TMR has grown, with numerous patients treated worldwide as sole therapy or in conjunction with CABG. Most studies suggested that surgical TMR used as sole therapy resulted in significant, long-term improvement of angina pectoris symptoms despite absence of clear evidence for improvement in myocardial perfusion.[12-24] A meta-analysis of seven randomized trials involving 1053 patients was performed to evaluate the effect of TMR as the sole procedural intervention on survival and angina relief. At 1 year, surgical TMR produced a significant improvement in angina class ($P < .0001$) but no improvement in survival ($P = .75$).[25] It is still remains to be determined whether there are any class I indications, as some would claim, for the use of TMR as a stand-alone therapy or class IIA indications for TMR as an adjunct to CABG.[26] Currently, surgical TMR is indicated for selected patients as a sole therapy. These are patients with refractory angina who are candidates for "alternative intervention" and also in patients who undergo CABG and have viable myocardial territories that cannot be effectively bypassed.

The goal of catheter-based TMR was to create nontransmural endomyocardial channels that are smaller in size but with comparable tissue effect to those generated by the surgical TMR.[27] The catheter-based approach for TMR was sought to provide equal effect without the need for surgical thoracotomy or general anesthesia. In addition, it enabled access to areas not approachable by surgical TMR (e.g., ventricular septum, posterior wall) and provided opportunities for multiple treatment sessions using a less invasive approach. Furthermore, in theory and practice, the catheter-based alternative for TMR was designed to lower procedural complications.

Laser Tissue Effects

Laser energy has specific tissue interactions that are fundamental for achieving controlled channel formation and tissue response, thereby avoiding unwarranted excessive myocardial damage.[28] In general, thermal injury leads to intense collagen deposition and scarring.[29,30] The myocardial tissue response to a laser energy source has been characterized acutely by sharply demarcated tracks appearing as open channels surrounded by a rim of necrotic tissue secondary to excessive heat (Fig. 57-1).[31] Tissue changes include sharply demarcated tracks surrounded by ablated

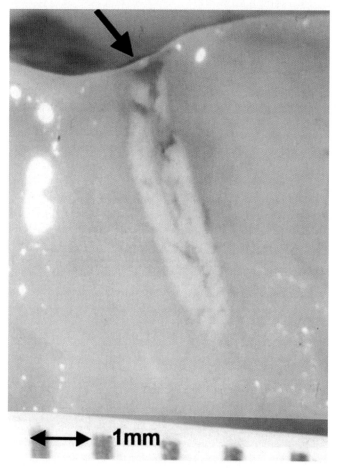

Figure 57-1. Endocardial surface and myocardium of an animal heart immediately after channel formation created using a catheter-based holmium: yttrium-aluminum-garnet (Ho: YAG) laser *(arrow)*.

tissue and profound local inflammatory reaction and cellular infiltrate of polymorphonuclear cells and macrophages, along with prominent dilated and damaged small blood vessels (Fig. 57-2). Adjacent zones show diffuse infiltration, with inflammatory cells, interstitial edema, and prominent vasodilation and extravasated red blood cells. Over time, extensive histologic evaluations of myocardium from 1 to 8 weeks after TMR failed to identify any persistently patent channels. This observation was independent of the laser source being used (holmium: yttrium-aluminum-garnet [Ho: YAG] or CO_2) and the tissue being treated (normal and ischemic myocardium). Channels are infiltrated with dense granulation tissue, which includes a high density of endothelium-lined vascular and sinusoidal structures with no detectable transmyocardial blood communications (see Fig. 57-2).[32] Similar histologic observations were made after the use of catheter-based TMR.[33] Months after TMR, the center of the channel was completely obliterated by collagen deposition.[34] The border zone was characterized by granulation tissue intersected by an abundance of capillaries.[35] Therefore, it appears that the original laser tracks do not remain patent and actually end as transendocardial scars.[36,37] It was suggested that, if indeed producing small scars in the myocardial wall is the mechanism of action, then lasers are probably not required, because this can be easily accomplished using heated needles or other less sophisticated energy sources.[38]

Several studies have suggested that TMR can enhance local angiogenesis in ischemic myocardium.[39,40] Experimental models demonstrated neovascularization and increased collateral flow possibly contributing to increased perfusion and myocardial salvage.[41,42] In other studies, immunohistochemical staining after TMR in ischemic hearts showed increased expression of angiogenic growth factors in laser-treated regions.[43-49] This phenomenon may also indicate a nonspecific tissue irritation associated with reparative response to mechanical myocardial injury of any kind.[50] In addition, clinical studies demonstrated a disturbing dichotomy between a favorable symptomatic response to TMR and lack of objective measures of myocardial perfusion.[38] This concern raises significant doubts as to whether any form of mechanical injury can induce a physiologically relevant angiogenesis as the predominant mechanism explaining the clinical response observed in patients.

Another mechanistic hypothesis concerning reduction of angina relates to cardiac denervation that may contribute to the rapid and significant symptomatic response after TMR. Compelling physiologic and biochemical evidence of denervation effects has been provided by some investigators.[49-53] It was proposed that laser injury causes damage to nerve fibers, resulting in an "anesthetic effect" without altered intramyocardial perfusion. It is possible, however, that the transendocardial approach, especially when lower energy is used, may induce more limited and reversible neuronal damage compared with surgical TMR. It is frequently stated that enthusiasm for TMR

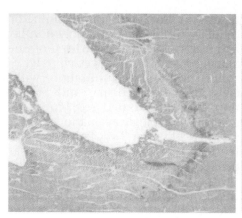
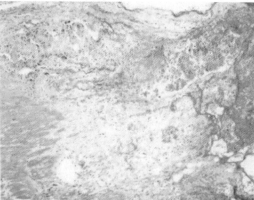

Figure 57-2. Histology of laser channel immediately *(left)*, and 2 weeks after *(right)* laser-induced myocardial injury. *Left,* Open laser channel with heat-damaged adjacent debris. (Trichrome stain, 12× magnification). *Right,* Typical granulation tissue in obliterated channel, with myofibroblasts and loose collagen matrix adjacent to viable myocytes and capillaries sprouting at the border zone (60×). See text for further details.

would wane if denervation were the dominant mechanism of benefit. Denervating the myocardium to produce cardiac sympathectomy and thus decrease the perception of anginal pain may provide clinical relief, but these patients may be exposed to severe silent ischemia with the undesirable consequences of repeated stunning and potential arrhythmia. Denervation effects would be of concern if associated with increased incidence of myocardial infarction, deterioration of cardiac function, and, more importantly, sudden death. Despite these concerns, currently available data from both surgical and catheter-based TMR clinical trials suggest no excess of mortality from sudden death. Moreover, a recent report indicated that neither surgical TMR nor percutaneous TMR induced significant silent ischemia, although surgical TMR more effectively suppressed pain during exercise and ischemic ST depression, compared with either medical treatment or catheter-based TMR.[54]

It remains to be determined whether these experimental findings pertain to the setting of human ischemic heart disease. Furthermore, it is likely that the effects of TMR are multifactorial, and the contribution of improved flow to the clinical effect remains a topic of active research and intense controversy.

Experience with Catheter-Based Laser Transmyocardial Revascularization

Three catheter-based laser TMR systems (Cardiogenesis, Eclipse, and Biosense) underwent extensive investigational clinical evaluation (Fig. 57-3).[55] The energy source for all three systems was a Ho:YAG laser. It is worth noting that, *as of mid-2006, none of these catheter-based TMR devices was approved for routine clinical use in the United States or elsewhere,* owing to reasons that are specified later. The results of four pivotal randomized efficacy studies comparing percutaneous TMR to "best" medical treatment were

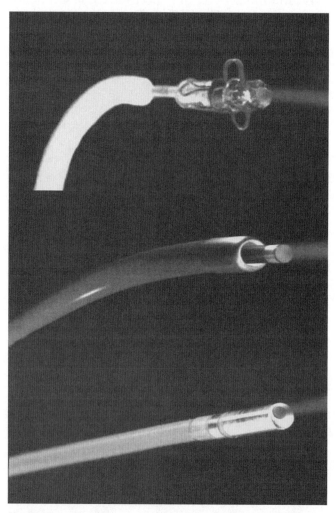

Figure 57-3. Close-up view of investigational holmium:yttrium-aluminum-garnet (Ho:YAG) laser-based catheter systems: Cardiogenesis *(top),* Eclipse *(middle),* Biosense *(bottom).*

Table 57-1. Design and Clinical Results of Catheter-Based Laser Transmyocardial Revascularization Randomized Trials

	PACIFIC[56]	Eclipse[57]	DIRECT[58]	BELIEF[59]
Design				
Laser source	Ho:YAG	Ho:YAG	Ho:YAG	Ho:YAG
Energy (Joule × pulse)	0.5 × 4	0.7 × 3	2 × 1	1 × 8
Number of channels	15	19	34/21/0*	20/0
Catheter guidance	X-ray	X-ray	LV mapping	X-ray
Blinding	No	No	Yes	Yes
Follow-up (mo)	12	12	12	6
Primary end points	ETT	ETT	ETT	CCS
Secondary end points	CCS, QOL	CCS, QOL	QOL, SPECT	ETT, QOL
Crossover	No	No	No	No
Patients				
Total (TMR group)	221 (110)	225 (64)	298 (196)	82 (40)
Age (yr)	62	63	63	66
CCS class III/IV (%)	61/39	60/40	67/33	86/14
Ejection fraction (%)	50	47	49	NA
Results				
Survival at 1 year (%), TMR vs. controls	93/97	93/96	79/86/89*	78/72
Angina relief (≥2 CCS), TMR vs. controls	42/8	55/31	41/48/41*	35/14
Change in ETT duration (sec), TMR vs. controls	89/12	100/−20	28/33/28*	10/7
Myocardial perfusion, TMR vs. controls	NA	NA	No change	NA
QOL assessment, TMR vs. controls	Improved	Improved	No change	Improved

*Indicates high-density vs. low-density vs. left ventricular mapping (placebo) groups.
CCS, Canadian Cardiovascular Society angina class; ETT, exercise tolerance test; Ho:YAG, holmium:yttrium-aluminum-garnet laser; LV, left ventricular; NA, not applicable; QOL, quality of life; SPECT, single-photon emission computed tomography; TMR, transmyocardial revascularization.

reported (Table 57-1).[56-59] Altogether, these studies dictated the doubtful "fate" of this technique as an alternative mode of myocardial revascularization that is no longer in routine clinical use.

The Potential Class Improvement From Intramyocardial Channels (PACIFIC) multicenter trial evaluated the potential of the Cardiogenesis TMR laser system to diminish angina and improve exercise tolerance in patients with refractory angina.[56] Patients (N = 221) with reversible myocardial ischemia of CCS angina class III or IV and incomplete response to other therapies were randomly assigned to percutaneous TMR with an Ho:YAG laser plus continued medical treatment or to continued medical treatment only. The primary end point was the exercise tolerance at 12 months. There were no procedure-related mortality or stroke events. Exercise tolerance at 12 months increased by an median of 89 seconds with TMR, compared to 12 seconds with medical treatment only (P = .008). Angina class was II or lower in 34% of percutaneous TMR treated patients compared to 13% of those medically treated. Angina decreased by two or more classes in 42% of TMR-treated patients versus 8% of controls. All indices of the Seattle Angina Questionnaire improved more with TMR than with medical care. By 12 months, there were eight deaths in the TMR group and three in the medical treatment group (P = .17), with similar survival rates in the two groups. Interestingly, there was no blinding or unmasked assessment of angina class by the study

investigators, which was suggested to contribute to 28% of the recorded subjective improvement in angina. Whitlow and coworkers reported similar findings from the Eclipse multicenter randomized trial investigating the potential of percutaneous TMR versus medical treatment to reduce angina and improve exercise tolerance in similar "no-option" patient cohorts.[57] A total of 225 patients were randomly assigned to percutaneous TMR plus medications (n = 64) or to continuing medications alone (n = 166). No attempt was made to blind the patient to the treatment status. One patient (0.6%) died from a procedure-related cause, and there was one (0.6%) additional stroke. Pericardial tamponade was noted in 5 patients (3%). Twelve months' follow-up revealed significant improvement in angina score and exercise tolerance for TMR-treated patients compared with the medication-treated controls. Fifty five percent of TMR-treated patients had improvement of two or more angina classes, compared with 31% of patients in the medical treatment arm (P < .05). Exercise time improved by 100 seconds in the TMR group but deteriorated by 20 seconds in the medical control group (P = .01). Exercise time improved by more than 60 seconds from baseline in 58% of patients who underwent TMR, compared with 33% of those treated with medication alone (P = .001). Mortality rates were similar in the TMR and medication-only groups (6.5% versus 6.0%, P = not significant [NS]), and freedom from mortality or myocardial infarction was not different between the two groups at 12 months ($P = .32$).

As mentioned earlier, results from randomized *nonblinded* studies indicated safety and feasibility, and suggested improvement in angina frequency and exercise duration in TMR-treated patients compared to those receiving "conservative" treatment alone. Based on these findings, a subsequent pivotal randomized blinded study was performed: the Direct Myocardial Revascularization (DMR) in Regeneration of Endomyocardial Channels Trial (DIRECT). This multicenter, *double-blinded* randomized trial included 298 patients who were randomized in a 2:1 fashion to either left ventricular guided "direct" Ho:YAG laser myocardial revascularization or Biosense-guided left ventricular NOGA mapping without laser ($n = 102$) followed by continued maximal medical management.[58] Treated patients were randomized to either (1) "low-density" treatment (10 to 15 laser channels per treated zone; $n = 98$), (2) "high-density" treatment (20 to 25 laser channels per zone; $n = 98$), or (3) "blinded" left ventricular mapping and medical management only.[58] Laser channels were applied to either one or two treatment zones with presumed myocardial ischemia. All patients underwent the diagnostic mapping procedure, allowing the patients to be blinded to treatment assignment. The primary end point of the study was change in exercise duration during standardized treadmill exercise tests from baseline to 6 and 12 months. Health status, angina pectoris symptoms, and myocardial radionuclide perfusion were assessed at baseline and up to 12 months. At 30 days, freedom from major adverse cardiac events was higher in the placebo group (100%) compared to the high-density (96%), and low-density (92%) laser treatment groups ($P = .014$). In the first 30 days, death, stroke, myocardial infarction, coronary revascularization, or left ventricular perforation occurred in two patients in the placebo group, eight patients in the low-dose group, and four patients in the high-dose group ($P = .12$); the 30-day myocardial infarction incidence was higher in patients receiving either low-dose or high-dose laser treatment (nine patients) compared with placebo (no patients) ($P = .03$).

There were no differences in exercise duration, time to symptom onset, or time to ST-segment changes at 6 and 12 months. In addition, angina improved by two or more classes at 1 year in 46% in the combined laser treatment groups and in 42% of the placebo group ($P =$ NS). Moreover, there were no differences in angina frequency or any other health status parameters that would indicate objective or subjective clinical benefit of the laser treatment. Importantly, however, there was a significant improvement in the control group in both exercise duration and angina frequency that persisted for 12 months, suggesting a substantial placebo effect. Also, there were no consistent changes in rest or stress nuclear perfusion imaging studies at follow-up to indicate improvement in myocardial perfusion. Despite the early increased adverse clinical events

associated with TMR in DIRECT, there was no significant difference in patients' survival during 1-year follow-up. The blinding process in DIRECT clearly demonstrated a profound placebo effect in "no-option" patients with severe angina.

The BELIEF trial (Blinded Evaluation of Laser PTMR Intervention Electively For angina pectoris study) used the Eclipse pecutaneous TMR system at higher laser energy output (8 J per treated Ho:YAG laser point) in a randomized, placebo-controlled study with a total of 82 patients, 40 of whom were treated by TMR.[59] Both the patient and physician were of *blinded* as to whether laser energy was actually applied. The results of this study showed a significant improvement in angina symptoms by 12 months among TMR-treated patients compared with controls (35% versus 14% improved by two or more angina classes; $P = .04$). Also, a trend toward improved quality-of-life and angina stability scores was noted among TMR-treated patients. Although no significant difference in total exercise tolerance was noted between the groups, the time to reported chest pain was increased by 76 seconds in TMR patients versus 12 seconds in control patients at 6-month follow-up ($P < .05$). No safety issues were noted in this trial, because the incidence of serious adverse events, as determined by cardiac event-free survival at 12 months, was similar between the groups. Currently, it is unknown whether differences among catheter-based TMR devices (Biosense, Cardiogenesis, or Eclipse), laser energy parameters (higher versus lower energy outputs), and/or catheter design may account for the differences in clinical outcomes observed in those pivotal trials. A graphic summary of the major end points in the four catheter-based TMR randomized trials is shown in Figure 57-4.

TMR FOR FAILED PERCUTANEOUS TOTAL OCCLUSION

Based on promising preliminary outcome data from the Eclipse trial,[60] a prospective multicenter, randomized, blinded trial was undertaken in which percutaneous TMR was conducted in patients with refractory angina caused by one or more chronic total occlusions of a native coronary artery. A total of 141 consecutive patients with class III or IV angina caused by one or more chronic total occlusions in which a percutaneous coronary intervention had failed were prospectively randomized, in the same procedure, to TMR plus maximal medical therapy ($n = 71$) or maximal medical therapy alone ($n = 70$). A median number of 20 laser channels were created in patients randomized to TMR. At 6 months, angina class had improved by two or more classes in 49% of patients assigned to TMR versus 37% of those assigned to medical treatment ($P = .33$). The median increase in exercise duration from baseline to 6 months was 64 seconds with TMR versus 52 seconds with medical treatment only ($P = .73$). There were no differences in the 6-month rates of death (8.6% versus 8.8%), myocardial infarction (4.3% versus 2.9%) or any

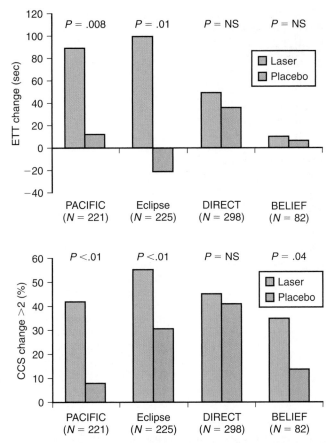

Figure 57-4. Change in total exercise duration compared to baseline *(upper panel)* and change in two or more angina classes *(lower panel)* in four randomized catheter-based transmyocardial revascularization trials after 12 months. See text, references 56-59, and Table 57-1 for further details.

revascularization (4.3% versus 5.9%) between the TMR and medicated groups (*P* = NS for each). It was therefore concluded that in patients with severe refractory angina caused by nonrecanalizable, totally occluded coronary vessels, the performance of percutaneous TMR does not result in a greater reduction in angina, improvement in exercise duration, or survival free of adverse cardiac events, compared with maximal medical treatment alone.

CATHETER-BASED TMR IN PERSPECTIVE

The history of treatments for angina pectoris has similar examples that underscore the importance of placebo effect. The DIRECT study is a characteristic example how phase II studies sometimes fail to prove the encouraging results of a similar nonrandomized phase I trial. It is important to recognize that in DIRECT the control group also improved significantly. This placebo effect may be due to the patient population being enrolled in those studies, who eagerly seek relief of their severe angina and improvement in quality of life and thus often have high expectations for improvement after new interventions.[61] Novel, sophisticated treatments have great

appeal to patients, especially when the term "laser" is used. Another factor that may contribute to the significant improvement observed in all phase I studies is the physician/investigator enthusiastic approach to the new treatment. Operators who were "enthusiasts" were shown to have better results than "skeptics," even in procedures having a nonspecific effect.[62] This "biased" approach may also explain why single-center phase I studies have better results than the corresponding treatment arms of multicenter phase II studies. This was true for laser TMR trials, and it is most probably a valid principle, considering the ongoing research in delivery of biologic compounds (discussed later).

In addition to these clinical results, recent animal and experimental human studies questioned the biologic effectiveness of TMR. As stated earlier, the myocardial tissue response to laser energy includes sharply demarcated channel tracks surrounded by a rim of necrotic tissue secondary to excessive heat.[31] Measurements performed on TMR-treated hearts failed to approve the original hypothesis of creating blood flow–conducting channels as in reptilian hearts.[37,42] Although several experimental studies have suggested that myocardial laser application may enhance angiogenesis and revascularization, clinical studies failed to show objective or consistent increase in myocardial perfusion.[12-24,56-60] Moreover, the effect of laser channeling on myocardial perfusion and denervation has not conclusively provided a mechanistic insight to support the clinical effect observed in patients after TMR. The microvascular responses occurring after percutaneous TMR may be undetectable by most conventional imaging modalities, or they simply may not be present. This raises significant doubts as to whether any form of mechanical injury can induce a physiologically relevant angiogenesis response.

Finally, one should consider that there are fundamental differences between the surgical and percutaneous TMR procedures. The transepicardial versus transendocardial approaches to energy delivery (e.g., full myocardial penetration using surgery versus limited endomyocardial access with catheters) may explain some of the differences in the biologic and clinical responses obtained by surgery compared to the percutaneous TMR technique. It is yet unknown whether those differences are key determinants of the adoption of surgical versus percutaneous TMR or merely the result of our ability to conduct a blinded randomization using catheters versus lack of such an aptitude using surgical techniques.

TRANSMYOCARDIAL DELIVERY OF BIOLOGIC COMPOUNDS

The delivery of biologic compounds (e.g., genetic sequences or progenitor cells) has been considered as an alternative and more "natural" approach for restoration of myocardial perfusion and/or mechanical function in the diseased heart. One of the fundamental biologic processes being explored is myocardial

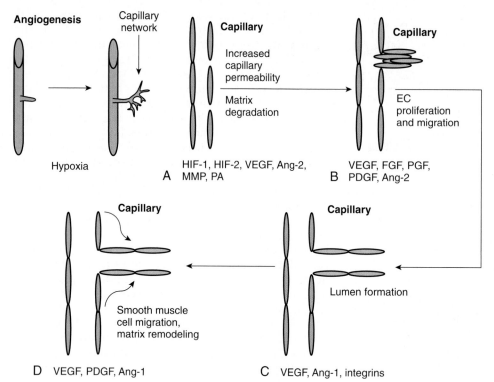

Figure 57-5. Schematic diagram of the various stages of angiogenesis attached to the formation of branching blood vessels over an existing vascular infrastructure. Ang, angiopoietin; EC, endothelial cells; FGF, fibroblast growth factor; HIF, hypoxia-inducible factor; MMP, matrix metalloproteinase; PA, plasminogen activator; PDGF, platelet-derived growth factor; PGF, placenta growth factor; VEGF, vascular endothelial growth factor.

angiogenesis. Angiogenesis is a complex biologic process of creation of new vascular structures branching out of existing blood vessels. This process involves secretion of multiple cytokines and matrix degradation along with cell proliferation and migration (Fig. 57-5).[63,64] Over the last few years, there have been multiple attempts by several groups of scientists over the world to develop meaningful gene and cell therapeutic approaches. This has included the development of angiogenic compounds and identification of potential cells along with delivery methods designed to improve myocardial perfusion and function and thus alleviate symptoms among patients with refractory coronary disease (Fig. 57-6).[65] The most tested catheter-based system is the Biosense-NOGA platform. This system uses a magnetic-based, nonfluoroscopic endocardial mapping system to identify the ischemic area and target it with the MyoStar injection catheter (Fig. 57-7).[66] Fluoroscopic guidance is also feasible using another delivery system, the Stolleto endocardial direct injection catheter (Fig. 57-8).

The role of the progenitor cells originating in the bone marrow, from which a few can be identified and isolated in the peripheral blood, has been studied over the last few years in relation to angiogenesis induction and/or myocardial regeneration.[67-70] It was found that progenitor cells that are carrying membranous indicators can react to systemic signals, multiply, and mobilize to areas with damaged tissue, such as in response to ischemia or myocardial infarction. The homing of these cells to "vulnerable myocardial regions" (or their mobilization by phar-

macologic means and/or cell delivery, as described later) may stimulate the cardiac regeneration and/or perfusion ability by: (1) secretion of cytokines that promote the generation of vessels from progenitor cells and/or (2) integration of the cells into the damaged tissue and transdifferentiation processes for myocardial cell regeneration. The latter process is still subjected to debate, and the scientific proofs are contradictory.[67-70]

Candidate Biologic Compounds

The genetic products used for transmyocardial transplantation belong to a family of compounds, termed "angiogenes" that may be capable of promoting collateral blood vessel formation, a process termed "neoangiogenesis" or "collateralization".[71] Among these are growth-promoting cytokines such as vascular endothelial growth factor (VEGF), fibroblast growth factor (FGF), and the vascular maturation factor termed angiopoietin 1 (Ang-1).[71] These cytokines are capable of promoting endothelial cell migration and proliferation and formation of branching vascular tubes in response to either physiologic or pathologic stimuli such as tissue ischemia or hypoxic insult secondary to occlusive vessel disease. The angiogenic response to hypoxia is mediated via a master gene encoding hypoxia-inducible factor 1 (HIF-1), which is activated locally and induces undermining of the angiogenic process by local upregulation of the VEGF pathway in its transcription and translation levels as well as the number of its receptors.[72] The current scientific findings support the

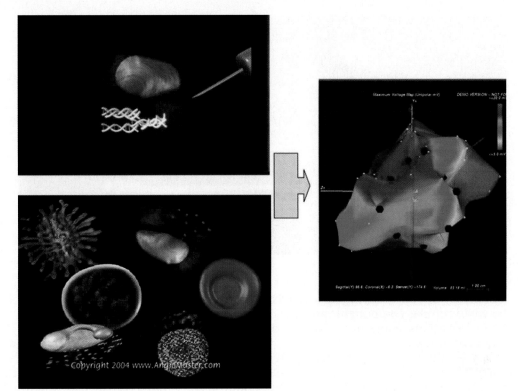

Figure 57-6. Representative scheme of the injection of therapeutic genetic compounds *(upper left)* or progenitor cells *(lower left)* into the myocardium using three-dimensional catheter-based myocardial imaging (Biosense-NOGA technology; *right*).

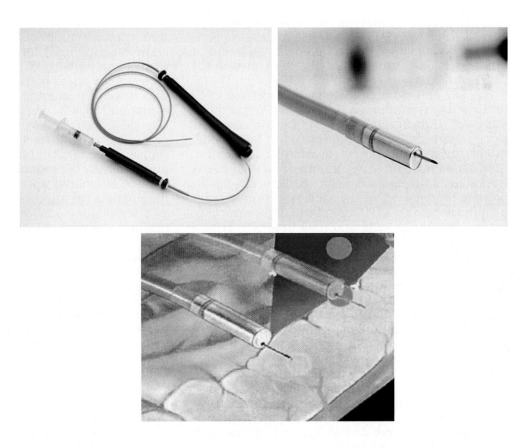

Figure 57-7. The MyoStar transendocardial injection catheter guided by endocardial mapping.

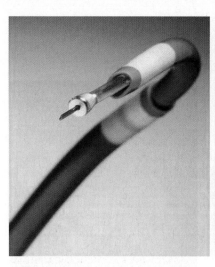
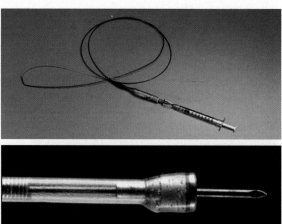

Figure 57-8. The Stolleto transendocardial injection catheter guided by fluoroscopy.

existence of and harmonic-synergistic processes between cellular components and the different cytokines in various stages of vascular and tissue regeneration processes.

For example, the bone marrow response to ischemic myocardial damage was investigated by Shintani and associates.[73] Circulating endothelial progenitor cells (EPCs) and bone marrow–derived cytokines were examined in 16 patients with recent myocardial infarction and 8 controls. The bone marrow response to myocardial damage was characterized by augmented EPCs in the peripheral circulation. EPC levels correlated to some degree with plasma levels of VEGF. The latter finding suggests that the bone marrow may respond via VEGF and/or other cytokine stimuli to ischemic myocardial damage by increasing circulating EPCs.

The fate and efflux of bone marrow–derived EPCs into infarct myocardium was studied by Yeh and colleagues.[74] Human progenitor cells expressing the surface marker CD34 were injected into immunodeficient mice afflicted by myocardial infarction. Animals were sacrificed at 2 months, and their hearts were stained for cardiac specific markers. The results propose the presence of transdifferentiation of adult peripheral blood CD34+ cells into cardiomyocytes, mature endothelial cells, and smooth muscle cells, a process that could be augmented by local tissue injury. Davani and colleagues[75] demonstrated in a rat model that mesenchymal stem cells transplanted into infarcted hearts appeared to differentiate into endothelial cells with loss of their smooth muscle phenotype. Thus, these studies may show that complex interactions exist between progenitor cells and cytokines, ensuing in fine modulation of biologic responses within the recipient ischemic heart tissue.

It is yet unclear to what extent the cardiac regeneration processes can actually decrease cardiac damage and/or reconstruct blood flow to extensive ischemic areas. In addition, there is a genetic diversity dependent on age and background diseases and medication intake in connection with angiogenesis processes. These are diverse biologic processes, and the pathophysiology response possibly varies among patients.[76,77]

Transmyocardial Gene Transfer

Preliminary clinical studies using angiogenic proteins have provided conflicting results: some studies have shown improvement in exercise tolerance and decrease in anginal symptoms, whereas in others (e.g., in phase II randomized trials) the improvement was modest or absent.[78-81] A potential drawback of these studies might be the short duration of action of the injected compound. It is conceivable that administration of genetic compounds would allow for prolonged local action of the angiogenic therapeutic protein. Whether this would result in a more robust effect is still questionable. In addition, the mode of administration of the angiogenic compound may be important for achieving optimal therapeutic effect. For that reason, over the last years, special catheters have been developed and cardiac imaging technologies implemented to enable direct delivery of proteins and genes into the myocardium.[82] Alternative approaches are the use of direct intramyocardial injection as an adjunct to CABG or as a stand-alone surgical treatment via "minithoracotomy." Another delivery method would be the use of transvenous access via the coronary sinus for retrograde infusion of biologic compounds.[83]

A group of scientists from St. Elizabeth's Medical Center in Boston (Isner, Losordo, and others) evaluated the safety and potential efficacy of direct intramyocardial injection of the gene encoding for VEGF-2 (i.e., the lymphatic isoform of VEGF) in 19 patients (12 in the treatment arm and 7 in the placebo-control arm).[84] After 1 year follow-up, it was found that the patients in the treatment arm demonstrated improvement in exercise tolerance and significant decrease in anginal symptoms (severity, intensity, and use of sublingual nitrates), as well as improvement of ischemic parameters in nuclear cardiac imaging performed in a subgroup of the patients.

Another study, the Euroinject One trial, has not demonstrated significant therapeutic advantage in 40 patients treated by direct NOGA-guided intramyocardial injection of the gene (plasmid) encoding for VEGF-165, compared to 40 control patients injected with an empty plasmid.[85] During this multisite European study, Kastrup and his colleagues reported minimal statistically significant improvement in parameters of myocardial perfusion in cardiac scintigraphy but clinically failed to demonstrate an advantage in reducing the severity of angina class (which showed significant improvement in both arms) or in improving exercise tolerance on bicycle.[85,86]

The REVASC study in Canada, headed by Stewart and coworkers, included 67 patients (32 in the treatment arm and 35 in the placebo-control arm).[87] Patients were randomized to receive either surgical direct intracardiac injection of a "sterilized" viral vector (i.e., a replication-deficient adenovirus) encoding for the VEGF-121 isoform or "best" medical treatment. The study demonstrated a significant advantage of VEGF-121 administration over medical treatment alone in relation to exercise tolerance at 12 and 26 weeks' follow-up. Although the severity of anginal symptoms improved significantly in treated patients over time, the study failed to demonstrate improvement in cardiac perfusion. The safety and feasibility of adeno-VEGF-121 in patients with refractory advanced coronary disease was tested among 10 patients in a phase I study that included a control arm (6 treated patients versus 4 injected with the viral diluent solution) using the NOGA/MyoStar injection device.[88] The results of this pilot evaluation indeed showed safety and feasibility and led to the conduction of a new study, named the NOVA trial (NOGA Delivery of VEGF for Angina). The NOVA study examined the safety and efficacy of the same replication-deficient ("sterilized") adenovirus encoding for the growth factor VEGF-121 administered by a catheter delivery in "no-option" patients with angina pectoris. This study enrolled 17 patients, and it was recently terminated prematurely owing to logistic reasons that were *not* related to safety issues.

Myocardial Cellular Delivery

Another therapeutic possibility being studied is the use of cells derived from different sources and by different techniques for the reconstruction of vascular-angiogenic properties and the mechanical-myogenic activity of the ischemic/infarcted heart.[89,90] As for gene transfer, the candidate patients for cardiac progenitor cell transplantation are those who have severe angina pectoris that is resistant to pharmacotherapy or myocardial damage and reduced ejection function.

Potential sources of cells for transplantation are diverse, and research groups focus particularly on the following candidates:

1. Autologous endothelial progenitor cells (EPCs) derived from the patient's bone marrow or from peripheral blood.[91] These cells can potentially be incorporated into emerging vascular structures and perhaps transdifferentiate into myocardial cells.[67]
2. Mesenchymal stem cells originating from the bone marrow that undergo ex vivo processing and selection and then are transplanted into the muscle of the left ventricle.[92] A preliminary clinical study is also assessing allogenic sources and intravenous administration of those cells.
3. Autologous cells derived from striated muscle biopsy taken from the patient's limb. Isolated satellite "immature" cells (i.e., myoblasts) are cultured ex vivo for 1 month, then implanted directly into cardiac scar tissue in order to improve cardiac function.[93]
4. Embryonic stem cells derived from hybridization and after laboratory culturing. It is possible to produce a colony of electrically active and beating myocardial cells constituting a potential reservoir for transplantation.[94]

Over the last few years, several studies have examined the feasibility, safety, and efficacy of these techniques. Some of the results are promising and demonstrate significant improvement in blood supply and cardiac function in infarcted areas, in dimensions that were not previously observed in laboratory experiments or with the use of other compounds. Clinical studies in humans have commenced in several locations over the globe. Generally speaking, three patient populations are being studied: (1) patients with refractory myocardial ischemia, (2) patients who sustained acute myocardial infarction, and (3) patients with old myocardial infarction lacking any viability in the damaged territory.

Bone marrow cells are the most studied cell source. The bone marrow contains cells and angiogenic substances that are capable of inducing the proliferation of endothelial cells. After a short bone marrow processing procedure carried out externally in a sterile environment, the cells are transplanted into the affected myocardium. The largest experience in patients with refractory myocardial ischemia was with the MyoStar catheter-based system, which was developed especially for the delivery of biologic compounds into the myocardium. This technique was tested in a study that involved 27 patients who had significant angina pectoris and were without any other option for treatment.[95,96] The patients' average age was 58 ± 9 years; 82% were males, 44% were diabetic, 93% had previously undergone CABG and 88% multiple coronary angioplasty procedures. The study showed that injection of nonmanipulated autologous bone marrow cells into the myocardium was a safe and practical procedure that was associated with no unusual side effects. Efficacy evaluation (i.e., in a nonrandomized and nonblinded study) demonstrated improvement in angina and exercise in 70% of patients and also improvement in regional myocardial perfusion as assessed by nuclear perfusion study. In the study under discussion, an average of

28 million cells were injected, of which 2.2% carried the phenotype CD34 as a positive indicator for progenitor cells.

A similar study was conducted in Brazil by the Texas Heart Institute group among 21 patients (14 in the treatment arm and 7 in the control arm) with severe ischemic cardiomyopathy (average LVEF, 20%).[97,98] The mononuclear cell subfraction was isolated from the bone marrow and then reinjected to the ischemic heart. The treatment arm demonstrated a significant early improvement in relation to the control arm in the severity of angina pectoris, extent of cardiac insufficiency, exercise tolerance, and degree of ischemia in perfusion tests (nuclear scintigraphy and cardiac mapping). However, at 12 months' follow-up, there were no differences in ventricular function, although differences in myocardial perfusion and clinical variables remain significant.

Preliminary data from Hong Kong were recently reported by Tse and colleagues.[99,100] Twenty-eight patients with refractory myocardial ischemia underwent NOGA-guided catheter-based myocardial delivery of bone marrow–derived mononuclear cells ($n = 19$) or saline injection ($n = 9$). On average, the results showed significant improvements in exercise time, nuclear scintigraphy assessment of myocardial ischemia, and anginal scores in treated patients compared with controls. This treatment strategy is therefore deserving an additional intensive inspection in controlled, wide-scale studies as a possible therapeutic option for patients with severe cardiac disease resistant to conventional pharmacotherapy.

The second patient population being studied comprises those patients who experience acute myocardial infarction. In this group of patients, intracoronary injection to the culprit artery of either bone marrow mononuclear fraction or peripheral blood enriched endothelial cells was performed 7 to 14 days after the acute event. Preliminary results from studies conducted in Germany demonstrated possible efficacy in achieving regional improvement of contractility and decreasing the area of the myocardium at risk.[101] In the BOOST (BOne marrOw transfer to enhance ST-elevation infarct regeneration) study, an average improvement in global ejection fraction of 12% compared to baseline was observed at 6 months, whereas no significant change was noted among controls.[102] However, at 18 months' follow-up, the average left ventricular function was similar between groups, owing to late improvement noted in the control arm.[103]

These results are encouraging but raise many questions about the efficacy of the therapeutic strategy discussed, its long-term effect, and the appropriate timing of the cell injection. In addition, it is unclear which cell population contributes most to the improvement demonstrated in these studies, and whether these cells can be isolated selectively to produce a homogeneous compound standing up to pharmacologic standards, including determination of therapeutic-toxicologic range, dosing, pharmacokinetics tests, and so on.

The third patient population is those with prior myocardial infarction and myocardial territory lacking viability. The aim among these patients is to regenerate the scarred area in order to improve regional and global left ventricular function.[104-106] The cells being studied are predominantly autologous myoblastic cells obtained from the quadriceps muscle and expanded ex vivo for 1 month. Intramyocardial injection was performed either as a stand-alone intervention or as an adjunct to CABG surgery. The clinical results obtained so far are contradictory.[104-106] In addition, there are a few cases of "malignant" ventricular arrhythmias reported soon after transplantation, indicating that the procedure may not be without significant risks.

Table 57-2 summarizes the current experimental clinical experiences using catheter-based transmyocardial delivery of biologic compounds.

ASSESSMENT OF THERAPEUTIC EFFICACY

In order to define the impact of experimental myocardial revascularization protocols among "no-option" patients, we propose the following criteria to assess clinical efficacy[7]:

1. A reproducible improvement in exercise capacity of 60 seconds or greater that is associated with a delay of at least 30 seconds in the time to ST-segment depression and/or level 2 (out of 4) grade angina chest pain symptoms
2. Reduced myocardial perfusion defects using myocardial SPECT, PET, or MRI perfusion imaging
3. Improved symptomatic angina (reduction by at least one CCS class, but ideally two or more classes)
4. Improvement in regional ischemic functional response (e.g., wall motion abnormalities), as measured by either dobutamine or stress echocardiography
5. Improvement on standard quality-of-life questionnaire parameters (e.g., Seattle Angina Survey)
6. Improved regional myocardial blush score, as measured by selective coronary angiography

The treatment of patients with very low LVEF (≤30%) may require the inclusion of additional end points, such as 6-minute walking distance, maximum oxygen consumption (VO_2 max), and *careful arrhythmia monitoring,* among other parameters. It is yet to be determined how many end points should be investigated and fulfilled in order to accept a new treatment modality as an effective approach. Moreover, the degree of improvement necessary to quantitatively demonstrate a treatment effect should be defined. Nonetheless, measures of improved perfusion, lowered ischemia, and reduced level of chest pain symptoms are the main goals ("major criteria") for angiogenesis-promoting interventions, whereas enhanced regional and/or global myocardial function and improved congestive heart failure symp-

Table 57-2. Design of Catheter-Based Intramyocardial Delivery of Biologic Compounds

Study (Ref. No.)	N*	Study Design	Angiogenic Compound	Delivery Mode	Injections No.	Injections Volume (mL)	Dosage	Follow-up (Mo)	ΔCCS	Other Angina Measures	ΔETT (Sec)	ΔNYHA	Myocardial Perfusion	Regional Global LV Function	LV Function	Adverse Events
Cell-based studies																
Tse (100)	8	Non R, P1	BM-MNC	Catheter-based (NOGA)	15.9 ± 5.4	0.1	$10\text{-}22 \times 10^6$ cells	3	NA	↓Anginal episodes ↓Nitro pills	NA	NA	Improved	NA	Improved	No
Perin (97,98)	21 (14 vs. 7)	Non R, P1	BM-MNC	Catheter-based (NOGA)	15 ± 2	0.2	$26\text{-}34 \times 10^6$ cells	2, 4, 12	↓1.4 class, sustained at 1 yr	NA	↑VO₂ max	—	Improved	Improved at 3 mo, no difference at 12 mo	NA	2 patients dead at follow-up
Fuchs (95,96)	27	Non R, P1	Unfractionated BM	Catheter-based (NOGA)	12	0.2	$4\text{-}109 \times 10^5$ cells	3, 12	↓1.2 class, sustained at 1 yr	Improved QOL measures, sustained at 12 mo	↑78	NA	Improved	No change	No change	No
Tse (99)	28 (19 vs. 9)	R, PC, P1	BM-MNC	Catheter-based (NOGA)	14.6 ± 0.7	0.1	Low dose: 10×10^6 cells High dose: 20×10^6 cells	6	↓−1.2 vs. ↓0.7 class	NA	↑−72 vs. 35	0.8 vs. −0.4	↓~1.2 vs. ↓0.7	Improved	NA	1 patient dead at 31-mo follow-up
Smits (105)	5	Non R, P1	Myoblasts	Catheter-based (NOGA)	16 ± 4	0.3	$196 \pm 105 \times 10^6$ cells	6	NA	NA	NA	NA	NA	Improved (36% to 45%)	Improved	VT (1 patient)
Siminiak (106)	10	Non R, P1	Myoblasts	Transcoronary venous	2-4	0.4-2.5	$\leq 100 \times 10^6$ cells	6	NA	NA	NA	↓1.3	NA	Improved (39% to 43%)	NA	VT (1 patient)
Gene-based studies																
Losordo (84)	19 (12 vs. 7)	R, PC, P1/2	VEGF-2 plasmid	Catheter-based (NOGA)	6	1	200, 800, 2000 µg	3	↓−1.3 vs. ↑0.1 in controls	Improved QOL parameters among treated patients	↓−92 vs. ↓4 in controls	NA	Improved among treated patients	NA	Improved electro-mechanical mapping parameters	1 treated patient underwent heart transplantation, 2 placebo-treated patients had CVA during follow-up
Fuchs (88)	10	Non R, PC, P1	VEGF₁₂₁ Gene-Ad	Catheter-based (NOGA)	10	0.3	0.5 mg	3, 12	↓1 vs. ↓2 in controls	Improved angina frequency in both groups	↓66 vs. ↓84 in controls	NA	NA	No change in both groups	NA	No
Kastrup (85)	80	R, PC, P2	VEGF₁₆₅ plasmid	Catheter-based (NOGA)	15	0.1	4×10^{10} pu	3, 6	↓0.7 vs. ↓1.2 in controls	No differences between groups	No differences between groups	NA	Improvement over time in treated patients	No change in both groups	Improved in treated patients only	Several complications in both groups, none related to the injected compound (one each tamponade, 3rd-degree AVB, AMI, CVA, sepsis)

*Numbers in parentheses indicated number treated versus number of controls.

AMI, acute myocardial infarction; AVB, atrioventricular block; BM-MNC, bone marrow mononuclear cells; ΔCCS, change in Canadian Cardiovascular Society angina class; CVA, cerebrovascular accident; ΔETT, change in exercise tolerance test; LV, left ventricular; NA, not available; NOGA, Biosense-NOGA mapping and delivery platform; ΔNYHA, change in New York Heart Association class; P1/2, phase 1/2 study; PC, placebo-controlled study; PU, particle units; QOL, quality of life; R, randomized; VEGF, vascular endothelial growth factor; VO₂ max, maximum oxygen consumption; VT, ventricular tachyarrhythmia.

toms should be the primary aims in myocardial regeneration (i.e., myogenesis) trials.

SUMMARY

Despite more than a decade of experimental studies and extensive clinical experiences employing both surgical and catheter-based systems, many fundamental questions remain unanswered, and the entire field of "direct" myocardial revascularization using lasers or other ablative sources is surrounded by controversy. Randomized, nonblinded clinical trials (i.e., TMR treatment alone versus medical treatment alone) have demonstrated improvement in angina symptoms and exercise tolerance in patients with refractory myocardial ischemia. For all the catheter-based TMR devices, there remains a poor correlation between clinical benefit and perfusion assessments using radionuclide imaging studies. The results of DIRECT, the first and largest blinded randomized clinical TMR trial, raised the disturbing possibility of important placebo effects contributing to the subjective benefits demonstrated in earlier surgical and catheter-based nonblinded studies. The blinding process clearly demonstrated a profound placebo effect in "no-option" patients with severe angina who were exposed to a new innovative technology with presumed therapeutic actions. Consequently, other clinical trials in this field should be viewed with caution and skepticism, unless proper attention is taken to account for placebo effects of those experimental therapies.

More rigorous assessments of objective and subjective end points derived from blinded and large randomized clinical trails are still required, and additional mechanistic insight is needed to determine whether surgical or catheter-based TMR strategies can be used in patients with refractory coronary artery disease.

The possibilities for the treatment of grave ischemic cardiac diseases may expand in the future along with the development of new methods for cardiac revascularization using the techniques of gene and/ or cell transplantation with the aim of improving cardiac function and relieving the symptoms of angina pectoris and/or cardiac insufficiency. This field is bringing new hope as well as raising ongoing skepticism regarding the efficacy and safety of these experimental treatments that continue to evoke much interest among the scientific and medical communities.

REFERENCES

1. Mukherjee D, Bhatt DL, Roe MT, et al: Direct myocardial revascularization and angiogenesis: How many patients might be eligible? Am J Cardiol 1999;84:598-600.
2. Mukherjee D, Ellis SG: New options for untreatable coronary artery disease: Angiogenesis and laser revascularization. Cleve Clin J Med 2000;67:577.
3. Jones JW, Schmidt SE, Richman BW: Lasers in the treatment of ischaemic heart disease. Ann Med 2000;32:113.
4. Lange RA, Hillis LD: Transmyocardial laser revascularization. N Engl J Med 1999;34:1075.
5. Horvath KA: Clinical results of sole therapy TMR treatment. Semin Thorac Cardiovasc Surg 2006;18:46-51.
6. Mukherjee D, Comella K, Bhatt DL, et al: Clinical outcome of a cohort of patients eligible for therapeutic angiogenesis or transmyocardial revascularization. Am Heart J 2001;142:72.
7. Kornowski R, Fuchs S, Zafrir N: Refractory myocardial ischemic syndromes: Current perspective on patients' characterization and treatment goal. Future Cardiol 2005;1:629.
8. Burkhoff D, Wesley MN, Resar JR, et al: Factors correlating with risk of mortality after transmyocardial revascularization. J Am Coll Cardiol 1999;34:55.
9. Burkhoff D, Kornowski R: An examination of potential mechanisms underlying transmyocardial laser revascularization: Channels, angiogenesis and neuronal effects. Semin Interv Cardiol 2000;5:71.
10. Allen KB, Shaar CJ: Transmyocardial laser revascularization: Surgical experience overview. Semin Interv Cardiol 2000;5:75.
11. Kornowski R, Fuchs S, Leon MB: Percutaneous transmyocardial laser revascularization: Overview of US clinical trials. Semin Interv Cardiol 2000;5:97.
12. Mirhoseini M, Muckerheide M, Cayton MM: Transventricular revascularization by laser. Lasers Surg Med 1982;2:187.
13. Mirhoseini M, Fisher JC, Cayton MM: Myocardial revascularization by laser: A clinical report. Lasers Surg Med 1982;3:241.
14. Mirhoseini M, Cayton MM, Shelgikar S, et al: Clinical report: Laser myocardial revascularization. Lasers Surg Med 1986;6:459.
15. Frazier OH, Cooley DA, Kadipasaoglu KA, et al: Myocardial revascularization with laser: Preliminary findings. Circulation 1995;92(Suppl II):II-58.
16. Cooley DA, Frazier OH, Kadipasaoglu KA, et al: Transmyocardial laser revascularization: Clinical experience with twelve-month follow-up. J Thorac Cardiovasc Surg 1996;111:791.
17. Horvath KA, Cohn LH, Cooley DA, et al: Transmyocardial laser revascularization: Results of a multicenter trial with transmyocardial laser revascularization used as sole therapy for end-stage coronary artery disease. J Thorac Cardiovasc Surg 1997;113:645.
18. Milano A, Pratali S, Tartrini G, et al: Early results of transmyocardial revascularization with a holmium laser. Ann Thorac Surg 1998;67:700.
19. Allen KB, Dowling RD, Fudge TL, et al: Comparison of transmyocardial revascularization with medical therapy in patients with refractory angina. N Engl J Med 1999;341:1029.
20. Frazier OH, March RJ, Horvath KA: Transmyocardial revascularization with a carbon dioxide laser in patients with end-stage coronary artery disease. N Engl J Med 1999;341:1021.
21. Schofield PM, Sharples LD, Caine N, et al: Transmyocardial laser revascularisation in patients with refractory angina: A randomised controlled trial. Lancet 1999;353:519.
22. Burkhoff D, Schmidt S, Schulman SP, et al: Transmyocardial laser revascularisation compared with continued medical therapy for treatment of refractory angina pectoris: A prospective randomised trial. ATLANTIC Investigators. Angina Treatments—Lasers and Normal Therapies in Comparison. Lancet 1999;354:885.
23. Aaberge L, Nordstrand K, Dragsund M, et al: Transmyocardial revascularization with CO_2 laser in patients with refractory angina pectoris: Clinical results from the Norwegian randomized trial. J Am Coll Cardiol 2000;35:1170.
24. Aaberge L, Rootwelt K, Smith HJ, et al: Effects of transmyocardial revascularization on myocardial perfusion and systolic function assessed by nuclear and magnetic resonance imaging methods. Scand Cardiovasc J 2001;35:8.
25. Liao L, Sarria-Santamera A, Matchar DB, et al: Meta-analysis of survival and relief of angina pectoris after transmyocardial revascularization. Am J Cardiol 2005;95:1243.
26. Bridges CR: Guidelines fr the clinical use of transmyocardial laser revascularization. Semin Thorac Cardiovasc Surg 2006;18:68-73.
27. Kornowski R, Bhargava B, Leon MB: Percutaneous transmyocardial laser revascularization: An overview. Catheter Cardiovasc Interv 1999;47:354.

28. Shehada RE, Mansour HN, Grundfest WS: Laser tissue interaction in direct myocardial revascularization. Semin Interv Cardiol 2000;5:63.

29. Cummins L, Nauenberg M: Thermal effects of laser radiation in biologic tissue. Biophys J 1983;43:99.

30. Kadipasaoglu KA, Frazier OH: Transmyocardial laser revascularization: Effect of laser parameters on tissue ablation and cardiac perfusion. Semin Thorac Cardiovasc Surg 1999; 11:4.

31. Kornowski R, Fuchs S, Leon MB: Mechanical approaches for myocardial angiogenesis. Curr Interv Cardiol Rep 1999;1: 199.

32. Fisher PE, Khomoto T, DeRosa CM, et al: Histologic analysis of transmyocardial channels: Comparison of CO_2 and holmium:YAG lasers. Ann Thorac Surg 1997;64:466.

33. Kornowski R, Hong MK, Haudenschild C, et al: Feasibility and safety of percutaneous direct myocardial revascularization using Biosens system in porcine hearts. Coron Artery Dis 1998;9:535.

34. Gassler N, Wintzer HO, Stubbe HM, et al: Transmyocardial laser revascularization: Histologic features in human non-responder myocardium. Circulation 1997;95:371.

35. Kohmoto T, DeRosa CM, Yamamoto N, et al: Evidence of vascular growth associated with laser treatment of normal canine myocardium. Ann Thorac Surg 1998;65:1360.

36. Burkhoff D, Fisher PE, Apfelbaum M, et al: Histologic appearance of transmyocardial laser channels after 4 1/2 weeks. Ann Thorac Surg 1996;61:1532.

37. Kohmoto T, Fisher PE, Gu A: Physiology, histology and 2-week morphology of acute transmyocardial laser channels made with a CO_2 laser. Ann Thorac Surg 1997;63: 1275.

38. Fuchs S, Kornowski R: Transepicardial or transendocardial injury: Controversies regarding angiogenic potential and mechanism of action. Cardiovasc Res 2001;16;49:582.

39. Kohmoto T, Fisher PE, Gu A, et al: Does blood flow through holmium:YAG transmyocardial laser channels? Ann Thorac Surg 1996;61:861.

40. Kohmoto T, Argenziano M, Yamamoto N, et al: Assessment of transmyocardial perfusion in alligator hearts. Circulation 1997;6:1585.

41. Whittaker P, Kloner RA, Przyklenk K: Laser-mediated transmural myocardial channels do not salvage acutely ischemic myocardium. J Am Coll Cardiol 1993;22:302.

42. Whittaker P, Kloner RA: Transmural laser channels as a source of blood flow to ischemic myocardium? Insights from the reptilian heart. Circulation 1997;95:1357.

43. Mack CA, Patel SR, Rosengart TK: Myocardial angiogenesis as a possible mechanism for TMLR efficacy. J Clin Laser Med Surg 1997;15:275.

44. Yamamoto N, Kohmoto T, Gu A, et al: Angiogenesis is enhanced in ischemic canine myocardium by transmyocardial laser revascularization. J Am Coll Cardiol 1998;31: 1426.

45. Hughes GC, Kypson AP, St Louis JD, et al: Improved perfusion and contractile reserve after transmyocardial laser revascularization in a model of hibernating myocardium. Ann Thorac Surg 1999;67:1714.

46. Pelletier MP, Giaid A, Sivaraman S, et al: Angiogenesis and growth factor expression in a model of transmyocardial revascularization. Ann Thorac Surg 1998;66:12.

47. Horvath KA, Chiu E, Maun DC, et al: Up-regulation of vascular endothelial growth factor mRNA and angiogenesis after transmyocardial laser revascularization. Ann Thorac Surg 1999;68:825.

48. Chu VF, Giaid A, Kuang JQ, et al: Angiogenesis in transmyocardial revascularization: Comparison of laser versus mechanical punctures. Ann Thorac Surg 1999;68:301.

49. Fuchs S, Baffour R, Vodovotz Y, et al: Laser myocardial revascularization modulates expression of angiogenic, neuronal, and inflammatory cytokines in a porcine model of chronic myocardial ischemia. J Card Surg 2002;17:413.

50. Spanier T, Smith CR, Burkhoff D: Angiogenesis: A possible mechanism underlying the clinical benefits of transmyocardial laser revascularization. J Clin Laser Med Surg 1997; 15:269.

51. Kwong KF, Kanellopoulos GK, Nickols JC, et al: Transmyocardial laser treatment denervates canine myocardium. J Thorac Cardiovasc Surg 1997;114:883.

52. Kwong KF, Schuessler RB, Kanellopoulos GK, et al: Nontransmural laser treatment incompletely denervates canine myocardium. Circulation 1998;98(Suppl 19):II-67.

53. Al-Sheikh T, Allen KB, Straka SP, et al: Cardiac sympathetic denervation after transmyocardial laser revascularization. Circulation 1999;100:135.

54. Myers J, Oesterle SN, Jones J, Burkhoff D: Do transmyocardial and percutaneous laser revascularization induce silent ischemia? An assessment by exercise testing. Am Heart J 2002;143:1052.

55. Smits PC, Serruys PW: Percutaneous direct myocardial revascularization: An overview of systems. Semin Interv Cardiol 2000;5:83.

56. Oesterle SN, Sanborn TA, Ali N, et al: Percutaneous transmyocardial laser revascularisation for severe angina: The PACIFIC randomised trial. Potential Class Improvement From Intramyocardial Channels. Lancet 2000;356:1705.

57. Whitlow PL, DeMaio SJ Jr, Perin EC, et al; Eclipse Investigators. One-year results of percutaneous myocardial revascularization for refractory angina pectoris. Am J Cardiol 2003;91: 1342.

58. Leon MB, Kornowski R, Downey WE, et al: A blinded, randomized, placebo-controlled trial of percutaneous laser myocardial revascularization to improve angina symptoms in patients with severe coronary disease. J Am Coll Cardiol 2005;46:1812.

59. Salem M, Rotevatn S, Stavnes S, et al: Usefulness and safety of percutaneous myocardial laser revascularization for refractory angina pectoris. Am J Cardiol 2004;93:1086.

60. Stone GW, Teirstein PS, Rubenstein R, et al: A prospective, multicenter, randomized trial of percutaneous transmyocardial laser revascularization in patients with nonrecanalizable chronic total occlusions. J Am Coll Cardiol 2002;39: 1581-1587.

61. Beecher HK: Surgery as placebo. JAMA 1961;176:1102.

62. Johnson AG: Surgery as placebo. Lancet 1994;344:1140.

63. Losordo DW, Dimmeler S: Therapeutic angiogenesis and vasculogenesis for ischemic disease. Part I: Angiogenic cytokines. Circulation 2004;109:2487.

64. Losordo DW, Dimmeler S: Therapeutic angiogenesis and vasculogenesis for ischemic disease. Part II: Cell-based therapies. Circulation 2004;109:2692.

65. Simons M, Post MJ: Coronary artery disease: Vascular endothelial growth factor and fibroblast growth factor. Curr Interv Cardiol Rep 2001;3:185.

66. Kornowski R, Leon MB, Fuchs S, et al: Electromagnetic guidance for catheter-based transendocardial injection: A platform for intramyocardial angiogenesis therapy. Results in normal and ischemic porcine models. J Am Coll Cardiol 2000;35:1031.

67. Kinnaird T, Stabile E, Burnett MS, Epstein SE: Bone-marrow-derived cells for enhancing collateral development: Mechanisms, animal data, and initial clinical experiences. Circ Res 2004;95:354.

68. Anversa P, Leri A, Kajstura J: Cardiac regeneration. J Am Coll Cardiol 2006;47:1769.

69. Stauer BE, Kornowski R: Stem cell therapy in perspective. Circulation 2003;107:929.

70. Laham RJ, Oettgen P: Bone marrow transplantation for the heart: Fact or fiction? Lancet 2003;361:11.

71. Epstein SE, Fuchs S, Zhou YF, et al: Therapeutic interventions for enhancing collateral development by administration of growth factors: Basic principles, early results and potential hazards. Cardiovasc Res 2001;49:532.

72. Conway EM, Collen D, Carmeliet P: Molecular mechanisms of blood vessel growth. Cardiovasc Res 2001;49:507.

73. Shintani S, Murohara T, Ikeda H, et al: Mobilization of endothelial progenitor cells in patients with acute myocardial infarction. Circulation 2001;103:2776.

74. Yeh ET, Zhang S, Wu HD, et al: Transdifferentiation of human peripheral blood CD34+-enriched cell population into cardiomyocytes, endothelial cells, and smooth muscle cells in vivo. Circulation 2003;108:2070.

75. Davani S, Marandin A, Mersin N, et al: Mesenchymal progenitor cells differentiate into an endothelial phenotype, enhance vascular density, and improve heart function in a rat cellular cardiomyoplasty model. Circulation 2003; 108(Suppl 1):II-253.

76. Urbich C, Dimmeler S: Endothelial progenitor cells: Characterization and role in vascular biology. Circ Res 2004;95:343.

77. Tirziu D, Simons M: Angiogenesis in the human heart: Gene and cell therapy. Angiogenesis 2005;8:241.

78. Epstein SE, Kornowski R, Fuchs S, Dvorak HF: Angiogenesis therapy: Amidst the hype, the neglected potential for serious side effects. Circulation 2001;104:115.

79. Henry TD, Rocha-Singh K, Isner JM, et al: Intracoronary administration of recombinant human vascular endothelial growth factor to patients with coronary artery disease. Am Heart J 2001;142.:872.

80. Simons M, Annex BH, Laham RJ, et al: Pharmacological treatment of coronary artery disease with recombinant fibroblast growth factor-2: Double-blind, randomized, controlled clinical trial. Circulation 2002;105:788.

81. Henry TD, Annex BH, McKendall GR, et al; VIVA Investigators. The VIVA trial: Vascular endothelial growth factor in Ischemia for Vascular Angiogenesis. Circulation 2003;107:1359.

82. Kornowski R, Fuchs S, Leon MB, Epstein SE: Delivery strategies to achieve therapeutic myocardial angiogenesis. Circulation 2000;101:454.

83. Fearon WF, Ikeno F, Bailey LR, et al: Evaluation of high-pressure retrograde coronary venous delivery of FGF-2 protein. Catheter Cardiovasc Interv 2004;61:422.

84. Losordo DW, Vale PR, Hendel RC, et al: Phase 1/2 placebo-controlled, double-blind, dose-escalating trial of myocardial vascular endothelial growth factor 2 gene transfer by catheter delivery in patients with chronic myocardial ischemia. Circulation 2002;105:2012.

85. Kastrup J, Jorgensen E, Ruck A, et al; Euroinject One Group. Direct intramyocardial plasmid vascular endothelial growth factor-A165 gene therapy in patients with stable severe angina pectoris: A randomized double-blind placebo-controlled study. The Euroinject One trial. J Am Coll Cardiol 2005;45:982.

86. Gyongyosi M, Khorsand A, Zamini S, et al: NOGA-guided analysis of regional myocardial perfusion abnormalities treated with intramyocardial injections of plasmid encoding vascular endothelial growth factor A-165 in patients with chronic myocardial ischemia: Subanalysis of the EUROIN-JECT-ONE multicenter double-blind randomized study. Circulation 2005;112(9 Suppl):I-157.

87. Stewart DJ, Hilton JD, Arnold JM, et al: Angiogenic gene therapy in patients with nonrevascularizable ischemic heart disease: A phase 2 randomized, controlled trial of AdVEGF(121) (AdVEGF121) versus maximum medical treatment. Gene Ther 2006;13:1503-1511. Epub 2006 June 22.

88. Fuchs S, Dib N, Cohen BM, et al: A randomized, double-blind, placebo-controlled, multicenter pilot study of the safety and feasibility of catheter-based intramyocardial injection of AdVEGF121 in patients with refractory advanced coronary artery disease. Catheter Cardiovasc Interv 2006;68:372-378.

89. Murasawa S, Asahara T: Endothelial progenitor cells for vasculogenesis. Physiology (Bethesda) 2005;20:36.

90. Leri A, Kajstura J, Anversa P: Cardiac stem cells and mechanisms of myocardial regeneration. Physiol Rev 2005;85:1373.

91. Fuchs S, Baffour R, Zhou YF, et al: Transendocardial delivery of autologous bone marrow enhances collateral perfusion and regional function in pigs with chronic experimental myocardial ischemia. J Am Coll Cardiol 2001;37:1726.

92. Amado LC, Saliaris AP, Schuleri KH, et al: Cardiac repair with intramyocardial injection of allogeneic mesenchymal stem cells after myocardial infarction. Proc Natl Acad Sci U S A 2005;102:11474.

93. Menasche P: Skeletal myoblast for cell therapy. Coron Artery Dis 2005;16:105.

94. Lev S, Kehat I, Gepstein L: Differentiation pathways in human embryonic stem cell-derived cardiomyocytes. Ann N Y Acad Sci 2005;1047:50.

95. Fuchs S, Satler LF, Kornowski R, et al: Catheter-based autologous bone marrow myocardial injection in no-option patients with advanced coronary artery disease: A feasibility study. J Am Coll Cardiol 2003;41:1721.

96. Fuchs S, Kornowski R, Weisz G, et al: Safety and feasibility of transendocardial autologous bone marrow cell transplantation in patients with advanced heart disease. Am J Cardiol 2006;97:823.

97. Perin EC, Dohmann HF, Borojevic R, et al: Transendocardial, autologous bone marrow cell transplantation for severe, chronic ischemic heart failure. Circulation 2003;107:2294.

98. Perin EC, Dohmann HF, Borojevic R, et al: Improved exercise capacity and ischemia 6 and 12 months after transendocardial injection of autologous bone marrow mononuclear cells for ischemic cardiomyopathy. Circulation 2004;110(11 Suppl 1):II-213.

99. Tse HF: Results from the PROTECT CAD trial. Presented at the American College of Cardiology Meeting, Atlanta, March 2006.

100. Tse HF, Kwong YL, Chan JF, et al: Angiogenesis in ischaemic myocardium by intramyocardial autologous bone marrow mononuclear cell implantation. Lancet 2003; 361:47.

101. Strauer BE, Brehm M, Zeus T, et al: Repair of infarcted myocardium by autologous intracoronary mononuclear bone marrow cell transplantation in humans. Circulation 2002; 106:1913.

102. Wollert KC, Meyer GP, Lotz J, et al: Intracoronary autologous bone-marrow cell transfer after myocardial infarction: The BOOST randomised controlled clinical trial. Lancet 2004;364:141.

103. Meyer GP, Wollert KC, Lotz J, et al: Intracoronary bone marrow cell transfer after myocardial infarction: eighteen months' follow-up data from the randomized, controlled BOOST (BOne marrow transfer to enhance ST-elevation infarct regeneration) trial. Circulation 2006;113:1287.

104. Hagege AA, Marolleau JP, Vilquin JT, et al: Skeletal myoblast transplantation in ischemic heart failure: Long-term follow-up of the first phase I cohort of patients. Circulation 2006;114(1 Suppl):I-108.

105. Smits PC, van Geuns RJ, Poldermans D, et al: Catheter-based intramyocardial injection of autologous skeletal myoblasts as a primary treatment of ischemic heart failure: Clinical experience with six-month follow-up. J Am Coll Cardiol 2003; 42:2063.

106. Siminiak T, Fiszer D, Jerzykowska O, et al: Percutaneous trans-coronary-venous transplantation of autologous skeletal myoblasts in the treatment of post-infarction myocardial contractility impairment: The POZNAN trial. Eur Heart J 2005;26:1188.

58 Stem Cell Therapy for Ischemic Heart Disease

Marc S. Penn

KEY POINTS

- Advances in reperfusion therapy have led to the development of a large population of patients with chronic heart failure who need new therapies such as stem cell therapy to experience improved outcomes.
- Strategies directed at optimizing cardiac function in the peri-infarct period do not necessarily translate to the heart failure setting owing to the differences in molecular signals between the two conditions.
- Recent studies have identified several different populations of stem cells that offer the potential to prevent and treat cardiac dysfunction.
- Well designed, randomized, blinded and controlled clinical studies have yielded conflicting results, the best of

which suggest only a modest benefit with current strategies of cell therapy in patients with acute myocardial infarction.
- Improvements in cardiac function with cell therapy do not necessarily imply improvements in electrical conduction or arrhythmogenic risk; in fact, in some circumstances the opposite could be true.
- Recently reported studies have included all patients with acute myocardial infarction; however, translation of preclinical studies to the clinic implies that we study only those patients with significant left ventricular dysfunction.

The many efforts to maximize therapy for patients with acute myocardial infarction (AMI) have yielded significant benefits. Beginning first with thrombolytic therapy for AMI, and more recently with the availability of primary percutaneous coronary intervention for ST-elevation MI, the mortality rates of this devastating ischemic event have decreased from almost 15% in clinical trials in the late 1980s[1] to less than 5% in recent primary percutaneous coronary intervention trials.[2] Before these advances, ischemic heart disease was the leading cause of chronic heart failure (CHF). Although further improvements in reperfusion are needed, the current advances have led to a growing epidemic of CHF, with many patients surviving what in the past might have been fatal events.

With these advances, the prevalence of congestive heart failure has increased dramatically over the preceding decade, with now more than 10% of the United States population older than 65 years of age carrying the diagnosis. Although the mechanisms are still under investigation,[3,4] the development of CHF after MI represents more than just the loss of contractile tissue; it is also determined, in part, by the ventricular remodeling that occurs in response to myocardial necrosis.[5] The inflammatory response to myocardial necrosis leads to infarct expansion, dila-

tion of the left ventricular (LV) cavity, and replacement of cardiomyocytes with fibrous tissue.[3,5] Currently available therapies to alter the remodeling process and the progression to CHF remain limited, and death rates from CHF continue to rise. Based on current trends, the problem is predicted to increase to affect more than 6 million people by the year 2030.

The increasing burden of CHF has been addressed with pharmacologic therapy, which in some cases can delay and improve the morbidity and mortality of CHF; by electrical therapy, including cardiac resynchronization therapy; by LV remodeling surgery; and by mechanical therapy, with the recent approval of the first LV assist device for destination therapy. Given the shortcomings of each of these strategies and the fact that none of them addresses the underlying problem—loss of cardiac myocytes due to ischemic death—many researchers have turned to molecular therapy, and more specifically to stem cell–based therapy, as the hope for the future.

APPROACHES TO CELL THERAPY

The field of cell transplantation for the treatment of LV dysfunction after ischemic injury is broad.[6] Theoretically, optimal cell therapy will use cell types that possess the capacity to incorporate into the recipient myocardium, survive, mature, and electromechanically couple to each other and to native cardiac myocytes.

In its simplest form, differentiated cell transplantation (Fig. 58-1A), the goal is to transplant autologous cells that are differentiated or committed to differentiate into specific cells into areas of myocardial scar, with the goal being to replace areas of scar tissue with living, viable cells. In perhaps its most futuristic form, stem cell mobilization (see Fig. 58-1B), cell therapy involves the pharmacologic mobilization of a patient's own bone marrow cells into the bloodstream, homing of these stem cells to engraft into areas of myocardial damage, and then differentiation of the engrafted stem cells into cardiac myocytes and vascular structures that fully integrate with the native myocardium. An in-between strategy, stem cell transplantation (see Fig. 58-1C) involves the removal of stem cells from the bone marrow of the patient, followed by injection of the whole bone marrow or a selected population of bone marrow–derived stem cells into the infarct zone.

Although each of these strategies has its own unique technologic and clinical challenges, they share a number of important questions:
1. What is the optimal cell type or class of cells for each strategy?
2. When is the earliest time after AMI that the cells would be available for transplantation?
3. Balancing safety and efficacy, when is the optimal time after AMI for initiation of cell therapy?
4. What is the mode of efficacy for a specific strategy (i.e., prevention of remodeling or regeneration of contractile tissue)?
5. Do the engrafted/transplanted cells represent an arrhythmogenic risk?

Although bench, animal and clinical research studies have significantly expanded our knowledge, no cell-based strategy to date has come close to meeting all of these challenges. That said, therapeutic strategies have emerged from animal studies into the phase I clinical trial arena,[7-10] and most recently into randomized, blinded, and placebo-controlled clinical trials.[11-13]

Differentiated cell transplantation

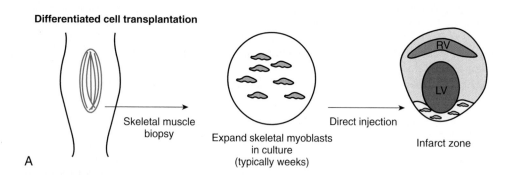

A

Stem cell mobilization

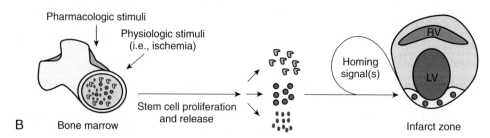

B

Stem cell transplantation

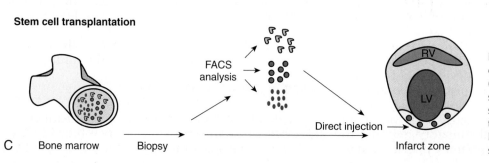

C

Figure 58-1. Schematic diagram of differentiated cell transplantation (**A**), stem cell mobilization (**B**), and stem cell transplantation (**C**) strategies of cell therapy for the treatment of cardiac dysfunction. FACS, fluorescence-activated cell sorting.

DIFFERENTIATED CELL TRANSPLANTATION

The goal of differentiated cell transplantation is the substitution of scarred myocardium with living, viable cells, ultimately leading to overall improvement of myocardial function. A number of cell types, including smooth muscle cells and skeletal myoblasts, have been studied as potential candidates for differentiated cell transplantation. The value of these cell types is their accessibility and their ability to be expanded in vitro before transplantation.

The majority of the animal work in this field has focused on the use of skeletal myoblasts (SKMB), and specifically on SKMB transplantation. In contrast to cardiac myocytes, SKMBs maintain their ability to regenerate and, during periods of stress, to proliferate and differentiate into myotubes, eventually forming new muscle fibers capable of contraction. In addition, skeletal muscle is much more resistant to ischemia than is cardiac muscle. Skeletal muscle can withstand many hours of ischemia without becoming irreversibly injured; in contrast, irreversible injury occurs within 20 minutes in cardiac muscle.[14]

Although SKMBs have desirable properties for cell therapy, the timing of their delivery before pathologic LV remodeling occurs after MI in clinical populations is problematic. It takes at least 2 to 3 weeks from skeletal muscle biopsy to the availability of a sufficient number of SKMBs for transplantation in humans. Therefore, if the main benefit of SKMB transplantation is to attenuate LV remodeling, then, unless patients who will benefit can be identified very early after MI and/or an off-the-shelf cell that is not immunogenic can be made available at the time

of MI, it is debatable whether SKMB transplantation alone can offer significant clinical benefit.

SKMB therapy is advancing through clinical trials (Table 58-1). Because of the above-mentioned limitations in the timing of SKMB therapy for patients with recent MI, the clinical studies to date have focused on patients with ischemic cardiomyopathy. Improvement in cardiac function using SKMB transplantation has been demonstrated in some studies in patients with late-stage ischemic cardiomyopathy (see Table 58-1). Transplantation of SKMBs has been performed at the time of LV device placement or as a stand-alone procedure in patients with end-stage congestive heart failure due to ischemic cardiomyopathy.[15,16] At the time of cardiac transplantation, SKMB engraftment has been demonstrated in patients at 3, 4, and 6 months after SKMB transplantation.[15,16]

Clinical trials to date suggest some potential benefits of this strategy; however, enthusiasm must be tempered by the recent discontinuation of the Myoblast Autologous Grafting in Ischemic Cardiomyopathy (MAGIC) trial. The purpose of this well designed, randomized trial was to determine whether SKMB transplantation at the time of coronary artery bypass grafting (CABG) would result in improved cardiac function without an increase in arrhythmogenic risk to patients. Although details have not yet been released, statements to date suggest that no benefit was seen after enrollment of almost 100 patients (from a planned enrollment of approximately 300 patients), leading the investigators and sponsors to prematurely stop the trial in the spring of 2006. Whether there was any arrhythmogenic risk to the

Table 58-1. Clinical Trials of Skeletal Myoblast (SKMB) Transplantation

Study (Ref. No.)	Clinical Population	No. Patients/Controls?	Cell No.	Comments
Direct Injection				
Menasche (7)	Adjunct to CABG	10/No	871×10^6	4 patients with VT 2 patients died unrelated to cell therapy
Herrores (53)	Adjunct to CABG	12/No	300×10^6	No VT reported
Siminiak (54)	Adjunct to CABG	10/No	300×10^6	4 patients with VT
Pagani (15)	Adjunct to LVAD placement	5/No	300×10^6	SKMB identified in explanted hearts of those patients who receive transplant
Dib (52)	Adjunct to CABG	30/No	Dose escalating: 10, 30, 100, and 300×10^6	1 death from VF 4 cases of nonsustained VT Ischemic cardiomyopathy (24) and LVAD patients (6)
Menasche (64)	Adjunct to CABG	97/Yes	Placebo/400 or 800×10^6 cells	Prematurely stopped; decreased LVEDD with high dose
Percutaneous Injection				
Smits (8)	Stand-alone Percutaneous	5/No	300×10^6	1 patient with VT
Serruys (65)	Stand-alone Percutaneous	15/No		1 patient with SCD 1 patient with VT storm
Siminiak (55)	Stand-alone Percutaneous	10/No	100×10^6	

CABG, coronary artery bypass grafting; LVAD, left ventricular assist device; LVEDD, left ventricular end diastolic dimension; SCD, sudden cardiac death; VF, ventricular fibrillation; VT, ventricular tachyarrhythmia.

patients who received SKMB awaits further analyses.

Further complicating the use of differentiated cells such as SKMBs is that the mechanism of functional LV improvement with SKMB transplantation is not clear. Transplanted SKMBs do not result[17] in the development of new cardiac myocytes, and the transplanted cells do not electromechanically integrate into the native myocardium.[18] However, the combined improvements in systolic and diastolic function that have been demonstrated ultimately appear to lead to overall improved cardiac performance. Despite the lack of definitive evidence, there is hope that SKMB transplantation can benefit clinical populations, even at times remote from MI,[16] and the therapy is under continued investigation.

MYOCARDIAL REGENERATION

Since the turn of the century, a significant body of literature has rewritten the once strongly held belief that the heart cannot repair itself. We have learned that, after MI in humans, there is a transient mobilization of stem cells and expression of stem cell homing factors that recruit these cells to the heart.[19,20] Human female hearts transplanted into males were found to have cardiac myocytes and vascular structures that stained positive for the Y chromosome, suggesting that these cells originated from the stem cells of the recipient.[21] These studies also demonstrated that stem cell engraftment and differentiation into cardiac myocytes is an infrequent event (0.02% cardiac myocytes, 3.3% endothelial cells). However, they did suggest that the normal physiologic response to myocardial injury is mobilization of stem cells, "homing" of these cells to the damaged myocardium, and differentiation of at least some of these stem cells into cardiac myocytes. Furthermore, if this natural repair mechanism can be potentiated, clinically meaningful myocardial regeneration may be achievable.

The excitement surrounding the use of stem cells is based on the unique biologic properties of these cells and their capacity to self-renew and regenerate tissue and organ systems. Figure 58-2 groups different stem cell populations of interest in myocardial regeneration based on their level of potency. It was once believed that all stem cell populations listed in Figure 58-2 could differentiate into cardiac myocytes,[22,23] but it is now quite clear that, although many of these cell populations may lead to improved cardiac function,[22,24] only a limited number of these cells become cardiac myocytes after transplantation.[25,26]

Bone Marrow–Derived Mononuclear Cells

The transplantation of bone marrow–derived mononuclear cell (BMC) preparations to the infarct-related vessel has progressed to the point where data from randomized controlled trials are now becoming available for patients with AMI (Table 58-2) and CHF (Table 58-3). The first randomized stem cell trial for

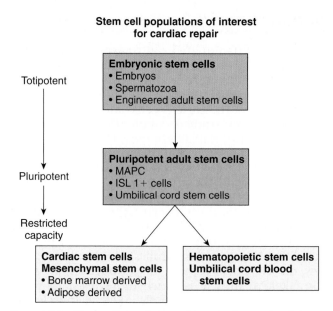

Stem cell populations of interest for cardiac repair

Figure 58-2. Stem cell populations of interest for myocardial repair stratified by the differentiation capacity of the given populations. ISL, islet; MAPC, multipotent adult progenitor cells.

patients with AMI was the Bone Marrow Transfer to Enhance ST-elevation Infarct Regeneration (BOOST) trial.[27] In this trial, all patients were emergently reperfused by primary percutaneous coronary intervention and received optimal medical care. One half of the patients were randomized to receive intracoronary infusion of a mononuclear preparation of cells from the marrow space of the iliac crest. The intracoronary infusion occurred between 4 and 5 days after MI. Six months after cell infusion, patients in the active arm of the trial demonstrated, on average, a 6.7% increase in ejection fraction, without significant changes in LV end-systolic or -diastolic volumes. Patients in the control arm exhibited only a 0.6% increase in ejection fraction. This unusually small increment in cardiac function with optimal medical therapy (see Table 58-2) resulted in statistical significance for the improvement seen with cell therapy. Of note, whereas the benefits seen with cell therapy were maintained, at 1 year there was no statistically significant benefit between the groups, because of further improvement in the control group. Therefore, this early trial and its subsequent follow-up suggested that infusion of BMCs accelerates healing of the heart but does not further improve it.[28]

The results seen in the BOOST population were recently reproduced by the Reinfusion of Enriched Progenitor Cells and Infarct Remodeling in Acute Myocardial Infarction (REPAIR-AMI) trial.[13] In this well designed, randomized, blinded, placebo-controlled study, patients with AMI received intracoronary infusion of BMCs 4 days after primary percutaneous coronary intervention. The absolute benefit seen in the REPAIR-AMI trial was small (6.0% versus 2.5%) but reached statistical significance.[13] Several important post hoc analyses were

Table 58-2. Stem Cell Transplantation in Acute Myocardial Infarction

Study (Ref. No.)	No. Patients/ Placebo Control?	Cell Type	Delivery Method	Time Since Infarct (Days)	Baseline LV Function (%)	Comments
Chen (56)	69/Yes	BM-derived MSC	Intracoronary	18.4±1.5	49-53	Improvement in perfusion, cardiac function; decreased LV dilation. No increase in restenosis noted.
BOOST (27, 57)	60/Yes	BM-derived mononuclear cells	Intracoronary	4.8	50-51	6 mo after MI, increase in EF (6.7%) with stem cell infusion vs. 0.6% with optimal medical management. Controls caught up; benefit not lost at 18 mo.
ASTAMI (11)	100/Yes	BM-derived mononuclear cells	Intracoronary	5-8	46	Noted chest pain and/or ECG changes with stem cell infusion. No improvement 6 mo after stem cell infusion.
REPAIR-AMI (13)	204/Yes	BM-derived mononuclear cells	Intracoronary	4	47-48	Modest improvement in EF 4 mo after stem cell infusion (5.5% vs. 3.0% for placebo). For baseline EF <49%, improvement was 7.5% with stem cell infusion vs. 2.5% for placebo.
Janssens (12)	66/Yes	BM-derived mononuclear cells	Intracoronary	4	46-49	First randomized, placebo-controlled, blinded study for cell therapy at the time of acute MI. No benefit seen.

BM, bone marrow; ECG, electrocardiogram; EF, ejection fraction; LV, left ventricular; MI, myocardial infarction; MSC, mesenchymal stem cells.

Table 58-3. Stem Cell Transplantation in Chronic Heart Failure

Study (Ref. No.)	No. Patients/ Placebo Control?	Cell Type	Delivery Method	Cause of Heart Failure	Effect on LV Function	Comments
Tse (58)	8/No	BMC	Stem cell transplantation (NOGA-guided catheter-basted intramyocardial injection)	Severe ischemic heart disease	Unchanged	Despite no change in EF, improvement in target wall thickening and wall motion was seen by MRI. No acute procedure-related complications.
Seiler (59)	21/Yes	Stem cells mobilized from the BM	GM-CSF, first dose intracoronary, then stem cells for 2 wk	Chronic ischemia	Unchanged, but decreased ischemia	Stem cell mobilization to induce angiogenesis as assessed by improved coronary collateral blood flow after 2 wk of daily GM-CSF administration.
Assmus (30)	75/Yes, with crossover	CPC or BMC	Intracoronary infusion	Ischemic cardiomyopathy	Improved with BMC only	For baseline EF ~40%, improvement was 2.9% with BMC, −1.2% without therapy, −0.4% with CPC
Perin (10)	21/Yes, nonrandomized	BMC	Stem cell transplantation (NOGA-guided catheter-based intramyocardial injection)	Severe ischemic cardiomyopathy	Improved	—
Fuchs (28)	10/No	BMC	Catheter-based intramyocardial delivery	Chronic ischemia	Unchanged, but decreased ischemia	Decreased stress-induced ischemia and CCS angina score

BMC, bone marrow–derived mononuclear cells; CCS, Canadian Cardiovascular Society; CPC, circulating progenitor cells; EF, ejection fraction; GM-CSF, granulocyte-macrophage colony-stimulating factor; MRI, magnetic resonance imaging.

performed that suggested directions for future trials; for example, the improvement observed was greater in patients with lower ejection fractions, and further improvement was observed in patients who received cell infusion at least 4 days after AMI.[13] The correlation with baseline ejection fraction is consistent with animal studies and is reassuring. The observation that therapy is more efficacious later after AMI suggests that there may be an interaction between inflammation and cell engraftment. Clearly, further basic, translational, and clinical trials are necessary before this strategy for cell therapy is optimized.

Whether this therapy has a real future was further brought into question by the recent release of the results of the Autologous Stem Cell Transplantation in Acute Myocardial Infarction (ASTAMI) trial (a randomized, nonblinded trial with no placebo)[11] and those of Janssens and colleagues (a randomized, blinded, and placebo-controlled trial).[12] The ASTAMI trial was an open-label study in patients with acute ST-elevation anterior wall MI. This was the first study to limit enrollment to patients with anterior wall MI, arguably the patient population that is at greatest risk for development of congestive heart failure and therefore the one that should be of most interest.[29] The ASTAMI trial showed no benefit with infusion of autologous BMCs. Although this was a well designed and executed study, there are some concerns regarding the viability of the cells at the time of cell infusion. The study by Janssens and colleagues failed to demonstrate a significant increase in ejection fraction, but the results did suggest a decrease in infarct size and improved regional function in those segments that demonstrated transmural involvement.[12]

Differences between the outcomes of these studies could be due to several factors, including number of cells infused (ASTAMI, 7×10^7; REPAIR-AMI, 2.4×10^8; Janssens, 3×10^8). It is also possible that cell viability may not have been similar, based on differences in harvesting and cell culture protocols between studies.

The strategy of infusing BMC preparations has recently been translated to patients with ischemic cardiomyopathy (see Table 58-3).[10,30] In an interesting crossover protocol design, patients received BMCs, circulating progenitor cells, or no infusion. Whereas the benefits observed were small, benefit was seen only after infusion of the BMCs (observed changes in ejection fraction: BMCs, 2.9%; circulating progenitor cells, –0.4%; and no infusion, –1.2%).[30] The fact that only BMCs yielded a significant benefit suggests that cells beyond simply hematopoietic stem cells need to be delivered to the myocardial tissue in order to obtain significant benefit. A discussion of other stem cells of interest, some of which are present in the bone marrow space, follows.

Mesenchymal Stem Cells and Multipotent Adult Progenitor Cells

Stromal progenitor cells make up less than 0.05% of the adult bone marrow. Mesenchymal stem cells

(MSC) and multipotent adult progenitor cells (MAPC) form subpopulations of bone marrow stromal progenitor cells that maintain the ability to differentiate along multiple lineages.[23,31] MSCs can be immunoselected via cell surface CD45 negativity and cultured through as many as 40 population doublings before attaining senescence. 5-Azacytidine or transforming growth factor-β (TGF-β) pretreatment can induce MSCs to increase expression of proteins in vitro that are normally expressed by cardiac myocytes. The benefits observed with MSC transplantation at the time of MI may have little to do with the cell itself, but rather how factors secreted by the MSCs alter the tissue microenvironment. This so-called paracrine effect of MSCs has been demonstrated,[32] showing that injection of the supernatant of MSC cell cultures at the time of the MI results in benefits similar to those associated with MSC transplantation. More recently, we demonstrated that the reestablishment of MSC recruitment months after a MI, through reestablishment of expression of monocyte chemotactic protein 3 (MCP-3), results in significant remodeling of the infarct zone and improved myocardial function, in the absence of any evidence of angiogenesis or cardiac myocyte regeneration.[26]

MAPCs are able to differentiate into endothelial, epithelial, and mesenchymal cell types.[33] They can be expanded in culture for more than 80 population doublings and still maintain their pluripotency by differentiating into most somatic cell types.[33] Other multipotent adult stem cells have recently been described that appear capable of differentiating into cardiac myocytes in vivo.[34] Whether these multipotent stem cells exist in vivo or are the result of serial cell passages in culture remains to be determined. However, the demonstration that multipotent cells can be significantly expanded and their benefit in early animal studies[34] bodes well for the development of future therapies.

Umbilical Cord Blood Stem Cells

The stem cell compartment in cord blood is less mature than that of adult bone marrow. Hematopoietic stem cells are less abundant in bone marrow than in cord blood, where they demonstrate greater proliferative potential associated with longer telomeres and an extended life span.[35,36] In addition to these benefits, cord blood is regularly harvested with little if any risk to the donor, it is abundantly accessible, and associated infectious agents are rare. Importantly, umbilical cord blood offers an abundant source of stem cells free of invasive techniques and ethical concerns. Administration of umbilical cord blood stem cells at the time of MI has been shown to improve cardiac function, but there is no evidence that these cells regenerate cardiac myocytes.[37]

Embryonic Stem Cells

Embryonic stem cells are continuously replicating cell lines derived from an embryonic origin isolated from the blastocyst inner cell mass.[38,39] The properties of embryonic stem cells include derivation from the preimplantation or peri-implantation embryo, prolonged undifferentiated proliferation with conditional constraints, and the ability to form tissues derived from all three germ layers. When they are properly cultured, embryonic stem cells expand at a rapid rate and group to form embryoidal bodies that have the ability to differentiate into a wide variety of specialized cells, including cardiomyocytes.

Great advances have been made in our understanding of embryonic stem cells, and it is becoming increasingly clear that, in order to regenerate cardiac myocytes, embryonic stem cells, at least in the bench or more likely as part of the therapy itself, will be necessary. Most exciting are the recent studies that have demonstrated the potential to derive cells with the properties of embryonic stem cells from adult cells.[40,41] Generation of embryonic stem cells from adult stem cells holds the potential to circumvent the ethical issues surrounding the acquisition of embryonic stem cells. Transplantation of human embryonic stem cells into immune-deficient rats has the potential to induce the formation of teratomas; and intramyocardial transplantation of cardiac myocytes derived from embryonic stem cells exhibits arrhythmic potential.

Embryonic stem cell commitment to the cardiac lineage promotes analysis of developing heart cells. In vitro differentiation of embryonic stem cells provides a powerful technique to investigate early cardiomyogenesis, differentiation of early cardiac precursor cells, the development of excitability, excitation-contraction coupling, and the molecular signals that occur in these processes. This line of research is critical, not only for our understanding of embryonic stem cells, but also to optimize adult stem cell therapies.

CYTOKINE-BASED STEM CELL THERAPY

The potential efficacy of stem cell mobilization as a noninvasive therapeutic strategy for the regeneration of the myocardium after MI has been demonstrated in animal models[42]; however, the majority of clinical trials to date have failed to demonstrate clinical efficacy (Table 58-4). There are several potential reasons that this strategy has failed in clinical trials.

The first potential reason is the timing of the stem cell mobilization relative to the heart's ability to recruit circulating stem cells. In the only trial that showed sustained improvement, granulocyte colony-stimulating factor (G-CSF) was administered within 1 hour after percutaneous coronary intervention.[43] Our group demonstrated that expression of stromal cell–derived factor-1 (SDF-1) is sufficient to induce stem cell homing to the heart in models of ischemic cardiomyopathy, and that transient and reestablishing expression of SDF-1 in the remodeled heart at a time remote for MI is sufficient to induce neovascularization and significant restoration of cardiac contractility.[19,44] Our data further showed that, by 7 days after MI, myocardial expression of SDF-1 has ceased. Therefore, timing is of the essence if hematopoietic stem cells are to be mobilized and engrafted in the heart.

Another reason this strategy failed may be that G-CSF-mobilized hematopoietic stem cells are unable to home due to dysfunctional expression of the chemokine receptor CXCR4 (the SDF-1 receptor). G-CSF mobilizes stem cells via the degradation of CXCR4, thus releasing the stem cell from its anchor in the

Table 58-4. Stem Cell Mobilization in Acute Myocardial Infarction (AMI)

Study (Ref. No.)	No. Patients/ Placebo Control?	Cell Type	Delivery Method	Time Since Infarct (Days)	LV Function	Comments
Kang (60)	27/Yes	Stem cells mobilized from the BM	G-CSF	3-270	Improved	Increased incidence of restenosis with G-CSF. Improved myocardial perfusion. Similar improvements seen with intracoronary infusion of peripheral blood stem cells
Valgimigli (61)	20/Yes	Stem cells mobilized from the BM	G-CSF		Trend towards improvement	No increase in restenosis with G-CSF. No improvement in myocardial perfusion.
Ellis (9)	18/Yes	Stem cells mobilized from the BM	G-CSF	1st dose ≤48 h from onset of symptoms	No Change	No benefit or harm with 5 or 10 μg/kg/day dose within 48 hr after AMI
Ince (43)	30/Yes	Stem cell mobilized from the BM	G-CSF	1 h	Improved	Control: EF 53 → 46% Treated: EF 52 → 56%
Ripa (62)	78/Yes	Stem cell mobilized from the BM	G-CSF		No Change	No significant changes in wall thickening or EF by echocardiography or MRI
Zohlnhofer (63)	114/Yes	Stem cell mobilized from the BM	G-CSF	5 d	No Change	No evidence of increased rate of restenosis with G-CSF

BM, bone marrow; EF, ejection fraction; G-CSF, granulocyte colony-stimulating factor; MRI, magnetic resonance imaging.

bone marrow. A recent clinical study demonstrated that stem cells mobilized using G-CSF are unable to home because of the loss of functional CXCR4.[45]

ELECTRICAL EFFECTS OF CELL THERAPY

While the field is moving forward in trying to identify strategies that either preserve or improve cardiac function in patients at the time of AMI or in patients with CHF, it is becoming clear that the mechanical and electrical effects of cell therapy are independent.[18,44] We recently demonstrated that either SKMB or MSC (1 million of each cell type) delivered in the peri-infarct period to the myocardium resulted in similar improvements in cardiac function (Fig. 58-3A); however, on electrophysiologic study of these hearts with the introduction of extrasystoles, the rate at which ventricular tachycardia is induced is significantly different depending on the cell type the animal received (see Fig. 58-3B). Animals that received SKMB were always inducible for ventricular tachycardia. As noted in Table 58-1, multiple studies have suggested an increased incidence of ventricular tachycardia in patients who received SKMB. This could be a spurious

result owing to the fact that all of the patients in these trials had a history of MI; however, whereas SKMB do express connexin 43 in culture, they do not express connexin 43 after transplantation, and SKMB do not electrically couple with the native myocardium.[18] These data, coupled with the clinical data to date, support the concept that cell therapy can separately modulate the functional and electrical size of the infarct zone. Future decisions that focus on the optimal cell populations for use in improving patient outcomes need to focus on improving both the electrical and the mechanical performance of the heart.

FUTURE DIRECTIONS AND CONTROVERSIES

A number of critical clinical and scientific issues need to be addressed before these therapies will become either optimized or part of the clinical armamentarium to arrest the development of congestive heart failure after MI. That said, the field continues to mature. It continues to be critical that the public be accurately informed and have realistic expectations. Given the pervasiveness of the disease, the pressure and interest from patients and special interest groups is significant.

We have already learned a great deal from those investigators who have performed either feasibility or placebo-controlled studies. The variety of approaches used in these studies highlights the need to eventually determine whether there is an optimal strategy for cell delivery. To date, intracoronary infusion and direct percutaneous delivery or direct visualization have all been shown to have some efficacy.

One key question and controversy facing the field is whether cardiogenesis can be truly achieved. There is little evidence that unmanipulated cardiac myocytes will divide and regenerate themselves after myocardial injury. However, genetic manipulation of cardiac myocytes using engineered murine models indicates that cardiac myocytes can be induced to divide and regress infarct size.[46,47] Whether pharmacologic strategies will be developed to allow these pathways to be activated after MI remains to be seen. Early animal studies suggested that a stem cell–based strategy for cardiogenesis might be possible[22,23,42,48,49]; however, more recent studies suggested that there is little potential for cardiogenesis with adult stem cells derived from the bone marrow.[19,25,26,44,50] Whether the heart has an endogenous cardiac stem cell population or, more likely, a population of stem cells that is replenished by the bone marrow[51] still needs to be determined; however, the cardiogenic potential of these cells is still unlikely. Similarly, it is clear that cardiogenesis is possible with embryonic cells, but how this strategy will be brought forward, including limiting the carcinogenic and immunologic consequences, is still under investigation.

What would cardiogenesis look like? Past studies suffered from the lack of specificity of immunohistochemical and immunofluorescent techniques. Although these are reasonable screening tools for

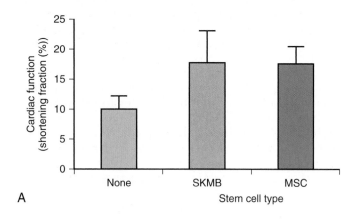

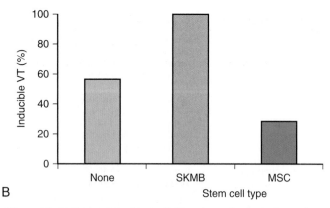

Figure 58-3. Frequency of inducibility of ventricular tachycardia (VT) (**A**) and cardiac function (**B**) 1 month after myocardial infarct induced by ligation of the left anterior descending coronary artery (LAD) in the Lewis rat. Animals received either no cells ($n=7$), 1 million skeletal myoblasts (SKMB, $n=5$) injected in the infarct zone at the time of LAD ligation, or 2 million mesenchymal stem cells (MSC, $n=7$) injected via tail vein 1 day after LAD ligation.

determining whether cardiogenesis might have occurred, they are not sufficient to validate the occurrence or frequency of cardiogenesis. Murine models using genetically engineered cell sources currently are state of the art.[25] Beyond that, cardiac myocytes, either differentiated in culture or isolated from hearts after cell therapy, need to demonstrate action potentials using patch clamp techniques.

If adult stem cell therapy does not result in cardiogenesis, should we be studying it in patients? After all, the impetus for taking these strategies to patients was their potential for cardiogenesis. Although these approaches are perhaps controversial, it is clear that these cells do offer significant therapeutic potential, either through paracrine effects or neovascularization or both. Given the relative safety that trials to date have shown, the lack of long-term toxicity, some evidence of short-term benefit, and the large unmet clinical need, further study of the effects of cell therapy in patients at risk for poor outcomes[29] appears reasonable.

Issues that need to be addressed include the following:

1. *Cardiogenesis*
   a. The appropriate source or identity of stem cell populations that can be expanded sufficiently to allow for clinical application as well as predictable differentiation into cardiac myocytes still remains to be identified. Most of the data suggest that only embryonic stem cells reliably differentiate into cardiac myocytes.
   b. We need to determine to what extent these novel strategies for generating embryonic stem cells from adult cells are valid options for generating cardiac myocytes.
   c. We need to determine the molecular pathways that control stem cell differentiation into cardiac myocytes and how to deliver those factors to injured myocardial tissue.
2. *Allogeneic source of appropriate stem cells for myocardial regeneration:* Based on current data, the maximal benefits of stem cell therapy for the preservation of myocardial function at the time of AMI require that a sufficient number of cells be available within days after the MI. Many of the cell types that are currently of interest require a significant amount of time (weeks) in order to obtain a sufficient number of cells for each person. The recent completion of a phase I clinical study in which allogeneic MSCs were infused into patients with AMI suggests that this important issue is being addressed.
3. *Stem cell delivery systems*
   a. Multiple catheter systems are being developed to deliver stem cells to myocardial tissue. Each of these approaches requires validation.
   b. Similarly, depending on the ability of the injected stem cell to migrate and respond to the local microenvironment, we will need to determine whether myocardial mapping (e.g.,

NOGA system) is required to optimize therapy.
   c. The science and clinical practicalities associated with timing of therapy and the dose of cells needs to be studied and optimized for each stem cell population of interest.
4. *Arrhythmogenic effects:* Early clinical studies with SKMB demonstrated that SKMB transplantation may increase the arrhythmogenic risk in patients who are already at significant risk.[7,52] These findings suggest that there could be adverse effects after cell therapy. Furthermore, they demonstrate that cardiac function is not the only parameter that should be studied. The electrical effects of cell therapy need to be addressed in clinical trials either through long-term monitoring of events using implantable devices or by assessing arrhythmogenic risk, possibly through T-wave alternans.
5. Arguably the greatest unknown facing the field of stem cell therapy for the treatment of MI is lack of knowledge regarding the *effects of stem cells on the underlying atherosclerosis* that ultimately caused the heart failure. Based on the current state of knowledge, it is theoretically possible that stem cells could decrease, have no effect, or increase the risk of plaque rupture and MI. Unfortunately, there is no reliable preclinical model to adequately study this problem before clinical trials are undertaken.

CONCLUSIONS

The simple conclusion is that we are on the verge of an extraordinary and exciting time in cardiovascular medicine. Basic and clinical studies continue along a path of discovery that allows for rapid translation of basic studies to the clinic. Further development and clinical fruition of these strategies for the treatment and/or prevention of congestive heart failure will continue to require a high level of collaboration between basic scientists and clinicians and a great deal of rigorous work on both sides. Given the current prevalence of patients with congestive heart failure and MI, combined with the economic burden of congestive heart failure, the potential human and societal benefits are great.

REFERENCES

1. Randomized factorial trial of high-dose intravenous streptokinase, of oral aspirin and of intravenous heparin in acute myocardial infarction. ISIS (International Studies of Infarct Survival) pilot study. Eur Heart J 1987;8:634-642.
2. Stone GW, Grines CL, Cox DA, et al: Comparison of angioplasty with stenting, with or without abciximab, in acute myocardial infarction. N Engl J Med 2002;346:957-966.
3. Askari A, Brennan ML, Zhou X, et al: Myeloperoxidase and plasminogen activator inhibitor-1 play a central role in ventricular remodeling after myocardial infarction. J Exp Med 2003;197:615-624.
4. Heymans S, Luttun A, Nuyens D, et al: Inhibition of plasminogen activators or matrix metalloproteinases prevents cardiac

rupture but impairs therapeutic angiogenesis and causes cardiac failure. Nat Med 1999;5:1135-1142.

5. Vasilyev N, Williams T, Brennan ML, et al: Myeloperoxidase-generated oxidants modulate left ventricular remodeling but not infarct size after myocardial infarction. Circulation 2005;112:2812-2820.

6. Penn MS, Francis GS, Ellis SG, et al: Autologous cell therapy for the treatment of damaged myocardium. Prog Cardiovasc Dis 2002;45:21-32.

7. Menasche P, Hagege AA, Vilquin JT, et al: Autologous skeletal myoblast transplantation for severe postinfarction left ventricular dysfunction. J Am Coll Cardiol 2003;41:1078-1083.

8. Smits PC, van Geuns RJ, Poldermans D, et al: Catheter-based intramyocardial injection of autologous skeletal myoblasts as a primary treatment of ischemic heart failure: Clinical experience with six-month follow-up. J Am Coll Cardiol 2003;42:2063-2069.

9. Ellis SG, Penn MS, Bolwell B, et al: Granulocyte colony stimulating factor in patients with large acute myocardial infarction: Results of a pilot dose-escalation randomized trial. Am Heart J 2006;152:1051.e9-e14.

10. Perin EC, Dohmann HF, Borojevic R, et al: Transendocardial, autologous bone marrow cell transplantation for severe, chronic ischemic heart failure. Circulation 2003;107:2294-2302. Epub 2003 Apr 21.

11. Lunde K, Solheim S, Aakhus S, et al: Intracoronary injection of mononuclear bone marrow cells in acute myocardial infarction. N Engl J Med 2006;355:1199-1209.

12. Janssens S, Dubois C, Bogaert J, et al: Autologous bone marrow-derived stem-cell transfer in patients with ST-segment elevation myocardial infarction: Double-blind, randomised controlled trial. Lancet 2006;367:113-121.

13. Schachinger V, Erbs S, Elsasser A, et al: Intracoronary bone marrow-derived progenitor cells in acute myocardial infarction. N Engl J Med 2006;355:1210-1221.

14. Campion DR: The muscle satellite cell: A review. Int Rev Cytol 1984;87:225-251.

15. Pagani FD, DerSimonian H, Zawadzka A, et al: Autologous skeletal myoblasts transplanted to ischemia-damaged myocardium in humans: Histological analysis of cell survival and differentiation. J Am Coll Cardiol 2003;41:879-888.

16. Dib N, Michler RE, Pagani FD, et al: Safety and feasibility of autologous myoblast transplantation in patients with ischemic cardiomyopathy: Four-year follow-up. Circulation 2005;112:1748-1755.

17. Askari A, Unzek S, Goldman CK, et al: Cellular, but not direct adenoviral delivery of VEGF results in improved LV function and neovascularization in dilated ischemic cardiomyopathy. J Am Coll Cardiol 2004;43:1908-1914.

18. Mills WR, Mal N, Kiedrowski M, et al: Stem cell therapy enhances electrical viability in myocardial infarction. J Mol Cell Cardiol 2006;42:304-314. Epub 2006 Oct 27.

19. Askari A, Unzek S, Popovic ZB, et al: Effect of stromal-cell-derived factor-1 on stem cell homing and tissue regeneration in ischemic cardiomyopathy. Lancet 2003;362:697-703.

20. Hofmann M, Wollert KC, Meyer GP, et al: Monitoring of bone marrow cell homing into the infarcted human myocardium. Circulation 2005;111:2198-2202.

21. Muller P, Pfeiffer P, Koglin J, et al: Cardiomyocytes of noncardiac origin in myocardial biopsies of human transplanted hearts. Circulation 2002;106:31-35.

22. Orlic D, Kajstura J, Chimenti S, et al: Bone marrow cells regenerate infarcted myocardium. Nature 2001;410:701-705.

23. Mangi AA, Noiseux N, Kong D, et al: Mesenchymal stem cells modified with Akt prevent remodeling and restore performance of infarcted hearts. Nat Med 2003;9:1195-1201.

24. Kocher AA, Schuster MD, Szabolcs MJ, et al: Neovascularization of ischemic myocardium by human bone-marrow-derived angioblasts prevents cardiomyocyte apoptosis, reduces remodeling and improves cardiac function. Nat Med 2001;7:430-436.

25. Murry CE, Soonpaa MH, Reinecke H, et al: Haematopoietic stem cells do not transdifferentiate into cardiac myocytes in myocardial infarcts. Nature 2004;428:664-668.

26. Schenk S, Mal N, Finan A, et al: MCP-3 is a myocardial mesenchymal stem cell homing factor. Stem Cells 2007;25:245-251. Epub 2006 Oct 19.

27. Wollert KC, Meyer GP, Lotz J, et al: Intracoronary autologous bone-marrow cell transfer after myocardial infarction: The BOOST randomised controlled clinical trial. Lancet 2004;364:141-148.

28. Schaefer A, Meyer GP, Fuchs M, et al: Impact of intracoronary bone marrow cell transfer on diastolic function in patients after acute myocardial infarction: Results from the BOOST trial. Eur Heart J 2006;27:929-935.

29. Penn MS: Stem-cell therapy after acute myocardial infarction: The focus should be on those at risk. Lancet 2006;367:87-88.

30. Assmus B, Honold J, Schachinger V, et al: Transcoronary transplantation of progenitor cells after myocardial infarction. N Engl J Med 2006;355:1222-1232.

31. Toma C, Pittenger MF, Cahill KS, et al: Human mesenchymal stem cells differentiate to a cardiomyocyte phenotype in the adult murine heart. Circulation 2002;105:93-98.

32. Gnecchi M, He H, Noiseux N, et al: Evidence supporting paracrine hypothesis for Akt-modified mesenchymal stem cell-mediated cardiac protection and functional improvement. FASEB J 2006;20:661-669.

33. Jiang Y, Jahagirdar BN, Reinhardt RL, et al: Pluripotency of mesenchymal stem cells derived from adult marrow. Nature 2002;418:41-49.

34. Yoon YS, Wecker A, Heyd L, et al: Clonally expanded novel multipotent stem cells from human bone marrow regenerate myocardium after myocardial infarction. J Clin Invest 2005;115:326-338.

35. Szilvassy SJ, Meyerrose TE, Ragland PL, et al: Differential homing and engraftment properties of hematopoietic progenitor cells from murine bone marrow, mobilized peripheral blood, and fetal liver. Blood 2001;98:2108-2115.

36. Vaziri H, Dragowska W, Allsopp RC, et al: Evidence for a mitotic clock in human hematopoietic stem cells: Loss of telomeric DNA with age. Proc Natl Acad Sci U S A 1994;91:9857-9860.

37. Leor J, Guetta E, Feinberg MS, et al: Human umbilical cord blood-derived CD133+ cells enhance function and repair of the infarcted myocardium. Stem Cells 2006;24:772-780.

38. Thomson JA, Itskovitz-Eldor J, Shapiro SS, et al: Embryonic stem cell lines derived from human blastocysts. Science 1998;282:1145-1147.

39. Reubinoff BE, Pera MF, Fong CY, et al: Embryonic stem cell lines from human blastocysts: somatic differentiation in vitro. Nat Biotechnol 2000;18:399-404.

40. Guan K, Nayernia K, Maier LS, et al: Pluripotency of spermatogonial stem cells from adult mouse testis. Nature 2006;440:1199-1203.

41. Takahashi K, Yamanaka S: Induction of pluripotent stem cells from mouse embryonic and adult fibroblast cultures by defined factors. Cell 2006;126:663-676.

42. Orlic D, Kajstura J, Chimenti S, et al: Mobilized bone marrow cells repair the infarcted heart, improving function and survival. Proc Natl Acad Sci U S A 2001;98:10344-10349.

43. Ince H, Petzsch M, Kleine HD, et al: Prevention of left ventricular remodeling with granulocyte colony-stimulating factor after acute myocardial infarction: Final 1-year results of the Front-Integrated Revascularization and Stem Cell Liberation in Evolving Acute Myocardial Infarction by Granulocyte Colony-Stimulating Factor (FIRSTLINE-AMI) Trial. Circulation 2005;112:I-73-I-80.

44. Deglurkar I, Mal N, Mills WR, et al: Mechanical and electrical effects of cell based gene therapy for ischemic cardiomyopathy are independent [Abstract]. Hum Gene Ther 2006;17:1144-1151.

45. Honold J, Lehmann R, Heeschen C, et al: Effects of granulocyte colony simulating factor on functional activities of endothelial progenitor cells in patients with chronic ischemic heart disease. Arterioscler Thromb Vasc Biol 2006;26:2238-2243.

46. Pasumarthi K B, Nakajima H, Nakajima HO, et al: Targeted expression of cyclin D2 results in cardiomyocyte DNA synthesis and infarct regression in transgenic mice. Circ Res 2005;96:110-118.

47. Nakajima H, Nakajima HO, Tsai SC, et al: Expression of mutant p193 and p53 permits cardiomyocyte cell cycle reentry after myocardial infarction in transgenic mice. Circ Res 2004; 94:1606-1614.

48. Dawn B, Guo Y, Rezazadeh A, et al: Postinfarct cytokine therapy regenerates cardiac tissue and improves left ventricular function. Circ Res 2006;98:1098-1105.

49. Urbanek K, Torella D, Sheikh F, et al: Myocardial regeneration by activation of multipotent cardiac stem cells in ischemic heart failure. Proc Natl Acad Sci U S A 2005;102:8692-8697.

50. Agbulut O, Mazo M, Bressolle C, et al: Can bone marrow-derived multipotent adult progenitor cells regenerate infarcted myocardium? Cardiovasc Res 2006;72:175-183.

51. Mouquet F, Pfister O, Jain M, et al: Restoration of cardiac progenitor cells after myocardial infarction by self-proliferation and selective homing of bone marrow-derived stem cells. Circ Res 2005;97:1090-1092.

52. Young JB, Abraham WT, Smith AL, et al: Combined cardiac resynchronization and implantable cardioversion defibrillation in advanced chronic heart failure: The MIRACLE ICD Trial. JAMA 2003;289:2685-2694.

53. Molkentin JD, Lin Q, Duncan SA, et al: Requirement of the transcription factor GATA4 for heart tube formation and ventral morphogenesis. Genes Dev 1997;11:1061-1072.

54. Donath S, Li P, Willenbockel C, et al: Apoptosis repressor with caspase recruitment domain is required for cardioprotection in response to biomechanical and ischemic stress. Circulation 2006;113:1203-1212.

55. Misao J, Hayakawa Y, Ohno M, et al: Expression of bcl-2 protein, an inhibitor of apoptosis, and Bax, an accelerator of apoptosis, in ventricular myocytes of human hearts with myocardial infarction. Circulation 1996;94:1506-1512.

56. Chen SL, Fang WW, Ye F, et al: Effect on left ventricular function of intracoronary transplantation of autologous bone marrow mesenchymal stem cell in patients with acute myocardial infarction. Am J Cardiol 2004;94:92-95.

57. Meyer GP, Wollert KC, Lotz J, et al: Intracoronary bone marrow cell transfer after myocardial infarction: Eighteen months' follow-up data from the randomized, controlled BOOST (BOne marrOw transfer to enhance ST-elevation infarct regeneration) trial. Circulation 2006;113:1287-1294.

58. Tse HF, Kwong YL, Chan JK, et al: Angiogenesis in ischaemic myocardium by intramyocardial autologous bone marrow mononuclear cell implantation. Lancet 2003;361:47-49.

59. Seiler C, Pohl T, Wustmann K, et al: Promotion of collateral growth by granulocyte-macrophage colony-stimulating factor in patients with coronary artery disease: A randomized, double-blind, placebo-controlled study. Circulation 2001;104: 2012-2017.

60. Kang HJ, Kim HS, Zhang SY, et al: Effects of intracoronary infusion of peripheral blood stem-cells mobilised with granulocyte-colony stimulating factor on left ventricular systolic function and restenosis after coronary stenting in myocardial infarction: The MAGIC cell randomised clinical trial. Lancet 2004;363:751-756.

61. Valgimigli M, Rigolin GM, Cittanti C, et al: Use of granulocyte-colony stimulating factor during acute myocardial infarction to enhance bone marrow stem cell mobilization in humans: Clinical and angiographic safety profile. Eur Heart J 2005;26:1838-1845.

62. Ripa RS, Jorgensen E, Wang Y, et al: Stem cell mobilization induced by subcutaneous granulocyte-colony stimulating factor to improve cardiac regeneration after acute ST-elevation myocardial infarction: Result of the double-blind, randomized, placebo-controlled stem cells in myocardial infarction (STEMMI) trial. Circulation 2006;113:1983-1992.

63. Zohlnhofer D, Ott I, Mehilli J, et al: Stem cell mobilization by granulocyte colony-stimulating factor in patients with acute myocardial infarction: A randomized controlled trial. JAMA 2006;295:1003-1010.

64. MAGIC (Myoblast Autologous Grafting in Ischemic Cardiomyopathy). Clin Cardiol 2007;30:98.

65. Smits PC, Nienaber C, Colombo A, et al: Myocardial repair by percutaneous cell transplantation of autologous skeletal myoblast as a stand alone procedure in post myocardial infarction chronic heart failure patients. EuroIntervention 2006;1: 417-424.

CHAPTER
59 Angiogenesis and Arteriogenesis

Michael Simons and Mark J. Post

KEY POINTS

- *Arteriogenesis,* a process of arterial/collateral growth, is functionally much more important than *angiogenesis,* a process of capillary growth.
- Arteriogenesis and angiogenesis are regulated in distinctly different manners. This has direct implication for selection of pro-arteriogenic versus pro-angiogenic agents.
- There are probably significant genetic differences that determine an individual patient's ability to develop collateral circulation and to respond to growth factor therapy.
- Currently, there are no biomarkers of collateral growth. This is a major need.
- Effective arteriogenesis requires the prolonged presence of the active agent, both to *induce* the growth of new arteries and to *stabilize* the newly formed vessels.

- No effective forms of sufficiently long gene expression in the heart currently exist. Therefore, existing attempts to induce functionally significant arteriogenesis in populations with coronary artery disease are likely to fail. In contrast, easy access to repeat administration of the same biologic agents in patients with peripheral artery disease is likely to translate into therapeutic successes in this area.
- The current means of device delivery of biologic agents to the myocardium remain rudimentary and inefficient. Much progress needs to occur in this area.
- To date, angiogenic therapies have not been associated with any significant side effects such as tumor induction, proliferative retinopathy, or progression of renal failure.

To date, treatment of obstructive coronary artery disease (CAD) relied on drugs designed to reduce, by various means, the oxygen requirements of the myocardium, and on mechanical revascularization procedures, including coronary artery bypass grafting (CABG) and various forms of percutaneous transcatheter-based approaches. Recent advances in understanding of the biologic processes underlying vessel growth and remodeling, combined with the ability to stimulate these processes in the coronary and peripheral vasculatures, have opened new possibilities for treatment of CAD. This chapter considers the biologic foundations of therapeutic neovascularization and its potential side effects, preclinical and clinical data that have formed the basis for ongoing clinical trials, issues surrounding effective delivery of angiogenic agents to the heart, and the current state of clinical research. For ease of presentation, only the most recent (from 2002 on) publications are cited, and we have referenced comprehensive reviews as often as possible. We apologize to all our colleagues whose important contributions to this field are not always acknowledged by name.

BIOLOGIC FOUNDATIONS OF THERAPEUTIC NEOVASCULARIZATION

Most of our knowledge of vessel growth and the role of various angiogenic factors in this process comes from studies of embryonic vascular development and tumor angiogenesis. Formation of mature vasculature in the course of normal embryonic development includes three distinct sequential steps: formation of primary capillary plexus from embryonic stem cells (vasculogenesis), sprouting of endothelium-lined vascular structures (angiogenesis), and, finally, remodeling, pruning, and maturation of these structures into fully fledged vessels (arteriogenesis) (Fig. 59-1). Such a complicated sequence of events involves multiple growth factors that drive various parts of the pathway as well as equally important proteins that regulate each of these steps, preventing excessive vascular growth or formation of defective vasculature.

Development of the primary vascular plexus depends on the appearance of embryonic endothelial stem cells (angioblasts). To date, little information is available with regard to the nature of these cells and the factors regulating their appearance and survival.

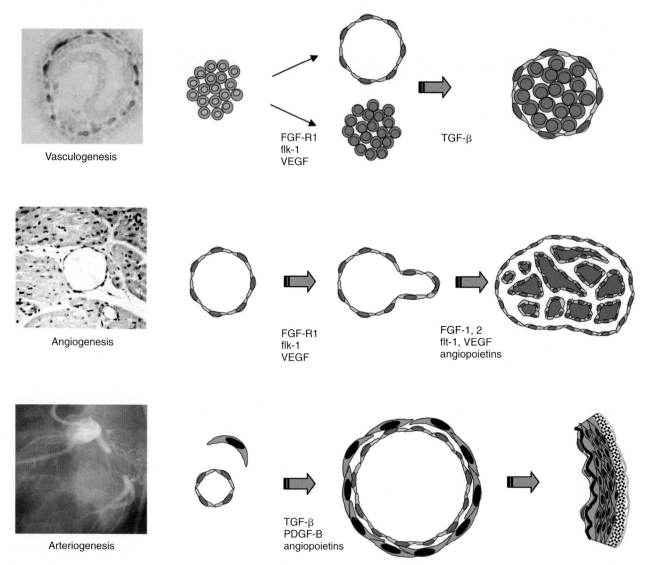

Figure 59-1. Three types of neovascularization. Vasculogenesis takes place during embryonic development and, to a smaller scale, in adult tissues. Hemangioblasts in extraembryonic regions develop into blood islands that differentiate into endothelial cells and blood cells. Angiogenesis is thought to be hypoxia driven. Under the influence of angiogenic cytokines, such as fibroblast growth factor-2 (FGF-2) and vascular endothelial growth factor (VEGF), capillaries sprout to form new vessels, eventually forming a plexus that subsequently prunes into a number of mature and persistent blood vessels. Arteriogenesis refers to a process of remodeling of preexisting collaterals which, under the influence of hemodynamic factors, enlarge and mature into fully functional arteries. The recruitment of pericytes under the influence of the BB homodimer of platelet-derived growth factor (PDGF-BB), angiopoietins, and transforming growth factor-β (TGF-β) is a crucial step in this sequence. FGF-R1, fibroblast growth factor receptor 1; flk-1, VEGF receptor.

They are thought to develop from a common blood cell/endothelial cell precursor, referred to as hemangioblast, and to express the vascular endothelial growth factor (VEGF) receptor Flk-1, as well as fibroblast growth factor (FGF) receptors.[1] The precise molecular characteristics of these cells are still, however, unknown. VEGF and transforming growth factor-β1 (TGF-β1) probably play key roles in vasculogenesis, because knockout of the gene for VEGF, Flk-1, or TGF-β1 results in embryonic lethality with a failure of endothelial precursors to differentiate and form the primary vascular plexus. In later stages of embryonic development, and perhaps in adult life, FGF-2, insulin-like growth factor-1 (IGF-1), and

granulocyte-macrophage colony-stimulating factor (GM-CSF) stimulate differentiation and mobilization of angioblasts from the bone marrow.[2]

Once formed, the primary plexus is then transformed by a process referred to as branching angiogenesis into a primitive vascular system. The failure of branching in *VEGF* heterozygote embryos with a single *VEGF* allele suggests that this process also heavily depends on VEGF. Other knockout experiments leading to embryonic lethality based on impaired angiogenesis show that a second VEGF receptor, Flt-1, and the angiopoietin-1 (Ang-1)/Tie-2 system are critical for undisturbed angiogenesis and vascular remodeling. The extent of sprouting (i.e., the total number of branches formed) is probably under the control of FGFs, because knockout of the only *FGF* gene in *Drosophila* results in markedly diminished branching of the trachea and bronchial tree, whereas overexpression of *FGF1* in mice leads to increased numbers of arterial branches.[3]

The primary vascular network then matures into adult vasculature by acquiring media and adventitia in a process termed arteriogenesis. Although our understanding of molecular events regulating this process is far from complete, platelet-derived growth factor (PDGF-B), TGF-β, Ang-1, and Ang-2 have all been implicated. Pericytes may play a particularly important role in this process. The formation of distinct arterial, venous, and lymphatic systems is a complicated and yet poorly understood process. A number of proteins are involved, including ephrins, Notch, sonic hedgehog, and VEGF. Nerve guidance plays a major role in arterial development through nerve-secreted VEGF as well as guidance receptors such as semaphorins, neuropilins, netrin, and plexins, among others.[4] One novel regulator of arterial development is a gene, *synectin,* that selectively regulates arterial but not venous formation, branching, and remodeling.[5]

In the case of tumor angiogenesis, VEGF again appears to be the primary growth factor, with the resultant vasculature consisting mainly of immature, endothelium-lined and leaky vessels, aptly called a "non-healing wound" by H. Dvorak. At the same time, the processes resulting in vessel growth in the setting of ischemia in adult tissues, and in particular in the adult heart, are much less well understood.[6]

Two different events can take place in ischemic tissues: capillary growth in the ischemic part of the muscle, a process called true angiogenesis, and the process leading to formation of epicardial collateral vessels, variously termed arteriogenesis or "collateralgenesis" (Table 59-1). The primary stimulus behind angiogenesis is tissue ischemia, which results in activation of hypoxia-inducible factor (HIF)-1α in cardiac myocytes, which in turn stimulates expression of VEGF, the VEGF receptor Flt-1, PDGF-B, Ang-2, and inducible nitric oxide synthase (iNOS).[7] As in the case of other VEGF-dependent processes, this results in increased capillary growth, which, under some as yet poorly understood circumstances, can be followed by maturation into functional arterial vessels, presumably through secondary involvement of PDGF and Ang-2. Numerous studies have demonstrated both increased VEGF and VEGF receptor expression in ischemic myocardial tissues as well as capillary proliferation.[6] However, it is doubtful that this process can effectively relieve tissue ischemia if the blood supply is compromised by occlusion of proximal coronary vessels.

In contrast to angiogenesis taking place in the ischemic areas of the heart, the formation of epicardial collaterals (arteriogenesis) occurs in nonischemic areas and, in some cases, may fully restore inflow of blood to the distal coronary bed, resulting in an effective "biologic bypass." Remarkably, there is still

Table 59-1. Principal Differences between Arteriogenesis and Angiogenesis

Parameter	Arteriogenesis	Angiogenesis
Vessel location	Intramyocardial	Epicardial
Primary stimulus	Tissue ischemia	Shear stress
		Inflammation
Primary sensor	HIF-1α	Unknown
Vessel wall layers	Intima	Intima
		Media
Cell types involved	Endothelial cells	Endothelial cells
		Smooth muscle cells
		Pericytes
		Blood-derived mononuclear cells
Primary growth factors	VEGF$_{165}$	PDGF-BB
	FGF	FGF
	HGF	HGF
	TNF-α	TGF-β
	Ang-1	PR39
	Ang-2	Ang-2
Functional impact	Minor	Major

Ang, angiopoietin; FGF, fibroblast growth factor; HGF, hepatocyte growth factor; HIF, hypoxia-inducible factor; PDGF, platelet-derived growth factor; PR39, proline/arginine-rich peptide 39; TNF, tumor necrosis factor; VEGF, vascular endothelial growth factor.

little understanding regarding stimuli that induce arterial growth and growth factors involved in development of these vessels. Accumulation of blood-derived monocyte-macrophages and other accessory cells appears to be critical,[8,9] because these cells secrete a number of growth factors and cytokines involved in the growth and differentiation of endothelial, pericyte, and smooth muscle cells, including VEGF, FGF-2, TGF-β, interleukin-8 (IL-8), and monocyte chemotactic protein-1 (MCP-1), as well as matrix metalloproteinases (MMPs) and other biologically active molecules. Among them is a proline/arginine-rich peptide, PR39, whose gene may serve as an angiogenesis master switch by increasing expression of HIF-1α and thereby mimicking hypoxic response and activating VEGF and VEGF receptor expression, while at the same time increasing expression of the FGF signaling molecules FGF-R1 and syndecan-4.[10]

Animal studies have demonstrated that activation of accumulations of monocyte-macrophages at the arterial occlusion sites, when stimulated by MCP-1, leads to a robust arteriogenic response that in turn can lead to significant restoration of distal tissue perfusion. At the same time, deficiency of a VEGF-related growth factor, PlGF, prevents collateral growth by impairing monocyte recruitment. Furthermore, the ability of monocytes to respond to hypoxic stress by increasing their HIF-1α protein level appears to correlate with the extent of coronary collateral development in patients with advanced CAD.[6] Although these observations clearly implicate monocytes as the primary cell type responsible for arteriogenic response, the factors that control monocyte recruitment to sites of arterial narrowing and subsequently regulate their adhesion, tissue invasion, and activation, have not been defined.

ANGIOGENIC REGULATORS

As the preceding discussion makes clear, many genes are involved in regulation of the angiogenic response. The major classes of these regulators include angiogenic growth factors, endothelial-specific genes regulating endothelial cell growth and migration (Table 59-2), and regulatory genes that control entire angiogenesis-related "cascades" (Table 59-3).

Vascular Endothelial Growth Factor Family

The six members of the VEGF family, including five VEGFs (A through E) and the closely related placental growth factor (PlGF), constitute perhaps the most intensively studied angiogenic growth factor family. The "founding" member, VEGF-A (commonly referred to as simply VEGF) was first isolated as a vascular permeability factor (VPF) and was subsequently shown to have endothelial cell growth stimulatory properties. It is the key angiogenic growth factor during embryonic vascular development.[11] Five different isoforms are generated by alternative splicing from a single *VEGFA* gene (subscript indicates the number of amino acids): $VEGF_{206}$, $VEGF_{189}$, $VEGF_{165}$, $VEGF_{145}$, and $VEGF_{121}$. $VEGF_{189}$ and $VEGF_{205}$ isoforms demonstrate very tight heparan sulfate binding and as a result are tightly bound to the cell surface once secreted. This property probably severely limits their utility as therapeutic agents. $VEGF_{165}$ and $VEGF_{145}$ also demonstrate heparan sulfate binding (significantly less than the other two), whereas $VEGF_{121}$ completely lacks the heparan sulfate binding site.

The heparan binding domain of $VEGF_{165}$ is required for its binding to a plasma membrane receptor, neuropilin-1, an interaction thought to be critical in arterial specification.[12] Binding to neuropilin-1 greatly increases VEGF concentration on the cell surface, and this interaction probably explains why $VEGF_{165}$ appears to be the most active isoform biologically in terms of the effects of gene disruption (i.e., disruption of $VEGF_{165}$ is lethal, whereas that of $VEGF_{121}$ is not), stimulation of growth of embryonic endothelial cells, and activation of the main VEGF signaling receptor Flk-1 ($VEGF_{165}$ is 10 times more active than $VEGF_{121}$ on a molar basis). Little is yet known about the activity of $VEGF_{145}$, but its inability to bind neuropilin-1 suggests that it should be less effective than $VEGF_{165}$ in activating Flk-1.

Angiogenic activity of VEGF requires the release of nitric oxide, and blockade of endothelial nitric oxide

Table 59-2. Angiogenic Growth Factors

Factor	Comments
VEGF Family	
VEGF-A (1)	
$VEGF_{121}$	Does not bind heparan sulfates or neuropilin-1
	Less effective than $VEGF_{165}$ in activating Flk-1 in vitro
$VEGF_{145}$	May be as active as $VEGF_{165}$
$VEGF_{165}$	Single-allele mutation is lethal in early development
$VEGF_{189,205}$	Strong heparan sulfate binding; not present in circulation
	Biologic function unclear
VEGF-C (2)	Predominantly involved in lymphogenesis
VEGF-B (3)	Predominantly found in pulmonary circulation
VEGF-D (4)	Function unknown
VEGF-E (5)	Function unknown
FGF Family	
FGF-1 and FGF-2	Lack classic leader sequence
	Probably involved in branching and vessel maturation
FGF-4 and FGF-5	Secreted FGF; demonstrated angiogenic activity
Other FGFs	Some may be angiogenic
PDGF Family	
PDGF-BB	Angiogenic in cardiac tissues
PDGF-AB	
HGF	Directly stimulates EC proliferation; may activate VEGF
Angiopoietin Family	
Ang-1	Activates Tie-2; involved in vascular remodeling and vessel maturation
Ang-2	Can both activate and inhibit Tie-2 receptor; plays a role in initiation of angiogenesis
Ang-3	Inhibits Tie-2; function unknown
Ang-4	Stimulates Tie-2; function unknown
Ephrin Family	
Ephrin-B1	
Ephrin B2	Present on arterial endothelium
EphB4	Ephrin-B2 receptor; present on venous endothelium
EphA1	

FGF, fibroblast growth factor; HGF, hepatocyte growth factor; PDGF, platelet-derived growth factor; VEGF, vascular endothelial growth factor.

Table 59-3. Angiogenesis Master Switch Genes and Other Agents

Factor	Comment
HIF-1α	Transcription factor activating expression of VEGF, Flt-1, and iNOS
	Protein levels controlled by proteasome-mediated degradation of the mature HIF-1α protein
	Sensitive to cellular oxygen levels
PR39	Proline/arginine-rich peptide produced by blood-derived macrophages and, potentially, granulocytes
	Inhibits proteasome degradation of HIF-1α
	Induces FGF-R1 and syndecan-4 expression
Relaxin	Circulating hormone produced in the ovaries
	Induces VEGF and FGF-2 expression at tissue injury sites
MCP-1	Endothelial adhesion protein
	Upregulated at sites of shear stress and ischemic injury
	Chemoattractant for circulating monocytes
Del1	Developmentally regulated endothelial locus
	Extracellular matrix protein capable of activation of $\alpha_v\beta_3$ signaling

FGF, fibroblast growth factor; HIF, hypoxia-inducible factor; iNOS, inducible nitric oxide synthase; MCP, monocyte chemotactic protein; VEGF, vascular endothelial growth factor.

synthase (eNOS) markedly reduces VEGF activity. The role of VEGF in the postnatal vasculature is less clear. Deactivation of the VEGF-A gene in Cre-loxP systems in mature animals does not lead to significant vascular defects. This may not be the case, however, for newly forming vasculature in adult tissues, where prolonged VEGF presence apparently is required for arterial maturation.[13] In addition, VEGF may play a vascular protective role in the adult vasculature.

Other VEGF genes include VEGF-C (also known as VEGF-2), VEGF-B (also known as VEGF-3), VEGF-D, and VEGF-E. VEGF-C appears to be involved predominantly in lymphangiogenesis,[14] whereas VEGF-B may play a role in the development of coronary capillaries. The functions of the VEGF-D and -E isoforms have not been fully established.

It is interesting to note that, despite clearly profound VEGF biologic effects, all isoforms are, by themselves, very weak mitogens. This observation alone strongly suggests that biologic effects of these molecules have a lot more to do with activities other than direct stimulation of endothelial cell growth. One such activity is the ability to induce a local inflammatory response by increasing vascular permeability. Others include stimulation of local production of nitric oxide, enhancement of monocyte and leukocyte adhesion to the endothelium, activation of tissue digesting enzymes such as MMPs, stimulation of expression of additional growth factors such as FGF2, and stimulation of bone marrow release of endothelial precursor cells.

Fibroblast Growth Factor Family

FGFs are members of a family of 22 closely related proteins. The complexity of this family and the apparent ability of its members to substitute for one another have limited the pace of inquiries and our knowledge of the roles played by individual isoforms. Disruptions of *FGF1*, *FGF2*, and *FGF5* genes produced subtle phenotypes, including, in the case of *FGF2*, abnormal vascular tone and delayed wound healing. Nevertheless, FGFs (FGF1 and possibly FGF2) have been shown to be critically involved in branching of both arterial and bronchial trees and may be involved in induction of angioblast differentiation and migration.[6]

One of the key differences among various FGFs is the presence or absence of the leader sequence required for conventional peptide secretion (absent in FGF1 and FGF2 but present in FGF4, FGF5, and most other FGFs) and differences in affinity for various isoforms of FGF receptors. The founding family members, FGF1 and FGF2, bind with high affinity to cellular heparan sulfates, and with even higher affinity to their own tyrosine kinase receptors. FGF2 binds predominantly to FGF receptors FGF-R1 and -R2, whereas FGF1 binds to all four FGF-Rs. A pattern of specific FGF-R interactions and tissue distribution probably accounts for differences in activity of various FGFs. However, for most FGFs, their ability to bind cell surface and matrix heparan sulfates serves both to prolong effective tissue half-life and to facilitate binding to corresponding high-affinity receptors.[15]

In cell culture as well as in in vivo studies, FGF1, FGF2, FGF4, and FGF5 are potent mitogens for cells of mesenchymal, neural, and epithelial origin, including all cell types found in the vascular wall (endothelial cells, smooth muscle cells, and pericytes). FGF2, and probably other FGFs, also is able to activate nitric oxide release, to induce synthesis of plasminogen activator and MMPs, and to stimulate chemotaxis. One interesting aspect of FGF2 biology is the synergy of its biologic activity with VEGF. A combination of FGF2 and VEGF is far more potent in inducing angiogenesis in vitro and in vivo than either growth factor alone. Furthermore, FGF2 induces VEGF expression in smooth muscle and endothelial cells.

Although both FGF1 and FGF2 are present in the normal myocardium, their expression is not significantly affected by hypoxia or hemodynamic stress, although their release into tissues is very inflammation- and copper-dependent. Despite significant levels of FGFs in normal tissues, the growth factors do not appear to be biologically active, as suggested by the lack of ongoing angiogenesis and the absence of baseline tyrosine phosphorylation of FGF receptors. Part of the explanation for this lack of activity of endogenous FGFs may be sequestration in the extracellular matrix by virtue of binding to the heparan sulfate–carrying proteoglycan perlecan, which would make them unavailable to cell surface receptors. In addition, very low levels of expression of both FGF-R1 and FGF-R2, as well as syndecan-4, another transmembrane protein involved in regulation of FGF-dependent signaling, probably also contribute to the lack of FGF activity in normal tissues. Thus, unlike VEGF, in which biologic activity appears to be driven by the amount of ligand present, FGF activity is controlled by level of expression of FGF receptors and their ability to bind the ligand.

Because FGFs, unlike VEGF, are potent mitogens with a broad spectrum of activity, this "nonspecific" stimulation of cell growth was initially held against them as potential therapeutic agents. However, new understanding of the fundamental biology of arteriogenesis makes them rather appealing, given the goal of creating functional arteries as opposed to endothelium-lined capillaries. Current understanding of the biology of FGFs suggests that we need to target enhanced signaling by FGF rather than supplementing the growth factor if we want to take advantage of the multiple biologic "abilities" of FGFs.

Angiopoietins and Ephrins

Angiopoietins were discovered during searches for ligands of the endothelial cell–specific Tie-2 receptor. The family currently consists of four members, and other related genes are likely to exist. The role played by Ang genes in vascular development has already been briefly addressed.[16] Overexpression of Ang-1 in the mouse leads to a striking increase in vascularization. The most prominent feature here is a pronounced increase in vessel size with only a modest increase in vessel number.[17] Combined VEGF/Ang-1 overexpression leads to a very pronounced increase in vascularity without the increased permeability seen with VEGF alone. Further, adenovirus-based gene transfer of Ang-1 into tissue can negate permeability increases induced by a number of inflammatory mediators. These findings suggest that Ang-1 plays a role in stabilizing the existing vessel in a yet undefined manner.

The role played by Ang-2 has proved to be even more elusive. Overexpression of Ang-2 during embryonic development leads to early mortality with morphologic defects resembling those of Ang-1 and Tie-2 knockouts, suggesting that Ang-2 acts as a Tie-2 antagonist. These and other observations suggest that Ang-2 might provide a destabilizing signal necessary for initiation of the angiogenic response. Because virtually nothing is known about Ang-3 and Ang-4, these will not be discussed further.

Ephrins and their corresponding Eph receptors constitute one of the largest tyrosine kinase signaling families that plays an important role in vascular development.[18] Knockouts of ephrin-B2 or its receptor, EphB4, result in early embryonic mortality due to failure of angiogenic remodeling. Further, this pair displays a remarkable complementary expression pattern during vascular development, with EphB4 present on the venous and ephrin-B2 on arterial endothelium. This observation has led to the suggestion that the ephrin and its receptor play a role in establishing arteriovenous identity and may regulate formation of arteriovenous junctions. These proteins also play a key role in arterial guidance regulating development of new arterial vasculature.[19] Ephrin-B2 continues to play this role in the adult circulation, selectively marking arterial vessels in neovascularization sites, although its expression is not limited to endothelial cells but extends to vascular smooth muscle and pericytes.

Other Angiogenic Growth Factors

In addition to the angiogenic growth factor families discussed previously, a number of other growth factors also possess angiogenic activity and may potentially be used as therapeutic agents. Most prominent of these are the hepatocyte growth factor (HGF) and the PDGF family.

PDGF was originally isolated from platelets, and this is still considered a major source of the protein. The PDGF family consists of four genes, PDGF-A, PDGF-B, PDGF-C, and PDGF-D. The A and B chains can form homodimers (AA or BB) or a heterodimer (AB), which have distinctly different properties and biologic activities. Likewise, PDGF receptors are composed of two chains, PDGF-Rα and PDGF-Rβ, which also form either homodimers (αα or ββ) or heterodimers (αβ). PDGF-AA binds only to PDGF-Rαα, whereas PDGF-BB binds to all three PDGF receptors, and

PDGF-AB is limited to αα or αβ. Knockout studies with either PDGF-B or the PDGF-β receptor have shown that PDGF-B is responsible for vascular maturation.[20] The knockout mice die late in gestation with abnormal kidney glomeruli and vascular wall abnormalities related to insufficient recruitment and organization of pericytes and smooth muscle cells, particularly in the brain and heart. The PDGF-A and PDGF-α knockouts show less overlapping phenotypes and have abnormalities related to patterning of somites, with less specific vascular pathology.

In adult tissues, PDGF-BB stimulates angiogenesis, which may be secondary to PDGF-β–mediated upregulation of VEGF-A expression. In the heart, a PDGF circuit has been described in which a myocyte-derived B-chain dimerizes with an endothelium-derived A-chain to form PDGF-AB, which then induces VEGF and Flk-1 expression through a PDGF-ββ receptor–mediated pathway, thus stimulating angiogenesis. Both PDGF-B and PDGF-Rβ are upregulated during hypoxia and in the setting of wound healing and inflammation. A key biologic activity of PDGF in angiogenesis seems to be attraction of pericytes and the formation of a mature arterial wall.[21]

PDGF-BB also promotes wound healing through various mechanisms, including promigratory and mitogenic effects on macrophages, fibroblasts, and keratinocytes, and it also demonstrates cytoprotective effect against ischemic injury in central nervous system tissue. PDGF-BB has also been widely implicated in the formation of intimal hyperplasia after arterial balloon injury and in the progression of atherosclerosis. In fact, PDGF receptor kinase inhibitors have been suggested as potential therapeutic agents for restenosis.[22] These aspects of PDGF's activity profile raise the concern that its therapeutic application in ischemic heart disease might be offset by stimulation of restenosis and atherosclerosis.

HGF, also known as the scatter factor (SF), has been identified as the ligand for the hepatocyte growth factor receptor *MET,* a well-known oncogene. Like FGF2 and VEGF, HGF has a high affinity for heparin, but unlike FGF2, this binding is not important for its signaling. The HGF peptide is a heterodimer, with the α chain having four kringle motifs and the β chain sharing homology with serine proteases without having actual enzymatic activity.[23] HGF and MET are essential for normal embryonic development, but they are not primarily involved in the development of the cardiovascular system. The HGF/MET system is upregulated in ischemic hearts, where it protects against ischemia-reperfusion injury, and HGF secretion is enhanced after myocardial infarction. In various in vivo models of angiogenesis and arteriogenesis, HGF has a robust angiogenic effect, which may at least in part be mediated by stimulation of VEGF expression.[24] In relation to their use as therapeutic agents, the definite pro-oncogenic properties of HGF and MET are a major concern. Transgenic overexpression of HGF leads to a variety of tumors of mesenchymal and epithelial origin, and mutations in the tyrosine kinase domain of MET that lead to its constitutive activation produce papillary renal carcinomas. Clinical studies of the therapeutic efficacy and safety of HGF are in progress in patients with peripheral vascular disease.

Master Switch Genes

In addition to the discussed major families of growth factors, several genes control entire cascades of angiogenic growth factors. The most extensively studied of these master switch genes is HIF-1α. HIF-1 was identified as a hypoxia-inducible response element binding activity in the erythropoietin gene. Further studies showed that HIF-1 was a heterodimer consisting of a labile protein, HIF-1α, and a stable protein, HIF-1β, which was previously isolated as an aryl hydrocarbon nuclear translocator protein. HIF-1 activity is directly related to HIF-1α expression, which in turn is rapidly induced by tissue hypoxia, with the magnitude of the response being inversely proportional to cellular O_2 concentration.[25]

The regulation of the cellular HIF-1α protein level is accomplished in an unusual fashion. Under normal oxygen tension conditions, the protein is very labile owing to presence of the PEST (polypeptide sequences enriched in proline, glutamate, serine, and threonine) domains, which serve as signals for rapid degradation by the ubiquitin-proteasome system. This degradation is so efficient that even significant acceleration of HIF-1α gene transcription does not result in an appreciable change in the cellular protein level. Once the cellular O_2 concentration is reduced, PEST domains are no longer recognized by the ubiquitin system, and HIF-1α protein accumulates in the cytoplasm. The newly translated HIF-1α protein is post-translationally modified by prolyl hydroxylase–containing enzymes that require oxygen as a cofactor. Once so modified, HIF-1α is immediately tagged for degradation by the Von Hippel-Lindau (VHL) protein. In the absence of oxygen, prolyl hydroxylation and the subsequent proteasome-mediated degradation of VHL-tagged HIF-1α is impaired, resulting in a rapid increase in its intracellular concentration.

Once cellular levels of HIF-1α increase, the protein is transported to the nucleus, where it can activate transcription of a wide range of angiogenesis-related genes, including VEGF, Flt-1 (VEGF-R1), iNOS (NOS3), heme oxygenase-1, and a broad spectrum of glycolytic enzymes.[26] The key role of HIF-1α in mediation of VEGF transcription and the subsequent angiogenic response was demonstrated in HIF-1α knockout mice. The deletion of both HIF-1α alleles resulted in early embryonic lethality, and embryonic stem cells derived from HIF-1α$^{-/-}$ embryos failed to induce VEGF expression in response to hypoxia. In adult mice, HIF-1α response is required for physiologic response to chronic hypoxia.

Another broad-spectrum regulator of angiogenic response is the PR39 peptide. This unusual, proline/arginine-rich peptide was initially isolated from the bone marrow and the intestine as a naturally occurring antibacterial peptide. More recently, it was shown to possess a strong angiogenic activity. Transgenic expression of the peptide in cardiac myocytes led to increased coronary vasculature and gene transfer in settings of myocardial ischemia with increased collateral growth.[27] Yet another peptide with a pronounced angiogenic activity is apelin (APLN), the ligand of the endothelial G protein–coupled receptor, AGTRL1 (formerly APJ).[28]

Other Genes Involved in Regulation of Angiogenic Response

Finally, a process as complex and as important as angiogenesis possesses an extensive array of additional regulators. These include circulating angiogenesis inhibitors (Table 59-4), enzymes that regulate the extracellular matrix breakdown necessary for angiogenic response (e.g. MMPs), and numerous genes that regulate endothelial cell adhesion (selectins, intercellular adhesion molecule [ICAM], and vascular cell adhesion molecule [VCAM], among others) and responsiveness to specific angiogenic growth factors (such as α_v integrins). Although a comprehensive review of these numerous gene families is outside the scope of this chapter, a brief discussion of circulating inhibitors of angiogenesis is included.

Endostatin, the first such inhibitor identified, is a 20-kd cleavage product of the C-terminal fragment of collagen XVIII derived through cleavage of an Ala-His linkage by an as yet unidentified elastase. It is a specific inhibitor of endothelial cell migration and proliferation that causes G_1 cell cycle arrest of endothelial cells and induces their apoptosis.[29] Although its activity has primarily been studied in oncologic settings, it also appears capable of inhibiting an-

Table 59-4. Derivation and Biologic Activities of Principal Angiogenic Inhibitors

Angiogenic Inhibitor	Source	Activity
Endostatin	Collagen XVIII	Inhibition of migration Inhibition of proliferation G_1 arrest EC apoptosis
Angiostatin	Plasminogen	Inhibition of migration
Canstatin	β2 chain collagen IV	Inhibition of migration Inhibition of proliferation EC apoptosis
Tumstatin	β3 chain collagen IV	Inhibition of proliferation EC apoptosis
Cleaved antithrombin	Antithrombin	Inhibition of EC migration
Type 2 repeats	Thrombospondin-1 and 2	Inhibition of migration Inhibition of proliferation

EC, endothelial cells.

giogenesis in the arterial wall, potentially reducing the size of atherosclerotic plaque.

Angiostatin, a 38-kd fragment derived from the enzymatic cleavage of plasminogen, is another circulating angiogenesis inhibitor. Similar to endostatin, it is a specific inhibitor of endothelial cell migration.[30]

A number of other angiogenesis inhibitors derived from various extracellular matrix or clotting cascade proteins have recently been identified. These include canstatin, a fragment of the α_2 chain of collagen IV, and tumstatin, a fragment of the β_2 chain of collagen IV and cleaved conformation of antithrombin. The physiologic roles of these molecules have not yet been established.

Thrombospondins are another class of extracellular matrix proteins that possess anti-angiogenic activity. Of particular interest, a knockout of the thromspondin-2 gene results in a generalized increase in capillary counts in mice and accelerated wound healing. At the same time, introduction of thrombospondin proteins is capable of inhibiting angiogenesis in a number of models. Although the mechanism of anti-angiogenic activity of thrombospondins is unknown, it may include inhibition of MMP activation.[31]

ANIMAL STUDIES

The concept of therapeutic angiogenesis as a treatment for occlusive CAD and peripheral vascular disease has been extensively tested in various animal models. In large animal (dog, swine) models of myocardial angiogenesis, local ischemia is created by gradual occlusion of a major epicardial artery, which leads to reduction in reversible regional blood flow and contractile function. Hydraulic occluder or repeat short-term coronary occlusions can be used to achieve similar effects, but the experience with these models is significantly more limited.

In these models, single-bolus intracoronary, periadventitial, or intrapericardial administration of FGF2 enhances neovascularization and restores blood flow in the ischemic territory to normal levels. This in turn improves regional contractile function.[32] At the same time, single-bolus intravenous injection is not effective, whereas prolonged systemic administration does restore flow.[32] Similar results have been obtained with sustained-release FGF1 mutant and VEGF proteins.[3] Gene therapy approaches have been used with equal success, including intracoronary injections of a number of FGF and VEGF isoforms (FGF4, FGF5, $VEGF_{121}$, $VEGF_{165}$).

These results stand in significant contrast to the so far less than spectacular results achieved in clinical trials (see later discussion). Many factors likely account for these differences, including age, atherosclerosis, diabetes, and selection of "end-stage" patients for these trials. One recent study demonstrated, for example, that both native arteriogenesis and arteriogenic response to a growth factor treatment were delayed and impaired in hypercholesterolemic versus normocholesterolemic mice.[33]

The second most popular animal model in this field is the ischemic hindlimb model. This model is mostly performed in rabbits, but it is currently scaled down to rats and mice. The femoral artery is occluded or excised, starting either distal or proximal to the deep femoral artery. The procedure results in ischemia in the adductor and calf muscles. Depending on the species, blood flow reserve to the ischemic territory typically recovers spontaneously in this model to 60% to 80% of the preligation value within 4 weeks. Treatment with angiogenic growth factors accelerates recovery but, depending on the growth factor, does not always augment the response beyond what is achieved spontaneously. The difference can be traced to whether the predominant effect is angiogenesis or arteriogenesis. For example, PlGF is very effective in selectively augmenting the arterial vasculature,[34] whereas VEGF has a predominant effect on capillary growth. Similarly, MCP-1, a cytokine that stimulates monocyte adhesion to the proximal artery and downstream to the collateral arteries, effectively mediates remodeling of collateral arteries, whereas its effect on small vessel angiogenesis is questionable.[35]

DELIVERY AND FORMULATIONS OF GROWTH FACTORS

Although the success of therapeutic angiogenesis in various animal models clearly establishes its theoretical viability, translation to clinical practice has been challenging, and there have been multiple clinical trial failures. This clinical experience has enlightened our understanding of therapeutic angiogenesis biology and has firmly focused attention on effective delivery and growth factor formulation. Safety of angiogenic therapy is also an important consideration in designing a delivery mode. Because the growth factor formulation plays an important role in dictating delivery strategy, these issues are discussed together.

To be effective, the application of any biologic therapeutic agent must satisfy three critical considerations: (1) the agent must get to the site of action; (2) the duration of action must be sufficient to generate the desired therapeutic response; and (3) the effect must persist after the biologic activity of the drug has dropped below a therapeutic level. We still have a very incomplete understanding of either the desired site of action for an angiogenic agent, the necessary duration of angiogenic response, or the fate of newly formed vasculature.

Delivery Site

A number of delivery sites are theoretically available for drug delivery, including the endocardium and the epicardium of the ischemic territory, the border zone, and the normal territory, as well as intracoronary infusion and retrograde infusion into the coronary veins (Fig. 59-2). On theoretical grounds, epicardium

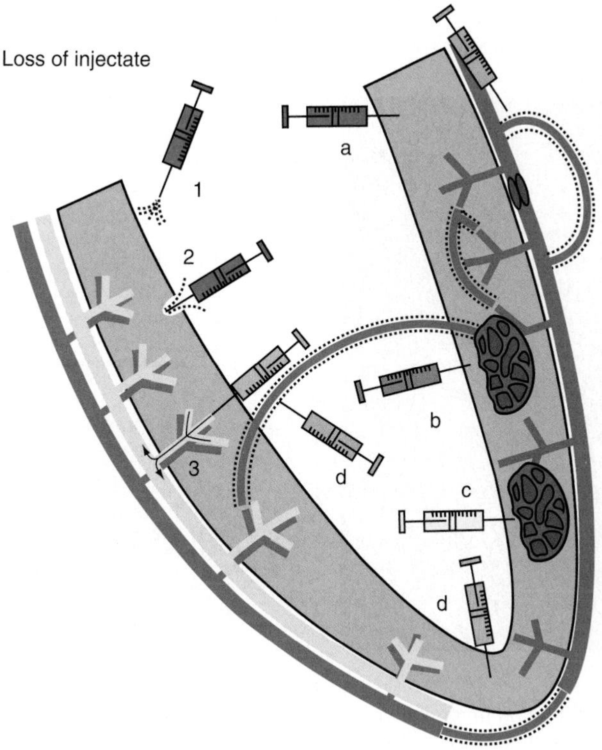

Figure 59-2. Potential sites of intramyocardial injection and losses of injectate. Growth factors can be injected into the healthy myocardium proximal from the occlusion to stimulate collateral genesis, either through an intramyocardial or a transvascular route (a). In the same philosophy, watershed areas from which projected collaterals may come can be targeted; the ameroid model, for instance, targets the posterior wall and the apex (d). To enhance angiogenesis, growth factors are injected in the border of the infarct (b) or the center of the ischemic zone (c). After intramyocardial injection, injectate can be lost because of inadvertent intraventricular injection (1), back leakage through the injection tract (2), or rapid washout through the venous and lymphatic systems (3).

of the normal territory upstream of the ischemic area is the most appealing site, because this is where native coronary collaterals form. However, this has never been demonstrated experimentally, either in animal models or in human trials.

Because the optimal site of administration has not been defined, the employed strategies tend to use either a "saturation" approach (i.e., intracoronary or intravenous administration) or a targeted approach. The first approach suffers from being systemic, with only small amounts (~1% in the case of FGF2 protein) of the administered agents being taken up by the myocardium and only trace amounts (0.01% in the case of FGF2) remaining in the heart after 24 hours. The uptake and retention of viral particles after intracoronary injection have not been defined very well, but a number of studies have demonstrated wide systemic distribution of injected adenoviruses, with the majority of the viral particles (and expressed transgenes) detected in liver, in spleen, and circulating monocytes.

Alternatively, intramyocardial injections into ischemic areas provide significant local concentration of the growth factor at the site of administration and minimize systemic distribution. A partial drawback of this approach is that, after injections of both growth factor proteins and protein-encoding adenoviruses, most of the injected material remains within approximately 1 cm of the injection site (Fig. 59-3).[27] Intramyocardial delivery may therefore be suboptimal, considering that the ultimate aim is induction of an arteriogenic response, a process taking place on the epicardial surface of the myocardium, and not stimulation of intramyocardial angiogenesis. A ratio-

nal site of delivery would be the "watershed" areas around ischemic regions or myocardium adjacent to the stenotic coronary artery. However, specific delivery to watershed areas has not yet been tested for efficacy.

A number of technical issues related to intramyocardial delivery need to be considered. Several factors play a role in the efficiency of injection: firm contact with the ventricular wall, angle of needle entry, depth of injection (needle length), rate of injection, and injection pressure. Preclinical studies have shown that most of the delivery losses are accounted for by injection into the left ventricular cavity, a rapid loss of injectate along the delivery needle track due to intramyocardial pressure, and rapid clearance from the extensive intramural vascular plexus. The latter can be a particularly important route of material loss, as suggested by real-time three-dimensional echocardiography.[36] The influence of the first two factors can be minimized with the use of optimal delivery techniques and catheter design.

Current intramyocardial injection devices utilize different technologies to address these issues. These include a screw-like tip that can minimize back-leak, contact detectors to control for the injection angle and stability of contact with the ventricular wall, or flexible tip designs that allow close contact with the wall during the cardiac cycle. One design includes a tip sensor that enables three-dimensional tracking of the tip in a magnetic field, enabling assessment of beat-to-beat stability of the tip as well as the angulation with the ventricular wall. In addition, it has an electronic sensor that transmits local electrocardiographic data, giving additional stability and contact

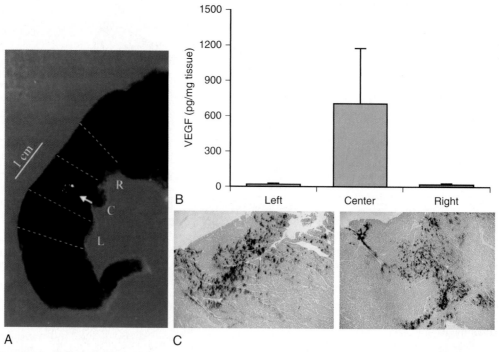

Figure 59-3. A, Protein distribution in the left ventricular (LV) wall after intramyocardial delivery of vascular endothelial growth factor (VEGF₁₂₁ adenovirus). One centimeter away from the injection site, protein expression is 50-fold lower than in the center. C, center; L, left; R, right. (From Kornowski R, Leon MB, Fuchs S, et al: Electromagnetic guidance for catheter-based transendocardial injection: A platform for intramyocardial angiogenesis therapy. Results in normal and ischemic porcine models. J Am Coll Cardiol 2000;35:1031.) **B,** Quantitative analysis of data from panel A. **C,** Gene expression along the needle injection track. (From Post MJ, Sato K, Murakami M, et al: Adenoviral PR39 improves blood flow and myocardial function in a pig model of chronic myocardial ischemia by enhancing collateral formation. Am J Physiol Regul Integr Comp Physiol 2006;290:R494-R500.)

information. Two other designs use either an ultrasound crystal at the end of the catheter or a conductance transducer that gives feedback on the axial force applied as well as the angulation. To further ensure intramyocardial position of the needle, the presence of premature ventricular excitations during needle penetration and injection are used as criteria for intramyocardial localization.

With induction of epicardial collateral growth as the goal, intrapericardial drug administration looks particularly appealing. This route provides access to the entire epicardial surface of the heart with a relatively favorable pharmacokinetic profile. Furthermore, the intrapericardial space can be safely accessed even in the absence of pericardial infusion, using either transthoracic or transatrial approaches. Specialized delivery catheters exist for both of these routes (Fig. 59-4). In animal studies, growth factor administration into the pericardial space, in the form of either protein or adenoviral constructs, resulted in increased angiogenesis and functional improvement in ischemic territories. The widespread application of this approach in patients is limited by the high frequency of prior CABG in patients referred for trials of angiogenic growth factor therapy and by the relatively minimal experience and low comfort levels of accessing normal pericardium on the part of the interventional community.

A related approach involves the insertion of polymers containing growth factor proteins along the epicardial surface of the occluded or severely narrowed coronary artery or injection of adenoviruses along the same territory. For protein therapy, variable release kinetics can be tailored from days to many weeks by adjusting the polymer of choice. When placed along the epicardial surface of the coronary, the growth factor is carried forward along the length of the artery, presumably via vasa vasorum. In preclinical studies, applications of polymers containing FGF1, FGF2, VEGF, or adenovirus- or plasmid-encoded VEGF resulted in significant arteriogenesis and functional improvement of ischemic tissues.[32] A limited clinical experience with this mode of delivery supports the utility of this approach.

Novel coronary transvenous and retroperfusion approaches, although potentially limited by venous anatomy, offer exciting prospects for gene, protein, and cell delivery, but data are still preliminary.[37]

Formulation and Duration of Action

The duration of action needed for an appropriate angiogenic response is closely related to the issue of delivery site. Large animal studies have routinely evaluated the angiogenic response to a single administration of a short-acting agent. However, it is reasonable to assume that the angiogenic process requires 2 to 3 weeks from initiation to completion. A critical consideration therefore is whether the growth factor presence is required for the entire dura-

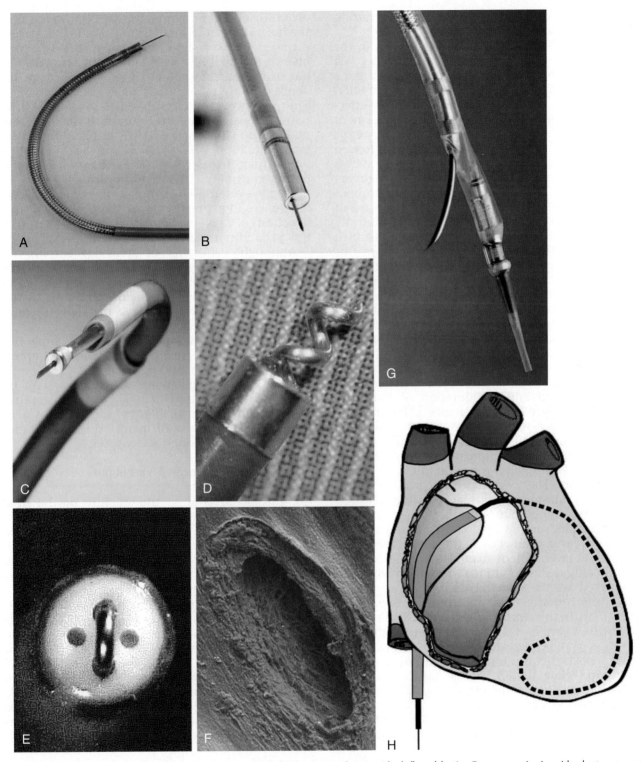

Figure 59-4. Types of delivery catheters: **A,** intramyocardial injection catheter with deflectable tip; **B,** same as in **A,** with electromagnetic sensor; **C,** coaxial design of intramyocardial injection system; **D,** corkscrew design to minimize back leak; and **E,** radiofrequency ablation catheter with two flush channels. **F,** Scanning electron micrograph of radiofrequency crater in endocardial surface. **G,** Transvenous access to the myocardium, guided by built-in ultrasound. **H,** Transatrial approach for intrapericardial delivery.

tion of angiogenic response or whether it may play a triggering role that initiates a self-replicating cascade. If triggering (which may, for example, include the release of a certain cell population from the bone marrow, which will then localize to the site of action) is sufficient, then even approaches that are very "ineffective" (from the standpoint of pharmacokinetics or local delivery) yet practical, such as intracoronary injections, may be sufficient. Indeed, the efficacy of single-bolus intracoronary FGF and VEGF protein infusions has been demonstrated in animals. However, clinical experience with this delivery mode has been very disappointing (see later discussion).

A prolonged presence of the growth factor in the desired location can be accomplished either via polymer-based protein administration or via gene therapy approaches (Table 59-5). Although polymer-based therapy is clearly feasible and probably effective,[38] a major drawback is the current requirement for open chest administration. Recently, however, needle-based delivery of gelatin microspheres loaded with FGF2 was successful in a preclinical model of hindlimb ischemia.[39] The development of delivery devices capable of safe administration of protein-containing polymers will greatly expand the reach of this mode of therapy. Gene therapy provides the only alternative to this approach. Whereas a detailed review of gene therapy is outside the scope of this chapter, and recent summaries of the field are available elsewhere,[40-43] we will briefly consider issues pertinent to angiogenic growth factor therapy.

The main perceived advantage of gene therapy over protein therapy is prolonged expression of the desired gene in a correct location, resulting in effective production of the therapeutic protein. Although in theory this assumption is correct, practical implementations have been difficult. The exact level of protein expression and the duration of transgene activity have been thorny issues. Naked DNA (plasmid) and adenoviruses have been the two most commonly employed vectors in cardiovascular studies. Plasmids have a surprising ability to achieve detectable expression after injection into cardiac and skeletal muscles. The magnitude of expression can be substantially improved by manipulating plasmid DNA sequences, methods of purification, and use of auxiliary factors such as lipid carriers and electrical current. However, even with all these improvements, the absolute level of gene expression achieved with plasmid-based delivery is much lower than what can be achieved with adenoviral vectors. More importantly, the duration of meaningful expression achieved with this form of gene transfer is fairly short, with a range of 3 to 5 days, although some expression can be detected several weeks later. It further appears that this form of gene transfer is more effective in skeletal than in cardiac muscle, with clinical trials suggesting some efficacy in PAD but not CAD (see later discussion).

At the same time, although the ability of adenoviruses to achieve significant gene expression after in vivo transduction in animal studies is unquestioned, the magnitude and duration of this effect in patients is uncertain. To a significant extent, this is a consequence of variability associated with virus delivery, but to even greater extent it reflects the high incidence of antiviral antibody titers found in patients. The presence of such antibodies severely shortens both expression level and duration. However, even under ideal circumstances, it is unlikely that meaningful duration of expression can be achieved for longer than 2 to 3 weeks. The delivery itself importantly contributes to variability of expression. Surprisingly, even in naïve animals, there are significant differences in expression levels after intramyocardial injections of a given adenovirus dose. The reasons for this variability have not been determined.[43]

Although a number of strategies employed in animal studies, such as increased intraventricular pressure after transient occlusion of the aortic root or injections of drugs capable of transiently disrupting endothelial integrity, have markedly increased transduction efficiency, the clinical utility of such techniques remains undefined. At the same time, gene therapy holds great potential, because improvements in vector technology promise the development of a fully regulatable expression system that could be turned on and off at will by pharmacotherapeutic means. The availability of such systems would make possible the use of many other gene transfer vectors, including long-lived viruses.

Stability of Newly Formed Vasculature

An unresolved issue is the stability of the newly formed vasculature once growth factor activity has ceased. Withdrawal of VEGF leads to prompt regression of the vessels induced by it.[13] However, this effect may depend on how long the VEGF was present to begin with and may not be applicable to other growth factors.

At the same time, addition of growth factors capable of attracting pericytes (PDGF-BB), stimulating growth of smooth muscle cells (FGF), or promoting cellular differentiation (Ang-2) has been shown to prolong the life of newly formed blood vessels. Therefore, it is likely that one set of growth factors will be needed to induce vessel growth and another will be required to stabilize, mature, and maintain these vessels. These concepts have not yet been tested in clinical trials.

Table 59-5. Comparison of Protein Therapy versus Gene Therapy

Protein Therapy	Gene Therapy
Direct introduction of the desired protein	Introduction of the genetic vector that will express the desired protein in situ
Defined dose	Dose (expression level) is variable
Defined duration of effect (limited by biologic and tissue half-life of the protein)	Variable duration of effect (limited by immune response, circulating antibodies, extinguishing of expression)
Duration of activity usually short (days)	Can produce prolonged expression (weeks)
Length of expression can be prolonged with use of sustained-release polymers	No ability at present to regulate duration and level of expression
Safety profile determined by the chosen protein	Gene transfect vectors may contribute to toxicity

CLINICAL TRIALS OF THERAPEUTIC ANGIOGENESIS

Patient Selection and Trial Design

The accumulating experience with a variety of clinical trials of angiogenic therapeutic agents over the last 5 to 7 years has led to identification of a number of issues common to all such trials.[6] These include trial design (randomization, blinding, choice of trial end point), patient selection, and choice of delivery modality. Perhaps one of the most striking lessons has been a most difficult translation from animal models, where virtually everything seems to work, to the clinical experience, where nothing seems to have worked.

Most initial open-label I phase I trials reported significant improvement in patients' symptoms, as well as in such objective measures of cardiac function as ejection fraction, regional wall motion, and myocardial perfusion. Yet the same agents were not nearly as effective in phase II trials. Interestingly, this lack of effectiveness was due to a combination of less dramatic improvement in treated patients and significant improvement in placebo-treated subjects. This combination suggests both the existence of a significant placebo effect and a genuine benefit from standard medical therapy that becomes manifest in the clinical trial setting in this patient population. The overall improvement in placebo-treated patients appears comparable to that seen in patients randomized to medical therapy in trials of coronary angioplasty. There is universal agreement now that blinding is required for any meaningful assessment of a therapeutic effect.

Another critical issue is the selection of an appropriate patient population. As with all radically new therapies, there is a tendency to initially restrict trials to the "no-option" population. Such patients tend to be older, with more extensive disease and with clinical evidence of not being responsive to standard therapies. Almost all of these individuals have had at least one bypass surgery and/or attempts at percutaneous catheter-based revascularization and remain significantly symptomatic. Clearly, this is a very heterogeneous group that most likely encompasses many biologic variations of a failure to elicit an effective endogenous angiogenic response. In some of these patients, this failure may be secondary to insufficient production of growth factors; in others, it may represent resistance to angiogenic simulation itself. Still others may possess an excess of local or systemic angiogenesis inhibitors or demonstrate growth factor resistance related to, for example, diabetes. Because of these variations, such a population may be particularly unsuitable for therapeutic angiogenesis trials. The availability of biomarkers predictive of neovascularization response would be highly desirable to improve patient selection.

A recent study documented significant differences in monocyte expression profile among patients with extensive versus minimal collateral development.[44] If this finding is confirmed in a larger sample, it would suggest that preexisting genetic differences may play an important role in the ability to develop collaterals and perhaps in the response to a therapeutic stimulation.

Yet another important nuance that has emerged from the clinical trial experience is the significant fluctuations in so-called "hard" end points, such as myocardial perfusion and function, in placebo-treated patients. Patients with advanced CAD demonstrate high variability on single-photon emission computed tomography (SPECT) perfusion studies even in the absence of any changes in therapy, with the percentage of myocardial ischemia varying by an average of 50%.[6] Similarly, large changes in ostensibly hard physiologic end points such as ankle-brachial index and transcutaneous partial oxygen pressure have been seen in the trials involving patients with PAD.[45] Such frequent and significant changes in physiologic parameters in these patients suggest a very heterogeneous population.

The choice of trial end points has been another vexing issue. Exercise testing has traditionally been used as a standard to evaluate the effectiveness of antianginal therapies. However, in such an advanced-disease population, it is much less reliable, because a significant number of patients discontinue exercise for reasons other then chest pain. It is likely that none of the studies completed to date has been large enough to conclusively demonstrate or reject an angiogenic therapeutic effect on the basis of this end point. Quality-of-life parameters offer another set of means for demonstration of patient benefits of antianginal therapy. In particular, semiquantitative indices such as the Seattle Angina Questionnaire (SAQ) and the Short Form 36 (SF36) questionnaire are less prone to variation than exercise testing and, therefore, may be more sensitive.

Protein Therapy Trials

The effectiveness of FGF and VEGF proteins in animal models led to early attempts at therapeutic use of these agents in clinical settings (Table 59-6). To simplify delivery issues, two initial FGF trials were conducted in the setting of CABG (see the detailed review by Annex and Simons[46]). Intramyocardial injection of FGF1 protein (10 µg/kg) was evaluated in 20 patients with three-vessel disease undergoing CABG in whom the growth factor or placebo was injected close to the anastomosis of the internal mammary artery and the left anterior descending coronary artery (LAD). The injections were well tolerated, and there were no systemic side effects. Subtraction angiography performed 3 months later suggested the presence of increased capillary filling in the growth factor–treated patients (Fig. 59-5). At follow-up 3 years later, dense capillary network was still present at the site of growth factor injection in 15 of 15 patients studied.

A double-blind, randomized trial of epicardially implanted FGF2 protein in sustained-release (heparin-

Table 59-6. Protein Therapy Trials of Therapeutic Angiogenesis in Coronary Artery Disease

Protein	Trial Type	N	Delivery	Results
FGF1	Phase I OL	20	IM injection	Safe Enhanced capillary blush at injection site
FGF2	Phase I/II DBR	24	Heparin-alginate capsules	Safe Improved symptoms Reduced SPECT defect size
FGF2	Phase I OL	30	IC infusion	Hypotension at high dosages Dilation of epicardial coronaries during infusion
FGF2	Phase I OL	52	IC infusion	Hypotension at high dosages Improved symptoms Reduced SPECT defect size
FGF2	Phase II DBR	337	IC infusion	Safe No effect on ETT or SPECT Improved symptoms compared with controls
VEGF-A$_{165}$	Phase I OL	15	IC infusion	Hypotension at low dosages Reduced SPECT defect size
VEGF-A$_{165}$	Phase I DBR	14	IV infusion	Safe No clear effects
VEGF-A$_{165}$	Phase II DBR	165	IC + IV infusion	Safe No improvement in ETT, symptoms, or SPECT defect size compared with controls

DBR, double-blind, randomized trial; ETT, exercise treadmill testing; FGF, fibroblast growth factor; IC, intracoronary; IM, intramuscular; IV, intravenous; OL, open-label trial; SPECT, single-photon emission computed tomography; VEGF, vascular endothelial growth factor.

alginate) beads was carried out in 24 patients undergoing CABG in whom one of the major arteries was supplying viable but ischemic myocardium that was considered not graftable for technical reasons (Fig. 59-6). The patients were randomized to receive 10 heparin-alginate beads containing FGF2 (total dose, 10 or 100 μg) or placebo.[46] After 90 days of follow-up, 7 of 7 patients in the group receiving 100 μg FGF2 were symptom-free, whereas 3 of 7 patients in the control group continued to experience angina, and 2 required additional revascularization procedures. Both nuclear and magnetic resonance (MRI) perfusion imaging demonstrated a significant reduction in the size of the target zone in 100-μg FGF2 group but not in 10-μg FGF2 group or the control group. The improvement in the 100-μg FGF2 group was maintained after 3 years of follow-up.

Single-bolus FGF2 infusion was tested in two open-label dose-escalation phase I studies. Thirty patients with stable and established CAD were randomized to infusions of increasing amounts of FGF2 (3 to100 μg/kg, $n=20$) or placebo ($n=10$). Coronary angiography demonstrated mild but significant dilation of epicardial coronary arteries (7.4%±2.5% mean diameter) during FGF2 infusion, and hypotension and bradycardia were seen at higher dosages (>30 μg/kg).[46]

In another study, 52 symptomatic (class III/IV angina) patients with severe coronary disease received

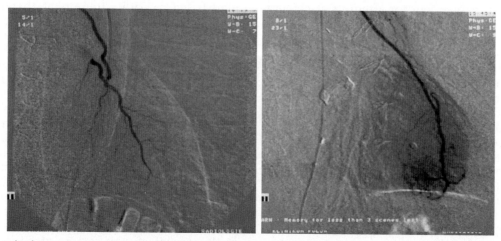

Figure 59-5. Digital subtraction angiograms of a patient 3 months after intramyocardial injection of FGF-1 *(right)* and saline injection *(left)*. Note the extensive capillary "cloud." (From Schumacher B, Pecher P, von Specht BU, Stegmann T: Induction of neoangiogenesis in ischemic myocardium by human growth factors: First clinical results of a new treatment of coronary heart disease. Circulation 1998;97:645-650.)

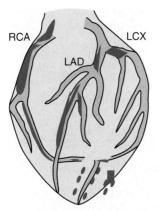
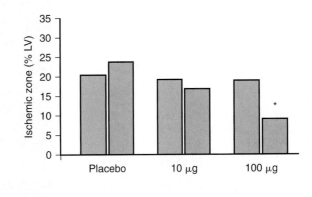

Figure 59-6. Heparin-alginate delivery of fibroblast growth factor 2 (FGF2). *Left,* Location of heparin-alginate beads inserted at the time of coronary artery bypass grafting (CABG). LAD, left anterior descending coronary artery; LCX, left circumflex coronary artery; RCA, right coronary artery. *Right,* Size of the myocardial perfusion defects before and 3 months after treatment, as defined by single-photon emission computed tomography. LV, left ventricle. (Redrawn from Laham RJ, Sellke FW, Edelman ER, et al: Local perivascular delivery of basic fibroblast growth factor in patients undergoing coronary bypass surgery: Results of a phase I randomized, double-blind, placebo-controlled trial. Circulation 1999;100:1865.)

a single intracoronary infusion of FGF2 in doses ranging from 0.33 to 48 μg/kg. Plasma concentration of FGF2 rose rapidly after injection and then gradually declined to baseline levels, with the plasma half-life demonstrating dependence on the amount of the injected growth factor (Fig. 59-7). FGF2 was well tolerated in doses up to 36 μg/kg. Higher doses resulted in systemic hypotension and central nervous system side effects (lethargy, fatigue, insomnia). In particular, a decline in the systolic blood pressure directly correlated with FGF2 dose (Fig. 59-8).

Efficacy evaluation demonstrated a significant reduction in SAQ angina frequency score and an increase in exercise treadmill test (ETT) time after 2 and 6 months, compared with baseline: 510±24 seconds at baseline, 609±26 seconds at day 57 (*P*<.001), and 633±24 seconds at day 180 (*P*<.001).

Blinded analysis of SPECT images demonstrated significant improvement after FGF2 therapy. Furthermore, in a subset of patients, MRI perfusion imaging demonstrated a significant reduction in the size of the ischemic territory and improved left ventricular wall thickening in this territory (Fig. 59-9); in several patients, positron emission tomographic (PET) scanning also demonstrated improvement in perfusion (Fig. 59-10). Taken together, these results suggested that intracoronary infusions of FGF2 are reasonably safe and may produce functionally significant benefits.

This conclusion was tested in a phase II trial (Pharmacological Treatment of Coronary Artery Disease with Recombinant Fibroblast Growth Factor-2 [FIRST] trial) involving 337 no-option/poor option patients with advanced angiographically confirmed CAD and class II/III angina (88% of the trial patients). The patients were randomized to receive, in a double-

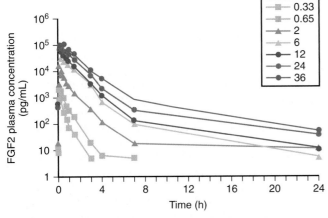

Figure 59-7. Mean plasma concentration of fibroblast growth factor-2 (FGF2) after intracoronary administration. Note a dose-dependent increase in plasma FGF2 levels and a zero-order kinetics washout. (From Bush MA, Samara E, Whitehouse MJ, et al: Pharmacokinetics and pharmacodynamics of recombinant FGF-2 in a phase I trial in coronary artery disease. J Clin Pharmacol 2001;41:378-385.)

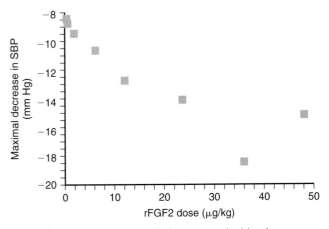

Figure 59-8. Dose-dependent decline in systolic blood pressure (SBP) after intracoronary (IC) infusion of recombinant fibroblast growth factor-2 (rFGF2). (From Bush MA, Samara E, Whitehouse MJ, et al: Pharmacokinetics and pharmacodynamics of recombinant FGF-2 in a phase I trial in coronary artery disease. J Clin Pharmacol 2001;41:378-385.)

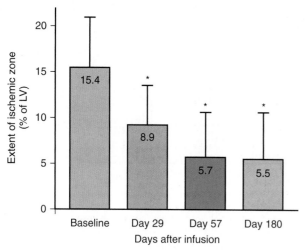

Figure 59-9. Time course of changes in the size of the left ventricular (LV) ischemic zone after intracoronary (IC) infusion of fibroblast growth factor-2 (FGF2), as determined by single-photon emission computed tomography (SPECT). (From Laham RJ, Chronos NA, Pike M, et al: Intracoronary basic fibroblast growth factor (FGF-2) in patients with severe ischemic heart disease: Results of a phase I open-label dose escalation study. J Am Coll Cardiol 2000;36:2132-2139.)

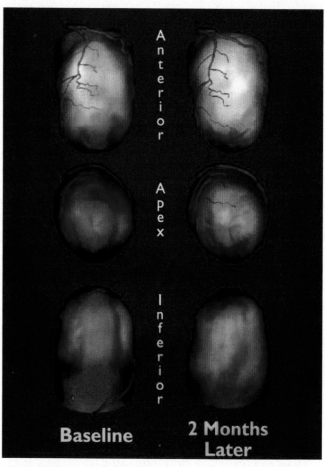

Figure 59-10. Example of positron emission tomographic (PET) image of a patient before (*left*) and 60 days after (*right*) intracoronary (IC) infusion of fibroblast growth factor-2 (FGF2). Purple areas represent ischemic segments. Note a significant reduction in the size of infero-apical defect. (Courtesy of Dr. N. Chronos, ACRI, Atlanta.)

blind manner, three different dosages of recombinant FGF2 (0.3, 3 and 30 µg/kg) or placebo given as a single intracoronary infusion divided between two arterial conduits. Ninety-day follow-up data demonstrated that all groups had a significant increase in exercise tolerance, and this increase was no greater in FGF2-treated patients than in control patients. This improvement in exercise tolerance was maintained at 6 months of follow-up in all four groups.[47]

At the same time, angina frequency, as measured by the SAQ (SAQ-AF scale), was significantly reduced by rFGF2 therapy at 90 days (overall $P=.035$; pairwise $P=.08$, .004, and .05 for the low-, middle-, and high-dose groups, respectively). However, this difference was lost at 180 days because of continued improvement in the placebo group. Symptom assessments using the Canadian Cardiovascular Society (CCS) angina class scale and the SF36 scale confirmed the results of the SAQ questionnaire. The improvement in CCS class reached statistical significance at 90 days for the middle-dose group ($P=.012$), and the physical component summary score of the SF36 form was significantly increased by rFGF2 infusion at 90 days in all groups (pairwise comparison of any FGF versus placebo $P=.033$). As with the SAQ-AF scale, the difference was lost at 180 days because of continued improvement in the control group. Subgroup analysis of the study suggested that benefits such as improvement in symptoms, increased exercise time, and reduced size of ischemic zone defect as measured by nuclear imaging were most prominent in "sicker" patients (i.e., those with lower baseline exercise capacity, higher baseline symptom frequency, and larger nuclear perfusion defects).[47] The validity of

these concepts will require further testing in a double-blind study format.

The companion Therapeutic Angiogenesis with Recombinant Fibroblast Growth Factor-2 for Intermittent Claudication (TRAFFIC) trial examined the utility of intra-arterial FGF2 in patients with peripheral vascular disease and also demonstrated a transient benefit in the rFGF2 group that disappeared by 6 months because of continued improvement in controls.[45] Taken together, these trials have demonstrated relative safety of FGF2; in particular, there was no excess mortality, sudden death, or cancer in FGF2-treated patients, and the observed overall mortality rate (2%) was significantly lower than that seen in laser revascularization trials.

VEGF$_{165}$ was initially evaluated in two small, open-label phase I trials of single intracoronary ($n=15$) and intravenous ($n=14$) infusions. Intracoronary VEGF was given as two 10-minute infusions into the right coronary artery and left main coronary artery ostia in doses ranging from 0.005 to 0.167 µg/kg/min. Radionuclide imaging was carried out before the growth factor infusion and again 30 and 60 days later. Severe hypotension was the dose-limiting toxicity, with a maximally tolerated dose of 0.05 µg/kg/min. SPECT imaging demonstrated a significant improvement in 7 of 14 patients, which correlated with a significant reduction in CCS angina class, and quantitative angiography demonstrated increased arterial density in 7 out of 7 patients having repeat coronary angiography. A trial of intravenous $VEGF_{165}$ infusion likewise suggested similar, but less pronounced, benefits (see review by Annex and Simons[46])

Nevertheless, when the efficacy of a combined intracoronary/intravenous $VEGF_{165}$ administration strategy was tested in a randomized, double-blind, placebo-controlled phase II trial (Vascular endothelial growth factor in Ischemia for Vascular Angiogenesis [VIVA] trial), the results were quite different. Two different dosages of VEGF were given, first by an intracoronary infusion, followed by two intravenous infusions 3 and 7 days later. The overall trial was negative with regard to exercise time, symptom improvement and nuclear imaging.[48] As in the FIRST study, placebo-treated patients demonstrated a significant improvement in exercise tolerance and angina class parameters. Several unusual features of this trial made interpretation of the therapeutic efficacy of $VEGF-A_{165}$ somewhat problematic, including the format of VEGF delivery (a combination of a single intracoronary and two intravenous infusions) and the fact that neither the highest intracoronary VEGF dose nor any of the intravenous VEGF administrations was found to be effective in the porcine ameroid model study. Furthermore, a high proportion of patients in the trial had class II angina, which, in light of the FIRST trial data, makes detection of efficacy much more difficult.

Taken together, the VIVA, FIRST, and TRAFFIC trials taught several very important lessons. Foremost is the high incidence of spontaneous improvement in this patient population, regard to not only such "soft" end points as frequency of angina or exercise tolerance but also "hard" end points such as MRI or PET perfusion. Indeed, profound improvement in MRI and PET images, as demonstrated in Figures 59-9 and 59-10 for open-label FGF2-treated patients, were similarly seen in placebo controls. The profound and very long-lasting placebo effect stipulates an absolute need for double-blind placebo-controlled trial design.

Gene Therapy Trials

A number of studies have used gene transfer approaches to VEGF and FGF therapy (see Tirziu and Simons[40] and Markkanen and colleagues[43] for recent reviews). As in the case of protein therapies, initial trials were open-label and relied on open-chest, direct-vision injections into the myocardium. Latter trials adopted catheter-based intracoronary and transendocardial injection approaches, in some cases supported by NOGA mapping and guidance (Table 59-7).

An initial open-label 20-patient study examined intramyocardial injection of $VEGF_{165}$ plasmid (125 or 250 mg) in patients with inoperable CAD. The plasmid DNA was injected via a minithoracotomy approach. Marked improvement in angina symptoms was observed in 16 patients at day 90, and a reduction in the number of SPECT defects was seen in 13 of 17 patients at 60 days. Plasmid injections were not associated with any acute toxicity, and only one death was reported on follow-up. Adenoviral intramyocardial transfer of $VEGF_{121}$ gene was tested in 21 patients. The adenovirus was injected into the myocardium as a sole therapy in 6 patients and in combination with CABG in 15 patients. In both groups, nuclear perfusion imaging and coronary angiography suggested some improvement at 30 days, whereas treadmill testing suggested improvement in the sole-therapy group. A 6 months' follow-up demonstrated no significant toxicity secondary to intramyocardial injection of adenoviral vectors, and the trends toward improvement in angina class and exercise performance were maintained. Intramyocardial injections of VEGF2 plasmid were studied in a six-patient, open-label, crossover study. A Cordis MyoStar delivery catheter was employed for plasmid injections after electromechanical mapping of the left ventricle. All

Table 59-7. Gene Therapy Trials of Therapeutic Angiogenesis in Coronary Artery Disease

Gene	Trial Type	N	Delivery	Results
$VEGF_{165}$	Phase I OL	5	Plasmid-IM	Reduced symptoms
		20	Plasmid-IM	Improved SPECT
		13	Plasmid-IM (NOGA)	Improved SPECT
	Phase II DBR	80	Plasmid-IM (NOGA)	Unchanged SPECT
$VEGF_{121}$	Phase I OL	21	Adeno-IM	No effect on SPECT
	Phase II OL	67	Adeno-IM	Improved symptoms; worse perfusion
VEGF2	Phase I OL	6	Plasmid-IM	Improved symptoms
				Reduced SPECT- and NOGA-defined defect size
$VEGF_{165}$	Phase I/II DBR	108	Adeno-Dispatch	No effect with plasmid; trend toward
			Plasmid-Dispatch	SPECT improvement with adenovirus
FGF-4	Phase I/II DBR	79	Adeno-IC	Safe
				Trend toward improvement in ETT in certain subgroups

Adeno, adenovirus vector; DBR, double-blind, randomized trial; ETT, exercise treadmill testing; FGF, fibroblast growth factor; IC, intracoronary; IM, intramuscular; OL, open-label trial; SPECT, single-photon emission computed tomography; VEGF, vascular endothelial growth factor.

patients (placebo- and VEGF2-treated) demonstrated a profound reduction in angina frequency for up to 90 days after injections. This reduction was maintained in the VEGF2 group, but the control group was not monitored because of the crossover study design.

On the basis of this and other experiences with VEGF$_{121}$, a randomized trial of open-chest adenoviral injections versus maximal medical treatment was carried out in 67 patients with severe angina.[49] Exercise time to 1-mm ST-segment depression was significantly increased in the open-chest VEGF$_{121}$-treated patients compared with medically treated controls at 26 weeks. However, the results of nuclear perfusion imaging favored the control group. Similarly, a double-blind, placebo-controlled trial of electromechanically guided intramyocardial injections of VEGF-A$_{165}$ plasmid in 80 patients showed similar improvements in symptoms in the VEGF and placebo groups and no differences in size of myocardial stress perfusion defects, although the VEGF-treated group demonstrated improvement in wall motion disturbance.[50]

Another strategy, involving myocardial gene transfer using intracoronary adenoviral injections, was pioneered in the Angiogenic Gene Therapy (AGENT) trials. In the AGENT 1 trial, adenoviral FGF4 (Ad-FGF4) was delivered by an intracoronary infusion to 79 patients with chronic stable CCS class II/III exertional angina. The participants were randomized to receive a single intracoronary infusion of either placebo ($n=19$) or FGF4 ($n=60$) in five ascending doses, from 3.2×10^8 to 3.2×10^{10} viral particles in 0.5-log steps.[51] Safety evaluation did not disclose any increase in serious adverse events associated with adenoviral FGF4 infusions. There were no acute hemodynamic effects, and the virus was not recovered from urine or semen. Three patients in the highest-dose group experienced fevers of less than 24 hours' duration. Most patients receiving active therapy demonstrated a rise in anti-adenoviral antibodies.

Improvement in exercise time at 4 and 12 weeks was used to evaluate anti-ischemic efficacy of Ad-FGF4 gene therapy. Overall, FGF4-treated patients (pooled dose groups) did not show a significant improvement in exercise duration compared to placebo controls at 4 weeks (1.3 versus 0.7 minutes, $P=$ not significant [NS]) or at 12 weeks (1.6 versus 0.8 minutes, $P=$ NS). There was a consistent relationship between the adenovirus dose and the change in ETT. However, subgroup analysis demonstrated significant benefit for FGF4 therapy in several patient subsets. Most meaningfully, patients with a low baseline anti-adenoviral antibody titer ($<1:100$, $n=46$) demonstrated significantly greater improvement in ETT compared to those with high baseline titer ($>1:100$, $n=14$). Equally important, FGF4 appeared to be effective in patients with a baseline ETT duration of less than 10 minutes ($P<.01$).[51]

The double-blind, randomized AGENT 2 trial used nuclear myocardial perfusion imaging to evaluate the efficacy of intracoronary Ad-FGF4 injections in 52 patients. There was a significant reduction of the ischemic defect size in the Ad-FGF4 group, whereas the control group demonstrated no changes. At the same time, the difference in defect size between the two groups was not significant at follow-up.[52] On the basis of these two trials, two large multicenter trials (AGENT 3 and AGENT 4), involving almost 1000 patients, were carried out. However, no significant differences were seen between groups in these trials, although some benefit appeared in various patient subsets (T. Henry, CRT presentation, 2005).

Another intracoronary gene transfer approach was used in the Kuopio Angiogenesis Trial (KAT) trial, in which plasmid- or adenovirus-based VEGF$_{165}$ or an empty vector control was delivered to the coronary wall at the site of angioplasty using a Dispatch catheter in 103 patients.[53] Local VEGF transfer had no effect on the incidence or severity of restenosis, contrary to early claims of efficacy of VEGF for this particular indication. However, patients receiving adenovirus-based, but not plasmid-based, VEGF gene transfer demonstrated smaller perfusion defects at follow-up.[53]

Summary: Current State of Clinical Trials and Future Directions

The current clinical trial experience with therapeutic angiogenesis, despite initial expectations, has not established the clinical utility of this novel form of therapy. Although a great deal has been learned, we are no closer to the goal of establishing therapeutic angiogenesis as a new form of therapy for advanced CAD then we were a decade ago.

Nevertheless, there are significant reasons for optimism, most important among them being improved understanding of angiogenesis biology. We have also convincingly demonstrated the safety of growth factor administration, in terms of both mechanical (delivery-related) and biologic side effects. The importance of the latter cannot be overemphasized. The key to success will be translating these new theoretical advances into useful practical applications. Given the history of interventional cardiology always meeting its challenges, we can be optimistic that these obstacles will be overcome as well.

Although, to paraphrase Yogi Berra, it is hard to make predictions, especially about the future, we suggest that the following are likely to be keys to success: (1) choice of agents stimulating arterial, not capillary growth (i.e., arteriogenesis, not angiogenesis), (2) effective local delivery, and (3) long duration of expression or repeat administrations.

Finally, in the last few years, the field of cell therapy has emerged as an important complement to protein and gene therapy approaches. In particular, much excitement has surrounded the potential presence of circulating endothelial precursor cells that can form new blood vessels in ischemic organs. The originating source of these precursors in adults has not been defined, but the cells themselves can be potentially

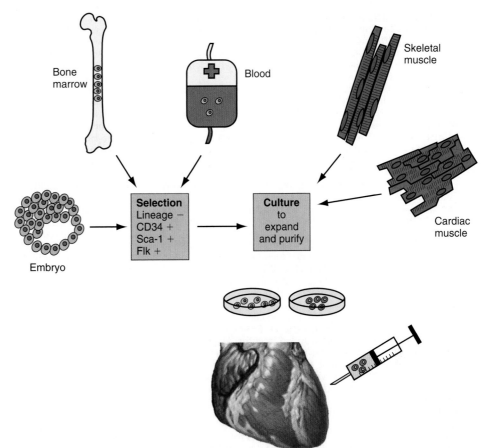

Figure 59-11. Cell-based therapies. Stem cells or endothelial cell precursors can be harvested from various sources, including embryonic tissues, adult bone marrow, and blood. Through various selection and culture methods, the number of cells are expanded and further selection steps are introduced to obtain the highest achievable purity. Muscle cells of skeletal (for gene transfer) or cardiac origin can potentially be harvested from adult tissues, expanded through de-differentiation and redifferentiation steps, and reintroduced in the heart.

obtained from either embryonic stem cells or blood- or bone marrow-derived cells.[54] Other strategies include fusion of adult target cells with denucleated embryonic stem cells. Conceivable, but not yet practical, is the harvesting of desired adult target cells (e.g., myocytes, endothelial cells) and their de-differentiation into a multipotent and proliferative phenotype. Subsequent differentiation steps in the desired direction would then follow (Fig. 59-11). Even if the initial hope of generating new vasculature from circulating or bone marrow-induced stem cells is not fulfilled, it is nevertheless clear that circulating cells play an important role in stimulating tissue neovascularization.[9]

REFERENCES

1. Luttun A, Carmeliet G, Carmeliet P: Vascular progenitors: From biology to treatment. Trends Cardiovasc Med 2002;12: 88-96.
2. Carmeliet P: Angiogenesis in life, disease and medicine. Nature 2005;438:932-936.
3. Simons M, Ware JA: Therapeutic angiogenesis in cardiovascular disease. Nat Rev Drug Discov 2003;2:863-871.
4. Weinstein BM: Vessels and nerves: Marching to the same tune. Cell 2005;120:299-302.
5. Chittenden TW, Claes F, Lanahan AA, et al: Selective regulation of arterial branching morphogenesis by synectin. Dev Cell 2006;10:783-795.
6. Simons M: Angiogenesis: Where do we stand now? Circulation 2005;111:1556-1566.
7. Semenza GL: Development of novel therapeutic strategies that target HIF-1. Expert Opin Ther Targets 2006;10:267-280.
8. Bergmann CE, Hoefer IE, Meder B, et al: Arteriogenesis depends on circulating monocytes and macrophage accumulation and is severely depressed in op/op mice. J Leukoc Biol 2006;80: 59-65.
9. Grunewald M, Avraham I, Dor Y, et al: VEGF-induced adult neovascularization: recruitment, retention, and role of accessory cells. Cell 2006;124:175-189.
10. Li J, Post M, Volk R, et al: PR39, a peptide regulator of angiogenesis. Nat Med 2000;6:49-55.
11. Ferrara N: Vascular endothelial growth factor: Basic science and clinical progress. Endocr Rev 2004;25:581-611.
12. Mukouyama YS, Gerber HP, Ferrara N, et al: Peripheral nerve-derived VEGF promotes arterial differentiation via neuropilin 1-mediated positive feedback. Development 2005;132: 941-952.
13. Dor Y, Djonov V, Abramovitch R, et al: Conditional switching of VEGF provides new insights into adult neovascularization and pro-angiogenic therapy. Embo J 2002;21:1939-1947.
14. Alitalo K, Tammela T, Petrova TV: Lymphangiogenesis in development and human disease. Nature 2005;438: 946-953.
15. Presta M, Dell'Era P, Mitola S, et al: Fibroblast growth factor/fibroblast growth factor receptor system in angiogenesis. Cytokine Growth Factor Rev 2005;16:159-178.
16. Yancopoulos GD, Davis S, Gale NW, et al: Vascular-specific growth factors and blood vessel formation. Nature 2000;407: 242-248.
17. Thurston G, Wang Q, Baffert F, et al: Angiopoietin 1 causes vessel enlargement, without angiogenic sprouting, during a critical developmental period. Development 2005;132: 3317-3326.
18. Pasquale EB: Eph receptor signalling casts a wide net on cell behaviour. Nat Rev Mol Cell Biol 2005;6:462-475.

19. Eichmann A, Makinen T, Alitalo K: Neural guidance molecules regulate vascular remodeling and vessel navigation. Genes Dev 2005;19:1013-1021.
20. Betsholtz C: Insight into the physiological functions of PDGF through genetic studies in mice. Cytokine Growth Factor Rev 2004;15:215-228.
21. Armulik A, Abramsson A, Betsholtz C: Endothelial/pericyte interactions. Circ Res 2005;97:512-523.
22. Levitzki A: PDGF receptor kinase inhibitors for the treatment of restenosis. Cardiovasc Res 2005;65:581-586.
23. Morishita R, Aoki M, Yo Y, Ogihara T: Hepatocyte growth factor as cardiovascular hormone: Role of HGF in the pathogenesis of cardiovascular disease. Endocr J 2002;49:273-284.
24. Morishita R, Aoki M, Hashiya N, et al: Therapeutic angiogenesis using hepatocyte growth factor (HGF). Curr Gene Ther 2004;4:199-206.
25. Lee JW, Bae SH, Jeong JW, et al: Hypoxia-inducible factor (HIF-1)alpha: Its protein stability and biological functions. Exp Mol Med 2004;36:1-12.
26. Vincent KA, Feron O, Kelly RA: Harnessing the response to tissue hypoxia: HIF-1 alpha and therapeutic angiogenesis. Trends Cardiovasc Med 2002;12:362-367.
27. Post MJ, Sato K, Murakami M, et al: Adenoviral PR39 improves blood flow and myocardial function in a pig model of chronic myocardial ischemia by enhancing collateral formation. Am J Physiol Regul Integr Comp Physiol 2006;290:R494-R500.
28. Cox CM, D'Agostino SL, Miller MK, et al: Apelin, the ligand for the endothelial G-protein-coupled receptor, APJ, is a potent angiogenic factor required for normal vascular development of the frog embryo. Dev Biol 2006;296:177-189.
29. Wickstrom SA, Alitalo K, Keski-Oja J: Endostatin signaling and regulation of endothelial cell-matrix interactions. Adv Cancer Res 2005;94:197-229.
30. Doll JA, Soff GA: Angiostatin. Cancer Treat Res 2005;126:175-204.
31. Roy R, Zhang B, Moses MA: Making the cut: Protease-mediated regulation of angiogenesis. Exp Cell Res 2006;312:608-622.
32. Hughes GC, Post MJ, Simons M, Annex BH: Translational physiology: Porcine models of human coronary artery disease. Implications for preclinical trials of therapeutic angiogenesis. J Appl Physiol 2003;94:1689-1701.
33. Tirziu D, Moodie KL, Zhuang ZW, et al: Delayed arteriogenesis in hypercholesterolemic mice. Circulation 2005;112:2501-2509.
34. Li W, Shen W, Gill R, et al: High-resolution quantitative computed tomography demonstrating selective enhancement of medium-size collaterals by placental growth factor-1 in the mouse ischemic hindlimb. Circulation 2006;113:2445-2453.
35. Voskuil M, van Royen N, Hoefer IE, et al: Modulation of collateral artery growth in a porcine hindlimb ligation model using MCP-1. Am J Physiol Heart Circ Physiol 2003;284:H1422-H1428.
36. Baklanov DV, de Muinck ED, Simons M, et al: Live 3D echo guidance of catheter-based endomyocardial injection. Catheter Cardiovasc Interv 2005;65:340-345.
37. Boekstegers P, Kupatt C: Current concepts and applications of coronary venous retroinfusion. Basic Res Cardiol 2004;99:373-381.
38. Zisch AH, Lutolf MP, Hubbell JA: Biopolymeric delivery matrices for angiogenic growth factors. Cardiovasc Pathol 2003;12:295-310.
39. Hosaka A, Koyama H, Kushibiki T, et al: Gelatin hydrogel microspheres enable pinpoint delivery of basic fibroblast growth factor for the development of functional collateral vessels. Circulation 2004;110:3322-3328.
40. Tirziu D, Simons M: Angiogenesis in the human heart: Gene and cell therapy. Angiogenesis 2005;8:241-251. Epub 2005 Nov 25.
41. Rissanen TT, Rutanen J, Yla-Herttuala S: Gene transfer for therapeutic vascular growth in myocardial and peripheral ischemia. Adv Genet 2004;52:117-164.
42. Yla-Herttuala S, Markkanen JE, Rissanen TT: Gene therapy for ischemic cardiovascular diseases: Some lessons learned from the first clinical trials. Trends Cardiovasc Med 2004;14:295-300.
43. Markkanen JE, Rissanen TT, Kivela A, Yla-Herttuala S: Growth factor-induced therapeutic angiogenesis and arteriogenesis in the heart: Gene therapy. Cardiovasc Res 2005;65:656-664.
44. Chittenden T, Sherman JA, Xiong F, et al: Transcriptional profiling in coronary artery disease: Indications for novel markers of coronary collateralization. Circulation 2006;114:1811-1820. Epub 2006 Oct 16.
45. Lederman RJ, Mendelsohn FO, Anderson RD, et al: Therapeutic angiogenesis with recombinant fibroblast growth factor-2 for intermittent claudication (the TRAFFIC study): A randomised trial. Lancet 2002;359:2053-2058.
46. Annex BH, Simons M: Growth factor-induced therapeutic angiogenesis in the heart: Protein therapy. Cardiovasc Res 2005;65:649-655.
47. Simons M, Annex BH, Laham RJ, et al: Pharmacological treatment of coronary artery disease with recombinant fibroblast growth factor-2: Double-blind, randomized, controlled clinical trial. Circulation 2002;105:788-793.
48. Henry TD, Annex BH, McKendall GR, et al: The VIVA trial: Vascular endothelial growth factor in Ischemia for Vascular Angiogenesis. Circulation 2003;107:1359-1365.
49. Stewart DJ, Hilton JD, Arnold JM, et al: Angiogenic gene therapy in patients with nonrevascularizable ischemic heart disease: A phase 2 randomized, controlled trial of AdVEGF(121) (AdVEGF121) versus maximum medical treatment. Gene Ther 2006;13:1503-1511. Epub 2006 Jun 22.
50. Kastrup J, Jorgensen E, Ruck A, et al: Direct intramyocardial plasmid vascular endothelial growth factor-A165 gene therapy in patients with stable severe angina pectoris: A randomized double-blind placebo-controlled study. The Euroinject One trial. J Am Coll Cardiol 2005;45:982-988.
51. Grines CL, Watkins MW, Helmer G, et al: Angiogenic Gene Therapy (AGENT) trial in patients with stable angina pectoris. Circulation 2002;105:1291-1297.
52. Grines CL, Watkins MW, Mahmarian JJ, et al: A randomized, double-blind, placebo-controlled trial of Ad5FGF-4 gene therapy and its effect on myocardial perfusion in patients with stable angina. J Am Coll Cardiol 2003;42:1339-1347.
53. Hedman M, Hartikainen J, Syvanne M, et al: Safety and feasibility of catheter-based local intracoronary vascular endothelial growth factor gene transfer in the prevention of postangioplasty and in-stent restenosis and in the treatment of chronic myocardial ischemia: Phase II results of the Kuopio Angiogenesis Trial (KAT). Circulation 2003;107:2677-2683.
54. de Muinck ED, Thompson C, Simons M: Progress and prospects: Cell based regenerative therapy for cardiovascular disease. Gene Ther 2006;13:659-671.

Evaluation of Interventional Techniques

60 Qualitative and Quantitative Coronary Angiography

Jeffrey J. Popma, Alexandra Almonacid, and Alexandra J. Lansky

---

KEY POINTS

- Although clinical outcomes after percutaneous coronary intervention (PCI) have substantially improved over the past decade with use of coronary stents, assessment of coronary lesion complexity remains valuable in estimating early and late procedural risk. Aggregate scores that consider both the vessel patency and underlying lesion morphology provide the most predictive information for estimating outcome. Longer lesions, thrombus-containing lesions, degenerated saphenous vein grafts, severe tortuosity and angulation, and total coronary occlusions hold the highest risk for failure with PCI.

- Assessment of both myocardial blood flow and myocardial perfusion is useful in predicting prognosis in patients with ST-segment elevation myocardial infarction (STEMI) and may also be valuable in predicting events in patients with non-ST-segment elevation myocardial infarction as well. More quantitative indices are preferred over more qualitative ones in order to assess the value of new drugs and devices in patients with STEMI.

- Interventional cardiologists remain firmly wedded to the coronary angiogram for the assessment of lesion severity before and after PCI, reserving the physiologic assessment of intermediate lesions to adjunct modalities such as fractional and coronary flow reserve measurements. However, more reliable and reproducible methods of severity assessment using quantitative angiography have provided important insights into the mechanism of benefit for new drugs and devices in patients undergoing coronary intervention.

- Late clinical restenosis can be predicted by the quantitative measurement of percent diameter stenosis and late lumen loss in patients undergoing drug-eluting stent placement compared with bare metal stent placement. More studies are needed to evaluate whether these angiographic measurements correlate with relevant differences in late clinical outcome when two drug-eluting stents are compared.

- Quantitative angiographic methods remain an extremely important tool for the assessment of outcome after new device and drug therapy in patients undergoing intervention for ischemic heart disease.

Percutaneous coronary intervention (PCI) has evolved dramatically over the past 2 decades, fundamentally altering the management of ischemic cardiovascular disease. Coronary stents and, more recently, drug-eluting coronary stents (DESs), are currently used in 80% to 90% of PCI procedures. Coronary arteriography is a fundamental component of PCI, providing prognostic information about the baseline lesion morphology and severity, quantification of antegrade perfusion, and adequacy of the final angiographic result. Conventional "visual" angiography has formed the cornerstone of clinical decision-making for patients undergoing cardiovascular intervention, but insights from more quantitative analysis of procedural and late angiograms have permitted a mechanistic understanding of the relative value of new devices and drugs developed for the treatment of ischemic cardiovascular disease. Refinements in the angiographic determinants of procedural complications, thrombosis, and restenosis have permitted more appropriate device evaluation and selection for patients undergoing these procedures.

The purposes of this review are threefold. First, the standard criteria used to stratify the baseline procedural risk in patients undergoing PCI are reviewed. These criteria have been modified since the availability of DESs, and a number of new predictive scores for early and late outcome after stent placement have been identified. Second, newer methods to assess myocardial perfusion beyond coronary flow that provide important prognostic information for patients with acute myocardial infarction (AMI) are reviewed. Third, the quantitative angiographic methods used for evaluating early and late procedural outcome after PCI are outlined, including a discussion of the value of these indices as surrogates for clinical outcome.

QUALITATIVE ANGIOGRAPHY

Assessment of procedural risk for PCI begins with accurate definition of the baseline coronary anatomy. Predictors for an adverse procedural outcome after balloon angioplasty were identified in early series, but a standardized approach to the assessment of lesion morphology in patients undergoing PCI was lacking until the late 1980s. Contemporary refinement of these criteria was necessary after the introduction of coronary stents in order to more appropriately estimate procedural risk in the new millennium of device intervention.

Update On The ACC/AHA Task Force on Lesion Morphology

A joint task force of the American College of Cardiology (ACC) and American Heart Association (AHA) established criteria in 1988 to estimate procedural success and complication rates after balloon angioplasty based on the presence or absence of specific high-risk lesion characteristics.[1] Although these criteria were developed based solely on the task force's clinical impressions (Table 60-1), their estimates of procedural success and complications were closely correlated with the procedural outcomes demonstrated in patients undergoing multivessel balloon angioplasty.[2] Lesion characteristics associated with an adverse outcome included chronic total occlusion, high-grade stenosis, stenosis on a bend of 60

degrees or more, and location in vessels with proximal tortuosity.[2] With improvements in equipment design and periprocedural anticoagulation, better outcomes were reported after balloon angioplasty, although the most complex lesion morphologies (i.e., "type C" lesions) were still associated with less satisfactory procedural outcomes.

Other composite risk scores were proposed as alternatives to the ACC/AHA score with the availablility of new coronary devices, including coronary stents.[3,4] The Society for Cardiac Angiography and Interventions (SCAI) Registry evaluated 61,926 patients (74.5% received stents) from the ACC National Cardiovascular Data Registry and classified their lesions into four groups: non-type C patent, type C patent, non-type C occluded, and type C occluded (Table 60-2).[3] These more simplified criteria provided better discrimination for success or complications than the ACC/AHA original classification with a c statistic of 0.69 for success using the ACC/AHA original classification system, 0.71 using the modified ACC/AHA system, and 0.75 for the SCAI classification.[3]

The Mayo Clinic Risk Score was constructed by adding integer scores for the presence of eight morphologic variables and was compared with the ACC/AHA risk score in 5064 patients undergoing PCI, of whom 183 (4%) experienced an adverse event (death, Q-wave myocardial infarction, stroke, emergency coronary artery bypass graft).[4] The Mayo Clinic risk score offered significantly better risk stratification than the ACC/AHA lesion classification for the development of cardiovascular complications, whereas the ACC/AHA lesion classification was a better system for determining angiographic success.[4]

Risk Assessment Using Specific Lesion Morphologic Criteria

Despite the value of risk scores in estimating aggregate procedural risk, there are several limitations of these criteria as applied to individual patients.

Table 60-1. ACC/AHA Characteristics of Type A, B, and C Coronary Lesions

Type A lesions—high success (>85%), low risk

Discrete (<10 mm)	Little or no calcium
Concentric	Less than totally occlusive
Readily accessible	Not ostial in location
Nonangulated segment (<45 degrees)	No major side branch involvement
Smooth contour	Absence of thrombus

Type B lesions—moderate success (60%-85%), moderate risk

Tubular (10-20 mm length)	Moderate to heavy calcification
Eccentric	Total occlusion <3 mo old
Moderate tortuosity of proximal segment	Ostial in location
Moderately angulated (45-90 degrees)	Bifurcation lesion requiring double guidewire
Irregular contour	Some thrombus present

Type C lesions—low success (<60%), high risk

Diffuse (>20 mm length)	Total occlusion >3 mo old
Excessive tortuosity of proximal segment	Inability to protect major side branches
Extremely angulated segment (>90 degrees)	Degenerated vein grafts with friable lesions

Modified from Ryan TJ, Faxon DP, Gunnar RP, et al: Guidelines for percutaneous transluminal coronary angioplasty: A report of the American College of Cardiology/American Heart Association Task Force on Assessment of Diagnostic and Therapeutic Cardiovascular Procedures (Subcommittee on Percutaneous Transluminal Coronary Angioplasty). J Am Coll Cardiol 1988;12:529-545.

Table 60-2. SCAI Lesion Classification System: Class I-IV Lesions

Type I lesion (highest success expected; lowest risk)
(1) Does not meet ACC/AHA criteria for type C lesion
(2) Patent

Type II lesion
1. Meets any of the following ACC/AHA criteria for type C lesion:
   Diffuse (>2 cm length)
   Excessive tortuosity of proximal segment
   Extremely angulated segments >90 degrees
   Inability to protect major side branches
   Degenerated vein grafts with friable lesions
2. Patent

Type III lesion
1. Does not meet ACC/AHA criteria for type C lesion
2. Occluded

Type IV lesion
1. Meets any of the following ACC/AHA criteria for type C lesion:
   Diffuse (>2 cm length)
   Excessive tortuosity of proximal segment
   Extremely angulated segments >90 degrees
   Inability to protect major side branches
   Degenerated vein grafts with friable lesions
2. Occluded

Modified from Krone R, Shaw R, Klein L, et al: Evaluation of the American College of Cardiology/American Heart Association and the Society for Coronary Angiography and Interventions lesion classification system in the current "stent era" of coronary interventions (from the ACC-National Cardiovascular Data Registry). Am J Cardiol 2003;92:389-394.

Identification of lesion characteristics, such as eccentricity, irregularity, angulation, and tortuosity, is limited by substantial interobserver variability. Agreement with ACC/AHA classification was noted in only 58% of lesions in one series, with disagreement by two classification grades noted in almost 10% of lesions.[2] Accordingly, rather than a composite score, description of individual morphologic features may be more predictive of early and late outcome after PCI. Some ACC/AHA morphologic features are associated with a complicated procedure (e.g., thrombus, saphenous vein graft [SVG] degeneration, angulated segments), whereas others are associated with an unsuccessful but uncomplicated procedure (e.g., chronic total occlusions, diffuse disease). As an alternative to providing a composite lesion complexity score, estimation of procedural risk based on the presence of one or more specific adverse morphologic features may be more useful (Table 60-3).

Irregular Lesions

With the advent of coronary stents, the prognostic importance of irregular lesions has been diminished substantially, although identification of an irregular plaque at angiography suggests the presence of an acute coronary syndrome and intracoronary thrombus. Semiquantitative and quantitative measurements of lesion irregularity were developed in the

Table 60-3. Definitions of Preprocedural Lesion Morphology

Feature	Definition
Eccentricity	Stenosis that is noted to have one of its luminal edges in the outer one-quarter of the apparently normal lumen
Irregularity	Characterized by lesion ulceration, intimal flap, aneurysm, or "sawtooth" pattern
Ulceration	Lesion with a small crater consisting of a discrete luminal widening in the area of the stenosis is noted, provided that it does not extend beyond the normal arterial lumen
Intimal flap	A mobile, radiolucent extension of the vessel wall into the arterial lumen
Aneurysmal dilation	Segment of arterial dilation larger than the dimensions of the normal arterial segment
"Sawtooth pattern"	Multiple, sequential stenosis irregularities
Lesion length	Measured "shoulder-to-shoulder" in an unforeshortened view
Discrete	Lesion length <10 mm
Tubular	Lesion length 10-20 mm
Diffuse	Lesion length ≥20 mm
Ostial location	Origin of the lesion within 3 mm of the vessel origin
Lesion angulation	Vessel angle formed by the centerline through the lumen proximal to the stenosis and extending beyond it and a second centerline in the straight portion of the artery distal to the stenosis
Moderate	Lesion angulation ≥45 degrees
Severe	Lesion angulation ≥90 degrees
Bifurcation stenosis	Present if a medium or large branch (>1.5 mm) originates within the stenosis and if the side branch is completely surrounded by stenotic portions of the lesion to be dilated
Lesion accessibility (proximal tortuosity)	
Moderate tortuosity	Lesion is distal to two bends ≥75 degrees
Severe tortuosity	Lesion is distal to three bends ≥75 degrees
Degenerated SVG	Graft characterized by luminal irregularities or ectasia comprising >50% of the graft length
Calcification	Readily apparent densities noted within the apparent vascular wall at the site of the stenosis
Moderate	Densities noted only with cardiac motion before contrast injection
Severe	Radiopacities noted without cardiac motion before contrast injection
Total occlusion	TIMI 0 or 1 flow
Thrombus	Discrete, intraluminal filling defect is noted with defined borders and is largely separated from the adjacent wall; contrast staining may or may not be present

SVG, saphenous vein graft; TIMI, Thrombolysis in Myocardial Infarction.

early 1990s to better characterize lesion morphology in patients with acute coronary syndromes, but these methods have not found clinical utility independent of other clinical risk factors.

Angulated Lesions

Vessel curvature at the site of maximum stenosis should be measured in the most unforeshortened projection using a length of curvature that approximates the balloon length used for coronary dilation. Although balloon angioplasty of highly angulated lesions is associated with an increased risk for coronary dissection, in the era of coronary stenting the greatest impediment of angulated lesions is inability to deliver the stent to the stenosis and straighten the arterial contour after stent placement, which may predispose to late stent fracture.

Lesion Calcification

Coronary artery calcium is an important marker for coronary atherosclerosis. Conventional coronary angiography has limited sensitivity for the detection of smaller amounts of calcium and is only moderately sensitive for the detection of extensive lesion calcium (60% and 85% sensitivity for three- and four-quadrant calcium, respectively).[5] The presence of coronary calcification reduces the compliance of the vessel and may predispose to dissection at the interface between calcified plaque and normal wall after balloon angioplasty. The presence of coronary calcification also reduces the ability to cross chronic total occlusions; moreover, in severely calcified lesions, stent strut expansion is inversely correlated with the circumferential arc of calcium.[6]

Rotational atherectomy is the preferred pretreatment method in patients with severe lesion calcification, particularly ostial lesions, and it facilitates the delivery and expansion of coronary stents by creating microdissection planes within the fibrocalcific plaque. Even with these contemporary methods, however, the presence of moderate or severe coronary calcification is associated with reduced procedural success and higher complication rates,[7] including stent dislodgement. In less severely calcified lesions, no difference in restenosis rate was found after paclitaxel-eluting stent implantation in calcified versus noncalcified vessels.[8] Calcification noted within SVGs is usually within the reference vessel wall rather than within the lesion and is associated with older graft age, insulin-dependent diabetes, and history of smoking.[9]

Degenerated Saphenous Vein Grafts

SVGs develop progressive degeneration over time, with 25% occluding within the first year after coronary bypass surgery[10] and 50% developing occlusion within 10 years after surgery. Although coronary stents and, more recently, DESs[11] reduce restenosis rates compared with balloon angioplasty, only embolic protection devices have reduced procedural complications.[12,13] One exception may be in patients treated for in-stent restenosis (ISR), where embolic protection may not be required. Self-expanding stents made with expanded polytetrafluoroethylene (ePTFE) provide no additional advantage over noncovered balloon-expandable stents on the development of early complications or late restenosis.[14]

The risk for embolic complications appears to be related to both the degree of overall graft degeneration and the length of the lesion.[15] Using angiographic assessments of the extent of graft degeneration and estimated volume of plaque in the target lesion, independent correlates of increased 30-day major adverse cardiac event rates were more extensive vein graft degeneration ($P = .0001$) and bulkier lesions (larger estimated plaque volume, $P = .0005$).

Thrombus

Conventional angiography is relatively insensitive for the detection of coronary thrombus. The presence of angiographic thrombus, usually identified by the appearance of discrete, intraluminal filling defects within the arterial lumen, is also associated with a higher, albeit widely variable (6% to 73%), incidence of ischemic complications after PCI. The primary complications related to PCI of thrombus-containing lesions are distal embolization and thrombotic occlusion, with the risk for complications with angiographic thrombus relating to the size of the coronary thrombus. Routine rheolytic thrombectomy provides no benefit in patients with AMI,[16] although it may be useful for patients with a large thrombus burden. A number of aspiration catheters have been used in patients with AMI and large thrombus burden, but large-scale studies are lacking.

Ostial Location

Ostial lesions are defined as those that begin within 3 mm of the origin of the coronary artery; they are classified as aorto-ostial and nonaorto-ostial. Balloon angioplasty of ostial lesions is limited by suboptimal procedural outcome, primarily due to technical factors such as difficulties with guide catheter support, lesion inelasticity precluding maximal balloon expansion, and early vascular recoil limiting the acute angiographic result. Debulking techniques such as directional and rotational atherectomy improve the compliance of the aorto-ostial lesion but have had limited effect on preventing late restenosis.

Coronary stenting, more recently with DESs, has become the default therapy for most aorto-ostial lesions, although there are unique challenges of stent placement in the aorto-ostial location, such as protrusion of the stent into the aorta precluding

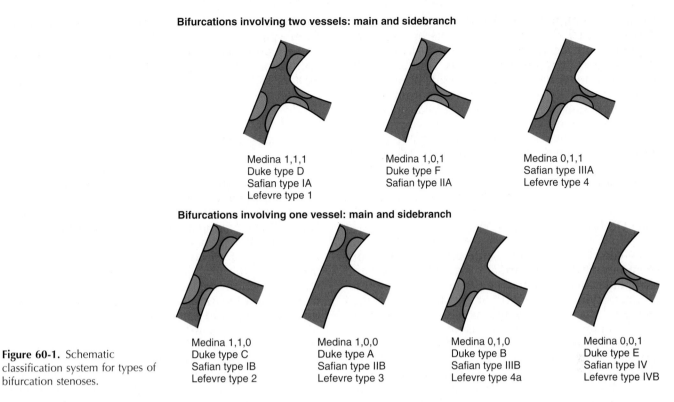

Bifurcations involving two vessels: main and sidebranch

Medina 1,1,1
Duke type D
Safian type IA
Lefevre type 1

Medina 1,0,1
Duke type F
Safian type IIA

Medina 0,1,1
Safian type IIIA
Lefevre type 4

Bifurcations involving one vessel: main and sidebranch

Medina 1,1,0
Duke type C
Safian type IB
Lefevre type 2

Medina 1,0,0
Duke type A
Safian type IIB
Lefevre type 3

Medina 0,1,0
Duke type B
Safian type IIIB
Lefevre type 4a

Medina 0,0,1
Duke type E
Safian type IV
Lefevre type IVB

Figure 60-1. Schematic classification system for types of bifurcation stenoses.

subsequent injection catheter engagement, compression, and avulsion of the stent struts into the aorta when new devices such as cutting balloon angioplasty are used to treat ISR.

Isolated nonaorto-ostial stenoses of the left circumflex and left anterior descending coronary arteries[17] and ostial side branch bifurcation lesions are also effectively treated with DES,[18] but they pose unique challenges regarding vessel wall geometry, adequate ostial branch coverage (particularly if there is a narrow angle with the adjacent branch), and plaque shifting causing compromise of the parent or adjacent branch vessels. Whereas stent protrusion into the parent vessel of less than 1 mm is usually well tolerated, stent protrusion to greater degrees precludes treatment of the parent branches.[18] Stent fractures have been reported with more advanced stenting techniques used to treat the parent vessel and ostial side branch stenoses.

Long Lesions

Lesion length may be estimated quantitatively as the "shoulder-to-shoulder" extent of atherosclerotic narrowing greater than 20%, although many clinicians estimate lesion length based on the identification of a "normal to normal" segment, which is usually longer than the length obtained with quantitative methods. Conventional balloon angioplasty of long lesions has been associated with reduced procedural success, particularly when the segment is diffusely diseased (i.e., >20 mm in length), primarily because of the more extensive plaque burden in long lesions.

Stents improve late outcome compared with balloon angioplasty, but stent and lesion length remain the most important predictors of restenosis in the stent era.[19] Coronary stents have been used to treat suboptimal angiographic results ("spot stenting") and dissections after balloon angioplasty of longer lesions, although the "full metal jacket" stent approach to diffuse disease is associated with a higher recurrence rate in the absence of complete stent expansion, particularly in smaller vessels. Overlapping sirolimus-eluting stents provide safe and effective treatment for long coronary lesions.[20]

Bifurcation Lesions

The risk of side branch occlusion in bifurcation lesions relates to the extent of atherosclerotic involvement of the side branch within its origin from the parent vessel, which ranges from 14% to 27% in side branches with ostial involvement. To accurately assess the risk of side branch occlusion and avoid conflicting definitions of side branch and ostial stenosis, a number of classification systems for bifurcation stenoses have been proposed (Fig. 60-1).[21-24]

One stent is preferable to stents in both the parent vessel and the side branch, because subacute thrombosis and restenosis remain higher in bifurcation disease treated with coronary stents in both branches.[25] If two stents are planned for the parent vessel and side branch, a number of stenting techniques are possible, including simultaneous kissing stents, crush, coulotte, and T stenting. To date, the optimal technique has not been identified, although the use of DESs appears to reduce restenosis compared with bare metal stents. The origin of the side branch is the most common location of failure (recurrence) after bifurcation stenting.[26] A number of dedicated bifurcation stents have been developed to provide adequate vessel coverage[27] and side branch access[28] during stent deployment. Common to all of these strategies is a final "kissing" balloon inflation in the parent vessel and side branch.[29]

Total Occlusion

Total coronary occlusion is identified as an abrupt termination of the epicardial vessel; anterograde and retrograde collaterals may be present and are helpful in quantifying the length of the totally occluded segment. Coronary occlusions are common findings[30] and often lead to the decision to perform coronary bypass surgery rather than PCI in the setting of multivessel disease.[31,32] The success rate for recanalization depends on the occlusion duration and on certain lesion morphologic features, such as bridging collaterals, occlusion length greater than 15 mm, and absence of a "nipple" to guide wire advancement. Although newer technologies and techniques have been used to recanalize refractory occlusions,[33,34] better guide wires and wire techniques have accounted for much of the improvement in crossing success over recent years.[35] Simultaneous coronary injections are sometimes useful for identifying the length of the total occlusion (Fig. 60-2). Once the occlusion has been crossed, coronary stents, including DES,[36,37] have been used to provide the best long-term outcomes.

A key component to the assessment of total occlusion is definition of the collateral grades that provide blood flow to the jeopardized myocardium.[38] The Rentrop classification system includes Rentrop grade 0 (no filling), Rentrop grade 1 (small side branches filled), Rentrop grade 2 (partial epicardial filling of the occluded artery), and Rentrop grade 3 (complete epicardial filling of the occluded artery). Anatomic collaterals summarized by the 26 potential pathways were consolidated into four groups: septal, intra-arterial (bridging), epicardial with proximal takeoff (atrial branches), and epicardial with distal takeoff.[39] Finally, the size of the collateral connection can be quantified as group 0 (no continuous connection between donor and recipient artery), group 1 (continuous threadlike connection ≤0.3 mm), or group 2 (continuous small, branch-like collateral through its course ≥0.4 mm).[39]

Angiographic Complications After Percutaneous Coronary Intervention

Although the frequency of angiographic complications during PCI has been reduced substantially with the use of coronary stents, untoward effects resulting from disruption of the atherosclerotic plaque and embolization of atherosclerotic debris, thrombus, and vasoactive mediators still occurs during 5% to 10% of PCI procedures.

Coronary Dissection

Plaque fracture is an integral component of balloon angioplasty, although significant vessel wall disruption resulting in reduced anterograde flow and lumen compromise is a relatively uncommon occurrence (<3%).[40] The National Heart, Lung, and Blood Institute (NHLBI) coronary dissection criteria categorize the severity of coronary dissection after PCI (Table 60-4), with the prognostic implications of the coronary dissection depending on extension into the media and adventitia, axial length, presence of contrast staining, and effect on anterograde coronary perfusion. It is sometimes difficult to assess the angiographic residual lumen in the presence of coronary dissection because of the frame-to-frame lumen diameter changes seen with two-dimensional imaging; in the setting, intravascular ultrasound (IVUS) may provide a more accurate reflection of the true circumference lumen dimensions. Dissections resulting in a residual area stenosis of 60% or greater by IVUS[41] and those extending more than 5 to 10 mm in axial length are associated with a worse prognosis.

"No-Reflow"

Reduced flow during PCI, also known as "no-reflow," is defined as a reduction in anterograde flow despite a patent lumen at the site of PCI. It occurs during 1% to 5% of PCI procedures. No-reflow is a strong predictor of mortality after PCI.[42] No-reflow is more common (15%) during primary angioplasty for AMI.[43] Predictors of no-reflow include a higher plaque burden, thrombus, lipid pools by IVUS, higher lesion elastic membrane cross-sectional area, preinfarction angina, and Thrombolysis in Myocardial Infarction (TIMI) flow grade 0 on the initial coronary angiogram, among other factors.[44-46] Compared to aspirates obtained from patients without no-reflow, aspirates obtained from patients who developed no-reflow contained more atheromatous plaque and significantly more platelet and fibrin complex, macrophages, and cholesterol crystals.[47] The 30-day mortality rate was significantly higher (27.5%) in patients with combined slow-flow and no-reflow phenomenon than in patients with normal coronary blood flow after PCI (5.3%; $P < .001$).[43] Intracoronary or intragraft nitroprusside,[48] adenosine,[49] verapamil,[50] and nicardipine[51] and aspiration of atherosclerotic debris have each been used to correct the episode of no-reflow.

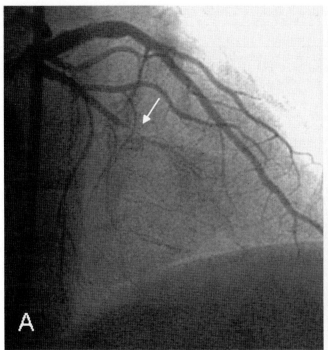

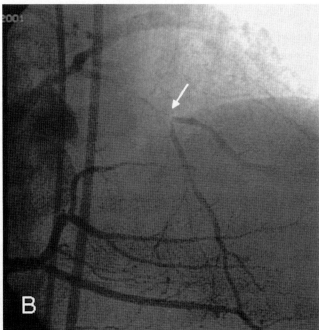

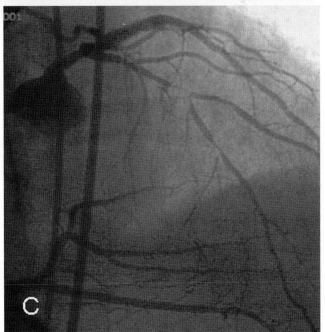

Figure 60-2. Simultaneous coronary injections to visual contralateral collaterals. **A,** A total occlusion of the middle left anterior descending artery (LAD) is visualized by contrast injection in the left coronary artery *(arrow)*. The distal portion of the LAD is not visualized.[52] **B,** Injection of the right coronary artery shows right-to-left collaterals that fill the LAD to the point of occlusion *(arrow)*. **C,** Simultaneous injection of the left and right coronary arteries provides sufficient visualization of the total occlusion to allow wire crossing.

Distal Embolization

Periprocedural myonecrosis provides clinical evidence of distal particulate embolization during PCI. Angiographic distal embolization is defined as the migration of a filling defect or thrombus to distally occlude the target vessel or one of its branches.[52] It occurs in approximately 10% of patients with an AMI undergoing PCI. Embolic complications occur more often in patients with AMI and in patients undergoing balloon angioplasty of SVG lesions, particularly those with recent occlusion.

Coronary Perforation

Coronary perforation is an uncommon (<1%) complication of PCI that is associated with significant morbidity and mortality.[53-57] Coronary perforations are infrequent in patients undergoing balloon angioplasty (0.1%) compared with patients undergoing atheroablative therapy (1.3%; $P < .001$).[54,58] Perforation due to coronary guide wires may manifest late after the procedure. Initial management strategies include prolonged balloon inflation, reversal of anticoagulation, and, in refractory cases, use of PTFE-covered stents.[59-61]

Table 60-4. Standardized Criteria for Postprocedural Lesion Morphology

Feature	Definition
Abrupt closure	Obstruction of contrast flow (TIMI 0 or 1) in a dilated segment with previously documented anterograde flow
Ectasia	A lesion diameter greater than the reference diameter in one or more areas
Luminal irregularities	Arterial contour that has a "sawtooth pattern" consisting of opacification but not fulfilling the criteria for dissection or intracoronary thrombus
Intimal flap	A discrete filling defect in apparent continuity with the arterial wall
Thrombus	Discrete, mobile angiographic filling defect with or without contrast staining
Dissection*	
A	Small radiolucent area within the lumen of the vessel
B	Linear, nonpersisting extravasation of contrast
C	Extraluminal, persisting extravasation of contrast
D	Spiral-shaped filling defect
E	Persistent lumen defect with delayed anterograde flow
F	Filling defect accompanied by total coronary occlusion
Length	Measure end-to-end for type B through F dissections
Staining	Persistence of contrast within the dissection after washout of contrast from the remaining portion of the vessel
Perforation	
Localized	Extravasation of contrast confined to the pericardial space immediately surrounding the artery and not associated with clinical tamponade
Nonlocalized	Extravasation of contrast with a jet not localized to the pericardial space, potentially associated with clinical tamponade
Side branch loss	TIMI 0, 1, or 2 flow in a side branch >1.5 mm in diameter that previously had TIMI 3 flow
Distal embolization	Migration of a filling defect or thrombus to distally occlude the target vessel or one of its branches
Coronary spasm	Transient or permanent narrowing >50% when a <25% stenosis was previously noted

*National Heart, Lung, and Blood Institute classification system for coronary dissection.
TIMI, Thrombolysis in Myocardial Infarction.

The prognosis after coronary perforation depends on the extent of extravasation into the pericardium.[58] A classification scheme has been developed based on angiographic appearance of the perforation, with type I perforations including an extraluminal crater without extravasation, type II perforations containing pericardial or myocardial blushing, and type III perforations having a diameter equal to or greater than 1 mm with contrast streaming and cavity spilling.[58] Type I perforations were associated with no deaths and cardiac tamponade in 8% of patients; type II perforations were associated with no deaths and cardiac tamponade in 13% of cases; and type III perforations were associated with death in 19% and cardiac tamponade in 63% of patients.[58]

Coronary Spasm

Coronary spasm is defined as a transient or sustained reduction in the diameter stenosis by more than 50% in an arterial segment with insignificant (<25%) baseline narrowing. Although coronary spasm may occur in approximately 5% of cases, its frequency has been reduced with the routine use of coronary vasodilators, such as nitroglycerin and calcium channel blockers. Wire straightening of the vessel can mimic coronary spasm.

Abrupt Closure

Abrupt closure during coronary intervention is defined as an abrupt cessation of coronary flow to TIMI 0 or 1; it occurs during 3% to 5% of balloon angioplasty procedures. Abrupt closure may be caused by coronary dissection, embolization, or thrombus formation within the vessel. Its incidence has been markedly reduced with the availability of coronary stents.[62]

Stent Thrombosis

With the addition of a thienopyridine derivative (i.e., ticlopidine or clopidogrel) to aspirin, the incidence of bare metal stent thrombosis within 30 days of the procedure is less than 1%. Predictive factors for stent thrombosis include persistent dissection NHLBI grade B or higher after stenting, greater total stent length, and a smaller final minimal lumen diameter within the stent.[63] DES administered with longer durations (3 to 6 months) of dual antiplatelet therapy have similar stent thrombosis rates to those found with bare metal stents,[64,65] although premature discontinuation of dual antiplatelet therapy has been associated with higher (6% to 29%) stent thrombosis rates.[25,66,67] In addition, diabetes, prior brachytherapy, bifurcation lesions with two stents, AMI, renal failure, lower ejection fraction, and longer stent length have been associated with stent thrombosis.[25,66,67] A recent concern is the occurrence of very late (>1 year) stent thrombosis with the use of DES[68] due to inflammation from the stent.[69,70] The estimated incidence of very late stent thrombosis ranges from 0.2% to 0.6% per year up to 3 years after stent placement. Long-term dual antiplatelet therapy may not be completely protective to prevent stent thrombosis.[66]

The Academic Research Consortium has proposed new criteria for the timing and definitions used to

Table 60-5. Academic Research Consortium (ARC) Stent Thrombosis Definitions

Stent Thrombosis	Definition
Definite	
Angiographic confirmation	TIMI flow grade 0 with occlusion originating in or within 5 mm of stent in the presence of a thrombus or TIMI flow grade 1, 2, or 3 originating in or within 5 mm of stent in the presence of a thrombus AND at least one of the following criteria within the last 48 hr:
	New acute onset of ischemic symptoms at rest (typical chest pain with duration >20 min)
	New ischemic ECG changes suggestive of acute ischemia
	Typical rise and fall in cardiac biomarkers
Pathologic confirmation	Evidence of recent thrombus within the stent determined at autopsy or via examination of tissue retrieved after thrombectomy
Probable	
	Any unexplained death within the first 30 days Irrespective of the time after the index procedure, any MI that is related to documented acute ischemia in the territory of the implanted stent without angiographic confirmation of stent thrombosis and in the absence of any other cause.
Possible	
	Any unexplained death >30 days after intracoronary stenting

ECG, electrocardiographic; MI, myocardial infarction; TIMI, Thrombolysis in Myocardial Infarction.

document stent thrombosis in clinical studies. Timing of stent thrombosis is defined as acute (<24 hours), subacute (24 hours to 30 days), late (30 days to 1 year), and very late (after one year).[71] The categories of definite stent thrombosis, probable stent thrombosis, and possible stent thrombosis have been proposed as a more inclusive and standardized way to characterize the occurrence of this event in patients undergoing stent implantation (Table 60-5).

Restenosis Pattern

When ISR occurs after bare metal stent implantation, the risk of recurrence can be predicted by the pattern of restenosis.[72,73] Using the Mehran classification system, pattern I includes focal (≤10 mm in length) lesions, pattern II is defined as ISR greater than 10 mm within the stent, pattern III includes ISR greater than 10 mm extending outside the stent, and pattern IV is totally occluded ISR.[72] Pattern I can be classified further by the location of the restenosis: Ia, within the stent; Ib, at the edge of the stent; Ic, at the articulation or gap; or Id, multifocal.[72] The need for recurrent target lesion revascularization (TLR) increased with increasing ISR class, from 19% to 35%, 50%, and 83% in classes I through IV, respectively ($P < .001$).[72] Restenosis after DES implantation is generally more focal than after bare metal stent placement,[19,74] and with the sirolimus-eluting stent, it is more commonly seen at the margin of the stent owing to balloon injury that is not covered with stent.[19,75]

Late Aneurysm Formation

Late vessel wall expansion of greater than 20% after PCI has been termed a coronary artery aneurysm. Coronary artery aneurysms, or, more precisely, pseudoaneurysms, are rare findings after balloon angioplasty, atheroablation, and coronary stenting.

Coronary artery aneurysms most likely arise from tears or dissection and incomplete healing that compromises vessel wall integrity and results in vessel wall expansion. Coronary artery aneurysms are also rarely (<1%) seen after DES placement, although the pathologic etiology of aneurysms in this setting may relate to expansion of all three layers of the arterial wall owing to inflammation and effects from the cytostatic or cytotoxic drugs and malapposition of the stent struts.[76,77] Under rare circumstances, coronary artery aneurysms can become infected, requiring surgical intervention.[78,79]

Coronary Perfusion

Evaluation of pharmacologic and mechanical methods to reperfuse coronary occlusions in patients with ST-segment elevation myocardial infarction (STEMI) is supported by the development of a reproducible angiographic method to assess the degree of coronary recanalization achieved with these therapies. The TIMI flow grade classification scheme characterizes the extent of coronary recanalization in patients with STEMI treated with systemic thrombolytic agents, and in patients presenting with non-ST-segment elevation myocardial infarction and unstable angina (Table 60-6).[80] The TIMI frame count[81] and the TIMI myocardial perfusion grade were developed to further quantify anterograde flow and assess distal microvascular perfusion.[82]

TIMI Flow Grade Classification Scheme

The TIMI Flow Grade System is a valuable tool for assessing the efficacy of reperfusion strategies in patients with STEMI and for identifying patients at higher risk for an adverse outcome with acute coronary syndromes or undergoing PCI. Several thrombolytic trials have identified an important relationship between 90-minute TIMI flow grade after

Table 60-6.   TIMI Flow Grade Classification

Grade	Characteristic
3 (complete reperfusion)	Anterograde flow into the terminal coronary artery segment through a stenosis is as prompt as anterograde flow into a comparable segment proximal to the stenosis. Contrast material clears as rapidly from the distal segment as from an uninvolved, more proximal segment.
2 (partial reperfusion)	Contrast material flows through the stenosis to opacify the terminal artery segment. However, contrast enters the terminal segment perceptibly more slowly than more proximal segments. Alternatively, contrast material clears from a segment distal to a stenosis noticeably more slowly than from a comparable segment not preceded by a significant stenosis.
1 (penetration with minimal perfusion)	A small amount of contrast flows through the stenosis but fails to fully opacify the artery beyond.
0 (no perfusion)	No contrast flow through the stenosis.

Modified from Sheehan FH, Braunwald E, Canner P, et al: The effect of intravenous thrombolytic therapy on left ventricular function: A report on tissue-type plasminogen activator and streptokinase from the Thrombolysis in Myocardial Infarction (TIMI) Phase I Trial. Circulation 1987;72:817-829.

thrombolysis and clinical outcome.[83] In the Global Utilization of Streptokinase and Tissue Plasminogen Activator for Occluded Coronary Arteries (GUSTO) angiographic substudy, the mortality rate for patients with TIMI 2 flow (7.4%) was similar to the mortality rate for those with TIMI 0 or 1 flow (8.9%). In contrast, the mortality rate was lowest (4.4%) in patients with TIMI 3 flow.[83]

Despite these important associations, there are a number of limitations of the TIMI classification system. Substantial observer variability has been noted with the TIMI flow grade, with the best agreement between the angiographic core laboratory and clinical centers occurring when the artery is graded as either open or closed (TIMI 0 or 1 flow; kappa value = 0.84).[81] Observer agreement is only moderate when assessing TIMI grade 3 flow (kappa value = 0.55) and is poor in the assessment of TIMI grade 2 flow (kappa value = 0.38). The lack of concordance for determining TIMI flow grade was also shown between experienced angiographic core laboratories. Another limitation of the TIMI flow grade is that it provides ordinal values rather than continuous ones, limiting its statistical power in clinical trials. Furthermore, although TIMI flow grade has classically compared flow in the infarct-related vessel to flow in the "normal" nonculprit artery, flow in the non-infarct-related artery in patients with STEMI is not truly normal compared with flow in patients without STEMI.[84] Difficulties in reproducibly assessing myocardial flow relative to other vessels (e.g., the right coronary artery, or in the setting of total occlusions of the contralateral vessel) led some investigators to modify the definition of "TIMI grade 3 flow" to include opacification of the distal coronary artery within three cardiac cycles.[85] The "three cardiac cycle" definition of TIMI 3 flow results in an absolute rate increase of approximately 10% compared with the original definition.[86] Accordingly, more quantitative measures of anterograde flow were developed.

TIMI Frame Count

The TIMI Frame Count (TFC) provides a quantitative assessment of the number of frames required for dye to reach standardized distal landmarks, and it may provide a more objective and precise method of estimating coronary blood flow than the TIMI flow grade.[81] The first frame used for TIMI frame counting is defined as the cineframe in which a column of dye touches both borders of the coronary artery and moves forward, and the last frame is characterized as the cineframe in which dye begins to enter (but does not necessarily fill) a standard distal landmark in the artery. The standard distal landmarks for epicardial vessels are the first branch of the posterolateral artery for the right coronary artery; the most distal branch of the obtuse marginal branch in the dye path through the culprit lesion in the circumflex system; and the distal bifurcation, which is also known as the "moustache," "pitch fork," or "whale's tail," in the left anterior descending coronary artery. These frame counts are corrected for the longer length of the left anterior descending coronary artery by dividing the TFC by 1.7 to arrive at the corrected TIMI frame count (CTFC).

The CTFC provides a number of advantages over TIMI flow grades. The CTFC is quantitative rather than qualitative, objective rather than subjective, and a continuous rather than a categorical variable. Observer variability is also substantially less with TFC measurements compared with TIMI flow grades.[81] Furthermore, although it has traditionally been assumed that basal flow in nonculprit arteries in the setting of AMI after thrombolysis is "normal," it is now appreciated that basal flow in the uninvolved artery is abnormal using the CTFC.[84]

The more objective CTFC has also been related to clinical outcomes.[82] Flow in the infarct-related artery in survivors of STEMI was significantly faster than in patients who died; mortality increased by 0.7% for every 10-frame rise in the CTFC ($P < .001$).[82] None of the patients in the TIMI studies who had a CTFC less than 14 (hyperemic or TIMI grade 4 flow) died within the first 30 days. In another series of patients undergoing PCI, none of the 376 patients with a CTFC less than 14 after angioplasty died, underscoring the fact that, within the subgroup of patients with "normal flow," there may be further subgroups with even better flow.

TIMI Myocardial Perfusion Grade

It is now apparent that epicardial flow does not necessarily imply tissue-level or microvascular perfusion. These findings led to the development of the TIMI Myocardial Perfusion Grade (TMPG) (Fig. 60-3; Table 60-7), which has been shown to be a multivariate predictor of mortality in AMI.[82] The TMPG permits risk stratification even within epicardial TIMI grade 3 flow. That is, despite achieving normal TIMI grade 3 flow after reperfusion therapy, patients with diminished microvasculature perfusion (TMPG 0 or 1) have a persistently elevated mortality rate of 5.4% compared with patients with both TIMI grade 3 flow and TMPG 3, who have a mortality rate less than 1%.[82] Accordingly, the TIMI flow grades and the TMPGs can be combined to identify a group of patients at "very low" or "very high" risk for mortality after STEMI. Those patients with both TIMI grade 3 flow and TMPG 3 flow had a mortality rate of 0.7%, whereas patients with both TIMI grade 0 or 1 and TMPG 0 or 1 flow had a mortality rate of 10.9%.

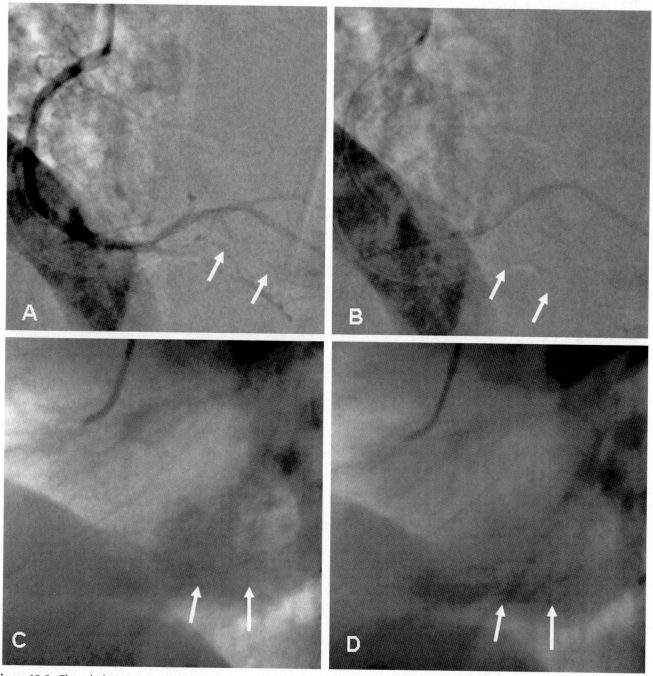

Figure 60-3. Thrombolysis in Myocardial Infarction (TIMI) myocardial perfusion grade using digital subtraction angiography. Perfusion grade 0 is characterized by the absence of the typical "ground-glass" filling of the distal vascular bed during coronary injection (**A**) and washout (**B**). Perfusion grade 1 is demonstrated by persistent contrast staining at the beginning (**C**) and end (**D**) of the coronary injection.

Continued

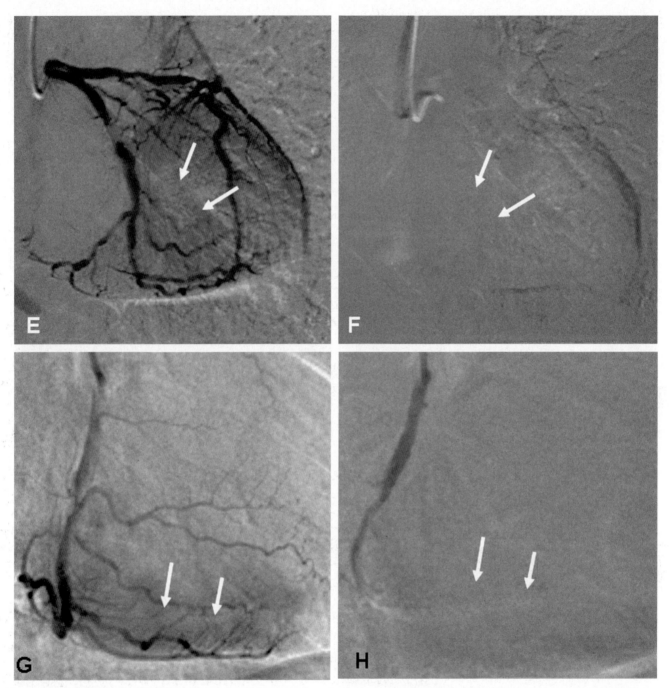

Figure 60-3, cont'd Perfusion grade 2 is manifested by a very prominent contrast appearance at the end of coronary injection **(E)** that washes out at the end of the contrast injection **(F)**. Perfusion grade 3 is shown as a normal ground-glass appearance of the distal vascular bed at the end of the contrast injection **(G)** that washes out at the end of the injection **(H).**

Another approach to assess myocardial perfusion is to use digital subtraction angiography (DSA) to quantitatively characterize the kinetics of dye entering the myocardium during contrast angiography. DSA is performed at end-diastole by aligning cine-frame images taken before dye fills the myocardium with those taken at the peak of myocardial filling to subtract spine, ribs, diaphragm, and epicardial artery. A representative region of the myocardium that is free of overlap by epicardial arterial branches is sampled to determine the increase in the gray-scale

brightness of the myocardium when it first reached its peak intensity. The circumference of the myocardial blush is measured using a hand-held planimeter. The number of frames required for the myocardium to first reach its peak brightness is converted into time (seconds) by dividing the frame count by 30 (for images acquired at 30 frames per second). The rate of rise in brightness (gray-scale change per second) and the rate of growth of blush in circumference (centimeters per second) can then be calculated. Using DSA, microvascular perfusion was reduced in

Table 60-7. TIMI Myocardial Perfusion Grades

Grade	Characteristic
3	Normal entry and exit of dye from the microvasculature. There is a ground-glass appearance ("blush") or opacification of the myocardium in the distribution of the culprit lesion that clears normally and is either gone or mildly or moderately persistent at the end of the washout phase (approximately three cardiac cycles), similar to an uninvolved artery. Blush that is of only mild intensity throughout the washout phase but fades normally is also classified as grade 3.
2	Delayed entry and exit of dye from the microvasculature. There is a ground-glass appearance ("blush") or opacification of the myocardium in the distribution of the culprit lesion that is strongly persistent at the end of the washout phase (i.e., dye is strongly persistent after three cardiac cycles of the washout phase and either does not diminish or only minimally diminishes in intensity during washout).
1	Slow entry of dye into but failure to exit the microvasculature. There is a ground-glass appearance ("blush") or opacification of the myocardium in the distribution of the culprit lesion that fails to clear from the microvasculature, and dye staining is present on the next injection (approximately 30 sec between injections).
0	Failure of the dye to enter the microvasculature. There is either minimal or no ground-glass appearance ("blush") or opacification of the myocardium in the distribution of the culprit artery, indicating lack of tissue-level perfusion.

AMI patients compared to normal patients, as demonstrated by a reduction in peak brightness (grayscale peak), the rate of rise in brightness, the blush circumference, and the rate of growth of blush in circumference.[87]

Coronary Flow Velocity

Absolute flow velocity can be measured using PCI guidewire velocity.[88] With this technique, the guidewire tip is placed at the coronary landmark after PCI, and a Kelly clamp is placed on the guidewire at the point at which it exits the Y-adapter. The guidewire tip is then withdrawn to the catheter tip, and a second Kelly clamp is placed on the wire where it exits the Y-adapter. The distance between the two Kelly clamps outside the body is measured as the distance between the catheter tip and the anatomic landmark inside the body. Velocity (centimeters per second) may be calculated as this distance (centimeters) divided by the product of the TFC (frames) and the film frame speed (frames per second). Flow (milliliters per second) may be calculated by multiplying velocity and the mean cross-sectional lumen area (square centimeters) along the length of the artery to the TIMI landmark. In a series of 30 patients undergoing PCI, velocity increased from 13.9 ± 8.5 cm/second before PCI to 22.8 ± 9.3 cm/second after PCI ($P < .001$). For all 30 patients, flow doubled from 0.6 ± 0.4 mL/second before PCI to 1.2 ± 0.6 mL/second after PCI ($P < .001$). In the 18 patients with TIMI grade 3 flow both before and after PCI, flow increased 86%, from 0.7 ± 0.3 to 1.3 ± 0.6 mL/second ($P = .001$).

QUANTITATIVE ANGIOGRAPHY

Quantitative coronary angiography (QCA) is most commonly performed using automated arterial contour detection, although videodensitometry and digital parametric imaging have also been tried with limited success. Whereas "online" QCA is somewhat cumbersome to use in the catheterization laboratory, "offline" QCA has proved to be valuable for research investigation in determining the effect of new drugs and devices on lumen dimensions early and late after PCI. Notably, for clinical decision-making in intermediate lesions, neither trained visual estimates or online quantitative angiography is a substitute for precise physiologic measurements of stenosis severity, such as fractional flow reserve or coronary Doppler measurements.[89]

Nonquantitative Estimates of Lesion Severity

Virtually every interventionalist uses an "eyeball" estimate for determining angiographic stenosis severity, although these visual estimations of lesion severity are of limited value for research studies because of substantial observer-to-observer variability. Blinded review of cineangiograms by experienced cardiologists found that the average visual diameter stenosis was 85% before PCI (versus 68% using quantitative methods) and 30% after PCI (versus 49% using quantitative methods); these differences correspond to a 200% error in the estimation of percent diameter stenosis.[90] Visual estimates of stenosis severity also result in some values (e.g., 90% to 99% diameter stenosis) that are physiologically untenable for anterograde flow. Inherent overestimation and underestimation visual stenosis severity can be overcome by retraining the clinician's eye.

A more quantitative approach to the assessment of lesion severity uses hand-held or digital calipers to estimate quantitative diameters and percent diameter stenosis. Angiographic images are magnified, and calibration is performed by measuring the known dimensions of the diagnostic or guiding catheter using digital calipers. The observer then visually identifies the lumen border using the calipers, and a calibration factor is obtained to determine absolute coronary dimensions. Properly applied, this method appears to correlate weakly with automated edge-detection algorithms. If caliper measurements are obtained from nonmagnified images, the correlation with automated edge-detection algorithms is less accurate.

Computer-Assisted Quantitative Coronary Angiography

QCA was initiated almost 30 years ago by Brown and colleagues, who magnified 35-mm cineangiograms obtained from orthogonal projections and hand-traced the arterial edges on a large screen. After computer-assisted correction for pincushion distortion, the tracings were digitized and the orthogonal projections were combined to form a three-dimensional representation of the arterial segment, assuming an elliptical geometry. Although the accuracy and precision were enhanced compared with visual methods, the time needed for image processing limited the clinical use of this method.

Several automated edge-detection algorithms were then developed and applied to directly acquired digital images or to 35-mm cinefilm digitized using a cine-video converter. Subsequent iterations of these first-generation devices used enhanced microprocessing speed and digital image acquisition to render the end-user interface more flexible and substantially shortened the time required for image analysis.

QCA is divided into several distinct processes, including film digitization (when applicable), image calibration, and arterial contour detection (Fig. 60-4). For processing 35-mm cinefilm, a cine-video converter is used to digitize images into a 512×512 (or larger) $\times$ 8-bit pixel matrix. Optical (preferably) or digital magnification results in an effective pixel matrix up to 2458×2458. For estimation of absolute coronary dimensions, the diagnostic or guiding catheter usually serves as the scaling device. In general, a nontapered segment of the catheter is selected, and a centerline through the catheter is drawn. Linear density profiles are then constructed perpendicular to the catheter centerline, and a weighted average of the first and second derivative functions is used to define the catheter edge points. Individual edge points are then connected using an automated algorithm, outliers are discarded, and the edges are smoothed. The diameter of the catheter is then used to obtain a calibration factor, expressed in millimeters per pixel. The injection catheter dimensions may be influenced by whether contrast or saline is imaged within the catheter tip and by the type of material used in catheter construction. As the high-flow injection catheters have been developed, more quantitative angiographic systems have been using contrast-filled injection catheters for image calibration. The automated algorithm is then applied to a selected arterial segment: absolute coronary dimensions are obtained from the minimal lumen diameter (MLD) reference diameter, and, from these, the percent diameter stenoses are derived. For most angiographic systems, interobserver variabilities are 3.1% for diameter stenosis and 0.10 to 0.18 mm for MLD for cineangiographic readings; variabilities are slightly higher (<0.25 mm) for repeated analyses of the digital angiograms owing to the slightly lower resolution compared with cineangiography. The two most commonly used QCA systems are described.

Cardiovascular Angiography Analysis System

The Cardiovascular Angiography Analysis System (CAAS, Pie Data Medical B.V., Maastricht, The Netherlands) is a QCA system developed for offline cineangiographic analysis (see Fig. 60-2). The edge-detection algorithm incorporates an optional correction for pincushion distortion; its edge detection uses a weighted (50%) sum of the first and second derivatives of the mean pixel density; and it applies minimal cost criteria for smoothing of the arterial edge contours. In addition to reporting a interpolated reference diameter and an MLD, a subsegment analysis provides mean, minimum, and maximum subsegment diameters. Specific reporting algorithms have been developed for DESs, for patients undergoing radiation brachytherapy, and for those undergoing peripheral intervention.

Coronary Measurement System

Specific features of the Coronary Measurement System (CMS, MEDIS, Leiden, The Netherlands) include two-point user-defined centerline identification, arterial edge detection using a weighted (50%) sum of the first and second derivatives of the mean pixel density, arterial contour detection using a minimal cost matrix algorithm, and an "interpolated" reference vessel diameter. One limitation of the minimal cost algorithm used with the first-generation CMS system (as well as the CAAS-II system) has been its inability to precisely quantify arterial lumen contours characterized by abrupt changes. The CMS-GFT is an algorithm that is not restricted in its search directions, incorporating multidirectional information about the arterial boundaries for construction of the arterial edge that is suitable for the analysis of complex coronary artery lesions. Specific reporting algorithms have been developed for bifurcation lesions (Fig. 60-5), for DESs (Fig. 60-6), patients undergoing radiation brachytherapy (Fig. 60-7), and for those undergoing peripheral intervention.

Factors Contributing to Variability Using Quantitative Coronary Angiography

Variability associated with measurements of MLD and reference diameter is affected by a number of factors, including (1) the biologic differences among lumen diameters (e.g., reference vessel size, vasomotor tone, thrombus); (2) inconsistencies in radiographic image acquisition parameters (e.g., quantum mottling, out-of-plane magnification, foreshortening); and (3) angiographic measurement variability (e.g., frame selection, factors affecting the edge-detection algorithm) (Table 60-8). These factors should be controlled in order to improve the overall diagnostic accuracy of QCA.

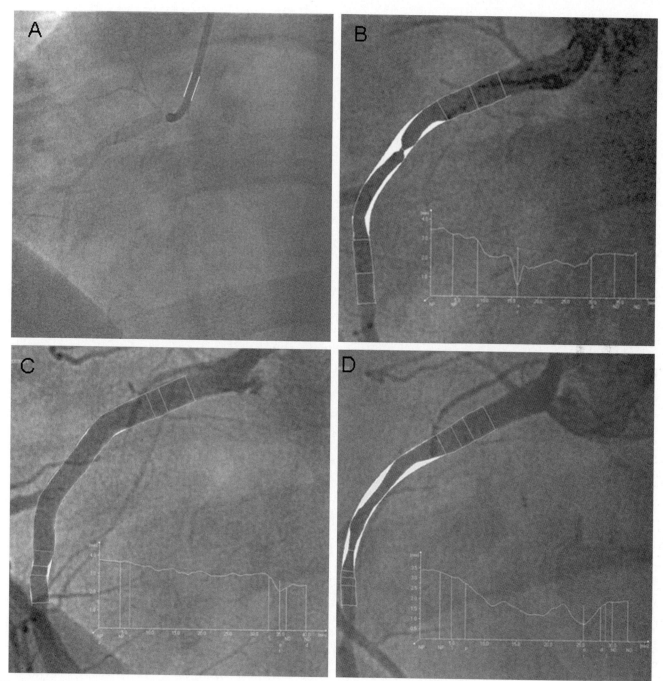

Figure 60-4. Quantitative coronary angiography. **A,** Image calibration is performed using the nontapered portion of the injection catheter as the calibration source. **B,** The automated edge detection algorithm (CMS, Leiden, The Netherlands) is applied to the arterial contour, and the minimal lumen diameter (MLD) is identified. A diameter function profile curve *(insert)* shows the diameters of the vessel along the length of the analysis segment. **C,** After coronary stent placement, the identical length of artery is analyzed to provide an assessment of the lumen improvement. **D,** At the time of angiographic follow-up, the location of late lumen loss along the length of the analysis segment is identified.

Biologic Variability

Studies that include a wide range of vessel sizes have more biologic variability in vessel diameter (as reflected in the standard deviation of the measurements) than those that are more restrictive in their inclusion criteria. Vasomotor tone may also affect the reference vessel size, resulting in distal vasoconstriction and vasospasm that dynamically affect the arterial diameter in paired measurements. Transient maximum coronary vasodilation may be achieved with intracoronary (50 to 200 μg), intravenous (>10 μg/min), or sublingual (0.4 to 0.8 mg) nitroglycerin.

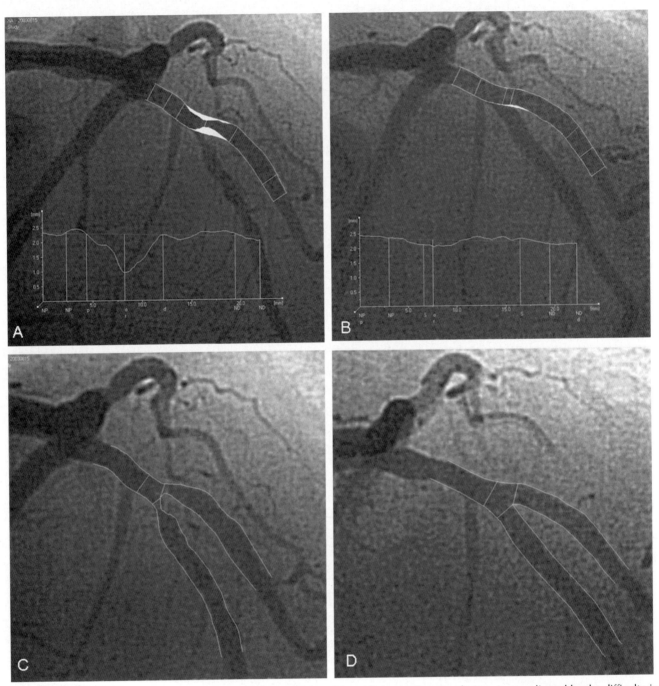

Figure 60-5. Bifurcation quantitative analysis. Quantitative angiographic analysis of bifurcation lesions is complicated by the difficulty in identifying minimal lumen diameter (MLD) at the site of vessel branching. Three methods of bifurcation analysis have been employed: conventional quantitative angiography separately applied to each branch (**A,** before intervention; **B,** after intervention); application of the edge algorithm to both branches (**C,** before intervention; **D,** after intervention); and beginning the analysis at the ostium of the branch (**E,** before intervention; **F,** after intervention).

Acquisition Variability

Acquisition factors that affect variability include cardiac and respiratory motion artifact, vessel foreshortening, inadequate filling of the coronary artery ("streaming"), overfilling of the aortic cusp with contrast, and failure to separate overlapping branch vessels from the stenosis. These factors may lead to either overestimation or underestimation of lesion severity. Out-of-plane magnification and pincushion distortion may also contribute to small errors in angiographic imaging. For sequential studies, use of the identical angiographic imaging laboratory allows replication of the x-ray generator, tube, and image intensifier parameters. With the introduction of digital imaging and archiving, image compression has raised potential problems with the quality of image quality for analysis. The standard Digital Imaging and Communications in Medicine (DICOM) 2:1 JPEG lossless compression has become the

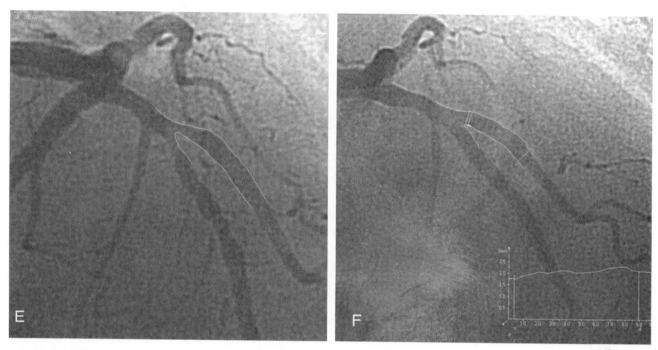

Figure 60-5, cont'd

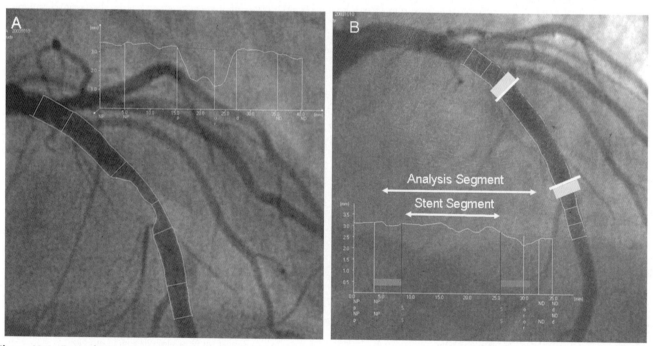

Figure 60-6. Drug-eluting stent quantitative angiographic analysis. **A,** Quantitative angiography is performed on a focal stenosis in the midportion of the left anterior descending coronary artery (LAD). **B,** After placement of a drug-eluting stent, the proximal and distal portions of the stent are identified *(solid bars)*. A 5-mm proximal and distal edge is also analyzed *(shaded boxes)*. From these measurements, the minimal lumen diameters within the stent ("stent" segment) and within the region of analysis ("analysis" segment) are identified.

industry standard for image storage and transfer and requires approximately 500 Mbytes of storage for each imaging study. The effect of image compression and decompression on image quality was evaluated by a joint task force of the American College of Cardiology and European Society of Cardiology using Joint Photographic Experts Group (JPEG) images at compression ratios of 1:1 (uncompressed), 6:1, 10:1, and 16:1.[91] The intraobserver analysis showed significant systematic and random errors in the calibration factor at JPEG compression ratios of 10:1 and higher, and therefore these should not be used in

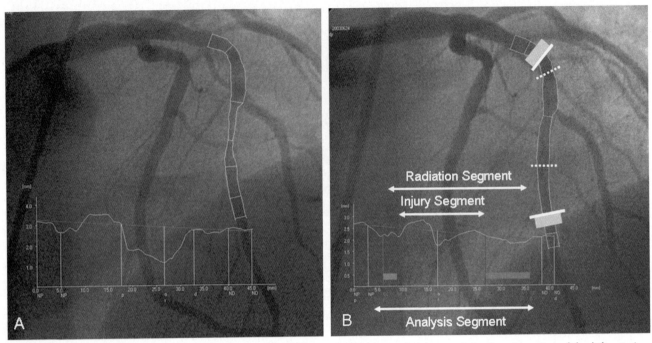

Figure 60-7. Brachytherapy analysis. **A,** Quantitative angiography is performed on a focal stenosis in the midportion of the left anterior descending coronary artery (LAD). **B,** After balloon angioplasty, the proximal and distal portions of the balloon injury are identified *(dashed lines).* After radiation brachytherapy, the proximal and distal portion of the radiation injury are identified *(solid lines).* A 5-mm proximal and distal edge of the radiation zone is also analyzed *(shaded boxes)* to identify the "edge effect." From these measurements, the minimal lumen diameters within the segment of balloon injury ("injury" segment), the segment of radiation injury ("radiation" segment), and within the region of analysis ("analysis" segment) are identified. The shaded portion in the diameter function profile curve *(insert)* represents the region of the artery that was treated with radiation but was not injured with the balloon.

Table 60-8. Correctable Sources of Imaging Error during Acquisition

Source of Error	Potential Corrections
Biologic variation in lumen diameter	
Vasomotor tone	Nitroglycerin, 100-200 µg intracoronary every 10 min
Variations in image acquisition	
Single Studies	
Vessel motion	
Cardiac	End-diastolic/end-systolic cineframe
Respiration	Breath-holding
Vessel foreshortening	Obtain multiple angiographic projections
Insufficient contrast injection	Use 7- or 8-Fr large, high-flow catheters
Branch vessel overlap	Obtain multiple angiographic projections
Pincushion distortion	Image objects in center of image
Sequential Studies	
X-ray generator (pulse width/dose/beam quality)	Repeat study in same imaging laboratory
X-ray tube (focal spot/shape/tube current)	As above
Image intensifier (magnification/resolution)	As above
Differences in angles and gantry height	Record gantry height/angle/skew on worksheet
Image calibration	Use measured catheter diameter
Errors in image analysis	
Electronic noise	Recursive digitization and frame averaging
Quantum noise	Spatial filtering of digital image data
Automated edge-detection algorithm	Minimize observer interaction
Selection of reference positions	Interpolated or averaged normal segment
Identification of lesion length	Use of side branches, other landmarks
Frame selection	End-diastolic frame showing "worst" view

QCA clinical research studies.[91] Similar issues exist for the analysis of S-VHS video tapes with substantial loss of image resolution. Flat panel image acquisition does not affect the quality of QCA.[92]

Measurement Variability

Analysis of two or more orthogonal projections permits a more accurate assessment of the physiologic significance of lesion severity, although a second, technically suitable projection in many cases is unavailable owing to vessel foreshortening, overlap, and poor image quality. If orthogonal projections are not available, analyses of the "worst-view" projection may provide sufficiently accurate information for clinical studies. Herrington and colleagues[93] used a components-of-variance model to show that the process of acquiring and performing QCA on selected cineframes accounted for 57% of the total measurement variability, whereas day-to-day variations in the patient, procedure, and equipment accounted for 30% of total variability. Frame selection accounted for the remaining 13% of total variability. When direct digital angiography is performed and random errors associated with noise in the cine-video pathway are eliminated, frame selection may be a much more important contributor to overall measurement variability. Frame selection has been associated with substantial interobserver variability, and the frame demonstrating the sharpest and tightest view of the stenosis should be used.

Automated QCA systems differ with respect to the preferred method of calibration, location of the arterial border, and construction of its contour; use of minimal cost or "smoothing" algorithms; and selection of normal "reference" segments. Edge-detection algorithms that identify the arterial edge using a 50% weighted threshold of the first- and second-derivative extrema may produce systematically larger reference and obstruction diameters than those using a 75% weighted value (weighted toward the first-derivative extremum) or the first-derivative extremum itself. These systematic differences may also affect the accuracy and reproducibility of the absolute and relative angiographic measurements. Accordingly, each angiographic core laboratory should independently determine its own variabilities during the performance of QCA studies, potentially permitting standardization of techniques among different core laboratories.

Quantitative Angiographic Indices

Early and late angiographic results after PCI have been described using a number of QCA criteria. Coronary stents provide a superior residual lumen compared with balloon angioplasty, but they may result in higher amounts of late intimal hyperplasia (and late lumen loss) than is seen after balloon angioplasty. The net balance is that stents provide a net larger late angiographic result.

Angiographic Success

The change in MLD that occurs immediately after PCI is called the *acute gain* (in millimeters), and the loss of MLD that occurs during the follow-up period is defined as the *late loss* (in millimeters). Relative changes that occur in the percent diameter stenosis are provided by the following relationship: % diameter stenosis = (1 − [MLD/Reference Diameter]) × 100. Traditionally, angiographic success after PCI has been defined as the achievement of a less than 50% residual diameter stenosis,[1] which is most often associated with at least 20% improvement from the baseline diameter stenosis as well as symptom improvement. With the advent of coronary stents and the determination that stent thrombosis was associated with a suboptimal initial angiographic result, a more contemporary definition of angiographic "stent success" was the attainment of a less than 20% residual diameter stenosis within the stent, although higher (up to 20% to 30%) "inflow" or "outflow" diameter stenosis may be present owing to residual plaque at the stent margins. Although the documented disparity between visual and quantitative estimates of angiographic success remains a challenge for self-reporting registries that describe procedural outcomes,[1] there has been documented improvement in angiographic success rates over the past decade with the more widespread use of coronary stents.[94]

Binary Angiographic Restenosis

A number of binary criteria have been used to describe angiographic restenosis after PCI. Binary angiographic restenosis is best defined as a 50% or greater diameter stenosis at follow-up, although a number of other dichotomous criteria have been used (e.g., loss of >50% of the initial gain, loss in MLD of ≥0.72 mm). Binary angiographic restenosis after DES placement may occur within the stent ("in-stent" restenosis), within the 5-mm margins of the stent ("edge" restenosis), or within the segment between the proximal and distal reference segments ("in-segment" or "in-lesion" restenosis).

Late Lumen Loss

The long-term success of PCI can be measured by several other QCA parameters. Serial QCA studies have shown that there is an approximate 0.50-mm reduction in lumen diameter that develops within 3 to 6 months after balloon angioplasty, although angiography cannot differentiate whether this reduction in lumen diameter is due to intimal hyperplasia or arterial remodeling (or constriction). Lumen loss after balloon angioplasty follows a near-gaussian distribution. Because there is little or no arterial remodeling after bare metal stent placement, late lumen loss after stent placement is primarily due to intimal hyperplasia, and angiographic estimates of volumetric percent volume obstruction have been well correlated with intravascular ultrasound measurements of intimal hyperplasia.[95]

The distribution of late luminal loss after placement of DES is unlike the distribution of late lumen loss noted after bare metal stent placement, with a narrowing variance (i.e., standard deviation) due to the reduced tissue growth and a rightward skewedness of the late lumen loss histogram,[96] suggesting an "all-or-none" response to the DES.[97] The patient-based relationship between late lumen loss and TLR was examined in 1314 patients with de novo lesions who were treated with bare metal or paclitaxel-eluting stents.[98] In this analysis, the relationship between late lumen loss and TLR was monotonic and curvilinear,[98] with the likelihood of TLR not exceeding 5% until the analysis segment late loss was greater than 0.5 mm, and not exceeding 10% until late loss was greater than 0.65 mm.[98] At lower magnitudes of late lumen loss, there was a very small incremental increase in the occurrence of TLR; with higher degrees of late lumen loss, the late loss–TLR relationship was steep and almost linear.[98] The rate of TLR was related not only to median late loss but also to measures of its statistical distribution. Specifically, TLR increased with lack of homogeneous biologic response, manifested by greater variance (i.e., higher standard deviations) and greater right skewedness of the late lumen loss histogram.[98]

To correct for the rightward skewedness and to develop better predictive models of restenosis, an optimized power transformation was applied to data from patients enrolled in two sirolimus-eluting stent trials to predict binary angiographic restenosis rates and compare them with observed restenosis rates.[99] The mean in-stent late loss was 0.17 ± 0.45 mm after sirolimus-eluting stent placement and 1.00 ± 0.70 mm after bare metal stent placement. If a normal distribution was assumed, late loss accurately estimated in-stent binary angiographic restenosis for the bare metal stent (predicted 35.4% versus observed 35.4%) but underestimated the binary restenosis rate in the sirolimus-eluting stent arm (predicted 0.6% versus observed 3.2%).[99] Power transformation improved the reliability of the estimate in the sirolimus arm (predicted 3.2% versus observed 3.2%).[99] In contrast, another study did not confirm the value of the power transformation as a predictor of binary angiographic restenosis.[100]

To formally evaluate four potential angiographic surrogate markers for TLR by applying well-defined criteria of surrogacy to an extensive database of randomized DES trials, Pocock and colleagues analyzed 11 multicenter, prospective randomized stent trials in 5381 patients with a single treated lesion and follow-up angiography.[101] Based on four surrogate criteria, late loss and percent diameter stenosis strongly predicted the risk of TLR, with in-segment percent diameter stenosis being the most highly predictive (c statistic ~0.95). Whereas late loss as a surrogate was dependent on vessel size, percent diameter stenosis was independent of vessel size. Differences in TLR rates for bare metal and drug eluting stents were fully explained statistically by their differences in late loss and percent diameter stenosis. However, because of the curvilinearity of the logistic model, trials comparing two effective DESs can have significant differences in mean late losses and percent diameter stenosis but negligible expected differences in TLR risk. Others have suggested a stronger relationship between late loss and TLR for comparative DES trials,[102] but whether late lumen loss will serve as a meaningful surrogate end point in DES comparative trials remains controversial.

Quantitative Coronary Angiography in Patients Undergoing Brachytherapy

New technologies, such as radiation brachytherapy, may cause injury at the margin of the treated segment, resulting in "edge" restenosis in regions that were not initially narrowed. Contemporary QCA analyses are performed to identify each of these regional changes in MLD to analyze the local biologic effects of therapy. Radiation coverage may be inadequate in regions of balloon injury ("geographic miss"), or it may have an independent effect on the lumen diameter in regions that are not injured with a balloon catheter ("geographic extension").[103] These quantitative methods have allowed elucidation of the biologic effects of radiation for the treatment of ISR.

Limitations of Quantitative Coronary Angiography

The ability of QCA to accurately detect the presence and severity of coronary atherosclerosis is limited by several factors. Compensatory arterial dilation occurs during the early stages of coronary atherosclerosis, resulting in a preserved coronary lumen despite the presence of significant coronary atherosclerosis. Routine coronary angiography can accurately measure the arterial lumen but is relatively insensitive for the detection of arterial wall atherosclerosis, circumferential plaque distribution, vessel wall calcification, or lumen dimensions after stent implantation.

Coronary angiography is limited to a lesser extent by radiographic factors, such as cardiac motion, pincushion distortion, and quantum mottling; most analysis systems have difficulty discriminating values less than 1.0 mm, owing to limitations of radiographic imaging of small objects (e.g., veiling glare, point spread function). Newer methods incorporating adaptive simultaneous coronary border detection have been developed to more accurately assess smaller vessel dimensions.

REFERENCES

1. Smith S, Feldman T, Hirshfeld J, et al: ACC/AHA/SCAI 2005 Guideline Update for Percutaneous Coronary Intervention: Summary article. A report of the American College of Cardiology/American Heart Association Task Force on Practice Guidelines (ACC/AHA/SCAI Writing Committee to Update

the 2001 Guidelines for Percutaneous Coronary Intervention). Circulation 2006;113:156-175.

2. Ellis SG, Roubin GS, King III SB, et al: Importance of stenosis morphology in the estimation of restenosis risk after elective percutaneous transluminal coronary angioplasty. Am J Cardiol 1989;63:30-34.

3. Krone R, Shaw R, Klein L, et al: Evaluation of the American College of Cardiology/American Heart Association and the Society for Coronary Angiography and Interventions lesion classification system in the current "stent era" of coronary interventions (from the ACC-National Cardiovascular Data Registry). Am J Cardiol 2003;92:389-394.

4. Singh M, Rihal CS, Lennon RJ, et al: Comparison of Mayo Clinic risk score and American College of Cardiology/American Heart Association lesion classification in the prediction of adverse cardiovascular outcome following percutaneous coronary interventions. J Am Coll Cardiol 2004;44:357-361.

5. Mintz GS, Popma JJ, Pichard AD, et al: Patterns of calcification in coronary artery disease: A statistical analysis of intravascular ultrasound and coronary angiography in 1155 lesions. Circulation 1995;91:1959-1965.

6. Vavuranakis M, Toutouzas K, Stefanadis C, et al: Stent deployment in calcified lesions: Can we overcome calcific restraint with high-pressure balloon inflations? Catheter Cardiovasc Interv 2001;52:164-172.

7. Wilensky RL, Selzer F, Johnston J, et al: Relation of percutaneous coronary intervention of complex lesions to clinical outcomes (from the NHLBI Dynamic Registry). Am J Cardiol 2002;90:216-221.

8. Moussa I, Ellis SG, Jones M, et al: Impact of coronary culprit lesion calcium in patients undergoing paclitaxel-eluting stent implantation (a TAXUS-IV sub study). Am J Cardiol 2005;96:1242-1247.

9. Castagna MT, Mintz GS, Ohlmann P, et al: Incidence, location, magnitude, and clinical correlates of saphenous vein graft calcification: An intravascular ultrasound and angiographic study. Circulation 2005;111:1148-1152.

10. Alexander JH, Hafley G, Harrington RA, et al: Efficacy and safety of edifoligide, an E2F transcription factor decoy, for prevention of vein graft failure following coronary artery bypass graft surgery: PREVENT IV: A randomized controlled trial. JAMA 2005;294:2446-2454.

11. Hoye A, Lemos PA, Arampatzis CA, et al: Effectiveness of the sirolimus-eluting stent in the treatment of saphenous vein graft disease. J Invasive Cardiol 2004;16:230-233.

12. Baim D, Wahr D, George B, et al: Randomized trial of a distal embolic protection device during percutaneous intervention of saphenous vein aorto-coronary bypass grafts. Circulation 2002;105:1285-1290.

13. Stone GW, Rogers C, Ramee S, et al: Distal filter protection during saphenous vein graft stenting: Technical and clinical correlates of efficacy. J Am Coll Cardiol 2002;40:1882-1888.

14. Turco MA, Buchbinder M, Popma JJ, et al: Pivotal, randomized U.S. study of the Symbiot™ covered stent system in patients with saphenous vein graft disease: Eight-month angiographic and clinical results from the Symbiot III trial. [In Process Citation]. Catheter Cardiovasc Interv 2006;68:379-388.

15. Giugliano GR, Kuntz RE, Popma JJ, et al: Determinants of 30-day adverse events following saphenous vein graft intervention with and without a distal occlusion embolic protection device. Am J Cardiol 2005;95:173-177.

16. Ali A, Cox D, Dib N, et al: Rheolytic thrombectomy with percutaneous coronary intervention for infarct size reduction in acute myocardial infarction: 30-Day results from a multicenter randomized study. J Am Coll Cardiol 2006;48:244-252.

17. Tsagalou E, Stancovic G, Iakovou I, et al: Early outcome of treatment of ostial de novo left anterior descending coronary artery lesions with drug-eluting stents. Am J Cardiol 2006;97:187-191.

18. Kini AS, Moreno PR, Steinheimer AM, et al: Effectiveness of the stent pull-back technique for nonaorto-ostial coronary narrowings. Am J Cardiol 2005;96:1123-1128.

19. Popma JJ, Leon MB, Moses JW, et al: Quantitative assessment of angiographic restenosis after sirolimus-eluting stent implantation in native coronary arteries. Circulation 2004;110:3773-3780.

20. Kereiakes DJ, Wang H, Popma JJ, et al: Periprocedural and late consequences of overlapping Cypher sirolimus-eluting stents: Pooled analysis of five clinical trials. J Am Coll Cardiol 2006;48:21-31.

21. Gobeil F, Lefevre T, Guyon P, et al: Stenting of bifurcation lesions using the Bestent: A prospective dual-center study. Catheter Cardiovasc Interv 2002;55:427-433.

22. Medina A, de Lezo J: A new classification of coronary bifurcation lesions. Rev Esp Cardiol 2006;59:183-184.

23. Lefevre T, Louvard Y, Morice MC, et al: Stenting of bifurcation lesions: Classification, treatments, and results. Catheter Cardiovasc Interv 2000;49:274-283.

24. Safian R: Bifurcation lesions. In Safian R: Manual of Interventional Cardiology. Royal Oak, MI, Physician' Press, 2001, pp 221-236.

25. Iakovou I, Schmidt T, Bonizzoni E, et al: Incidence, predictors, and outcome of thrombosis after successful implantation of drug-eluting stents. JAMA 2005;293:2126-2130.

26. Colombo A, Moses JW, Morice MC, et al: Randomized study to evaluate sirolimus-eluting stents implanted at coronary bifurcation lesions. Circulation 2004;109:1244-1249.

27. Lefevre T, Ormiston J, Guagliumi G, et al: The Frontier stent registry: Safety and feasibility of a novel dedicated stent for the treatment of bifurcation coronary artery lesions. J Am Coll Cardiol 2005;46:592-598.

28. Ikeno F, Kim YH, Luna J, et al: Acute and long-term outcomes of the novel side access (SLK-View) stent for bifurcation coronary lesions: A multicenter nonrandomized feasibility study. Catheter Cardiovasc Interv 2006;67:198-206.

29. Ge L, Airoldi F, Iakovou I, et al: Clinical and angiographic outcome after implantation of drug-eluting stents in bifurcation lesions with the crush stent technique: Importance of final kissing balloon post-dilation. J Am Coll Cardiol 2005;46:613-620.

30. Christofferson RD, Lehmann KG, Martin GV, et al: Effect of chronic total coronary occlusion on treatment strategy. Am J Cardiol 2005;95:1088-1091.

31. Stone GW, Reifart NJ, Moussa I, et al: Percutaneous recanalization of chronically occluded coronary arteries: A consensus document. Part II. Circulation 2005;112:2530-2537.

32. Stone GW, Kandzari DE, Mehran R, et al: Percutaneous recanalization of chronically occluded coronary arteries: A consensus document. Part I. Circulation 2005;112:2364-2372.

33. Baim DS, Braden G, Heuser R, et al: Utility of the Safe-Cross-guided radiofrequency total occlusion crossing system in chronic coronary total occlusions (results from the Guided Radio Frequency Energy Ablation of Total Occlusions Registry Study). Am J Cardiol 2004;94:853-858.

34. Orlic D, Stankovic G, Sangiorgi G, et al: Preliminary experience with the Frontrunner coronary catheter: Novel device dedicated to mechanical revascularization of chronic total occlusions. Catheter Cardiovasc Interv 2005;64:146-152.

35. Saito S, Tanaka S, Hiroe Y, et al: Angioplasty for chronic total occlusion by using tapered-tip guidewires. Catheter Cardiovasc Interv 2003;59:305-311.

36. Rahel BM, Laarman GJ, Suttorp MJ: Primary stenting of occluded native coronary arteries II—Rationale and design of the PRISON II study: A randomized comparison of bare metal stent implantation with sirolimus-eluting stent implantation for the treatment of chronic total coronary occlusions. Am Heart J 2005;149:e1-e3.

37. Suttorp MJ, Laarman GJ, Rahel BM, et al: Primary Stenting of Totally Occluded Native Coronary Arteries II (PRISON II): A randomized comparison of bare metal stent implantation with sirolimus-eluting stent implantation for the treatment of total coronary occlusions. Circulation 2006;114:921-928.

38. Seiler C: The human coronary collateral circulation. Heart (England) 2003;89:1352-1357.

39. Werner GS, Ferrari M, Heinke S, et al: Angiographic assessment of collateral connections in comparison with invasively determined collateral function in chronic coronary occlusions. Circulation 2003;107:1972-1977.

40. Laskey WK, Williams DO, Vlachos HA, et al: Changes in the practice of percutaneous coronary intervention: A compari-

son of enrollment waves in the National Heart, Lung, and Blood Institute (NHLBI) Dynamic Registry. Am J Cardiol 2001;87:964-969; A3-A4.

41. Nishida T, Colombo A, Briguori C, et al: Outcome of nonobstructive residual dissections detected by intravascular ultrasound following percutaneous coronary intervention. Am J Cardiol 2002;89:1257-1262.

42. Resnic FS, Wainstein M, Lee MK, et al: No-reflow is an independent predictor of death and myocardial infarction after percutaneous coronary intervention. Am Heart J 2003;145: 42-46.

43. Yip HK, Chen MC, Chang HW, et al: Angiographic morphologic features of infarct-related arteries and timely reperfusion in acute myocardial infarction: Predictors of slow-flow and no-reflow phenomenon. Chest 2002;122:1322-1332.

44. Iijima R, Shinji H, Ikeda N, et al: Comparison of coronary arterial finding by intravascular ultrasound in patients with "transient no-reflow" versus "reflow" during percutaneous coronary intervention in acute coronary syndrome. Am J Cardiol 2006;97:29-33.

45. Tanaka A, Kawarabayashi T, Nishibori Y, et al: No-reflow phenomenon and lesion morphology in patients with acute myocardial infarction. Circulation 2002;105:2148-2152.

46. Iwakura K, Ito H, Kawano S, et al: Predictive factors for development of the no-reflow phenomenon in patients with reperfused anterior wall acute myocardial infarction. J Am Coll Cardiol 2001;38:472-477.

47. Kotani J, Nanto S, Mintz GS, et al: Plaque gruel of atheromatous coronary lesion may contribute to the no-reflow phenomenon in patients with acute coronary syndrome. Circulation 2002;106:1672-1677.

48. Hillegass WB, Dean NA, Liao L, et al: Treatment of no-reflow and impaired flow with the nitric oxide donor nitroprusside following percutaneous coronary interventions: Initial human clinical experience. J Am Coll Cardiol 2001;37: 1335-1343.

49. Barcin C, Denktas AE, Lennon RJ, et al: Comparison of combination therapy of adenosine and nitroprusside with adenosine alone in the treatment of angiographic no-reflow phenomenon. Catheter Cardiovasc Interv 2004;61: 484-491.

50. Michaels AD, Appleby M, Otten MH, et al: Pretreatment with intragraft verapamil prior to percutaneous coronary intervention of saphenous vein graft lesions: Results of the randomized, controlled Vasodilator Prevention on No-Reflow (VAPOR) trial. J Invasive Cardiol 2002;14:299-302.

51. Huang RI, Patel P, Walinsky P, et al: Efficacy of intracoronary nicardipine in the treatment of no-reflow during percutaneous coronary intervention. [In Process Citation]. Catheter Cardiovasc Interv 2006;68:671-676.

52. Ishizaka N, Issiki T, Saeki F, et al: Predictors of myocardial infarction after distal embolization of coronary vessels with percutaneous transluminal coronary angioplasty: Experience of 21 consecutive patients with distal embolization. Cardiology 1994;84:298-304.

53. Fasseas P, Orford JL, Panetta CJ, et al: Incidence, correlates, management, and clinical outcome of coronary perforation: Analysis of 16,298 procedures. Am Heart J 2004;147: 140-145.

54. Dippel EJ, Kereiakes DJ, Tramuta DA, et al: Coronary perforation during percutaneous coronary intervention in the era of abciximab platelet glycoprotein IIb/IIIa blockade: An algorithm for percutaneous management. Catheter Cardiovasc Interv 2001;52:279-286.

55. Javaid A, Buch AN, Satler LF, et al: Management and outcomes of coronary artery perforation during percutaneous coronary intervention. Am J Cardiol 2006;98:911-914.

56. Klein LW: Coronary artery perforation during interventional procedures. [In Process Citation]. Catheter Cardiovasc Interv 2006;68:713-717.

57. Stankovic G, Orlic D, Corvaja N, et al: Incidence, predictors, in-hospital, and late outcomes of coronary artery perforations. Am J Cardiol 2004;93:213-216.

58. Ellis SG, Ajluni S, Arnold AZ, et al: Increased coronary perforation in the new device era: Incidence, classification, management, and outcome. Circulation 1994;90:2725-2730.

59. Ly H, Awaida JP, Lesperance J, Bilodeau L: Angiographic and clinical outcomes of polytetrafluoroethylene-covered stent use in significant coronary perforations. Am J Cardiol 2005;95:244-246.

60. Gercken U, Lansky AJ, Buellesfeld L, et al: Results of the Jostent coronary stent graft implantation in various clinical settings: Procedural and follow-up results. Catheter Cardiovasc Interv 2002;56:353-360.

61. Lansky AJ, Yang YM, Khan Y, et al: Treatment of coronary artery perforations complicating percutaneous coronary intervention with a polytetrafluoroethylene-covered stent graft. Am J Cardiol 2006;98:370-374.

62. Suh WW, Grill DE, Rihal CS, et al: Unrestricted availability of intracoronary stents is associated with decreased abrupt vascular closure rates and improved early clinical outcomes. Catheter Cardiovasc Interv 2002;55:294-302.

63. Cutlip D, Baim D, Ho K, et al: Stent thrombosis in the modern era: A pooled analysis of multicenter coronary stent clinical trials. Circulation 2001;103:1967-1971.

64. Urban P, Gershlick AH, Guagliumi G, et al: Safety of coronary sirolimus-eluting stents in daily clinical practice: One-year follow-up of the e-Cypher registry. Circulation 2006;113: 1434-1441.

65. Moreno R, Fernandez C, Hernandez R, et al: Drug-eluting stent thrombosis: Results from a pooled analysis including 10 randomized studies. J Am Coll Cardiol 2005;45: 954-959.

66. Park DW, Park SW, Park KH, et al: Frequency of and risk factors for stent thrombosis after drug-eluting stent implantation during long-term follow-up. Am J Cardiol 2006;98: 352-356.

67. Kuchulakanti PK, Chu WW, Torguson R, et al: Correlates and long-term outcomes of angiographically proven stent thrombosis with sirolimus- and paclitaxel-eluting stents. Circulation 2006;113:1108-1113.

68. Ong AT, McFadden EP, Regar E, et al: Late angiographic stent thrombosis (LAST) events with drug-eluting stents. J Am Coll Cardiol 2005;45:2088-2092.

69. Virmani R, Guagliumi G, Farb A, et al: Localized hypersensitivity and late coronary thrombosis secondary to a sirolimus-eluting stent: Should we be cautious? Circulation 2004;109: 701-705.

70. Joner M, Finn AV, Farb A, et al: Pathology of drug-eluting stents in humans: Delayed healing and late thrombotic risk. J Am Coll Cardiol 2006;48:193-202.

71. Cutlip DE, Windecker S, Mehran R, et al: Clinical end points in coronary stent trials: A case for standardized definitions. Circulation 2007;115:2344-2351.

72. Mehran R, Dangas G, Abizaid A, et al: Angiographic patterns of in-stent restenosis: Classification and implications for long-term outcome. Circulation 1999;100:1872-1878.

73. Alfonso F, Cequier A, Angel J, et al: Value of the American College of Cardiology/American Heart Association angiographic classification of coronary lesion morphology in patients with in-stent restenosis: Insights from the Restenosis Intra-stent Balloon angioplasty versus elective Stenting (RIBS) randomized trial. Am Heart J 2006;151:681-689.

74. Colombo A, Orlic D, Stankovic G, et al: Preliminary observations regarding angiographic pattern of restenosis after rapamycin-eluting stent implantation. Circulation 2003;107: 2178-2180.

75. Lemos PA, Saia F, Ligthart JM, et al: Coronary restenosis after sirolimus-eluting stent implantation: Morphological description and mechanistic analysis from a consecutive series of cases. Circulation 2003;108:257-260.

76. Stabile E, Escolar E, Weigold G, et al: Marked malapposition and aneurysm formation after sirolimus-eluting coronary stent implantation. Circulation 2004;110:e47-e48.

77. Gupta RK, Sapra R, Kaul U: Early aneurysm formation after drug-eluting stent implantation: An unusual life-threatening complication. J Invasive Cardiol 2006;18:E140-E142.

78. Alfonso F, Moreno R, Vergas J: Mycotic aneurysms after sirolimus-eluting coronary stenting. Catheter Cardiovasc Interv 2006;67:327-328.

79. Singh H, Singh C, Aggarwal N, et al: Mycotic aneurysm of left anterior descending artery after sirolimus-eluting stent

implantation: A case report. Catheter Cardiovasc Interv 2005;65:282-285.

80. Group TS: The Thrombolysis in Myocardial Infarction (TIMI) trial: Phase I findings. N Engl J Med 1985;312:932-936.

81. Gibson CM, Cannon CP, Daley WL, et al: TIMI frame count: A quantitative method of assessing coronary artery flow. Circulation 1996;93:879-888.

82. Gibson C, Cannon C, Murphy S, et al: Relationship of TIMI myocardial perfusion grade to mortality following thrombolytic administration. Circulation 2000;101:125-130.

83. The GUSTO Angiographic Investigators: The effects of tissue plasminogen activator, streptokinase, or both on coronary artery patency, ventricular function, and survival after acute myocardial infarction. N Engl J Med 1993;329:1615-1622.

84. Gibson C, Ryan K, Murphy S, et al: Impaired coronary blood flow in non-culprit arteries in the setting of acute myocardial infarction. J Am Coll Cardiol 1999;34:974-982.

85. Stone GW, Brodie BR, Griffin JJ, et al: Prospective, multicenter study of the safety and feasibility of primary stenting in acute myocardial infarction: In-hospital and 30-day results of the PAMI stent pilot trial. Primary Angioplasty in Myocardial Infarction Stent Pilot Trial Investigators. J Am Coll Cardiol 1998;31:p23-p30.

86. Gibson C, Ryan K, Sparano A, et al: Methodologic drift in the assessment of TIMI grade 3 flow and its implications with respect to the reporting of angiographic trial results. Am Heart J 1999;137:1179-1195.

87. Gibson CM, Cannon CP, Murphy SA, et al: Relationship of the TIMI myocardial perfusion grades, flow grades, frame count, and percutaneous coronary intervention to long-term outcomes after thrombolytic administration in acute myocardial infarction. Circulation 2002;105:1909-1913.

88. Gibson CM, Dodge JT, Goel M, et al: Angioplasty guidewire velocity: A new simple method to calculate absolute coronary blood velocity and flow. Am J Cardiol 1997;80:1536-1539.

89. Fischer JJ, Samady H, McPherson JA, et al: Comparison between visual assessment and quantitative angiography versus fractional flow reserve for native coronary narrowings of moderate severity. Am J Cardiol 2002;90:210-215.

90. Fleming RM, Kirkeeide RL, Smalling RW, Gould KL: Patterns in visual interpretation of coronary arteriograms as detected by quantitative coronary arteriography. J Am Coll Cardiol 1991;18:945-951.

91. Tuinenburg JC, Koning G, Hekking E, et al: American College of Cardiology/European Society of Cardiology International Study of Angiographic Data Compression. Phase II: The effects of varying JPEG data compression levels on the quantitative assessment of the degree of stenosis in digital coronary angiography. Joint Photographic Experts Group. J Am Coll Cardiol 2000;35:1380-1387.

92. Tuinenburg JC, Koning G, Seppenwoolde Y, Reiber JH: Is there an effect of flat-panel-based imaging systems on quantitative coronary and vascular angiography? [In Process Citation]. Catheter Cardiovasc Interv 2006;68:561-566.

93. Herrington DM, Siebes M, Walford GD: Sources of error in quantitative coronary angiography. Cathet Cardiovasc Diagn 1993;29:314-321.

94. Peterson ED, Lansky AJ, Anstrom KJ, et al: Evolving trends in interventional device use and outcomes: Results from the National Cardiovascular Network Database. Am Heart J 2000;139:198-207.

95. Tsuchida K, Garcia-Garcia HM, Ong AT, et al: Revisiting late loss and neointimal volumetric measurements in a drug-eluting stent trial: Analysis from the SPIRIT FIRST trial. Catheter Cardiovasc Interv 2006;67:188-197.

96. Mauri L, Orav EJ, Kuntz RE: Late loss in lumen diameter and binary restenosis for drug-eluting stent comparison. Circulation 2005;111:3435-3442.

97. Lemos PA, Mercado N, van Domburg RT, et al: Comparison of late luminal loss response pattern after sirolimus-eluting stent implantation or conventional stenting. Circulation 2004;110:3199-3205.

98. Ellis SG, Popma JJ, Lasala JM, et al: Relationship between angiographic late loss and target lesion revascularization after coronary stent implantation: Analysis from the TAXUS-IV trial. J Am Coll Cardiol 2005;45:1193-1200.

99. Mauri L, Orav EJ, O'Malley AJ, et al: Relationship of late loss in lumen diameter to coronary restenosis in sirolimus-eluting stents. Circulation 2005;111:321-327.

100. Agostoni P, Valgimigli M, Abbate A, et al: Is late luminal loss an accurate predictor of the clinical effectiveness of drug-eluting stents in the coronary arteries? Am J Cardiol 2006;97:603-605.

101. Pocock S, Lansky A, Mehran R, et al: Angiographic surrogate endpoints in drug-eluting stent trials: A systematic evaluation based on individual patient data from eleven randomized controlled trials. Personal communication, October 2006.

102. Mauri L, Orav EJ, Candia SC, et al: Robustness of late lumen loss in discriminating drug-eluting stents across variable observational and randomized trials. Circulation 2005;112:2833-2839.

103. Lansky AJ, Dangas G, Mehran R, et al: Quantitative angiographic methods for appropriate end-point analysis, edge-effect evaluation, and prediction of recurrent restenosis after coronary brachytherapy with gamma irradiation. J Am Coll Cardiol 2002;39:274-280.

61 Intracoronary Pressure and Flow Measurements

Morton J. Kern and Michael J. Lim

Andreas Grüntzig performed the first percutaneous transluminal coronary angioplasty (PTCA) in 1977, using 4-Fr balloon dilation catheters with a double lumen, allowing on one side balloon inflation and on the other side pressure recordings. Because of the limitations of angiography, transstenotic pressure gradient measurements were used as a guide to the progress of the dilation. With improvements in imaging capabilities and the introduction of drug-eluting stents to reduce restensosis rates, many interventional cardiologists currently believe that angiographic information alone is sufficient for patient care decision-making and that attempts to perform physiologic pressure and flow recordings can be reserved for research purposes.

The limitations of coronary angiography for the physiologic assessment of intermediate coronary lesions in unselected patients with extensive coronary atherosclerosis have been well recognized. This has been repeatedly documented by intravascular ultrasound (IVUS) imaging and ischemia stress testing. Coronary angiography produces a silhouette image and cannot identify intraluminal detail nor provide the angiographer with information about the characteristics of the vessel wall. Furthermore, the accurate identification of both normal and diseased vessel segments is complicated by diffuse disease and by angiographic artifacts of contrast streaming, image foreshortening, or calcification. Bifurcation or ostial lesion locations may be obscured by overlapping branch segments. Even with numerous angiographic angulations to reveal the lesion in its best view, the physiologic significance of a coronary stenosis, especially for an intermediately severe luminal narrowing (approximately 40% to 70% diameter narrowing), cannot be accurately determined. The use of electronic calipers or quantitative coronary angiography (QCA) does not universally allow the operator to circumvent these pitfalls of angiography, especially after angioplasty, when the borders of the vessel may be hazy and not well visualized.

In a manner similar to stress imaging, invasive measurements of coronary pressure and flow provide complementary information to the anatomic characterization of coronary disease obtained by both angiographic and IVUS examinations. Such physiologic data acquired during the angiographic procedure can facilitate timely decision-making regarding therapy. Thus, the rationale for using coronary physiologic measurement is to overcome the limitations of coronary angiography and provide the angiographer with an objective indicator of clinically relevant lesion significance.

FUNDAMENTAL CONCEPTS OF CORONARY BLOOD FLOW

Coronary blood flow can increase from a resting level to a maximum depending on increases in myocardial oxygen demand or in response to neurogenic or pharmacologic hyperemic stimuli. Normally, large epicardial vessel resistance to blood flow is trivial. Most coronary flow is regulated by the myocardial precapillary arteriolar resistance vessels. In a normal adult artery supplying normal myocardium, coronary blood flow can increase more than threefold. However, several conditions, including left ventricular hypertrophy, myocardial ischemia, and diabetes, can affect the microcirculation, blunting the maximal absolute increase in coronary flow or increasing resting flow above the expected level for myocardial oxygen demand at rest. The regulation of coronary vasomotor tone and the influence of several mechanisms such as α-adrenoreceptor-mediated vasoconstriction have been extensively reviewed elsewhere and are beyond the scope of this chapter.[1]

Significant atherosclerotic stenosis produces epicardial conduit resistance. In response to the loss of perfusion pressure and flow to the distal (poststenotic) vascular bed, the small resistance vessels dilate to maintain satisfactory basal flow appropriate for myocardial oxygen demand. Viscous friction, flow separation forces, and flow turbulence at the site of the stenosis produce energy loss at the stenosis (Fig. 61-1). Energy (heat) is extracted, reducing pressure distal to the stenosis and thereby producing a pressure gradient between proximal and distal artery regions. The pressure loss or gradient increases with increasing coronary flow.[2] There exists an absolute poststenotic myocardial perfusion pressure threshold below which myocardial ischemia may be easily induced.

Coronary Flow and Flow Reserve

As stenosis severity increases, maximal coronary flow becomes attenuated and coronary flow reserve (CFR) decreases. CFR is a combined measure of the capacity of the major resistance components (the epicardial coronary artery and supplied vascular bed) to achieve maximal blood flow in response to hyperemic stimulation. A normal CFR implies that both epicardial and microvascular bed resistances are low (normal) (Fig. 61-2). However, if they are abnormal, CFR does not indicate which component is affected, a fact that limits the clinical applicability of this measurement. Although early studies in animals and patients indicated an absolute normal value for CFR of 3.5 to 5, the CFR in adult patients with chest pain syndromes and coronary artery disease (CAD) risk factors undergoing cardiac catheterization with angiographically normal vessels was 2.7 ± 0.6, suggesting a degree of patient variability and microvascular disease. In patients with essential hypertension and normal coronary arteries and in those with aortic stenosis

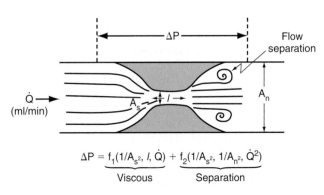

Figure 61-1. Total pressure loss across a stenosis is derived from two sources: frictional losses along the leading edge of the stenosis and inertial losses stemming from the sudden expansion, which causes flow separation and eddies (exit losses). Frictional losses are linearly related to flow, $\dot{Q}$, by the law of Poiseuille, and exit losses increase with the square of the flow (law of Bernoulli). The total change in pressure gradient (ΔP) is the sum of the two: $\Delta P = f_1 * \dot{Q} + f_2 * \dot{Q}^2$. The loss coefficients, f_1 and f_2, are functions of stenosis geometry and rheologic properties of blood (viscosity and density). The graphic representation of this equation results in a quadratic relationship, in which the curvilinear shape demonstrates the presence of nonlinear exit losses. If no stenosis is present, the second term is zero and the curve becomes a straight line (with a positive slope that depends on the diameter of the vessel, based on the law of Poiseuille). A_n, area of the normal segment; A_s, area of the stenosis; L, length. (Redrawn from Kern MJ: Coronary physiology revisited: Practical insights from the cardiac catheterization laboratory. Circulation 2000; 101:1344-1351.)

In the figure:

$$\Delta P = \underbrace{f_1(1/A_{s}^2, l, \dot{Q})}_{\text{Viscous}} + \underbrace{f_2(1/A_{s}^2, 1/A_{n}^2, \dot{Q}^2)}_{\text{Separation}}$$

? Turbulence (beyond or within stenosis)

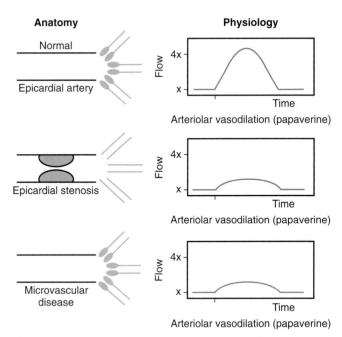

Figure 61-2. Schematic representation of coronary flow reserve findings. In the top panel, a normal artery without any epicardial stenosis or microvascular disease demonstrates the ability to significantly increase coronary flow when a hyperemic agent is given. The middle panel depicts an artery with a significant epicardial stenosis that blunts the ability to increase flow over baseline. The bottom panel depicts the same finding of an artery unable to increase its flow rate. However, the reason in this case is not epicardial stenosis but severe microvascular disease. (Redrawn from Wilson RF, Lascon DD: A clinician's guide to assessing the physiologic significance of arterial stenoses. Cathet Cardiovasc Diagn 1993; 29:93-98.)

and normal coronary arteries, CFR may be reduced, in part related to myocardial hypertrophy and an abnormal microvasculature. Furthermore, CFR can be altered by changes in either basal or hyperemic flow that are influenced by hemodynamics, loading conditions, and contractility. For example, tachycardia increases basal flow and decreases hyperemic flow, thus reducing CFR by 10% for each 15-beat increase in heart rate.

Because CFR is a summed response of both epicardial and microvascular flow, operators should be reluctant to use it as the sole indicator of lesion significance except when it is normal. To increase confidence in CFR as a measure of lesion severity, the determination of relative CFR (rCFR) has been proposed. rCFR is defined as the ratio of maximal flow in the coronary artery with a stenosis ($\dot{Q}^S$) to maximal flow in a normal coronary artery without a stenosis ($\dot{Q}^N$). It was shown that rCFR is independent of the aortic pressure and of the rate-pressure product and is well suited to assess the physiologic significance of coronary stenoses when an adjacent nondiseased coronary artery is available. For invasive catheterization laboratory flow studies, rCFR was defined as the ratio of CFR_{target} to $CFR_{normal\ reference\ vessel}$: $rCFR = (\dot{Q}^S/\dot{Q}\,base)/(\dot{Q}^N/\dot{Q}\,base) = (CFR_{target}/CFR_{reference})$. The normal range for rCFR is 0.8 to 1.0. Because of the variability of CFR and the inherent limitations in patients with multivessel CAD, rCFR is not commonly used. Likewise, rCFR relies on the assumption that the microvascular circulatory response is uniformly distributed among the myocardial beds; therefore, rCFR is of no value in patients with myocardial infarction or left ventricular regional dysfunction, nor in patients in whom the microcirculatory responses may be heterogeneous (e.g., myocardial fibrosis, asymmetric hypertrophy).

In clinical terms, CFR is best used to assess the microcirculation in the absence of epicardial artery narrowings. CFR should not be used to assess stenosis significance, because of the influence of hemodynamics and the unknown impact of the microcirculation. A further discussion of the principles and potential research implications of CFR can be found later in this chapter.

Intracoronary Pressure Measurements and Fractional Flow Reserve

As the limitations of CFR were recognized, the field returned to better characterizing the translesional pressure gradient used by Grüntzig. Pressure measurements made with a guidewire transducer across a lesion during maximal hyperemia, termed the myocardial fractional flow reserve (FFR_{myo}), were introduced.[3] When blood flows from the proximal to the distal part of the normal epicardial coronary artery, virtually no energy is lost; therefore, the pressure remains constant throughout the conduit. In the case of epicardial coronary narrowing, potential energy is transformed into kinetic energy and heat when blood traverses the lesion. The resultant pressure drop reflects the total loss of energy. In order to maintain resting myocardial perfusion at a constant level, a decrease in myocardial resistance compensates for any resistance of flow caused by the epicardial narrowing. The decrease in myocardial resistance reserve is proportional to the resistance that can be computed from the pressure gradient-flow relation; therefore, the pressure at constant maximal flow can represent an index of the physiologic consequences of a given coronary narrowing on the myocardium.

The maximal myocardial blood flow in the presence of a stenosis is reduced relative to expected normal flow in the absence of a stenosis and can be expressed as a fraction of its normal expected value if there were no lesion. This value can be derived from pressure data alone for the myocardium (FFR_{myo}), the epicardial coronary artery (FFR_{cor}), and the collateral supply (FFR_{coll}), based on several assumptions regarding translesional pressure measured during maximal hyperemia (Fig. 61-3).[3,4] The proposed equations have been derived from a theoretical model of the coronary circulation and have been validated experimentally in instrumented dogs, and later in humans, by comparison with myocardial flow measured by positron emission tomography (PET).[5] During maximal hyperemia (using papaverine or adenosine), coronary resistance is at the lowest level and remains constant, so that flow is directly related to the measured pressure gradient. The total myocardial blood flow ($\dot{Q}$) in an area served by a coronary artery with a stenosis is the sum of the flow through the stenosis ($\dot{Q}^S$) and the collateral flow ($\dot{Q}^C$). FFR_{myo} is defined as the ratio of the measured flow ($\dot{Q}$) to the maximal flow that should be present without any stenosis ($\dot{Q}^N$):

$$FFR_{myo} = \dot{Q}/\dot{Q}^N = \frac{(P_d - P_v)/R}{(P_a - P_v)/R}$$

where P_a = mean arterial pressure; P_v = mean venous pressure; P_d = mean pressure distal to the stenosis; and R = resistance of the myocardial vascular bed. Because this resistance is assumed to be constant,

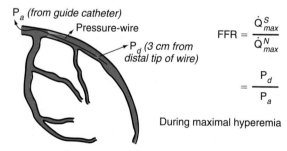

$$FFR = \frac{\dot{Q}^S_{max}}{\dot{Q}^N_{max}} = \frac{P_d}{P_a}$$

During maximal hyperemia

Figure 61-3. Schematic representation showing how to measure fractional flow reserve (FFR) to assess the significance of stenosis of a proximal left anterior descending coronary artery. The proximal pressure (P_a) is the mean pressure taken from the guiding catheter during maximal hyperemia. The distal pressure (P_d) is measured by the guide wire sensor placed distal to the stenosis. FFR is calculated as P_d divided by P_a. $\dot{Q}^N_{max}$, maximal flow of normal vessel; $\dot{Q}^S_{max}$, maximal flow of stenotic vessel.

$$FFR_{myo} = \frac{(P_d - P_v)}{(P_a - P_v)} = 1 - \frac{\Delta P}{(P_a - P_v)} \cong \frac{P_d}{P_a}$$

where P_v is assumed to be low and constant. FFR_{myo} can thus be estimated as the ratio of the mean distal coronary blood pressure (using ultrathin pressure transducers) to the mean aortic blood pressure (measured by the guiding catheter). Because each myocardial territory serves as its own control, FFR is a lesion-specific index. Furthermore, it is independent of the microcirculation, heart rate, blood pressure, and other hemodynamic variables and can be applied in multivessel disease.

FFR_{coll} and FFR_{cor} are calculated with similar equations:

$$FFR_{cor} = 1 - \Delta P/(P_a - P_w)$$
$$FFR_{coll} = FFR_{myo} - FFR_{cor}$$

where P_w = the coronary wedge pressure measured distally when the PTCA balloon is inflated in the artery.

Unlike most other physiologic indexes, FFR has a normal value of 1.0 for every patient and every coronary artery. FFR has high reproducibility and low intra-individual variability (Fig. 61-4). Moreover, FFR, unlike CFR, is independent of gender or CAD risk factors such as hypertension and diabetes and has less variability with common doses of adenosine. De Bruyne and associates demonstrated that, in humans, FFR_{myo} is independent of hemodynamic conditions: changes in heart rate effected by pacing, in contractility by dobutamine infusion, and in blood pressure by nitroprusside infusion did not alter FFR_{myo} (see Fig. 61-4).[6] The coefficient of variation between two consecutive measurements was 4.2%, lower than the 17.7% for CFR measured with a Doppler wire.

METHODOLOGY OF CORONARY PRESSURE MEASUREMENT

General Setup and Guide Wire Manipulation

The measurement of coronary pressure is similar to performing an angioplasty in that a sensor guide wire is passed through an angioplasty Y connector attached to a guiding catheter, with anticoagulation (intravenous [IV] heparin 70 U/kg) given beforehand. To minimize measurement variability due to vessel spasm, intracoronary (IC) nitroglycerin (100 to 200 µg) is given before the guide wire is advanced into the artery.

For coronary pressure measurements, two pressure wire systems are available at this time: Pressure Wire (Radi Medical Systems, Uppsala, Sweden) and Smart Wire (Volcano Therapeutics, Rancho Cardova, CA). Both can be used as angioplasty guide wires with mechanical properties close to standard "workhorse" guide wires. For both wires, a pressure sensor is located 3 cm from the tip, at the junction of the radio-opaque and radiolucent portions of the wire, and the tip can be shaped to facilitate delivery to the distal vessel.

Before inserting the guide wire into the patient, the sensor-wire and guide catheter pressure signals are calibrated and zeroed. The sensor wire is then introduced and positioned at the tip of the guiding catheter, where the guiding catheter and wire pres-

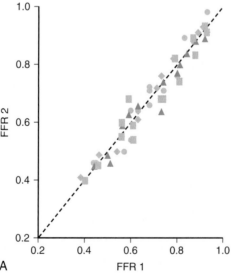

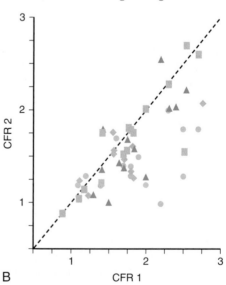

A   FFR 1

B   CFR 1

Figure 61-4. A, Reproducibility of fractional flow reserve (FFR) by serial measurements in a multicenter study of 325 patients in whom FFR was measured twice within a 10-minute interval. **B,** Reproducibility of coronary flow reserve (CFR) in the same patients. *Blue boxes* represent baseline conditions. *Violet diamonds* represent changes in blood pressure induced by infusion of nitroprusside. *Blue triangles* represent changes in heart rate induced by pacing. *Pink circles* represent changes in contractility induced by infusion of dobutamine. Despite variations in heart rate of 40%, blood pressure of 35%, and contractility of 50%, FFR but not CFR was unaffected by these changes. (Data from De Bruyne B, Bartunek J, Sys SU, et al: Simultaneous coronary pressure and flow velocity measurements in humans: Feasibility, reproducibility and hemodynamic dependence of coronary flow velocity reserve, hyperemic flow versus pressure slope index and fractional flow reserve. Circulation 1996;94:1842-1849.)

sures are equalized (assuming an accurate baseline before advancing down the artery). The wire is then advanced across the stenosis, or to the most distal part of the coronary artery for assessment of serial lesions or diffuse disease. Ideally, the sensor should be at least 3 cm distal to the coronary stenosis being assessed.

A pharmacologic hyperemic stimulus is then administered through the guide catheter (IC or IV). The mean and phasic pressure signals are continuously recorded, and at peak hyperemia (represented by the nadir or lowest distal pressure), the FFR is calculated as the ratio between the mean distal coronary pressure (measured by the pressure wire) and the mean aortic pressure (measured by the guiding catheter):

$$FFR = P_d/P_a$$

To study the distribution of abnormalities along a diseased coronary artery (with serial lesions or diffuse disease), the pressure wire can be pulled back slowly during intravenously induced hyperemia. Simutaneously observing the location of the wire and the pressure curves can precisely indicate at which particular locations hemodynamically significant abnormalities are present. Pressure loss due to diffuse atherosclerosis is gradual, whereas a focal stenosis can be differentiated by an abrupt increase in pressure proximal to the lesion. By moving the sensor back and forth, the exact location of a pressure drop representing a focal obstruction to flow can be determined.

After pressures are measured, the interface coupler is disconnected, and the pressure wire can be used to deliver a balloon catheter or stent, or other interventional equipment can be advanced over the pressure guide wire. 6-Fr guiding catheters are commonly used for FFR assessment, but diagnostic catheters as small as 4-Fr have been used.

At the end of the procedure, the wire should be withdrawn and the sensor positioned again at the tip of guiding catheter to verify equal guiding catheter and guide wire pressures, thus ensuring that no pressure signal drift has occurred. A more complete description of the application and pitfalls of coronary pressure measurements can be found elsewhere.[7]

Safety of Intracoronary Sensor Wire Measurements

Qian and coworkers[8] examined the safety of IC Doppler wire measurements in 906 patients. Fifteen patients (1.7%) had severe transient bradycardia after administration of IC adenosine (14 in the right coronary artery [RCA] and 1 in the left coronary artery [LCA]). Nine patients (1%) had coronary spasm during passage of the Doppler guide wire (5 in the RCA and four in the left anterior descending coronary artery [LAD]). Two patients (0.2%) had ventricular fibrillation during the procedure. Hypotension with bradycardia and ventricular asystole occurred in one patient. Transplant recipients had more of these complications than did patients undergoing either diagnostic or interventional procedures. All complications were managed medically without long-term adverse consequences. These data support the safe clinical practice of sensor wire measurements with IC adenosine.

Pharmacologic Hyperemic Stimuli

Stenosis severity should always be assessed using measurements obtained during maximal hyperemia (Table 61-1). The most widely used maximal vasodilator agents are dipyridamole, papaverine, and adenosine. The hyperosmolar ionic and low-osmolar non-ionic contrast media do not produce maximal vasodilation. Nitrates increase volumetric flow, but, because these agents also dilate epicardial conductance vessels, the increase in coronary flow velocity is less than with adenosine or papaverine.

IC papaverine increases coronary blood flow velocity four to six times over resting values in patients with normal coronary arteries. Papaverine (8 to 12 mg) produces a response equal to that of an IV infusion of dipyridamole in a dose of 0.56 to 0.84 mg/kg of body weight, but it can occasionally cause

Table 61-1.   Pharmacologic Characteristics of Agents Used for Induction of Hyperemia

Drug	Dose	Plateau (sec)	Half-life (min)	Side Effects	Comments
Papaverine IC	15 mg LCA 10 mg RCA	30-60	2	Transient QT prolongation Torsades de pointes	
Adenosine IV	140 µg/kg/min	60-120	1-2	Decreased blood pressure (10%-15%), chest burning	Avoid in patients with history of bronchospasm
Adenosine IC	>30 µg LCA 24-36 µg RCA	5-10	0.5-1	Transient AV block when injected into the dominant artery	Must repeat with escalating doses to ensure that maximal hyperemia is reached
Dobutamine IV	20-40 µg/kg/min	60-120	3-5	Tachycardia, increase in blood pressure	
Nitroprusside IC	0.3-0.9 µg/kg	20	1	Decreased blood pressure (20%)	

AV, atrioventricular; IC, intracoronary; IV, intravenous; LCA, left coronary artery; RCA, right coronary artery.

QT prolongation and ventricular tachycardia or fibrillation.

Adenosine

Both IC and IV adenosine have the advantage of a short half-life. The total duration of the hyperemic response to IC adenosine is only 25% that seen with papaverine or dipyridamole. Adenosine is benign in the appropriate dosages (18 to 24 µg in the RCA or 24 to 48 µg in the LCA, or infused IV at 140 µg/kg/minute), although many have reported safety at much higher dosages. As described earlier, transient atrioventricular block and bradycardia may occur. IV administration tends to have a higher incidence of flushing, chest tightness, and atrioventricular block than IC dosing.

Jeremias and colleagues[9] examined differences in FFR between IC adenosine (15 to 20 µg in the RCA or 18 to 24 µg in the LCA) and IV adenosine (140 µg/kg/minute) in 52 patients with 60 lesions. Mean percent stenosis was 56%±24% (range, 0% to 95%). The mean FFR was 0.78±0.15, with a range of 0.41 to 0.98. There was a strong and linear relationship between IC and IV adenosine (r=.978 and P<.001). The mean measurement difference for FFR was −0.004±0.03. A small random scatter in both directions of FFR was noted in 8.3% of stenoses, where the IC adenosine FFR value was 0.05 greater than the IV adenosine FFR value, suggesting a suboptimal IC hyperemic response. Changes in heart rate and blood pressure were significantly greater with IV adenosine. Two patients with IV, but none with IC, adenosine had side effects of bronchospasm and nausea. These data indicated that IC adenosine is equivalent to IV infusion for determination of FFR in most patients. However, in a small percentage of cases, coronary hyperemia was suspected to be suboptimal with IC adenosine, suggesting that a repeated, higher IC adenosine dose may be helpful.

Intracoronary Adenosine Triphosphate

Although it is unavailable in the United States, adenosine triphosphate (ATP) may also be used to stimulate maximal hyperemia. Coronary flow velocity, hemodynamics, electrocardiography, and myocardial lactate metabolism before and after administration of 50 µg of IC ATP and 10 mg of papaverine into the LCA were examined in 18 patients with normal coronary arteries. Dose responses were obtained with IC ATP doses of 0.5, 5, 15, 30, and 50 µg and compared to the papaverine response in an additional seven patients. ATP did not produce significant hemodynamic or electrocardiographic changes. CFR was similar between ATP and papaverine. All patients showed lactate production after papaverine; only three patients showed lactate production after ATP (P<.001). There was a significant correlation between CFR with ATP and with papaverine, indicating that maximal coronary vasodilation is safely obtained with IC ATP doses greater than 15 µg.

Dobutamine Hyperemia

Bartunek and associates[10] examined FFR in response to IC adenosine and IV dobutamine (10 to 40 µg/kg/minute) in 22 patients with single-vessel CAD. Peak dobutamine infusion produced similar distal coronary pressures and pressure ratios (P_d/P_a, 60±18 and 59±18 mm Hg; FFR, 0.68±0.18 and 0.68±0.17, respectively; all P=not significant [NS]). An additional bolus of IC adenosine given at peak dobutamine in nine patients failed to change the FFR. By angiography, high-dose IV dobutamine did not modify the area of the epicardial stenosis and, much like adenosine, fully exhausted myocardial resistance regardless of inducible left ventricular dysfunction.

Sodium Nitroprusside

IC nitroprusside may be an alternative to IC adenosine. Parham and associates[11] examined coronary blood flow velocity, heart rate, and blood pressure in unobstructed LADs in 21 patients at rest, after IC adenosine (boluses of 30 to 50 µg), and after three serial doses of IC nitroprusside (boluses of 0.3, 0.6, and 0.9 µg/kg). IC nitroprusside produced equivalent coronary hyperemia with a longer duration (about 25%) compared with IC adenosine. IC nitroprusside (0.9 µg/kg) decreased systolic blood pressure by 20% with minimal change in heart rate, whereas IC adenosine had no effect on these parameters. FFR measurements with IC nitroprusside were identical to those obtained with IC adenosine (r=.97). IC nitroprusside, in doses commonly used for the treatment of the no-reflow phenomenon, can produce sustained coronary hyperemia without detrimental systemic hemodynamics. Sodium nitroprusside also appears to be a suitable hyperemic stimulus for coronary physiologic measurements.

CLINICAL VALIDATION OF INTRACORONARY PRESSURE MEASUREMENTS

A summary of physiologic threshold values for common clinical applications is provided in Table 61-2.

In order to define the threshold of FFR_{myo} below which inducible ischemia is present, Pijls[12] and De Bruyne[13] and their colleagues conducted independent but parallel and complementary investigations. Pijls' group studied 60 patients accepted for a single-vessel PTCA who had a positive exercise test in the preceding 24 hours. FFR_{myo} was measured before and 15 minutes after PTCA, and the exercise test was repeated after 1 week. If the second exercise test had reverted to normal after PTCA, FFR_{myo} values were associated with inducible ischemia. All except two FFR_{myo} measurements greater than 0.74 were not associated with ischemia, and all FFR_{myo} measure-

Table 61-2. Physiologic Criteria Associated with Clinical Applications

Indication	CFR	rCFR	FFR
Ischemia detection	<2.0	<0.8	<0.75
Deferred angioplasty	>2.0	—	>0.75
End point of angioplasty	>2.0-2.5*	—	>0.90
End point of stenting	—	—	>0.90

*With a <35% diameter stenosis.
CFR, coronary flow reserve; FFR, fractional flow reserve; rCFR, relative coronary flow reserve.
Modified from Kern MJ: Coronary physiology revisited: Practical insights from the cardiac catheterization laboratory. Circulation 2000;101:1344-1351.

Table 61-3. Summary of Correlation between Noninvasive Stress Test Results and Physiologic Measurements

Index	Ischemic Test	N	BCV	Accuracy (%)
FFR	SPECT	763	0.74-0.78	75-95
	DSE	58	0.67-0.75	90
CFR	SPECT	704	1.7-2	75-92
	DSE	58	2	87-88
rCFR	SPECT	260	0.64-0.75	75-92
	DSE	28	0.75	81

BCV, best cutoff value (defined as the value with the highest sum of sensitivity and specificity); CFR, coronary flow reserve; DSE, dobutamine stress echocardiography; FFR, fractional flow reserve; rCFR, relative coronary flow reserve; SPECT, single photon emission tomography.

ments of 0.74 or less were related to inducible ischemia. In normal coronary arteries, FFR_{myo} was 0.98±0.03. De Bruyne's group studied FFR_{myo} in 60 patients with one isolated lesion in one major coronary artery who had a maximal exercise test 6 hours before catheterization. ST-segment depression was compared to FFR_{myo}, ΔP_{max}, and ΔP_{rest}. Intersections of sensitivity and specificity curves were at 87%, 83%, and 75%, respectively, for FFR_{myo}=0.66, ΔP_{max}=31 mm Hg, and ΔP_{rest}=12 mm Hg. No abnormal test was present for FFR_{myo} greater than 0.72. FFR_{myo} has also been compared with the results of dobutamine echocardiography in 75 patients with normal left ventricular function and single-vessel CAD; the degree of dobutamine-induced dyssynergy correlated significantly with the QCA data, but the correlation was markedly better with FFR_{myo}. All but one patient with a FFR_{myo} greater than 0.75 had a normal stress test result.

Among the most important reports of FFR_{myo} is that of Pijls and colleagues,[14] who compared FFR_{myo} with the unique ischemic standard of common noninvasive testing modalities in 45 patients with moderate coronary stenoses and chest pain syndromes. When the FFR_{myo} was lower than 0.75 (21 patients), reversible myocardial ischemia was demonstrated unequivocally on at least one noninvasive test (bicycle exercise testing, thallium scintigraphy, stress echocardiography with dobutamine), and all these positive test results were reversed after PTCA or coronary artery bypass graft (CABG) surgery. In 21 of 24 patients with a FFR_{myo} greater than 0.75, all of the tests showed no demonstration of ischemia, and no revascularization procedure was performed. Importantly, no revascularization was required after 14 months of follow-up. The sensitivity of FFR_{myo} in the identification of reversible ischemia was 88%, the specificity was 100%, the positive predictive value was 100%, the negative predictive value was 88%, and the accuracy was 93%.

INTRACORONARY PRESSURE AND FLOW MEASUREMENTS AND MYOCARDIAL PERFUSION IMAGING

Strong correlations exist between myocardial stress testing and FFR_{myo} or CFR. A FFR_{myo} of less than 0.75

identifies physiologically significant stenoses associated with inducible myocardial ischemia with high sensitivity (88%), specificity (100%), positive predictive value (100%), and overall accuracy (93%). An abnormal CFR (<2.0) corresponds to reversible myocardial perfusion imaging defects with high sensitivity (86% to 92%), specificity (89% to 100%), predictive accuracy (89% to 96%), and positive and negative predictive values (84% to 100% and 77% to 95%, respectively). A summary of ischemic stress testing and coronary physiologic measurements is provided in Table 61-3.

INTRACORONARY PHYSIOLOGIC MEASUREMENTS AND INTRAVASCULAR ULTRASOUND MEASUREMENTS

As another method of assessing a coronary artery beyond coronary angiography, IVUS offers a high degree of anatomic detail that can aid the operator in making clinical decisions. A study comparing IVUS, QCA, and FFR in 42 patients with 51 stenoses also demonstrated that QCA alone was not accurate in determining physiologic lesion significance assessed by either IVUS or FFR.[15] There was, however, a strong correlation of minimal lumen area (MLA) IVUS less than 3.0 mm^2 and cross-sectional area (CSA) IVUS stenosis greater than 60% with a measured FFR less than 0.75 (IVUS sensitivity 83%, specificity 92%).

Briguori and colleagues[16] related anatomy and physiology in 53 lesions. The percent area stenosis and lesional length had a significant inverse correlation with FFR (r=−.58, P<.001 and r=−.41, P<.004, respectively). Minimal lumen diameter (MLD) and MLA showed significant positive correlation with FFR. By receiver operating characteristic (ROC) curves, a percent area stenosis greater than 70%, MLD less than 1.8 mm, MLA less than 4.0 mm^2, and lesional length greater than 10 mm were the best cutoff values to fit FFR less than 0.75.

Thus, from these studies, some general IVUS measurements have been shown to be associated with functionally significant coronary stenoses and may guide appropriate revascularization.

CLINICAL UTILITY OF FRACTIONAL FLOW RESERVE IN DAILY PRACTICE

Determining the Need for Revascularization in Single-Vessel Disease with an Intermediate Stenosis

Determining the clinical significance of intermediate coronary stenoses on angiography frequently requires adjunctive noninvasive stress testing. Direct translesional flow measurements now available correlate well with myocardial perfusion imaging studies and may assist in clinical decision-making. The clinical outcomes of deferring coronary intervention for intermediate stenoses with normal physiology are remarkably consistent, with clinical event rates of less than 10% over a 2-year follow-up period. No study has deferred treatment in symptomatic patients with abnormal translesional physiology. Bech and colleagues recently reported the results of a large, randomized study (Deferral of PTCA versus performance of PTCA [DEFER]) of 325 patients for whom PTCA was planned who did not have documented ischemia.[17] The FFR of the stenosis was measured, and, if it was greater than 0.75, patients were randomly assigned to deferral of PTCA (deferral group; *n*=91) or performance of PTCA (performance group; *n*=90). If the FFR was less than 0.75, PTCA was performed as planned (reference group; *n*=144). Clinical follow-up was obtained at 1, 3, 6, 12, and 24 months. Event-free survival was similar in the deferral and performance groups (92% versus 89%, respectively, at 12 months and 89% versus 83% at 24 months) but was significantly lower in the reference group (80% at 12 months and 78% at 24 months) (Fig. 61-5). In addition, the percentage of patients free from angina was similar in the deferral and performance groups (49% versus 50% at 12 months and 70% versus 51% at 24 months) but was significantly higher in the reference group (67% at 12 months and 80% at 24 months). It was concluded that, in patients with a coronary stenosis without evidence of ischemia, coronary pressure–derived FFR identifies those who will benefit from PTCA.

Despite excellent safety, some patients with deferred procedures may still have recurrent angina, requiring continued medical therapy. Nonetheless, if they are physiologically normal, the functional and clinical impact of angiographically intermediate stenoses is associated with an excellent clinical outcome. Like other tests at a single point in time, in-laboratory translesional hemodynamics may not reflect the episodic ischemia-producing conditions of daily life, particularly those related to vasomotor changes during exercise or emotional stress. Fortunately, most dynamic conditions are highly responsive to medical therapy. Physiologic thresholds validated by ischemic stress testing and clinical outcomes support decisions to defer intervention while continuing medical therapy for endothelial dysfunction, hypertension, hyperlipidemia, and episodic coronary vasoconstriction. Table 61-4 summarizes

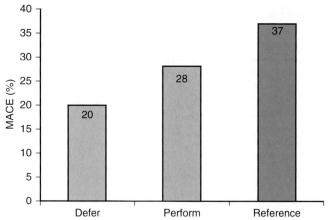

Figure 61-5. Graph showing the 5-year results from the Deferral of PTCA versus performance of PTCA (DEFER) trial. The *y*-axis depicts the percentage of patients with major adverse cardiac events (MACE): death, myocardial infarction, coronary artery bypass surgery, or percutaneous intervention. The "DEFER" group (*n*=91) consisted of those patients found to have an intermediate coronary stenosis in whom the measured FFR was greater than 0.75 and no angioplasty was performed (MACE=20%). The "PERFORM" group (*n*=90) consisted of those patients with an intermediate coronary stenosis with FFR values greater than 0.75 in whom angioplasty was performed (MACE=28%). The "REFERENCE" group (*n*=144) comprised patients whose lesions had measured FFR values of less than 0.75 in whom angioplasty was performed (MACE=37%). (From Van Schaardenburgh P, Bech GJW, De Bruyne B, et al: Is it necessary to stent non-ischaemic stenoses? Five year follow-up of the DEFER study. Eur Heart J 2005;26[Suppl 1]:3747).

the results of studies deferring PCI of intermediate lesions based on physiologic end points.

Multivessel Disease

With the increasing use of coronary stents in an ever more complex patient population, a frequent application of physiologic assessment involves lesion selection in patients with multivessel disease. Accurate lesion selection is important, because noninvasive studies have demonstrated that technetium 99m sestamibi single-photon emission computed tomography (MIBI-SPECT) failed to correctly indicate all ischemic areas in 90% of patients.[18] In 35% of such patients, no perfusion defect was present, possibly owing to balanced ischemia. Often, one ischemic area was masked by another, more severely underperfused area. Furthermore, when several stenoses or diffuse disease are present within one coronary artery, an abnormal MIBI-SPECT hypoperfusion image cannot discriminate among the different stenoses along the length of that vessel. For clinical practice, these observations highlight the fact that regions that may not appear responsible for ischemia can contain significant appearing narrowings, whereas other, more severe-appearing lesions may not be hemodynamically important. Coronary pressure measurements are particularly useful to localize regions of suspected ischemia.

Table 61-4. Outcomes after Deferral of Coronary Intervention for Intermediate Coronary Artery Disease

Index	Author	Reference	N	Defer Value	MACE (%)	Follow-up (mo)
FFR	Bech	17	100	0.75	8	18
	Bech	32	150	0.75	8	24
	Hernandez Garcia	54	43	0.75	12	11
	Bech*	21	24	0.75	21	29
	Rieber	55	47	0.75	13	12
	Chamuleau	56	92	0.75	9	12
	Rieber	57	24	0.75	8	12
	Lessar†	29	34	0.75	9	12
CFR	Kern	58	88	2.0	7	9
	Ferrari	59	22	2.0	9	15
	Chamuleau‡	60	143	2.0	6	12

*Patients with left main coronary artery disease.
†Patients with unstable angina.
‡Patients with multivessel disease.
CFR, coronary flow reserve; Defer Value, cutoff value used by study for decision-making; FFR, fractional flow reserve; MACE, major adverse cardiac events.

Several small, nonrandomized studies have reported the use of coronary physiology in multivessel disease. Recently, in patients with multivessel disease referred for CABG, patients who underwent selective PCI of hemodynamically significant stenoses, with medical therapy for all other nonsignificant lesions, had a prognosis similar to that of patients who underwent CABG of all angiographic diseased vessels.[19] In a similar study, 150 patients with multivessel disease reffered for CABG had FFR performed.[20] If three vessels were significant (FFR<0.75) or two vessels were significant with one being the proximal LAD, CABG was performed; otherwise, significant lesions were treated with stenting. After a 2-year follow-up, there was no difference in event-free survival, including repeat revascularization, showing that a tailored approach to patients with multivessel disease can be accomplished by deteriming the hemodynamic significance of each lesion.

Left Main Coronary Artery Disease

FFR can be used to assess narrowings of the left main coronary artery with specific technical considerations regarding guiding catheter seating and use of IV adenosine. Because of the potential of guiding catheter obstruction to blood flow across an ostial narrowing, FFR measurements should be performed with the guiding catheter disengaged from the coronary ostium and hyperemia induced with IV adenosine. Initially, the guiding catheter and wire pressures should be matched (equalized) before the guiding catheter is seated. Then, the guiding catheter is seated and the pressure wire is advanced into the LAD or left circumflex artery. The guiding catheter is then disengaged, and IV adenosine infusion is initiated. After 1 to 2 minutes, the FFR is calculated, and thereafter the wire can be pulled back slowly to identify the exact location of the pressure drop. In case of a distal narrowing of the left main coronary artery, this procedure may be performed twice, once with the pressure wire in the LAD and then again in the circumflex artery.

The use of FFR in left main stenosis was examined in 54 patients.[21] In the 30 patients who had an FFR of less than 0.75, surgery was performed, and in the 24 patients with an FFR of 0.75 or greater, medical therapy was chosen. After a follow-up of 3 years, there was no difference in event-free survival or functional class between the groups. None of the patients in the medical group experienced myocardial infarction or died. Similar results were recently shown by Lindstaedt and colleagues,[22] who monitored 51 patients with intermediate left main disease. The decision to perform CABG was based on FFR measurement of the left main coronary artery. In this patient population, 27 received CABG. After an average of 19 months of follow-up, there was no difference in event-free survival between those who underwent CABG and those who were treated medically.

Serial (Multiple) Lesions in a Single Vessel

If more than one discrete stenosis is present in the same vessel, the hyperemic flow and pressure gradient through the first stenosis will be attenuated by the presence of the second one, and vice versa. Each stenosis will mask the true effect of its serial counterpart by limiting the achievable maximum hyperemia. This fluid dynamic interaction between two serial stenoses depends on the sequence, severity, and distance between the lesions as well as the flow rate. If the distance between two lesions is greater than 6 times the vessel diameter, the stenoses generally behave independently and the overall pressure gradient is the sum of the individual pressure losses at any given flow rate.

When addressing two stenoses in series, equations have been derived to predict the FFR (FFR_{pred}) of each stenosis separately (i.e., as if the other one were removed), using arterial pressure (P_a), pressure

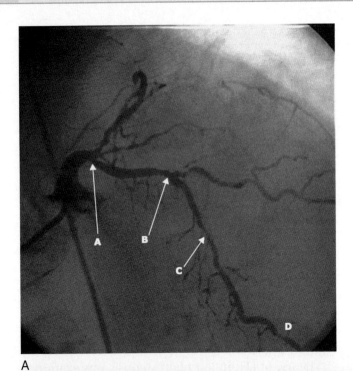

A

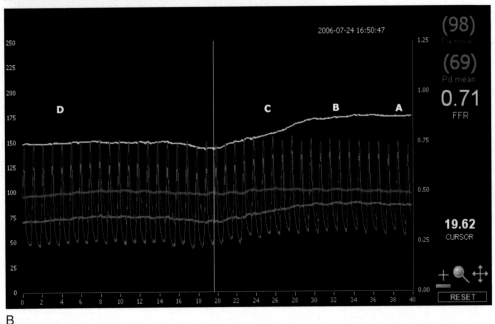

B

Figure 61-6. Case example of a patient who presented to the catheterization laboratory complaining of angina-like symptoms. **A,** Right anterior oblique (RAO)-cranial angiogram shows multiple lesions (A through D) within the left anterior descending coronary artery (LAD). **B,** A pull back curve through the LAD during intravenous adenosine administration (points A through D represent the lesions identified in **A**).

between the two stenoses (P_m), distal coronary pressure (P_d), and coronary occlusive pressure (P_w). FFR_{app} (ratio of the pressure just distal to that just proximal to each stenosis) and FFR_{true} (ratio of the pressures distal and proximal to each stenosis but after removal of the other one) have been compared in instrumented dogs[23] and in patients.[24] FFR_{true} was more overestimated by FFR_{app} than by FFR_{pred}. It was clearly demonstrated that the interaction between two stenoses is such that the FFR of each lesion separately cannot be calculated by the equation for isolated stenoses applied to each separately; however, the FFR

for each lesion can be predicted by more complete equations that take into account P_a, P_m, P_d, and P_w.

Although calculation of the exact FFR for each lesion separately is possible, it remains academic. In clinical practice, the use of the pressure pull back recording is particularly well suited to identify the several regions of a vessel with large pressure gradients that may benefit by treatment. The one stenosis with the largest gradient can be treated first, after which the FFR can be remeasured for the remaining stenoses to determine the need for further treatment (Fig. 61-6).

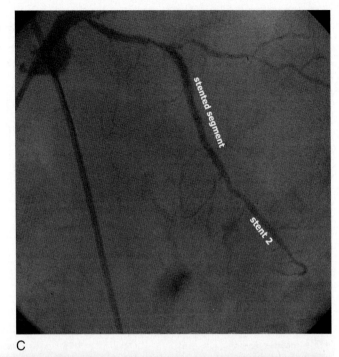

C

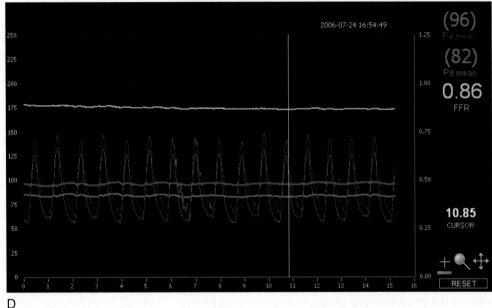

D

Figure 61-6, cont'd C, RAO-cranial angiogram after treatment of lesions D and C with stents. **D,** Fractional flow reserve (FFR) of the LAD after stenting, with the wire distal to the last stent. The FFR of 0.86 reflects the fact that the ostial and middle lesions (A and B) did not need to be treated.

Diffuse Coronary Disease

A diffusely diseased atherosclerotic coronary artery can be viewed as a series of branching units diverting and gradually distributing flow along the longitudinally narrowing conduit length. The perfusion pressure gradually diminishes along this artery. CFR is reduced but is unassociated with a focal stenotic pressure loss. Therefore, mechanical therapy directed at a presumed "culprit" plaque to reverse such abnormal physiology would be ineffective in restoring normal coronary perfusion. With the use of FFR_{myo} during continuous-pressure wire pull back from a distal to a proximal location, the impact of a specific area of angiographic narrowing can be examined and the presence of diffuse atherosclerosis can be documented.

Diffuse atherosclerosis, as opposed to a focal narrowing, is characterized by a continuous and gradual pressure recovery without localized abrupt increase in pressure related to an isolated region. De Bruyne and coworkers demonstrated the influence of diffuse atherosclerosis that often remains invisible at angiography.[25] FFR_{myo} measurements were obtained from 37 arteries in 10 individuals without atherosclerosis (group I) and from 106 nonstenotic arteries in 62 patients with arteriographic stenoses in another coronary artery (group II). In group I, the pressure

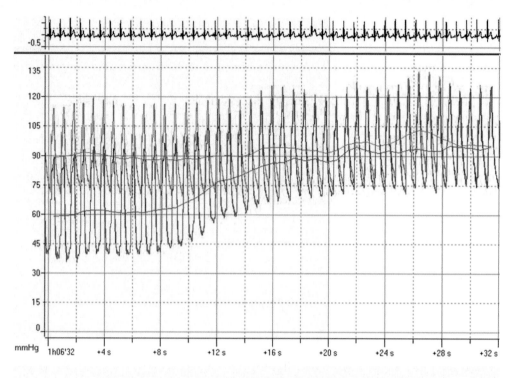

Figure 61-7. A pull back curve created in a patient with diffuse disease throughout the left anterior descending coronary artery (LAD). The fractional flow reserve (FFR) for this vessel is 0.67, reflecting ischemia-producing lesions. However, the gradual decrease in gradient from pressure distal to the stenosis (P_d) to arterial pressure (P_a) is reflective of severe, diffuse narrowing in the major portion of the vessel. This gradual change in the pressure curve shows that an extremely long segment is responsible for the ischemia and is most likely not best treated with multiple stents (i.e., "full metal jacket"). (Courtesy of B. De Bruyne.)

gradient between aorta and distal coronary artery was minimal at rest (1±1 mm Hg) and during maximal hyperemia (3±3 mm Hg). Corresponding values were significantly larger in group II (5±4 and 10±8 mm Hg, respectively; both $P < .001$). The FFR_{myo} was near unity (0.97±0.02; range, 0.92 to 1) in group I, indicating no resistance to flow in truly normal coronary arteries, but it was significantly lower (0.89±0.08; range, 0.69 to 1) in group II, indicating a higher resistance to flow. This resistance to flow contributes to myocardial ischemia and has consequences for decision-making during PCI.

As for patients with several discrete stenoses within one coronary artery, similar considerations can be applied for patients with diffuse CAD or long lesions. The pressure pull back recording at maximum hyperemia provides the necessary information to decide whether and where stent implantation may be useful. The location of a focal pressure drop superimposed on the diffuse disease can be identified as an appropriate location for treatment. In some cases, the gradual decline of pressure along the vessel occurs over a very long segment, such that interventional treatment is not possible (Fig. 61-7). Medical treatment (or CABG) can then be elected.

Ostial Lesions and "Jailed" Side Branches

The ability to determine the physiologic significance of ostial lesions, particularly in side branch vessels, remains difficult with current angiographic techniques and equipment. This is particularly problematic after the side branch has been "jailed" by a stent in the parent vessel. Koo and coworkers[26] examined the physiologic assessment of jailed side branches and compared the FFR with the QCA of stenosis severity. Ninety-seven jailed side branch lesions in vessels larger than 2.0 mm with a percent stenosis greater than 50% by visual estimation after stent implantation underwent FFR, measuring the pressure 5 mm distal and proximal to the ostial side branch lesion.

In 94 lesions, the mean FFR was 0.94±0.04 at the main branch and 0.85±0.11 at the jailed side branch. There was a negative correlation between percent stenosis and FFR ($r = .41$, $P < .001$). However, no lesion with less than 75% stenosis had an FFR less than 0.75. Among 73 lesions with greater than 75% stenosis, only 20 lesions were functionally significant (Fig. 61-8). The authors concluded that measurement of FFR in jailed side branch lesions is both safe and feasible, and, as with other intermediate lesions, QCA is unreliable. Moreover, the measurement of FFR suggested that most of these lesions do not have functional significance and that intervention on these nonsignificant lesions may not be necessary (see example in Fig. 61-9). Similar findings have been reported for native ostial and branch lesions not "jailed" with intracoronary hardware that were found during routine coronary angiography.[27,28]

Unstable Angina and Non-ST-Segment Elevation Myocardial Infarction

After stabilization of patients with unstable angina or non-ST-segment elevation myocardial infarction (NSTEMI), traditional management involves instituting maximal medical therapy and performing risk stratification by stress testing before coronary angiography and intervention based on the results. As an alternative approach, Leesar and colleagues used FFR to risk-stratify patients with acute coronary syndrome

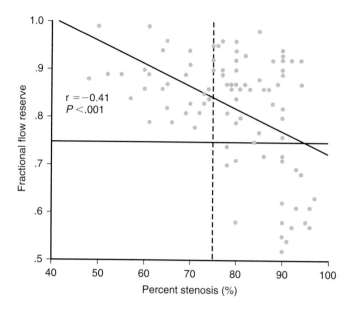

	% stenosis	
	≥50, <75	≥75
All lesions (n = 94)		
FFR <0.75	0	20 (27%)
FFR ≥0.75	20	53
Vessel size ≥2.5 mm (n = 28)		
FFR <0.75	0	8 (38%)
FFR ≥0.75	7	13

Figure 61-8. *Top,* Graph comparing percent diameter stenosis (by quantitative coronary angiography) to fractional flow reserve (FFR) across jailed side branches. Despite the statistical significance of the correlation, one should note the frequency of severely narrowed side branches without significant FFR values (indicated by points in the upper right corner). *Bottom,* Table showing the relationship between percent stenosis and FFR values across jailed side branches. (From Koo BK, Kang HJ, Youn TJ, et al: Physiologic assessment of jailed side branch lesions using fractional flow reserve. J Am Coll Cardiol 2005;46;633-637.)

in the laboratory at the time of catheterization after medical stabilization.[29] Seventy patients were randomly assigned to either early in-hospital invasive evaluation (*n*=35) with FFR or noninvasive evaluation by perfusion scintigraphy (*n*=35). The decision to revascularize was based on abnormal FFR or MIBI-SPECT scans. The early invasive FFR-guided approach was equally effective as the standard of care with noninvasive risk stratification. The rate of major adverse cardiac events at 1 year follow-up were similar between the groups. The FFR-guided approach was also associated with a shorter hospital stay and a significant decrease in total costs of the hospitalization. For patients who cannot be medically stabilized, current guidelines recommend urgent angiography with appropriate revascularization as indicated, without FFR. Nonetheless, FFR could be useful to assess other intermediately severe non-culprit lesions for consideration of complete revascularization.

Recent ST-Segment Elevation Myocardial Infarction

After an acute myocardial infarction, the predictive ability of FFR has some theoretic limitations, because the microvascular bed in the infarct zone does not necessarily have a uniform and constant resistance. However, DeBruyne and associates demonstrated that a threshold of 0.75 was also valid in 57 patients who had sustained a myocardial infarction more than 6 days earlier.[30] Myocardial perfusion SPECT imaging and FFR_{myo} were obtained before and after angioplasty. The sensitivity and specificity of the 0.75 value of FFR_{myo} to detect flow maldistribution on SPECT imaging were 82% and 87%, respectively. The concordance between the FFR and SPECT imaging was 85% (*P*<.001). When only truly positive and truly negative SPECT imaging results were considered, the corresponding values were 87%, 100%, and 94% (*P*<.001). Patients with positive SPECT imaging before angioplasty had a significantly lower FFR_{myo} than did patients with negative SPECT imaging (0.52±0.18 versus 0.67±0.16; *P*=.0079); they also had a significantly higher left ventricular ejection fraction (LVEF, 63%±10% versus 52%±10%; *P*=.0009) despite a similar percent diameter stenosis (67%±13% versus 68%±16%; *P*=NS). A significant inverse correlation was found between LVEF and FFR_{myo} (*R*=.29, *P*=.049). It appears that, for a similar degree of stenosis, the value of FFR_{myo} depends on the mass of viable myocardium. The possibility of analyzing truly positive and negative SPECT imaging in this study confirmed the validity of the 0.75 threshold, which could not be derived from a study based only on angiographic parameters.[31]

PROGNOSTIC VALUE OF INTRACORONARY PHYSIOLOGIC MEASUREMENTS AFTER PERCUTANEOUS CORONARY INTERVENTION

The use of coronary pressure or flow to guide coronary interventions was of value when stenting was considered difficult and was associated with marginally improved restenosis rates. Since the introduction of drug-eluting stents with their excellent long-term outcomes, the concept of employing physiologic measurements to achieve optimal interventional results has become obsolete. FFR, and in some studies CFR after PTCA, can identify patients with stent-like results, but the practice has not been accepted for evident reasons. The technology required for provisional stenting is more time-consuming than that needed for routine stenting. Although QCA, IVUS, Doppler, and FFR are valuable on an individual basis, the universal application of these devices is thought to be neither time- nor cost-effective. In some analyses, routine stenting appears less costly than provisional stenting, and any cost differential is offset by the increased procedure time required for adjunctive technology.

A normal FFR after PTCA is associated with stent-like late outcomes. Bech and colleagues[32] reported 2-year clinical follow-up data using FFR in 60 patients

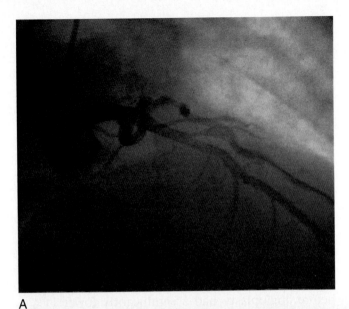

A

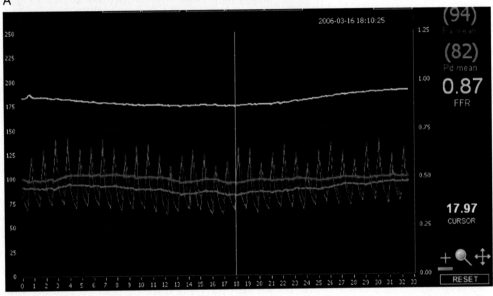

B

Figure 61-9. **A,** Right anterior oblique (RAO)-cranial angiogram showing a left anterior descending coronary artery (LAD) without significant angiographic stenosis but a diagonal artery that appears to have a high-grade stenosis. **B,** Measurement of fractional flow rate (FFR) across the diseased ostial diagonal shows a value of 0.87, reflecting a nonsignificant ostial lesion despite its angiographic appearance.

after single-vessel angioplasty. In the 43% of angioplasty patients (26 of 60) with optimal QCA residual diameter stenosis less than 35% and functional results (FFR>0.90), event-free survival rates were significantly better at 6 months (92% versus 72%; $P=.047$), 12 months (92% versus 69%; $P=.028$), and 24 months (88% versus 59%; $P=.014$), compared with those patients who had an FFR of less than 0.90. No improvement in clinical outcome was gained by additional stenting. From these studies, a suboptimal functional angioplasty, reflected by an FFR of less than 0.90 or impaired rCFR/CFR, suggests that further intervention may be needed to improve the result with stenting.

A normal FFR after stenting should indicate near-complete elimination of epicardial resistance after stent deployment. However, analyzing FFR, QCA, and IVUS measurements of stents implanted in vitro in a hydraulic bench, we showed that FFR cannot

discriminate between suboptimally and optimally deployed stents.[33] Struts that appear clearly malapposed by IVUS do not influence the pressure gradient, whereas FFR can increase by 15% to 20% owing to changes in blood flow from 50 to 150 mL/minute.

Similar data were reported in a large prospective, multicenter trial that evaluated the use of FFR to optimize stenting by comparing it with standard IVUS criteria.[34] A total of 84 stable patients with isolated coronary lesions underwent coronary stent deployment, starting at 10 atm and increasing serially by 2 atm until the FFR was 0.94 or greater or 16 atm was achieved. IVUS was then performed. Over a range of IVUS criteria, the highest sensitivity, specificity, and predictive accuracy of FFR were 80%, 30%, and 42%, respectively. ROC analysis defined an optimal FFR cutpoint at 0.96 or greater. At this threshold, the sensitivity, specificity, and predictive accuracy of FFR were 75%, 58%, and 62%, respectively.

The negative predictive value was 88%. An FFR of less than 0.96 after stenting predicts an IVUS suboptimal result well. However, an FFR of 0.96 or greater does not reliably predict an optimal stent result.

INTRACORONARY PHYSIOLOGIC MEASUREMENTS AS A RESEARCH TOOL FOR THE STUDY OF CORONARY CIRCULATION

Study of Collateral Circulation

The collateral circulation can be described by intracoronary pressure and flow relationships. Ipsilateral collateral flow and contralateral arterial responses have been described in numerous studies that used both pressure and flow to provide new information regarding mechanisms, function, and clinical significance of collateral flow[35] and to improve the conventional angiographic assessment of collateral supply, according to the research of Rentrop and colleagues.[36] The coronary collateral flow velocity response is characterized by flow reversal or persistent antegrade flow during coronary balloon occlusion. The phasic nature of the reversed flow pattern appears to be related to the source artery and the pathways of the collateral channels. Large, completely epicardial collaterals with grade 3 Rentrop angiographic flow have the most clearly demarcated phasic components. Figure 61-10 illustrates a typical evaluation of collateral flow during balloon occlusion. However, the reader is referred to excellent works elsewhere for details of these methods that are beyond the scope of this chapter.[37]

Microvascular Disease and Chest Pain with Normal Coronary Arteries

As part of the Women's Ischemic Syndrome Evaluation (WISE) study, Reis and associates[38] examined 48 women with chest pain, normal coronary arteries, or minimal luminal irregularities with CFR. Sixty percent of women with CFR of less than 2 had a hyperemic velocity 89% of baseline but no change in cross-sectional vessel area. Forty percent of women with normal microcirculation, with average CFR of 3.24, had associated increases in coronary flow velocity and CSA of 179% and 17%, respectively. A CFR of 2.2 provided a high sensitivity (90%) and specificity (89%) for the diagnosis of microvascular dysfunction. Failure of the epicardial coronary artery to dilate at least 9% was also a sensitive (79%) and specific (79%) surrogate marker of microvascular dysfunction. The attenuated epicardial coronary dilatory response likely represents significant microvascular dysfunction in women with chest pain and no obstructive CAD.

Similar data were reported by Hasdai and colleagues[39] in 203 patients with angiographically normal coronary arteries. CFR and endothelial vasodilatory response to IC acetylcholine and adenosine were measured. Ninety-two percent of patients had at least one risk factor for atherosclerosis. Abnormal CFR was found in 59% of patients; 11% had impaired response to adenosine with CFR less than 2.5, and 29% had impaired response to acetylcholine with CFR less than 1.5; 18% had a combined abnormality. There was no correlation between endothelium-dependent and endothelium-independent flow response. The authors concluded that most patients with chest pain syndromes and nonobstructive CAD had risk factors for CAD with diverse abnormalities and endothelium-dependent and -independent function.

Assessment of Endothelial Function

Acetylcholine is the prototype and the most frequently used pharmacologic stimulus, with a primary endothelium-independent contractile action on the vascular smooth muscle cells and an opposite endothelium-mediated vasodilatory activity that is predominant in normal conditions and at physiologic concentrations. Atherosclerotic experimental animals show an abnormal endothelium-dependent vasodilation of the coronary resistance arteries despite the absence of structural atherosclerotic lesions.[40] Comparison of the flow response to acetylcholine in patients with CAD and in control subjects has confirmed an impaired flow increase in the patients with CAD, despite the absence of significant lesions of the epicardial coronary arteries.[41]

Using two-dimensional intracoronary ultrasound and Doppler measurements, Reddy and coworkers[42] demonstrated that patients with one or more risk factors had an abnormal epicardial artery CSA vasoconstriction response to acetylcholine infusion. However, patients presenting with minimal disease on ultrasound (intimal thickening or small eccentric plaque) did not respond differently from those patients without demonstrable disease on ultrasound. Using a similar methodology, Suwaidi and colleagues demonstrated that severe endothelial dysfunction was associated with a high incidence of cardiac events.[43] A total of 157 patients with mildly diseased coronary arteries were monitored after coronary vascular reactivity evaluation by graded administration of IC acetylcholine, adenosine, and nitroglycerin and intracoronary ultrasound at the time of diagnostic study. Patients were divided on the basis of their response to acetylcholine into three groups: group 1 (n=83), patients with normal endothelial function; group 2 (n=32), patients with mild endothelial dysfunction; and group 3 (n=42), patients with severe endothelial dysfunction. Over an average 28-month follow-up (range, 11 to 52 months), none of the patients from group 1 or 2 had cardiac events. However, six (14%) of the patients with severe endothelial dysfunction had 10 cardiac events (myocardial infarction, percutaneous or surgical coronary revascularization, and/or cardiac death; $P<.05$ versus groups 1 and 2).

In humans, beneficial effects on endothelial function, evaluated by a reduction of acetylcholine-induced vasoconstriction, have been demonstrated

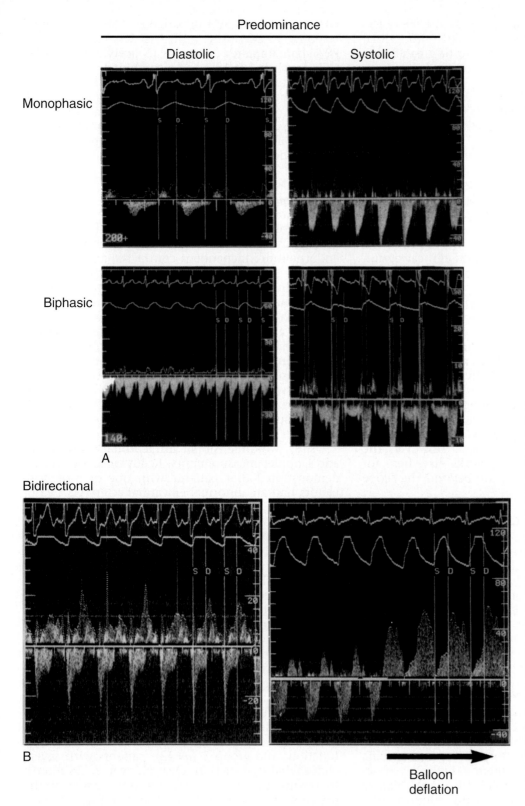

Figure 61-10. A, Changes in coronary flow velocity before, during, and after balloon occlusion in a patient undergoing angioplasty of the right coronary artery. The left panel shows bidirectional collateral flow during the occlusion. The right panel shows large retrograde flow that quickly changes to antegrade flow on deflation of the balloon. **B,** The four types of phasic epicardial collateral flow velocity seen during balloon occlusion. Top panels show monophasic signals with systolic and with diastolic predominance. Bottom panels show systolic and diastolic biphasic signals. The direction of flow depends on the location of the wire relative to the input source of collateral flow. (From Tron C, Donohue TJ, Bach RG, et al: Differential characterization of human coronary collateral blood flow velocity Am Heart J 1996;132:508-515.)

for inhibitors of hydroxymethylglutaryl-coenzyme A reductase and with angiotensin-converting enzyme inhibitor. The possibility of delaying or even reversing the atherosclerotic process and improving endothelial function is being studied in ongoing trials by the combined use of IVUS, QCA, and flow measurements with Doppler wire. There remains some controversy, with no effect found by some investigators[44] and improvements reported by others.[45] The beneficial effect of exercise on endothelium-dependent vasodilation of both epicardial coronary vessels and resistance vessels has also been recently reported.[46]

SIMULTANEOUS MEASUREMENT OF FLOW VELOCITY AND TRANSSTENOTIC PRESSURE GRADIENT

Although the maximal flow and, consequently, the maximal transstenotic gradient is determined also by factors independent of the stenosis resistance, the pressure gradient–flow velocity relation is intimately correlated with the stenosis hemodynamics. Study of the instantaneous pressure gradient–flow velocity relation during the progressive flow decrease in middle to late diastole has the advantage of an assessment based on instantaneous instead of mean gradient-flow changes during the cardiac cycle. The phases of acceleration/deceleration of flow, influenced by factors not related to stenosis resistance, can be eliminated from the analysis. The pressure gradient–flow velocity relation can also be studied during a prolonged cardiac arrest induced with a high-dose IC bolus of adenosine during papaverine-induced maximal hyperemia. In principle, however, the pressure gradient–flow velocity relation is independent of the hemodynamic conditions of assessment, including the maximal level of flow and pressure gradient, and could give sufficient information to characterize stenosis severity in resting conditions also.

Mancini and associates[47,48] validated in dogs the slope of the instantaneous pressure-flow relation as an index of coronary stenosis. This relation was compared to a microsphere-derived index of myocardial conductance. The instantaneous hyperemic flow-versus-pressure index demonstrated no dependence on heart rate, left ventricular end-diastolic pressure, mean aortic pressure, or inotropic changes.[49,50] The decrease in flow-pressure slope with the presence of stenoses of increasing severity correlated well with the transmural and subendocardial microsphere-derived measurements.

The feasibility and reproducibility of assessment of the slope of the instantaneous diastolic relation between coronary flow velocity and aortic pressure during maximal hyperemia (instantaneous hyperemic diastolic pressure-velocity slope, or IHDPVS) was investigated in 95 patients.[51] It was postulated that the changes in coronary blood velocities recorded by the Doppler wire were related directly, and only, to changes in flow (assuming a constant velocity profile and a constant coronary diameter), to derive Mancini's index from the velocity-pressure relation. The Doppler signal was acquired distal to the stenosis using a Doppler guide wire. The proximal coronary pressure was measured through the guiding catheter. Linear regression analysis was used to assess the slope of the digitized pressure-velocity relation (mm Hg versus cm/second) in four consecutive beats during maximal coronary vasodilation. Among those patients with greater than 30% diameter stenosis, five (21%) had a CFR greater than 2 and three (12%) had an IHDPVS greater than 1. In the normal group, a CFR of 2 or less was observed in four arteries (7%) and an IHDPVS of 1 or less in eight (14%) arteries.

Using these arbitrarily defined cutoff values, CFR and IHDPVS correctly identified 79% and 88%, respectively, of the arteries with greater than 30% diameter stenosis and excluded the presence of a stenosis in 93% and 86% of the 55 control arteries, respectively (P=NS).

A possible limitation of IHDPVS is the dependence of the hyperemic pressure-velocity slope on the CSA, as would be expected for an index reflecting coronary conductance. The inability to normalize coronary flow for the perfused myocardial mass limits the comparability of measurements performed in vessels of different dimensions.

De Bruyne and colleagues[6] compared the feasibility and variability of IHDPVS, CFR, and FFR$_{myo}$. Both CFR and FFR$_{myo}$ could be calculated in all cases, but IHDPVS could be calculated in only 82 (79%) of the 104 investigated patients. CFR was sensitive to hemodynamic changes (atrial pacing, dobutamine infusion), but IHDPVS and FFR$_{myo}$ were not influenced. Coefficients of variation between two consecutive measurements were 4.2% for FFR$_{myo}$, significantly lower than the 17.7% and 24.7% for CFR and IHDPVS, respectively.

With combined distal measurements, a clinician has all relevant hemodynamic information to make an informed decision about the physiologic condition of the entire coronary circulation. Combined simultaneous measurement of the phasic pressure and Doppler velocity distal to a stenosis permits the calculation of stenosis and microvascular resistances and has been applied clinically. With the use of distal pressure and velocity measured during hyperemic conditions, a hyperemic stenosis resistance (by velocity, v) index (HSR) is calculated as follows: HSR=ΔP/v, where ΔP equals the hyperemic pressure gradient ($P_a - P_d$) and v equals the average peak velocity at hyperemia. This index purportedly provides a refined physiologic measurement quantifying the impediment to maximal flow caused exclusively by the stenosis. Like FFR, HSR has a normal reference value (HSR=0) and is independent of basal hemodynamic conditions, with high reproducibility and low variability. Simultaneous measurement of distal pressure and flow velocity also allows the separate assessment of microvascular resistance[52] and the construction of stenosis pressure gradient-velocity curves that uniquely characterize the hemodynamics of any lesion and associated physiologic responses. The pressure drop-velocity relations are also well suited to visualize the effect of percutaneous intervention. An HSR value greater than 0.8 mm Hg/cm/second is the threshold for prediction of reversible ischemia when compared to noninvasive stress testing. HSR had a higher diagnostic accuracy than either pressure (FFR) or flow velocity (CFR) alone, especially in cases where outcomes of FFR and CFR did not agree. HSR requires the use of both a distal pressure and a flow velocity signal, which can be obtained with a dual-sensor (pressure and Doppler velocity) guide wire.

Another method uses distal pressure and thermodilution flow, as assessed by the inverse of the arrival

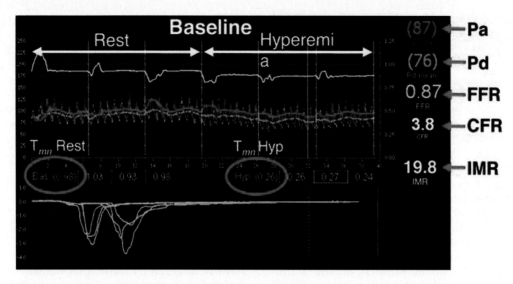

Figure 61-11. Simultaneous measurement of pressure and flow (by thermodilution). The upper portion of the figure shows proximal (P_a) and distal (P_d) pressures at rest (*left*) and during hyperemia (*right*). The lower portion of the figure depicts the thermodilution curves at rest and during hyperemia with the associated average transit times at baseline and hyperemia circled. These values are used to calculate the coronary flow reserve (CFR) and the index of microcirculatory resistance (IMR), as seen on the right side of the panel. FFR, fractional flow reserve. (From Martin KC, Yeung AC, Fearon WF: Invasive assessment of the coronary microcirculation. Circulation 2006;113:2054-2061.)

(transit) time of a room-temperature saline bolus to the distal coronary artery segment. By measuring the mean transit time at rest and comparing it with the mean transit time at peak hyperemia, a thermodilution CFR can be calculated. Experimental animal and human studies have validated the thermodilution CFR (CFR$_{thermo}$) against the CFR measure by Doppler technique (CFR$_{Doppler}$). The ability to measure distal pressure and estimate flow using the thermodilution technique with a single wire also allows independent assessment of the microvasculature by calculating the index of microcirculatory resistance (IMR).[53] Although principally a research tool, the simultaneous measurement of FFR, CFR, IMR, and HSR permits a unique characterization of the epicardial and microvascular resistances (example shown in Figure 61-11).

CONCLUSIONS

The field of interventional cardiology continues to see rapid advances in technology, and the use of coronary physiology continues to provide valuable assistance for the catheterization laboratory operator to make meaningful patient care decisions. Although routine assessment of coronary flow reserve has largely been abandoned, the integration of physiologic assessment of intermediate stenoses in patients with complex CAD, including left main coronary artery disease and multivessel disease, has increased the utility of FFR. This is especially useful with the replacement of surgical revascularization by percutaneous revascularization in recent years: FFR can help operators achieve complete resolution of coronary ischemia, similar to complete surgical revascularization.

It is hoped that future advances in coronary physiology will give practitioners the ability to independently evaluate the contribution of microvascular disease to a patient's symptoms, target therapies that can improve microvascular dysfunction, and to evaluate endothelial dysfunction as a precursor to the atherosclerotic process. However, technology alone cannot improve patient care, and careful consideration of all available information during the catheterization, coupled with evidence-based decision-making by the operator, continues to be the cornerstone of practical interventional cardiology.

ACKNOWLEDGEMENT

The authors recognize and thank Sherry Karstens for her work in preparing this chapter.

REFERENCES

1. Duncker DJ, Bache RJ: Regulation of coronary vasomotor tone under normal conditions and during acute myocardial hypoperfusion. Pharmacol Ther 2000;86:87-110.
2. Gould KL, Kirkeeide RL, Buchi M: Coronary flow reserve as a physiologic measure of stenosis severity. J Am Coll Cardiol 1990;15:459-474.
3. Pijls NHJ, van Son JAM, Kirkeeide RL, et al: Experimental basis of determining maximum coronary, myocardial, and collateral blood flow by pressure measurements for assessing functional stenosis severity before and after percutaneous transluminal coronary angioplasty. Circulation 1993;86:1354-1367.
4. Pijls NHJ, Van Gelder B, Van der Voort P, et al: Fractional flow reserve: A useful index to evaluate the influence of an epicardial coronary stenosis on myocardial blood flow. Circulation 1995;92:318-319.
5. De Bruyne B, Baudhuin T, Melin JA, et al: Coronary flow reserve calculated from pressure measurements in humans:

Validation with positron emission tomography. Circulation 1994;89:1013-1022.

6. De Bruyne B, Bartunek J, Sys SU, et al: Simultaneous coronary pressure and flow velocity measurements in humans: Feasibility, reproducibility and hemodynamic dependence of coronary flow velocity reserve, hyperemic flow versus pressure slope index and fractional flow reserve. Circulation 1996;94:1842-1849.

7. Pijls NH, Kern MJ, Yock PG, De Bruyne B: Practice and potential pitfalls of coronary pressure measurements. Cath Cardiovasc Intervent 2000;49:1-16.

8. Qian J, Ge J, Baumgart D, et al: Safety of intracoronary Doppler flow measurement. Am Heart J 2000;140:502-510.

9. Jeremias A, Whitbourn RJ, Filardo SD, et al: Adequacy of intracoronary versus intravenous adenosine-induced maximal coronary hyperemia for fractional flow reserve measurements. Am Heart J 2000;140:651-657.

10. Bartunek J, Wijns W, Heyndrickx GR, de Bruyne B: Effects of dobutamine on coronary stenosis physiology and morphology: Comparison with intracoronary adenosine. Circulation 1999;100:243-249.

11. Parham WA, Bouhasin A, Ciaramita JP, et al: Coronary hyperemic dose responses to intracoronary sodium nitroprusside. Circulation 2004;109:1236-1243.

12. Pijls NHJ, Van Gelder B, Van der Voort P, et al: Fractional flow reserve: A useful index to evaluate the influence of an epicardial coronary stenosis on myocardial blood flow. Circulation 1995;92:3183-3193.

13. De Bruyne B, Bartunek J, Sys SU, Heyndrickx GR: Relation between myocardial fractional flow reserve calculated from coronary pressure measurements and exercise-induced myocardial ischemia. Circulation 1995;92:39-46.

14. Pijls NHJ, de Bruyne B, Peels K, et al: Measurement of fractional flow reserve to assess the functional severity of coronary-artery stenoses. N Engl J Med 1996;334:1703-1708.

15. Abizaid A, Mint GS, Pichard AD, et al: Clinical, intravascular ultrasound, and quantitative angiographic determinants of the coronary flow reserve before and after percutaneous transluminal coronary angioplasty. Am J Cardiol 1998;82:423-428.

16. Briguori C, Anzuini A, Airoldi F, et al: Intravascular ultrasound criteria for the assessment of the functional significance of intermediate coronary artery stenoses and comparison with fractional flow reserve. Am J Cardiol 2001;87:136-141.

17. Bech GJ, De Bruyne B, Bonnier HJ, et al: Long-term follow-up after deferral of percutaneous transluminal coronary angioplasty of intermediate stenosis on the basis of coronary pressure measurement. J Am Coll Cardiol 1998;31:841-847.

18. Lima RS, Watson DD, Goode AR, et al: Incremental value of combined perfusion and function over perfusion alone by gated SPECT myocardial perfusion imaging for detection of severe three-vessel coronary artery disease. J Am Coll Cardiol 2003;42:64-70.

19. Berger A, Botman KJ, MacCarthy PA, et al: Long-term clinical outcome after fractional flow reserve-guided percutaneous coronary intervention in patients with multivessel disease. J Am Coll Cardiol 2005;46:438-442.

20. Botman KJ, Pijls N, Bech JW, et al: Percutaneous coronary intervention or bypass surgery in multivessel disease? A tailored approach based on coronary pressure measurement. Catheter Cardiovasc Interv 2004;63:184-191.

21. Bech GJ, Drouste H, Pijls NH, et al: Value of fractional flow reserve in making decisions about bypass surgery for equivocal left main coronary artery disease. Heart 2001;86:547-552.

22. Lindstaedt M, Yazar A, Germing A, et al: Clinical outcome in patients with intermediate or equivocal left main coronary artery disease after deferral of surgical revascularization on the basis of fractional flow reserve measurements. Am Heart J 2006;152:156.e1-156.e9.

23. De Bruyne B, Pijls NH, Heyndrickx GR, et al: Pressure-derived fractional flow reserve to assess serial epicardial stenoses: Theoretical basis and animal validation. Circulation 2000;101:1840-1847.

24. Pijls NH, De Bruyne B, Bech GJ, et al: Coronary pressure measurement to assess the hemodynamic significance of serial

stenoses within one coronary artery: Validation in humans. Circulation 2000;102:2371-2377.

25. De Bruyne B, Hersbach F, Pijls NH, et al: Abnormal epicardial coronary resistance in patients with diffuse atherosclerosis but "normal" coronary angiography. Circulation 2001;104:2401-2406.

26. Koo BK, Kang HJ, Youn TJ, et al: Physiologic assessment of jailed side branch lesions using fractional flow reserve. J Am Coll Cardiol 2005;46:633-637.

27. Lim MJ, Kern MJ: Utility of coronary physiologic hemodynamics for bifurcation, aorto ostial and ostial branch stenoses to guide treatment decisions. Cath Cardiovasc Intervent 2005;65:461-468.

28. Ziaee A, Parham WA, Herrmann SC, et al: Lack of relationship between imaging and physiology in ostial coronary artery narrowings. Am J Cardiol 2004;93:1404-1407.

29. Leesar MA, Abdul-Baki T, Akkus NI, et al: Use of fractional flow reserve versus stress perfusion scintigraphy after unstable angina: Effect on duration of hospitalization, cost, procedural characteristics, and clinical outcome. J Am Coll Cardiol 2003;44:1115-1121.

30. De Bruyne B, Pijls NH, Bartunek J, et al: Fractional flow reserve in patients with prior myocardial infarction. Circulation 2001;104:157-162.

31. Caymaz O, Tezcan H, Fak AS, et al: Measurement of myocardial fractional flow reserve during coronary angioplasty in infarct-related and non-infarct related coronary artery lesions. J Invasive Cardiol 2000;12:236-241.

32. Bech GJ, Pijls NH, De Bruyne B, et al: Usefulness of fractional flow reserve to predict clinical outcome after balloon angioplasty. Circulation 1999;99:883-888.

33. Matthys K, Carlier S, Segers P, et al: In vitro study of FFR, QCA, and IVUS for the assessment of optimal stent deployment. Cathet Cardiovasc Interv 2001;54:363-375.

34. Fearon WF, Luna J, Samady H, et al: Fractional flow reserve compared with intravascular ultrasound guidance for optimizing stent deployment. Circulation 2001;104:1917-1922.

35. Piek JJ, van Liebergen RA, Koch KT, et al: Clinical, angiographic and hemodynamic predictors of recruitable collateral flow assessed during balloon angioplasty coronary occlusion. J Am Coll Cardiol 1997;29:275-282.

36. Rentrop KP, Thornton JC, Feit F, Van Buskirk M: Determinants and protective potential of coronary arterial collaterals as assessed by an angioplasty model. Am J Cardiol 1988;61:677-684.

37. Lim M, Ziaee A, Kern M: Collateral vessel physiology and functional impact: In vivo assessment of collateral channels. Coronary Artery Disease 2004;15:379-388.

38. Reis SE, Holubkov R, Lee JS, et al: Coronary flow velocity response to adenosine characterizes coronary microvascular function in women with chest pain and no obstructive coronary disease: Results from the pilot phase of the Women's Ischemia Syndrome Evaluation (WISE) study. J Am Coll Cardiol 1999;33:1469-1475.

39. Hasdai D, Holmes DR Jr, Higano ST, et al: Prevalence of coronary blood flow reserve abnormalities among patients with nonobstructive coronary artery disease and chest pain. Mayo Clin Proc 1998;73:1133-1140.

40. Selke FW, Armstrong ML, Harrison DG: Endothelium-dependent vascular relaxation is abnormal in the coronary microcirculation of atherosclerotic primates. Circulation 1990;81:1586-1593.

41. Zeiher AM, Drexler H, Wollschläger H, Just H: Endothelial dysfunction of the coronary microvasculature is associated with impaired coronary blood flow regulation in patients with early atherosclerosis. Circulation 1991;84:1984-1992.

42. Reddy KG, Nair RN, Sheehan HM, Hodgson JM: Evidence that selective endothelial dysfunction may occur in the absence of angiographic or ultrasound atherosclerosis in patients with risk factors for atherosclerosis. J Am Coll Cardiol 1994;24:833-843.

43. Suwaidi JA, Hamasaki S, Higano ST, et al: Long-term follow-up of patients with mild coronary artery disease and endothelial dysfunction. Circulation 2000;101:948-954.

44. Vita JA, Yeung AC, Winniford M, et al: Effect of cholesterol-lowering therapy on coronary endothelial vasomotor function

in patients with coronary artery disease. Circulation 2000;102:846-851.

45. Hamasaki S, Higano ST, Suwaidi JA, et al: Cholesterol-lowering treatment is associated with improvement in coronary vascular remodeling and endothelial function in patients with normal or mildly diseased coronary arteries. Arterioscler Thromb Vasc Biol 2000;20:737-743.

46. Hambrecht R, Wolf A, Gielen S, et al: Effect of exercise on coronary endothelial function in patients with coronary artery disease. N Engl J Med 2000;342:454-460.

47. Mancini GB, Cleary RM, DeBoe SF, et al: Instantaneous hyperemic flow-versus-pressure slope index: Microsphere validation of an alternative to measures of coronary reserve. Circulation 1991;84:862-870.

48. Mancini GB, McGillem MJ, DeBoe SF, Gallagher KP: The diastolic hyperemic flow versus pressure relation: A new index of coronary stenosis severity and flow reserve. Circulation 1989;80:941-950.

49. Cleary RM, Moore NB, DeBoe SF, Mancini GBJ: Sensitivity and reproducibility of the instantaneous hyperemic flow versus pressure slope index compared to coronary flow reserve for the assessment of stenosis severity. Am Heart J 1993;126:57-65.

50. Cleary RM, Ayon D, Moore NB, et al: Tachycardia, contractility and volume loading alter conventional indexes of coronary flow reserve, but not the instantaneous hyperemic flow versus pressure slope index. J Am Coll Cardiol 1992;20:1261-1269.

51. Di Mario C, Krams R, Gil R, Serruys PW: Slope of the instantaneous hyperemic diastolic coronary flow velocity-pressure relation: A new index for assessment of the physiological significance of coronary stenosis in humans. Circulation 1994;90:1215-1224.

52. Ofili EO, Kern MJ, Labovitz AJ, et al: Analysis of coronary blood flow velocity dynamics in angiographically normal and stenosed arteries before and after endoluminal enlargement by angioplasty. J Am Coll Cardiol 1993;21:308-316.

53. Fearon WF, Balsam LB, Farouque HM, et al: Novel index for invasively assessing the coronary microcirculation. Circulation 2003;107:3129-3132.

54. Hernandez Garcia MJ, Alonso-Briales JH, Jimenez-Navarro M, et al: Clinical management of patients with coronary syndromes and negative fractional flow reserve findings. J Interv Cardiol 2001;14:505-509.

55. Rieber J, Schiele TM, Koenig A, et al: Long-term safety of therapy stratification in patients with intermediate coronary lesions based on intracoronary pressure measurements. Am J Cardiol 2002;90:1160-1164.

56. Chamuleau SAJ, Meuwissen M, van Eck-Smit BLF, et al: Fractional flow reserve, absolute and relative coronary blood flow velocity reserve in relation to the results of technetium-99m sestamibi single-photon emission computed tomography in patients with two-vessel coronary artery disease. J Am Coll Cardiol 2001;37:1316-1322.

57. Rieber J, Jung P, Schiele TM, et al: Safety of FFR-based treatment strategies: The Munich experience. Z Kardiol 2002;91:III115-III119.

58. Kern MJ, Donohue TJ, Aguirre FV, et al: Clinical outcome of deferring angioplasty in patients with normal translesional pressure-flow velocity measurements. J Am Coll Cardiol 1995;25:178-187.

59. Ferrari M, Schnell B, Werner GS, Figulla HR: Safety of deferring angioplasty in patients with normal coronary flow velocity reserve. J Am Coll Cardiol 1999;33:83-87.

60. Chamuleau SAJ, Tio RA, de Cock CC, et al: Prognostic value of coronary blood flow velocity and myocardial perfusion in intermediate coronary narrowings and multivessel disease. J Am Coll Cardiol 2002;39:852-858.

62 Intravascular Ultrasound

Yasuhiro Honda, Peter J. Fitzgerald, and Paul G. Yock

KEY POINTS

- Intravascular ultrasound (IVUS) has provided significant insights into biologically mediated processes of the vasculature, such as the extent of plaque burden, vascular remodeling, and restenosis.
- IVUS has proved to be a practically useful tool in the evaluation and guidance of interventional techniques, including balloon angioplasty, debulking techniques, conventional stenting, brachytherapy, and, most recently, drug-eluting stents.

- Improvements in core IVUS technology have allowed for higher-resolution images and greater operator convenience.
- Advanced technical developments currently being explored may further enhance the utility of IVUS in both research and clinical arenas of future interventional cardiology, particularly with sophisticated therapeutic technologies to modify local vascular biology.

Intravascular ultrasound (IVUS) imaging has provided, for the first time, a clinical method to directly visualize atherosclerosis and other pathologic conditions within the walls of blood vessels. Because the ultrasound signal is able to penetrate below the luminal surface, the entire cross-section of an artery—including the complete thickness of a plaque—can be imaged in real time. This offers the opportunity to gather diagnostic information about the process of atherosclerosis and to directly observe the effects of various interventions on the plaque and arterial wall.

The first ultrasound imaging catheter system was developed by Bom and colleagues in Rotterdam in 1971 for intracardiac imaging of chambers and valves.[1,2] In the early to mid-1980s, several groups began work on different catheter systems designed to image plaque and facilitate balloon angioplasty and other catheter-based interventions.[3-7] The first images of human vessels were recorded by Yock and colleagues in 1988,[8] with coronary images produced the next year by the same group[9] and by Hodgson and colleagues.[10] The intervening period has seen rapid technical improvements of the systems, with significant enhancement in image quality and miniaturization of the imaging catheters.

IMAGING SYSTEMS AND PROCEDURES

IVUS imaging systems use reflected sound waves to visualize the vessel wall in a two-dimensional, tomographic format, analogous to a histologic cross-section. These systems use significantly higher frequencies than noninvasive echocardiography, achieving greater radial resolutions at the expense of limited beam penetration. The resolution, depth of penetration, and attenuation of the acoustic pulse by tissue are dependent on the geometric and frequency properties of the transducer. Current IVUS catheters used in the coronary arteries have center frequencies ranging from 20 to 45 MHz, providing theoretical lower limits of resolution (calculated as half the wavelength) of 31 and 19 μm, respectively. In practice, the radial resolution is at least two to five times poorer, determined by factors such as the length of the emitted pulse and the position of the imaged structures relative to the transducer.

Catheter Design and Imaging Procedures

There are two basic catheter designs, based on solid-state or mechanical approaches (Fig. 62-1). Both types of catheters generate a 360-degree, cross-sectional image plane that is perpendicular to the catheter tip.

Solid-State Dynamic Aperture System

In the solid-state approach, the individual elements of a circumferential array of transducer elements mounted near the tip of the catheter are activated with different time delays, to create an ultrasound

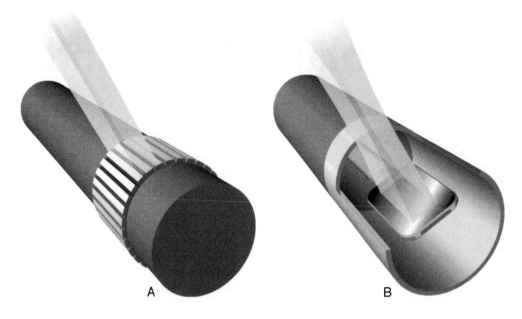

Figure 62-1. Diagrams of the two basic imaging catheter designs, solid state (**A**) and mechanical (**B**).

beam that sweeps the circumference of the vessel. As the number of elements has increased, there have been progressive improvements in lateral resolution. Complex miniaturized integrated circuits in the catheter tip control the timing and integration of the transducer activation and route the resulting echocardiographic information to a computer, where cross-sectional images are reconstructed and displayed in real time. In addition to the absence of any moving parts, one of the advantages of the multielement approach is the ability to manipulate the beam electronically—achieving, for example, the ability to focus at different depths.

The current solid-state coronary catheter system (Volcano Therapeutics, Inc., Rancho Cordova, CA) has 64 transducer elements arranged around the catheter tip and uses a center frequency of 20 MHz. The latest coronary catheters in a rapid-exchange configuration are 2.9 Fr and thus compatible with a 5-Fr guiding catheter. Larger peripheral imaging catheters are produced in both over-the-wire and rapid-exchange configurations. As an exception, a phased-array catheter (8-Fr or 10-Fr) for intracardiac echocardiographic imaging (Siemens Medical Solutions USA, Malvern, PA) uses a different technology, adapted from transesophageal echocardiography, that provides a sector ultrasound image with color and spectral Doppler capabilities. The catheter is compatible with multiple-frequency imaging (5.0 to 10 MHz) so that the operator can determine the desired tradeoff between resolution and penetration (up to 15 cm).

Setup of the solid-state catheter is straightforward: A thin cable connector is passed off the sterile field to attach to a pole-mounted remote unit. This, in turn, is connected to the system cart with a monitor, videotape recorder, and digital storage capacity. Before IVUS imaging, an intravenous injection of 5,000 to 10,000 U heparin or equivalent anticoagula-tion should be administered, as well as intracoronary nitroglycerine (100 to 300 μg), to reduce the potential for spasm. Because the solid-state transducer has a zone of "ring-down artifact" encircling the catheter, an extra step is required to form a mask of the artifact and subtract this from the image. The mask is usually acquired by disengaging the guiding catheter from the ostium and positioning the tip of the imaging catheter free in the aorta. The imaging element is then advanced distal to the area of interest, and the length of the target vessel is scanned by a motorized or manual withdrawal of the entire catheter over a standard 0.014-inch angioplasty guide wire.

Mechanically Rotating Single-Transducer System

In the mechanical approach, a single transducer element is rotated inside the tip of a catheter via a flexible torque cable spun by an external motor drive unit attached to the proximal end of the catheter. Images from each angular position of the transducer are collected by a computerized image array processor, which synthesizes a cross-sectional ultrasound image of the vessel.

The mechanical IVUS system is available commercially from two manufacturers in the United States and one in Japan. The imaging catheters use a 40- or 45-MHz transducer with a distal crossing profile of 3.2 Fr (compatible with 6-Fr guiding catheters). Larger catheters with lower center frequencies are also available for peripheral and intracardiac echocardiographic imaging. The catheters are advanced over a standard guide wire using a short rail section at the catheter tip. The length of the target vessel is scanned by retracting the rotating transducer manually or mechanically within a stationary outer sheath at the distal end of the catheter (Boston Scientific

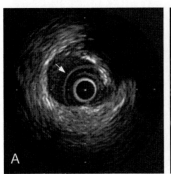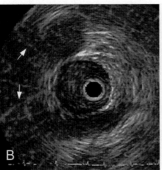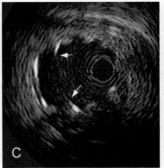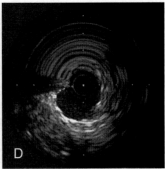

Figure 62-2. Common image artifacts. **A,** A "halo" or a series of bright rings immediately around the mechanical intravascular ultrasound (IVUS) catheter (*arrow*) is usually caused by air bubbles that need to be flushed out. **B,** Radiofrequency noise (*arrows*) appears as alternating radial spokes or random white dots in the far-field. The interference is usually caused by other electrical equipment in the catheterization laboratory. **C,** "White cap" artifacts caused by side lobe echoes (*arrows*) originate from a strong reflecting surface, such as metal stent struts or calcification. The smearing of the strut image can lead to the mistaken impression that the struts are protruding into the lumen, potentially interfering with area measurements and the assessment of apposition, dissection, and so on. **D,** Non-uniform rotational distortion (NURD) results in a wedge-shaped, smeared appearance in one or more segments of the image (between 9 and 4 o'clock in this example).

Corporation, Natick, MA; Volcano Therapeutics) or by moving the catheter itself (Terumo Corporation, Tokyo, Japan). The fact that the guide wire runs outside the catheter, parallel to the imaging segment, results in a shadow artifact in the image (the so-called guide wire artifact).

Use of mechanical catheters is similar to the use of solid-state catheters, except that mechanical catheters require flushing with saline before insertion to eliminate any air in the path of the beam. Incomplete flushing can leave microbubbles adjacent to the transducer, resulting in poor image quality once the catheter is inserted (Fig. 62-2). Non-uniform rotational distortion (NURD) can occur when bending of the drive cable interferes with uniform transducer rotation, causing a wedge-shaped, smeared image to appear in one or more segments of the image. This may be corrected by straightening the catheter and motor drive assembly, lessening tension on the guiding catheter, or loosening the hemostatic valve of the Y-adapter.

Head-to-Head Comparisons

Mechanical transducers have traditionally offered advantages in image quality compared with the solid-state systems, although this gap has narrowed in recent years. In general, mechanical catheters have excellent near-field resolution and do not require the subtraction of a mask. At the procedure, the short rail design of the mechanical systems may not track as well as the longer rapid-exchange, solid-state catheter. On the other hand, mechanical catheters with a stationary outer sheath are easy to use with a motorized pullback device, allowing the transducer to be moved through a segment of interest in a precise and controlled manner. The use of motorized pullback is important for two reasons: it gives the ability to measure the length of a given segment or register the

position of a given cross-section for repeat studies,[11] and it provides the potential for a reasonably accurate longitudinal or three-dimensional representation of a segment. With both systems, still frames and video images can be digitally archived on local storage memory or a remote server using Digital Imaging and Communications in Medicine (DICOM) Standard 3.0.

IMAGE INTERPRETATION

Three-Layered Appearance of Arterial Wall

The interpretation of IVUS images relies on the fact that the layers of a diseased arterial wall can be identified separately. Particularly in muscular arteries, such as the coronary tree, the media of the vessel stands out as a dark band compared with the intima and adventitia (Fig. 62-3).[12,13] Media are less distinctly seen by IVUS in elastic arteries such as the aorta and carotid, so differentiation of the layers in those vessels can be problematic.[14] However, most of the vessels currently treated by catheter techniques are muscular or transitional, and identification of the medial layer is usually possible (this includes the coronary, iliofemoral, renal, and popliteal systems).

The relative echolucency of media compared with intima and adventitia gives rise to a three-layered appearance (bright-dark-bright), first described in vitro by Meyer and colleagues[15] and subsequently confirmed in vivo.[16] The lower ultrasound reflectance of the media is due to the presence of less collagen and elastin than in the neighboring layers. Because the intimal layer reflects ultrasound more strongly than the media, a spillover effect, known as "blooming," is seen in the image. This results in a slight overestimation of the thickness of the intima and a corresponding underestimation of the medial thickness. On the other hand, the media/adventitia border

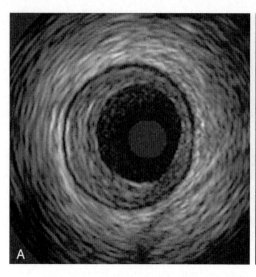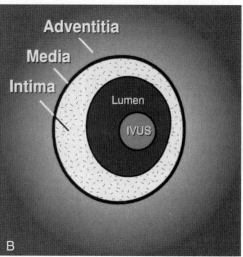

Figure 62-3. Intravascular ultrasound (IVUS) image **(A)** and schematic diagram **(B)** demonstrate the classic three-layered appearance of intima (plaque), media, and adventitia. In many cases, the media can be difficult to resolve clearly in some portion of the image, but in this particular image, it stands out in all sectors. Note the speckled appearance of the blood within the lumen, particularly near the luminal border.

is accurately rendered, because a step-up in echo reflectivity occurs at this boundary and no blooming appears. The adventitia and periadventitial tissues are similar enough in echoreflectivity that a clear outer adventitial border cannot be defined.

Several deviations from the classic three-layered appearance are encountered in practice. In truly normal coronary arteries from young patients, echoreflectivity of the intima and internal lamina may not be sufficient to resolve a clear inner layer.[17] This is particularly true when the media has a relatively high content of elastin.[18] However, most adults seen in the cardiac catheterization laboratory have enough intimal thickening to show a three-layered appearance, even in angiographically normal segments (Fig. 62-4). At the other end of the spectrum, patients with a significant plaque burden have thin-

ning of the media underlying the plaque,[5,19,20] often to the degree that the media is indistinct or undetectable in at least some part of the IVUS cross-section. This problem is exacerbated by the blooming phenomenon. Even in these cases, however, the inner adventitial boundary (at the level of the external elastic lamina) is always clearly defined. For this reason, most IVUS studies measure and report the plaque-plus-media area as a surrogate measure for plaque area alone. Adding in the media represents only a tiny percentage increase of the total area of the plaque.

Unlike coronary angiograms, IVUS images have an intrinsic distance calibration, which is usually displayed as a grid on the image. Electronic caliper (diameter) and tracing (area) measurements can be performed at the tightest cross-section, as well as at

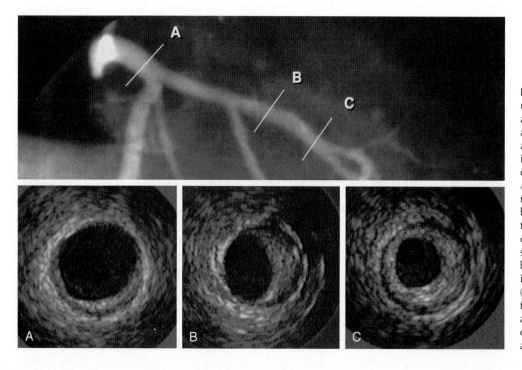

Figure 62-4. Intravascular ultrasound (IVUS) images from a transplantation patient with an almost normal-appearing angiogram *(top)*. **A,** The IVUS image from the left main coronary artery (cross-section A on the angiogram) shows minimal plaque accumulation between 2 and 9 o'clock. **B,** In the left anterior descending coronary artery, the IVUS image shows an eccentric plaque between 12 and 6 o'clock that is not evident on the angiogram (cross-section B). **C,** The image from cross-section C on the angiogram shows a more concentric plaque that also is angiographically undetected.

reference segments located proximal and distal to the lesion.[21] In general, the reference segment is selected as the most normal-looking cross-section (i.e., largest lumen with smallest plaque burden) occurring within 10 mm of the lesion with no intervening major side branches.

Vessel and lumen diameter measurements are important in everyday clinical practice, where accurate sizing of devices is needed. The maximum and minimum diameters (i.e., the major and minor axes of an elliptical cross-section) are the most widely used dimensions. The ratio of maximum to minimum diameter defines a measure of symmetry. Area measurements are performed with computer planimetry; lumen area is determined by tracing the leading edge of the blood/intima border, whereas vessel (or external elastic membrane [EEM]) area is defined as the area enclosed by the outermost interface between media and adventitia. Plaque area (or plaque-plus-media area) is calculated as the difference between the vessel and lumen areas; the ratio of plaque to vessel area is termed percent plaque area, plaque burden, or percent cross-sectional narrowing. With the use of motorized pullback, area measurements can be added to calculate volumes using Simpson's rule.

Plaque Composition

In addition to demonstrating the extent and distribution of plaque within the vessel wall, IVUS provides information about the composition of plaque.[22,23] Regions of calcification are very brightly echoreflective and create a dense shadow more peripherally from the catheter (Fig. 62-5).[5,24-26] Shadowing prevents determination of the true thickness of a calcific deposit and precludes visualization of structures in the tissue beyond the calcium. Another characteristic finding with calcification is reverberation, which causes the appearance of multiple ghost images of the leading calcium interface, spaced at regular intervals radially (see Fig. 62-5C). Like calcium, densely fibrotic tissue gives a bright appearance on the ultrasound scan and can cause shadowing. The brightness is less intense, however, and the beam penetrates a short distance into the tissue beyond the initial interface. The extent of shadowing depends on both the thickness and the density of the fibrotic region as well as the transducer strength. Fatty plaque is less echogenic than fibrous plaque. The brightness of the adventitia can be used as a gauge to discriminate predominantly fatty from fibrous plaque. An area of plaque that images darker than the adventitia is fatty. In an image of extremely good quality, the presence of a lipid pool can be inferred from the appearance of a dark region within the plaque.[5,7] However, not all hypoechoic zones within plaque represent lipid. False channels within the plaque can give a similar appearance, and, occasionally, shadowing from an adjacent region of calcification or fibrosis may look much like a lipid pool.[27]

One of the major limitations of IVUS in terms of identifying tissue is the difficulty in discriminating thrombus from soft plaque.[28] This is a complementary strength for angioscopy, whose color capability makes identification of thrombus at the luminal surface relatively easy. On ultrasound scanning, clues to the presence of thrombus are useful in some cases. Fresh thrombus can exhibit a scintillating tissue appearance that is fairly characteristic. Thrombus is much more likely than soft plaque to have the appearance of clefts or microchannels. In favorable cases, a thrombus has an undulating motion during the pulse cycle that is not seen with plaque. Computer-enhanced processing of the raw ultrasound signal promises to help in the discrimination between thrombus and plaque.[29-33]

Image Orientation

One important aspect of image interpretation is determining the position of the imaging plane within the artery. The IVUS beam penetrates beyond the artery, providing images of perivascular structures, including the cardiac veins, myocardium, and pericardium.[34] These structures have a characteristic

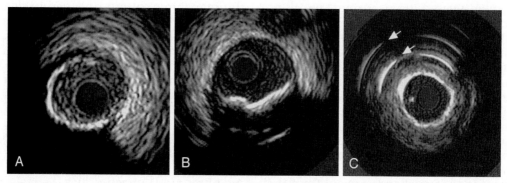

Figure 62-5. Examples of coronary calcification. **A,** A rim of calcium is seen between 5 and 10 o'clock, located beneath a fibrofatty plaque that tightly surrounds the catheter. Note the shadowing beyond the calcium. **B,** Superficial calcium (between 3 and 7 o'clock) at the luminal surface. The speckles within the lumen are signals from blood. **C,** Circumferential, "napkin ring" calcification. Two arcs of reverberation are seen *(arrows)*, and another pair of reverberations is seen to the right of the arrows. The small bright point adjacent to the catheter at 8:30 o'clock is the guide wire artifact from this mechanical catheter.

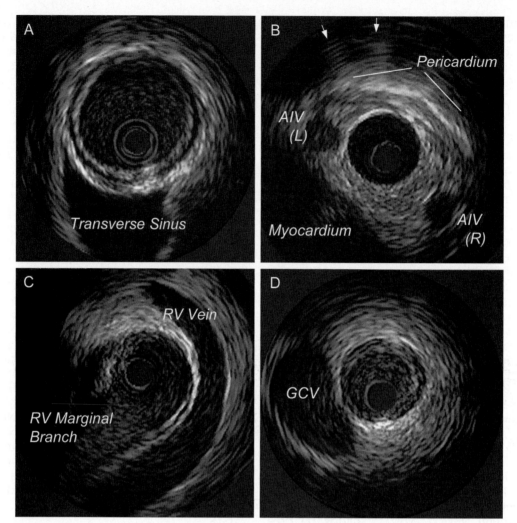

Figure 62-6. Perivascular landmarks. **A,** In the proximal portion of the left main coronary artery, a clear echo-free space filled with pericardial fluid, called the transverse sinus, is found adjacent to the artery, immediately outside of the left lateral aspect of the aortic root. **B,** In this distal cross-section from the left anterior descending coronary artery (LAD), the right (R) and left (L) branches of the anterior interventricular vein (AIV) are seen to straddle the coronary artery. The pericardium appears as a typical bright stripe with rays emitting from it *(arrows)*. **C,** At the level of the middle right coronary artery, the veins arc over the artery, typically at a position just adjacent to the right ventricular (RV) marginal branches. **D,** The great cardiac vein (GCV), running superiorly to the left circumflex coronary artery (LCx), appears as a large, low-echoic structure with fine blood speckle. The recurrent atrial branches emerge from the LCx in an orientation directed toward the GCV, whereas the obtuse marginal branches emerge opposite the GCV and course inferiorly to cover the lateral myocardial wall.

appearance when viewed from various positions within the arterial tree, so they provide useful landmarks regarding the position of the imaging plane (Fig. 62-6). The branching patterns of the arteries are also distinctive and help identify the position of the transducer. In the left anterior descending (LAD) coronary artery system, for example, the septal perforators usually branch at a wider angle than the diagonals; on the IVUS scan, the septals appear to bud away from the LAD much more abruptly than the diagonals. The combination of perivascular landmarks and branching patterns allows the experienced operator to identify the vessel and segment from the IVUS image alone. It is also important to understand that, with current systems, the rotational orientation of an IVUS image as presented on the screen is arbitrary and can vary between imaging runs. Here again,

the branching pattern and perivascular landmarks, once understood, can provide a reference to the actual orientation of the image in space. Some operators prefer to have a standard rotational orientation for each imaging run and take the time to adjust the presentation on the screen by rotating it electronically, so that the branches always appear in a uniform position.

INSIGHTS INTO PLAQUE FORMATION AND DISTRIBUTION

As ultrasound imaging has actively entered the cardiac catheterization laboratory, some of the classic pathologic findings in arterial disease have been "rediscovered" in vivo by interventionalists. The single most impressive finding from IVUS, in most cases, is the sheer bulk of plaque present in the artery.[35-40] In a vessel that appears to have a discrete stenosis by angiography, IVUS almost invariably shows considerable plaque burden throughout the entire length of the vessel. In fact, several IVUS studies have shown that the reference segment for an intervention—which by definition is normal or nearly normal angiographically—has, on average, 35% to 51% of its cross-sectional area occupied by plaque.[41] IVUS has also demonstrated significant limitations in the ability of angiography to characterize the degree of plaque eccentricity.[38,42] Phase I of the Guidance by Ultrasound Imaging for Decision Endpoints (GUIDE) trial compared the assessment of concentricity and eccentricity by angiography to an IVUS-determined eccentricity ratio of the thinnest to the thickest segment of plaque. In plaques that were judged to be concentric by angiography, there was a broad distribution of actual eccentricity ratios, from plaques with a ratio near 1:1 (truly concentric) to plaques with a ratio as low as 1:5 (highly eccentric). Conversely, many plaques judged to be eccentric by angiography were relatively concentric when viewed directly by IVUS. These findings may have important clinical implications, particularly when considering atherectomy, intracoronary brachytherapy, or other new catheter-based biologic treatment techniques targeting the plaque or adventitia of coronary arteries.

The phenomenon of remodeling, first described in human coronary specimens by the pathologist Glagov, is well illustrated in vivo by IVUS (Fig. 62-7A).[43-45] This classic form of remodeling is a localized expansion of the vessel wall in areas of high plaque burden—as if the vessel has stretched to accommodate the accumulation of plaque. IVUS studies have also added to the original descriptions in the pathology literature by demonstrating that the remodeling response is in fact bidirectional, with some segments showing the positive remodeling of the typical Glagov paradigm and others showing negative remodeling, or constriction, in the area of lumen stenosis (see Fig. 62-7B).[45-50] One important issue in evaluating this heterogeneous process by IVUS is the methodology used to quantify and categorize arterial remodeling. Although remodeling was originally conceptualized as a change in vessel size in response to plaque accumulation over time, most histomorphometry or IVUS studies have relied on measurements of reference sites as a surrogate for the size of the vessel before it became diseased. Therefore, results can vary distinctly according the choice of reference site as well as the manner of dealing with vessel tapering.[51] Theoretically, the use of the proximal reference, rather than the distal reference or the average of proximal and distal references, should preclude the potential influence of distal flow and pressure disturbance due to the presence of the IVUS catheter in the stenotic site. A remodeling index (the ratio of vessel area at the lesion site to that at the reference site) as a continuous variable may be also preferable to categorical classifications, because arte-rial remodeling is considered to be a continuous biologic process. In fact, this remodeling index has been shown to conform to the normal frequency distribution in patients with chronic stable angina.[48]

The assessment of remodeling is clinically important, not only for optimal therapeutic device sizing but also for risk stratification regarding plaque rupture or procedural and long-term outcomes of intervention. The "hot" lesions responsible for unstable angina or acute coronary syndromes have usually undergone extensive positive remodeling.[52-57] A histopathologic study by Pasterkamp and colleagues supported these clinical IVUS observations by demonstrating that positive remodeling is frequently associated with large, soft, lipid-rich plaques with increased inflammatory cell infiltrate.[58] In addition, remodeling appears to have specific relevance to interventional procedures. One IVUS study reported an association between preinterventional positive remodeling and creatine kinase elevation after intervention—a marker of distal embolization and future adverse cardiac events.[59] Furthermore, several other investigators directly showed that preinterventional positive remodeling assessed by IVUS predicts target lesion revascularization after coronary interventions.[60-64] Although the predictive values of these parameters in the context of stenting have not been established with certainty,[63-69] preinterventional IVUS may identify lesions with significant positive remodeling, providing triage information for increased risk of unfavorable outcomes and possible need of adjunctive biologic modalities for antirestenosis therapy.

INTERVENTIONAL APPLICATIONS

Preinterventional Imaging

Preinterventional IVUS has been used to clarify situations in which angiography is equivocal or difficult to interpret (especially in ostial lesions or tortuous segments in which the angiogram may not lay out the vessel well for interpretation). For intermediate lesions, careful IVUS measurement is made of the minimum lumen area (MLA) compared to the proximal and distal reference lumen areas. The ischemic MLA threshold is 3 to 4 mm^2 for major epicardial coronary arteries[70-73] and 5.5 to 6 mm^2 for the left main coronary artery,[74] based on physiologic assessment with coronary flow reserve, fractional flow reserve, or stress scintigraphy. The mere presence of plaque in coronary arteries by IVUS does not justify coronary revascularization, because plaque burden can be high in areas of minimal stenosis that do not warrant treatment.

Preinterventional IVUS imaging is also useful in determining the appropriate catheter-based intervention strategy. With current IVUS catheters, most of the significant stenoses can be safely imaged before intervention, providing detailed information about the circumferential and longitudinal extent of plaque as well as the character of the tissue involved. This can lead to a change in interventional strategy in

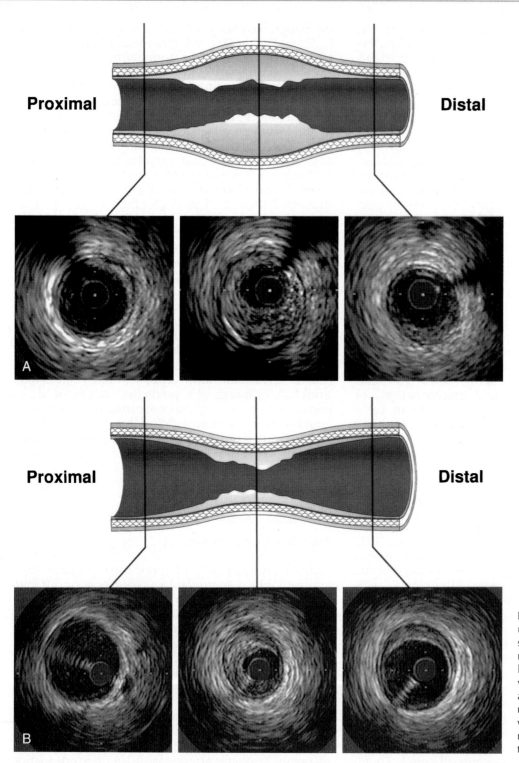

Figure 62-7. Intravascular ultrasound (IVUS) images showing remodeling. **A,** Glagov remodeling, in which there is localized expansion of the vessel in the area of plaque accumulation. **B,** Negative remodeling or shrinkage, in which the lesion has a smaller media-to-media diameter than the adjacent, less diseased sites.

20% to 40% of cases.[75,76] In particular, the presence, location, and extent of calcium can significantly affect the results of balloon angioplasty, atherectomy, and stent deployment. The amount and distribution of plaque can be accurately determined and may favor atheroablative procedures as primary or adjunctive treatment. Precise measurements of lesion length and vessel size can guide the optimal sizing of devices to be employed. Detailed assessment of target lesion anatomy in the coronary tree is also useful to prevent major side branch encroachment by intervention.

Balloon Angioplasty

Insights into Mechanism of Action

IVUS imaging of percutaneous transluminal coronary angioplasty (PTCA) sites demonstrates plaque

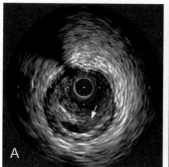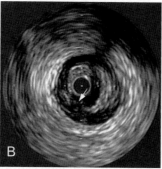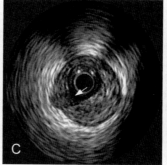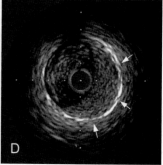

Figure 62-8. Four examples of dissections. **A,** A superficial (intimal) dissection starting at 6 o'clock and extending clockwise. The dissection flap does not extend far into the lumen. **B,** A deeper (medial) dissection with a flap extending into the lumen may compromise flow or precede abrupt closure. Injection of contrast in this setting can demonstrate free fluid flow behind the flap to better define the extent of tear. **C,** Eccentric plaque with a deep (adventitial) dissection at 8 o'clock that penetrates the external elastic lamina and extends into the adventitia. **D,** Intramural hematoma appears as an accumulation of blood within the medial space, displacing the internal elastic membrane inward and the external elastic membrane outward.

disruption or dissection more often than angiography does (40% to 70% of cases, versus 20% to 40% by angiography).[42,77-81] IVUS is able to characterize the depth and extent of dissections created by balloon inflation with relatively high accuracy.[77,81,82] Although the extent of dissections is relatively unpredictable,[83] it is frequently possible to predict where tears will occur, based on certain morphologic features shown by IVUS. If a plaque deposit is eccentric, tears usually occur at the junction between the plaque and the normal wall (Fig. 62-8). This is presumably because the nondiseased wall is more elastic than the plaque, and, with balloon inflation, it stretches away from the plaque, creating a cleavage plane running either within the media or within the plaque substance, close to the media. Another important factor in determining the location of tears is the presence of localized calcium deposits.[84] During balloon inflation, shear forces are highest at the junction between the calcium and softer, surrounding plaque.[85,86] This creates an "epicenter" for the start of a tear, which then extends out to the lumen. Interestingly, one IVUS study suggested that the size and location of dissections after cutting balloon angioplasty were relatively independent of calcium deposits, compared with those produced by conventional balloon angioplasty.[87] In lesions with localized calcification, cutting balloon angioplasty may be preferable, owing to its controlled tearing, to avoid the risk of unfavorable large dissections. Creating dissections in a controlled manner may also be beneficial to lessen acute elastic recoil after balloon angioplasty. Data from phase I of the GUIDE trial showed that the lesions with tears had less recoil than lesions that had not torn, suggesting that plaque tearing may effectively act to release the diseased segment from the mechanical constriction process caused by the plaque.[42]

Guidance of Procedures

A direct approach to balloon sizing, based on IVUS images, was pursued by the Clinical Outcomes with Ultrasound Trial (CLOUT) investigators, who reasoned that more aggressive balloon sizing might be more safely accomplished using the "true" vessel size and plaque characteristics as determined by IVUS.[88] In this prospective, nonrandomized study, balloon sizes were chosen to equal the average of the reference lumen and media-to-media diameters for cases in which the plaques were not extensively calcified. This led to an average 0.5-mm "oversizing" of the balloon, compared with sizing based on the standard angiographic criteria, and resulted in a significant decrease in postprocedure residual stenoses (from 28% to 18%). Importantly, there was no increase in clinically significant complications from this aggressive balloon sizing approach. One-year follow-up of this trial showed a late adverse event rate (death, myocardial infarction, or target lesion revascularization) of 22%.[89] More recently, this IVUS-guided aggressive PTCA strategy was expanded and confirmed by two single-center studies of provisional stenting, wherein balloon sizing was performed based on IVUS measurements of media-to-media diameter at the lesion site.[90,91] Angiographic or clinical follow-up of these studies also showed long-term outcomes equivalent to those of elective stenting.

Insights into Long-Term Outcomes

Several clinical trials have addressed IVUS predictors of outcome after PTCA. In the Post-Intracoronary Treatment Ultrasound Result Evaluation (PICTURE) trial, morphometric IVUS parameters were significantly related to angiographic minimum lumen diameter (MLD) at follow-up, but these factors were not statistically related to a 50% or greater categorical restenosis threshold.[92] Interestingly, in this 200-patient trial, angiographic MLD and percent diameter stenosis were strongly related to categorical restenosis. The authors pointed out in the discussion that the relatively large size and limited imaging quality of the first-generation IVUS catheters used in this study may have influenced the results. In a single-center study of 360 nonstented native coronary lesions, Mintz and colleagues showed that the percent plaque area (plaque area divided by vessel area × 100), as assessed by IVUS, was strongly related to binary restenosis, follow-up diameter stenosis, and late lumen loss.[93] Phase II of the GUIDE trial confirmed the potential significance of these findings by the analysis of 524 follow-up studies obtained from 22 institutions in the United States and Europe.[94] Six-month follow-up of this trial revealed that no morphologic variable (e.g., presence or type of dissection, calcification) was predictive of outcome. On the other hand, the percent plaque area after intervention was the *single* most powerful predictor of outcome among all of the angiographic and ultrasound variables tested. IVUS-determined MLD was also significantly predictive of restenosis. In combination, these studies suggest that residual plaque burden may be a more powerful predictor of restenosis after PTCA or atherectomy than standard clinical or angiographic variables.

Atherectomy

Insights into Mechanism of Action

Initial studies from our group suggested that there is a large residual plaque detected by IVUS after angiographically successful directional coronary atherectomy (DCA).[95] The discrepancy between the angiographic and IVUS assessment of plaque burden after atherectomy is largely due to two of the factors mentioned earlier: the remodeling phenomenon (with expansion of the vessel in the area of the lesion) and the fact that the angiographically "normal" reference segment has a significant plaque burden (causing the percent stenosis comparison to underestimate plaque burden in the lesion). In addition to these factors, it has been shown that the lumen expansion seen with DCA occurs partly as a result of mechanical expansion or "Dottering" of the lesion as well as extraction of plaque. This Dotter effect has been estimated to account for 50% of lumen expansion by angiographic studies[96,97] and between 30% and 40% by IVUS studies.[98,99]

As in the case of balloon angioplasty, the presence and location of calcium within the lesion has a powerful impact on the performance of the DCA device. Severe calcification seen on fluoroscopy, within and proximal to the lesion, is a well-recognized relative contraindication for DCA, in part because device delivery to the target lesion may be difficult. What is striking from IVUS studies, however, is that the *level* of the calcium deposition within the lesion is a major determinant of the success of tissue retrieval. Calcium that is located superficially (see Figs. 62-5B,C) is difficult for the conventional DCA device to remove. In a study comparing tissue weights extracted from lesions with no calcification, deep calcium, or superficial calcium, tissue retrieval was shown to be reduced by almost half in the presence of superficial calcification.[100-102] Improvements in the latest DCA device

with a titanium nitride–coated cutter—as well as the advent of a completely redesigned atherectomy device—may translate into greater success rates in this lesion subset.

On the other hand, rotational atherectomy is highly effective in treating superficial calcification. Studies from Mintz and colleagues showed that, in hard plaque, the neolumen created by the device is round and regular, with essentially the same diameter as the definitive burr.[103-105] Conversely, in soft plaque, the postprocedure lumen is typically less round and may be significantly smaller than the burr used, perhaps owing to some combination of less effective debulking and spasm. In our day-to-day experience with rotational ablation, the choice of burr size is frequently influenced by the images, usually in the direction of more aggressive burrs earlier in the procedure. IVUS is also useful in clarifying the issue of guide wire bias, in which the burr cuts a trough in one side of the vessel wall.

Guidance of Procedures

The ability of IVUS to directly assess the extent and distribution of plaque provides a natural link to the guidance of DCA. One practical issue in applying imaging to DCA is how to orient the atherectomy catheter toward the maximal accumulation of plaque seen with IVUS.[106] In practice, the location of branches on the ultrasound scan is the most useful cue for orienting the device. A branch near the plaque is identified on the ultrasound image, and the rotational orientation of the deepest portion of the plaque is gauged, relative to the branch. Once the atherectomy device is inserted, the housing is rotated the corresponding number of degrees clockwise or counterclockwise from the branch. Serial IVUS examination with repeated orientation is required for aggressive debulking.

Insights into Long-Term Outcomes

DCA trials conducted with IVUS investigation provide an interesting composite picture of the impact of residual plaque burden on the long-term outcome of the procedure. During the Coronary Angioplasty Versus Excision Atherectomy Trial (CAVEAT) era of atherectomy, the relatively conservative approach to plaque removal was associated with residual plaque areas by IVUS of 60% or greater. The angiographic restenosis rates were correspondingly high at 50%.[107] In the Optimal Atherectomy Restenosis Study (OARS), more aggressive atherectomy was performed, to an angiographic end point of 10% residual stenosis, yet with a residual percent plaque area of 58% and a restenosis rate of 29%.[99] In a third study, the Adjunctive Balloon Angioplasty following Coronary Atherectomy Study (ABACAS), even lower plaque residuals were achieved using IVUS guidance (46% in the DCA group and 43% in the adjunctive balloon group), with a resulting restenosis rate of 21%.[108] These findings were confirmed in the contemporary series of the Stent versus Directional Coronary Atherectomy Randomized Trial (START).[109] When considered together, these studies suggest that a technique that could effectively remove relatively large amounts of plaque (with a residual of 50% or less) would have restenosis rates that are competitive with stenting. The ABACAS trial also provided some new insight into the impact of deep wall cutting (i.e., cutting into media or adventitia) on restenosis.[110] Segments with deep wall cuts on average had *lower* rates of recurrence than did lesions without deep wall invasion. However, some of the patients with subintimal cuts had local aneurysm formation.

IVUS studies after atherectomy and angioplasty have provided some other key insights into the mechanisms of restenosis. In addition to intimal proliferation, there is a second major process causing late lumen loss: shrinkage of the treated segment (Fig. 62-9), which is a form of remodeling similar to the process illustrated in Figure 62-7B.[111-114] By performing serial IVUS examinations at multiple intervals after DCA, Kimura and colleagues demonstrated that, overall, more than 60% of lumen loss at 6 months was caused by shrinkage, with the remainder caused by intimal proliferation.[114] It is unclear which factors may predispose a treated segment to restenosis, although remodeling, seen as an important mechanism of restenosis, has opened a new line of investigation into molecular mechanisms and potential therapies. Clearly, the shrinkage process is directly preventable by stenting. This probably accounts for the favorable restenosis rates seen with this technique, despite even greater degrees of intimal proliferation than with non-stent interventions.[112] A recent study of intracoronary radiation therapy (ICRT) also showed beneficial effects on remodeling at non-stented lesions.[115]

Bare Metal Stents

Insights into Mechanism of Action

Stent struts are easily visualized on IVUS examination as a collection of bright, distinct echoes, characteristic for each stent type. In contrast, the proliferative tissue within the stent struts has low echoreflectivity, similar to thrombus, so that optimal instrument settings are required to visualize the restenotic material clearly. Stents essentially provide a rigid scaffold against the force of vessel recoil. During stent implantation, axial extrusion of noncalcified plaque into the adjacent reference zones can occur (Fig. 62-10).[116-119] Mintz and colleagues demonstrated a similar phenomenon in balloon angioplasty.[120] However, the extrusion effect in stenting may be more prominent than for balloon angioplasty, commensurate with the increased ability of the stent to enlarge and hold open the treated segment. Extrusion of plaque may also contribute to the step-up/step-down appearance seen on angiography, as well as some of the side branch encroachment after stent deployment.

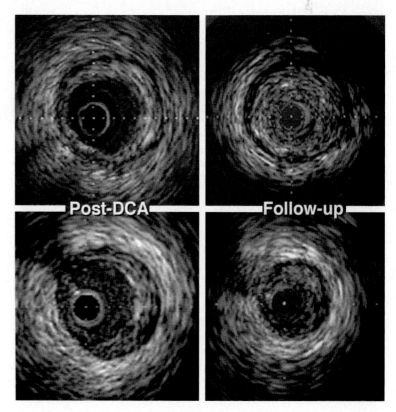

Figure 62-9. Two different mechanisms of restenosis as demonstrated by serial IVUS after non-stent intervention. *Top,* Extensive plaque proliferation leading to late lumen loss without a substantial change in the overall (media-to-media) dimensions of the vessel. *Bottom,* Negative remodeling or shrinkage is the major contributor to lumen loss.

Plaque Proliferation

Vessel Shrinkage

Post-DCA

Follow-up

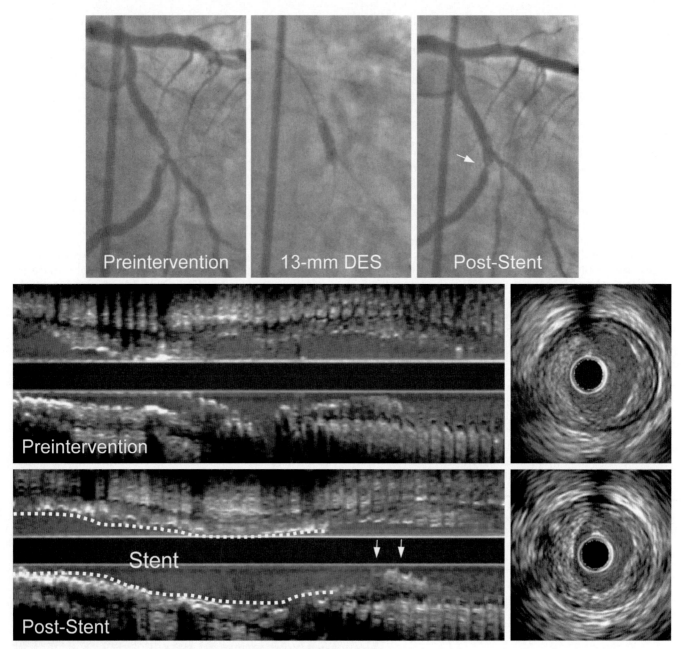

Figure 62-10. Plaque extrusion occurring as a result of stenting. The coronary angiogram taken immediately after stenting showed a new stenosis *(arrow)* at the distal adjacent segment to the implanted stent. Although spasm, dissection, and/or hematoma was suspected by angiography, intravascular ultrasound (IVUS) revealed that the secondary lesion was caused by a significant plaque increase *(arrows)*, presumably resulting from axial plaque redistribution, otherwise known as "plaque shift" from the stented segment into this region.

Guidance of Procedures

IVUS has identified several stent deployment issues, including incomplete expansion and incomplete apposition (Fig. 62-11). Incomplete expansion occurs when a portion of the stent is inadequately expanded compared with the distal and proximal reference dimensions, as may occur where dense fibrocalcific plaque is present. Incomplete apposition (seen in 3% to 15% of stent cases) occurs when part of the stent structure is not fully in contact with the vessel wall, possibly increasing local flow disturbances and the potential risk for subacute thrombosis in certain clin-

ical settings. The collaboration of Tobis and Colombo in the early 1990s demonstrated an unexpectedly high percentage of these stent deployment issues, leading to their development of the current high-pressure stent deployment techniques.[121,122]

After stent implantation, tears at the edge of the stent (marginal tears or pocket flaps) occur in 10% to 15% of cases (see Fig. 62-11).[123-125] These tears have been attributed to the shear forces created at the junction between the metal edge of the stent and the adjacent, more compliant tissue, or to the effect of balloon expansion beyond the edge of the stent (the "dog-bone" phenomenon). Although minor

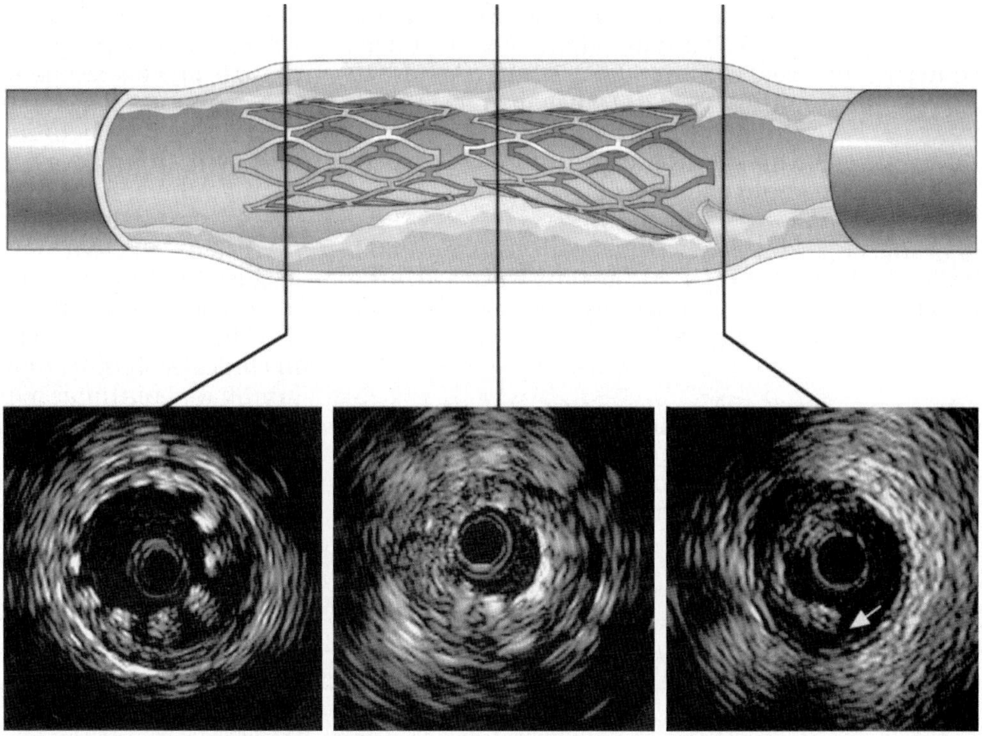

Figure 62-11. Problems with stent deployment detected by intravascular ultrasound (IVUS). The diagram indicates the cross-sections shown in the IVUS images. *Left,* Incomplete apposition, in which there is a gap between a portion of the stent and the vessel wall (between 12 and 7 o'clock on the IVUS image). The apparent thickness of the stent struts in this area is due to reverberations. *Middle,* Incomplete expansion relative to the ends of the stent and the reference segments. *Right,* An edge tear or "pocket flap" with a disruption of plaque at the stent margin *(arrow).*

non-flow-limiting edge dissections may not be associated with late angiographic in-stent restenosis, significant residual dissections can lead to an increased risk of early major adverse cardiac events.[126,127] The current practice in our laboratory is to make a determination from the IVUS image as to whether the tear appears to be flow-limiting (i.e., whether there is an extensive tissue arm projecting into the lumen). If this is the case, an additional stent is placed to cover this region.

Over the past decade, a number of studies have shown that IVUS-guided stent placement improves the clinical outcome of bare metal stents.[128-137] In the Multicenter Ultrasound-guided Stent Implantation in Coronaries (MUSIC) trial, IVUS-guided stenting required: (1) complete apposition over the entire stent length; (2) in-stent minimum stent area (MSA) greater than or equal to 90% of the average of the reference areas or 100% of the smallest reference area; and (3) symmetric stent expansion with the minimum/maximum lumen diameter ratio greater than or equal to 0.7.[138] Subacute thrombosis of less than 2% was believed to represent a reduction compared with nonguided deployment, although, with current antiplatelet regimens, similar results can usually be achieved by high-pressure postdilation without IVUS confirmation. Nevertheless, a number of studies have suggested a link between suboptimal stent implantation and stent thrombosis, including the Predictors and Outcomes of Stent Thrombosis (POST) registry, which demonstrated that 90% of thrombosis patients had suboptimal IVUS results (incomplete apposition, 47%; incomplete expansion, 52%; and evidence of thrombus, 24%), even though only 25% of patients had abnormalities on angiogra-

phy.[139] These observations were replicated in a more recent study by Cheneau and colleagues, which suggested that mechanical factors continue to contribute to stent thrombosis, even in this modern stent era, with optimized antiplatelet regimens.[140] Although the use of IVUS in all patients for the sole purpose of reducing thrombosis is clearly not warranted from a cost standpoint, IVUS imaging should be considered in patients who are at particularly high risk for thrombosis (e.g., slow flow) or in whom the consequences of thrombosis would be severe (e.g., left main coronary artery or equivalent).

MSA, as measured by IVUS, is one of the strongest predictors for both angiographic and clinical restenosis after bare metal stenting.[66,141-144] Kasaoka and colleagues indicated that the predicted risk of restenosis decreases 19% for every 1-mm^2 increase in MSA and suggested that stents with MSA greater than 9 mm^2 have a greatly reduced risk of restenosis.[143] In the Can Routine Ultrasound Improve Stent Expansion (CRUISE) trial, IVUS guidance by operator preferences increased MSA from 6.25 to 7.14 mm^2, leading to a 44% relative reduction in target vessel revascularization at 9 months, compared with angiographic guidance alone.[133] In the Angiography versus IVUS-Directed stent placement (AVID) trial, IVUS-guided stent implantation resulted in larger acute dimensions than angiography alone (7.54 versus 6.94 mm^2), without an increase in complications, and lower 12-month target lesion revascularization rates for vessels with angiographic reference diameter less than 3.25 mm, severe stenosis at preintervention (>70% angiographic diameter stenosis), and vein grafts.[132] However, controversial results were also reported in some IVUS-guided stent trials,[145,146] presumably due to differing procedural end points for IVUS-guided stenting, as well as various adjunctive treatment strategies that were used in these trials in response to suboptimal results (Table 62-1). Overall, a meta-analysis of 9 clinical studies (2972 patients) demonstrated that IVUS-guided stenting significantly lowers 6-month angiographic restenosis (odds ratio [OR] = 0.75, 95% confidence interval [CI], 0.60 to 0.94; P = .01) and target vessel revascularizations (OR = 0.62; 95% CI, 0.49 to 0.78; P = .00003), with a neutral effect on death and nonfatal myocardial infarction, compared to an angiographic optimization.[147]

Insights into Long-Term Outcomes

In-stent restenosis is primarily caused by intimal proliferation rather than chronic stent recoil.[112,148]

Growth of neointima is usually greatest in the areas with the largest plaque burden,[64,149,150] and the intimal growth process seems to be more aggressive in diabetic patients.[151] In the treatment of in-stent restenosis, IVUS can be helpful to differentiate pure intimal ingrowth from poor stent expansion, especially if ablative therapies are being considered. Using serial IVUS immediately before and after balloon angioplasty for in-stent restenosis, Castagna and colleagues[152] showed, in 1090 consecutive in-stent restenosis lesions, that 38% of lesions had an MSA of less than 6.0 mm². Stent underexpansion can result in clinically significant lumen compromise even with minimal neointimal hyperplasia. For this type of in-stent restenosis, mechanical optimization is appropriate in most cases.

IVUS can also track the response to treatment, with evidence that angioplasty of in-stent restenosis

Table 62-1. IVUS Versus Angiographic Guidance of Bare Metal Stent Implantation

Study* (Ref. No.)	N	Population	Study Design	IVUS Criteria for Optimal Expansion	Criteria Fulfilled	End Points	Results
Albiero et al. (128)	312	De novo, native	Multicenter, registry	Complete apposition, no ref disease, MSA ≥60% of average ref VA (early phase) or MSA ≥ distal ref LA (late phase)	NA	6-mo angiography	IVUS better (early phase)
Blasini et al. (129)	212	De novo and restenotic, native and SVG	Single center, registry	Complete apposition, no residual dissection, MSA >8 mm² and/or 90% of average ref LA	50%	6-mo angiography	IVUS better
Choi et al. (130)	278	De novo, native	Single center, registry	Complete apposition, no residual dissection, MSA ≥80% of distal ref LA	NA	Acute closure, 6-mo MACE	IVUS better
Gaster et al. (131)	108	De novo and restenotic, native	Single center, randomized	MUSIC criteria	64%	6-mo angiography, CFR, FFR, TVR; 2.5-yr MACE	IVUS better
AVID (132)	759	De novo, native and SVG	Multicenter, randomized	MUSIC criteria	NA	12-mo TLR	IVUS better (subset analysis)
CRUISE (133)	499	De novo and restenotic, native	Multicenter, nonrandomized	Discretion of individual institutional practice	—	9-mo TVR	IVUS better
OPTICUS (145)	550	De novo and restenotic, native	Multicenter, randomized	MUSIC criteria	56%	6-mo angiography, 12-mo MACE	No difference
PRESTO (146)	9070	De novo and restenotic, native	Multicenter, nonrandomized	Discretion of individual institutional practice	—	9-mo MACE	No difference
RESIST (134, 135)	155	De novo, native	Multicenter, randomized	MSA >80% of average ref LA	80%	6-mo angiography, 18-mo MACE	IVUS better (nonsignificant reduction)
SIPS (136)	269	De novo and restenotic, native	Single center, randomized	MLA >65% of average ref LA	69%	6-mo angiography, 2-yr TLR	IVUS better (2-year TLR)
TULIP (137)	144	Long lesions (>20 mm)	Single center, randomized	Complete apposition, MLD ≥80% of average ref diameter, MSA ≥ distal ref LA	89%	6-mo angiography, 12-mo MACE	IVUS better

*AVID, Angiography versus IVUS-Directed stent placement trial; CRUISE, Can Routine Ultrasound Influence Stent Expansion study; MUSIC, Multicenter Ultrasound guided Stent Implantation in Coronaries; OPTICUS, Optimization with ICUS to Reduce Stent Restenosis; PRESTO, Results of Prevention of REStenosis with Tranilast and its Outcomes Trial; RESIST, REStenosis after Intravascular ultrasound STenting; SIPS, Strategy for IVUS-Guided PTCA and Stenting; TULIP, Thrombocyte activity evaluation and effects of Ultrasound guidance in Long Intracoronary Stent Placement.
CFR, coronary flow reserve; FFR, fractional flow reserve; IVUS, intravascular ultrasound; LA, lumen area; MACE, major adverse cardiac events; MLD, minimum lumen diameter; MSA, minimum stent area; ref, reference vessel; SVG, saphenous vein graft; TLR, target lesion revascularization; TVR, target vessel revascularization; VA, vessel area.

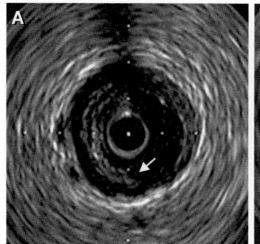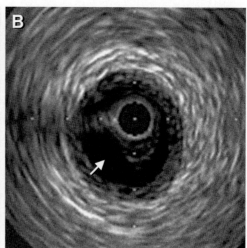

Figure 62-12. Arrows indicate unhealed dissection **(A)** and echolucent neointimal tissue, so-called acoustic hole or "black hole" **(B),** observed at follow-up after intracoronary radiation therapy.

is followed by early lumen loss due to decompression[153] and/or reintrusion[154] of tissue immediately after intervention. This phenomenon was more prominent in longer lesions and in those with greater in-stent tissue burden, which may partially account for the worse long-term outcomes in diffuse versus focal in-stent restenosis. Direct tissue removal, rather than tissue compression/extrusion through the stent struts, may help minimize early lumen loss due to this phenomenon. Several investigators have reported a considerable reduction in angiographic and/or clinical recurrence of in-stent restenosis in patients with diffuse in-stent restenosis treated with ablative therapies (DCA, rotational atherectomy, or laser angioplasty) compared with PTCA alone.[155-161]

Intracoronary Radiation Therapy

Insights into Mechanism of Action

ICRT, the first biologic treatment targeting excessive proliferative response of vascular smooth muscle cells to mechanical intervention, has undergone extensive clinical testing with IVUS characterization. Regardless of radiation source or delivery platform, most IVUS studies of ICRT in PTCA, stenting, and treatment of in-stent restenosis showed significant in-lesion or in-stent efficacy.[162-171] Serial IVUS investigations confirmed that these beneficial effects are primarily derived from decreased neointimal hyperplasia, but there is also an effect from accelerated positive remodeling at the irradiated segment.[115,162]

Guidance of Procedures

IVUS revealed that a combination of increased neointimal hyperplasia and either absence of positive remodeling or negative remodeling accounts for the unfavorable edge effect of ICRT.[172-174] Because, in catheter-based ICRT (not radioactive stents), most edge effects are related to inadequate coverage of injured edge segments (so-called geographic miss),[175]

IVUS guidance may greatly enhance the safety and efficacy of this highly geographically specific technique. A combined ICRT/imaging device was developed to facilitate the fine-tuning of catheter positioning.[176] This device also forms an asymmetric dose distribution to compensate for the eccentricity of the target plaque as well as the off-center position of the catheter in response to on-line IVUS guidance. Other investigator groups have developed detailed dosimetric analysis algorithms, based on dose-volume histograms derived from three-dimensional IVUS,[177-183] for optimal dose prescription.

Insights into Long-Term Outcomes

Unusual IVUS observations related to ICRT include unhealed dissections, late-acquired incomplete stent apposition, and acoustic holes (or "black holes")—that is, echolucent neointimal tissue. Delayed healing is commonly seen after brachytherapy in general. A substudy from the Beta Energy Restenosis Trial (BERT) reported that 8 (50%) of 16 dissections identified immediately after PTCA were still present at 6-month follow-up.[184] Similarly, an IVUS analysis from the Stents and Radiation Therapy (START) 40/20 trial showed that 43% of dissections had partially healed and 7% were unchanged over time (Fig. 62-12A).[185] Of note, previous nonradiation trials indicated that dissections seen after intervention normally heal within a 6-month follow-up period.[186-188] Late-acquired incomplete stent apposition was reported with both catheter-based ICRT (beta and gamma radiation) and radioactive stents (Fig. 62-13). Detailed serial IVUS examination revealed that this phenomenon is a result of excessive positive remodeling of the underlying vessel wall combined with significant neointimal inhibition.[189,190] Okura and colleagues also reported that late-acquired incomplete stent apposition appears to occur in segments with relatively little peri-stent plaque burden but high radiation dose exposure.[190] Late-acquired incomplete stent apposition can also be seen after mechanical vessel injury in nonradiation interventions (e.g.,

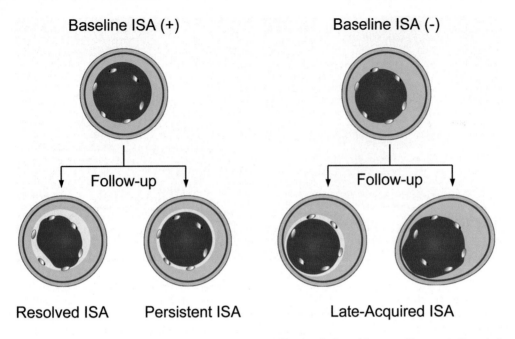

Baseline ISA (+)   Baseline ISA (-)

Follow-up   Follow-up

Resolved ISA   Persistent ISA   Late-Acquired ISA

Remodeling (-)   Remodeling (+)

Figure 62-13. Classification of incomplete stent apposition (ISA). Baseline ISA can either be resolved (resolved ISA) or remain (persistent ISA) at follow-up. Late-acquired ISA without vessel expansion is typically seen in thrombus-containing lesions, whereas late-acquired ISA with focal, positive vessel remodeling is more characteristic with brachytherapy and drug-eluting stents.

atherectomy plus stenting),[191] although delayed endothelialization by ICRT may lead to different clinical implications. The acoustic hole or "black hole" consists of echolucent neointimal tissue and has been seen in all types of ICRT (see Fig. 62-12B).[192] Post-ICRT specimens retrieved with DCA show large myxoid areas, with interspersed smooth muscle cells, scattered in a proteoglycan-containing extracellular matrix—findings that are compatible with a weak backscattering of echoes and a dark appearance on IVUS. These IVUS findings after ICRT are unique, but their exact clinical implications remain unknown.

Drug-Eluting Stents

Insights into Mechanism of Action

IVUS observations from the clinical experience with antiproliferative drug-eluting stents (DES) have shown a striking inhibition of in-stent neointimal hyperplasia, whereas the mechanical performances of these new stents are similar to those of conventional bare metal stents.[193-197] Additionally, both statistical and geographic distributions of neointimal hyperplasia can be significantly different between the biologic (DES) and mechanical (bare metal) stents. In general, neointimal volume (as a percentage of stent volume) within bare metal stents follows a near-Gaussian or normal frequency distribution, with a mean value of 30% to 35%. The standard deviation of this statistical distribution represents biologic variability in vascular response to acute and chronic vessel injury by interventions. In contrast, biologic modifications by DES often result in a non-Gaussian

frequency distribution, with variable degrees of the tail ends. Because restenosis corresponds to the right tail end of the distribution curve, a discrepancy between mean neointimal volume and binary or clinical restenosis can occur in DES trials.[194,198,199] Similarly, bare metal stents show a wide individual variation in geographic distribution of neointima along the stented segment,[200] whereas some types of DES demonstrate predilection of in-stent neointimal hyperplasia for specific locations (e.g., proximal stent edge).[201] In serial IVUS studies with multiple long-term follow-ups, neointima within nonrestenotic bare metal stents showed mild regression after 6 months.[202] In contrast, both sirolimus- and paclitaxel-eluting stents showed a slight but continuous increase in neointimal hyperplasia for up to 4 years.[203-206]

Guidance of Procedures

In DES, the fact that the drugs dramatically reduce the variability of the biologic response (neointimal proliferation) further strengthens the prognostic value of the MSA as a powerful predictor for in-stent restenosis.[207-211] This was well illustrated in recent IVUS work by Sonoda and colleagues, in which sirolimus-eluting stents showed a stronger positive relation, with a greater correlation coefficient between baseline MSA and 8-month MLA, compared to control bare metal stents (0.8 versus 0.65 and 0.92 versus 0.59, respectively).[207] The utility of IVUS to ensure adequate stent expansion cannot be overemphasized, particularly if there are clinical risk factors for DES failure (e.g., diabetes, renal failure).

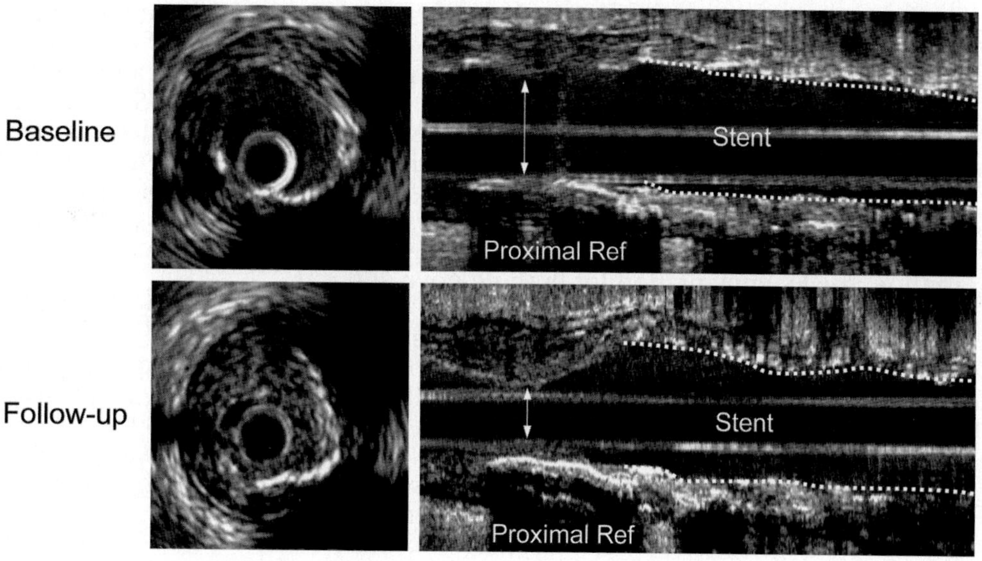

Figure 62-14. Proximal disease development 8 months after drug-eluting stent implantation. In this example, the new stenosis at the proximal stent margin is primarily caused by plaque proliferation, despite minimal neointimal hyperplasia observed inside the stent. Baseline intravascular ultrasound (IVUS) reveals a significant residual plaque at the corresponding uncovered segment.

In this context, preinterventional IVUS can also provide useful information about plaque composition. In particular, calcified plaque is important to identify, because the presence, degree, and location of calcium within the target vessel can substantially affect the delivery and subsequent deployment of coronary stents (see Fig. 62-5).[212,213] One important advantage of online IVUS guidance is the ability to assess the extent and distance from the lumen of calcium deposits within a plaque. For example, lesions with extensive superficial calcium may require rotational atherectomy before stenting.[213,214] Conversely, apparently significant calcification on fluoroscopy may subsequently be found by IVUS to be distributed in a deep portion of the vessel wall or to have a lower degree of calcification (calcium arc <180 degrees). In these cases, stand-alone stenting is usually adequate to achieve a lumen expansion large enough for a DES.

The discovery of "edge effects" associated with ICRT raised the concern of lumen narrowing in adjacent reference segments as a potential limitation of DES. However, current clinical experience with sirolimus- and paclitaxel-eluting stents has shown no accelerated edge restenosis overall, compared with conventional bare metal stents. A detailed serial IVUS analysis from the SCORE trial revealed that the favorable edge effect was primarily due to lack of vessel shrinkage, despite similar amounts of plaque proliferation, compared with the control group.[215] Similar vessel responses were reported in the Asian Paclitaxel-Eluting Stent Clinical Trial (ASPECT), TAXUS-II, and TAXUS-IV.[196,216,217] On the other hand, some DES trials demonstrated less effective suppression of late lumen loss at the proximal stent edge segment compared with the distal edge, possibly providing an important clue for optimal deployment of DES. In an IVUS substudy of the Sirolimus-Eluting Stent in De Novo Coronary Lesions (SIRIUS) trial, lesions with stent edge stenosis (>50% diameter stenosis) at 8 months had greater reference plaque burden (61% versus 49%; $P = .03$) (Fig. 62-14) and a higher overexpansion index (maximum stent area/reference MLA, 1.8 versus 1.5; $P = .03$) at baseline, compared to those without edge stenosis.[218]

More recently, the Stent Deployment Techniques on Clinical Outcomes of Patients Treated with the Cypher Stent (STLLR) trial also demonstrated that geographic miss (defined as the length of injured or stenotic segment not fully covered by DES) had a significant negative impact on both clinical efficacy (target vessel and lesion revascularization) and safety (myocardial infarction) at 1 year after sirolimus-eluting stent implantation.[219] These findings suggest that less aggressive stent dilation and complete coverage of reference disease may be beneficial, as long as significant underexpansion and incomplete strut apposition are avoided. On-line IVUS guidance can facilitate both the determination of appropriate stent size and length and the achievement of optimal procedural end points, with the goal being to cover significant pathology with reasonable stent expansion while anchoring the stent ends in relatively plaque-free vessel segments.

Insights into Long-Term Outcomes

Because of the low incidence of DES failure, clarification of its exact mechanisms awaits the cumulative analysis of large clinical studies. Nevertheless, suboptimal deployment or mechanical problems appear to contribute to the development of both restenosis and thrombosis. Particularly, the most common mechanism is stent underexpansion, the incidence of which has been reported as 60% to 80% in DES failures.[210,211,220] In a study of 670 native coronary lesions treated with sirolimus-eluting stents, the only independent predictors of angiographic restenosis were postprocedural final MSA and IVUS-measured stent length (OR = 0.586 and 1.029, respectively).[208] Recurrent restenosis after DES implantation for bare metal stent restenosis was also recently investigated using IVUS. In a series of 48 in-stent restenosis lesions treated with sirolimus-eluting stents, 82% of recurrent lesions had an MSA of less than 5.0 mm², compared with only 26% of nonrecurrent lesions (P = .003).[220] In addition, a gap between sirolimus-eluting stents was identified in 27% of recurrent lesions versus 5% of nonrecurrent lesions. These observations emphasize the importance of procedural optimization at DES implantation for both de novo and in-stent restenosis lesions.

Although published data on DES thrombosis are further limited, one single-center IVUS study reported stent underexpansion (P = .03) and a significant residual reference segment stenosis (P = .02) as independent multivariate predictors of sirolimus-eluting stent thrombosis (median time, 14 days after implantation).[221] For very late DES thrombosis (>12 months), another investigator group also suggested smaller stent expansion and incomplete stent apposition as possible risk factors.[222]

Late-acquired incomplete stent apposition with DES has been reported in both experimental (paclitaxel)[223] and clinical (sirolimus and paclitaxel) studies (see Fig. 62-13).[193,196,224,225] Several IVUS studies indicated that the main mechanism is focal, positive vessel remodeling, as in the case of brachytherapy.[193,224] In addition, there is a strong suggestion that incompletely apposed struts are seen primarily in eccentric plaques, and that the gaps develop mainly on the disease-free side of the vessel wall. The combination of mechanical vessel injury during stent implantation and biologic vessel injury with pharmacologic agents or polymer in the setting of little underlying plaque may predispose the vessel wall to chronic, pathologic dilation. At present, however, no data directly link this finding with subsequent unfavorable clinical events such as late stent thrombosis.[226] Nevertheless, the potential impact of this finding on long-term outcomes needs to be carefully assessed over an extended period.

Other IVUS-detected conditions that may be of importance in DES include non-uniform stent strut distribution and strut fractures after implantation (Fig. 62-15).[227-230] Theoretically, both abnormalities can reduce the local drug dose delivered to the arterial wall, as well as mechanical scaffolding of the affected lesion segment. A recent IVUS study of 24 sirolimus-eluting stent restenoses identified the number of visualized struts (normalized for the number of stent cells) and the maximum interstrut angle as independent multivariate IVUS predictors of both neointimal hyperplasia and MLA.[228] In contrast, the exact incidence and clinical implications of strut fractures remain to be investigated.[231,232]

SAFETY

As with other interventional procedures, the possibility of spasm, dissection, and thrombosis exists when intravascular imaging catheters are used. In a retrospective study of 2207 patients, Hausmann and colleagues identified spasm in 2.9% of patients, and other complications, including dissection, thrombosis, and abrupt closure with "certain relation" to IVUS, in 0.4%.[233] This study was performed with first-generation catheters in the early 1990s, and it is likely (although not documented) that the incidence of spasm and other complications is substantially lower with the current generation of catheters.

COSTS

In the United States, current retail sales prices for the stand-alone single-use imaging catheters range between $600 and $850. The retail price of the IVUS imaging consoles is between $150,000 and $250,000, although the actual prices paid by hospitals vary widely depending on "bundling" deals and other special purchase arrangements. The U.S. Health Care Financing Administration approved reimbursement for the IVUS procedure and interpretation for Medicare patients in 1997, based on the number of vessels imaged. A number of other carriers have also approved reimbursement for IVUS, although payment is on a region-by-region basis. In most places, the total reimbursement is less than the cost of the catheters.

ONGOING AND ANTICIPATED TECHNICAL DEVELOPMENTS

Three-Dimensional Transducer Tracking

Compared with external imaging methods, one technical disadvantage common to catheter-based imaging modalities is difficulty in obtaining accurate spatial orientation of the investigated vessel segment. To overcome this limitation, three-dimensional transducer navigation or tracking techniques have been introduced by several investigator groups. In IVUS, this can be accomplished by reconstructing the three-dimensional pull back trajectory, using biplane x-ray recordings of the transducer,[234] or by real-time tracking of a miniaturized electromagnetic position sensor mounted in the catheter tip.[235] Computational algorithms and instrumentation have been developed to reduce significant artifacts induced by respiratory and cardiac motions.

The geometrically correct three-dimensional IVUS reconstruction of vessel wall structure may not only facilitate routine percutaneous interventions in complex coronary anatomy, but also allow detailed in vivo profiling of intracoronary hemodynamics and endothelial shear stress.[236,237] A number of pathologic and experimental studies have shown that inhomogeneities and irregularities of these factors play an important role in the initiation, localization, growth, composition, remodeling, and destabilization of atheromatous plaque.[238] A recent human in vivo study with the spatially correct three-dimensional IVUS partly confirmed these observations in a clinical setting, directly relating local endothelial

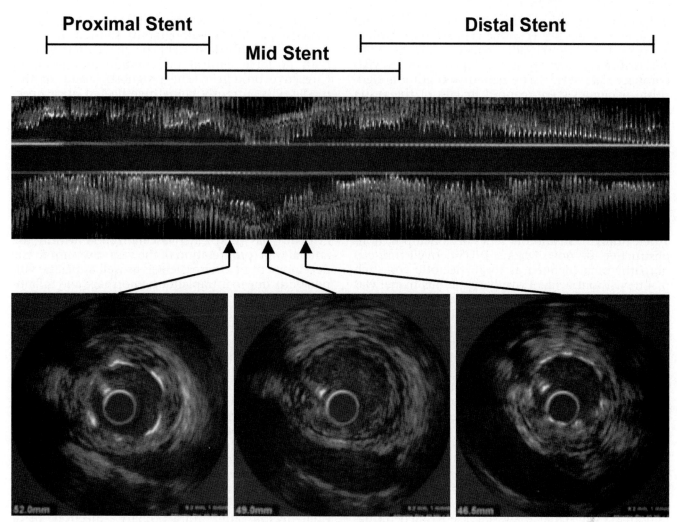

Figure 62-15. Stent strut discontinuity (fracture) observed 8 months after deployment of three overlapping drug-eluting stents. On the cross-sectional intravascular ultrasound (IVUS) image *(bottom, middle)*, an abnormal paucity of stent struts, not seen at implantation, is detected at a portion of the mid stent. The longitudinal IVUS image *(top)* shows an acute-angled bend at the corresponding segment. In this particular case, the strut discontinuity is not associated with increased intimal hyperplasia, at least at this time point.

shear stress at baseline to subsequent plaque progression and arterial remodeling at 6 months.[237] Although the predictive value of this parameter in the context of vulnerable plaque requires further investigation, this technique, particularly if combined with advanced catheter-based diagnostic modalities, may offer further insight into the natural history of native coronary artery disease. In addition, vascular response to stent implantation is another potentially important field to investigate with this technology,[239-241] because anatomically complex lesions, such as bifurcation and long lesions, are being more actively treated with DES that can significantly alter the vascular geometry and, consequently, local endothelial shear stress.

Tissue Characterization

Another intriguing area of current IVUS development is the attempt to identify tissue components using computer-assisted analysis of raw radiofrequency signals in the reflected ultrasound beam. This is pri-marily based on the fact that there is greater information contained in the backscattered ultrasound signal than is revealed by the conventional amplitude-based image presentation alone. To date, a variety of signal parameters and mathematical modeling techniques have been proposed and have been shown to enhance the tissue discrimination. One investigator group demonstrated that integrated backscatter values, calculated as the average power of the backscattered ultrasound signal from a sample tissue volume, were significantly different among tissue types (calcification, fibrous tissue, mixed lesion, lipid core or intimal hyperplasia, and thrombus).[242,243] Other investigators, including our own group, used unique ultrasound wave properties from different tissue types (e. g., signal attenuation slopes, statistical frequency distribution, angle-dependent echo-intensity variation).[244-248] Wavelet analysis, a mathematical model for assessing local wave patterns within a complex signal, has also been proposed and has demonstrated accurate in vitro and in vivo discrimination of lipid-rich from fibrous plaques.[249]

To date, one system (Virtual Histology, Volcano Therapeutics) has been commercialized in the United States. It uses spectral radiofrequency analyses with a classification algorithm developed from ex vivo coronary data sets.[250] The pattern recognition algorithm generates color-mapped images of the vessel wall, with a distinct color for each of the fibrous, necrotic, calcific, and fibrofatty categories. Combined use with automated pull back and border detection techniques enables quantitative assessment of each tissue category over a three-dimensional volume of a coronary artery. An initial clinical study showed significant correlation between IVUS-determined plaque compositions and corresponding histopathology of the coronary specimens obtained by directional atherectomy.[251] In another series of nonculprit, nonobstructive, de novo lesions, IVUS-derived thin-cap fibroatheroma (defined as focal, necrotic core–rich plaque without evident overlying fibrous tissue) was a more prevalent finding in acute coronary syndrome than in stable angina.[252] Current technical limitations include limited spatial resolution (100 to 250 μm); no classifications for thrombus, blood, or intimal hyperplasia; and potential errors due to poor ultrasound penetration through extensive calcification. Several multicenter studies have been initiated worldwide, and the role of this system in the detection of rupture-prone plaques is yet to be established.

Mechanical Strain Assessment

IVUS elastography, which measures the mechanical strain property of the arterial wall, is an extension of radiofrequency signal analysis. Local tissue deformation is determined with the use of cross-correlation analysis of radiofrequency signals recorded at two different intravascular pressures during near end-diastole.[253,254] The calculated local radial strain is displayed on the IVUS image, color coded on the plaque area (elastography) or the luminal boundary (palpography), on the IVUS image. An initial in vitro validation study with diseased human coronary and femoral arteries revealed different mean strain values among fibrous, fibrofatty, and fatty plaque components.[253] A subsequent animal study using peripheral arteries demonstrated a high sensitivity to identify fatty plaque material from its increased mean strain value.[255] These results were confirmed by a postmortem human coronary study that demonstrated 88% sensitivity and 89% specificity to detect histologic vulnerable plaque, defined as a high strain region at the plaque surface with adjacent low strain regions in elastography.[256] In this study, the strain in caps also showed a high positive correlation with the amount of macrophages ($P < .006$), as well as an inverse relation with the amount of smooth muscle cells ($P < .0001$). One hypothesis for these observations is that active macrophage infiltration can cause local weakening of a fibrous cap, because macrophages play a key role in degradation of the extracellular matrix by secreting proteolytic enzymes.

Accordingly, a recent clinical study using three-dimensional IVUS palpography showed that the number of highly deformable plaques correlated with both unstable clinical presentation and levels of C-reactive protein.[257] The prognostic value of this modality is currently being investigated in prospective multicenter studies.

Contrast Intravascular Ultrasound for Neovascular and Molecular Imaging

The application of contrast ultrasound technology for catheter-based coronary imaging may add another dimension to the arena of atherosclerotic plaque assessment. For the past several decades, mounting evidence has linked neovascularization within the arterial wall (proliferation of the vasa vasorum) to the development of atherosclerosis as well as plaque vulnerability due to intraplaque hemorrhage and inflammation.[258-261] Recent animal studies have also shown that suppression of plaque neovascularization with angiogenesis inhibitors or statins can significantly attenuate the progression of atherosclerosis.[259,262] These pioneering works, however, were reported using histopathology, in vitro microcomputed tomography, or preclinical targeted-magnetic resonance imaging. Contrast-enhanced IVUS with microbubble agents may offer, for the first time, in vivo quantification of vasa vasorum density and plaque perfusion in a clinical setting.

A preliminary human study using conventional IVUS systems demonstrated the feasibility to track the distribution and dynamic changes in the echo density within the coronary plaque and adventitial region after intracoronary injection of a clinically available microbubble agent.[263] In this series, one case also showed persistent plaque enhancement (an IVUS "blush sign"), suggesting pathologic extravasation of microbubbles due to increased porosity of the neoangiogenic vessels. Although this analysis currently relies on the processing of gray-scale, phase-correlated IVUS images, use of raw radiofrequency signals may further improve the detection and quantification of subtle changes in the backscattered ultrasound intensity within the arterial wall.

The utility of contrast IVUS imaging can be significantly enhanced by the introduction of contrast agents targeted to specific tissue components, cells, molecules, or biologic processes. This biomedical imaging technique, so-called molecular imaging, is also potentially applicable to site-targeted delivery of therapeutic agents with visual verification and quantification of the treatment. To date, several industrial and university-based research groups are developing molecular imaging agents for ultrasound applications. In addition to the traditional microbubble-based technology, nongaseous acoustically reflective nanoparticles have shown significant potentials,[264] owing to their smaller particle sizes and greater in vivo stability.[265] Whereas passive targeting uses primarily nonspecific uptake of the acoustic particles by

Site-Targeted Contrast Agent

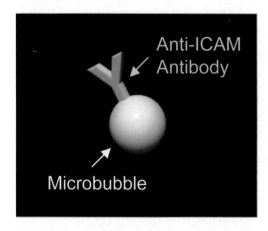

Endothelial Layer

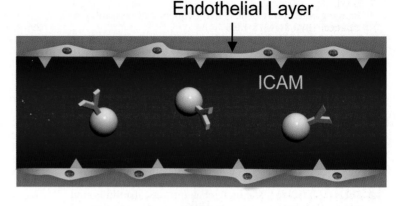

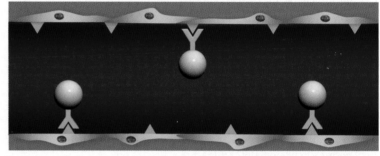

Figure 62-16. Conceptual diagrams of an active site-targeted ultrasound contrast agent. A variety of ligands conjugated to the particle surface can be used to provide site-specific ultrasound enhancement, offering the ability to detect and quantify the various cell-surface molecular signatures (e.g., intercellular adhesion molecule [ICAM]) of endothelium and atheroma components.

macrophages, active targeting agents provide site-specific enhancement using a variety of ligands conjugated to the particle surface (Fig. 62-16). In a study using biotinylated, lipid-coated, perfluorocarbon emulsion nanoparticles, Lanza and colleagues first demonstrated marked acoustic enhancement of in vivo thrombi in a canine model.[266] In a more recent animal study, the nanoemulsion was targeted to tissue factor (a 43-kDa transmembrane glycoprotein responsible for initiating coagulation cascade), confirming that the acoustic nanoparticles can infiltrate into arterial walls after balloon injury and detect the localized expression of tissue factor with conventional IVUS.[267] Several other investigator groups have also developed echogenic liposomes conjugated with anti-intercellular adhesion molecule-1 (ICAM-1), anti-vascular cell adhesion molecule-1 (VCAM-1), anti-fibrin, anti-fibrinogen, and anti-tissue factor (TF) and have proven the in vivo feasibility of IVUS to detect and quantify the various cell-surface molecular signatures of endothelium and atheroma components.[265,268] Furthermore, extended efforts are ongoing to integrate therapeutic agents, such as antiproliferative drugs and gene transfection agents, into these ligand-targeted ultrasound contrast systems.[269]

ACKNOWLEDGMENTS

We appreciate Heidi N. Bonneau, RN, MS, for her expert review and editing advice, as well as Ichizo Tsujino, MD, PhD, and Atsushi Hirohata, MD, for their professional work with the figures.

REFERENCES

1. Bom N, Lancee CT, Van Egmond FC: An ultrasonic intracardiac scanner. Ultrasonics 1972;10:72-76.
2. Bom N, ten Hoff H, Lancee CT, et al: Early and recent intraluminal ultrasound devices. Int J Card Imaging 1989;4:79-88.
3. Yock PG, Johnson EL, Linker DT: Intravascular ultrasound: Development and clinical potential. Am J Cardiac Imag 1988;2:185-193.
4. Mallery JA, Tobis JM, Griffith J, et al: Assessment of normal and atherosclerotic arterial wall thickness with an intravascular ultrasound imaging catheter. Am Heart J 1990;119:1392-1400.
5. Gussenhoven EJ, Essed CE, Lancee CT, et al: Arterial wall characteristics determined by intravascular ultrasound imaging: An in vitro study. J Am Coll Cardiol 1989;14:947-952.
6. Pandian NG, Kreis A, Brockway B, et al: Ultrasound angioscopy: Real-time, two-dimensional, intraluminal ultrasound imaging of blood vessels. Am J Cardiol 1988;62:493-494.

7. Potkin BN, Bartorelli AL, Gessert JM, et al: Coronary artery imaging with intravascular high-frequency ultrasound. Circulation 1990;81:1575-1585.

8. Yock P, Linker D, Saether O, et al: Intravascular two-dimensional catheter ultrasound: Initial clinical studies [Abstract]. Circulation 1988;78:II-21.

9. Marco J, Fajadet J, Robert G, et al: Intracoronary ultrasound imaging: Initial clinical trials [Abstract]. Circulation 1989;80:II-374.

10. Graham SP, Brands D, Sheehan H, et al: Assessment of arterial wall morphology using intravascular ultrasound in vitro and in patients [Abstract]. Circulation 1989;80:II-565.

11. Fuessl RT, Mintz GS, Pichard AD, et al: In vivo validation of intravascular ultrasound length measurements using a motorized transducer pullback system. Am J Cardiol 1996;77:1115-1118.

12. Tobis JM, Mallery J, Mahon D, et al: Intravascular ultrasound imaging of human coronary arteries in vivo: Analysis of tissue characterizations with comparison to in vitro histological specimens. Circulation 1991;83:913-926.

13. Siegel RJ, Chae JS, Maurer G, et al: Histopathologic correlation of the three-layered intravascular ultrasound appearance of normal adult human muscular arteries. Am Heart J 1993;126:872-878.

14. Nishimura RA, Edwards WD, Warnes CA, et al: Intravascular ultrasound imaging: In vitro validation and pathologic correlation. J Am Coll Cardiol 1990;16:145-154.

15. Meyer CR, Chiang EH, Fechner KP, et al: Feasibility of high-resolution, intravascular ultrasonic imaging catheters. Radiology 1988;168:113-116.

16. Yock PG, Linker DT, Angelsen BA: Two-dimensional intravascular ultrasound: Technical development and initial clinical experience. J Am Soc Echocardiogr 1989;2:296-304.

17. Fitzgerald PJ, St Goar F, Connolly AJ, et al: Intravascular ultrasound imaging of coronary arteries: Is three layers the norm? Circulation 1992;86:154-158.

18. Maheswaran B, Leung CY, Gutfinger DE, et al: Intravascular ultrasound appearance of normal and mildly diseased coronary arteries: Correlation with histologic specimens. Am Heart J 1995;130:976-986.

19. Gussenhoven EJ, Frietman PA, The SH, et al: Assessment of medial thinning in atherosclerosis by intravascular ultrasound. Am J Cardiol 1991;68:1625-1632.

20. Isner JM, Donaldson RF, Fortin AH, et al: Attenuation of the media of coronary arteries in advanced atherosclerosis. Am J Cardiol 1986;58:937-939.

21. Mintz GS, Nissen SE, Anderson WD, et al: American College of Cardiology Clinical Expert Consensus Document on Standards for Acquisition, Measurement and Reporting of Intravascular Ultrasound Studies (IVUS): A report of the American College of Cardiology Task Force on Clinical Expert Consensus Documents. J Am Coll Cardiol 2001;37:1478-1492.

22. Rasheed Q, Dhawale PJ, Anderson J, et al: Intracoronary ultrasound-defined plaque composition: Computer-aided plaque characterization and correlation with histologic samples obtained during directional coronary atherectomy. Am Heart J 1995;129:631-637.

23. Di Mario C, The SH, Madretsma S, et al: Detection and characterization of vascular lesions by intravascular ultrasound: An in vitro study correlated with histology. J Am Soc Echocardiogr 1992;5:135-146.

24. Mintz GS, Popma JJ, Pichard AD, et al: Patterns of calcification in coronary artery disease: A statistical analysis of intravascular ultrasound and coronary angiography in 1155 lesions. Circulation 1995;91:1959-1965.

25. Mintz GS, Douek P, Pichard AD, et al: Target lesion calcification in coronary artery disease: An intravascular ultrasound study. J Am Coll Cardiol 1992;20:1149-1155.

26. Tuzcu EM, Berkalp B, De Franco A, et al: The dilemma of diagnosing coronary calcification: Angiography versus intravascular ultrasound. J Am Coll Cardiol 1996;27:832-838.

27. Yock PG, Fitzgerald PJ, Linker DT, et al: Intravascular ultrasound guidance for catheter-based coronary interventions. J Am Coll Cardiol 1991;17:39B-45B.

28. Pandian NG, Kreis A, Brockway B: Detection of intraarterial thrombus by intravascular high frequency two-dimensional ultrasound imaging in vitro and in vivo studies. Am J Cardiol 1990;65:1280-1283.

29. Nailon WH, McLaughlin S, Spencer T, et al: Can statistical texture analysis of unprocessed intravascular ultrasound (IVUS) signal discriminate red and white thrombi and plasma? [Abstract]. Circulation 1996;94:I-612.

30. Fitzgerald PJ, Connolly AJ, Watkins RD, et al: Distinction between soft plaque and thrombus by intravascular tissue characterization [Abstract]. J Am Coll Cardiol 1991;17:111A.

31. Metz JA, Preuss P, Komiyama N, et al: Discrimination between soft plaque and thrombus based on radiofrequency analysis of intravascular ultrasound [Abstract]. J Am Coll Cardiol 1996;27:200A.

32. Komiyama N, Chronos NA, Uren NG, et al: The progression of thrombus in an ex-vivo shunt model evaluated by intravascular ultrasound radiofrequency analysis. Ultrasound Med Biol 1999;25:561-566.

33. Ramo MP, Spencer T, Kearney PP, et al: Characterisation of red and white thrombus by intravascular ultrasound using radiofrequency and videodensitometric data-based texture analysis. Ultrasound Med Biol 1997;23:1195-1199.

34. Fitzgerald PJ, Yock C, Yock PG: Orientation of intracoronary ultrasonography: Looking beyond the artery. J Am Soc Echocardiogr 1998;11:13-19.

35. Ge J, Liu F, Gorge G, et al: Angiographically "silent" plaque in the left main coronary artery detected by intravascular ultrasound. Coron Artery Dis 1995;6:805-810.

36. Hausmann D, Johnson JA, Sudhir K, et al: Angiographically silent atherosclerosis detected by intravascular ultrasound in patients with familial hypercholesterolemia and familial combined hyperlipidemia: Correlation with high density lipoproteins. J Am Coll Cardiol 1996;27:1562-1570.

37. Kimura BJ, Russo RJ, Bhargava V, et al: Atheroma morphology and distribution in proximal left anterior descending coronary artery: In vivo observations. J Am Coll Cardiol 1996;27:825-831.

38. Mintz GS, Popma JJ, Pichard AD, et al: Limitations of angiography in the assessment of plaque distribution in coronary artery disease: A systematic study of target lesion eccentricity in 1446 lesions. Circulation 1996;93:924-931.

39. Sheikh KH, Harrison JK, Harding MB, et al: Detection of angiographically silent coronary atherosclerosis by intracoronary ultrasonography. Am Heart J 1991;121:1803-1807.

40. St. Goar F, Pinto FJ, Alderman EL, et al: Intravascular ultrasound imaging of angiographically normal coronary arteries: An in vivo comparison with quantitative angiography. J Am Coll Cardiol 1991;18:952-958.

41. Mintz GS, Painter JA, Pichard AD, et al: Atherosclerosis in angiographically "normal" coronary artery reference segments: An intravascular ultrasound study with clinical correlations. J Am Coll Cardiol 1995;25:1479-1485.

42. Fitzgerald PJ, Yock PG: Mechanisms and outcomes of angioplasty and atherectomy assessed by intravascular ultrasound imaging. J Clin Ultrasound 1993;21:579-588.

43. Glagov S, Weisenberg E, Zarins CK, et al: Compensatory enlargement of human atherosclerotic coronary arteries. N Engl J Med 1987;316:1371-1375.

44. Hermiller JB, Tenaglia AN, Kisslo KB, et al: In vivo validation of compensatory enlargement of atherosclerotic coronary arteries. Am J Cardiol 1993;71:665-668.

45. Schoenhagen P, Ziada KM, Vince DG, et al: Arterial remodeling and coronary artery disease: The concept of "dilated" versus "obstructive" coronary atherosclerosis. J Am Coll Cardiol 2001;38:297-306.

46. Nishioka T, Luo H, Berglund H, et al: Absence of focal compensatory enlargement or constriction in diseased human coronary saphenous vein bypass grafts: An intravascular ultrasound study. Circulation 1996;93:683-690.

47. Nishioka T, Luo H, Eigler NL, et al: Contribution of inadequate compensatory enlargement to development of human coronary artery stenosis: An in vivo intravascular ultrasound study. J Am Coll Cardiol 1996;27:1571-1576.

48. Mintz GS, Kent KM, Pichard AD, et al: Contribution of inadequate arterial remodeling to the development of focal

coronary artery stenoses: An intravascular ultrasound study. Circulation 1997;95:1791-1798.

49. Pasterkamp G, Wensing PJ, Post MJ, et al: Paradoxical arterial wall shrinkage may contribute to luminal narrowing of human atherosclerotic femoral arteries. Circulation 1995;91:1444-1449.

50. Pasterkamp G, Borst C, Post MJ, et al: Atherosclerotic arterial remodeling in the superficial femoral artery: Individual variation in local compensatory enlargement response. Circulation 1996;93:1818-1825.

51. Hibi K, Ward MR, Honda Y, et al: Impact of different definitions on the interpretation of coronary remodeling determined by intravascular ultrasound. Catheter Cardiovasc Interv 2005;65:233-239.

52. Schoenhagen P, Ziada KM, Kapadia SR, et al: Extent and direction of arterial remodeling in stable versus unstable coronary syndromes: An intravascular ultrasound study. Circulation 2000;101:598-603.

53. Smits PC, Pasterkamp G, Quarles van Ufford MA, et al: Coronary artery disease: Arterial remodelling and clinical presentation. Heart 1999;82:461-464.

54. Kaji S, Akasaka T, Hozumi T, et al: Compensatory enlargement of the coronary artery in acute myocardial infarction. Am J Cardiol 2000;85:1139-1141, A1139.

55. Jeremias A, Spies C, Herity NA, et al: Coronary artery compliance and adaptive vessel remodelling in patients with stable and unstable coronary artery disease. Heart 2000;84:314-319.

56. Gyongyosi M, Yang P, Hassan A, et al: Arterial remodelling of native human coronary arteries in patients with unstable angina pectoris: A prospective intravascular ultrasound study. Heart 1999;82:68-74.

57. Nakamura M, Nishikawa H, Mukai S, et al: Impact of coronary artery remodeling on clinical presentation of coronary artery disease: An intravascular ultrasound study. J Am Coll Cardiol 2001;37:63-69.

58. Pasterkamp G, Schoneveld AH, van der Wal AC, et al: Relation of arterial geometry to luminal narrowing and histologic markers for plaque vulnerability: The remodeling paradox. J Am Coll Cardiol 1998;32:655-662.

59. Mehran R, Dangas G, Mintz GS, et al: Atherosclerotic plaque burden and CK-MB enzyme elevation after coronary interventions: Intravascular ultrasound study of 2256 patients. Circulation 2000;101:604-610.

60. Dangas G, Mintz GS, Mehran R, et al: Preintervention arterial remodeling as an independent predictor of target-lesion revascularization after nonstent coronary intervention: An analysis of 777 lesions with intravascular ultrasound imaging. Circulation 1999;99:3149-3154.

61. Okura H, Hayase M, Shimodozono S, et al: Impact of pre-interventional arterial remodeling on subsequent vessel behavior after balloon angioplasty: A serial intravascular ultrasound study. J Am Coll Cardiol 2001;38:2001-2005.

62. Okura H, Morino Y, Oshima A, et al: Preintervention arterial remodeling affects clinical outcome following stenting: An intravascular ultrasound study. J Am Coll Cardiol 2001;37:1031-1035.

63. Endo A, Hirayama H, Yoshida O, et al: Arterial remodeling influences the development of intimal hyperplasia after stent implantation. J Am Coll Cardiol 2001;37:70-75.

64. Shiran A, Weissman NJ, Leiboff B, et al: Effect of preintervention plaque burden on subsequent intimal hyperplasia in stented coronary artery lesions. Am J Cardiol 2000;86:1318-1321.

65. Hoffmann R, Mintz GS, Kent KM, et al: Serial intravascular ultrasound predictors of restenosis at the margins of Palmaz-Schatz stents. Am J Cardiol 1997;79:951-953.

66. Hoffmann R, Mintz GS, Mehran R, et al: Intravascular ultrasound predictors of angiographic restenosis in lesions treated with Palmaz-Schatz stents. J Am Coll Cardiol 1998;31:43-49.

67. Dangas G, Mintz GS, Mehran R, et al: Stent implantation neutralizes the impact of preintervention arterial remodeling on subsequent target lesion revascularization. Am J Cardiol 2000;86:452-455.

68. Hong MK, Park SW, Lee CW, et al: Preintervention arterial remodeling as a predictor of intimal hyperplasia after intracoronary stenting: A serial intravascular ultrasound study. Clin Cardiol 2002;25:11-15.

69. Mintz GS, Kimura T, Nobuyoshi M, et al: Relation between preintervention remodeling and late arterial responses to coronary angioplasty or atherectomy. Am J Cardiol 2001;87:392-396.

70. Abizaid A, Mintz GS, Pichard AD, et al: Clinical, intravascular ultrasound, and quantitative angiographic determinants of the coronary flow reserve before and after percutaneous transluminal coronary angioplasty. Am J Cardiol 1998;82:423-428.

71. Takagi A, Tsurumi Y, Ishii Y, et al: Clinical potential of intravascular ultrasound for physiological assessment of coronary stenosis: relationship between quantitative ultrasound tomography and pressure-derived fractional flow reserve. Circulation 1999;100:250-255.

72. Briguori C, Anzuini A, Airoldi F, et al: Intravascular ultrasound criteria for the assessment of the functional significance of intermediate coronary artery stenoses and comparison with fractional flow reserve. Am J Cardiol 2001;87:136-141.

73. Nishioka T, Amanullah AM, Luo H, et al: Clinical validation of intravascular ultrasound imaging for assessment of coronary stenosis severity: Comparison with stress myocardial perfusion imaging. J Am Coll Cardiol 1999;33:1870-1878.

74. Jasti V, Ivan E, Yalamanchili V, et al: Correlations between fractional flow reserve and intravascular ultrasound in patients with an ambiguous left main coronary artery stenosis. Circulation 2004;110:2831-2836.

75. Mintz GS, Pichard AD, Kovach JA, et al: Impact of preintervention intravascular ultrasound imaging on transcatheter treatment strategies in coronary artery disease. Am J Cardiol 1994;73:423-430.

76. Gorge G, Ge J, Erbel R: Role of intravascular ultrasound in the evaluation of mechanisms of coronary interventions and restenosis. Am J Cardiol 1998;81:91G-95G.

77. Tobis JM, Mallery JA, Gessert J, et al: Intravascular ultrasound cross-sectional arterial imaging before and after balloon angioplasty in vitro. Circulation 1989;80:873-882.

78. Baptista J, Umans VA, Di Mario C, et al: Mechanisms of luminal enlargement and quantification of vessel wall trauma following balloon coronary angioplasty and directional atherectomy. Eur Heart J 1995;16:1603-1612.

79. Baptista J, Di Mario C, Ozaki Y, et al: Impact of plaque morphology and composition on the mechanisms of lumen enlargement using intracoronary ultrasound and quantitative angiography after balloon angioplasty. Am J Cardiol 1996;77:115-121.

80. Braden GA, Herrington DM, Downes TR, et al: Qualitative and quantitative contrasts in the mechanisms of lumen enlargement by coronary balloon angioplasty and directional coronary atherectomy. J Am Coll Cardiol 1994;23:40-48.

81. Honye J, Mahon DJ, Jain A, et al: Morphological effects of coronary balloon angioplasty in vivo assessed by intravascular ultrasound imaging. Circulation 1992;85:1012-1025.

82. Buller CE, Davidson CJ, Virmani R, et al: Real-time assessment of experimental arterial angioplasty with transvenous intravascular ultrasound. J Am Coll Cardiol 1992;19:217-222.

83. Athanasiadis A, Haase KK, Wullen B, et al: Lesion morphology assessed by pre-interventional intravascular ultrasound does not predict the incidence of severe coronary artery dissections. Eur Heart J 1998;19:870-878.

84. Fitzgerald PJ, Ports TA, Yock PG: Contribution of localized calcium deposits to dissection after angioplasty: An observational study using intravascular ultrasound. Circulation 1992;86:64-70.

85. Lee RT, Richardson SG, Loree HM, et al: Prediction of mechanical properties of human atherosclerotic tissue by high-frequency intravascular ultrasound imaging: An in vitro study. Arterioscler Thromb 1992;12:1-5.

86. Richardson PD, Davies MJ, Born GV: Influence of plaque configuration and stress distribution on fissuring of coronary atherosclerotic plaques. Lancet 1989;2:941-944.

87. Shimodozono S, Okura H, Hayase M, et al: Influence of calcium on coronary dissection following cutting balloon angioplasty: An intravascular ultrasound study. J Am Coll Cardiol 2000;35:A18.

88. Stone GW, Hodgson JM, St Goar FG, et al: Improved procedural results of coronary angioplasty with intravascular ultrasound-guided balloon sizing: The CLOUT pilot trial. Circulation 1997;95:2044-2052.

89. Stone GW, Frey A, Linnemeier T, et al: 2.5 Year follow-up of the CLOUT study: Long-term implications for an aggressive IVUS guided balloon angioplasty strategy. J Am Coll Cardiol 1999;33:81A.

90. Schroeder S, Baumbach A, Haase KK, et al: Reduction of restenosis by vessel size adapted percutaneous transluminal coronary angioplasty using intravascular ultrasound. Am J Cardiol 1999;83:875-879.

91. Abizaid A, Pichard AD, Mintz GS, et al: Acute and long-term results of an intravascular ultrasound-guided percutaneous transluminal coronary angioplasty/provisional stent implantation strategy. Am J Cardiol 1999;84:1298-1303.

92. Peters RJ, Kok WE, Di Mario C, et al: Prediction of restenosis after coronary balloon angioplasty: Results of PICTURE (Post-IntraCoronary Treatment Ultrasound Result Evaluation), a prospective multicenter intracoronary ultrasound imaging study. Circulation 1997;95:2254-2261.

93. Mintz GS, Popma JJ, Pichard AD, et al: Intravascular ultrasound predictors of restenosis after percutaneous transcatheter coronary revascularization. J Am Coll Cardiol 1996;27:1678-1687.

94. The GUIDE trial investigators: IVUS-determined predictors of restenosis in PTCA and DCA: Final report from the GUIDE trial, phase II [Abstract]. J Am Coll Cardiol 1996;27:156A.

95. Yock PG, Fitzgerald PJ, Sykes C, et al: Morphologic features of successful coronary atherectomy determined by intravascular ultrasound imaging [Abstract]. Circulation 1990;82:III-676.

96. Safian RD, Gelbfish JS, Erny RE, et al: Coronary atherectomy: Clinical, angiographic, and histological findings and observations regarding potential mechanisms. Circulation 1990;82:69-79.

97. Sharaf BL, Williams DO: "Dotter effect" contributes to angiographic improvement following directional coronary atherectomy [Abstract]. Circulation 1990;82:III-310.

98. Nakamura S, Mahon DJ, Leung CY, et al: Intracoronary ultrasound imaging before and after directional coronary atherectomy: in vitro and clinical observations. Am Heart J 1995;129:841-851.

99. Simonton CA, Leon MB, Baim DS, et al: "Optimal" directional coronary atherectomy: final results of the Optimal Atherectomy Restenosis Study (OARS). Circulation 1998;97:332-339.

100. Matar FA, Mintz GS, Pinnow E, et al: Multivariate predictors of intravascular ultrasound end points after directional coronary atherectomy. J Am Coll Cardiol 1995;25:318-324.

101. Popma JJ, Mintz GS, Satler LF, et al: Clinical and angiographic outcome after directional coronary atherectomy: A qualitative and quantitative analysis using coronary arteriography and intravascular ultrasound. Am J Cardiol 1993;72:55E-64E.

102. Umans VA, Baptista J, di Mario C, et al: Angiographic, ultrasonic, and angioscopic assessment of the coronary artery wall and lumen area configuration after directional atherectomy: The mechanism revisited. Am Heart J 1995;130:217-227.

103. Dussaillant GR, Mintz GS, Pichard AD, et al: Effect of rotational atherectomy in noncalcified atherosclerotic plaque: A volumetric intravascular ultrasound study. J Am Coll Cardiol 1996;28:856-860.

104. Kovach JA, Mintz GS, Pichard AD, et al: Sequential intravascular ultrasound characterization of the mechanisms of rotational atherectomy and adjunct balloon angioplasty. J Am Coll Cardiol 1993;22:1024-1032.

105. Mintz GS, Potkin BN, Keren G, et al: Intravascular ultrasound evaluation of the effect of rotational atherectomy in obstructive atherosclerotic coronary artery disease. Circulation 1992;86:1383-1393.

106. Kimura BJ, Fitzgerald PJ, Sudhir K, et al: Guidance of directed coronary atherectomy by intracoronary ultrasound imaging. Am Heart J 1992;124:1365-1369.

107. Topol EJ, Leya F, Pinkerton CA, et al: A comparison of directional atherectomy with coronary angioplasty in patients with coronary artery disease. The CAVEAT Study Group. N Engl J Med 1993;329:221-227.

108. Suzuki T, Hosokawa H, Katoh O, et al: Effects of adjunctive balloon angioplasty after intravascular ultrasound-guided optimal directional coronary atherectomy: The result of Adjunctive Balloon Angioplasty After Coronary Atherectomy Study (ABACAS). J Am Coll Cardiol 1999;34:1028-1035.

109. Tsuchikane E, Sumitsuji S, Awata N, et al: Final results of the STent versus directional coronary Atherectomy Randomized Trial (START). J Am Coll Cardiol 1999;34:1050-1057.

110. Honda Y, Yock PG, Fitzgerald PJ: Impact of residual plaque burden on clinical outcomes of coronary interventions. Catheter Cardiovasc Interv 1999;46:265-276.

111. Mintz GS, Popma JJ, Pichard AD, et al: Arterial remodeling after coronary angioplasty: A serial intravascular ultrasound study. Circulation 1996;94:35-43.

112. Mintz GS, Popma JJ, Hong MK, et al: Intravascular ultrasound to discern device-specific effects and mechanisms of restenosis. Am J Cardiol 1996;78:18-22.

113. Lansky AJ, Mintz GS, Popma JJ, et al: Remodeling after directional coronary atherectomy (with and without adjunct percutaneous transluminal coronary angioplasty): A serial angiographic and intravascular ultrasound analysis from the Optimal Atherectomy Restenosis Study. J Am Coll Cardiol 1998;32:329-337.

114. Kimura T, Kaburagi S, Tamura T, et al: Remodeling of human coronary arteries undergoing coronary angioplasty or atherectomy. Circulation 1997;96:475-483.

115. Sabate M, Serruys PW, van der Giessen WJ, et al: Geometric vascular remodeling after balloon angioplasty and beta-radiation therapy: A three-dimensional intravascular ultrasound study. Circulation 1999;100:1182-1188.

116. Honda Y, Yock CA, Hermiller JB, et al: Longitudinal redistribution of plaque is an important mechanism for lumen expansion in stenting [Abstract]. J Am Coll Cardiol 1997;29:281A.

117. Ahmed JM, Mintz GS, Weissman NJ, et al: Mechanism of lumen enlargement during intracoronary stent implantation: An intravascular ultrasound study. Circulation 2000;102:7-10.

118. Maehara A, Takagi A, Okura H, et al: Longitudinal plaque redistribution during stent expansion. Am J Cardiol 2000;86:1069-1072.

119. von Birgelen C, Mintz GS, Eggebrecht H, et al: Preintervention arterial remodeling affects vessel stretch and plaque extrusion during coronary stent deployment as demonstrated by three-dimensional intravascular ultrasound. Am J Cardiol 2003;92:130-135.

120. Mintz GS, Pichard AD, Kent KM, et al: Axial plaque redistribution as a mechanism of percutaneous transluminal coronary angioplasty. Am J Cardiol 1996;77:427-430.

121. Nakamura S, Colombo A, Gaglione A, et al: Intracoronary ultrasound observations during stent implantation. Circulation 1994;89:2026-2034.

122. Colombo A, Hall P, Nakamura S, et al: Intracoronary stenting without anticoagulation accomplished with intravascular ultrasound guidance. Circulation 1995;91:1676-1688.

123. Goldberg SL, Colombo A, Nakamura S, et al: Benefit of intracoronary ultrasound in the deployment of Palmaz-Schatz stents. J Am Coll Cardiol 1994;24:996-1003.

124. Metz JA, Mooney MR, Walter PD, et al: Significance of edge tears in coronary stenting: Initial observations from the STRUT registry [Abstract]. Circulation 1995;92:I-546.

125. Schwarzacher SP, Metz JA, Yock PG, et al: Vessel tearing at the edge of intracoronary stents detected with intravascular ultrasound imaging. Cath Cardiovasc Diagn 1997;40:152-155.

126. Hong MK, Park SW, Lee NH, et al: Long-term outcomes of minor dissection at the edge of stents detected with intravascular ultrasound. Am J Cardiol 2000;86:791-795, A799.

127. Nishida T, Colombo A, Briguori C, et al: Outcome of nonobstructive residual dissections detected by intravascular ultrasound following percutaneous coronary intervention. Am J Cardiol 2002;89:1257-1262.

128. Albiero R, Rau T, Schluter M, et al: Comparison of immediate and intermediate-term results of intravascular ultrasound versus angiography-guided Palmaz-Schatz stent implantation in matched lesions. Circulation 1997;96:2997-3005.

129. Blasini R, Neumann FJ, Schmitt C, et al: Restenosis rate after intravascular ultrasound-guided coronary stent implantation. Cathet Cardiovasc Diagn 1998;44:380-386.

130. Choi JW, Goodreau LM, Davidson CJ: Resource utilization and clinical outcomes of coronary stenting: A comparison of intravascular ultrasound and angiographical guided stent implantation. Am Heart J 2001;142:112-118.

131. Gaster AL, Slothuus Skjoldborg U, Larsen J, et al: Continued improvement of clinical outcome and cost effectiveness following intravascular ultrasound guided PCI: Insights from a prospective, randomised study. Heart 2003;89:1043-1049.

132. Russo RJ, Attubato MJ, Davidson CJ, et al: Angiography Versus Intravascular ultrasound-Directed stent placement: Final results from AVID [Abstract]. Circulation 1999;100: I-234.

133. Fitzgerald PJ, Oshima A, Hayase M, et al: Final results of the Can Routine Ultrasound Influence Stent Expansion (CRUISE) study. Circulation 2000;102:523-530.

134. Schiele F, Meneveau N, Seronde MF, et al: Medical costs of intravascular ultrasound optimization of stent deployment. Results of the multicenter randomized "REStenosis after Intravascular ultrasound STenting" (RESIST) study. Int J Cardiovasc Intervent 2000;3:207-213.

135. Schiele F, Meneveau N, Vuillemenot A, et al: Impact of intravascular ultrasound guidance in stent deployment on 6-month restenosis rate: A multicenter, randomized study comparing two strategies—with and without intravascular ultrasound guidance. RESIST Study Group. REStenosis after Ivus guided STenting. J Am Coll Cardiol 1998;32: 320-328.

136. Frey AW, Hodgson JM, Muller C, et al: Ultrasound-guided strategy for provisional stenting with focal balloon combination catheter: Results from the randomized Strategy for Intracoronary Ultrasound-guided PTCA and Stenting (SIPS) trial. Circulation 2000;102:2497-2502.

137. Oemrawsingh PV, Mintz GS, Schalij MJ, et al: Intravascular ultrasound guidance improves angiographic and clinical outcome of stent implantation for long coronary artery stenoses: Final results of a randomized comparison with angiographic guidance (TULIP Study). Circulation 2003;107: 62-67.

138. de Jaegere P, Mudra H, Figulla H, et al: Intravascular ultrasound-guided optimized stent deployment: Immediate and 6 months clinical and angiographic results from the Multicenter Ultrasound Stenting in Coronaries Study (MUSIC Study). Eur Heart J 1998;19:1214-1223.

139. Uren NG, Schwarzacher SP, Metz JA, et al: Predictors and outcomes on stent thrombosis: An intravascular ultrasound registry. Eur Heart J 2002;23:124-132.

140. Cheneau E, Leborgne L, Mintz GS, et al: Predictors of subacute stent thrombosis: Results of a systematic intravascular ultrasound study. Circulation 2003;108:43-47.

141. Ziada KM, Tuzcu EM, De Franco AC, et al: Absolute, not relative, post-stent lumen area is a better predictor of clinical outcome [Abstract]. Circulation 1996;94:I-453.

142. Moussa I, Moses J, Di Mario C, et al: Does the specific intravascular ultrasound criterion used to optimize stent expansion have an impact on the probability of stent restenosis? Am J Cardiol 1999;83:1012-1017.

143. Kasaoka S, Tobis JM, Akiyama T, et al: Angiographic and intravascular ultrasound predictors of in-stent restenosis. J Am Coll Cardiol 1998;32:1630-1635.

144. Morino Y, Honda Y, Okura H, et al: An optimal diagnostic threshold for minimal stent area to predict target lesion revascularization following stent implantation in native coronary lesions. Am J Cardiol 2001;88:301-303.

145. Mudra H, di Mario C, de Jaegere P, et al: Randomized comparison of coronary stent implantation under ultrasound or

146. Orford JL, Denktas AE, Williams BA, et al: Routine intravascular ultrasound scanning guidance of coronary stenting is not associated with improved clinical outcomes. Am Heart J 2004;148:501-506.

147. Casella G, Klauss V, Ottani F, et al: Impact of intravascular ultrasound-guided stenting on long-term clinical outcome: A meta-analysis of available studies comparing intravascular ultrasound-guided and angiographically guided stenting. Catheter Cardiovasc Interv 2003;59:314-321.

148. Hoffmann R, Mintz GS, Dussaillant GR, et al: Patterns and mechanisms of in-stent restenosis: A serial intravascular ultrasound study. Circulation 1996;94:1247-1254.

149. Prati F, Di Mario C, Moussa I, et al: In-stent neointimal proliferation correlates with the amount of residual plaque burden outside the stent: An intravascular ultrasound study. Circulation 1999;99:1011-1014.

150. Hibi K, Suzuki T, Honda Y, et al: Quantitative and spatial relation of baseline atherosclerotic plaque burden and subsequent in-stent neointimal proliferation as determined by intravascular ultrasound. Am J Cardiol 2002;90:1164-1167.

151. Kornowski R, Mintz GS, Kent KM, et al: Increased restenosis in diabetes mellitus after coronary interventions is due to exaggerated intimal hyperplasia: A serial intravascular ultrasound study. Circulation 1997;95:1366-1369.

152. Castagna MT, Mintz GS, Leiboff BO, et al: The contribution of "mechanical" problems to in-stent restenosis: An intravascular ultrasonographic analysis of 1090 consecutive in-stent restenosis lesions. Am Heart J 2001;142:970-974.

153. Albertal M, Abizaid A, Munoz JS, et al: A novel mechanism explaining early lumen loss following balloon angioplasty for the treatment of in-stent restenosis. Am J Cardiol 2005;95:751-754.

154. Shiran A, Mintz GS, Waksman R, et al: Early lumen loss after treatment of in-stent restenosis: An intravascular ultrasound study. Circulation 1998;98:200-203.

155. Dauerman HL, Baim DS, Cutlip DE, et al: Mechanical debulking versus balloon angioplasty for the treatment of diffuse in-stent restenosis. Am J Cardiol 1998;82:277-284.

156. Mehran R, Mintz GS, Satler LF, et al: Treatment of in-stent restenosis with excimer laser coronary angioplasty: Mechanisms and results compared with PTCA alone. Circulation 1997;96:2183-2189.

157. Mahdi NA, Pathan AZ, Harrell L, et al: Directional coronary atherectomy for the treatment of Palmaz-Schatz in-stent restenosis. Am J Cardiol 1998;82:1345-1351.

158. Lee SG, Lee CW, Cheong SS, et al: Immediate and long-term outcomes of rotational atherectomy versus balloon angioplasty alone for treatment of diffuse in-stent restenosis. Am J Cardiol 1998;82:140-143.

159. Sharma SK, Kini A, Mehran R, et al: Randomized trial of Rotational Atherectomy Versus Balloon Angioplasty for Diffuse In-stent Restenosis (ROSTER). Am Heart J 2004; 147:16-22.

160. Radke PW, Klues HG, Haager PK, et al: Mechanisms of acute lumen gain and recurrent restenosis after rotational atherectomy of diffuse in-stent restenosis: A quantitative angiographic and intravascular ultrasound study. J Am Coll Cardiol 1999;34:33-39.

161. Dahm JB, Kuon E: High-energy eccentric excimer laser angioplasty for debulking diffuse in-stent restenosis leads to better acute- and 6-month follow-up results. J Invasive Cardiol 2000;12:335-342.

162. Kay IP, Sabate M, Costa MA, et al: Positive geometric vascular remodeling is seen after catheter-based radiation followed by conventional stent implantation but not after radioactive stent implantation. Circulation 2000;102:1434-1439.

163. Albiero R, Adamian M, Kobayashi N, et al: Short- and intermediate-term results of (32)P radioactive beta-emitting stent implantation in patients with coronary artery disease: The Milan Dose-Response Study. Circulation 2000;101:18-26.

164. Bhargava B, Mintz GS, Mehran R, et al: Serial volumetric intravascular ultrasound analysis of the efficacy of beta irradiation in preventing recurrent in-stent restenosis. Am J Cardiol 2000;85:651-653, A610.

165. Mintz GS, Weissman NJ, Teirstein PS, et al: Effect of intracoronary gamma-radiation therapy on in-stent restenosis: An intravascular ultrasound analysis from the gamma-1 study. Circulation 2000;102:2915-2918.

166. Raizner AE, Oesterle SN, Waksman R, et al: Inhibition of restenosis with beta-emitting radiotherapy: Report of the Proliferation Reduction with Vascular Energy Trial (PREVENT). Circulation 2000;102:951-958.

167. Sabate M, Marijnissen JP, Carlier SG, et al: Residual plaque burden, delivered dose, and tissue composition predict 6-month outcome after balloon angioplasty and beta-radiation therapy. Circulation 2000;101:2472-2477.

168. Popma JJ, Suntharalingam M, Lansky AJ, et al: Randomized trial of 90Sr/90Y beta-radiation versus placebo control for treatment of in-stent restenosis. Circulation 2002;106:1090-1096.

169. Silber S, Popma JJ, Suntharalingam M, et al: Two-year clinical follow-up of 90Sr/90Y beta-radiation versus placebo control for the treatment of in-stent restenosis. Am Heart J 2005;149:689-694.

170. Teirstein PS, Massullo V, Jani S, et al: Catheter-based radiotherapy to inhibit restenosis after coronary stenting. N Engl J Med 1997;336:1697-1703.

171. Waksman R, White RL, Chan RC, et al: Intracoronary gamma-radiation therapy after angioplasty inhibits recurrence in patients with in-stent restenosis. Circulation 2000;101:2165-2171.

172. Albiero R, Nishida T, Adamian M, et al: Edge restenosis after implantation of high activity (32)P radioactive beta-emitting stents. Circulation 2000;101:2454-2457.

173. Ahmed JM, Mintz GS, Waksman R, et al: Serial intravascular ultrasound analysis of edge recurrence after intracoronary gamma radiation treatment of native artery in-stent restenosis lesions. Am J Cardiol 2001;87:1145-1149.

174. Okura H, Lee DP, Handen CE, et al: Contribution of vessel remodeling to "edge effect" following intracoronary beta-radiation therapy: A serial volumetric intravascular ultrasound study [Abstract]. Circulation 1999;100:I-511.

175. Sabate M, Costa MA, Kozuma K, et al: Geographic miss: A cause of treatment failure in radio-oncology applied to intracoronary radiation therapy. Circulation 2000;101:2467-2471.

176. Ciezki JP: Brachytherapy guided by ultrasound. In Waksman R, Serruys PW (eds): Handbook of Vascular Brachytherapy, 2nd ed. London, Martin Dunitz, 2000, pp 153-162.

177. Kirisits C, Wexberg P, Gottsauner-Wolf M, et al: Dose-volume histograms based on serial intravascular ultrasound: A calculation model for radioactive stents. Radiother Oncol 2001;59:329-337.

178. Carlier SG, Marijnissen JP, Coen VL, et al: Guidance of intracoronary radiation therapy based on dose-volume histograms derived from quantitative intravascular ultrasound. IEEE Trans Med Imaging 1998;17:772-778.

179. Kozuma K, Costa MA, Sabate M, et al: Relationship between tensile stress and plaque growth after balloon angioplasty treated with and without intracoronary beta-brachytherapy. Eur Heart J 2000;21:2063-2070.

180. Crocker I, Fox T, Carlier SG: IVUS based dosimetry and treatment planning. J Invasive Cardiol 2000;12:643-648.

181. Morino Y, Kaneda H, Fox T, et al: Delivered dose and vascular response after beta-radiation for in-stent restenosis: Retrospective dosimetry and volumetric intravascular ultrasound analysis. Circulation 2002;106:2334-2339.

182. Kaneda H, Honda Y, Morino Y, et al: Safety of beta radiation exposure to the non-target segment: An intravascular ultrasound dosimetric analysis. J Invasive Cardiol 2006;18:309-312.

183. Maehara A, Patel NS, Harrison LB, et al: Dose heterogeneity may not affect the neointimal proliferation after gamma radiation for in-stent restenosis: A volumetric intravascular ultrasound dosimetric study. J Am Coll Cardiol 2002;39:1937-1942.

184. Kay IP, Sabate M, Van Langenhove G, et al: Outcome from balloon induced coronary artery dissection after intracoronary beta radiation. Heart 2000;83:332-337.

185. Morino Y, Bonneau HN, Fitzgerald PJ: Vascular brachytherapy: What have we learned from intravascular ultrasound? J Invasive Cardiol 2001;13:409-416.

186. Alfonso F, Hernandez R, Goicolea J, et al: Coronary stenting for acute coronary dissection after coronary angioplasty: Implications of residual dissection. J Am Coll Cardiol 1994;24:989-995.

187. Di Mario C, Gorge G, Peters R, et al: Clinical application and image interpretation in intracoronary ultrasound. Study Group on Intracoronary Imaging of the Working Group of Coronary Circulation and of the Subgroup on Intravascular Ultrasound of the Working Group of Echocardiography of the European Society of Cardiology. Eur Heart J 1998;19:207-229.

188. Meerkin D, Tardif JC, Bertrand OF, et al: The effects of intracoronary brachytherapy on the natural history of postangioplasty dissections. J Am Coll Cardiol 2000;36:59-64.

189. Kozuma K, Costa MA, Sabate M, et al: Late stent malapposition occurring after intracoronary beta-irradiation detected by intravascular ultrasound. J Invasive Cardiol 1999;11:651-655.

190. Okura H, Lee DP, Lo S, et al: Late incomplete apposition with excessive remodeling of the stented coronary artery following intravascular brachytherapy. Am J Cardiol 2003;92:587-590.

191. Shah VM, Mintz GS, Apple S, et al: Background incidence of late malapposition after bare-metal stent implantation. Circulation 2002;106:1753-1755.

192. Kay IP, Ligthart JM, Virmani R, et al: The black hole: Echolucent tissue observed following intracoronary radiation. Int J Cardiovasc Intervent 2003;5:137-142.

193. Serruys PW, Degertekin M, Tanabe K, et al: Intravascular ultrasound findings in the multicenter, randomized, double-blind RAVEL (RAndomized study with the sirolimus-eluting VElocity balloon-expandable stent in the treatment of patients with de novo native coronary artery Lesions) trial. Circulation 2002;106:798-803.

194. Moses JW, Leon MB, Popma JJ, et al: Sirolimus-eluting stents versus standard stents in patients with stenosis in a native coronary artery. N Engl J Med 2003;349:1315-1323.

195. Tanabe K, Serruys PW, Degertekin M, et al: Chronic arterial responses to polymer-controlled paclitaxel-eluting stents: Comparison with bare metal stents by serial intravascular ultrasound analyses. Data from the randomized TAXUS-II trial. Circulation 2004;109:196-200.

196. Weissman NJ, Koglin J, Cox DA, et al: Polymer-based paclitaxel-eluting stents reduce in-stent neointimal tissue proliferation: A serial volumetric intravascular ultrasound analysis from the TAXUS-IV trial. J Am Coll Cardiol 2005;45:1201-1205.

197. de Ribamar CJ Jr, Mintz GS, Carlier SG, et al: Intravascular ultrasound assessment of drug-eluting stent expansion. Am Heart J 2007;153:297-303.

198. Stone GW, Ellis SG, Cox DA, et al: A polymer-based, paclitaxel-eluting stent in patients with coronary artery disease. N Engl J Med 2004;350:221-231.

199. Fajadet J, Wijns W, Laarman GJ, et al: Randomized, double-blind, multicenter study of the Endeavor zotarolimus-eluting phosphorylcholine-encapsulated stent for treatment of native coronary artery lesions: Clinical and angiographic results of the ENDEAVOR II trial. Circulation 2006;114:798-806.

200. Weissman NJ, Wilensky RL, Tanguay JF, et al: Extent and distribution of in-stent intimal hyperplasia and edge effect in a non-radiation stent population. Am J Cardiol 2001;88:248-252.

201. Hirohata A, Morino Y, Ako J, et al: Comparison of the efficacy of direct coronary stenting with sirolimus-eluting stents versus stenting with predilation by intravascular ultrasound imaging (from the DIRECT Trial). Am J Cardiol 2006;98:1464-1467.

202. Kuroda N, Kobayashi Y, Nameki M, et al: Intimal hyperplasia regression from 6 to 12 months after stenting. Am J Cardiol 2002;89:869-872.

203. Sousa JE, Costa MA, Abizaid A, et al: Four-year angiographic and intravascular ultrasound follow-up of patients treated

with sirolimus-eluting stents. Circulation 2005;111:2326-2329.

204. Sousa JE, Costa MA, Abizaid AC, et al: Sustained suppression of neointimal proliferation by sirolimus-eluting stents: One-year angiographic and intravascular ultrasound follow-up. Circulation 2001;104:2007-2011.

205. Sousa JE, Costa MA, Sousa AG, et al: Two-year angiographic and intravascular ultrasound follow-up after implantation of sirolimus-eluting stents in human coronary arteries. Circulation 2003;107:381-383.

206. Aoki J, Colombo A, Dudek D, et al: Peristent remodeling and neointimal suppression 2 years after polymer-based, paclitaxel-eluting stent implantation: Insights from serial intravascular ultrasound analysis in the TAXUS II study. Circulation 2005;112:3876-3883.

207. Sonoda S, Morino Y, Ako J, et al: Impact of final stent dimensions on long-term results following sirolimus-eluting stent implantation: Serial intravascular ultrasound analysis from the sirius trial. J Am Coll Cardiol 2004;43:1959-1963.

208. Hong MK, Mintz GS, Lee CW, et al: Intravascular ultrasound predictors of angiographic restenosis after sirolimus-eluting stent implantation. Eur Heart J 2006;27:1305-1310.

209. Cheneau E, Pichard AD, Satler LF, et al: Intravascular ultrasound stent area of sirolimus-eluting stents and its impact on late outcome. Am J Cardiol 2005;95:1240-1242.

210. Takebayashi H, Kobayashi Y, Mintz GS, et al: Intravascular ultrasound assessment of lesions with target vessel failure after sirolimus-eluting stent implantation. Am J Cardiol 2005;95:498-502.

211. Kim SW, Mintz GS, Escolar E, et al: An intravascular ultrasound analysis of the mechanisms of restenosis comparing drug-eluting stents with brachytherapy. Am J Cardiol 2006;97:1292-1298.

212. Hodgson JM: Oh no, even stenting is affected by calcium! Cathet Cardiovasc Diagn 1996;38:236-237.

213. Hoffmann R, Mintz GS, Popma JJ, et al: Treatment of calcified coronary lesions with Palmaz-Schatz stents: An intravascular ultrasound study. Eur Heart J 1998;19:1224-1231.

214. Henneke KH, Regar E, Konig A, et al: Impact of target lesion calcification on coronary stent expansion after rotational atherectomy. Am Heart J 1999;137:93-99.

215. Kataoka T, Grube E, Honda Y, et al: Three-dimensional IVUS assessment of edge effects following drug-eluting stent implantation. J Am Coll Cardiol 2002;39:70A.

216. Hong MK, Mintz GS, Lee CW, et al: Paclitaxel coating reduces in-stent intimal hyperplasia in human coronary arteries: A serial volumetric intravascular ultrasound analysis from the ASian Paclitaxel-Eluting Stent Clinical Trial (ASPECT). Circulation 2003;107:517-520.

217. Serruys PW, Degertekin M, Tanabe K, et al: Vascular responses at proximal and distal edges of paclitaxel-eluting stents: Serial intravascular ultrasound analysis from the TAXUS II trial. Circulation 2004;109:627-633.

218. Sakurai R, Ako J, Morino Y, et al: Predictors of edge stenosis following sirolimus-eluting stent deployment (a quantitative intravascular ultrasound analysis from the SIRIUS trial). Am J Cardiol 2005;96:1251-1253.

219. Costa MA. Impact of stent deployment techniques on long-term clinical outcomes of patients treated with sirolimus-eluting stents: Results of the multicenter prospective S.T.L.L.R. trial. Transcatheter Cardiovascular Therapeutics Convention. Washington, DC, 2006.

220. Fujii K, Mintz GS, Kobayashi Y, et al: Contribution of stent underexpansion to recurrence after sirolimus-eluting stent implantation for in-stent restenosis. Circulation 2004;109:1085-1088.

221. Fujii K, Carlier SG, Mintz GS, et al: Stent underexpansion and residual reference segment stenosis are related to stent thrombosis after sirolimus-eluting stent implantation: An intravascular ultrasound study. J Am Coll Cardiol 2005;45:995-998.

222. Cook S, Wenaweser P, Togni M, et al: Incomplete stent apposition and very late stent thrombosis after drug-eluting stent implantation. Circulation 2007;115:2426-2434.

223. Drachman DE, Edelman ER, Seifert P, et al: Neointimal thickening after stent delivery of paclitaxel: Change in composi-

tion and arrest of growth over six months. J Am Coll Cardiol 2000;36:2325-2332.

224. Ako J, Morino Y, Honda Y, et al: Late incomplete stent apposition after sirolimus-eluting stent implantation: A serial intravascular ultrasound analysis. J Am Coll Cardiol 2005;46:1002-1005.

225. Tanabe K, Serruys PW, Degertekin M, et al: Incomplete stent apposition after implantation of paclitaxel-eluting stents or bare metal stents: Insights from the randomized TAXUS II trial. Circulation 2005;111:900-905.

226. Hong MK, Mintz GS, Lee CW, et al: Late stent malapposition after drug-eluting stent implantation: An intravascular ultrasound analysis with long-term follow-up. Circulation 2006;113:414-419.

227. Sano K, Mintz GS, Carlier SG, et al: Volumetric intravascular ultrasound assessment of neointimal hyperplasia and nonuniform stent strut distribution in sirolimus-eluting stent restenosis. Am J Cardiol 2006;98:1559-1562.

228. Takebayashi H, Mintz GS, Carlier SG, et al: Nonuniform strut distribution correlates with more neointimal hyperplasia after sirolimus-eluting stent implantation. Circulation 2004;110:3430-3434.

229. Lemos PA, Saia F, Ligthart JM, et al: Coronary restenosis after sirolimus-eluting stent implantation: Morphological description and mechanistic analysis from a consecutive series of cases. Circulation 2003;108:257-260.

230. Halkin A, Carlier S, Leon MB: Late incomplete lesion coverage following Cypher stent deployment for diffuse right coronary artery stenosis. Heart 2004;90:e45.

231. Aoki J, Nakazawa G, Tanabe K, et al: Incidence and clinical impact of coronary stent fracture after sirolimus-eluting stent implantation. Catheter Cardiovasc Interv 2007;69:380-386.

232. Lee MS, Jurewitz D, Aragon J, et al: Stent fracture associated with drug-eluting stents: Clinical characteristics and implications. Catheter Cardiovasc Interv 2007;69:387-394.

233. Hausmann D, Erbel R, Alibelli CM, et al: The safety of intracoronary ultrasound: A multicenter survey of 2207 examinations. Circulation 1995;91:623-630.

234. Evans JL, Ng KH, Wiet SG, et al: Accurate three-dimensional reconstruction of intravascular ultrasound data: Spatially correct three-dimensional reconstructions. Circulation 1996;93:567-576.

235. Solomon SB, Dickfeld T, Calkins H: Real-time cardiac catheter navigation on three-dimensional CT images. J Interv Card Electrophysiol 2003;8:27-36.

236. Feldman CL, Ilegbusi OJ, Hu Z, et al: Determination of in vivo velocity and endothelial shear stress patterns with phasic flow in human coronary arteries: A methodology to predict progression of coronary atherosclerosis. Am Heart J 2002;143:931-939.

237. Stone PH, Coskun AU, Kinlay S, et al: Effect of endothelial shear stress on the progression of coronary artery disease, vascular remodeling, and in-stent restenosis in humans: In vivo 6-month follow-up study. Circulation 2003;108:438-444.

238. Stone PH, Coskun AU, Yeghiazarians Y, et al: Prediction of sites of coronary atherosclerosis progression: In vivo profiling of endothelial shear stress, lumen, and outer vessel wall characteristics to predict vascular behavior. Curr Opin Cardiol 2003;18:458-470.

239. Wentzel JJ, Krams R, Schuurbiers JC, et al: Relationship between neointimal thickness and shear stress after Wallstent implantation in human coronary arteries. Circulation 2001;103:1740-1745.

240. Gijsen FJ, Oortman RM, Wentzel JJ, et al: Usefulness of shear stress pattern in predicting neointima distribution in sirolimus-eluting stents in coronary arteries. Am J Cardiol 2003;92:1325-1328.

241. Carlier SG, van Damme LC, Blommerde CP, et al: Augmentation of wall shear stress inhibits neointimal hyperplasia after stent implantation: Inhibition through reduction of inflammation? Circulation 2003;107:2741-2746.

242. Kawasaki M, Takatsu H, Noda T, et al: Noninvasive quantitative tissue characterization and two-dimensional color-coded map of human atherosclerotic lesions using ultrasound integrated backscatter: Comparison between histology and

integrated backscatter images. J Am Coll Cardiol 2001;38: 486-492.

243. Kawasaki M, Sano K, Okubo M, et al: Volumetric quantitative analysis of tissue characteristics of coronary plaques after statin therapy using three-dimensional integrated backscatter intravascular ultrasound. J Am Coll Cardiol 2005;45: 1946-1953.

244. Wilson LS, Neale ML, Talhami HE, et al: Preliminary results from attenuation-slope mapping of plaque using intravascular ultrasound. Ultrasound Med Biol 1994;20: 529-542.

245. Spencer T, Ramo MP, Salter DM, et al: Characterisation of atherosclerotic plaque by spectral analysis of intravascular ultrasound: An in vitro methodology. Ultrasound Med Biol 1997;23:191-203.

246. Komiyama N, Berry GJ, Kolz ML, et al: Tissue characterization of atherosclerotic plaques by intravascular ultrasound radio-frequency signal analysis: An in vitro study of human coronary arteries. Am Heart J 2000;140:565-574.

247. Hiro T, Fujii T, Yasumoto K, et al: Detection of fibrous cap in atherosclerotic plaque by intravascular ultrasound by use of color mapping of angle-dependent echo-intensity variation. Circulation 2001;103:1206-1211.

248. Nair A, Kuban BD, Obuchowski N, et al: Assessing spectral algorithms to predict atherosclerotic plaque composition with normalized and raw intravascular ultrasound data. Ultrasound Med Biol 2001;27:1319-1331.

249. Murashige A, Hiro T, Fujii T, et al: Detection of lipid-laden atherosclerotic plaque by wavelet analysis of radiofrequency intravascular ultrasound signals: In vitro validation and pre-liminary in vivo application. J Am Coll Cardiol 2005;45: 1954-1960.

250. Nair A, Kuban BD, Tuzcu EM, et al: Coronary plaque classifi-cation with intravascular ultrasound radiofrequency data analysis. Circulation 2002;106:2200-2206.

251. Nasu K, Tsuchikane E, Katoh O, et al: Accuracy of in vivo coronary plaque morphology assessment: A validation study of in vivo virtual histology compared with in vitro histopa-thology. J Am Coll Cardiol 2006;47:2405-2412.

252. Rodriguez-Granillo GA, Garcia-Garcia HM, McFadden EP, et al: In vivo intravascular ultrasound-derived thin-cap fibro-atheroma detection using ultrasound radiofrequency data analysis. J Am Coll Cardiol 2005;46:2038-2042.

253. de Korte CL, Pasterkamp G, van der Steen AF, et al: Charac-terization of plaque components with intravascular ultra-sound elastography in human femoral and coronary arteries in vitro. Circulation 2000;102:617-623.

254. de Korte CL, van der Steen AF, Cepedes EI, et al: Characteriza-tion of plaque components and vulnerability with intra-vascular ultrasound elastography. Phys Med Biol 2000;45: 1465-1475.

255. de Korte CL, Sierevogel MJ, Mastik F, et al: Identification of atherosclerotic plaque components with intravascular ultra-sound elastography in vivo: A Yucatan pig study. Circulation 2002;105:1627-1630.

256. Schaar JA, De Korte CL, Mastik F, et al: Characterizing vulner-able plaque features with intravascular elastography. Circula-tion 2003;108:2636-2641.

257. Schaar JA, Regar E, Mastik F, et al: Incidence of high-strain patterns in human coronary arteries: assessment with three-dimensional intravascular palpography and correlation with clinical presentation. Circulation 2004;109:2716-2719.

258. Barger AC, Beeuwkes R, 3rd, Lainey LL, et al: Hypothesis: Vasa vasorum and neovascularization of human coronary arteries. A possible role in the pathophysiology of atheroscle-rosis. N Engl J Med 1984;310:175-177.

259. Wilson SH, Herrmann J, Lerman LO, et al: Simvastatin pre-serves the structure of coronary adventitial vasa vasorum in experimental hypercholesterolemia independent of lipid lowering. Circulation 2002;105:415-418.

260. Kolodgie FD, Gold HK, Burke AP, et al: Intraplaque hemor-rhage and progression of coronary atheroma. N Engl J Med 2003;349:2316-2325.

261. Moreno PR, Purushothaman KR, Fuster V, et al: Plaque neo-vascularization is increased in ruptured atherosclerotic lesions of human aorta: Implications for plaque vulnerabil-ity. Circulation 2004;110:2032-2038.

262. Moulton KS, Vakili K, Zurakowski D, et al: Inhibition of plaque neovascularization reduces macrophage accumula-tion and progression of advanced atherosclerosis. Proc Natl Acad Sci U S A 2003;100:4736-4741.

263. Carlier S, Kakadiaris IA, Dib N, et al: Vasa vasorum imaging: A new window to the clinical detection of vulnerable athero-sclerotic plaques. Curr Atheroscler Rep 2005;7:164-169.

264. Alkan-Onyuksel H, Demos SM, Lanza GM, et al: Develop-ment of inherently echogenic liposomes as an ultrasonic contrast agent. J Pharm Sci 1996;85:486-490.

265. Hamilton AJ, Huang SL, Warnick D, et al: Intravascular ultra-sound molecular imaging of atheroma components in vivo. J Am Coll Cardiol 2004;43:453-460.

266. Lanza GM, Wallace KD, Scott MJ, et al: A novel site-targeted ultrasonic contrast agent with broad biomedical application. Circulation 1996;94:3334-3340.

267. Lanza GM, Abendschein DR, Hall CS, et al: In vivo molecular imaging of stretch-induced tissue factor in carotid arteries with ligand-targeted nanoparticles. J Am Soc Echocardiogr 2000;13:608-614.

268. Demos SM, Alkan-Onyuksel H, Kane BJ, et al: In vivo target-ing of acoustically reflective liposomes for intravascular and transvascular ultrasonic enhancement. J Am Coll Cardiol 1999;33:867-875.

269. Crowder KC, Hughes MS, Marsh JN, et al: Sonic activation of molecularly-targeted nanoparticles accelerates transmem-brane lipid delivery to cancer cells through contact-mediated mechanisms: Implications for enhanced local drug delivery. Ultrasound Med Biol 2005;31:1693-1700.

63 Atherothrombosis and the High-Risk Plaque: Definition, Diagnosis, and Treatment

Pedro R. Moreno, Javier Sanz, and Valentin Fuster

KEY POINTS

- Plaque instability can now be detected through a number of invasive and noninvasive technologies.
- It is unclear which of these technologies will emerge as the most pragmatic and useful.

- Validation of plaque instability imaging via clinical follow-up to determine natural history will be quite important.

Independent of social status, race, or economical income, cardiovascular disease is by far the first cause of death, as shown in Figure 63-1.[1] In the United States alone, someone is experiencing a heart attack every 30 seconds, on average, with more than 1 million attacks per year.

Despite its deadly manifestations, coronary atherosclerosis is a condition that can remain asymptomatic for decades. The transition from asymptomatic, nonobstructive disease to symptomatic, occlusive disease is related to coronary thrombosis. This condition, known as atherothrombosis,[2] is related mostly to plaque rupture or plaque erosion. Atherosclerotic plaques at increased risk for rupture are characterized by specific features suitable for proper identification by novel imaging techniques. Therefore, it is easy to understand why the high-risk, vulnerable plaque[3] is considered by some the "holy grail" of cardiology today.[4] However, several high-risk plaques can be present in the same patient, making it difficult for the interventionalist to identify and treat the single plaque that would trigger thrombosis. This fundamental issue may limit the scope of this field in the future. Nevertheless, tremendous advances are being made in the diagnosis and therapy of high-risk plaques. Therefore, it is crucial for interventional cardiologists to develop a comprehensive approach to plaque vulnerability.

This chapter provides a systematic approach to high-risk vulnerable plaques and is divided into four sections. The first section is devoted to definition, incidence, location, risk factors, and clinical presentation. The second section is devoted to plaque composition, setting up the foundations for understanding plaque vulnerability. The third section summarizes the evolving field of invasive plaque imaging. The final section is devoted to therapy, from conservative, pharmacologic options to aggressive percutaneous coronary intervention (PCI) alternatives.

CLINICAL CHARACTERISTICS

Definition and Clinical Evidence

The concept of high-risk plaques evolved from pathologic studies that evaluated lesions responsible for thrombosis. Muller and colleagues originally introduced the term "vulnerable plaque" in 1985 to describe the potential of certain vessels to become vulnerable to thrombotic occlusion after plaque disruption in a circadian pattern.[5]

The adoption of the term "vulnerable plaque" by most investigators relies on the temporal associations among acute coronary thrombosis and certain types of morphologic features contained in the culprit atherosclerotic plaques (thin fibrous cap, large lipid core,

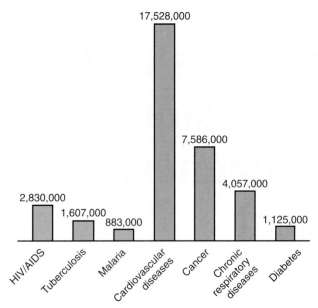

17,528,000

7,586,000

4,057,000

2,830,000

1,607,000

883,000

1,125,000

HIV/AIDS

Tuberculosis

Malaria

Cardiovascular diseases

Cancer

Chronic respiratory diseases

Diabetes

Figure 63-1. Projected global deaths according to the World Health Organization. (Redrawn from Fuster V, Moreno PR, Fayad ZA, et al: Atherothrombosis and high-risk plaque. Part I: Evolving concepts. J Am Coll Cardiol 2005;46:937-954.)

macrophages),[6] which are discussed later in this chapter. However, in daily practice in the cardiac catheterization laboratory, these morphologic features cannot be visualized. As a result, a histologic definition does not meet clinical standards. Therefore, we need a definition that can be useful in daily practice. For the interventionalist, the high-risk, vulnerable plaque is defined as a nonobstructive, silent coronary lesion that suddenly becomes obstructive and symptomatic, as shown in Figure 63-2. The clinical evidence of this disease was developed by Ambrose and Fuster in 1988, when they studied the baseline characteristics of lesions that evolved to produce acute myocardial infarction (AMI).[7] The investigators found that, at baseline, the majority of these lesions were nonobstructive, with mean diameter stenosis of 48%. Multiple investigators reproduced this finding, creating the concept that most of the lesions responsible for infarction originate from nonobstructive coronary artery disease (CAD).

Incidence

In line with the Ambrose and Fuster criteria, the number of nonobstructive, asymptomatic lesions

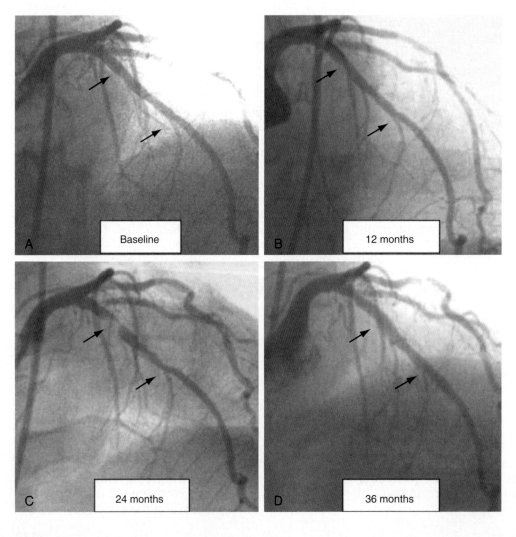

Figure 63-2. Rapid progression from nonobstructive, asymptomatic to severely obstructive and symptomatic disease, fulfilling the clinical definition of vulnerable plaques. Sequential coronary angiograms of the left anterior descending coronary artery (LAD) were performed at 12-month intervals. Arrows indicate locations of stenosis. **A,** Baseline angiogram showing 10% to 20% stenosis in the LAD in the proximal and middle segments. **B,** Progression to 30% to 40% stenosis in both segments, 12 months after the baseline angiogram. **C,** At 24 months, there is further progression to severe, 95% stenosis in the proximal segment and 50% stenosis in the middle segment. At that time, the patient was treated with a single drug-eluting stent covering both lesions (angiogram not shown). **D,** Stenosis is 10% to 20% in the same segments 12 months after local therapy with stent (36 months after baseline angiogram). (Courtesy of the cardiac catheterization laboratory at Mount Sinai Medical Center, New York, New York.)

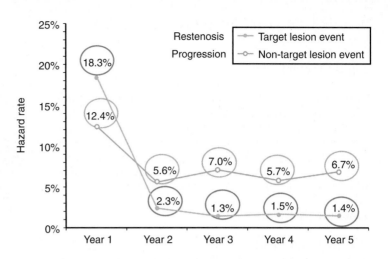

Figure 63-3. Hazard rates per year for target-lesion (*blue*) and nontarget-lesion (*red*) events derived from life table survival analysis. Target-lesion events include any repeat revascularization, death, myocardial infarction (MI), acute coronary syndrome (ACS), or congestive heart failure (CHF) attributed to the target lesion. Nontarget-lesion events include all repeat revascularizations involving the target vessel outside the target lesion, any nontarget-vessel revascularization, and any death, MI, ACS, or CHF that was clearly not attributable to the target lesion. (Adapted and redrawn from Cutlip DE, Chhabra AG, Baim DS, et al: Beyond restenosis: Five-year clinical outcomes from second-generation coronary stent trials. Circulation 2004;110:1226-1230.)

that progress to obstructive, symptomatic lesions can indicate the incidence of vulnerable plaques in patients with established CAD. Two studies have carefully addressed this issue. The first study included 1228 patients who underwent PCI for symptomatic CAD. The incidence of nonobstructive (also called nontarget) lesions that required additional PCI was 12.4% in the first year and 5% to 7% per year in years 2 to 5 after the initial procedure (Fig. 63-3).[8] The second study included 3747 post-PCI patients from the National Heart, Lung, and Blood Institute (NHLBI) registry.[9] The incidence of nonobstructive (nontarget) lesions that required additional PCI was 6% in the first year, ranging from 4.4% to 12.8% according to the number of vessels involved (Fig. 63-4).

Risk Factors

The risk factors associated with nonobstructive, silent lesions evolving into obstructive, symptomatic lesions requiring PCI were identified using multiple regression analysis and included multivessel CAD at baseline (three- and two-vessel CAD), previous PCI, and age younger than 65 years. Of note, treatment with statins failed to protect patients within the first year.[9] Regarding biomarkers, a 2007 review by Koening and Khuseyinova summarized the current view of this field.[10] Biomarkers per se cannot predict plaque instability but provide only likelihood ratios, c statistics, area under the curve data, and receiver operating characteristic analysis. Further research is needed to completely elucidate the role of

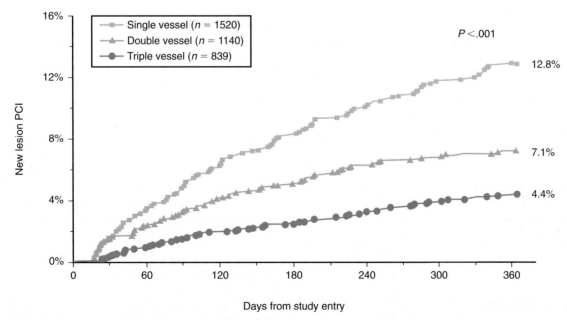

Figure 63-4. Kaplan-Meier analysis of repeat coronary intervention for rapid progression of nontarget lesions one year after coronary intervention. Note that the increased incidence of repeat intervention is related to the number of epicardial vessels involved during the first percutaneous revascularization. (Redrawn from Glaser R, Selzer F, Faxon DP, et al: Clinical progression of incidental, asymptomatic lesions discovered during culprit vessel coronary intervention. Circulation 2005;111:143-149.)

biomarkers in predicting plaque rupture and coronary events.[10]

Clinical Presentation

Nonobstructive, silent lesions evolving into obstructive, symptomatic lesions requiring PCI trigger acute coronary events in 68.5% of the cases, the majority of patients presenting with unstable angina pectoris and 9.3% presenting with nonfatal myocardial infarction.[9] Of note, because these studies excluded death, fatal events are probably underestimated.

Anatomic Distribution

The anatomic distribution of lesions evolving into acute coronary events was initially evaluated by Ambrose and Fuster, who identified proximal location as the only independent predictor for progression to AMI.[7] More recently, Wang and associates properly characterized the anatomic distribution of coronary lesions responsible for AMI.[11] As previously reported by other trials of AMI, the right coronary artery was the vessel most commonly involved (45%), followed by the left anterior descending coronary artery (LAD, 39%) and the left circumflex coronary artery (16%). The location within the vessel was dominated by the proximal segment, which harbored 80% of the lesions responsible for myocardial infarction in all three major vessels. For example, in the LAD, 90% of the high-risk plaques that evolved into AMI were located within the first 40 mm of the vessel. For all lesions, with each 10-mm increase in distance from the ostium, the risk of an acute coronary occlusion was significantly decreased, by 30% in the LAD, 26% in the left circumflex artery, and 13% in the right coronary artery. These data were recently reproduced by other investigators.[12] As a result, proper evaluation and treatment of high-risk plaques in the proximal segments of the coronary tree has the potential of preventing 80% of AMIs.

For the interventionalist, the incidence of high-risk, vulnerable plaques evolving into clinical events ranges from 4% per year, in patients with single-vessel disease, up to 13% in patients with triple-vessel disease. The lesions are usually located in the proximal segment of the coronary arteries, and the most common presentation is acute coronary syndrome (ACS).

After a review of the clinical characteristics, the next section of this chapter provides the basis for understanding the pathophysiology of the disease. Most importantly, this offers the foundation to critically evaluate novel imaging techniques that claim effectiveness in the diagnosis of high-risk, vulnerable plaques.

PLAQUE COMPOSITION

As discussed earlier, the mechanisms responsible for rapid progression to occlusion in atherothrombosis include plaque rupture and plaque erosion.[2] Plaque

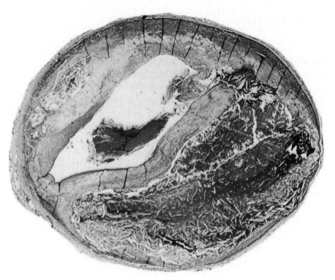

Figure 63-5. Cross-sectioned coronary artery containing a ruptured plaque at the shoulder of the fibrous cap with a nonocclusive thrombus superimposed. The large necrotic core can be identified by cholesterol crystals and extensive intraplaque hemorrhage secondary to plaque rupture. (Trichrome stain, rendering thrombus red, collagen blue, and lipid colorless.) (Courtesy of Dr. K-Raman Purushothaman, Mount Sinai Hospital, New York, New York.)

rupture is by far the most common cause of atherothrombosis, responsible for 70% to 75% of all events and up to 85% of events in hypercholesterolemic white males. In plaque rupture, disease progresses through lipid core expansion and macrophage accumulation at the edges of the plaque, leading to fibrous cap disruption (Fig. 63-5). As a result, identifying plaques at risk for rupture offers the possibility of preventing the most common substrate for coronary thrombosis. The second cause of atherothrombosis is plaque erosion. Included initially as "other causes of coronary thrombosis," plaque erosion gained attention in the last decade as a significant substrate for coronary thrombosis and sudden cardiac death in premenopausal female patients.[13] In contrast to plaque rupture, erosion occurs in plaques with no specific features suitable for detection. Most of these plaques exhibit histologic patterns similar to those of plaques responsible for stable angina. They are characterized by a thick, smooth muscle cell–rich, fibrous cap; reduced necrotic core areas; and a low degree of inflammation[13] (Fig. 63-6). Plaque erosion is also associated with cigarette smoking, suggesting that thrombosis in these patients may be related to a systemic, prothrombogenic pathway rather than a local, atherothrombotic mechanism.

Considering that plaques at risk for erosion cannot be differentiated from stable plaques, the imaging field has focused its attention on characterizing plaques at risk for rupture. In the absence of prospective, natural history studies, investigators have extrapolated the structural and chemical features of ruptured plaques to study this disease. The characteristic lesion is the thin-cap fibroatheroma (TCFA),

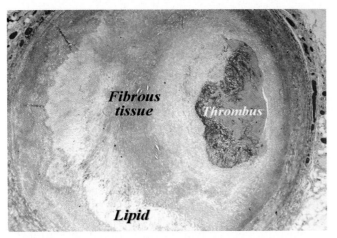

Figure 63-6. Plaque erosion. Cross-section of a coronary artery containing a stenotic atherosclerotic plaque with an occlusive thrombosis superimposed. The endothelium is missing at the plaque-thrombus interface, but the plaque surface is otherwise intact. (Trichrome stain, rendering thrombus red, collagen blue, and lipid colorless.) (Courtesy of Dr. Erling Falk, Aarhus, Denmark.)

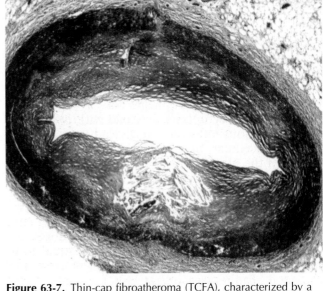

Figure 63-7. Thin-cap fibroatheroma (TCFA), characterized by a very thin fibrous cap and a large necrotic core. (Trichrome stain.) (Courtesy of Dr. K-Raman Purushothaman, Mount Sinai Hospital, New York, New York.)

which is considered the hallmark of high-risk, vulnerable plaques[14] (Fig. 63-7). The classic histologic patterns of TCFA include, but are not limited to (1) thin fibrous cap with increased stress/strain relationship; (2) large necrotic core with increased free-to-esterified cholesterol ratio; (3) increased plaque inflammation; (4) positive vascular remodeling; (5) increased vasa vasorum neovascularization; and (6) intraplaque hemorrhage (IPH).

Thin Fibrous Cap with Increased Stress/Strain Relationship

Autopsy studies have shown that ruptured plaques are characterized by a very thin fibrous cap, measuring $23 \pm 19\,\mu m$ (microns) in thickness. Most importantly, 95% of ruptured caps measured $64\,\mu m$ or less in the coronary arteries[15] and $60\,\mu m$ or less in the

aorta.[16] As a result, the first and probably most important histologic feature of TCFA is a fibrous cap $65\,\mu m$ or less in thickness. These thin caps are unable to withstand the circumferential tensile stress applied by the oscillations of arterial blood pressure. The ratio of the circumferential tensile stress to the radial strain of the fibrous cap equals the stiffness of the tissue. Hence, soft (fatty) tissue will be more strained than stiff (fibrous) tissue when equally stressed.[17] Furthermore, as caps become thinner, the stress increases in an exponential pattern[18] (Fig. 63-8). In addition, as lipid pools become larger, stress also increases. Therefore, the strength of a cap may be as important as the actual thickness of a fibrous cap. This stress/strain relation in the fibrous cap is considered a feature for plaque vulnerability.[17]

New technology aiming at detecting TCFAs should have a radial resolution less than $65\,\mu m$ and the

Figure 63-8. Relationship between circumferential stress (vertical axis) and fibrous cap thickness (horizontal axis). Note the exponential increase in circumferential stress when cap thickness is reduced to less than 200 μm. (Redrawn from Loree HM, Kamm RD, Stringfellow RG, Lee RT: Effects of fibrous cap thickness on peak circumferential stress in model atherosclerotic vessels. Circ Res 1992;71:850-858.)

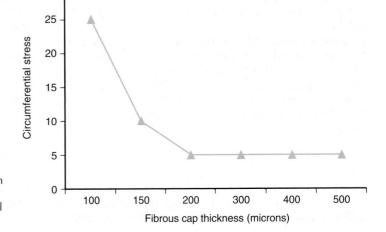

ability to quantify the stress/strain relationship in the fibrous cap.

Large Necrotic Core with Increased Free-to-Esterified Cholesterol Ratio

Modified oxidized low-density lipoprotein (oxLDL) is avidly taken up by macrophages via scavenger receptors, leading to cytoplasm overload with lipid droplets. Continuous inflow of oxLDL leads to cell death, with extracellular lipid accumulation within the matrix of the plaque. This is the basic mechanism of the necrotic core, which is formed after cell death by necrosis or apoptosis of lipid-laden macrophages, foam cells, and erythrocytes.[19] Active collagen dissolution by metalloproteinases contributes to core expansion, which plays a major role in plaque vulnerability. Dr. Michael Davies suggested that coronary plaques with necrotic cores larger than 50% of the total plaque area are at risk for rupture and thrombosis.[20] In the aorta, TCFAs exhibit necrotic core areas of 40%, and ruptured plaques up to 50%, of total plaque area.[16] However, other studies in coronary arteries have shown lower necrotic areas, down to 24% and 34% in TCFAs and ruptured plaques, respectively.[14]

The composition of the core may influence the propensity to develop plaque rupture and thrombosis. A necrotic core with an increased free-to-esterified cholesterol ratio favors plaque rupture.[21] The composition of fatty acids at the rupture site may also determine the likelihood of local platelet thrombus and fibrin formation. Increased concentrations of pro-aggregatory saturated fatty acids and oxidized derivatives of polyunsaturated fatty acids favor thrombus formation. Most importantly, tissue factor activity within the necrotic core is currently considered the major source of thrombin generation leading to arterial thrombosis in humans.[22] Of interest, the percentage of cholesterol clefts within the necrotic core is increased in ruptured plaques,[23] and these clefts may even exert a direct local effect by tearing the fibrous cap, as recently documented by electron microscopy.[24] Finally, the degree of calcification in the necrotic core is variable in TCFA. In a series of sudden coronary death cases, more than 50% of TCFAs showed a lack of calcification or only speckled calcification on postmortem radiographs of coronary arteries. In the remaining lesions, calcification was either fragmented or diffuse, suggesting a large variation in the degree of calcification within TCFAs.[25] In contrast, 65% of acute ruptures demonstrated speckled calcification, with the remainder showing fragmented or diffuse calcification.[25] To evaluate the role of necrotic core calcification in plaque instability, our group quantified the incidence of calcification in human aortic TCFAs ($n=42$), compared with non-TCFA plaques ($n=128$), using Von-Kossa staining.[26] The incidences of early (speckled) and advanced (coarse) calcification were 62% and 82%, respectively ($P=.006$), suggesting that a significant number of TCFAs may not exhibit necrotic core calcification. As

a result, calcification is an equivocal variable in TCFA and may not be used as a surrogate for high-risk necrotic cores.[27,28]

New technology aiming at detecting TCFAs should precisely quantify necrotic core areas, which should be at least 24% of total plaque area. It should also provide free cholesterol and tissue factor content, independent of the degree of calcification.

Increased Plaque Inflammation

Macrophages and T cells play a major active role in the pathophysiology of TCFA. These cells are capable of degrading extracellular matrix by phagocytosis or secretion of proteolytic enzymes; thus, enzymes such as plasminogen activators and matrix metalloproteinases (MMPs)—including collagenases, elastases, gelatinases, and stromelysins—weaken the already thin fibrous cap and predispose it to rupture.[29,30] The continuing entry, survival, and replication of monocyte-macrophages within plaques is mediated by a defense mechanism aimed to remove oxLDL and reduce the deleterious effects related to oxidation and reactive oxygen generation (ROS) products. Cytokines regulate oxLDL uptake, modulating the macrophage scavenger receptors. Most importantly, in situations where the macrophage scavenger capacity is overloaded, these cytokines also activate cell death by apoptosis, releasing MMPs and tissue factor.[31,32] This link was elegantly documented by Hutter and colleagues, who showed excellent correlations between macrophage density, apoptosis, and tissue factor expression in human and mouse atherosclerotic lesions.[33] Thus, macrophages, following what appears to be a defensive mechanism protecting the vessel wall, may eventually fail and undergo apoptosis, leading to plaque rupture and thrombosis.[31,34,35] Of clinical relevance, multiple studies have shown that macrophage content is increased in plaques from patients with ACS, compared to plaques from patients with stable angina.[36] Therefore, plaque inflammation is a pivotal feature of plaque vulnerability.[2,37,38]

New technology aiming at detecting TCFAs should have the resolution to identify and quantify macrophages in the fibrous cap and shoulders of the atherosclerotic plaque.

Positive Vascular Remodeling

The eccentric growth of atheroma away from the lumen was described by Glagov and colleagues in 1987.[39] The vessel wall can expand significantly to harbor large atheromas without obstructing the lumen (Fig. 63-9). Since then, remodeling has been consistently identified in lesions responsible for ACS. Varnava and Davies studied the relationship between remodeling and plaque vulnerability. Of 108 coronary plaques analyzed, 64 (59%) had undergone no remodeling or positive remodeling, and 44 (41%) had undergone negative remodeling (vessel shrinkage).[40] Lesions with positive remodeling, compared

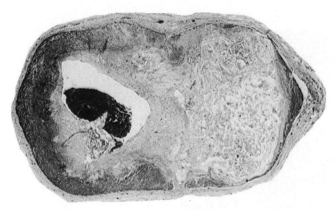

Figure 63-9. Large human thrombotic left main coronary artery plaque with extensive remodeling containing a large necrotic core. (Courtesy of Dr. K-Raman Purushothaman, Mount Sinai Hospital, New York, New York.)

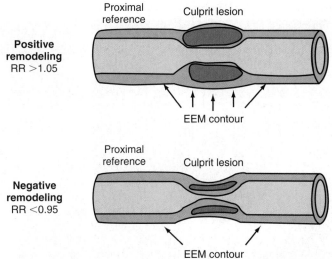

Remodeling ratio (RR) = EEM area lesion / EEM area proximal reference

Figure 63-10. Diagram of remodeling explaining the direction of positive and negative remodeling. See text for details. EEM, external elastic membrane; RR, remodeling ratio. (Redrawn from Schoenhagen P, Ziada KM, Kapadia SR, et al: Extent and direction of arterial remodeling in stable versus unstable coronary syndromes: An intravascular ultrasound study. Circulation 2000;101:598-603.)

to lesions with vessel shrinkage, had a larger lipid core (mean, 39%±21% versus 22%±23%; $P<.0001$) and a higher macrophage count (16±12 versus 9±11; $P=.005$), explaining the common link between compensatory remodeling and plaque rupture.

The mechanisms responsible for remodeling involve an inflammatory process at the base of the plaque, which leads to digestion of the internal elastic lamina (IEL) and involvement of the deeper layers of the vessel wall, including the tunica media and the adventitia. Several studies have shown increased expression of MMPs within the intimomedial interface of remodeled plaques.[41] Furthermore, disruption of the IEL is associated with medial and adventitial inflammation.[16] Concordantly, Burke and coworkers demonstrated that marked expansion of the IEL occurred also in plaque hemorrhage with or without rupture.[42] Based on multivariate analysis, independent predictors of remodeling included macrophage infiltration, calcification, and lipid core area, providing further evidence linking remodeling to plaque vulnerability.

The clinical relevance of remodeling was pioneered by Schoenhagen and colleagues, who studied 85 patients with unstable and 46 with stable coronary syndromes using intravascular ultrasound (IVUS) before coronary intervention.[43] The remodeling ratio (RR) was defined as the area of the external elastic membrane at the lesion divided by the same area at the proximal reference site. Positive remodeling was defined as an RR greater than 1.05, and negative remodeling as an R lower than 0.95 (Fig. 63-10). The RR was higher at target lesions in patients with ACS than in patients with stable angina. As a result, positive remodeling was more frequent in ACS (51.8% versus 19.6%), whereas negative remodeling was more frequent in stable angina (56.5% versus 31.8%) ($P=.001$), confirming the histopathologic associations between plaque remodeling and vulnerability.[43]

New technology aiming at detecting TCFAs should provide exact measurements to quantify the degree of vascular remodeling.

Of clinical relevance, Corti and colleagues were the first to document the same eccentric pattern for plaque regression after aggressive lipid therapy.[44] Multiple studies have confirmed this observation[45-47] (Fig. 63-11). Considering that lipid is the main plaque component that can be reversed with therapy, this eccentric pattern of plaque regression suggests an effective reverse lipid transport system through the deeper layers of the vessel wall, probably mediated by vasa vasorum neovascularization.[2,48]

Increased Vasa Vasorum Neovascularization

Neovascularization is the process of generating new blood vessels to nurture the atherosclerotic plaque.[48] Angiogenesis, the predominant form of neovascularization in atherosclerosis,[49] is mediated by progenitor and/or endothelial cell sprouting from postcapillary venules, leading mostly to new capillaries.[50] Atherosclerotic neovascularization evolves in early atherogenesis as a defense mechanism against hypoxia, which is generated by thickening of the tunica intima.[51] In advanced disease, neovessels may play a defensive role, allowing for lipid removal from the plaque through the adventitia, leading to plaque regression, as described earlier. The adventitial vasa vasorum is the main source of neovascularization in atherosclerotic lesions (Fig. 63-12). Coronary vasa originate from bifurcation segments of epicardial vessels and selectively respond to sympathetic activity.[51] Coronary plaque neovascularization in humans

Baseline Follow-up

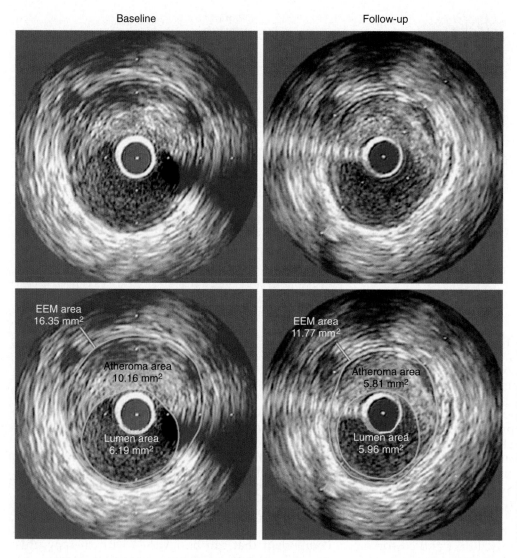

Figure 63-11. The top panels show the baseline and follow-up intravascular ultrasound (IVUS) images of a single coronary cross-section after 24 months of rosuvastatin treatment. The bottom two panels illustrate measurements superimposed on the same cross-sections, demonstrating the reduction in atheroma area. EEM, external elastic membrane. (From Nissen SE, Nicholls SJ, Sipahi I, et al: Effect of very high-intensity statin therapy on regression of coronary atherosclerosis: The ASTEROID trial. JAMA 2006;295:1556-1565.)

was elegantly delineated by Barger and colleagues[52] using cinematography (Fig. 63-13). Neovascularization was distributed from the epicardial fat to the plaque throughout vessel wall.[52] A decade later, Kumamoto and associates identified the vessel lumen as another source for microvessels.[53] Nevertheless, neovessels from adventitial vasa were 28 times more numerous (96.5%) than those from luminal side (3.5%). Neovessels from adventitial vasa characterized severely stenotic lesions and correlated with the extent of inflammatory cell infiltration and lipid core size. On the other hand, neovessels from lumen origin were found in plaques with 40% and 50% stenosis and were associated more often with IPH or hemosiderin deposits.[53]

Neovessels may also serve as a pathway for leukocyte recruitment to high-risk areas of the plaque, including the cap and shoulders.[54] The pivotal work of O'Brien and colleagues documented the mechanisms underlying neovessel recruitment of plaque leukocytes in human atherosclerosis. The expressions of vascular cell adhesion molecule-1 (VCAM-1), intercellular adhesion molecule-1 (ICAM-1), and E-selectin were twofold to threefold higher on neoves-

sels compared to the arterial luminal endothelium, confirming the predominant role for neovessels as a pathway for leukocyte infiltration in human coronary plaques.[55,56] More recently, our group documented histologic evidence of atherosclerotic neovascularization as a pathway for macrophage infiltration in advanced, lipid-rich plaques[57] (Fig. 63-14). Of clinical relevance, neovessel content was significantly increased in plaques with severe inflammation. Moreover, ruptured plaques exhibited the highest degree of neovascularization.[58] Further analysis of plaque angiogenesis in diabetes documented a complex morphology including sprouting, red blood cell (RBC) extravasation, and perivascular inflammation.[59]

New technology aimed at detecting TCFAs should quantify vasa vasorum neovascularization in the adventitia, in the tunica media, and within the atherosclerotic plaque.

In summary, plaque neovascularization, in what appears to be a defensive mission to provide oxygen and remove lipid from the atherosclerotic lesion, may eventually fail, leading to extravasation of RBCs, perivascular inflammation, and IPH.

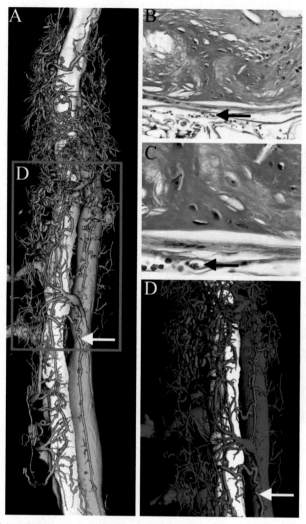

Figure 63-12. A, Volume-rendered high-resolution, three-dimensional microcomputed tomographic image of the descending aorta vasa vasorum. **B,** Histologic cross-section demonstrates atherosclerotic lesion in the inferior vena cava (*black arrow*). **C,** Enlargement of microphotograph shown in **B. D,** Highlighted differentiated arterial (*red*) and venous (*blue*) vasa vasorum (box and white arrow correspond to same areas on **A**). (Masson Trichrome stain, bar 500 μm).

Intraplaque Hemorrhage

Neovessel leakage leads to extravasation of plasma content and RBCs into the plaque, also known as IPH. Two main events occur after IPH. The first event includes ceroid accumulation, RBC membrane lysis, and lipid deposition. Perivascular foam cells frequently contain RBCs (hemoglobin [Hb], iron), suggesting that IPH initiates erythrocyte phagocytosis, leading to iron deposition and macrophage activation.[60] In addition, the erythrocyte membrane is very rich in cholesterol, promoting lipid core expansion and increasing plaque vulnerability for rupture.[61,62]

The second event after IPH includes macrophage activation by free Hb. After RBC membrane lysis, extracorpuscular Hb can induce oxidative tissue damage by virtue of its heme iron,[63] with subsequent production of reactive oxygen species (ROS). Extracorpuscular Hb can also activate the pro-inflammatory transcription factor, nuclear factor-κB (NF-κB),[64] leading to inflammation and angiogenesis.[65] The primary defense mechanism against free Hb is haptoglobin (Hp), which rapidly and irreversibly binds to free Hb to form a Hp-Hb complex. In the vascular compartment, the Hp-Hb complex is cleared by two pathways, via the liver (90%) or the monocyte (10%).[66,67] However, in extravascular sites such as atherosclerotic plaques, the only route for clearance of the Hp-Hb complex is via the macrophage.[67] Most importantly, the ultimate effect of the Hp-Hb complex on iron deposition and macrophage activation may be determined by the Hp genotype.[68] Two classes of alleles (Hp-1 and Hp-2) have been identified at the Hp locus at chromosome 16q22,[66,69] The protein products of the two Hp alleles are structurally different,[66,69] and the cardiovascular effects of this Hp polymorphism play a major role in patients with diabetes mellitus.[70-73] Multiple independent epidemiologic studies examining incident cardiovascular disease have demonstrated that diabetic individuals who are homozygous for the Hp-2 allele have four to five times the risk for cardiovascular events as those individuals who are homozygous for the Hp-1 allele. An intermediate risk was found in individuals who were heterozygous.[70,74-76] Remarkably, these studies demonstrated that the cardiovascular risk of Hp 1 homozygosity in individuals with diabetes mellitus was not significantly different from that found in individuals without diabetes; apparently the homozygous genotype mitigates the effect of diabetes on the development of cardiovascular disease.

New technology aimed at detecting TCFAs should identify IPH, iron deposition, RBC membranes, and hemosiderin deposits in macrophages. In diabetic patients, Hp genotyping may offer additional prognostic value.

Summary of Plaque Composition

Atherosclerotic plaques at high risk for rupture and thrombosis are characterized by several features, including large lipid core, thin fibrous cap, macrophage infiltration, positive remodeling, vasa vasorum neovascularization, and increased IPH. These concepts apply only to lesions at risk for plaque rupture and thrombosis (i.e., TCFAs). Plaques at risk for erosion and thrombosis do not exhibit any specific morphologic feature, limiting their detection by any imaging technique. This is a significant limitation of the individual, lesion-oriented approach to the high-risk, vulnerable plaque hypothesis. Nevertheless, even if only TCFAs can be identified and treated, a significant reduction of clinical events can be achieved.

PLAQUE IMAGING

Having reviewed the key features of plaque vulnerability, it is now easy for the clinician to understand

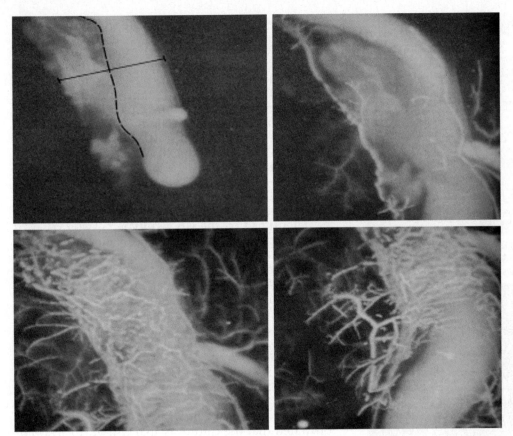

Figure 63-13. Color prints taken during the injection of silicone polymer into the coronary arteries of cleared hearts, demonstrating regions of vessels with abundant neovascularization. The positive regions are composed of networks of small-caliber vessels coming from the adventitia and penetrating the tunica media into the atherosclerotic plaque. (From Barger AC, Beeuwkes R 3rd, Lainey LL, Silverman KJ: Hypothesis: Vasa vasorum and neovascularization of human coronary arteries. A possible role in the pathophysiology of atherosclerosis. N Engl J Med 1984;310:175-177. Copyright 1984 Massachusetts Medical Society. All rights reserved.)

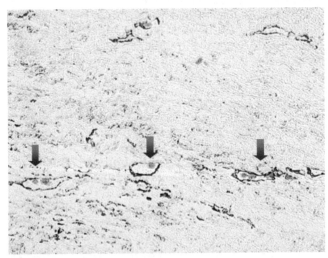

Figure 63-14. Histologic evidence of atherosclerotic neovascularization as a pathway for macrophage infiltration in human aortic plaques obtained at autopsy. Bicolor, contrasting immunohistochemical technique showing microvessels in cross-sections (*red arrows*) identified with the monoclonal endothelial cell marker CD34 linked to a blue chromogen and inflammatory cells identified with a combined macrophage/T-cell marker, CD68-CD3, linked to a red chromogen. (From Fuster V, Moreno PR, Fayad ZA, et al: Atherothrombosis and high-risk plaque. Part I: Evolving concepts. J Am Coll Cardiol 2005;46:937-954.)

the basic needs of any given technique to identify TCFA. Both noninvasive and invasive techniques are evolving rapidly. The noninvasive techniques were recently updated by our group and are beyond the scope of this review.[77] This section concentrates in the invasive imaging techniques, as understood in 2007. Multiple intracoronary imaging techniques are under development to identify TCFAs. Of pivotal importance, every imaging technique should have proper validation by histologic investigation. Considering that most atherosclerotic plaques (TCFA and non-TCFA) have a certain degree of fibrous cap thickness, necrotic core area, macrophage area, positive remodeling, and vasa vasorum neovascularization, simply determining the presence or absence of these features (sensitivity and specificity) is not enough. Proper histologic validation must include the accuracy of the technique to predict the extent or degree of these components, which involves linear regression analysis. These validation processes should be confirmed in animal models of TCFA before being introduced in human coronary arteries, with the ultimate test being a natural history study showing that specific plaque components detected by the technique are associated with increased clinical events.

Seven novel intracoronary techniques to detect TCFA are clinically relevant: IVUS, virtual histology

(VH), palpography, optical coherence tomography (OCT), intravascular magnetic resonance imaging (ivMRI), angioscopy, and spectroscopy. A summary of these techniques, the component detected, and the resolution or accuracy[6] is presented in Table 63-1. The first five techniques, IVUS, VH, palpography, OCT, and ivMRI, are already available in the catheterization laboratory or are under active evaluation in humans. As a result, these five techniques require a critical approach. For the remaining two techniques, angioscopy and spectroscopy, a summarized, evidence-based approach is presented.

The interventionalist must develop a critical approach to evaluate these novel techniques, understanding their potential but most importantly discerning their multiple limitations before considering them for clinical use.

Intravascular Ultrasound

After almost 40 years of evaluating the disease by lumen obstruction (angiography), IVUS allowed proper visualization the disease itself, and provided cross-sectional imaging of atherosclerotic plaques in vivo.[48-50] IVUS is based on transmitting and receiving high frequency sound waves from tissue through a low profile catheter (~1 mm), reaching a radial resolution between 100 and 250 μm.[51] With the years, IVUS became a very friendly tool; it is safe, quick, and easy. Most importantly, IVUS allows you to identify hemodynamically significant lesions that may be underestimated by angiography. This is the most common indication for IVUS in clinical practice. In addition, it provides the degree of calcification, plaque density, and most importantly, the degree of arterial remodeling. In addition, IVUS can document and provide information about plaque regression. As a result, IVUS is a fundamental tool for the interventionalist interested in vulnerable plaque.

Several studies have reported the IVUS characteristics of culprit lesions,[78] and the presence of multiple ruptured plaques in patients with acute coronary events.[79]

Now we will review the ability of IVUS to identify TCFA, which can be summarized as follows.

Fibrous Cap Thickness

Considering that the resolution of IVUS is greater than that needed to detect TCFA, IVUS-based efforts at quantifying cap thickness will always provide information that overestimates the expected values by histology. For example, Ge and coworkers carefully quantified IVUS-derived fibrous cap thickness in ruptured and nonruptured plaques from 144 consecutive patients with angina pectoris.[80] IVUS-derived ruptured plaques showed thinner caps compared with nonruptured plaques, with a mean cap thickness of 0.47 mm (470 μm), as shown in Figure 63-15. However, when ruptured plaques were evaluated by histology, the mean cap thickness was about 20 times lower, 23 ± 19 μm in the coronary arteries[15] and 34 ± 16 μm in the aorta.[16] As discussed earlier, this significant overestimation of cap thickness by IVUS is related to its poor axial resolution (100 to 200 μm), an inherent limitation impossible to overcome. As a result, it is very unlikely that IVUS or any IVUS-related technology will detect TCFA, the more common form of high-risk, vulnerable plaque.

Necrotic Core Area

Peters and colleagues evaluated the ability of IVUS to detect human coronary necrotic cores using in vitro video densitometry with a 30-MHz ultrasound catheter. Pixel gray-level distributions were represented as frequency histograms. The sensitivity of IVUS for necrotic core was 46%, and the specificity was 97%.[81] Several studies were then performed in attempts to improve these results with the use of an integrated backscatter approach.[82] The most recent study, by Sano and associates, showed encouraging results.[83] Of clinical relevance, a three-vessel prospective IVUS study evaluated the association between large echolucent areas (possible necrotic cores) and risk of future coronary events in 106 patients, 80% of whom had chronic stable angina.[84] Twelve patients had events 4 ± 3 months after IVUS evaluation. Most of these events (93%) occurred in plaques with large echolucent areas, suggesting a prognostic value for IVUS to predict future coronary events. Nevertheless, the total number of echolucent areas detected at baseline was not reported in the study, limiting the interpretation of the results.[84] We conclude that,

Table 63-1.   Summary of Current Invasive Detection Technologies

Technology	Component Detected	Resolution/Accuracy
Intravascular ultrasound (IVUS)	Remodeling, calcium	100-250 μm
IVUS-Virtual Histology	Calcific necrotic core, fibrous tissue, fibrofatty tissue, calcium	240-480 μm
Optical coherence tomography (OCT)	Necrotic core, fibrous cap thickness, macrophages	5-20 μm
IVUS-Elastography	Plaque strain	100-250 μm
Spectroscopy	Necrotic core, fibrous cap thickness, macrophages	NA
Thermography	Metabolic activity of the plaque	0.05°C accurate
Angioscopy	Surface appearance of the plaque	In vivo surface evaluation

NA, not applicable.
Modified from Granada JF, Kaluza GL, Raizner AE, Moreno PR: Vulnerable plaque paradigm: Prediction of future clinical events based on a morphological definition. Catheter Cardiovasc Interv 2004;62:364-374.

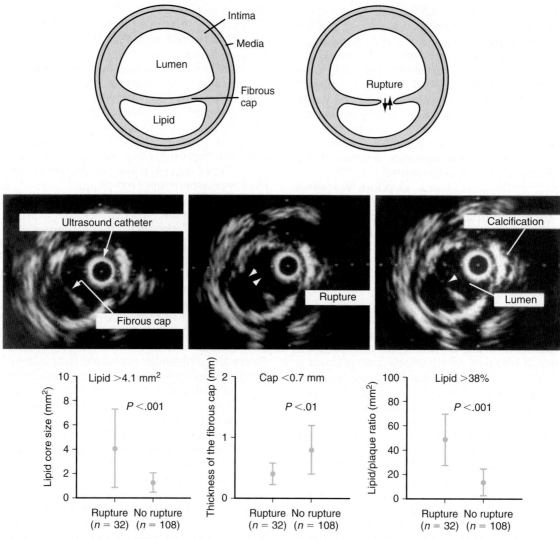

Figure 63-15. Intravascular ultrasound (IVUS) images of ruptured plaques, highlighting the fibrous cap and a large echolucent area under the cap suggestive of a large necrotic core (*upper panel*). Lipid area, cap thickness, and lipid percent area in ruptured versus nonruptured plaques are shown (*lower panel*). (Redrawn from Ge J, Chirillo F, Schwedtmann J, et al: Screening of ruptured plaques in patients with coronary artery disease by intravascular ultrasound. Heart 1999;81;621-627.)

although IVUS provides useful information about plaque echogenicity, the exact sensitivity and accuracy to identify necrotic cores are still unclear. The overall sense is that the resolution may not be enough to properly quantify this important feature of plaque vulnerability.

Plaque Inflammation
Detection of macrophages within the fibrous cap requires a resolution within 10 to 20 µm. Considering that IVUS resolution is 10 to 20 times higher than that, it is impossible for IVUS to detect macrophages in atherosclerotic plaques.

Degree of Positive Remodeling
Contrary to the previous features of plaque composition, IVUS is an excellent tool to detect remodeling, a major feature of plaque vulnerability. Multiple studies have documented an increased prevalence of

positive remodeling in culprit lesions responsible for acute coronary events.[85] IVUS-derived arterial remodeling allows understanding of the paradoxical relation between lumen and plaque size in ACS. It is clear that ruptured plaques are larger than fibrocalcific nonruptured plaques.[16,78] However, the degree of arterial remodeling is so pronounced that even large plaques can appear as nonobstructive, "mild" stenosis on angiography.[78] No other imaging modality can quantify remodeling better than IVUS. Therefore, IVUS will stand high in the search for the ideal combination technique that eventually can detect all features of plaque composition in the search for TCFAs.

Plaque Neovascularization
IVUS has the potential to detect flow within the plaque and therefore to identify functional neovessels. Whereas real-time IVUS is limited in the evalu-

ation of plaque perfusion, recent developments with contrast agents have dramatically improved the quality of Doppler ultrasound. Intravascular injection of microbubbles (i.e., small encapsulated air or gas bubbles) can boost the Doppler signal from blood vessels. Microbubbles can help in visualizing flow in smaller vessels, even at the capillary level, as previously shown within the myocardium using contrast-enhanced echocardiography (CEE).[86,87] Direct visualization of atherosclerotic plaque microvessels using CEE was successfully done by Feinstein in carotid lesions before endarterectomy.[88] In coronary arteries, IVUS-CEE successfully identified plaque neovessels with spatiotemporal changes and enhancement-detection techniques[89,90] (Fig. 63-16). To improve resolution, an IVUS prototype using "harmonic" imaging with transmission of ultrasound at 20 MHz (fundamental) and detection of contrast signals at 40 MHz (second harmonic) was developed.[91] Experiments showed improved detection of small vessels in harmonic mode relative to fundamental mode. Harmonic imaging improved contrast resolution outside the aortic lumen in atherosclerotic rabbits, consistent with the detection of adventitial microvessels.[91] Most importantly, these microvessels were not detected in fundamental imaging mode, suggesting that harmonic imaging is needed for detection and quantification of atherosclerotic neovascularization.

Virtual Histology

Considering the significant limitations of traditional IVUS imaging for identification of necrotic cores, Nair and Vince at The Cleveland Clinic decided to evaluate the ultrasound scattered reflection wave as a possible alternative to improve tissue characterization by IVUS.[92,93] This backscattered reflection wave is received by the transducer, where it is converted into voltage. This voltage is known as the backscattered radiofrequency (RF) data. Using a combination of previously identified spectral parameters, the researchers developed a classification scheme to construct an algorithm to test plaque composition ex vivo. Four major plaque components were tested: fibrotic tissue, fibrofatty tissue, calcific-necrotic core, and calcium. A color was assigned for each of these components and was displayed on the IVUS image (Fig. 63-17). Initial validation was performed on ex vivo human coronary specimens using 30-MHz, 2.9-Fr, mechanically rotating IVUS catheters (Boston Scientific Corp, Natick, MA). The Movat-stained histologic images identified homogeneous regions representing each of the four plaque components (Fig. 63-18). The unit of analysis (also called the "box") was initially composed of 64 backscattered RF data samples 480 μm in length.[93] In 2007, the unit of analysis comprises 32 backscattered RF data samples 240 μm in length (D.G. Vince, personal communication). The algorithm developed was validated ex vivo, with sensitivities and specificities between 79%

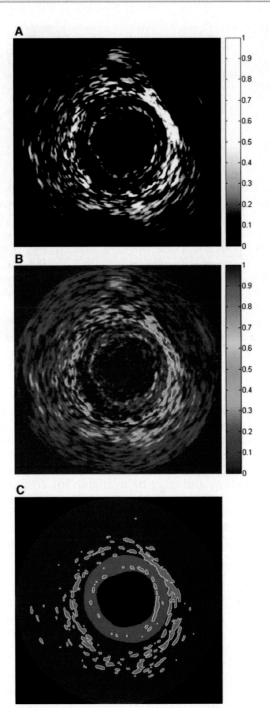

Figure 63-16. Differential intravascular ultrasound images to identify vasa vasorum, showing the subtraction of postinjection signals from baseline signals. **A,** Black and white image. **B,** Color coding applied to the image in panel **A. C,** Thresholding shows the most significant areas of enhancement. (Adapted from Vavuranakis M, Kakadiaris IA, O'Malley SM, et al: Images in cardiovascular medicine: Detection of luminal-intimal border and coronary wall enhancement in intravascular ultrasound imaging after injection of microbubbles and simultaneous sonication with transthoracic echocardiography. Circulation 1005;112:e1-e2.)

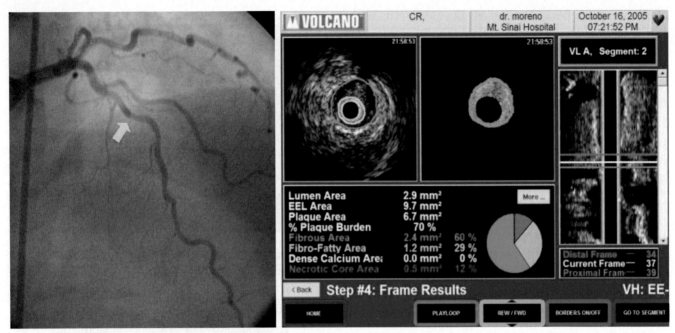

Figure 63-17. Color-coded reproduction of intravascular ultrasound Virtual Histology (IVUS-VH) plaque composition displayed in vivo in the cardiac catheterization laboratory at Mount Sinai Hospital, New York, New York.

and 93% for all four-plaque components.[93] Even though the initial work was performed with a 30-MHz catheter, the current Food and Drug Administration (FDA)-approved catheter (Eagle-Eye Gold) is a 20 MHz device. Nevertheless, a 45-MHz catheter is under testing and may be available for commercial use soon. VH gained a lot of attention recently because of the Providing Regional Observations to Study Predictors of Events in the Coronary Tree (PROSPECT) Trial, the first prospective natural history study designed to evaluate the prognostic value of IVUS-VH-derived plaque composition in nonobstructive segments. Seven hundred patients with ACS underwent three-vessel IVUS-VH after successful PCI. Enrollment was completed by mid-2006 and a preliminary report on follow-up will be available by the end of 2007. Despite all of these promising facts on IVUS-VH, the interventionalist needs objective information regarding the ability to detect TCFA, which can be summarized as in the following paragraphs.

Fibrous Cap Thickness
Considering that the resolution of IVUS-VH is greater than that needed to detect TCFA, IVUS-VH is limited in cap thickness evaluation. This was elegantly addressed in the initial publication by Nair and Vince[93]: "The window size currently applied for selection of regions of interest and eventual tissue map reconstructions is 480 microns in the radial direction. Therefore, detection of thin fibrous caps (≤65 microns below the resolution of IVUS) would be compromised, restricting the detection of vulnerable atheromas." Despite this inherent limitation, investigators have proposed a classification of "IVUS-VH-derived TCFA."[94,95] As a result, lesions with fibrous cap thickness greater than 65 μm will be incorrectly

classified as TCFAs, and the total number per patient will be overestimated. Still, if these data demonstrate prognostic value, we may have a useful tool for potential clinical use.

Necrotic Core Area
IVUS-VH was initially developed to identify calcific necrotic cores. However, the incidence and degree of calcification in necrotic cores is variable, and necrotic cores without calcification may not be properly identified.[28] Most importantly, the majority of advanced atherosclerotic lesions display a certain degree of necrotic core. As a result, when validating necrotic core using IVUS-VH, not only the presence/absence of the necrotic core is important (sensitivity/specificity)[96] but also the area. IVUS-VH routinely reports necrotic core area (mm²) and percent of total plaque area when used in patients. However, as of yet, no proper validation of these areas in patients (linear regression analysis) has been published. The only study that performed correlations between necrotic core areas by IVUS-VH and histology was done in the swine model, and the regression curves showed no correlations at all.[97]

As discussed earlier, multiple pathologic studies have established the concept that necrotic core areas from patients with ACS are larger than those from patients with chronic stable angina.[2,14,20] Conversely, fibrous plaque areas (collagen) have been found to be significantly lower in ACS patients.[22] Recently, Surmely and coworkers quantified necrotic core and fibrous areas in patients with ACS using IVUS-VH and compared them with those of patients with chronic stable angina.[98] Necrotic core areas were significantly lower in patients with ACS (6.8 mm²±6% versus 11 mm²±8%; $P=.02$). In addition, fibrous areas were

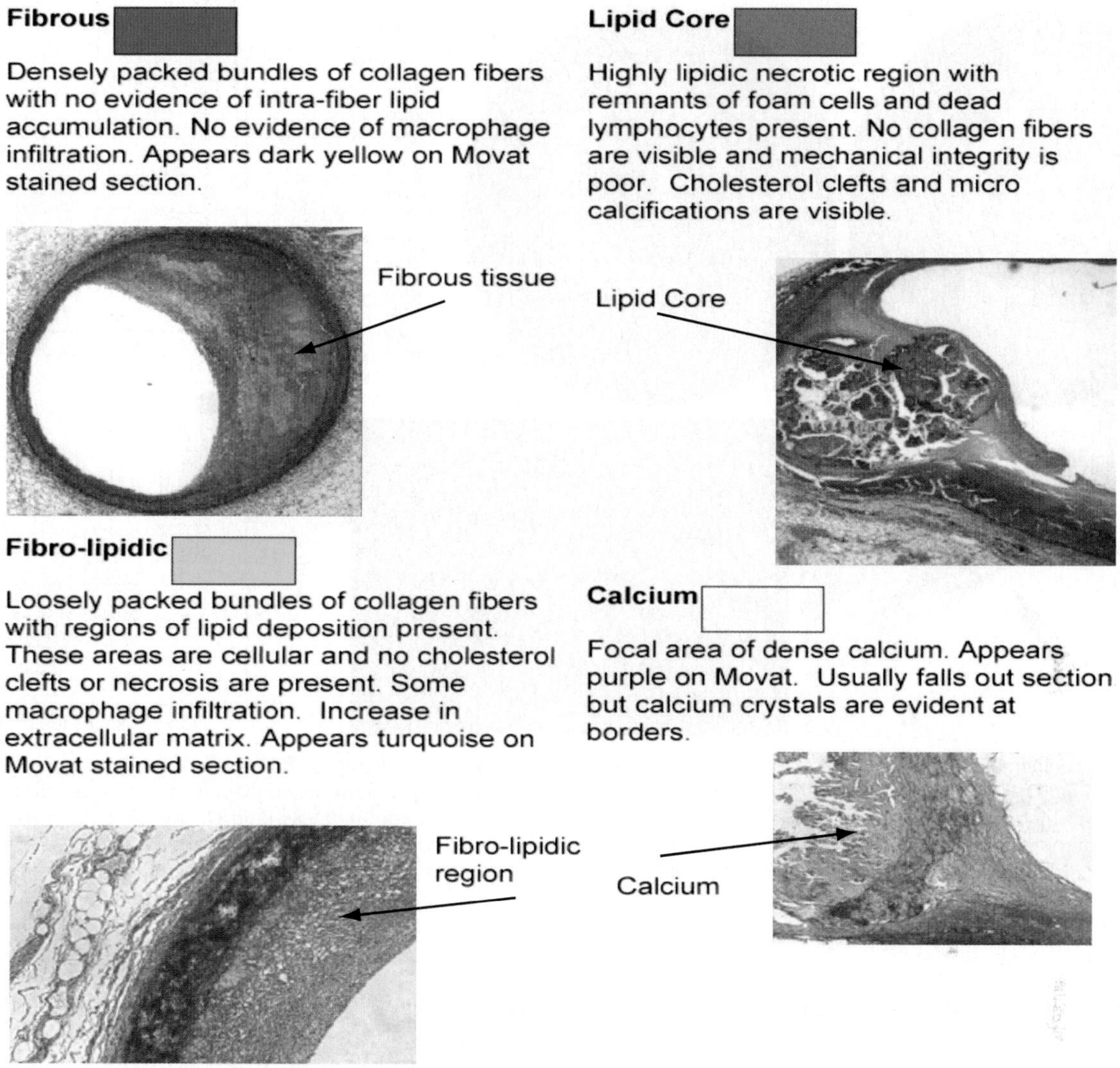

Fibrous

Densely packed bundles of collagen fibers with no evidence of intra-fiber lipid accumulation. No evidence of macrophage infiltration. Appears dark yellow on Movat stained section.

Fibrous tissue

Fibro-lipidic

Loosely packed bundles of collagen fibers with regions of lipid deposition present. These areas are cellular and no cholesterol clefts or necrosis are present. Some macrophage infiltration. Increase in extracellular matrix. Appears turquoise on Movat stained section.

Fibro-lipidic region

Lipid Core

Highly lipidic necrotic region with remnants of foam cells and dead lymphocytes present. No collagen fibers are visible and mechanical integrity is poor. Cholesterol clefts and micro calcifications are visible.

Lipid Core

Calcium

Focal area of dense calcium. Appears purple on Movat. Usually falls out section but calcium crystals are evident at borders.

Calcium

Figure 63-18. Definitions of the various plaque components obtained with intravascular ultrasound Virtual Histology (IVUS-VH). (Courtesy of D.G. Vince, The Cleveland Clinic, 2006).

higher in patients with ACS ($66 \, mm^2 \pm 11\%$ versus $61 \, mm^2 \pm 9\%$; $P = .03$). The authors concluded that plaque composition obtained by IVUS-VH is in contradiction to previously published histopathologic data.[98] Contrary to this observation, Rodriguez-Granillo and colleagues identified larger necrotic areas in ruptured plaques[99] and in nonculprit lesions[100] from patients with ACS. No IVUS-VH coronary autopsy studies have characterized lesions by clinical syndrome, and proper histopathologic validation of IVUS-VH by clinical syndrome is urgently needed to elucidate this controversy.

Plaque Inflammation

As discussed earlier, detection of macrophages within the fibrous cap requires a resolution within 10 to 20 μm. Considering that IVUS-VH resolution is at least 10 to 20 times higher, it is impossible for VH to detect macrophages in the fibrous cap of the plaque.

Degree of Positive Remodeling

IVUS is an excellent tool to detect remodeling, and IVUS-VH should preserve this advantage. As reviewed earlier, positive remodeling is related to large necrotic core areas, more frequently seen in patients with ACS. Plaques with negative or constrictive remodeling are associated with smaller necrotic core areas, usually seen in patients with chronic stable angina. Recent studies evaluated IVUS-VH necrotic core areas in plaques with positive and negative remodeling and found lower necrotic core areas in positively remodeled plaques.[78] Other investigators[101] confirmed these data. However, Rodriguez-Granillo and colleagues published opposite data showing larger IVUS-VH necrotic core areas in positively remodeled plaques, with an impressive correlation ($r = .83$; $P < .0001$).[102] It is difficult to reconcile these controversial findings and therefore impossible to elucidate, at this time, the real clinical value of IVUS-VH-derived plaque composition in clinical practice. Finally, vasa vasorum neovascularization and IPH require very

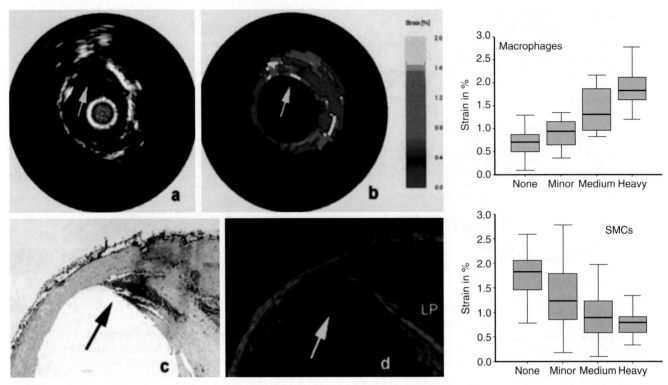

Figure 63-19. Vulnerable plaque (*arrows*) marked by intravascular ultrasound (**A**), elastography (**B**), macrophage staining (**C**), and collagen staining (**D**). In the elastogram, a vulnerable plaque is indicated by a high strain on the surface. In the corresponding histologic images, a high number of macrophages are visible in **C**, with a thin cap and a lipid pool (LP) visible in **D**. Box plots correlate the amount of macrophages (*upper right*) and the smooth muscle cell (SMC) content (*lower right*) with the level of strain. High levels of strain are associated with significant increases in macrophage content and significant decreases in SMC content. (Redrawn from Schaar JA, De Korte CL, Mastik F, et al: Characterizing vulnerable plaque features with intravascular elastography. Circulation 2003;108:2636-2641.)

sophisticated technology and cannot be identified by IVUS-VH.

Palpography

The stress/strain relationship on coronary lesions may play a significant role in plaque rupture and can be identified by another IVUS-derived technique called elastography or palpography.[17] Changes in blood pressure (stress) can induce deformation of the fibrous cap (strain) that can be quantified and displayed in a color-coded scale. Purple indicates a low-strain region that is hard, stiff, and rigid, whereas yellow indicates a region of high strain that is soft, deformable, and therefore potentially suitable for plaque rupture.[95] Studies at The Thoraxcenter have documented high sensitivity and specificity of this technique, with a deformation of more than 2% reflecting increased macrophage infiltration and reduced smooth muscle cell and collagen content[3] (Fig. 63-19). Therefore, this technique may provide valuable information to detect TCFAs. To risk-stratify patients, The Thoraxcenter developed a scale called the Rotterdam Classification, which divides the strain into four subclasses, the worst being ROC IV, with a deformation of greater than 1.2%. Three clinical observations are consistent[95]: (1) the number of high-

strain spots rises in parallel with the level of C-reactive protein; (2) strain is higher in ST-segment elevation myocardial infarction than in unstable or stable angina; and (3) aggressive treatment using statins, angiotensin-converting enzyme inhibitors, clopidogrel, and aspirin can reduce, over a period of 6 months, the intensity and frequency of these high-strain spots.

This specific technique was not designed to evaluate any of the other components of TCFA. As a result, fibrous cap thickness, necrotic core, degree of remodeling, neovascularization, and IPH are not suitable for evaluation by palpography.

Optical Coherence Tomography

A novel high-resolution intravascular imaging technique, optical coherence tomography (OCT), offers great promise to identify TCFAs. It is catheter-based, measures back-reflected infrared light, and provides the highest resolutions of all invasive modalities (5 to 20 μm).[103] Excellent histopathologic correlations have been performed, both for human coronary tissue and for animal models, highlighting a sensitivity and specificity of 92% and 94%, respectively, for lipid-rich plaque; 95% and 100% for fibrocalcific plaque; and 87% and 97% for fibrous plaque.[103]

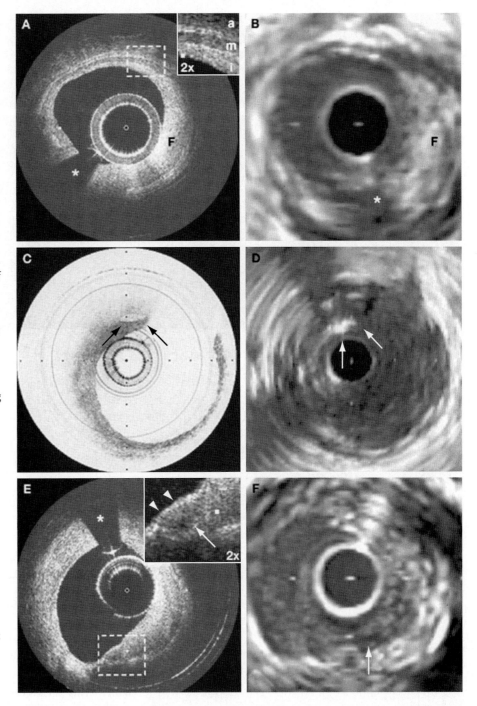

Figure 63-20. In vivo optical coherence tomography (OCT) images of various coronary plaque types compared with intravascular ultrasound (IVUS) images of the same sites. **A,** Fibrous plaque. From 9 o'clock to 2 o'clock, the three-layer structure of a typical intimal hyperplasia is shown, and a magnified area is shown in the inset. A homogeneous, signal-rich pattern indicates fibrous plaque (F), which is partly obscured by a guidewire artifact (*). a, adventitia; i, intima; m, media. **B,** The IVUS image corresponding to **A. C,** Calcific plaque. A signal-poor region surrounded by sharp borders represents calcific plaque, which is clearly delineated on the OCT image (*arrows*). **D,** On the corresponding IVUS image, calcium is easily identified (*arrows*), but the strong signal obscures the structure in front of the calcium deposit, and a back-shadow artefact obscures that behind the deposit. **E,** Lipid-rich plaque. A signal-poor region (*arrow* in inset) surrounded by diffuse borders and separated by a thin cap (*arrowheads* in inset) is consistent with thin-cap fibroatheroma (TCFA). **F,** The corresponding IVUS image suggests a superficial echolucent region. (From Low AF, Tearney GJ, Bouma BE, Jang IK: Technology Insight: Optical coherence tomography—current status and future development. Nat Clin Pract Cardiovasc Med 2006;3:154-162.)

Superb resolution allows for detailed imaging (Fig. 63-20). The major limitation of OCT is the need to displace blood in the vessel with saline flush, which makes this technique difficult in the evaluation of long segments. However, recent advances using optical frequency domain imaging (OFDI) allow for high-speed comprehensive imaging, scanning up to 5 cm with a single saline flush (Fig. 63-21).[104]

Considering all these promising facts, the interventionalist needs objective information regarding the ability of OCT to detect TCFAs, which can be summarized as in the following paragraphs.

Fibrous Cap Thickness

OCT is the only imaging tool that can identify plaques with cap thickness of 65 μm or less. This was demonstrated with histologic studies using proper linear regression analysis, which showed excellent correlations between OCT and ocular micrometry (light microscopy; r=.89)[105] as shown in Figure 63-22. Subsequently, in vivo studies with patients were performed to identify TCFA. Fibrous cap thickness was lowest in patients with AMI, intermediate in those with ACS, and highest in those with chronic stable angina[106] (Fig. 63-23). Using this analysis, OCT can

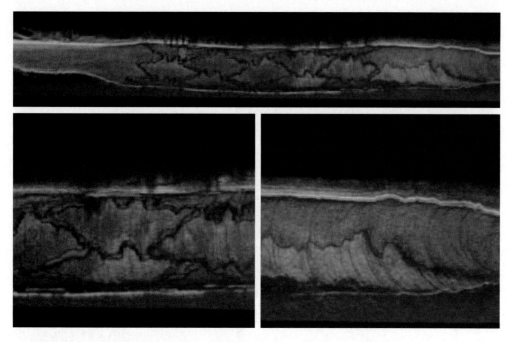

Figure 63-21. In vivo optical frequency domain images (OFDI) of a coronary stent deployed in the swine model. Normal endothelium is seen in red, dissections induced by the balloon during stent deployment in white, and stent struts in blue. Two sections of the image are enlarged below. (From Yun SH, Tearney GJ, Vakoc BJ, et al: Comprehensive volumetric optical microscopy in vivo. Nat Med 2006;12:1429-1433.)

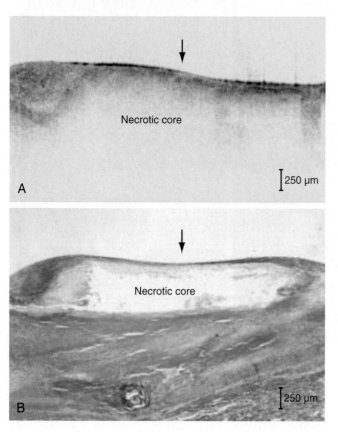

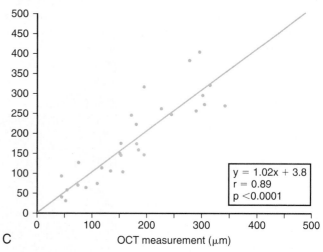

Figure 63-22. Optical coherence tomography (OCT) evaluation of fibrous cap thickness. **A,** Minimal fibrous cap thickness measuring 44.1 μm by OCT (*black arrow*), obtained from plaque illustrated in **B. B,** Minimal fibrous cap thickness measuring 40.4 μm by histology (*black arrow*). Necrotic core is visualized underneath the fibrous cap. **C,** Linear regression analysis showing an excellent correlation between OCT and histology measurements in 29 human atherosclerotic plaques. (From Jang IK: Optical coherence tomography: Studies at MGH. Presented to the Transcatheter Cardiovascular Therapeutics Convention, Washington, DC, 2002.)

estimate the incidence of TCFA according to the clinical syndrome, as also illustrated in Figure 63-23.

Necrotic Core Area

Because lipid pool and necrotic core are signal-poor, they are poorly delineated with respect to the sur-

rounding tissue. The lipid-rich plaque can be recognized, therefore, by the presence of large areas of ill-defined, signal-poor regions that are evident to the naked eye, as seen in Figure 63-20E, F. On the other hand, when the cap is thick and the signal is strong, the operator can tell that the signal is coming from a fibrous plaque composed mostly of collagen, as

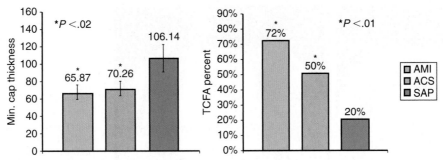

Figure 63-23. In vivo quantification of fibrous cap thickness by optical coherence tomography (OCT). Cap thickness was lowest in patients with acute myocardial infarction (AMI), intermediate in patients with acute coronary syndrome, and highest in patients with chronic stable angina. As a result, the incidence of thin-cap fibroatheroma was highest in AMI and lowest in chronic stable angina. (Redrawn from Jang IK, Tearney GJ, MacNeill B, et al: In vivo characterization of coronary atherosclerotic plaque by use of optical coherence tomography. Circulation 2005;111:1551-1555.)

illustrated in Figure 63-24 (see also Figs. 63-20A,B and 63-22). Of note, linear correlations of human coronary plaque collagen were recently performed, showing regression plots between OCT and measured collagen with a correlation value of 0.475 (P<.002); the predictive values for collagen were between 89% and 93%.[107] Nevertheless, it is important to highlight that OCT has not validated necrotic core areas as well as cap thickness and collagen.

Plaque Inflammation

As discussed for cap thickness, OCT resolution allows for proper identification of macrophages in the atherosclerotic plaques.[103] The first correlation in vitro was performed by Tearney and colleagues,[108] who identified multiple strong back-reflections from caps with abundant macrophage infiltration, resulting in a relatively high OCT signal variance. This signal variance was processed using logarithmic transfor-

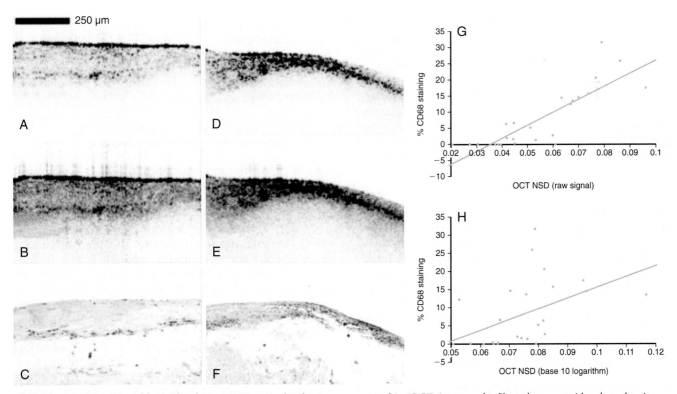

Figure 63-24. Raw (**A**) and logarithm base 10 (**B**) optical coherence tomographic (OCT) images of a fibroatheroma with a low density of macrophages within the fibrous cap. **C,** Histologic section corresponding to **A** and **B** (CD68 immunoperoxidase stain; original magnification ×100). Raw (**D**) and logarithm base 10 (**E**) OCT images of a fibroatheroma with a high density of macrophages within the fibrous cap. **F,** Histologic section corresponding to **D** and **E** (CD68 immunoperoxidase; original magnification ×100). Correlation between the raw (**G**) and logarithm base 10 (**H**) OCT NSD and CD68 percent area staining (*diamonds,* NSD data; *solid line,* linear fit). (From Tearney GJ, Yabushita H, Houser SL, et al: Quantification of macrophage content in atherosclerotic plaques by optical coherence tomography. Circulation 2003;107:113-119.)

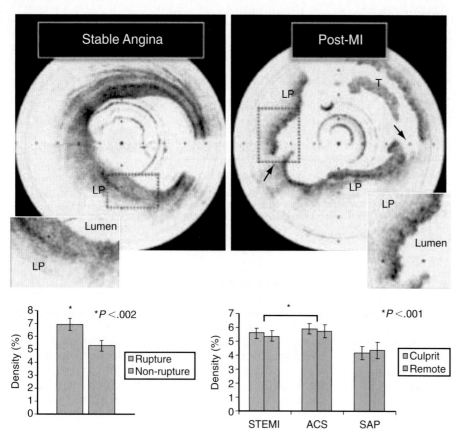

Figure 63-25. *Top,* Optical coherence tomographic (OCT) images of plaques from patients with stable angina and postmyocardial infarction (post-MI). LP, lipid pool. Note increased signal area at the fibrous cap in post-MI figure (*inset detail*), highlighting areas of increased macrophage density. *Bottom left,* Increased macrophage density in ruptured versus nonruptured plaques. *Bottom right,* Macrophage density in culprit versus remote plaques from patients with ST-segment elevation myocardial infarction (STEMI), acute coronary syndromes (ACS), and stable angina pectoris (SAP). Macrophage density is higher in both plaques (culprit and remote) among patients with STEMI and ACS, compared to patients with SAP. (From MacNeill BD, Jang IK, Bouma BE, et al: Focal and multi-focal plaque macrophage distributions in patients with acute and stable presentations of coronary artery disease. J Am Coll Cardiol 2004;44:972-979.)

mation (see Fig. 63-24A-F). Linear regression analysis then showed correlations for raw and logarithmic OCT-derived and immunostained macrophages of 0.84 (*P*<.0001) and 0.47 (*P*<.05), respectively (see Fig. 63-24G,H). In vivo studies subsequently showed increased macrophage density in ruptured plaques from patients with ACS (at both culprit and nonculprit lesions), when compared with nonruptured plaques from patients with chronic stable angina[109] (Fig. 63-25).

Degree of Positive Remodeling

OCT has limited penetration and requires a bloodless field to obtain good images. Proper quantification of remodeling results from multiple images with precise identification of normal vessel wall segments proximal and distal to the stenosis, as discussed earlier. Considering that OCT images are difficult to obtain and plaque penetration is limited, OCT may not properly quantify remodeling. This is a significant limitation of OCT.

Plaque Neovascularization and Intraplaque Hemorrhage

OCT is the gold standard to quantify neovascularization and the effects of novel anti-angiogenic therapies in other common diseases such as age-related macular degeneration, extrafoveal choroidal neovascularization, and proliferative diabetic retinopathy.[110-112] However, at the present time, no studies have tested OCT in the evaluation of athero-

sclerotic neovascularization or IPH. Nevertheless, it is likely that OCT will reproduce its resolution and clinical value in ophthalmology if tested to quantify atherosclerosis neovascularization in the cardiac catheterization laboratory.

Intravascular Magnetic Resonance Imaging

MRI is being increasingly recognized as a potential approach for the quantitation of atherosclerotic plaque burden and lesion composition.[77] MRI allows for three-dimensional evaluation of vascular structures with outstanding depiction of various components of the atherothrombotic plaque, including lipid, fibrous tissue, calcium, and thrombus formation.[113] In addition, MRI combined with cellular and molecular targeting is providing important data on the biologic activity of high-risk, vulnerable plaques, especially for carotid and aortic lesions.[114] However, MRI characterization of coronary plaques is considerably more difficult. The deep intrathoracic position of the coronary arteries (4 to 10 cm from the surface), the smaller dimensions, and the tortuous and irregular course of these vessels under continuous movement further exacerbate the problem, resulting in a reduction in image quality.[115]

Whereas conventional MRI resolution is approximately 460 μm, the resolution of intravascular MRI (ivMRI) is improved to 250 μm. As a result, ivMRI may provide valuable information in plaque characterization of coronary lesions. Pursuing this effort, ivMRI has undergone successful testing and is currently under aggressive clinical testing in the United States and Europe, with more than 100 patients enrolled. Therefore, MRI requires careful attention regarding the ability to detect TCFA, which can be summarized as in the following paragraphs.

Fibrous Cap Thickness and Necrotic Core

As stated earlier, the resolution of ivMRI is higher than 65 μm. As a result, ivMRI is limited in the identification of TCFA. To overcome this limitation, the luminal surface of the plaque was simultaneously evaluated in two separate bands: a superficial, luminal band of 0 to 100 μm and a deeper band of 100 to 250 μm.[116] TCFA was defined as the presence of an increased lipid fraction within the superficial band, which in turn denotes the presence of a thin fibrous cap, and increased lipid in the deep band, which indicates the presence of a necrotic core or an increased concentration of lipid-rich cells. Absence of lipid within the superficial band may be indicative of a thick fibrous cap, which is associated with more stable lesions.[116] With the aid of a partially inflated balloon, the MRI catheter obtains images in four quadrants (Fig. 63-26). Within each quadrant, the percentage of lipid is assessed in both the superficial and deep bands simultaneously, and the data are integrated to produce a circular, color-coded display. The resulting image represents the sum of the four superficial and four deep bands from the four quadrants. Validation studies were performed using a total of 34 human plaques (aortic and coronary). Examples are shown in Figure 63-27. Results of histologic analysis in addition to the aortic data resulted in a sensitivity of 100% and a specificity of 89%.[116]

Plaque Inflammation

With the advantage of molecular targeting, MRI can image macrophages using various pathways.[117] Several compounds, contrast agents, and nanoparticles are now available to target different molecules within macrophages.[118] The ultrasmall superparamagnetic particles of iron oxide compounds (USPIOs, SPIOs), also called magnetic nanoparticles, are internalized by macrophage-receptors and can be properly imaged by MRI, as shown in Figure 63-28. In addition to macrophage-receptor uptake, inflammatory cells can be imaged by targeting metabolic and proteolytic activity. The combination of MRI and [18]fluorodeoxyglucose positron emission tomography (FDG-PET) successfully images metabolic activity of plaque macrophages in patients with symptomatic carotid atherosclerosis (Fig. 63-29).[119,120] Proteolytic activity can be identified by MRI targeting cathepsin-B, MMPs, and myeloperoxidase, as recently reviewed.[118] Contrast agents including gadolinium-containing immunomicelles can also identify inflammatory cells in atherosclerosis.[121] Finally, imaging of interleukin-2 presence[122] and of apoptosis[123] may also provide an estimation of macrophage content in atherosclerotic plaques. Of note, macrophage imaging by MRI is available only as a noninvasive tool. To become useful for coronary plaque imaging, ivMRI will require higher resolution and signal-to-noise ratios than can be obtained with ivMRI coils.[116] Alternatively, newer magnetic nanoparticles, such as those that permit concomitant near-infrared fluorescence imaging,[124] may allow for sequential optical imaging of coronary macrophages, also via intravascular catheters.[118]

Degree of Positive Remodeling

The evaluation of remodeling requires perfect delineation of the external elastic lamina, both at the site

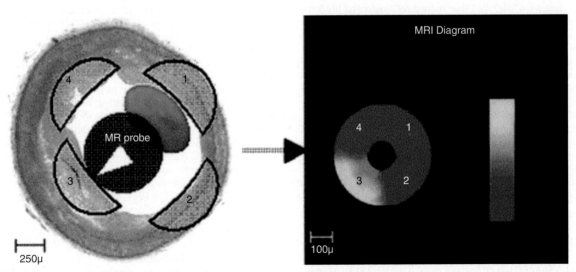

Figure 63-26. *Left,* Depiction of the magnetic resonance (MR) imaging catheter with imaging areas superimposed on a cross-section of a human coronary artery. Interrogation of the arterial wall takes place in four quadrants, each comprising a field of view. A single field of view is denoted by the white arrowhead. *Right,* The magnetic resonance imaging (MRI) diagram displays the lipid fraction in each quadrant assessed by the catheter. In this particular illustration, an increased lipid concentration is noted only in quadrant 3, which displays yellow. Quadrants 1, 2, and 4 are shown in blue, indicating a low lipid content or increased fibrous content.

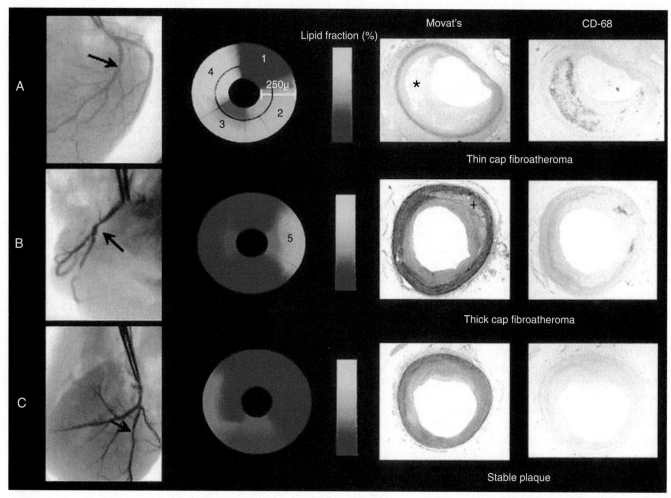

Figure 63-27. The magnetic resonance imaging (MRI) scan demonstrates excellent correlation with histology. Coronary angiograms, MRI scans, and histologic cross-sections of three intermediate coronary lesions are shown. An arrow on each angiogram marks the site of interrogation. The corresponding MRI is shown in the second column, and histologic sections of the interrogated sites are shown in the third and fourth columns, with Movat's pentachrome and anti-CD68 antibody staining, respectively. **A,** *left to right,* Thin-cap fibroatheroma in the proximal left anterior descending artery. The MRI display shows the presence of a high lipid content within three quadrants (2 to 4). Quadrant 1 has little lipid within the wall, as indicated by the lack of foam cells by Movat's staining or macrophages by CD68 staining. Quadrant 2 has moderately increased lipid concentrations, as noted by an approximate lipid fractional index of 60%. Quadrant 3 has increased lipid only in the deep layer, whereas quadrant 4 has high lipid fractional indexes (±100%) within the superficial and deep layers. Approximately 75% of the arterial circumference is lipid-rich. The MRI display corresponds well with subsequent histology, because the Movat-stained section shows a large necrotic core (*) and a thin fibrous cap, and the adjoining immunohistochemical staining is markedly positive for CD68 in the area corresponding to quadrant 4 of the MRI display. **B,** Thick-cap fibroatheroma in the right coronary artery. The MRI display shows no lipid content within the superficial layer (*blue*); however, a mild degree of increased lipid concentration is observed within the deep band (>100 μm from the lumen) in quadrant 5 only. The lipid fractional index is about 50%. The corresponding histologic section shows a thick-cap fibroatheroma with a small, deep necrotic core (+), which is confirmed by the anti-CD68 staining, corresponding with the MRI image. Because there is little to no lipid within the superficial layer, this lesion is considered a thick fibroatheroma. **C,** Stable lesion in the intermediate branch of the left coronary artery. A mild stenosis is seen by angiography. The MRI display of the lesion shows no increased lipid concentration in the shallow or deep bands of any quadrant, indicating the presence of a fibrous lesion (hence, blue display). This diagnosis was confirmed by histology to be adaptive intimal hyperplasia, and the corresponding anti-CD68 staining was negative for foam cells or a necrotic core. (From Schneiderman J, Wilensky RL, Weiss A, et al: Diagnosis of thin-cap fibroatheromas by a self-contained intravascular magnetic resonance imaging probe in ex vivo human aortas and in situ coronary arteries. J Am Coll Cardiol 2005;45:1961-1969.)

of the plaque and at the reference segment. The current stage of ivMRI does not provide this degree of delineation and therefore cannot quantify remodeling. However, ongoing coronary studies with ivMRI document the degree of remodeling using concomitant IVUS.

Plaque Neovascularization

As a general principle, molecular imaging for angiogenesis targets the endothelial cell. Proliferating endothelial cells respond to signaling by adhesion molecules, including integrins and cadherins, along with signals generated by secreted growth factors.[125]

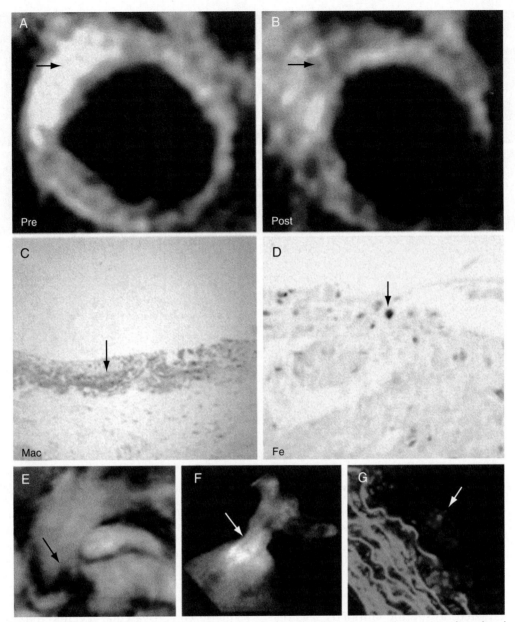

Figure 63-28. A through **D,** Cellular magnetic resonance images (MRI) of macrophage (Mac) endocytosis in clinical and experimental atherosclerosis using magnetic nanoparticles. MRIs obtained before (**A**) and after (**B**) injection of dextrinated magnetic nanoparticles (ferumoxtran, 2.6 mg/kg) show focal signal loss (*arrow*) within a carotid plaque of a neurologically symptomatic patient. Histologic examination of the carotid endarterectomy specimen demonstrated colocalization of macrophages, revealed by anti-CD68 macrophage antibody staining (original magnification ×100) (**C**), and of iron (Fe), indicated by Perls iron stain with neutral red counterstain (original magnification ×400) (**D**). **E** through **G,** Multimodality MRI and near-infrared fluorescent imaging of murine atherosclerosis using magnetofluorescent nanoparticles. **E,** In vivo 9.4-T electrocardiogram- and respiratory-gated MRI of an apolipoprotein E-deficient (apoE–/–) mouse. Injection of a clinical-type near-infrared fluorescent dextrinated magnetic nanoparticle (15 mg/kg of iron, 24-hour circulation time) produced focal signal loss (*arrow*) in the aortic root, a known site of atherosclerosis in the apoE–/– mouse. **F,** Fluorescence reflectance imaging of the resected aorta confirms a focal near-infrared fluorescent signal within the aortic root (*arrow*). **G,** On fluorescence microscopy, the near-infrared magnetofluorescent nanoparticles accumulate in intimal macrophages (*red, arrow*) within aortic root plaque sections (original magnification ×200). In contrast, smooth muscle cells (stained here with a spectrally distinct α-actin fluorescent antibody, *green*) modestly colocalize with the magnetofluorescent nanoparticles. (From Jaffer FA, Libby P, Weissleder R: Molecular and cellular imaging of atherosclerosis: Emerging applications. J Am Coll Cardiol 2006;47:1328-1338.)

As a result, molecular imaging can target these molecules, such as the integrin $a_v\beta_3$, which promotes angiogenesis by signaling basic fibroblast growth factor (FGF), or $a_v\beta_5$, which promotes angiogenesis by signaling vascular endothelial growth factor (VEGF).

Winter and colleagues evaluated atherosclerotic neovessels using $a_v\beta_3$-targeted paramagnetic nanoparticles in hypercholesterolemic rabbits[126] (Fig. 63-30). Other molecular targets have been successfully labeled for imaging of atherosclerosis. Matter and

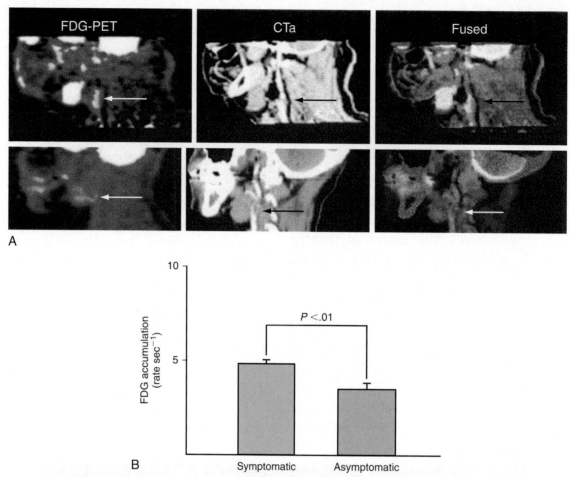

Figure 63-29. ^{18}F-fluorodeoxyglucose positron emission tomography (FDG-PET) and computed tomography angiography (CTa) images from patients with unstable carotid disease. **A,** FDG-PET (*left*), CTa (*middle*) images are combined to produce a fused image (*right*). *Top row,* Patient with symptomatic carotid stenosis. *Bottom row,* Patient with contralateral asymptomatic carotid stenosis. The arrows highlight areas of FDG uptake, corresponding to stenotic carotid plaque. **B,** A graph showing FDG accumulation rate in symptomatic versus asymptomatic carotid plaques. Note that FDG uptake into symptomatic plaque was significantly higher. (From Davies JR, Rudd JH, Weissberg PL, Narula J: Radionuclide imaging for the detection of inflammation in vulnerable plaques. J Am Coll Cardiol 2006;47: C57-C68.)

colleagues[127] targeted a specific antibody against the fibronectin extradomain B, which was labeled with radioiodine and infrared fluorophores and injected intravenously into atherosclerotic ApoE-knockout mice. Immunohistochemical studies revealed increased expression of extradomain B, not only in murine but also in human plaques, where it was found predominantly around vasa vasorum.[127] Finally, VCAM-1, a critical component of the leuko-cyte-endothelial adhesion cascade, was successfully targeted using phage display-derived peptide sequences and multimodal nanoparticles for MRI and fluorescence molecular imaging in ApoE-knock-out mice, adding an additional method to interrogate angiogenesis in atherosclerotic plaques.[128]

Intraplaque Hemorrhage

The evaluation of human carotid IPH was elegantly performed by Takaya and associates,[129] as shown in Figure 63-31. Of clinical relevance, IPH detected by MRI is associated with a significant increase in sub-sequent cerebrovascular events (hazard ratio, 5.2; *P*=.005).[130] Other investigators have confirmed these findings,[131] highlighting the value of MRI-detected IPH in complex atherosclerosis.

Angioscopy

Direct visualization of atherosclerotic plaques can provide information about plaque composition. Angioscopic classification of coronary lesions is performed by noting the color of plaques in a bloodless field. White, yellow, and glistening yellow plaques have been observed and studied in patients with CAD. Of significant clinical value, Uchida and coworkers evaluated the clinical prospective value of these three different types of plaques in a prospective, three-vessel angioscopic study including 157 patients with chronic stable angina.[132] The incidence of ACS was evaluated 12 months later. The majority of patients (75%) had white plaques, which were

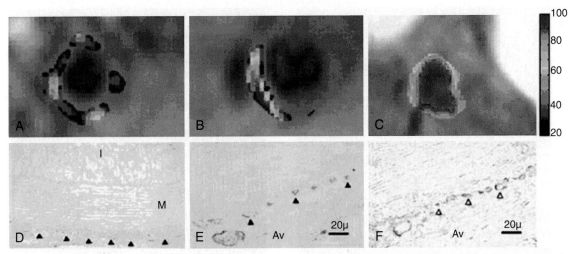

Figure 63-30. Molecular magnetic resonance images of arterial neovessels in cholesterol-fed rabbits. Percent enhancement of adventitial signal (false-colored from blue to red) is shown in aortic segments at the renal artery (**A**), in mid-aorta (**B**), and at the diaphragm (**C**) 2 hours after administration of $\alpha_v\beta_3$-targeted gadolinium-loaded nanoparticles. **D,** Immunohistochemistry of $\alpha_v\beta_3$ integrin demonstrates thickened intima (I) and $\alpha_v\beta_3$ integrin staining in adventitial neovessels (*black arrowheads*). Immunostaining in aorta from the cholesterol-fed animal in **A** (×600) delineates neovascular $\alpha_v\beta_3$ integrin (**E,** *solid arrows*) and expression of platelet and endothelial cell adhesion molecules (**F,** *open arrows*) at the interface between media (M) and adventitia (Av). (From Winter PM, Morawski AM, Caruthers SD, et al: Molecular imaging of angiogenesis in early-stage atherosclerosis with alpha(v)beta3-integrin-targeted nanoparticles. Circulation 2003;108:2270-2274.)

associated with a low incidence of ACS (3.3%). The second group of patients (18%) had yellow plaques, which were associated with an intermediate incidence of ACS (7.6%). Finally, the third group of patients (8%) had *glistening* yellow plaques, which were associated with an impressive incidence of ACS (68%), including death in 22% of the cases. Using autopsy information, Uchida evaluated fibrous cap thickness for each of the three plaque types (Fig. 63-32). White plaques were associated with thick caps (400 μm), yellow plaques with thinner caps (80 μm), and glistening yellow plaques with the thinnest caps (10 to 20 μm).[132]

Of note, Uchida also studied patients with chronic stable angina, who had a rather low incidence of yellow plaques. Other angioscopic studies in patients with ACS have shown a higher incidence of yellow plaques. Asakura and colleagues performed three-vessel angioscopy in patients 1 month after myocardial infarction.[133] Yellow plaques were detected in 90% of 21 culprit lesions. Yellow plaques were equally prevalent in infarct-related and noninfarct-related coronary arteries (3.7±1.6 versus 3.4±1.8 plaques per artery), suggesting a diffuse rather than a localized process in patients with myocardial infarction.

To evaluate the predictive value of yellow plaques in clinical practice, Ohtani and associates performed culprit vessel angioscopy in 552 patients with chronic stable angina, ACS, or AMI.[134] Yellow color intensity was also graded. The number of yellow plaques varied from 0 to more than 5 (Fig. 63-33). After 5 years, 7.1% of the patients developed ACS. The mean number of yellow plaques was higher in patients with an ACS event than in those without such an event (3.1±1.8 versus 2.2±1.5; *P*=.008). However,

the yellow color intensity scale was similar and not predictive.

Spectroscopy

Spectroscopy is a nondestructive optical technology by which the chemical composition of plaque components can be analyzed. After irradiation of tissue with a laser beam, scattered photons are acquired to identify specific features of plaque vulnerability.[135] Two different modalities are currently under active evaluation for intravascular detection of high-risk, vulnerable plaques: near-infrared and Raman spectroscopy. Both techniques have good correlations with histologic analysis of coronary and aortic tissue.[136,137] However, the complexity of signal analysis may force investigators to focus on only one or two features of plaque vulnerability. Both techniques face technological challenges in obtaining reliable signals through blood in the beating heart. Although this technique is promising, spectroscopy will require a significant effort to successfully overcome its limitations. Efforts are ongoing,[138] and in the near future it will be possible to know whether spectroscopy can stand as a useful clinical tool in the catheterization laboratory.

Before completing the imaging section of this review, it is important to mention that thermography was extensively evaluated in multiple settings with promising results.[139] However, the cooling effect of the blood and other limitations significantly reduced the enthusiasm for thermography as a potentially useful tool for intravascular detection of high-risk plaques.

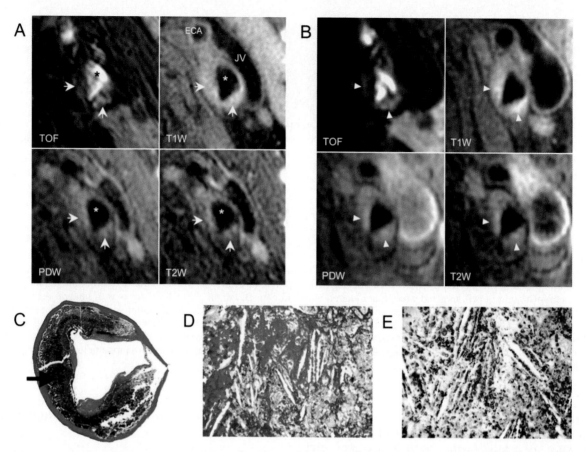

Figure 63-31. A, Signal intensity of type II hemorrhage at baseline examination. Type II hemorrhage is identified by hyperintense signals on time of flight (TOF), T1-weighted (T1W), protein density weighted (PDW), and T2-weighted (T2W) magnetic resonance images of left internal carotid artery (*arrows*). Asterisks show location of lumen. ECA, external carotid artery; JV, jugular vein. **B,** Images from 18-month follow-up scans showed a similar signal intensity pattern in the same regions (*arrowheads*). **C,** Matched Mallory's trichrome-stained sections from excised carotid endarterectomy specimen. **D,** High-power (×400) field taken from region (*arrow* in **C**) deep within necrotic core, shows hemorrhagic debris and cholesterol clefts. **E,** Glycophorin A immunostaining of the same region (×400) in an adjacent section shows extensive staining of hemorrhagic debris, indicating the presence of erythrocyte membranes. (From Takaya N, Yuan C, Chu B, et al: Presence of intraplaque hemorrhage stimulates progression of carotid atherosclerotic plaques: A high-resolution magnetic resonance imaging study. Circulation 2005;111:2768-2775.)

Summary of Intracoronary Imaging

The development of new technologies for the purpose of detection of high-risk plaques is progressing rapidly. Although individual devices have reached a certain degree of technological sophistication, a combination these modalities may have a better future (e.g., OCT plus backscattered IVUS,[140] IVUS plus Raman spectroscopy[141]). In the recently completed PROSPECT trial, three-vessel coronary imaging was performed in patients with ACS; the findings of this trial will certainly provide prognostic information related to invasive plaque imaging in CAD. If the event rate at follow-up is higher than expected with pharmacologic therapy, the scientific community will need to consider additional therapeutic strategies.

A comprehensive approach regarding invasive therapy is becoming mandatory for the interventionalist who is interested in prevention of recurrent coronary events. The next section of this review summarizes current and future therapies for high-risk, vulnerable plaques.

THERAPY

Systemic Therapy

The treatment of high-risk, vulnerable plaques relies on aggressive medical therapy, which has been shown to reduce coronary events and improve survival. As a result, systemic therapy is the cornerstone of plaque stabilization, with documented reductions in lipid content, inflammation, and vasa vasorum neovascularization.[142] Intensive statin therapy has produced a significant decrease in coronary events in patients with stable disease (Treating New Targets study [TNT] and Incremental Decrease in Clinical Endpoints Through Aggressive Lipid Lowering [IDEAL]) and in patients with ACS (Aggrastat to Zocor study [A to Z] and Pravastatin or Atorvastatin Evaluation and Infection Therapy [PROVE IT-TIMI-22]), not only in the

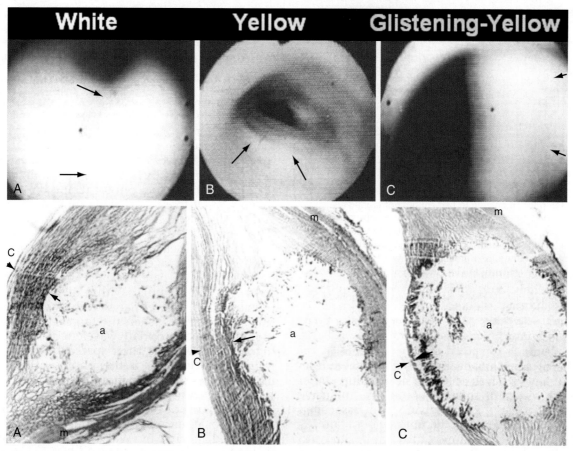

Figure 63-32. Angioscopic (*top row*) and histologic (*bottom row*) appearance of plaques at the time of autopsy. **A,** White plaque, associated with a thick cap. **B,** Yellow plaque, associated with a thinner cap. **C,** Glistening yellow plaque, associated with the thinnest cap. See text for details. (From Uchida Y, Nakamura F, Tomaru T, et al: Prediction of acute coronary syndromes by percutaneous coronary angioscopy in patients with stable angina. Am Heart J 1995;130:195-203.)

Figure 63-33. Angioscopic detection and grading of color of yellow plaques. **A,** Representative case in which no yellow plaque was detected in the right coronary artery (RCA): number of yellow plaques, 0; maximum color grade of yellow plaques, 0. **B,** Representative case in which multiple yellow plaques were detected in the RCA: number of yellow plaques, 3; maximum color grade of yellow plaques, 3. (From Ohtani T, Ueda Y, Mizote I, et al: Number of yellow plaques detected in a coronary artery is associated with future risk of acute coronary syndrome: Detection of vulnerable patients by angioscopy. J Am Coll Cardiol 2006;47:2194-2200.)

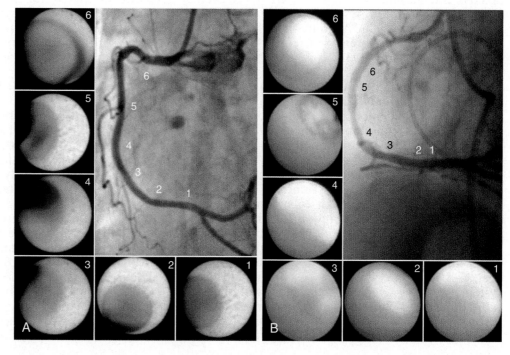

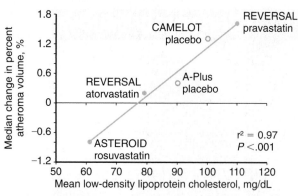

Figure 63-34. Median change in percent atheroma volume according to the type of statin used. A-Plus, Avasimbe and Progression of Lesions on UltraSound; ASTEROID, A Study to Evaluate the Effect of Rosuvastatin on Intravascular Ultrasound-Derived Coronary Atheroma Burden; CAMELOT, Comparison of Amlodipine versus Enalapril to Limit Occurrences of Thrombosis; REVERSAL, Reversal of Atherosclerosis with Aggressive Lipid Lowering Therapy trial. (Redrawn from Nissen SE, Nicholls SJ, Sipahi I, et al: Effect of very high-intensity statin therapy on regression of coronary atherosclerosis: The ASTEROID trial. JAMA 2006;295:1556-1565.)

incidence of coronary death or myocardial infarction[143] but also in development of heart failure, independent of recurrent infarct.[144] Similarly, intensive statin therapy early after an ACS was associated with clinical benefits that became evident after 4 to 12 months.[145] Most importantly, in A Study to Evaluate the Effect of Rosuvastatin on Intravascular Ultrasound-Derived Coronary Atheroma Burden (ASTEROID),[47] aggressive therapy with rosuvastatin (40 mg/day) led to an absolute regression of atheroma volume (Fig. 63-34). Another potent anti-atherogenic therapy is increasing high-density lipoprotein (HDL). Studies using bezafibrate, a peroxisome proliferator-activated receptor (PPAR)-α agonist, and fenofibrate demonstrated reduced events and plaque regression, respectively.[146,147] These beneficial effects may be due not only to HDL augmentation and reverse cholesterol transport,[148] but also to recruitment of endothelial progenitor cells into damaged endothelium.[149]

In addition to high-dose statin therapy, angiotensin-converting enzyme (ACE) inhibitors, β-blockers, and aspirin have demonstrated reductions in death and myocardial infarction and therefore are mandatory therapy in the stabilization of high-risk, vulnerable plaques.[142,150]

Despite the tremendous value of systemic therapy, patients still come back with recurrent events, and therefore prove to be resistant to systemic therapy. For example, the combination of ACE inhibitors, β-blockers, aspirin, and high doses of atorvastatin (80 mg per day), still yields a 22% recurrent event rate within 2 years, as was shown in the PROVE IT trial.[151] As a result, even the best combination of systemic therapy available today does not successfully prevent all episodes of plaque rupture and thrombosis. Therefore, new therapies are urgently needed as coadjuvants to systemic therapy in high-

risk patients. Classified as regional and local therapies, these new options are under aggressive investigation and will need prospective, placebo-controlled, randomized trials before being considered for clinical use.

Regional Therapy

Regional therapy is defined as the intravascular treatment of coronary segments with therapeutic agents that will stabilize high-risk, vulnerable plaques. Regional therapy includes photodynamic therapy (PDT),[152] endoluminal phototherapy,[153,154] and cryotherapy.[155] Of these, PDT has gained more attention and is discussed here. PDT uses photosensitizing (light-sensitive) drugs, light, and tissue oxygen to treat targeted diseases, mostly in the field of cancer.[156] Photosensitizing agents (porphyrins) are administered locally or parenterally. They are selectively absorbed and retained within tissues for targeted therapy. This differential selectivity offers selective therapeutic effects when the target tissue is exposed to light at an appropriate wavelength; the surrounding normal tissue is then spared from therapeutic injury.[153] Activation of the photosensitizer within tissue induces the production of free radicals, leading to selective cytotoxic effects, mostly apoptosis (DNA fragmentation) or delayed necrosis. The application of PDT to atherosclerotic plaques was successfully performed in vivo by Waksman and colleagues in hypercholesterolemic rabbits.[157] PDT induced a significant reduction (92%±6%) in the population of nuclei of all cell types in plaques relative to controls (P<.01). This effect was partly due to reduction of smooth muscle cells (α-actin) and macrophages (RAM-11), as shown in Figure 63-35. These results suggest that PDT can almost eliminate macrophages from atherosclerotic plaques and may provide a therapeutic alternative for high-risk, vulnerable plaques refractory to aggressive systemic therapy. The other two therapies, endoluminal phototherapy and cryotherapy, are also under investigation, but the experience is limited and escape the scope of this review.

Local Therapy

Coronary stents offers the possibility of stabilizing high-risk, vulnerable plaques by thickening the fibrous cap through the formation of neointimal hyperplasia. As predicted by Libby almost a decade ago,[158] and more recently highlighted by Serruys,[95] "If we could identify potentially unstable atheroma before they are evident, clinically we might even contemplate angioplasty on nonsignificant stenosis to induce smooth muscle cell proliferation and reinforce the plaque fibrous cap."[158] On the same subject, Davies wrote in an editorial, "the time for prophylactic angioplasty has not come yet, but it may."[159] There are some doubts, however, that better understanding of vulnerable plaques will do much to improve preventive therapy, particularly with stents. Atherosclerosis attacks the entire coronary system,

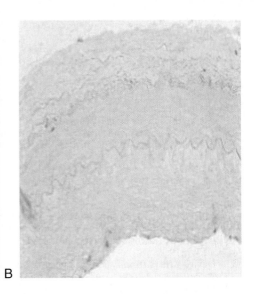

Figure 63-35. Histologic micrographs of the effects of photodynamic therapy on atherosclerotic plaques from hypercholesterolemic rabbits. **A,** Control, showing macrophages (*black arrow*). **B,** Seven days after photodynamic therapy, few macrophages are seen. (From Waksman R: Photodynamic Therapy. New York, Taylor & Francis, 2004.)

and there may be multiple TCFA plaques in the same patient. As a result, local therapy to reinforce TCFA may lead to a losing game of fixing one trouble spot, then finding many others.[4] The controversy associated with late stent thrombosis is another disadvantage for the potential application of coronary stents in vulnerable plaques.[160]

On the other hand, proponents of the stent hypothesis argue that the clinical event rate associated with TCFA (4% to 13% per year, as discussed previously) will always be higher than the clinical event rate associated with stenting (4% to 6% for the first year and approximately 1% to 2% per year thereafter). Furthermore, new stent designs including biodegradable materials[161] and self-expanding delivery systems, may reduce the long-term risk of stent thrombosis and preserve the integrity of the fibrous cap, with further reinforcement by neointimal tissue.[162] The prediction of how we will treat vulnerable plaques resistant to aggressive medical therapy in the future is still a matter of great controversy, but it provides a wonderful opportunity for interventional cardiologists. Only prospective, randomized clinical trials can completely elucidate this issue.

SUMMARY AND FUTURE PREDICTIONS

Atherosclerosis continues to evolve in diagnosis, imaging, and therapy. The concept of a high-risk, vulnerable plaque with specific histologic features continues to be the focus of many investigators, who are developing multiple imaging modalities for invasive diagnosis and therapy. This chapter reviews the state of the art in these techniques. However, the concept of vulnerable plaques may be outdated. The fact that many lesions exhibit the same morphology simultaneously in the same patient suggests that a single-plaque approach is narrow-minded and difficult to prove in clinical practice. A broader concept of disease burden is currently evolving, leading toward quantification by noninvasive imaging techniques. Only randomized clinical trials will help to elucidate the risks and benefits of the proper approach, either invasive with local devices or noninvasive with aggressive systemic therapy.

REFERENCES

1. Fuster V, Voute J. MDGs: Chronic diseases are not on the agenda. Lancet 2005;366:1512-1514.
2. Fuster V, Moreno PR, Fayad ZA, et al: Atherothrombosis and high-risk plaque. Part I: Evolving concepts. J Am Coll Cardiol 2005;46:937-954.
3. Schaar JA, De Korte CL, Mastik F, et al: Characterizing vulnerable plaque features with intravascular elastography. Circulation 2003;108:2636-2641.
4. Feder B: In Quest to Improve Heart Therapies: Plaque Gets a Fresh Look. New York Times. November 27, 2006:A1.
5. Muller JE, Stone PH, Turi ZG, et al: Circadian variation in the frequency of onset of acute myocardial infarction. N Engl J Med 1985;313:1315-1322.
6. Granada JF, Kaluza GL, Raizner AE, Moreno PR: Vulnerable plaque paradigm: Prediction of future clinical events based on a morphological definition. Catheter Cardiovasc Interv 2004;62:364-374.
7. Ambrose JA, Tannenbaum MA, Alexopoulos D, et al: Angiographic progression of coronary artery disease and the development of myocardial infarction. J Am Coll Cardiol 1988;12:56-62.
8. Cutlip DE, Chhabra AG, Baim DS, et al: Beyond restenosis: Five-year clinical outcomes from second-generation coronary stent trials. Circulation 2004;110:1226-1230.
9. Glaser R, Selzer F, Faxon DP, et al: Clinical progression of incidental, asymptomatic lesions discovered during culprit vessel coronary intervention. Circulation 2005;111:143-149.
10. Koenig W, Khuseyinova N: Biomarkers of atherosclerotic plaque instability and rupture. Arterioscler Thromb Vasc Biol 2007;27:15-26. Epub 2006 Nov 2.
11. Wang JC, Normand SL, Mauri L, Kuntz RE: Coronary artery spatial distribution of acute myocardial infarction occlusions. Circulation 2004;110:278-284.
12. Valgimigli M, Rodriguez-Granillo GA, Garcia-Garcia HM, et al: Distance from the ostium as an independent determinant of coronary plaque composition in vivo: An intravascular ultrasound study based radiofrequency data analysis in humans. Eur Heart J 2006;27:655-663.
13. Farb A, Burke AP, Tang AL, et al: Coronary plaque erosion without rupture into a lipid core: A frequent cause of coro-

nary thrombosis in sudden coronary death. Circulation 1996;93:1354-1363.

14. Virmani R, Burke AP, Farb A, Kolodgie FD: Pathology of the vulnerable plaque. J Am Coll Cardiol 2006;47:C13-C18.

15. Burke AP, Farb A, Malcom GT, et al: Coronary risk factors and plaque morphology in men with coronary disease who died suddenly. N Engl J Med 1997;336:1276-1282.

16. Moreno PR, Purushothaman KR, Fuster V, O'Connor WN: Intimomedial interface damage and adventitial inflammation is increased beneath disrupted atherosclerosis in the aorta: Implications for plaque vulnerability. Circulation 2002;105:2504-2511.

17. Schaar JA, van der Steen AF, Mastik F, et al: Intravascular palpography for vulnerable plaque assessment. J Am Coll Cardiol 2006;47:C86-C91.

18. Loree HM, Kamm RD, Stringfellow RG, Lee RT: Effects of fibrous cap thickness on peak circumferential stress in model atherosclerotic vessels. Circ Res 1992;71:850-858.

19. Oliver MF, Davies MJ: The atheromatous lipid core. Eur Heart J 1998;19:16-18.

20. Davies MJ: Pathophysiology of acute coronary syndromes. Indian Heart J 2000;52:473-479.

21. Felton CV, Crook D, Davies MJ, Oliver MF: Relation of plaque lipid composition and morphology to the stability of human aortic plaques. Arterioscler Thromb Vasc Biol 1997;17:1337-1345.

22. Moreno PR, Bernardi VH, Lopez-Cuellar J, et al: Macrophages, smooth muscle cells, and tissue factor in unstable angina: Implications for cell-mediated thrombogenicity in acute coronary syndromes. Circulation 1996;94:3090-3097.

23. Virmani R, Kolodgie FD, Burke AP, et al: Lessons from sudden coronary death: A comprehensive morphological classification scheme for atherosclerotic lesions. Arterioscler Thromb Vasc Biol 2000;20:1262-1275.

24. Abela GS, Aziz K: Cholesterol crystals rupture biological membranes and human plaques during acute cardiovascular events: A novel insight into plaque rupture by scanning electron microscopy. Scanning 2006;28:1-10.

25. Burke AP, Weber DK, Kolodgie FD, et al: Pathophysiology of calcium deposition in coronary arteries. Herz 2001;26:239-244.

26. Moreno PR, Purushothaman KR, Fuster V, et al: Lack of association between aortic calcification and histologic signs of plaque rupture. J Am Coll Cardiol 2000;35:303A.

27. Moreno P: The Role of Calcification in Plaque Vulnerability and Disruption. New York, Futura, 2002.

28. Burke AP, Joner M, Virmani R: IVUS-VH: A predictor of plaque morphology? Eur Heart J 2006;27:1889-1890.

29. Shah PK, Falk E, Badimon JJ, et al: Human monocyte-derived macrophages induce collagen breakdown in fibrous caps of atherosclerotic plaques: Potential role of matrix-degrading metalloproteinases and implications for plaque rupture. Circulation 1995;92:1565-1569.

30. Shah PK, Galis ZS: Matrix metalloproteinase hypothesis of plaque rupture: Players keep piling up but questions remain. Circulation 2001;104:1878-1880.

31. Steinberg D, Witztum JL: Is the oxidative modification hypothesis relevant to human atherosclerosis? Do the antioxidant trials conducted to date refute the hypothesis? Circulation 2002;105:2107-2111.

32. Seshiah PN, Kereiakes DJ, Vasudevan SS, et al: Activated monocytes induce smooth muscle cell death: Role of macrophage colony-stimulating factor and cell contact. Circulation 2002;105:174-180.

33. Hutter R, Valdiviezo C, Sauter BV, et al: Caspase-3 and tissue factor expression in lipid-rich plaque macrophages: Evidence for apoptosis as link between inflammation and atherothrombosis. Circulation 2004;109:2001-2008.

34. Rosenfeld ME: Leukocyte recruitment into developing atherosclerotic lesions: The complex interaction between multiple molecules keeps getting more complex. Arterioscler Thromb Vasc Biol 2002;22:361-363.

35. Mallat Z, Hugel B, Ohan J, et al: Shed membrane microparticles with procoagulant potential in human atherosclerotic plaques: A role for apoptosis in plaque thrombogenicity. Circulation 1999;99:348-353.

36. Moreno PR, Falk E, Palacios IF, et al: Macrophage infiltration in acute coronary syndromes: Implications for plaque rupture. Circulation 1994;90:775-778.

37. Galis ZS: Vulnerable plaque: The devil is in the details. Circulation 2004;110:244-246.

38. Libby P: Inflammation and cardiovascular disease mechanisms. Am J Clin Nutr 2006;83:456S-460S.

39. Glagov S, Weisenberg E, Zarins CK, et al: Compensatory enlargement of human atherosclerotic coronary arteries. N Engl J Med 1987;316:1371-1375.

40. Varnava AM, Mills PG, Davies MJ: Relationship between coronary artery remodeling and plaque vulnerability. Circulation 2002;105:939-943.

41. Tronc F, Mallat Z, Lehoux S, et al: Role of matrix metalloproteinases in blood flow-induced arterial enlargement: Interaction with NO. Arterioscler Thromb Vasc Biol 2000;20:E120-E126.

42. Burke AP, Kolodgie FD, Farb A, et al: Morphological predictors of arterial remodeling in coronary atherosclerosis. Circulation 2002;105:297-303.

43. Schoenhagen P, Ziada KM, Kapadia SR, et al: Extent and direction of arterial remodeling in stable versus unstable coronary syndromes: An intravascular ultrasound study. Circulation 2000;101:598-603.

44. Corti R, Fayad ZA, Fuster V, et al: Effects of lipid-lowering by simvastatin on human atherosclerotic lesions: A longitudinal study by high-resolution, noninvasive magnetic resonance imaging. Circulation 2001;104:249-252.

45. Schoenhagen P, Tuzcu EM, Apperson-Hansen C, et al: Determinants of arterial wall remodeling during lipid-lowering therapy: Serial intravascular ultrasound observations from the Reversal of Atherosclerosis with Aggressive Lipid Lowering Therapy (REVERSAL) trial. Circulation. 2006;113:2826-2834.

46. Sipahi I, Nicholls SJ, Tuzcu EM, Nissen SE: Coronary atherosclerosis can regress with very intensive statin therapy. Cleve Clin J Med 2006;73:937-944.

47. Nissen SE, Nicholls SJ, Sipahi I, et al: Effect of very high-intensity statin therapy on regression of coronary atherosclerosis: The ASTEROID trial. JAMA 2006;295:1556-1565.

48. Moreno PR, Purushothaman KR, Zias E, et al: Neovascularization in human atherosclerosis. Curr Mol Med 2006;6:457-477.

49. Simons M: Angiogenesis: Where do we stand now? Circulation 2005;111:1556-1566.

50. Carmeliet P: Angiogenesis in health and disease. Nat Med 2003;9:653-660.

51. Moreno PR, Purushothaman KR, Sirol M, et al: Neovascularization in human atherosclerosis. Circulation 2006;113:2245-2252.

52. Barger AC, Beeuwkes R 3rd, Lainey LL, Silverman KJ: Hypothesis: Vasa vasorum and neovascularization of human coronary arteries. A possible role in the pathophysiology of atherosclerosis. N Engl J Med 1984;310:175-177.

53. Kumamoto M, Nakashima Y, Sueishi K: Intimal neovascularization in human coronary atherosclerosis: Its origin and pathophysiological significance. Hum Pathol 1995;26:450-456.

54. de Boer OJ, van der Wal AC, Teeling P, Becker AE: Leucocyte recruitment in rupture prone regions of lipid-rich plaques: A prominent role for neovascularization? Cardiovasc Res 1999;41:443-449.

55. O'Brien KD, Allen MD, McDonald TO, et al: Vascular cell adhesion molecule-1 is expressed in human coronary atherosclerotic plaques. J Clin Invest 1993;92:945-951.

56. O'Brien KD, McDonald TO, Chait A, et al: Neovascular expression of E-selectin, intercellular adhesion molecule-1, and vascular cell adhesion molecule-1 in human atherosclerosis and their relation to intimal leukocyte content. Circulation 1996;93:672-682.

57. Moreno PR, Fuster V: New aspects in the pathogenesis of diabetic atherothrombosis. J Am Coll Cardiol 2004;44:2293-2300.

58. Moreno PR, Purushothaman KR, Fuster V, et al: Plaque neovascularization is increased in ruptured atherosclerotic

lesions of human aorta: Implications for plaque vulnerability. Circulation 2004;110:2032-2038.

59. Moreno PR, Purushothaman KR, O'Connor WN, et al: Microvessel sprouting, red blood cell extravasation, and perivascular inflammation is increased in plaques from patients with diabetes mellitus. J Am Coll Cardiol 2005;45:430A.

60. Kockx MM, Cromheeke KM, Knaapen MW, et al: Phagocytosis and macrophage activation associated with hemorrhagic microvessels in human atherosclerosis. Arterioscler Thromb Vasc Biol 2003;23:440-446.

61. Arbustini E, Morbini P, D'Armini AM, et al: Plaque composition in plexogenic and thromboembolic pulmonary hypertension: The critical role of thrombotic material in pultaceous core formation. Heart 2002;88:177-182.

62. Kolodgie FD, Gold HK, Burke AP, et al: Intraplaque hemorrhage and progression of coronary atheroma. N Engl J Med 2003;349:2316-2325.

63. Vlodavsky I, Friedmann Y: Molecular properties and involvement of heparanase in cancer metastasis and angiogenesis. J Clin Invest 2001;108:341-347.

64. Brownlee M: Biochemistry and molecular cell biology of diabetic complications. Nature 2001;414:813-820.

65. De Martin R, Hoeth M, Hofer-Warbinek R, Schmid JA: The transcription factor NF-kB and the regulation of vascular cell function. Arterioscler Thromb Vasc Biol 2000;20:e83-e88.

66. Langlois MR, Delanghe JR: Biological and clinical significance of haptoglobin polymorphism in humans. Clin Chem 1996;42:1589-1600.

67. Graversen JH, Madsen M, Moestrup SK: CD163: A signal receptor scavenging haptoglobin-hemoglobin complexes from plasma. Int J Biochem Cell Biol 2002;34:309-314.

68. Schaer DJ: The macrophage hemoglobin scavenger receptor CD163 as a genetically determined disease modifying pathway in atherosclerosis. Atherosclerosis 2002;163:199-201.

69. Bowman BH, Kurosky A: Haptoglobin: The evolutionary product of duplication, unequal crossing over, and point mutation. Adv Hum Genet 1982;12:189-261, 453-454.

70. Levy AP: Haptoglobin: A major susceptibility gene for diabetic cardiovascular disease. Isr Med Assoc J 2004;6:308-310.

71. Asleh R, Marsh S, Shilkrut M, et al: Genetically determined heterogeneity in hemoglobin scavenging and susceptibility to diabetic cardiovascular disease. Circ Res 2003;92:1193-1200.

72. Asleh R, Guetta J, Kalet-Litman S, et al: Haptoglobin genotype- and diabetes-dependent differences in iron-mediated oxidative stress in vitro and in vivo. Circ Res 2005;96:435-441.

73. Levy AP, Roguin A, Hochberg I, et al: Haptoglobin phenotype and vascular complications in patients with diabetes. N Engl J Med 2000;343:969-970.

74. Levy AP, Hochberg I, Jablonski K, et al: Haptoglobin phenotype is an independent risk factor for cardiovascular disease in individuals with diabetes: The Strong Heart Study. J Am Coll Cardiol 2002;40:1984-1990.

75. Roguin A, Koch W, Kastrati A, et al: Haptoglobin genotype is predictive of major adverse cardiac events in the 1-year period after percutaneous transluminal coronary angioplasty in individuals with diabetes. Diabetes Care 2003;26:2628-2631.

76. Suleiman M, Aronson D, Asleh R, et al: Haptoglobin polymorphism predicts 30-day mortality and heart failure in patients with diabetes and acute myocardial infarction. Diabetes 2005;54:2802-2806.

77. Fuster V, Fayad ZA, Moreno PR, et al: Atherothrombosis and high-risk plaque. Part II: Approaches by noninvasive computed tomographic/magnetic resonance imaging. J Am Coll Cardiol 2005;46:1209-1218.

78. Fujii K, Mintz GS, Carlier SG, et al: Intravascular ultrasound profile analysis of ruptured coronary plaques. Am J Cardiol 2006;98:429-435.

79. DeMaria AN, Narula J, Mahmud E, Tsimikas S: Imaging vulnerable plaque by ultrasound. J Am Coll Cardiol 2006;47:C32-C39.

80. Ge J, Chirillo F, Schwedtmann J, et al: Screening of ruptured plaques in patients with coronary artery disease by intravascular ultrasound. Heart 1999;81:621-627.

81. Peters RJ, Kok WE, Havenith MG, et al: Histopathologic validation of intracoronary ultrasound imaging. J Am Soc Echocardiogr 1994;7:230-241.

82. Komiyama N, Berry GJ, Kolz ML, et al: Tissue characterization of atherosclerotic plaques by intravascular ultrasound radiofrequency signal analysis: An in vitro study of human coronary arteries. Am Heart J 2000;140:565-574.

83. Sano K, Kawasaki M, Ishihara Y, et al: Assessment of vulnerable plaques causing acute coronary syndrome using integrated backscatter intravascular ultrasound. J Am Coll Cardiol 2006;47:734-741.

84. Yamagishi M, Terashima M, Awano K, et al: Morphology of vulnerable coronary plaque: Insights from follow-up of patients examined by intravascular ultrasound before an acute coronary syndrome. J Am Coll Cardiol 2000;35:106-111.

85. Schoenhagen P, Nissen SE, Tuzcu EM: Coronary arterial remodeling: From bench to bedside. Curr Atheroscler Rep 2003;5:150-154.

86. Kaul S, Ito H: Microvasculature in acute myocardial ischemia. Part I: Evolving concepts in pathophysiology, diagnosis, and treatment. Circulation 2004;109:146-149.

87. Kaul S, Ito H: Microvasculature in acute myocardial ischemia. Part II: Evolving concepts in pathophysiology, diagnosis, and treatment. Circulation 2004;109:310-315.

88. Feinstein SB: Contrast ultrasound imaging of the carotid artery vasa vasorum and atherosclerotic plaque neovascularization. J Am Coll Cardiol 2006;48:236-243.

89. O'Malley SM, Vavuranakis M, Naghavi M, Kakadiaris IA: Intravascular ultrasound-based imaging of vasa vasorum for the detection of vulnerable atherosclerotic plaque. Med Image Comput Comput Assist Interv Int Conf Med Image Comput Comput Assist Interv 2005;8:343-351.

90. Carlier S, Kakadiaris IA, Dib N, et al: Vasa vasorum imaging: A new window to the clinical detection of vulnerable atherosclerotic plaques. Curr Atheroscler Rep 2005;7:164-169.

91. Goertz DE, Frijlink ME, Tempel D, et al: Contrast harmonic intravascular ultrasound: A feasibility study for vasa vasorum imaging. Invest Radiol 2006;41:631-638.

92. Nair A, Kuban BD, Obuchowski N, Vince DG: Assessing spectral algorithms to predict atherosclerotic plaque composition with normalized and raw intravascular ultrasound data. Ultrasound Med Biol 2001;27:1319-1331.

93. Nair A, Kuban BD, Tuzcu EM, et al: Coronary plaque classification with intravascular ultrasound radiofrequency data analysis. Circulation 2002;106:2200-2206.

94. Rodriguez-Granillo GA, Garcia-Garcia HM, McFadden EP, et al: In vivo intravascular ultrasound-derived thin-cap fibroatheroma detection using ultrasound radiofrequency data analysis. J Am Coll Cardiol 2005;46:2038-2042.

95. Serruys PW: Fourth annual American College of Cardiology international lecture: A journey in the interventional field. J Am Coll Cardiol 2006;47:1754-1768.

96. Nasu K, Tsuchikane E, Katoh O, et al: Accuracy of in vivo coronary plaque morphology assessment: A validation study of in vivo virtual histology compared with in vitro histopathology. J Am Coll Cardiol 2006;47:2405-2412.

97. Granada JF: In vivo plaque characterization using intravascular ultrasound-virtual histology in a porcine model of complex coronary lesions. Arterioscler Thromb Vasc Biol 2007;27:387-393. Epub 206 Nov 30.

98. Surmely JF, Nasu K, Fujita H, et al: Coronary plaque composition of culprit/target lesions according to the clinical presentation: A virtual histology intravascular ultrasound analysis. Eur Heart J 2006;27:2939-2944. Epub 2006 Oct 13.

99. Rodriguez-Granillo GA, Garcia-Garcia HM, Valgimigli M, et al: Global characterization of coronary plaque rupture phenotype using three-vessel intravascular ultrasound radiofrequency data analysis. Eur Heart J 2006;27:1921-1927.

100. Rodriguez-Granillo GA, McFadden EP, Valgimigli M, et al: Coronary plaque composition of nonculprit lesions, assessed by in vivo intracoronary ultrasound radiofrequency data analysis, is related to clinical presentation. Am Heart J 2006;151:1020-1024.

101. Surmely JF, Nasu K, Fujita H, et al: Association of coronary plaque composition and arterial remodeling: A virtual histology intravascular ultrasound analysis. Heart 2007;93:928-932.

102. Rodriguez-Granillo GA, Serruys PW, Garcia-Garcia HM, et al: Coronary artery remodelling is related to plaque composition. Heart 2006;92:388-391.

103. Low AF, Tearney GJ, Bouma BE, Jang IK: Technology insight: Optical coherence tomography. Current status and future development. Nat Clin Pract Cardiovasc Med 2006;3:154-162; quiz 172.

104. Bouma BE: New insights from OCT, polarization-sensitive OCT, and the emergence of OFDI. Presented at The Vulnerable Plaque Session: Pathophysiology, Detection, and Therapeutic Intervention. Transcatheter Therapeutic Intervention (TCT) Meeting, Washington, DC, 2006.

105. Jang IK: Optical coherence tomography: Studies at MGH. In Transcatheter Cardiovascular Therapeutics Convention, Washington, DC, 2002.

106. Jang IK, Tearney GJ, MacNeill B, et al: In vivo characterization of coronary atherosclerotic plaque by use of optical coherence tomography. Circulation 2005;111:1551-1555.

107. Giattina SD, Courtney BK, Herz PR, et al: Assessment of coronary plaque collagen with polarization sensitive optical coherence tomography (PS-OCT). Int J Cardiol 2006;107:400-409.

108. Tearney GJ, Yabushita H, Houser SL, et al: Quantification of macrophage content in atherosclerotic plaques by optical coherence tomography. Circulation 2003;107:113-119.

109. MacNeill BD, Jang IK, Bouma BE, et al: Focal and multi-focal plaque macrophage distributions in patients with acute and stable presentations of coronary artery disease. J Am Coll Cardiol 2004;44:972-979.

110. Jonas JB, Harder B, Spandau UH, et al: Bevacizumab for occult subfoveal neovascularization in age-related macular degeneration. Eur J Ophthalmol 2006;16:774-775.

111. Moon SJ, Wirostko WJ: Photodynamic therapy for extrafoveal choroidal neovascularization associated with choroidal nevus. Retina 2006;26:477-479.

112. Avery RL, Pieramici DJ, Rabena MD, et al: Intravitreal bevacizumab (Avastin) for neovascular age-related macular degeneration. Ophthalmology 2006;113:363-372.

113. Fuster V, Corti R, Fayad ZA, et al: Integration of vascular biology and magnetic resonance imaging in the understanding of atherothrombosis and acute coronary syndromes. J Thromb Haemost 2003;1:1410-1421.

114. Sirol M, Fuster V, Fayad ZA: Plaque imaging and characterization using magnetic resonance imaging: Towards molecular assessment. Curr Mol Med 2006;6:541-548.

115. Wilensky RL, Song HK, Ferrari VA: Role of magnetic resonance and intravascular magnetic resonance in the detection of vulnerable plaques. J Am Coll Cardiol 2006;47:C48-C56.

116. Schneiderman J, Wilensky RL, Weiss A, et al: Diagnosis of thin-cap fibroatheromas by a self-contained intravascular magnetic resonance imaging probe in ex vivo human aortas and in situ coronary arteries. J Am Coll Cardiol 2005;45:1961-1969.

117. Lipinski MJ, Frias JC, Fayad ZA: Advances in detection and characterization of atherosclerosis using contrast agents targeting the macrophage. J Nucl Cardiol 2006;13:699-709.

118. Jaffer FA, Libby P, Weissleder R: Molecular and cellular imaging of atherosclerosis: Emerging applications. J Am Coll Cardiol 2006;47:1328-1338.

119. Rudd JH, Warburton EA, Fryer TD, et al: Imaging atherosclerotic plaque inflammation with [18F]-fluorodeoxyglucose positron emission tomography. Circulation 2002;105:2708-2711.

120. Davies JR, Rudd JH, Weissberg PL, Narula J: Radionuclide imaging for the detection of inflammation in vulnerable plaques. J Am Coll Cardiol 2006;47:C57-C68.

121. Lipinski MJ, Amirbekian V, Frias JC, et al: MRI to detect atherosclerosis with gadolinium-containing immunomicelles targeting the macrophage scavenger receptor. Magn Reson Med 2006;56:601-610.

122. Fayad ZA, Amirbekian V, Toussaint JF, Fuster V: Identification of interleukin-2 for imaging atherosclerotic inflammation. Eur J Nucl Med Mol Imaging 2006;33:111-116.

123. Sosnovik DE, Schellenberger EA, Nahrendorf M, et al: Magnetic resonance imaging of cardiomyocyte apoptosis with a novel magneto-optical nanoparticle. Magn Reson Med 2005;54:718-724.

124. Jaffer FA, Sosnovik DE, Nahrendorf M, Weissleder R: Molecular imaging of myocardial infarction. J Mol Cell Cardiol 2006;41:921-933.

125. Purushothaman KR, Sanz J, Zias E, et al: Atherosclerosis neovascularization and imaging. Curr Mol Med 2006;6:549-556.

126. Winter PM, Morawski AM, Caruthers SD, et al: Molecular imaging of angiogenesis in early-stage atherosclerosis with alpha(v)beta3-integrin-targeted nanoparticles. Circulation 2003;108:2270-2274.

127. Matter CM, Schuler PK, Alessi P, et al: Molecular imaging of atherosclerotic plaques using a human antibody against the extra-domain B of fibronectin. Circ Res 2004;95:1225-1233.

128. Kelly KA, Allport JR, Tsourkas A, et al: Detection of vascular adhesion molecule-1 expression using a novel multimodal nanoparticle. Circ Res 2005;96:327-336.

129. Takaya N, Yuan C, Chu B, et al: Presence of intraplaque hemorrhage stimulates progression of carotid atherosclerotic plaques: A high-resolution magnetic resonance imaging study. Circulation 2005;111:2768-2775.

130. Takaya N, Yuan C, Chu B, et al: Association between carotid plaque characteristics and subsequent ischemic cerebrovascular events: A prospective assessment with MRI—Initial results. Stroke 2006;37:818-823.

131. Puppini G, Furlan F, Cirota N, et al: Characterisation of carotid atherosclerotic plaque: Comparison between magnetic resonance imaging and histology. Radiol Med (Torino) 2006;111:921-930.

132. Uchida Y, Nakamura F, Tomaru T, et al: Prediction of acute coronary syndromes by percutaneous coronary angioscopy in patients with stable angina. Am Heart J 1995;130:195-203.

133. Asakura M, Ueda Y, Yamaguchi O, et al: Extensive development of vulnerable plaques as a pan-coronary process in patients with myocardial infarction: An angioscopic study. J Am Coll Cardiol 2001;37:1284-1288.

134. Ohtani T, Ueda Y, Mizote I, et al: Number of yellow plaques detected in a coronary artery is associated with future risk of acute coronary syndrome: Detection of vulnerable patients by angioscopy. J Am Coll Cardiol 2006;47:2194-2200.

135. Moreno PR, Muller JE: Detection of high-risk atherosclerotic coronary plaques by intravascular spectroscopy. J Interv Cardiol 2003;16:243-252.

136. van de Poll SW, Kastelijn K, Bakker Schut TC, et al: On-line detection of cholesterol and calcification by catheter based Raman spectroscopy in human atherosclerotic plaque ex vivo. Heart 2003;89:1078-1082.

137. Moreno PR, Lodder RA, Purushothaman KR, et al: Detection of lipid pool, thin fibrous cap, and inflammatory cells in human aortic atherosclerotic plaques by near-infrared spectroscopy. Circulation 2002;105:923-927.

138. Caplan JD, Waxman S, Nesto RW, Muller JE: Near-infrared spectroscopy for the detection of vulnerable coronary artery plaques. J Am Coll Cardiol 2006;47:C92-C96.

139. Madjid M, Willerson JT, Casscells SW: Intracoronary thermography for detection of high-risk vulnerable plaques. J Am Coll Cardiol 2006;47:C80-C85.

140. Kawasaki M, Bouma BE, Bressner J, et al: Diagnostic accuracy of optical coherence tomography and integrated backscatter intravascular ultrasound images for tissue characterization of human coronary plaques. J Am Coll Cardiol 2006;48:81-88.

141. Romer TJ, Brennan JF 3rd, Puppels GJ, et al: Intravascular ultrasound combined with Raman spectroscopy to localize and quantify cholesterol and calcium salts in atherosclerotic coronary arteries. Arterioscler Thromb Vasc Biol 2000;20:478-483.

142. Ambrose JA, D'Agate DJ: Classification of systemic therapies for potential stabilization of the vulnerable plaque to prevent

acute myocardial infarction. Am J Cardiol 2005;95:379-382.

143. Cannon CP, Steinberg BA, Murphy SA, et al: Meta-analysis of cardiovascular outcomes trials comparing intensive versus moderate statin therapy. J Am Coll Cardiol 2006;48:438-445.

144. Scirica BM, Morrow DA, Cannon CP, et al: Intensive statin therapy and the risk of hospitalization for heart failure after an acute coronary syndrome in the PROVE IT-TIMI 22 study. J Am Coll Cardiol 2006;47:2326-2331.

145. Hulten E, Jackson JL, Douglas K, et al: The effect of early, intensive statin therapy on acute coronary syndrome: A meta-analysis of randomized controlled trials. Arch Intern Med 2006;166:1814-1821.

146. Goldenberg I, Goldbourt U, Boyko V, et al: Relation between on-treatment increments in serum high-density lipoprotein cholesterol levels and cardiac mortality in patients with coronary heart disease (from the Bezafibrate Infarction Prevention trial). Am J Cardiol 2006;97:466-471.

147. Corti R, Osende J, Hutter R, et al: Fenofibrate induces plaque regression in hypercholesterolemic atherosclerotic rabbits: In vivo demonstration by high-resolution MRI. Atherosclerosis 2007;190:106-113. Epub 2006 Apr 5.

148. Naik SU, Wang X, Da Silva JS, et al: Pharmacological activation of liver X receptors promotes reverse cholesterol transport in vivo. Circulation 2006;113:90-97.

149. Tso C, Martinic G, Fan WH, et al: High-density lipoproteins enhance progenitor-mediated endothelium repair in mice. Arterioscler Thromb Vasc Biol 2006;26:1144-1149.

150. Dagenais GR, Pogue J, Fox K, et al: Angiotensin-converting-enzyme inhibitors in stable vascular disease without left ventricular systolic dysfunction or heart failure: A combined analysis of three trials. Lancet 2006;368:581-588.

151. Cannon CP, Braunwald E, McCabe CH, et al: Intensive versus moderate lipid lowering with statins after acute coronary syndromes. N Engl J Med 2004;350:1495-1504.

152. Waksman R, Leitch IM, Roessler J, et al: Intracoronary photodynamic therapy reduces neointimal growth without suppressing re-endothelialisation in a porcine model. Heart 2006;92:1138-1144.

153. Waksman R: Photodynamic Therapy. New York, Taylor & Francis, 2004.

154. Kipshidze N: Endoluminal phototherapy with low-power red light laser for vulnerable plaque passivation. Presented to the Transcatheter Cardiovascular Therapeutics Convention, Washington, DC, October 2006.

155. Dorval JF, Geoffroy P, Sirois MG, Tanguay JF: Endovascular cryotherapy accentuates the accumulation of the fibrillar collagen types I and III after percutaneous transluminal angioplasty in pigs. J Endovasc Ther 2006;13:104-110.

156. Triesscheijn M, Baas P, Schellens JH, Stewart FA: Photodynamic therapy in oncology. Oncologist 2006;11:1034-1044.

157. Waksman R: Photodynamic therapy. In Virmani R, Narula J, Leon MB, Willerson JT (eds): The Vulnerable Atherosclerotic Plaque: Strategies for Diagnosis and Management. Malden, MA, Blackwell Futura, 2007, pp. 321-330.

158. Lafont A, Libby P: The smooth muscle cell: Sinner or saint in restenosis and the acute coronary syndromes? J Am Coll Cardiol 1998;32:283-285.

159. Davies MJ: Detecting vulnerable coronary plaques. Lancet 1996;347:1422-1423.

160. Serruys PW, Kukreja N: Late stent thrombosis in drug-eluting stents: Return of the "VB syndrome." Nat Clin Pract Cardiovasc Med 2006;3:637.

161. Waksman R: Biodegradable stents: They do their job and disappear. J Invasive Cardiol 2006;18:70-74.

162. Moreno PR: First report of a vulnerable plaque specific stent capable of focal passivation without fibrous cap rupture. Presented to the Transcatheter Cardiovascular Therapeutics Convention, Washington, DC, October 2006.

64 Cardiovascular Interventional Magnetic Resonance Imaging

Robert J. Lederman

KEY POINTS

- Interventional cardiovascular magnetic resonance imaging (MRI) remains investigational.
- Because it makes soft tissue and blood conspicuous, interventional MRI may enable nonsurgeons to conduct novel minimally invasive procedures.
- Potential applications include radiation-sparing conventional catheter procedures, image-guided myocardial ablation or targeted drug or cell delivery, and catheter-based surgical procedures such as valve implantation.
- Interventional XMR suites can be configured from MRI and X-ray systems that can be operated together or fully independently.

- Fusion of prior MRI datasets with real-time X-ray, an intermediate step, may provide enhanced image guidance for conventional interventional procedures.
- Coronary artery interventional procedures are not possible under MRI guidance, barring unforeseen technology breakthroughs.
- The lack of availability of clinical-grade MRI catheter devices poses the chief obstacle to wider clinical translation of this technology.

As this textbook attests, a remarkable range of minimally invasive procedures can be conducted safely and effectively under the guidance of X-ray imaging. For the most part, these procedures are confined to existing vascular lumens and chambers, and they are effective even though soft tissues such as myocardium are not readily conspicuous. Alternative image guidance modalities such as magnetic resonance imaging (MRI) may further broaden the range of therapeutic possibilities for catheter-based interventions. This may prove useful to avoid ionizing radiation, as during pediatric procedures; to view the tissue response to treatment interactively, as during myocardial ablation to treat rhythm disorders; and to cross ordinary tissue boundaries, as during extra-anatomic bypass.

Interventional MRI remains in its infancy. Provocative initial demonstrations have been conducted in animals. Initial human testing is underway throughout the world. This chapter reviews the challenges and future applications of this exciting new technology for interventional catheterization.

HOW MRI CREATES PICTURES FOR INTERVENTION

A brief review of MRI follows, but better introductions can be found elsewhere.[1] An image is a two-dimensional (2D) grid of pixels, each having numeric values that correspond to brightness, color, or both. Ultrasound, computed tomography (CT), and MRI images usually represent flattened tomographs (slices), and each contributing pixel actual represents a 3D volume (voxel) within that slice. Three-dimensional matrices can be acquired that contain image data, but usually these are computer-reconstructed into viewable images that are either thin-slice samples (such as 2D echocardiography) or projections (such as shadows). MRI technology and terminology can be offputting to cardiologists, but it should be remembered that cardiac ultrasound has comparable complexity and terminology and is merely in a more advanced stage of clinical development.

Interventional cardiologists are accustomed to using images that are X-ray projections (shadows), in which there is a direct relationship between the position in space of X-ray beam attenuation and the position in the image of the features (bone, tissue, catheter) that caused the beam attenuation. Unlike X-ray projections, images in MRI are acquired in the form of frequency information that corresponds to image features only after a complex mathematical transformation. These frequency datasets are not interpretable as images (Fig. 64-1).

Such frequency encoding of information is similar in many ways to human hearing: audio information is encoded as an amalgam of sound frequencies with varying amplitudes that are decoded by the cochlea and transmitted to the brain. Similarly, video information in MRI is encoded as an amalgam of frequencies that are decoded by Fourier transformation into spatial equivalents that constitute an image.

MRI exploits the phenomenon of nuclear magnetic resonance (NMR, or MR). Protons within the hydrogen atoms of water have an intrinsic magnetism that causes them to interact with external magnetic fields. Because water is ubiquitous in biologic tissues, proton NMR is most widely used for MRI. For hydrogen protons in water, at a given magnetic field (e.g., 1.5 Tesla [T]), there is a characteristic Larmor frequency (63.87 MHz at 1.5 T) at which the protons absorb energy. Once energized, these protons "decay" and emit radiofrequency (RF) energy at the same Larmor frequency. Most important, if the magnetic field strength is altered, the Larmor frequency is also altered proportionately.

MR images are created by exploiting this fundamental relationship between the Larmor frequency and the strength of the magnetic field. Specifically, a

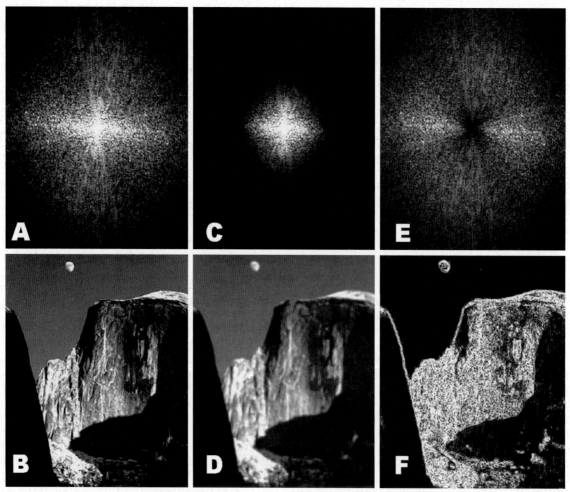

Figure 64-1. Frequency characteristics of a classic image, Ansel Adams' *Moon Over Half Dome*. Images in magnetic resonance imaging (MRI) are sampled as frequency or *k-space* data, then usually converted using a Fourier transformation into spatial representations. **A,** The Fourier transformation of the full-spectrum image **(B)**. The starburst pattern indicates that most of the information is contained by the center frequencies. If the same frequency data are filtered to retain only the low frequencies **(C)**, the image appears mostly intact but devoid of detail **(D)**. The low frequencies are said to contain most of the image contrast data. One approach to real-time MRI is to sample only center frequencies, so as to create low-resolution images quickly. If the same frequency data are filtered to retain only the high frequencies **(E)**, the resulting image **(F)** contain only the edges or spatial detail of the original image. (Source: U.S. Government work [Lederman, NHLBI], public domain.)

linear magnetic field gradient is created (i.e., the magnetic field strength changes according to position in space) at specific times. The position in space of excited spins is "encoded" onto their frequency by creating known magnetic field values in different positions. The RF frequency of the spins corresponds exactly to their position within the artificially created magnetic field.

This characteristic is generally exploited to create images using a repeated two-step process. The 2D position is encoded onto spins, first when spins are *excited* using RF (one dimension) and second when spins *emit* RF. Each cycle creates a line in a 2D image. Repeated cycles generate multiple lines to create a complete 2D image. A computer coordinates the timing of RF excitation and "readout" of RF emissions, along with excitation magnetic field gradients and readout magnetic fields, so that the exact position of these lines is known in advance. More specifically, for every line contributing to a 2D image, MRI excites a slice of the patient in space by creating a known gradient and exposing the body to RF energy precisely tuned to the Larmor frequency of the desired slice. Once a 2D slice is excited, the entire slice begins to emit RF energy. During that emission, the MRI scanner rapidly creates a new magnetic field gradient so that an individual line within that slice can be "read" using a high-sensitivity radio receiver tuned to the characteristic (Larmor) frequency of spins within that selected line. Because the gradient strength is known, the location of the line is also known, using the Larmor relationship. The process is repeated for the additional lines within the selected slice, until sufficient frequency information is accumulated to create a complete 2D image.

The computer "program" used to accumulate these image data is called a pulse-sequence. Manipulation of the timing, strength, speed, and phase of the RF energy and magnetic field gradients in different pulse-sequences can dramatically alter the appearance of different tissues. Other features can be imaged apart from the position of tissues in space, such as the velocity of excited spins using "phase-contrast" or "velocity-encoded" MRI. Exogenous contrast agents can be administered to alter image contrast; for example, to create contrast-enhanced MR angiograms or to enhance the MRI appearance of scarred or infarcted myocardium.

Certain pulse-sequences are particularly useful for cardiovascular and interventional MRI. Steady-state free precession (SSFP, also known as Fiesta, TrueFISP, and balanced fast field echo) is a popular workhorse pulse-sequence because of high signal-to-noise, speed, and versatility. In SSFP, blood appears bright and myocardium appears gray.

CONFIGURING AND OPERATING AN iCMR LABORATORY

An interventional cardiovascular magnetic resonance imaging (iCMR) laboratory can be configured and installed by commercial vendors with only minor modification.[2,3] Usually these are configured as "XMR" suites with adjoining X-ray and MRI bays. The two otherwise ordinary systems can be used independently as in any other hospital. Alternatively, they can be used together during interventional MRI procedures. Compared with two separate suites, the incremental capital cost is fairly low and consists primarily of the intermodality patient transfer system and the barrier doors.

Hardware

Real-time MRI hardware requires highly homogeneous magnetic fields that usually are available only on "closed-bore" systems. At higher field strengths, tissues yield stronger MRI signals. However, higher field strengths pose additional engineering challenges. For example, at 3 T, minor magnetic field inhomogeneities are amplified during rapid imaging in a way that dramatically degrades images. As a result, most interventional MRI applications today seem best addressed at field strengths limited to approximately 1.5 T. Indeed, contemporary gradient systems have approached a plateau in price-performance ratio and have approached physiologic limits of heating or peripheral nerve stimulation. Vendors are introducing shorter and wider closed-bore MRI systems (one system is only 120 cm long, with a bore inner diameter of 70 cm). These are attractive for interventional MRI procedures, because the systems induce less claustrophobia, patients can more readily be monitored visually, and operators' arms can directly reach the center "suite spot" of the magnet.

Most interventional MRI investigators ensure that X-ray fluoroscopy systems are readily available if not adjoining, both to use for emergency bailout and for simple procedural steps such as vascular access.

Conventional X-ray image intensifier systems are subject to image distortion by the high magnetic fields, but they usually operate satisfactorily if situated more than 4 or 5 m away from the MRI bore. Newer flat-panel detector systems are relatively insensitive to this distortion and have significant advantages when combining or "fusing" image data from the two modalities at once.

One vendor introduced a 1.0-T MRI system in a "double-doughnut" configuration so that the central imaging field is exposed and directly accessible for interventional procedures.[4] The Stanford team integrated a retractable flat-panel X-ray into this system, so that conventional fluoroscopy could be conducted without moving the patient.[5]

MRI systems are enclosed in an RF barrier so that ambient RF noise, including ordinary communication signals as well as noise emitted by the X-ray and other electronics systems, does not interfere with the high-sensitivity MR system. Merely opening these RF doors creates significant artifacts during MRI. The Kings College London laboratories have implemented a double-door RF barrier entrance, analogous to an "air lock," so that staff can enter and exit the laboratory without disturbing the MRI system (Video 64-1).[6]

Modifications for Interventional MRI

Traditional MRI is designed around diagnostic applications, wherein the rate-limiting step usually is image acquisition, not image display. Diagnostic MRI workflows afford the "luxury" of slower image reconstruction for later off-line review by the clinician.

Interventional MRI requires almost instantaneous or "real-time" MRI. This acquisition-to-display delay is barely noticeable when it is less than about 250 msec, compared with X-ray systems, which have a delay of about 100 msec. Real-time MRI also has utility in diagnostic settings with much nonperiodic motion, such as atrial fibrillation, noncooperative patients, or cardiac stress testing. Most commercial systems provide real-time MRI functionality, but we have found it more useful to extract raw data from the commercial MRI system during acquisition and to reconstruct and display it to the operator on an inexpensive, fast external computer. Indeed at least one vendor is using this approach in commercializing an interventional MRI package as an external computer add-on to their diagnostic MRI systems, attached conveniently via high-speed network.

MRI requires a compromise between spatial resolution and speed; interventional MRI usually sacrifices image quality in favor of speed. Projection X-ray imaging uses a pixel matrix as large as 1024×1024 at 15 to 30 frames per second. Our typical interventional MRI pulse-sequences generate 192×128 pixels at 8 to 10 frames per second. The soft tissue content often makes the images comparably information-rich (Fig. 64-2).

Many techniques are combined to accelerate MRI for intervention. *Undersampling* refers to the creation of images using incomplete data. This is analogous to video compression for Web broadcasts. For example, the frequency data contributing to images have intrinsic symmetries that can be undersampled and computer-regenerated. Similar approaches exploit the fact that the low-frequency center of frequency space (*k*-space) is more information-rich than the higher frequency data. These data can be sampled radially so that each line intersects the center frequency. An image created using such radial sampling may contain information comparable to that of an image created using more lines in classic rectilinear ("Cartesian") fashion but can be faster. Various research groups (e.g., Stanford) advocate other approaches to sampling frequency data, including "spiral" trajectories. Commercial MRI systems are beginning to employ so-called parallel imaging techniques (with commercial names such as SENSE, SMASH, GRAPPA, and BLAST) to increase speed. These exploit the unique differences between multiple surface receiver coils, analogous to the way that binoculars provide more information than monoculars. Parallel imaging requires optimized MRI surface coil hardware.

Another popular image acceleration technique is echo-sharing, wherein lines are recycled over multiple images. This technique is used for broadcast television in the United States, in which updates of odd and even lines are alternated on images. Imaging speed is effectively doubled, but temporal resolution is not.

Michael Guttman and Elliot McVeigh at the National Heart, Lung, and Blood Institute (NHLBI) have developed numerous additional features that we have found valuable in interventional MRI applications. Perhaps most important is the ability to process signals independently from "active" catheters containing embedded antennae (see later discussion). When so attached to separate MRI receiver channels,

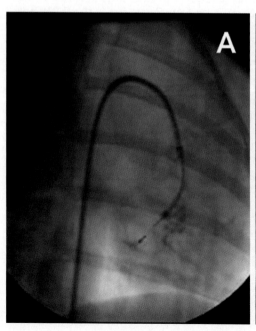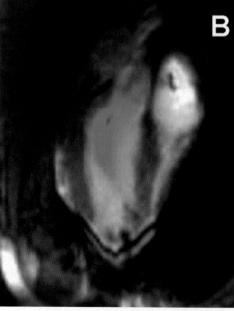

Figure 64-2. A comparison of the information content of X-ray images (**A**) and real-time magnetic resonance images (MRI) (**B**) using a transaortic myocardial injection catheter. The X-ray pixel matrix is greater (512×512) than that of the MRI (192×128). Even at this reduced spatial resolution, the soft-tissue display in MRI can provide superior information. (Source: U.S. Government work [Lederman, NHLBI], public domain.)

the device-related images can be displayed in color, and their brightness can be adjusted independently. Other useful features include the ability to toggle electrocardiographic (ECG) gating to "suspend" cardiac motion and the ability to toggle "saturation" MRI pulses that turn the image dark except for gadolinium contrast used to enhance myocardial infarction or injected during procedures. They also have developed real-time multislice acquisitions, with instantaneous rotating display of the slices in their true 3D relation. Finally, Guttman developed a "projection-mode" feature that is useful when catheters are manipulated during tomographic imaging. As catheter parts move outside the selected slice, they become invisible. Projection-mode imaging resembles X-ray imaging, so that the catheter can be manipulated back into the desired slice.

The groups from Case Western Reserve and Johns Hopkins University have pioneered automated slice prescription features such as the ability to have the MR imaging plane automatically track the position of active-tracking catheter devices (see later discussion). Similar techniques automatically create rapid low-resolution pictures when these catheters are moved rapidly and slower high-resolution pictures when the catheters are adjusted finely. This has created competing philosophies about how to select images during interventional procedures: some advocate images created in relation to the catheter; we advocate images focused on target pathology. Ideally both approaches should be available.

Image Display

Interventional images can be displayed to the operators inside the MRI laboratory using either RF-shielded liquid crystal diode (LCD) displays, which are expensive, or more affordable custom RF-shielded LCD projectors onto aluminum-framed screens. The screens and the LCDs can be mounted on movable booms, as in X-ray laboratories. Usually, separate screens are necessary for MRI system control, for real-time MRI, and for invasive hemodynamics.

Communications

MRI systems are almost as loud as airplanes, especially during rapid imaging. Most of the noise is generated when rapidly fluctuating magnetic fields force gradient coil elements inside the scanner to strike each other. Even newer "acoustically-shielded" MRI systems are loud enough to preclude verbal communications. Patients and staff must wear ear protection for safety and for comfort.

Fiberoptic, pneumatic, and wireless transmission systems are available with noise cancellation technology to permit staff to communicate even during MRI. We recommend systems that permit "open" audio communication without speakers first needing to switch on their microphones. We also recommend a second audio channel to permit staff independently to communicate with or monitor the patient.

Patient Monitoring

Commercial MRI patient monitoring systems are designed for use in diagnostic imaging. Available systems usually have limited display capability, with display tracings from only one ECG lead, one or two invasive blood pressure channels, noninvasive blood pressure monitoring, pulse-oximetry, and exhaled carbon dioxide and anesthesia gas concentrations. Because these are "monitoring" systems, they do not provide high-fidelity "recording" signals used in conventional cardiovascular catheterization suites. These are, however, safe for operation during interventional MRI.

Absent commercial interventional MRI hemodynamics recording systems, we recommend that operators substitute biomedical research hemodynamics equipment (e.g., Powerlab, ADInstruments) and operate under Institutional Review Board supervision, which in the United States constitutes the Investigational Device Exemption in this setting. Such systems are easily configured to display high-fidelity signals in a format that resembles commercial clinical hemodynamics recording systems. We prefer to use our commercial monitoring system in tandem with a research recording system; most can be configured to output monitoring signals such as oximetry and noninvasive blood pressure data to the research recording system.

ECG is intrinsically limited during MRI. Blood flowing through the heart and aorta carries a charge that generates current in the high magnetic field, the so-called magnetohydrodynamic effect. This makes the ST-T wave segments of the ECG uninterpretable inside the MRI bore. The MRI RF and gradient systems contribute additional noise to the ECG signal. As a result, ECG cannot be used to detect myocardial ischemia or injury during MRI and is useful primarily for rhythm detection.

Patient Transfer

In an XMR configuration, patients are transferred bidirectionally between the X-ray and MRI systems for combined or bailout procedures (Fig. 64-3). Transfer systems are available from all major vendors that convey the patient between imaging systems while protecting from significant decelerations. The patient lies on a transfer shell that also carries the operators' sterile field, interventional equipment, and transducers.

A surprisingly large number of lines and devices may be attached to patients during interventional procedures: (1) oxygen gas; (2) endotracheal tube; (3) pulse oximetry and capnography probes; (4) multiple intra-arterial pressure lines and transducers; (5) multiple intravenous catheters and extension lines; (6) interventional catheterization manifold including contrast, flush, waste, pressure transducer, and catheter extension lines; (7) urinary catheter and collection bag; (8) ECG leads for MRI; (9) ECG leads for X-ray; (10) intravascular MRI coil connectors; and

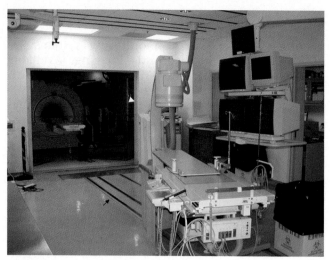

Figure 64-3. A combined X-ray and magnetic resonance imaging ("XMR") interventional suite. A standard single-plane X-ray system has its table pedestal mounted on floor rails. With the X-ray and radiofrequency barrier door open, patients can be transferred rapidly and smoothly between the two modalities. With the barrier doors closed, the laboratories function independently. (Source: U.S. Government work [Lederman, NHLBI]) public domain.)

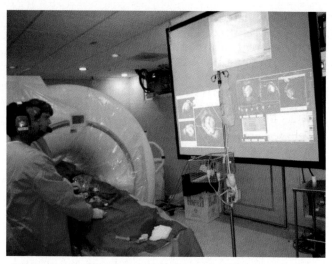

Figure 64-4. Inside the interventional magnetic resonance imaging (MRI) laboratory. The operators communicate with the use of sound-suppressing headsets and fiberoptic microphones. In-room projectors display (clockwise from top) hemodynamics, scanner control, and real-time MRI data. (Source: U.S. Government work [Lederman, NHLBI] public domain.)

(11) surface MRI coils and connectors. These should be secured and organized at the beginning of the procedure in case emergency intermodality transfer is required. The operators should verify that conductive cables do not form loops and are kept away from the inner wall of the magnet bore (near the body/transmit coil); both predispose to heating during MRI.

Safety and Sterility Practices

Patient care practices during interventional MRI procedures combine standard practices from X-ray and from MRI suites.

The MRI bore and surface are draped with sterile adhesive drapes. Before intermodality transfer, the sterile field is covered with an additional sterile drape. Depending on the field to be imaged (i.e., pelvis or chest), the MRI surface coils can be placed under the sterile drapes or can be enclosed in sterile bags and positioned on top of the sterile field. Intravascular receiver coil transmission lines are covered with sterile sheaths marketed for intravascular ultrasound probes (Fig. 64-4).

Inside the MRI laboratory, ferrous materials can become missiles that endanger both patients and staff. This risk is highest during emergencies, and therefore emergency practices must be planned and rehearsed. All staff must be trained about MRI safety, including removal of ferrous materials before entering the laboratory. Some laboratories issue pocketless uniforms to further reduce this risk.[6] Cardiac defibrillation is hazardous within the high magnetic field, because the high currents generate sufficient force to displace the electrodes and the operators (literally knocking staff off their feet). By convention,

the magnetic field is considered clinically negligible outside the 5 Gauss (0.0005 T) magnetic field line, which many laboratories mark on the floor and which should not encroach on the neighboring X-ray laboratory.

Adjunctive patient care devices are marketed specifically for operation within the high magnetic field and include mechanical ventilators, intravenous pumps, oxygen tanks, and mobile aluminum tables. These should be specifically labeled as "MRI-safe"; all other equipment should be assumed not to be safe for use in the MRI laboratory. All other ferrous materials that are deemed essential must be tethered to the wall and kept outside the 5-Gauss line. When equipment appears interchangeable, such as catheter preparation tables, it is prudent to use MRI-safe selections for both X-ray and MRI rooms.

CATHETER DEVICES FOR INTERVENTIONAL CARDIOVASCULAR MRI

Catheter devices for X-ray procedures are usually conspicuous because they readily attenuate incident X-rays. X-ray catheter development primarily focuses on mechanical performance. MRI catheters, however, are not as simple and must be engineered not only for mechanical performance but also (1) to be conspicuous, (2) to avoid magnetic attraction and displacement, (3) to avoid distorting the image because of magnetic susceptibility effects of metal components, and (4) to avoid heating during exposure to the high RF energy required to create MR images. Most off-the-shelf clinical catheter devices suffer limitations in one of these areas. Indeed, these challenges pose the chief limitation to clinical development of interventional cardiovascular MRI.

Materials Considerations

Ferrous materials are incompatible with MRI. The most common, 316L stainless steel, is not significantly attracted by magnetic fields. However, 316L and other steel stents create large (susceptibility) signal voids because they disrupt the nearby magnetic field during MRI. As a result, most commercial braided diagnostic and guiding catheters, most balloon-expandable stents, most guidewires, and most device delivery systems are not suitable for MRI. Other metals are better suited, including nitinol, many nickel-cobalt-chromium alloys (e.g., MP35N, L605), copper, gold, tungsten, and platinum, in that they create comparably minor magnetic susceptibility artifacts. Not all of these materials are biocompatible.

Long conductive structures are prone to inductive heating during MRI, especially during RF excitation, and especially if longer than 50 to 80 cm, at 1.5T. This is similar to metal heating in a microwave oven. As a result, even unmodified nitinol guidewires can cause thrombosis or tissue damage during MRI interventional procedures. Various modifications can render conductive guidewires safe. Shorter metallic structures, including stents, are unlikely to heat in this way.

MRI catheter devices have two basic designs. *Passive* catheters are conspicuous based on their intrinsic materials properties. *Active* catheters are conspicuous because they contain embedded electronics that interact with the MRI system. The various approaches are summarized in Table 64-1 and Figure 64-5.

Passive Catheter Devices

The simplest passive catheters are unbraided polymers and are visible based on the absence of water. These are intrinsically safe. Unfortunately, such catheters appear "dark" under MRI, which makes them poorly conspicuous for a number of reasons. First, the darkness, or absence of signal, is easily diluted by water signal ("volume-averaged") within the voxels constituting the picture. Second, many imaging artifacts also appear dark, so simple passive catheters do not necessarily have a specific "signature" on images. As a result, although simple passive catheters appear acceptably well when depicted in ex vivo imaging phantoms, they can be hard to see in vivo. Finally, magnetic susceptibility artifacts are usually much larger than the devices that generate them, so the "blooming" signal voids may obscure nearby tissue or other features of interest.

Catheters filled with dilute gadolinium-based contrast agents appear bright and can be tracked under MRI. However, interventional devices displace the contrast agent and reduce catheter visibility using this approach. Unal and colleagues[7] have reported effective hydrophilic catheter coatings that render devices bright under MRI by permitting a great deal

Table 64-1. Approaches to Make Catheters Conspicuous on MRI

Approach	Advantages	Disadvantages	Examples
Passive catheters, visible based on intrinsic materials properties	Simple, inexpensive Can be used in combination with other approaches	Usually visible based on absence of water, generating dark signals Dark signals are easily diluted on MRI "Compatible" conductive wires can heat Must not contain ferrous braids	Gadolinium-filled balloon dilatation catheters Nonbraided angiography catheters
Active "imaging" catheters, incorporating MRI antennae	Highly conspicuous Catheters can be depicted in color Versatile imaging approaches, including projection-mode	Complex, expensive Conductive wires can heat Blurry profile compared with X-ray catheters Dipole designs have poor distal tip visibility	Surgi-Vision Intercept 0.030" dipole guide wire coil Boston Scientific MRI Stilletto endomyocardial injection system
Active "tracking" catheters, incorporating MRI antennae	Simple, inexpensive Marker points can be tracked without imaging, to increase speed or reduce heating Marker points can be used to automate scan plane adjustments	MRI pulse sequence must be modified Catheter locations are computer-synthesized on image Conductive wires can heat	General Electric Massachusetts General/ St. Jude electrophysiologic catheter mapping system[26]
Wireless devices	Requires no physical connection	Embeds electronics that might interfere with mechanical performance (i.e., on stents) Imaging compromises, such as reduced flip angle	Essen wireless stents[38] and catheters[8]
Multispectral devices	Non-proton MRI species can be displayed in different colors from target tissue Passive imaging that does not require transmission lines or embedded electronics	Additional hardware required to excite and detect the alternate compounds Hyperpolarized ^{13}C requires constant replenishment using specialized generator hardware	^{13}C selective coronary arteriography[10] ^{19}F catheter tracking[9]

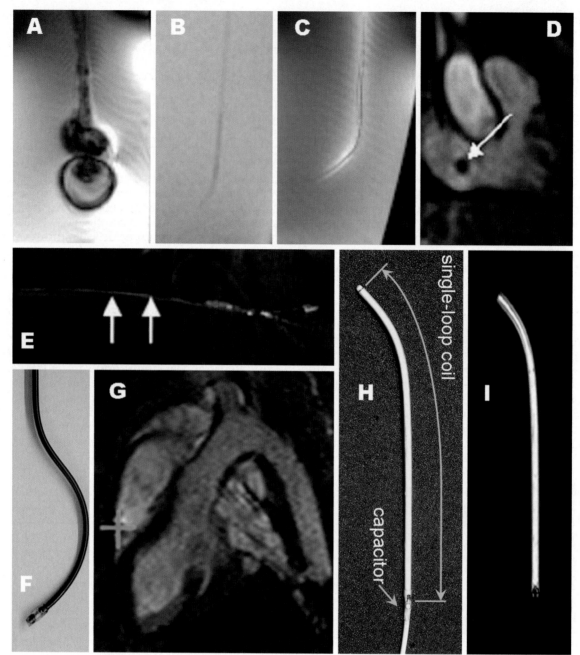

Figure 64-5. A comparison of representative catheter designs for interventional cardiovascular magnetic resonance imaging (iCMR). **A,** Magnetic resonance imaging (MRI) of a typical steel-braided X-ray catheter. The ferrous material destroys the MRI image, may generate force inside the high magnetic field, and may heat during MRI. **B,** The same catheter is shown without the steel braids. It is difficult to see even in vitro. **C,** An "imaging-active" version of the same catheter contains MRI antennae and is attached to the scanner hardware. Signal from excited spins can be depicted in color. Note that the signal "falls off" toward the tip of this simple dipole design. **D,** A CO_2-filled balloon catheter in a human right atrium during real-time MRI. It is visible only as a signal void *(arrow)*. **E,** A 4-Fr catheter *(arrows)* coated with a hydrophilic gadolinium paint. It can be seen as a white line within the aorta of a large mammal. **F,** A "tracking-design" active catheter has a microcoil embedded near the tip. **G,** The position of the microcoil catheter in **F** is displayed as green crosshairs inside the right ventricle of an animal. **H,** A "wireless" catheter is tuned to resonate passively because of embedded electronics. It appears bright **(I)** during low-flip-angle MRI pulse-sequences. (**A-C,** From U.S. Government work [Lederman, NHLBI], public domain. **D,** Courtesy of Reza Razavi. From Miquel ME, Hegde S, Muthurangu V, et al: Visualization and tracking of an inflatable balloon catheter using SSFP in a flow phantom and in the heart and great vessels of patients. Magn Reson Med 2004;51:988-995. **E,** Courtesy of Orhan Unal. From Unal O, Li J, Cheng W, et al: MR-visible coatings for endovascular device visualization. J Magn Reson Imaging 2006;23:763-769. **F** and **G,** Courtesy of Michael Bock and Sven Zuehlsdorff, DKFZ Heidelberg. Original work. Distinct from Figure 3G in Bock M, Muller S, Zuehlsdorff S, et al: Active catheter tracking using parallel MRI and real-time image reconstruction. Magn Reson Med 2006;55:1454-1459. **H** and **I,** Courtesy of Harald H. Quick. From Quick HH, Zenge MO, Kuehl H, et al: Interventional magnetic resonance angiography with no strings attached: Wireless active catheter visualization. Magn Reson Med 2005;53:446-455, Figure 2A&B.)

of gadolinium agent to interact with excited water spins (see Fig. 64-5). Simpler passive devices have been tracked under MRI based on their dark appearance, including polymer guidewires with embedded dysprosium markers (which create disproportionate signal voids), gas-filled balloon catheters (see Fig. 64-5D), and various nitinol and platinum implants. Such polymer devices also are resistant to RF-induced heating during MRI. Special MRI pulse-sequences can enhance the appearance of metal-induced susceptibility artifacts in passive catheters, but at present these compromise the imaging in other ways.

Active Catheter Devices

Active catheter devices contain integrated MRI receiver coils, or antennae, and are connected to the MRI system hardware. They are visualized using two general approaches. *Imaging*-active catheters are intrinsically visible on images because they contribute information used to create the image displayed to the operator. This approach is called "profiling," because usually a length of the catheter "profile" also is visualized. An alternative is to embed point-markers on the active catheter, use special MRI pulse-sequences to detect the location of these points, and synthesize the location markers electronically on the image. These catheters are known as *tracking*-design active devices. We advocate the former, but compelling in vivo experiments have been conducted using both approaches.

Imaging-active catheters detect nearby excited spins and usually appear as a nebulous bright field surrounding the catheter device, unlike the sharp profiles generated by catheters in X-ray images (see Fig. 64-5C). More importantly, because imaging-active catheters can be attached to separate RF receiver channels on the MRI system, they can be processed separately and displayed in color. We have found this method to be particularly helpful (Fig. 64-6B). The simplest imaging-active catheter design is the loop-

less dipole antenna. One iteration is approved for marketing as a 0.030-inch intravascular MRI guidewire (Intercept, Surgi-Vision, Baltimore, MD); it uses external detuning and decoupling circuitry to prevent heating. The dipole design, however, suffers sensitivity falloff near the guidewire distal tip, which limits its suitability for interventional procedures (see Fig. 64-5C). More sophisticated designs, with conspicuous tips, are under development. Imaging-active catheters are especially helpful when used in tandem with passive devices. For example, balloon angioplasty catheters filled with dilute gadolinium contrast are far more conspicuous when delivered over an imaging-active guidewire coil, especially when signal from that coil is color-coded (see Fig. 64-6).

Tracking-design active catheters contain embedded point-marker receiver microcoils that also detect nearby excited spins. Usually, the MRI pulse-sequence is modified for short periodic RF pulses used to find these microcoils in space. Computer synthesized point- or line-markers are overlaid on the MR image to indicate the position of the catheter (see Fig. 64-5F,G). Active-tracking catheters are also useful when used with automated MRI pulse-sequences that interact with the catheter, for example to keep the imaged slice aligned with the catheter as it moves, or to speed up imaging when the catheter is moved rapidly. A simple extension of the active-tracking microcoil design, with two opposed solenoids wound in opposite directions, can be used for high-sensitivity MRI of nearby structures. Related approaches incorporate miniature magnetic field detectors into the catheter device and use the active microcoils to generate blinking susceptibility artifacts (dark spots).

The transmission lines connecting active catheter devices to the MRI hardware are themselves conductive and prone to heating. This can be addressed using electronic decoupling and detuning circuitry, alternative transmission line designs that incorporate transformer devices, or nonconductive approaches such as fiberoptic lines.

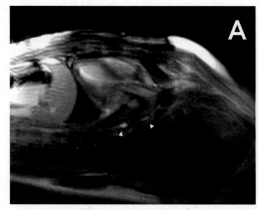
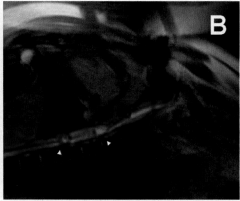

Figure 64-6. The utility of combining active and passive devices. **A,** A platinum stent is premounted on a partially inflated balloon with dilute gadolinium contrast and advanced over a nitinol guidewire. The guidewire is not visible, and only the balloon "dumbbells" *(arrowheads)* are conspicuous. **B,** The same balloon and stent are advanced over an active-imaging guidewire. The devices are brighter and more conspicuous, and their signal can be displayed in color. (Source: U.S. Government work [Lederman, NHLBI], public domain.)

Other Novel MRI Catheter Designs

One particularly attractive approach is to use *wireless* catheter devices or even stents, which couple inductively to the MRI system using embedded electronics.[8] Present designs work best when imaging at low flip angles, which may otherwise compromise image quality (see Fig. 64-5H,I). Most designs also are not detected on separate receiver channels, so catheter signals cannot be depicted in separate colors from anatomic structures.

Another creative approach is to coat or fill catheter devices or contrast media with non-proton materials such as [19]fluorine[9] or hyperpolarized [13]carbon.[10] Multispectral MRI techniques can image water proton spins and these other species either simultaneously or in alternating fashion. These solutions combine the safety and simplicity of passive designs with the ability to use color to distinguish catheter components from target tissues.

The Topspin medical device is a wholly self-contained MRI catheter device intended for intravascular atherosclerosis imaging. It operates within a conventional X-ray suite without a traditional MRI system. The catheter incorporates strong static magnets and radio transmitter-receiver coils and uses a technology called rotating-frame zeugmatography to create MRI. It can distinguish nearby plaque components.[11]

APPLICATIONS

Atherosclerosis Imaging

The earliest invasive MRI devices were developed to improve imaging of atherosclerotic lesions. The rationale was to improve signal-to-noise ratio, and thereby spatial resolution or speed, by bringing receiver coils closer to the tissue of interest. Larose and colleagues at Brigham and Women's Hospital positioned active dipole guidewire coils under X-ray in iliac artery lesions before conducting MRI.[12] Other laboratories have reported similar work using the same guidewire,[3,13] but none has convincingly demonstrated the value of MRI in imaging atheromata. Higher-sensitivity devices are actively being developed.[14] Macrophage uptake of iron-based contrast agents can be detected in patients using MRI,[15,16] but such examinations can be accomplished noninvasively.

Coronary Artery Interventions Are Not Feasible Using Interventional Proton MRI

In healthy swine, Speuntrup and associates[17] delivered stainless steel stents into normal coronary arteries using passive visualization. Both devices and the widely-patent coronary arteries were well visualized using SSFP MRI at 1.5 T, in spite of cardiac and respiratory motion. Similar work has not been reported in diseased coronary arteries. Active invasive devices are unlikely to help, because, as presently envisioned, they would need to be navigated through coronary arteries before they can be expected to enhance spatial resolution.

X-ray fluoroscopy can resolve points as close as 200 µm, with a frame rate up to 30 frames per second (33 msec/frame). Operators can navigate 0.014-inch guidewires through tortuous, even occluded, coronary arteries under X-ray based on subtle visual feedback. Proton-based MRI cannot approach this performance, because signal-to-noise is too low. Meaningful MRI-guided transluminal coronary artery interventional procedures would require a technical breakthrough not anticipated at present.

Cell and Drug Delivery to the Myocardium

Endoluminal catheter procedures on heart muscle are particularly well suited for interventional MRI applications. Despite significant cardiac and respiratory motion, hearts are sufficiently large and thick-walled that they can be imaged with good spatial resolution in real time. Workhorse pulse-sequences such as SSFP depict blood as bright, so the endocardial border is highly conspicuous. Thinner-wall structures such as the atria, however, are difficult to visualize under real-time MRI.

Our laboratories[3,18] and many others[19-23] have conducted targeted cell delivery into specified targets in diseased heart models in swine. This has been particularly successful using two-channel active devices. A steerable guiding catheter system and a separate injection needle are attached to different receiver channels and displayed in color (Fig. 64-7). This can target delayed gadolinium hyperenhancement (infarcts), infarct borders, wall motion abnormalities, subvalvular or papillary structures, perfusion maps, strain maps, and other features of interest.

Multiple cell preparations can be made conspicuous under MRI by labeling with iron, yet without apparently disturbing in vitro functional assessments. Labeled cells can be seen to accumulate within target territories interactively during injection. This can be useful to confirm successful delivery, to visualize previous injections and avoid inadvertent overlap, or to ensure confluence of treatment targets if desired.

Operationally, we have found it useful to image multiple slices simultaneously and to render their 3D volumetric relationship during device manipulation. This provides superior imaging of the beating heart during catheter-based procedures. To date, MRI-guided cell and drug delivery has advanced ahead of development of suitable agents that might require targeted delivery.

Therapeutic Electrophysiology Procedures

Catheter-based therapeutic cardiac electrophysiology procedures are traditionally conducted under functional guidance of local electrograms, with adjunctive projection X-ray imaging. Several guidance systems combine functional contact or noncontact maps with electromagnetic catheter positioning systems (e.g., CARTO [Biosense-Webster]), increas-

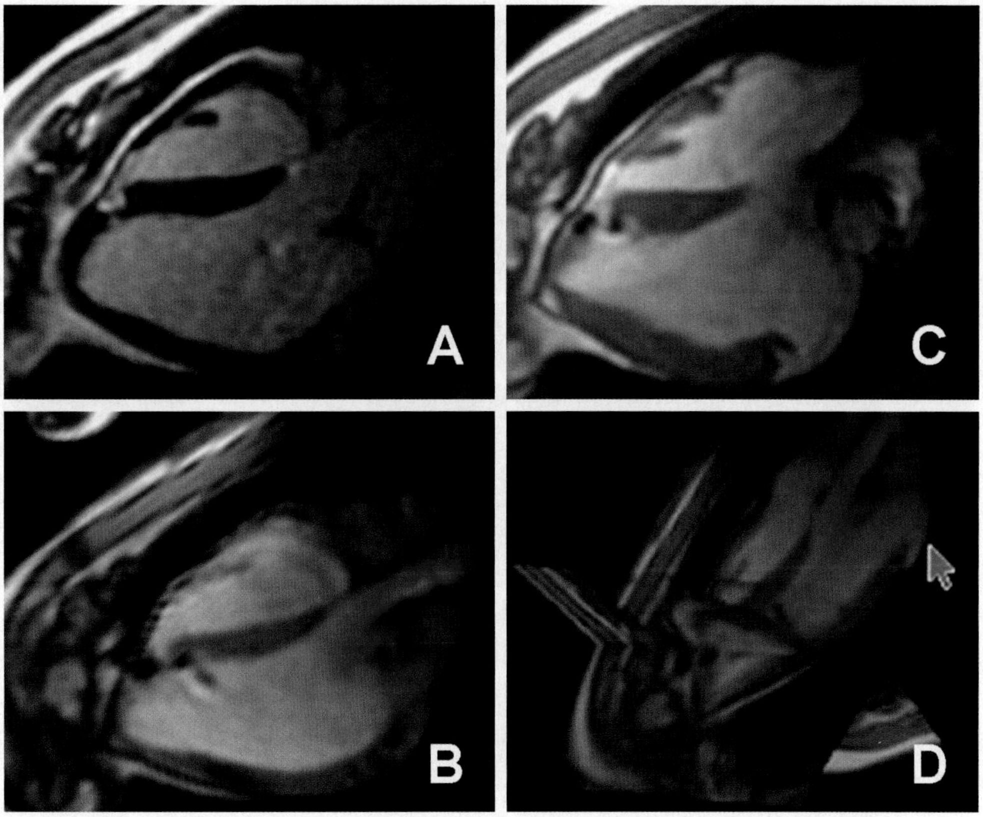

Figure 64-7. Magnetic resonance imaging (MRI)-guided cell delivery to the borders of a small myocardial infarct. **A,** A small infarct is visualized in the distal septum based on delayed gadolinium enhancement. **B,** A two-channel active endomyocardial injection guiding catheter *(green)* and needle *(red)* are used to inject iron-labeled stromal cells *(black)* to the target. **C,** The two cell injections are visible as black spots along the proximal and distal borders of the infarct. **D,** View of the real-time multislice imaging used during this procedure. (Source: U.S. Government work [Lederman, NHLBI], public domain.) (See Video 64-2.)

ingly overlaid with static roadmaps imported from prior MRI or X-ray CT acquisitions. However, few such electrophysiology procedures are conducted under imaging guidance. By contrast, numerous effective therapeutic electrophysiology procedures are conducted fairly rapidly under direct *visual* guidance after surgical exposure. MRI might have value in specifying the instantaneous position of devices in relation to actual anatomic structures or in identifying tissue response to treatment (e.g., myocardial edema after RF ablation). In particular, MRI might be useful in identifying lines of continuity created by ablative energy, which might represent functional electrophysiologic block.

Henry Halperin and colleagues at Johns Hopkins University successfully tracked active dipole catheters and acquired intracardiac electrograms during real-time MRI.[24] They also characterized the MRI appearance of fresh RF ablation lesions.[25] Vivek Reddy, Ehud Schmidt, Charles Dumoulin, and colleagues[26] reported instantaneous positioning of cardiac electrophysiology catheters overlaid on high-resolution ECG-gated moving cardiac images. The cardiac images could be updated intermittently as needed.

Valve Interventions and MRI-Guided Cardiac Surgery

MRI might have value in positioning valve prostheses delivered from a transcatheter or minimally invasive approach. Kuehne and colleagues[27] used MRI to deliver and position a passive nitinol-based valve prosthesis in the aortic position from a transfemoral approach in healthy swine. This demonstrated the value of combined device and tissue imaging using MRI.

At present, the chief limitations to catheter-based prosthetic valve implantation relate to impaired performance of devices miniaturized for transcatheter deployment. One exciting application of MRI is to guide minimally invasive *surgical* deployment of valve prostheses. McVeigh, Horvath, and colleagues[28] used minimally invasive access to the left ventricular apex (via a pursestring suture) with MRI-guided implantation of an aortic prosthesis in swine (Fig. 64-8). The apical access provided large-bore access to deliver a large-profile stent-mounted commercial bioprosthesis. MRI permitted precise orientation, axial positioning, and deployment of the prosthesis. Their subsequent work demonstrated the incremental value of active catheter devices over solely passive devices. Whether MRI has value in other minimally invasive cardiac valve annulus and leaflet interventions remains untested.

Connecting and Disconnecting Chambers and Vessels

Several groups have deployed passive nitinol occluder devices across atrial septal defects in swine using MRI guidance.[29-31] MRI is useful for intraprocedural assessment of outcomes. Whether it has incremental value for this procedure over transesophageal or intracardiac ultrasound remains uncertain. MRI may prove

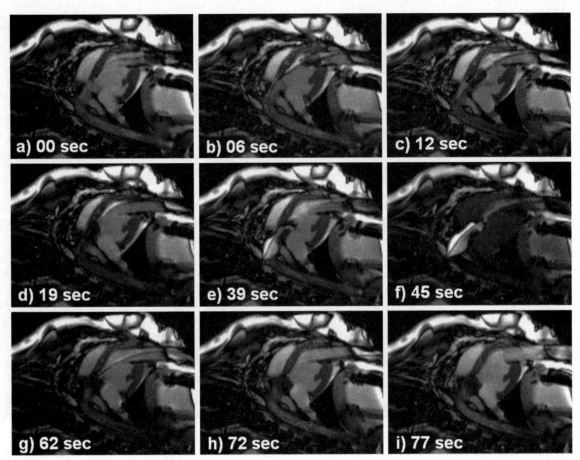

Figure 64-8. Magnetic resonance imaging (MRI)-guided transapical aortic valve implantation. **A,** With a trocar inserted across the left ventricular apex, a passive guidewire is advanced across the aortic valve. **B,** The prosthetic valve is introduced into the trocar, then into the left ventricular outflow tract **(C),** and is then positioned across the native aortic valve **(D)** and aligned with respect to the coronary ostia (not shown). The balloon-expandable stent is inflated with gadolinium contrast agent **(E),** and "saturation" imaging is toggled **(F)** to highlight this agent. The balloon is deflected **(G)** and withdrawn **(H),** along with the guidewire **(I).** (Source: U.S. Government work [McVeigh, NHLBI], public domain.) (See Videos 64-3 through 64-6.)

useful to deploy occlusion devices in more complex lesions such as ventricular septal defects, but few data are available.

Interventional cardiovascular MRI starts to get interesting when it can enable operators to defy the normal confines of vascular chambers. A simple step in this direction is to connect adjacent vascular structures during atrial septal puncture. The interatrial septum in swine is easily and safely punctured and enlarged under MRI guidance using active Brockenbraugh-style needles and guidewires.[32]

Arepally and colleagues at Johns Hopkins University used a similar active needle to effect a transcatheter mesocaval shunt, connecting the vena cava and the superior mesenteric vein using a nitinol connector.[33] The Stanford team, using the "double-doughnut" MRI system described earlier, conducted effective transjugular intrahepatic portosystemic shunts (TIPS) in patients.[34] MRI guidance reduced the number of unsuccessful punctures, which can be hazardous.

MRI might enable nonsurgeons to establish connections between other nonadjacent vascular struc-

tures, for example connecting the subclavian and pulmonary arteries, or the aorta and femoral arteries. Catheter-based extra-anatomic bypass might be an attractive alternative to open-surgical bypass and is under active development. MRI should permit inspection of vascular and extravascular spaces and the trajectory of connecting devices, as well as instantaneous assessment of the adequacy of catheter-based anastomoses.

Chronic Total Occlusion

Another attractive application is to use MRI to negotiate intravascular trajectories that cannot be visualized by X-ray techniques. Chronic total occlusion (CTO) of peripheral arteries is one such setting. X-Ray fluoroscopic angiography with radiocontrast identifies the occluded inflow artery and possibly collateral-dependent outflow beyond the occlusion, but it cannot discriminate CTO arterial wall and lumen. In these cases, the entire occluded arterial segment remains invisible to the operator. Virtually "blind" device manipulation risks procedural failure and arterial perforation. MRI can visualize even the occluded arterial segment, including arterial wall, lumen content, and adjacent structures, and therefore could guide recanalization of CTO.

Raval and colleagues created an animal model of peripheral artery CTO in swine. They were able to recanalize these lesions, using homemade active devices under MRI guidance, but were largely unsuccessful using X-ray guidance and high-performance contemporary clinical guidewires.[35] Clinical-grade devices are currently under development to translate this experience to human subjects.

Aortic and Other Peripheral Artery Interventions

Endovascular repair for abdominal aortic aneurysm (AAA) is limited in part by endoleak due to inflow or outflow malapposition. X-ray alone is imperfect in visualizing complex 3D aneurysms. Raman and colleagues[36] used MRI to guide simple endograft repair of AAA in pig models. Homemade, temporarily active tube endograft devices, which appeared in color until they were disconnected after deployment, were more useful and successful than comparable passive endograft devices. MRI afforded precise positioning as well as immediate anatomic and functional evaluation of success by visualizing stent apposition, flow contours, and contrast exclusion.

Eggebrecht and colleagues in Essen, Germany, demonstrated a wonderful application of MRI to guide deployment of unmodified passive, self-expanding Gore endografts in an animal model of descending thoracic aortic dissection.[37] MRI distinguished the true from the false lumen, guided device

positioning and deployment, and demonstrated obliteration of the dissection (Fig. 64-9).

Straightforward clinical peripheral angioplasty and stenting is not likely to be a high-priority application for interventional MRI. MRI has been used to conduct angioplasty and stenting in animal models of iliac, renal, and carotid arteries[38-40]; to deploy vena cava stents[41] and image captured embolic material; and to guide visceral embolization such as in kidney segments.[42] These and many other applications reflect important technical advances. The team at the University of Regensberg have conducted MRI-guided angioplasty and stenting, using only passive devices, of human iliac[43] and of femoropopliteal[44] atherosclerotic lesions. Other laboratories are beginning similar work using passive and active devices.

Pediatric and Other Congenital Applications

There are settings where interventional MRI may have value even in straightforward catheter-based procedures. The advantages of MRI might include avoiding radiation or iodinated radiocontrast or reducing operator musculoskeletal injury from lead aprons. Children with congenital cardiovascular abnormalities are subjected to multiple catheter procedures during their lifetime and may accumulate a large radiation exposure with excess malignancy risk. Schalla, Higgins, Moore, and colleagues at the University of California San Francisco conducted comprehensive diagnostic cardiac catheterization procedures in swine with atrial septal defect (Fig. 64-10), using active-tracking catheters containing microcoils. They traversed right-sided and left-sided

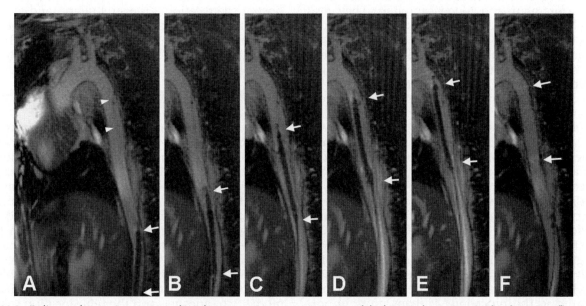

Figure 64-9. Delivery of a passive aortic endograft *(arrows)* to treat a porcine model of aortic dissection. **A,** The dissection flap is visible *(arrowheads).* **B** through **E,** The endograft is positioned over the dissection origin. **F,** The dissection is obliterated by the self-expanding endograft. (Courtesy of Harald H. Quick. Modified slightly from Eggebrecht H, Kuhl H, Kaiser GM, et al: Feasibility of real-time magnetic resonance-guided stent-graft placement in a swine model of descending aortic dissection. Eur Heart J 2006;27:613-620, by permission of Oxford University Press.) (See Video 64-7.)

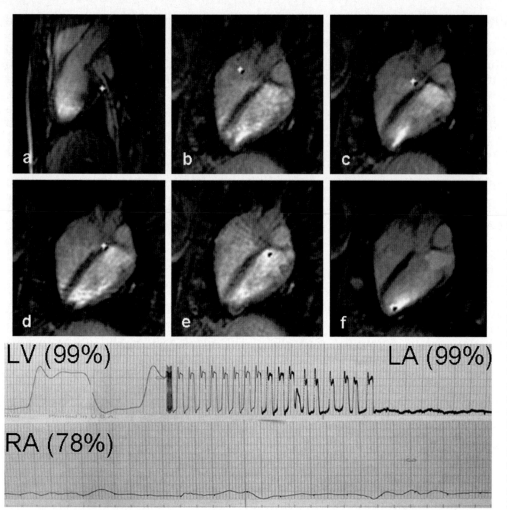

Figure 64-10. Diagnostic cardiac catheterization using magnetic resonance imaging (MRI) and tracking-design active catheters in swine. The distal microcoil receiver is displayed as a dot as the catheter traverses from the inferior vena cava (**A**) to the right atrium (**B** and **C**) and across an atrial septal defect (**D**) into the left atrium (**E**) and left ventricle (**F**). Continuous pressure recordings are displayed during pull back at the bottom of the image, along with hemoglobin saturation values. (Courtesy of Simon Schalla. From Schalla S, Saeed M, Higgins CB, et al: Magnetic resonance-guided cardiac catheterization in a swine model of atrial septal defect. Circulation 2003;108:1865-1870.)

heart chambers with continuous intracavitary pressure measurement and blood sampling. They also used velocity-encoded MRI to make measurements such as shunt ratios.

In landmark work, the team at Kings College London tested these techniques in humans using a combined XMR suite. They used MRI and passive gas-filled balloon-tipped catheters to conduct diagnostic cardiac catheterization in children, to avoid radiation exposure.[6] In this and subsequent reports, they used MRI to make hemodynamic measurements after provocation, for selective gadolinium arteriography, and for measuring pulmonary artery compliance.[45]

We deployed stents to treat an animal model of aortic coarctation using commercially available clinical devices, including an active guidewire.[46] Using a passive balloon filled with dilute gadolinium and an active guidewire, MRI provided continuous display of stent and target tissue during deployment (Fig. 64-11). Phase-contrast MRI provided hemodynamic results during the procedure. Perhaps more importantly, during deliberate balloon overstretch of the animal coarctation lesion, MRI provided instantaneous feedback about life-threatening aortic perforation. This might have incremental value over X-ray,

which would require contrast administration to demonstrate perforation. Krueger, Kuehne, and colleagues in Berlin performed balloon angioplasty of aortic coarctation lesions in patients during MRI in an important clinical first step toward wholly MRI-guided treatment of this congenital lesion.[47]

X-RAY FLUOROSCOPY FUSED WITH MRI

Clinical interventional MRI remains inaccessible to most clinicians, yet MRI acquisitions are readily available. One obvious intermediate step would be to combine prior MRI datasets with real-time X-ray fluoroscopy to guide therapeutic procedures (X-ray fused with MRI, or XFM). The challenge is to ensure that the images are properly aligned or "registered."

Images are registered by aligning common points of reference. There are two general approaches. The simpler approach is to assume a common image space; for example, in relation to a patient table. The table, bearing the patient, is moved from one imaging modality to another, and the table location is known precisely to the registration computer. As long as the patient does not move or change, images from one modality can be registered and combined precisely with images from another. The second general

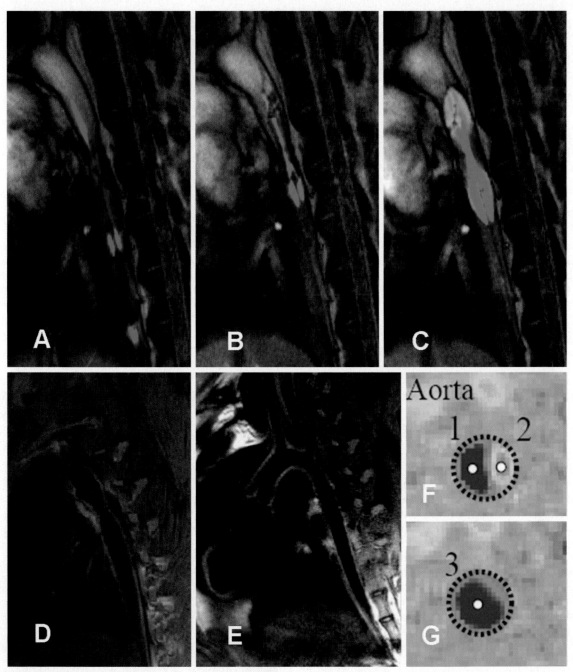

Figure 64-11. Delivery of a platinum stent into a porcine model of aortic coarctation.[46] **A,** A platinum stent is hand-crimped on a delivery balloon that is partially inflated with dilute gadolinium. The balloon is advanced over an active-imaging guidewire using real-time magnetic resonance imaging (MRI). The signal from the active guidewire is colored green, which makes the balloon also appear green. The system is positioned in the coarctation **(B),** and the balloon is inflated **(C).** Both the devices and the target tissue are visible with the use of real-time MRI. Conventional (non-real-time) black-blood MRI shows the hourglass deformity of the coarctation lesion before **(D)** and after **(E)** stenting. **F,** Through-plane phase-contrast MRI just below the coarctation lesion shows turbulence-induced flow reversal. **G,** After stenting, laminar flow is restored. *1* and *3* indicate antegrade flow and *2* indicates flow reversal. (Source: U.S. Government work [Lederman, NHLBI], public domain.) (See Videos 64-8 through 64-10.)

approach uses so-called "fiducial" markers, which are uniquely identified in both imaging modalities. After corresponding fiducial markers are identified using each modality, computerized transformations can register and combine images from both. Fiducial markers may be simple beads attached to patients' skin; better fiducial markers can be endogenous, such as bones or vascular bifurcations. Motion of the fidu-

cial markers causes misregistration. Combining X-ray fluoroscopy and MRI requires further computer manipulation in 3D-to-2D transformation.

The Kings College London team used the first approach, optically tracking the patient transport shell.[2,6] They overlaid MRI-derived endocardial surfaces with electrograms from contact mapping catheters during therapeutic electrophysiology procedures

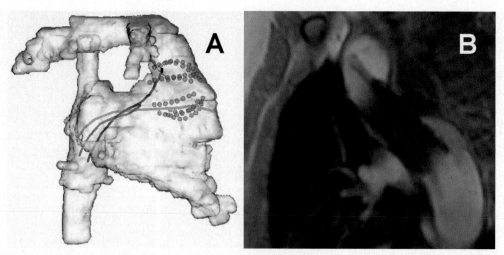

Figure 64-12. Two examples of X-ray fused with magnetic resonance imaging (XFA). **A,** Magnetic resonance angiography (MRA) contours of cavae, right atrium, right ventricle, and pulmonary arteries are combined with colored, computer-segmented X-ray images obtained with the use of an electrophysiology basket catheter. **B,** X-ray stent implantation for aortic coarctation under XFM, combining a magnetic resonance roadmap image. **A,** Adapted from Rhode KS, Sermesant M, Brogan D, et al: A system for real-time XMR guided cardiovascular intervention. IEEE Transactions on Medical Imaging 2005;24:1428-1440. **B,** Original work, courtesy of Reza Razavi, Kings College London.)

to enhance image guidance. They also have overlaid MR images with real-time X-ray during vascular interventions such as coarctation stenting (Fig. 64-12).

Our laboratories use the second approach, affixing multimodality beads (containing X-ray and MRI contrast agents) to the skin of animals and patients during catheter procedures. These beads serve as fiducial markers to register prior MRI datasets, even ECG-gated cinematic ones, with real-time X-ray images. Once registered, the combination of 2D (X-ray) and 3D (MRI) data is automatic irrespective of gantry or table motion. The combined XFM images can display features of interest, such as myocardial infarcts or zones of thinned myocardium. Using beating-heart endomyocardial cell injections to test the geometric accuracy of the XFM guidance system in vivo, we found a mean target registration error of about 3 mm (Fig. 64-13).[48] An obvious next step is to combine ECG and respiratory gating for even finer combination of the two image datasets. Many other laboratories are developing combined MRI, CT, electroanatomic maps, and fluoroscopic images registered in many different ways to guide therapeutic procedures.

CONCLUSION

This chapter outlined how an XMR facility can be configured during installation of two independent X-ray and MRI systems. The incremental cost of an intermodality transportation system and of barrier doors is relatively low. Existing technology already provides excellent real-time MR imaging sufficient to guide an array of investigational therapeutic procedures and to care for patients in this environment. The only barrier to clinical development of interven-

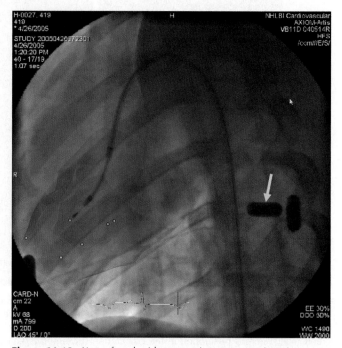

Figure 64-13. X-ray fused with magnetic resonance imaging (XFM) of myocardial cell injection in swine. Multimodality external fiducial markers *(yellow arrows)* are used to establish a common frame of reference to combine images from MRI onto X-ray. Electrocardiographic (ECG)-gated moving features of interest from MRI can be combined with real-time X-ray images to provide some of the best capabilities of each independent modality. The red surface represents the MRI-derived left ventricular endocardium, blue the left ventricular epicardium, and green a large myocardial infarction. A transfemoral endomyocardial injection needle is shown delivering cells to desired targets *(yellow dots)*. (Source: U.S. Government work [Lederman, NHLBI], public domain.)

tional cardiovascular MRI is the commercial unavailability of clinical-grade active catheter devices.

Competing technologies are available but suffer important limitations. Electromagnetic position mapping relies on prior (roadmap) anatomic information. CT provides superb soft tissue imaging but requires prohibitive ionizing radiation exposure to guide interventional cardiovascular procedures. Three-dimensional ultrasound suffers limited acoustic windows and acoustic shadowing from interventional devices but will benefit from continued engineering development.

MRI may prove superior because it provides "one-stop shopping" in a single imaging modality, combining 3D anatomy, biochemical characterization, mechanical function, and hemodynamics. Real-time MRI provides surgical exposure to nonsurgeons conducting minimally invasive procedures and has the potential to revolutionize interventional cardiology.

REFERENCES

1. NessAiver M: All You Really Need to Know about MRI Physics. Baltimore, MD, Simply Physics, 1997.
2. Rhode KS, Sermesant M, Brogan D, et al: A system for real-time XMR guided cardiovascular intervention. IEEE Transactions on Medical Imaging 2005;24:1428-1440.
3. Dick AJ, Raman VK, Raval AN, et al: Invasive human magnetic resonance imaging during angioplasty: Feasibility in a combined XMR suite. Catheter Cardiovasc Interv 2005;64:265-274.
4. Fahrig R, Butts K, Wen Z, et al: Truly hybrid interventional MR/X-ray system: Investigation of in vivo applications. Acad Radiol 2001;8:1200-1207.
5. Rieke V, Ganguly A, Daniel BL, et al: X-ray compatible radiofrequency coil for magnetic resonance imaging. Magn Reson Med 2005;53:1409-1414.
6. Razavi R, Hill DL, Keevil SF, et al: Cardiac catheterisation guided by MRI in children and adults with congenital heart disease. Lancet 2003;362:1877-1882.
7. Unal O, Li J, Cheng W, et al: MR-visible coatings for endovascular device visualization. J Magn Reson Imaging 2006;23:763-769.
8. Quick HH, Zenge MO, Kuehl H, et al: Interventional magnetic resonance angiography with no strings attached: Wireless active catheter visualization. Magn Reson Med 2005;53:446-455.
9. Kozerke S, Hegde S, Schaeffter T, et al: Catheter tracking and visualization using 19F nuclear magnetic resonance. Magn Reson Med 2004;52:693-697.
10. Olsson LE, Chai CM, Axelsson O, et al: MR coronary angiography in pigs with intraarterial injections of a hyperpolarized 13C substance. Magn Reson Med 2006;55:731-737.
11. Schneiderman J, Wilensky RL, Weiss A, et al: Diagnosis of thin-cap fibroatheromas by a self-contained intravascular magnetic resonance imaging probe in ex vivo human aortas and in situ coronary arteries. J Am Coll Cardiol 2005;45:1961-1969.
12. Larose E, Yeghiazarians Y, Libby P, et al: Characterization of human atherosclerotic plaques by intravascular magnetic resonance imaging. Circulation 2005;112:2324-2331.
13. Hofmann LV, Liddell RP, Eng J, et al: Human peripheral arteries: Feasibility of transvenous intravascular MR imaging of the arterial wall. Radiology 2005;235:617-622.
14. Hillenbrand CM, Elgort DR, Wong EY, et al: Active device tracking and high-resolution intravascular MRI using a novel catheter-based, opposed-solenoid phased array coil. Magn Reson Med 2004;51:668-675.
15. Kooi ME, Cappendijk VC, Cleutjens KB, et al: Accumulation of ultrasmall superparamagnetic particles of iron oxide in human atherosclerotic plaques can be detected by in vivo magnetic resonance imaging. Circulation 2003;107:2453-2458.
16. Trivedi RA, U-King-Im J, Graves MJ, et al: In vivo detection of macrophages in human carotid atheroma: Temporal dependence of ultrasmall superparamagnetic particles of iron oxide-enhanced MRI. Stroke 2004;35:1631-1635.
17. Spuentrup E, Ruebben A, Schaeffter T, et al: Magnetic resonance-guided coronary artery stent placement in a swine model. Circulation 2002;105:874-879.
18. Lederman RJ, Guttman MA, Peters DC, et al: Catheter-based endomyocardial injection with real-time magnetic resonance imaging. Circulation 2002;105:1282-1284.
19. Karmarkar PV, Kraitchman DL, Izbudak I, et al: MR-trackable intramyocardial injection catheter. Magn Reson Med 2004;51:1163-1172.
20. Rickers C, Gallegos R, Seethamraju RT, et al: Applications of magnetic resonance imaging for cardiac stem cell therapy. J Intervent Cardiol 2004;17:37-46.
21. Krombach GA, Pfeffer JG, Kinzel S, et al: MR-guided percutaneous intramyocardial injection with an MR-compatible catheter: Feasibility and changes in T1 values after injection of extracellular contrast medium in pigs. Radiology 2005;235:487-494.
22. Corti R, Badimon J, Mizsei G, et al: Real time magnetic resonance guided endomyocardial local delivery. Heart 2005;91:348-353.
23. Saeed M, Martin AJ, Lee RJ, et al: MR guidance of targeted injections into border and core of scarred myocardium in pigs. Radiology 2006;240:419-426. Epub 2006 Jun 26.
24. Susil RC, Yeung CJ, Halperin HR, et al: Multifunctional interventional devices for MRI: A combined electrophysiology/MRI catheter. Magn Reson Med 2002;47:594-600.
25. Lardo AC, McVeigh ER, Jumrussirikul P, et al: Visualization and temporal/spatial characterization of cardiac radiofrequency ablation lesions using magnetic resonance imaging. Circulation 2000;102:698-705.
26. Reddy V, Malchano Z, Dukkipati S, et al: Interventional MRI: Electroanatomical mapping using real-time MR tracking of a deflectable catheter [Abstract]. Heart Rhythm 2005;2:S279-S280.
27. Kuehne T, Yilmaz S, Meinus C, et al: Magnetic resonance imaging-guided transcatheter implantation of a prosthetic valve in aortic valve position: Feasibility study in swine. J Am Coll Cardiol 2004;44:2247-2249.
28. McVeigh ER, Guttman MA, Lederman RJ, et al: Real-time interactive MRI-guided cardiac surgery: Aortic valve replacement using a direct apical approach. Magn Reson Med 2006;56:958-964.
29. Buecker A, Spuentrup E, Grabitz R, et al: Magnetic resonance-guided placement of atrial septal closure device in animal model of patent foramen ovale. Circulation 2002;106:511-515.
30. Rickers C, Jerosch-Herold M, Hu X, et al: Magnetic resonance image-guided transcatheter closure of atrial septal defects. Circulation 2003;107:132-138.
31. Schalla S, Saeed M, Higgins CB, et al: Balloon sizing and transcatheter closure of acute atrial septal defects guided by magnetic resonance fluoroscopy: Assessment and validation in a large animal model. J Magn Reson Imaging 2005;21:204-211.
32. Raval AN, Karmarkar PV, Guttman MA, et al: Real-time MRI guided atrial septal puncture and balloon septostomy in swine. Catheter Cardiovasc Interv 2006;67:637-643.
33. Arepally A, Karmarkar PV, Weiss C, Atalar E: Percutaneous MR imaging-guided transvascular access of mesenteric venous system: Study in swine model. Radiology 2006;238:113-118.
34. Kee ST, Ganguly A, Daniel BL, et al: MR-guided transjugular intrahepatic portosystemic shunt creation with use of a hybrid radiography/MR system. J Vasc Interv Radiol 2005;16(2 Pt 1):227-234.
35. Raval AN, Karmarkar PV, Guttman MA, et al: Real-time magnetic resonance imaging-guided endovascular recanalization of chronic total arterial occlusion in a swine model. Circulation 2006;113:1101-1107.
36. Raman VK, Karmarkar PV, Guttman MA, et al: Real-time magnetic resonance-guided endovascular repair of experimental

abdominal aortic aneurysm in swine. J Am Coll Cardiol 2005;45:2069-2077.

37. Eggebrecht H, Kuhl H, Kaiser GM, et al: Feasibility of real-time magnetic resonance-guided stent-graft placement in a swine model of descending aortic dissection. Eur Heart J 2006; 27:613-620.

38. Quick HH, Kuehl H, Kaiser G, et al: Inductively coupled stent antennas in MRI. Magn Reson Med 2002;48:781-790.

39. Elgort DR, Hillenbrand CM, Zhang S, et al: Image-guided and -monitored renal artery stenting using only MRI. J Magn Reson Imaging 2006;23:619-627.

40. Omary RA, Gehl JA, Schirf BE, et al: MR imaging versus conventional X-ray fluoroscopy-guided renal angioplasty in swine: Prospective randomized comparison. Radiology 2006;238:489-496.

41. Bartels LW, Bos C, van Der Weide R, et al: Placement of an inferior vena cava filter in a pig guided by high-resolution MR fluoroscopy at 1.5 T. J Magn Reson Imaging 2000;12: 599-605.

42. Fink C, Bock M, Umathum R, et al: Renal embolization: Feasibility of magnetic resonance-guidance using active catheter tracking and intraarterial magnetic resonance angiography. Invest Radiol 2004;39:111-119.

43. Manke C, Nitz WR, Djavidani B, et al: MR imaging-guided stent placement in iliac arterial stenoses: A feasibility study. Radiology 2001;219:527-534.

44. Paetzel C, Zorger N, Bachthaler M, et al: Magnetic resonance-guided percutaneous angioplasty of femoral and popliteal artery stenoses using real-time imaging and intra-arterial contrast-enhanced magnetic resonance angiography. Invest Radiol 2005;40:257-262.

45. Muthurangu V, Atkinson D, Sermesant M, et al: Measurement of total pulmonary arterial compliance using invasive pressure monitoring and MR flow quantification during MR-guided cardiac catheterization. Am J Physiol 2005;289:H1301-H1306.

46. Raval AN, Telep JD, Guttman MA, et al: Real-time magnetic resonance imaging-guided stenting of aortic coarctation with commercially available catheter devices in swine. Circulation 2005;112:699-706.

47. Krueger JJ, Ewert P, Yilmaz S, et al: Magnetic resonance imaging-guided balloon angioplasty of coarctation of the aorta: A pilot study. Circulation 2006;113:1093-1100.

48. de Silva R, Gutierrez LF, Raval AN, et al: X-ray fused with magnetic resonance imaging (XFM) to target endomyocardial injections: Validation in a swine model of myocardial infarction. Circulation 2006;114:2342-2350.

49. Miquel ME, Hegde S, Muthurangu V, et al: Visualization and tracking of an inflatable balloon catheter using SSFP in a flow phantom and in the heart and great vessels of patients. Magn Reson Med 2004;51:988-995.

50. Bock M, Muller S, Zuehlsdorff S, et al: Active catheter tracking using parallel MRI and real-time image reconstruction. Magn Reson Med 2006;55:1454-1459.

51. Schalla S, Saeed M, Higgins CB, et al: Magnetic resonance-guided cardiac catheterization in a swine model of atrial septal defect. Circulation 2003;108:1865-1870.

Outcome Effectiveness of Interventional Cardiology

65 Medical Economics in Interventional Cardiology

Daniel B. Mark

KEY POINTS

- The most important determinant of the results of an economic analysis is the absolute magnitude of the clinical benefits being produced by the new therapy or strategy relative to the comparison therapy or strategy.
- An economic analysis should examine the full spectrum of incremental clinical and cost outcomes of the therapy or strategy being studied over a time horizon, typically the lifetime of the cohort, that reasonably reflects the long-term consequences of that technology for the patients being treated.
- Cost-effectiveness analysis assesses the extra or incremental cost for a new therapy or strategy to produce an incremental or extra unit of health benefits, such as an extra life-year or quality-adjusted life-year. The focus is on the assessment of efficiency of a particular investment relative to alternative ways to spend health care dollars.
- Therapies with large up-front costs and delayed incremental clinical benefits, such as coronary artery bypass grafting (CABG), can be economically attractive if applied to sufficiently high-risk populations (and if the analysis examines an appropriately long time horizon).
- Infrequently, a new therapy or strategy is so effective at reducing complications that it fully offsets its cost (a therapy that offers better clinical outcomes with lower cost is referred to as a "dominant therapy"), but most new therapies that improve outcomes are also more costly in the long run, necessitating cost-effectiveness analysis.

According to American Heart Association estimates, percutaneous coronary intervention (PCI) is now performed in the United States about 1,244,000 times each year on more than 600,000 patients.[1] Despite this astonishing level of adoption into mainstream cardiovascular practice, many controversies persist about the appropriate indications for PCI and about its value provided for money spent. The purpose of the present chapter is to review the latter question. The first part of the chapter provides a brief overview of key economic concepts and approaches. The second part reviews empirical research data on the economics of interventional cardiology.

MEDICAL ECONOMICS CONCEPTS AND METHODS

Medical Cost Definitions and Terminology

The traditional economic view of "cost" is that it represents the consumption of societal resources that could have been used for another purpose.[2] The term "opportunity cost" is sometimes used to indicate this particular meaning of cost. Society consumes resources to satisfy its wants, including those for food, housing, and recreation as well as health care.

However, because resources are ultimately finite, society cannot satisfy all wants and is obliged to choose from among the potential alternative uses of its resources. Economics provides a set of tools and approaches to assist with the decisions regarding what health care to produce, in what quantity, and for whom. The classic illustration of the constrained resources concept is the "guns-versus-butter" example from freshman economics. Resources expended in the production of weapons cannot also be applied to the production of food; therefore, in a world of limited resources, more weapons may mean less food. At the societal level, more health care may ultimately translate into less investment in education, transportation, housing, or other societal priorities.

In most businesses or industries, the market price of a product or service is equal to the cost of producing that item plus some amount of profit (typically reflecting a fair return on investment). In the U.S. medical sector, the discrepancy almost universally observed between *prices* (or charges) and *costs* (the true cost of providing a given medical service) is largely attributable to "cost shifting," a set of accounting practices designed to shift costs from a variety of sources (Table 65-1) onto whichever group of payers is most willing and able to absorb them. The net

Table 65-1. Major Components of Hospital Charges for Medical Services

Cost for given hospital service
True costs to hospital of resources consumed (e.g., disposable supplies, personnel, equipment, allocated overhead)

Charge or price for given hospital service
Cost-shifting accounting maneuvers
  Bad debts
  Free services (e.g., indigent care, employees)
  Disallowed costs by third-party payers
Replacement of existing equipment
Acquisition of new technologies (e.g., magnetic resonance imaging)
Budgeting for expansion of services (e.g., more inpatient beds, more outpatient clinics)

From Mark DB, Jollis J: Economic aspects of therapy for acute myocardial infarction. In Bates ER (ed): Adjunctive Therapy for Acute Myocardial Infarction. New York, Marcel Dekker, 1991, 471-496.

Table 65-2. Major Methodological Issues in Medical Cost Studies

Measurement of cost
Categories of cost items to be included
  Disposable supplies
  Personnel (direct cost component)
  Department overhead (e.g., departmental administration, maintenance, equipment depreciation, utilities)
  Allocated hospital or clinic overhead (e.g., hospital administration, admissions, medical records)
Focus for cost analysis
  Resources consumed/service provided ("bottom-up")
  Billed charges/fees ("top-down")
  Episode of care
  Historical data
Structural framework of this study
  Randomized controlled trial
  Observational study
  Cost-effectiveness model
Possible perspectives of the cost analysis
  Societal
  Medicare, managed care, other third-party payers
  Hospitals, clinics, physicians, other providers
  Patients
Time effects on medical costs
  Inflation
  Discounting of future costs
Geographic effects on medical costs
  Different practice settings
  Different geographic locations within a country

effect of these cost-shifting practices is to distort the relationship between U.S. medical prices or charges and medical resource consumption.

The concepts of marginal and incremental costs are commonly used in medical economics. Strictly speaking, *marginal cost* is defined as the cost of producing *one* additional (or *one* less) unit of product, such as a PCI or bypass surgery procedure. However, although the notion of one more or one less test or procedure is useful for some types of (usually theoretical) economic analyses, the more practical questions usually center on examining the costs of shifting *groups* of patients from one diagnostic or therapeutic strategy to another. For this type of analysis, the term *incremental* is often substituted for marginal. (Unfortunately, some leading medical economics researchers use "marginal" and "incremental" synonymously, whereas others do not, leading to potential confusion for those outside the field.) Incremental cost analysis is an important component of cost-effectiveness analysis and is central to the economic notion of cost as a measure of alternative uses of scarce resources introduced at the beginning of this chapter. In the next section, we consider how incremental costs are actually measured and some of the problems involved in translating economic theory into practice.

Induced costs (or *savings*) are the costs of the tests or therapies added or averted as a consequence of some initial management decision and/or resource use. A few examples will make the concept clear. The institution of an aggressive program of intravenous thrombolytic therapy in patients with acute myocardial infarction (MI) by a given hospital or physician practice group may be accompanied by a rise in the number of patients with major disabling strokes who need long-term care. That latter cost is a cost *induced* by the initial therapeutic decision. In the same way, performance of PCI induces the cost of repeat revascularization procedures to treat symptomatic restenosis. Use of statin therapy for secondary prevention induces a cost savings over the long term owing

to reduced need for cardiac procedures and hospitalizations.

Finally, the term *indirect costs* is often used by health service researchers to discuss the societal costs associated with loss of employment or productivity due to morbidity. Because of the potential for confusion with the accounting meaning of indirect costs, the alternative term *productivity costs* is used by some.

Methodologic Issues in Medical Cost Studies

To perform a medical cost study, it is necessary to consider five major issues (Table 65-2): (1) the way cost is to be conceptualized and measured, (2) the type of study to be performed (the structural framework in which the cost analysis will be accomplished, discussed later), (3) the perspectives of the analysis, (4) the importance of cost variations over time, and (5) the importance of cost variations due to geographic and market factors.

Cost Measurement

In any clinical cost study, the investigators must decide at an early stage what categories of cost items they need to include in the analysis and at what level of detail they wish to focus (see Table 65-2). In practice, the types of detailed data required for marginal or incremental cost analysis are difficult to obtain unless the hospital involved has a computerized cost-accounting system, and they are impractical (if not

Table 65-3.   Five Estimates of Cost Savings Available by Shifting Patients from CABG to PTCA

Component	Cost Accounting Method*				
	1	**2**	**3**	**4**	**5**
Total Difference ($)[†]	1,935	4,593	5,346	7,837	10,087
Room	283	2,323	1,939	3,052	3,277
Procedure	28	334	1,014	876	1,348
Blood Bank	342	390	466	532	749
Electrocardiography	3	16	33	47	70
Laboratory	65	146	368	1,035	1,392
Pharmacy	1,061	1,115	682	1,076	1,727
Respiratory	48	120	358	463	529
Supplies	68	68	93	135	271
Radiology	38	78	263	459	555

From Hlatky MA, Lipscomb J, Nelson C, et al: Resource use and cost of initial coronary revascularization: Coronary angioplasty versus coronary bypass surgery. Circulation 1990;82(Suppl IV):IV-208-IV-213.
*Method 1, disposable supplies only; Method 2, supplies plus personnel; Method 3, costs from charges using department-level cost/charge ratios; Method 4, costs from charges using Medicare cost/charge ratios; Method 5, charges.
[†]Cost differences are given in 1986 U.S. dollars.
CABG, coronary artery bypass graft surgery; PTCA, coronary angioplasty.

impossible) to obtain for all participants in the typical large multicenter trial. Therefore, rather than adding up the individual resources being consumed (which might be termed the *bottom-up approach*), most U.S. cost studies start with an aggregated measure of costs, such as can be obtained from hospital or physician bills (a *top-down analysis*). Although the top-down approach is much more practical for many cost studies, especially multicenter studies, it does reduce the ability of the investigator to control the factors that are included as costs in the analysis.

To evaluate the practical impact of using top-down versus bottom-up cost estimates, Hlatky and colleagues at Duke compared the magnitude of cost savings available by shifting from a more expensive treatment (i.e., coronary artery bypass grafting [CABG]) to a less expensive one (i.e., percutaneous transluminal coronary angioplasty [PTCA]) in 389 patients with coronary artery disease (CAD). Two bottom-up and three top-down cost estimates were examined (Table 65-3). Using only hospital charges (method 5), the cost savings was estimated at $10,000 per patient shifted to PTCA. However, if no hospital or departmental overhead is to be saved from this change in practice, then the true cost savings would be that estimated by method 1 or 2: 20% to 46% of the amount estimated from charges. Methods 3 and 4, which include varying amounts of overhead, overestimate the short-term cost savings from the CABG to PTCA shift; they are more correctly viewed as providing an estimate of the difference in *average* cost. On the other hand, methods 1 and 2 indicate the *marginal* or *incremental* difference.

Note that the difference between costs using the Medicare correction factors (method 4) and using charges (method 5) is due at least in part to the hospital's shifting of costs from nonpaying patients to the paying segment. This "surtax" would, of course, never be recoverable by changes in patient management. For this reason alone, charges represent a poor

choice for evaluating the cost implications of different clinical strategies.

A true bottom-up cost analysis, sometimes referred to as *microcosting*, is a complex, time-consuming process that requires identification of all the inputs into a health care service and the assignment of an appropriate cost to each. This is easiest for a relatively simple service, such as the administration of an antibiotic, the performance of a radiograph, or a laboratory test. A more complex hospital laboratory procedure, such as a coronary angioplasty, is a considerably greater challenge because of the large variability of inputs from one case to the next. Most complicated of all is an entire episode of care from admission to discharge, because this requires detailed cost and resource-use data from virtually every major hospital department.

Of the top-down strategies for estimating costs, the most widely used in the United States involves converting hospital charges (taken from the hospital bill) to costs using the correction factors or ratios of costs to charges (RCCs) included in each hospital's annual Medicare Cost Report. Medicare RCCs are largely a holdover from the era before prospective payment, when Medicare reimbursed hospitals on the basis of costs incurred. To do so, Medicare developed a method of deciding how to reimburse hospitals for the reasonable and necessary costs of providing care to its beneficiaries (i.e., true hospital cost), rather than paying the full charged amount. This method involved an elaborate reporting system that required each hospital to file with Centers for Medicare and Medicaid Services (CMS) each year. In this report, which is still required, the hospital details how expenses for direct patient care, overhead, capital equipment, and so forth relates to billed charges. To provide CMS with a means of converting charges to costs for its various ancillary services, each hospital includes in its report a set of ratios, the RCCs. Although not designed for research, the Medicare

RCCs represent a moderately standardized means of estimating cost across all the hospitals in the United States that file a Medicare Cost Report. Although no longer used for reimbursement, the Medicare Cost Report still serves as the primary source of government data on hospital costs. In addition, costs calculated with the RCC method are used to recalibrate diagnosis-related group (DRG) weights. Therefore, this method represents a valuable tool for multicenter cost research.

There are three important limitations to the RCC method of cost estimation that should be noted. First, this approach does not separate out overhead and most other fixed costs and therefore provides an estimate of average rather than marginal cost; hence, it may overestimate potential cost savings. Second, Medicare Cost Reports have complex, detailed instructions for how they are to be filled out; as with the complex federal income tax reporting system, this means that hospitals may choose to interpret the instructions differently (just as different people choose to fill out their income tax forms differently). For this reason, the goal of uncovering a hospital's true cost of providing care may be accomplished to a varying degree using this method. Finally, RCCs are themselves averages of all the cost/charge relationships within a large hospital revenue (ancillary) center such as the radiology, pharmacy, or laboratory departments. If an individual patient's resource consumption pattern in a given cost center is not "average," the Medicare RCCs may not be particularly accurate in converting those charges to costs. For the same reason, conversion of charges to costs for individual items on a detailed hospital bill may not be particularly accurate if the RCC for that item is not close to the average RCC of that cost center. By extension, the practice some have advocated of using one average RCC for an entire hospital may also be less accurate.

Medicare DRG reimbursement rates provide an alternative top-down cost estimation method that does not depend on the vagaries of hospital bills. Once the patient's DRG assignment is known, it becomes a simple matter to calculate the "hospital costs." This system of cost estimation has a number of limitations, however. First, it is not sensitive to variations in resource-use intensity within a DRG. Thus, DRG reimbursement rates are averages in the sense that they represent the "average cost" for a particular DRG among all (elderly) patients in that DRG. Second, if CMS decides not to increase reimbursement to cover the costs of new technology, which has been the case with many new, expensive drug therapies, the DRG reimbursement is insensitive to large differences in resource costs. To take a more complex example, a patient who is admitted for unstable angina and undergoes a diagnostic cardiac catheterization, a PCI, a repeat PCI for abrupt closure, and then CABG will likely be coded out as DRG 106 (CABG with catheterization); from CMS's point of view, the cost of the two PCIs is the hospital's problem. For all these reasons, DRG reimbursement

is not a particularly good way of estimating costs in an economic analysis unless the analysis is being done from CMS's perspective.

The most approximate cost-estimation method used in clinical research involves counting only big-ticket items consumed (such as number of coronary angioplasties, cardiac catheterizations, or CABGs; days in the intensive care unit; and total hospital length of stay) and assigning arbitrary unit prices to each item. The prices assigned are usually charges derived from a single institution or estimated from expert opinion. The resulting linear formula:

$$\text{Total cost} = \Sigma \text{ price} \times \text{quantity}$$

is simple and inexpensive to use (hence its appeal in clinical research), but it suffers from some important drawbacks. First, this approach has almost never been empirically validated within a given institution or (even more important) across institutions. Second, the appropriate set of big-ticket items necessary to estimate costs accurately using this method has never been rigorously defined. Third, the method usually treats the big-ticket inputs as though they were homogeneous. For example, an uncomplicated single-vessel PCI would typically be assigned the same price as a complex three-vessel PCI procedure complicated by abrupt closure. The true costs of these two procedures may in fact differ substantially.

Assignment of costs to physician services in a cost analysis is usually done in one of two ways. In the past, physician fees (which are charges, analogous to hospital charges) have been used. Because most patients receive care from a variety of practitioners (each billing out of a separate office), collecting actual physician bills is several times more complicated than collecting hospital bills. Increasingly, however, physician fees have become a distorted measure of true resource inputs, because physicians have been forced to employ the same types of cost shifting used by hospitals to cover unreimbursed and underreimbursed services. Furthermore, it can be reasonably argued that physician fees in the "fee-for-service" era have never properly reflected a true market price for physician services. Unlike the situation for hospitals, however, Medicare has never required physicians to disclose their true costs in a cost report.

Because of these distortions, the Medicare Fee Schedule—based on the resource-based relative-value scale (RBRVS) of Hsiao and colleagues[3]—has been adopted as a more appropriate method for assigning costs to physician services. The basic concept of the RBRVS is that the price of a service should reflect the (long-term) cost of providing that service. Medicare fees are tied to the American Medical Association Physician's Current Procedural Terminology (CPT) classification system, so that to estimate physician costs from these fees, some map must be created between the CPT codes and the data available in the study database about physician services.

Although the Medicare Fee Schedule is not an ideal measure of the consumption of physician work in health care, it has the advantage of being more objective and consistent than charges or fees. Furthermore, the Medicare RBRVS payment schedule is now being used by many private insurers and managed care organizations, although with variations. Therefore, it represents the best available national fee schedule for physician work.

Importance of Perspective in Cost Analysis

Cost is always defined (either explicitly or implicitly) in terms of specific buyers and sellers (or consumers and producers). Table 65-2 lists the different perspectives that can be used for a medical cost analysis. Most commonly, economists and health policy analysts advocate the use of a societal perspective, in which total health expenditures (public and private) are examined as a function of the benefits produced and the opportunities forgone across the economy. Such an analysis ideally includes hospital costs, physician fees, outpatient testing, outpatient drug therapy costs, non-medical direct expenses (e.g., transportation to the medical facility, child care, housekeeping), and the economic impact of lost productivity due to illness.

In contrast, analysis from the perspective of specific payers or providers typically includes only a portion of the costs listed for a societal analysis. For CMS, for example, hospital costs are defined by the payments specified by the relevant DRG regardless of the amount of services provided (or their cost to the provider). The Medicare Fee Schedule performs a similar function for physician services. For payers other than CMS, costs are the amount they are actually required to pay (or agree to reimburse providers) for health care services. Large insurance companies and managed care plans usually are able to obtain significant discounts off the list price, whereas the individual or the small company that is self-insured may be required to pay total charges. As a practical matter, payer perspectives other than societal and that of CMS are infrequently used in cost studies in the medical literature.

Time Effects in Cost Analysis

Time effects are important to medical cost analyses for two major reasons (see Table 65-2). First, inflationary forces in the economy cause the value of money to diminish over time, so that cost studies from different years should not be directly compared until differences due solely to inflation are accounted for. Although there are several ways to make this adjustment (none of them ideal), perhaps the most widely used is the medical care component of the Producer Price Index (available at http://www.bls.gov/ppi/).

Independent of the effects of inflation, future medical expenditures are considered less costly than current ones, because current expenditures take the money out of your pocket right away, whereas future expenditures allow you to hold onto your money for a period and invest it at the market rate of return. Assuming that the inflation-adjusted price for medical care does not change over time (i.e., no technologic advances that increase or decrease true costs), one can buy more medical care with a given nominal sum of money in 5 or 10 years than is possible in the present. For this reason, cost studies using a long-term perspective employ a technique called *discounting* to account for the differences between the present and future value of money.

Geographic and Market Factors

Geographic and market economic factors also have important effects on medical care costs, although these have received little study in empirical medical cost research. Different practice settings (e.g., within a particular region of the country) can affect the cost of providing a given type of care owing to variations in case mix, different practice patterns of the health care team (e.g., physicians, nurses, administrators), and different levels of efficiency within each setting. For example, for a given patient, care in an academic tertiary care center and care in a large private community hospital in the same city may be associated with quite different hospital costs. First, the teaching hospital must add at least part of the cost of its resident staff, and because the latter must be supervised by an attending physician, total physician time is usually increased per unit of care in a teaching hospital. Furthermore, residents typically order more tests per patient encounter. Other cost differences could arise from differing levels of nursing intensity at each stage in the hospitalization, differing use of intensive and intermediate care beds, and different typical lengths of stay for particular problems. A comparison of patients in the Thrombosis in Myocardial Infarction (TIMI) II trial conservative arm initially admitted to a tertiary versus a community hospital revealed that tertiary centers used more coronary angiography, coronary angioplasty, and CABG for medically equivalent patients.[4]

The costs of material and labor inputs to medical care can vary substantially from one part of the country to another, creating true differences in the cost of providing a given medical service according to geographic factors. Labor costs (e.g., nursing salaries) are probably the most important of the geographic determinants of health care cost variations. Thus, comparison of cost studies from different regions of the country or different practice settings should include an adjustment for geographic cost differences. Several geographic adjustment indices are available, including the Medicare area wage index (for adjusting DRG reimbursement) and the Medicare Fee Schedule geographic adjustment factor.

Table 65-4. Cost Effectiveness, Cost Utility, and Cost Benefit: Sample Calculations

Strategy	Treatment Costs	Effectiveness (Life Expectancy)	Utility (Quality of Life)	QOL-Adjusted Life-Expectancy	Benefits*
Rx A	$20,000	4.5 Years	0.80	3.60 QALYs	$4000
Rx B	$10,000	3.5 Years	0.90	3.15 QALYs	$2000

$$\text{Incremental Cost-Effectiveness Ratio} = \frac{\$20,000 - \$10,000}{4.5 \text{ years} - 3.5 \text{ years}} = \text{per Life Year Saved}$$

$$\text{Incremental Cost-Utility Ratio} = \frac{\$20,000 - \$10,000}{3.6 \text{ QALYs} - 3.15 \text{ QALYs}} = \text{per QALY Saved}$$

$$\text{Incremental Cost-Benefit Ratio} = \frac{\$20,000 - \$10,000}{\$4,000 - \$2,000} = 5$$

*Shows health benefits valued in dollars.
QALY, quality-adjusted life year; QOL, quality of life; Rx, treatment.
From Detsky AS, Naglie IG: A clinician's guide to cost-effectiveness analysis. Ann Intern Med 1990;113:147-154, with permission.

Cost Study Structures

Cost studies generally fall into one of three categories: randomized, controlled trials; observational studies; and cost-effectiveness models. *Cost-effectiveness models* are discussed in the next section. A cost study in a *randomized clinical trial* is usually ancillary to the primary objective of the trial. Typically, cost or resource consumption patterns are a secondary end point in a trial that has either a composite clinical or (preferably) a mortality primary end point. Some have argued that because randomized trials are rarely performed with cost as a primary end point, the trials are usually not optimized to answer the economic questions of greatest interest, except in so far as these questions parallel the primary clinical ones. In addition, requirements of the clinical portion of the study may distort the economic substudy. For example, follow-up protocol angiography to define restenosis leads to repeat revascularization procedures that would not otherwise have been done.

Observational cost studies include both nonrandomized treatment comparisons and descriptive series without an intrinsic comparison group. Descriptive cost studies are useful in areas in which few empirical cost data have been published. Such data can be used to make sample size projections for randomized trials or to inform cost-effectiveness and other health policy studies (in conjunction with appropriate sensitivity analyses). Little has been done to date with observational treatment comparisons involving cost data. As with observational comparisons of medical outcomes, statistical adjustment techniques to "level the playing field" are critical. However, because medical costs are subject to variations over time and over geographic location and practice setting, it is still uncertain what boundaries exist for defining when a nonrandomized cost comparison can be appropriately performed and when it cannot.

Cost-Effectiveness Analysis

In clinical medicine, the term *cost-effective* is frequently used synonymously with *worthwhile* to indicate an intuitive, unspecified threshold between useful and wasteful medical expenditures. In addition, the term *cost-effective* has a specific technical (and not particularly intuitive) meaning. Cost-effectiveness analysis involves the explicit comparison of one option or program with at least one alternative investment of dollars, and it never indicates whether a given expenditure is worthwhile in an absolute sense but rather how it stands relative to other potential expenditures. Therefore, it is incorrect to speak of any medical practice in isolation as cost-effective. The primary objective of cost-effectiveness analysis is to evaluate disparate health care expenditures in common terms so that policy and other decision-makers can choose the most efficient method of producing extra health benefits from among the alternative ways that health care dollars can be distributed.

The general term *cost-effectiveness analysis* actually refers to a family of methods for economic analysis (Table 65-4). For all methods, the final measure is expressed in ratio form, with incremental costs in the numerator and incremental health care benefits or outcomes in the denominator. The distinction among the methods derives primarily from how health benefits are measured. In cost-effectiveness analysis, the measure of incremental health effects chosen is typically the difference in life expectancy between the alternative strategies being evaluated (see Table 65-4). This is the most common type of economic health care analysis performed. In *cost-utility analysis,* remaining survival is adjusted for less than full quality (quality-adjusted life-years [QALYs]). Used much less often in medicine is *cost-benefit analysis,* probably because it requires measuring all health-related benefits of a program in monetary terms (see Table 65-4). Cost-benefit analysis permits comparison of medical care expenditures with societal expenditures on education, defense, transportation, and so forth, whereas cost-effectiveness analysis is useful only in comparison of expenditures that produce the same type of outcome (e.g., QALYs).

Table 65-4 compares two hypothetical treatment strategies (A and B) for a particular disease and summarizes the calculations involved in the different analyses. Treatment A costs twice as much as treatment B but also improves average life expectancy by 1 year. Thus, the cost-effectiveness ratio for A relative to B is $10,000 per life-year saved. Whether switching from B to A is "worthwhile" depends on the alternative health care expenditures (aside from A) available for $10,000 or less. This is the most common sort of problem faced in cost-effectiveness analysis: whether to fund a new program that provides more health benefits than the standard therapy but at a substantially increased cost. (It is theoretically possible to go in the other direction—to give up health benefits to save substantial health care dollars—but this is rarely politically viable.)

QALYs allow us to factor in the *value* of the extended survival offered by a new program or alternative therapy to the patient, as well as its quantity. In the example in Table 65-4, strategy A improves life expectancy relative to B, but the average quality of life for survivors is lower. This could come about in several ways. For example, with strategy B the sickest patients could die, leaving a relatively healthier group of survivors. In contrast, strategy A saves these sick patients from dying but cannot restore them to the same level of health as other patients with lower disease severity. These sicker surviving patients lower the average quality of life for the group. Alternatively, there could be something about strategy A that negatively affects quality of life, such as the need for chronic medication that is associated with significant side effects and that is not required with strategy B. In this example, moving from cost-effectiveness to cost-utility analysis more than doubles the cost of an additional unit of (quality-adjusted) survival with strategy A.

The underlying tenet of all these forms of economic analysis is that the analyst desires to determine the most efficient means of maximizing the net health benefits for a particular group or population under the constraint of limited resources (i.e., where it is not possible to provide every beneficial service to every potential recipient). Note that such economic analyses are neutral to the specific patients and diseases under study; the health benefits being maximized are abstractly conceptualized as belonging to a large group or population. In actual practice, however, political and other forces may play a large role in deciding where societal dollars are to be invested.

The ultimate problem for economic analysis is that individual patients (and their physicians) wish to obtain all the health benefits that are available from modern medical technology. However, the collection of all patients taken together (i.e., society), does not have enough resources to provide this for everyone, thereby forcing the need for difficult and potentially divisive choices. The more we do for selected segments of the population (e.g., chronic renal failure patients receiving dialysis, AIDS patients, patients with acute MI), the less we are able to do for the remainder. In the next section, we examine the costs of various coronary disease therapies. We then return to the issue of cost-effectiveness at the end of this chapter and examine the ways in which this tool can be applied (and misapplied) in the analysis of these difficult choices.

General Issues

An economic analysis comparing a new drug, device, or strategy with "conventional" or "usual" care starts with an exploration of the ways in which the new approach will alter costs for the patients involved. At the most basic level, this involves understanding the resource consumption patterns and associated incremental costs of the new approach or technology. For a new interventional procedure, this includes the costs of the equipment and supplies used and the personnel changes required. A careful economic analysis also must determine what diagnostic or therapeutic procedures and what complications are added or averted, along with the cost effects of these changes in practice and outcome. Understanding these relationships is often difficult in practice, and one of the major advantages of empirical data collection over armchair models for cost studies is the frequency with which actual medical practices and outcomes diverge from the expected ideal.

In general, three major patterns of cost outcomes are possible when comparing alternative medical strategies or technologies (Fig. 65-1).
1. The new strategy or technology is associated with net higher costs but also provides additional clinical benefits. For example, CABG saves more lives than medical therapy in patients with severe CAD, but it costs more money. In such cases, economic analysis attempts to define the relationship between incremental costs and incremental health benefits, so that policy judgments can be made about whether the new strategy should be adopted. Cost-effectiveness analysis is the technique used to formalize this assessment. In some cases, the new strategy or technology may recoup some of its costs by reducing or preventing costly complications that occur with the comparison approach. For example, coronary stenting reduces the need for repeat revascularization procedures relative to conventional balloon angioplasty. These follow-up benefits provide at least a partial offset to the initially higher costs of stenting. However, because the total costs of the new strategy are often higher, cost-effectiveness analysis is still required to define its economic attractiveness.

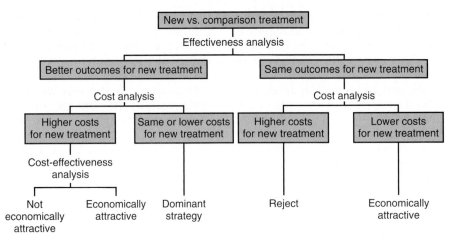

Figure 65-1. Schematic representation of patterns of outcome and cost differences that may result when a new therapy or strategy is compared with an existing standard. Effectiveness is always considered first, because if the new therapy is less effective, its cost is rarely of concern. If effectiveness is better, or at least equivalent, then costs are prepared. If the outcomes are better but the net costs are higher, cost-effectiveness analysis is then performed. If the costs are equivalent or lower, the therapy is said to be *dominant* (i.e., it becomes the preferred option). If outcomes are equivalent, cost analysis is used to select the more efficient, less costly option. This form of cost analysis is sometimes referred to as *cost minimization* or *cost-efficiency analysis.*

2. The new strategy or technology produces better outcomes and has lower net costs. Use of enoxaparin for patients with acute coronary syndrome (ACS) in the Low Molecular Weight Heparin (Enoxaparin) in the Management of Unstable Angina (ESSENCE) trial is an example. Such strategies are referred to by economists as *dominant.*

3. The new strategy or technology provides a less expensive, more efficient alternative to conventional therapy with the same benefits. For example, to the extent that PCI provides an equivalent revascularization option to CABG for some CAD patients, it may substantially reduce costs.

Coronary Revascularization

In 2003, approximately 1.4 million diagnostic cardiac catheterization procedures were done in the United States, followed by over 1.2 million PCIs and almost half a million CABG surgeries.[1] Because a hospitalization for PCI costs from $8000 to $12,000 and a hospitalization for CABG costs $30,000 or more, coronary revascularization costs in aggregate probably exceed $30 billion per year. Although the procedures may be more efficient now than in the past owing to shortened hospital stays and lower complication rates, use in patients with more complex disease and advances in technology, especially for PCI, have tended to push costs back up. In this portion of the chapter, we review the available data addressing two key questions: First, what information do we have about how much these procedures cost? Second, what is the value of these procedures, where *value* refers to the balance between incremental costs and benefits? The literature on interventional cardiology tends to be divided into studies focused on the procedure, which may include both stable and

unstable patients, and studies focused on a portion of the clinical spectrum of CAD, which typically examine strategies of care. Therefore, this section starts with a general review of economics of coronary revascularization.

Percutaneous Coronary Intervention

The costs of PCI have changed considerably over time, as have the clinical and technical aspects of the procedures. Stenting is now used in more than 80% of PCI cases in the United States, and a similar proportion of patients also receive an intravenous glycoprotein (GP) IIb/IIIa inhibitor. Similar trends have been observed in Canada and Europe, although absolute rates are often lower, depending on the countries considered.

Kugelmass and colleagues performed an analysis of the cost of Medicare beneficiaries undergoing PCI and observed the average cost of hospitalization in patients who did not develop complications to be $13,861, whereas patients undergoing PCI who developed complications had costs of $26,807.[5] This analysis was based on the fiscal year 2002 Medicare Provider Analysis and Review file containing 336,373 hospital admissions with an International Classification of Diseases (ICD-9) procedure code indicating a PCI procedure during that admission.

To understand what determines or "drives" these costs, we must examine four major categories of determinants: patient-specific, hospital-specific, treatment-specific, and geographic-economic. Patient-specific factors such as disease severity affect costs by influencing the type of procedure needed to treat the patient's CAD, the associated likelihood of success, and the risks of short- and long-term complications (e.g., abrupt closure, restenosis). (Note that this discussion pertains to the cost of an episode of care, not simply the procedural costs in the catheterization laboratory.) Procedures in patients with complex lesions (e.g., chronic total occlusions) are more costly, for example, because success rates are lower and long-term durability of successful dilations is reduced. The extent of CAD is also an important cost determinant: Costs are lowest in single-vessel disease and highest in three-vessel disease. In addition, diabetes and older age have been associated with higher costs. Among 1258 patients treated at the Cleveland Clinic from 1992 to 1993, costs of percutaneous revascularization were increased with acute MI (91% increase), recent MI (17% increase), more complex lesion morphology (≥12% increase), diabetes (12% increase), and number of diseased vessels (9% increase per vessel).[6]

Treatment-related factors include decisions made in the catheterization laboratory as well as management decisions before and after the procedures. In the large Cleveland Clinic series, physician decision delay (i.e., delay between admission and diagnostic catheterization or between catheterization and revascularization) increased hospital costs by 86%, and weekend delay (procedure postponed because of a weekend) increased costs by 61%.[6] The cost of a combined diagnostic catheterization/coronary angioplasty procedure at University of California, San Francisco (UCSF) was $850 higher than when these two procedures were performed separately.[7] An unsuccessful procedure, particularly with abrupt closure and need for bailout stenting or emergency CABG, is also associated with significantly higher costs. In the Cleveland Clinic series, need for urgent CABG increased costs by 83%, and need for intra-aortic balloon pumping increased costs by 42%.[6] Newer revascularization technologies are associated with significantly higher costs than those of balloon angioplasty. In addition, use of adjunctive pharmacotherapy also increases costs. In the Evaluation of Platelet IIb/IIIa Inhibitor for Stenting (EPISTENT) trial, use of bare metal stents added $2200 to the hospital costs and use of both abciximab and stents added $3600.[8] In Evaluation in Percutaneous Transluminal Coronary Angioplasty to Improve Long-Term Outcome with Abciximab GP IIb/IIIa Blockade (EPILOG), use of abciximab added about $600 net to the hospital costs for balloon angioplasty. In Enhanced Suppression of the Platelet IIb/IIIa Receptor with Integrilin Therapy (ESPRIT), use of eptifibatide added about $300 net to the hospital costs for PCI.[9]

Less work has been done to define important provider-related cost determinants. In a large-claims database, Topol and colleagues found that care at a teaching hospital resulted in lower charges.[10] In 250 patients treated at UCSF, the physician operator was a major cost determinant, with the highest-cost physician averaging $4400 more than the lowest-cost physician.[7] This difference was due to a more resource-intensive style of practice and not to disease severity or procedure outcome differences. Another study found that high-volume operators (i.e., ≥50 cases per year) had slightly lower hospital costs than low-volume operators (approximately $300 difference, $P=.07$) despite performing more complex procedures on a higher-risk population.[11]

Finally, geographic factors have been infrequently studied but appear to explain modest differences in cost on a national level. In one study, costs in the West were highest and costs in the Midwest were lowest.[10]

Coronary Artery Bypass Graft Surgery

In the recently completed Pexelizumab for the Reduction of Infarction and Mortality in Coronary ARtery Bypass Graft Surgery (PRIMO-CABG) trial, the hospital cost of a CABG was almost $30,000, with an additional $4000 in physician fees.[12] As with the costs of PCI described in the previous section, the costs of CABG can be analyzed to identify their major determinants. A recent comparison of costs of CABG at five U.S. and four Canadian hospitals using the same cost accounting system showed that U.S. hospital costs were substantially higher ($20,673 versus $10,373; $P<.001$).[13] These differences were not explained by clinical differences, and length of stay in Canada was 17% longer.

Patient characteristics typically account for 25% or less of the variance in hospital costs. In 12,807 patients in New York State who underwent CABG in 1992, patient characteristics accounted for 23% of the variance in log costs.[14] In a cohort of patients receiving their operation at Emory University, the major determinants of higher costs included worse angina class, previous MI, older age, heart failure, and more extensive CAD, with diabetes being a marginally significant predictor ($P=.07$).[15] In contrast, in the Bypass Angioplasty Revascularization Investigation (BARI) study, CABG in diabetic patients had 5-year costs that were $15,000 higher than in non-diabetics.[16] In the New York state data referred to earlier, the major predictors of extremely high costs of CABG included older age, nonelective procedure, ejection fraction less than 50%, repeat heart surgery, diabetes, chronic obstructive pulmonary disease, hepatic failure, chronic renal insufficiency, and transfer from another acute care facility.

Three major procedural factors increase CABG costs: use of an internal mammary artery graft, use of cardiopulmonary bypass, and need for additional procedures such as valvular repair or replacement. Complications that occur after the operation (which may reflect a combination of patient, treatment-related, and provider factors) substantially increase costs. In the Emory study, important cost drivers of this sort included adult respiratory distress syndrome, septicemia, pneumonia, bleeding requiring re-exploration, major arrhythmias, and neurologic events. Patients without any of these complications averaged hospital costs of $16,776 (1990 U.S. dollars); patients with one complication averaged $17,794; those with three complications, $23,624; and those with five complications, $50,609.[15] Similar findings were reported from 6791 CABG patients in the Massachusetts Health Data Consortium database.[17]

Hospital-level provider-related factors "explain" about 40% of the variance in the initial costs of CABG.[14] In a Duke analysis, the attending surgeon was the most important determinant of cost among all factors examined.[18] The most expensive surgeon had a median cost that was $4200 higher than the least expensive surgeon. As with PCI costs, the explanation for this appears to lie in a more resource-intensive style of practice rather than in a difference in disease severity or in complication rates.

Use of the minimally invasive approaches to CABG and valvular surgery is now established as a viable alternative to standard operative approaches for selected patients. These procedures are performed by a subset of heart surgeons. Initial economic work in this area suggested that a minimally invasive direct coronary artery bypass (MIDCAB) procedure has costs that are about half those of a conventional CABG.[19] Full sternotomy off-pump CABG is a recently developed variant of CABG that seeks to protect patients from complications attributed to cardiopulmonary bypass. At the Minneapolis Heart Institute, both MIDCAB and off-pump CABG required less operating room time than conventional CABG.[20] Mean hospital costs were $17,000 for 44 MIDCAB procedures, $15,000 for 62 off-pump CABGs, and $19,000 for 243 conventional CABGs.

In a trial conducted at a single academic medical center to assess clinical, economic, and quality-of-life outcomes, 200 patients were randomized to either elective off-pump CABG or CABG with pulmonary bypass.[21] Follow-up out to 1 year showed similar graft patency; rates of death, MI, angina, stroke, and reintervention procedures; and quality-of-life measures. Initial hospitalization costs were $2272 higher in the CABG with bypass arm, and 1-year costs in this arm were $1955 higher. In the Canadian Off-pump CABG Registry, involving 1657 consecutive off-pump patients and 1693 consecutive on-pump patients, the initial hospital costs for off-pump CABG were significantly lower ($11,744 versus $13,720; $P < .01$).[22] These differences persisted out to 1 year.

Comparisons of Treatment Options for Coronary Artery Disease

Revascularization versus Medical Therapy

For any CAD patient, medical therapy without revascularization is one important therapeutic option that must be considered. In the most recent meta-analysis on the trial data making this comparison, PCI demonstrated no prognostic advantage over initial medical therapy.[23] Two recent trials have compared the costs of these two strategies. In the Trial of Invasive versus Medical therapy in Elderly patients (TIME) (which was not included in the previously described meta-analysis), a predefined subgroup of 188 chronic symptomatic CAD patients 75 years or older were

randomized to optimized medical therapy or coronary angiography followed by PCI or CABG at four hospitals in Northern Switzerland and monitored for resource utilization and quality-of-life status.[24] At 1 year of follow-up, the rate of death or nonfatal MI was similar in the two arms, whereas the rate of major adverse cardiovascular events was significantly reduced in the invasive strategy arm. These outcomes were similar to the overall trial cohort. The invasive arm was found to have nonsignificantly increased total 1-year costs compared to the medical therapy arm and yielded an economically attractive cost-effectiveness ratio.

Sculpher and colleagues prospectively collected resource utilization data on 1018 patients in the second Randomized Intervention Treatment of Angina (RITA-2) trial.[25] Patients with proven CAD were randomized to an initial strategy of PTCA or continued medical management, and follow-up was conducted out to 3 years. The composite end point of death or MI was higher in patients randomized to the PTCA arm (7.3% versus 4.1%; $P = .025$). Patients in the PTCA arm were also more likely to undergo subsequent coronary angiograms, whereas those in the medical therapy arm were more likely to undergo a nonrandomized PTCA procedure and use more antianginal medication. Mean resource utilization costs were £2685 higher per patient in the PTCA arm at 3 years.

Although interventional therapy is expensive, especially initially, the cost involved with decades of medical therapy should not be underestimated. In the Women's Ischemia Syndrome Evaluation (WISE), 833 women referred for angiography to evaluate chest pain were followed and their long-term costs were modeled.[26] The 5-year cost averaged about $50,000, and patients with three-vessel disease had modestly higher costs than those with single-vessel disease. More than half of the expense was due to cost of hospital-based care, with outpatient medications accounting for an additional 25% to 30% of costs (Fig. 65-2).

An important trial, the Clinical Outcomes Utilizing Revascularization and Aggressive DruG Evaluation (COURAGE) trial, randomized 2287 patients with evidence of ischemia and significant coronary artery disease to undergo either PCI with optimal medical therapy or optimal medical therapy alone. The patients were followed for a period of 2.5 to 7 years, with median follow-up of 4.6 years. In this cohort, the addition of PCI to optimal medical therapy did not reduce the risk of death, MI, or other major cardiovascular events. An economic analysis of this trial is forthcoming.[27,28,28a] The Bypass Angioplasty Revascularization Investigation 2 Diabetes (BARI 2D) is testing whether coronary revascularization added to state-of-the-art medical therapy in 2800 diabetics improves all-cause mortality. Collection of cost data out to 5 years and performance of a cost-effectiveness analysis are integral parts of the study program.[29] The study is currently completing its follow-up phase.

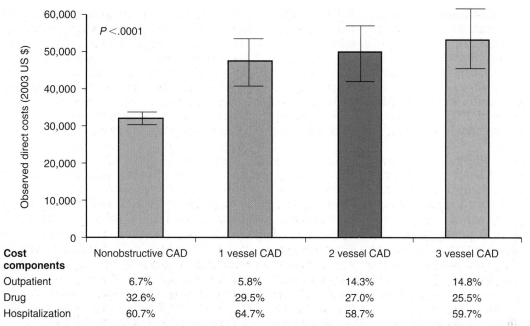

Cost components	Nonobstructive CAD	1 vessel CAD	2 vessel CAD	3 vessel CAD
Outpatient	6.7%	5.8%	14.3%	14.8%
Drug	32.6%	29.5%	27.0%	25.5%
Hospitalization	60.7%	64.7%	58.7%	59.7%

Figure 65-2. Five-year cardiovascular costs for women with nonobstructive and one- to three-vessel coronary artery disease in the Women's Ischemia Syndrome Evaluation (WISE) study. (From Shaw LJ, Merz CN, Pepine CJ, et al: The economic burden of angina in women with suspected ischemic heart disease: Results from the National Institutes of Health–National Heart, Lung, and Blood Institute–sponsored Women's Ischemia Syndrome Evaluation. Circulation 2006;114:894-904.)

PTCA versus CABG

Two major randomized trials have compared PTCA and CABG costs in U.S. patients. The Emory Angioplasty Surgery Trial (EAST) enrolled 392 multivessel CAD patients between 1987 and 1990. For the initial hospitalization, the PTCA patients averaged $11,684 ($16,223 including physician fees), whereas the CABG patients averaged $14,579 ($24,005 with physician fees) (all 1987 dollars).[30] At the end of 3 years, the PTCA arm had cumulative costs of $23,734 versus $25,310 for the CABG arm (P<.001). Thus, PTCA was initially 32% less expensive than CABG, but after 3 years it was only 6% less expensive in this population of multivessel CAD patients. Between 3 and 8 years, the PTCA arm averaged $4700 in additional hospital-related costs compared with $2700 for the CABG arm. Thus, at the end of 8 years, cumulative costs were $44,491 for PTCA and $46,348 for CABG (P=.37).[31]

Of the trials comparing PTCA and CABG, BARI was the largest, enrolling 1829 multivessel CAD patients at 18 centers between 1988 and 1991. The BARI Substudy of Economics and Quality of Life (SEQOL) enrolled 934 of these patients at the seven largest enrolling sites.[16] Initial costs for the PTCA arm were $14,415 in hospital costs and $6698 in physician fees. For the CABG arm, initial hospital costs were $21,534, with physician fees of $10,813. Total inpatient follow-up costs (hospital and physician fees) were $27,439 for PTCA and $19,529 for CABG. Outpatient follow-up care was equivalent in the two arms. The cumulative 5-year cost for medications was higher in the PTCA arm ($4948 versus $3670). Thus, at the end of 5 years, total discounted costs in the PTCA arm were 5% lower than in the CABG arm ($56,225 versus $58,889). Five-year costs in the patients with two-vessel disease were significantly lower with angioplasty ($52,390 versus $58,498 for CABG), whereas in three-vessel disease, angioplasty was actually more expensive ($60,918 versus $59,430). At 12 years of follow-up in the BARI SEQOL study, cumulative costs had narrowed to $120,750 for the PTCA arm versus $123,000 in the CABG arm, and the difference was no longer significant (P=.55). CABG yielded a cost-effectiveness ratio of $14,300 per life year added when compared to PTCA at 12 years.[32]

The British Randomized Intervention Treatment of Angina (RITA) compared the costs of PTCA and CABG (using U.K. costs) in 1011 patients and confirmed the results of EAST and BARI.[33] Initial costs of PTCA were half those of CABG, but at the end of 2 years, PTCA costs had risen to 80% of CABG costs.

The Angina With Extremely Serious Operative Mortality Evaluation (AWESOME) trial randomized 454 high risk patients with medically refractory angina to either PCI or CABG.[34] Costs out to 5 years were estimated using Medicare reimbursement rates. At 5 years, the PCI arm was $18,732 less expensive than the CABG arm. Survival at 5 years was 0.75 for PCI and 0.70 for CABG (P=.21). Bootstrap analysis demonstrated that the PCI arm was more effective clinically and less costly in 89% of repetitions.

Bare Metal Stenting versus Balloon PTCA

Several randomized trials have compared primary coronary stenting with conventional balloon PTCA in native coronary vessels of stable patients. Meta-analysis of these data showed no evidence of a reduction in deaths or MIs with stenting.[35] The trials also showed equivalent 8- to 12-month reduction in anginal symptoms. The major clinical advantage of stenting is a reduction in the need for repeat revascularization, primarily repeat percutaneous procedures, due to a reduced clinical restenosis rate. In the Belgium Netherlands Stent (BENESTENT) II trial, by 6 months, 14% of PTCA patients and 9% of stent patients had received a repeat revascularization procedure.[36]

Cohen and colleagues performed an economic analysis of BENESTENT II using U.S. costs along with the resource consumption patterns observed in the trial, which was conducted in Europe.[37] They found that initial procedural costs were approximately $1900 higher with stenting and that post-procedure costs were equivalent. Follow-up costs were reduced by half in the stent arm, so that at the end of 6 months, stenting had a net incremental cost of $900 over PTCA.

The Optimum Percutaneous Transluminal Coronary Angioplasty Compared with Routine Stent Strategy (OPUS) trial enrolled 479 patients with single-vessel disease.[38] In the optimum PTCA arm, 37% of patients required stents. Use of abciximab was low in both arms (13% to 14%). Length of stay averaged 2.5 days and was similar in the two arms. The procedural costs were higher in the routine stenting arm ($5455 versus $4219; $P<.001$). Total hospital costs showed a similar pattern: $9234 for the stent arm versus $8434 for the PTCA arm ($P<.001$). However, in follow-up, the PTCA arm had a 15% repeat revascularization rate out to 6 months, compared with 5% in the stent arm. Thus, at 6 months, cumulative costs were $10,206 for stent and $10,490 for PTCA. In 1000 bootstrap replications, the routine stenting arm was less expensive by 6 months 69% of the time.

Bare Metal Stenting versus CABG

Although comparisons of stenting with balloon PTCA provide useful information about the value that stents add to the interventionalist's armamentarium, the more important comparison is between a primary percutaneous strategy and a primary surgical one for coronary revascularization. The Arterial Revascularization Therapies Study (ARTS) compared PCI with stenting versus CABG in 1205 multivessel disease patients.[39] By 1 year, the major difference between the two arms was a higher repeat revascularization rate in the stent arm (21.2% versus 3.8% in the CABG arm), a difference that persisted at 3-year follow up (26.7% versus 6.6% in the CABG arm). One-year total costs were €11,117 for the stent group versus €13,896 for the CABG group, a difference of €2779. This difference in costs had narrowed to €1798 at the 3-year follow-up, with the stent group showing €14,302 in total costs versus €16,100 for the surgery group. These cost estimates, which were calculated from limited resource use data and European cost weights, appear to underestimate costs as typically seen in the United States. At 5 years, there was no difference in survival or freedom from death, MI, or stroke between the

two strategies, but repeat revascularization remained higher in the PCI arm (30% versus 9%; $P<.001$).[40] The diabetic subgroup (208 patients) showed a non-significant trend toward higher mortality with PCI (13.4% versus 8.3%; $P=.27$).

Between 1996 and 1999, the Canadian/European Surgery or Stent (SoS) trial randomly assigned 988 patients with typical angina and multivessel disease to either stent-assisted PCI or CABG. In an economic analysis of this trial, initial hospitalizations costs were higher in the CABG arm, and follow-up costs were higher in the PCI arm, consistent with previous trials.[41] Total 1-year follow-up costs in the subgroup of patients with ACS were $6435 for the PCI arm and $8870 for the CABG arm. Total 1-year costs in the non-ACS subgroup were $5069 for the PCI arm and $7487 for the CABG arm. Patients with ACS had significantly higher initial costs and total 1-year costs.

A meta-analysis of four trials comparing CABG versus PCI with mutivessel stenting showed no difference in the composite end point of death, MI, or stroke at 1 year.[42] Repeat revascularization was more common among the PCI patients and freedom from angina was better in the CABG patients (82% versus 77%; $P=.002$).

Drug-Eluting Stents versus Bare Metal Stents

Drug-eluting stents (DES) were received with much fanfare at the 2001 European Society of Cardiology meetings, where initial results were reported from the Randomized Study with the Sirolimus-Eluting Velocity Balloon-Expandable Stent (RAVEL) trial. Five years and millions of implanted stents later, at the 2006 European Society of Cardiology meetings a major subject of debate was the emerging reports of a late risk of catastrophic thrombosis with drug-eluting stents. During the intervening years, DES have become the de facto standard of care for PCI in many parts of the world. The recognition of a small but important late risk attached to these devices has stimulated a re-evaluation of the incremental benefits of the technology. Meta-analyses have repeatedly shown that DES, compared with bare metal stents, have no effect on death or nonfatal MI.[43] The only end point consistently modified by DES is the need for repeat target lesion revascularization. Further, data from Emory showed that the occurrence of restenosis had no discernible effect on late survival.[44]

Several of the earlier DES trials have published an economic analysis. Van Hout and colleagues studied the economics of the RAVEL trial.[45] RAVEL compared a sirolimus-eluting stent (SES) with a bare metal stent for single de novo coronary lesions in 238 symptomatic patients in Europe and Latin America. At 6 months, restenosis was 0% in the SES arm and 26% in the bare stent arm. The SES arm also had a substantially lower rate of major adverse clinical events. In the economic analysis, although the additional initial procedural cost of the SES was €1286, this difference had been reduced to €54 at 1 year owing to the reduced need for repeat revascularization.

In the Sirolimus-Eluting Balloon Expandable Stent in the Treatment of Patients With De Novo Native Coronary Artery Lesions (SIRIUS) trial, 1058 patients with complex coronary stenosis were randomized to receive either an SES or a bare metal stent. Cohen and colleagues performed a prospective economic analysis of this trial.[46] They found initial hospital costs to be $2881 per patient higher in the SES arm, but this additional cost had attenuated to $309 at 1 year as costs in the SES arm were reduced because of significant reductions in repeat revascularization rates. The incremental cost-effectiveness ratio for SES versus bare metal stent was $1650 per repeat revascularization avoided. One important caveat about these results is that they were substantively influenced by the protocol 8-month repeat coronary angiography, which led to a doubling in the rate of late repeat revascularization procedures in the bare metal stent arm and a consequent narrowing in the cost difference between the two arms. If the extra procedures induced by the protocol angiograms are deleted from the calculations, the net cost of the DES strategy in this trial was $1300.

The cost effectiveness of paclitaxel-eluting stents (PES) was prospectively examined by Bakhai and colleagues in the TAXUS-IV trial.[47] In this study, 1314 patients undergoing PCI were randomly assigned to either PES or a bare metal stent, with follow-up out to 1 year. The PES arm index hospitalization costs were $2028 per patient higher when compared with the BMS arm. Cost savings of $1456 per patient in the PES arm were realized at 1-year follow-up, primarily owing to reductions in repeat revascularization procedures. The incremental cost effectiveness of PES was $4678 per target vessel revascularization avoided and $47,798 per QALY gained.

In the randomized Basel Stent Kasten Effekivitäts Trial (BASKET), 826 consecutive, unselected patients were treated with a DES (both SES and PES were used) or a bare metal stent.[48] After 6 months of follow-up, total costs in the DES arm were €10,544, compared with €9639 in the bare metal stent arm ($P<.00001$). The incremental cost-effectiveness ratio to avoid one major event (cardiac death, MI, or target vessel revascularization) was €18,311.

Reperfusion and Revascularization of Acute Coronary Disease

Thrombolytic Therapy

In the United States, more than 200,000 patients each year get acute reperfusion therapy for ST-elevation acute myocardial infarction (STEMI). The use of thrombolytic therapy has diminished in recent years in favor of primary PCI, and the use of streptokinase is particularly uncommon. In contrast, in the remainder of the world, streptokinase continues to be the most commonly used thrombolytic. With regard to the cost of thrombolytic therapy relative to conventional therapy, the major variable costs are those of the drug itself, the pharmacy costs to ready the drug for administration, and the labor costs of administra-

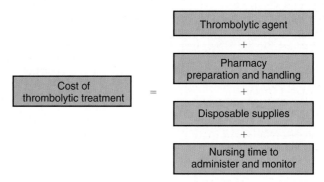

Figure 65-3. Cost components of thrombolytic therapy.

tion and monitoring (Fig. 65-3). The drug costs of thrombolytic therapy are now well known: the average wholesale price for 1.5 million U of streptokinase is about $590, for 100 mg of tissue plasminogen activator (t-PA) it is about $2800, and the same price applied to both 30 mg of recombinant tissue plasminogen activator (rt-PA) and 50 mg of tenecteplase (TNK).[49]

From a research point of view, the most controversial aspect of the cost of thrombolytic therapy pertains to the induced costs and savings: the cost of those aspects of medical care that are added or averted specifically because the patient received thrombolytic therapy. No prospective empirical comparison of thrombolytic therapy versus no reperfusion therapy in the United States has been published. Therefore, although it is possible that the use of streptokinase induces cost savings relative to no reperfusion therapy by reducing postinfarction complications, no empirical data are available to support this hypothesis. In fact, Naylor and Jaglal found in pooled analysis of several small, blinded trials that use of thrombolytic therapy was associated with higher revascularization rates.[50] In the absence of adequate empirical data on this question, most economic analysts have chosen to assume that thrombolytic therapy does not influence medical resource use, either in the short term (e.g., length of stay for the acute MI) or in the long term (e.g., rehospitalization). Naylor and colleagues calculated a cost-effectiveness ratio for streptokinase of $2000 to $4000 per life-year added relative to no reperfusion therapy, under the assumptions that each additional survivor produced by streptokinase would live an average of 10 years.[51] In summary, these analyses show that the use of streptokinase in lieu of a management strategy without reperfusion therapy is quite economically attractive and might be reasonably considered one of medicine's "best buys." Although the cost-effectiveness of treating anterior MIs is most favorable, treatment of inferior MIs and treatment in elderly patients is also economically attractive using conventional benchmarks.

In the Global Use of Strategies to Open Occluded Coronary Arteries (GUSTO) I trial, t-PA (alteplase) was shown to save one extra life per 100 patients with acute MI shifted from streptokinase and to produce a higher proportion of TIMI grade 3

Table 65-5. Cost-Effectiveness Ratios for t-PA Compared with Streptokinase in the Primary Analysis and Selected Subgroups of Patients in GUSTO I

| Patient Groups | Increased Life Expectancy with t-PA (Years of Life Saved) | | Cost Effectiveness Ratio (Dollars per LY Saved) |
	Undiscounted	Discounted	
Primary Analysis	0.14	0.09	32,678
Inferior MI ≤40 yr	0.03	0.01	203,071
Inferior MI 41-60 yr	0.07	0.04	74,816
Inferior MI 61-75 yr	0.16	0.10	27,873
Inferior MI >75 yr	0.26	0.17	16,246
Anterior MI ≤40 yr	0.04	0.02	123,609
Anterior MI 41-60 yr	0.10	0.06	49,877
Anterior MI 61-75 yr	0.20	0.14	20,601
Anterior MI >75 yr	0.29	0.21	13,410

GUSTO, Global Use of Strategies to Open Occluded Coronary Arteries trial; LY, life year; MI, myocardial infarction; t-PA, tissue plasminogen activator.
Data from Mark DB, Hlatky MA, Califf RM, et al. Cost effectiveness of thrombolytic therapy with tissue plasminogen activator as compared with streptokinase for acute myocardial infarction. N Engl J Med 1995;332:1418-1424.

coronary flow in the infarct vessel. In the prospective GUSTO I economic substudy, substitution of an accelerated t-PA regimen for intravenous streptokinase was economically attractive, with a cost-effectiveness ratio of $27,000 to $33,000, depending on the specific assumptions used in the calculations.[52] Subgroup analysis showed that t-PA was modestly more cost effective in anterior MIs but was considerably more effective in older patients (Table 65-5). These results were not substantially altered after taking into account the 1 per 1000 extra nonfatal disabling strokes produced by t-PA.

In an effort to improve the efficacy of pharmacologic reperfusion, two studies have examined regimens that combine lower-dose thrombolytic therapy with intravenous GP IIb/IIIa inhibitors and with low-molecular-weight heparin. GUSTO V compared half-dose rt-PA plus full-dose abciximab against full dose rt-PA in 16,588 patients.[53] There was no difference in 30-day mortality, but nonfatal MIs were reduced by the combination regimen, as was urgent revascularization.

The Assessment of the Safety and Efficacy of a New Treatment Strategy for Acute Myocardial Infarction 3 (ASSENT 3) trial randomized 6095 patients with acute MI to receive one of three regimens: TNK with unfractionated heparin, TNK with enoxaparin, or half-dose TNK with full-dose abciximab. Mortality at 30 days was 5.4% in the enoxaparin arm, 6.6% in the abciximab arm, and 6.0% in the unfractionated heparin arm (P=.25). Corresponding in-hospital reinfarction rates were 2.7%, 2.2%, and 4.2%, respectively (P=.0009). Both experimental arms also decreased in-hospital refractory ischemia (P<.0001) and increased major bleeding other than intracranial hemorrhage (P=.0005). Kaul and associates performed a prospective economic analysis of the ASSENT 3 study and found a trend toward lower costs in the TNK plus enoxaparin group at 30 days, but the difference was not significant.[54]

Another approach to improving the results of thrombolysis is to couple it with rescue PCI. In the recently published Rescue Angioplasty versus Conservative Treatment or Repeat Thrombolysis (REACT) trial, 427 patients with clinically failed thrombolysis were randomized to rescue PCI or conservative therapy.[55] The rescue PCI arm had significantly improved event-free survival but no difference in all-cause mortality. In a meta-analysis of five trials of rescue PCI, mortality risk was reduced but risk of heart failure and stroke were increased.[56] No modern comparison of the economic consequences of these strategies is available.

Primary Percutaneous Coronary Reperfusion

Between 1990 and 2002, a total of 25 randomized trials compared primary PCI with thrombolysis. Pooling of patient-level data from 22 of these trials revealed that primary PCI was associated with a 37% reduction in 30-day mortality rates.[57] This advantage was evident both in patients who presented early and in those who presented longer than 4 hours after symptom onset. Angiographic comparisons showed a higher early reperfusion rate and a higher proportion of patients achieving TIMI grade 3 flow. In addition, two early randomized trials suggested that direct PTCA might actually be a less expensive reperfusion strategy than t-PA.[58]

The contemporary economic consequences of primary PCI versus thrombolysis have not been studied. The Stenting versus Thrombolysis in Acute Myocardial Infarction (STAT) trial, a small Canadian study of 123 patients, reported initial hospital costs (in 1999 U.S. dollars) of $6354 for primary PCI and $7893 for t-PA (P<.01).[59] The cost of t-PA in Canada at the time of the trial was about $1800, whereas the cost of the PCI using bare metal stents was approximately $2100. The study is difficult to interpret, both because it was unblended and small and also because 64% of the patients in the t-PA arm had an unscheduled coronary angiogram during the index hospitalization. An economic analysis of the Comparison of Angioplasty and Pre-hospital Thrombolysis in Acute Myocardial Infarction (CAPTIM) trial found no dif-

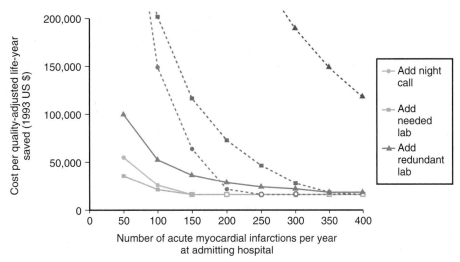

Figure 65-4. Cost per quality-adjusted life-year saved (1993 U.S. dollars) by employing a policy of direct angioplasty. Solid symbols indicate comparison with thrombolysis. Open symbols indicate comparison with no reperfusion therapy (angioplasty dominant over thrombolysis at those points). Solid lines give three hospital scenarios, with most favorable assumption of efficacy based on pre-GUSTO IIb randomized trials. Dashed lines give three hospital scenarios using effectiveness data from community-based observational studies. GUSTO IIb, Global Use of Strategies To Open Occluded Arteries in Acute Coronary Syndromes trial IIb. (From Lieu TA, Gurley J, Lundstrom RJ, et al: Projected cost-effectiveness of primary angioplasty for acute myocardial infarction. J Am Coll Cardiol 1997;30:1741-1750. Reprinted with permission from the American College of Cardiology.)

ference between the two reperfusion strategies in 1-year outcomes but costs were lower for primary PCI.[60] The thrombolysis strategy in this trial included the use of rescue PCI as needed. A model-based analysis of these two therapies using European costs concluded that primary PCI had both improved health benefits and lower long-term costs.[61] In contrast, a model-based analysis from the U.K. perspective found that primary PCI improved clinical outcomes at a modest increase in cost and was economically attractive in cost-effectiveness analysis.[62]

Lieu and colleagues demonstrated that the costs of a primary PTCA strategy vary importantly with the structural details of individual hospital programs.[63] Using a spreadsheet-based model and cost data obtained from a Kaiser Permanente Hospital, they showed that procedural costs varied from $1600 to $14,300, depending on extra costs for night call, annual procedural volume, and (particularly) the need to construct a new catheterization laboratory to handle the extra volume.

Using these data in a decision analytic model along with effectiveness data from published clinical trials and other studies, Lieu and colleagues examined the cost-effectiveness of primary angioplasty.[64] In the base case analysis, they considered the case of a hospital with an existing catheterization laboratory with night and weekend coverage that admitted 200 acute MI patients each year. Under these assumptions, direct PTCA was cost-saving compared with thrombolysis (either t-PA or streptokinase regimens) and had a cost of $12,000 per QALY relative to no reperfusion therapy. In sensitivity analyses, the need to build a new catheterization laboratory, the need to add the costs of night call, and a diminution of laboratory volume all significantly increased the cost-

effectiveness ratio (Fig. 65-4). This model demonstrates that the economic attractiveness of primary PTCA relative to thrombolysis depends not only on its incremental effectiveness in improving health outcomes but also on the availability of regional high-volume laboratories with experienced operators. Redundant low-volume laboratories led to worse outcomes and higher costs and made the procedure much less economically attractive.

More recent trials have examined the use of stenting versus balloon PCI for acute MI as well as the benefits of adjunctive therapies with balloon- or stent-based PCI. The Primary Angioplasty in Myocardial infarction stent trial (PAMI-STENT) randomized 900 acute MI patients who had a native infarct-related artery suitable for stenting to routine stenting or balloon PCI. Use of a GP IIb/IIIa inhibitor was low in both arms (5%). At 30 days, the stent arm had a trend toward increased mortality and decreased reinfarction. By 6 months, the stent arm had a 10 per 100 lower rate of target vessel repeat revascularization. In the economic analysis of this trial, the stent arm had a higher index hospitalization cost of about $2000 (due primarily to the cost of the stents used in PCI).[65] Over the 12-month follow-up, reduced need for repeat procedures saved about half that amount, leaving a net cost for the stent arm of $1000. The higher mortality trend for stenting makes estimation of cost-effectiveness problematic.

In order to improve the early patency associated with the primary PCI strategy, researchers have examined adjunctive use of both GP IIb/IIIa inhibitors and low-dose thrombolytics. Adding abciximab to primary stenting for acute MI improved early (pre-PCI) TIMI grade 3 flow and reduced target vessel repeat revascularization in Abciximab before Direct Angioplasty and Stenting in Myocardial Infarction Regarding Acute and Long-term Follow-up study (ADMIRAL), a 300-patient trial. These results, including no differences in mortality or reinfarction, persisted out to 3 years.[66]

In the larger Controlled Abciximab and Device Investigation to Lower Late Angioplasty Complications (CADILLAC) trial, abciximab plus stenting showed a trend toward lower mortality and a reduction in ischemia and ischemic-driven repeat revascularization. Bakhai and coworkers performed a prospective cost-utility analysis in this study, with follow-up out to 1 year.[67] Although initial procedural and hospitalization costs were higher in the stent arm compared with PTCA, at 1 year the total costs in both arms were similar, primarily owing to fewer repeat revascularizations in the stent arm. Stenting compared to PTCA produced a cost-effectiveness ratio of $11,237 per QALY gained in this acute MI cohort. Initial costs in the abciximab arm were comparable to those of the standard therapy arm, but abciximab had $1244 higher total costs at 1 year, and the cost-effectiveness of this therapy was uncertain.

Early Invasive Versus Early Conservative Strategies

In the United States, angiography is frequently performed after acute MI. In the GUSTO I trial, 71% of 21,772 U.S. STEMI patients had a diagnostic catheterization, whereas in the more recent GUSTO III trial, the rate was 78%.[68,69] In the non-STEMI portion of the ACS spectrum, the rate is even higher: In the Platelet Glycoprotein IIb/IIIa in Unstable Angina: Receptor Suppression Using Integrilin Therapy (PURSUIT) trial, 88% of such patients underwent catheterization in the United States during their initial hospitalization. In a managed care environment, rates are lower and surprisingly variable, ranging from 30% to 77% in one study.[70] A recent study from the Can Rapid risk stratification of Unstable angina patients Suppress ADverse outcomes with Early implementation of the ACC/AHA guidelines (CRUSADE) registry found that only 45% of high risk non-STEMI ACS patients received the early invasive strategy.[71] The decision to refer for diagnostic catheterization in acute coronary disease is at best modestly influenced by clinical factors but is substantially influenced by structural aspects of the practice environment, such as the availability of catheterization facilities at the admitting hospital, being admitted by a cardiologist rather than a generalist, and having an attending cardiologist who performs invasive procedures.

A systematic review of invasive versus noninvasive management of uncomplicated STEMI identified six clinical trials published between 1988 and 2002.[72] In aggregate, these trials did not demonstrate a prognostic benefit for the early invasive strategy. In addition, most of the trials reflected management that is no longer current. Observational studies of the same issue suggest that the early invasive approach may improve quality-of-life end points, particularly functional status. The durability of that effect is uncertain.

Kuntz and colleagues used a decision model to compare routine coronary angiography in the convalescent phase of acute MI hospitalization with medical therapy and exercise testing.[73] Because of the lack of clinical trial data in acute coronary disease, the estimates needed for this analysis were collected from trials in chronic coronary disease and from a variety of literature and expert opinion sources. Long-term survival was projected using the Coronary Heart Disease Policy Model of Weinstein and colleagues. Cost data (given in 1994 U.S. dollars) were obtained from Medicare data. In this model-based analysis, routine coronary angiography increased quality-adjusted life expectancy (through its effect on subsequent revascularization) in almost all MI subgroups examined. Only women aged 35 to 44 years with normal ejection fractions, no post-MI angina, and a negative treadmill test appeared not to benefit. When costs were factored into the model, however, the cost to produce an extra unit of benefit varied substantially among subgroups. The most economically attractive cost-effectiveness ratios were obtained in patients with a history of a prior MI (presumably a surrogate marker for greater cumulative left ventricular dysfunction) and in those with inducible myocardial ischemia (Fig. 65-5). Cost-effectiveness ratios with both of these factors ranged between $44,000 and $17,000 per QALY added.[73] Conversely, most patients with negative exercise tests had ratios exceeding $50,000 per added QALY.

Several major randomized trials have compared early invasive with early conservative management strategies for ACS. The Treat Angina with Aggrastat and Determine Cost of Therapy with an Invasive or Conservative Strategy (TACTICS-TIMI 18) trial reflects contemporary management, with coronary stents used in more than 80% of patients undergoing PCI and all patients receiving an intravenous GP IIb/IIIa inhibitor (tirofiban).[74] Diagnostic catheterization was performed in 51% of patients receiving early conservative management and 97% of those receiving early invasive management. At 6 months, the early invasive arm had 2 per 1000 fewer deaths and 20 per 1000 fewer MIs. Economic analysis of this trial found that the early invasive arm had higher initial costs ($15,714 versus $14,047) and lower follow-up costs out to 6 months ($6098 versus $7180).[75] Cumulative 6-month costs were very similar. Cost per life year added was estimated at $13,000.

Fragmin and Revascularization during Instability in Coronary Artery Disease II (FRISC II) compared an invasive strategy (diagnostic catheterization rate, 96%) with a noninvasive strategy (diagnostic catheterization rate, 10%) in 2457 patients with ACS. At 1 year, the invasively treated group had a mortality rate of 2.2%, compared with 3.9% in the noninvasive strategy group (P=.016); the corresponding rates for MI were 8.6% and 11.6%, respectively (P=.015).[76]

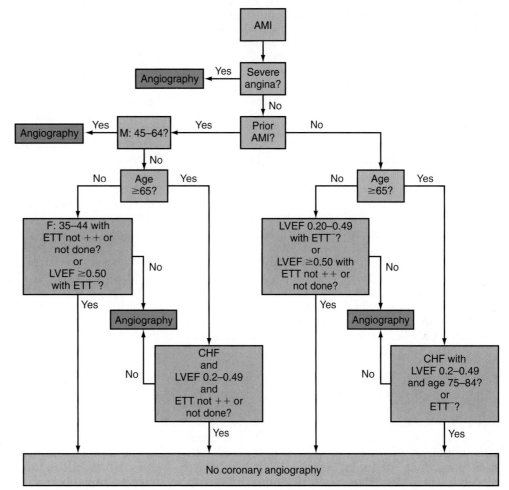

Figure 65-5. Cost-effective use of diagnostic coronary angiography after acute myocardial infarction (AMI). Angio, angiography; CHF, congestive heart failure; ETT, exercise treadmill test; F, female; LVEF, left ventricular ejection fraction; M, male. (From Kuntz KM, Tsevat J, Goldman L, Weinstein MC: Cost-effectiveness of routine coronary angiography after acute myocardial infarction. Circulation 1996;94:957-965.)

The invasive strategy was also associated with a reduction in readmissions (37% versus 57%; $P<.001$) and (repeat) revascularization (7.5% versus 31%; $P<.001$). An economic analysis of FRISC II from the Swedish perspective has been published. At the end of 1 year, cumulative costs in the invasive arm were SEK 201,622 (US $20,072) versus SEK 177,746 (US $16,939) for the noninvasive arm, leaving the invasive arm with a $3133 cost at the end of 1 year. Five-year follow-up from this trial has recently been published.[77] Mortality was 9.7% in the invasive group and 10.1% in the noninvasive group ($P=.69$). Nonfatal MI rates were 12.9% in the invasive group and 17.7% in the noninvasive group ($P=.002$).

In contrast with TACTICS-TIMI 18 and FRISC II, the Invasive versus Conservative Treatment in Unstable Coronary Syndromes (ICTUS) trial of 1200 ACS patients with an elevated troponins failed to find any benefit in hard cardiac events for the early invasive strategy.[78] A meta-analysis of seven trials involving 8,375 patients and a mean follow-up of 2 years reported a 25% reduction in all-cause mortality and a 17% reduction in nonfatal MI for early invasive management.[79] However, these results did not take account of the heterogeneous varieties of "early invasive" management represented in the seven trials, with hospital angiography rates ranging from 10% to more than 50%. The more aggressive the "early conservative" arm, the more difficult it is to demonstrate any incremental benefit to routine early angiography. The most optimistic estimates of benefit for the early invasive strategy were seen in the smallest trial and in the trial with the most conservative version of the early conservative management strategy.

Antiplatelet Therapy

One of the most important advances in interventional cardiology has been the development of platelet GP IIb/IIIa receptor blockers. These drugs have been studied in three types of populations: acute MI, as an adjunct to thrombolytic therapy; non-STEMI ACS; and PCI. The GUSTO V and ASSENT 3 trials, which combined abciximab with thrombolytic therapy, were discussed earlier in this chapter.

Use of intravenous GP IIb/IIIa blockers in ACS has now been extensively studied. Among the largest trials, two, Platelet Receptor Inhibition for Ischemic Syndrome Management (PRISM) and Platelet Receptor Inhibition for Ischemic Syndrome Management in Patients Limited by Unstable Signs and Symptoms (PRISM-PLUS), studied tirofiban, while PURSUIT used eptifibatide and GUSTO IV tested abciximab. Of these, only PURSUIT has published an economic analysis.[80] In the 3522 U.S. patients enrolled in the trial there was no evidence that eptifibatide use altered resource use or costs through either a positive or a negative effect on clinical course. The absence of an effect on resource use despite reduced ischemic complications may be related to the very high (85%) rate of routine diagnostic catheterization in the U.S. cohort. The cost of the eptifibatide regimen was $1014, and the 3.5% absolute reduction in death or MI at 30 days in the U.S. cohort translated into an incremental life expectancy of 0.11 life years per patient added by eptifibatide. The resulting cost-effectiveness ratio was $13,700 per added life year.

In PCI populations, five trials with prospective economic analysis have been concluded, three with abciximab and one each with tirofiban and eptifibatide. In the Evaluation of 7E3 for the Prevention of Ischemic Complications (EPIC) trial, abciximab reduced 30-day ischemic endpoints after high-risk coronary angioplasty by 35% but increased in-hospital bleeding. Six-month ischemic episodes were reduced by 23%. A prospective economic substudy was conducted as part of the EPIC research effort.[81] During the initial hospitalization, reduced ischemic events generated a potential cost savings of $622 per patient, but this was canceled out by an equivalent ($521) rise in costs due to care required for major bleeding episodes. Baseline medical costs (hospital plus physician) averaged $14,984 for the abciximab arm (which included $1407 for the bolus and infusion abciximab regimen) versus $13,434 for the placebo arm. During the 6-month study follow-up, the abciximab arm had a 23% decrease in rehospitalizations and a 22% decrease in repeat revascularizations, generating a mean cost savings of $1207 per patient (P=.02). Combining baseline and follow-up costs for each treatment arm yielded a net incremental 6-month cost for the abciximab strategy of $293 per patient.

The Evaluation in Percutaneous Transluminal Coronary Angioplasty to Improve Long-Term Outcome with Abciximab GP IIb/IIIa Blockade (EPILOG) trial was conducted to validate and extend the findings of EPIC in a broader PTCA population. It also examined the benefits of using a weight-adjusted low-dose heparin regimen to reduce the early bleeding complications seen in EPIC. In 2792 patients, EPILOG demonstrated a 58% reduction in ischemic complications (death, MI, urgent revascularization) in the abciximab arm by 30 days, with elimination of excess major bleeding episodes by the modified heparin dosing regimen. Prospective cost analysis showed total baseline medical costs for the abciximab arm of $10,125 (including a $1457 cost for the abciximab regimen), compared with $9632 for placebo, resulting in a $583 excess cost for the abciximab strategy.[82] EPILOG confirmed the prediction by EPIC that a reduction in ischemic complications without an excess of major bleeds would produce a cost offset of about $600 (EPIC estimate, $622; EPILOG cost saving, $583).

Follow-up data from EPILOG did not show the reduction in subsequent hospitalizations and procedures that had been observed in EPIC: Costs for the abciximab low-dose heparin arm to 6 months were $4221, compared with $3568 for placebo (P=.43). Cumulative 6-month incremental costs for the abciximab arm were $1236.

The EPISTENT trial extended the EPILOG results to the use of stenting. Patients were randomized to stenting with abciximab, stenting with placebo, or balloon angioplasty with abciximab. Prospective economic analysis in the 1438 U.S. patients showed that costs for the baseline hospitalization differed only in the costs of the stents and abciximab used: $13,228 for stent plus abciximab, $11,923 for stent plus placebo, and $11,357 for balloon plus abciximab.[8] Thus, stent plus abciximab therapy was $1300 more expensive than stent plus placebo and almost $1900 more expensive than balloon plus abciximab arm.

In follow-up, the two stent groups had similar costs, whereas the balloon plus abciximab group exceeded these groups by more than $900. Therefore, at 1 year, the stent plus abciximab arm was $930 more expensive than balloon plus abciximab. At 1 year, 1.0% of the stent plus abciximab group had died, compared with 2.4% of the stent plus placebo patients and 2.1% of balloon plus abciximab patients. Incremental life expectancy was projected from these data and used to calculate cost-effectiveness ratios. For stent plus abciximab relative to stent plus placebo, the cost to add a life year was $6200; relative to balloon plus abciximab, the cost to add a life year was $5300.

The Randomized Efficacy Study of Tirofiban for Outcomes and Restenosis (RESTORE) trial randomized 2212 patients with an ACS referred for PCI to tirofiban or placebo.[83] At 30 days, the primary end point (death, MI, urgent revascularization) was reduced 16% by tirofiban (P=.16). The treatment effect was greatest within the first 48 hours and appeared to attenuate somewhat thereafter. There was no excess of major bleeding seen with tirofiban. Economic analysis of 820 patients at 30 U.S. sites showed a hospital cost of $12,145 for placebo versus $12,230 for tirofiban.[83] The cost of the tirofiban regimen itself was estimated at $700, which was largely offset by a reduced need for repeat PTCA or for CABG.

The ESPRIT trial (1999-2000) randomized 2064 patients undergoing PCI with stenting to either eptifibatide or placebo. The eptifibatide arm had reduced ischemic complications. The cost of the eptifibatide regimen was $495. Total hospital costs (including eptifibatide) were $10,721 for the eptifibatide arm versus $10,430 for placebo, an incremental cost of $291 per patient.[9] Follow-up costs out to 1 year were $2121 for eptifibatide versus $2254 for placebo. Therefore, the net 1-year costs of the eptifibatide strategy were $146. At 1 year, eptifibatide was associated with 6 per 1000 fewer deaths (P=.28) and 35 per 1000 fewer MIs (P=.004). This translated into

0.104 added life years per patient (discounted at 3%) and a cost-effectiveness ratio of $1407 per added life year.

Several studies have examined the economics of clopidogrel use after PCI. In the PCI-CURE substudy of the Clopidogrel in Unstable angina to Prevent Recurrent Events (CURE) trial (1998-2000), 2658 patients were randomized to clopidogrel or placebo after PCI. Clopidogrel reduced the rate of cardiovascular death or MI by 25% but had no effect on cardiovascular death alone. The cost per day of the clopidogrel therapy was $3.22, which was largely offset by reductions in complications, so that, at the end of 1 year, the net cost of the clopidogrel strategy was between $250 and $425.[84] Incremental cost effectiveness was less than $5000 per life year gained, making clopidogrel use in this setting highly economically attractive. Two decision-model-based analyses of the use of clopidogrel for 1 year after PCI came to similar conclusions with a cost of US $15,696 per life year saved in the United States and €10,993 in Sweden.[85,86]

Antithrombin Therapy

Based on several small trials showing a reduction in death and nonfatal MI, heparin has been standard therapy for moderate- or high-risk patients with unstable angina. Several studies have been conducted with low-molecular-weight heparins in patients with ACS. Enoxaparin was the first low-molecular-weight heparin to be tested in a clinical trial that incorporated a prospective economic analysis. The Efficacy and Safety of Subcutaneous Enoxaparin in Non-Q Wave Coronary Events (ESSENCE) trial randomized 3171 patients with non-STEMI ACS in North and South America and Europe. At the end of 14 days, the enoxaparin therapy had resulted in a significant 15% lower rate of death, MI, or refractory angina (the primary end point) relative to standard unfractionated heparin therapy. Economic analysis of this trial, performed in the 923 patients randomized in the United States, showed that the enoxaparin regimen cost $75 more than standard heparin therapy. At the end of the initial hospitalization, the enoxaparin arm had not only recouped this cost difference but had also produced a cost savings of more than $700 owing to reduced invasive cardiac procedures and a small concurrent reduction in length of stay. At 30 days, the cost advantage for the enoxaparin arm had risen to $1100.

The Superior Yield of the New Strategy of Enoxaparin Revascularization and Glycoprotein IIb/IIIa Inhibitors (SYNERGY) trial compared subcutaneous enoxaparin versus intravenous heparin in 10,027 patients with non-STEMI ACS (2001-2003).[87] No difference was observed in the primary end point of death or nonfatal MI. In addition, enoxaparin was associated with a moderate increase in major bleeding. Compared with earlier trials making this same comparison, the SYNERGY patients were older and both the medical and interventional therapies were more aggressive. Whether these differences explain the lack of superiority for enoxaparin in SYNERGY remains unclear.

The FRISC II investigators prospectively examined the cost-effectiveness of extended treatment with dalteparin in 2267 patients with unstable coronary artery disease.[88] After a minimum of 5 days' open label dalteparin treatment, patients were randomized to 3 months of subcutaneous dalteparin twice daily or placebo. The dalteparin arm produced a significant reduction in death or MI at 1 month, at an additional cost of SEK 849. The cost-effectiveness ratio was SEK 30,300 per death or MI avoided. Despite these early gains, no significant difference was detected in death or MI between the two arms at 3 months.

Several newer and more potent antithrombin agents have been tested in clinical trials. At present, bivalirudin appears the most promising. Bivalirudin plus provisional GP IIb/IIIa inhibition was found to provide similar cardiac event rates out to 1 year while reducing the risk of severe bleeding events when compared with routine GP IIb/IIIa inhibition plus heparin in the Randomized Evaluation in PCI Linking Angiomax to Reduced Clinical Events (REPLACE)-2 trial, a randomized, double-blind trial of 4651 U.S. patients undergoing nonemergent PCI.[89] Cohen and colleagues conducted a prospective economic evaluation of this study and found that bivalirudin produced a cost savings of $375 to $400 per patient at 30 days, primarily because of the reduction in bleeding episodes.[90]

Preventive Therapies

A number of secondary prevention programs have been shown to be effective in large-scale clinical trials and have also been shown to be economically attractive. These include statin therapy for hypercholesterolemia, smoking cessation interventions, aspirin therapy, β-blockers for post-MI patients, and angiotensin-converting enzyme inhibitors for post-MI survivors with depressed left ventricular function. These data have been reviewed.[2]

COST EFFECTIVENESS AND HEALTH POLICY

From 1994 to 1999, managed care had an almost unprecedented inhibitory effect on the growth of health care spending in the United States. During this period, the proportion of the Gross Domestic Product (GDP) devoted to health care remained stable at 13% to 13.3%. The era of managed care as a restraining influence on health care spending now appears finished. Growth in annual medical spending has gone back up, and current estimates are that the United States is devoting 16% of its GDP to health care. As of 2007, no significant federal efforts to control health care spending have been proposed. Nonetheless, experience from the last 40 years suggests that employers (who pay for much of the health insurance in the United States) and the federal government (who pays for the rest through the Medicare and Medicaid programs) will not tolerate unchecked growth in medical spending.

Any future health care reform that succeeds in restraining total annual U.S. medical care spending (public and private) will indirectly force patients to compete for health care resources and will directly force providers and policy makers to make more explicit decisions about which types of care are worthwhile. For example, should all PCI patients receive the next generation of more expensive DES? What about uncomplicated inferior MIs? Should patients older than 80 years of age be offered revascularization procedures or receive medical therapy only? As described in this chapter, defining the cost of medical care is an important first step. But when the overall goal is to decide which types of care to provide from among the available alternatives, cost must be explicitly tied to the health benefits produced, and the benefits must be valued in some uniform, comparable currency.

A host of controversial and complex allocation decisions will be required if providers can no longer count on payers to cover all the care they believe is appropriate for their patients. In the view of some, cost-effectiveness analysis provides the soundest and most logical method for making decisions about health care allocation. Canada, the United Kingdom, and other countries that seek to maximize health benefits within a fixed budget are actively debating the use of cost-effectiveness as a decision aid. The Oregon Medicaid reform plan attempted to make cost-effectiveness the primary criterion for determining what to cover in the program. One important lesson from the Oregon experience is that current methodology and data are insufficient to permit a comprehensive cost-effectiveness ranking of all health care services.

The insufficient database on cost-effectiveness is not a critical limitation; if desired, an aggressive empirical research program could rapidly improve the available information base. In addition, policy decisions would not depend on an encyclopedia covering all possible health care expenditures, as was attempted in Oregon. Some therapies would clearly be cost-effective (e.g., aspirin for acute MI), whereas others would clearly not be (e.g., a treatment that is both less effective and more costly than "usual care").

More serious challenges to the use of cost-effectiveness analysis as the primary tool for health care spending decisions come from methodologic considerations. Principal among these is the absence of any uniform method for measuring either health care benefits or costs for use in cost-effectiveness analysis. On the effectiveness side, several major problems face the analyst. Chief among these is the difficulty in accurately estimating the change in life expectancy attributable to a new therapeutic strategy. Unless the disease process under study is rapidly fatal, it is virtually impossible to obtain timely empirical life-expectancy data for use in cost-effectiveness calculations. Most commonly, analysts use survival or mortality rate measures at selected times, such as 30 days, 1 year, or 5 years, and attempt to project life expectancy from these figures with the aid of simple parametric survival modes. Examples include the Markov model and the declining exponential approximation of life expectancy (DEALE). Other, more empirical approaches have recently been developed.[80,91]

Problems also arise in interpreting statistical survival estimates in life-expectancy terms. For example, consider a therapy that lowers 30-day mortality rates for acute MI patients by 1%, with no additional therapeutic effect (i.e., survival curves are parallel after 30 days). Many would conclude that the therapy saves an average of 1 life per 100 treated. However, the "saved patient" is a statistical patient and cannot be clinically identified. Furthermore, it is uncertain whether only one patient benefits from therapy (by having his or her life prolonged) and 99 receive no benefits or whether some or all treated patients receive benefits, the average effect of which is to decrease the mortality rate by 1%. The distinction is relevant because life-expectancy projections must assume either that one patient is being saved and has some estimated number of life-years remaining or that all patients are being benefited somewhat and the additional life expectancy should be estimated for the group. Because there is no current way of validating such projections and no gold standard to aid in choosing from among competing methods for making them, different analysts may come to substantially different conclusions about the effects on life expectancy of a given therapy.

Substantial additional difficulties arise if the analyst wishes to move from survival (cost-effectiveness analysis) to quality-adjusted survival (cost-utility analysis). No standard approach has been agreed on for quality adjustment of life expectancy figures, although QALYs have been used most often. One of the major assumptions of the QALY construct is that, for a given person, it is possible to identify some point of indifference between living x years with some disease state or health impairment and living y years (where $y < x$) in full health. Another assumption is that improving the quality of life for one type of patient may provide more societal "value" than saving the life of another type of patient. Three main approaches have been used to derive the quality weights or utilities employed in calculating QALYs: the standard reference gamble, the time trade-off technique, and category rating scales. In each case, the resulting measure is presumed to reflect patient preferences in a way that would allow prediction of their future economic behavior (specifically, their purchase of future health care).

The advantage of the QALY for economic analysis is that it permits reduction of all survival, quality-of-life, and patient preference issues to a single measure. Whether such a reduction is valid or even appropriate continues to be vigorously debated among health policy investigators. Critics of the QALY construct have pointed out that some of its major assumptions are probably invalid. For example, none of the current estimation methods take into account that good health is likely to be more highly valued at some stages in life (e.g., childrearing years) than at others. In addition, calculation of QALYs requires the assumption that patient preferences for different health states do not depend on the length of time spent in those states. Important technical issues relating to QALYs remain unsettled. For example, should ratings of disease states be obtained from patients who actually have the disease, from members of the general public asked to imagine that they have the disease, or from members of the medical profession familiar with the disease and its manifestations? Some data suggest that patient preferences (and consequently QALYs) may not be stable over time and that they are strongly influenced by the context of the assessment in which they are measured. Some have argued that QALYs and other utility scales are uniquely personal and cannot be averaged across a population, as is required in cost-effectiveness analysis. Furthermore, use of average utilities in cost-effectiveness analyses maximizes community preferences over those of the individual and raises important ethical questions. As might be expected, recent research has shown that different approaches to calculating quality-adjusted survival may yield significant differences in resulting cost-effectiveness ratios.

Finally, cost-effectiveness studies may differ substantially in the methodology used to estimate costs. Some use carefully measured data obtained from randomized trials or observational studies, whereas others use expert opinion. As discussed earlier in the chapter, actually two factors must be estimated: what resources were consumed in what quantities and the associated unit costs. Often, none of the cost data

used in cost-effectiveness models is derived from empirical research. In addition, substantial assumptions are required to project the lifetime health care costs of a cohort of patients. Although the importance of such assumptions can be examined through sensitivity analyses, as with life expectancy estimates, these data are rarely tested against empirical observations.

Thus, cost-effectiveness ratios are calculated by multiplying two imprecise measures—life expectancy gained and utilities of those years—and dividing the result by a third imprecise measure, the lifetime incremental costs. The resulting measure is necessarily imprecise. Despite these substantial limitations, which can severely limit the validity of comparing cost-effectiveness ratios from different studies, "league tables" providing such comparisons are common (Table 65-6). These figures, which are usually presented without any variability or distributional information, appear misleadingly precise and rigorous.

Several groups have proposed standards for cost-effectiveness analysis, thereby addressing some of the potential weaknesses described earlier. The Panel on Cost Effectiveness in Health and Medicine convened by the U.S. Public Health Service, in particular, has generated a carefully researched monograph that should help to advance work in this area.[92] A number of commentators have noted that if cost-effectiveness assessment were an expensive new technology (which, in a sense, it is), health policy analysts would demand rigorous evaluations before it was unleashed on the public. Cost-effectiveness analysis is extremely useful when it focuses and informs professional and public debate, and much additional research is needed in this area. To use it as the *primary* method of medical resource allocation, however, implies that it possesses

Table 65-6. Cost-Effectiveness and Use of Selected Interventions in the Medicare Population*

Intervention	Cost-Effectiveness (Cost/QALY)[†]
Influenza vaccine	Cost saving
Pneumococcal vaccine	Cost saving
β-Blockers after myocardial infarction	<$10,000
Mammographic screening	$10,000-$25,000
Colon-cancer screening	$10,000-$25,000
Osteoporosis screening	$10,000-$25,000
Management of antidepressant medications	Cost saving up to $30,000
Hypertension medication (DBP>105 mm Hg)	$10,000-$60,000
Cholesterol management, as secondary prevention	$10,000-$50,000
Implantable cardioverter-defibrillator	$30,000-$85,000
Dialysis in end-stage renal disease	$50,000-$100,000
Lung-volume-reduction surgery	$100,000-$300,000
Left ventricular assist devices	$500,000-$1.4 million
Positron emission tomography in Alzheimer's disease	Dominated[‡]

*Ranges are provided, rather than point estimates, because the actual cost effectiveness will vary according to the target populations and the strategies used.
[†]Calculation based on 2002 U.S. dollars.
[‡]Benefits are lower and costs are higher than with the use of the standard workup.
DBP, diastolic blood pressure; QALY, quality-adjusted life year.
Modified from Sanders GD, Hlatky MA, Owens DK. Cost-effectiveness of implantable cardioverter-defibrillators. N Engl J Med 2005;353:1471-1480, with permission.

a rigor it currently lacks and shifts the locus of decision-making to a bureaucracy without appropriate policy guidance from the political and moral arenas.

SUMMARY

The question of how much of societal resources to devote to health care is not one that can be settled by economic analysis. Rather, it is a political and ethical question that reflects, at least in part, the type of society we are (or purport to be) and our willingness to accept the necessity of trade-offs in a world of finite resources. In this context, the role of medical economic analysis is to define the relationship between dollars expended and benefits gained. Although the primary goal of economic analysis is theoretically to maximize efficient use of available health care resources, many pitfalls, both technical and ethical, separate theory from practice. Uncritical acceptance by medical professionals of the results of economic analyses does not serve the interests of patients any more than does uncritical acceptance of the dictates of any one clinical randomized trial. On the other hand, uninformed skepticism applied uniformly to all economic analyses serves no useful purpose. Much remains to be done to improve the empirical base and methodology of health care economic research. For this to happen, cost outcomes (with all their shortcomings) must become as much a routine part of clinical research as mortality and morbidity outcomes are now.

REFERENCES

1. Thom T, Haase N, Rosamond W, et al: Heart disease and stroke statistics—2006 update: A report from the American Heart Association Statistics Committee and Stroke Statistics Subcommittee. Circulation 2006;113:e85-e151.
2. Mark DB: Medical economics in cardiovascular medicine. In Topol EJ (ed): Textbook of Cardiovascular Medicine. Philadelphia, Lippincott Williams & Wilkins, 2006, pp 736-756.
3. Hsiao WC, Braun P, Dunn D, et al: Results and policy implications of the resource-based relative-value study. N Engl J Med 1988;319:881-888.
4. Feit F, Mueller HS, Braunwald E, et al; The TIMI Research Group: Thrombolysis in Myocardial Infarction (TIMI) Phase II trial: Outcome comparison of a "conservative strategy" in community versus tertiary hospitals. J Am Coll Cardiol 1990;16:1529-1534.
5. Kugelmass AD, Cohen DJ, Brown PP, et al: Hospital resources consumed in treating complications associated with percutaneous coronary interventions. Am J Cardiol 2006;97: 322-327.
6. Ellis SG, Miller DP, Brown KJ, et al: In-hospital costs of percutaneous coronary revascularization: Critical determinants and implications. Circulation 1995;92:741-747.
7. Heidenreich PA, Chou TM, Amidon TM, et al: Impact of the operating physician on costs of percutaneous transluminal coronary angioplasty. Am J Cardiol 1996;77:1169-1173.
8. Topol EJ, Mark DB, Lincoff AM, et al; for the EPISTENT Investigators: Outcomes at 1 year and economic implications of platelet glycoprotein IIb/IIIa blockade in patients undergoing coronary stenting: results from a multicentre randomised trial. Lancet 1999;354:2019-2024.
9. Cohen DJ, O'Shea JC, Pacchiana CM, e al: In-hospital costs of coronary stent implantation with and without eptifibatide

10. (the ESPRIT Trial). Enhanced Suppression of the Platelet IIb/IIIa Receptor with Integrilin. Am J Cardiol 2002;89:61-64.
10. Topol EJ, Ellis SG, Cosgrove DM, et al: Analysis of coronary angioplasty practice in the United States with an insurance-claims data base. Circulation 1993;87:1489-1497.
11. Shook TL, Sun GW, Burstein S, et al: Comparison of percutaneous transluminal coronary angioplasty outcome and hospital costs for low-volume and high-volume operators. Am J Cardiol 1996;77:331-336.
12. Chen JC, Kaul P, Levy JH, et al; PRIMO-CABG Investigators: Myocardial infarction following coronary artery bypass graft surgery increases healthcare resource utilization. Crit Care Med 2007;35:1296-1301.
13. Eisenberg MJ, Filion KB, Azoulay A, et al: Outcomes and cost of coronary artery bypass graft surgery in the United States and Canada. Arch Intern Med 2005;165:1506-1513.
14. Cowper PA, DeLong ER, Peterson ED, et al: Variability in cost of coronary bypass surgery in New York State: Potential for cost savings. Am Heart J 2002;143:130-139.
15. Mauldin PD, Becker ER, Phillips VL, Weintraub WS: Hospital resource utilization during coronary artery bypass surgery. J Interventional Cardiol 1994;7:379-384.
16. Hlatky MA, Rogers WJ, Johnstone I, et al: Medical care costs and quality of life after randomization to coronary angioplasty or coronary bypass surgery. Bypass Angioplasty Revascularization Investigation (BARI) Investigators. N Engl J Med 1997;336:92-99.
17. Hall RE, Ash AS, Ghali WA, Moskowitz MA: Hospital cost of complications associated with coronary artery bypass graft surgery. Am J Cardiol 1997;79:1680-1682.
18. Smith LR, Milano CA, Molter BS, et al: Preoperative determinants of postoperative costs associated with coronary artery bypass graft surgery. Circulation 1994;90:II-124-II-128.
19. Doty JR, Fonger JD, Nicholson CF, et al: Cost analysis of current therapies for limited coronary artery revascularization. Circulation 1997;69:II-16-II-21.
20. Arom KV, Emery RW, Flavin TF, Petersen RJ: Cost-effectiveness of minimally invasive coronary artery bypass surgery. Ann Thorac Surg 1999;68:1562-1566.
21. Puskas JD, Williams WH, Mahoney EM, et al: Off-pump vs conventional coronary artery bypass grafting: Early and 1-year graft patency, cost, and quality-of-life outcomes. A randomized trial. JAMA 2004;291:1841-1849.
22. Lamy A, Wang X, Farrokhyar F, Kent R: A cost comparison of off-pump CABG versus on-pump CABG at one-year: The Canadian off-pump CABG registry. Can J Cardiol 2006;22: 699-704.
23. Katritsis DG, Ioannidis JP: Percutaneous coronary intervention versus conservative therapy in nonacute coronary artery disease: A meta-analysis. Circulation 2005;111:2906-2912.
24. Claude J, Schindler C, Kuster GM, et al: Cost-effectiveness of invasive versus medical management of elderly patients with chronic symptomatic coronary artery disease: Findings of the randomized trial of invasive versus medical therapy in elderly patients with chronic angina (TIME). Eur Heart J 2004;25: 2195-2203.
25. Sculpher M, Smith D, Clayton T, et al: Coronary angioplasty versus medical therapy for angina: Health service costs based on the second Randomized Intervention Treatment of Angina (RITA-2) trial. Eur Heart J 2002;23:1291-1300.
26. Shaw LJ, Merz CN, Pepine CJ, et al: The economic burden of angina in women with suspected ischemic heart disease: Results from the National Institutes of Health–National Heart, Lung, and Blood Institute–sponsored Women's Ischemia Syndrome Evaluation. Circulation 2006;114:894-904.
27. Boden WE, O'Rourke RA, Teo KK, et al: Design and rationale of the Clinical Outcomes Utilizing Revascularization and Aggressive DruG Evaluation (COURAGE) trial. Veterans Affairs Cooperative Studies Program no. 424. Am Heart J 2006;151: 1173-1179.
28. Weintraub WS, Barnett P, Chen S, et al: Economics methods in the Clinical Outcomes Utilizing percutaneous coronary Revascularization and Aggressive Guideline-driven drug Evaluation (COURAGE) trial. Am Heart J 2006;151: 1180-1185.

28a. Boden WE, O'Rourke RA, Teo KK, et al: Optimal medical therapy with or without PCI for stable coronary disease. N Engl J Med 2007;356:1503-1516.

29. Hlatky MA, Melsop KA, Boothroyd DB: Economic evaluation of alternative strategies to treat patients with diabetes mellitus and coronary artery disease. Am J Cardiol 2006;97:59G-65G.

30. Weintraub WS, Mauldin PD, Becker E, et al: A comparison of the costs of and quality of life after coronary angioplasty or coronary surgery for multivessel coronary disease: Results from the Emory Angioplasty Versus Surgery Trial (EAST). Circulation 1995;92:2831-2840.

31. Weintraub WS, Becker ER, Mauldin PD, et al: Costs of revascularization over eight years in the randomized and eligible patients in the Emory Angioplasty versus Surgery Trial (EAST). Am J Cardiol 2000;86:747-752.

32. Hlatky MA, Boothroyd DB, Melsop KA, et al: Medical costs and quality of life 10 to 12 years after randomization to angioplasty or bypass surgery for multivessel coronary artery disease. Circulation 2004;110:1960-1966.

33. Sculpher MJ, Seed P, Henderson RA, et al; for the RITA trial participants. Health service costs of coronary angioplasty and coronary artery bypass surgery: The Randomised Intervention Treatment of Angina (RITA) trial. Lancet 1994;344:927-930.

34. Stroupe KT, Morrison DA, Hlatky MA, et al: Cost-effectiveness of coronary artery bypass grafts versus percutaneous coronary intervention for revascularization of high-risk patients. Circulation 2006;114:1251-1257.

35. Nordmann AJ, Hengstler P, Leimenstoll BM, et al: Clinical outcomes of stents versus balloon angioplasty in non-acute coronary artery disease: A meta-analysis of randomized controlled trials. Eur Heart J 2004;25:69-80.

36. Serruys PW, van Hout B, Bonnier H, et al: Randomised comparison of implantation of heparin-coated stents with balloon angioplasty in selected patients with coronary artery disease (BENESTENT II). Lancet 1998;352:673-681.

37. Cohen DJ, van Hout B, Juliard JMJ, et al: Economic outcomes after coronary stenting or balloon angioplasty in the BENESTENT II trial: The US perspective. Circulation 1997;96:455A.

38. Weaver WD, Reisman MA, Griffin JJ, et al: Optimum percutaneous transluminal coronary angioplasty compared with routine stent strategy trial (OPUS-1): A randomised trial. Lancet 2000;355:2199-2203.

39. Legrand VM, Serruys PW, Unger F, et al: Three-year outcome after coronary stenting versus bypass surgery for the treatment of multivessel disease. Circulation 2004;109:1114-1120.

40. Serruys PW, Ong AT, van Herwerden LA, et al: Five-year outcomes after coronary stenting versus bypass surgery for the treatment of multivessel disease: The final analysis of the Arterial Revascularization Therapies Study (ARTS) randomized trial. J Am Coll Cardiol 2005;46:575-581.

41. Zhang Z, Spertus JA, Mahoney EM, et al: The impact of acute coronary syndrome on clinical, economic, and cardiac-specific health status after coronary artery bypass surgery versus stent-assisted percutaneous coronary intervention: 1-Year results from the Stent or Surgery (SoS) trial. Am Heart J 2005;150:175-181.

42. Mercado N, Wijns W, Serruys PW, et al: One-year outcomes of coronary artery bypass graft surgery versus percutaneous coronary intervention with multiple stenting for multisystem disease: A meta-analysis of individual patient data from randomized clinical trials. J Thorac Cardiovasc Surg 2005;130:512-519.

43. Roiron C, Sanchez P, Bouzamondo A, et al: Drug eluting stents: An updated meta-analysis of randomised controlled trials. Heart 2006;92:641-649.

44. Weintraub WS, Ghazzal ZM, Douglas JS Jr, et al: Long-term clinical follow-up in patients with angiographic restudy after successful angioplasty. Circulation 1993;87:831-840.

45. van Hout BA, Serruys PW, Lemos PA, et al: One year cost effectiveness of sirolimus eluting stents compared with bare metal stents in the treatment of single native de novo coronary lesions: An analysis from the RAVEL trial. Heart 2005;91:507-512.

46. Cohen DJ, Bakhai A, Shi C, et al: Cost-effectiveness of sirolimus-eluting stents for treatment of complex coronary stenoses: Results from the Sirolimus-Eluting Balloon Expandable Stent in the Treatment of Patients With De Novo Native Coronary Artery Lesions (SIRIUS) trial. Circulation 2004;110:508-514.

47. Bakhai A, Stone GW, Mahoney E, et al: Cost effectiveness of paclitaxel-eluting stents for patients undergoing percutaneous coronary revascularization: Results from the TAXUS-IV Trial. J Am Coll Cardiol 2006;48:253-261.

48. Kaiser C, Brunner-La Rocca HP, Buser PT, et al: Incremental cost-effectiveness of drug-eluting stents compared with a third-generation bare-metal stent in a real-world setting: Randomised Basel Stent Kosten Effektivitäts Trial (BASKET). Lancet 2005;366:921-929.

49. 2004 Drug Topics Red Book. Montvale, NJ, Medical Economics Data, 2004.

50. Naylor CD, Jaglal SB: Impact of intravenous thrombolysis on short-term coronary revascularization rates: A meta-analysis. JAMA 1990;264:697-702.

51. Naylor CD, Bronskill S, Goel V: Cost-effectiveness of intravenous thrombolytic drugs for acute myocardial infarction. Can J Cardiol 1993;9:553-558.

52. Mark DB, Hlatky MA, Califf RM, et al: Cost effectiveness of thrombolytic therapy with tissue plasminogen activator as compared with streptokinase for acute myocardial infarction. N Engl J Med 1995;332:1418-1424.

53. Topol EJ: Reperfusion therapy for acute myocardial infarction with fibrinolytic therapy or combination reduced fibrinolytic therapy and platelet glycoprotein IIb/IIIa inhibition: The GUSTO V randomised trial. Lancet 2001;357:1905-1914.

54. Kaul P, Armstrong PW, Cowper PA, et al: Economic analysis of the Assessment of the Safety and Efficacy of a New Thrombolytic Regimen (ASSENT-3) study: Costs of reperfusion strategies in acute myocardial infarction. Am Heart J 2005;149:637-644.

55. Gershlick AH, Stephens-Lloyd A, Hughes S, et al: Rescue angioplasty after failed thrombolytic therapy for acute myocardial infarction. N Engl J Med 2005;353:2758-2768.

56. Patel TN, Bavry AA, Kumbhani DJ, Ellis SG: A meta-analysis of randomized trials of rescue percutaneous coronary intervention after failed fibrinolysis. Am J Cardiol 2006;97:1685-1690.

57. Boersma E: Does time matter? A pooled analysis of randomized clinical trials comparing primary percutaneous coronary intervention and in-hospital fibrinolysis in acute myocardial infarction patients. Eur Heart J 2006;27:779-788.

58. Grines CL, Browne KF, Marco J, et al: A comparison of immediate angioplasty with thrombolytic therapy for acute myocardial infarction. N Engl J Med 1993;328:673-679.

59. Le May MR, Davies RF, Labinaz M, et al: Hospitalization costs of primary stenting versus thrombolysis in acute myocardial infarction: cost analysis of the Canadian STAT Study. Circulation 2003;108:2624-2630.

60. Machecourt J, Bonnefoy E, Vanzetto G, et al: Primary angioplasty is cost-minimizing compared with pre-hospital thrombolysis for patients within 60 min of a percutaneous coronary intervention center: The Comparison of Angioplasty and Pre-hospital Thrombolysis in Acute Myocardial Infarction (CAPTIM) cost-efficacy sub-study. J Am Coll Cardiol 2005;45:515-524.

61. Selmer R, Halvorsen S, Myhre KI, et al: Cost-effectiveness of primary percutaneous coronary intervention versus thrombolytic therapy for acute myocardial infarction. Scand Cardiovasc J 2005;39:276-285.

62. Hartwell D, Colquitt J, Loveman E, et al: Clinical effectiveness and cost-effectiveness of immediate angioplasty for acute myocardial infarction: Systematic review and economic evaluation. Health Technol Assess 2005;9:i-iv.

63. Lieu TA, Lundstrom RJ, Ray GT, et al: Initial cost of primary angioplasty for acute myocardial infarction. J Am Coll Cardiol 1996;28:882-889.

64. Lieu TA, Gurley J, Lundstrom RJ, et al: Projected cost-effectiveness of primary angioplasty for acute myocardial infarction. J Am Coll Cardiol 1997;30:1741-1750.

65. Cohen DJ, Taira DA, Berezin RH, et al; on behalf of the Stent PAMI Investigators: Cost-effectiveness of coronary stenting in acute myocardial infarction: Results from the Stent Primary

Angioplasty in Myocardial Infarction (Stent-PAMI) Trial. Circulation 2001;104:3039-3045.

66. ADMIRAL Investigators: Three-year duration of benefit from abciximab in patients receiving stents for acute myocardial infarction in the randomized double-blind ADMIRAL study. Eur Heart J 2005;26:2520-2523.

67. Bakhai A, Stone GW, Grines CL, et al: Cost-effectiveness of coronary stenting and abciximab for patients with acute myocardial infarction: Results from the CADILLAC (Controlled Abciximab and Device Investigation to Lower Late Angioplasty Complications) trial. Circulation 2003;108:2857-2863.

68. The GUSTO III Investigators: A comparison of reteplase with alteplase for acute myocardial infarction. N Engl J Med 1997;337:1118-1123.

69. Pilote L, Miller DP, Califf RM, et al: Determinants of the use of coronary angiography and revascularization after thrombolysis for acute myocardial infarction. N Engl J Med 1996;335:1198-1205.

70. Selby JV, Fireman BH, Lundstrom RJ, et al: Variation among hospitals in coronary angiography practices and outcomes after myocardial infarction in a large health maintenance organization. N Engl J Med 1996;335:1888-1896.

71. Bhatt DL, Roe MT, Peterson ED, et al: Utilization of early invasive management strategies for high-risk patients with non-ST-segment elevation acute coronary syndromes: Results from the CRUSADE Quality Improvement Initiative. JAMA 2004;292:2096-2104.

72. Beck CA, Eisenberg MJ, Pilote L: Invasive versus noninvasive management of ST-elevation acute myocardial infarction: A review of clinical trials and observational studies. Am Heart J 2005;149:194-199.

73. Kuntz KM, Tsevat J, Goldman L, Weinstein MC: Cost-effectiveness of routine coronary angiography after acute myocardial infarction. Circulation 1996;94:957-965.

74. Cannon CP, Weintraub WS, Demopoulos LA, et al: Comparison of early invasive and conservative strategies in patients with unstable coronary syndromes treated with the glycoprotein IIb/IIIa inhibitor tirofiban. N Engl J Med 2001;344:1879-1887.

75. Mahoney EM, Jurkovitz CT, Chu H, et al: Cost and cost-effectiveness of an early invasive vs conservative strategy for the treatment of unstable angina and non-ST-segment elevation myocardial infarction. JAMA 2002;288:1851-1858.

76. Wallentin L, Lagerqvist B, Husted S, et al: Outcome at 1 year after an invasive compared with a non-invasive strategy in unstable coronary-artery disease: The FRISC II invasive randomised trial. FRISC II Investigators. Fast Revascularisation during Instability in Coronary artery disease. Lancet 2000;356:9-16.

77. Lagerqvist B, Husted S, Kontny F, et al: 5-Year outcomes in the FRISC-II randomised trial of an invasive versus a non-invasive strategy in non-ST-elevation acute coronary syndrome: A follow-up study. Lancet 2006;368:998-1004.

78. de Winter RJ, Windhausen F, Cornel JH, et al: Early invasive versus selectively invasive management for acute coronary syndromes. N Engl J Med 2005;353:1095-1104.

79. Bavry AA, Kumbhani DJ, Rassi AN, et al: Benefit of early invasive therapy in acute coronary syndromes: A meta-analysis of contemporary randomized clinical trials. J Am Coll Cardiol 2006;48:1319-1325.

80. Mark DB, Harrington RA, Lincoff AM, et al: Cost effectiveness of platelet glycoprotein IIb/IIIa inhibition with eptifibatide in patients with non-ST elevation acute coronary syndromes. Circulation 2000;101:366-371.

81. Mark DB, Talley JD, Topol EJ, et al; for the EPIC Investigators: Economic assessment of platelet glycoprotein IIb/IIIa inhibition for prevention of ischemic complications of high risk coronary angioplasty. Circulation 1996;94:629-635.

82. Lincoff AM, Mark DB, Tcheng JE, et al: Economic assessment of platelet glycoprotein IIb/IIIa receptor blockade with abciximab and low-dose heparin during percutaneous coronary revascularization: Results from the EPILOG randomized trial. Circulation 2000;102:2923-2929.

83. Weintraub WS, Culler S, Boccuzzi SJ, et al: Economic impact of GPIIB/IIIA blockade after high-risk angioplasty: Results from the RESTORE trial. J Am Coll Cardiol 1999;34:1061-1066.

84. Mahoney EM, Mehta S, Yuan Y, et al: Long-term cost-effectiveness of early and sustained clopidogrel therapy for up to 1 year in patients undergoing percutaneous coronary intervention after presenting with acute coronary syndromes without ST-segment elevation. Am Heart J 2006;151:219-227.

85. Cowper PA, Udayakumar K, Sketch MH Jr, Peterson ED: Economic effects of prolonged clopidogrel therapy after percutaneous coronary intervention. J Am Coll Cardiol 2005;45:369-376.

86. Lindgren P, Stenestrand U, Malmberg K, Jonsson B: The long-term cost-effectiveness of clopidogrel plus aspirin in patients undergoing percutaneous coronary intervention in Sweden. Clin Ther 2005;27:100-110.

87. Ferguson JJ, Califf RM, Antman EM, et al: Enoxaparin vs unfractionated heparin in high-risk patients with non-ST-segment elevation acute coronary syndromes managed with an intended early invasive strategy: Primary results of the SYNERGY randomized trial. JAMA 2004;292:45-54.

88. Janzon M, Levin LA, Swahn E: Cost effectiveness of extended treatment with low molecular weight heparin (dalteparin) in unstable coronary artery disease: Results from the FRISC II trial. Heart 2003;89:287-292.

89. Lincoff AM, Bittl JA, Harrington RA, et al: Bivalirudin and provisional glycoprotein IIb/IIIa blockade compared with heparin and planned glycoprotein IIb/IIIa blockade during percutaneous coronary intervention: REPLACE-2 randomized trial. JAMA 2003;289:853-863.

90. Cohen DJ, Lincoff AM, Lavelle TA, et al: Economic evaluation of bivalirudin with provisional glycoprotein IIB/IIIA inhibition versus heparin with routine glycoprotein IIB/IIIA inhibition for percutaneous coronary intervention: Results from the REPLACE-2 trial. J Am Coll Cardiol 2004;44:1792-1800.

91. Mark DB, Nelson CL, Anstrom KJ, et al: Cost-effectiveness of defibrillator therapy or amiodarone in chronic stable heart failure: Results from the Sudden Cardiac Death in Heart Failure Trial (SCD-HeFT). Circulation 2006;114:135-142.

92. Weinstein MC, Siegel JE, Gold MR, et al: Recommendations of the Panel on Cost-Effectiveness in Health and Medicine. JAMA 1996;276:1253-1258.

66 Quality of Care in Interventional Cardiology

Ralph G. Brindis

KEY POINTS

- In the present era of increasing state regulations, consumer demands for quality, and pressures from payers for cost-efficiency, quality in the cardiac catheterization laboratory is being examined more closely than ever before.

- The invasive cardiologist must lead the initiative to assess quality, because physician expertise in interventional cardiology and cardiovascular outcomes is best suited to define and determine "quality" in the delivery of cardiac catheterization care.

- Donabedian's triad describes the programmatic features needed to achieve quality in the cardiac catheterization laboratory: structure, process, and outcomes.

- Continuous Quality Improvement (CQI), an organized, scientific process for evaluating, planning, improving, and controlling quality, has been demonstrated to reduce variation and improve overall performance in the cardiac catheterization laboratory.

- Registries such as the American College of Cardiology–National Cardiovascular Data Registry (ACC-NCDR) CathPCI Registry can not only form the cornerstone for both local and national hospital quality initiatives, but

also can: (1) provide important feedback to influence ACC/American Heart Association (AHA) clinical guidelines and recommendations, (2) lead to the generation of new concepts for additional clinical trials, and (3) help set state and national regulatory standards and policies based on quality assessment rather than simple "volume criteria" or limited administrative data.

- Volume criteria provide an inadequate surrogate for defining quality in the cardiac catheterization laboratory, particularly with the ability to actually measure and benchmark percutaneous coronary intervention (PCI) process and performance measures in addition to PCI outcomes including morbidity and risk-adjusted mortality.

- Significant challenges exist for "Pay-for Performance" programs and state and national hospital and physician public reporting initiatives. These efforts should be cautiously implemented with close scrutiny and oversight to ensure promotion of the intended purpose of improving quality in patient care rather than the real potential of causing negative unintended consequences.

The potential to deliver high-quality care in the cardiac catheterization laboratory centers on the core values espoused in the Institute of Medicine's (IOM's) report, *Crossing the Quality Chasm*, which defines quality as "the degree to which health care systems, services and supplies for individuals and populations increase the likelihood for desired health outcomes in a manner consistent with current professional knowledge."[1] The IOM further states that health care should be safe, effective, evidence-based, timely, equitable, and patient-centered. In the present era of increasing state regulations, consumer demand for quality, pressures from payers to be cost-efficient, and increasing implementation of the public reporting of mortality and morbidity rates, quality in the cardiac catheterization laboratory is being examined more closely than ever before.

The cardiac catheterization laboratory has evolved from an investigational facility that provided much of our knowledge of cardiac pathophysiology to its preeminence as the central arena for cardiovascular diagnostic and therapeutic procedures. Invasive cardiovascular procedures have become a cornerstone for the evaluation and management of many cardiovascular diseases, with more than 1 million cardiac catheterization studies performed annually in the United States.[2] Although there are no formal national standards to judge cardiac catheterization laboratory quality, some states have used clinical practice guidelines and expert consensus documents published by the American College of Cardiology Foundation (ACCF), the American Heart Association (AHA), and the Society for Cardiovascular Angiography and Interventions (SCAI) to develop quality standards.[3-5]

Although these consensus documents and relevant clinical guidelines were never intended to serve primarily as state or national standards, they have often become the de facto basis for licensure regulations imposed by state health departments in an attempt to improve quality.

The assessment of quality should not be likened to the mere identification of an isolated patient complication. There are data from the American College of Cardiology–National Cardiovascular Data Registry (ACC-NCDR CathPCI) documenting a fairly wide range in the risk-adjusted in-hospital mortality rate for percutaneous coronary intervention (PCI) that cannot be explained solely by the clinical status of the patient, suggesting a substantial variation in cardiac catheterization quality in the United States.[6,7] In addition, the marked variation of utilization rates of PCI throughout the United States in the Medicare population, well documented by the *Dartmouth Atlas of Cardiovascular Health Care,* is also receiving increasing scrutiny.[8,9] Quality of care not only encompasses risk-adjusted mortality and procedure-related adverse outcomes, but also must include assessment of the appropriateness of the test or procedure and other metrics, such as patient satisfaction and issues evaluating efficiency.

EVALUATING QUALITY IN THE CARDIAC CATHETERIZATION LABORATORY

The invasive cardiologist must lead the initiative to assess quality. Payers, purchasers, consumers, and an entire industry of health care performance and outcomes graders may seek to compare and shape the quality of cardiac catheterization care. However, physician expertise in interventional cardiology and cardiovascular outcomes is best suited to define and determine "quality" in the delivery of cardiac catheterization care, as opposed to Web-based health graders' "report cards" or other various insurance industry–derived metrics, which often rely primarily on administrative data.[10,11] Nevertheless, collaborations and partnerships that take into consideration each of various stakeholders' perspectives can represent an important platform for improving cardiac care.

Quality of care in the cardiac catheterization laboratory is not an assessment of outcomes alone. In Redding, California, allegations of inappropriate patient selection combined with inaccurate image acquisition and interpretation led to unnecessary coronary artery bypass grafting (CABG) surgeries. By 2001, Redding demonstrated a CABG utilization rate of more than 12 per 1000 Medicare patients per year, whereas the state of California had utilization rates for CABG of approximately 5/1000.[9,12,13] Clearly, the assessment of outcomes alone therefore does not adequately assess cardiac catheterization laboratory quality. Inappropriate referral of patients for either PCI or CABG substantially compromises quality, even if the actual outcomes of the unnecessary PCI or CABG include a low frequency of mortality or adverse events.

Components for Quality Assessment: Structure, Process, and Outcomes

Although there are many approaches to guide evaluation of care in the cardiac catheterization environment, Donabedian's triad provides an ideal model for identifying the major domains of health care that best describe the programmatic features needed to achieve quality: structure, process, and outcomes (Fig. 66-1; Table 66-1).[14]

Structure

Structure refers to the infrastructure needed to provide ideal care. In addition to personnel, equipment, facilities, training, and laboratory protocols, structural components include oversight of training and certification for physicians, cardiovascular and radiology technicians, and nurses.

Since 1999, The American Board of Internal Medicine (ABIM) has administered an additional qualification (AQ) examination for board certification in interventional cardiology. This added proficiency examination for interventional cardiology has been well received by the cardiology community and hospital privileges committees, and there are now more than 5020 ABIM certified interventional cardiologists.[15] Extensive knowledge is required of the interventionalist, encompassing concepts of radiation physics and radiation safety, vascular biology, and

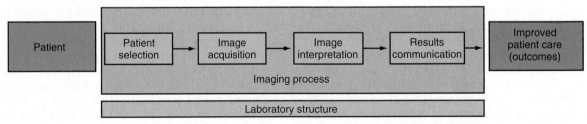

Figure 66-1. "Dimensions of Care" framework for evaluating quality of cardiovascular imaging (From Douglas PS, Iskandrian A, Krumholz H, et al: Achieving quality in cardiovascular imaging: Proceedings from the American College of Cardiology-Duke University Medical Center Think Tank on Quality in Cardiovascular Imaging. J Am Coll Cardiol 2006;48:2141-2151. Epub 2006 Nov 1. Review.

Table 66-1. Cardiac Catheterization Laboratory Quality Measures

Domain	Description
Laboratory structure	Laboratory accreditation: The Joint Commission
	American Board of Internal Medicine Certification in Interventional Cardiology
	Registry participation
Patient selection	Assess: % cardiac Cath/PCI meeting Cath/PCI appropriateness criteria through appropriateness criteria evaluation
Image acquisition	Measure radiation dosage (patient and physician)
	Annual radiation safety training
	Contrast volume utilization
	Quarterly image quality assessment
	Weekly cardiac catheterization conferences
Image interpretation	Inter-reader and intra-reader variability assessment
Results communication	Define key report data elements
	Develop timeliness guidelines for reports
	% studies with critical parameters (e.g., LVEF)
Improved patient care (outcomes)	Normal coronary angiography rates
	Data collection/outcomes assessment/benchmarking via ACC-NCDR, use CQI implementation (CathKit)

ACC-NCDR, American College of Cardiology–National Cardiovascular Data Registry; CQI, continuous quality improvement; LVEF, left ventricular ejection fraction; PCI, percutaneous coronary intervention.
Data from Douglas PS, Iskandrian A, Krumholz H, et al: Achieving quality in cardiovascular imaging: Proceedings from the American College of Cardiology-Duke University Medical Center Think Tank on Quality in Cardiovascular Imaging. J Am Coll Cardiol 2006;48:2141-2151.

the response to vessel wall injury and thrombosis, including the intimate roles of platelets, thrombin, and fibrinolytics. Proficiency in the breadth of the interventional armamentarium and its proper use, such as atherectomy, complex multivessel PCI, rotablation, extraction catheters, embolic protection devices, flow and pressure wires, and intravascular ultrasound (IVUS), is assessed. Currently, the ABIM AQ examination is a written test evaluating key concepts and interpretation of clinical decisions in the interventional catheterization laboratory related to patient management and patient selection. To qualify to sit for the ABIM examination, the applicant must first receive certification from the interventional program director of his or her fourth-year interventional training program as to interventional proficiency and training, along with documentation of direct participation in 250 coronary interventional procedures.[15]

Laboratory accreditation by The Joint Commission (formerly known as the Joint Commission on Accreditation of Healthcare Organizations [JCAHO]) is an integral part of the general hospital accreditation process. Assessment of cardiac catheterization laboratory structure is an important aspect of a Joint Commission review. Education, in the form of cardiac catheterization conferences that encompass both case review and morbidity and mortality reviews as part of a peer review quality improvement program, is an important cardiac catheterization laboratory structural component.[16] In order to be effective, these programs must emphasize improving performance and not punishing individual physicians as potential one-time outliers.

Participation in national data collection and quality improvement programs offers additional infrastructure to accurately assess clinical outcomes. Examples include programs focusing on acute myocardial infarction (AMI), such as the American Heart Association's Get with the Guidelines Program (AHA-GWTG), the National Registry for Myocardial Infarction (NRMI), and the national quality improvement initiative and registry known as CRUSADE (Can Rapid Risk Stratification of Unstable Angina Patients Suppress Adverse Outcomes with Early Implementation of the ACC/AHA Guidelines—A CQI Initiative). Other programs focus directly on performance of cardiac catheterization and PCI, such as the ACC-NCDR CathPCI registry.[17-19]

Participation in such programs provides caregivers both the standardized tools for data collection and important information risk-adjustment of patient outcomes, such as mortality based on relevant individual patient clinical factors. Registries also offer feedback on how a given hospital or clinician's practice compares with that of peers through benchmarking performance against aggregate national or like hospital outcomes. Such feedback systems are known to be a critical element in quality improvement.[20-23] Not only does feedback of outcomes data to clinicians offer the infrastructure engine to determine opportunities to improve clinical performance and quality, but, when fed back into the "Cycle of Clinical Therapeutic Effectiveness" (Fig. 66-2), it also can lead to new hypotheses and concepts for disease treatment, eventually resulting in new clinical trials and the generation of new clinical guidelines, recommendations, and performance indicators.

Process

Process refers to actions performed in the delivery of patient care, including the timing and technical competency of their delivery. Additionally, process includes methodology surrounding patient selection, image acquisition, interpretation, and reporting of data.

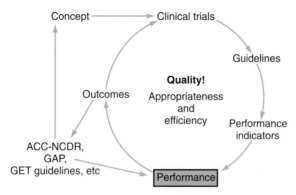

Quality in the cycle of clinical therapeutic effectiveness

Figure 66-2. Quality in the Cycle of Clinical Therapeutic Effectiveness. ACC-NCDR, American College of Cardiology-National Cardiovascular Data Registry, GAP, Guidelines Applied in Practice; GET Guidelines, American Heart Association's Get with the Guidelines Program. (Redrawn from Califf RM, Peterson ED, Gibbons RJ, et al: Integrating quality into the cycle of therapeutic development. J Am Coll Cardiol 2002;40:1895-1901.)

Patient Selection: The Role of Appropriateness Criteria

Proper patient selection for PCI therapy is undergoing increasing scrutiny by all health care stakeholders. Wennberg's *Dartmouth Atlas* demonstrated substantial variability in PCI utilization within the Medicare population of the United States. For example, a hospital in Elyria, Ohio, had a PCI utilization rate in 2003 of 42/1000 Medicare enrollees; in comparison, the national utilization rate was 11.3/1000 Medicare enrollees (Figs. 66-3 and 66-4).[9,24] The high rate might reflect an overuse at this particu-

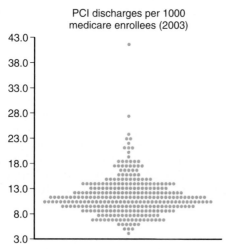

PCI discharges per 1000 medicare enrollees (2003)

Figure 66-3. Graph showing frequency of percutaneous coronary interventions (PCIs) among Medicare enrollees by hospital referral region. PCI rates varied more than 10-fold across the United States. (From Dartmouth Atlas of Cardiovascular Health Care, Regional Variations in Rates of Percutaneous Coronary Interventions in Medicare Enrollees. Center for the Evaluative Clinical Sciences, Dartmouth Medical School, 2003.)

lar hospital or, instead, an appropriate use, with the implication of a widespread underuse nationally of PCI. This variation in utilization might also simply reflect the reasonable options available among treatment choices based on evidenced-based medicine combined with patient- and family-centered preferences.[25]

In 2005, the ACCF established the Appropriateness Criteria Working Group to determine a methodology for establishing the appropriate use of imaging procedures to generate information that has positive consequences for a patient's care.[26] Since the Working Group's inception, the ACCF, in partnership with relevant specialty and subspecialty societies, has been developing an increasing portfolio of Appropriateness Criteria in cardiovascular diagnostic imaging, and there are similar plans to develop Appropriateness Criteria for PCI.[27,28]

Appropriateness Criteria have been defined by the ACCF as follows: "An appropriate imaging study is one in which the expected incremental information, combined with clinical judgment, exceeds the expected negative consequences by a sufficiently wide margin for a specific indication that the procedure is generally considered acceptable care and a reasonable approach for the indication."[28] The ACCF defined negative consequences in this context, as follows: "Negative consequences include the risks of the procedure (e.g., radiation or contrast exposure) and the downstream impact of poor test performance, such as delay in diagnosis (false-negatives) or inappropriate diagnosis (false-positives)."

By this definition, Appropriateness Criteria can provide a guide as to whether an imaging procedure is a "reasonable" approach for a given clinical circumstance. Although many acceptable indications outside these developed Appropriateness Criteria exist, measuring the degree of adherence to the clinical situations covered by such criteria would be valuable for assessing quality of patient selection. Application and assessment of appropriateness of care requires collection of the relevant patient clinical variables. For example, benchmarking the assessment of percentage of patients found to have normal coronary arteries may be one measurement to assess appropriate cardiac catheterization rates. Before the creation of PCI Appropriateness Criteria, the ACC/AHA/SCAI guidelines for coronary angiography can serve as a foundation for developing cardiac catheterization laboratory appropriateness criteria.[29]

Image Acquisition

Image quality is a key component for accurate diagnosis and appropriate interventional therapy in the cardiac catheterization laboratory.[30] Assessing image quality and radiation dosimetry with the use of the National Electrical Manufacturers Association (NEMA) SCAI XR-21 Imaging Phantom, for example, can allow a cardiac catheterization laboratory to evaluate objectively the performance of the imaging equipment. This information provides both an initial evaluation and the potential to follow performance over

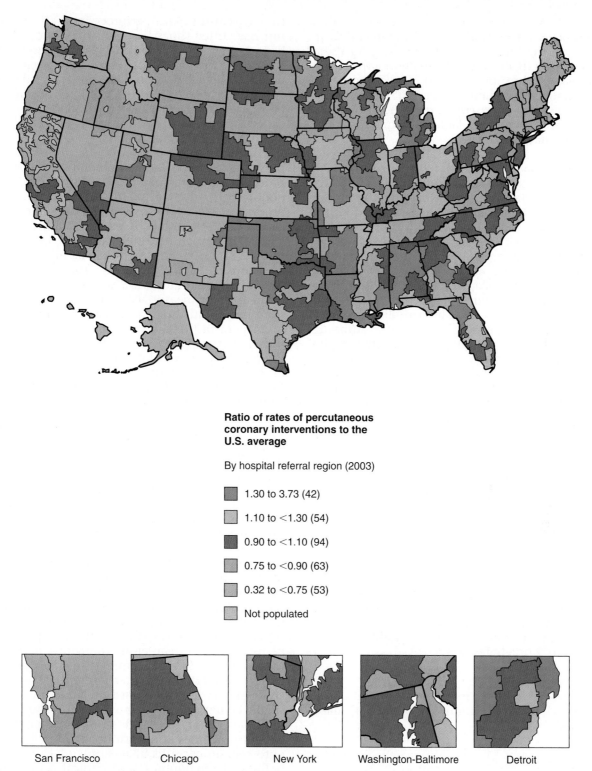

Ratio of rates of percutaneous coronary interventions to the U.S. average

By hospital referral region (2003)

- 1.30 to 3.73 (42)
- 1.10 to <1.30 (54)
- 0.90 to <1.10 (94)
- 0.75 to <0.90 (63)
- 0.32 to <0.75 (53)
- Not populated

San Francisco   Chicago   New York   Washington-Baltimore   Detroit

Figure 66-4. United States map demonstrating the regional variations in rates of percutaneous coronary interventions among Medicare enrollees, 2003. (From Dartmouth Atlas of Cardiovascular Health Care, Regional Variations in Rates of Percutaneous Coronary Interventions in Medicare Enrollees. Center for the Evaluative Clinical Sciences, Dartmouth Medical School, 2003.)

time, in relation to the same or other laboratories' past performance.[31] This provides for a vendor-independent equipment assessment that may provide useful information regarding subjective operator issues, as well as both quality and safety information,

to justify appropriate equipment retention or replacement.[32]

Measuring patient radiation exposure and providing for radiation safety education for the cardiac catheterization laboratory physicians and staff is mandatory.[5] Although education is a structure rather than a process component, educational materials are available on the International Committee on Radiation Protection (ICRP) Web site, including the ACCF/AHA/Heart Rhythm Society (HRS)/SCAI clinical competence statement,[5] published in 2005, and an educational PowerPoint presentation on radiation safety for patients and staff (available at: http://www.icrp.org/educational_area.asp.)

Image Interpretation

Interventional cardiology board certification has established a certain knowledge base required for an interventional cardiologist, but this alone does not ensure accurate, high-quality acquisition and interpretation of coronary angiography. To ensure quality acquisition and interpretation in cardiac imaging, the cardiac catheterization laboratory should provide objective evidence of accuracy and reproducibility of image assessment.[30] Accurate image interpretation of coronary angiograms is aided by periodic assessment of both intra- and inter-reader variation.[30] Although it is not routinely utilized in general practice, digital quantification of coronary artery stenoses, compared to subjective interpretation, can reduce variation and improve accuracy. Similar attention should be directed to assessing the quality of interpretation of all imaging adjuncts that direct clinical decision-making in the cardiovascular suite, such as coronary IVUS and flow and pressure wire measurements.

Results Communication

The quality of the procedure, as perceived by the requesting physician, is only as good as the information made available to the requesting health care personnel. Periodic assessment of the completeness of cardiac catheterization procedure reports, the effectiveness in report turnaround times and communication with referring individuals, and other associated processes ensures quality. It is essential to verify that the reports contain all the relevant key data elements and that they are produced and communicated to the relevant clinicians and health care personnel in a timely fashion.[30]

Outcomes Assessment

The final component of process is assessment of outcomes, which is also the third component of Donabedian's triad.

Outcomes

Outcomes refers to tangible measures of the consequences of diagnostic cardiac catheterization and PCI care, including risk-adjusted mortality rates and related adverse outcomes, such as groin and vascular complications, stroke, contrast nephropathy, cardiac tamponade, periprocedural myocardial infarction (MI), and the rate of emergency CABG.

Many outcome metrics have their own intrinsic challenges, however. There are debates not only as

to what constitutes a periprocedural MI (any troponin rise? three times baseline? five times baseline?) but whether there is actually clinical significance to such a rise in a cardiac marker in the periprocedural period. There are also substantial challenges in consistency of the data definitions of such complications, particularly bleeding and vascular complications, despite the creation of ACC/AHA ACS Data Standards and Definitions.[33] Outcomes assessment in the cardiac catheterization laboratory often encompass other Donabedian components of the structure, process, and outcomes triad, such as the so-called door-to-balloon time, volume of contrast use, and procedural radiation doses. Evaluation and quantification of patient health status measures, such as anginal burden, functional status, and quality of life, offers clinicians and researchers alike important mechanisms to truly evaluate the benefits of PCI therapy.[34] Ideal outcomes assessment would not only be an episodic measure based on PCI hospital admissions but would also include a longitudinal follow-up assessment of the clinical impact of a PCI intervention. For example, the clinical concerns surrounding the true frequency of late subacute thrombosis (SAT) of drug-eluting stents requires such longitudinal patient outcomes data. Issues surrounding patient compliance with medications such as clopidogrel, with its demonstrated importance in preventing SAT, could also be longitudinally tracked.[35] Outcome assessment can also consider the impact of care on indirect health-related measures, such as patient satisfaction related to the overall care process itself, along with quantifying the actual cost of the care delivery, including cost-effectiveness and cost-efficiency calculations. Outcomes measures may also explore potential unanticipated consequences of care changes.

Outcomes, therefore, represent the aggregate effect of all of the structure and care processes. Improving this end product is the ultimate evaluation of the success of medical care. However, the use of outcome metrics also has substantial challenges. Many PCI adverse events rates, particularly mortality, tend to be uncommon. Therefore, outcome performance measures can often be seemingly unstable, with year-to-year or quarter-to-quarter substantial variations of crude outcomes when measured at the level of a single center or physician operator. Additionally, multiple factors beyond provider quality affect patient outcomes and must be accounted for before outcome comparisons are meaningful. Patient comorbidities, demographics, and clinical acuity all play huge, if not the predominant roles, in determining patient outcome, independent of the quality of care actually provided. Therefore, there is a need for collection of accurate and detailed clinical data, as well as use of a rigorous risk-adjustment methodology to truly and accurately describe provider outcome measurements.[11] In addition to the ACC-NCDR CathPCI registry, there are many superb state and regional data collection programs in place to aid clinicians and hospitals in PCI outcome assessments. These include the national Veterans Administration program, along with other excellent well-established and rigorous programs in New York, Massachusetts, Michigan, Pennsylvania, Washington State, West Virginia, Virginia, and elsewhere.

Continuous Quality Improvement in the Cardiac Catheterization Laboratory

Continuous quality improvement (CQI) is a methodology to improve the processes associated with providing a product or service to meet or exceed consumer expectations.[1] Based on the work of pioneers in industrial management, specifically Deming and Juran, the CQI process is a collection of techniques borrowed from the fields of systems theory, statistics, engineering, and psychology.[36] CQI is an organized, scientific process for evaluating, planning, improving, and controlling quality. The goal of CQI is to reduce variation and improve overall performance. Positive experiences in other industries led to the application of CQI methods in health care, in the hope that reduced variation and better performance would improve patient outcomes and also result in cost savings.

CQI is fundamentally different from quality assurance (QA), which typically is geared to identifying so-called low-end performers or outliers. CQI, promoted by individuals such as Donabedian, Berwick and colleagues, and Jencks and Wilensky, builds on traditional QA methods to develop programs that will reduce variation and improve overall performance.[37-39] CQI efforts in cardiovascular care have shown benefits such as attaining a high level of adherence to evidence-based performance and process measures in the management of acute coronary syndromes (ACS). Through this improvement in care, CQI has been associated with better clinical outcomes, with emerging data demonstrating decreased cardiovascular mortality.[22] The core of most CQI programs includes the following:[40]

1. The collection of data containing relevant patient variables that allows assessment of clinical processes, performance, and outcomes.
2. Feedback of these performance and outcomes results to the clinicians, ideally with risk adjustment and benchmarking of the data.
3. Implementation of appropriate interventions to promote reduction in wasteful and inefficient variation of care while simultaneously improving performance.

The actual interventions can be varied and multiple, but they typically include grand rounds dissemination of evidenced-based guidelines, "pocket guides" of PCI critical pathways, and other reminder tools, such as preprinted order sheets. The key ingredients of these potential tools to best ensure successful CQI programs are not fully understood. However, there are several known predictors of success for CQI programs, and they invariably focus on the presence or absence of local physician champions, in conjunction with an administrative and financial commitment from the parent organization.[18,21]

Moscucci and colleagues[41] provided convincing evidence that implementing a statewide CQI PCI initiative in Michigan led to substantial improvement in a number of process and outcomes measures. The investigators used a wide range of CQI strategies, particularly relying on a quarterly feedback report to clinicians on their adherence to process and performance measures, along with crude and risk-adjusted outcomes. Various bedside clinical tools to assess the risk of in-hospital PCI mortality, along with aids for prediction and prevention of contrast nephropathy and the need for blood transfusions, were distributed as part of this study.

Other instituted interventions included nursing protocols for assessment of preprocedure medications, routine preprocedure hydration protocols, modification of emergency room protocols for patients with ACS, and efforts for limiting contrast administration in high-risk patients. Moscucci demonstrated that the application of this PCI CQI program resulted in decreases in bleeding, transfusion requirements, vascular complications, and contrast utilization, leading to a trend toward reduction of contrast nephropathy.[41] Temporal improvement in major clinical outcomes included lower rates of crude and risk-adjusted in-hospital death, emergency CABG, contrast-induced nephropathy requiring dialysis, MI, and stroke. Although this Michigan project was not a true randomized study, and appreciating that many of the improvements in care could reflect temporal improvement in PCI practice, the decrease in contrast-induced nephropathy requiring dialysis strongly supports the benefit of the CQI intervention. Comparing 2002 data from the hospitals using the CQI intervention with data from their cohort control hospitals, the authors found statistically significantly better clinical outcomes, defined by a quadruple end point of death, emergency bypass surgery, stroke, and repeated PCI.[41] Rihal and coworkers also identified the benefit of CQI intervention for PCI delivery with demonstration of improvement in both clinical and economic outcomes in a temporal observational study at the Mayo Clinic.[42]

CathKit for Quality Improvement

Physicians and catheterization laboratory directors and managers typically are not trained or versed in CQI methodology, nor have they the inherent skill set to fully implement CQI initiatives into laboratory operations. To fill this unmet need, ACCF and SCAI created a cardiac catheterization laboratory improvement quality tool called CathKit, which was launched in 2003.[43] CathKit is a Web-based up-to-date cardiac catheterization and PCI tool kit devised to help clinicians, managers, and hospitals to develop their own CQI initiatives in the cardiac catheterization laboratory (Fig. 66-5). CathKit offers instruction in CQI methodology, provides examples of relevant CQI projects (e.g., management and avoidance of groin

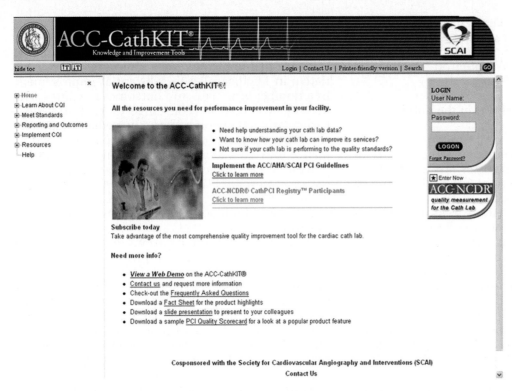

Figure 66-5. American College of Cardiology-National Cardiovascular Data Registry (ACC-NCDR) CathKit Home Page. Available at: http://www.accncdr.com.

complications), and has downloadable templates for catheterization protocols and PCI pathways. Major sections of CathKit include the following:

1. Learn about CQI—principles, analytical tools, benchmarking and comparative data, change management, and peer review.
2. Meeting Standards—facilities and environment, management considerations, personnel, and patient care.
3. Reporting and Outcomes—self-evaluation summary, quality scorecard.
4. Implement CQI—using FOCUS Plan-Do-Study-Act (PDSA) methodology with case examples, such as door-to-balloon time.
5. Resources—with state licensure requirements and contact information, tools and templates, case studies, a bibliography, and a discussion board.

Individual NCDR participants' hospital presentations at ACC-NCDR user group meetings have confirmed the positive changes in aspects of cardiac catheterization care, along with associated cost savings to their institution.[40,43]

National Percutaneous Coronary Intervention Registries

The role of national registries focusing on PCI and cardiac catheterization has grown substantially, particularly since the launching of the ACC-NCDR CathPCI registry in 1998 (Fig. 66-6). This registry, created under the auspices of the ACCF, was developed to respond to clinicians' and hospitals' needs for standardized elements to accurately describe clinical outcomes; it offers risk-adjusted quarterly data reports with comparisons against national and "like" hospital benchmarks.[44] Table 66-2 displays 2005 ACC-NCDR cardiac catheterization and PCI data, composed of diagnostic cardiac catheterizations and interventional (PCI) procedures harvested from participating facilities across the nation. Listed are aggregated data of 604,042 diagnostic cardiac catheterizations and 293,775 PCI procedures performed on patients discharged in 2005 from 462 participating facilities. Figure 66-7 represents the Key Performance Measures executive summary page that is supplied to every NCDR hospital each quarter, and the explanation of the benchmarking methodology is shown in Figure 66-8. Table 66-3 delineates the relative importance of the clinical descriptors used in the PCI mortality risk-adjustment methodology. Figure 66-9 displays various performance measures from the ACC-NCDR CathPCI of the results of individual participating hospitals in a benchmarked format.

The NCDR now has more than 5 million patient records, collecting patient cardiac catheterization data from more than 850 United States hospitals. The NCDR also has developed registries for carotid stenting and endarterectomy (CARE), Implantable Cardiac Defibrillators (ICD Registry), and Acute Coronary Syndromes (ACTION). Efforts are underway at the NCDR to develop longitudinal modules for the ICD registry and the PCI registry, as well as a registry for the management of coronary artery disease in the ambulatory setting. The enhanced value of collecting longitudinal patient follow-up data on these registries is that the data can be used to further evaluate the true benefits and effectiveness of treatment strategies. To promote and ensure data veracity and

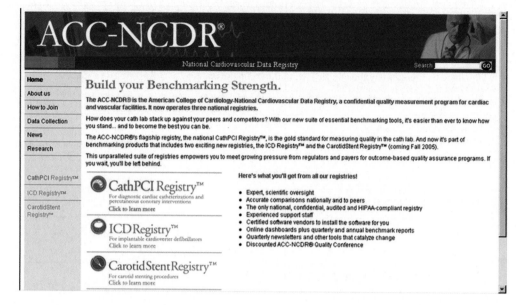

Figure 66-6. American College of Cardiology-National Cardiovascular Data Registry (ACC-NCDR) Web site home page. Available at: http://www.accncdr.com.

quality, internal quality checks of the data are ensured by data quality reports on the submitted quarterly data and an external on-site auditing program.

These registries have huge potentials, not only in forming the cornerstone for local hospital quality initiatives, but also through the valuable information that can be gleaned from the large numbers of patients in the "real-world" environment. The registries can (1) provide important feedback to influence ACC/AHA Clinical Guidelines recommendations, (2) lead to the generation of new concepts for additional clinical trials, and (3) help set state and national regulatory standards and policies based on quality

assessment rather than simple "volume criteria" or limited administrative data.

Anderson, for example, assessed the PCI risk-adjusted mortality data in relation to the indication class assignment based on ACC/AHA PCI Clinical Guidelines recommendations from the patient records of the ACC-NCDR CathPCI Registry. Increasing frequencies of risk components were observed across the ACC/AHA PCI guidelines indications for classes I, IIa, IIb, and III. Observed mortality rates for each guidelines indication class were 0.49%, 0.63%, 1.88%, and 1.60%, respectively which also correlated closely to the expected risk-adjusted mortality

Table 66-2. ACC-NCDR Cardiac Catheterization and PCI Data*

Parameter	Overall Mean	"Leading" Centers (Top 25%)	"Lagging" Centers (Bottom 25%)
Diagnostic Cardiac Catheterization			
In-lab mortality (%)	0.06	0.00	0.08
Major complications (%)\†	1.87	0.24	1.98
Percutaneous Coronary Intervention (PCI)			
Major complications (%)†	2.31	0.96	3.21
Vascular complications (%)‡	1.73	0.83	2.34
Antiplatelet drug administration (%)§	95.81	98.09	94.80
Emergency coronary artery bypass grafting (%)	0.39	0.00	0.56
Door-to-balloon time (DBT)¶			
Average DBT (min)	142.88	92.00	144.12
DBT ≤90 min (%)	50.66	64.28	37.15
DBT ≤120 min (%)	73.33	85.70	65.90
Risk-adjusted mortality (%)¶	1.14	0.77	1.44

*The American College of Cardiology maintains a number of clinical data registries as part of the National Cardiovascular Data Registry (ACC-NCDR). Among them is the CathPCI registry, which is composed of diagnostic cardiac catheterizations and interventional (PCI) procedures harvested from participating facilities across the nation. Listed here are aggregated data of 604,042 diagnostic cardiac catheterizations and 293,775 PCI procedures performed on patients discharged in 2005 from 462 participating facilities. Only records with valid responses to indicators were considered, and not all procedures qualified for every indicator.

†Contrast media reaction, cardiogenic shock, cerebrovascular accident, congestive heart failure, cardiac tamponade, renal failure.

‡Bleeding at entry site (femoral approach), vascular access occlusion at entry site, peripheral embolization, vascular dissection, pseudoaneurysm, arteriovenous fistula.

§Percentage of patients receiving antiplatelet therapy such as clopidogrel (Plavix) or ticlopidine (Ticlid) during admission.

¶Elapsed time between entry to facility and reperfusion of the affected coronary vessel for patients with acute myocardial infarction treated with primary PCI.

¶PCI mortality rate adjusted by ACC-NCDR Risk Adjustment Algorithm.

From American Heart Association Heart and Stroke Fact Book 2006. Dallas, TX, American Heart Association 2006.

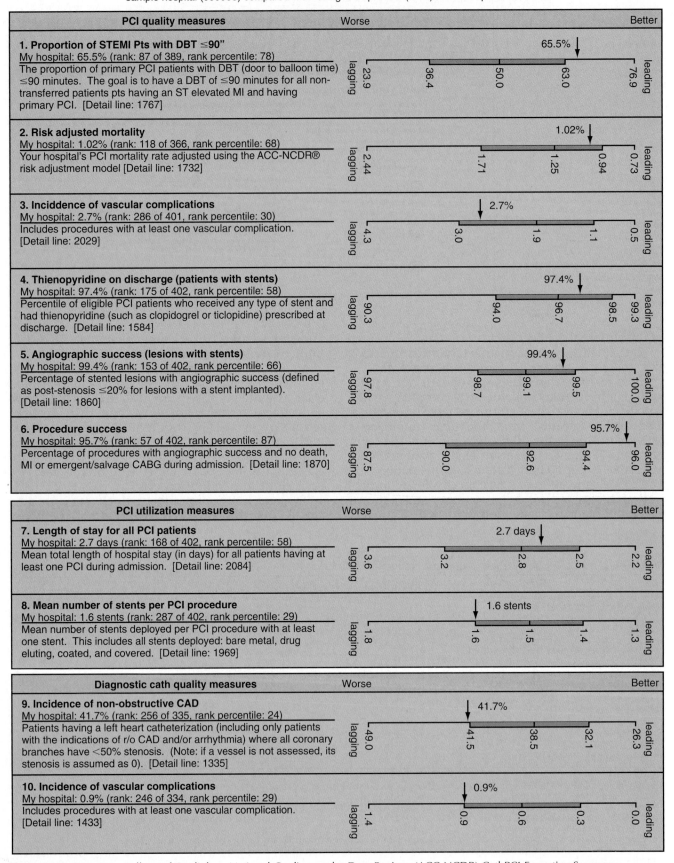

Executive summary
PCI and diagnostic catheterization performance measures
sample hospital (999998) compared with rolling four quarters (R4Q) for all hospitals - 2005Y3

Figure 66-7. American College of Cardiology-National Cardiovascular Data Registry (ACC-NCDR) CathPCI Executive Summary Performance Measures. Sample hospital executive summary page of the ACC-NCDR CathPCI (version 3) 2005 Quarterly Report displaying 10 performance measures surrounding percutaneous coronary intervention (PCI) quality, PCI utilization, and diagnostic catheterization quality. Available at: http://www.accncdr.com.

CathPCI™ report: executive summary

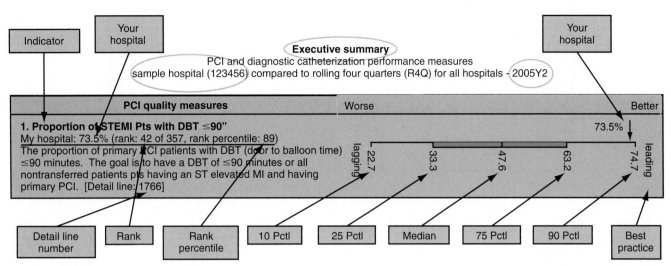

Figure 66-8. American College of Cardiology–National Cardiovascular Data Registry (ACC-NCDR) CathPCI Executive Performance Measure description. Explanation of the performance measure benchmarking methodology of the ACC-NCDR CathPCI (version 3) 2005 Quarterly Report. Available at: http://www.accncdr.com.

rates[45,46] (Fig. 66-10). Klein and colleagues reported PCI mortality data from more than 8800 octogenarians from the ACC-NCDR CathPCI Registry. The overall in-hospital PCI mortality rate was 3.77%, whereas the mortality rate among NCDR octogenarians undergoing elective PCI was 1.35%. In-hospital mortality in NCDR octogenarians with an AMI less than 6 hours before PCI was 13.8%.[47] Registry studies such as these can not only help guide physicians, patients, and families to make difficult treatment decisions at the bedside but offer valuable information to guidelines committees, because octogenarians usually are excluded from clinical trials. Similarly of value for clinicians, patients, and their families are

the data, also published by Klein and colleagues, on a risk prediction model for performance of emergent PCI in the setting of cardiogenic shock associated with AMI.[48]

Postmarket device and drug surveillance is also ideally suited to using the high-volume and good-quality data available through the NCDR, particularly because low-frequency adverse events are best discovered via a registry format. Because of the large number of patients tracked, the registries can identify important signals against the background of random noise. For example, the ACC-NCDR CathPCI has published safety and efficacy data concerning vascular closure devices, in partnership with the U.S. Food

Table 66-3.   ACC-NCDR CathPCI Risk-Adjusted PCI Mortality*

Factor	Odds (Coefficient)	95% CI	P Value
Shock	8.49 (2.139)	6.99 to 10.87	<.0001
Salvage vs. elective	13.38 (2.594)	8.38 to 21.34	<.0001
Emergent-stable vs. elective	5.75 (1.676)	4.37 to 7.57	<.0001
Urgent vs. elective	1.78 (0.548)	1.39 to 2.28	<.0001
IABP placed pre-PCI	1.68 (0.470)	1.08 to 2.63	<.05
Age (per 10 yr)	2.61, 11.25 (0.98, 2.43)	1.63 to 17.82	<.0001
LVEF (10% higher)	0.87, 3.93 (−0.17, 1.43)	0.66 to 15.41	<.0001
Acute MI within 24 hr	1.31 (0.270)	1.05 to 1.64	<.01
Lesion classification (SCAI II, II, IV)	1.64, 2.11 (0.49, 0.75)	1.28 to 2.70	<.0001
Left main disease	2.04 (0.680)	1.56 to 2.66	<.0001
Proximal LAD lesion	1.97 (0.263)	1.51 to 2.58	<.01
Renal failure	3.04 (1.113)	2.33 to 3.98	<.0001
Chronic lung disease	1.33 (0.287)	1.09 to 1.68	<.01
Diabetes	1.41 (0.340)	1.10 to 1.91	<.001
Use of non-stent device	1.64 (0.497)	1.38 to 2.00	<.0001
Use of thrombolytic	1.39 (0.344)	1.09 to 1.78	<.01

*Constant (intercept) = −4.464; C-index = 0.89.
ACC-NCDR, American College of Cardiology–National Cardiovascular Data Registry; CI, confidence interval; IABP, intra-aortic balloon pump; LAD, left anterior descending coronary artery; LVEF, left ventricular ejection fraction; MI, myocardial infarction; PCI, percutaneous coronary intervention; SCAI, Society for Cardiac Angiography and Interventions.
Data from Shaw RE, Anderson HV, Brindis RG, et al: Development of a risk adjustment mortality model using the American College of Cardiology-National Cardiovascular Data Registry (ACC-NCDR) Experience: 1998-2000. J Am Coll Cardiol 2002;39:1104-1112.

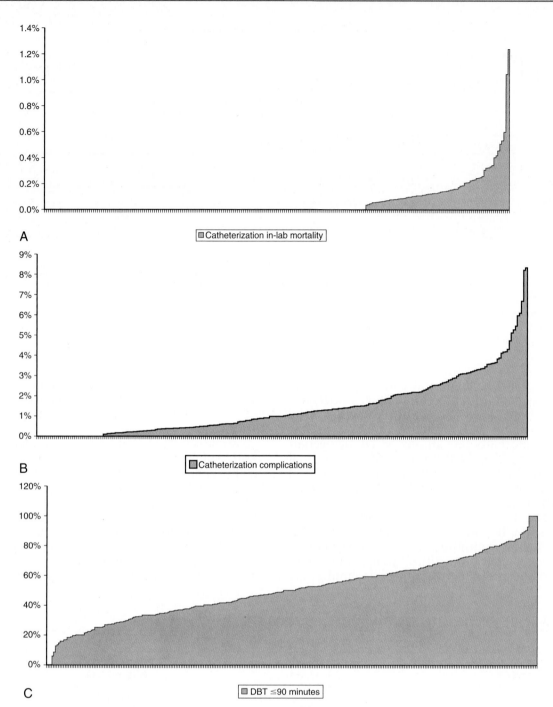

Figure 66-9. American College of Cardiology–National Cardiovascular Data Registry (ACC-NCDR) cardiac catheterization and percutaneous coronary intervention (PCI) data, 2005, displayed by hospital benchmarking. Vertical axis shows percentile; horizontal axis shows individual NCDR hospital data points. **A,** Diagnostic cardiac catheterization (Cath) in-lab mortality. **B,** Diagnostic cardiac catheterization (Cath) complications. **C,** Door-to-balloon time (DBT) <90 minutes for ST-segment elevation myocardial infarction (STEMI).

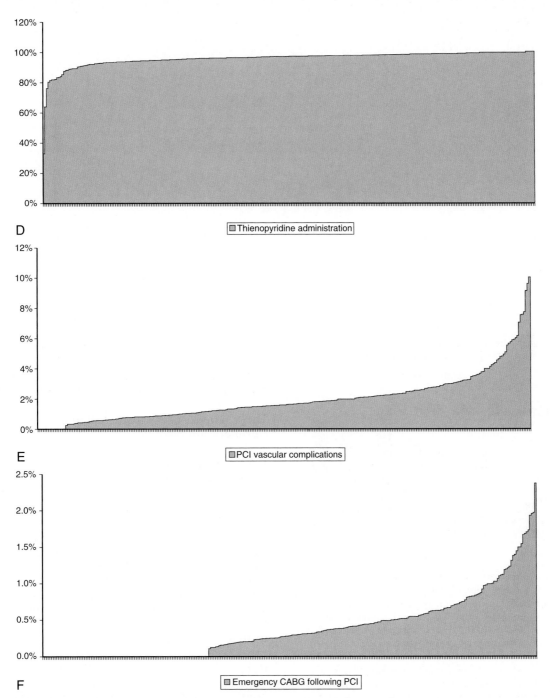

Figure 66-9, cont'd D, Thienopyridine use for PCI stent implantation. **E,** PCI vascular complications. **F,** Emergency coronary artery bypass surgery after PCI.

Continued

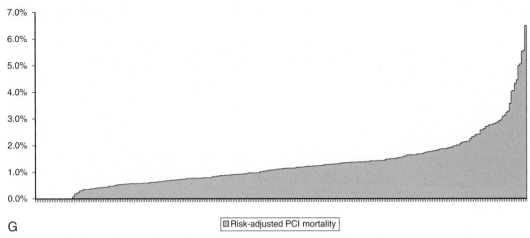

G

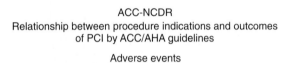

Figure 66-9, cont'd G, Risk-adjusted PCI in-hospital mortality rate (PCI RAM). Available at: http://www.accncdr.com.

ACC-NCDR
Relationship between procedure indications and outcomes
of PCI by ACC/AHA guidelines

Adverse events

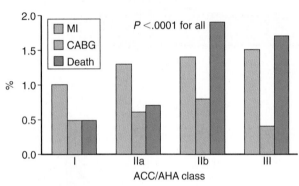

Figure 66-10. Adverse events (death, myocardial infarction [MI], and emergency coronary artery bypass grafting [CABG]) associated with percutaneous coronary interventions (PCI). From the American College of Cardiology–National Cardiovascular Data Registry (ACC-NCDR) CathPCI, stratified by American College of Cardiology/American Heart Association (ACC/AHA) Recommendation Classification. (Redrawn from Anderson HV, Shaw RE, Brindis RG, et al: Relationship between procedure indications and outcomes of percutaneous coronary interventions by American College of Cardiology/American Heart Association Task Force Guidelines. Circulation 2005;112:2786-2791.)

and Drug Administration[49] (Fig. 66-11). Long-term effectiveness of drug-eluting stents (e.g., morbidity, mortality, quality of life through assessment of angina burden) could provide important "real-world" experience regarding the effectiveness of these new innovations, with insights that could supplement the efficacy established in clinical trials. Issues surrounding recent concerns of late SAT with drug-eluting stents can be assessed in the large-patient-volume longitudinal registry format.

Data from registries can also provide performance metrics to payers to help implement "Pay for Perfor-

mance" programs (discussed later). The Virginia Quality In-Sights Hospital Incentive Program (QHIP) is using performance metrics derived from the ACC-NCDR CathPCI Registry to quantify and differentially reward cardiovascular performance quality.[50]

The Volume-Quality Relationship in Percutaneous Coronary Intervention

Until recently, many of state regulations focused on the perceived validity of the volume-quality relationship, both for individual physician operators and for a given hospital. Although there has been historical data suggesting a relationship between higher operator procedure volumes and improved outcome for PCI, similar data do not exist for diagnostic cardiac catheterization. The 2005 ACC/AHA/SCAI PCI guidelines offer a class I recommendation of a operator minimum volume of 75 PCI procedures per year and a hospital volume of 400 PCI procedures. These 2005 PCI guidelines offer a class IIa recommendation for individuals with operator volumes of less than 75 cases per year if they were performed in an institution performing more than 600 cases and if the low-volume operator has a defined, ongoing mentoring relationship with a high-volume operator at that institution. In addition, an institution performing 200 to 400 PCI procedures per year was given a class IIa recommendation if the operator was actually performing a volume of more than 75 cases per year.[3]

Using data from 1998-2000 obtained from the New York State registry, Hannan and colleagues examined the impact of hospital and operator volume on risk-adjusted in-hospital PCI mortality and same-day CABG surgery. Using a hospital volume threshold of 400 procedures per year, the odds ratio for low-volume versus high-volume hospitals was 1.98 for in-hospital mortality and 2.07 for same-day CABG surgery. Evaluating an operator volume threshold of 75 cases per year, there was no association of low-volume versus high-volume operators for mortality,

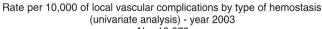

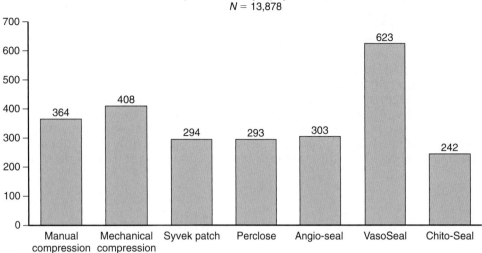

Rate per 10,000 of local vascular complications by type of hemostasis
(univariate analysis) - year 2003
$N = 13,878$

Figure 66-11. Rate per 10,000 patients of local vascular complications by type of hemostasis: Data from the American College of Cardiology–National Cardiovascular Data Registry (ACC-NCDR) CathPCI. (Redrawn from Tavris DR, Dey S, Weintraub WS, et al: Risk of local adverse events following cardiac catheterization by hemostasis device and gender. J Am Coll Cardiol 2005;45:40A.)

but there was an odds ratio of 1.65 for same-day CABG surgery based on operator volume threshold. The relationship between volume and quality was accentuated by analysis of the combined presence of both a low-volume hospital (<400 procedures per year) and a low-volume operator (<75 procedures per year) threshold, which demonstrated an odds ratio of 5.92 for mortality and 4.02 for same-day CABG surgery.[51]

However, the use of volume alone as a surrogate for quality in invasive cardiology is substantially flawed. Low-volume operators or low-volume hospitals can deliver high-quality care, while at the same time high-volume operators or high-volume hospitals can practice substandard care.[52-55] Use of advanced statistics with hierarchical modeling minimizes false inferences that traditional statistical techniques risk by ignoring the structure of the data.[56] In addition, much of the historical data supporting the volume-quality relationship is from the pre-stent era and also does not account for other technological advances in PCI procedures, nor for the advances in adjunctive medical therapy, such as platelet glycoprotein IIb/IIIa inhibitors, direct thrombin inhibitors, and pretreatment with clopidogrel. The actual measurement of PCI quality through data collection vehicles such as

the ACC-NCDR CathPCI Registry and the New York State PCI reporting system clearly is a preferable method to assess quality, compared with the use of the volume surrogate alone. Recent data from the ACC-NCDR CathPCI covering participating NCDR hospitals from 2001 to 2004 did not demonstrate a significant difference in in-hospital mortality based on hospital procedure volume[53] (Table 66-4).

Percutaneous Coronary Intervention without Onsite Surgical Backup

The 2005 PCI ACC/AHA/SCAI clinical guidelines state that primary PCI without cardiovascular surgery on-site (SOS) backup is a class IIb indication further requiring a minimum hospital caseload of 36 primary PCI cases per year performed by operators with an individual minimum PCI caseload of 75 cases per year. Furthermore, to meet this class IIb indication recommendation, a suggested minimum for an individual operator of 11 acute PCI interventions per year is described. The 2005 PCI ACC/AHA/SCAI clinical guidelines furthermore state that elective PCI without SOS is considered a class III recommendation. Nevertheless, there has been a noticeable and documented increasing trend in not only the number of

Table 66-4. In-Hospital Mortality Rate by Hospital PCI Volume and Type of Procedure, ACC-NCDR CathPCI, 2001-2004

Hospital PCI Volume (No. of Patients)	Odds Ratio (95% Confidence Interval)		
	STEMI ($n = 90,256$)	Non-STEMI ($n = 94,587$)	Elective ($n = 482,960$)
≤200 vs. >800	0.99 (0.75,1.31)	0.64 (0.38,1.06)	1.17 (0.81,1.71)
201-400 vs. >800	0.96 (0.83,1.12)	0.87 (0.68,1.10)	1.12 (0.96,1.31)
401-800 vs. >800	0.95 (0.85,1.07)	0.96 (0.81,1.14)	1.10 (0.99,1.22)
Mortality (%)	4.83	2.09	0.41

ACC-NCDR, American College of Cardiology–National Cardiovascular Data Registry; PCI, percutaneous coronary intervention; STEMI, ST-segment elevation myocardial infarction.
Data from Zhang Z, Veledar E, Foster J, et al: Relationship between Hospital Coronary Angioplasty Volume and In-Hospital Mortality: Results from the ACC-NCDR. Circulation 2005;112(Suppl II):792.

centers in the United States performing these procedures without SOS, but also the percentage of total PCIs being performed in the United States without SOS[57] (Fig. 66-12).

A number of state regulatory agencies already endorse or are exploring the institution of demonstration hospital sites to meet the perceived needs for an increased availability of primary PCI for management of ST-segment elevation myocardial infarction (STEMI). In some instances, states allow both primary PCI and elective PCI without SOS or are having these options evaluated through state-sponsored demonstration projects. The close scrutiny and accurate assessment of the quality of PCI without SOS should be incumbent on all cardiovascular stakeholders, because many of these hospitals are low-volume PCI centers and may also have low-volume operators.[58] Utilization of outcomes collection tools, such as those contained in the ACC-NCDR CathPCI, will be key in accurate quality assessment of this strategy of PCI delivery. Evaluation of the individual hospitals participating can be accomplished through the strength of the NCDR's PCI risk-adjusted mortality methodology and also by benchmarking outcomes with the national PCI data and that of similar hospitals that perform PCI without SOS.

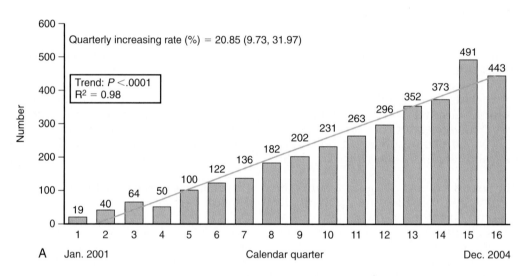

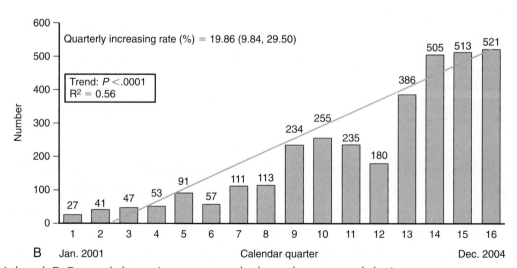

Figure 66-12. A through **D,** Temporal changes in percentage and volume of emergent and elective percutaneous coronary interventions (PCI) among hospitals participating in American College of Cardiology–National Cardiovascular Data Registry (ACC-NCDR) CathPCI™ from 2001 to 2004. (Redrawn from Dehmer GJ, Kutcher M, Dey SK, et al: Frequency of percutaneous coronary interventions at facilities without on-site cardiac surgical backup is increasing: A report from the American College of Cardiology–National Cardiovascular Data Registry (ACC-NCDR®). Am J Cardiol 2007;99:329-332. Epub 2006 Nov 29.

67 Regulatory Issues

Andrew Farb, Ashley B. Boam, David Buckles,
Wolf Sapirstein, and Daniel G. Schultz

KEY POINTS

- The mission of the U.S. Food and Drug Administration's Center for Devices and Radiological Health (CDRH) is to protect and promote the public health by ensuring that safe and effective medical devices reach the American public in a timely and efficient manner.
- CDRH regulates medical devices based on the Total Product Life Cycle, which encompasses every phase in the life of a medical device, from early inception through preclinical testing, clinical trials, marketing application, and postmarket monitoring of device performance.
- High-risk (class III) interventional cardiology devices such as intravascular stents and stent grafts, heart valves, and intracardiac shunt occlusion devices require submission of a Premarket Approval Application (PMA). PMA approval of new class III devices is based on valid scientific evidence that demonstrates that the device is both safe and effective for its intended uses.
- The PMA review and approval process of a new class III device consists of a comprehensive assessment of all relevant information, including device components and their manufacture, principles of operation and mechanism of action, proposed indications for use, preclinical studies, and all human clinical investigations.

- The rapid development and clinical use of interventional cardiac devices present multiple regulatory challenges to accommodate expeditious review and approval. Regulatory issues common to many innovative devices include (1) randomized versus nonrandomized trials and superiority versus noninferiority trials, (2) clinical trial sample size considerations for completely novel and next-generation devices, (3) study end points (clinical versus surrogate end points and appropriate study duration), (4) postmarket surveillance of approved devices, and (5) proof of concept versus clinical utility of novel devices, as well as the balance of safety and effectiveness for a percutaneous alternative to a surgical standard of care.
- It can be expected that interventional medical devices will continue their rapid development and use by interventional cardiologists. CDRH remains committed to working interactively with industry and academic sponsors in the design and execution of trials that collect valid scientific evidence, encompass real-world device utilization, and provide an assessment of clinically meaningful outcomes.

The Center for Devices and Radiological Health (CDRH) of the U.S. Food and Drug Administration (FDA) is tasked by Congress with ensuring that new medical devices demonstrate a reasonable assurance of safety and effectiveness before they are approved for commercial distribution in the United States. CDRH also monitors the performance of medical devices, once approved, to assess the continuing risk-benefit profile in the interests of protecting the public health.

FDA traces its origins as an organization to the Food and Drugs Act of 1906. In 1938, the Federal Food, Drug and Cosmetic (FD&C) Act was passed, extending coverage for the first time to devices and making it illegal to sell therapeutic devices that were dangerous or were being marketed with false claims. The first case prosecuted under the FD&C Act was in 1950 for a device marketed as an effective treatment for, among other ailments, insomnia, rheumatism, heart attack, dandruff, and paralysis. In this landmark case, the defendant was fined $1000, setting the precedent for future enforcement actions.

In the years between 1938 and 1969, the primary focus of medical device regulation was on radiation-emitting devices such as x-ray machines. In 1969, President Nixon called on Congress to set minimum performance standards and for the establishment of premarket clearance procedures for certain medical devices. The Department of Health, Education and Welfare formed The Cooper Committee, an advisory group that calculated that approximately 10,000 injuries and 700 deaths occurred annually due to so-called "therapeutic devices." The Committee recommended the inventory and classification of all existing medical devices as a precursor to legislation intended to regulate medical devices for the protection of the public health.

The landmark legislation that led directly to the formation of CDRH was the Medical Device Amendments of 1976 ("the Amendments"). The Amendments required that all medical devices be classified based on risks to patients (class I, II or III, discussed later) and mandated that all devices be subject to Federal Government regulation. In the years since 1976, FDA has steadily developed and refined the regulations to reflect the law enacted in the Amendments and in subsequent federal legislation such as the Safe Medical Devices Act of 1990.

CDRH has developed an integrated approach to medical device regulation based on the principles of the Total Product Life Cycle (TPLC) (Fig. 67-1). This approach encompasses every phase in the life of a medical device, from early inception through preclinical testing, clinical trials, marketing application, postmarket monitoring of device performance, and eventual withdrawal from the market due to obsolescence. By applying appropriate risk management strategies at each stage of product development and marketing, CDRH is able to promote innovative measures for assessing safety and effectiveness while ensuring the protection of public health. FDA in general, and CDRH in particular with medical devices, takes a measured approach to device regulation to ensure an optimal balance between expeditious approval of needed devices, especially if a significant treatment benefit is expected or if there are no viable alternatives, with a thorough evaluation of all aspects of device performance. The mission of CDRH is to protect and promote the public health by ensuring that safe and effective medical devices reach the American public in a timely and efficient manner. Further information about the history and mission

of CDRH can be found on the CDRH Web site (http://www.fda.gov/cdrh/centennial/devices.html).

ROLE OF CDRH IN DEVICE DEVELOPMENT, EVALUATION, AND APPROVAL

Regulatory Terminology and Device Development Paradigms

FDA plays a critical role in multiple stages of device development. As a manufacturer begins the process of device design, produces a prototype, and initiates bench and animal testing, various regulations apply. For example, manufacturers comply with design controls, an interrelated set of practices and procedures, throughout the device development process. Generally, design controls are intended to ensure that device characteristics and performance are measured against a clear set of design inputs to increase the likelihood that the design can translate into a product appropriate for its intended use. This is addressed in Good Manufacturing Practice (GMP) requirements (outlined in the *Code of Federal Regulations, 21 CFR Part 820*), which require manufacturers to have a Quality System for the design, manufacture, packaging, labeling, storage, installation, and servicing (where applicable) of finished medical devices intended for commercial distribution in the United States. The Quality System includes such aspects as manufacturing standard operating procedures, quality controls, complaint-handling procedures, and clearly defined roles for company management to ensure appropriate employee training and accountability. Each device manufacturer undergoes an FDA inspection to evaluate compliance. The manufacturer's design control procedures and Quality System are considered critical components of GMPs to ensure that safe and effective devices can be and are reproducibly manufactured. The FDA's guidance docu-

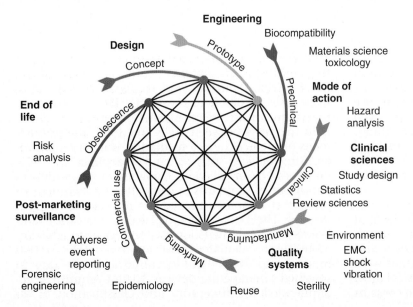

Figure 67-1. The total product life cycle (TPLC) as viewed by U.S. Food and Drug Administration's FDA's Center for Devices and Radiological Health (CDRH). Medical devices follow a continuum of development phases. Product risk and benefit assessments occur at all stages of the product life cycle.

ment, "Design Control Guidance For Medical Device Manufacturers" (http://www.fda.gov/cdrh/comp/designgd.pdf) is a valuable resource for additional information.

The facility performing nonclinical testing on a new class III device should be in compliance with Good Laboratory Practices (GLP; see 21 CFR 58). If clinical testing is conducted in humans, regulations intended to protect the welfare of those subjects apply, including the requirements for informed consent, Institutional Review Board (IRB) approval, and, if the study presents a significant risk and is to be conducted in the United States, an FDA-approved Investigational Device Exemption (IDE) (21 CFR Parts 50, 56, and 812).

FDA regulates the marketing of medical devices using a risk-based approach, categorizing devices into three categories. The requirements for marketing are then commensurate with the level of risk. Class I devices are the lowest-risk devices and are subject only to General Controls. General Controls are the baseline requirements of the Food, Drug and Cosmetic Act (as amended) that apply to all medical devices. They consist of registration and listing requirements, GMPs, labeling requirements banning provisions, medical device reporting (MDR) requirements, and submission of a premarket notification (called a "510[k]" after the section of the Act in which it is described). The vast majority of class I devices are exempt from the requirement to submit a 510(k) before marketing. Elastic bandages and certain manual hand-held surgical instruments are examples of class I devices.

Moderate-risk devices are termed class II, and most require the submission of a 510(k) application before the device can be cleared for marketing. In addition to General Controls, class II devices must also comply with Special Controls, which may consist of device-specific labeling requirements, performance standards, or postmarket surveillance. Examples of class II cardiovascular devices are guidewires, guide catheters and introducers, hemostasis devices, and embolic protection devices.

The highest-risk devices are categorized as class III; they are those devices for which insufficient information exists to ensure safety and effectiveness solely through General or Special Controls. A class III device is one for which General and Special Controls are insufficient to provide reasonable assurance of the device type and is purported or represented to be for a use in supporting or sustaining human life or for a use that is of substantial importance in preventing impairment of human health or presents a potential unreasonable risk of illness or injury. An IDE application is required to conduct clinical studies when the device (1) is intended as an implant and presents a potential for serious risk to the health, safety, or welfare of a subject; (2) is for use in supporting or sustaining human life and represents a potential for serious risk to the health, safety, or welfare of a subject; (3) is for a use of substantial importance in diagnosing, curing, mitigating, or treating disease or otherwise preventing impairment of human health and presents a potential for serious risk to the health, safety, or welfare of a subject; or (4) otherwise presents a potential for serious risk to a subject (21 CFR 812.3[m]). Many IDE applications involve class III devices and should contain basic information about the device and the planned study, such as a detailed device description, proposed indications for use, a report of prior investigations including reports of all nonclinical studies (bench and animal), previous clinical experience, a summary of the manufacturing process, the proposed investigational plan, and proposed labeling and informed consent documents to be used in the study (see 21 CFR 812 for full requirements). In most cases, marketing of class III devices requires the submission and approval of a Premarket Approval Application (PMA, discussed later) before marketing. Class III cardiovascular devices include intravascular stents, abdominal aortic aneurysm grafts, surgically and percutaneously deployed heart valves, and intracardiac shunt occlusion devices.

For those devices that require a 510(k) submission before marketing, the manufacturer must demonstrate that the new device is "substantially equivalent" to one or more legally marketed devices. A legally marketed device is (1) a device that was legally marketed before May 28, 1976 and does not require PMA approval; (2) a device that has been reclassified from class III to class II or I; (3) a device that has been found to be substantially equivalent to a marketed device through the 510(k) process; or (4) one established through Evaluation of Automatic Class III Designation. The legally marketed device (or devices) to which equivalence is drawn is known as the "predicate" device. To make a claim of substantial equivalence to a predicate device, the manufacturer must show that the intended use and the technological characteristics of the new device and the predicate device are the same. If the new device has different technological characteristics, the differences must not raise new safety and effectiveness concerns, and the manufacturer must demonstrate that the new device is at least as safe and effective as the predicate. This is typically accomplished through a comparison of device descriptive characteristics, proposed labeling, and performance data, which may include bench, animal, and/or clinical testing (although fewer than 10-15% of class II devices require clinical data).

PMA-approval of new class III devices is based on valid scientific evidence that demonstrates that the device is both safe and effective for its intended uses. Valid scientific evidence is defined in the regulations as a hierarchy of data ranging from well-controlled investigations, partially controlled studies, studies without matched controls, well-documented case histories conducted by qualified experts, to reports of significant human experience with a marketed device. These data, assessed by qualified experts, are intended to provide a reasonable assurance of the safety and effectiveness of a device under its conditions of use (see 21 CFR 814 or http://www.fda.gov/cdrh/

devadvice). A PMA application (Table 67-1) should contain full information about the device and its intended uses, including a complete and detailed description of the device, its components and principles of operation; the proposed indications for use; alternative treatments for the disease or condition; technical sections describing nonclinical studies; the results of all human clinical investigations (e.g., studies conducted under an IDE and any other clinical studies of the device); a description of the methods, facilities, and controls used in the manufacture, processing, packing, storage, and, where appropriate, installation of the device; marketing history (if the device has been previously marketed either within the United States under a previous marketing approval or clearance, or outside of the United States); a bibliography of any relevant published information; proposed labeling; and a Summary of Safety and Effectiveness Data, which summarizes the device, studies conducted on the device, and conclusions drawn from those studies (see 21 CFR 814 for full application requirements). A schematic overview of the regulatory pathways for new device introduction into the U.S. market is presented in Figure 67-2.

The Office of Device Evaluation (ODE) consists of five system-specific divisions, including the Division of Cardiovascular Devices (DCD), each further subdivided into organ- and device-related branches. FDA encourages manufacturers to contact the specific branch responsible for review of a particular device for guidance during all stages of the device regulatory process. Through the pre-IDE process, a manufacturer can submit proposed test protocols for nonclinical (bench and/or animal testing) or clinical evaluations of a new device for informal feedback within 60 days, by telephone, fax, e-mail, or in an in-person meeting. This process can be used more than once during development. For example, it may be helpful to have FDA provide initial informal comments on animal studies to be conducted, then have a later meeting to discuss planned clinical studies once some nonclinical testing on the device has been completed. For more on the pre-IDE process, please see "Guidance on IDE Policies and Procedures" at http://www.fda.gov/cdrh/ode/idepolicy.pdf.

Total Product Life Cycle

CDRH's commitment to the TPLC encompasses all phases of the life of a device (from concept to obsolescence) and provides a means for comprehensive, integrated medical device regulation. In practice, TPLC has meant that traditional barriers within the Center among premarket assessment teams, postmarket surveillance efforts, and compliance enforcement actions and inspections have been superseded by an integrated approach to medical device regulation. Although the implementation of TPLC has depended primarily on coordination of effort across multiple offices within the Center aimed at a balance among premarket, postmarket, and enforcement strategies,

Table 67-1. Required Elements for a Premarket Approval Application (PMA)

1. Applicant's name and address
2. Table of contents
3. Summary of safety and effectiveness data
   a. Indications for use
   b. Device description
   c. Alternative practices and procedures
   d. Marketing history
   e. Summary of nonclinical studies
   f. Summary of clinical studies
   g. Conclusions drawn from the studies
4. Complete descriptions of:
   a. The device, including pictures
   b. Each device component
   c. The properties of the device relevant to the diagnosis, treatment, prevention, cure, or mitigation of a disease or condition
   d. The principles of operation of the device
   e. The methods, facilities, and controls used in the manufacture, processing, packing, storage, and, where appropriate, installation of the device
5. Reference to any performance standard or voluntary standard
6. Technical sections containing data and information in sufficient detail to permit FDA to determine whether to approve or deny the application
   a. Results of nonclinical laboratory studies such as microbiology, toxicology, immunology, biocompatibility, stress, wear, shelf life, and other laboratory or animal testing
   b. Results of clinical investigations involving human subjects including
      (1) Clinical protocols
      (2) Number of investigators and subjects per investigator
      (3) A discussion of subject selection and exclusion criteria
      (4) Study population demographics
      (5) Study period
      (6) Safety and effectiveness data
      (7) Adverse reactions and complications
      (8) Patient discontinuation
      (9) Patient complaints
      (10) Device failures and replacements
      (11) Tabulations of data from all individual subject reporting forms and copies of such forms for each subject who died or did not complete the study
      (12) Results of statistical analyses
      (13) Contraindications and precautions for use of the device
      (14) Any other information from the clinical studies as appropriate
7. For a PMA supported solely by data from one investigator, a justification showing why data and other information from a single investigator is sufficient to demonstrate the safety and effectiveness of the device and to ensure reproducibility of test results
8. Bibliography of all published reports that are known to or should be reasonably known to the applicant and concern the safety or effectiveness of the device
9. One or more samples of the device
10. Copies of all proposed labeling
11. Environmental assessment or environmental impact statement
12. Financial certification or disclosure statement or both (see 21 CFR 54)
13. Such other information as FDA may request.

CFR, *Code of Federal Regulations*; FDA, Food and Drug Administration.

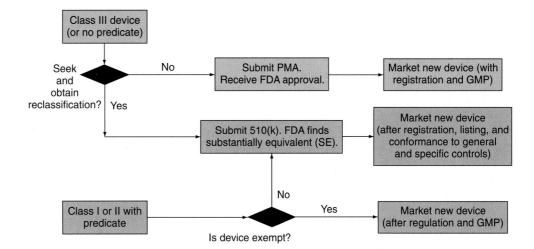

Figure 67-2. Regulatory pathways for new device introduction into the U.S. market. FDA, Food and Drug Administration; GMP, Good Manufacturing Practice; PMA, Premarket Approval Application.

successful implementation of this plan has also involved a broad range of related initiatives. A network of internal and external partners, active on the leading edge of medical device development, provides a means for accelerating the review of priority devices to address areas of high public health need. Further information regarding TPLC can be found at http://www.fda.gov/cdrh/strategic/tplc.html.

Premarket Versus Postmarket Considerations

FDA utilizes an integrated approach to medical device regulation, which is evident in the interactions between the areas of premarket assessment and postmarket surveillance within the Center. The premarket assessment teams within the ODE and the postmarket surveillance analysts in the Office of Surveillance and Biometrics (OSB) were originally developed to handle separate aspects of device regulation, with ODE conducting device assessments before allowing devices on the market and OSB monitoring device performance. TPLC has fostered closer collaboration between the ODE and OSB teams, and this has led to the development of more innovative approaches to balance premarket assessment and postmarket surveillance. For example, the overall performance of a given medical device may reflect short-term factors such as deployability and stability, combined with long-term factors such as resistance to wear and corrosion. Additionally, in contrast to drugs, most devices are continuously modified in an effort to improve their performance, and preclinical and clinical studies may be needed to detect consequences (intended and unintended) of these changes. The TPLC approach has allowed the Center to spread the management of risks associated with medical devices across the premarket and postmarket phases, and this in turn has promoted faster time to market for innovative devices while still ensuring protection of the public health. Communication with medical device developers and manufacturers has become more efficient and effective because closer collaboration among offices has led to more consistent regulation across the product life cycle.

CDRH INTERACTIONS WITH THE MEDICAL COMMUNITY

In recent years, CDRH has undertaken a renewed effort to increase contact and cooperation with a wide variety of stakeholders. Effective communication with the medical device industry has always been a key element in the Center's mission to protect and promote public health. In most cases, CDRH does not specify the exact parameters of clinical trial protocols, preferring instead to develop protocols collaboratively with industry sponsors, with the goal of promoting well-designed clinical studies that can lead to innovative and successful products reaching the market in a timely fashion. Moreover, CDRH has also focused on collaborative interactions with industry trade groups to identify topics for guidance development, provide educational opportunities (e.g., Vendor Day and site visit programs), and cosponsor public workshops on issues of mutual interest including premarket evaluation, postmarket surveillance, and risk communication.

Representatives of the Center frequently attend and give presentations at academic meetings. These forums educate medical device regulators about issues associated with currently marketed devices, identify trends in new device development and innovative medical procedures, provide access to expertise within the academic community, and allow attendees to interact with regulators so that the Agency's responsibilities and actions can be better understood by health care providers. CDRH's interactions with academic medicine also include review of sponsor-investigator IDEs; in these clinical investigations, an individual, rather than a company, initiates and conducts the study. Clinical studies funded by the National Institutes of Health (NIH) that involve certain types of investigational devices must have an approved IDE *before* the study is initiated. FDA collaboration in studies funded by NIH can address safety and effectiveness questions relevant to device review regarding broad treatment strategies affecting several interventional devices (e.g., percutaneous catheter-based intervention versus coronary bypass surgery). The Center has also developed effective relationships with a number of professional societies, such as the Heart Rhythm Society (HRS) and the American College of Cardiology (ACC). A collaboration between CDRH and HRS regarding risks associated with implantable cardioverter-defibrillators provided an understanding of the issues associated with device recalls and risk communication with health care providers and the public. This type of collaboration enhances the Center's ability to protect and promote public health.

One of the major issues confronting medical device developers is reimbursement for procedures that employ innovative devices. Traditionally, there has been a separation between premarket assessment and regulation of devices by FDA and reimbursement of medical procedures as established by the Centers for Medicare and Medicaid Services (CMS). Although both of these organizations reside within the Department of Health and Human Services (HHS), the missions of each differ. The mission of CDRH is to ensure that medical devices are safe and effective, whereas CMS is charged with reimbursing medical procedures that are reasonable and necessary. As a consequence, medical device developers have typically been required to interact first with FDA and then, separately, with CMS. In an effort to streamline the introduction of innovative devices and medical procedures that are important to the public health, FDA and CMS have begun to work together in selected areas to explore the implications of new medical technologies, particularly with regard to identification of appropriate target patient populations and opportunities for data sharing.

KEY TOPICS IN CARDIOVASCULAR DEVICE REGULATION: CASE STUDIES

The rapid development and clinical use of interventional cardiac devices present multiple regulatory challenges to accommodate expeditious review and approval. The following case studies address regulatory issues common to many devices, including trial design considerations, study end points, label expansion and off-label use, proof of concept versus clinical utility, and the balance of safety and effectiveness.

Moving a Breakthrough Technology to the Next Generation: Regulatory Approaches to DES

Historical Background of the Initially Approved DES

The development and clinical adoption of percutaneous coronary intervention (PCI) procedures for atherosclerotic disease have evolved over the last 3 decades from balloon angioplasty (percutaneous transluminal coronary angioplasty, PTCA), to bare metal stents (offering improved acute outcomes, an enhanced ability to treat acute arterial complication, and a modest reduction in restenosis rates compared with PTCA), to drug-eluting stents (DES) (providing a significant reduction in restenosis rates compared with bare metal stents).

Based on the results of large randomized controlled trials (RCTs), FDA has approved two DESs: the CYPHER Sirolimus-Eluting Coronary Stent (PMA approved April 24, 2003) and the TAXUS Express Paclitaxel-Eluting Coronary Stent (PMA approved March 4, 2004). In the pivotal clinical trials for both devices (the SIRIUS study for the CYPHER stent and the TAXUS IV study for the TAXUS stent), both DES met their primary end points (a significant reduction in 9-month target vessel failure [TVF] for CYPHER and 9-month target vessel revascularization [TVR] for TAXUS compared to control bare metal stents). Additionally, the rates of TVF or major adverse cardiac events (MACE; composites of TVR, myocardial infarction [MI], and cardiac death) were reduced for both devices. The clinical benefit of the DES was demonstrated by reduced target lesion and target vessel revascularization rates; there was no reduction in the rate of death or MI. The dramatic reduction in restenosis rates associated with DES use resulted in the enthusiastic adoption of DES in the United States, which led to DES use in more than 80% of PCI procedures.

General Regulatory Considerations for the Next Generation of DESs

Medical devices commonly undergo modifications during the product life cycle. In the case of DES, these developments may consist of new combinations of stent metal alloys (e.g., 316L stainless steel, cobalt chromium, nitinol), configurations (open and closed ring designs with a variety of linkers between rings and struts with laser cut wells for drug deposition), coatings (polymeric and nonpolymeric, basecoats and topcoats, erodable versus nonerodable), antiproliferative agents (including sirolimus analogues and others), elution pharmacokinetics (initial burst phase, extended drug release, lipophilic properties), and completely biodegradable stent systems. The amount of preclinical and clinical data needed to support FDA approval of a new DES depends on the novelty of the device components and their mechanisms of action.

A comprehensive set of preclinical bench testing and in vivo animal studies are required to fully characterize the drug-device combination product, including pharmacology and toxicology of the eluted drug, coating evaluation, drug release kinetics, and biocompatibility. Preclinical animal studies of coronary DES implantation typically show operator handing features of the device and evidence of device effectiveness in reducing in-stent neointimal thickening; however, the major focus of these in vivo implants is to demonstrate an acceptable level of safety so that initiation of a clinical trial in humans may be considered. Preclinical safety assessment includes an evaluation of stent endothelialization, thrombus deposition, inflammation, arterial injury and necrosis, arterial remodeling, and aneurysm formation. Because the mechanism of inhibition of in-stent neointimal growth by a DES often involves a delay in arterial healing, long-term animal studies, with stent analysis at least through 180 days, are particularly useful. Separate studies of overlapping stents and stents with drug dosages in multiples of the intended clinical dose (which expose the arterial wall to an "overdose" of eluted drug) are important to simulate clinical practice, and the overlapped region provides the opportunity to evaluate a drug overdosage safety margin.

A PMA application for a completely new DES or a DES that incorporates major changes from an approved device commonly includes a staged clinical development plan to establish a reasonable assurance of device safety and effectiveness. Relatively small feasibility trials (which may be performed in the United States or outside the United States) are typically completed to support initiation of a larger, pivotal, randomized, controlled trial of the new DES compared with an FDA-approved DES. Pivotal trials typically involve several hundred patients and include a clear statement of the product's intended use, a study hypothesis, primary and secondary end points, criterion for study success, well-defined clinical and angiographic inclusion and exclusion criteria, case report forms, risk-benefit analyses, and informed consent documents. The inclusion criteria should be sufficiently broad so that the demographic and clinical characteristics of the enrolled subjects are representative of a typical patient population with symptomatic coronary atherosclerosis (with a sufficient number of women and patients with traditional coronary risk factors, often in combination). Enrollment commonly requires documentation of clinical ischemia based on symptoms with a positive function study (cardiac stress test) or a recent acute coronary ischemic syndrome. Subjects may have stable symptoms or may have been stabilized after an acute coronary ischemic syndrome. Special clinical presentations that may be expected to have heightened safety and effectiveness concerns, such as acute ST-segment elevation myocardial infarction (STEMI), are usually considered in an independent trial that is specific for that clinical indication.

The angiographic inclusion criteria identify the intended anatomic target of the DES (e.g., denovo lesions with at least 50% stenosis, with specified reference vessel diameters and lesion lengths). A trial of new DES compared to an FDA-approved device may exclude highly complex lesions that are known to be associated with elevated adverse event rates during PCI and which are beyond the intended use of the approved DES (see later). However, inclusion criteria that are so restrictive with respect to common patient and lesion characteristics may lead to trial results that are not particularly relevant to current interventional cardiology practice.

Independent monitoring of clinical trials is critically important to patient protection and the integrity of study outcomes. It is recognized that coronary stents are permanent implants, and DESs are novel combination products for which long-term risks are not completely known. Therefore, data safety and monitoring boards (DSMB) are established to track MACE events (including stent thrombosis episodes) as study enrollment progresses. Ideally, the independent DSMB sets, prior to study initiation, the expected number of meetings, timing of reports, and appropriate study stopping rules. For DES with novel components, the DSMB may provide periodic safety updates to FDA, which provide the Agency with real-time safety information and facilitate a more continuous patient enrollment, rather than enrollment of a limited number of patients and submission of initial data prior to study expansion. An independent clinical events committee adjudicates events among study subjects. Independent core laboratories provide expert and reproducible interpretation of special studies (e.g., coronary angiography, intravascular ultrasound [IVUS]).

Randomized Versus Nonrandomized Trials and Superiority Versus Noninferiority Trials

RCTs offer distinct statistical and interpretive advantages compared to other trial designs. However, completion of RCTs may be precluded by sample size and enrollment challenges especially during the maturation phase of device development where clinical equipoise may no longer exist. An RCT would be appropriate for a novel DES, which uses a completely new stent design, a new molecular entity (NME) drug (a drug that contains no active moiety that has been approved by FDA in any other application submitted under section 505(b) of the Federal Food, Drug, and Cosmetic Act [FFDCA]), and/or unique elution kinetics. A single-arm clinical study in a limited number of subjects with an historical control may be a reasonable choice for a serial iteration of an approved DES (e.g., a smaller-diameter stent that uses an identical stent platform, drug, polymer coating, drug density, and elution kinetics as a previously approved stent with a larger diameter). For a new DES that has significant differences from an approved device but is not completely novel (e.g., a change in stent coating that affects elution kinetics), either an RCT or a single-arm study with historical controls may be considered, depending on the nature of the modifications and expected impact on device effectiveness and patient safety.

Given the demonstrated superiority of the current FDA-approved DESs (compared with bare metal stents) with respect to their reduction in repeat revascularization rates and their high penetrance into interventional cardiology practice, it may no longer be feasible in the United States to test a new DES against a bare metal stent (control) in a randomized superiority clinical trial. Therefore, if randomized studies are indicated, a noninferiority (or equivalence) trial design may be the study design of choice with an approved DES serving as the "active" control. A noninferiority design is *not* the same as finding a nonsignificant probability value in a typical superiority trial (which may be due insufficient statistical power), and true equivalence cannot be proven statistically (because it would require a study of infinite size). Instead, a noninferiority trial uses a clinically relevant numerical margin (or "delta") that sets a boundary for finding two treatments equivalent if the treatment outcome falls within the delta.[1] The noninferiority margin is selected in consultation with the FDA and is prespecified before the initiation of the trial.

An important consideration for noninferiority trials is the potential for *outcome drift* after several noninferiority studies. In this scenario, each subsequent new, slightly inferior DES is deemed statistically noninferior to its immediate predecessor (i.e., differences in the primary end point fall within the allowable range of delta), raising the possibility that, after serial trials, a later-generation DES could be no better or even inferior to the original placebo treatment (i.e., a bare metal stent). To prevent outcome drift, one can perform statistical sensitivity testing to demonstrate the robustness of study outcome, include an imputed placebo, and/or apply "upper bound" constraints on DES performance. Although noninferiority trials are widely utilized during the evolutionary phases of DES development, this does not preclude a superiority trial proposal with a clinically relevant margin of superiority.

Clinical Versus Angiographic Study End Points and Study Duration for End Point Determination

For a pivotal DES trial, an emerging consensus within the clinical cardiology community appears to support a clinical, rather than an angiographic, primary end point. The most commonly used primary clinical end point is MACE (a safety and effectiveness composite of cardiac death, nonfatal MI, and ischemia-driven TVR) or TVF (a composite of cardiac death, nonfatal MI attributable to the target vessel, and TVR). For non-complex de novo lesions in clinically stable patients, rates of death and MI in current DES trials are sufficiently low that differences between the new DES and an FDA-approved device (noninferiority trial) or a bare metal stent (superiority trial) are expected to be driven by TVR rates.

Important secondary end points include the rates of the individual components of MACE and TVF and acute procedural outcomes such as stent deliverability, deployment, and stenosis reduction without the need for adjunctive dilation therapies. For a new DES, angiographic follow-up in a subset of subjects is useful to assess local biologic responses such as in-stent neointimal proliferation (percent stent diameter stenosis, late loss, and late loss index), and angiography can be used to determine the binary restenosis rate (>50% diameter stenosis at follow-up). IVUS is particularly useful in evaluating stent volume obstruction by neointimal tissue and stent strut malapposition to the underlying arterial wall. Both angiography and IVUS can identify aneurysm formation and adverse edge effects proximal and distal to the stent.

Although follow-up coronary angiography can provide important DES mechanistic insights, it may also introduce potentially confounding data in regard to TVR rates. Patients who undergo follow-up angiography are significantly more likely to have repeat revascularization procedures based on the "oculo-stenotic reflex." In these circumstances, repeat PCI procedures may be performed irrespective of whether clinical signs and/or symptoms of ischemia are present. Strategies used to mitigate TVR rate inflation as a result of the oculo-stenotic reflex are assessment of the clinical end point before per-protocol angiographic follow-up or angiographic follow-up in a cohort of patients separate from the pivotal study subjects. Additionally, one could propose specific criteria for "ischemia-driven TVR"; for example, only TVRs that are associated with a significant stenosis, anginal symptoms, and objective evidence of ischemia would count toward the primary end point.

Study duration is determined to reflect the mechanism of action for the device and be sufficiently long to ensure that safety and effectiveness outcomes are relevant to the underlying disease process. For DESs, the clinical outcomes for the primary end point have been assessed at least 9 to 12 months after the index stent placement. This study duration, substantially longer than in previous trials of bare metal stents, is based on the time course of neointimal growth inhibition associated with DES use. The trial must be suitably long so as to provide a reasonable degree of assurance that there is no significant worsening in MACE rates over time (i.e., the DES merely delays rather than prevents TVR over the near term) and that there are no major unanticipated safety concerns (see also postmarket considerations, discussed later). In general, assessment of the primary end point at 12 months with subject follow-up through 5 years (to be continued, in part, following marketing approval) appears to be an appropriate model for the evaluation of DES across the product life cycle.

Sample Size Considerations

For a pivotal trial, sample size reflects overall study design (superiority, noninferiority, or both) and estimates of differences in outcomes between the treatment groups. Pivotal trials are also sized to provide a robust evaluation of device safety. DES program submissions to date, inclusive of feasibility studies, the large pivotal trial, and other clinical experience with device (e.g., side registry studies), have included a total of at least 2000 patients implanted with the new DES. The 2000 subject cohort is based on an ability to identify low-frequency, clinically severe events such as death or stent thrombosis; data on a population of 2000 subjects provides the ability to detect catastrophic safety events that occur at a 1% rate, with an upper 95% confidence bound of 1.4%.

To fulfill the general recommendation of the need for large study sample sizes, it should be understood that not all patients need to be part of randomized trials. Further, the FDA is permitted to consider studies performed outside the United States as supportive evidence for U.S. product approval (21 CFR 814.15). The use of multiple study sites both within and outside the United States offers the potential benefit of enhanced generalizability of the study results. However, when data are collected outside of the United States to support PMA approval, it is important to demonstrate that they are applicable to the U.S. population. This may include an assessment of differences in patient demographic and clinical characteristics and standards of medical care (including the availability of testing and availability of adjunctive medications). Statistical analyses can evaluate comparability of study results across treatment centers and across geographic locations.

Label Expansion and Off-Label Use: The Case of DES

Like many innovative and promising drugs and devices that are widely adopted by health care providers, clinical use of DES may expand beyond the labeled indication that was established in selected patient populations or lesions present in the preapproval clinical trials submitted to FDA. It is instructive to review the restricted anatomic features stated in the indications for use statements for the currently approved DESs as of July 2007 (http://www.fda.gov/cdrh/pdf2/P020026.html and http://www.fda.gov/cdrh/pdf3/P030025.html):

- The CYPHER Sirolimus-Eluting Coronary Stent is indicated for improving coronary luminal diameter in patients with symptomatic ischemic disease due to discrete de novo lesions of length ≤30 mm in native coronary arteries with reference vessel diameter of 2.5 mm to 3.5 mm.
- The TAXUS Express Paclitaxel-Eluting Coronary Stent System is indicated for improving luminal diameter for the treatment of de novo lesions ≤28 mm in length in native coronary arteries 2.5 to 3.75 mm in diameter.

These basic lesion descriptions do not address the wide heterogeneity of coronary atherosclerotic lesions that are commonly subjected to PCI, including bifurcations, chronic total occlusions, thrombus-containing acutely ruptured lesions (in acute MI), post-PTCA or in-stent restenosis, ostial lesions, left main coronary artery disease, and coronary bypass grafts. In addition, subjects with important cardiovascular and noncardiovascular comorbidities (e.g., significant left ventricular or renal dysfunction, recent MI) were excluded from the pivotal DES trials.

Use of the FDA-approved DESs in more complex lesion and patient subsets is considered to be off-label use. Off-label use is defined as use of a medical product for treatments other than explicitly included in product labeling. This does not mean that off-label use by an individual physician for an individual patient is inappropriate or represents substandard clinical practice. However, in many cases, it does mean that clinical data from well-designed trials has not been collected to establish a reasonable assurance of safety and effectiveness for these off-label uses. It should be noted that FDA does not regulate the practice of medicine: "Nothing in this Act [FDAMA § 906 (21 USC § 396)] shall be construed to limit or interfere with the authority of a health care practitioner to prescribe or administer any legally marketed device to a patient for any condition or disease within a legitimate health care practitioner-patient relationship." Practice of medicine activities include discussing treatments with patients, using treatments on patients, and discussing treatments with other physicians in the course of professional activity.

While FDA recognizes the importance of allowing individual physicians to use legally marketed devices according to their best clinical judgement, there are multiple off-label use issues that may potentially compromise optimal evidence-based medical care. As noted, off-label uses are not subject to a rigorous premarket approval process, and widely applied off-label use may diminish or eliminate the incentive for a manufacturer to study or seek FDA approval for the indication for which the therapy is being applied. Because rigorous clinical trial data for off-label use may not be collected, it may be difficult to fairly evaluate and correct device problems that emerge. Off-label use may also expose physicians to potential medical-legal questions if complications occur, and data may be insufficient for patients to provide fully informed consent decisions.

The likelihood of unexpected outcomes is likely to be increased when devices are deployed to treat lesions that are inherently more complex than those treated in the preapproval clinical trials and for which only limited data are available. In the case of DES, single-arm studies in complex lesions may demonstrate reduced effectiveness and/or safety compared with more "straightforward" lesions, but it can be difficult to interpret the significance of outcome differences in the absence of a valid control group. For example, if a registry study of DES used in thrombus-containing lesions (in the setting of acute MI) showed a doubling of the rate of observed periprocedural MIs when compared with stable coronary lesions, it would be difficult to appreciate the significance of this difference without a well-matched, valid control group such as subjects treated with bare metal stents or thrombolytic therapy.

Completion of scientifically sound studies to define the optimal role of DES in complex lesion and patient subsets is clearly a desirable goal. To this end, FDA has worked collaboratively with DES manufacturers, the NIH, and investigators in the design, initiation, and review of novel clinical trials to address widely used treatment strategies for which there is an established standard of care, and FDA is willing to consider other creative trial designs within the framework of an RCT. For example, CABG is the standard of care for patients with left main disease or proximal three-vessel disease. Currently, multivessel revascularization (including left main disease) with DES versus

CABG is being explored in the TAXUS Drug-Eluting Stent Versus Coronary Artery Bypass Surgery for the Treatment of Narrowed Arteries (SYNTAX) trial using a noninferiority design. Additionally, a randomized controlled superiority design of multivessel stenting versus CABG focused on diabetics is being employed in the Future Revascularization Evaluation in Patients with Diabetes Mellitus: Optimal Management of Multivessel Disease (FREEDOM) trial. PCI with bare metal stents is the standard treatment for most individuals with acute STEMI, but the safety and efficacy of deploying a DES in a thrombus-containing lesion associated with an acutely disrupted plaque has not been established. To investigate this issue, STEMI subjects in the Harmonizing Outcomes with Revascularization and Stents (HORIZONS) acute MI trial are randomized to either the TAXUS stent or the bare metal EXPRESS stent.

Whereas RCTs may be desirable, FDA recognizes that alternative study designs may be necessary for label expansion studies for specific lesion subsets. In the case of DESs, it is generally recognized that, given the high penetrance of DESs in the U.S. clinical practice of PCI procedures, a trial that requires subjects to be randomized to a control bare metal stent may not be feasible due to reluctance of patients to enroll. For example, if a sponsor wished to expand the DES label to treat long coronary lesions, the absence of a device approved for this indication (typically due to the lack of a comprehensive supportive dataset) would raise safety and informed consent concerns for individuals randomized to the control group. Therefore, to meet the issues associated with some label expansion studies, the use of a control derived from previous studies with patient-level data or the establishment of an optimal performance criterion historical control based on a broad-based literature review may be considered.

Postmarket Surveillance: The Case of DES Thrombosis

Postmarket surveillance is particularly relevant to the field of cardiovascular devices in view of the rapidity of technology advancement and shortened product life cycles. Therefore, extended follow-up of subjects enrolled in the pivotal randomized and registry preapproval studies (e.g., through 5 years for DES and other interventional cardiology implants), in addition to postmarket clinical studies, is critical to establishing, primarily, the long-term device safety and, secondarily, the long-term effectiveness of implanted devices.

A large database of patient exposure to the device as part of a PMA submission, supplemented by clinical experience via continued access registries that may be ongoing during the PMA review and approval process, provide valuable additional information regarding device performance. In recognition that the real-world safety and effectiveness experience with any new device may be different from that observed in premarket clinical trials, and particularly

for devices like DES when market penetrance has been extremely rapid, it is imperative that postapproval surveillance studies initiate enrollment at the time of PMA approval. Although the intended use and indications for use of an approved device are clearly described in the product's labeling and instructions for use, it is expected that these postapproval studies will include more complex patient and lesion subsets that were not part of the preapproval clinical trials. An appreciation of the true rate of rare but serious adverse events may emerge from the expanded database provided by these postapproval studies. These data can greatly enhance clinical decision-making by individual physicians by providing a balance of the risks and benefits of the expanded device use compared with alternative therapies.

A vexing issue that draws together the recommendation for large databases (from preapproval, continued access, and postapproval studies), off-label use, and need for well-designed clinical trials for label expansion is DES thrombosis and the optimal duration of dual antiplatelet therapy. Stent thrombosis, occurring after either bare metal stenting or DES placement, is often a catastrophic clinical event leading to sudden death or acute MI. In the randomized controlled pivotal trials for the two FDA-approved DES, the stent thrombosis rates through 9 to 12 months were less than 1% and were similar in the DES cohorts and in their respective control bare metal stent treatment groups.[2] However, a general consensus has emerged that the duration of risk for stent thrombosis is longer for DES than for bare metal stents, based on the DES mechanism of action; the inhibition of in-stent neointimal thickening is accompanied by a delay in or incomplete endothelial coverage of the DES. Hypersensitivity to a component of the DES (polymer or drug) may also be associated with prolonged local inflammatory reactions and stent thrombosis.

Identifying cases of DES thrombosis to determine the true frequency of this adverse event is problematic. In-stent luminal thrombosis detected during coronary angiography or at autopsy is unequivocal evidence, but many patients do not undergo follow-up angiography, and autopsy rates in the United States are exceedingly low, both among hospitalized patients and in cases of out-of-hospital sudden death. Counting only cases of unequivocal stent thrombosis (confirmed by angiography or autopsy) underestimates the true rate. Conversely, ascribing all new MIs or sudden cardiac deaths to stent thrombosis would inflate the rate of DES thrombosis, because coronary atherosclerosis is a multifocal, often progressive disease, and patients may have events secondary to rupture of a de novo plaque or die suddenly owing to a lethal arrhythmia in the absence of stent thrombosis. Because of these limitations, it has been proposed to separate stent thrombosis cases into general categories, such as definitive, probable, and possible: autopsy or angiography is required for a definitive stent thrombosis; an acute MI in the coronary artery distribution of a previously deployed DES constitutes probable stent thrombosis; and unexplained sudden death is considered a possible stent thrombosis.[3]

Higher rates of stent thrombosis than those observed in the pivotal randomized trials have been reported in several published studies of DES use in more complex lesion and patient subsets.[4-6] Independent predictors of DES thrombosis (including underlying renal dysfunction, reduced ejection fraction, bifurcation lesions, and in-stent restenosis lesions) reflect patient and lesion subsets of increased complexity compared to those enrolled in the preapproval DES pivotal trials.[4,5] It is noteworthy, however, that published data on DES thrombosis in real-world use are currently limited to relatively small, nonrandomized registry studies, so the true rate of DES thrombosis has not been established.

Compounding the uncertainty of the rare but relatively elevated DES thrombosis rates in increasingly complex lesion and patient subsets are questions regarding optimal dual antiplatelet therapy. There is general agreement based on small registry studies and anecdotal reports that noncompliance with or premature discontinuation of dual antiplatelet therapy is an important risk factor for DES thrombosis.[4,5] FDA has actively disseminated information to health care providers and patients regarding the need to seek guidance from cardiologists whenever changes in antiplatelet therapy are contemplated. An appreciation of the costs of prolonged dual antiplatelet therapy, particularly for individuals with limited financial resources, may influence the decision to deploy a DES versus a bare metal stent (for which 1 month of clopidogrel treatment is typically sufficient). Postintervention patient education programs that strongly convey the need for uninterrupted antiplatelet medication use may be particularly useful before hospital discharge.

With regard to the duration of dual antiplatelet therapy, in the pivotal SIRIUS trial of the CYPHER stent, patients were treated with clopidogrel or ticlopidine for 3 months, and in the TAXUS IV trial of the TAXUS Express stent, clopidogrel or ticlopidine was administered for 6 months. These antiplatelet regimens are reflected in the current DES labeling (as of July 2007). As noted earlier, however, the pivotal DES trial enrolled clinically stable patients with selected anatomically straightforward lesions; these patient and lesion types represent only a portion of real-world DES use. The causes of DES thrombosis are likely to be multifactorial, involving lesion characteristics (lumen diameter, lesion length, bifurcations, total occlusions, presence of thrombus), procedural characteristics (stent diameter and length, stent overlap), and patient characteristics (presence or absence of renal insufficiency, diabetes mellitus). It is conceivable that the optimal duration of dual antiplatelet therapy varies based on patient and lesion characteristics and that extended administration (e.g., 12 months or longer) may be beneficial in complex lesions that are inherently more prone to thrombosis. Physicians may choose to empirically extend dual antiplatelet coverage in response to DES thrombosis concerns, but this approach is not without an increased risk of bleeding and substantial cost considerations.

Concerns regarding DES thrombosis led to the convening of the FDA Circulatory System Devices Advisory Panel on December 7 and 8, 2006. In this public forum, clinical data relevant to the issue of DES thrombosis (both when DESs are used according to their label and in more complex patients beyond their labeled indication) were presented and questions regarding the appropriate duration of antiplatelet therapy (aspirin plus clopidogrel) in DES patients were addressed. A comprehensive review of the data presentations and panel deliberations is beyond the scope of this chapter and is discussed elsewhere in this textbook. The notable conclusions from this panel meeting included: (1) both approved DESs (when used in accordance with their labeled indications) are associated with a small increase in the rates of stent thrombosis compared to bare metal stents that emerges 1 year post–stent implantation; (2) based on available data, the increased risk of DES thrombosis with on-label use was not associated with an increased risk of death or MI compared to bare metal stents; (3) off-label use of DES is associated with an increased risk of stent thrombosis, death, or MI compared to on-label use; and (4) the labeling for both approved DESs should include reference to the ACC/AHA/SCAI PCI Practice Guidelines, which recommend that patients receive aspirin indefinitely plus a minimum of 3 months (for CYPHER patients) or 6 months (for TAXUS patients) of clopidogrel, with therapy extended to 12 months in patients at a low risk of bleeding.[7]

The FDA Panel Meeting on DES Thrombosis is an example of public collaboration among the FDA, device manufacturers, investigators, professional societies, interventional and non-interventional cardiologists, cardiovascular surgeons, and biostatisticians to address an important public health issue. Postmarket clinical studies designed for label expansion to more complex patient and lesion subsets and which have a sufficiently large sample size to capture low frequency events may provide valuable data to better characterize the balance between the primary clinical benefit of DES (reduced restenosis rates) with the potentially increased risk of stent thrombosis.

Surrogate End Points

A surrogate end point is a marker that is intended to substitute for a clinical end point and is expected to predict clinical outcomes based on epidemiologic, therapeutic, pathophysiologic, or other scientific evidence.[8] A surrogate end point must fulfill two critical criteria to be considered valid: (1) the surrogate must be highly predictive of the clinical outcome, and (2) the surrogate must fully reflect the treatment effect, both positive and negative, on the clinical outcome.[9,10] In cardiovascular drug trials, blood pressure reduction and lipid lowering have been proposed as physiologic and biochemical markers, respectively, to serve as valid surrogate end points for coronary heart disease and stroke.

For devices, a relevant surrogate end point characterizes the mechanical/physical performance of a device, which is intrinsic to the device and independent of its biological and clinical effects.[8] For DES, particularly the next generation of iterative and novel devices, attention has focused on the use of surrogate end points in clinical trials. Not unexpectedly, given the high frequency of DES use for a highly prevalent disease process, DES development is a rapidly evolving field, both in the design of totally novel stent platforms, coatings, and drugs and in proposed improvements of currently approved stents. There are clearly logistic challenges in bringing a promising innovative DES to the market with deliberate speed with the current expectations of 2000 patients (inclusive of a randomized trial plus single-arm registry studies) exposed to a new DES; it would not be unusual for trial enrollment and follow-up to require at least 2 years to complete. This raises the possibility that the stent might be considered obsolete by the time it is approved for marketing. Further, cardiac event rates (including cardiac death, MI, and target lesion revascularization [TLR]) associated with the current approved DES are sufficiently low so that sample sizes required to show clinically relevant differences between test and control DESs can become prohibitively large.

The relatively low clinical event rates observed in DES trials of non–highly complex coronary lesions has led the consideration of surrogate end points that rely on coronary artery imaging to provide a reasonable assurance of device effectiveness. Meta-analyses of large datasets of multiple randomized PCI studies of DES and bare metal stents suggest that angiographic late loss and percent stent diameter stenosis are highly correlated with TLR and TVR rates, the primary DES effectiveness outcome parameters.[11] As quantitative measurements, angiographic late loss and percent stent stenosis may discern statistically significant differences between test and control devices with far fewer patients compared with traditional *clinical* outcome measurements (i.e., MACE or TVF). As a consequence, superiority or noninferiority studies could be completed expeditiously, allowing promising devices to come to the market at a more rapid pace and/or fewer individuals to be exposed to less effective devices.

However, there are multiple issues regarding the adoption of an exclusive surrogate end point strategy based on angiographic late loss or percent stent diameter stenosis. Angiographic surrogate end points require optimal image quality with consistent views from the index procedure to follow-up and standardized core laboratory protocols and software. By definition, angiographic surrogate end points require a high degree of subject compliance with follow-up angiography. Given the expected low event rates, patients may be reluctant to undergo a protocol-driven (rather than symptom-driven) repeat invasive imaging study. The acceptability of study results could be compromised owing to data loss secondary to a substantial subject dropout. Further, patients who undergo follow-up angiography may be subject to the oculo-stenotic reflex, resulting in increased rates of revascularization procedures (of both target and nontarget lesions), which may not be clinically driven. Although analyses of large angiographic stent databases from randomized studies indicate that late loss and percent stent diameter stenosis are strong predictors of repeat revascularization, most trial data are derived from relatively straightforward, noncomplex lesions; it is uncertain whether imaging-based surrogate end point models would apply to more complicated patient and lesion subsets. It can be anticipated that most current trials will be constructed as test DES versus control DES noninferiority designs using a noninferiority margin (delta) for either late loss or percent stenosis. Although the noninferiority margin can be based on well-established device performance data, the choice of delta remains arbitrary. Therefore, there is a risk that a new DES will fail to meet its noninferiority angiographic end point in comparison with the control DES but will appear to be "similar" to the control device with respect to an important clinical end point (e.g., MACE), with the trial underpowered (insufficient sample size) to show statistically significant noninferiority for the clinical end point.

Although the use of a valid surrogate may result in studies of reasonable size to demonstrate device effectiveness, it must be recognized that FDA is tasked to comprehensively assess device safety performance (with MACE or a similar clinical composite as a primary end point). For DES applications that involve NMEs or completely novel polymer, elution kinetics, and/or stent platforms, at least one sufficiently large study that has a clinical (nonsurrogate) primary end point, statistically powered for superiority or noninferiority, has been the norm. Alternative trial design strategies that combine conventional clinical outcome measures with a surrogate parameter (potentially as coprimary end points), adequately controlled for correlation and type I error inflation, may be considered. Because of these considerations, surrogate end points may be most useful for primary effectiveness end points for second-generation devices (i.e., iterative changes in an approved device). Continued exploration of scientifically valid surrogate end points and innovative trial designs may aid in the development of helpful strategies in the assessment of an evolving novel technology.

Proof of Concept Versus Clinical Utility Considerations: Regulatory Approaches to Vulnerable Plaque Detection Devices

Ruptured atherosclerotic plaques are responsible for 60% to 70% of fatal coronary thrombi. Numerous pathologic studies have demonstrated that the thin-cap fibroatheroma is the precursor lesion of plaque rupture and has been commonly referred to as the "vulnerable plaque."[12,13] Studies demonstrating that culprit lesions responsible for acute coronary events were often non–flow-limiting on previous angiograms have provided clinical evidence in support of the concept of the vulnerable plaque.[14-16] Reliable identification of vulnerable plaques before they become disrupted, leading to acute coronary ischemic syndromes or sudden coronary death, would have the clinical utility of identifying individuals who are at high cardiovascular risk and who might benefit from close clinical follow-up and aggressive coronary risk factor modification.

Vulnerable plaques offer multiple potential targets for device assessment of plaque instability. Among the various structural atherosclerotic plaque elements, a device might be designed to measure fibrous cap thickness, concentration of activated inflammatory cells in the fibrous cap, fibrous cap smooth muscle cell and type 1 collagen content, lipid core area, positive arterial remodeling, plaque neovascularization and hemorrhage, and adventitial vasa vasorum. Probes for nonstructural factors associated with plaque vulnerability may assay for proinflammatory cytokines, matrix metalloproteinases, adhesion molecules, myeloperoxidase, C-reactive protein, and evidence of cellular apoptosis. Physical properties such as increased plaque temperature (a marker of inflammation) and focally increased intraplaque strain may be markers for plaque instability. Although the multitude of potentially measurable parameters provide a rich research environment for device development, it must be recognized that to date there is no single accepted definition of what essential elements constitute a vulnerable plaque.

Insights into the regulatory approaches to vulnerable plaque detection devices require an understanding of the differences between a "tool claim" and a "diagnostic claim." A tool simply measures a physiologic parameter, such as plaque temperature, lesion lipid content, fibrous cap thickness, inflammatory cell content, or arterial compliance. The output of a "diagnostic" device has predictive capability or obvious clinical utility; potential diagnostic indications for vulnerable plaque detection devices include identification of thin-cap fibroatheromas and prediction of a future acute coronary syndrome within a specific arterial segment.

As with other intracoronary devices, a comprehensive battery of bench testing is important in the evaluation of vulnerable plaque detection devices, including assessment of mechanical safety, electrical safety, electromagnetic compatibility, biocompatibility, shelf life, sterilization, and software. Preclinical animal studies are useful to demonstrate a likely acceptable level of device safety during intracoronary use. Proof of concept testing for vulnerable plaque detection devices to support tool indications (e.g., measurement of plaque lipid content) are particularly challenging, because coronary arteries cannot be excised from living subjects and directly examined by other methods (e.g., histology) to confirm the accuracy of the measured parameter. Therefore, the validation vulnerable plaque tools indications may rest on combined evidence from benchtop phantoms, ex vivo human atherosclerotic arteries, and animal models of atherosclerotic disease. These preclinical "proof of concept" studies may be used to develop algorithms to detect plaque features of interest. Because coronary plaques from human patients are not readily available for direct analysis, preclinical testing provides the initial demonstration of device efficacy (i.e., the device accurately measures what it claims to measure). Accurate pathologic definitions that are relevant to the device's tool or diagnostic indications, precise registration of histologic sections with device acquisition data, a large lesion library reflecting the wide heterogeneity of atherosclerotic plaque morphology, and an acceptable degree of lesion characteristic sensitivity and specificity are fundamental to preclinical device evaluation so that device output can be reliably extrapolated to in vivo use in living patients.

It can be anticipated that identification of vulnerable plaque features in patients might result in treatment decisions (e.g., aggressive medical therapy, invasive interventions). Therefore, although attention is appropriately focused on a device's sensitivity to detect a vulnerable plaque marker, it is highly desirable that there be an acceptable level of negative predictive accuracy. Preclinical animal and ex vivo human arterial studies can be instrumental in demonstrating that a device can accurately identify the *absence* of vulnerable lesion characteristics (i.e., demonstrating normal arterial architecture or an absence of vulnerable plaque features).

Device safety is the primary focus of initial proof of concept human studies, in addition to providing information about device handling and output algorithms. Because no gold standard validation method to assess device efficacy is available, proof of concept relies on the robustness of the preclinical testing program and how closely the device measurements fall within the expected range of the predicted lesion characteristic parameters. It should be noted, however, that there will always be limitations in extrapolating findings from ex vivo and preclinical animal studies to real-time in vivo human use; such limitations include registration of regions of interest with device-derived data, sampling errors, tissue processing and fixation artifacts, and tissue shrinkage secondary to dehydration.

Vulnerable plaque detection devices may provide the critical link between the various markers of plaque instability and coronary risk assessment and treatment. However, to move these devices beyond an academic research environment into general interventional cardiology practice, larger and longer natural history studies will provide the clinical relevance of the measured lesion feature(s). Natural history studies can address questions such as (1) does a particular lesion characteristic have prognostic value for future events?; (2) does a vulnerable plaque detection device provide value added to other traditional lesion features or other, perhaps less invasive, clinical markers?; (3) is vulnerable lesion detection beneficial for all patients, or only for those at intermediate or high risk at baseline? and (4) is it worth the time, effort, and cost to measure parameters of plaque vulnerability and does the potential benefit outweigh the risk of additional coronary artery instrumentation?

An approach to a natural history study for a vulnerable plaque detection device could establish "local" proof of the device's utility in clinical practice by assessing whether subsequent clinical events occur because of a specific culprit plaque that had a vulnerable plaque feature identified at baseline. Multiple challenges associated with this type of natural history study should be recognized, the most important of which is the need for repeat imaging soon after the subsequent coronary event. The study size will have to be large enough and of sufficient duration to capture an adequate number of patients with subsequent events, and fatal events may not provide much additional data owing to low autopsy rates. Alternatively, one could consider a natural history trial to show that the detection of vulnerable plaque features identifies patients at a generally increased risk for future coronary events. Although this study design would not necessarily show that a specific vulnerable plaque identified at baseline was responsible for the subsequent event, results could provide valuable risk stratification data.

Natural history studies that confirm that a vulnerable plaque detection device can reliably identify asymptomatic lesions at high risk of future destabilization would provide the necessary foundation for follow-up trials of systemic or local (catheter-based) therapies specifically directed toward vulnerable lesions. Ultimately, one could envision surrogate end point development based on changes in features of plaque vulnerability (e.g., reduction in lesion lipid concentration, increased thickness of the fibrous cap, decreased plaque inflammation) after local or systemic treatment.

Effectiveness Versus Safety Considerations in the Regulation of a Percutaneous Alternative to a Surgical Standard of Care: Regulatory Approaches to Percutaneous Heart Valve Repair and Replacement

The exponentially increasing pace of device treatment for cardiovascular disease is readily apparent in the management of valvular heart disease. The earliest widely applied interventions were beating-heart commissurotomy, performed during the 1950s for relief of aortic, mitral, and pulmonic stenosis.[17] The introduction of extracorporeal heart and lung bypass circulatory support in the late 1950s permitted these procedures to be performed under direct vision. There was, however, surprisingly little improvement in results until the successful introduction of a mechanical valve prosthesis in 1960, pioneered by the collaboration of Starr and Edwards, and the use of allograft aortic replacements in 1962 by Barret-Boyes.[18,19] This was also the period when Carpentier demonstrated that repair of a mitral valve was feasible, and in 1967 he initiated the use of xenografts for

biologic tissue replacement of both the mitral and aortic valves.[20,21] This period of rapid change covered about 2 decades and was followed by 35 years of improvement in devices but relative stagnation in surgical technique. With the new millennium came a renewed interest in research in the management of cardiac valve disease. Starting with adaptation of minimally invasive methods of performing conventional open heart surgery, the focus changed to a search for entirely catheter-based treatments that aimed at duplicating established and successful open surgical procedures with totally closed, percutaneous methods.

Cribier introduced the earliest percutaneous treatment for valve disease in 1984 with balloon valvuloplasty based on the model of angioplasty successfully employed in the coronary vasculature.[22] Bonhoeffer's report of the transvenous deployment of a prosthetic valve in a failed pulmonary conduit in 2000 and Cribier's transvascular implantation of a stented biologic valve prosthesis after balloon valvuloplasty of calcific aortic stenosis in 2002 set the stage for a marked increase in research and development of devices directed at this type of valve treatment.[23,24] Although no new device has been approved for marketing by the FDA as yet, some 24 different catheter-based percutaneous heart valve (PHV) devices were described in various stages of development at recent professional meetings.

PHV prostheses are Class III devices for which a rigorous evaluation is required to provide reasonable assurance of safety and effectiveness (21 CFR Part 814). PMA approval, necessary for commercial distribution of a PHV cardiac prosthesis, rests on valid scientific evidence to support device safety and effectiveness. Such evidence can be obtained from an FDA-approved IDE clinical study of the experimental PHV that can begin enrollment after a demonstration of acceptable device performance in preclinical and feasibility studies. A limited observational pilot or feasibility study can provide initial safety information and help to clarify aspects of the pivotal study trial. While single arm studies using universally accepted objective performance criteria (OPC) are generally acceptable for the evaluation of open surgical replacement of cardiac valves with mechanical and biologic prostheses, FDA believes that an RCT is the appropriate pivotal study design for novel technologies such as PHVs. This difference reflects that fact that there is over five decades of experience with open surgical replacement of cardiac heart valves. The stages in the approval process are strictly monitored by the Agency, and an advisory panel of nongovernment experts may be utilized to provide additional scientific insight and recommendations to FDA.

Indesigning a clinical trial for PHV therapy, the goal is to establish a risk-benefit ratio appropriate for the intended use in a target population. For example, a percutaneous aortic valve device intended for use in patients who are not surgical candidates should provide both reasonable safety and significant benefit compared to a concurrent control, which may be medical management and balloon valvuloplasty. A similar device used in patients at higher than usual surgical risk may provide evidence of superior safety while perhaps accepting a reduction in effectiveness to the standard surgical control. For example, mild-to-moderate valvular regurgitation may be clinically well tolerated. A PHV intervention for severe valvular regurgitation that was slightly less effective than total resolution of regurgitation could be proposed if there were a potentially important benefit with respect to safety. Acceptable degrees of safety and effectiveness of the PHV compared to its control are prespecified before the trial is initiated. As with all novel interventional cardiology procedures, the durability of a PHV treatment is an important consideration that can be addressed through long-term follow-up studies continued in the postmarketing phase. Characterization of failure modes of PHVs and the clinical consequences of device failures are critical components of the device's safety profile. A suboptimal result after PHV deployment might increase the risk and adversely affect any open surgery required, for example precluding valve repair in favor of valve replacement.

This discussion emphasizes the value of close cooperation between interventional cardiologists and cardiac surgeons in configuring a strategy for evaluating PHV therapy. The importance of such collaboration is particularly apparent when determining criteria for patients who are deemed inoperable or who have higher surgical risk. The study hypotheses determine the indication and target population for which these devices can seek FDA regulatory approval. It is therefore important that sponsors and their investigators engage in early and frequent consultation with the FDA to ensure that the study will generate the necessary data to address these hypotheses.

OTHER KEY REGULATORY TOPICS

Combination Products

A combination product is a product that involves two or more regulated products (device, drug, biologic) that are either combined physically or chemically (as in DESs or hormone-releasing skin patches), packaged together in a single unit (as in an asthma inhaler plus cartridge), or packaged separately but with labeling stating that both products (either approved or investigational) are needed to achieve the intended effect (Table 67-2).

Because the FDA has historically been divided into separate centers for device, drug, and biologic products, defining a consistent and appropriate process for the review of a combination product has been challenging. In response to the recognition of these issues and substantial growth in the number of combination products under development and coming to market, the Medical Device User Fee and Modernization Act of 2002 established a formal FDA Office of Combination Products (OCP). OCP's many respon-

---

Table 67-2. Definitions of Combination Products

According to the *Code of Federal Regulations*, 21 CFR Part 3.2(e), a combination product is:

(1) a product comprised of two or more regulated components, i.e., drug/device, biologic/device, drug/biologic, or drug/device/biologic, that are physically, chemically, or otherwise combined or mixed and produced as a single entity;

(2) two or more separate products packaged together in a single package or as a unit and comprised of drug and device products, device and biological products, or biological and drug products;

(3) a drug, device, or biological product packaged separately that according to its investigational plan or proposed labeling is intended for use only with an approved individually specified drug, device, or biological product where both are required to achieve the intended use, indication, or effect and where upon approval of the proposed product the labeling of the approved product would need to be changed (e.g., to reflect a change in intended use, dosage form, strength, route of administration, or significant change in dose); or

(4) any investigational drug, device, or biological product packaged separately that according to its proposed labeling is for use only with another individually specified investigational drug, device, or biological product where both are required to achieve the intended use, indication, or effect.

---

sibilities include assigning an FDA Center to have primary jurisdiction for review of a combination product, ensuring timely and effective premarket review by overseeing reviews involving more than one Center, ensuring consistency and appropriateness of postmarket regulation of combination products, and updating agreements, guidance documents, or practices specific to the assignment of combination products.

In the case of DES, FDA's approach was directed through the Request for Designation process, which determined that the primary mode of action was the mechanical support of the vessel wall provided by the stent, with the drug acting to enhance this action by potentially reducing restenosis. Because the device component was found to be most responsible for the therapeutic effect of the product, CDRH was named the lead Center, with significant consultation to be provided by the Center for Drug Evaluation and Research. The official Request for Designation for DES is available on the OCP website (http://www.fda.gov/oc/combination/stents.html).

Assessment of combination products poses numerous challenges for both premarket and postmarket evaluation. The premarket review requires the participation of numerous scientific experts from multiple Centers, and, in many cases, decisions regarding how to apply standard policies related to testing recommendations differs between Centers. Once a combination product is approved, analysis of adverse events can also be problematic, because it may not be clear whether a single component or the combination of components is responsible for the reported event. For example, a small number of reports of hypersensitivity reactions have been received for DES, but it is difficult to discern whether the reactions were due to the metal stent, the polymer coating, the drug in the coating, and/or adjunctive medications.

Role of the Advisory Panel

FDA employs scientists, engineers, and clinicians to review marketing applications, but for first-of-a-kind technologies, or for controversial applications, an Advisory Panel of experts may also be consulted for a recommendation regarding approvability of the application. Advisory Panels are usually composed of a combination of physicians, statisticians, ethicists, biomedical engineers, and patient advocates with expertise relevant to the application being considered and no financial and/or intellectual conflict of interest with either the subject device or competing devices. To be considered for participation as an Advisory Panel member, an expert must have the training and experience necessary to evaluate information objectively and to interpret its significance. The Panel is considered to be advisory only; FDA has responsibility for making final decisions.

Labeling

Labeling is defined as "display of written, printed, or graphic matter upon the immediate container of any article . . . [and] all labels and other written, printed, or graphic matter" (Sections 201(k) and (m) of FFDCA). Practically, FDA views device labeling as a means to communicate to physicians and patients a description of the device, how and in whom the device should be used, situations in which the device should not be used or should be used with caution, and the safety and effectiveness outcomes associated with use of the device in one or more clinical studies. The "indication for use" statement identifies the target population, in a significant portion of which sufficient valid scientific evidence has demonstrated that the device as labeled will provide clinically effective results and at the same time does not present an unreasonable risk of illness or injury associated with the use of the device.

Product Recall and CDRH

The Center is responsible for managing recalls of medical devices. A recall is an action that is taken to address a problem with a medical device when the problem violates FDA regulation, a situation that is termed "violative." Devices are violative and subject to recall if the device is defective and/or poses a risk to public health. Recalls are subject to FDA oversight to ensure that the actions taken by the recalling company are appropriate to protect the public health. This may include audits to ensure that the recall is completed in a timely manner as well as follow-up with the company to minimize the likelihood of a recurrence of the problem.

A recall does not necessarily imply that the device can no longer be used or that it must be returned to the responsible manufacturer. In some instances, a recall simply indicates that the device must be checked or repaired or that the labeling must be changed or replaced to ensure the continued safe operation of the device. Implanted devices such as pacemakers and heart valves may or may not be required to be replaced, depending on the nature of the defect or risk. On occasion, a recall can be completed by notifying the public of the situation so that individuals affected by the recall can contact their physician for appropriate follow-up. A recall may be either a "correction," wherein the problem can be addressed with the device in place, or a "removal," in which the device must be physically removed from the place where it is used or sold.

Recalls are classified based on the potential risk to public health imposed by the device problem. Class I recalls represent the highest risk, with class II posing a less serious risk and class III the lowest risk. Classification of the recall helps to inform the public regarding the seriousness of the problem and also determines the nature and extent of audits and other regulatory follow-up actions. More information on recalls and the relationship between FDA, industry, and the public in the event of a recall can be found at the FDA Web site (http://www.fda.gov/cdrh/recalls/learn.html).

CONCLUSIONS

Based on the experience of the past decade, it can be expected that interventional medical devices will continue their rapid development and use by interventional cardiologists. The brisk pace of change presents special challenges to FDA's Center for Devices and Radiological Health in its mission to protect public health via the assessment of device safety and effectiveness. To this end, CDRH remains committed to working interactively with industry and academic sponsors through all phases of product development and approval for use. Well-designed trials that collect valid scientific evidence, encompass real-world device utilization, and provide an assessment of clinically relevant outcomes are critical elements in the balance between expeditious approval of promising novel therapies and protection of the public from unanticipated serious adverse events.

REFERENCES

1. Muni NI, Califf RM, Foy JR, et al: Coronary drug-eluting stent development: Issues in trial design. Am Heart J 2005;149: 415-433.
2. Moreno R, Fernandez C, Hernandez R, et al: Drug-eluting stent thrombosis: Results from a pooled analysis including 10 randomized studies. J Am Coll Cardiol 2005;45:954-959.
3. Cutlip DE, Windecker S, Mehran R, et al: Clinical end points in coronary stent trials: A case for standardized definitions. Circulation 2007;115:2344-2351.
4. Iakovou I, Schmidt T, Bonizzoni E, et al: Incidence, predictors, and outcome of thrombosis after successful implantation of drug-eluting stents. JAMA 2005;293:2126-2130.
5. Kuchulakanti PK, Chu WW, Torguson R, et al: Correlates and long-term outcomes of angiographically proven stent thrombosis with sirolimus- and paclitaxel-eluting stents. Circulation 2006;113:1108-1113.

6. Hoye A, Iakovou I, Ge L, et al: Long-term outcomes after stenting of bifurcation lesions with the "crush" technique: Predictors of an adverse outcome. J Am Coll Cardiol 2006;47:1949-1958.

7. Farb A, Boam AB: Stent thrombosis redux—the FOA perspective. N Eng J Med 2007;356:984-987.

8. Biomarkers Definition Working Group: Biomarkers and surrogate endpoints: Preferred definitions and conceptual framework. Clin Pharmacol Ther 2001;69:89-95.

9. Prentice RL: Surrogate endpoints in clinical trials: Definition and operational criteria. Stat Med 1989;8:427-430.

10. DeMets DL: The role of surrogate outcome measures in evaluating medical devices. Surgery 2000;128:379-385.

11. Mauri L, Orav EJ, Candia SC, et al: Robustness of late lumen loss in discriminating drug-eluting stents across variable observational and randomized trials. Circulation 2005;112:2833-2839.

12. Farb A, Burke AP, Tang AL, et al: Coronary plaque erosion without rupture into a lipid core: A frequent cause of coronary thrombosis in sudden coronary death. Circulation 1996;93:1354-1363.

13. Virmani R, Kolodgie FD, Burke AP, et al: Lessons from sudden coronary death: A comprehensive morphological classification scheme for atherosclerotic lesions. Arterioscler Thromb Vasc Biol 2000;20:1262-1275.

14. Ambrose JA, Tannenbaum MA, Alexopoulos D, et al: Angiographic progression of coronary artery disease and the development of myocardial infarction. J Am Coll Cardiol 1988;12:56-62.

15. Little WC, Constantinescu M, Applegate RJ, et al: Can coronary angiography predict the site of a subsequent myocardial infarction in patients with mild-to-moderate coronary artery disease? Circulation 1988;78(5 Pt 1):1157-1166.

16. Giroud D, Li JM, Urban P, et al: Relation of the site of acute myocardial infarction to the most severe coronary arterial stenosis at prior angiography. Am J Cardiol 1992;69:729-732.

17. Bailey CP: The surgical treatment of mitral stenosis (mitral commissurotomy). Dis Chest 1949;15:377.

18. Starr A, Edwards ML: Mitral replacement: Clinical experience with a ball-valve prosthesis. Ann Surg 1961;154:726-740.

19. Barratt-Boyes BG: Long-term follow-up of aortic valvar grafts. Br Heart J 1971;33(Suppl):60-65.

20. Carpentier A, Lemaigre G, Robert L, et al: Biological factors affecting long-term results of valvular heterografts. J Thorac Cardiovasc Surg 1969;58:467-483.

21. Carpentier A, Deloche A, Dauptain A, et al: A new reconstructive operation for correction of mitral and tricuspid insufficiency. J Thorac Cardiovasc Surg 1971;61:1-13.

22. Cribier A, Savin T, Berland J, et al: Percutaneous transluminal balloon valvoplasty of adult aortic stenosis: Report of 92 cases. J Am Coll Cardiol 1987;9:381-386.

23. Bonhoffer P, Boudjemline Y, Saliba Z, et al: Percutaneous replacement of pulmonary valve in right ventricle to pulmonary artery prosthetic conduit with valve dysfunction. Lancet. 2000;356:1403-1405.

24. Cribier A, Eltchaninoff H, Bash A, et al: Percutaneous transcatheter implantation of an aortic valve prosthesis for calcific aortic stenosis: First human case description. Circulation 2002;106:3006-3008.

Index

Note: Page numbers followed by f and t indicate figures and tables, respectively.